SAUNDERS
MANUAL OF PHYSICAL
THERAPY PRACTICE

Rose Sgarlat Myers, PT, PhD, CAE

Managing Partner, Myers Associates; President, Corporation for Health Education and Careers, Charlottesville, Virginia; Vice President, American College of Continuing Education, Hunt Valley, Maryland; Former Director, Department of Education, American Physical Therapy Association, Alexandria, Virginia

W.B. SAUNDERS COMPANY
A Division of Harcourt Brace & Company

Philadelphia London Toronto Montreal Sydney Tokyo

SAUNDERS
MANUAL OF PHYSICAL
THERAPY PRACTICE

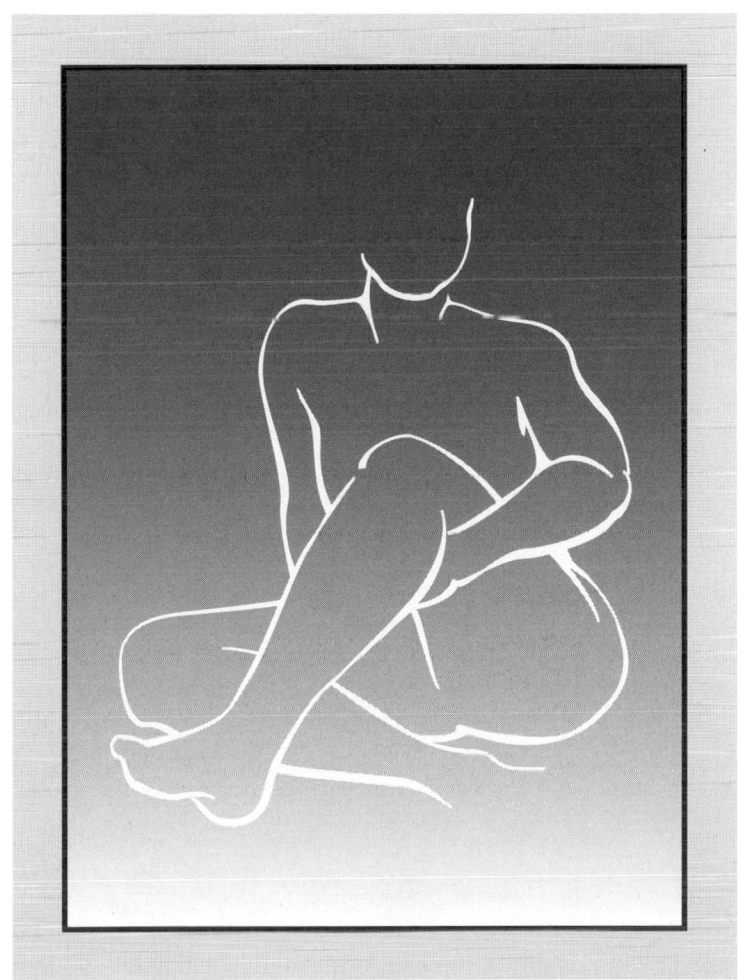

W.B. SAUNDERS COMPANY
A Division of Harcourt Brace & Company

The Curtis Center
Independence Square West
Philadelphia, Pennsylvania 19106

Library of Congress Cataloging-in-Publication Data

Saunders manual of physical therapy practice / [edited by] Rose Sgarlat Myers.—1st ed.
    p.   cm.
    ISBN 0–7216–3671–3
    1. Physical therapy—Handbooks, manuals, etc. I. Myers, Rose Sgarlat. II. Title:
Saunders manual of physical therapy practice.
    [DNLM: 1. Physical Therapy.   WB 460 S257 1995]
    RM700.S363   1995
    615.8′2—dc20
    DNLM/DLC   94-452

SAUNDERS MANUAL OF PHYSICAL THERAPY PRACTICE   ISBN 0–7216–3671–3

Printed in the United States of America.

Last digit is the print number: 9   8   7   6   5   4   3   2   1

This book is dedicated to all of the following:

My husband and best friend, Snuffy; my daughters, Jessica and Gabrielle; my sister, Sara; and Virginia and Chuck, my in-laws, whose love, encouragement, and support made this book possible.

My teachers and mentors from high school through adulthood for their indelible influences and encouragement: Mary Catherine Egan, Margaret Fetch, John Mills, Dorothy Baethke, E. Jane Carlin, and Eugene "Mike" Michels.

My deceased parents, Micheline and Samuel, who taught me the value of hard work and perseverance.

My contributors for sharing their expertise and love for our profession.

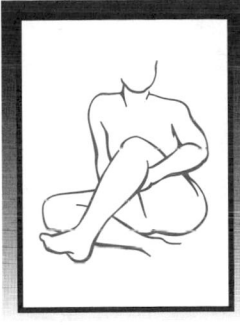

Contributors

CARA C. ADAMS, PT, MS
Associate Professor, Department of Physical Therapy, School of Health Related Professions, University of Alabama at Birmingham, Birmingham, Alabama

Genitourinary System

MARGARET ANDERSON, PT, GDMT, MApplSci
Senior Faculty, Kaiser-Hayward Physical Therapy Residency Program in Advanced Manual Therapy, California; Private Practitioner, Marin Orthopedic Rehabilitation, Mill Valley, California

Cervical Spine

CHERYL APPEL, PT, ACCE
Guest Lecturer, University of Wisconsin—Madison; Perinatal Specialist, Meriter Hospital, Madison, Wisconsin

Obstetrical Considerations

DOLORES B. BERTOTI, PT, MS, PCS
Assistant Professor, Alvernia College, Reading, Pennsylvania; Adjunct Professor, Beaver College, Glenside, Pennsylvania; Research Associate, Shriners Hospital, Philadelphia, Pennsylvania

Age-Related Considerations: Pediatric

BARBARA M. BOURBON, PT, PhD
Assistant Professor, Philadelphia College of Pharmacy and Science, Philadelphia, Pennsylvania

Craniomandibular Examination and Treatment

SUSAN K. BRENNEMAN, PT, MS
Education/Development Coordinator, Physical Therapy Department, University of Pennsylvania Medical Center, Philadelphia, Pennsylvania

Age-Related Considerations: Pediatric

NANCY BYL, PT, MPH, PhD
Associate Professor and Director, Graduate Program in Physical Therapy, University of California, San Francisco, San Francisco, California

Introduction: Anatomical and Physiological Considerations; Integumentary System Screening, Examination, and Assessment; Systemic Issues and Skin Conditions: Wound Healing, Oxygen Percutaneous Drug Delivery, Burns, and Desensitized Skin; Treatment and Prevention: Goals and Objectives

MICHELLE H. CAMERON, PT, BS
Guest Lecturer, University of California, San Francisco—San Francisco State University Graduate Program in Physical Therapy; Physical Therapist, Private Practice, San Francisco, California

Treatment and Prevention: Goals and Objectives

CATHERINE CERTO, PT, ScD
Chairman and Associate Professor, Department of Physical Therapy, Sargent College of Allied Health Professions, Boston University, Boston, Massachusetts

Cardiovascular System

SUSAN CROMWELL, PT, MS
Advanced Clinician, Physical Therapy Department, Medical Center Hospital of Vermont, Burlington, Vermont

Neurological Evaluation and Assessment; Treatment Planning; Balance Instability; Patients with Quadriplegia

ANTHONY DELITTO, PT, PhD
Assistant Professor, Chair, Department of Physical
Therapy, School of Health and Rehabilitation
Sciences, University of Pittsburgh; Director, Acute
Physical Therapy Services, Comprehensive Spine
Center, University of Pittsburgh Medical Center,
Pittsburgh, Pennsylvania
Lower Extremity: Knee

MIRIAM C. DEPRETIS, MSPT, BS, MS
Senior Staff Therapist, Department of Physical
Therapy, North Penn Hospital, Lansdale, Pennsyl-
vania
Lower Extremity: Hip

WAYNE DIAMOND, PT, GDMT, OCS
Clinical Faculty, University of California, San Fran-
cisco, Graduate Program in Physical Therapy, San
Francisco, California; Clinical Specialist, Orthopae-
dics/Sports Medicine, Kaiser Permanente Medical
Center, Oakland, California
Upper Extremity: Shoulder

JOAN E. EDELSTEIN, PT, MA
Associate Professor, Clinical Physical Therapy and
Director, Program in Physical Therapy, Columbia
University, New York, New York
Orthoses

PETER I. EDGELOW, PT, MA
Co-Director, Physiotherapy Associates, Haywood,
California
Trunk

JANE M. FRAHM, BS, PT
Obstetrics/Gynecology Coordinator and Co-man-
ager, Rehabilitation Services, Hutzel Hospital, Detroit, Michigan
Genitourinary System

LISA M. GIALLONARDO, PT, MS, OCS
Senior Clinical Specialist Faculty, Northeastern Uni-
versity, Bouvé, College of Pharmacy and Health
Sciences, Boston, Massachusetts; Private Practi-
tioner, Natick, Massachusetts
*Lower Extremity: Ankle; Lower Extremity: Foot; Posture;
Gait*

JEAN M. HELD, PT, EdD
Associate Professor, Physical Therapy, Coordinator,
Graduate Program in Physical Therapy, University
of Vermont, Burlington, Vermont
*Theories and Principles of Therapeutic Intervention Based
on Contemporary Models of Motor Control*

SUZANNE P. HICKLIN, MPT
Clinical Education Coordinator, North Penn Hospi-
tal, Lansdale, Pennsylvania
Lower Extremity: Hip

TERRY R. HOLLEY, PT, MHS, GCS
Geriatric Clinical Specialist, Salem, Oregon
Age-Related Considerations: Geriatric

GAIL JENSEN, PT, PhD
Associate Professor, Department of Physical Ther-
apy, Creighton University, Omaha, Nebraska
Cervical Spine

MARTHA J. JEWELL, PT, PhD
Associate Professor and Chairperson, Department
of Physical Therapy, Samuel Merritt College, Oakland, California
Trunk

LUTHER C. KLOTH, PT, MS
Professor in Physical Therapy, Marquette Univer-
sity, Milwaukee, Wisconsin
Treatment and Prevention: Goals and Objectives

ANNA CONAWAY LESCAK, MPT
Clinical Coordinator, Orthopedics and Job Care,
Kaiser Foundation Hospital, Honolulu, Hawaii
Trunk

KATHRYN P. MEDLIN, PT, MS, GCS
Supervisor, Inpatient Physical Therapy, St. Mar-
garet's Memorial Hospital, Pittsburgh, Pennsylvania
Age-Related Considerations: Geriatric

POLLY MENENDEZ, MS, PT
Senior Physical Therapist, Medical Center Hospital of Vermont, Burlington, Vermont

Neurological Evaluation and Assessment; Patients with Hemiparesis/Hemiplegia; Orthotic Management for Lower Extremity Dysfunction; Evaluation and Prescription for Wheelchairs and Seating

ROSE SGARLAT MYERS, PT, PhD, CAE
Managing Partner, Myers Associates, President, Corporation for Health Education and Careers, Charlottesville, Virginia; Vice President, American College of Continuing Education, Hunt Valley, Maryland; Former Director, Department of Education, American Physical Therapy Association, Alexandria, Virginia

Historical Perspective, Assumptions, and Ethical Considerations for Physical Therapy Practice

LEE NELSON, PT, MS
Clinical Associate Professor, Department of Physical Therapy, University of Vermont; Assistant Manager, Department of Physical Therapy, Medical Center Hospital of Vermont, Burlington, Vermont

Critical Frameworks for Evaluation, Assessment, and Treatment Planning; Longitudinal Pediatric Considerations

BARBARA J. NORTON, BSPT, MHS/PT
Instructor and Associate Director for Postprofessional Education, Program in Physical Therapy, Washington University School of Medicine, St. Louis, Missouri

Clinical Decision Making in Physical Therapy Practice

MARIANNE OREST, PT, MEd
Advanced Clinician, Medical Center Hospital of Vermont, Burlington, Vermont

Screening a Patient with Neurological Damage; Patients with Hemiparesis/Hemiplegia; Patients with a Low Level of Responsiveness; Determining the Need for Skilled Physical Therapy

PEGGY OWEN, PT, MS
Assistant Academic Coordinator of Clinical Education, Department of Physical Therapy, University of Vermont; Staff Therapist, Associates in Physical and Occupational Therapy, Inc., Burlington, Vermont

Screening a Patient with Neurological Damage; Neurological Evaluation and Assessment; Treatment Planning; Children with a Variety of Problems; Longitudinal Pediatric Considerations; Determining the Need for Skilled Physical Therapy

DAVID G. PATRICK, PT, MS, CPO
Assistant Professor, Department of Physical Therapy, College Misericordia, Dallas, Pennsylvania

Prosthetics

LUCINDA A. PFALZER, PT, PhD
Associate Professor, Director of Research and the Post-Professional Masters in Physical Therapy Program, Physical Therapy Department, School of Health Professions and Studies, University of Michigan–Flint, Flint, Michigan

Oncology: Examination, Diagnosis, and Treatment. Medical and Surgical Considerations; Oncology: Examination, Diagnosis, and Treatment. Physical Therapy Considerations; Integumentary System Screening, Examination, and Assessment; Systemic Issues and Skin Conditions: Wound Healing, Oxygen Percutaneous Drug Delivery, Burns, and Desensitized Skin; Treatment and Prevention: Goals and Objectives

JAN RICHARDS, PT, MS
Clinical Faculty, Kaiser-Hayward Physical Therapy Residency Program in Advanced Manual Therapy; Clinical Specialist, Kaiser Permanente Medical Center, Oakland, California

Cervical Spine

BEVERLY J. SCHMOLL, PT, PhD
Associate Professor, Physical Therapy, Interim Director, Graduate and Special Programs, University of Michigan—Flint, Flint, Michigan

Behavioral and Social Science: Considerations for Current Practice

MEG STANGER, PT, MS, PCS
Director of Program Services, Easter Seal Society of Lancaster County, Lancaster, Pennsylvania

Age-Related Considerations: Pediatric

JULIE ANN STARR, PT, MS
Clinical Assistant Professor, Department of Physical Therapy, Sargent College of Allied Health Professions, Boston University, Boston, Massachusetts

Pulmonary System

BARBARA STEVENS, PT, GDMT

Coordinator of Rehabilitative Services, Oklahoma Neurosurgical Institute, Oklahoma City, Oklahoma

Cervical Spine

CAROLYN T. WADSWORTH, PT, MS, CHT

Owner and Practitioner, Heartland Physical Therapy, Cedar Rapids, Iowa

Elbow, Forearm, Wrist, and Hand

MARY ANN WHARTON, PT, MS

Geriatric Physical Therapy Consultant, Pittsburgh; Associate Professor, School of Physical Therapy, Slippery Rock University, Slippery Rock, Pennsylvania

Age-Related Considerations: Geriatric

LINDA ROSENBERG ZELLERBACH, PT, MS

Guest Lecturer, University of California, San Francisco–San Francisco State University Graduate Program in Physical Therapy; Physical Therapy Clinical Specialist: Burns, St. Francis Memorial Hospital, San Francisco, California

Systemic Issues and Skin Conditions: Wound Healing, Oxygen Percutaneous Drug Delivery, Burns, and Desensitized Skin; Treatment and Prevention: Goals and Objectives

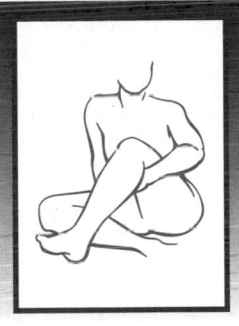

Preface

Before our very eyes the United States health care system is in the midst of the most dramatic and rapid change in our history. The very structures of delivery and reimbursement are changing overnight and indeed hourly. Hospitals are buying outpatient clinics, rehabilitation centers, and nursing homes and are either buying or merging with other hospitals. Health Maintenance Organizations (HMOs) and Managed Care Corporations are contracting with networks of physicians and physical therapists. In several short years, previously owner-managed physical therapy practices have been bought by large corporations. What was once private or independent practice is now corporate practice. Change, it seems, will only continue to accelerate as state governments, the US Congress, the health care insurance industry, and health care providers try to streamline to reduce costs in striving for a more efficient and cost-effective health care delivery system. Whether or not the United States establishes a National Health Service System, the ensuing events in the anticipation of this change have created a great deal of uncertainty for patients and health care practitioners alike.

The subsequent changes in physical therapy practice will be inherent in and dependent on the roles that physical therapists carve out of the current chaos. If physical therapists are assertive and successful in communicating the benefits and positive outcomes of physical therapy treatment and the cost-effectiveness of the physical therapist as the "gate keeper" for musculoskeletal problems, then physical therapy will continue to grow exponentially. The successful transition will require an effective team member, a professional who is able to put forward the best aspects of physical therapy care with the best overall integrated treatment for the resolution of the patient's problems. The physical therapist must become an integral part of the patient-centered team and cannot practice in isolation. Additionally, physical therapists must more often involve technical personnel, the patient, and the family in treatment. The education of these assistants in physical therapy care will in the long run reduce costs by reducing the length of treatment episodes.

The challenges will remain with examination, diagnosis, and treatment and will not center only on the challenge of documentation for further treatments and for reimbursement. This focus will require a sound knowledge of physical therapy foundations and proven methods of examination, diagnosis, and treatment. The improvement of patient care is every physical therapist's responsibility. The imperative to continue to discover and develop new methods of treatment for specific patient diagnoses will require that the physical therapist read, attend professional meetings, and contribute to the scientific base of physical therapy and health care, perhaps in multiple disciplines.

Physical therapy has developed and grown rather dramatically over the last few years, the scope of practice has expanded, and the physical therapist's responsibility for clinical decision making has increased. The number of state practice acts that include direct access of patients to physical therapists has increased and, concomitantly, the responsibility of physical therapists to make prudent decisions is becoming more important. Physical therapists are responsible for deciding what to include in the physical therapy screening, for evaluating and assessing patients, for making diagnoses within our scope of knowledge and practice, and for deciding whether to treat or to refer patients to other practitioners. If physical therapists decide to treat, they must decide on the treatment goals and plans, what treatment methods to include, and when to discharge patients. The level of a physical therapist's responsibilities will increase whether or not the number of states with direct access increases. Therefore, this book includes discussions of the art and science of clinical decision making to assist the practitioner in incorporating more advanced clinical decision making into his/her practice and to stimulate the teacher and researcher to look at practice more pragmatically.

This "manual" was designed as a comprehensive resource book of physical therapy practice written for the experienced physical therapist–clinician. The majority of the book is written in "outline form," with a body systems approach to material presentation that allows the clinician to quickly find and comprehend the information. We are aware that a patient's signs and symptoms often reflect multiple and complex etiologies involving several body systems. Therefore, it is appropriate to examine and evaluate the total patient, or at least more than one system, regardless of the patient's initial complaint. The decision to present the material as indicated was justified on the basis that this book is not an entry-level text; therefore, the reader should know the total evaluation process.

The book is divided into seven major sections with six directly dealing with patient examination, diagnosis, and treatment. The assumption has been made that the experienced physical therapist will have already integrated basic concepts studied during entry-level education. However, the contributors have provided a brief review of the relevant information such as anatomy if it is necessary to the discussion of the system or the philosophy of the evaluation and treatment approach. Each section covers examination (history and physical), assessment and diagnosis, treatment, and age-related concerns and contains a number of clinical decision-making cases that illustrate the decision-making process for patients presenting with different types of problems.

Part I: Foundations for the Future. A brief history of the profession and some ethical and legal issues are presented in the first chapter. Next, Barbara Norton discusses clinical decision making, including diagnosis as defined in medicine and in relation to terms in other classification systems such as the World Health Organization's (WHO) International Classification of Impairments, Disabilities, and Handicaps (ICIDH) and the system of categories proposed by Nagi. Norton provides a cogent discussion of the diagnostic process, including test selection, treatment management, and prognosis with respect to the parameters of clinical research. In the last chapter of this section, Beverly Schmoll presents her new theory for understanding physical therapist and patient interactions. The theory is based on an individual's frame of refer-

ence. The discussion provides new information for dealing with the complex interrelationships encountered in physical therapy practice.

Part II: General Considerations for Practice. Lucinda Pfalzer provides an example of a complex, sometimes unisystem and often multisystem disease—cancer. The first chapter describes the medical and surgical aspects of the various cancers, and the second is an in-depth discussion of the physical therapist's examination, assessment, and treatment issues.

Part III: Cardiopulmonary Systems. This section is divided into two chapters. Catherine Certo discusses anatomy, physiology, assessment, laboratory and physiological tests, major conditions, and physical therapy treatment with principles of exercise prescription and special consideration for the cardiovascular system. Julie Starr presents a comprehensive approach to the evaluation and treatment of patients with pulmonary problems.

Part IV: Neurological/Neuromuscular System. This section contains 14 chapters that are based on theories and principles of contemporary models of motor control, a relatively new approach, in the evaluation and treatment of patients with neurological system problems. Jean Held coordinated the work in this section, accompanied by Lee Nelson, Marianne Orest, Peggy Owen, Susan Cromwell, and Polly Menendez.

Part V: Genitourinary System. Cara Adams and Jane Frahm collaborated to provide physical therapists with a reference resource for the evaluation and treatment of incontinence, which is the most comprehensive presentation to appear in the physical therapy literature. Other genitourinary system disorders are also discussed. Cheryl Appel has contributed a chapter on the evaluation and treatment of patients with normal and complicated pregnancies.

Part VI: Integumentary System. Nancy Byl and colleagues Linda Zellerbach, Luther Kloth, Michelle Cameron, and Lucinda Pfalzer have written perhaps the most comprehensive presentation on the integumentary system to appear in the physical therapy literature. Burns, wounds, ulcers, and other skin disorders are discussed with respect to etiology (eg, mechanical, chemical, autoimmune, and metabolic), evaluation, and treatment.

Part VII: Musculoskeletal System. The last and final section consists of 15 chapters providing where appropriate reviews of anatomy, physiology, and other basic principles and concepts. Each chapter stands alone, but of course several may apply in the examination, diagnosis, and treatment of patients with musculoskeletal signs and symptoms. Barbara Bourbon ("Craniomandibular Examination and Treatment"); Margaret Anderson, Jan Richards, Barbara Stevens, and Gail Jensen ("Cervical Spine"); Wayne Diamond ("Upper Extremity: Shoulder"), Carolyn Wadsworth ("Elbow, Forearm, Wrist, and Hand"); Peter Edgelow, Anna Conaway Lescak, and Martha Jewell ("Trunk"); Suzanne Hicklin and Miriam DePretis ("Lower Extremity: Hip"); Anthony Delitto ("Lower Extremity: Knee"); Lisa Giallonardo ("Lower Extremity: Ankle"; "Lower Extremity: Foot"; "Posture"; "Gait"); David Patrick ("Prosthetics"); Joan Edelstein ("Orthoses"); Susan Brenneman, Meg Stanger, and Dolores Bertoti ("Age-Related Considerations: Pediatric"); and Mary Ann Wharton, Terry Holley, and Kathryn Medlin ("Age-Related Considerations: Geriatric") have brought a unique blending and interpretation of research and extensive clinical experience to their respective subjects in a detailed presentation of each musculoskeletal area.

My goal in editing this book was to provide physical therapists with a useful reference for physical therapy practice that combined the *available* scientific evidence with current practice for rational clinical decision making. Whether the contributors and I have met this goal satisfactorily will depend on the readers' abilities to improve patient care based on the information contained within the covers of the book. Concomitant confirmation of our achievement will be evident in research (theoretical, basic, and clinical) stimulated by the ideas presented. We hope that this is the first of many editions documenting the evolution of physical therapy practice.

Rose Sgarlat Myers

Editor

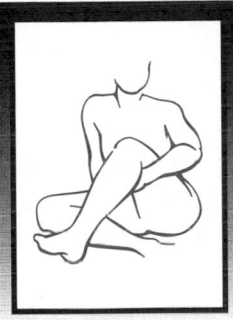

Acknowledgments

I would like to thank the following for their assistance in the early formulation of this book: Beverly Schmoll, Rebecca Craik, and Nancy Byl; my editors, Margaret Biblis and Scott Weaver, for their encouragement, assistance, and support; and Judith Forrest for help in editing and typing.

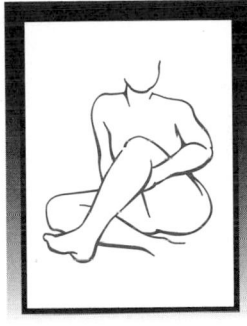

Contents

PART ONE

Foundations for the Future

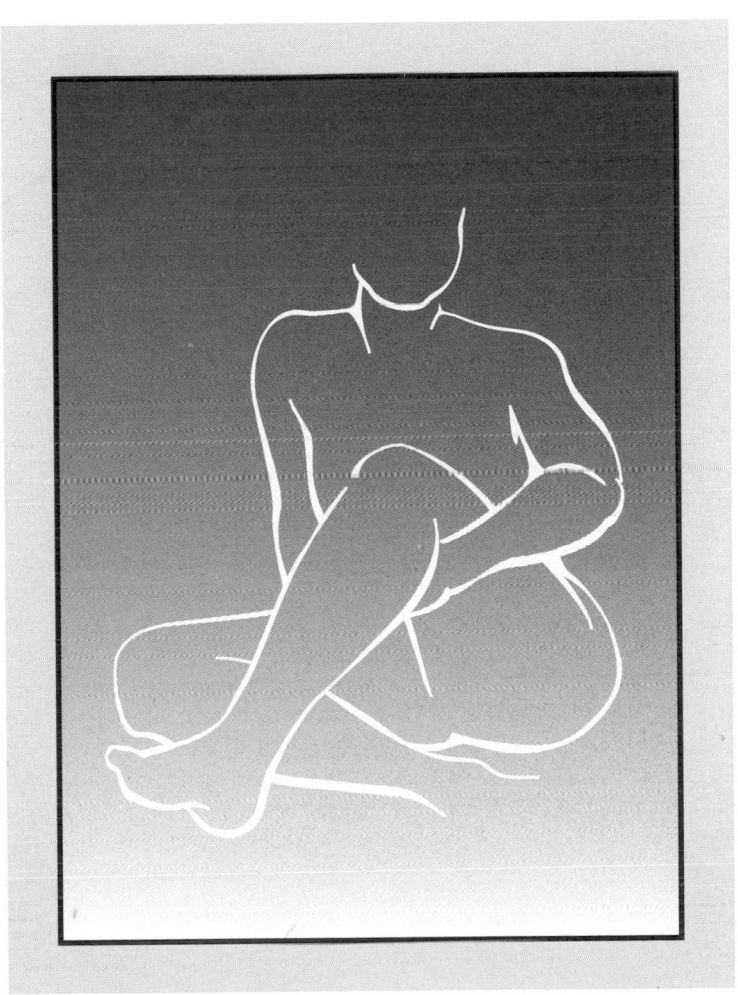

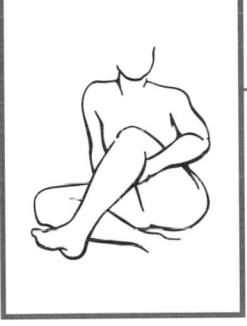

CHAPTER 1

Historical Perspective, Assumptions, and Ethical Considerations for Physical Therapy Practice

Rose Sgarlat Myers

HISTORICAL PERSPECTIVE

Organized physical therapy began during World War I, starting with 800[1,2] trained Reconstruction Aides and expanding to include approximately 80,000 licensed physical therapists in 1993.[3] * Four major growth periods illustrate the growth of the physical therapy profession and merit discussion.

Major Growth Periods

The First Major Growth Period: World War I (1918) to 1940

In 1917, the United States was entrenched in World War I. There was a tremendous need to rehabilitate wounded soldiers to help them overcome movement dysfunction and return to a productive life. Unfortunately, there were very few people trained in physical therapy in the United States at that time. The few who existed were women trained as physical educators who worked in physician's offices instructing patients in corrective exercises. Therefore, a new profession was created by volunteers—women who were physical educators or nurses. Education programs were quickly established, first at Reed College in Oregon, and later at 14 other institutions.[1,2] These were postgraduate programs, but no degree was given on completion.

Three physicians, Brackett, Goldthwait, and Granger, and a physical educator from Boston, Margaurite Sanderson, established a reconstruction unit in the US Army Medical Corps.[1,2] Mary McMillan, the first president of the national physical therapy association, helped establish this fledgling service of Reconstruction Aides. McMillan trained in England in the basic sciences and in corrective and remedial exercise and worked there for several years before returning to the United States. At the 25th anniversary of the professional

---

* These estimates are based on the number of licensees with a correction factor for physical therapists with multiple licenses. Data are from the *American Physical Therapy Association State Licensure Reference Guide*, Alexandria, American Physical Therapy Association, 1993. The formula is from Michels E: *Development of Manpower Requirements Estimates for Physical Therapists: Final Summary Report*, Rockville, MD, Bureau of Health Professions, and Alexandria, American Physical Therapy Association, 1984.

association McMillan reflected on its inauspicious beginning:

The US Army Medical Corps knew nothing about physical therapy and I knew nothing about about the US Army Medical Corps. Through the kindness of one of the physicians I was initiated into Army ways and learned how to go through Army channels to get the necessary requirements. First I asked for a place to work, for there was no place provided. After some time a sun porch was allotted as a workroom for physical therapy. Then I thought I would show where physical therapy stood, so I had some prescription blanks printed. I made personal calls upon the different department heads and tried to sell physical therapy and to sell myself—it was a hard job; they had little time for the likes of me.[4]

McMillan, like many women entering professional fields at that time, faced a staunch male bastion. After establishing the first physical therapy service program at Walter Reed Army Hospital, McMillan taught at Reed College. Her first class consisted of 208 women; her second included only 60. Altogether, McMillan and others trained 800 women who worked during the war in army hospital reconstruction physical therapy departments in both the United States and Europe.

After the war ended, approximately 245 of the Reconstruction Aides joined together to establish our nation's first physical therapy association, the American Women's Physical Therapeutic Association. In 1921, the Association's constitution stated that its purpose would be

1. To establish and maintain a professional and scientific standard for those engaged in the profession of physical therapeutics.
2. To increase efficiency among its members by encouraging them in advanced study.
3. To disseminate information by the distribution of medical literature and articles of personal interest.
4. To make available efficiently trained women to the medical profession.
5. To sustain social fellowship and intercourse upon grounds of mutual interest.[5]

In 1922, the Association changed its name to the American Physiotherapy Association so that men could join, and in 1927, the constitution was revised. The Association's goals were as follows:

1. To form a nationwide organ to establish and maintain a professional and scientific standard for those engaged in physical therapy.
2. To promote the science of physical therapy by cooperating in the establishment of standardized schools of physical therapy and by encouraging scientific research in the profession.
3. To cooperate with, or under the direction of, the medical profession and to provide a central registry which will make available to the medical profession efficiently trained assistants in physical therapy.[6]

In the early years, the American Physiotherapy Association aligned itself very closely with the medical profession. To prevent physical therapy from being mistaken for a cult, the Association demanded that physical therapists work only under the referral of the physician. Individual physical therapists were not to diagnose or to comment on a patient's prognosis.[7]

Those in the profession recognized the importance of high standards for the education and training of physiotherapists and for patient care. However, after a few years, the professional association found the approval process for education, although important, to be somewhat of a burden for an organization run by volunteers. Subsequently, the Association enlisted the professional and financial assistance of the American Medical Association in 1933. Listed in Table 1–1 is the chronology of accreditors of physical therapy education programs. In 1936, ''The Essentials for an Acceptable School for Physical Therapy Technicians,'' criteria for accrediting programs, was developed by the Council on Medical Education and Hospitals of the American Medical Association and the American Physiotherapy Association. The ''Essentials,''

Table 1–1. ACCREDITING AGENCIES FOR PHYSICAL THERAPY EDUCATION PROGRAMS

Agency	Years
American Physiotherapy Association	1928–1933
Council on Medical Education and Hospitals of the American Medical Association	1933–1959
American Medical Association in conjunction with the American Physical Therapy Association	1959–1976
Council on Allied Health Education Accreditation, American Medication Association*	1976–1983
Commission on Accreditation of Physical Therapy Education, American Physical Therapy Association*	1976–present

* From 1976 to 1983 the Council on Allied Health Education Accreditation of the American Medical Association only accredited a few programs. The vast majority were accredited by the Commission on Accreditation of Physical Therapy Education of the American Physical Therapy Association. After 1983, all programs were accredited by the Commission on Accreditation of Physical Therapy Education of the American Physical Therapy Association.

which were adopted by the American Medical Association's House of Delegates, stated that candidates for admission to accredited physical therapy programs must meet at least one of the following requirements:

- Two years or 60 semester hours of college, including courses in physics and biology.
- Graduation from an accredited school of nursing.
- Graduation from an accredited school of physical education.[8]

Education for the physical therapist was conducted in hospital programs and institutions of higher education. The "Essentials" stated that affiliation with a college, university, or medical school was desirable but not an absolute requirement. Early in the profession's history, two significant trends developed: a preference for postgraduate candidates and a preference for locating programs in institutions of higher education.

Physical therapy practice was concentrated in military hospitals, childrens' hospitals, civilian hospitals, and outpatient clinics. At least one physical therapist, Hazel Furscott, practiced independently as early as 1918.[9]*

The Second Major Growth Period: World War II (1940 to 1946)

In 1941, the United States, in the midst of yet another world war, found that the country needed a substantial increase in the number of qualified physical therapists to treat the wounded.[10] Emergency training programs were conducted in three civilian installations and in 10 army hospitals. Walter Reed, one of the army schools, once again became a focal point for the profession.[11] During the war, the number of physical therapists who served in the army increased from 250 to 1632. These numbers included the additional physical therapists who volunteered and those newly trained by the Army.[10,11]

The Third Major Growth Period: The Polio Epidemic (1948 to 1970)

Following World War II, the polio epidemic increased the need for physical therapists in this country and abroad. Physical therapists treated the victims of polio in many different settings, not just

hospitals. When gamma globulin and vaccines were developed, physical therapists helped conduct controlled studies in multiple sites to determine the effectiveness of the treatments.[2] The physical therapists who participated in the first study of gamma globulin were Miriam Jacobs, Carmella Gonnella, and Georgianna Harmon. Thirty-eight additional physical therapists participated in the follow-up study in 35 states. This was one of the first multicenter clinical research trials involving physical therapists. Later, in 1954, when the Salk vaccine was developed and tested, an additional 35 physical therapists participated in the multicenter study. These clinical trials benefited physical therapy as well as medicine. The abridged muscle grading system, developed by Jessie Wright, PT, MD, and her staff at the DT Watson School of Physiatrics, was produced at the same time in conjunction with the studies.[2]

The Fourth Major Growth Period: Social Forces[12]† (1970 to 1993)

Between the beginning of the polio epidemic in the 1950s and 1970, the number of physical therapists and physical therapy education programs increased very gradually. Since 1970, the number of schools, and concomitantly the number of physical therapists, has risen dramatically (see Figure 1–1). No single event accounts for the increase in the demand for physical therapy services. Rather, it

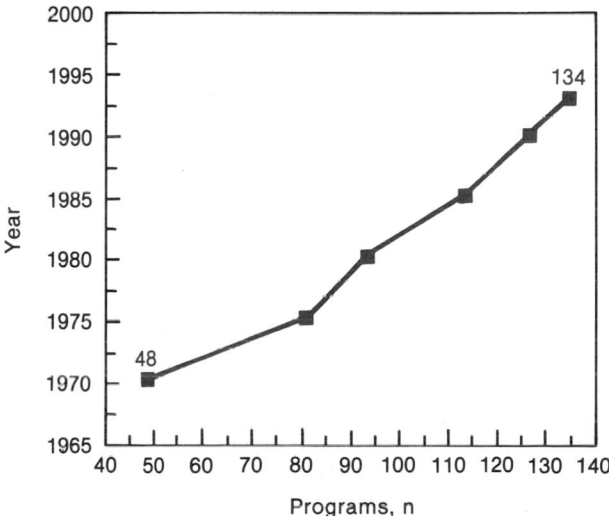

FIGURE 1–1 The growth of physical therapist education programs from 1970 to the present.

---

* Furscott, the fifth president of the American Physiotherapy Association (1928–1930), started an independent practice at 384 Post Street, San Francisco 2 weeks after Armistice Day in 1918.

---

† The author attributes M. J. Delehanty with the name for this period.

reflects the public's growing realization that physical therapy makes a difference in the lives of those afflicted with hereditary diseases, birth defects, athletic injuries, traumatic injuries, surgical interventions, infectious diseases, and acute and chronic diseases affecting most of the body's systems. Legislative acts reflecting the increase in concern for infants and children (Education of All Handicapped Act) and the elderly (Medicare Act) and the dramatic increase in health care for people who are between childhood and old age reflects the nation's concern for our physical health. The increased interest in sports and other activities that aid in cardiovascular fitness and the increase in the number of Americans participating in various organized and unorganized sports also are signs of this focus on health. For the first time, physical therapists are examining and treating substantial numbers of people who are injured but not sick. Another factor in the increased demand for physical therapists is the change in reimbursement for health services—namely, Diagnostic Related Groups (DRGs). This change necessitates earlier discharge of patients from hospitals, which has two effects: (1) physical therapy is needed earlier in a patient's hospital stay to improve function as quickly as possible; and (2) the need for home physical therapy services has increased because patients who are discharged from hospitals earlier are in many cases sicker, weaker, and not as functional as patients were in the past when discharged.

Despite the tremendous increase in the number of education programs for physical therapists and the addition of education programs for physical therapy assistants (see Figure 1–2), as well as the immigration of foreign physical therapists, the demand for services far outweighs the supply. The American Physical Therapy Association (APTA) estimates that of the approximately 80,000 licensed physical therapists, 77,500 are practicing.[3] Based on projections made in 1992 by the US Bureau of Labor Statistics,[13] approximately 93,000 physical therapist positions existed in the United States in 1993, resulting in a shortage of 15,400.[3] Whether the demand for physical therapy services will continue to increase at its current rate is a matter of dispute.

The health care delivery system and the methods of reimbursement are changing in response to technological advances, the urgent need to control costs, and the political impetus to provide health care for all citizens. The effects of a national health care system may result in changes in the location, method, and content of physical therapy services and the frequency of treatment. Given the

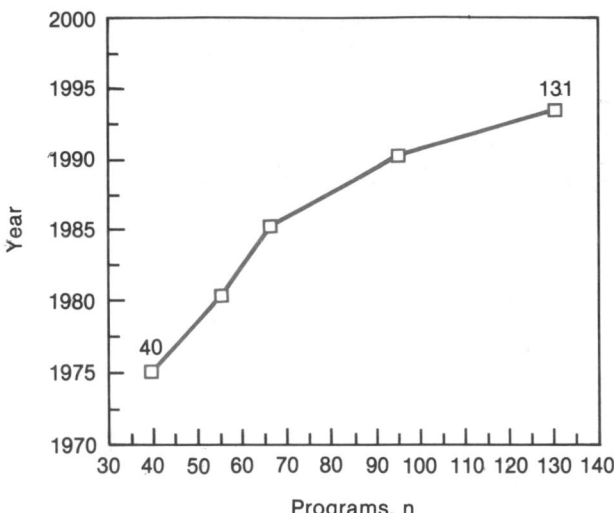

FIGURE 1–2   The growth of physical therapist assistant education programs from 1970 to the present.

projected increases in the elderly population and in the number of patients with human immunodeficiency virus, as well as the possible extension of health care coverage to those not currently covered and the other influences mentioned here, it reasonably can be presumed that the demand for physical therapists will only increase in the future. Demand may plateau or even decrease for a few years before a new health care system is truly established. However, demand should increase once again to levels similar to those experienced in the early 1990s.

Brown has suggested that physical therapists should know, participate in forming, and provide services in concert with the *mission* of the health care institution, because the impending changes in health care delivery may be quite radical.[14] The author further predicts that all health care services will be judged, paid for, and continued to be offered based on the following criteria:

1. Cost-effectiveness.
2. Contribution that they make to overall patient outcomes.
3. Alternative procedures and their cost effectiveness and benefits compared with those of physical therapy services.

ASSUMPTIONS

Practice Environments

When the profession began, physical therapists practiced mainly in hospitals and occasionally in physicians' offices. During the 75-year history of the profession, the settings became more diverse, and the percentage of physical therapists practicing in certain settings has shifted significantly. For example, during the past 15 years, the percentage of physical therapists practicing in hospitals has decreased by 46%, and the percentage practicing in independent physical therapy offices has increased by 176%.[15] Other changes include an increase of 42% in rehabilitation hospitals with and without inpatient beds, an increase of 31% in home health agencies, an increase of 182% in prepaid health care organizations, a decrease of 10% in extended-care facilities, and a decrease of 19% in academic institutions (see Table 1–2). Other types of settings include industrial settings, freestanding outpatient clinics, physicians' offices, and health maintenance and prevention programs.

Physical therapists often practice in more than one setting, combining both a primary and a secondary practice setting. In the APTA's *"1993 Active Membership Profile Report,"* 53% of the respondents indicated that they practice in a secondary setting in addition to their primary setting (see Table 1–3).[15]

When viewed in conjunction, the primary and secondary physical therapy practice settings indicate that a significant number of physical therapists practice in settings in which they are relatively autonomous. This is not to say that physical therapy practice is without referral from another practitioner in all of these settings, but rather that, on

Table 1–2. PRIMARY PHYSICAL THERAPY PRACTICE SETTINGS: 1978 TO 1993

Setting	Distribution in 1978, %	Distribution in 1993, %	Percent Change
Hospital	47.10	25.4	−46.0
Private physical therapy office	9.92	27.4	176.0
Rehabilitation center	9.24	13.1	42.0
Extended-care facility	8.20	7.4	−10.0
Home health agency	5.88	7.7	31.0
School	5.65	3.5	−38.0
Academic institution	5.20	4.2	−19.0
Prepaid health care organization	0.39	1.1	182.0
Research center	0.19	0.2	5.0
Other	8.23	8.2	22.0

(Calculated from American Physical Therapy Association: *1993 Active Membership Profile Report.* Alexandria, American Physical Therapy Association, 1994.)

Table 1–3. SECONDARY PHYSICAL THERAPY PRACTICE SETTINGS: 1993

Secondary Setting	Distribution, %
Home health agency	12.3
Extended-care facility or nursing home	8.6
Hospital	8.6
Research center	6.2
Rehabilitation center	5.9
Prepaid health care organization	3.0
Private physical therapy office	0.7
School	0.6
Academic institution	0.4
Other	8.3

(Calculated from American Physical Therapy Association: *1993 Active Membership Profile Report.* Alexandria, American Physical Therapy Association, 1994.)

a day-to-day basis, physical therapists make independent decisions about the treatment of their patients.

This author assumes that the diversity of practice settings will increase as the health care delivery system evolves and changes. Brown speaks of the continual "unbundling" of services, evidenced by many free-standing, loosely coupled services. In addition to the settings listed in Tables 1–2 and 1–3, other settings include surgical centers and ambulatory health care centers.[14]

Direct Access, Diagnosis, and Referral to Other Practitioners

Direct access is the evaluation and treatment without referral from another health care practitioner. Traditionally, physical therapists evaluated and treated patients only on the basis of written referral from a practitioner such as a physician, osteopath, dentist, or podiatrist. In fact, most physical therapist state practice acts contained language limiting practice to written referrals. (The exceptions were those of Nebraska and California.) Additionally, from 1935 to 1977, the APTA's *Code of Ethics* and *Guide for Professional Conduct* contained similar limitations.[16–21]

In the 1970s, the Australian Physiotherapy Association, the Canadian Physiotherapy Association, and the World Confederation for Physical Therapy changed their codes of ethics to allow for practice without a referral.[22] In 1979, changes in a physical therapist's ethical and legal right to evaluate and treat a patient without a referral from another practitioner began to evolve in the United States. Maryland was the first state in 11 years to change the Physical Therapist Practice Act to include evaluation and treatment without referral.[23,24]*

In 1979 and 1981, the APTA House of Delegates adopted the following policies:

- Physical therapists may ethically provide evaluation and consultation without practitioner referral where permitted by law (RC 17-79).[25]
- Physical therapists may be a point of entry into the health care system for evaluation, treatment, and prevention (RC 60-81).[26]
- Physical therapists may ethically treat patients, within the limits of their knowledge, experience, and expertise, without practitioner referral where permitted by law (RC 52-81).[26]

''Practice only on referral'' was deleted from the APTA's *Code of Ethics and Guide for Professional Conduct* in 1981.[27] The publication contained the following language:

PRINCIPLE 2

Physical therapists comply with the laws and regulations governing the practice of physical therapy.
2.1 Professional Practice

Physical therapists are to provide consultation, evaluation, treatment, and preventative care, in accordance with the laws and regulations of the jurisdiction(s) in which they practice.

PRINCIPLE 3

Physical therapists accept responsibility for the exercise of sound judgment.
3.1 Acceptance of Responsibility

A. Upon accepting an individual for provision of physical therapy services, physical therapists are to assume the responsibility for evaluating that individual; planning, implementing, and supervising the therapeutic program; reevaluating and changing that program; and maintaining adequate records of the case, including progress reports.
   B. When the individual's needs are beyond the scope of the physical therapist's expertise, the individual is to be so informed and assisted in identifying a qualified person to provide the necessary services.[27]

---

* Nebraska's physical therapy practice act never contained the referral restrictions. Therefore, in 1957 Nebraska was the first state to allow direct access to physical therapy services without referral.

California was actually the first state to change an existing practice act to allow direct access (1968).

Principles 2 and 3 in the current *Code and Guide* read essentially the same with the exception of the revision of 3.1 B, which now reads as follows:

When the individual's needs are beyond the scope of the physical therapist's expertise, or when additional services are indicated, the individual shall be so informed and assisted in identifying a qualified provider.[28]

The current APTA policy, which was adopted in 1985, reads as follows:

Entry Point into Health Care:
A physical therapist may be the entry point into the health care system for evaluation, treatment, and prevention. External recognition and acceptance of this policy shall serve as a goal for the Association (RC 33-85).[29]

The number of states permitting direct access grew from 2 in 1968 to 30 in 1993. The greatest increase occurred during the period between 1985 and 1990 (see Table 1–4).[30] Fourteen additional states allow the physical therapist to evaluate the patient without a referral; however, in these states, a written referral must be obtained to treat a patient.

These changes in the *Code of Ethics* and in state licensure regulations have had profound implications for physical therapy practice. The physical therapist currently enjoys a different level of professional responsibility and stature in the health care system in the states that permit direct access. Physical therapy can be a point of entry for the patient into the health care system, thereby reducing the amount of time before the patient is treated by the physical therapist and, additionally, decreasing the cost of medical care by eliminating an unnecessary consultation. Of course, as usually is the case when changes occur, reimbursement for direct access lags behind the changes in the

Table 1–4. CUMULATIVE NUMBER OF STATES HAVING A PRACTICE ACT THAT PERMITTED DIRECT ACCESS TO PHYSICAL THERAPY SERVICES

Years	States, n	Increase, n
1975–1979	3	1
1980–1984	6	3
1985–1990	24	18
1991–1993	30	6

(From American Physical Therapy Association: *States Which Permit Physical Therapy Treatment Without Referral.* Alexandria, American Physical Therapy Association, 1993.)

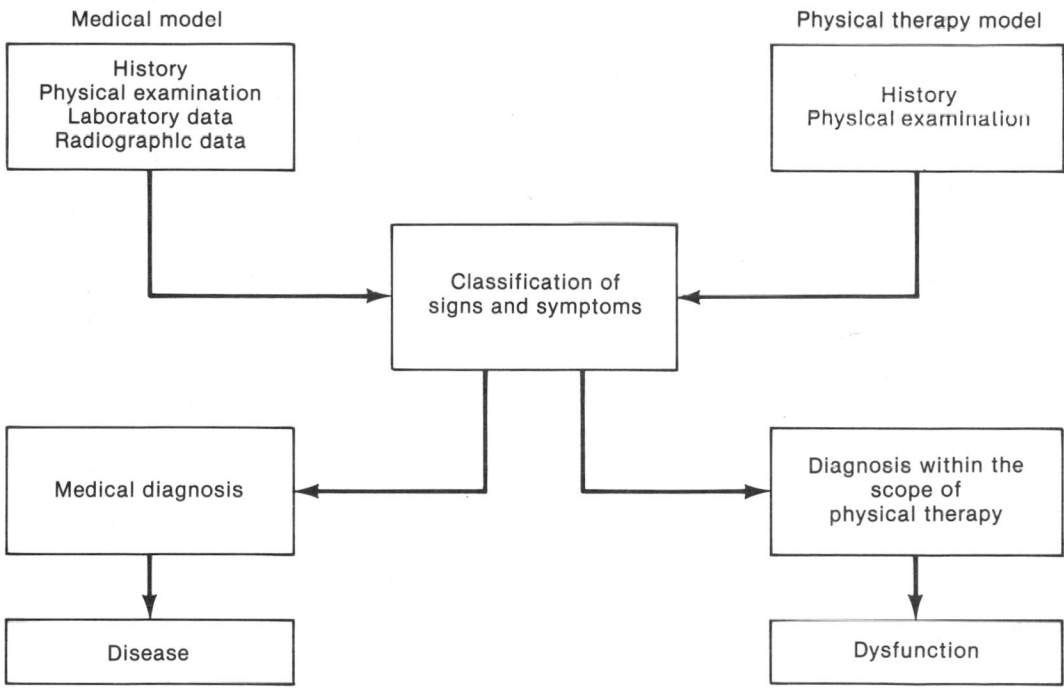

FIGURE 1–3   A comparison of the diagnostic process in physical therapy and medicine. (Redrawn from Domholdt E, Clawson AL, Flech PW, Taylor TK: *Direct Access to Physical Therapy Services.* Alexandria, American Physical Therapy Association, 1991, p 22 with the permission of the American Physical Therapy Association.)

law. Slowly, insurance companies are recognizing the right of the patient to seek physical therapy care first when a problem is evident, and they realize that there are cost savings when the patient seeks such care.

Diagnosis and Prognosis

Concomitant with the change to direct access is the growing realization that physical therapists should establish a diagnosis before beginning physical therapy treatment. The level of professional responsibility should be evident if the physical therapist is the patient's first contact in the health care system. It is the physical therapist's responsibility to examine the patient and diagnose the condition or dysfunction for which the patient will be treated. This does not mean that the physical therapist may establish a medical or dental diagnosis. The physical therapist should establish a diagnosis "within the scope of physical therapy, within the physical therapist's knowledge, experience, and expertise."[31] The diagnosis established by the physical therapist should assist in determining the dysfunction's treatment and, presumably, the prognosis (see Figures 1–3 and 1–4).

Shirley Sahrmann, a professor in physical therapy at Washington University, has proposed the following:

Physical therapists should have a clear statement of the meaning of the diagnostic word and the context in which they will responsibly and legally use it. A generic definition will also help to guide the development of diagnostic classification schemes:

. . . Diagnosis is the term that names the primary dysfunction toward which the physical therapist directs treatment. The dysfunction is identified by the physical therapist based on the information obtained from the history, signs, symptoms, examination, and tests the therapist performs or requests.[32]

Sahrmann further stipulates that the proposed definition is broad enough to provide for future growth and to include specialty practice. She argues against a "*physical therapy diagnosis* which would imply that it would be unique to physical therapy."[32]

For some, the word "diagnosis" evokes apprehension. However, diagnosis, in the practical sense, simply implies the recognition of signs and symptoms as a pattern. Diagnosis is the classification of conditions based on a fit with a recognizable pattern.

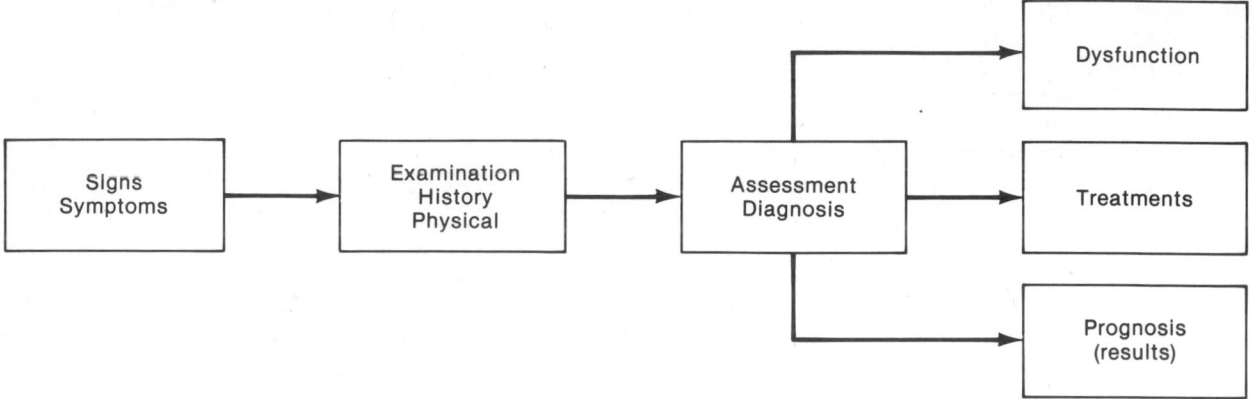

FIGURE 1–4   The diagnosis established by the physical therapist should assist in determining what to treat (dysfunction), which treatments to use, and what result to expect (prognosis).

Diagnosis, then, basically involves pattern recognition and indentification of diagnostic categories. Physical therapists are developing new categories, but their number is not yet sufficient for our diverse practice. We are challenged to increase these diagnostic categories and use them universally in our practice.

Physical therapy has come a long way since 1935, when the profession's *Code of Ethics* flatly stated the following:

I. Professional practice

a. *Diagnosing, stating of the prognosis of a case, and prescribing of treatment shall be entirely the responsibility of the physician. Any assumption of this responsibility by one of our members shall be considered unethical.*
b. *The patient shall be referred back to the physician for periodical examinations.*
c. *A member shall not attempt to criticize the physician or dictate technique or procedure.[16]*

Until 1969, the *Code* remained essentially unchanged on diagnosis, prognosis, and referral. In 1969, the language on diagnosis and prognosis was eliminated, signaling that the profession had taken a significant step in recognizing the growing knowledge and independence of the physical therapist. This change in the *Code* on diagnosis and prognosis, however, preceded by 12 years the elimination of the requirement to treat patients only on the referral of another practitioner. The importance of diagnosing patients before treating them became evident, and in fact necessary, with the change to direct access. However, others may argue that these changes in diagnosis merely reflect the maturation of the profession, which is exhibited in our growing sophistication in examination and treatment. Direct access and diagnostic

sophistication are obvious signs of growing autonomy and therefore are inextricably intertwined.

In Chapter 2, the concepts and the process of diagnosis and its relevance in physical therapy practice are further developed.

The Referral Process and Responsibilities

The ability to discern which cases exceed the therapist's training is an inherent responsibility of direct-access practice. The emphasis on discernment closely parallels one of the basic philosophical tenets of the participants of the consensus development conference, Impact I on the Content of Postbaccalaureate Degree Entry-Level Education. The participants noted that "Above all else, graduates are expected to do no harm."[33] But of course, the responsibilities of the physical therapist go beyond doing no harm; as professionals, they must provide good care and advice to their patients. The *Guide for Professional Conduct*'s interpretation of the *Code of Ethics* "Principle 3" is as follows: "Physical therapists accept responsibility for the exercise of sound judgement." The guide clearly states that physical therapists have a responsibility to inform the patient as well as to provide assistance in identifying a qualified provider.[28] Of course, the responsibility to refer the patient is really independent of whether it is a referral or direct-access patient.

The physical therapist's responsibility goes beyond assistance in identifying a qualified provider for the patient. The physical therapist's major responsibility in referral is to provide the physical therapist, physician, or other health care professional with adequate information based on the examination (history and physical), assessment and diagnosis, and recommendations. Goodman and Snyder[34] and Boissonnault[35] have provided a process for identifying the signs and symptoms that indicate that the case exceeds the professional capacity of the practitioner. All of these authors suggest that the physical therapy examination should contain four major components:

1. Subjective examination.
2. Objective examination.
3. Specific review of symptoms.
4. Assessment[35] (Figure 1–5).

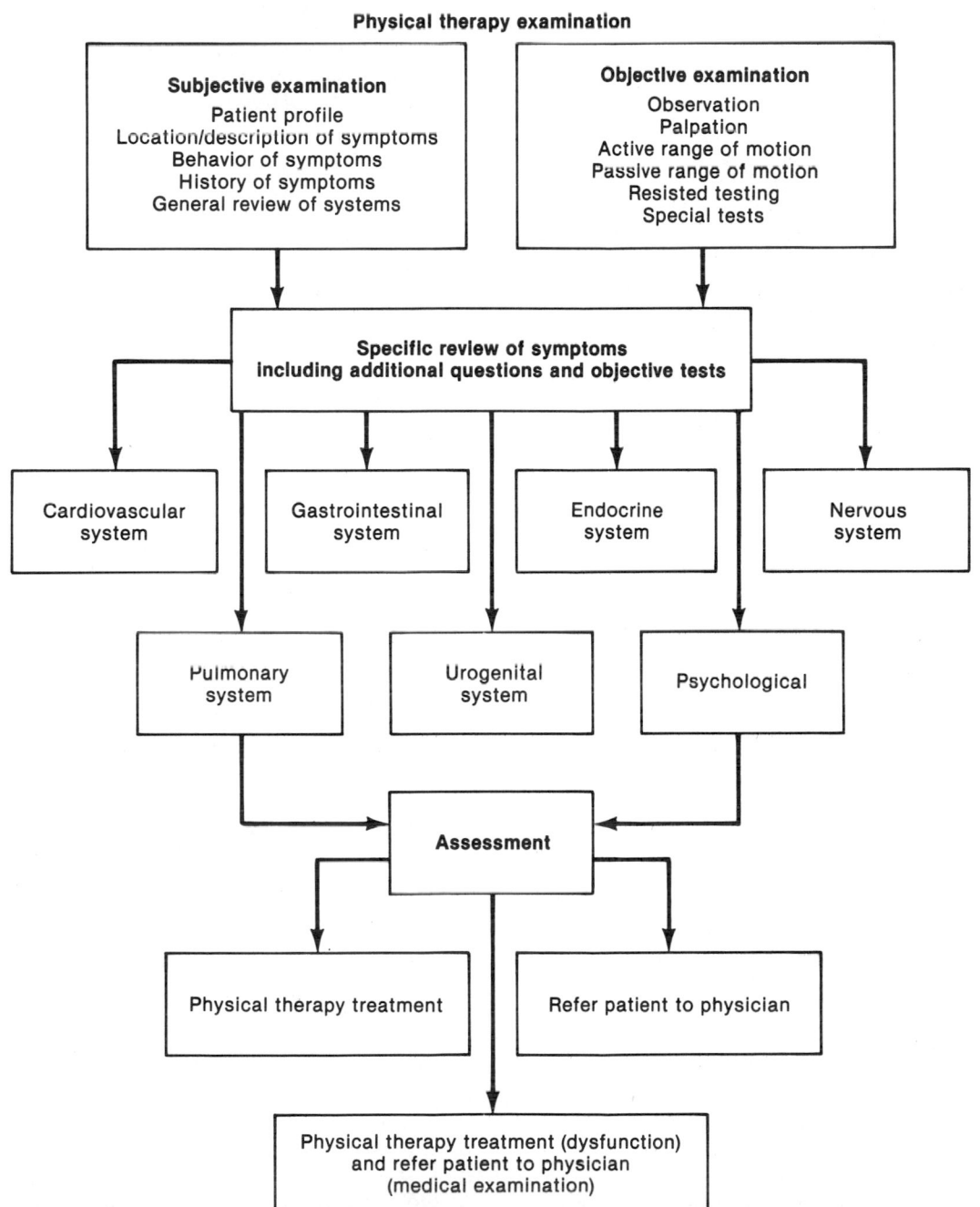

FIGURE 1–5 Components of a physical therapy evaluation that may provide the clinical information that leads to referring the patient to a physician. (From Boissonnault WG: *Examination in Physical Therapy Practice: Screening for Medical Disease.* New York, Churchill Livingstone, 1991, p 3.)

The information that should be contained in a written referral from the physical therapist to a physician or other practitioner is listed in Table 1–5. The referral provides the physical therapist with two additional opportunities, one of which is to educate the practitioner about physical therapy, and the other, to develop a collegial relationship. Adequate written and oral communication is essential in the physical therapist's referral relationships with other practitioners and, of course, with their patients.

The Scientific and Theoretical Basis of Physical Therapy Practice

For years, physical therapists based their approaches on the philosophy, "if it works use it," regardless of whether the tests and treatments had been subjected to rigorous study or whether they were based on theoretical constructs. Certain methods of treatment were used, and later, physical therapists tried to establish why these methods worked or on what basis they should work. An example is the Bobath method for treating individuals with cerebral palsy. Research was not conducted in the early days to ascertain whether this approach was more effective in treating neurological disorders than the conventional treatment. We in fact relied on the testimony of individuals who used the newer approach. Ironically, a requirement for employment in certain institutions was certification in the unsubstantiated neuromuscular developmental treatment.

Table 1–5. SUMMARY OF INFORMATION INCLUDED IN A REFERRAL TO ANOTHER PRACTITIONER

A. Date of patient examination
B. Presenting complaints
   1. Signs
   2. Symptoms
C. History
D. Physical therapy examination
   1. Differential examination
   2. Tests and results
E. Assessment and diagnosis
   1. Dysfunction (diagnosis)
   2. Findings requiring referral
F. Recommendations:
   1. Medical or other type of follow-up
      a. Return to physical therapy
         (1) Specific information requested before physical therapy treatment is initiated
      b. No return to physical therapy for this set of signs, symptoms, and diagnosis

Perhaps the first physical therapist to raise concerns in the profession about failure to adhere to scientific standards in the choice of treatments was Catherine Worthingham. In her 1959 speech to the New York Chapter of the APTA, she stated

Many of you fail to realize that to call yourselves professional does not of itself entitle you to such a designation. To be professional, members of a group must possess a body of knowledge that is both identifiable and different from that of other professionals. They must also assume responsibility for adding to that body of knowledge and for developing their own standards of education and practice.

If we agree that a craftsman becomes a professional when he possesses an identifiable body of knowledge built on basic principles and not just a set of techniques, we must also agree that the rate of growth of the profession will be in proportion to the rate at which that body of knowledge and basic principles grows.

How, then, is any body of knowledge and set of basic principles developed? In one form or another (depending on the kind of material one deals with) the answer is: through research.[36]

This address was given 32 years after the adoption of the APTA's constitution, which stated that one of its purposes was "encouraging scientific research in the profession." In 1959, very few physical therapists were educated at the doctoral level.[37] In recent years, considerably greater numbers of physical therapists have obtained the academic preparation necessary to conduct good research.[15,38] Research in the early years did not always focus on clinical trials; therefore, the profession has developed its own unique body of knowledge very slowly.

In her landmark 1975 speech, "The Not-So-Impossible Dream," Helen Hislop suggested that the profession should define its body of knowledge as *pathokinesiology*.[39] She challenged the profession to achieve greatness through the development of its unique science of pathokinesiology, the development of absolute standards of clinical performance, and the production of scholars in human pathokinesiology. She stated that "Not every therapist can become a scholar in the true sense, but every therapist can be imbued with an understanding of science as it is applied to physical therapy."[39]

In the subsequent years, academic education programs included research design in the curriculum. Indeed, many programs required a completed research project for graduation. Student research projects represent a significant number of research articles reported in our journal, *Physical Therapy*. In addition, research today is often conducted by clinicians who have not necessarily completed doctoral programs. They usually do not have knowledge of intricate clinical trial design or the theoretical base to conduct coherent large-scale research projects.

In 1988 and 1990, two articles were published in *Physical Therapy* that argued that physical therapy research should be *theoretically* based.[40,41] In the 1990 article, Tammivaara and Shepard noted that there had been a significant increase in the number of research articles published and reported at physical therapy conferences in a struggle to develop a core of knowledge for basic practice. However, the authors asked how physical therapists differed from other specialists, such as exercise physiologists: "Are their research programs leading them to develop and test knowledge that is unique to physical therapy practice?"[41] They suggested that many studies lack an underlying explanatory framework and thus do not lead to new areas of research. The conclusion can be made that much of our research is piecemeal and does not represent a coherent whole for the clinician. Studies should not only examine the reliability and validity of our measurement instruments but should also address basic and advanced theories of practice.

The majority of this book is devoted to the examination and treatment of the patient. Subsequent chapters discuss the state of the art and science as we know it today. The authors have written their chapters based on current literature and their clinical expertise. Books such as this manual document an ever-increasing scientific core of knowledge. In the next few years, an integrated model of physical therapy practice based on theoretical frameworks for clinical practice will be refined, and preliminary testing begun.[42]

Two significant publications, *Movement Science: Foundation for Physical Therapy in Rehabilitation*[43] and *Contemporary Management of Motor Control Problems: Proceedings of the II Step Conference,*[44] have recently steered the profession in new directions. Both publications suggest that a new theoretical basis for physical therapy should be movement science combined with the study of motor control and motor learning. The term *movement science,* which includes developmental, behavioral, anatomical, physiological, biochemical, and biomechanical theories and their influences on movement, appears to have supplanted the term *pathokinesiology* in physical therapy literature.

It is imperative that a partnership between clinicians and researchers be created for the development of tests and treatments based on theoretical constructs. This partnership is crucial not only for establishing the profession's core of knowledge but also for the survival and future growth of the profession. This author mentioned earlier that the health care system is undergoing dramatic changes and that these changes are often based on cost. If the profession is to survive the reconstruction, physical therapy practice must have sound foundations and demonstrate functional outcomes at an effective cost. Physical therapists must know what they are treating, what works, why it works, and how long it will take to reach certain functional outcomes. They will be required to demonstrate that their research base for clinical practice is credible. They can no longer say "I use this method because it works for me" but will be required to produce the scientific literature substantiating their choice of examinations and treatments rather than relying on their past experience.

Additionally, what is practiced must go hand in hand with how physical therapists interact with those in their environment. The physical therapist cannot practice in a vacuum but must interact effectively with the patient, the family, and, of increasing importance, other health care professionals, technicians, administrators of institutions, third-party payers, and personnel of managed health care. The ability to communicate effectively may determine which tests and treatments will be reimbursed and how many treatments will be funded for each patient.

ETHICAL CONSIDERATIONS

The APTA's *Code of Ethics and Guide for Professional Conduct* (see Appendix A), and *Standards of Practice for Physical Therapy* provide an ethical and good-practice basis for physical therapy. As illustrated in the preceding pages, aspects of these documents have been revised to reflect changes in the evolving practice and ethical behavior of the profession. In addition to other aspects of ethical behavior contained in the *Code of Ethics*, physical therapy professionals recognize the need to obtain informed consent before evaluating and treating patients. Informed consent has been a critical component in the conduct of research.[45–50] However, from an ethical and legal standpoint, consent is now more important in patient treatment.[51–65] In the United States, the APTA's *Standards of Practice for Physical Therapy* contains the mandate to obtain informed consent, with the *Code of Ethics and Guide for Professional Conduct*[28] providing the background for the *Standards.* However, the Canadian Physiotherapy Association's *Code of Ethics: Rules of Conduct*[66] directly addresses the need for informed consent.

Following are definitions, background information, and elements of informed consent:

Definitions

Ethics. The philosophical study of morality.
Law. The system of principles governing conduct; law is enforced by courts.
Beneficence. The act of producing good outcomes or doing what is good for an individual.
Paternalism. In ethics, the making of decisions for the patient without allowing the patient to choose the evaluations or treatments (or no treatment) based on the information provided by the health care professional. It implies that the health care professional knows exactly what is best for the patient and also that what is done protects the patient. In some cases, the health care professional may override or distort the information to coerce the patient to choose one treatment or evaluation over another. This is usually done for the patient's benefit.
Battery. Simply the act of touching a patient directly or with an object without that person's consent. The touching may or may not be offensive. It may be done for the patient's benefit. The important element is that it is done without the patient's permission.
Autonomy. The right of self-determination. A competent person always has the right to decide what will or will not be done to them. This term implies that the person will be involved in the decision.
Disclosure. Information provided to the patient. Various types of disclosure are:

- Patient preference (providing the patient with information that the person requests).
- Customary professional information (telling the patient what is usually told to patients in a given situation).
- Prudent person (providing the patient with the information that a prudent, reasonable person would want before making a decision about treatment or refusing treatment)[67]
- Subjective substantial disclosure (providing the patient with everything that is material or important to an individual patient, not a fictitious patient, in making a decision).[67]

Surrogate. Usually a family member who decides whether treatment will be accepted when patients are not competent to decide for themselves. Ethical and legal competence may differ. For example, a minor is not legally responsible for his/her actions but may be judged ethically competent whether to accept or refuse treatment.

Informed Consent

Historically, physicians and physical therapists evaluated a patient and subsequently decided which treatment option had the best outcome potential for him/her. Little if any information on the diagnosis, prognosis, and treatment options was given to the patient. It was understood that the patient would submit to any tests or treatments the health care professional determined best. Both physician and physical therapist were paternalistic.

The patient's right of self-determination has become legally and ethically more important as technology has enhanced treatment options and as patients are better informed about health, ethical, and legal issues. Changes to direct access and independent practice should spur the physical therapist to obtain the patient's informed consent before treatment is given.[51,52,55,60,62] However, acquiring informed consent is important in all practice settings. Additionally, seeking the patient's informed consent may enhance patient compliance.[57]

Obtaining Informed Consent

The written information provided to the patient or surrogate should contain the following:[51,55,59,60,62,65,68,69]

1. Diagnosis and description of the patient's status.
2. Description and purpose of the proposed examination or treatment procedures.
3. Rationale for the recommended examination or treatment procedures.
4. Description of the potential risks and consequences associated with the examination or treatment procedures. Exclude eventualities too remote or improbable to bear significantly on the decision process of a reasonable person. Include the provider and the institution's success or failure rate with the proposed procedures.
5. Explanation of benefits resulting from the examination or treatment procedures.
6. Prospects for the examination's or treatment procedure's success.
7. Reasonable alternative forms of examination or treatment procedures. Repeat Steps 2 through 7 for the alternatives.
8. Prognosis if examination or treatment is rejected.
9. All costs, including the amount and duration of pain generally involved, the potential impact on lifestyle and ability to resume work, and the economic costs of both the treatment and the

follow-up care. The patient also should be told if insurance will cover the bills.

The information provided to the patient should be tailored to him/her in language that is not overly technical. This, of course represents a challenge for the physical therapist who must acquaint himself/herself with the patient reasonably well in the first one or two visits. In preparing the informed consent forms, physical therapists must compile materials on many different examinations and treatments and should review their own personal records and the institutions' records of success.

The informed consent process provides several unique benefits for the patient and the physical therapist, including:

1. Respect for the patient's autonomy and dignity.
2. Enhanced communication between the patient and the physical therapist, which may lead to

   • A better understanding of the patient's goals by both the physical therapist and the patient.
   • More consistent patient compliance with the treatment if the patient decides to accept the recommendations.

3. The fact that the physical therapist will review alternatives to the proposed examinations or treatment procedures, perhaps leading to a better understanding of these methods.
4. The need to explain in writing should clearly illustrate which procedures are documented and supported by well-designed and well-executed research.
5. The inability to provide adequate documentation for a favorite treatment may prompt the physical therapist to look for better-supported treatments. More importantly, the lack of documentation may be the stimulus to participate in research to find the answers not now available.

The informed consent process certainly should lead to effective and, hopefully, cost-effective, treatment while complying with the law and ethical professional behavior.

Acknowledgement

I appreciate the assistance of Jessica L. Myers in editing this chapter.

References

1. Hazenhyer IM: A history of the American Physiotherapy Association: prelude. *Phys Ther Rev* 1946, 26:3–17.
2. Beard G: Foundations of growth: a review of the first forty years in terms of education, practice, and research. *Phys Ther Rev* 1961, 41:843–861.
3. American Physical Therapy Association: *Human Resources Estimates for Physical Therapists in the United States*. Alexandria, American Physical Therapy Association, 1993.
4. McMillan M: Physical therapy from the embryo on three continents. *Phys Ther Rev* 1946, 26:254–257.
5. American Women's Physical Therapeutic Association: *Constitution*. New York, American Women's Physical Therapeutic Association, 1921.
6. American Physiotherapy Association: Constitution. *Phys Ther Rev* 1927, 7:31.
7. American Physiotherapy Association: *Code of Ethics*. New York, American Physiotherapy Association, 1935.
8. The essentials for an acceptable school for physical therapy technicians. *Phys Ther Rev* 1936, 16:202–204.
9. Hislop HJ, Winters Schottstaedt D: Personal communication, November, 1993.
10. Hazenhyer IM: A history of the American Physiotherapy Association: Part IV. Maturity, 1939–1946. *Phys Ther Rev* 1946, 26:174–184.
11. Vogel ME: The status of medical department physical therapists from World War I to V-J Day. *Phys Ther Rev* 1946, 26:259–261.
12. Delehanty MJ: Personal communication, August, 1993.
13. US Department of Labor, Bureau of Labor Statistics: *Occupational Outlook Handbook [Bulletin 2400]*. Washington, DC, US Department of Labor Bureau of Labor Statistics, 1992.
14. Brown GD: Changing health care environments: Implications for physical therapy research, education, and practice. *Phys Ther Rev* 1986, 66:1242–1245.
15. American Physical Therapy Association: *1993 Active Membership Profile Report*. Alexandria, American Physical Therapy Association, 1995.
16. American Physiotherapy Association: *Code of Ethics*. Alexandria, American Physical Therapy Association, 1935.
17. American Physical Therapy Association: *Code of Ethics*. Alexandria, American Physical Therapy Association, 1948.
18. American Physical Therapy Association: *Code of Ethics*. Alexandria, American Physical Therapy Association, 1952.
19. American Physical Therapy Association: *Code of Ethics*. Alexandria, American Physical Therapy Association, 1957.
20. American Physical Therapy Association: *Code of Ethics*. Alexandria, American Physical Therapy Association, 1968.
21. American Physical Therapy Association: *Code of Ethics and Guide for Professional Conduct*. Alexandria, American Physical Therapy Association, 1977.
22. Teager DPG: Referral. *Physiotherapy* 1983, 69:49–51.
23. Taylor TK, Domholdt E: Legislative change to permit direct access to physical therapy services: a study of process and content issues. *Phys Ther* 1991, 71:382–389.
24. Chesin L: Personal communication, August, 1993.
25. American Physical Therapy Association: *House of Delegates Minutes*. Alexandria, American Physical Therapy Association, 1979, p 13.
26. American Physical Therapy Association: *House of Delegates Minutes*. Alexandria, American Physical Therapy Association, 1981, pp 9, 10.
27. American Physical Therapy Association: *Code of Ethics and Guide for Professional Conduct*. Alexandria, American Physical Therapy Association, 1981.
28. American Physical Therapy Association: *Code of Ethics and Guide for Professional Conduct*. Alexandria, American Physical Therapy Association, 1991.
29. American Physical Therapy Association: *House of Delegates Policies: Entry Point into Health Care*. Alexandria, American Physical Therapy Association, 1993, p 30.

30. American Physical Therapy Association: *States Which Permit Physical Therapy Treatment Without Referral.* Alexandria, American Physical Therapy Association, 1993.

31. American Physical Therapy Association: *House of Delegates Policies: Diagnosis by Physical Therapists.* Alexandria, American Physical Therapy Association, 1993, p. 27.

32. Sahrmann SA: Diagnosis by the physical therapist: prerequisite for treatment. A special communication. *Phys Ther* 1988, 68:1703–1706.

33. Myers RS, Wilkinson CP (eds): *Working Papers: Content of Postbaccalaureate Degree Entry-Level Curricula. Impact I Conference.* Alexandria, American Physical Therapy Association, 1992, p 9.

34. Goodman CC, Snyder TEK: *Differential Diagnosis in Physical Therapy: Musculoskeletal and Systemic Conditions.* Philadelphia, W.B. Saunders Company, 1990.

35. Boissonnault WG: *Examination in Physical Therapy Practice: Screening for Medical Disease.* New York, Churchill Livingstone, 1991.

36. Worthingham C: The development of physical therapy as a profession through research and publication. *Phys Ther Rev* 1959, 40:573–577.

37. Hislop HJ, Worthingham C: An analysis of physical therapy education and careers. *Phys Ther Rev* 1958, 38:228–241.

38. American Physical Therapy Association: *Physical Therapy Education.* Alexandria, American Physical Therapy Association, 1992.

39. Hislop HJ: The not so impossible dream: the tenth Mary McMillan lecture. *Phys Ther* 1975, 55:1069–1080.

40. Krebs D, Harris SR: Elements of theory presentations in physical therapy. *Phys Ther* 1988, 68:690–693.

41. Tammivaara J, Shepard KF: Theory: the guide to clinical practice and research. *Phys Ther* 1990, 70:578–582.

42. *The Clinical Practice of Phyiscal Therapy in the 21st Century.* Pittsburgh, Executive Communications, Inc, 1992.

43. Carr JH, Sheperd RB, Gordon J, et al.: *Movement Science: Foundations for Physical Therapy Rehabilitation.* Rockville, Aspen Publishers, Inc, 1987.

44. Lister MJ (ed): *Contemporary Management of Motor Control Problems: Proceedings of the II Step Conference.* Alexandria, Foundation for Physical Therapy, 1991.

45. American Physical Therapy Association: Standards for test and measurements in physical therapy practice. *Phys Ther* 1991, 71:589–622.

46. Michels E: Research and human rights: Part I. *Phys Ther* 1976, 56:407.

47. Michels E: Research and human rights: Part II. *Phys Ther* 1976, 56:546.

48. Payton OD: *Research: The Validation of Clinical Practice,* 2nd ed. Philadephia, F. A. Davis Company, 1988.

49. Currier DP: *Elements of Research in Physical Therapy,* 3rd ed. Baltimore, Williams & Wilkins, 1990.

50. Bork CE: *Research in Physical Therapy.* Philadelphia, J. B. Lippincott Company, 1993.

51. Dumholdt E: *Physical Therapy Research: Principles and Applications.* Philadelphia, W. B. Saunders Company, 1993.

52. Purtilo RB: Applying the principles of informed consent to patient care: legal and ethical considerations for physical therapy. *Phys Ther* 1984, 64:934–937.

53. Purtilo R: Professional responsibility in physiotherapy: old dimensions and new directions. *Physiotherapy* 1986, 72:579–583.

54. Sim J: Informed consent: ethical implications for physiotherapy. *Physiotherapy* 1986, 72:584–587.

55. Bruckner J: Physical therapists as double agents: ethical dilemma of divided loyalties. *Phys Ther* 1987, 67:383–387.

56. Banja JD, Wolf SL: Malpractice litigation for uninformed consent: implications for physical therapists. *Phys Ther* 1987, 67:1226–1229.

57. Purtilo RB: Ethical considerations in physical therapy. In Scully RM, Barnes MR (eds): *Physical Therapy.* Philadelphia, J. B. Lippincott Company, 1989, pp 36–40.

58. Coy JA: Autonomy-based informed consent: ethical implications for patient noncompliance. *Phys Ther* 1989, 69:826–833.

59. Purtilo R: *Health Professional and Patient Interaction,* 4th ed. Philadelphia, W. B. Saunders Company, 1990.

60. Scott RW: *Health Care Malpractice: A Primer on Legal Issues for Professionals.* Thorofare, NJ, Slack, Inc, 1990.

61. Scott RW: Informed consent: Legal briefs. *Clin Management* 1991, 11:12–14.

62. Guccicone AA: Are ethics of clinical research the same as the ethics of clinical practice? *APTA Research Section Newsletter* 1992, 25:2–4.

63. Garrett TM, Baille HW, Garrett RM: *Health Care Ethics: Principles and Problems,* 2nd ed. Englewood Cliffs NJ, Prentice-Hall, 1993.

64. Purtilo R: *Ethical Dimensions in the Health Professions,* 2nd ed. Philadelphia, W. B. Saunders Company, 1993.

65. Lewis CB, Jensen J, Wagner M: The right to choose & refuse. *PT Magazine* 1993, 1:60–63, 91.

66. Canadian Physiotherapy Association: *Code of Ethics: Rules of Conduct.* Toronto, Canadian Physiotherapy Association, 1989.

67. Scott RW: Informed consent: a reminder. *PT Magazine* 1993, 1:63.

68. Meisel A: *The Right to Die.* New York, John Wiley & Sons, 1989.

69. Faden R, Beauchamp TL: *A History and Theory of Informed Consent.* New York, Oxford University Press, 1986.

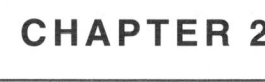

CHAPTER 2

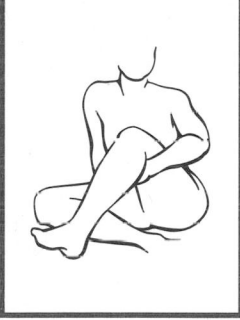

Clinical Decision Making in Physical Therapy Practice

Barbara J. Norton

This manual presents detailed information viewed as germane to physical therapy practice. Each chapter in the sections related to the major body systems incorporates relevant contemporary knowledge from a variety of basic and applied sciences as well as descriptions of (1) specific disorders, (2) relevant examination and test procedures, and (3) treatment options. Therefore, to the extent that the authors have succeeded in their task, this manual reflects the current state of physical therapy practice in each specialty area. Presumably, the practical use of the content-specific information in this manual will benefit physical therapy clients.

When the reader goes back to the beginning of the last statement in the previous paragraph, he/she might notice that the term *presumably* rather than *undoubtedly* was used. This is because at least two assumptions regarding this manual and the reader should be questioned before conclusions are drawn about the impact of the information in this manual on patients and clients. First, can it be assumed that the information in this manual is true? Second, can it be assumed that the reader will apply it correctly? Hopefully now the reader is thinking, "Isn't that true for anything I hear or read?" to which this author would reply "Of course!" The reason it is important to examine these issues now is because two of the general purposes of this chapter are to offer some guidelines for assessing both the credibility and usefulness of information and to ensure the appropriate application of useful information in the clinical setting. To adapt a phrase from Sackett and colleagues,[1] the topics to be covered in this chapter can be said to be part of "the science of the art" of clinical practice.

What is the "science of the art" of clinical practice? The title of the book by Sackett *et al.*, *Clinical Epidemiology: A Basic Science for Clinical Medicine,*[1] reveals one perspective. The science referred to as "clinical epidemiology" by the authors draws on theories and principles from the literature in a variety of areas, such as epidemiology, judgement and decision making, economics, cognitive psychology, social psychology, measurement, research design, statistics, and computer science. At first glance, it may seem odd that none of the basic biomedical and clinical sciences, namely anatomy, physiology, biochemistry, and pathology, are included in the list. The exclusion is not meant to imply that the biomedical and clinical sciences are irrelevant to clinical physical therapy practice but to emphasize the fact that optimal patient care is dependent on the ability of the clinician to apply the most appropriate knowledge in the most useful way to each patient situation. Therefore, clinical epidemiology may be viewed as encompassing the "rules of the game" for selecting and applying information from the basic biomedical and clinical sciences to patient care.

What are some of the major aspects of clinical practice to which "the science of the art" can be applied? According to Sackett and colleagues,[1] there are "three challenges that face every clinician every day: reaching the correct diagnosis, selecting the management that does more good than harm, and keeping up to date with useful advances in medicine." Although many other challenges exist in clinical practice to which every clinician must attend, these three are the focus of this chapter. The organization of this chapter was adapted from the book by Sackett *et al.*; its content is divided into two major sections, the first focusing on diagnosis and classification, and the second on selecting an optimal management strategy. Issues related to keeping oneself informed about current developments are embedded within the sections on diagnosis, classification, and management.

The purpose of this chapter is to draw together a wide variety of topics applicable to physical therapy practice and to present them in a manner that helps clinicians appreciate their relevance. Given the wide range of topics included, none is covered in sufficient depth to provide the reader with a thorough understanding. For a more complete treatment of topics introduced in this chapter, please refer to the "Recommended Reading" section at the end of this chapter.

DIAGNOSIS AND CLASSIFICATION

Evolution in Physical Therapy

Traditional Role of Physical Therapists

Historically, treatment procedures performed by a physical therapist were prescribed by a physician based on the diagnosis of the patient's problem.[2] The physical therapist was trained to perform tests and provide treatments, not to render diagnoses.

Relevance of Physician's Knowledge

Today, much more information is available regarding the effects at cellular and subcellular levels of both disease and pharmacological agents; physicians must be familiar with this information to practice medicine optimally. In addition, the knowledge base specific to movement-related problems amenable to intervention by physical therapists has grown.

Given the modest degree of overlap in knowledge required to manage disease and movement dysfunction, it is unlikely that most physicians have the knowledge required to prescribe the optimal physical therapy treatment for each patient. For example, a prescription from the physician that directs the physical therapist to apply hot packs to the back of a patient with a herniated intervertebral disc may not be appropriate.

Furthermore, it is unlikely that the disease-specific diagnoses rendered by physicians can direct physical therapy treatment. For example, the diagnosis of right cerebrovascular accident on a referral from a physician should give the physical therapist some indication of potential problems but does not serve to delineate a specific focus of and approach to treatment for that particular patient.

Adoption of a New Policy

Recognizing the inadequacy of most physician referrals to direct physical therapy management, in 1984 the House of Delegates (HOD) of the American Physical Therapy Association (APTA) adopted a policy permitting physical therapists to "establish a diagnosis within the scope of their knowledge, experience and expertise."[3] Extreme care was taken in the wording of the policy to ensure that physical therapists would not be either unwittingly encouraged to attempt or understood as attempting to practice medicine.

Since 1984, the increased emphasis on the obligation of physical therapists to assume responsibility for selection of the appropriate physical therapy treatment for each patient based on their examination of the patient and categorization of a patient's condition has been reflected in the professional literature.[2,4–11]

Current Issues

Despite the careful wording of the 1984 HOD policy[3] and the increased emphasis on the need to classify problems before selecting treatment options, the policy and concepts related to the policy still evoke considerable comment and discussion among physical therapists.[9–11]

Applicability of the Term "Diagnosis." One major issue is whether the term "diagnosis" is applicable in the practice of physical therapy.[10,11] One way to approach the issue is to consider the meanings of several inter-related terms in detail; *eg,* as is evident in the definitions provided in Table 2–1, the word "diagnosis" has multiple meanings, and as noted by Guccione,[8] each of the

Table 2–1. DEFINITIONS OF TERMS USED IN CLASSIFICATION AND DIAGNOSIS*

Term	Definition
Classification	1. The act or process of classifying 2. A systematic arrangement in groups or categories according to established criteria; taxonomy, class, category
Classify	1. To arrange in classes 2. To assign to a category
Diagnosis	1. The art or act of identifying a disease from its signs and symptoms; the decision reached by diagnosis 2. A concise technical description of a taxon 3. An investigation or analysis of the cause or nature of a condition, situation, or a problem; a statement or conclusion from such an analysis
Disease	1. Trouble 2. A condition of the living animal or plant body or of one of its parts that impairs the performance of a vital function

* Definitions from *Webster's Ninth New Collegiate Dictionary.* Springfield, MA, Merriam-Webster, Inc, 1990.

meanings is important in the development of the concept of "diagnosis" in physical therapy.

In the following subsection, "Diagnosis: The Label," a line of reasoning is presented that leads to the conclusion that the term diagnosis *is* applicable in physical therapy practice. Because there appears to be some agreement within the profession[2,6–8] that impairments are within the "scope of [the physical therapist's] knowledge, skill, and experience,"[3] the primary objective of this subsection is to demonstrate that the term diagnosis applies not only to diseases but also to impairments.

Diagnosis: The Label. In Table 2–1, the second definition and the second part of the third definition of the term diagnosis refer to the result of the diagnostic process, *ie*, the label or category name given to the condition that traditionally has been referred to in medicine as a "disease." An essential issue is whether disease is the only category of conditions with which the term "diagnosis" can be associated.

Adequacy of the Term "Disease" in Medicine. A related issue that evokes debate in the medical community is the adequacy of the term "disease" for characterizing all of the conditions addressed by physicians. Dictionary definitions of the term "disease" (see Table 2–1) do not refer explicitly to the causes of the conditions referred to as diseases. In common usage, however, the term seems to apply mainly to conditions associated with specific

pathogens (*eg*, bacterial endocarditis and streptococcal pneumonia). Unfortunately, restriction of usage in the manner described excludes a host of clinical entities commonly referred to as diseases, such as multiple sclerosis, rheumatoid arthritis, and diabetes.

As an alternative, Sackett and colleagues[1] suggested that what usually is meant by disease is "the anatomic, biochemical, physiologic, or psychologic derangement whose etiology (if known), maladaptive mechanisms, presentation, prognosis, and management we read about in medical texts." As the authors noted, however, the usefulness of the term is limited by its ambiguity, which is reflected in disagreements over whether "common problems such as hypertension, hay fever and hemorrhoids are diseases,"[1] even though these are conditions for which physicians render diagnoses.

Because of the ambiguity and limitations of the term "disease," Sackett and colleagues[1] recommend using the following two terms:

Target Disorder. This term refers to any one of a broad range of conditions, including diseases, when they become the "element of a patient's sickness," which is the "objective of the diagnostic process."[1]

Illness. This term refers to the "cluster of symptoms and signs"* exhibited by the patient (*eg*, fever, headache, coughing, and sneezing) due to the presence of a target disorder.[1]

Sackett and colleagues also suggest that the purpose of the act of diagnosis is to "recognize the class or group to which a patient's *illness* belongs . . . ."[1]

One implication of the framework of Sackett and colleagues is that the term "diagnosis" may be applicable as a label not only for a disease or target disorder but also for an illness.[1] In fact, it seems safe to assume that many clinical entities were named and were considered diseases when the full extent of knowledge regarding these conditions consisted of a recognizable collection of symptoms and signs, *ie*, an illness. For example, consider Australian X disease. Given the vagueness of the name, at the time the disease was named, it apparently was identifiable only as a distinct cluster of symptoms and signs, *ie*, an illness. Nonetheless, it was labeled a disease.

_____

* As used in this context, "symptoms" refer to manifestations of the problem that a patient perceives; *eg*, pain, stiffness, and difficulty in moving. In contrast, "signs" refer to manifestations of the problem that the clinician observes or measures during the clinical examination; *eg*, limited range of motion, decreased strength, and instability. Emphasis is placed on *clusters* of signs and symptoms, because it rarely is possible to identify a problem on the basis of a single characteristic.

Table 2–2. THE WHO'S ICIDH CATEGORY DEFINITIONS

Category	Definition
Disease	Any pathological process associated with a characteristic and identifiable set of symptoms and signs defined in morphological, chemical, microbiological, and physiological terms*
Impairment	Any loss or abnormality of psychological, physiological, or anatomical structure or function†
Disability	Any restriction or lack (resulting from an impairment) of ability to perform an activity in the manner or within the range considered normal for a human being†
Handicap	A disadvantage for a given individual, resulting from an impairment or a disability, that limits or prevents the fulfillment of a role that is normal (depending on age, sex, and social and cultural factors) for that individual†

* Data from Jette AM: Diagnosis and classification by physical therapists: a special communication. *Phys Ther* 1989, 69:967–969.

† Data from Wood PHN: Appreciating the consequences of disease: the International Classification of Impairments, Disabilities, and Handicaps. *WHO Chronicle* 1980, 34:376–380.

Therefore, even in medicine, the use of the term "diagnosis" is not limited strictly to the labeling of diseases but also seems to be used with illnesses.

Relationship to Terms in Other Classification Systems. The definition of disease in the International Classification of Impairments, Disabilities, and Handicaps (ICIDH), a classification system developed by the World Health Organization (WHO), is noted in Table 2–2. Because the ICIDH definition of disease[12] appears similar to the one offered by Sackett and colleagues,[1] the ICIDH definition also might be viewed as inadequate for encompassing all conditions diagnosed by physicians. In an effort "to expand the concept of disease to cover other conditions of interest to physical therapists," Guccione[8] suggested that "*medical syndromes* which are recognized clusters of signs and symptoms" should be included at the same level as disease in the system of categories proposed by Nagi[8] * (see Table 2–3).

It is interesting to note at least three things about the suggestions offered by Sackett and colleagues[1] and by Guccione[8] for addressing the inad-

* As indicated, Guccione's suggestion relates to the system of categories proposed by Nagi.[8] Presumably, his suggestion also would be applicable to the ICIDH system, because disease is defined essentially the same both in the ICIDH system and in the Nagi model. Please refer to Tables 2–2 and 2–3 for definitions of the categories in the respective models.

equacy of the term "disease" in the two different systems of terminology. First, all of the authors attempted to enlarge the scope of the term "disease." However, the two suggestions could be viewed as being diametrically opposed. Specifically, Sackett and colleagues[1] enlarged the scope of the collective term used to describe the category by substituting the term target disorder for the term disease, whereas Guccione[8] elected to increase the number of collective terms used by adding another (medical syndromes). Second, the fact that Sackett and coauthors are physicians, whereas Guccione is a physical therapist, lends support to the assertion that not only physical therapists but also physicians question the adequacy of the term "disease" for dealing with the variety of conditions encountered in clinical medicine and physical therapy practice. Finally, all of the authors assign a different label to the same concept, *ie,* "cluster of symptoms and signs"; Sackett and colleagues use the term illness,[1] whereas Guccione uses the term medical syndrome.[8] If, as Guccione suggests, medical syndromes should be included at the level of disease, then perhaps illness also should be included at that level. However, because the terminology introduced by Sackett and colleagues[1] specifically distinguishes between "disease" or "target disorder" and "illness," it may not be appropriate to include "illness" at the level of "disease."

This author suggests that both syndromes and illnesses are more consistent with the impairment level of the ICIDH system (see Table 2–2) and the Nagi model (see Table 2–3) than with the disease level, because most typically, "loss or abnormality of function" is made manifest as symptoms and signs. If, as suggested earlier, the term "diagnosis" is applicable to illnesses, as well as to diseases, and if illnesses are considered to be at the level of

Table 2–3. NAGI'S CATEGORY DEFINITIONS*

Category	Definition
Disease	Equivalent to ICIDH definition
Impairment	Equivalent to ICIDH definition
Functional limitations	Inability to perform a task or obligation of usual roles and typical daily activities as the result of impairment
Disability	Overall patterns of behavior in situations of long-term or continued impairments that result in functional limitations

* Data from Guccione AA: Physical therapy diagnosis and the relationship between impairments and function. *Phys Ther* 1991, 71:499–503.

impairments, then it follows that the term "diagnosis" also may be applicable at the level of impairments.

Summary

- Because the term "disease" does not appear to encompass adequately all of the conditions addressed even by physicians, restricting the use of the term "diagnosis" strictly to the act of identifying disease does not appear to serve the purpose of demarcating the boundaries of practice for either physicians or physical therapists.
- The label "diagnosis" appears to be applicable at both the disease and impairment levels of two major contemporary classification systems, the ICIDH system and the Nagi model.
- Physical therapists are considered qualified to identify and manage problems related to movement dysfunction at the impairment level.[2,6-8] Therefore, it seems justifiable for physical therapists to use the term "diagnosis" in reference to conditions at the level of impairment, as long as recognition of the particular *cluster* of symptoms and signs is "within the scope of their knowledge, experience, and expertise."[3]

Diagnosis: The Process. The preceding subsection focused on the use of the term "diagnosis" as a label for conditions of patients. This section addresses another use of the term "diagnosis"—namely, the process of diagnosing a condition. The question in physical therapy is whether physical therapists should engage in the diagnostic process.

Definitions. The first definition and the first part of the third definition of the term "diagnosis" (see Table 2-1) refer to the act of investigating and identifying the cause or nature of a condition. According to Sackett et al.,[1] "the act of clinical diagnosis focuses on the patient's *illness*," ie, the cluster of signs and symptoms exhibited by the patient "as the result of having, and responding to, the target disorder." The act of clinical diagnosis also is classification for the purpose of recognizing the category "to which a patient's illness belongs, so that, based on [the clinician's] prior experience with that" category, he/she will know how to proceed.

Applicability to Physical Therapy. Given the perspective expressed by Sackett et al.,[1] it seems reasonable to conclude that when physical therapists classify a patient's condition on the basis of signs, symptoms, and test results for the purpose of directing subsequent clinical decisions and actions, they are engaged in the act of clinical diagnosis.

Support for View. As noted earlier, support for the view that physical therapists should engage in diagnostic activity within the scope of their knowledge, experience, and expertise has been expressed repeatedly in the physical therapy literature.[2,4-9] Perhaps Jette[7] made the point most clearly when he noted that "What differentiates diagnosis by the physical therapist from diagnosis by the physician is not the process itself but the *phenomena* that are being observed and classified."

One of the most recent affirmations of the need to classify emanated from a consensus development forum (Project Focus '93, Alexandria, VA, August 28 and 29, 1993) sponsored by the Foundation for Physical Therapy. This forum was held for the purpose of establishing priorities for research funding in the area of work-related injuries. The consensus of the forum's group focusing on low back pain was that the development and validation of classification systems that could be used to direct physical therapy treatment should be given the highest priority. Therapists would have to engage in what would be considered diagnostic activity to use the systems.

In summary, there seems to be general acceptance of the notion that physical therapists must engage in diagnostic activity to classify their patients' conditions in a manner that helps direct the therapists' choices and actions more specifically than does the medical diagnosis.

Specification of the Diagnoses. In addition to the applicability of the term "diagnosis" in physical therapy, another major issue is that implementation of the 1984 HOD policy is contingent on the ability of physical therapists to specify the diagnoses that are "within the scope of their knowledge, experience, and expertise."[3] Two different but complementary perspectives have been serving as guideposts for the interrelated tasks of defining the scope of practice and of specifying the diagnoses within the scope of physical therapy practice.

Movement Dysfunction. One perspective on the scope of physical therapy practice and diagnosis is that the unique focus of physical therapy practice is movement dysfunction, and therefore, the diagnoses physical therapists identify should relate to movement dysfunction. As is evident from the following list, many individuals have contributed to the evolution of this view over the past two decades.

- Hislop first introduced the term "pathokinesiology" to describe the body of knowledge of physical therapy.[13]

- In 1986, Rose offered a description of potential links between the "science of pathokinesiology" and clinical practice based on the use of movement-related concepts and terminology in the development of clinical diagnostic classification schemes.[4]
- In 1987, the APTA's HOD adopted a philosophical statement that specified movement dysfunction as the primary content area of physical therapy.[14]
- In the context of her article regarding diagnosis by physical therapists, Sahrmann not only discussed the issues surrounding diagnosis but also provided numerous specific examples of movement dysfunction diagnoses that could be made by physical therapists to help direct their decisions and actions.[2]

Functional Ability. The other perspective on physical therapy practice and diagnosis is based on the belief that any classification system promoted for use by physical therapists must incorporate categories related not only to movement dysfunction but also to the patient's functional ability.

International Classification of Impairments, Disabilities, and Handicaps System. Jette[7] has urged physical therapists to consider using the WHO's ICIDH system as a framework for the diagnoses that they develop.[12] Note that the ICIDH system, outlined in Table 2–2, provides a means for organizing clinical data at four different levels—not just at the level of disease. Because disease is not the focus of physical therapy practice, the advantage of the ICIDH system is that it provides a framework for the development of categories within the scope of practice that, according to Jette,[7] are at the levels of impairment, disability, and handicap.

Nagi's Model. Guccione[8] has presented arguments in favor of adopting Nagi's model of the process of disablement (see Table 2–3) instead of the ICIDH system to serve as a framework for the development of diagnostic classification systems. Within his discussion of the Nagi model, Guccione notes that "Recognition of 'physical impairment' and 'functional limitations' as the core categories of physical therapy classification is long overdue."

As the reader may have noted, there are some differences between the Nagi and ICIDH systems with respect to terminology used and between the views of Jette and Guccione regarding the levels at which physical therapists should play a role. The most important points, however, are that (1) both schemes reflect the importance of factors beyond disease in specifying the status of a patient and that (2) both authors posit a substantial role for physical therapists in the development and use of the systems.

Summary. In light of the two perspectives noted in this section and of the discussion in previous sections regarding use of the terms "disease," "illness," "impairments," and "diagnosis," it seems reasonable to assume the following:

- Clusters of symptoms and signs associated with specific subtypes of movement dysfunction can be viewed as diagnoses that are within the scope of practice of physical therapists.
- Movement dysfunction diagnoses based on clusters of symptoms and signs can be considered consistent with the impairment level of the ICIDH and Nagi systems of classification.
- Classification of a patient's status at the third level of the ICIDH and Nagi systems (disability and functional limitation, respectively) is within the scope of practice of physical therapists, but the term "diagnosis" does not seem to be applicable.
- Classification of a patient's status at the fourth level of the ICIDH and Nagi systems (handicap and disability, respectively) may be within the scope of physical therapists.

Summary of Evolution in Physical Therapy

The evolution of the concept of diagnosis and classification in physical therapy is progressing. Issues related to philosophy and terminology are being discussed, a unique focus for the practice of physical therapy has been specified, and examples of the type of broad framework into which diagnoses relevant to physical therapy practice might be incorporated have been identified. As noted by Guccione, however, "The development of a classification system for physical therapy diagnosis has been delayed by excessive, albeit understandable, concern over the boundaries of diagnosis and scant attention to the categories and content of diagnosis."[8] Perhaps the progress of the profession in the area of diagnosis and classification can be gauged by considering the contents of the bulk of this manual in light of the focus and schemes just discussed.

Strategies for Making Clinical Diagnoses or Classifications

Assume for a moment that the problem of describing a substantial number of diagnoses and classifications within the scope of our practice has been solved. Now a new problem exists—namely, making the correct diagnosis or classification for each patient's condition. The purpose of this section is to give the reader a brief overview of the various ways investigators from a number of different disciplines have attempted to characterize and to enhance the diagnostic activity of clinicians. Because the reader is a physical therapist and not a psychologist, economist, or computer scientist, the concepts and terminology used in this section may be unfamiliar. In the case that this material seems difficult, read the section entitled "Artificially Aided Approaches" for some examples of practical applications and then skip to the summary at the end of this section for the main points. Most importantly, keep in mind that "Clinical Examination" is the next major section.

Historical Perspective

Although diagnosis has been a focus of medicine for approximately 150 years,[15] reports of studies designed to examine either the clinicians' diagnostic accuracy or the processes involved in arriving at a diagnosis did not begin to appear until about 40 years ago.

The diagnostic performance of clinical psychologists was the first target of researchers.[16] Based on his review of the literature on clinical judgement* through 1967, Goldberg[16] summarized that clinical judgements tend to be "(1) rather unreliable, (2) only minimally related to the confidence and amount of experience of the judge, (3) relatively unaffected by the amount of information available to the judge, and (4) rather low in validity on an absolute basis."

Given the suboptimal performance of clinicians, alternatives were sought. Meehl[18] compared clinical approaches, also referred to as "intuitive" approaches, with statistical and actuarial approaches and suggested that clinical judgments based on statistical models are as accurate, if not more accurate, than those based on clinical intuition. Meehl's claim sparked a major controversy known

as the "clinical versus statistical prediction controversy."

Over the 20 years following Meehl's work, additional studies on the clinical judgement accuracy of various types of clinicians, such as physicians and nurses, appeared; however, the findings provided no reason to reverse the original conclusions.[17]

By the middle of the 1960s, the mounting negative evidence regarding the diagnostic accuracy of clinicians served as an impetus to shift the focus of research on clinical judgement from one exclusively aimed at examining outcome accuracy in validity studies to two new foci:

1. Developing techniques to improve a clinician's judgements, referred to collectively as "prescriptive approaches."
2. Describing and understanding the cognitive processes of the clinician, referred to as "descriptive approaches."

Prescriptive Approaches. Much of the work related to the prescriptive approach deals with the application of decision-making theories (eg, expected utility theory, subjective expected utility theory) and mathematical techniques (eg, Bayes's theorem, regression analysis, decision analysis) to clinical practice.[15] One could view the prescriptive approaches as similar to the statistical or actuarial approach noted by Meehl[18] and as sharing some of the same problems:

- It has been demonstrated that the behaviors of subjects do not always conform to those prescribed by the theories.[19,20]
- As Elstein noted, clinicians are reluctant to use the techniques in actual clinical practice.[15]
- The theories do not explain how clinicians actually make clinical judgements.[21,22]

Therefore, although the prescriptive approaches may be more accurate, the nature of the problems encountered with them suggests that another approach to improving the diagnostic performance may be to identify and understand what clinicians actually do before prescribing a remedy.

Descriptive Approaches. In contrast to prescriptive approaches, descriptive approaches emphasize description of the cognitive processes (mental activity) underlying the diagnostic task.

Problem Solving. One line of investigation has focused on the analysis of problem-solving behavior of clinicians within the framework of the information-processing model of cognition.

In the problem-solving tradition of Newell and Simon, medical diagnosis is considered to be an

---

* As described by Arkes and Hammond,[17] "clinical judgment is the name given to the cognitive activity of skilled professionals (e.g., clinical psychologists, medical doctors, nurses, social workers), who review a large amount of clinical data (signs, symptoms, laboratory reports, etc.) regarding a patient's or client's situation, organize the information in their minds according to their training and experience, and offer a diagnosis or prognosis." In concert with Arkes and Hammond's description, the term "clinical judgement" will be used in this chapter in reference only to the diagnostic task—not the treatment-selection task—of clinicians.

"inductive task" aimed at "infer[ring] the cause of . . . malfunction." [23] Medical diagnosis is considered an inductive, rather than a deductive, task because typically the conclusions drawn on the basis of evidence available are only possibly, not positively, correct. For example, it is possible that a person with a fever has a bacterial infection, but it is also possible that the person has any of a number of different problems that could cause fever.

Although induction generally is considered a form of reasoning, it also can be regarded as a problem for which the problem solver must find a general principle or structure that is consistent with the data; in clinical practice, the diagnosis corresponds to the principle or structure, and the collection of signs and symptoms corresponds to the data.

Elstein and colleagues[24] were the first to apply the problem-solving model of Newell and Simon to the study of clinical judgement by physicians. The primary investigative approach used was process tracing based on analysis of verbal reports—so-called "thinking aloud" reports—produced by subjects engaged in a diagnostic task. One of the principal findings of Elstein's group, consistent with a top-down, hypothetico-deductive method of problem solving, was that "medical problem solving proceeds by selecting a number of diagnostic hypotheses as possible goals, and then testing to see whether one or more of the hypotheses selected can be justified." [24] This finding also is considered consistent with Elstein's view that "rationality is desirable and necessary in medicine."

Two of Elstein's other findings, however, did not appear to be as confirmatory of the existence of a complex rational thought process. In a study using 4- to 6-minute filmed patient interviews, Elstein's group demonstrated that experienced clinicians generated their initial diagnosis within the first 30 seconds of viewing the film in 35% of the cases and within the first 60 seconds in 96% of the cases. They also showed that in 53% of the cases, the first hypothesis was based on the statement of the patient's presenting complaint. The authors concluded that "generation of problem formulations appears to be primarily a process of direct associative retrieval, rather than one of strategy-guided search."

The automaticity of the behavior suggests that the generation of the initial hypothesis may be a function primarily of the contents of memory rather than of complex information-processing strategies. The implication of memory content and retrieval as the primary factors in generation of the initial hypothesis is consistent with Elstein's finding that "knowledge of [case-specific] content is more critical than mastery of a generic problem-solving process." [24] Given these results, reliance solely on diagnostic strategies based on the information-processing model of cognition seems unwarranted.

Categorization. More recently, the view that "medical diagnosis is primarily a categorization task" [25] has received increased attention. Generally, categorization behavior is thought to be a function of the organization of memory rather than of complex problem-solving processes.

Categorization "involves determining that a specific instance is a member of a concept" (*eg*, patient X has a lumbar flexion syndrome) "or that one particular concept is a subset of another" (*eg*, lumbar flexion syndrome is a type of low back pain syndrome).[26]

The general assumption is that an individual must have some information about the properties of the members of a category in his/her memory to be able to categorize an instance as a member of the category. For the clinician, the *properties* of interest may include the signs, symptoms, results of special tests, presence of risk factors, other patient characteristics, and relevant patient history items. The *categories* of interest for the clinician are diagnoses associated with a specific set of the properties noted previously.

Three major types of models have been proposed to account for a person's ability to categorize the members of categories: classical models, independent cues model, and exemplar models. The majority of recent evidence supports exemplar and mixed models, the basis of which is a clinician's dependence on memory of previous experiences with specific category members. One of the most recent models of categorization is based on an artificial neural (or connectionist) network, which combines aspects of both the independent cues model and exemplar model.[27]

The implication for clinicians is that the ability to diagnose the problems of new patients (or at least the generation of the first tentative diagnosis) simply may be a function of their memory of experiences with previous similar patients being triggered by the salient characteristics of the new patients. For example, almost immediately on observation of pill-rolling tremor and masked facies, a physical therapist thinks of Parkinson's disease.

Organization and Content of Memory. Closely related to the work of those who view diagnosis as a categorization task is a line of investigation that has focused on describing the organization and content of the clinician's memory. As an example, Patel and Groen[28] and Patel and colleagues[29] have used a technique called "propositional analysis" to study the relationships between basic biomedical knowledge and clinical knowledge. The propositional networks derived from their analyses of verbal reports of a clinician's thoughts during a diagnostic task represent the collection of separate ideas generated and of the specific relationships among the separate ideas. Schmidt and colleagues[30] have proposed a stage theory of clinical reasoning. One of the main assumptions underlying their theory is that experienced physicians rely on knowledge structures referred to as "illness scripts" in diagnosing common problems. The illness scripts develop as the result of exposure to patients and contain primarily the clinical, not pathophysiological, information associated with the different types of patients. Some of the types of clinical information included in illness scripts are the patient's complaint, symptoms, signs, predisposing factors, history items, patient characteristics, and complications to be expected. According to this theory, the diagnostic problem is solved by finding the script (collection of clinical information) that matches the current situation.

Artificially Aided Approaches. Several types of artificially aided approaches are algorithms and flowcharts, production rules, and computer-aided diagnostic (CAD) systems.

Algorithms and Flowcharts. An algorithm is a step-by-step procedure for solving a problem.* A flowchart is a diagram constructed from a set of geometric symbols (*eg,* rectangles, circles, and diamonds) and connecting lines that represents an algorithm. Algorithms and their accompanying flowcharts explicitly specify all possible conditions at each stage of the diagnostic problem. Algorithms and flowcharts are especially useful for triage (screening) situations, training novices, and handling uncommon problems. Figure 2–1 is an example of a simple flowchart† that could be used in conjunction with the "Client Checklist" for screening medical conditions and its companion "Guidelines for Interpretation" represented in Figures 2–2 and 2–3, respectively.

Production Rules. A production rule is a statement such as

If {condition A exists},
  then {do action X}.

The following is a simple clinical example:

If {patient cannot bear weight},
  then {do not use a standing-pivot transfer}.

Like the algorithm or flowchart, production rules provide explicit, unambiguous instructions. Systems of production rules are major elements of some types of computerized expert systems and are inherent in guidelines for practice that specify a set of alternative actions (*ie,* treatment options) viewed to be reasonable in light of a specified condition (diagnosis or classification), even though guidelines typically are not represented explicitly as production rules.

CAD Systems. In a sense, CAD systems contain a very large number of relatively small but interrelated algorithms and production rules. CAD systems have the potential to reduce the number of diagnostic errors.

Although the number of CAD systems for medicine continues to increase, development of the systems has been slow compared with early expectations, and the systems that have been developed are not used widely. One of the major difficulties in developing CAD systems is extracting the relevant set of correct rules from the experts. As suggested earlier, experts are not infallible when attempting to specify the information and processes they use in making a diagnosis. To date, most systems have been built on the basis of prespecified information in the form of either prediction equations or sets of production rules. As indicated at the 15th Annual Meeting of the Society for Medical Decision Making (Durham, NC, October 24–27, 1993), artificial neural networks are being developed to assist in the making of clinical judgements. One of the advantages of artificial neural networks is that they do not require prior definition of rules. Some of the factors that may adversely affect acceptance are clinicians' limited access to computers, computer illiteracy, lack of confidence in the systems, egoism, limited applicability (specificity) of the systems available, and difficulties using the systems.

Some efforts have been made to develop a CAD system for use in physical therapy.[32] Given the relative immaturity of diagnostic systems in physical therapy, however, it would seem prudent to devote more resources and effort to the dual tasks of developing classification systems and accumulating systematized clinical data.

Summary of Strategies for Making Clinical Diagnoses or Classifications. Many theories designed to characterize the cognitive (thinking) processes of clinicians engaged in the task of diagnosing

---

* For an example of an algorithm designed for clinical use, refer to the article by Echternach and Rothstein.[31]

† The flowchart in Figure 2–1 is presented simply as an illustration of the use of a flowchart. The actual flowchart developed for use by our students is more fully elaborated.

Screening flowchart

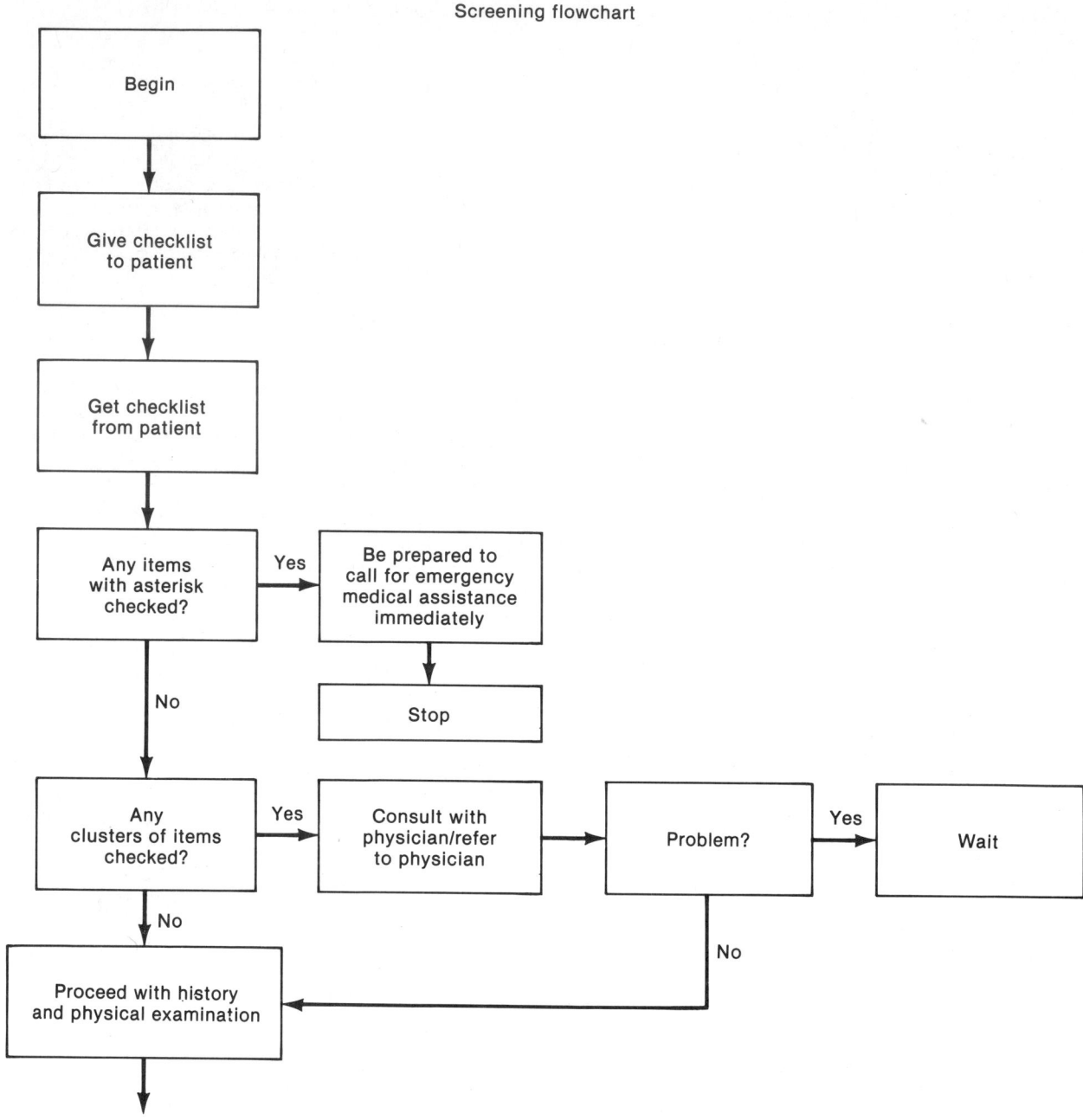

FIGURE 2–1   Sample flowchart that illustrates the clinical screening technique.

health-related conditions have been proposed. Although some evidence exists to support each of the theories, no single existing theory is accepted universally as providing a full account of the clinician's cognitive activity. The hypothetico-deductive, problem-solving approach has received the most attention in medicine[33–37] and in physical therapy.[31,38–41] Although this approach may be use- ful, it should be recognized that it may not accurately describe what is really going on in a clinician's mind. Pattern recognition based on similarity of a current patient's presentation to that of other patients represented in the clinician's memory may be a dominant factor. Caution should be exercised in adopting a particular model of cognition because the model should guide the approach

Client checklist

Date: _____

Name: _____

Reason for seeking physical therapy:

Have you had a complete medical check-up within the last year? _____

Do you now have anything contagious? _____ Yes   _____ No
    If yes, please specify:

Do you now have or have you recently had any of the following complaints?

_____ Shortness of breath
_____ Pain or a feeling of heaviness in your chest
_____ Pulsating pain anywhere in your body
_____ Constant and severe pain in lower leg (calf)
_____ Discolored or painful feet
_____ Dizziness
_____ Swelling

_____ Persistent pain at night
_____ Constant pain anywhere in your body
_____ Unexplained weight loss (10–15 lb in 2 weeks)
_____ Loss of appetite
_____ Unusual lumps or growths
_____ Fatigue

_____ Frequent or severe abdominal pain
_____ Frequent heartburn or indigestion
_____ Frequent nausea or vomiting

_____ Change or problems with bladder function
        (ie, urinary tract infection)
_____ Change or problems with bowel function
_____ Unusual menstrual irregularities

_____ Changes in hearing
_____ Frequent or severe headaches
_____ Problems with swallowing or changes in speech
_____ Changes in vision (ie, blurred vision or loss of sight)
_____ Problems with balance or falling
_____ Fainting spells
_____ Problems with coordination
_____ Sudden weakness

_____ Fever or night sweats
_____ Recent severe emotional disturbances
_____ Swelling or redness in any joints
_____ Pregnant

FIGURE 2–2 Checklist designed to screen for possible medical conditions. (Redrawn from a checklist developed and used by members of the faculty of the Program in Physical Therapy, Washington University School of Medicine, St. Louis, MO. Project Coordinator, Nancy B. Woolsey.)

Guidelines for interpretation of
client checklist for screening medical conditions

Cardiovascular

  Shortness of breath
* Pain or a feeling of heaviness in your chest
* Pulsating pain anywhere in your body
* Constant and severe pain in lower leg (calf)
  Discolored or painful feet
  Swelling

Cancer

  Persistent pain at night
  Constant pain anywhere in your body
  Unexplained weight loss (10–15 lb in 2 weeks)
  Loss of appetite
  Unusual lumps or growths
  Fatigue

Genitourinary or gastrointestinal

* Frequent or severe abdominal pain
  Frequent heartburn or indigestion
  Frequent nausea or vomiting
  Change or problems with bladder function
     (ie, urinary tract infection)
  Change or problems with bowel function
  Unusual menstrual irregularities

Neurological

  Changes in hearing
  Frequent or severe headaches
  Problems with swallowing or changes in speech
  Changes in vision (ie, blurriness or loss of sight)
  Problems with balance or falling
  Fainting spells
  Problems with coordination
  Sudden weakness

Miscellaneous

  Fever or night sweats
  Recent severe emotional disturbances
  Swelling or redness in any joints
  Pregnant

Rules for use:

1. IF any of the items with an asterisk are checked by the patient, THEN be prepared to call for emergency medical assistance immediately.

2. IF several items within a group are checked by the patient, THEN consult with a physician before proceeding.

FIGURE 2–3 Companion document used for teaching students how to interpret the screening checklist. (Redrawn from the document developed and used by members of the faculty of the Program in Physical Therapy, Washington University School of Medicine, St. Louis, MO. Project Coordinator, Nancy B. Woolsey.)

to education. Emphasis on the process of problem solving at the expense of extended repetition with content-specific information may not be warranted. Artificial aids, such as flowcharts and production rules, may be useful ways to present content-specific information within the context of related content. The development of expert systems within physical therapy has just begun. Artificial neural networks seem to offer an alternative approach for developing computer-aided systems.

Clinical Examination

Screening

Definition. Like most words, the word "screening" is used and understood in many different ways. In the context of this section, screening refers to the process of obtaining information about a client for the purpose of deciding whether or not the client should be referred to another practitioner. Specifically, the focus of this section is on screening for the presence of medical conditions.*

Need for Screening. The issue of screening for the presence of medical conditions has received increased attention recently because of a concern expressed by opponents of "direct access" practice (*ie*, the provision of care by a physical therapist without physician referral). The concern is that in direct access situations, clients with serious medical conditions may suffer needlessly because the physical therapist may not recognize the need to refer the patient.[42] The following are at least two ways that this concern can be addressed:

- Concede that the problem is insurmountable, and support efforts to deny patients the opportunity to be seen by a physical therapist without a physician's referral.
- Recognize that physical therapists have the responsibility to refer patients with problems outside the scope of their expertise to other practitioners, *regardless of the referral situation,* and make sure that sufficient information is available to aid in the clinical judgement process.

Assume that the latter approach is taken. The next major problem is to delineate the amount and type of information required to minimize the likelihood that a therapist will fail to recognize the need to refer a patient to the appropriate practitioner.

Focus of Screening. Screening must focus on two major categories of medical conditions: those that require immediate emergency medical attention, such as unconsciousness; and those that may mimic mechanical musculoskeletal dysfunction, such as cancer.

Conditions that require immediate emergency medical attention typically can be detected by observing a patient's level of consciousness and distress, asking the patient about a few critical symptoms, and checking the patient's vital signs. Figure 2–2 is an example of the type of checklist that can be used to survey critical symptoms. The scheme underlying the checklist is represented in Figure 2–3. Items marked with an asterisk require immediate medical attention.

In conditions that mimic mechanical musculoskeletal dysfunction, delineating the amount and type of information required to make a judgement depends on whether it is deemed necessary to rule out specific medical diagnoses or simply to recognize that the problem falls outside the scope of the therapist's expertise.

One approach is to recommend that the physical therapist be skilled in performing a complete physical examination of all body systems that is similar to the examination a physician would perform to rule out specific medical conditions. Another approach is to rely primarily on the patient's responses to a series of questions designed to detect the possible presence of most serious medical conditions, *ie*, any of the items on the screening checklist—not only the ones indicated by an asterisk in Figure 2–3; the physical therapist can rely secondarily on the degree of similarity between the patient's presentation and the criteria for a diagnosis within the scope of his/her expertise. Finally, the physical therapist can rely on the response of the patient's condition to the management strategy of choice for the specific movement dysfunction diagnosis made by him/her.

The emphasis placed on specific medical conditions and examination of structures that are not part of the musculoskeletal system required by the first approach may be perceived as advocating a major role for physical therapists in the differential diagnosis of specific medical conditions. Clearly, the identification of specific medical conditions is not within the scope of physical therapy practice.

Proposed Emphasis. In the opinion of this author, the physical therapist's task is to delineate

---

* Although the focus of this section is on screening for medical conditions, similar issues must be considered for any condition outside the scope of physical therapy.

the knowledge and skills required to *detect* the possible existence of conditions that may manifest signs and symptoms otherwise attributable to movement dysfunction—not to engage in differential diagnosis of specific medical conditions.

History and Physical Examination

Importance of Clinical Examination.* Implementation of each of the strategies noted in the section "Strategies for Making Clinical Diagnoses or Classifications" is dependent on the acquisition of information about the patient.

The following quote from Sackett and colleagues illustrates the importance of history taking and physical examination as sources of data: "Clinical examination is far more powerful than laboratory evaluation in establishing diagnoses, prognoses, and therapeutic plans for most patients in most places." Partial justification for their statement is the report of a study of general practice in which "88% of diagnoses were established by the end of a brief history and physical exam subroutine."[1]

Relevance and Accuracy of Clinical Data. Given the importance of data derived from the history and physical examination, it is imperative that the information obtained is both relevant and accurate.

Relevance of Clinical Data. Inherent in the use of the term "relevant" is the notion that information should not be obtained just for the sake of amassing a comprehensive description of the patient. Instead, information gathering should be aimed at decreasing the number of plausible diagnoses. This does not mean, however, that the physical therapist should only seek information that confirms a suspected diagnosis, because the tendency to do so increases the likelihood that a mistake will be made. Just as in any investigative endeavor, it is important to seek evidence that both confirms and disconfirms a suspected diagnosis. Confirming evidence typically supports the favored hypothesis, whereas disconfirming evidence serves to reduce the plausibility of alternative hypotheses.

Accuracy of Clinical Data. The accuracy of clinical data is dependent in large measure on the reliability of the clinician in making judgements about the presence, absence, and severity of signs (*eg*, excessive lordosis, increased tendon jerks) in obtaining measurements manually (*eg*, of muscle strength, joint range of motion).

Reliability of Clinical Data. Because the accuracy of diagnoses is dependent on the accuracy of clinical data, every clinician must assume responsibility for ensuring the reliability of the judgements and measurements they use in making diagnoses. The purpose of this section is to highlight some of the major issues.†

Definition. Typically, the term "reliability" is associated with the notion of the reproducibility of judgements or measurements. In the simplest case, if a judgement or measurement is performed twice and the result is the same, the judgement or measurement is considered reliable.‡

Judgements or measurements do not reflect the true state or score of the subject, and they are not reliable if they contain error.

Sources of Error. Efforts to improve reliability should focus on minimizing the error that can arise from each of three major potential sources of error: the observer, the patient, and the examination.

General Elements of Reliability Studies. At a minimum, the plan for a reliability study should include the following:

- A description of the measurement scale to be used (*ie*, names and definitions of categories or units of measure).
- Rules for making judgements (assigning observations to categories) and for measuring variables (assigning numbers to observations).
- Detailed instructions on the acts to perform and the order in which to perform them.
- The number of observers and the order in which observers perform their observations or measurements.
- The interval between repeated observations or measurements.
- The technique to be used for assessing reliability (*ie*, statistical analysis).

Types of Reliability. Primarily, two types of reliability are important in the clinical setting: intraobserver and interobserver. *Intraobserver* reliability refers to the reproducibility of repeated measurements on the same set of subjects performed by the *same* observer (examiner). *Interobserver* reliability refers to the reproducibility of repeated measurements on the same set of subjects performed

---

* Sackett *et al*.[1] use the term clinical examination to refer to the combined activities of history taking and physical examination.

† As implied, the information presented in this section does not constitute a comprehensive treatment of the topic. Additional detailed information may be found in sources cited in the "Recommended Readings" list at the end of this chapter.

‡ Implicit in this definition is the notion that measurements must be performed at least twice on the same set of subjects to assess reliability.

by a minimum of two *different* observers (examiners).

Statistical Analysis Issues. In clinical literature, the statistics most commonly used to assess observer agreement or reliability are Cohen's kappa statistic,[43] the weighted kappa statistic,[44] and the intraclass correlation coefficient (ICC).[45–47]

All three statistics serve a similar purpose but are used with different types of data. The *Cohen's kappa statistic* is used with nominal type (also called categorical) data. Side of hemiplegia, gender, diagnosis, and shape of back are some examples of variables that conform to a nominal data type. The *weighted kappa statistic* is used with nominal scale data, which essentially is treated as ordinal data because of the weighting scheme. Examples of variables that are treated as being on an ordinal scale are the following:

- Muscle strength, as determined by manual testing.
- Severity of condition.
- Amount of assistance required to transfer.

The *ICC** is used most legitimately with ratio data, but it is also used frequently with interval-type data. Examples of ratio or interval-type data include measures of range of motion, leg length, Q-angle, limb circumference, and blood pressure.

In general, the range of legitimate values for all three types of reliability coefficients is from 0 to 1. The closer the values are to 1, the better the agreement between repeated measurements.

The size of all three types of coefficients is diminished if too many subjects share the same score (inadequate variability among subjects). Therefore, interpretation of reliability data must be based both on the value of the reliability coefficient *and* on a measure of variability among subjects. If variability among subjects is inadequate, then the reliability coefficient is essentially uninterpretable.

Summary. One of the most important functions of clinicians is to gather clinical data for the purpose of defining the condition to which treatment should be aimed. Clinicians must assume the responsibility for ensuring the accuracy and rele-

vance of the data that they gather in their own practice.

Selection and Interpretation of Tests

General Principles† and Selection of Tests

Definition. In general, a test is a procedure used for acquiring data about subjects. In medicine, the term "test" typically refers to a special procedure ordered by a physician and conducted by a laboratory technician with the aid of special equipment. In physical therapy, special equipment may be involved, but the physical therapist typically conducts the test.

Uses of Tests. Test results can be used to help do the following:

- Confirm or disconfirm diagnostic hypotheses.
- Rate the severity of a patient's problem.
- Estimate a patient's prognosis.
- Monitor a patient's response to treatment.

Criteria for Tests. The results of a test will be helpful and should be used *only* if the test meets certain criteria.

Is the test *reliable?* Typically, the reliability of a test is demonstrated by repeating the test at least twice on a number of people and by subjecting the results to statistical analysis and interpretation. In many cases, the design and analysis are similar to those described for assessing the reliability of clinical judgement. If the test is not reliable, its use may lead to erroneous inferences.

Is the test *valid?* In simplest terms, does the test really measure what it is supposed to measure? It seems relatively certain that a ruler can be used to measure the length of a line, but does a tendon jerk really measure spasticity? If the results of the test compare favorably to those of a "gold standard," the validity of the test is supported. However, if the new test offers no advantage over the gold standard in terms of cost, discomfort to the patient, practicality, and reliability, then the new test may not be useful.

In the case of diagnostic tests, do the results of the test serve to *discriminate* those who have the diagnosis from those who do not have the diagnosis? Were the test results described as "normal" values obtained by actually testing individuals without the target disorder (disease)? Is the test "sensitive," *ie,* is the test result positive when the

---

* Actually, there are several different versions of the formula used to calculate the estimates of reliability referred to as ICCs. Each version of the formula is based on a different set of assumptions regarding the following: the method used for selection of observers, the intended generalizability of the results, and the number of observations on which each score is based. For each analysis, selection of a specific formula should be based on matching the assumptions for the formula with the conditions of the study.

† Please refer to the article "Standards for tests and measurements in physical therapy practice" for additional details.[48]

disorder (disease) is present? Is the test "specific," *ie*, is the test result negative when the target disorder (disease) is absent? Is the test useful for both mild and severe cases as well as for commonly confused disorders?

Based on the description of the procedures for conducting the test provided by those who examined the reliability, validity, sensitivity, and specificity of the test, is it possible to *replicate* the test?

In the case of tests used to monitor the effect of treatment, are there any published reports of the values for the test associated with specific levels of functional performance?

Cautions Regarding the Criteria for Tests. It is difficult to justify using a test that does not meet the criteria for a test. At best, time and money will be wasted. At worst, erroneous inferences may be drawn, and a patient may suffer additional discomfort needlessly. It is the responsibility of every clinician who uses a test to know the status of the test with respect to the criteria discussed here.

Tests that meet all the technical criteria for a test should be used only if a patient will benefit from it. In other words, if the cost, possible complications, discomfort to a patient, and other potentially harmful effects of the test are outweighed by the anticipated benefit of knowing the test result, then the patient's *utility* for the test should be high enough to warrant using the test.

Information Derived from Tests. Diagnostic test results are not uniformly informative for all cases. One way to think about the amount of information gained from a test result is reflected in the question "How much does it decrease your uncertainty about the diagnosis?" * For example, if the likelihood that a patient has a particular diagnosis is 95%, performing an additional diagnostic test cannot increase the likelihood by very much. Therefore, the results of the test would be relatively uninformative. On the other hand, if the likelihood that a patient has a particular diagnosis is only 40% to 60%, performing an additional diagnostic test could potentially produce a relatively large increase or decrease in the likelihood that the patient has the diagnosis. Therefore, the

results of the same test would be very informative in this situation, compared with the previous situation. In conclusion, one of the key factors that should guide the selection of diagnostic tests is the degree of certainty in the diagnostic hypothesis before any test is performed.

Epilogue. In the preceding section, "General Principles and Selection of Tests," the characteristics of tests, rather than the strategies for selecting specific tests in unique situations, were emphasized primarily for the following two reasons:

- If a test does not meet the criteria for a test, it is very difficult to justify using the test in any situation.
- Although some strategies for selecting tests have been identified, most require the use of information that generally does not exist in physical therapy, *eg*, criteria for inclusion in specific diagnostic categories, sensitivity and specificity of the tests, and prevalence of the conditions.

Although this section focuses on tests, virtually everything noted is applicable to data derived from the clinical examination (*ie*, clinical signs and symptoms). Therefore, the principles guiding selection of questions and clinical examination items could be the same as those used for tests.

Interpretation of Tests

Interpretation of diagnostic tests would be quite simple if all test results were one of two possible values, if all subjects with one value had the problem, and if all subjects with the other value did not have the problem. Typically, however, test results can have many possible values, and overlap between the values obtained from subjects with and without the problem may exist. Consequently, interpretation of test results can become complicated.

The sensitivity and specificity of a test as well as the prevalence of a "disease" in the population have a major impact on the interpretation of the test's results. Techniques for interpreting diagnostic test results that take into account sensitivity, specificity, and prevalence have been described in the medical literature.[1,49-51] Physical therapists would be able to use the same techniques to assist in making diagnoses if information concerning the sensitivity and specificity of tests for specific diagnostic categories as well as the prevalence of each diagnostic category existed.

It seems clear that as the work of physical therapists on defining the categories within the scope of

---

* Often, the use of a quantitative approach to solving diagnostic problems, based on estimating the likelihood (probability) of a particular diagnosis early in the process and then revising the estimates on the basis of new information, such as clinical signs, symptoms, and test results is emphasized in the medical literature.[1,47] The probabilities reflect the degree of uncertainty in the diagnosis. Very low and very high probabilities are associated with little uncertainty; midrange probabilities are associated with relatively great uncertainty.

the practice progresses, information about the sensitivity and specificity of tests for specific diagnostic categories also must be accumulated. This would allow physical therapists to determine the prevalence of the categories and to use the techniques for interpreting test results that already have been elaborated in the medical literature.

MANAGEMENT

Making a Prognosis

Physical therapists often must estimate the likely outcome for their patients relative to remediation of impairments, recovery of functional abilities, and resumption of role. Commonly, the basis for a physical therapist's estimate is the recollection of personal experience with previously encountered similar patients. In some areas of practice, information about the natural history of the disease and the expected clinical course in response to medical treatment also can be used to assist the therapist in forming estimates.

The source of information most likely to improve the accuracy of outcome estimates made by physical therapists is the literature that reports the results of studies designed to describe the natural history and the clinical course of the specific problems (diagnoses) to which therapists direct their treatment. Currently, there are very few reports of this type in the clinical literature owing, at least in part, to the limited development and use of diagnostic classification schemes specific to the problems managed by physical therapists.

As a starting point, systematic retrospective review of multiple patient records may provide a more accurate description of time course and level of recovery for various types of patients than a therapist's unaided recollection of past experiences.

Selecting Appropriate Treatment Approaches

Preliminary Decisions

Before selecting a specific treatment, the following two preliminary decisions must be made: whether to treat and how to direct treatment.

Treat or Not Treat. The first decision concerns the appropriateness of providing *any* treatment. Some of the factors to consider are

- The possible benefit of treatment to the patient.
- The possible negative effects of treatment on the patient.
- The cost of the treatment in relation to the possible benefit.

Although the factors noted undoubtedly are obvious to every clinician, the issue of deciding whether to provide *any* treatment was raised to emphasize the point that the option to *not* treat should be exercised when appropriate.

Focus of Treatment. The second decision concerns the level or levels at which treatment should be focused. These levels are represented in the terms proposed by Nagi[8]—namely, disease, impairment, functional limitation, and disability.

An assumption underlying Nagi's theoretical model is that the process of disablement is a continuum in which problems at each lower level lead to problems at the higher levels. For example, disease leads to impairment, which leads to functional limitations, which leads to disability. Although it may be true theoretically that impairments can lead to functional limitations, the relationship between specific impairments and functional limitations has not been studied systematically to any great extent. Therefore, it cannot be assumed that the best way to improve function is to focus attention on impairments. Although optimal function may not be possible in the presence of impairments, prolonged efforts to remediate impairments in the hope that function will improve may not be warranted in all cases.

Studies that compare relationships among impairments (both the type and severity) and functional limitations seen early in the course of a problem with those seen at the end of recovery are needed so that a physical therapist can make an informed decision regarding the level at which treatment should be focused. For example, if a particular type of patient with hemiplegia never regains useful voluntary movement of the hand but does regain the ability to transfer independently, emphasis placed on retraining the hand in similar patients may be unwarranted.

Selection and Justification

When a decision has been made to treat a specific problem, the next critical step is to select an appropriate treatment approach or approaches. Based on the premise that the most appropriate approaches are the ones that are most justifiable, the emphasis in this section is on sources of justification.*

Clinical Research Literature

The Gold Standard. The most legitimate way for a clinician to select and to justify the selection of a specific treatment approach is to cite credible, clinical research–based evidence regarding the beneficial effects of a treatment approach that may be useful in patients with similar problems.

Credibility. Evidence regarding the effect of treatment is *credible* to the extent that it meets the criteria for a true experiment, also known in the clinical literature as a *randomized clinical trial* (RCT). The criteria for an RCT[52] are exemplified by the following questions:

- Were the subjects *selected* from the population *randomly* or at least *assigned* to separate experimental groups *randomly?*
- Were *at least two* different groups of subjects included in the study?
- Did the *investigators apply the treatment* intervention they wanted to examine in a *controlled* manner?

If the answer to all three questions is "Yes" based on information found in the "Methods" section of an article, then the study reported was an RCT.

Usefulness. Evidence regarding the effect of treatment is *useful* if the following is true:

- The patients studied are similar to the physical therapist's current patients.
- The amount of difference between the groups after treatment is clinically important, not just statistically significant.[53]
- The treatment procedure is practical to use in a clinical setting.

Acceptable Alternatives. Some other types of studies used in clinical research are the following:

- Prospective cohort study.
- Retrospective case-control study.
- Interrupted time series study.
- Single case study.

Regardless of the type of research, however, keep the following in mind:

---

* Admittedly, many other important factors must be considered before finalizing decisions about the approach to treatment for a particular patient, including the wishes of the patient. Owing to space constraints, however, discussion of other factors is not included in this chapter.

- The results of the research should not be ignored.
- The results should be considered carefully, because it may be difficult to discern whether differences attributed to treatment are actually due to treatment rather than something else. For example, the time of day at which ROM in a patient with arthritis is measured may have a large effect on range of motion, which might erroneously be attributed to treatment.
- The credibility of evidence provided by one study in support of a particular approach to treatment is increased if either the results are consistent with the results of other studies, the results are replicated, or the results are consistent with the assumptions of a theory.

Review of Accumulated Clinical Observations. Another way to select and justify selection of a treatment approach is to review systematically the results recorded for similar patients.

Every time a patient is diagnosed and treated, evidence is produced. Systematic recording of a physical therapist's observations and measurements make it possible for him/her to tabulate and summarize the responses of a series of patients to a particular treatment approach. Whenever possible, construct simple tables and graphs of the data to enhance the analysis of the accumulated evidence.

As the accumulated evidence is examined, make a concerted effort to draw conclusions based only on the evidence—not on personal bias. As a physical therapist becomes more experienced at reviewing accumulated evidence, he/she may consult any of several sources on single case design research for information on techniques that may enhance data analysis.

 NOTE: Some sources are listed in the "Suggested Reading" list at the end of this chapter.

Decision Analysis. A technique called "decision analysis"[54–57] may be useful for selecting and justifying selection of a treatment approach in situations in which the choice among treatment alternatives is especially difficult, either because reported evidence does not clearly favor one alternative or because the treatments have potentially serious negative, as well as positive, effects.

One of the essential elements of decision analysis is the explicit specification of all relevant treatment options and their consequences. Typically, the information is depicted in a graphic form referred to as a "decision tree," which contains

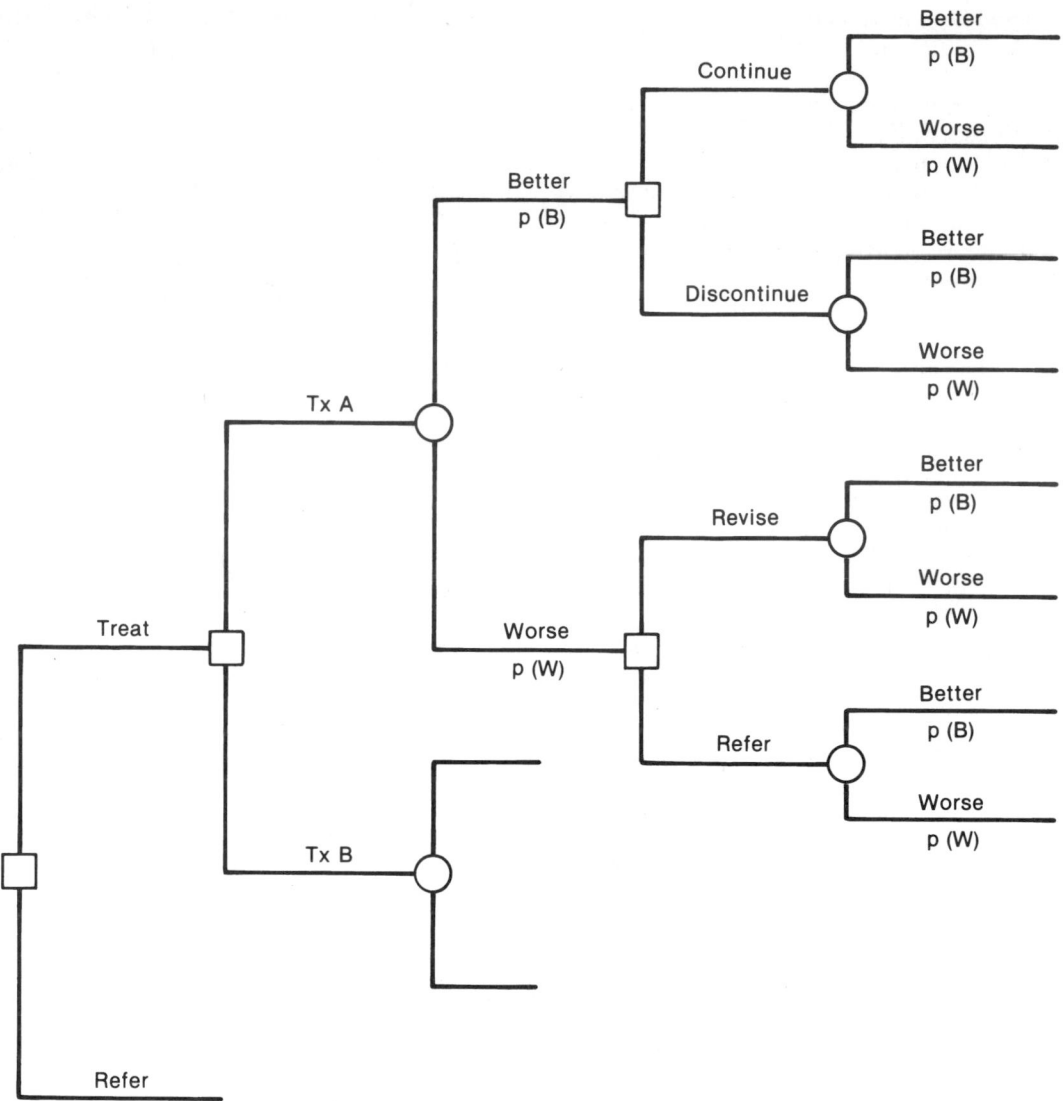

FIGURE 2–4   Hypothetical partially elaborated decision tree for treatment option decisions. *Squares* indicate choice points; *circles* indicate chance points. *Abbreviations:* p(B) = probability getting better; p(W) = probability getting worse; Tx A = treatment option A; Tx B = treatment option B.

branches for each of the options (see Figure 2–4). Another major element of decision analysis is the attachment of probabilities associated with the various options on each branch of the tree and then the carrying out of the mathematical operations required to generate estimates of the probability of each possible outcome.

The main advantages of decision analysis are that all options are made explicit, and the final decision is based on numbers that take into account a patient's preferences. One of the practical problems facing those who wish to use decision analysis in physical therapy is the lack of data regarding the probabilities associated with various treatment options.

Theories. For at least the past 30 years, considerable emphasis has been placed on the use of theories underlying the mechanisms of function and dysfunction for justification of treatment selection. Although the use of theories is acceptable for identifying approaches worth considering, justification for the continued use of an approach must rest upon the credible clinical evidence of effectiveness.[58]

Summary

Selection of appropriate treatment approaches must be based on the specific problem and circumstances of a patient. The most credible source of justification for the selection is the clinical research literature. In the absence of relevant research findings, alternative sources of justification, such as reviews of systematically accumulated clinical observations, must be considered. Decision analysis is a mathematical technique that can be used for selecting among alternative approaches, provided the probabilities associated with the various options are available. Perhaps theories regarding pathophysiological mechanisms have been relied on too much for the justification of treatment selection. Undoubtedly, expert opinion not substantiated by credible clinical evidence has been relied on excessively.

SUMMARY

Most of this manual contains information regarding specific clinical conditions and treatment options. The focus of this chapter has been on issues related to the application of the type of information presented in this manual to the clinical situation. The notion of the "science of the art" of clinical practice[1] was introduced to provide an alternative to basic biomedical science as the primary underpinning of clinical practice. Special emphasis was placed on issues related to diagnosis and classification and to justification of treatment selection based on credible evidence because of their great importance in the future growth of the profession. Concepts drawn from a wide range of disciplines were noted because of their potential for application to physical therapy. Sources for additional detailed information are listed in the "Recommended Reading" section.

References

1. Sackett DL, Haynes RB, Guyatt GH, Tugwell P: *Clinical Epidemiology: A Basic Science for Clinical Medicine*, 2nd ed. Boston, Little, Brown and Company, 1991.
2. Sahrmann SA: Diagnosis by the physical therapist: a prerequisite for treatment. *Phys Ther* 1988, 68:1703–1706.
3. Diagnosis by physical therapists [HOD 06-84-19-78]. In *Applicable House of Delegates Policies*. Alexandria, American Physical Therapy Association, 1989, p 28.
4. Rose SJ: Description and classification: the cornerstones of pathokinesiological research. *Phys Ther* 1986, 66:379–381.
5. Rose SJ: Musing on diagnosis: editor's note. *Phys Ther* 1988, 68:1665.
6. Rose SJ: Physical therapy diagnosis: role and function. *Phys Ther* 1989, 69:535–547.
7. Jette AM: Diagnosis and classification by physical therapists: a special communication. *Phys Ther* 1989, 69:967–969.
8. Guccione AA: Physical therapy diagnosis and the relationship between impairments and function. *Phys Ther* 1991, 71:499–503.
9. Behr DW, Katz ME, Krebs DE: Diagnosis enhances, not

impedes, boundaries of physical therapy practice. *J Orthop Sports Phys Ther* 1991, 13:218–219.
10. Reynolds JP (ed): Diagnosis in physical therapy: a roundtable discussion. *PT Magazine* 1993, 1:58–65.
11. Rothstein JM: Patient classification: editor's note. *Phys Ther* 1993, 73:214–215.
12. Wood PHN: Appreciating the consequences of disease: the International Classification of Impairments, Disabilities, and Handicaps. *WHO Chronicle* 1980, 34:376–380.
13. Hislop HJ: The not so impossible dream: the tenth Mary McMillan lecture. *Phys Ther* 1975, 55:1069–1080.
14. Philosophical statement on physical therapy [HOD 06-83-03-05]. In *Applicable House of Delegates Policies*. Alexandria, American Physical Therapy Association, 1987, p 17.
15. Schwartz S, Griffin T: *Medical Thinking: The Psychology of Medical Judgment and Decision Making*. New York, Springer-Verlag, 1986.
16. Goldberg LR: Simple models or simple processes? Some research on clinical judgments. *Am Psychol* 1968, 23:483–496.
17. Arkes HR, Hammond KR (eds): *Judgment and Decision Making: An Interdisciplinary Reader*. Cambridge, England, Cambridge University Press, 1986, pp 333, 334.
18. Meehl PE: *Clinical Versus Statistical Prediction: A Theoretical Analysis and a Review of the Evidence*. Minneapolis, University of Minnesota Press, 1954.
19. Lichtenstein S, Slovic P: Reversal of preferences between bids and choices in gambling decisions. *J Exp Psychol* 1971, 89:46–55.
20. Kahneman D, Slovic P, Tversky A (eds): *Judgment Under Uncertainty: Heuristics and Biases*. Cambridge, England, Cambridge University Press, 1982.
21. Lichtenstein S, Earle T, Slovic P: Cue utilization in a numerical prediction task. *J Exp Psychol Hum Percept Perform* 1975, 104:77–85.
22. Birnbaum MH: Intuitive numerical prediction. *Am J Psychol* 1976, 89:417–429.
23. Greeno JG, Simon, HA: Problem solving and reasoning. In Atkinson RC, Herrnstein RJ, Lindzey G, Luce RD (eds): *Stevens' Handbook of Experimental Psychology*, 2nd ed. New York, John Wiley & Sons, 1988, pp 589–672.
24. Elstein AS, Shulman LS, Sprafka SA: *Medical Problem Solving: An Analysis of Clinical Reasoning*. Cambridge, MA, Harvard University Press, 1978.
25. Brooks LR, Norman GR, Allen SW: Role of specific similarity in a medical diagnostic task. *J Exp Psychol Gen* 1991, 120:278–287.
26. Smith EE, Medin D: *Categories and Concepts*. Cambridge, MA, Harvard University Press, 1981.
27. Kruschke JK: ALCOVE: An exemplar-based connectionist model of category learning. *Psychol Rev* 1992, 99:22–44.
28. Patel VL, Groen GJ: Knowledge based solution strategies in medical reasoning. *Cogn Sci* 1986, 10:91–116.
29. Patel VL, Evans DA, Kaufman DR: Reasoning strategies and the use of biomedical knowledge by medical students. *Med Educ* 1990, 24:129–136.
30. Schmidt HG, Norman GR, Boshuizen HPA: A cognitive perspective on medical expertise: theory and implications. *Acad Med* 1990, 65:611–621.
31. Echternach JL, Rothstein JM: Hypothesis-oriented algorithms. *Phys Ther* 1989, 69:559–564.
32. Weed LL, Zimny NJ: The problem-oriented system, problem-knowledge coupling, and clinical decision making. *Phys Ther* 1989, 69:565–568.
33. Barrows HS, Bennett K: The diagnostic (problem solving) skill of the neurologist: experimental studies and their implications for neurological training. *Arch Neurol* 1972, 26:273–277.

34. Barrows JS, Tamblyn RM: *Problem-Based Learning: An Approach to Medical Education.* New York, Springer Publishing Company, 1980.

35. Barrows JS, Feltovich PJ: The clinical reasoning process. *Med Educ* 1987, 21:86–91.

36. Elstein AS, Bordage G: Psychology of clinical reasoning. In Dowie J, Elstein AS (eds): *Professional Judgment: A Reader in Clinical Decision Making.* Cambridge, England, Cambridge University Press, 1988, pp 109–129.

37. Elstein AS, Shulman LS, Sprafka SA: Medical problem solving: a ten-year retrospective. *Evaluation Health Sci* 1990, 31:5–36.

38. May BJ: An integrated problem-solving curriculum design for physical therapy education. *Phys Ther* 1977, 57:807–813.

39. Payton OD: Clinical reasoning process in physical therapy. *Phys Ther* 1985, 65:924–928.

40. Burnett CN, Pierson FM: Developing problem-solving skills in the classroom. *Phys Ther* 1988, 68:1381–1385.

41. Slaughter DS, Brown DS, Gardner DL, Perritt LJ: Improving physical therapy students' clinical problem-solving skills: an analytical questioning model. *Phys Ther* 1989, 69: 441–447.

42. Boissonnault WG (ed): *Examination in Physical Therapy Practice: Screening for Medical Disease.* New York, Churchill Livingstone, 1991, pp xv–xvi.

43. Cohen J: A coefficient of agreement for nominal scales. *Educ Psychol Measurement* 1960, 20:37–46.

44. Cohen J: Weighted kappa: nominal scale agreement with provision for scaled disagreement or partial credit. *Psychol Bull* 1968, 70:213–220.

45. Bartko JJ, Carpenter WT: On the methods and theory of reliability. *J Nerv Ment Dis* 1976, 163:307–317.

46. Bartko JJ: On various intraclass correlation reliability coefficients. *Psychol Bull* 1976, 83:762–765.

47. Lahey MA, Downey RG, Saal FE: Intraclass correlation: there's more to it than meets the eye. *Psychol Bull* 1983, 93:586–595.

48. Task Force on Standards for Measurement in Physical Therapy: Standards for tests and measurements in physical therapy practice. *Phys Ther* 1991, 71:589–622.

49. Sox HC Jr, Blatt MA, Higgins MC, Marton KI: *Medical Decision Making.* Boston, Butterworth Publishers, 1988.

50. Feinstein AR: *Clinical Epidemiology: The Architecture of Clinical Research.* Philadelphia, W. B. Saunders Company, 1985, pp 434–439.

51. Feinstein AR: Clinical biostatistics: XXXIX. The haze of Bayes, the aerial palaces of decision analysis, and the computerized Ouija board. *Clin Pharmacol Ther* 1977, 21:482–496.

52. Norton BJ, Strube MJ: Making decisions based on group designs and meta-analysis. *Phys Ther* 1989, 69:594–600.

53. Michels E: *Design of Research and Analysis of Data in the Clinic: An Introductory Manual for Clinical Research.* Alexandria, American Physical Therapy Association, 1985.

54. Watts N: Clinical decision analysis. *Phys Ther* 1989, 69:569–576.

55. Weinstein MC, Fineberg JV: *Clinical Decision Analysis.* Philadelphia, W. B. Saunders Company, 1980.

56. Kassirer J: The principles of clinical decision making: an introduction to decision analysis. *Yale J Biol Med* 1976, 49:149–164.

57. Pauker S, Kassirer J: Therapeutic decision making: a cost-benefit analysis. *N Engl J Med* 1975, 293:229–234.

58. Michels E: Evaluation and research in physical therapy. *Phys Ther* 1982, 62:828–834.

Suggested Reading

CLINICAL EPIDEMIOLOGY

Feinstein AR: *Clinical Epidemiology: The Architecture of Clinical Research.* Philadelphia, W. B. Saunders Company, 1985, pp 434–439.

Sackett DL, Haynes RB, Guyatt GH, Tugwell P: *Clinical Epidemiology: A Basic Science for Clinical Medicine,* 2nd ed. Boston, Little, Brown and Company, 1991.

JUDGEMENT AND DECISION MAKING

Arkes HR, Hammond KR (eds): *Judgment and Decision Making.* Cambridge, England, Cambridge University Press, 1986.

Dowie J, Elstein AS (eds): *Professional Judgment: A Reader in Clinical Decision Making.* Cambridge, England, Cambridge University Press, 1988.

Elstein AS, Shulman LS, Sprafka SA: *Medical Problem Solving: An Analysis of Clinical Reasoning.* Cambridge, MA, Harvard University Press, 1978.

Kahneman D, Slovic P, Tversky A (eds): *Judgment Under Uncertainty: Heuristics and Biases.* Cambridge, England, Cambridge University Press, 1982.

Sox HC Jr, Blatt MA, Higgins MC, Marton KI: *Medical Decision Making.* Boston, Butterworth Publishers, 1988.

Schwartz S, Griffin T: *Medical Thinking: The Psychology of Medical Judgment and Decision Making.* New York, Springer-Verlag, 1986.

RELIABILITY

Anastasi A: *Psychological Testing,* 4th ed. New York, Macmillan, 1976.

Cronbach LJ, Gleser GC, Nanda H, Rajaratnam N: *The Dependability of Behavioral Measurements: Theory of Generalizability for Scores and Profiles.* New York, John Wiley & Sons, 1972.

Ghiselli EE, Campbell JP, Zedeck S: *Measurement Theory for the Behavioral Sciences.* New York, Freeman, 1981

Shavelson RJ, Webb NM, Rowley GL: *Generalizability Theory: A Primer.* Newbury Park, CA, Sage, 1991.

RESEARCH DESIGN AND STATISTICS

Barlow DH, Hersen M: *Single Case Experimental Designs: Strategies for Studying Behavior Change,* 2nd ed. New York, Pergamon Press, 1984.

Cook TD, Campbell DT. *Quasi-experimentation: Design and Analysis Issues for Field Settings.* Boston, Houghton Mifflin Company, 1979.

Domholdt E: *Physical Therapy Research: Principles and Applications.* Philadelphia, W. B. Saunders Company, 1993.

Neale JM, Liebert RM: *Science and Behavior: An Introduction to Methods of Research,* 3rd ed. Englewood Cliffs, Prentice-Hall, 1986.

Ottenbacher KJ: *Evaluating Clinical Change: Strategies for Occupational and Physical Therapists.* Baltimore, Williams & Wilkins, 1986.

Payton OD: *Research: The Validation of Clinical Practice,* 3rd ed. Philadelphia, F. A. Davis Company, 1994.

Portney LG, Watkins MP: *Foundations of Clinical Research: Applications to Practice.* Norwalk, Appleton & Lange, 1993.

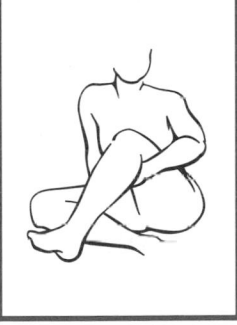

CHAPTER 3

Behavioral and Social Science: Considerations for Current Practice

Beverly J. Schmoll

PHYSICAL THERAPY: AN ART AND A SCIENCE

Physical therapy is both an art and a science. It is the special blending of knowledge about the science of the discipline with knowledge of the behavioral aspects of the discipline that results in optimal interactions with clients and leads to the outcomes desired for those clients. Physical therapy practice is influenced by the behavior of the physical therapist and by the behavior of the patient or client.

FRAMES OF REFERENCE DEFINE PERSPECTIVES FOR INTERACTION

The physical therapist and patient each bring a unique frame of reference that influences the therapeutic interaction. Effective therapeutic inter-

actions rest in large measure with the physical therapist's capacity to be sensitive and alert to a patient's frame of reference.

Common factors influence the behavior of all persons. These factors are depicted in Figure 3–1 as parts of a "picture frame." Each person brings his/her own particular picture frame to any interaction with another human being or to any situation of which he/she is a part. It is through each person's unique frame that he/she views events, situations, and interactions. This can be regarded as the person's "frame of reference."

The frame of reference for each person shares common components with those of other persons. The specific aspects of each component, however, are unique for each person. The commonalities bind human beings, whereas the differences make each person unique. It is the uniqueness of each person that makes working with a variety of persons interesting; however, this uniqueness also presents particular challenges to physical therapists.

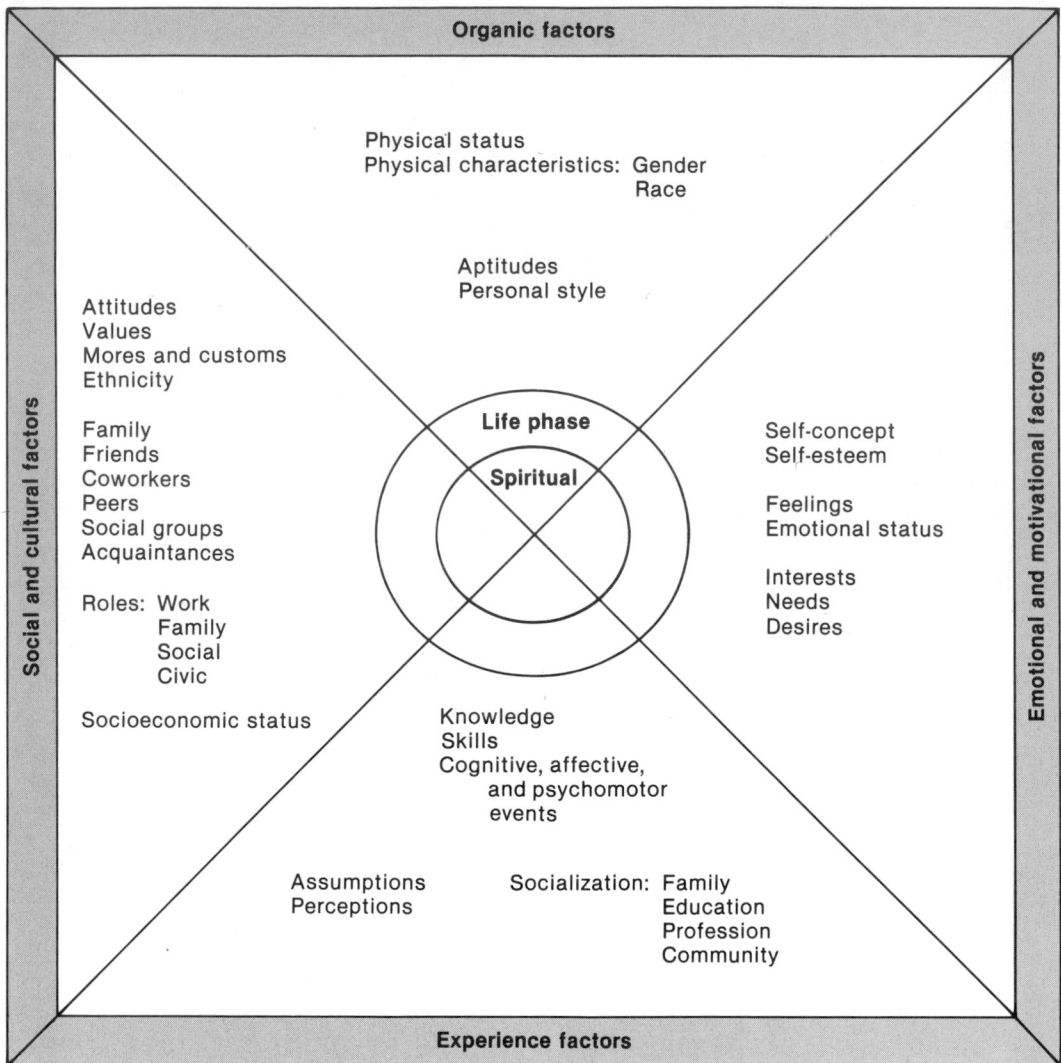

FIGURE 3–1 Components of a person's frame of reference.

Each person's frame of reference is composed of four distinct parts. These are (1) organic factors, (2) emotional or motivational factors, (3) experience factors, and (4) social or cultural factors. The four components are influenced and linked by each person's life phase and spirituality. These influences cause changes in each of the quadrants of the frames of reference so that a frame of reference is dynamic and ever changing. A change in any part of a person's frame of reference, whether caused by aging or any one of a multitude of life events, has an impact on the other components of that person's frame of reference.

A person's frame of reference represents her/his "system" and thus changes when there is a change in any part of the system. It is the very dynamic nature of each individual that makes him/her so fascinating. However, the infinite number of possible composites of clients presents a particular challenge for those in a helping profession such as physical therapy. The challenge is to glean some sense of the frame of reference of each person served so that therapeutic interactions can be optimally effective.

COMPONENTS OF A FRAME OF REFERENCE

The four main components of a frame of reference described earlier are common to all persons and are concomitantly influenced by a person's life phase and spirituality. Each component is comprised of several subcomponents that lead to the unique qualities of each person.

Organic Factors

Organic factors represent innate characteristics and the anatomical or physiological status of an individual at any point in time.

Physical Characteristics

Physical characteristics include gender, race, skeletal structure, physiological status, and facial appearance.

Gender. Gender influences a person's frame of reference in a number of ways. First, anatomy and physiological functions vary with gender. Anatomical characteristics commonly are used as the basis for defining the gender of a person. Caution must be exercised, however, in relying solely on anatomical characteristics for making determinations of expected gender behavior or frames of reference.

Studies on prenatal and perinatal hormonal influences suggest that some differences in sex behaviors are hormonal in origin.[1] Other studies suggest that different preferences for behavior relate to the nature of a person's interactions with their parents.[2]

There is a significant body of research describing the differences in male and female behavior.[2-4] Although it may remain debatable as to whether the differences are purely genetic, purely environmental, or a combination of the two, it is widely agreed that boys and girls are socialized differently. Girls are socialized in many cultures to be passive, nonaggressive, self-disclosing, and nurturing. Boys on the other hand are socialized to be active and aggressive, to withhold expression of feelings, and to be in roles of power.[5] Differences in socialization often result in different styles of communication. These differences often lead to different interpretations of conversations, events, and situations.[6]

Race. The color of a person's skin has a marked influence on how he/she is perceived by others and how he/she perceives others. Evidence of racial stereotyping is apparent in the news media. Often, cultural influences are closely associated with race—particularly if race and ethnicity are strongly linked. As health care practitioners, physical therapists have a responsibility to be aware of trends that relate to groups that may have bearing on our interactions; however, physical therapists must avoid behaving as though trends are general-

izable to every person from a given racial or ethnic group.

Skeletal Structures. A person's skeletal structure determines his/her height, may influence the presence or absence of deformity, contributes to postural status, and tends to be associated with body type. Although studies have attempted to correlate body type with personality, this link has not been substantiated. A study by Brodsky[7] and more recent studies by Strongman and Hart[8] and by Wells and Siegel[9] suggest that persons have stereotypic manners of responding to various types of male physiques. For example, men with endomorphic body types are regarded as being physically weak, loving to eat and drink, and being happy-go-lucky and talkative. Men with mesomorphic body types are regarded as being muscular, athletic, able to be leaders, and self-confident. Ectomorphic men are regarded as being fragile, tense, quiet, and ambitious. A person's body type seems to evoke a response from others that is likely to influence how a person perceives himself/herself and thus how he/she interacts with others.

Skeletal status influences appearance and how others perceive an individual. Tall people tend to be viewed as holding more authority, power, and status.[2] Persons who stand erect project a persona of self-confidence, whereas persons who slouch and look down at their feet project an image that they lack self-esteem, power, or influence. Feelings of fear, curiosity, or pity may emerge when viewing persons with skeletal deformities or absence of limbs. Each person's frame of reference is influenced by the reactions of others toward his/her appearance; that person's frame of reference also influences how he/she perceives others. Tall people "see" the world differently than short people by virtue of their greater height.

Physiological Status. A person's physiological status relates to his/her state of health or disease, which is discussed later. A person's metabolic rate and various human rhythms also influence his/her behavior and frame of reference at any point in time. The more active an individual, the higher his/her metabolic rate. A higher metabolic rate results in a higher level of energy consumption and influences a person's actual and perceived level of energy. Many human rhythms tend to influence behavior during the course of a day, month, year, or many years.[10] For example, degree of alertness relates to circadian temperature cycle; lunar rhythms are similar to the menstrual cycles of women; and 1-year and 11-year electrical and magnetic-field rhythms of the earth correlate with incidence patterns of disease.[10]

Facial Appearance. A person's facial features, hair and eye color, and amount of facial hair all have an influence on interactions with others. A person's appearance is a reflection of the individual and provides cues to others about the individual's frame of reference. The cues may or may not be accurate but are being conveyed. Rightly or wrongly, appearance communicates a great deal about people. The way a person perceives his/her appearance influences how he/she relates to others.[2]

Health Status

Health status relates to both body and mind. The brain masterminds or indirectly influences body functions and reactions to a whole array of stressors.[11,12] Ideally, the body and mind are healthy. Physical therapy patients do not enjoy this state of physical and mental health. Although they present themselves for therapy with problems of the body, physical therapists should be cognizant of the role of the mind in contributing to both the problem and the resolution of the problem. The mind and body are inseparable.

Four combinations of mind and body status exist; they are

Healthy mind and healthy body.
Healthy mind and unhealthy body.
Unhealthy mind and healthy body.
Unhealthy mind and unhealthy body.

If physical therapists accept the premise that the mind and body are inseparable, then they can appreciate that the problems patients present themselves with may emerge from injuries or diseases, and that such manifestations are linked closely with the patient's mindset for being vulnerable to injury or disease.

When a person has a healthy mind and a healthy body, he/she can be said to be in a state of equilibrium or hemostasis. The person's "body system" is in harmony. It is only when a person becomes unbalanced or is in a state of disequilibrium that either the body or mind is in an unhealthy state.

A healthy mind and unhealthy body is the most desirable state of disequilibrium. Ferguson emphasizes the power of mind in healing in her presentation of a "new paradigm of health."[11] Studies on the effects of placebo show the strong influence that the mind has in countering disease and promoting health.[10]

An unhealthy mind and healthy body is a state of disequilibrium that results in mental illness in any of its many forms. Mental illness can be as debilitating as physical illness. The body often shows signs of mild mental illness as manifested in the posture; in extreme circumstances, the person may enter a catatonic state. Emotional or psychological disease can result in physical symptoms. Such symptoms are labeled "psychosomatic" and exist in the absence of organic findings to support their presence. In healing, the body cannot do for the mind what the mind can do for the body.

An unhealthy mind and an unhealthy body is the most severe state of disequilibrium. It is unlikely that physical therapists can be optimally effective with a patient in this state. Specialists with expertise beyond that of physical therapists are required to intervene to bring about a healthier mental state. Achievement of a healthy body or a level of optimal body function requires a reasonably healthy mind.

Teaching and Learning Styles

Several learning inventories are commonly used to identify learning-style preferences. Knowledge of one or more of these inventories can be highly useful to a physical therapist. Such inventories provide insight regarding the physical therapist's preference for learning, which typically is reflected in his/her style of teaching. Knowledge of learning styles enables the physical therapist to identify the learning preferences of patients. This is important in facilitating optimal patient learning and patient-therapist interactions.

Kolb has developed the Learning-Style Inventory (LSI).[13] The inventory is available for purchase. It is based on research that the author conducted during the 1970s and 1980s. Normative values have been established for four learning scales, based on 1446 adults ranging in age from 18 to 60 years.

Kolb's LSI identifies one of four learning-style types. The four learning-style types identified in the LSI are "assimilator," "accommodator," "converger," and "diverger."[13] The *assimilator* and *accommodator* types are based in part on a theory of Jean Piaget. Piaget described the processes of assimilation and accommodation.[14] *Assimilation* refers to integrating knowledge or observations into one's existing knowledge base, *ie*, new knowledge is consistent with one's existing knowledge. *Accommodation* refers to making adjustments in one's existing knowledge base to include new knowledge or observations. This is more than adding to or affirming existing knowledge. It requires changes in one's knowledge base.

The *converger* and *diverger* types are based on

work by Guilford.[13] These types emerge from the structure-of-intellect model developed by Guilford. *Convergence* and *divergence* are processes that are essential to creativity.

Kolb described an experiential learning model that comprises four stages.[13] Kolb stated that a learner needs four types of learning capabilities to be an effective learner. These are as follows:

1. Ability to learn by feeling or through specific experiences, which Kolb labeled "concrete experience."
2. Ability to learn by watching and listening without judging from different perspectives, which Kolb labeled "reflective observation."
3. Ability to learn by thinking logically, by problem solving, and by developing theories, which Kolb labeled "abstract conceptualization."
4. Ability to learn by doing, risk taking, and getting things done, which Kolb labeled "active experimentation."

These four abilities combine to form the four learning-style types just named (converger, diverger, assimilator, and accommodator).[13]

The converger combines the abilities of abstract conceptualization and active experimentation. Persons with this learning-style preference enjoy putting ideas and theories to practical use and are comfortable with problem solving and decision making.

The diverger combines the abilities of concrete experience and reflective observation. Persons with this learning-style preference are effective in idea generation and brainstorming sessions. They view concrete situations from many points of view and prefer to observe and exercise creativity rather than to take action.

The assimilator combines the abilities of abstract conceptualization and reflective observation. Persons with this learning-style preference enjoy synthesizing a wide array of information into a concise and logical format. They regard logical soundness of a theory more highly than its practical value.

The accommodator combines concrete experience and active experimentation. Persons with this learning-style preference enjoy "hands-on" experiences. They are risk takers who act on "gut" feelings more than on systematic, logical processes.

Ideally, a person would possess all four abilities and have the capacity to combine the abilities to be an effective learner using any one of the four learning-style types. Although this is rarely the case, an understanding of these different preferences can help people understand some of the differences in the frames of reference of those with whom they work and interact. Recognition of how others may be similar or different from them can assist physical therapists in planning therapeutic activities that are more effective for their patients and can help them to engage in more effective interpersonal interactions with all persons with whom they come in contact.

Personal Style

According to Jung's theory of psychological types, each person has inherent preferences for perceiving and judging.[15] Each person may perceive or acquire information in a realistic or practical manner or through his/her intuition, imagination, and possibilities. Judgements and decisions are made based on the information people obtain through logical processes or from the priorities that they or others set. Environmental factors enhance or impede the expression of psychological type. Type is dynamic rather than stable. Although people have preferences for their behavior, they occasionally may choose to behave differently. Nonetheless, inborn preferences persist. All psychological types are equally valuable. There is no good or bad preference type.[16]

Jung's theory of psychological type was extended, modified, and translated into the Myers-Briggs Type Indicator (MBTI) by Myers and her mother, Briggs. The MBTI helps to identify or indicate a person's type preferences.[16] The MBTI indicates a person's preferences on four scales: the extraversion-introversion (EI), the sensing-intuition (SN), the thinking-feeling (TF), and the judging-perceptive (JP) scales. Each scale represents two opposite preferences for behavior. Therefore, eight possible preferences that contribute to a person's type exist.[17]

The EI scale describes two opposite preferences for whether a person's attention is focused on the outer or inner world: extraversion (E) and introversion (I).[18]*

"People who prefer extraversion tend to focus on the outer world of people and the external environment. When you are extraverting, you are energized by what goes on in the outer world, and this is where you tend to

---

* Modified and reproduced by special permission of the publisher, Consulting Psychologists Press, Inc, Palo Alto, CA 94303 from *Introduction to Type* by Isabel Briggs Myers. Copyright 1987 by Consulting Psychologists Press, Inc. All rights reserved. Further reproduction is prohibited without the publisher's written consent.

direct your own energy. Extraverts usually prefer to communicate more by talking than by writing. They need to experience the world in order to understand it and thus tend to like action.

People who prefer introversion focus more on their own inner world. When you are introverting, you are energized by what goes on in your inner world, and this is where you tend to direct your own energy. Introverts tend to be more interested and comfortable when their work requires a good deal of their activity to take place quietly inside their heads. They like to understand the world before experiencing it, and so often think about what they are doing before acting."

The SN scale describes opposite ways people acquire information: through senses (S) and intuition (N).[18]

"One way to find out is to use your sensing function. Your eyes, ears, and other senses tell you what is actually there and actually happening, both inside and outside of yourself. Sensing is especially useful for appreciating the realities of a situation. Sensing types tend to accept and work with what is given in the here-and-now, and thus become realistic and practical. They are good at remembering and working with a great number of facts.

[Another] way to find out is through intuition, which shows you the meanings, relationships, and possibilities that go beyond the information from your senses. Intuition looks at the big picture and tries to grasp the essential patterns. If you like intuition, you grow expert at seeing new possibilities and new ways of doing things. Intuitive types value imagination and inspirations."

The TF scale describes how people prefer to make decisions or judgements about things: through thinking (T) and feeling (F). Feeling does not refer to a person's emotions but to his/her values.[18]

"One way to decide is through your thinking. Thinking predicts the logical consequences of any particular choice or action. When you use thinking you decide objectively, on the basis of cause and effect, and make decisions by analyzing and weighing the evidence, even including the unpleasant facts. People with a preference for thinking seek an objective standard of truth. They are frequently good at analyzing what is wrong with something.

[Another] way to decide is through your feeling. Feeling considers what is important to you or to other people (without requiring that it be logical), and decides on the basis of person-centered values. When making a decision for yourself, you ask how much you care, or how much personal investment you have, for each of the alternatives. Those with a preference for feeling like dealing with people and tend to become sympathetic, appreciative, and tactful."

The fourth scale, the JP scale, describes how a person is oriented or orients himself/herself to the outer world; *ie,* from a judging (J) attitude (thinking or feeling) or from a perceptive (P) attitude (sensing or intuition).[18]

"Those who take a judging attitude (either thinking or feeling) tend to live in a planned, orderly way, wanting to regulate life and control it. When you use your judging function, you like to make decisions, come to closure, and then carry on. People with a preference for judging prefer to be structured and organized and want things settled. [Note: judging doesn't mean judgemental. Any of the types can be judgemental.]

Those who prefer a perceptive process when dealing with the outer world (either sensing or intuition) like to live in a flexible, spontaneous way. When using your perception, you are gathering information and keeping your options open. People with a preference for perceiving seek to understand life rather than control it. They prefer to stay open to experience, enjoying and trusting their ability to adapt to the moment."

These 4 preference scales describe the basic possible dimensions of a person's type. The 8 preferences can combine to form 1 of 16 types. The understanding of each of these 16 types requires extensive study and understanding of the combinations of preferences for behavior.

It is important for a physical therapist to recognize different personal types so he/she can adjust to clients with different personal styles and recognize how differences in personal style can influence therapist-patient interactions. The preferences physical therapists and patients have concerning focusing on the outer or inner world, acquiring information through their senses or intuition, making decisions, or dealing with the outer world influence the therapeutic relationship. The dynamic interaction of two people of similar or different types has great bearing on the success of a therapeutic encounter.

Emotional and Motivational Factors

Emotional and motivational factors include a person's self-concept, self-esteem, emotional status, interests, needs, desires, and support systems.

Self-concept

A person's self-concept refers to how he/she perceives himself/herself. It is the cognitive view a person has of himself/herself, which culminates from his/her entire frame of reference at any given moment in time.[2] This perception relies in great measure on the feedback an individual receives from others.

Self-concept also is derived from a culture's or society's expectations for certain persons or groups of persons. For example, American society sends many messages through advertisements about the desirability for persons to be thin. This causes many individuals to hold a negative self-concept if, in their view, they do not weigh what they perceive to be socially appropriate. Unfortunately, some individuals misinterpret these apparent expectations from society and behave in a manner that is not ordinarily regarded as acceptable or desirable. An example of a person with a skewed self-concept is the anorexic or bulemic individual. Such an individual is so obsessed with being thin that he/she puts his/her health at risk.

Persons with disabilities also find themselves existing outside the bounds of what society generally regards as "normal." Therefore, their self-concept may exaggerate their disabilities, causing them to impose limitations on themselves that are neither emotionally or psychologically healthy. Evidence of such skewed self-concepts among people with a disability often can be seen in their self-portraits, which tend to exaggerate the nature of the disability.

Self-esteem

Self-esteem refers to how an individual values himself/herself or deems himself/herself as worthy of giving or receiving caring. It is the affective part of a person that reflects his/her feelings about himself/herself.

People often cite low self-esteem as a reason for poor performance; in contrast, high self-esteem is believed to lead to productive or meaningful levels of performance. Like self-concept, self-esteem seems to develop from how a person views his/her own behavior, accomplishments, and capacities. These views emerge from feedback from others and from self-imposed expectations that come from the media, life experiences, and interactions with other people.

Self-esteem is a critical variable in the therapeutic relationship. Glasser[19] described the role of self-esteem in chronic pain: eg, a person with low self-esteem may rely on the presence of a chronic back problem to foster certain types of relationships with family or friends that bolster his/her self-esteem. A very real barrier to the success of physical therapists may rest with a patient's reliance on a "disability" to maintain a semblance of self-esteem. In spite of effective measures to treat a

condition with physical therapy, a patient may not show improvement if the condition is closely linked to the patient's capacity to maintain a level of self-esteem that he/she sees as desirable.

Patients with high levels of self-esteem, on the other hand, are ideal. Persons who believe in themselves tend to believe they can improve and are motivated to work during therapy and between therapy sessions. They also tend to be willing to accept and receive support from other people. This combination of valuing oneself and deeming oneself as worthy of receiving support and caring from other people results in an optimal circumstance for having a positive outcome in physical therapy.

Current Emotional Status

A person's emotional status has an impact on his/her performance in a therapeutic relationship. Stress often has an impact on a person's emotional status. Emotional stress can be a major factor that contributes to a state of disequilibrium. "Common medical guesstimates indicate that approximately 75 percent of all diseases have their origins in stress."[20] The link between stress and emotion is one to which a physical therapist must be acutely attuned. To the degree that stress and disequilibrium of emotional origin contribute to a patient's condition, a physical therapist must be cognizant of these factors and anticipate barriers to recovery. A physical therapist's interactions with a patient may compound self-limiting situations or facilitate positive changes that result in a more positive therapeutic outcome.

Selye claims that "Stress is essentially reflected by the rate of all the wear and tear caused by life."[21] Furthermore, he regards stress as a "disease of adaptation." Any stimulus to the body and mind creates a response to the "stress" of the stimulus. When individuals are unable to respond adaptively to an accumulation of stimuli, their inability to adaptively respond to stress manifests itself as a disease or sign of stress.

Whether stress is caused by physical or emotional situations, it results in three successive stages of bodily response. Initially, the body responds to stress with a general "call to arms." This is followed by a persistent stage of resistance. Finally, the third stage—exhaustion—occurs, which ultimately leads to death.[22]

The first two reactions to stress are common. People often experience a "fight or flight" response to situations. Presented with challenging situations, people adapt and move beyond the fight or flight response to one of affronting the stress and its origins, if possible. Physical therapists desire that their patients manage stress in a manner that allows them to resist debilitating stress but to use the energy from a stressful situation to work on their behalf.

Recent past events may have a significant bearing on the interaction between the physical therapist and patient. Joyous occasions tend to have a positive impact on behavior, whereas negative events tend to have a negative impact on behavior.

Interests, Needs, and Desires

Maslow described motivation as being rooted in a hierarchy of needs that are successive and interactional.[23] The needs range from those basic to survival to safety needs, belongingness needs, self-esteem needs, and finally, to the highest and most advanced level of need, ''self-actualization.''

Basic needs refer to the physiological needs that are necessary to maintain a level of homeostasis sufficient to sustain survival. For example, these needs include food and water. Anyone who has been extraordinarily thirsty or hungry can relate to how these basic needs dominate to the exclusion of all others when the thirst or hunger is severe. Even when not so severe, these needs interfere with concentration and other activities if they are not adequately satisfied.

Safety needs refer to a person's needs for being secure, feeling safe, having freedom from fear, having protection, and having law and order and rules and regulations. In general, these needs are satisfied if a person does not fear bodily harm or falling victim to arbitrary and capricious behavior. Most people have their safety needs satisfied. However, many people who live in unsafe neighborhoods or find themselves homeless operate at this level of need. It is difficult to focus on higher levels of need when a person's well-being is perceived as being endangered.

Belongingness and love needs emerge when the physiological and safety needs are reasonably fulfilled. For example, people need to have friends and they have a desire to be part of a family, social group, or work group. Most people experience intense feelings when separated from loved ones. Each person also can probably remember the discomfort he/she experienced as the new child in the class, part of the new family in the neighborhood, or the new employee in a department. This discomfort can persist until a person begins to feel like a part of the group. Importantly, these needs require a person to both give of himself/herself and have a willingness to receive from others if he/she expects to be satisfactorily fulfilled. Mas-

low[23] and, later, Glasser[19] cited the role that the lack of the satisfaction of these needs plays in the malfunction of many individuals. Delinquency, alcoholism, and even chronic pain, for example, can relate to an individual's lack of feeling cared for by others and his/her inability to care for others.

Esteem needs refer to how a person values himself/herself and how he/she perceives that others value him/her. People desire achievement, adequancy, mastery of skills and knowledge, competence, and independence. They also desire a positive reputation, and they seek prestige, status, recognition, attention, appreciation, and often dominance or power. When a person's esteem needs are fulfilled, he/she feels self-confident, capable, useful, and worthwhile as a human being.

Self-actualization is the highest order of need, according to Maslow. This need refers to a person's striving for self-fulfillment by being all that he/she can be as a human and by feeling at peace. As Maslow described, a painter must paint and a musician must play music if their needs for self-fulfillment are to be satisfied.

Support Systems

To flourish as human beings, each of us must believe that a person or persons care for us. It is the belief that others care that often enables people to withstand tragedy and adversity in their lives.

The importance of being loved and cared for by others has been addressed in the section ''Interests, Needs, and Desires.'' This caring or support system has particular relevance to physical therapists. In large measure, a patient's progress relies on his/her perceptions of being cared for and valued by the physical therapist or significant others in his/her life.

Support from others also is vital for the continued growth and success of physical therapists as professionals. Much is written about the possible positive impact of a mentor on a person's career development. Undoubtedly, everyone can benefit from supporters or cheerleaders who provide occasional shots of reaffirmation for his/her sense of worth. People are strengthened in their belief of self when they perceive that others also believe in them.

Experience Factors

Experience factors include attained knowledge and skills, socialization and perceptions, and assumptions derived from life experiences.

Knowledge and Skills

A person's knowledge and skills have a great bearing on the frame of reference and the behavior of that individual as well as on the behavior of others toward him/her or in his/her presence.

Physical therapists are regarded as the "experts" by their patients. Therefore, patients look to their therapists for help and generally convey a respect for their expertise and afford them a level of authority in the management of their care. However, physical therapists may not be regarded as possessing expert knowledge in other areas of their lives. In those situations, they may not behave as assertively as when they are in their professional role. Therefore, others are not as likely to afford them the same degree of respect and authority.

A particular problem for many physical therapy patients is that when they are not in the role of "patient," they are held in high regard for their knowledge and expertise. Because of the hectic pace of the physical therapy clinics, therapists often do not become aware of a patient's area of expertise or perhaps lack the time to acknowledge his/her expertise. Although the therapist does not expect most patients to share his/her level of expertise, the physical therapist can enhance the therapeutic relationship by conveying a sense of value and worthiness to the patient by recognizing, acknowledging, and using his/her expertise.

Socialization

The socialization process refers in general terms to how people are "groomed" or prepared to assume certain roles, *eg*, in the family, community, society, or profession. Socialization of a person occurs through interactions with many people and groups throughout his/her life. If socialization is successful, it results in the adoption of values, attitudes, mores, and customs common to the person or group that has actively engaged in the socialization process.

Most people are subject to socialization as part of a family unit, during education, via peer groups, and through their work or in their professions. This socialization process influences the development of values, attitudes, and expectations for appropriate behavior.

The socialization of a person who is to become a physical therapist involves three phases.[24] First, socialization begins with formal education in the classroom and laboratories. Second, it continues during clinical education experiences. Third, socialization is completed during initial work experiences. This socialization is reflected in how physical therapists address their patients, in the nature of their conversations, and in appropriate and inappropriate forms of touch. Physical therapists also are socialized to behave in an ethical manner by abiding by the American Physical Therapy Association's *Code of Ethics and Guide for Professional Conduct*.[25]

Physical therapy patients undergo similar types of socialization processes that influence their interactions with their therapists. If a physical therapist and the patient are socialized similarly, their interactions are likely to be more effective because they are on the same "wavelength," so to speak. If, on the other hand, their socialization experiences were quite different, effective communication is more difficult.

People's perceptions about things, events, and circumstances derive from their experiences or lack of experiences. Concrete experiences, in combination with the many socialization processes that people undergo, have considerable influence on their perceptions and often lead to the formation of assumptions about expected relationships and behavior. As professionals, physical therapists must clearly differentiate between fact and assumption. It is important to label assumptions as such. Physical therapy patients may not differentiate between fact and assumption and thus act on assumptions rather than reality. As health practitioners, physical therapists are faced not only with sorting out their own perceptions, assumptions, and factual basis for actions but also with helping to clarify those of their patients. Great pains must be taken to acquire knowledge about patients' frames of reference to promote effective therapeutic relationships.

Consider a situation in which a patient from Brazil is to be treated. The physical therapist may give the patient an "okay" sign by placing the thumb and index finger together in a circle to convey the message "good job!" This sign in Brazil, however, is a vulgar sexual invitation and may be perceived as very insulting.[26]

Physical therapists must be alert to the perceptions, assumptions, values, and attitudes about behavior that emerge from the many socialization processes that they experience throughout life. The culmination of life experiences has a powerful impact on each person's frame of reference.

Social and Cultural Factors

Values, Attitudes, Mores, and Customs

In the discussion of experience factors, the impact of values, attitudes, and the mores and customs that evolve through socialization processes were identified as having a powerful influence on the nature of interpersonal relationships. These social and cultural factors form the basis for all communication—verbal, nonverbal, and symbolic as well as for expectations of acceptable and unacceptable behavior.

Culture represents the totality of beliefs and behaviors that have been learned through various socialization processes and that is common to a group whether it be a society, community, ethnic group, family unit, profession, or workplace. Many values, attitudes, mores, and customs derive from ethnic orientation. An ethnic group may represent a religious, racial, national, or cultural group.

Values, attitudes, mores, and customs are established through a complex set of interactions and life experiences. In her book *Caring for Patients from Different Cultures: Case Studies from American Hospitals,* Galanti emphasizes the distinction between "stereotype" and "generalization" when applied to cultural and ethnic beliefs and behaviors.[26] She defines *stereotype* as an ending point. A *stereotype* represents a person's assumptions about the beliefs and behaviors of a particular group of people that are automatically applied to each individual from a particular group. *Generalization,* on the other hand, is a beginning point. It represents beliefs and behaviors generally associated with a particular cultural or ethnic group but does not assume that those beliefs and behaviors are applicable to every member of the group. As those in the field are well aware, to know one physical therapist is to know *one* physical therapist! Therefore, physical therapists may begin with generalizations about various groups of individuals, but they must not assume that the generalizations apply to all persons they encounter from that group. It is the obligation of physical therapists to ascertain whether the generalization about beliefs and behaviors is true for the specific patients they encounter.

Roles

Every person wears several "hats" as a function of his/her carrying out multiple roles. Commonly, people assume family, work, social, and civic roles. These roles are interactive, and each is more or less of a priority for a person, depending on the individual's values and attitudes regarding these roles. At times, roles associated with family may be dominant and thus place work, social, and civic roles in a lower order of priority. It is not uncommon for these roles to place people in situations of conflict.

Many adults find themselves a part of the "sandwich" generation. They are sandwiched between responsibilities for children and aging parents while they attempt to consolidate their careers. When such people find themselves sidetracked by disease or injury, they may experience considerable stress, guilt, and concern for younger and older family members while trying to sustain a level of energy necessary for their own recovery or rehabilitation.

Recognition of the multiple roles assumed by patients provides therapists with greater insights about issues, ranging from compliance with home programs to mind-body states that may influence the patient's prognosis.

Socioeconomic Status

Many behaviors, values, and attitudes are associated with various levels of socioeconomic status (SES). Daily news accounts reflect the beliefs of many that people with money can buy almost anything, including better health care. Many such monied people do indeed behave in a way to support such a generalization. The debates regarding systems of health care delivery typically describe a system that provides access to all persons, but varying degrees of care and convenience can be obtained if persons wish to purchase privately more personalized forms of service.

Attitudes about health, fitness, severity of disease, and willingness to engage in therapeutic regimens also have been found to vary with SES. For example, lower compliance in keeping appointments may be more common among people of a lower SES because they may lack transportation or childcare.

Life Phase

A person's life phase permeates all components of his/her frame of reference. As people progress through life phases, their frames of reference change. Physical therapists can better relate to their patients and have greater insights about their behaviors if they are aware of common tasks associated with each life phase.

It must be emphasized that although approximate ages are offered for each life stage, considerable variation exists among individuals. One stage of development is not more or less important or more or less desirable than any other stage of development (although parents of 2-year-old children may think otherwise). Additionally, much of the research on adult development has been limited to men.

Each stage of life development encompasses one or more primary tasks. Successful completion of these tasks enables an individual to fully move on to yet another life stage and another set of tasks. The succession from one stage to the next is not, however, clear-cut. An individual may be working on tasks associated with more than one life stage simultaneously. Whatever tasks are not mastered or fully achieved do influence subsequent development and become part of the "baggage" a person carries throughout life. Such tasks may or may not be fully resolved. People's continued development is not blocked by unachieved or unresolved life tasks, but they are not likely to be all that they could be when they continue to carry baggage throughout life. On the other hand, people are never too old to resolve pending life tasks.

Life stages are characterized as stable and transitional. Approximately every 10 years from adolescence on, people experience a time of transition as they move from one major life phase to the next. The times of transition are unsettling and often downright stormy. These are times when people engage in review and determine whether they are satisfied or dissatisfied with their lives up to that point in time. Generally, times of transition result in some degree of change that is essential for continued growth and development. Transitions are times of disequilibrium. They are times when people experience "growing pains," so to speak, that are made more tolerable when they recognize that significant growth occurs only with some degree of disequilibrium. The stable times lie between the times of transition. During stable times, people may feel some degree of complacency and pursue their life tasks with vigor and energy.

Major life phase tasks can be related to career development. The summary in Table 3–1 is based on studies by Levinson,[27] Gould,[28] Sheehy,[29] and Vaillant.[30] Erikson described major stages of life development.[31] His description of life stages provides an overview of life development. His eight stages of development are as follows:

1. **Basic trust versus basic mistrust.** This earliest life task is the cornerstone for a person's achieving a sense of well-being. Success in this stage of development results in a sense of trust in others and in oneself.
2. **Autonomy versus shame and doubt.** This life phase deals with holding on and letting go. Ideally, children learn to exercise self-control over their free choices and experience a sense of good will and pride rather than feel doubt and shame because of a sense of lost control.
3. **Initiative versus guilt.** This stage is characterized by taking delight in the initiation of activities in a manner that does not misuse or overstep the

Table 3–1. THE LINK BETWEEN ADULT DEVELOPMENT AND CAREERS

Life Phase (y)	Characteristics Related To Work
Leaving family (16–24)	Initial decisions about what to study, work, or career
Entering adult world (20s)	Provisional commitment to work or career; first job; adjusting to work world; working toward competence, testing; building a dream; finding or gaining a niche; forming supportive relationships; developing intimacy
Age 30 transition (27–33)	Re-examining life, revising or reaffirming career goals, going back to school
Settling down (early 30s)	Focusing on work (career consolidation); looking or preparing for promotion, recognition; seeking increased responsibility; breaking or establishing supportive relationships
Becoming one's own person (35–42)	Strong focus on work; becoming more senior; establishing expertise; promotion, recognition; breaking with mentor
Midlife transition (early 40s)	Reassessing, reordering priorities, exploring; assisting others; desiring to unite and balance personal and professional goals
Midlife (40s)	Assisting others; sharing knowledge or skills; developing new interests, hobbies
50s transition (late 40s, early 50s)	Re-examining life, accomplishing whatever has been put on "hold"
50s–early 60s	Accomplishing important goals, broader perspective
Life review (60s and beyond)	Accepting or being dissatisfied with accomplishments, life; retirement (for some)

appropriate boundaries of the activities. Ideally, the child attaches his/her dreams to the goals of an active adult life.
4. **Industry versus inferiority.** This phase focuses on learning to desire and derive pleasure from completion of a task. This coincides with the advent of formal education. Ideally, the child believes in his/her capacity to complete tasks and does not feel inadequate and inferior because of an inability to complete tasks.
5. **Identity versus role confusion.** With the entrance of puberty and adolescence, young people must revisit their sense of self as they have come to know it in childhood. They seek to

integrate childhood and their feelings about self with the feedback they receive from their peers. It is now that the young person identifies tentatively his/her career plans and further establishes his/her identity.

6. **Intimacy versus isolation.** This stage focuses on the young adult's capacity to commit himself/herself to relationships, even if these demand compromise or sacrifice. Avoidance of intimacy may lead to isolation and self-absorption.

7. **Generativity versus stagnation.** This is a vital stage of adulthood that is concerned with establishing and guiding the next generation. "Mature man needs to be needed, and maturity needs guidance as well as encouragement from what has been produced and must be taken care of."[31]

8. **Ego integrity versus despair.** This last stage, when experienced successfully, is exemplified with the joy of a person's accomplishments, contributions to others, and a general sense of well-being with his/her life. Erikson brings full circle the stages of human life when he states, "healthy children will not fear life if their elders have integrity enough not to fear death."[31]

Spirituality

Spirituality refers to life principles that permeate a person's being. Spirituality is not religion but rather the "essence" of a human being that is intangible and difficult to describe. It is a force that is present in each person. It influences values, beliefs, and behavior. Spirituality is the innermost core from which each person seeks meaning and purpose for his/her existence.

INTERACTIONS BETWEEN PATIENT AND THERAPIST

The components of a person's frame of reference and the influence of life phase and spirituality set the stage for interactions with others. Given the complexity of people's frames of reference and the infinite number of possible composites, it is truly astonishing that people experience as much success in communication as they do. It also becomes obvious why people often find themselves in less than satisfactory interpersonal relationships, or, at very least, it is quite understandable why people may not be on the same wavelength as are other people.

The therapist and patient interaction can be enhanced if physical therapists first become attuned to the specific aspects of their own frames of reference. Such an introspective review helps them to identify the values, attitudes, strengths, weaknesses, characteristics, aptitudes, and biases that influence their interactions with others. Such an assessment also helps them to better identify the specific aspects of the frames of reference of others. If therapists know themselves, they can better learn about others and modify their behavior to result in an optimally effective therapeutic relationship.

The following is a section in which the reader should ask himself/herself a number of questions to assess his/her own frame of reference. As you, the reader, embark on this self-assessment, you are encouraged to do so with an open mind, allowing yourself to ponder questions not asked herewith; you should give yourself time to ponder those questions that undoubtedly will be triggered as you proceed. Throughout, ask, "How can I modify my behavior to achieve an optimal therapeutic relationship if my patients do not share my frame of reference?"

ASSESSMENT OF FRAME OF REFERENCE

Organic Factors

Physical Characteristics

- What are your views about femininity and masculinity?
- How does your family or ethnic group view your gender? Do you agree? Do you believe society, your community, your profession, and your workplace view your gender as you do? If not, how does this make you feel? How do you feel about your gender? How do you feel about the opposite gender?
- How do you feel about your race? Do you believe others feel the same way? If so, who shares your feelings and why? Who do you believe feels different than you about your race? Why do you think others feel differently? How do you feel about other races? Can you recall how your feelings about yourself and others developed?
- How would you describe yourself from the perspective of physical characteristics? What is your height? What is your weight? What is your body type? Are you pleased with your physical appearance? If yes, why? If not, why not? What physical characteristics do you find appealing in others? What physical characteristics do you find unappealing or repulsive?

- How would you describe your physiological status? Are you satisfied with your physiological status? If so, why? If not, why not?

Health Status

- How would you classify your mind-body status?
- Do you feel in balance? Or do you feel a bit "out of kilter?" "Out of sorts?"
- Have you been ill in the past year? Have you had any of the following?

  Colds or influenza?
  Respiratory problems?
  Ear, nose, or throat problems?
  Cardiovascular or blood pressure problems?
  Endocrine system problems?
  Allergies?
  Gastrointestinal problems?
  Genitourinary problems?
  Liver disease?
  Nervous system disease?
  Musculoskeletal disease?
  Skin or connective tissue disorders?
  Metabolic disturbances?
  Gynecologic or obstetric problems?

- Have you been injured during the past year?
- Do you have a chronic condition?
- Do you have chronic pain?
- If you have been ill, injured, or have a chronic disorder, can you recall the circumstances of its onset? Was it during a happy time in your life? A sad time in your life? A stressful time in your life?
- Do you have a history of mental illness?
- Do you experience symptoms of stress?
- Do you feel "burnout"?
- Do you like your work?
- In general, do you feel contented? satisfied? angry? frustrated?

Teaching or Learning Preferences

- Do you prefer to seek the deeper meaning of relationships or events?
- Do you like to be told what to learn?
- Do you like to learn all you can learn about a subject or limit the information to that which is useful to you?
- Do you prefer learning about things that have direct relevance for you? Or, do you enjoy learning about hypothetical circumstances and possibilities?
- Do you prefer to learn from specific experiences?

- Do you prefer learning from hands-on experience?
- Do you prefer listening and watching to learn?
- Do you like to read and learn on your own? With others? In groups? In pairs?
- Do you prefer self-discovery?
- Do you prefer self-paced learning?
- Do you prefer fast-paced learning?
- Do you thrive on problem solving and decision making?
- Do you like to contemplate many possibilities and explore a topic from several points of view?
- Do you enjoy gathering several pieces of information and bringing them together in a meaningful manner, like an investigator?
- Do you learn better by reading? listening? watching? through hands-on experience?

The reader is encouraged to take a learning inventory to best understand his/her learning preferences. This also provides insight into his/her teaching-style preference.

Personal Style

The reader is encouraged to take a personal style inventory. The information about personal style is based on the MBTI. Often, people in human resource management or in career planning and placement services are qualified to administer this inventory. Another option is for the reader to take a self-assessment of his/her temperament. Such an assessment appears in the book *Please Understand Me*,[32] which is available in area bookstores.

Many tools are available for self-assessment; these tools provide insight into a person's personal style and manner of interacting in the world. What is important is for the reader to take one or more inventories to gain insight into his/her own style and to become well aware of styles different from his/her own, so that the reader may become more effective in working with clients who have different styles.

Emotional and Motivational Factors

Self-concept or Self-image

- How do you rate your physical appearance?
- Does your appearance match your expectations? others' expectations? If not, how does it matter to you? Does it matter because of what others think? Does it matter for health reasons?
- Is your body image consistent with your actual

appearance? with feedback you receive from others?

- What would you change to have the self-image you desire? Why? What difference might it make? If you can't change your image, what is terrific about yourself?

Self-esteem

- Do you feel a sense of self-esteem when you behave authentically?
- Do you feel a sense of self-esteem when you behave responsibly?
- Do you feel a sense of self-esteem when you behave ingeniously?
- Do you feel a sense of self-esteem when you behave gracefully?
- Do you feel good about yourself when you perform competently?
- Do you feel good about yourself when you act boldly?
- Do you feel good about yourself when you act unselfishly?
- Do you feel good about yourself when you behave benevolently?
- Do you believe you can do a good job at work? at home? with family?
- Do you believe you have earned a promotion? a raise in pay? recognition for what you do? merit an award or special recognition?
- Do you believe you are up to the next challenge that awaits you?
- Do you believe you can reach your dreams?

Current Emotional Status

The following questions are based on early symptoms of stress as described by Selye.[22]

- Do you feel irritable? depressed?
- Do you have high blood pressure?
- Do you experience a dry mouth or throat?
- Do you experience an overpowering urge to cry or hide?
- Do you have trouble concentrating?
- Do you feel weak or dizzy?
- Do you feel fatigued?
- Do you experience a sense of anxiety without knowing why you feel anxiety?
- Do you feel tense or keyed up?
- Do you tremble or have nervous tics?
- Do you tend to be startled by small sounds?
- Do you have a high-pitched laugh?
- Do you stutter or have difficulty with articulation?
- Do you grind your teeth?

- Do you experience insomnia?
- Do you have difficulty relaxing?
- Do you sweat under stressful situations?
- Do you experience urinary or gastrointestinal symptoms such as frequent urination, diarrhea, indigestion, queasiness in the stomach, or frequent vomiting?
- Do you have migraine headaches?
- Do you experience premenstrual tension or missed menstrual cycles?
- Do you experience chronic neck or back pain?
- Do you have an excessive loss of appetite?
- Do you quit smoking and then resume or smoke more?
- Do you take tranquilizers or amphetamines routinely?
- Do you consume excessive amounts of alcohol?
- Do you experience nightmares?
- Do you tend to be accident prone?
- Do you believe you exhibit any neurotic behavior?

If you, the reader, wish to further explore your current emotional status, you are referred to an article by Dohrenwend, Krasnoff, and Askenasy,[33] who have developed a 102-item list of life events that may produce stress and contribute to the onset of physical or emotional illness. The general areas relate to the following:

- Health.
- Work.
- Financial status.
- Home and family life.
- Personal and social events or circumstances.

Interests, Needs, and Desires

- Are your basic needs for food and water being met?
- Is there a reason you are unable to eat certain foods that you like very much?
- Do you have a comfortable living residence?
- Do you feel free from fear and harm in your neighborhood?
- Do you feel you have adequate police and fire protection?
- Are you comfortable with your status in your family?
- Do you feel comfortable with the roles you assume in your family?
- Do you feel part of the group at work?
- Do you feel like a valued member of your church or of organizations in which you participate?
- Do you feel that you are competent to practice in the setting you desire?

- Do you feel that you are up to date with respect to your skills and with respect to recent advancements in your field?
- Do you receive the recognition for your efforts that you deserve?
- Do you feel self-confident in your abilities?
- In general, do you feel valued by most people with whom you come into contact?
- Do you feel that you are fulfilling your dreams?
- Do you feel that you are pursuing your "chosen" field or responding to a "calling?"

Support Systems

- Do you have the support of your family? friends? colleagues?
- Do you have significant others in your life?
- Do you have one or more persons in your life with whom you can talk about any subject, problem, or situation?
- Do you have cheerleaders in your life? a coach?
- Do you have a mentor? people who inspire you?

Experience Factors

Knowledge and Skills

- What are your areas of expertise?
- In what areas of practice do you deem yourself inadequate?
- What are your career goals? Do you have the knowledge and skills necessary to fulfill your career goals? If not, what knowledge and skills do you need to obtain?

Professional Socialization

- Are you knowledgeable about the APTA's *Code of Ethics and Guide for Professional Conduct?*[25]
- Are you familiar with the American Physical Therapy Association's *Standards of Practice for Physical Therapy?*[34]
- Are you at ease with the pervading values of the physical therapy profession? If not, with what values do you have a problem?
- Do you feel torn between two or more sets of expectations for professional behavior? If so, why?

Social and Cultural Factors

Values, Attitudes, Mores, and Customs

- What are your most cherished beliefs? What are you willing to fight for?

- What messages did you receive over and over again as you grew up?
- What behavior do you believe all persons should exhibit? What behavior do you deem unacceptable under any circumstances? If some behavior is acceptable only under specific circumstances, what is the behavior and what are the circumstances?
- What are the common beliefs held by your family? church? ethnic group? community? region? country?
- What customs are an integral part of your life? Which customs accompany holidays? Which are routine in nature?

Roles

- How many roles do you assume on a daily basis? weekly basis? monthly basis?
- Are you a daughter? son? sister? brother? aunt? uncle?
- Are you a parent? Are you an in-law?
- Are you a spouse or significant other for another person?
- What are your household roles?
- What is your work role? professional? student?
- Are you a volunteer?
- Do you participate in civic organizations? If so, how?
- Do you belong to social groups? What is your role in these groups?
- Are you part of a religious group? If so, what is your role?

Socioeconomic Status

- How would you describe your SES?
- Do you belong to the lower fourth, lower-middle fourth, upper-middle fourth, or upper fourth of the population from an economic point of view?
- Do you have adequate financial resources to live comfortably? To send children to college? To pursue advanced education for yourself?
- Do you support parents or others with insufficient means to sustain themselves?
- Do you have any concerns about insurance coverage? house? car? health care? life insurance?

Life Phase

- At what life stage do you find yourself?
- What are your priorities for family?
- What are your priorities for work?
- What are your priorities for intimate or casual relationships?

- What role does leisure play in your life?
- What are your dreams? Have any of your dreams been fulfilled? How will you pursue your dreams?

Spirituality

- Do you feel whole as a human being?
- Do you feel connected with others? the universe? a power greater than life?
- Do you feel you are living in a totality that permits you to be all that you can be?

These many questions have been posed to assist you, the reader, in examining yourself so that you can have greater insight into the specific aspects of your frame of reference. This is also intended to heighten your awareness of the degree of variation that exists among individuals and to provide you with a starting point for learning more about the frames of reference of those with whom you live and work, and of those for whom you provide service.

VARIATIONS IN FRAMES OF REFERENCE THAT IMPACT ON PATIENT AND THERAPIST INTERACTIONS

There are many variables that can influence the patient and therapist relationship. This text cannot possibly address them all nor shall it attempt to do so. The intent of the prior description of the components of a person's frame of reference is to provide a conceptual basis for regarding similarities and differences among persons and to emphasize the complexity of a given person's frame of reference. The complexity of a single person's frame of reference thus leads one to appreciate the exponential challenge for two or more people to effectively interact.

This section focuses on the Health Belief Model and how different frames of reference mesh with the model. Cultural differences in regard to illness and health also will be addressed.

Health Belief Model

The Health Belief Model was initially developed in the 1950s based on a survey conducted by Hochbaum.[35] The impetus for the survey was to explain why people did not take actions to prevent or detect disease. The model is based on the premise that individuals take action to prevent illness if they believe that serious consequences exist,

that action will be beneficial, and that the action is beneficial in relation to effort and costs.

The basic components of the model as described by Rosenstock include the following:[36]

1. **Perceived susceptibility.** This component refers to whether a person perceives that he/she can contract an illness or believes that he/she has or is otherwise susceptible to an illness.
2. **Perceived severity.** This reflects a person's feelings about the seriousness of contracting a disease or of an existing disease or condition.
3. **Perceived benefits.** Even if a person regards a condition as serious or believes himself/herself to be highly susceptible to a disease or condition, willingness to take preventive measures or to seek intervention depends on whether he/she deems such action as beneficial.
4. **Perceived barriers.** A person's choice to take preventive measures or to seek intervention for an existing disease or condition also depends on his/her perception about the cost and benefits of such action. If, for example, the side effects are deemed to be too costly in relation to possible benefits, an individual is unlikely to take action.

The Health Belief Model as originally conceptualized focused on outcome expectations. More recently, Bandura's concept of self-efficacy has been added to the Health Belief model.[37,38] The outcome focus reflected a person's cognitive perceptions about whether a behavior or change in behavior would have a desired or worthwhile outcome. The addition of self-efficacy to the model provides information about a person's belief about his/her success in changing a behavior or maintaining a desirable behavior. Self-efficacy adds an affective dimension to the model. For example, if a person believes that regular exercise will reduce the likelihood of cardiac disease *and* believes that he/she is capable of executing the exercise regime, it is more likely that the individual will engage in an exercise program. An adage often used in relation to change process ("If a person who must change does not choose to change, there will be no change!") also is applicable to the Health Belief model.

A review of studies related to the Health Belief model was done by Janz and Becker.[39] They developed a "significance ratio" that represents the number of studies with statistically significant findings. The authors found that studies indicated a high significance ratio for "perceived susceptibility" and prevention behaviors and for "perceived benefits" and sick-role behavior. "Perceived barriers" were found to be the most predictive dimension of the Health Belief Model, whereas "perceived severity" was found to be the least predictive dimension of the model.

Other Models of Health Behavior

The Health Belief Model has been emphasized because of its widespread use and general acceptability to date. Several other models of health behavior also have been developed that have uses in various contexts. Rimer provided an excellent description and critique of several such models.[40] Briefly, other models appearing in the literature include the following:

The **Theory of Reasoned Action** predicts a person's intent to engage in a specific behavior.[41,42] This theory states that a person's intent is the best predictor of future behavior. In a review of studies on health behavior, Kaplan and Simon concluded that self-reports of intent to comply with various regimens were highly correlated with actual compliance.[43]

The **Multiattribute Utility Theory** predicts individual perceptions of possible outcomes or consequences of behaving in compliant or noncompliant manners through extensive interviews. At present, the models based on this theory are cumbersome for practitioners, but they may become more prevalent in simplified versions in the future.[39]

The **Attribution Theory** explains how people attribute their state of health or disease to various events or circumstances. Views held by people regarding the causes or events that lead to the onset of disease or an injury have considerable influence on their acceptance or rejection of various types of intervention. It is important to learn about these views during a therapist's initial interview when he/she records the patient's history and complaints.[40]

The **Protection Motivation Theory** is based on a cognitive process that describes health behavior in terms of a person's perception of the severity of a threat and the perceived cost and benefits of maintaining unhealthy lifestyles or making adaptations in his/her lifestyle. The "threat" provides a person with motivation to act if the severity of the threat is sufficient in relation to his/her degree of vulnerability. "Coping" leads to action based on what is perceived to be an effective response.[40,44]

The **Self-Regulation Theory** focuses on problem solving, reflecting both cognitive and affective perspectives of an individual. The patient's perceived extent of a health threat, identification of an appropriate or acceptable coping or action plan, and the likelihood of the individual believing compliance with the action plan will achieve success are the basis of this theory.[45–47]

The **Transtheoretical Model** focuses on the change process. It is a circular model that allows a person to enter or leave at any of the stages of change, depending on the stage of the person. The change stages include contemplating a change in behavior, determining to in fact change behavior, taking action to change behavior, and maintaining the change in behavior.[48,49]

The **Relapse Prevention Theory** addresses strategies for preventing relapses of addictions or unhealthy behaviors. Self-control techniques and expectations of positive outcomes are central to assisting people's continued success in changing behavior during the maintenance stage of change.[50]

Common threads exist among all of the health behavior theories and models described. These are as follows:

They all conceptually rely on the perceptions of individuals and the totality of their being, as reflected in their frames of reference.

All of the theories and models rely on communication. A thorough understanding of the elements of effective communication in concert with an in-depth knowledge of a person's own frame of reference is required for effective patient and therapist interactions.

All of these theories and models incorporate the concepts of motivation and change. Influences on motivation vary for each person. Although all people may share some forms of motivation, given the uniqueness of each person's frame of reference, no two sets of motivating factors are exactly the same. Motivation to change is an essential precursor for change to take place. The phases of a change process seem to be similar for all persons in all contexts.

Health behaviors rely in great measure on knowledge and information. It is important to make information available to people to inform and persuade them to adopt or maintain healthy behaviors. Studies such as that by Fleetwood and Packa[51] show that a higher level of health-promoting behavior exists when greater levels of knowledge about risk behaviors are present. Their study focused on coronary artery disease. However, because each person brings a different "knowledge" and "experience" frame of reference to the introduction of information, it cannot be assumed that each person interprets the information or attaches the same meaning to the information as do others or as is intended by the sender of the information. Again, this emphasizes the importance of effective communication and the need for physical therapists to try to get on the same wavelength as those with whom they communicate.

Given the reliance of compliance and the adaptation of healthy lifestyles on the change process, physical therapists must think of themselves as "change agents." The change process and the roles physical therapists may assume as change agents are discussed as part of the roles of physical therapists later in this chapter.

Cultural Influences on Health Beliefs

Time orientations differ among various cultural groups. An individual may emphasize the past, present, or future, depending on his/her time orientation. This has implications for patient and therapist interactions, particularly when the time orientation between the two differs.

A **past time orientation** focuses on tradition. Many people from countries such as China, Austria, and England cherish tradition and tend to exemplify a past orientation to time.[26] When a physical therapist is confronted with a person whose frame of reference includes a belief in "home remedies," it may be difficult to introduce "contemporary" measures for intervention.

A **present time orientation** focuses on the here and now; the events and circumstances of the moment take precedence. Many Latin Americans, Native Americans, black Americans, and Middle Easterners tend to hold a present time orientation.[26] This frame of reference does not lend itself to prevention of disease. Individuals in these groups may not place the highest priority on an appointment because other "present" events take a higher priority.

A **future time orientation** is common for many middle-class white Americans.[26] These individuals are engaged in planning for the future and tend to regard time as a valued "commodity." This orientation lends itself to health promotion and prevention of illness.

Social structures also vary among cultures. Different groups have varying beliefs about the roles and status of people based on age, gender, and occupation. Some cultures are relatively egalitarian, such as American culture. The United States *Bill of Rights* proclaims that all persons are created equally and equally share in certain unalienable rights as human beings in this country. Although this is the case, it is well known that some Americans have differing views about the roles of men and women, appropriate behavior for children versus adults, and different levels of regard given to persons that depend on occupation or community status. Other cultures more openly hold different levels of regard for people with different roles, ages, and gender. A caste system is present in India and is an accepted hierarchial differentiation among people and other groups in many Asian cultures. This author recalls a physical therapy student who did not become a physical therapist after having nearly completed the entire curriculum because the man her family had arranged for her to marry did not approve of such a role for her.

Disease attribution varies among cultural groups. Some people believe that germs cause disease, but others attribute the onset of disease to an imbalance in the body, a loss of the soul, possession by an evil spirit, a breach of taboo, or the intrusion of an object that causes one to become ill.[26] Western medicine emphasizes that germs are the cause of disease. Eastern culture emphasizes lack of balance as the origin of disease. Other beliefs regarding the cause of disease exist in Latin American and Third World countries. It is important for physical therapists to identify from the patient's frame of reference why he/she is ill or suffered an injury. Therapists must allow the cause to be "treated" by the appropriate intervention. To impose their own frame of reference as the only one that can explain disease may result in an unsuccessful therapeutic relationship.

Communication protocols vary among cultural groups. This includes who may be told or not told various types of information, the appropriate or inappropriate personal space for communicating with others, and the appropriate or inappropriate use of eye contact.

It is not uncommon for women, for example, to be uncomfortable with describing "female" types of problems to men or for men to refrain from discussing female anatomy. For example, a woman once whispered in the ear of this author in the presence of the author's husband about an infection of her pelvic bone. This was deemed as too "private" for her to discuss in the presence of a man. This was so much the case that she refused to explain the condition even to her male employer after a 3-week absence from work.

Galanti described a situation in which a Hispanic son was asked to explain a surgical procedure to his mother for completion of an informed consent form. The mother was scheduled to have a hysterectomy performed, and the son described it to his mother as the removal of a tumor, because it is inappropriate for a Hispanic man to discuss female anatomy with his mother.[26]

Acceptable space between people varies according to the nature of relationships and circumstances.[52] Hall described four levels of personal distance:

1. **Intimate distance** is that which occurs during lovemaking, comforting, or close physical contact sports, such as wrestling. In each case, there is much close physical contact and a heightened awareness of the physical presence of the other person.
2. **Personal distance** is that which represents an arm's length between two people. This is the space that is deemed comfortable and appropriate during personal conversations. Europeans tend to have a greater degree of comfort with less personal space than do Americans.
3. **Social distance** is the distance deemed appropriate for business or acquaintance interactions. This is the distance maintained in talking with colleagues over a cup of coffee or while chatting with a store clerk.
4. **Public distance** is that in which no physical contact and little, if any, eye contact is allowed. This is the distance people maintain while walking on sidewalks. It is also the distance people desire while on an elevator; however, this distance is difficult to exercise because of the limited space available, particularly if the elevator is crowded.

Physical therapists interact at intimate and personal distances with their patients. Because of the variety in patients' frames of reference, interactions may violate or stress comfortable and acceptable distances for interaction. Physical therapists must be mindful of these perceptions and prepare their patients for interventions that demand touching and "near space."

Eye contact is regarded in many different ways, depending on a person's frame of reference. Eye contact can mean "paying attention." Some people do not give eye contact out of respect. This author had a colleague who did not make eye contact during the serious discussion of issues. Rather, he closed his eyes and tended to bob his head while this author spoke. Although this could be interpreted as a lack of interest in what I was saying, from his frame of reference, he was giving his undivided attention. He closed his eyes to focus solely on what was being said. Asians consider it disrespectful to look someone directly in the eye, especially if the other person holds a superior status. Middle Eastern men regard direct eye contact from a woman as an invitation for sexual activity.[26]

Certain expressions of speech can be interpreted in different ways. The use of the word "boy" by a white person when addressing a black person is likely to be deemed offensive. Blacks may use that expression among themselves without offense, but it is inappropriate for others to use the expression.[26] The use of a first name is regarded differently, depending on a person's frame of reference. People in certain racial groups may be offended by the use of a first name when used by people in certain other racial groups. Older people may regard the use of their first name by younger people as inappropriate. Physical therapists should not assume that all people are comfortable nor deem it appropriate to use first names in their interactions.[26]

The desire of many people spanning many cultures is to please or fulfill the expectations of others. This desire leads people to say things or agree with statements in an effort to appear as meeting the expectations and desires of physical therapists. Patients may claim compliance with an exercise regime in an effort to please the therapist with their performance when in fact they have not been compliant at all. Such behavior is not meant to deceive but rather to please. Therapists must always exercise caution in attributing their frames of reference and meaning to those of others.

Grieving

People grieve for all types of losses. Physical therapists find themselves in the role of grieving for a loss and in the role of providing support to others who are grieving a loss. The physical therapist's loss may be that of a patient whom he/she has treated. The patients grieve for their loss of function. The patients' families and significant others also grieve. Often a therapist grieves as he/she attempts to provide support for a patient or family that grieves. If physical therapists understand the process of grieving and the importance of coming to terms with losses, they can be more effective as practitioners.

The stages of the grieving process described by

Kubler-Ross often are referred to in discussions of the grieving process.[53] The five stages of grieving are denial, anger, bargaining, depression, and acceptance.

Denial is the initial stage of grieving in which a person cannot believe that there is a loss. He/she feels numb, and the reality of loss does not seem to exist. As the numbness subsides, he/she may say something like, "This can't be happening to me."

Anger is the stage during which a person realizes that the loss is real. A person may lash out at himself/herself or at others in response to the loss. It is most typical to be angry with others and to blame others for the loss. The displacement of anger on others is difficult for the family and health care workers who often are the recipients of such anger.

Bargaining is the stage at which a person says that if what was lost can be regained, then he/she is willing to do X, Y, or Z. This stage also may be characterized as one of hope, but the hope may not be realistic.

Depression occurs as a person comes to realize that nothing will bring back what has been lost. He/she is beyond denial, beyond being angry, and beyond coming to the realization that bargaining will not bring back function or bring back life.

Acceptance is the final stage of the grieving process. It is during this stage that a person accepts the reality of the loss and begins to adapt to it. He/she accepts the loss and begins to live with the disability or loss of function or begins to re-establish life without the presence of another.

Although discrete stages of grieving have been identified, a person may not proceed through the stages in an orderly manner. It is not uncommon for a person to experience two or more stages imultaneously. Patients may fluctuate from denial to anger to bargaining within a given treatment session. The intensity of the stages varies as the person works through the entire grieving process. It is important for physical therapists to be sensitive to the cues they receive about "where" the patient is at any point in time. It also is important not to assume that a patient is at a certain stage of grieving based on just a single encounter or a few remarks. This process evolves in a dynamic fashion.

As patients progress through the grieving process, they have a number of needs that require sensitivity from helping professionals. Physical therapists serve people well by being honest within their scope of practice. They must provide emotional support for existing or anticipated losses. Acknowledge a patient's fear of loss and reinforce his/her value as a human being. Accept and value the patient's right to make decisions about physicians, seeking second opinions, seeking opinions or services from other physical therapists, refusing treatment, or seeking forms of therapy that physical therapists may not support. This does not mean therapists should not share their professional expertise as is appropriate, but they must think in terms of the patient's frame of reference and provide support that allows the patient to progress through the grieving process in a manner that allows him/her to accept his/her physical or life status.

COMMUNICATING IN A THERAPEUTIC RELATIONSHIP

Nature of Therapeutic Relationships

Therapeutic relationships are human relationships. Several elements of human interaction impact on the relationship between the therapist and the patient. Optimal therapeutic relationships are attained only if therapists convey certain attitudes through their verbal, nonverbal, and symbolic forms of communication.

At the core of an effective therapeutic relationship is the capacity of the therapist to convey to his/her patients that he/she values them as human beings and regards them worthy as human beings to receive the very best care. The other elements that contribute to establishing optimal therapeutic partnerships emerge and manifest themselves from these core attitudes.

Ideally, therapeutic relationships are partnerships between the physical therapist and the patient. Elements of human behavior that contribute positively to these partnerships include:

The physical therapist should know himself/herself. The self-assessment presented earlier in the chapter assists one in gaining greater clarity about a person's beliefs, values, and attitudes. If therapists develop self-awareness, they can better recognize when attitudes, beliefs, or values that they hold may interfere with an optimal therapeutic relationship. This recognition allows them to make adjustments in their behavior that may otherwise be detrimental to interactions with patients.

The physical therapist should learn about his/her patients. The more they learn about their patients through review of medical records, initial interviews, and ongoing information gathering, the better they can appreciate their frames of reference. This knowledge enables therapists to communicate more effectively and to better meet the real and perceived needs of their patients. Knowledge of the patients provides therapists with a sense of where to begin their patients' therapeutic journeys. It also allows therapists to build on the skills, knowledge, and life experiences of the patients as they build their therapeutic partnerships.

The establishment of trust is essential for an effective therapeutic partnership. Trust develops in an environment in which physical therapists convey a sense of value and regard for their patients. The environment also should include the involvement of patients in an active and participatory manner.

Therapists should develop a tolerance for difference. A challenge that all therapists face as they encounter a heterogeneous patient population is recognizing and tolerating differences between themselves and those they serve. Distinguishing between the concepts of acknowledgement and agreement can help in this process. Although therapists acknowledge the presence of differences between themselves and others and accept the context of these differences, it does not mean that they must agree to adopt the differences. This distinction often helps to fully engage in a therapeutic relationship even when great differences exist between therapists and their patients.

A physical therapist must distinguish between empathetic behavior and sympathy and pity. Empathy is desirable in a therapeutic relationship. Empathy is an intersubjective process that happens to therapists when they briefly proceed through the stages of cognitively relating to another person's frame of reference, crossing over into that frame of reference, and returning to their own frame of reference. Davis describes this experience as "a momentary merging with another person in a unique moment of shared meaning." Sympathy, on the other hand, is sharing or understanding the feelings of another person. The expression of sympathy is appropriate in a therapeutic relationship. Pity is aroused by the misfortune of others but lacks emotional investment. Pity may convey disinterest or condescension, which is inappropriate for a therapeutic relationship.[54]

Therapists should have a wholistic concern for patients. Recognition of the many facets of patients' lives and their frames of reference enables physical therapists to form therapeutic partnerships characterized by wholistic concern for their patients. Wholistic concern does not imply that physical therapists are all things for all patients. Rather, it means that they engage in the therapeutic process with emphasis on their particular role and expertise but in the context of the "whole" person with whom they are working. A wholistic concern facilitates the therapist's capacity to be optimally effective with his/her patients and to help them realize their therapeutic goals.

Patients are partners. Patients must be regarded as partners in the therapeutic relationship. Optimal effectiveness requires that patients actively engage in the therapeutic process by being fully informed of their options and their possible consequences and by helping to establish the therapeutic goals and plan of action to the degree that they can participate in such decision making. Obviously, some patients are not able to fully participate as described, but caretakers, family members, or other significant persons to the patients can be involved in the decision making on the behalf of the patients. Shared decision making is vital for establishing an environment that encourages patient motivation and changes in patient behavior.

Modes of Communication

Three modes of communicating exist: verbal, nonverbal, and symbolic. Each of these modes of communication is in action at all times during interactions with patients. Communication is central to establishing an effective therapeutic relationship and to promoting changes in patients' health behaviors.

Verbal Communication

Verbal communication refers to the use of formal language in oral or written forms. Physical therapists engage in verbal communication through talking, listening, writing, and reading. Nearly half of their work day is spent listening. The other half is spent collectively talking, reading, and writing.

Active Listening. *Active listening* is listening as a fully engaged person who desires to understand the meaning of a message conveyed by another person. Active listening means listening to the words spoken and to the tone of voice and inflection, observing body language in its many forms, and noticing the presence or absence of tension, for example, when touching a patient. Active listening means to listen and gain meaning through all of the senses. Rogers and Farson describe the four following prerequisites for effective active listening:[55]

1. People must want to listen.
2. People must be willing to suspend judgement.
3. People must allow and encourage statements of feelings by others.
4. People must be aware of their own personal feelings.

Therapists must also use listening behaviors that convey their sincere attention to the speaker. Maintain good eye contact, maintain an open and relaxed posture with the arms and hands, and provide oral responses such as "uh huh" or "I see" or gestures such as a head nod to indicate that attention is being devoted to what is being said. It is important to stress the use of these behaviors in a sincere manner, because many people use the responses in a rather mechanical style and thus do not convey engagement in active listening. When the physical therapist restates a message sent by another in his/her own words, this also shows interest and helps to make sure that the therapist understands what is being said.

Speaking. As therapists speak, they should be cognizant of their tone of voice. A familiar adage states that "90% of the problems in the course of a day are due to the wrong tone of voice." It is not always the words spoken that are problematic but rather the tone of voice used in speaking these words. Consider the various meanings a therapist can convey with the words "Sure, OK." Voice fluctuations also add meaning by placing emphasis on various words or phrases.

Writing. Therapists often present themselves to others through the written word. It is important to pay heed to spelling and grammar, even during hectic times of note writing.

Nonverbal Communication

Nonverbal communication is always taking place when people are in the presence of others. Nonverbal communication is regarded as the most reliable form of communication. Nonverbal communication has been estimated to carry four to three times the weight of verbal messages[56] (thus, the adage "actions speak louder than words"). Nonverbal communication occurs alone and in combination with verbal communication. In fact, nonverbal communication always accompanies verbal communication. Many examples of nonverbal communication (eg, tone of voice, fluctuations in voice, eye contact, spelling, and grammar) represent nonverbal components of verbal communication.

Another major component of nonverbal communication includes "body language" in the forms of posture, nature of movement, space, and various gestures. The meaning of some types of nonverbal language is described in the discussion of the impact of variations in frames of reference on therapist and patient interactions. Physical therapists communicate a great deal through their facial expressions, arm and hand gestures, and touch. Their smile or frown does not go unnoticed by their patients. The therapist must exercise caution to avoid exhibiting nonverbal behavior that is not relevant to his/her interaction with a patient. A patient may interpret a therapist's furrowed brow over a recent verbal exchange with a colleague as displeasure with his/her performance. Open arms and hands convey a therapist's acceptance of his/her patients. Folded arms convey that he/she is bored. Hands on hips express impatience. A therapist's touch may convey that he/she is relaxed, confident, and professional, or that he/she is tense, unsure, and thus less competent from the patient's perspective.

Symbolic Communication

Symbolic communication refers to the many ways people communicate through appearance, possessions, affiliations, titles, and other measures of status. This is the least reliable form of communication, but it is a powerful form of communication nonetheless. It is powerful because it often is concrete, visual, and readily apparent to others.

Ideally, verbal, nonverbal, and symbolic modes of communication are consistent and congruent. Communication becomes ineffective when people say one thing through words and another through actions, whether they be nonverbal or symbolic. Therapists must strive to avoid sending mixed messages.

Establishing Rapport with Patients

The capacity of physical therapists to engage in a therapeutic relationship in concert with their communication skills provides the basis for their establishing rapport with their patients. The adage "There is no second chance at making a first impression" certainly applies to the initial encounters of therapists with their patients. The first encounter sets the stage for future sessions together.

Establishing rapport with patients requires attention to the factors discussed for developing a therapeutic relationship and effective communication in its many forms. Key elements for establishing patient rapport include the following:

1. Be ready to greet the patient when he/she enters the clinic, or arrange for someone else to warmly greet the patient. Provide a non-threatening environment for the patient so that he/she feels welcome and valued as a human being.
2. The initial exchange with the patient is important. Position yourself to greet the patient eye to eye. Introduce yourself and refer to the patient by his/her title. Avoid using first names until initial rapport is established and then only if deemed appropriate by the patient. Be sure your tone of voice and gestures convey your welcome and valuing of the patient.
3. Explain to the patient what your role is in this therapeutic relationship. Inform the patient about what you plan to do initially. For example, state that you will ask some questions, perform an examination, and provide the patient with information about a possible course or courses of action.
4. Interview the patient to determine the patient's perceptions about his/her problem and the various factors relating to the problem.
5. Determine the patient's goals for treatment.
6. Inform the patient of the tests you plan to perform and of any consequences of the tests that may be expected. Obtain informed consent for the examination you plan to perform.
7. Inform the patient of the examination results. Provide your recommendations for treatment and relate the recommendations to the findings and to the patient's goals.
8. Mutually establish therapeutic goals.
9. Advise the patient in regard to options for therapeutic intervention. If more than one option exists, share possibilities, and invite the patient to give his/her input on the final decision.
10. Obtain informed consent from the patient for the treatment that is to be rendered.
11. Actively involve the patient in therapeutic interventions. Mutually determine levels of patient responsibility and accountability for behavior between treatment sessions.
12. Readily respond to patient questions and concerns throughout interactions.
13. Promote greater degrees of patient autonomy and responsibility for care and behavior as the patient progresses through the therapeutic regimen.
14. Prepare for the termination of the therapeutic relationship.

The Teaching and Learning Process

The teaching and learning process is central to interactions with patients. As yet another adage states, "If I treat you, it is only for today. If I teach you, it is for a lifetime." Therapists must regard the therapeutic relationship as a teaching and learning interaction if they strive to change patient behavior to achieve successful adaptations to disease and injury or to prevent further injury or aggravations to injury.

The relationship between change process and learning informs therapists of the stages of patient behavior they should expect and provides them with a frame of reference for planning therapeutic interventions and their progression. The stages of change in the context of the learner include the following:[57]

1. The learner (patient) must be aware of a need to change behavior or to learn something new.
2. The learner (patient) seeks information and asks questions. This aspect of patient behavior is common today. It is important for the physical therapist to determine the level of knowledge of his/her patients, to encourage questions, and to make sure that his/her patients' information is accurate based on current research and knowledge.
3. When a strategy for new behavior or for adaptations is introduced, the learner "tries it on for size." The learner (patient) thinks about the change and determines from a cognitive point of view whether the change in behavior that is introduced is acceptable.
4. If a learner (patient) cognitively accepts the new information, the patient will attempt to change behavior. The acceptance of a change in behavior or compliance with a therapeutic regimen rests with the patient's cognitive willingness to change behavior and emotional acceptance to change behavior. Although changes in behavior may make sense from a cognitive point of view, if a person does not accept change from an emotional point of view, then there is no change. People must embrace change with brain and heart for it to become realized.
5. A patient does not demonstrate success in

changing a behavior until he/she demonstrates the behavior as a matter of routine. Physical therapists must make themselves available to provide support and encouragement to their patients during their transition from trying a new behavior to incorporating the new behavior into their usual mode of daily activity.

Physical therapists must possess a sufficient level of therapeutic competence to provide interventions for problems that originate from a cellular, tissue, organ, or systemic context. Any of these contexts alone is insufficient. The behavioral dimensions of interaction are ever present and interact with the interventions of physical therapists at various levels of anatomical and physiological systems. Therapists must encounter their therapeutic relationships with an appreciation for the special blending of the art and science of the practice if they hope to achieve optimal therapeutic interactions and ultimately optimal therapeutic outcomes.

References

1. Stone LJ, Smith HT, Murphy LB: Prenatal and perinatal development: editor's introduction. In Stone LJ, Smith HT, Murphy LB (eds): *The Competent Infant Research And Commentary.* New York, Basic Books, Inc, 1973, pp 109–117.
2. Hamachek DE: *Encounters with the Self,* 2nd ed. New York, Holt, Rinehart and Winston, Inc, 1978.
3. Goldberg S, Lewis M: Play behavior in the year-old infant: early sex differences. In Stone LJ, Smith HT, Murphy LB (eds): *The Competent Infant Research and Commentary.* New York, Basic Books, Inc, 1973, pp 1244–1251.
4. Murphy LB, *et al.:* Sex differences in coping and development. In Stone LJ, Smith HT, Murphy LB (eds): *The Competent Infant Research and Commentary.* New York, Basic Books, Inc, 1973, pp 1268–1274.
5. Henley NM: Power, sex and nonverbal communication. In Thorne B, Henley NM (eds): *Language and Sex Difference and Dominance.* Rowley, MA, Newbury House Publishers, Inc, 1975, pp 184–203.
6. Tannen D: *That's Not What I Meant! How Conversational Style Makes or Breaks Relationships.* New York, Ballantine Books, 1987.
7. Brodsky CM: *A Study of Norms for Body Form–Behavior Relationships.* Washington DC, The Catholic University of America Press, 1954.
8. Strongman KT, Hart CJ: Stereotyped reactions to body build. *Psychol Rep* 1968, 23:1175–1178.
9. Wells W, Siegel B: Stereotyped somatotypes. *Psychol Rep* 1961, 8:77–78.
10. Milsum JH: *Health, Stress, and Illness: A Systems Approach.* New York, Praeger Publishers, 1984.
11. Ferguson M: *The Aquarian Conspiracy: Personal and Social Transformation in the 1980s.* Los Angeles, J. P. Tarcher, Inc 1980, pp 241–277.
12. Neuman B: *The Neuman Systems Model.* Norwalk, Appleton-Century-Crofts, 1982.
13. Kolb DA: *Learning Style Inventory. Revised.* Boston, McBer and Company, 1985.
14. Piaget J: *The Origins of Intelligence in Children.* New York, W. W. Norton & Company, Inc, 1952.
15. Lawrence G: *People Types and Tiger Stripes.* Gainesville, Center for Applications of Psychological Type, 1982.
16. Myers IB, Myers PB: *Gifts Differing.* Palo Alto, Consulting Psychologists Press, Inc, 1980.
17. Myers IB, McCaulley MH: *Manual: A Guide to the Development and Use of the Myers-Briggs Type Indicator.* Palo Alto, Consulting Psychologists Press, Inc, 1985.
18. Myers IB: *Introduction to Type.* Palo Alto, Consulting Psychologists Press, Inc 1987, p 5.
19. Glasser W: *Reality Therapy.* New York, Harper & Row, 1965.
20. Applebaum SH: *Stress Management for Health Care Professionals.* Rockville, Aspen Systems Corporation, 1981.
21. Selye H: *Stress in Health and Disease.* Reading, MA, Butterworth Publishers, 1976.
22. Selye H: *The Stress of Life.* New York, McGraw-Hill, 1956.
23. Maslow AH: *Motivation And Personality,* 2nd ed. New York, Harper & Row, 1970.
24. Yarbrough P: *An Ethnography of Physical Therapy Practice.* Atlanta, Georgia State University, 1980. Doctoral dissertation.
25. American Physical Therapy Association: *Code of Ethics and Guide for Professional Conduct.* Alexandria, American Physical Therapy Association, 1991.
26. Galanti GA: *Caring for Patients from Different Cultures: Case Studies from American Hospitals.* Philadelphia, University of Pennsylvania Press, 1991.
27. Levinson DJ: *The Seasons Of A Man's Life.* New York, Ballantine Books, 1978.
28. Gould RL: *Transformations.* New York, Simon & Schuster, 1978.
29. Sheehy G: *Passages.* New York, E. P. Dutton, 1976.
30. Vaillant GE: *Adaptation To Life.* Boston, Little, Brown and Company, 1977.
31. Erikson EH: *Childhood and Society.* New York, W. W. Norton & Company, 1963.
32. Kiersey D, Bates M: *Please Understand Me,* 3rd ed. Del Mar, CA, Prometheus Books, 1978.
33. Dohrenwend BS, Krasnoff L, Askenasy AR: Exemplification of a method for scaling life events: the PERI Life Events scale. *J Health Soc Behav* 1978, 19:205–229.
34. American Physical Therapy Association: *Standards of Practice for Physical Therapy.* Alexandria, VA, American Physical Therapy Association, June 1992.
35. Hochbaum GM: *Public Participation in Medical Screening Programs: A Sociopsychological Study [PSH publication #572].* Public Health Service, 1958.
36. Rosenstock IM: The Health Belief model: explaining health behavior through expectancies. In Glanz FM, Rimer BK (eds): *Health Behavior and Health Education: Theory, Research and Practice.* San Francisco, Jossey-Bass Publishers, 1990, pp 39–62.
37. Bandura A: *Social Learning Theory.* Englewood Cliffs, Prentice-Hall, 1977.
38. Bandura A: Self-efficacy: toward a unifying theory of behavior change. *Psych Rev* 1977, 84:191–215.
39. Janz NK, Becker MH: The Health Belief model: a decade later. *Health Educ Q* 1984, 11:1–47.
40. Rimer BK: Perspectives on intrapersonal theories in health education and health behavior. In Glanz K, Lewis FM, Rimer BK (eds): *Health Behavior and Health Education: Theory, Research and Practice.* San Francisco, Jossey-Bass Publishers, 1990, pp 140–160.

41. Fishbein M, Ajzen I: *Belief, Attitude, Intention Behavior: An Introduction to Theory and Research.* Reading, MA, Addison Wesley, 1975.

42. Ajzen I, Fishbein M: *Understanding Attitudes and Predicting Social Behavior.* Englewood Cliffs, NJ, Prentice-Hall, 1980.

43. Kaplan RM, Simon HJ: Compliance in medical care: reconsideration of self-predictions. In *The Cardiac Family Recovery Program Training Manual.* Heartmates Inc, 1990, pp 168–175.

44. Prentice-Dunn S, Rogers RS: Protection Motivation theory and preventive health: beyond the Health Belief model. *Health Educ Res* 1986, 1:153–161.

45. Leventhal H, Zimmerman R, Gutmann M: Compliance: a self-regulation perspective. In Gentry WD (ed): *Handbook of Behavioral Medicine.* New York, Guilford Press, 1984.

46. Leventhal H, Cameron L: Behavioral theories and the problem of compliance. *Patient Educ Couns* 1987, 10:117–138.

47. Leventhal H: Emotional and behavioural processes. In Johnston J, Wallace L (eds): *Stress and Medical Procedures.* Oxford, England, Oxford Science and Medical Publications, 1989.

48. Prochaska JO, Crimi P, Lapsanski D, et al.: Self-change processes, self-efficacy and self-concept in relapse and maintenance of cessation of smoking. *Psych Rep* 1982, 51:983–990.

49. Prochaska JO, DiClemente CC: Common processes of self-change in smoking, weight control, and psychological distress. In Shiffman S, Wills T (eds): *Coping and Substance Use.* Orlando, Academic Press, 1985, pp 345–364.

50. Marlatt GA, Gordon JR: *Relapse Prevention.* New York, Guilford Press, 1985.

51. Fleetwood J, Packa DR: Determinants of health-promoting behaviors in adults. *J Cardiovasc Nurs* 1991, 5:67–79.

52. Hall E: *Hidden Dimensions.* Garden City, NY, Doubleday & Company, 1966.

53. Kubler-Ross E: *On Death and Dying.* New York, Macmillan, 1969.

54. Davis CM: *Patient Practitioner Interaction.* Thorofare, NJ, Slack, Inc, 1989.

55. Rogers CR, Farson RE: *Active Listening.* Chicago, Industrial Relations Center, University of Chicago, 1955.

56. Argyle M, et al. The communication of inferior and superior attitudes by verbal and nonverbal signals. *Br J Soc Clin Psychol* 1970, 9:222–231.

57. Robinson RD: *An Introduction to Helping Adults Learn and Change.* Milwaukee, Omnibook Company, 1979.

PART TWO

General Considerations for Practice

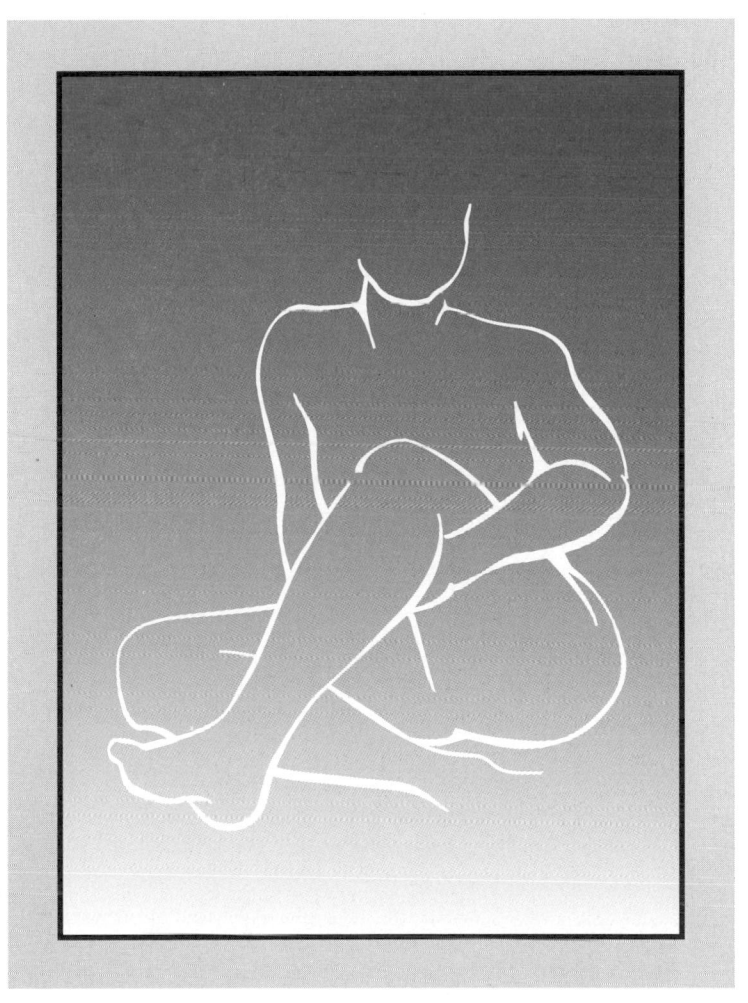

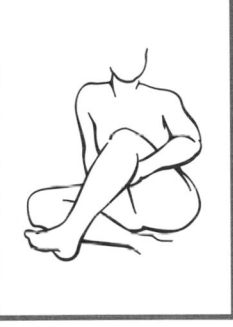

Oncology: Examination, Diagnosis, and Treatment. Medical and Surgical Considerations

Lucinda A. Pfalzer

Cancer is a large group of diseases characterized by uncontrolled growth and spread of abnormal cells. In a malignant or cancerous tumor, the normal controls on cell growth are ineffective, resulting in rapid cellular proliferation. The genetic changes within a cell's deoxyribonucleic acid (DNA) that result in cancer are a mystery that is slowly being unraveled. Current research focuses on the factors that "turn on" oncogenes, the cancer-causing genes that produce a protein that leads to abnormal cellular growth, converting normal cells to cancer cells.

There are more than 100 different types of cancer. More than 95% of cancers occur in adults. Organs are the most common site of adult cancer, four of which account for more than 50% of all cancers: breast, lung, bowel, and uterus.[1,2] Tissues such as reticuloendothelial tissue in leukemia and Ewing's sarcoma are common sites of childhood cancers.[3,4] If the spread of cancer is not controlled or checked, it results in death and remains the second leading cause of death (Fig. 4–1) and disability in the United States (Table 4–1).[2,5–7] About 83 million Americans now living will have cancer eventually; about 33% of the U.S. population, according to present rates.[1] Minorities with different cultural backgrounds and health beliefs consistently represent to a greater degree the populations with cancer (Fig. 4–1).[6,7] This difference is often not statistically significant when other factors are controlled in the United States. In 1982 and 1986, 50% of all diagnosed cancer occurred in individuals older than 65 years.[3,4] Cancer is, however, the largest disease-related killer of young adults from 15 to 34 years of age, and these rates have continued to rise through the 1980s into the 1990s.[3,4] Cancer is surpassed only by accidents as the leading cause of death in young females, and cancer is the leading cause of death in women between the ages of 25 and 44 years (Fig. 4–2).[8] Only accidents, suicide, and homicide surpass cancer as the leading causes of deaths among young men (Fig. 4–3).[8] Leukemia is the leading cause of cancer deaths in young males aged 15 to 34 years.[3,4] Acute lymphocytic leukemia accounts for 85% of all pediatric leukemia, and acute nonlymphocytic leukemia (ANLL) accounts for the other 15%.[2,3] The most common forms of leukemia in adults are chronic leukemia and ANLL.[1,2] In 1993, human immunodeficiency virus/acquired immunodeficiency syndrome (HIV/AIDS) became the leading cause of death in men between the ages of 25 and 44 years (Fig. 4–3) and the ninth leading cause of death overall.[8] The most significant improvement in survival rates has been in the pediatric cancers.[1,3,4]

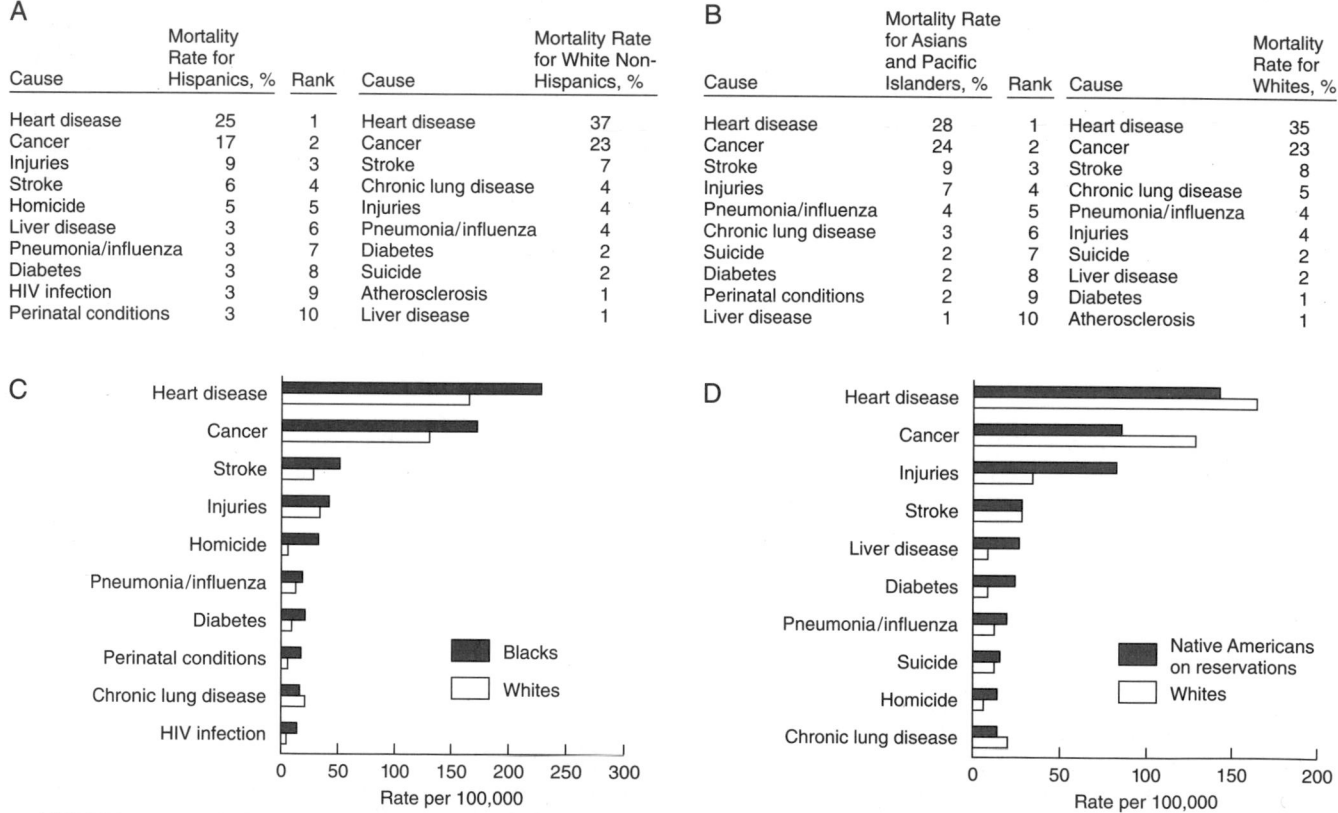

A

Cause	Mortality Rate for Hispanics, %	Rank	Cause	Mortality Rate for White Non-Hispanics, %
Heart disease	25	1	Heart disease	37
Cancer	17	2	Cancer	23
Injuries	9	3	Stroke	7
Stroke	6	4	Chronic lung disease	4
Homicide	5	5	Injuries	4
Liver disease	3	6	Pneumonia/influenza	4
Pneumonia/influenza	3	7	Diabetes	2
Diabetes	3	8	Suicide	2
HIV infection	3	9	Atherosclerosis	1
Perinatal conditions	3	10	Liver disease	1

B

Cause	Mortality Rate for Asians and Pacific Islanders, %	Rank	Cause	Mortality Rate for Whites, %
Heart disease	28	1	Heart disease	35
Cancer	24	2	Cancer	23
Stroke	9	3	Stroke	8
Injuries	7	4	Chronic lung disease	5
Pneumonia/influenza	4	5	Pneumonia/influenza	4
Chronic lung disease	3	6	Injuries	4
Suicide	2	7	Suicide	2
Diabetes	2	8	Liver disease	2
Perinatal conditions	2	9	Diabetes	1
Liver disease	1	10	Atherosclerosis	1

FIGURE 4–1   Mortality rates across the lifespan for minority populations in the United States. **A,** Leading causes of death for Hispanics and white non-Hispanics in 18 states and the District of Columbia, as a percentage of total deaths in 1987. (National death rate data were not available for Hispanics.) **B,** Leading causes of death for Asians and Pacific Islanders and whites. (California's published data [1987] on Asians and Pacific Islanders included 93% Asians and 7% other [Native Americans, Eskimos, and Aleuts]. National death rate data were not available for Asians and Pacific Islanders.) **C,** Leading causes of death for blacks and whites (1987, age-adjusted rates). **D,** Leading causes of death for Native Americans on reservations and whites (1987, age-adjusted rates). (**A**–**D** Adapted from *Healthy People 2000: National Health Promotion and Disease Prevention Objectives* [DHHS Pub. No. (PHS) 91-50212]. Washington D.C., US Government Print Office, 1990, pp 32, 35, 37, and 38.)

Table 4–1. LIMITATIONS IN FUNCTION ACROSS THE LIFESPAN RELATED TO CANCER

Causes of Limitations	All Ages		Younger than 18 Years		18–44 Years		45–69 Years		70–84 Years		85 + Years	
	*No.**	*%†*	*No.**	*%†*	*No.**	*%†*	*No.**	*%†*	*No.**	*%†*	*No.**	*%†*
Cancer, lung/bronchial	125	0.2	—		4	0.0	81	0.3	39	0.4	2	0.1
Leukemia	58	0.1	9	0.2	7	0.1	29	0.1	13	0.1	1	0.0
Cancer, female breast	159	0.3	—		19	0.2	101	0.4	34	0.3	5	0.2
Cancer, genitourinary	173	0.3	2	0.1	20	0.2	96	0.4	48	0.4	8	0.4
Cancer, digestive	185	0.4	1	0.0	14	0.1	114	0.5	48	0.4	9	0.4
Cancer of all other sites, NEC	190	0.4	10	0.3	96	0.9	240	1.0	96	0.9	13	0.6
Skin cancer	44	0.1	—		8	0.1	20	0.1	13	0.1	3	0.1
Bone cancer	52	0.1	1	0.0	5	0.0	24	0.1	20	0.2	2	0.1
All cancers	986	1.8	23	0.6	173	1.6	705	2.9	311	2.8	43	1.9

Adapted from Cole TM, Edgerton VR: Report on the task force on medical rehabilitation research. Presented to Hunt Valley, MD, June 28–29, 1990.
* Number of conditions per 1000.
† Percentage distribution

There are more than 8 million cancer survivors in the United States, 4 million of them with a diagnosis made 5 or more years ago.[1] Cancer is a leading cause of morbidity; many survivors have impairments and dysfunctions (see Table 4–1).[5] Although the initial calls for rehabilitation services to manage these impairments and disabilities was during the 1970s, many of these short-term and long-term disabilities continue to be unrecognized and untreated.[9–55] Cancer has become a chronic disease for many survivors. Most of these 4 million

individuals can be considered cured.[1,2] They have no evidence of cancer and have the same life expectancy as a person who has never had cancer; however, late physical[56–99] and psychosocial[100–135] complications of disease and treatment are now being recognized. In their study of 805 cancer patients, Lehman et al.[15] reported problems encountered at different cancer sites; the need for rehabilitation services; and gaps in the delivery of rehabilitation care. Significant numbers of rehabilitation problems were found that could be im-

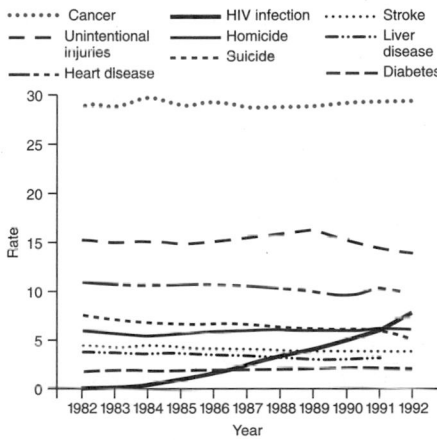

FIGURE 4–2   Death rates (per 100,000 population) from leading causes of death among women 25 to 44 years of age, by years in the United States, 1982–1992. (National vital statistics based on underlying cause of death, using final data for 1982 to 1991 and provisional data for 1992. Data for liver disease in 1992 were unavailable.) (Redrawn from *MMWR* 1993, 42.)

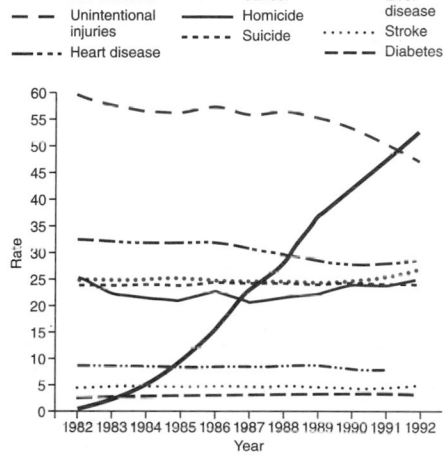

FIGURE 4–3   Death rates (per 100,000 population) from leading causes of death among men 25 to 44 years of age, by years in the United States, 1982–1992. (National vital statistics based on underlying cause of death, using final data for 1982 to 1991 and provisional data for 1992. Data for liver disease in 1992 were unavailable.) (Redrawn from *MMWR* 1993, 42.)

proved by rehabilitation care, and psychological problems were commonly encountered. The problems seemed more severe in patients with physical disabilities.[15] For those who still have evidence of cancer, the trend is clear: Statistics show that 51% or more of these people will be cancer-free 5 years after their diagnosis.[1] Behind the higher survival rates are better treatment technologies, including tracking of data. The National Cancer Institute's computer system known as Physician Data Query contains up-to-date-treatment information for more than 80 types of cancer. Furthermore, people are more alert to symptoms and are reporting them earlier, increasing the likelihood that their treatment will succeed. With early detection, 89% will survive.[1] About 80% of these cancer survivors — currently, more than 2.5 million people—are now receiving their cancer medical treatment in their own community hospitals. More physical therapists will encounter patients currently with or a history of cancer irrespective of practice setting.

Increased risk of mortality and morbidity in patients with cancer relates to cachexia: anorexia and weight loss, paraneoplastic syndrome signs and symptoms, age, initial functional status, and other disease- and treatment-related changes.[136–151] Cancer is frequently asymptomatic in the early stages. In cancer, metabolic demand increases and the protein-sparing mechanisms are essentially absent (see clinical manifestations for more detail on anorexia and cancer cachexia).[136,137] Normally during starvation, the body decreases its metabolic demand and uses protein-sparing mechanisms to preserve muscle mass and energy levels. Deweys et al. analyzed the prognostic effect of weight loss before chemotherapy using data from 3047 patients enrolled in 12 chemotherapy protocols of the Eastern Cooperative Oncology Group. Their findings included the following:

1. The frequency of weight loss ranged from 31% for favorable non-Hodgkin's lymphoma to 87% in gastric cancer. The frequency of weight loss increased with increasing number of anatomical sites involved with metastases, but within categories of anatomical involvement, weight loss was associated with decreased median survival.
2. Median survival was significantly shorter in nine protocols for the patients with weight loss compared with the patients with no weight loss.
3. Chemotherapy response rates were lower in the patients with weight loss, but this difference was significant only in patients with breast cancer.
4. Decreasing weight was correlated with decreasing performance status except for patients with pancreatic and gastric cancer.

5. Within performance status categories, weight loss was associated with decreased median survival.

Reuben et al., in a National Hospice Study, examined the correlation of 14 easily assessable clinical symptoms with survival in patients with terminal cancer.[144] Performance status was the most important clinical factor in estimating survival time, but five other symptoms had independent predictive value as well (shortness of breath, problems eating or anorexia, trouble swallowing, dry mouth, and weight loss). A model was developed to predict survival; the model was unaffected by patient age, sex, primary tumor type, and site. The prevalence of a similar constellation of symptoms among patients with cancer of various primary and metastatic sites supports the concept of a common final clinical pathway in patients with advanced cancer. In addition, the value of "soft" clinical data in predicting survival in patients with terminal cancer was validated.

Even with nutritional support such as enteral, parenteral, and hyperalimentation, cachexia may fail to be completely reversed.[142–149] Many of the previous studies of nutritional support in cancer survivors have applied parenteral techniques for relatively short periods. In their comparison of patients with inoperable squamous carcinoma of the nasopharynx and oropharynx with patients who received optimal oral nutrition, Daly et al.[149] found the following:

1. Improved mean weight maintenance
2. Improved mean caloric and protein intake
3. Improved mean serum albumin levels
4. Unchanged tumor response to radiation therapy

Sarna et al. described the relationship of nutritional intake to weight change, symptom distress, and functional status over a 6-month period.[150] The majority of patients had progressive non–small-cell lung cancer and had lost less than 10% of their body weight at the time of study entry. The percentage of weight loss over time was greater in subjects younger than 65 years, in those with small-cell lung cancer, and in those who received chemotherapy. Functional status related inversely to kilocalorie intake. Brown's subjects also had a diagnosis of non–small-cell lung cancer and had had postradiotherapy at least 1 month before.[151] Partial correlations, controlling for stage of disease, indicated that gender, age, and current smoking correlated significantly with cancer-related weight loss and decreased food intake. Gender, age, and current smoking accounted for 21% of the variance of weight loss postradiotherapy over and above stage of disease. Nutritional assessment and early intervention were enhanced for men, the elderly, and current smokers, who are at higher risk for weight loss. Prior weight loss was significantly associated with base-line functional status. Age was not significantly associated with degree of functional disruption, although 42% of the sample was 65 years of age or older. The greatest disruptions in physical activity were noted in ambulation. One third of the sample had difficulty walking one block or more. Serious fatigue was experienced by 79% of the subjects, and 44% had difficulty with household chores. Only 21% were completely satisfied with their level of activity. Pain improved in the treated subjects over time. Despite no significant differences at base line, untreated subjects had more limitations in physical activities than did treated subjects over time. Brown[151] studied prospectively a series of 578 patients after surgery for colorectal carcinoma. The factors that most significantly affect operative mortality are the age of the patient, a history of loss of weight, limited preoperative patient mobility, and the presence of intestinal obstruction with perforation of the bowel. By identifying high-risk patients, attention may be focused on particular patients at risk to reduce operative mortality. Further research needs to clarify the role of nutritional support specific to weight loss, cancer diagnosis and stage, and functional status.

About 70% to 80% of cancer survivors report feelings of fatigue during radio- or chemotherapy.[52,53,55,152] Fatigue is considered to be a multidimensional concept; however, fatigue has been assessed mostly by single items in general symptom check lists. A few specific instruments have been used in cancer populations. Patients with several types of cancer remain fatigued long after treatment ended.[55,152] Weight loss, decreased strength and endurance, impaired functional status, and fatigue are major contributors to the mortality and morbidity of cancer survivors.

Maintaining and restoring function are challenges for the cancer survivor undergoing long months of complex, multimodal treatment. The physical therapy profession has a responsibility to meet the needs of these cancer survivors with disease- and treatment-related dysfunctions and disabilities. Both "cured" and "controlled" patients have a frequent need for treatment of dysfunction and disability.[2,5,9,14–16,20,21,25,30–55] The physical therapist is increasingly called to contribute in the rehabilitation of persons with both acute and chronic cancer-related dysfunctions and dis-

abilities.[2,12,13–21,25,29–34,39–51,154–164] O'Hara et al. reported that personal care and home activity needs were not being met adequately in their sample of low-income, urban-dwelling, black patients with cancer.[9] Patients had significantly greater symptom distress related to frequency of nausea, intensity of pain, and difficulty breathing, whereas patients with breast and gynecological cancers reported the highest levels of symptom distress. Women who were elderly, black, living alone, poor, and chronically ill were likely to have unmet needs and high levels of symptom distress. General unmet needs have been consistently reported in many cancer survivor populations, with several site specific needs also reported.[9–11,15] Primary barriers to optimal delivery of rehabilitation care identified in 1978 were a lack of identification of patient problems and a lack of appropriate referral by physicians unfamiliar with the concept of rehabilitation.

An elderly population living in six counties in New Mexico diagnosed with breast, prostate, or colorectal cancer had the following variables associated significantly with nonreceipt of definitive therapy for cancer:

1. Advanced age
2. Impairment in activities of daily living
3. Low physical activity
4. Decreased mental status
5. Impaired access to transportation
6. Poor social support

Goodwin et al.[11] concluded that an age-related decline in the percentage of adults with cancer who received definitive therapy was independent of other potentially explanatory factors such as comorbidity. In addition, decisions about radiation may be influenced by nonmedical, potentially correctable factors such as impaired access to transportation. They found that subjects with functional limitations were more likely to have poorer social support networks than those without such limitations. The deleterious combination of impaired functional status and a limited social support network may explain why elderly cancer patients are at increased risk for not receiving appropriate therapy. Studies of job security and insurability among cancer survivors of an employable age demonstrated significant problems of and biases against cancer survivors.[165–167]

Since the late 1970s and early 1980s, many preliminary studies in oncology, physical therapy, and rehabilitation described or demonstrated efficacy of treatment interventions for cancer survivors, for example, after mastectomy.[157,159,163,168–210] In addi-

Table 4–2. GENERAL TREATMENT GOALS FOR PATIENTS SUSTAINING
PERIODS OF INACTIVITY, BED REST, IMMOBILITY OR DISUSE

1. Improve the functional status of the patient.
2. If active motion not possible of all joints or body segments or segments for which motion is contraindicated, prevent loss of joint alignment and motion by active motion and movement or passive mobilization as indicated.
3. Prevent loss of muscle flexibility by active motion and movement or passive mobilization if active motion not possible of all joints or body segments that are not immobilized or for which motion is contraindicated.
4. Stimulate peripheral and central circulation by active motion and exercise.
5. Increase stimulation or intensity of pulmonary and ventilatory function by implementing breathing exercises, active exercise, and frequent position changes.
6. Prevent loss of motor control, muscle strength, endurance, and cross-sectional area (volume) by resistive exercise.
7. Prevent thrombosis by active exercise and prophylactic support wraps or hose as indicated.
8. Prevent pressure areas or sores by active exercise and frequent position changes as possible.
9. Promote normal myoarthrokinetic reflexes and orthostatic reflexes by active exercise and frequent position changes as possible.
10. Reduce the rate of loss of bone density by active and resistive exercise.
11. Slow the reduction in metabolic processes, *eg,* in basal metabolic rate and glucose tolerance by active exercise.
12. Promote patient motivation and prevent sensory deprivation by active exercise.
13. Anticipate and treat psychological disturbances, behavioral and mood changes such as depression, hostility, anger, anxiety, insomnia, agitation, confusion, irritability, nervousness, hallucinations, and euphoria.
14. Prevent loss of bone density, or osteoporosis, bone metastasis, and pathological fracture.
15. Prevent loss of tissue, including muscle, nerve, connective tissue, and adipose tissue (surgery, radiation fibrosis, local or metastatic tumor invasion, and tissue compression)
16. Monitor signs or symptoms, *ie,* nausea, vomiting, and diarrhea or weakness, fatigue, or lethargy, dyspnea, pallor, dizziness, blurred vision, fever and chills, facial flushing, confusion or disorientation, claudication, or cramping. Many other superimposed problems may lead to these signs and symptoms, requiring assessment to rule out other problems.
17. Monitor intravenous chemotherapy received within the past day (increase in heart rate greater than 8 to 10 bpm is considered significant).
18. Monitor consequences of inactivity, bed rest, or disuse such as orthostatic hypotension

tion, several promising epidemiological reports were published on the positive effects of physical activity and fitness as a cofactor, with decreased dietary fat intake, decrease in weight, and smoking cessation, and as an independent factor in reducing or preventing colorectal and reproductive cancers.[211–247] Physical therapists help cancer survivors recuperate and return to productive lifestyles. They improve their quality of life by increasing their physical independence and level of function and by reducing their pain, physical impairments, and dysfunctions. Patients may find recovery harder and less successful without the assistance of therapists. Therapists help cancer survivors overcome the significant dysfunctions, physical impairments, and psychosocial and emotional stress of the disease and its often aggressive medical treatments.

Many of these impairments and dysfunctions may relate to inactivity and disuse. The deconditioning interacts with disease- and treatment-related side effects to compromise severely the person's ability to function independently. General preventive and intervention goals for any patient sustaining periods of inactivity, disuse, and bed rest are reviewed in Table 4–2. Many patients with cancer undergo surgical tumor resection such as mastectomy, neck dissection, thoracotomy, amputation, and limb salvage. General postsurgical management guidelines specific to the surgical site are used. The overall goal of physical therapy and rehabilitation for the cancer survivors is to return them to their maximal function, *eg,* return to work, domestic activities, caregiving, school, or social activities.

I. Health Care Team

Rehabilitation of cancer survivors is a dynamic, problem-centered team approach. Cancer, as a chronic illness, requires that all health care professionals view the patient from a perspective of functional abilities rather than from a disease process.

The health care team used in addressing different patient problems may vary considerably. Members of the health care team are listed in Table 4–3. The relationships of the interdisciplinary team including the patient and family as the care unit are

Table 4–3. HEALTH CARE TEAM USED IN ADDRESSING DIFFERENT PATIENT PROBLEMS

1. Oncology and hematology	12. Radiologist
2. Psychiatry	13. Psychiatrist
3. Neurology	14. Physical therapist
4. Neurosurgery	15. Nurse
5. Endocrinology	16. Social worker
6. Hematology	17. Registered dietitian
7. Cardiology	18. Occupational therapist
8. Pulmonary	19. Vocational rehabilitation counselor
9. Nephrology	20. Medical technician
10. Speech pathologist	
11. Chaplain	

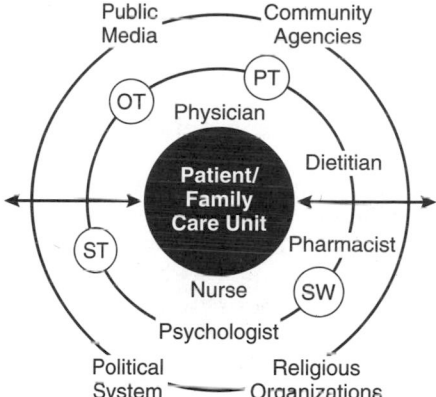

FIGURE 4–4   Using the interdisciplinary treatment team and including the family with the patient as the care unit, a "circle of care" is provided for the patient with cancer. *Abbreviations:* OT = occupational therapist; PT = physical therapist; ST = speech therapist; SW = social worker. (Reprinted from Toot J: Tapestry of Care. *Clin Man Phys Ther* 1992, 4:9–10 with the permission of the American Physical Therapy Association.)

illustrated in Figure 4–4.[164] The most important members of the team are the patient and family. The patient involved in the team approach helps to identify specific needs throughout the course of cancer diagnosis and treatment. The spouse and friends of the cancer survivor make up an important support system. Rehabilitation goal setting is generally based on the patient's goals and prognosis such as whether the patient will (1) experience progression of cancer, (2) be "controlled" with cancer, or (3) be a "cured," noncancer patient. The patient's age, functional status, and weight loss also need to be considered. Dietz described four levels of rehabilitation[248–251] and prevention used for goal setting for cancer survivors.

1. **Restorative:** The patient will have little or no residual disability.

2. **Supportive:** The patient will have ongoing disease and persistent disability; however, the patient can make gains toward reducing disability or controlling problems.

3. **Palliative:** The patient will have advanced progressive disease and disabilities cannot be corrected.

4. **Preventive:** The patient will have a predictable disability that, with appropriate prior training, is minimized. (This fourth category was added to Dietz's original classification.)

II. Prevention

As more emphasis is placed on preventive services during this era of health care reform, physical therapists must become more involved in routine preventive health care. The role of the physical therapist in prevention and risk reduction for clients may include incorporating cancer prevention screening and education into daily practice by implementing the following:[1–5,252–264]

1. Making available information on current recommendations for routine screening, cancer prevention materials, and guidelines to establish a safe environment, *ie*, smoke-free environment for clean air
2. Conducting routine screening of cancer survivors at high risk for disease- or treatment-related impairments and dysfunctions requiring

further assessment to determine the type and severity of their dysfunctions (screening only high-risk individuals will reduce the cost of such activities while maximizing the benefits)
3. A general goal for the physical therapist is to educate clients about their risks, preventive measures, and early detection and screening (self-care and self-examination practices and screening for cancer); some specific goals may include the following:

• Monitor client's weight, body mass index, or percentage of body fat, and give feedback
• Encourage appropriate diet, exercise, and rest patterns
• Identify risk factors, *ie*, stressors and lack of coping tools available to patient, tobacco usage and

smoking, occupational and home exposures for chemical and radiation exposure

- Provide the recommendations for routine cancer screening
- Provide the recommendations for exercise for health (American Heart Association and American College of Sports Medicine guidelines)[172,265]
- Make available American Dietetic Association and U.S. dietary recommendations[261,266]
- Consider providing tips to help reduce the risk for impairments and dysfunctions, *eg*, tips to reduce the risk of falling at home to those at high risk
- Provide information on the role of physical activity in reducing risk of reproductive and colorectal cancers

Exercise, a low-fat and high-fiber diet, avoiding obesity, and smoking cessation are important in reducing not only cancer mortality and morbidity but also cancer incidence; therefore, longevity can be increased. These factors are also important in reducing the incidence of cardiovascular disease, *ie*, strokes and coronary heart disease, emphysema (chronic obstructive pulmonary disease [COPD]), and lung and oropharyngeal cancers. In addition to prognosis with cancer, diet is linked to the etiology of about 50% of all cancers, acting as a promoter, in the multistep pathogenesis of cancer. The Kockum study of risk factors for coronary heart disease (CHD) included a sample of 464 individuals—one third white-collar workers, one third heavy workers, and one third well-trained firefighters—all of whom have now been observed for 22 years.[216] A high cholesterol value was found to predict an increased death rate not only from CHD but also from malignant disease, with a markedly decreased life expectancy in multi-risk factor patients as a result of not only CHD but also of cancer.[216]

Research indicates that a high-fat, low-fiber diet increases the risk for some cancers. Dietary modifications may reduce the risk for CHD and of some types of cancers, breast, colon, and prostate in particular. Dietary modification clinical trials are currently being sponsored by the National Cancer Institute such as a low-fat dietary intervention as an adjunct to breast cancer treatment.[213] The goal is to have people eat a low-fat diet of 25% or less of total daily calories and a high-fiber diet of 20 to 30 g daily. Research also indicates that a lack of immune surveillance increases the risk for cancer, acting as a promoter. Vitamins A, B_6, C, and E and the minerals selenium and zinc have shown some evidence of being able to restore or maintain im-

munocompetence; they may be recommended as dietary supplements. Evidence that physical activity protects against certain forms of cancer continues to mount from studies of experimental animals, former athletes, people employed in active occupations, and people with an active, recreational lifestyle.

Exercise is also a prognostic factor for cancer. The effect of exercise on tumor-bearing animals was investigated as early as the 1940s.[137-141] This line of research continues to demonstrate some promise for the role of physical activity and exercise in the prevention of select cancers such as the reproductive cancers and assisting in control of side effects of treatment.[138-141,213-247] Sturgeon *et al.* demonstrated, in a case-control study of middle-aged British women, that physically inactive women may be at increased risk of endometrial cancer because they are more likely to be overweight or obese and that inactivity per se may be associated with an increased risk of endometrial cancer.[243] They recommended that future studies obtain more detailed assessments of physical activity, including the intensity with which an individual engaged in an activity and the actual time involved in exertion.[243]

Albanes *et al.* found that, among 5138 men and 7407 women aged 25 to 74 years, nonrecreational activity increased the risk of cancer among inactive individuals compared with very active persons.[245] These findings were unchanged after adjusting for cigarette smoking, body mass index (BMI), and other potential confounders. Sites that demonstrated stronger inactivity–cancer associations included the colorectum and the lung among men and breast (postmenopausal) and cervix among women, although these findings for women were based on relatively few cases. The association between inactivity and cancer was greater among persons of moderate (or lower) BMI and, in women, those older than 60 years. In contrast, recreational exercise showed little relation to cancer, with the exception of prostate cancer, suggesting that inactive individuals are at increased risk of cancer.[245] In a British population of middle-aged men, Wannamethee *et al.* found a strong positive association between increased resting heart rate and all noncardiovascular mortality, cancer mortality, and other noncardiovascular mortality, even after adjusting for age, blood cholesterol, BMI, heavy alcohol consumption, physical activity, pre-existing ischemic heart disease, smoking, social class, and systolic blood pressure; that persisted even after further adjustment for lung function (forced expiratory volume in 1 second) and exclusion of men with underlying ill health and of deaths occurring within the first 5 years of follow-up.[228] A significant inverse association was seen between physical activity and risk of cancer death, even after adjustment for these factors and heart rate; a significant reduction was only found in those engaged in high levels of usual physical activity, suggesting that resting heart rate and physical activity are independent prognostic factors for cancer mortality.

Slattery et al. examined the development of colon cancer in a Utah sample using a case-control design with 204 females and 180 males controls and 119 females and 110 males cases.[247] Total physical activity was protective against the development of colon cancer for both males and females. Intense physical activity was the component of activity that had the greatest protective effect for males and females. The relationship between physical activity and colon cancer was not confounded by dietary intake of calories, fat, or protein, nor was the diet and colon cancer relationship confounded by physical activity.

Assessment of the interrelationships among physical activity, diet, and colon cancer suggests that physical activity modifies colon cancer risk associated with diet. Severson et al. evaluated several direct measurements of physical activity and also resting heart rate as determined from an electrocardiogram.[242] Increased activity was consistently associated with a decreased relative risk of colon cancer for each measure of activity. Relative risk of colon cancer increased significantly with increasing resting heart rate. Relative risks associated with physical activity were also evaluated for cancers of the stomach, rectum, lung, prostate, and urinary bladder. An increased relative risk of stomach cancer was associated with several measures of increased activity. A similar finding was reported for prostate cancer and requires further investigation.

Brownson et al. conducted a case-control study to investigate occupational risks for colon cancer.[244] The subject sample included 1993 white males who served as cases and 9965 age-matched cancer controls from Missouri whose cancer was diagnosed between 1984 and 1987. Elevated risks were identified for workers in several occupations and industries including printing machine operators, workers in food manufacturing, communications workers, and workers employed in the petroleum product trade. Previous findings of excess risk among selected occupations of higher socioeconomic status were confirmed. Analyses by anatomical subsite showed that excess risk for an occupational group was usually confined to a single

subsite, which suggests some specificity of effect. For example, elevated risk among males employed in manufacturing-related industries was shown primarily for cancer of the cecum. The findings by level of occupational physical activity corroborated reports of increased colon cancer risk associated with employment in sedentary occupations with an inverse linear trend in risk according to level of occupational physical activity.

Blair et al.[246] and Thompson[222] made several recommendations for further investigation of the relationship between exercise and breast cancer; however, these recommendations are generalizable to many cancers. These authors advocated investigation of the following:

1. Effects of timing of exercise relative to the phases of carcinogenesis
2. The precise dose of activity that is required for specific benefits
3. The role (if any) of intensity of effort
4. Frequency of exercise on the tumorigenic response in the mammary gland
5. Spectrum of exercise conditions that exert differential effects on measures of physical fitness, energy intake, body composition, and/or the efficiency of utilization of carbohydrate, fat, and protein as energy substrates
6. Elucidation of biological pathways whereby activity contributes to health

This should facilitate identification of critical relationships between physical activity and the risk for cancer.

Ultimately, investigations of the type proposed should allow for determination of whether the quantity and quality of exercise needed to attain health-related benefits for chronic diseases such as cancer differ from what is recommended for fitness benefits. This should also permit formulation of a specific set of recommendations about the amount and type of physical activity that, in concert with appropriate dietary practices, can significantly reduce the risk for cancer.[222] One such series of preliminary studies by Cohen et al.[223] found that voluntary activity suppresses the development of chemically and virally induced primary mammary tumors in rats and mice fed high-fat diets. The diets used were chosen to mimic the current U.S. fat consumption of approximately 40% of calories as fat. It remains to be seen whether activity exerts a similar suppressive effect on animals fed their customary low-fat diet (10% calories as fat). The suppressive effect of activity on the MMTV-induced mouse mammary tumor was of particular interest because it raised the possibility that activity may exert effects on the process of provirus insertion and/or oncogene activation, an area of great promise in cancer prevention. Activity appeared to enhance the volume and to a lesser degree the number of metastatic foci in the lungs of F-344 retired breeders under high-fat but not medium-fat conditions. In addition, the most active animals in the high-fat group exhibited the greatest volume of metastases. These results, together with those from another animal model, the NMU model, point to the critical importance of the quantity of voluntary activity an animal engages in and its relationship to both primary and secondary cancer prevention. The results imply that, beyond a certain point of either frequency or intensity, the beneficial effect of exercise may be nullified by competing deleterious effects.[223] The metastases study has also brought to light the importance of dietary fat as a potential intervening variable.

There are probably 40 million adults in the United States whose sedentary habits place them at considerable increased risk of morbidity and mortality from several diseases including cancer.[246]

These same individuals also are more likely to have functional limitations, especially as they move into the later years of life. The sizable independent relative risk for impaired health in sedentary persons, and the large number at risk, leads to a substantial public health burden. Blair et al.[246] reviewed the epidemiological studies and concluded that the data supported the following:

1. A linear dose-response relationship, at least up to a point, between physical activity and health and functional effects
2. Public health recommendations directed toward the most sedentary and unfit stratum of the population and emphasizing at least moderate physical activity
3. Most sedentary adults who accumulate 30 minutes of walking per day (or the equivalent energy expenditure in other activities) would receive clinically significant health benefits
4. It does not matter what type of physical activity is performed: sports, planned exercise, household or yard work, and occupational tasks are all beneficial. The key factor is total energy expenditure; if that is constant, improvements in fitness and health will be comparable

III. Etiology, Stages, and Types of Cancer Development

A. **Normal (mitosis) and abnormal cell renewal.**[267–270] **Normal tissues contain cells of uniform shape, maturity, nuclear structure, differentiation, and size**

1. Alterations of tissue growth and cell biology with carcinogenesis may be as follows:
   a. Anatomical changes
   b. Biochemical changes (metabolism, growth factors, and prostaglandins)
   c. Cellular dedifferentiation and kinetics (cell cycle)
2. Rate of cell turnover leading to tissue changes: labile (clonogenic) versus stable (nonclonogenic) tissues
   a. Precancerous
      (1). Hypertrophy (increased size of cell)
      (2). Neoplastic hyperplasia (increased number of cells are due to tumor formation)
      (3). Dysplasia (replacement of mature

cell type by another less mature type; may reverse, persist, or transform and progress) is often due to chronic irritation
      (4). Metaplasia (early dysplasia-reversible replacement of mature cell type by another cell type not normally found in that tissue, ie, vitamin deficient, irritation, inflammation, or other pathology)
      (5). Anaplasia (cellular disorganization commonly found in dysplasia and is an advanced form of metaplasia found in cancerous cells)
   b. Neoplasia (nonrandom autonomous tissue growth)
      (1). Invasion
      (2). Metastatic process (major cause of death by neoplasm) and spread of tumors
         (a). Occur by seeding, transplanta-

tion, lymphatic, and blood vessels (hematogenous spread)

(b). Factors that may increase risk of metastasis are heat, radiation, chemotherapy, trauma (biopsy, massage of tumor), primary tumor of long duration or high mitotic rate, and dead normal or tumor cells

(c). Factors that may decrease risk of metastasis are radiation, chemotherapy, large primary tumors, ascites, fibrinolytic agents (aspirin, heparin, dicumarol, plasmin)

(d). Tumors vary in their capacity to metastasize, and the number, size and distribution of metastatic tumors all vary; some disseminate widely, others disseminate preferentially to selected sites

(e). A variable portion of metastatic disease is likely to be occult and remain undetected during life

(f). There often is no orderly progression in malignant tumors; the disease may first be diagnosed through signs of metastasis rather than primary tumor such as unexplained anemia, lymphadenopathy, or pathological fracture

(3). Escape of malignant cells from immune surveillance appears to be an important predisposition in the development of cancer; a multitude of factors turn on oncogenes, leading to formation of malignant cells throughout life that normally are recognized and destroyed by the following:

(a). Immune surveillance (inefficient in young and old, in the early and late stages of cancer, in immunocompetent or immune-suppressed individuals such as patients with AIDS, those who underwent organ and tissue transplant, those with chronic disease and malnutrition (see chapter on nutrition, the immune system, and HIV/AIDS)

(b). Formation of tumor antigens (tumor antigens are recognized by the immune system)

B. Stages of cancer development[267-270]

1. Initiators irreversibly alter DNA (route of exposure by mouth, inhalation, injection, or skin, and exposure occurs through environment, occupation, medicine, or home)

   a. Ionizing radiation (diagnostic and therapeutic x-ray films, cosmic radiation, radioactive ground minerals, other radioactive materials)

   b. Ultraviolet radiation (sunlight, industrial sources)

   c. Chemical agents (tobacco products, aromatic hydrocarbons, aromatic amines, alkylating agents, organic and inorganic compounds such as benzene, chromium, vinyl chloride, asbestos, alcohol, hormones such as testosterone and estrogen, and plant products)

   d. Viruses (slow acting and fast acting)

   e. Oncogenes (genes regulating cell proliferation)

2. Transforming factors (multistep process of increasing cell dedifferentiation that is poorly understood)

3. Promoters (substances that enhance transformation)

   a. Biological properties of promoting factors

      (1). Exert an effect only after initiating factor has irreversibly altered DNA

      (2). Require prolonged exposure before altering cell

      (3). Can be reversed in the early stages of transformation

4. Reversing factors (inhibit promoting factors effects)

   a. Oxygen free-radical scavengers (antioxidants enzymes)

   b. Dietary factors (vitamin C, E, A, selenium and beta carotene, indoles such as broccoli, Brussels sprouts, other antioxidant food additives)

   c. Drugs (see chemotherapy, drugs that inhibit ribonucleic acid synthesis)

C. Types of cancer

The types of cancer are classified according to the following:

1. Histogenesis: tissue of origin and cell types
2. Anatomical location
   a. Local
   b. Regional

c. Distant or disseminated (common sites of metastatic spread are lung, liver, central nervous system, bone, and marrow)

3. Biological behavior (benign or malignant)
   a. Benign: suffix "oma"; cysts or polyps, such as *lipoma*
   b. Malignant: suffix "sarcoma" or "carcinoma," such as *liposarcoma*
      (1). Sarcoma: tumors of connective tissue; prefix describes specific tissue (osteo-, bone; lipo-, fat; chondro-, cartilage; rhabdo-, skeletal muscle)
      (2). Carcinoma: tumors from the epithelium; prefix describes specific epithelium (adeno-, glandular epithelium; squamous-, squamous epithelium); such as squamous cell carcinoma of the skin that tends to be solid tumors
      (3). Lymphoma: cancer originating in lymph tissue
      (4). Mixed
      (5). Many exceptions to rules exist, particularly in nervous, lymph, bone marrow (hemopoietic tissue), and epithelial tissue

4. Group classification of tumors
   a. Group 1: epithelial tumors
   b. Group 2: connective tissue tumors
   c. Group 3: hematopoietic tumors
   d. Group 4: peripheral and central nervous system tumors
   e. Group 5: tumors of more than one tissue type
   f. Group 6: miscellaneous tumors

5. Degree of dedifferentiation (*ie*, blastoma-; suffix used when tissue resembles embryonic tissues)

D. Susceptibility to carcinogens

Carcinogens do not cause cancer in all persons exposed; some people are more resistant, whereas others are more susceptible.

1. Sex (some cancers are sex dependent and only appear in males or females, *eg*, breast cancer is a leading cause of death in women but is rare in men)
2. Age (cancer occurrence is low in persons younger than 30 years but increases steadily thereafter)
3. Race (little statistical difference for most cancers between white and nonwhite populations except for skin cancer, which is higher among whites; the increased rates in nonwhites may represent recent improved reporting, geographical variations that are difficult to demonstrate except for skin cancer, which is more prevalent in southern, sunny climates, and cultural and social differences in factors influencing the development of cancer such as diet, level of stress, urban environment, smoking and alcohol consumption, and sexual habits)
4. Metabolical and immunological differences (ability to keep the agent from entering the body; ability to look for, recognize, and remove the agent)
5. Inheritance or genetic predisposition (susceptibility transmitted from parent to child by biological laws of reproduction)

IV. Clinical Manifestations

Clinical presentations and course (usually begin to have symptoms when a tumor mass of 1×10^{11} cells are present, clinically visible when 1×10^8 or 1 g in weight, in remission when fewer than 1×10^8 cells) are dependent on tumor type, site, and presence of metastatic disease. The most common warning signs are as follows:[1,2]

1. Change in bowel or bladder habits
2. Sore that does not heal
3. Unusual bleeding or discharge
4. Thickening or lump in the breast or elsewhere
5. Indigestion or difficulty swallowing
6. Obvious change in a wart or mole
7. Nagging cough or hoarseness

These signs and symptoms may be caused by many other problems, but a person should be referred to a physician if any problem lasts as long as 2 weeks. Educate patients not to wait for symptoms to become painful; pain is not an early sign of cancer.

A. Gastrointestinal (GI)[301–305]

Gastrointestinal signs and symptoms include vomiting, nausea, constipation, diarrhea, signs of GI obstruction, irritation, or malabsorption and cachexia.[69] Cachexia is manifested as anorexia, early satiety and food aversions, change in dietary patterns, weight loss, anemia, and asthenia. The only effective management of cachexia is by controlling or curing the disease.[142-152] Nutritional support can help reduce the severity of the cachexia but will not cure it.[144,146] Endurance exercise has modified cachexia in rats.[138-140] Weight loss is often a better predictor of functional outcome than stage or grade of disease.[142-152] Breast cancer is an exception as is metastasis, both of which do not usually lead to significant weight loss or cachexia.[276-279]

1. Anorexia leading to weight loss is often an early sign of malignant disease that continues until the tumor is removed or tumor cell load is significantly decreased and returns with recurrence of tumor growth or metastases. Anorexia may be secondary to local, systemic, or remote effects. Local effects include stenosis, obstruction, or dysphagia from primary tumors, such as head and neck tumors, stomach and pelvic tumors, and metastatic GI tumors (hepatic metastases), and surgical treatment or radiation therapy. Systemic effects may be from chemotherapy and radiation therapy such as difficulty eating secondary to stomatitis, mucositis, taste disorders, systemic illness such as infection, endocrinopathies, pancreatitis or hepatitis, or nausea and vomiting with resulting malabsorption. Remote effects of the neoplasm include taste disorders, food aversions, and early satiety.
2. Food aversions are common with a change in taste and smell as the disease progresses and includes aversions to meats, coffee, and chocolate. If food aversions are present, patients will often present with anorexia, weight loss, and early satiety.
3. Early satiety or filling is a less frequent symptom. The patient feels hungry but after a few mouthfuls of food is completely full.
4. Changes in dietary patterns are common; cancer manipulates the diets in half of all patients. Change in diet may lead to an unbalanced nutrition intake. Specific nutritional deficiencies also develop such as loss of intrinsic factor, vitamin B_{12} deficiency, bile salt deficiency, and electrolyte and fluid disorders.

B. Acute and chronic pain

Pain is rarely present during the early stages of cancer, with the exception of bone cancer of which pain is often the first symptom. Pain is a major problem in a small number of patients with cancer. Some patients with the same cancer will present with severe pain, others have little pain, and a few have no pain. Pain may originate for many reasons in a patient with cancer, including any of the usual causes such as the following:[280-282]

1. Cancer-related pain (see later discussion)
2. Treatment, ie, surgical resection of tumor (postsurgical pain), postchemotherapy pain, and postradiation pain
3. Associated with a debilitating disease
4. Unrelated to disease or treatment such as trauma
5. Psychological and cultural factors

Chronic pain lacks positive meaning, usually gets worse rather than better, and frequently expands to occupy the patient's whole attention, and it is impossible to predict when pain will end (see Tables 4–4 to 4–6 and sections on pain assessment).

Table 4–4. CHARACTERISTICS OF ACUTE AND CHRONIC PAIN

Function	Acute *First, Rapid Pain*	Chronic *Second, Slow*
Adequate stimulus	Pinprick, heat	Tissue damage
Nerve fibers	A-delta (small myelinated)	C (unmyelinated)
Conduction velocity	5–15 m/s (11.0–33.5 mph)	0.5–2.0 m/s (1.0–4.5 mph)
Distribution	Body surface (including mouth and anus)	All tissues except brain and spinal cord
Reflex response	Withdrawal (flexion), muscle contraction	Spasm, rigidity, tonic phasic muscle contraction*
Biological value	Causes organism to avoid possible tissue damage	Brings about enforced rest of damaged part, so promoting natural healing
Effect of morphine	Very little	Suppression of pain sensation, abolition of spasm

Adapted from Bowsher D: Acute and chronic pain and assessment. In Wells PE, Frampton V, Bowsher D (eds): *Pain Management in Physical Therapy.* Norwalk, CT, Appleton & Lange, 1988, 2nd ed.

* Note that this reflex involves agonists and antagonists, which is part of the definition of spasm or rigidity, as a pathological rather than a physiological reaction.

Table 4–5. FACTORS THAT MODULATE PAIN THRESHOLD

Threshold Elevated	Threshold Lowered
Fatigue	Sleep
Insomnia	Rest
Discomfort	Relief of symptoms
Fear	Sympathy
Anxiety	Understanding
Anger	Companionship
Depression	Reduction in anxiety
Boredom	Elevation of mood
Mental isolation	Antidepressants
Social abandonment	Analgesics
Introversion	Anxiolytics
Sadness	Diversional activities
Hypercalcemia	Relaxation

If related to the cancer, the pain is usually the result of the following:

1. Tissue destruction such as bone
2. Obstruction
3. Infiltration or compression or pressure
4. Infiltration, distention, or stretching of viscera
5. Inflammation, infection, and tissue necrosis
6. Previous cultural and psychophysiological perceptions of pain

The pain associated with cancer is often caused by more than one of these factors. Bone pain may be caused by pathological fracture, medullary pressure, or periosteal irritation. Chest pain may be caused by stretching or distention of the pleura secondary to pleural effusion or by local infection or irritation of the parietal pleura in lung cancer. A common perception of cancer is often one of pain, hopelessness, and death, although pain is often a late symptom of cancer;[167–178] how these attitudes and feelings are expressed may vary considerably among individuals, family units, and cultures.

Table 4–6. TREATMENT OF ACUTE PAIN VERSUS CANCER PAIN WITH ANALGESICS

Variable	Acute Pain	Cancer Pain
Goal	Pain relief	Pain relief
Desired effect (duration)	2–4 hours	As long as possible
Timing	On demand (as required)	In anticipation (regularly)
Dose	Standardized	Individualized
Route	Injection	By mouth
Adjuvant medication	Uncommon	Common
Sedation	Often wanted	Undesirable (usually)

For a comprehensive review of acute pain management, see U.S. Department of Health and Human Services' *Clinical Practice Guidelines.*[280]

PLEASE NOTE: More than 40% of late-stage patients with cancer do not receive adequate pain relief, although existing methods of pain control are available. As long as pain persists in late-stage patients, functional activities are limited. Strang[283] studied the emotional and social consequences of pain in 93 consecutive inpatients, 44 males and 49 females, suffering from cancer-related pain. Visual analogue scales, standardized interviews, and comprehensive self-questionnaires were used to collect data. Forty-seven patients (51%) experienced certain or pronounced anxiety because of their pain, and 66 patients (71%) expressed depressive pain-associated symptoms, which was highly correlated with the intensity of their pain. Physical activities such as movements, dressing/undressing, washing, and cooking were hampered in about 66% of the patients, and mental activities such as reading were significantly disturbed in 48%. For every social activity listed in the questionnaires (hobbies, seeing friends, and so on), most patients reported a decreased activity because of pain, and in most cases the decrease correlated significantly with the intensity of the pain. The family roles had changed because the patient could not participate in a usual manner. The results demonstrate the profound consequences of pain: physical suffering, emotional distress, dependency, social handicap, and altered family roles.[283] In 1990, Strang *et al.* achieved similar results using the same data-collection methods in a prospective study of 84 consecutive patients with cancer-related pain.[284] Sixty-one (73%) patients experienced two or more different types of pain, and anxiety and depressive feelings correlated with the intensity of pain. Pain had a negative influence on activities of daily living and on concentration in 76% and 56% of the patients, respectively. Social activities such as visits and conversations decreased significantly with increasing pain. They concluded that effective pain control is achievable in most cases with already existing analgesics and complementary methods; pain control should be a high-priority matter in palliative care.

C. Neurological and psychological symptoms

Symptoms include fatigue and generalized weakness, pain, specific muscle weakness, paralysis, and other lower motor neuron changes (spinal cord compression including some upper motor neuron changes dependent on the level of compression or peripheral nerve involvement), cranial nerve changes and other upper motor neuron changes (brain tumors or increases in intracranial pressure), paresthesia, numbness, changes in balance, changes in mental status and affect such as confusion, anxiety, depression, anger, hostility, insomnia, restlessness, behavior and mood changes related to paraneoplastic syndrome, and signs and symptoms of the following:[26,52,53,55,69,267,270, 276,280,285-302]

1. Neuromuscular disorders, including weakness (asthenia), atrophy, loss of stretch reflexes, sensory and sensory motor neuropathy (polyneuropathy), myasthenia gravis or myasthenic syndrome, Guillain-Barré syndrome, dermatomyositis, and polymyositis
2. Spinal cord involvement, including cerebellar degeneration, dementia, encephalitis, and optic neuritis
3. Central nervous system (CNS) involvement, including motor neuropathy, necrotic myelopathy, and amyotrophic lateral sclerosis

In paraneoplastic syndrome, the incidence of neurological disorders may be higher than 7%, running a course similar to but independent of the tumor. Neurological changes can complicate advanced cancer, with stroke as the most common complication from emboli, hemorrhage, or infarction. More than half of the strokes are caused by events uncommon in the general population. Strokes occur from emboli, tumor-related or subarachnoid hemorrhage, and disseminated intravascular coagulation.[303] Fatigue and generalized muscle weakness can be secondary to the following: (1) disease such as paraneoplastic syndrome and hormonal changes, (2) treatment such as chemotherapy, ie, type II muscle fiber myopathy secondary to prednisone administration or anemia secondary to bone marrow suppression from chemotherapy or radiation, and (3) inactivity and bed rest.[26,52,53,55,64,85,96,137,139,141,153,271-275,285,288,291,292] Localized weakness may be secondary to surgical resection of muscle and soft tissue, nerve compression, nerve resection, and radiation fibrosis.[275,287,293,304-315] Cardiac autonomic nerve involvement after chemotherapy with anthracyclines has been demonstrated[63,67,76,99]

D. Hematological effects

These effects often present as fatigue, opportunistic infection, and, occasionally, bleeding disorders.[64,96,270-275,288,303,315,316]

1. Anemia may be secondary to many causes such as blood loss, severe malnutrition, treatment, or cancer of the bone marrow and hemopoietic tissues. Anemia also occurs often with paraneoplastic syndrome presenting as a complaint of fatigue.
2. Erythrocytosis occurs with kidney and adrenal tumors and some lung, ovarian, and thymus tumors.
3. Thrombocytosis also occurs with paraneoplastic syndrome.
4. Thrombocytopenia is rare, with paraneoplastic syndrome occurring in patients not presenting with anemia and with cancers of the lung, breast, rectum, testes, gallbladder, several types of leukemia, and Hodgkin's disease; it presents as thrombocytopenia purpura.
5. Granulocytosis presents with infection and leukemia and with paraneoplastic syndrome in lung, brain, pancreatic, gastric cancer, lymphoma, and melanoma; opportunistic infection is common, such as the following: (1) secondary bacterial infections, ie, Staphylococcus and Streptococcus, (2) upper respiratory infections, (3) tuberculosis (pulmonary TB), and (4) Pneumocystis carinii pneumonia.
6. Granulocytopenia is uncommon with paraneoplastic syndrome.
7. Eosinophilia is associated with mycosis fungal infections, Hodgkin's disease, and some lymphomas, brain tumors, and melanomas.

E. Metabolic and endocrine effects

Hypercalcemia, other changes with paraneoplastic syndrome, and uremia are common (see Table 4-7).[64,69,270-275,276,279,286,288,291,317] Hormone levels are usually elevated and do not respond to normal mechanisms of physiological regulation.

1. Hypercalcemia occurs as an indirect humoral effect on bone in 10% to 20% of patients with advanced cancer and to a greater extent in patients with breast and lung cancer. Humoral effects are from osteolytic stimulating factor, prostaglandins, calcitonin, vitamin D resistance, osteomalacia, and corticotropin and parathyroid hormone. The cranium is involved 22% of the time, the long bones (extremities) 34% of the time, and the bones of the thorax 50% of the time. It can be life threatening and requires immediate treatment. Signs and symptoms include weakness, lethargy, nausea, vomiting, diarrhea, depression, constipa-

Table 4–7. COMPLICATIONS OF DISEASE AND TREATMENT REQUIRING A SCREEN BEFORE PHYSICAL THERAPY

1. CNS and cerebellar syndromes, cerebral atrophy, encephalopathies, cranial and peripheral neuropathies and fibrosis, plexopathies, myelopathies (chemo- and radiotherapy, surgical resection, poor dietary intake, tumor invasion with tissue compression) resulting in ptosis, footdrop, visual disturbances (double vision, blurred vision, decreased visual acuity) and retinopathy, tinnitus, hearing loss (high frequency), dizziness/vertigo, paresthesia, problems with motor coordination and gait, changes in mood and level of consciousness, constipation
2. Erosion and changes in skin such as hair loss (see Table 4–4) and wound closure problems, including incisional wounds resulting in fissures and fistulas
3. Lymphedema
4. DVTs, venous stasis, and emboli
5. Hepatotoxicity and nephrotoxicity with dysfunction such as acute renal failure
6. Arthralgia and joint edema and other pain related or unrelated to disease and treatment
7. Bone marrow suppression leading to anemia and fatigue, low platelet counts, bleeding disorders such as epistaxis or bleeding from any orifice, ecchymosis, petechiae, signs of occult bleeding, and immune function compromise with opportunistic infections
8. Cachexia, anorexia, poor nutritional intake, electrolyte imbalances and acid-base disturbances, and dehydration
9. Erosion of mucous membranes and lining of GI tract resulting in stomatitis, pharyngitis, diarrhea, and ulceration
10. Cardiomyopathy, pericarditis, endocarditis, CHF, and arrhythmia (early changes may be within 6 months of therapy; late changes may occur years after therapy, with some agents specifically cardiotoxic such as antibiotic agents)
11. Nonproductive cough, dyspnea (exertional and nocturnal), decreased forced vital capacity and diffusion capacity, infiltration and respiratory distress, interstitial pulmonary fibrosis and pneumonitis
12. Loss of muscle, myopathies, myalgia, and weakness (corticosteroid and inactivity, surgical)

Abbreviations: CNS = central nervous system; DVTs = deep vein thromboses; GI = gastrointestinal; CHF = congestive heart failure.

---

tion, increased pain, coma, and serious cardiac arrhythmia, leading to death.

2. Corticotropin elevation is common with cancer of the lung, ovary, pancreas, adrenal, and thymus glands. The presentation is atypical for elevated corticotropin, lacking the appearance of moon face, buffalo hump, centripedal obesity, and cutaneous striae and pigmentations, but often includes hypertension, muscle weakness, hyperglycemia, hypokalemia, edema, and weight loss. As many as 90% of the corticotropin-producing cancers are beyond the stage of cure when initially detected.

3. Insulin elevation presenting as insulin shock is most often seen in bronchial cancer and liposarcoma.

4. Antidiuretic hormone (ADH) elevation presenting as hemodilution produces hyponatremia secondary to decreased water excretion. Increased ADH initially presents with neurological changes, eventually leading to serious electrical conduction deficits in the heart and brain.

5. Gonadotropin (human chorionic gonadotropin [HCG]), luteinizing hormone, follicle-stimulating hormone often are elevated in lung and mediastinal tumors and liver tumors; however, HCG is the most commonly elevated.

6. Parathyroid hormone elevations found in cancer of the lung, colon, uterus, bladder, kidney, liver, and pancreas. The result is hypercalcemia with its signs and symptoms (see previous discussion).

7. Increased metabolism is typical in patients with cancer in spite of decreased caloric intake. A negative nitrogen balance resulting in loss of muscle mass and decreased serum albumin levels in more than 90% of patients with cancer cachexia. Patients, especially those with advanced cancer, may experience edema secondary to the elevation in intra- and extracellular water content and hyponatremia with the hypoalbuminemia.

8. Asthenia has a pattern of increasing weakness and levels of fatigue from morning to evening; metabolic acidosis from an increased glycolytic rather than oxidative metabolism was implicated in animal studies.

F. Effects on bone leading to pathological fracture (see discussion of musculoskeletal tumors)

1. Indirect humoral effects from disease and treatment (see hypercalcemia) with decreases in bone density and/or metabolic effects are from surgical side effects or spinal cord compression mechanically unloading bone or metastatic tumors of lung, breast,

prostate, pancreatic, stomach, and bladder cancer and Hodgkin's disease.[286,288,290,291,307]

2. Direct effects from primary and metastatic biopsy and radiotherapy on bone, inactivity and disuse effects on bone, high risk of falls secondary to disease and treatment, and other comorbidities in an aged population such as being postmenopausal or having a history of long-term corticosteroid use.

G. Effects on peripheral vascular and lymph system

Effects include compression with venous stasis, increased risk of infection and lymphedema. Risk increases significantly after treatment compression is relieved; however, resection of tumor and fibrosis lead to complications such as deep vein thromboses (DVTs), emboli, thrombophlebitis, ischemia, and lymphedema, with signs and symptoms in the involved extremity of edema, pain, cyanosis or hyperemia in the extremity, tenderness, warmth or coolness on palpation, and reduced or absent peripheral pulses (see sections on hematological effects, radiation therapy, and lymphedema).[271-275]

H. Effects on skin[64,69,270-275,286,288,313-317,321,337-341]

1. Direct effect of tumor such as with primary

skin cancers (see chapter on the integument); effect of radiotherapy resulting in radiation fibrosis and burns that lead to signs and symptoms of blistering and dermatitis, irritation and itching, ulceration and bedsores, fistulas; or secondary to surgical excision, grafting, and reconstruction.

2. Indirect effects secondary to opportunistic infection, paraneoplastic effects, indirect humoral effects, genetic effects, and treatment effects such as mucositis. There is an exhaustive number of extremely rare to occasionally seen skin lesions related to paraneoplastic syndrome. The lesions are erythema, bulbous and urticarial lesions, acquired ichthyosis, endocrine and metabolic disorders, pigmented lesions, hereditary and miscellaneous lesions. Often the cause is unknown. Table 4–8 lists skin lesions that may occur as direct and indirect effects of cancer.[203-206]

I. Cardiopulmonary effects[54,56,58-65,67,71-79,81,83,84,87,90-99,151,271-275,342-362]

1. Direct effects of space-occupying primary mediastinal and pulmonary tumors, ie, bronchogenic carcinoma that are usually a late symptom of disease such as dyspnea, coughing, hemoptysis, and chest pain

Text continued on page 85

Table 4–8.   SKIN LESIONS OCCURRING WITH CANCER

Variable	Description	Predominant Malignancy	Cause	Comments
Erythema and Pigmented Lesions				
Acanthosis nigricans*	Hyperkeratosis and pigmentation, especially of axillae, neck, flexes, and anogenital region	Gastric, 60%; abdominal, 90%; other	Unknown	Most important to distinguish benign forms present from birth and benign forms associated with various syndromes
Leser-Trelat*	Sudden showing of large numbers of seborrheic (wartlike) keratoses	NHL, miscellaneous GI adenocarcinomas	Unknown	Must be distinguished from multiple seborrheic keratoses, which are common and may not be associated with malignancy; occasionally associated with acanthosis nigricans

Table continued on following page

Table 4–8. SKIN LESIONS OCCURRING WITH CANCER *Continued*

Variable	Description	Predominant Malignancy	Cause	Comments
Erythema and Pigmented Lesions continued				
Bowen's disease	Persistent progressive non-elevated red, scaly, or crusted plague caused by intraepidermal neoplasm	Lung, GI, GU, skin	Generally unknown; arsenic exposure in some cases	One fourth acquire systemic cancers an average of 5 years after initial skin lesions but significance of association has been questioned
Chronic arsenism	Cornlike, punctate keratosis more profuse on the extremities and characteristically affecting palms and feet	Lung, miscellaneous	Chronic exposure to arsenic	Not a true paraneoplastic lesion
Generalized melanosis	Diffuse darkening of the skin with a ruddy gray color secondary to chronic liver disease; generalized blue-gray appearance			
Paget's disease	Erythematous keratotic patch over areola, nipple, or accessory breast tissue	Breast	Paget cells are either migrants from the carcinoma or Langerhans' cells	Occurs in less than 3% of breast cancers
Bazex's disease	Erythema hyperkeratosis with scales and pruritus predominantly on palms and soles	Head and neck, GI, lung	Unknown	Males only
Erythema gyratum	Responds rapidly, changing and advancing gyri with scaling and pruritus	Breast, lung, other	Unknown	Almost always associated with malignancy
Erythema annulare centrifugum	Slowly migrating annular and configurate erythematous lesions	Prostate, myeloma, other	Unknown	Occurs also with infections and other disorders
Necrolytic migratory erythema (glucagonoma)	Circinate and gyrate areas of blistering and erosive erythema on limbs; stomatitis	Islet cell on pancreas	Glucagonoma or other metabolic product	
Flushing*	Episodic flushing of face and neck	Carcinoid; medullary carcinoma of thyroid	Serotonin or other vasoactive peptide	
Exfoliative dermatitis*	Progressive erythema followed by scaling	Cutaneous T-cell lymphomas, Hodgkin's disease, non-Hodgkin's lymphoma	Unknown	Account for 10%–20% of all exfoliative dermatitis
Erythema multiforme	Distinctive target lesions in symmetrical distribution sometimes with plaques or bullae			

Table 4–8.　SKIN LESIONS OCCURRING WITH CANCER *Continued*

Variable	Description	Predominant Malignancy	Cause	Comments
Metabolic and Endocrine Disorders				
Systemic nodular pan- niculitis* (nodular re- lapsing fat necrosis) (Weber-Christian dis- ease)*	Recurrent crops of ten- der erythematous subcutaneous nod- ules; may be accom- panied by abdominal pain, fat necrosis in bone marrow, lungs, and other organs	Adenocarcinoma pan- creas	Effect of pancreatic en- zymes released into circulation on fatty tis- sues	
Porphyria cutanea tarda*	Photosensitive skin le- sions, often painful or pruritic	Liver	Increased porphyrin in skin tissues	Rare
Cushing's syndrome	Broad purple striae, at- rophy hyperpigmen- tation (uncommon), plethora, telangiecta- sias, mild hirsutism	Ectopic lung (small cell), thyroid, testes, ovary, adrenal tumors; pan- creatic islet cell, pitui- tary	Increased corticotropin	
Addison's syndrome	Generalized hyperpig- mentation, especially scars, pressure points, points of fric- tion	Adrenal gland invasion, lymphomas, or carci- nomas	Decreased glucocorti- coids rarely caused by tumors invading the adrenal	
Hirsutism	Increased amounts of hair	Adrenal tumors, ovarian tumors	Increased glucocorticoid; increased tetosterone	Associated with virilism
Bulbous and Urticarial Lesions				
Pemphigoid	Large, tense bullae with histologically ab- sent acantholysis	Miscellaneous	Unknown	Although the clinical as- sociation of bullous pemphigoid and ma- lignancy was once accepted, recent age- matched studies have failed to support the association
Dermatitis herpetiformis	Symmetrical subepider- mal bullae, particu- larly with scarring	Lymphomas, miscella- neous	Related to autoanti- bodies	
Hereditary Disorders				
Gardner's syndrome	Epidermal cyst, se- baceous cysts, der- moid tumors, lipo- mas, fibromas	Adenocarcinoma of large or small bowel	Autosomal dominant	Associated with polypo- sis of colon and bony exostoses
Peutz-Jeghers syn- drome				
Tylosis (palmaris and plantaris)	Hyperkeratosis of palms and soles after age 10 years	Esophageal carcinoma	Autosomal dominant	95% incidence of carci- noma by age 65 years
Multiple mucosal neuro- mas	Neuromas of eyelids, lips, tongue, and oral mucosa	Pheochromocytoma, medullary carcinoma of thyroid (MEA II)	Autosomal dominant	Parathyroid adenomas, hypertension com- mon

Table continued on following page

Table 4–8.   SKIN LESIONS OCCURRING WITH CANCER *Continued*

Variable	Description	Predominant Malignancy	Cause	Comments
Hereditary Disorders continued				
Cowden's disease– multiple hamartoma syndrome	Fibromas of oral mucosa, acral papulas, facial trichilemmomas	Thyroid, breast carcinomas	Autosomal dominant	Associated with multiple hamartomas, lipomas, neuromas, hemangiomas, thyroid adenomas
Multiple basal cell neuromas syndrome	Multiple basal cell carcinomas, pits on soles and palms	Medulloblastoma fibrosarcoma (jaw)	Autosomal dominant	Infrequent, associated with internal malignancy
Phakomatoses neurofibromatosis (von Recklinhausen)	Neurofibromas, café au lait	Pheochromocytoma	Autosomal dominant	Malignancies develop in a minority of patients
Tuberous sclerosis (Bourne-Ville)	Lipopigmented maculas, adenomas, fibromas	Neurological malignancies	Autosomal dominant	Malignancies develop in a minority of patients
Cerebelloretinal hemangioblastoma (von Hippel-Lindau)	Retinal malformation, papilledema	Neurological malignancies	Autosomal dominant	Malignancies develop in a minority of patients
Encephalotrigeminal syndrome (Sturge-Weber)	Capillary or cavernous hemangiomas within the cutaneous distribution of the trigeminal nerve	Neurological malignancies	Autosomal dominant	Malignancies develop in a minority of patients
Ataxia telangiectasia	Telangiectasias	Lymphomas, leukemia	Autosomal recessive	IgA± IgE deficiency; sinopulmonary infections, tumors in <10%
Bloom's syndrome	Photosensitivity, telangiectasias, erythema of face	Leukemia	Autosomal recessive	Stunted growth, high incidence
Fanconi's anemia	Patchy hyperpigmentation	Leukemia	Autosomal recessive	High incidence
Chédiak-Higashi syndrome	Recurrent pyoderma, giant melanosomes, dilution of skin and hair color	Lymphomas	Autosomal recessive	High incidence
Wiskott-Aldrich syndrome	Eczematous dermatitis, pyoderma	Lymphomas	Sex linked (males)	>10% incidence
Bruton's sex-linked agammaglobulinemia	Recurrent infections	Lymphoma, leukemia	Sex linked	>5% incidence

Table 4–8. SKIN LESIONS OCCURRING WITH CANCER *Continued*

Variable	Description	Predominant Malignancy	Cause	Comments
Miscellaneous Lesions				
Dermatomyositis*	Purplish pink erythema especially of eyelids, neck, and hands	Miscellaneous	Unknown	Malignant disease reported in 7%–50%; precedes carcinoma by days–years with an average of 6 months
Hypertrichosis languginosa*	Rapid development of fine, long, silky hair, especially on ears, forehead; may involve the entire body	Lung, colon, bladder, uterus, gallbladder	Unknown	High association
Acquired icthyosis*	Generalized dry crackling skin, hyperkeratotic palms and soles, rhomboidal scales	Hodgkin's disease, other lymphomas, multiple myeloma, other	Unknown	Should be distinguished from hereditary form, which occurs before age 20 years
Pachydermoperiostosis*	Thickening of skin and creation of new folds; Thickened lips, ears, lids; macroglossia; thick forehead and scalp; clubbing; excessive sweating	Lung, uterus	Unknown	Occurs also in lung abscess and benign tumors
Pruritus*	Failure to determine an overt or covert cutaneous cause of generalized pruritus necessitates evaluation for a possible underlying systemic disease	Lymphomas, leukemia, multiple myelomas, CNS tumors, abdominal tumors	Unknown	Also associated with many benign diseases
Amyloid deposits	Macroglossia, pinch purpura, superficial waxy yellow and pink elevated nodules	Multiple myeloma, Waldenström's macroglobulinemia	Amyloid deposition in blood vessels and dermis	Also associated with primary systemic amyloid and other benign conditions
Herpes zoster	Vesicular eruption in a dermatomal distribution	Hodgkin's disease, non-Hodgkin's lymphomas, CLL, SCLC cancer	Immunosuppression	Increased incidence in cancers associated with immunosuppression and after severely immunosuppressive therapy

Adapted from DeVita V, Hellman S, Rosenberg S: *Cancer Principles and Practice of Oncology.* Philadelphia, J. B. Lippincott Company, 1986.
* True paraneoplastic syndrome.
Abbreviations: CLL = chronic lymphocytic leukemia; CNS = central nervous system; GI = gastrointestinal; GU = genitourinary; IgA = immunoglobulin A; IgE = immunoglobulin E; NHL = non-Hodgkin's lymphoma; SCLC = small cell lung cancer.

2. Indirect effects from systemic tumor changes in metabolism, from secondary opportunistic infection, and from side effects of treatment such as cardiomyopathy and pulmonary fibrosis (see chemo- and radiotherapy)

J. **Genitourinary signs and symptoms: These include urinary frequency and incontinence, urinary retention, infertility, impotence, pain with urination, pain with intercourse, amenorrhea in the childbearing years, hematuria, and fistulas.**[42,43,57,363–371]

V. Diagnosis of Cancer [1,3,161,199,263,264,267–270,276,297–299,326,337]

A. Three stages of diagnostic process

1. Screen to identify those individuals with a high probability of developing cancer
2. Screen high-risk individuals to determine whether cancer is present or absent
3. Diagnose an individual with disease to determine the extent of the cancer

B. Assessment

A treatment plan and prognosis are based on these assessments. The types of tests used during assessment depend on the type and stage of the cancer and recognition of clinical manifestations of disease but generally include the following:

1. History and systems review
   a. General health
   b. Skin
   c. Head and neck
   d. Breasts
   e. Pulmonary and cardiovascular systems
   f. GI system
   g. Genitourinary systems (male and female)
   h. Peripheral and CNS
   i. Hematological system
   j. Endocrine system
   k. Psychiatric
2. Biopsies (needle or punch, incisional, and excisional) and fluid aspirations
3. Genetic markers and radiological studies (computed tomographic [CT] scans, x-ray films, positron emission tomography, radioactive scans such as bone scans, magnetic resonance imaging [MRI])
4. Optical exams such as endoscopy
5. Laboratory and blood tests (urine, blood, and stool)
6. Cytological study of sloughed-off tissues such as cell samples or smears
7. Tumor markers such as alpha-fetoprotein, carcinoembryonic antigen, alkaline phosphatase
8. Classification of tumors

C. Grades and stages

The information obtained is used to determine the nature and extent (grade and stage) of the cancer. The grades and stages are used to quantify the extent of the disease and spread, aid in planning treatment and rehabilitation, estimate prognosis, and evaluate results of treatment. Specific staging criteria are organ-site dependent.

1. General TNM classification (T = primary tumor, N = regional lymph node involvement, M = metastasis) is as follows:
   a. T: T_0, no evidence of tumor; TX, tumor cannot be assessed; T_1–T_4, progressive increase in tumor size; Tis, carcinoma in situ
   b. N: N_0, regional lymph nodes are not demonstrably abnormal; NX, regional lymph nodes cannot be assessed; N_1–N_4 progressive increase in abnormality of regional lymph nodes
   c. M: M_0, no known distant metastasis; MX, metastasis cannot be assessed; M_1–M_3, increasing degrees of distant metastasis

PLEASE NOTE: These categories are grouped into different combinations to create several stages of disease.

2. Stages I (in situ) through IV (distant) for solid tumors and its relationship with TNM classification system varies based on site
   a. Stage I: T_1, $N_{0 \text{ or } 1}$, $M_{0 \text{ or } 1}$—(Tis or in situ, 2 cm) cancer limited to local site, resectable, with best chance of survival (70–90%)
   b. Stage II: T_2, $N_{0 \text{ or } 1}$, $M_{0 \text{ or } 1}$—(locally invasive, 2 to 4 or 5 cm) invasion into organ or adjacent tissue, regional with microinvasion into lymphatic, resectable but uncertain of complete removal, with about a 50% or more chance of survival
   c. Stage IIIA or IIIB (A or B used in Hodgkin's disease to indicate absence (A) or presence (B) of unexplained fever, night sweats, weight loss, and so on): T_3, N_2, $M_{1 \text{ or } 2}$—(extensive primary lesions, 4–5 cm, with regional spread) an extension of Stage II with invasion of the lymphatic; operable but not resectable, with some chance of survival around 20% to 25%; varies based on site and size of regional spread
   d. Stage IV: T_4, N_3, $M_{2 \text{ or } 3}$—(extensive primary lesion, 10 cm, with metastatic or distant lesions) regional and metastatic

spread evident beyond local site, inoperable for resection with little chance of survival, around 5% or less

3. Grades are a histological or cytological characteristic of cell- and site-dependent classification system (Broders system), which is as follows:

a. GX: grade cannot be assessed

b. G1: well differentiated; 75% or more of cells differentiated (the greater the re-semblance to normal cell, the better the prognosis)

c. G2: slight to moderate dysplasia and metaplasia; 75% to 50% of cells differentiated

d. G3–G4: poorly to very poorly differentiated: G3, 50% to 25% of cells differentiated, marked dysplasia and atypical cells, and cancer in situ; G4, 25% to 0% of cells differentiated

VI. Diagnosis of Selected Specific Cancers

A. Assessment

To find the cause of any symptoms that may be a warning sign of cancer, the physician obtains the patient's personal and family medical history, performs a complete physical exam, and checks the general signs of health.

B. Musculoskeletal tumors

1. Bone tumors[1,2,6,289,290,318,319,322–331,333,336,340,341, 372–375]

a. Bone cancers are rare, with about 2000 new cases diagnosed each year[1]

b. Males are more likely than females, and children and adolescents more likely than adults, to acquire bone cancer

c. The most common bone tumors are osteosarcoma, Ewing's sarcoma, and chondrosarcoma

d. Osteosarcoma and Ewing's sarcoma usually occur between the ages of 10 and 25 years

e. Chondrosarcoma usually occurs in adults

f. Fibrosarcoma, chondroma, and malignant giant cell tumor are rare, mainly affecting persons older than age thirty years

g. Types of bone tumors

(1). Bone cortex tumors

(a). Benign bone tumors: osteochondroma, chondroma, and osteoclastoma (benign giant cell tumor) are examples; osteochondroma is the most common of the benign bone tumors, occurring mainly during adolescence and affecting the metaphysis at the elbow and knee most often. Osteoclastomas, or giant cell tumor, make up 4% to 5% of bone tumors most often occurring between the ages of 20 and 40 years; they are located in the epiphysis of long bones such as the distal femur and radius and proximal tibia; osteoid osteoma and osteoblastoma are similar types of benign bone tumors that occur more commonly in young boys; osteoblastoma occurs in the spine in 34% of all cases, presenting as neurological symptoms 50% of the time; malignant transformation occurs with some of these tumors

(b). Malignant bone tumors: chondrosarcoma, Ewing's sarcoma, and osteosarcoma are examples of primary malignant bone tumors; osteosarcoma is the most common bone cancer, making up 25% of all cases; it is twice as common in boys compared with girls; usually found near the metaphysis of long bones such as the distal femur, proximal tibia, and proximal humerus; hematogenous spread to the lung; Ewing's sarcoma arises from the reticuloendothelial tissue of the bone marrow in persons between the ages of 5 and 30 years; the tumor is often located in the diaphysis of the femur but is also found in the pelvis, tibia, and humerus; as it is rapidly growing, cortical thinning is common, leading to pathological fracture; it tends to metastasize rapidly, and metastatic disease develops in 25% of patients

(c). Metastatic bone tumors: these are most frequently associated with cancers of the breast, prostate, and lung (primary malignancy site) and often first present as pain; many other cancers also give rise to bone metastases such as renal and thyroid cancers, lymphomas, and melanoma; spinal cord compression from epidural disease may only have transient symptoms with medical treatment; however, involvement of the vertebrae can result in compression, leading to paraplegia or quadriplegia

(2). Bone marrow tumors: multiple myeloma, lymphoma, and leukemia are malignant neoplasms arising from the bone marrow and are discussed under hemopoietic tumors; they usually present as disseminated cancer

h. Clinical manifestations

(1). Bone cancer is an exception to the rule that pain is not an early sign of cancer: Pain is usually the first noticeable symptom

(2). Tenderness and stiffness occur if the tumor is near a joint

(3). Bowel and bladder function can be affected if the tumor is in the pelvis or at the base of the spine

(4). A palpable mass of soft tissue attached to bone may be found on palpation

(5). Osteoporosis or cortical bone erosion is found

(6). An abnormally high alkaline phosphatase level is found in half of the patients with osteosarcoma

(7). Pathological fracture of long bones occurs in less than 1% of patients with advanced cancer; however, when it occurs considerable loss of function often accompanies the fracture; almost all fractures occur proximal to the knee or elbow

i. Diagnosis: Tests such as bone scans, CT scans, and surgical biopsy are done to diagnose and stage the tumor; they include the following:

(1). X-ray films, bone scan, or CT scan will usually reveal bone tumor; may show increased or decreased bone density

(2). Bone scan is helpful in detecting initial extent of malignancy, in planning therapy, in defining level of amputation, and after radiation or chemotherapy

(3). Serum alkaline phosphatase is usually increased

(4). Biopsy of bone confirms suspected diagnosis

(5). Chest x-ray film and lung scan determine whether metastasis is present

(6). Arteriography assesses soft tissue

2. Soft-tissue sarcomas in adults:[1,3,4,307,324,340,373-383] Sarcomas are rare; about 4500 cases of all types of soft-tissue sarcoma are diagnosed in both adults and children each year in the United States, with survival rates of 70% to 80%; there are no racial or gender differences in the total incidence of soft-tissue sarcomas, although differences do exist for specific types.

a. Risk factors

(1). Exposure to phenoxyacetic acids in herbicides and chlorphenols in wood preservatives

(2). Work-related exposure to vinyl chloride, a substance used in the manufacture of certain plastics (results in a rare blood vessel tumor, angiosarcoma of the liver; the plastics themselves are not a cancer hazard)

(3). High doses of radiation

(4). Certain viruses were shown to cause sarcomas in laboratory animals, but there is no evidence that viruses are a direct cause of human sarcomas; researchers believe that a retrovirus plays an indirect role in the development of Kaposi's sarcoma, a rare cancer of the cells that line blood vessels, when it occurs in patients with AIDS

(5). There are a few families in which more than one member in the same generation has developed sarcoma or in which relatives of children with sarcoma have acquired other forms

Table 4–9. MAJOR TYPES OF SOFT-TISSUE SARCOMAS IN ADULTS

Tissue of Origin	Types of Cancer	Usual Locations in Body
Fibrous tissue	Fibrosarcoma	Arms, legs, trunk
	Malignant fibrous hystiocytoma	Legs
Fat	Liposarcoma	Arms, legs, trunk
Muscle		
Striated muscle	Rhabdomyosarcoma	Arms, legs
Smooth muscle	Leiomyosarcoma	Uterus, digestive tract
Blood vessels	Hemangiosarcoma	Arms, legs, trunk
	Kaposi's sarcoma	Legs, trunk
Lymph vessels	Lymphangiosarcoma	Arms
Synovial tissue	Synovial sarcoma	Legs
(linings of joint cavities, tendon sheaths)		
Peripheral nerves	Neurofibrosarcoma	Arms, legs, trunk
Cartilage and bone-forming tissue	Chondrosarcoma	Legs

of cancer at an unusually high rate; sarcomas in these family clusters represent a very small fraction of all cases and appear to be related to a rare genetic defect

(6). Some inherited diseases are associated with an increased risk of soft-tissue sarcomas, approximately 15% of people who have neurofibromatosis (von Recklinghausen's disease) acquire neurofibrosarcoma

b. Sites of sarcomas

(1). Soft-tissue sarcomas can arise almost anywhere in the body (see Table 4–9), with about 40% occurring in the legs; most develop at or above the knee, but sometimes they occur in the feet; 15% develop in the arms and hands, an additional 15% in areas of the head and neck, and another 30% in tissues of the trunk

(2). Physical impairments and dysfunctions are dependent on the site and stage of the tumor and its treatment; until the 1980s, amputation was common

(3). Soft-tissue sarcomas rarely invade bone or spread to regional lymph nodes; they tend to spread outward from the original tumor along tissues of muscle, blood vessels, and nerves

(4). When sarcomas metastasize, the cancer cells generally travel through the bloodstream to the lungs

(5). Some more common malignant tumors of soft tissue include fibro-sarcoma, malignant fibrous histiocytoma, synovial sarcoma, rhabdomyosarcoma, liposarcoma, and leiomyosarcoma

c. Types of soft-tissue tumors

(1). Fibrosarcomas (fibrous tissue tumors) are common in men in their mid-40s to early 50s; fibrosarcomas are often located deep in the thigh, and these tumors are usually large when diagnosed

(2). Malignant fibrous histiocytomas (fibrous connective tissue and muscle tumors) are most common in people in their 50s and 60s; men have about a two times greater risk compared with women for these tumors; they usually develop in the legs or arms but also occur in the lining of the lower abdomen

(3). Synovial sarcomas arise close to joints (synoviomas in tendons and in bursae); adults in their 20s and 30s are usually affected and may be more common among men than women; the most common site is the leg, often between the thigh and knee; they also may arise in the hands and feet

(4). Rhabdomyosarcomas (skeletal [striated] muscle tumors) are equally common in men and women in their 40s and 50s; they usually occur in the thigh, shoulder, and upper arm and are usually large when diagnosed

(5). Liposarcomas (fatty tissue tumors)

usually occur in the thigh; they are usually found in middle-aged men

(6). Leiomyosarcomas (smooth-muscle tumors) can arise in the walls of blood vessels; these very rare tumors most often occur in the uterus and in the back part of the abdominal cavity

d. Clinical manifestations: Soft-tissue sarcomas seldom cause symptoms in the early stage of the disease because soft tissue is elastic. Tumors can grow large, compressing or stretching normal tissue such as nearby nerves and muscles, before they cause any symptoms or signs; the first noticeable sign usually is a painless lump

e. Diagnosis: surgical biopsy to determine whether the tumor is benign or malignant and the type and grade or degree of differentiation of the cancer cells; x-ray films and scans of the affected area show the exact location and dimensions of a tumor and how normal tissue around the tumor is being affected by its growth; the following tests are used in staging soft-tissue sarcomas:

(1). A xerogram, or soft-tissue radiograph, is an x-ray film that gives detailed images of muscles, fat, blood vessels, and other soft tissues

(2). CT scans and tomogram: tomogram is similar to a standard x-ray film except shadows of body structures in front of and behind the tissue being examined do not show

(3). Arteriogram assesses soft-tissue involvement

(4). MRI

(5). Ultrasonogram

(6). Chest x-ray film and lung scan determine whether metastasis is present

f. Simplified staging system: A simplified description for the current staging system for soft-tissue sarcomas is as follows:

(1). Stage I (has two subgroups) means the sarcoma is localized; it has not spread to regional lymph nodes or to other parts of the body: Stage IA, tumors that are smaller than 5 cm in diameter (G1, T1, N0, M0); Stage IB, tumors that are larger than 5 cm in diameter (G1, T2, N0, M0)

(2). Stage II (has two subgroups) describes localized sarcomas that have not spread to lymph nodes or other sites: Stage IIA, tumors smaller than 5 cm in diameter (G2, T1, N0, M0); Stage IIB, tumors larger than 5 cm in diameter (G2, T2, N0, M0)

(3). Stage III (has three subgroups) refers to invasive sarcomas that have not spread or to sarcomas of any grade that have spread to nearby lymph nodes but not to other parts of the body: Stage IIIA, tumors smaller than 5 cm in diameter that have not spread (G3, T1, N0, M0); Stage IIIB, tumors larger than 5 cm in diameter that have not spread (G3, T2, N0, M0); Stage IIIC, tumors of any grade and size that have spread to regional lymph nodes but not to other organs (G1–3, T1–2, N1, M0)

(4). Stage IV sarcomas: Stage IVA, tumors of any grade or size that have invaded bone, a major blood vessel, or a major nerve; they may or may not have spread to lymph nodes but have not spread to other sites (G1–3, T1–3, N0–1, M0); Stage IVB, tumors that have spread to other sites in the body (G1–3, T1–3, N0–1, M1)

3. Head and neck cancer[24,37,149,308–313,338,384–392]

a. Head and neck cancers are some of the easiest cancers to detect, accounting for about 5% of all cancers with about a 66% survival rate[1,2,7]; approximately 59,000 new cases a year

b. The stage of disease remains the major prognostic indicator for head and neck cancer

c. Five-year survival declines as the disease stage progresses

d. The most common head and neck cancer is squamous cell carcinoma with specific cancers including a basal cell carcinoma (BCC) of the cheek, multiple BCC of the forehead and scalp, sarcoma of the cheek, adenosarcoma of the cheek, squamous cell carcinoma of the tongue and retromolar area, tumor of the larynx, and squamous cell carcinoma of the buccal mucosa

e. The most common sites in descending order are larynx, oral cavity, pharynx, and salivary glands

f. Signs and symptoms are color changes in the mouth and tongue, a lump in the mouth or neck, a sore that does not heal within 2 weeks, persistent and unexplained bleeding, persistent dysphagia, numbness of the mouth or lips, recent onset of nasal obstruction

g. Currently, only Stage I and Stage II head and neck cancers are curable; therefore, early detection is imperative

h. Treatment for Stage III and Stage IV disease is only palliative

i. Early detection is promoted by educating high risk populations (older patients who drink and smoke have 2.5 times greater risk than nondrinkers/nonsmokers) and monitoring their use of nonprescription medications for palliation of symptoms

(1). Oral cancer

    (a). More than 90% of all oral cancers are found in people older than 45 years, but oral cancer can occur at any age[1]

    (b). Tobacco users (smoking, chewing, or dipping) are 4 to 15 times more likely than nonusers to acquire these cancers

    (c). Almost all oral cancers are squamous cell carcinomas (cancers that begin in the flat, scale-like cells that line the oral cavity

    (d). Pain is usually not a symptom of oral cancer

    (e). Individuals can spot symptoms by doing a monthly oral self-exam

    (f). This exam should include a check for the following symptoms, which are some of the warning signs of oral cancer:

        (i). A sore in the mouth that bleeds easily and does not heal

        (ii). A lump or thickening in the cheek that can be felt with the tongue

        (iii). A white or red patch on the gums, tongue, or lining of the mouth

        (iv). Soreness or a feeling that something is caught in the throat

        (v). Difficulty chewing or swallowing

        (vi). Difficulty moving the jaw or tongue

        (vii). Numbness of the tongue or other areas of the mouth

        (viii). Swelling of the jaw that causes dentures to fit poorly or become uncomfortable

■ PLEASE NOTE: These symptoms are not sure signs of cancer; however, it is important to refer the patient to a dentist or physician if any of these problems lasts more than 2 weeks.

    (g). Diagnosis: To diagnose oral cancer, a dentist or physician carefully checks the mouth for lumps, swelling, or abnormal-looking areas; when a problem is found, a biopsy specimen is examined to confirm the diagnosis; staging generally includes the following tests:

        (i). Dental x-ray films and x-ray films of the head and chest

        (ii). Palpation of the lymph nodes in the front and back of the neck to check for swelling or other changes

        (iii). Endoscopy using a flexible, lighted instrument to look for tumors in the throat

        (iv). CT scan

        (v). Ultrasonography

        (vi). MRI

(2). Esophageal cancer

    (a). Approximately 11,000 cases of esophageal cancer are diagnosed each year[1]

    (b). It occurs in persons mainly older than 55 years and affects men twice as often as women

    (c). Heavy users of both alcohol and tobacco are much more likely to get esophageal cancer than nonusers; also, chronic irritation of the esophagus, esophageal reflux, increases the risk

    (d). Cancer that occurs in the middle or upper part of the esophagus is usually squamous cell carcinoma (e). When cancer develops at the lower end of the esophagus, near the stomach, it is usually adenocarcinoma

(f). Very small tumors in the esophagus usually do not cause symptoms

(g). Problems with swallowing may come and go; at first, they may be noticed mainly when the person eats meat, bread, and coarse foods such as raw vegetables; as the tumor grows larger and the pathway to the stomach becomes narrower, other foods—even liquids—may be hard to swallow, and swallowing may be painful

(h). Signs and symptoms include the following:
  (i). Dysphagia, difficulty swallowing, is the most common symptom as the tumor grows
  (ii). A feeling of fullness, pressure, or burning as food goes down the esophagus
  (iii). Feeling as though food gets stuck behind the breastbone
  (iv). Indigestion, heartburn, vomiting
  (v). Frequent choking on food
  (vi). Weight loss common secondary to clinical manifestations
  (vii). Coughing and hoarseness
  (viii). Pain behind the breastbone or in the throat

PLEASE NOTE: Any of these symptoms may be caused by cancer or by other, less serious conditions. People with symptoms like these are referred to a gastroenterologist, a specialist in diseases of the digestive tract.

(i). Diagnosis
  (i). X-ray films
  (ii). Esophagram (also called a barium swallow in which the patient drinks a barium solution that coats the inside of the esophagus, showing changes in the shape of the esophagus on a series of x-ray films of the esophagus)
  (iii). A special x-ray machine called a fluoroscope can be used to watch the barium move down the esophagus to the stomach as the patient swallows
  (iv). Esophagoscopy (a thin, flexible, lighted instrument called an endoscope through the mouth and down the throat into the esophagus imaging the lining of the esophagus and the juncture of the esophagus and stomach)
  (v). If an abnormal area is found, a biopsy specimen is taken through the endoscope (also, cells can be brushed or washed from the walls of the esophagus through the scope)

(j). Staging usually involves the following:
  (i). A physical exam, with special attention to the neck and chest
  (ii). Blood tests
  (iii). Additional x-ray films
  (iv). CT scans of the chest and upper abdomen
  (v). MRI
  (vi). If metastatic spread is a concern, additional tests to examine the organs near the esophagus are done such as laryngoscopy to see whether the cancer has spread to the larynx or a bronchoscopy to examine the trachea and bronchi
  (vii). If lymph nodes near the esophagus are enlarged, the surgeon may perform a biopsy to determine whether the cells are cancerous

(3). Cancer of the larynx
  (a). Cancer of the larynx occurs most often in men between 50 and 70 years of age
  (b). Approximately 12,000 cases of

laryngeal cancer are diagnosed each year[1]

(c). This cancer is four times more common in men than women

(d). As with esophageal cancer, persons who smoke are at greater risk, particularly in combination with heavy alcohol use

(e). Cigarette smoking and alcohol consumption are responsible for more than 75% of cases

(f). Workers exposed to asbestos are also at greater risk for this cancer

(g). Almost all cancers of the larynx are squamous cell carcinomas

(h). This type of cancer begins in the flat, scalelike cells that line the epiglottis, vocal cords, and other parts of the larynx

(i). Hoarseness is the most common presenting complaint; if hoarseness persists for more than 2 weeks, largyngoscopy is indicated

(j). Clinical staging uses direct laryngoscopy, esophagoscopy, and bronchoscopy to exclude synchronous malignancies

(k). The 5-year cure rate, with preservation of voice and glottic function, is as high as 90% if the lesions of the vocal cords are found in an early stage

(l). Total laryngectomy is required for more extensive disease

(m). The symptoms of cancer of the larynx depend mainly on the size and location of the tumor:
  (i). Tumor on the vocal cords (most cancers of the larynx) are seldom painful, but they almost always cause hoarseness or other changes in the voice
  (ii). Tumor in the area above the vocal cords may cause a lump on the neck, a sore throat, or an earache
  (iii). Tumor in the area below the vocal cords are rare and can lead to dyspnea; breathing may be noisy

(n). Additional signs and symptoms common as the tumor enlarges are as follows:

  (i). A cough that does not go away or the feeling of a lump in the throat
  (ii). Pain
  (iii). Weight loss
  (iv). Bad breath
  (v). Frequent choking on food
  (vi). Difficulty swallowing

PLEASE NOTE: Any of these symptoms may be caused by cancer or by other, less serious problems. Patients should be referred to an ear, nose, and throat specialist (otolaryngologist).

(o). Diagnosis: The exam includes palpation of the neck to check for lumps, swelling, tenderness, or other changes; further examination includes either of the following:
  (i). Indirect laryngoscopy, in which the throat is examined with a small, long-handled mirror to check for abnormal areas and to determine whether the vocal cords move as they should; this test is painless, but a local anesthetic may be sprayed in the throat to prevent gagging
  (ii). Direct laryngoscopy with a laryngoscope inserted through the patient's nose or mouth to image areas that cannot be seen with a simple mirror; a local anesthetic eases discomfort and prevents gagging; patients may also be given a mild sedative to help them relax
  (iii). If abnormal areas are found, a biopsy through a laryngoscope is the only sure way to determine whether cancer is present; if cancer is found, to determine the size of the tumor and whether the cancer has spread, additional tests are done such as x-ray films, a CT scan, and/or MRI

(4). Breast cancer[1,2,6,7,25,26,39,40,45,47,61,63,66,67,70, 75,84,86,89,100,101,111,114,122,124,127,181,186–192, 199,201,207,277–279,287,291,293,305,319,339,393–405]

(a). Carcinoma of the breast is one of the most common forms of cancer in white women older than 40 years; approximately 183,000 new cases are diagnosed annually;[1] only cancers of the lung and skin are more common

(b). About 1 of 9 women will have breast cancer sometime during her life, with a high rate of reoccurrence[1] accounting for 43,000 deaths per year

(c). Seventy-five percent of all breast cancers occur in women older than 50 years[1]

(d). It is the leading cause of death in women between the ages of 40 and 60 years; the disease is rare in women younger than 20 years

(e). Women who are at greater risk have any of the following:
  (i). A positive family history
  (ii). A history of breast cancer
  (iii). First menstrual period at an early age
  (iv). Menopause at a late age
  (v). Had their first child after age 30 or have never had children

(f). Research has also implicated diets high in fat as increasing risk

(g). Four of five breast lumps are not cancer

(h). If a woman has a fluid-filled cyst, it most likely can be drained by fine-needle aspiration; if the lump is a benign tumor, it often can be removed by surgery with no further problems; some lumps may not need any treatment except regular examination

(i). Fibrocystic breast disease refers to a constellation of breast changes observed in premenopausal women, and 90% of all women experience evidence of pathophysiological changes in the breast during their lifetime[393]

(j). Tumors that are detected early and are localized can be successfully treated by partial (lumpectomy) or complete (mastectomy) surgical resection of breast tissue and adjuvant therapy

(k). Breast cancer is the most common cause of bone metastases, and the common sites are the pelvis, ribs, spine, or proximal femur

(l). Breast cancer can cause many symptoms and warning signs, including the following:
  (i). A lump or thickening in the breast or under the arm
  (ii). A change in the size or shape of the breast
  (iii). Discharge from the nipple
  (iv). A change in the color or feel of the skin of the breast or areola (such as dimpling, puckering, or scaliness)

PLEASE NOTE: Pain is usually not an early warning sign of breast cancer; however, a woman should see her physician if she notices any changes in her breasts. Changes may be caused by cancer or by other less serious problems such as fibrocystic disease. Early diagnosis is important because breast cancer is treated best before it has spread. The earlier breast cancer is found and treated, the better the chances for complete recovery.

(m). Diagnosis: Examination includes the following:
  (i). Palpation of the breast to feel whether a breast lump is present: its size, texture, and whether it is movable
  (ii). Needle aspiration to remove fluid or a small amount of tissue from a breast lump to determine whether the lump is a fluid-filled cyst (not cancer) or a solid mass

(which may or may not be cancer)

(iii). Mammography, x-ray films of the breast can show tumors too small to be felt

(iv). Other tests called imaging techniques such as ultrasonography, thermography (heat patterns in the breast), diaphanoscopy (shining a bright light through the breast); however, at this time, these tests are not reliable enough to be used alone

(v). Biopsy

(vi). Hormone receptor tests are laboratory tests called estrogen and progesterone receptor tests usually done on the cancer cells; these tests determine whether hormones promote the growth of the cancer; this information helps decide whether hormone treatment is likely to be useful

(o). If the biopsy shows that the lump is cancer, other special laboratory tests are done to stage the cancer such as chest x-ray films and blood tests; because later stage breast cancer often may spread to the bones, liver, lungs, or brain, special exams to examine these areas are frequently done; these tests help determine the extent, or stage of breast cancer:

(i). The tumor is carcinoma in situ when cancer is found in a local area, in only a few layers of cells, and is a very early stage of breast cancer

(ii). In Stage I, the tumor is no larger than 2 cm and has not spread beyond the breast

(iii). In Stage II, the tumor is from 2 to 5 cm and/or has spread to the axillary lymph nodes

(iv). In Stage III, the cancer is larger than 5 cm; it involves more of the axillary lymph nodes and/or has spread to other lymph nodes or tissues in the region

(v). In Stage IV, the cancer has metastasized to other organs of the body, most often the bones, liver, lungs, or brain

C. Neurological tumors (brain and spinal cord)[1,2,6,7,285,289–297,406–422]

1. Approximately 17,000 brain tumors are diagnosed annually in the United States[1]

2. They occur commonly in two age groups: children between the ages of 3 and 12 years and adults between the ages of 40 and 70 years

3. Clear causes of primary brain cancer have been identified, and, although frequently it is an invasive cancer, rarely do metastases occur outside the CNS

4. Research has identified increased incidence of brain tumors with certain occupational exposures such as oil refining, rubber manufacturing, drug manufacturing, chemical manufacturing, and embalming; viruses and heredity are under current research as potential risks

5. The most common type of brain tumors are gliomas in the supporting glial cells of the brain

6. Spinal cord cancers are similar to brain cancers because the spinal cord and brain contain similar types of tissue from which the tumors grow; however, tumors grow less often in the spinal cord than in the brain

7. Types of brain and spinal cord cancer are as follows:

a. Benign tumors

(1). Meningiomas are usually benign, occurring primarily in women between the ages of 30 and 50 years; because these tumors arise from the meninges and are slow growing, they are often large before the person presents with symptoms, leading to diagnosis

(2). Schwannomas occur in adults and twice as frequently in women compared with men; these tumors arise from the Schwann cells, *eg,* an acoustic neuroma

(3). Craniopharyngiomas occur most often in children and adolescents; they are occasionally malignant because they arise near the pituitary gland and hypothalamus and can damage the hypothalamus

b. Malignant tumors

(1). Gliomas

  (a). In children, astrocytomas occur usually in the brain stem, cerebellum, and cerebrum; in adults, they occur in the cerebrum (Grade III: anaplastic astrocytoma, Grade IV: glioblastoma multiform

  (b). Brain-stem gliomas are usually late-stage astrocytomas that cannot be resected

  (c). Ependymomas are most common in children and adolescents, developing in the lining of the ventricles and spinal cord

  (d). Oligodendrogliomas are rare, occurring most often in middle-aged adults; these tumors arise in the cerebrum from myelin tissue and usually do not spread

(2). Medulloblastomas occur in children and are more common in males than females; they usually arise in the cerebellum and are also called primitive neuroectodermal tumors because they develop from primitive nerve cells that are normally not in the body after birth

(3). Germinoma is the most common germ cell tumor arising from germ cells (primitive or developing sex cell)

(4). Pineocytoma (slow growing) and pineoblastoma (fast growing) tumors occur in the region of the pineal gland near the center of the brain; these tumors are, therefore, often not resectable

c. Metastatic tumors

(1). Treatment of secondary brain tumors is dependent on the type of primary cancer, extent of spread, and other factors such as the person's age, general health, and previous response to treatment

(2). Metastases occur by spread through direct extension or the cerebrospinal fluid, resulting in nerve root and spinal cord compression

(3). The brain is a common site of metastatic spread

(4). Direct growth of a tumor usually compresses the anterior spinal cord

(5). Fifty percent of all metastatic brain tumors are related to primary lung cancer, and 15% are related to primary breast cancer

(6). Most cancers found in the spinal cord have spread from other parts of the body

(7). Pain is a common symptom because of pressure on the spinal cord within the backbone

(8). Sensory-motor loss in the arms and legs may follow, sometimes with hemiparalysis on one side of the body and loss of sensation on the other

(9). The spinal compression occurs in 5% of persons with metastatic brain cancer

(10). Prostate, kidney, lymphoma, and multiple myeloma also result in spinal compression

d. Clinical manifestations: Brain cancer symptoms are varied and depend on the part of the brain that is involved; any of the symptoms may be caused by a condition other than cancer; symptoms are caused by the following:

(1). Invasion or compression of vital tissue of the brain as the tumor grows within the limited space in the cranium

(2). Edema and a buildup of fluid around the tumor

(3). Hydrocephalus occurring when the tumor blocks the flow of cerebrospinal fluid and causes it to build up in the ventricles

(4). Depending on the location and size of the tumor, the most frequent symptoms of brain tumors include the following:

  (a). Headaches are most common and tend to be worse in the morning and ease during the day

  (b). Seizures (convulsions in about one third of brain cancer patients)

  (c). Nausea and vomiting

(d). Weakness or loss of feeling in the arms or legs

(e). Stumbling or lack of balance or coordination in walking (ataxic gait)

(f). Abnormal eye movements or changes in vision

(g). Drowsiness

(h). Changes in personality, memory, or mood such as increasing irritability, a feeling of laziness, or unusual sleepiness

(i). Changes in speech

(5). Disturbance or loss of hearing, sight, taste, smell or any change in control of movement are less common; if a tumor grows slowly, its symptoms may appear so gradually that they are scarcely noticed and are overlooked for a long time

(6). Other symptoms may be increasing irritability, a feeling of laziness, or unusual sleepiness; they may indicate a growing tumor's increasing pressure on normal brain tissues; when a tumor grows quickly, symptoms are more noticeable and tend to be more disturbing

(7). A patient with any new severe or persistent headache should be referred promptly to a physician; these symptoms may be caused by brain tumors or other problems; a patient should be referred to a neurologist for examination.

e. Diagnosis: Examination of the eye with an ophthalmoscope allows visualization of the retina and the optic nerve; a tumor pressing anywhere along the route of this nerve swells it, causing a visible condition called papilledema; a neurological exam will be conducted, including tests of muscle function (key myotome), reflexes, ability to feel pinpricks for response to pain, alertness and memory, muscle strength, coordination, and cranial nerve examination

f. Examination: If distinctive characteristics of cancer are detected, microscopic examination of a specimen of tissue from the suspected area is done; careful physical examination and x-ray films of the affected spinal areas are required for diagnosis of spinal tumors; examination of spinal fluid may be necessary to confirm the diagnosis; depending on the re-

sults of the physical and neurological examinations, further testing may be indicated such as CT scan and/or MRI; other tests include the following:

(1). A cranial x-ray film can show changes in the bones of the skull caused by a tumor; it can also show calcium deposits, which are present in some types of brain tumors

(2). In a brain scan, areas of abnormal growth in the brain are revealed and recorded on special film; a small amount of radioactive material is injected into a vein, this dye is absorbed by the tumor, and the growth shows up on the film (the radiation leaves the body within 6 hours and is not dangerous)

(3). An angiogram, or arteriogram, is a series of x-ray films taken after a special dye is injected into an artery (usually in the area where the abdomen joins the top of the leg); these x-ray films can show the tumor and the blood vessels that lead to it

(4). A myelogram is an x-ray film of the spine; a special dye is injected into the cerebrospinal fluid in the spine, and the patient is tilted to allow the dye to mix with the fluid; this test may be done when the physician suspects a tumor in the spinal cord

(5). Electroencephalography

(6). Pneumoencephalography: an x-ray picture of the brain is taken after air or gas is injected into the space around the segments of the brain; the examination may also be called ventriculography

(7). Echoencephalography: an image of the brain is produced

PLEASE NOTE: Careful physical examination and x-ray films of the affected spinal areas are required for diagnosis of spinal tumors. Examination of fluid taken from the spine may be necessary to confirm the finding.

D. Genitourinary cancers[1,2,6,7,369,370]

1. Prostate cancer[1,2,6,7,42,332,363–367,371]

   a. Prostate cancer is the second most common cause of cancer deaths in men (20% of all cancers in men) and the most common in men older than 50 years of age; 99% of all cases occur after age 50. One of every 11 men receives such a diagnosis; 200,000 new cases are diagnosed each year

b. Advances in medical care have produced cures; approximately 71% of all patients diagnosed with prostate cancer survive for more than 5 years

c. Prostate cancer is the leading cause of cancer deaths in men

d. Fifty percent of the metastatic spread is to bone, and common sites of spread are the lumbar spine and pelvis, proximal femurs, thoracic spine and ribs, and sternum

e. Early prostate cancer often does not cause symptoms; when symptoms of prostate cancer do occur, they may include any of the following problems:
    (1). A need to urinate frequently, especially at night
    (2). Difficulty starting urination or holding back urine
    (3). Inability to urinate
    (4). Weak or interrupted flow of urine
    (5). Painful or burning urination
    (6). Painful ejaculation
    (7). Blood in urine or semen
    (8). Frequent pain or stiffness in the lower back, hips, or upper thighs

f. A man who has these symptoms should be referred to a urologist (specialist in diseases of the genitourinary system), who will determine whether such symptoms are caused by prostate cancer, benign prostatic hypertrophy (BPH), or some other condition, such as an infection or stones in the prostate

g. The consequences of cancer and its treatment can produce side effects varying from inconsequential to severely debilitating

h. One study identified several factors associated with poorer quality of life after a prostate cancer diagnosis, including a poorer quality of life for patients with active disease than for those with no evidence of disease (NED); the widespread group had significantly poorer quality of life than patients with NED or localized disease

i. Contrary to prediction, the local group's quality of life was not significantly different from the NED group; also, there was no significant difference between the different phases of disease and problems interacting with the health care team

j. It was concluded the rehabilitation needs are more significant for patients with widespread metastatic disease

k. Although there is the consistent and significant impact on sexual functioning at all phases of the disease, the physical and psychosocial problems are more profound in patients with advanced disease[367]

l. Diagnosis: The rectal exam involves palpating the prostate to check for hard or lumpy areas; often blood tests to measure substances called prostate-specific antigen (PSA) and prostatic acid phosphatase (PAP) are done because this tumor may be hormone sensitive; the level of PSA in the blood may rise in men who have prostate cancer or benign prostatic hypertrophy; elevated PAP levels are found in many prostate cancer patients, especially if the cancer has spread beyond the prostate; additional tests to help distinguish between benign and malignant conditions of the prostate include the following:
    (1). Transrectal ultrasonography: probe is inserted into the rectum to create an image called a sonogram
    (2). Intravenous pyelogram (IVP): a series of x-ray films of the organs of the urinary tract
    (3). Urine tests
    (4). Cystoscopy: a thin, lighted tube inserted into the urethra and bladder to image those structures
    (5). Biopsy: usually with a needle

m. If the diagnosis is cancer, the pathologist determines whether cells are likely to grow slowly or quickly; even if the physical exam and test results do not suggest cancer, surgery may be recommended to relieve problems with urination; the surgery used in such cases is transurethral resection (TUR) of the prostate: An instrument is inserted through the penis to remove prostate tissue that is compressing the upper part of the urethra; sometimes, a small cancer is found when the tissue is examined; treatment decisions depend on the stage of the cancer. The following tests are used to stage the disease:
    (1). Laboratory tests to check the levels of PSA and PAP in the blood may be repeated

(2). If transrectal ultrasonography was not done earlier, this procedure may be part of the staging process

(3). CT scan to check for swollen lymph nodes, which might mean the cancer has spread

(4). MRI to image the prostate and nearby lymph nodes

(5). Bone scan shows areas of rapid growth in bones and may be a sign of cancer that has spread, or it may be the result of other problems in the bones

(6). Chest x-ray can show whether cancer has spread to the lungs.

n. The results of these tests help determine which of the following stages best describes a patient's disease:

(1). Stage A: cancer not detected by rectal exam but is found during surgery to relieve problems with urination; Stage A tumors have not spread beyond the prostate

(2). Stage B: tumor palpated in a rectal exam, but the cancer has not spread beyond the prostate

(3). Stage C: cancer extended outside the prostate to adjacent tissues

(4). Stage D: cancer cells spread to regional lymph nodes or to other parts of the body, most commonly to the bones

2. Renal Cancers[1,2,6,7]

a. Approximately 27,000 cases of kidney cancer are diagnosed each year

b. Kidney cancer primarily affects persons older than 50 years, and it affects men twice as often as women

c. Renal cell carcinoma is the most common kidney cancer; it rarely occurs before the age of 30 and has a peak incidence during the sixth decade of life

d. Metastatic spread is most often to the lungs, liver, and bones

e. Smokers have an increased risk of renal cell carcinoma compared with nonsmokers

f. Symptoms may develop suddenly; however, as with other types of cancer, kidney cancer can cause a general feeling of poor health; the signs and symptoms of kidney cancer are as follows:

(1). Blood in the urine (most common sign): Traces of blood may be found in urine; in some cases, a person can actually see the blood;

it may be present one day and not the next

(2). A lump or mass palpated in the kidney area

(3). A dull ache or pain in the back or side

(4). Hypertension

(5). Abnormal red blood cell count

(6). Constitutional signs such as fatigue, loss of appetite, and weight loss; some have a fever that comes and goes

(7). These symptoms may be caused by cancer or by other, less serious problems such as an infection or a fluid-filled cyst

b. Diagnosis: Typical testing includes the following:

(1). Blood and urine tests

(2). IVP

(3). CT scan

(4). Ultrasonography: Healthy tissues, cysts, and tumors produce different echoes

(5). An arteriogram of the smaller blood vessels around and in the kidney

(6). MRI of the kidney

(7). A nephrotomogram (series of x-ray films of cross-sections of the kidney after an injection of a dye that outlines the kidney)

(8). Confirm the diagnosis with a needle biopsy

(9). Kidney cancer may spread to the bones, lungs, liver, or brain; if transitional cell carcinoma is suspected, other tests may be used

3. Bladder cancer[1,2,6,7]

a. There are approximately 51,000 cases of bladder cancer each year, and it is the fifth most common cause of cancer deaths in men, the second most common genitourinary cancer

b. Bladder cancer is a disease of middle-aged men, usually older than 55 years, but can develop in younger adults

c. It is three to six times more common in men than in women

d. Smokers acquire bladder cancer two to three times more often than nonsmokers

e. Work exposures have been identified for those employed in the chemical, rubber, and leather industries and for painters, textile workers, truck drivers, machinists, metal workers, and hairdressers

f. Work continues on the development of effective screening methods

g. Prevention is the key to managing this disease; public health campaigns on the hazards of smoking should include information on smoking's link to bladder cancer

h. Workers in high-risk industries should be made aware of the risk and practice good work habits; in industries in which workers handle known bladder carcinogens, protective clothing should be worn

i. The most common sites of metastatic spread are the lungs, liver, and bones. Often bladder tumors cause no symptoms; when symptoms do occur, they are not always signs of cancer; they may also be caused by infections, benign tumors, bladder stones, or other problems; patients should be referred to a urologist to determine the cause of the symptoms; any illness should be diagnosed and treated as early as possible; the warning signs of bladder cancer are as follows:

(1). Blood in the urine (most common sign); depending on the amount of blood present, the color of the urine can turn faintly rusty to deep red

(2). Pain during urination

(3). A need to urinate often or urgently

j. Diagnosis: Sometimes a large tumor can be palpated during a rectal or vaginal exam; typical tests include the following:

(1). Urinalysis

(2). IVP

(3). Cystoscopy

(4). Biopsy

4. Testicular cancer[1,2,6,7,57,368,425,426]

a. Although relatively rare overall in men, testicular cancer is an important disease because it is the first disseminated solid tumor occurring in adults for which truly effective therapy was developed, and it is one of the more common cancers in young men between the ages of 15 and 34 years

b. The disease also occurs in other age groups, so all men should be aware of its symptoms

c. More than 90% of testicular neoplasms are of germ cell origin; about 40% of cases involve pure seminoma; and nonseminoma include 15% to 20% that are pure embryonal (choriocarcinoma, embryonal carcinoma, teratoma, and yolk sac tumors), and the rest are of mixed types

d. Each of these two major types of testicular cancer grows and spreads differently, and they are treated differently

e. Most testicular cancers are detected by men themselves, by accident or when doing testicular self-examination; any changes in the way they feel from month to month should be reported to a doctor; most men with testicular neoplasms initially complain of a painless testicular mass; testicular cancer can cause a number of symptoms; listed next are warning signs for testicular cancer:

(1). A lump in either testicle

(2). Any enlargement of a testicle

(3). A feeling of heaviness in the scrotum

(4). A dull ache in the lower abdomen or the groin

(5). A sudden collection of fluid in the scrotum

(6). Pain or discomfort in a testicle or in the scrotum

(7). Enlargement or tenderness of the breasts

PLEASE NOTE: These symptoms are not sure signs of cancer. They can also be caused by other conditions and the patient should be referred to a physician if these symptoms last as long as 2 weeks. Any illness should be diagnosed and treated as soon as possible. There is a 95% cure rate with Stage 1 cancer.

f. Diagnosis: Examine the scrotum, have chest x-ray film taken, take blood and urine tests

(1). If the physical exam and lab tests do not show an infection or another disorder, cancer is likely to be suspected because most tumors in the testicles are cancer; biopsy is the next step

(2). To obtain the tissue, the affected testicle is removed through the groin by an operation called inguinal orchiectomy (the surgeon does not cut through the scrotum and does not remove just a part of the testicle because, if the problem is cancer, cutting through the outer layer of the testicle might cause local spread of the disease)

g. Staging procedures
   (1). Physical exam
   (2). Blood tests
   (3). X-ray films and scans and, in some cases, additional surgery
   (4). CT scan
h. Staging can include IVP, lymphangiography, or ultrasonography; special lab tests can reveal certain tumor markers because they often are found in abnormal amounts in patients with some types of cancer and can help the physician determine what types of testicular cancer the patient has
i. Surgery may be recommended to remove the lymph nodes deep in the abdomen
j. For patients with nonseminoma, removing the nodes helps stop the spread of their disease; seminoma patients do not need this surgery because cancer cells in their lymph nodes can be destroyed with radiation therapy

5. Cancer of the cervix[1,2,6,7,43,369,370,427,428]
   a. Carcinoma in situ of the cervix most often develops in women between the ages of 30 and 40 years, whereas invasive cervical cancer occurs most often in women between the ages of 40 and 60 years (15,000 new cases a year)
   b. Several risk factors of cervical cancer are as follows:
      (1). Women who began having sexual intercourse before 18 years of age
      (2). Women who have had multiple sexual partners
      (3). Women whose mothers were given diethylstilbestrol (DES) during pregnancy
      (4). History of smoking
   c. In addition, oral contraceptives are implicated, and some research indicates viruses may play a role such as genital herpes and papillomaviruses
   d. Dysplasia and early cervical cancer seldom cause symptoms; they can only be detected by a pelvic exam and a Papanicolaou (Pap) smear
   e. Pain is not an early warning sign of the disease; symptoms generally do not appear until cervical cancer becomes invasive; signs and symptoms of cancer of the cervix are as follows:
      (1). Abnormal bleeding (the most common sign): Bleeding may start and stop between regular menstrual periods, or it may occur after sexual intercourse, douching, or a pelvic exam; menstrual bleeding may last longer and be heavier than usual
      (2). Increased vaginal discharge

PLEASE NOTE: These symptoms are not sure signs of cancer; however, it is important for a woman to be referred to a gynecologist if any symptom lasts longer than 2 weeks.

   f. Diagnosis: If the pelvic exam or the Pap smear shows any abnormality, further testing is indicated; when a vaginal infection is the suspected cause of an abnormal Pap smear, the infection is treated and then the Pap smear is repeated; if an infection is not the reason for the abnormal Pap smear, a biopsy is done; additional tests include the following:
      (1). Schiller test: an iodine solution is applied to the cervix and healthy cells turn brown; abnormal cells turn white or yellow
      (2). A colposcope is used to visualize the cervix and biopsy abnormal tissue
      (3). Conization (cone biopsy) or dilatation and curettage (D&C) are used when larger samples of tissue are needed to make a diagnosis; in a conization, a cone-shaped piece of tissue is removed from the cervix and cervical canal. In a D&C, the cervix is dilated and a curette is inserted to scrape tissue from the cervical canal and the lining of the uterus
   g. Staging procedures include the following:
      (1). A physical exam that is done under anesthesia
      (2). Blood and urine tests
      (3). A chest x-ray film
      (4). Because cancer of the cervix can spread to the bladder, colon, and rectum, special exams of those areas may also be requested

6. Ovarian cancer[1,2,6,7,43,970]
   a. Ovarian cancer is diagnosed in approximately 20,000 women each year
   b. The risk factors for developing this cancer are as follows:
      (1). Women who have had breast cancer (twice the risk of women who have not had breast cancer)

(2). Women who have never been pregnant are at greater risk and the more often a woman has been pregnant, the less likely she is to acquire ovarian cancer

(3). Women with a positive family history are more likely to acquire this cancer, whereas a woman who uses oral contraceptives is less likely to do so

c. Ovarian cancer is difficult to detect because cancer limited to the ovary usually does not cause symptoms; a tumor in the ovary can grow for some time before it causes pressure, pain, or other problems; even when symptoms appear, they may be so vague that they are ignored; symptoms of ovarian cancer, in order of decreasing occurrence, are as follows:

(1). Swelling
(2). Bloating
(3). Discomfort in the lower abdomen
(4). Loss of appetite and a feeling of fullness, even after a light meal
(5). Gas
(6). Indigestion
(7). Nausea
(8). Weight loss
(9). Constipation and frequent urination as the tumor grows and compresses nearby organs such as the bowel and bladder
(10). Fluid buildup in the abdomen (ascites) from ovarian cancer that has spread to other parts of the abdomen may result in swelling and discomfort
(11). Bleeding from the vagina can be a symptom of ovarian cancer

PLEASE NOTE: These symptoms may be caused by cancer or by other, less serious conditions, and patients should be diagnosed and treated as early as possible.

d. Diagnosis: Physical exam includes a pelvic exam; the vagina, rectum, and lower abdomen are palpated for masses or growths; a Pap smear may be done as part of the regular exam, but it is not a reliable way to diagnose ovarian cancer; diagnostic tests are listed next:

(1). Ultrasonogram

(2). CT scan
(3). Lower GI series or barium enema
(4). IVP

e. The only sure way to know whether cancer is present is examination of a biopsy

f. To obtain the tissue, the entire affected ovary is removed because, if the problem is cancer, cutting through the outer layer of the ovary can cause spread of the disease

g. In addition, the second ovary, the uterus, and the fallopian tubes are nearly always removed if the biopsy is positive for cancer

h. The cancer is staged by sampling nearby lymph nodes, the diaphragm, and fluid from the abdomen to determine whether the cancer has spread

i. Careful staging is needed to determine the extent of the cancer so that follow-up treatment can be planned

6. Cancer of the uterus[1,2,6,7,43,243,369,370]

a. Uterine cancer accounts for 13% of all cancers in women and occurs most often in women between the ages of 55 and 75 years (this represents approximately 31,000 new cases a year in addition to the 15,000 new cases of cancer of the cervix)

b. Cancer of the uterus does not often occur before menopause, but it does occur around the time menopause begins

c. The reappearance of bleeding should not be considered simply part of menopause.

d. Risk factors for uterine cancer include the following:

(1). Obesity
(2). Women with few or no children
(3). Women who began menstruating at a young age
(4). Women who had a late menopause
(5). Women of high socioeconomic status

e. Most of the risk appears related to excess estrogen, with the highest risk occurring with at least 2 to 4 years of use of estrogen replacement therapy (ERT) and large-dose therapy

f. Abnormal bleeding after menopause is the most common symptom of cancer of the uterus; bleeding may begin as a watery, blood-streaked discharge; later, the discharge may contain more blood; abnormal bleeding is not always a sign of cancer, and referral should be made because that is the only way to determine the problem

g. Early diagnosis is especially important for cancer of the uterus

h. Diagnosis: One or more of the following exams are conducted for diagnosis:

(1). Pelvic exam: Thorough examination of the uterus, vagina, ovaries, bladder, and rectum; palpation of these organs for any abnormality in shape or size; a speculum is used to widen the opening of the vagina so that the upper portion of the vagina and the cervix can be examined

(2). Biopsy

(3). D&C

(4). Pap smear (not a reliable test for uterine cancer because it cannot always detect abnormal cells from endometrium)

i. If cancer cells are found, other tests are used to determine whether the disease has spread from the uterus to other parts of the body, including the following:

(1). Blood tests

(2). Chest x-ray films

(3). CT scan of the abdomen

(4). Ultrasonogram

(5). Patients also may have exams of the bladder, colon, and rectum

E. GI cancers. Cancer of the digestive organs accounts for approximately 233,000 new cases of cancer a year. Colorectal cancer alone accounts for over half of all newly diagnosed cases, approximately 149,000 cases a year.

Stomach and pancreatic cancer accounts for 24,000 and 27,000 new cases a year, respectively. (Esophageal cancer—see "Head and Neck Cancer.")

1. Cancer of the colon and rectum[1,2,6,7,152, 238,244,247,429,430]

a. Occur most often in persons older than 40 years and are one of the most common cancers in the aged

b. Risk factors include the following:

(1). Positive family history, especially of familial polyposis

(2). Diets high in fat (diets high in fiber appear to reduce risk)

(3). Residence in urban, industrialized areas

c. When an illness affects the colon or rectum, a number of symptoms occur, including the following:

(1). Diarrhea or constipation

(2). Blood in or on the stool

(3). Stools that are narrower than usual

(4). General stomach discomfort (bloating, fullness, cramps)

(5). Frequent gas pains

(6). A feeling that a bowel does not empty completely

(7). Loss of weight for no known reason

(8). Constant fatigue

d. These symptoms can be caused by a number of problems such as the flu, ulcers, an inflamed colon, or cancer

PLEASE NOTE: If any of these symptoms lasts as long as 2 weeks, the patient should be referred to a physician.

e. Early diagnosis is especially important for cancer of the colon and rectum

f. Liver metastases are a sign of advanced cancer from the GI tract such as colon, rectal, stomach, and pancreatic cancers secondary to the liver receiving venous drainage from the GI tract

g. Diagnosis: Exams frequently used in diagnosis are as follows:

(1). Rectal exam

(2). Proctoscopy: sigmoidoscope is inserted into the rectum to examine the rectum and the lower end of the colon; some scopes are rigid; others are flexible, allowing the physician to see higher up in the colon; about 50% of colon and rectal cancers can be found by a proctoscopic exam

(3). Lab tests such as a stool sample to determine whether there is blood in the stool

(4). Colonoscopy to see the entire length of the colon; if an abnormal growth is found, the physician will remove a biopsy sample for examination or, in many cases, use the colonoscope to remove the whole growth

(5). Lower GI series or barium enema

F. Respiratory cancers. (Laryngeal cancer—see "Head and Neck Cancer.")

1. Lung cancers[1,2,6,7,65,87,147,150,151,257,286,344–362,379,431,432]

a. Lung cancer remains the leading cause of cancer death in the U.S. adult population, and the American Cancer Society estimates that cigarette smoking is responsible for about 83% of all lung cancer cases[1]
b. Approximately 152,000 cases of lung cancer are diagnosed annually[1]
c. The risk factors identified to date are as follows:
   (1). Cigarette smoking (causes about 85% lung cancer deaths)
   (2). Work-related hazards
   (3). Air pollution
   (4). Other environmental factors such as asbestos exposure
d. Significant reductions in incidence and mortality associated with lung cancer unlikely without effective antismoking campaigns
e. Coronary artery disease, emphysema, and lung cancer often occur together and have cigarette smoking as a common etiological contributor[432]
f. Lung cancer is usually divided into two types: small-cell lung cancer (oat cell, SCLC) and non–small-cell lung cancer (NSCLC) such as squamous cell carcinoma, adenocarcinoma, and large-cell carcinoma
   (1). SCLC occurs in about 20% to 25% of all cases, is rapidly growing, spreads early to other organs and adjacent tissues, including bronchial, mediastinal, and hilar lymph nodes, and is usually found in persons who are heavy smokers; approximately 70% of patients have extensive disease at diagnosis; SCLC is responsive to combination chemotherapy regimens; although many different agents are effective in this disease, most SCLCs eventually become refractory to chemotherapy and most patients do not survive longer than 2 years
   (2). The three main types of NSCLC are as follows:
      (a). Epidermoid or squamous cell carcinoma occurs in about 33% of all cases and is the most common type of lung cancer, is slower to spread usually originating in the bronchi

      (b). Adenocarcinoma occurs in about 25% of all cases, growing in the periphery of the lungs and under the tissue lining the bronchi
      (c). Large-cell carcinomas occur in about 16% of all cases, most often originating in the small bronchi
g. At present NSCLC is generally curable only if it is diagnosed while the tumor is small and localized and can be surgically removed
h. Pulmonary metastases are the most common of all metastatic tumors secondary to venous return to the heart and then circulated through the lungs
i. Early diagnosis is again important in lung cancers
j. Although progress has been made in the understanding and management of lung cancer, effective therapies that consistently produce effective responses are still lacking (see section on treatment)
k. Lung cancer causes a number of signs and symptoms, usually in the latter stages:
   (1). Extrapulmonary signs, such as lower extremity weakness, and fatigue, loss of appetite, loss of weight
   (2). Cough is likely to occur when a tumor grows and blocks a bronchiole
   (3). Chest pain, which feels like a constant ache that may or may not be related to coughing
   (4). Dyspnea (shortness of breath) and wheezing
   (5). Repeated pneumonia or bronchitis
   (6). Coughing up blood
   (7). Hoarseness
   (8). Swelling of the neck and face
l. Additional extrapulmonary signs and symptoms do not appear to be related to the lungs; these may be caused by the spread of lung cancer to other parts of the body; depending on which organs are affected, symptoms can include the following:
   (1). Headache
   (2). Weakness and fatigue
   (3). Pain
   (4). Pathological fractures
   (5). Bleeding
   (6). Thrombi and emboli

(7). Loss of appetite

(8). Insomnia

m. Sometimes symptoms may be caused by hormones that are produced by the cancer cells such as a sharp drop in the level of sodium in the body and quadriceps weakness[291]

n. Decrease in sodium level can produce many symptoms, including confusion and sometimes even coma; pain and fatigue frequently occur as comorbidities[344]

o. Concurrent respiratory disease, previous chemotherapy, recurrent lung cancer, no surgical treatment, and low income were associated with a high level of symptom distress in a sample of 69 women with lung cancer;[344] treatment was not a significant factor relating to distress because distress was strongly correlated to quality of life and functional status; poverty-level income was a weak predictor of distress among demographical and disease/treatment variables, accounting for 17% of the variance; combined with recurrence, the model accounted for 26% of the variance

PLEASE NOTE: The symptoms related to lung cancer may be caused by a number of problems and are not a sure sign of cancer; however, patients should be referred to a physician if any of these symptoms lasts as long as 2 weeks.

p. Diagnosis: A routine exam and work histories and chest x-ray films are the first steps followed by needle biopsy, surgery, or other methods; additional tests include the following:

(1). Lung tomogram

(2). CT scan (useful in determining whether the tumor spread from the lung to other parts of the chest or more distant organs such as the brain or liver)

(3). Bronchoscopy (visualization of the breathing passages through a thin, hollow, lighted tube inserted through the patient's nose or mouth into the lung; cells may be collected from the bronchial walls or a biopsy sample taken)

(4). Needle aspiration biopsy guided by fluoroscopy (new procedure used to collect cells that are difficult to reach with the bronchoscope; fluoroscopy is an x-ray test that uses a television screen so that internal organs, such as the heart, can be viewed while they are in motion; using the picture on the screen as a guide, a needle is inserted into the tumor to withdraw cells for examination)

(5). Mediastinoscopy (incision in the chest) may be used to determine whether cancer cells have spread to lymph nodes in the mediastinum

(6). Mediastinotomy is similar to mediastinoscopy, except the incision is made in another part of the chest

(7). Scans to locate lung cancer cells that may have spread to the brain, bone, or liver

G. Hematological cancers

PLEASE NOTE: Many of the hematological cancers are being cured by or in clinical trials for treatment by bone marrow transplant (BMT)[74,78,80,82,117,292,342,434-437]

1. Lymphomas[1-4]

a. Lymphomas account for about 3% of all cancers

(1). Hodgkin's disease[90,91,95,98,425]

(a). Rare (less than 1% of all cancers) and occur most often between the ages of 15 and 34 years and after 55 years

(b). Approximately 8000 cases are diagnosed annually; more than 75% of newly diagnosed cases are curable because of treatment advances in radiation and chemotherapy

(c). As lymphomas progress, the body is less able to fight infection, and opportunistic infections occur such as herpes zoster and *Pneumocystis carinii*

(d). Viral transmission and infection, family history, and genetics have been linked to possible risk of disease, although the cause of Hodgkin's lymphoma is unknown

(e). Signs and symptoms of Hodgkin's disease are as follows:
  (i). Painless swelling in the lymph nodes in the neck, underarm, or groin (most common signs)
  (ii). Fevers
  (iii). Night sweats
  (iv). Fatigue
  (v). Weight loss
  (vi). Itching skin

PLEASE NOTE: These symptoms are not sure signs of cancer and may also be caused by many common illnesses, such as flu, or other infections, such as TB. The patient should be referred to a physician if any of these symptoms lasts longer than 2 weeks.

(f). Diagnosis: If Hodgkin's disease is suspected, diagnostic tests include the following:
  (i). X-ray films of the chest, bones, liver, and spleen
  (ii). Biopsy of an enlarged lymph node to look for presence of Reed-Sternberg cells (abnormal cells that are usually found with Hodgkin's disease)
(g). When Hodgkin's disease is diagnosed, staging is conducted by determining the following:
  (i). Number and location of affected lymph nodes
  (ii). Whether the affected lymph nodes are above, below, or on both sides of the diaphragm
  (iii). Whether the disease has spread to the bone marrow or to places outside the lymphatic system, such as the liver
(h). In staging, the tests include the following:
  (i). Biopsies of the lymph nodes, liver, and bone marrow
  (ii). Lymphangiograms, x-ray films of the lymphatic system
  (iii). CT scans
  (iv). Ultrasonography

(2). Non-Hodgkin's lymphoma (NHL)[1-4]
  (a). There are at least 10 types of NHL; about 45,000 cases diagnosed annually; these are the most common hematological cancers
  (b). Often they are grouped by how fast they grow: low grade (slow growing, accounting for 40% of cases), intermediate grade (accounting for 40%–45% of cases), and high grade (rapidly growing, accounting for 15%–20% of cases)
  (c). NHL tends to occur later in life, with 25% of the cases diagnosed between the ages of 50 and 59 years, peaking in incidence between 60 and 69 years of age
  (d). Men are at a slightly greater risk than women
  (e). Most relapses occur within 2 years of treatment, leading to approximately 13,000 deaths per year
  (f). Chronic immunosuppressive therapy in organ transplants was linked to lymphocytic cancers
  (g). Signs and symptoms include the following:
    (i). Painless swelling in the lymph nodes in the neck, underarm, or groin (most common sign)
    (ii). Fevers and night sweats
    (iii). Fatigue
    (iv). Weight loss
    (v). Itching and reddened patches on skin
    (vi). Nausea, vomiting, or abdominal pain sometimes present

PLEASE NOTE: As with Hodgkin's disease, these symptoms are not sure signs of cancer and may also be caused by many common illnesses, such as the flu or other infections. Patients should be referred to a physician if any of these symptoms lasts longer than 2 weeks.

(h). Diagnosis: See prior section on Hodgkin's disease

2. Multiple myeloma[1,2,6,7]
   a. Approximately 12,000 cases of multiple myeloma diagnosed each year
   b. Often occurs in persons 50 to 70 years of age and men more often than women; 90% of cases occur after age 40.
   c. Prognosis poor; disease is a lymphoproliferative disorder of plasma cells
   d. Risk factors include the following:
      (1). Positive family history
      (2). Exposure to chemicals in the petroleum industry
      (3). Exposure to large amounts of radiation
   e. Symptoms of multiple myeloma depend on how advanced the disease is; in earliest stage, there may be no symptoms; symptoms and signs include the following:
      (1). Bone pain, often in the back or ribs (most common symptom secondary to osteolytic lesions with frequent fracture)
      (2). Pathological fracture with spinal cord compression with pain
      (3). Hypercalcemia
      (4). Fatigue and weakness
      (5). Weight loss
      (6). Repeated infections secondary to leukopenia, such as pneumonia
   f. When the disease is advanced, symptoms may include the following:
      (1). Nausea and vomiting
      (2). Constipation
      (3). Problems with urination and urinary tract infections and renal failure
      (4). Weakness or numbness in the legs
      (5). Signs of increased blood viscosity such as headache, drowsiness, irritability, visual disturbances, anginal pain, congestive heart failure
      (6). Coagulation disorders
      (7). Carpal tunnel syndrome

PLEASE NOTE: These are not sure signs of multiple myeloma; they can be symptoms of other types of medical problems, and a patient should be referred to a physician.

   g. Diagnosis
      (1). Multiple myeloma may be found as part of a routine physical exam before patients have symptoms of the disease

      (2). When patients do have symptoms, a number of tests to determine the cause of these symptoms are performed, including the following:
         (a). X-ray films if a patient has bone pain
         (b). Blood and urine tests are examined for high levels of antibody proteins called M proteins
         (c). Bone marrow needle aspiration and/or a bone marrow biopsy to check for myeloma cells
         (d). Biopsy using a larger gauge needle to remove a sample of solid tissue from the marrow
3. Leukemia[1,2–4,6,7,58,72–74,78,80,82,117,292,316,342,434–437]
   a. Generalized proliferative disorder of white blood cell production in which abnormal white blood cells accumulate in the blood and bone marrow; approximately 28,500 new cases a year
   b. In children, cells appear suddenly in the same bone marrow that previously formed only normal, healthy, mature white cells
   c. Cause of leukemia is unknown; however, genetic and immunological factors, viral factors, and radiation exposure are implicated
   d. Leading cause of cancer deaths in young males aged 15 to 34 years
   e. Most significant improvement in survival rates, however, has been in childhood cancers such as acute lymphocytic leukemia (ALL; also named acute lymphatic leukemia and acute lymphoblastic leukemia); approximately 12,500 new cases a year
      (i). ALL is primary type of leukemia affecting children, accounting for about 83% of all pediatric leukemia cases; its onset is quick and severe in children compared with most adult leukemias, in which the onset is slow and insidious; abnormal cells resemble lymphocytes
      (ii). Acute myelocytic leukemia (also named acute granulocytic or myelogenous leukemia or acute non-lymphoblastic leukemia) occurs less commonly, in approximately 8000 adults per year and 15% of cases of pediatric leukemia per year

f. This leukemia has a poor prognosis greater than 5 years and involves neutrophils

g. Chronic myelogenous leukemia is rare before the age of 20 years and increasing with age

h. It is a translocation defect on the long arm of chromosome 22, which leads to proliferation of myeloid precursors and cells

i. Men have a greater incidence than women, and initially the disease may be stable and then transform to a more aggressive disease.

j. Although acute myelocytic leukemia, chronic lymphocytic leukemia, and chronic myelocytic leukemia are occasionally seen in children, they primarily appear in adults and, therefore, are much less common and are not discussed here

k. Signs and symptoms of acute lymphocytic leukemia in the early stages are identical to those that accompany many common childhood diseases; some are even less specific and resemble the day-to-day fluctuations in energy level; fatigue and malaise, change in appetite and temperament, and headache are seen in healthy children

l. During early stages, it may be difficult to identify the condition as anything more than one of the many minor illnesses that children always seem to be passing through

m. Usual presentation with acute leukemia in children, however, is that it appears suddenly and progresses rapidly as follows:
 (1). Lymph nodes, spleen, testicles, and liver become infiltrated with white blood cells and may be enlarged with abdominal discomfort
 (2). Bone and joint pain (common symptom)
 (3). Cyanosis
 (4). Bleeding disorders indicated by a tendency to bleed or bruise on the arms and legs easily, bleed from the gums or nose, or have tiny red dots on the skin
 (5). Frequent infections
 (6). Occasionally leukemic meningitis or CNS disease with signs and symptoms such as headache, diplopia

and papilledema, cranial nerve palsy, and changes in mental status

n. Diagnosis
 (1). Can be diagnosed only by microscopic examination of the blood and the bone marrow
 (2). If abnormal white cells characteristic of leukemia are present, they can be identified and the diagnosis made
 (3). Additional signs on the blood test are low hemoglobin concentrations, low white cell counts with a particular paucity of granulocytes, an increase in lymphocytes, and a low platelet level
 (4). Blast cells may also be present in the blood
 (5). Because these findings suggest leukemia, a bone marrow biopsy may be done; the biopsy establishes the specific type of leukemia, which is essential in determining the best form of treatment; it is also later used as a measure of the progress of therapy
 (6). ALL has three subtypes (L1, L2, L3) based on a cytological classification system, with 85% of ALL of the L1 subtype

o. CNS involvement
 (1). Possible cause of treatment failure in leukemia is the tendency of leukemic cells to accumulate in the brain; here, because of properties of the blood vessel walls, "blood-brain barrier," chemotherapeutic drugs cannot generally penetrate CNS
 (2). Leukemic cells may be reactively safe from chemical attack
 (3). In the past, approximately 75% of children with ALL eventually had infiltration of the CNS with leukemia cells; in about 25% the CNS served as the primary site of relapse
 (4). For this reason, patients with this disease are now being treated early, before CNS symptoms appear, with drugs administered directly into the spinal fluid and in some cases with radiation therapy to the brain as well, with a 90% to 95% crisis remission rate

VII. Medical Treatment

PLEASE NOTE: Most of the treatments for cancer are aggressive such as chemotherapy, radiotherapy, and biological therapy. The side effects during cancer treatment vary for each person. Fortunately, most side effects are temporary and resolve gradually after therapy is discontinued.

A. Goals of medical treatment[69,267,326,337]

1. Cure
2. Control
3. Palliation
4. Prophylaxis

B. Sequence of medical treatment (determined by type, location of primary tumor, grade and stage)

1. Primary
2. Salvage (for recurrent disease)
3. Adjuvant (in addition to primary therapy)

C. Surgical management[65,66,69,86,87,103–106,152,157,359,186,257,307–311,318,323,325,327–331,334,336,338,340,341,354–359,372,375]

1. Local: Optimal for slow-growing tumors; impairments and loss of function relate directly to the extent of tissue or organ resected such as a wide excision to resect rhabdomyosarcoma of the vastus lateralis, requiring an orthotic to assist in stabilizing the knee
   a. Local excision
   b. Block dissection
      (1). En bloc, debulking, radical
      (2). Extended (wide excision)
   c. Limb salvage (see musculoskeletal tumors)[340,376]
2. Curative, palliative (for the patient with incurable disease), preventive/prophylactic (ablative), and reconstructive surgery
3. Diagnostic surgical techniques (see biopsy previously discussed[324])
4. Complications (Tables 4–7 and 4–10): physical and psychological complications common to any surgical procedure and the following: bed rest or reduced activity such as postsurgical incision pain, DVTs, impaired wound healing, phantom sensation or lymphedema, and impairment and loss of function related to tissue or organ resection
   a. Psychosocial effects such as changes in appearance with amputation

D. Radiation therapy[42,61,69,73,90–95,97,98,149,201,257,267,271–273,275,282,287,299,302–306,312–314,326,333,397,339,363,381,399,403,407–411,416,417,422,423,428,445]

1. An estimated 50% of all Americans with cancer will receive radiation therapy during their disease
2. Radiation at high levels destroys the ability of cells to grow and divide
3. Both normal cells and cancer cells are affected, but most normal cells are able to recover quickly
4. During radiation therapy, the side effects that patients notice most often are unusual fatigue, especially in the latter weeks of treatment, and skin reactions in the area being treated
5. This is usually a local treatment without systemic effects unless the tissue or organ in the treatment area is severely impaired
   a. Delivery of radiotherapy and blocking (locoregional, total body irradiation, internal or external [most common form of delivering radiotherapy since 1960s])
      (1). Internal radiation therapy: patient must be hospitalized to have radioactive materials implanted; implant may be temporary or permanent; because radiation is most active during hospital stay, patient may not be able to have visitors or may have visitors for only a short time
      (2). External radiation therapy is usually given 5 days a week for 5 to 6 weeks; this schedule helps protect normal tissue by spreading out the total dose of radiation; patient does not need to stay in the hospital for external radiation therapy
      (3). For tumors close to vital organs, such as the heart or liver, high-dose radiation therapy may be difficult because of the risk of damaging these organs; a new technique, intraoperative radiation therapy, is being studied as a solution to this problem; radiation is delivered through a specially designed cone-shaped device during surgery when vital organs can be moved out of range
   b. Radiation terminology (i.e., types of radiation): At cancer centers, new forms of radiation therapy are being compared

Table 4–10. GUIDELINES FOR PT PROGRAM, EXERCISE PRESCRIPTON, AND LEVEL OF ACTIVITY FOR PATIENTS WITH CANCER

Goals	Palliation and Support	Support and Restoration	Restoration and Prevention
Restrictions	Severe	Moderate	Mild to none
Platelet counts	<5000–10,000/mm³ No antigravity exercise No resistive exercise	10,000–20,000/mm³ Active ROM Submax isometrics Isotonic—light weights No prolonged stretching No heavy resistive exercise No low-speed isokinetics	>20,000/mm³ Most programs OK
Hct/Hb	<25%/8 g/dl	>25%/8–10 g/dl	>25%/>10 g/dl
WBC	<500/mm³ and fever ROM No aerobics Submax isometrics No isotonics	>500/mm³ Low-impact and intensity aerobics (bike ergometer) Isometrics Modified isotonic	>500/mm³ Most programs OK
PFTs	>50% capacity Light aerobic	50%–75% Low-intensity aerobics	>75% Most programs OK
Metastatic* or bone tumor	>50% cortex eroded No exercise Non–weight-bearing*	25%–50% cortex eroded ROM (no stretching) PWB* to FWB Submax isometrics	0–25% cortex eroded Most programs OK FWB Maximal isometrics Low-impact aerobics
Osteoporosis*	Severe: ROM	Moderate: Submaximal isometrics Light isotonics	Mild: Most exercise OK
ECG	Recent PVCs Fast atrial arrhythmia Ventricular arrhythmia Ischemic pattern	No exercise	Consult cardiologist
Chest x-ray film	Large pleural effusions Pericardial effusions Multiple metastasis	ROM and submaximal isometrics	Consult pulmonary specialist/cardiologist, primary care physician Consult internist before exercise
K + /NA	Na+ below 130 K + 3.0 or below		
Osmolality	Low serum osmolality		

* Note that if the site of bony metastasis or severe osteoporosis is stabilized, these precautions are modified.
Abbreviations: ROM = range of motion; Hct = hematocrit; Hb = hemoglobin; WBC = white blood cell; PFT = pulmonary function tests; PWB = partial weight bearing; FWB = full weight bearing; PVC = premature ventricular contractions.

with standard radiation treatment (cobalt-60 gamma rays, electron beams from a linear accelerator, and so on); two new forms are neutron-beam therapy and heavy-particle therapy, which use neutrons or ions stripped from individual atoms; known as atomic particles, these neutrons or ions are beamed into a patient's body, where they break apart the atoms in tumor cells, destroying the cells

c. Radiosensitivity of tumors: Radiosensitizers, substances that can make cancer cells more sensitive to the effects of radiation therapy, also are being investigated

d. Indications for and goals of radiation therapy

(1). Cure: radiation therapy is used in some cases both before and after surgery to shrink a tumor preoperatively and improve the chances for successful surgery and postoperatively to destroy cancer cells that remain in the area; adjuvant radiation therapy and chemotherapy are used in addition to surgery to treat Stage III and IV tumors

(2). Control: when a tumor cannot be removed surgically, well-planned, high-dose radiation therapy may be able to control the primary tumor

(3). Palliative (*ie*, bony metastasis, spinal cord compression, symptoms from brain metastasis, and tumor obstructions)

(4). Prophylactic radiation therapy to

prevent metastatic spread of the tumor

e. Combined approaches, *ie,* radiation therapy and surgery or chemotherapy

PLEASE NOTE: Protective skin care is important for these patients. It is common for the skin in the treated area to become red or dry. The skin should be exposed to the air but protected from the sun, and patients should avoid wearing clothes that rub the area. During radiation therapy, hair usually does not grow in the treated area. If it does, for example on the face, men should not shave. Patients are shown how to keep the area clean. They should not put anything on the skin before their radiation treatments, and they should not use any lotion or cream at other times without approval from their physician.

f. Side effects of radiation on normal tissue in field of treatment: increased risk of sunburn, irritation, fibrosis (see Tables 4–7 and 4–10) (The National Cancer Institute [NCI] booklets *Radiation Therapy and You* and *Eating Hints* have helpful information about cancer treatment and coping with side effects)[438]
   (1). Acute and chronic local effects in irradiated field and adjacent tissue are dependent on the following:
      (a). Type of radiation
      (b). Area of field exposure
      (c). Length of time of exposure/total cumulative exposure
   (2). Acute and chronic systemic effects (organ and tissue such as connective and epithelial tissue changes, *ie,* skin, hair, and mucosal membranes, bone marrow aplasia, neurological, metabolic and endocrine, and cardiopulmonary changes); other examples of complications include radiation myelopathy and burns or mucositis often with secondary infection
   (3). Genetic effects
   (4). Late carcinogenic effects, which are greater with combined therapies, such as pulmonary interstitial fibrosis, which may develop over 2 years after treatment has been discontinued; fibrosis around nerves such as the brachial, lumbar, and sacral plexus often appears 8 months to 3 years after treatment
   (5). Psychosocial effects such as changes

in appearance with alopecia (hair loss)

g. Low-level radiation: *Safety Measures and Low-Level Radiation Exposure,* from American Cancer Society, reviews low-level radiation exposure

E. Chemotherapy[10,36,39,64,68,69,71–85,94,96,97,99,124,143,147, 168,191,201,257,267,271,274,315,321,326,337,339,360,361,380,399,439]

Chemotherapy means treatment with drugs that usually have a systemic effect. It is used to attempt to destroy cancer cells that have spread beyond the original, local tumor.

1. Methods and routes of administration: A Hickman catheter is used for long-term intravenous administration; some researchers are testing another method, regional chemotherapy, for control of local disease, which involves giving drugs through a major blood vessel in the region of the tumor; in this way, a more concentrated dose can be directed to the area of the tumor
2. Indications: regional and systemic disease; chemotherapy is administered before and after surgery and is used in combination with radiation therapy
3. Goals of treatment
   a. Cure
   b. Control: chemotherapy also being explored in cases in which the tumor cannot be completely removed surgically
   c. Palliative
   d. Prophylactic therapy
4. Normal cell cycle and effects on cell growth
   a. In general, chemotherapy affects rapidly growing and dividing cells, such as hair follicles, mucosal cells, epidermal cells, and hemopoietic cells, resulting in hair loss, skin or mucosal membrane thinning, irritation or ulceration, nausea, vomiting, loss of appetite, anemia, fatigue, and decreased resistance to infection
   b. Cells that are slower dividing will present with symptoms later during the course of treatment such as renal and neural cells, resulting in kidney damage and paresthesia, tinea, and difficulty hearing
   c. Cells that are even slower to divide can present as symptoms after chemotherapy is completed

5. Side effects tend to be systemic (see Tables 4–7 and 4–10) (The NCI booklets *Chemotherapy and You* and *Eating Hints* have helpful information about cancer treatment and coping with side effects)[439]
   a. Early
      (1). Local (infusion site may have phlebitis or extravasation at injection site when given intravenously, intrathecally, or by Hickman catheter)
      (2). Systemic (dependent on extent of impairment of organ and tissue function such as acute and chronic weakness and fatigue secondary to anemia, hypoxia, and myopathy or psychological changes may involve any of the tissues or organ systems (see Tables 4–7 and 4–10); these effects may include steroid pseudorheumatism secondary to withdrawal of steroids, including myalgia, arthralgia, joint effusion, exaggerated neurological symptoms, and occasional fever, aseptic necrosis of the femoral or humeral heads with steroid therapy; mucositis; polyneuropathy secondary to agents such as vincristine, vinblastine, or procarbazine; or cardiomyopathy secondary to agents such as doxorubicin (Adriamycin) or daunorubicin
   b. Late, such as pulmonary fibrosis or secondary malignancy
6. Contraindications/precautions based on family of drugs' side effects, single-drug agent use, high-dose therapy, and total cumulative dose
7. Classification of anticancer agents (specific or nonspecific)
8. Families of drugs (alkylating agents, nitrosoureas, antimetabolites, antibiotics, hormonal and antihormonal agents such as tamoxifen or antiestrogen agents [see Biological Response Modifiers], corticosteroid agents, plant alkaloids, miscellaneous agents): drugs from the same family will tend to have similar side effects
9. Combination chemotherapy to achieve a greater patient response at a lower toxicity rate and to reduce potential problems of drug resistance; combinations of chemotherapeutic agents from different families of drugs or drug mechanisms of action are given in varying courses separated by rest periods
10. Adjuvant chemotherapy in addition to other treatments is used when regional spread of a tumor is suspected to prevent cancer cell growth and metastasis

F. Therapy with blood products[286,303,315,316,434,437]

1. Purpose is to support absolute and relative hemopoietic cells and concentrations
   a. Plateletpheresis is a technique in which platelets are removed from normal whole blood by centrifugation and the red blood cells are returned to the donor or patient promptly; an individual may be able to donate platelets as frequently as twice a week for periods up to 3 months (in contrast, donors can give whole blood only once every 6 to 8 weeks)
      (1). Transfusions of blood platelets have proved effective in preventing or stopping hemorrhage
      (2). Plateletpheresis enables a single adult donor, often a parent or other family member, to provide the major portion of the platelets required by a child with leukemia
      (3). Use of platelet transfusions has reduced the occurrence of hemorrhage during the last decade, making it possible to use effective chemotherapeutic agents even though platelet production is depressed
      (4). Patients may become resistant to platelets obtained from persons of different platelet histocompatibility "types"; when this occurs, the donated platelets are rapidly destroyed, and the patient is in danger of hemorrhage
      (5). Fortunately, platelets can be typed according to a histocompatibility system (human lymphocyte antigen [HLA]), and HLA-matched platelets often survive normally in patients who have become resistant to nonmatched platelets; HLA typing can frequently identify a suitable donor
      (6). Platelets obtained from a patient (while in remission) can be frozen and reinfused during relapse; these platelets are often effective when

the patient is resistant to random donor platelets

b. Granulocyte (white blood cell) replacement: the success achieved with platelet transfusion prompted the attempt to treat infection in leukemia patients

    (1). Granulocyte transfusions are given with beneficial effects to some patients with bacterial infections, but it has been difficult to obtain these cells in adequate amounts from normal blood donations

    (2). A continuous-flow centrifuge was developed to increase the availability of granulocytes; the centrifuge is used to separate granulocytes from other blood elements, which are returned to the donor

    (3). It is possible to obtain as many granulocytes from one normal donor at one sitting as are contained in 30 to 40 units of blood collected by standard methods; investigators have shown that a suitable donor can effectively support the granulocyte levels of otherwise granulocytopenic patients (patients with a deficiency of granulocytes in the blood) for several weeks, and that repeated white blood cell transfusions to certain infected granulocytopenic patients permit control of infection

    (4). Simpler methods of procuring granulocytes for transfusion are being developed

2. Side effects include constitutional symptoms, fever, nausea, fluid overload, transfusion reactions, and so on

G. Biological response modifiers (immunotherapy/hormonal therapy)[44,88,337,364,430,439]

1. Indications: regional and systemic disease
   a. Hormone therapy is used to prevent cancer cells from receiving the hormones they need to grow
   b. These agents are used when a tumor is hormone sensitive as indicated by being receptor positive, such as breast and prostate tumors
   c. Immunotherapy is the use of agents to try and boost or enhance immune surveillance functions
   d. Biological response modifiers (BRM) include tamoxifen, DES, interferon (IFN),

interleukin-2 (IL-2), tumor necrosis factor (TNF), colony-stimulating factors (CSF), and bacille Calmette-Guérin (BCG); many of these agents are in use in ongoing clinical trials

2. Route of administration is orally or intravenously; can have infusion site complications

3. Side effects tend to be systemic and constitutional, flulike symptoms such as the following (see musculoskeletal-soft-tissue sarcomas and reactions to and side effects of treatment, Tables 4–7 and 4–10):
   a. Chills
   b. Fever
   c. Muscle aches
   d. Weakness and fatigue are common
   e. Loss of appetite, nausea, vomiting, or diarrhea
   f. Rash with dry, itching skin in some patients

PLEASE NOTE: In addition, IL-2 can cause the patient to retain fluid. These problems can be severe, and most patients having biological therapy must stay in the hospital so that the effects of their treatment can be monitored.

H. Hyperthermia and treatment indications

1. Not a physical therapy therapeutic heat modality; intended to kill target cells[399,411,423,440–444]

2. Clinical studies showing heat to be effective in treating cancer in humans

3. Given at an intensity and duration of heat needed to kill cancer cells

4. Heat is an important adjunct to conventional radiotherapy and chemotherapy in cancer treatment

5. Several types of heat modalities are used in cancer treatment such as ultrasonography and diathermy

I. New technologies for treatment

1. BMT[72–74,78,80,82,117,292,342,434–437,460] (see discussion of hematopoietic tumors)

2. Limb salvaging[340,374,376,519] (see discussion of musculoskeletal tumors)

3. BRM (see prior discussion of BRM, TNF, IL-2, and so on)

4. Electricity is being explored for use in treating cancer using a similar approach to that used in hyperthermia

VIII. Medical Treatment of Specific Cancers

A. Musculoskeletal tumors

Treatment for musculoskeletal tumors such as bone tumors, soft-tissue sarcomas, and breast, head, and neck cancers is often radical and may compromise the patient's appearance, function, and quality of life. The most common treatment modalities used include chemotherapy, radiation, surgery, hormone therapy, or a combination. Each treatment involves general and unique complications and compromises, many of which are responsive to rehabilitation and physical therapy techniques

1. Bone tumors[289,290,318,319,322–324,326–331,333,336,340, 341,372–374,376,445,446,519]

Surgery remains the primary treatment for bone cancer (except for Ewing's sarcoma). If a patient has no signs of metastatic spread, treatment by adjuvant chemotherapy along with surgery has a 60% to 80% 5-year survival rate or longer. Ewing's sarcoma is radio- and chemosensitive; therefore, it is treated by combined radio- and chemotherapy. The basic objective is to halt the progression of the tumor by destroying or removing the lesion.

a. Surgery with tumor resection with bone grafting is the primary treatment; surgical ablation of tumor may require amputation, or disarticulation, or a limb salvage of affected extremity

(1). Until fairly recently, amputation was nearly always the treatment recommended for a bone tumor in an arm or a leg; however, with treatment advances amputation is the last choice of treatment today

(2). Radiation therapy before or after surgery has made less radical, bone grafting, and limb-sparing surgery possible in most cases involving Stages I and II tumors as well as many tumors of higher grade

(3). Surgery and radiation therapy can also control many bone cancers in the head and neck area and in the trunk

(4). Use of chemotherapy is also being explored in cases in which the tumor cannot be completely removed surgically

(5). Some centers are performing limb-salvaging procedures: resection of affected bone and surrounding normal muscle tissue and reconstruction using metallic prostheses or allografts for bone/joint replacement (usually performed at cancer centers)

(i). Tikhoff-Linberg procedures are used to salvage the proximal humerus in place of a forequarter amputation

(ii). Other common sites for limb-salvage procedures are the distal femur and proximal tibia

(iii). Partial pelvic resections are used in place of hemipelvectomy

(6). The need for a standardized system of reporting results of various surgical alternatives after limb-salvaging and ablative procedures for musculoskeletal tumors was clearly recognized during the 1981 International Symposium on Limb Salvage (ISOLS); during the ensuing symposia, there was ongoing development of a system extensively field tested in 1989 by the Musculoskeletal Tumor Society (MSTS); this system of functional evaluation was adopted by the MSTS and ISOLS for their joint studies and program presentation

(i). The system assigns numerical values (0–5) for each of six categories: pain; function and emotional acceptance in upper and lower extremities; supports; walking and gait in the lower extremity; hand positioning; dexterity and lifting ability in the upper extremity[340]

(ii). Demographical information and a patient satisfaction component is included

(iii). Numerical score and percentage rating are calculated to allow for comparison of results

(iv). The system has been field tested in 220 patients with low (+/−) interobserver variability; it was well accepted by the participants, and its usage is recommended by the MSTS to facilitate valid comparative end-result studies of musculoskeletal tumor reconstructions[340]

b. Chemotherapy used in combination (multimodal therapy) to achieve a greater patient response at a lower toxicity rate and to reduce potential problems of drug resistance; combinations of chemotherapeutic agents are given in varying courses separated by rest periods; chemotherapy is administered before and after surgery or in combination with radiation therapy; the usefulness of adding chemotherapy to the treatment plan is in clinical trial; multimodal chemotherapy in combination with radiotherapy has improved 5-year survival rates in Ewing's sarcoma to 60% to 80%

c. Radiation therapy in several cases may be given both before and after surgery to preoperatively shrink a tumor and improve the chances for successful surgery and postoperatively to destroy cancer cells that remain in the area. Osteosarcoma is radioresistant, whereas Ewing's sarcoma is radiosensitive; prophylactic lung irradiation is carried out to suppress metastasis such as Ewing's sarcoma

d. Immunotherapeutic approach may be selected, or hormone therapy is used with bone metastatic tumors of the breast and prostate (hormone-sensitive tumors)

e. BMT is in clinical trials for patients with disseminated disease or a poor prognosis

■ PLEASE NOTE: If pathological fracture of long bones occurs, the fracture is managed with open reduction and internal fixation, insertion of a prosthesis, or other fracture treatment method. Pain is either completely relieved or significantly reduced, and the need for prolonged bed rest is removed. Prophylactic internal fixation is considered when 50% or more of the bone cortex is destroyed. If half the bone cortex is eroded, deformation occurs on weight bearing, resulting in pain and risk of spontaneous fracture. Spontaneous fracture is common when 75% of the bone cortex is eroded. Fracture is unlikely when 25% or less of the bone cortex is eroded (see Table 4–9). Side effects of treatment are common (see discussion of radiotherapy, chemotherapy, BRMs); wide excision, salvage procedures, and amputation sur-

gical procedures may result in many musculoskeletal deficits specific to the location and extent of the procedure, and neurological deficits may result from treatment

2. Soft-tissue sarcomas

Because soft-tissue sarcomas are rare and often require wide excision or limb-salvage procedures, experienced teams provide treatment at cancer centers. The type of sarcoma is not as important in selecting treatment as are its size, location, extent, and grade. The basic objective is to halt the progression of the tumor by destroying or removing the lesion. Current treatment includes the following:

a. Surgery is the primary treatment for sarcomas with multimodal adjuvant chemotherapy

(1). Most patients have an excellent chance of cure if all of the tumor is removed plus at least 2 cm of surrounding cancer-free tissue

(2). Stages I and II tumors usually are curable by surgery

(3). Sarcomas of a Stage III or Stage IV tumor are more likely to recur in the area of the original tumor, and they are more likely to spread

(4). Until recently, amputation was nearly always the treatment recommended for a sarcoma in an arm or a leg (see discussion of osteosarcoma under bone tumors)

(5). Radiation and chemotherapy before or after surgery has now made less radical, limb-sparing surgery possible in most cases involving Stage I and Stage II tumors as well as many tumors of higher grade

(6). Surgery plus radiation therapy can also control many sarcomas in the head and neck area and in the trunk

b. Radiation therapy is used (see discussion of radiation therapy)

(1). When a sarcoma cannot be removed surgically, well-planned, high-dose radiation therapy may be able to control the primary tumor by as much as 99%, thus enabling surgery

(2). Adjuvant radiation therapy and chemotherapy are used in addition to surgery to treat Stage III and Stage IV tumors

(3). Prophylactic lung irradiation may be done to suppress metastasis in late-stage or high-grade soft-tissue sarcomas when metastasis occurs, because the secondary tumors are likely to occur in the lungs; these metastatic tumors sometimes can be removed surgically

c. Chemotherapy

(1). The usefulness of adding chemotherapy to the treatment plan is in clinical trial

(2). Use of chemotherapy is also being explored in cases in which the tumor cannot be completely removed surgically

(3). Doxorubicin (Adriamycin) currently is the most widely used drug for soft-tissue sarcomas; doxorubicin is given alone or in combination with other agents such as vincristine, methotrexate, actinomycin D, decarbazine (DTIC), cisplatin (Platinol), and cyclophosphamide (Cytoxan)

(4). Regional chemotherapy, for control of sarcomas that are local, is being tested; this approach involves giving drugs through a major blood vessel in the region of the tumor; a more concentrated dose of the agents can then be directed to the area of the tumor to enable limb-salvage procedures

d. Immunotherapeutic agents in clinical trial include IFN, IL-2, TNF, CSF, and BCG; side effects of treatment are common (see discussion of radiotherapy, chemotherapy, and BRMs), and wide-excision surgical procedures may result in many musculoskeletal deficits specific to the extent of tissue excised, location of resection, and whether nerve resection is required

3. Head and neck cancer

• Treatment of head and neck cancer often includes intravenous (IV) methotrexate and bleomycin; side effects of chemotherapy may include ulceration of the oral and digestive tract, cachexia, depression of the bone marrow, hair loss, hypotension, pulmonary fibrosis, muscle weakness, fatigue

• Activities must be modified to stress safety and hygiene

• Radiation therapy will cause lifelong tissue changes; tissue fibrosis, skin damage, xerostomia, altered taste, and rapid caries formation are common and require treatment

• Nutritional supplementation is often necessary because altered taste, dry mouth, loss of teeth, and nausea may result in anorexia

• Disabilities associated with surgery include cosmetic deformity; oral, pharyngeal, and laryngeal disabilities; and head, neck, and shoulder dysfunction

• The prognosis is good, however, if the side effects are aggressively managed

• Skin flaps and prosthesis are often used for reconstruction secondary to the wide excisions that are frequently necessary to resect the tumor

• Two types of reconstructive surgery are used: myocutaneous pectoralis major flap procedure and reconstruction of the mandible using a trapezius osteomyocutaneous flap

a. Oral cancer: Patients with oral cancer often are treated by a team including an oral surgeon; ear, nose, and throat surgeon; medical oncologist; radiation therapist; plastic surgeon; prosthodontist; dietitian; physical therapist and speech therapist.

(1). Surgery: Most patients with oral cancer have surgery to remove the tumor in the mouth; if there is evidence that the cancer has spread, the surgeon may remove lymph nodes in the neck; the surgeon will attempt to resect only cancerous lymph nodes and an adjacent amount of tissue; if the disease involves muscles and other tissues in the neck, the resection is more extensive, and a radical dissection is done; reconstruction is an option after radical dissection to repair function such as swallowing and cosmesis

(2). Radiation therapy: May be used instead of surgery for small tumors in the mouth; patients with larger tumors often receive both surgery and radiation

(3). Chemotherapy: To date, chemotherapy has not been very effective in treating oral cancers; researchers are still looking for effective drugs or drug combinations to treat oral cancers

(4). Side effects of treatment

    (a). Treatments for oral cancers may injure healthy tissues of the mouth; therefore, it is important for patients to have a dental checkup and any needed dental work before cancer treatment begins.

    (b). Surgery and radiation therapy often cause side effects that may be short term or permanent; surgery to remove small tumors in the oral cavity usually does not cause any major problems; for a larger tumor, side effects are common because the surgeon may need to remove parts of the pharynx, palate, or jaw; side effects include the following:

        (i). Difficulty chewing, swallowing, or speaking

        (ii). Altered appearance

        (iii). Drooling and difficulty controlling the lip if surgery affects the innervation to the muscles of the bottom lip

        (iv). Facial edema after surgery, which usually resolves within a few weeks; however, if the lymphatic system has been damaged, lymph may collect in the tissues and edema may persist for a long time

    (c). Radiation to the mouth reduces the amount of saliva, and the saliva becomes thicker and contains more acid than is normal; the mouth may be very dry and some patients use the following:

        (i). Special sprays to help relieve dryness

        (ii). Iced beverages

        (iii). Special chewing gum

        (iv). Frequent rinsing also can help keep the mouth moist

    (d). Other side effects include the following:

        (i). Tooth decay begins because the saliva is thicker, food remains in contact with the teeth longer

        (ii). Tenderness in the tissues of the mouth; many patients are unable to floss or brush their teeth thoroughly

        (iii). Gums shrink during radiation treatment, dentures may not fit properly, and after treatment patients may need to have dentures refitted or replaced

        (iv). Mucositis and stomatositis; the mouth sores heal slowly, and often good mouth care can prevent sores

    (e). Good mouth care can help keep the teeth and gums healthy and can make the patient feel more comfortable

        (i). Patients should do their best to keep their teeth clean

        (ii). If it is hard to floss or brush the teeth in the usual way, patients can use gauze, a soft toothbrush, or a special toothbrush that has a spongy tip instead of bristles

        (iii). A mouthwash made with diluted peroxide, saltwater, and baking soda can keep the mouth fresh and help protect the teeth from decay; do not use commercial mouthwashes that contain alcohol (a drying agent)

        (iv). It also may be helpful to

use a fluoride toothpaste and/or a fluoride rinse to reduce the risk of cavities

   (v). The dentist usually suggests a special fluoride program to keep the mouth healthy (see discussion of side effects of radiation therapy)

b. Esophageal cancer

   Cancer of the esophagus usually cannot be cured unless it is found in the earliest stages before it has begun to spread. Unfortunately, early esophageal cancer causes few symptoms, and the disease is usually advanced when the diagnosis is made. However, advanced esophageal cancer can be treated and symptoms relieved. Esophageal cancer is usually treated with surgery or radiation therapy.

   (1). Surgery is the primary treatment, and many patients with esophageal cancer have an esophagectomy

   (a). Surgery for cancer of the esophagus is a major operation; generally, the tumor is resected along with a portion of the esophagus, nearby lymph nodes, and adjacent tissue; usually, the stomach is connected to the remaining part of the esophagus

   (b). Occasionally, the surgeon must form a new passageway from the throat to the stomach, using tissue from another part of the digestive tract (such as the colon) to replace the esophagus

   (c). If the tumor blocks the esophagus but cannot be removed, a by-pass can be created: a new pathway to the stomach

   (d). In some cases, the esophagus can be dilated; this procedure may have to be repeated as the tumor grows

   (e). Sometimes a tube in the esophagus is used to maintain patency

   (f). A laser has been used to destroy cancerous tissue and relieve blockages

   (2). Radiation therapy primarily affects cells in the treated area (see discussion of radiation therapy)

   (3). Chemotherapy clinical trials are underway to determine whether these drugs are effective in treating patients with this disease

   (4). Side effects of treatment

   (a). Surgery: Patients with difficulty eating and drinking may need IV feedings and fluids and antibiotics to prevent or treat infection; patients are taught special coughing and breathing exercises to keep lungs clear; discomfort or pain after surgery can be controlled with acute pain-management techniques

   (b). See previous sections for side effects of radiation therapy and chemotherapy

c. Cancer of the larynx

   Cancer of the larynx is usually treated with radiation therapy or surgery; therefore, the side effects will tend to be local in the area treated. Speech rehabilitation has been revolutionized by tracheoesophageal speech techniques.

   (1). Surgery

   (a). Surgery is the usual treatment if a tumor does not respond to radiation therapy or grows back after radiation therapy

   (b). The type of surgery depends on the size and location of the tumor

   (c). If a tumor on the vocal cord is very small, a laser may be used to remove the tumor

   (d). Surgery to remove part or all of the larynx is a partial or total laryngectomy

   (e). A tracheostomy is done to keep the new airway open

   (f). A partial laryngectomy preserves the voice, and only part of the voice box is removed—just one vocal cord, part of a cord, or just the epiglottis—and the stoma is temporary; in some cases, however, the voice may be hoarse or weak

   (g). In a total laryngectomy, the voice box is removed, and the stoma is permanent (h). The patient, called a laryngectomee, breathes through the stoma; a laryngectomee must learn to communicate verbally in a new way

(i). If the cancer may have spread, a neck dissection may be done with removal of the lymph nodes in the neck and adjacent tissue

(2). Radiation therapy: treatment of choice because it spares the vocal cords

(3). Chemotherapy: drugs usually given by IV

(4). Side effects of treatment

(a). Radiation therapy: See discussion of oral cancer side effects of radiation

(i). Radiation to the larynx can change the way patient's voice sounds, voice may be weak at the end of the day, and it is not unusual for voice to be affected by changes in weather

(ii). Voice changes, sore throat, and the feeling of a lump in the throat may come from local edema in the larynx from the radiation

(iii). Patients may want to try soft, bland foods moistened with sauces or gravies, thick soups, puddings, and high-protein milk shakes

(iv). Dietitian will help patient choose the right kinds of food

(v). Many patients find that eating several small meals and snacks during the day works better than trying to have three large meals

(b). Surgery

(i). For a few days after surgery, the patient is unable to eat or drink, and an IV supplies fluids

(ii). Within a day or 2, the digestive tract is returning to normal, but the patient still cannot swallow because the throat has not healed

(iii). Fluids and nutrition are given through a nasogastric feeding tube (put in place during surgery); the feeding tube is removed after healing

(iv). The patient gradually returns to a regular diet; some patients find liquids easier to swallow and others do better with solid foods

(v). After surgery, the lungs and trachea produce a large amount of mucus, which is removed by suctioning; acutely, it may also be necessary to suction saliva from the mouth because swelling in the throat prevents swallowing; learning to swallow again may take some practice with the help of a nurse or speech pathologist

(vi) For several days after a partial laryngectomy, the patient breathes through the stoma; however, within a few weeks, the stoma closes after removal of the tracheal tube

(vii). After a complete laryngectomy, the stoma is permanent; the patient breathes, coughs, and "sneezes" through the stoma and has to communicate verbally in a new way

(viii). The tracheal tube stays in place for at least several weeks (until the skin around the stoma heals), and some people continue to use the tube all or part of the time (ix). If the tube is removed, it is usually replaced by a smaller tracheostomy button (also called a stoma button)

(x). After a while, some laryngectomees get along without either a tube or a button

(xi). After a laryngectomy, parts of the neck and throat may be numb because nerves have been cut, and the shoulder and neck may be weak and have loss of motion

(c). Chemotherapy (see discussion of chemotherapy side effects): Loss of appetite can be a problem for patients treated for laryngeal cancer; they

(i). May not feel hungry when they are uncomfortable or tired

(ii). May lose their interest in food because the surgery changes the way things smell and taste

(iii). May have side effects of chemotherapy that can also make it difficult to eat such as nausea, vomiting, or mucositis

PLEASE NOTE: Patients who have good nutrition are better able to withstand the side effects of their treatment, so good nutrition is important. Eating well means getting enough calories and protein to prevent weight loss, to regain strength, and to rebuild normal tissues.

3. Breast cancer

Breast cancer is treated with surgery, radiation therapy, chemotherapy, and hormone therapy. Bornstein et al. used hyperthermia in combination with radiation therapy and chemotherapy as part of a Phase I and II trial in patients with locally or regionally recurrent or advanced adenocarcinoma of the breast.[399] Cisplatin alone or cisplatin with etanidazole or bleomycin was delivered just before hyperthermia once weekly. After hyperthermia, radiation was given. A statisti-

cally significant association between the likelihood of complications and the total radiation therapy dose (previous radiation and present radiation) was found. Persistent ulceration lasting longer than 1 month after completing treatment was seen in 67% of previously irradiated fields compared with 21% of fields that had not been previously treated, and surgical wound repair was needed for 38% of fields with a history of irradiation versus 6% of those without prior treatment. None of the hyperthermia temperature parameters studied correlated with an increased risk of complication. Bornstein et al. concluded that patients who were treated with prior radiation therapy had more locally toxic side effects than did those treated with hyperthermia or radiation therapy alone.[399] Surgery is the most common treatment.

a. Surgery: The different types of surgery used to treat breast cancer are described next:

(1). Modified radical mastectomy removes the entire breast, the axillary lymph nodes (they are one of the primary sites where breast cancer spreads), and the fascia over the chest muscles (but leaves the pectoralis muscles intact)

(a). This reduces cosmetic deformity and muscular weakness

(b). This is the most common surgery for breast cancer

(c). Although the use of less invasive and deforming surgical procedures, such as the lumpectomy and quadrectomy, is increasing, mastectomy is still the most common procedure used to prevent metastasis and, depending on the stage of the cancer, to ensure a high rate of survival

(2). Radical mastectomy (also called the Halsted radical mastectomy) removes the breast, chest fascia and muscles, primarily the pectoralis muscles, all of the ipsilateral axillary lymph nodes, some additional fat and skin, and often some of the innervation to the chest wall and shoulder girdle; radiation therapy to the involved area follows surgery (a). Radical mastectomy was the treatment of choice until the 1970s; this operation was the standard for many years

(b). It is still used on occasion, but, for most patients, less extensive surgery is just as effective

(c). It has the highest rate and severity of complications because it is the most invasive

(d). Lymphedema, upper extremity weakness, and significant disfigurement result

(3). Lumpectomy removes the breast lump only and is followed by radiation therapy; most surgeons also remove the axillary lymph nodes

(4). Total or simple mastectomy removes the entire breast; the lymphatic system and pectoralis muscles are preserved; sometimes the axillary lymph nodes adjacent to the breast also are removed; postoperative radiation therapy is usually used to decrease the regional recurrence of the cancer

(5). Partial or segmental mastectomy removes the tumor, some of the normal breast tissue around it, and the fascia over the chest muscle below the tumor; usually some of the axillary lymph nodes are removed; in most cases, radiation therapy follows the surgery to decrease regional recurrence of the cancer

b. Prosthetic fitting is frequently used to improve cosmesis after mastectomy; breast implants are still used for cosmesis; however, the complications from silicone implants have led to the development of other types of implants, and breast reconstructive surgery is becoming a more common choice for cosmesis with the use of a myocutaneus flap usually from the anterior abdominal wall[106,405]

PLEASE NOTE: **The length of stay after surgical treatment for primary breast cancer is often only 2 days.** The effects of early discharge from hospital on women undergoing surgery for primary breast cancer was evaluated in 169 consecutive self-selected patients in Sweden; 118 of 169 patients participated in the data collection.[447]

Twenty-eight subjects (24%) chose early discharge with the drain still in place and were compared with the 90 patients (76%) who were discharged without a drain. The median stay in the hospital for those who chose early discharge was 2 days; for those who remained in hospital until the drain was removed, it was 6 days. Those who opted for early discharge were significantly younger than those who did not. There were no differences between the groups in type or incidence of complications, and the groups were equally satisfied with their length of hospital stay and their treatment in the hospital. Early discharge with the drain still in place after surgery for primary breast cancer was not found to be associated with any untoward events.[447]

c. See previous sections for radiation therapy and chemotherapy treatment and side effects; radiation therapy may lead to fibrosis with the formation of scar tissue in the axilla and obstruct lymphatic vessels; ulceration and wound healing in irradiated fields may be a frequent problem (see discussion of hyperthermia complications of Phase I and Phase II clinical trial[399])

d. Hormone therapy, such as use of the drug tamoxifen, or removal of the ovaries: this treatment is also being proposed for prevention of breast cancer; tamoxifen provides endocrine control of estrogen-regulated breast tumor growth; breast cancer chemoprevention trials using tamoxifen among postmenopausal women have been proposed, and pilot studies are under way

e. Side effects of treatment

(1). High rates of physical and psychological impairments are demonstrated in patients with breast cancer

(2). **Axillary dissection and radiotherapy are probably the major risks for posttreatment lymphedema as opposed to the surgical procedure, with the exception of radical mastectomy, and many women have long-term impairments**

(3). Sixty-three women participated in a study in Canada to assess the rate of arm recovery and factors affecting it up to 1 year after axillary node dissection for breast cancer;[448] approximately 42% had residual impairment of at least one type 1 year after surgery, the most being pain (16%) and reduced grip strength (16%)

(4). Except for lymphedema, measurements 1 year after surgery showed little change from measurements at 6 months, suggesting that the shorter follow-up may be appropriate for assessing the long-term effects of axillary dissection; lymphedema was the only sequela that increased over time[448]

(5). Conservative breast surgery for early-stage breast cancer treatment results in improved body image and sexual functioning compared with mastectomy but appears to have little impact on psychological adjustment to the cancer

(6). Kiebert *et al.* reviewed the literature on treatment of early-stage breast cancer, investigating the impact of breast-conserving treatment versus mastectomy on quality of life;[449] 18 studies were examined with respect to medical issues (treatment modality, stage of disease), methodological issues (design, measurement moment, sample size), and results (psychological discomfort, changes in life patterns, fears, and concerns); they concluded that there was no evidence to support better psychological adjustment after breast-conserving treatment; however, with respect to body image and sexual functioning, use of breast-conserving treatment is favored[449]

(7). A case-control study in Japanese women with breast cancer examined mass screening;[451] the control group had more early-stage patients; chest wall pain was observed in 35.2% of the study group and in 46.5% of the control group ($P < .05$); although control patients were more optimistic than study group patients, disturbed daily life and anxiety about recurrence were a little more frequent in the control group than in the study group; in particular, shoulder stiffness was frequently seen in the control group

(8). Early detection and information do not create anxiety in mass-screening patients. Yokoe *et al.*[451] concluded that mass screening should be recommended to patients to detect early-stage breast cancer and provide better quality of life

f. Surgery: After a mastectomy and the accompanying excision or radiation of adjacent axillary lymph nodes, a patient is at risk for upper extremity lymphedema and loss of shoulder motion; therapists often become involved in the postoperative management of patients who have undergone a mastectomy; therapeutic exercise is an important part of the patient's postoperative plan of care to prevent or minimize lymphedema or loss of shoulder motion (see discussion of physical therapy management); additional side effects of mastectomy include the following:

(1). Weight shift resulting in a change in balance after removal of a breast with postural deformity of the trunk, especially if a woman has large breasts

(2). Postoperative incisional pain secondary to the transverse incision across the chest wall that is made to remove the breast tissue

(3). Skin in the breast area is tight after surgery, and the muscles of the arm and shoulder feel stiff

  (a). Secondary chest wall adhesions can result in increased risk of postoperative pulmonary complications, impaired and reduced range of motion of the shoulder on the involved side, postural deformity of the trunk, pain and discomfort in the neck and back

  (b). Chest wall adhesions may develop because of this restrictive scarring, radiation fibrosis of overlying tissue on the chest wall, or wound infection after surgery and previous course of radiotherapy with shoulder stiffness

  (c). All of these factors contribute to decreased function and range of motion in the involved upper extremity

(4). Some permanent loss of strength with a radical mastectomy, but for most women, reduced strength and impaired movement are temporary (see section on physical therapy management for recommended exercises to help regain movement and strength)

(a). Weakness of the involved upper extremity often involves weakness of the horizontal adductors of the shoulder

(b). If a radical mastectomy is performed, the pectoralis major muscle is removed; this results in a decrease in strength and function of the upper extremity on the involved side

(c). Weakness of the serratus anterior also occurs when the long thoracic nerve is temporarily traumatized during axillary dissection and removal of the axillary lymph nodes, resulting in weakness of the serratus anterior and compromised shoulder stabilization and function; without the stabilization during arm elevation movement and upward rotation of the scapula that the serratus anterior normally supplies, active flexion and abduction of the arm will be limited

(d). Impingement of the subacromial space may develop secondary to muscle guarding and substitution by the posterior shoulder girdle musculature by the levator scapulae and trapezius during arm elevation movement patterns with impaired scapulothoracic-glenohumeral motion and reduced active shoulder movement

(5). Pain and muscle spasm may occur in the posterior cervical region and shoulder girdle as a result of muscle guarding; the levator scapulae, teres major and minor, and the infraspinatus are often tender with palpation and often impair scapulotho-racic-glenohumeral motion and reduce active shoulder movement

(6). Patients may have numbness and tingling in the chest, axilla, shoulder, and arm because nerves are injured or resected during surgery, radiation fibrosis, or chemotherapy toxicity; these symptoms usually resolve within a few weeks after surgery or cessation of chemotherapy, but some numbness may be permanent

(7). Lymphedema secondary to removing the axillary lymph nodes because the flow of lymph slows collecting in the arm and hand; it is difficult for the body to fight infection after the lymph nodes have been removed

(a). After surgery, a woman will tend to decrease the use of the involved upper extremity; this sets the stage for the development of a chronic frozen shoulder and increases the likelihood of lymphedema in the hand and arm

(b). Early intervention to increase usage within prescribed limitations is important

(c). With edema, there is an increased size of the extremity, sensory disturbances in the hand, stiffness, and impaired active and passive range of motion in the fingers; this results in decreased function of the involved upper extremity

PLEASE NOTE: Women need to protect the arm or hand on the treated side from injury for the rest of their lives. Good skin care is necessary to prevent wounds and secondary infection.

g. Hormone therapy side effects include some of the symptoms of menopause when treatment interferes with the body's production or use of estrogen (number of symptoms depends on the specific drug or surgical procedure but usually are not severe):

(1). Hot flashes
(2). Interrupted periods
(3). Vaginal dryness

PLEASE NOTE: Reach to Recovery, a one-to-one patient education program sponsored by the American Cancer Society, usually sends representatives of this program to provide emotional support to the patient and family as well as to supply current information on breast prostheses and reconstructive surgery.

B. Neurological tumors

Benign or cancerous brain tumors may be treated by surgery, radiation, or chemotherapy. Before treatment begins, most patients are given corticosteroids to reduce edema and anticonvulsant drugs to prevent or control seizures. If hydrocephalus is present, a shunt may be placed to drain the cerebrospinal fluid. (A shunt is a long, thin tube placed in a ventricle of the brain and then threaded under the skin to another part of the body, usually the abdomen. Fluid is carried away from the brain and is absorbed in the abdomen. Occasionally, the fluid is drained into the heart.) A recurring theme in the current literature on malignant glioma is the importance of prognostic factors other than medical treatment in determining patient outcome;[423] this may also be the case with several other neurological tumors and requires further research. Bleehen and Ford[423] reviewed the results of trials with several new techniques and reported that interesting results are emerging from stereotactic radiotherapy, brachytherapy, and photodynamic therapy, although authors who report these results acknowledge that they have often reviewed patients with intrinsically good prognoses.[407–410,416,417,422,423]

1. Surgery is the usual treatment for most brain tumors and is the oldest method of treating brain tumors
   a. Steady advances have been made since modern techniques were introduced in the 1930s
   b. A benign tumor or cancer that is encapsulated may be able to be completely removed
   c. If the cancer cannot be removed completely, a partial resection may be done to relieve signs and symptoms of increased intracranial pressure that the growing tumor is causing within the cra-

nium and to reduce the amount of tumor to be treated by radiation therapy or chemotherapy
   d. To resect a brain tumor, a neurosurgeon performs a craniotomy by making an opening in the cranium
   e. If the tumor cannot be completely removed without damaging vital brain tissue, as much of the tumor as possible is resected
   f. Some tumors cannot be removed, and in such cases only a biopsy may be performed with a needle
   g. CT scans or MRI are used to locate the tumor, a special head frame (like a halo) holds the head while a small hole is made in the cranium; the needle is then directed to the tumor; this technique is called stereotaxis and can be used for treatment; when used for a biopsy, this helps decide which treatment to use
2. Radiation therapy is used to kill benign or cancerous brain tumor cells that cannot be removed completely by surgery
   a. External radiation therapy under study is being given twice a day instead of once using radiosensitizers to increase the effectiveness of treatments
   b. Implant radiotherapy is also used
   c. Stereotaxic radiosurgery, also called a gamma knife, is done by using the methods described under surgery as stereotaxic biopsy
   d. Treatment is done by high-energy rays during a single session with the radiation focused on the tumor from several angles
3. Chemotherapy is the most recent approach to treatment of brain cancers
   a. Most anticancer agents cannot get through the blood-brain barrier; however, a group of anticancer drugs called nitrosoureas are effective in reaching brain cancers; these can be delivered by mouth or injection
   b. Drugs that do not cross the barrier are delivered by intrathecal chemotherapy
   c. Therapy by placing tiny wafers containing anticancer drugs directly into the tumor is also being studied (the wafers dissolve over time)
4. Side effects of treatment
   a. Surgery: A craniotomy can result in the following:
      (1). Damage to normal brain tissue and edema

(2). Weakness and impaired coordination

(3). Personality changes, difficulty in speech and thinking, headaches, and memory loss

(4). Seizures

PLEASE NOTE: For a short time after surgery, symptoms may be worse than before surgery. Most of the side effects of surgery lessen or disappear with time.

b. Radiation therapy

(1). Sometimes brain cells killed by radiation form a mass in the brain; the mass may look like a tumor and may cause similar symptoms, such as headaches, memory loss, or seizures

(2). Suggested treatment includes surgery or corticosteroid to relieve these problems

(3). Children who have had radiation therapy for a brain tumor may have learning difficulties or partial loss of eyesight

(4). If the pituitary gland is damaged, children may not grow or develop normally

(5). In addition to the normal side effects of radiation therapy, radiation to the scalp usually causes hair loss (alopecia), which is occasionally permanent

c. Chemotherapy (see previous sections for side effects of chemotherapy)

d. Hyperthermia (heating the tumor to increase the effect of radiation therapy); immunotherapy; and high-dose chemotherapy followed by BMT are also under investigation

e. Spinal cord compression from primary neurological and bone tumors are more common with secondary metastatic tumor from breast, prostate, and lung cancers[415,452]

(1). Hacking et al. tried to develop a method to predict the survival and the functional outcome following neoplastic spinal cord injury (SCI); six of the factors showed a positive relationship with prolonged survival (>1 year after discharge) and improved functional level: tumor biology (lymphoma, myeloma, breast and kidney tumors); SCI as the presenting symptom of the malignancy; slow (>1 week) progression rate of neurological symptoms; tumors treated with a combination of surgery and radiotherapy; (partial) bowel control at admission; and (partial) independence regarding transfer activities at admission; a sum score (range, 0–6) of these indicators was used to predict survival; a patient with a sum score of 0 to 1 had zero probability of living longer than 1 year after discharge and 0.19 of functional improvement during stay at the spinal cord unit (SCU); a patient with a score of 5 or 6 had probabilities of 0.77 for living longer than 1 year after discharge and 0.92 for functional improvement during a stay at the SCU; the authors concluded that the sum score could be helpful when selecting patients for an intensive inpatient rehabilitation program or when modifying such a program, and further validation of the model is needed[452]

f. Patients being treated for a brain tumor may acquire DVTs or emboli and inflammation in a vein (thrombophlebitis); a patient who notices swelling in the leg, leg pain, or redness in the leg should be referred to a physician

C. Genitourinary cancers

1. Prostate cancer

Benign prostatic hyperplasia (BPH) is a very common condition, affecting more than 800,000 men in the United States each year. Prostatectomy is a well-proven surgical procedure used in the United States to treat approximately 400,000 BPH patients annually.[364] Major treatment benefit is expected in 70% to 80% of patients. Complications are seen in 20% of the surgically treated patients. Because of the advanced age of BPH patients and the presence of other serious, coexisting medical problems, surgical therapy may be difficult. Those patients who present a high risk for surgery, such as BPH patients with clinically important symptoms and signs of urinary outflow obstruction, need alternative treatments such as pharmacological agents, balloon dilatation, laser-beam therapy, transurethral thermal therapy, transrectal microwave hyperthermia, and transurethral microwave hyperthermia. These new treatment modalities must be compared with the standard treatment, which is prostatectomy. Because of the unpredictable natural history of BPH, it is desirable that each Phase III study should contain a no-treatment, observation-only arm.[364] Adenocarcinoma of the prostate is first in frequency and second in mortality among cancers in American men.[1]

A small (Stage A) prostate cancer may be found as a result of surgery performed to relieve problems with urination. Many men whose cancer is found in this way do not need treatment but are followed closely with tests and exams. Prostate cancer patients who do require treatment have surgery, radiation therapy, or hormone therapy. Sometimes, patients receive a combination of these treatments. In addition, other methods of treatment are under investigation to determine whether they are effective against this disease. Surgery and radiation therapy appear to be equally effective for men who require treatment for early-stage prostate cancer (some Stage A patients and most Stage B patients). Decisions about which treatment to use are made on an individual basis; depending on the patient, the urologist may prefer one approach over the other. For example, radical prostatectomy is a major operation that may not be recommended for an older man, especially one who has other health problems.[364] Men with Stage C prostate cancer usually receive radiation therapy. Sometimes, surgery alone or a combination of surgery and radiation therapy is used. The main form of treatment for men with Stage D prostate cancer is hormone therapy to prevent the prostate cancer cells from receiving the male hormones they need to grow. In Fossa et al.'s study of 58 patients with progressive hormone-resistant metastatic prostate cancer, a PSA greater than 100 μg/L, hemoglobin less than 12.0 g/dl, and pronounced fatigue were found to be independent adverse prognostic factors.[453] These risk factors discriminated a subgroup of patients with a median survival of 9 months (none or only one risk factor present) from a subgroup with a median survival of 4 months (greater than or equal to two risk factors present). Fossa et al. con-

cluded that clinicians should be reluctant to enter patients from the second group into complicated and resource-demanding clinical studies.[453] Although there is little evidence that sexual behavior causes prostate cancer, men with prostate cancer often have sexual dysfunction before the cancer diagnosis is made. Each treatment for prostate cancer increases the prevalence of sexual problems.

a. Surgery to remove the entire prostate is called radical prostatectomy; it is done in one of two ways
 (1). In retropubic prostatectomy, the prostate and nearby lymph nodes are removed through an incision in the abdomen
 (2). In perineal prostatectomy, an incision is made between the scrotum and the anus to remove the prostate
 (3). Nearby lymph nodes sometimes are removed through a separate incision in the abdomen
 (4). Local tumor control rates and long-term survival rates, with radical prostatectomy or radiation therapy, have been excellent
b. Radiation therapy
 (1). Sometimes, both external and internal radiation therapy are used
 (2). For external radiation therapy for prostate cancer, treatment generally is given 5 days a week for 5 to 7 weeks
 (3). This schedule helps protect healthy tissues by spreading out the total dose of radiation; the rays are aimed at the pelvic area
 (4). At the end of treatment, an extra "boost" of radiation is often given to a smaller area of the pelvis, where most of the tumor was located (see discussion of methods of radiotherapy)
 (5). There was concern regarding a high incidence of microscopic local tumor recurrence after a definitive course of irradiation
 (6). Deep regional or intracavitary hyperthermia with phase steering may be of value as an adjuvant treatment to radiotherapy and Phase I and II clinical studies are currently underway[363,364,453]
c. Hormone therapy is used to treat pros-

tate cancer that has spread because it is systemic therapy
  (1). Use of hormone therapy may depend on whether a patient's cancer has spread only to nearby lymph nodes or disseminated to other parts of the body
  (2). Some physicians do not recommend hormone therapy unless the man has symptoms, such as bone pain, that are caused by the spread of the cancer
  (3). With hormone therapy, patients take estrogen to stop the testicles from producing testosterone
  (4). Luteinizing hormone-releasing hormone (LHRH) agonist is another type of hormone therapy; LHRH normally controls the production of sex hormones; an LHRH agonist is like LHRH but has a different effect on the body's functions; LHRH agonists are given by daily or monthly injection and prevent the testicles from producing testosterone; initially, an LHRH agonist tends to increase tumor growth and make the patient's symptoms worse, but gradually the drug causes testosterone level to diminish
  (5). Tumor growth slows down without testosterone and the patient's condition improves. Another form of hormone therapy is surgery to remove the testicles; this operation, called orchiectomy, eliminates the main source of male hormones
  (6). After orchiectomy or treatment with estrogen or an LHRH agonist, testosterone is no longer produced by the testicles; however, the adrenal glands still produce small amounts of male hormones
  (7). Sometimes the patient takes an antiandrogen, a drug that blocks the effect of any remaining male hormones
  (8). Eventually, prostate cancer cells are able to grow with very little or no male hormones; when this happens, hormone therapy is no longer effective; other forms of treatment are under study
d. Side effects of treatment
  (1). Surgery
    (a). Before the 1990s, surgery to remove the prostate often caused permanent impotence and urinary incontinence
    (b). These side effects do not occur as often as in the past
    (c). New techniques are used primarily when treating fairly small tumors; these techniques avoid permanent injury to the nerves that control erection and damage to the sphincter of the bladder
    (d). Potency and total urinary control may require several months to a year after surgery to be restored
    (e). Men who have had prostatectomy no longer produce semen, so they have dry orgasms; however, it need not affect sexual pleasure
    (f). After nerve-sparing radical prostatectomy, the chance of recovering erections is better for men who are younger and in whom both neurovascular bundles can be spared
    (g). Definitions of ''potency'' after nerve-sparing surgery have not specified the rigidity of the erections achieved; some men classified as ''potent'' may desire additional sexual rehabilitation[366]

PLEASE NOTE: See clinical practice guidelines for the management of urinary incontinence in adults (AC HC PR Pub# 92-0038 ns DHHS PHS AHCPR, March 1992).

  (2). Radiation therapy
    (a). May cause impotence in some men; this does not occur as often with internal radiation therapy as with external radiation therapy[363]
    (b). Internal radiation therapy is less likely to damage the nerves that control erection; this treatment is suitable only for patients with early-stage cancer

and is used only at a few cancer centers

(c). Patients also may have diarrhea or frequent and uncomfortable urination; often the urologist can suggest ways to reduce these problems

(d). The chance that definitive radiation therapy will cause erectile dysfunction probably has been overestimated, with the prevalence rate closer to 25% of men with new problems as compared with the 50% often cited in the literature;[363,366] men are more at risk to have erection problems after radiation therapy if the quality of erections before treatment was borderline (see discussion of side effects of radiation therapy for the other general effects of therapy)

(3). Hormone therapy

(a). Orchiectomy, LHRH agonists, and estrogen frequently cause loss of sexual desire, impotence, and hot flashes

(b). Patients who receive estrogen or an antiandrogen may have nausea, vomiting, or tenderness and swelling of the breasts (estrogen is used less today because it increases the risk of heart disease; this form of treatment is not appropriate for men who have a history of heart disease)

(c). Hormonal therapy has an impact on the central mechanisms mediating sexual desire and arousability; therefore, with most treatment methods, approximately 20% of men remain sexually functional

(d). Newer antiandrogenic drugs in clinical trials interfere less with sexual function[364,366]

(e). Their long-term ability to control prostate cancer is yet to be determined

(4). Chemotherapy (see discussion of side effects of chemotherapy) and BRM therapy for advanced prostate cancer have other side effects (see discussion of side effects of BRM)

■ PLEASE NOTE: Sexual rehabilitation should be addressed by the primary care team. Sexual partners should be included in brief sexual counseling, even when a mechanical treatment for erectile dysfunction is prescribed.[366] There has been a growing recognition of the need to include parameters representing the patients' view of their conditions and quality of life.[365,367,454,455] The European Organization for Research and Treatment of Cancer (EORTC) Genitourinary Group, in cooperation with the EORTC Quality of Life Group, examine quality of life in untreated patients with Stage M+ disease.[454,455] Psychological distress, fatigue, social and family life, and pain are the most important issues to the patient on a subjective basis, and these were confirmed in relationship to objective parameters. There was a discrepancy between the physicians' evaluations and the patients' opinions about subjective morbidity, namely, in regard to sexual status and pain. The researchers concluded that the trial revealed the reluctance of clinicians to perform quality of life research and that quality of life assessment should become a mandatory part of clinical trials in prostatic cancer.

2. Kidney cancer[1-3,337]

Kidney cancer is treated with surgery, embolization, radiation therapy, hormone therapy and BRM, chemotherapy, or a combination. Surgery, embolization, and radiation therapy are forms of local therapy and primarily affect only the cells in the treated area. Hormone and BRM therapy and chemotherapy are types of systemic therapy.

a. Surgery

(1). Most patients with kidney cancer have surgery: a nephrectomy

(2). In some cases, the whole kidney is resected or just the part of the kidney that contains the tumor

(3). More often, the whole kidney along with the adrenal gland and the fat around the kidney is removed; also, nearby lymph nodes may be removed

(4). For several days before and after surgery, IV feedings and fluids are given, and the fluid intake and the amount of urine produced are monitored

(5). The remaining kidney assumes the work of both kidneys

(6). In embolization, a substance is injected to block the renal blood vessels; the tumor shrinks because of a lack of nutrient supply; in some cases, embolization makes surgery easier; when surgery is not possible, this treatment may help reduce pain and hemorrhage; patients require IV fluid replacement

b. Radiation therapy (see discussion of side effects of radiotherapy)

c. Some kidney cancers may be treated with hormones, *eg,* advanced kidney cancer, especially when the disease has spread to the lungs

  (1). Progesterone is the hormone most often used to treat kidney cancer

  (2). Biological therapy using IL-2 and INF are being studied for treatment of advanced kidney cancer and after surgery for early-stage kidney cancer; this additional treatment, adjuvant therapy, may prevent the cancer from recurring by killing undetected cancer cells that may remain in the body

d. Chemotherapy has not been effective against kidney cancer, but new drugs and multimodal combinations that may prove to be useful are under investigation

e. Side effects of treatment

  (1). Surgery

    (a). After nephrectomy most patients need pain medication

    (b). Discomfort may make it difficult to breathe deeply, and patients have to do special coughing and breathing exercises to help keep their lungs clear

    (c). Some of these difficulties may be secondary to inadequate pain control

    (d). Embolization can cause the following, which are treated pharmacologically:

      (i). Pain

      (ii). Fever

      (iii). Nausea or vomiting

  (2). Radiation therapy (see discussion of side effects of radiation therapy)

  (3). Hormone therapy side effects are usually mild; drugs containing progesterone generally cause few side effects; some patients may retain fluid and gain weight (see discussion of side effects of BRMs)

3. Bladder cancer[1–3,337,424]

a. Surgery is the most common method of treatment

  (1). Early (superficial) bladder cancer (in which the tumors are found on the surface of the bladder wall) generally are treated by a TUR

  (2). The cystoscope can remove all or part of a tumor or destroy it with an electric current

  (3). When the cancer involves much of the bladder wall surface or has grown into the bladder wall, standard treatment is a radical cystectomy

  (4). The bladder and nearby organs are removed

  (5). In women, the uterus, fallopian tubes, ovaries, and part of the vagina are removed

  (6). In men, the prostate and seminal vesicles are removed

  (7). Researchers are attempting to find treatments that spare the bladder

b. Chemotherapy and BRM

  (1). TUR is often followed by BRM such as BCG when several tumors are present in the bladder or when there is a risk that the cancer will recur

  (2). A solution containing BCG is directly administered into the bladder

  (3). Chemotherapy may also be administered directly into the bladder

  (4). Chemotherapy is used when cancer involves the pelvis or has metastatic spread

c. Radiation therapy may be needed to control the cancer when it is too large an area of the bladder to be removed with TUR

d. Side effects of treatment

  (1). Surgery

    (a). Radical cystectomy causes infertility in both men and women and can also lead to sexual problems; nearly all men were impotent after this procedure in the past, but surgical improvements have prevented this in many men

    (b). In women, the vagina may be narrower or shallower, and intercourse may be difficult or painful

    (c). Various methods are used after the bladder is removed to store and pass urine:

      (i). A piece of the person's

small intestine is used to form a new pipeline, and the ureters attach to one end, and the other end is brought out through a stoma in the abdominal wall (it is also called an ostomy or urostomy); an enterostomal therapist will show the patient how to care for the ostomy; a flat bag fits over the stoma to collect urine

(ii). A newer method uses part of the small intestine to make a new storage pouch (a continent reservoir with an ileal conduit); the urine collects there, and a catheter is used to drain the urine through a stoma

(d). To improve quality of life of patients requiring urinary diversion, several surgical techniques were developed including those using a continent urinary reservoir (CUR), such as Kock pouch or Indiana pouch, and those using the conventional ileal conduit

(e). A Japanese study had CUR patients complete a questionnaire relating to the quality of life during the disease-free period;[456] physical abilities related to exercise were not significantly hampered by this operation; 80% were not bothered by having a stoma; the operation had a negative impact in 20% to 30% on their interaction with friends and hobbies; and males suffered impotence at a very high rate, but only 26% of the patients lost interest in sex; 22% who had a job before operation stopped working; however, only a few patients abandoned traveling; symptoms related to the operation were mild; overall, 94% of the patients would choose the same operation again if it were required[456]

(2). See previous sections for discussion of side effects of BRMs, radiation therapy, and chemotherapy

4. Testicular cancer[1–3,57,337,368,425,426]

Major advances have been made over the last two decades in curing patients with testicular cancer. Testicular cancer can be treated with surgery, radiation therapy, and chemotherapy. Surgery is done to remove the testicle in most cases and lymph nodes in the abdomen in some cases. In addition, metastatic tumors may be partly or entirely removed by surgery. After surgery, men with seminomas generally have radiation therapy to their abdominal lymph nodes because seminomas are highly sensitive to radiation. Overall cure rates with a diagnosis of seminoma now approach 95% to 98%[368]

Nonseminomas are somewhat less sensitive to radiation. Patients with this type of cancer usually have other types of treatment to control the cancer. Surgical exploration follows, with orchiectomy and complete excision of the spermatic cord if a neoplasm is documented. Patients with nonseminomatous testicular cancer who do not have metastases are treated with a traditional orchiectomy and retroperitoneal lymph node dissection; about 10% of patients will relapse and must be treated with antineoplastic agents.[368]

Patients with disseminated disease require systemic treatment with cisplatin-based combination drug therapy, and it has been effective in treating patients with extensive disease. Reduction of toxicity and identification of patients who can be spared extensive treatment are currently being investigated; treatment outcomes are excellent for several regimes.

a. Side effects of treatment

(1). Surgery

(a). Resection of one testicle does not make a patient impotent and seldom interferes with fertility; a man with one healthy testicle can still have a normal erection and produce sperm; many men worry that losing one testicle will affect their ability to have sexual intercourse or make them sterile

(b). Men can also have a prosthetic implant, an artificial testicle, placed in the scrotum that has the weight and feel of a normal testicle (c). Lymph node dissection does not change a man's ability to have an erection or an orgasm, but sterility can occur because it interferes with ejaculation

(d). Some men gradually recover the ability to ejaculate without treatment, and medication may help others

(e). A special surgical technique that may protect the ability to ejaculate should be discussed when removing the lymph nodes

(2). See previous sections for discussion of side effects of radiation therapy and chemotherapy; most men who receive chemotherapy for testicular cancer can continue to function sexually; although some agents interfere with sperm production, many patients recover their fertility over time; however, this effect is permanent for some patients

5. Cancer of the cervix

Treatment for cervical cancer may involve surgery, radiation therapy, or chemotherapy.[1–3,43,337,369,427]

a. Surgery may remove only a small area of abnormal tissue, or it may remove the cervix, uterus, and other nearby tissues (hysterectomy)

(1). Moderate dysplasia usually is treated by cryosurgery (freezing) or cauterization (burning), destroying abnormal areas of the cervix without harming surrounding healthy tissues

(2). Conization is the usual treatment for severe dysplasia and lasers have been used[369,427]

b. Radiation therapy is used for patients with cancer that has spread to the pelvis, to the lower parts of the vagina, or to the ureters

c. Chemotherapy, in addition to surgery or radiation therapy, is used for patients with cervical cancer that has spread to the bladder, rectum, or distant parts of the body

d. Side effects of treatment

(1). Hysterectomy is major surgery and the hospital stay may last about 1 week

(2). Postoperatively, patients may have problems, including the following:

(a). Lower abdomen discomfort

(b). Urinary retention

(c). Constipation

(3). Normal activities, including sexual intercourse, usually can be resumed in 4 to 8 weeks

(4). Women who have had their uterus removed no longer have menstrual periods

(5). Women do not go through menopause when the ovaries are not removed because their ovaries still produce hormones; menopause will occur if the ovaries are removed or damaged by radiation therapy

(6). Sexual desire and the ability to have intercourse usually are not affected by hysterectomy

(7). Many women have an emotionally difficult time after a hysterectomy, with feelings of deep emotional loss because they are no longer able to become pregnant

(8). Functional limitations have been reported after treatment by radiation therapy[43] (see previous sections for discussion of side effects of radiation therapy and chemotherapy)

6. Ovarian cancer

Ovarian cancer may be treated with surgery, chemotherapy, radiation therapy, or a combination.[1–3,43,337,370]

a. Surgery is part of the treatment for almost all patients with ovarian cancer and includes removal of the ovaries, uterus, and fallopian tubes; if a woman has an early, slow-growing tumor and wants to be able to have a child, only the affected ovary is removed

b. Chemotherapy is given when the cancer has spread or when the entire tumor cannot be removed by surgery

c. Radiation therapy is used in addition to surgery to kill cancer cells that may remain in the pelvic area

d. Biological therapy is being studied for effectiveness in patients with recurrent or advanced ovarian cancer[370]

e. Side effects of treatment

(1). Surgery for ovarian cancer is a major operation, and the hospital stay may last for about a week

(a). Postoperatively, drugs are given to relieve pain and to prevent or treat infection (b). A woman may have problems with urinary retention and constipation for several days after surgery

(c). Patients are advised not to have sexual intercourse for about 6 to 8 weeks after surgery

(d). Menopause starts immediately when the ovaries are removed, and the symptoms such as hot flashes are more severe than when menopause happens naturally

(e). Although ERT may be prescribed for many women during natural menopause, it is not used for women with ovarian cancer

(2). See previous sections for discussion of side effects of radiation therapy and chemotherapy

7. Cancer of the uterus

Surgery, radiation therapy, hormone therapy, and chemotherapy may be used to treat uterine cancer.[43,369,427] Early-stage cancer of the uterus usually is treated with surgery. The uterus and cervix are removed (hysterectomy) as are the fallopian tubes and ovaries (salpingo-oophorectomy).

a. Side effects of treatment

(1). Surgery: see discussion of cancer of the cervix and ovarian cancer for side effects of surgery

(2). Radiation therapy causes some patients to have diarrhea, frequent and uncomfortable urination, dryness, itching, and burning in the vagina with pain on intercourse; some women are advised not to have intercourse at this time: however, most women can resume sexual activity after a few weeks once treatment is completed

(3). See previous discussions of side effects of chemotherapy and radiation therapy; functional impairments have been reported after treatment with radiation therapy[43]

D. GI cancers

1. Colorectal cancer

There are three main ways to treat cancer of the colon and rectum: surgery, radiation therapy, and chemotherapy; a combination also may be used.[1-3,152,238,337,429,430] Immunotherapy is being studied in clinical trials. The standard treatment for most colon and rectal cancers is surgery.[430]

a. Surgery procedures are described next:

(1). Bowel resection is removal of only the part of the bowel that contains the cancer and then rejoining the healthy sections together; the lymph nodes near the tumor are also removed; often, this is all that is needed

(2). Colostomy performed (temporary or permanent) if the cancer is blocking the bowel; the cancerous bowel is resected and an opening created in the abdomen for the body's wastes to be removed, by-passing the lower colon and rectum

(a). Temporary colostomy allows the lower colon and rectum to heal; when healed, a second operation closes the stoma; normal bowel functions return

(b). Permanent colostomy is needed when the entire lower rectum is removed; only about 15% of patients with colorectal cancer need a permanent colostomy

(3). After surgery for a colostomy, an appliance (a special collecting bag) is attached to the stoma to collect waste matter; the appliance does not show under most clothing; an enterostomal therapist teaches patients with a colostomy how to care for the stoma and appliance

b. See previous sections for radiation therapy and chemotherapy treatments

E. Lung cancer

Lung cancer is treated by surgery, radiation therapy, and chemotherapy or a combination of these methods.[1-3,65,147,257,337,344,345,348,354-356,358-361,431,432,457,458] The type of surgery that the physician recommends depends on the size and location of the tumor. Many of these patients have comorbidities such as coronary artery disease (CAD) and emphysema (COPD), and their management is complex.[211,432] The patient with significant CAD should undergo coronary artery by-pass before or concurrently with pulmonary resection. Only proven carcinomas should be resected at the time of by-pass grafting because immunosuppression secondary to cardiopulmonary by-pass can result in the life-threatening infection such as fungal infections.[432] The risk of pulmonary resection is increased in the patient with COPD because of decreased efficiency of the lungs and chest wall.

1. Treating SCLC

   SCLC spreads quickly to distant parts of the body, and frequently the metastatic tumors cannot be found by routine tests. Local treatments (surgery or radiation therapy to the chest) are usually not effective in controlling SCLC. Patients with SCLC are commonly treated with multimodal drug therapy or with multimodal therapy and radiation to the primary tumor in the lungs, whereas the chemotherapy is used to reach the disseminated cancer. SCLC is responsive to a combination of chemotherapy regimens. Although many different agents are effective in this disease, most SCLCs eventually become refractory to chemotherapy, and most patients do not survive longer than 2 years.

2. Treating NSCLC

   a. Patients with NSCLC generally can be divided into three groups:

      (1). Patients whose cancer is only in the lung and whose tumor can be removed by a wedge resection (portion of lung), lobectomy (entire lobe of the lung), or pneumonectomy (entire lung); radiation therapy may be used to treat patients in this group who cannot have surgery because of other medical problems; radiation therapy may also be effective in localized cases

      (2). Patients whose cancer has spread regionally to nearby tissue or lymph nodes; usual treatment for these patients is radiation therapy to the chest and is sometimes combined with other forms of treatment such as surgery

      (3). Patients whose cancer has disseminated to distant parts of the body; radiation therapy and chemotherapy are used to shrink the cancer and palliation is used to relieve symptoms; combination chemotherapy regimens have not consistently produced quality responses in patients with advanced tumors; however, newer regimens using high doses of cisplatin, mitomycin and vinca alkaloids, or cisplatin and etoposide have produced encouraging results

PLEASE NOTE: Although progress has been made in the treatment of lung cancer, effective therapies that consistently produce responses are still lacking. Clinical trials must continue to evaluate therapeutic modalities for all types of lung cancer. Several promising research studies on the use of preoperative physiological variables to predict postoperative complications have been reported.[348–353,359,362] In 117 patients undergoing thoracotomy for possible or definite lung cancer, 37% experienced at least one respiratory complication (*eg*, pneumonia, atelectasis prompting bronchoscopy, pulmonary embolism).[349] Twofold or greater increases in respiratory complications were associated with current smoking, cancer as the final pathological condition, at least moderate dyspnea, forced expiratory volume in 1 second of less than 60% of predicted, ventilatory reserve less than 25 L, and maximal oxygen consumption (Vo_{2max}) less than 1.25 L. Twofold increases in the incidence of any complication (respiratory, cardiac, and so on) were associated with age greater or equal to 75 years and cancer as the final pathological condition. Dales *et al.* concluded that simple historical information (age, smoking status, cancer status, dyspnea) indicated risk of postoperative morbidity, but general quality of life measures were not good predictors of morbidity.[349] A few studies confirmed the increased morbidity with increasing age.[355,357]

   1. Side effects of treatment

      Complications can occur after surgery to remove cancer in the lungs, such as blood loss which may be greater than during other types of surgery or damage to or removal of lung tissue that may lead to difficulty breathing and drowsiness. (See discussion of side effects of chemotherapy and radiation therapy.) Postoperative incisional pain is present at the thoracotomy site.

PLEASE NOTE: Impaired cardiopulmonary function and arrhythmias are a frequent postoperative complication and require careful monitoring of signs and symptoms during physical therapy. A preliminary study on the effects of pulmonary lobectomy on cardiopulmonary function were investigated in 9 patients with lung cancer. Hemodynamic studies at rest and during exercise were performed before and 4 to 6 months after the operation. Heart rate, pulmonary arterial pressure, and pulmonary vascular resistance index were significantly increased after operation, whereas stroke volume index was significantly decreased. It appears cardiac index was preserved by the increase in heart rate despite a decrease in stroke volume index associated with the decreased pulmonary vascular bed after the operation. These results suggest a significant deterioration in cardiopulmonary function after lobectomy. The patient characteristics were heterogeneous (five lobectomies and four bilobectomies) and their findings are limited.[457] In a larger study of 598 patients after undergoing thoracic surgical procedures for lung cancer, charts were reviewed for occurrence of cardiac arrhythmias and myocardial ischemic (MI) events.[458] Atrial tachycardias occurred in 16% (94 patients); atrial fibrillation occurred in 87% (520 patients) followed by supraventricular tachycardia and atrial flutter. An abnormal preoperative exercise test result and intraoperative hypotension were strongly associated with both arrhythmia and ischemia. Pneumonectomy, ischemic changes on the electrocardiogram (ECG), and cardiac enlargement were also associated with arrhythmias. Patients with recurrent episodes of arrhythmia had a significantly higher mortality rate than those without episodes or with a single episode only (17% vs. 2.4%). Transient ischemic ECG changes were documented in 23 patients (3.8%) and MI in 7 (1.2%). A weaker association was found between postoperative arrhythmias and old MI (greater than 6 months), arterial hypertension, and heart failure. A history of angina or old MI was predictive of transient postoperative MI but not MI. In the last decade, improved anesthetic and monitoring techniques and more frequent use of the intensive care unit postoperatively have not reduced the incidence of arrhythmias after thoracotomy.[458]

Several studies reported reduced functional states and quality of life with increased symptoms in patients with lung cancer related to weight loss, fatigue, dyspnea, smoking history, preoperative functional status, and so on.[52,53,147,150,151,344-346] One study of 69 women with primary or recurrent NSCLC for more than 12 months who had limited disease and were not currently receiving treatment reported on diminished quality of life.[344] The typical subject was younger than 65 years and married. Subjects had greater disruptions in global quality of life and its dimensions compared with a normative heterogeneous female cancer sample. The most common serious disruptions were fatigue, difficulty with household chores, worry about ability to care for self, and worry about cancer progression. The quality of life score was moderately correlated to functional status ($r = .69$, $P < .001$) and to symptom distress ($r = .72$, $P < .001$). Symptom distress was associated strongly with the physical subscale of quality of life ($r = .80$, $P = .001$) and significantly but less strongly with all other dimensions of quality of life. Significantly greater differences in disruptions of quality of life occurred in women younger than 65 years, women with recurrent disease, and women with low income. Symptom distress predicted 53% of the variance followed by functional status (59%) and recurrence (63%) when quality of life was the outcome variable.[344]

F. Hematological cancers

1. Lymphoma

Treatment planning takes into account the type of lymphoma, the stage of disease, whether it is likely to grow slowly or rapidly, and the general health and age of the patient. For low-grade lymphomas (usually grow very slowly and cause few symptoms), treatment is often held until the disease shows signs of spreading. Treatment for intermediate- or high-grade lymphomas usually involves chemotherapy with or without radiation therapy.[433] In addition, surgery may be needed to remove a large tumor.

a. Hodgkin's disease[1-3,90,91,95,98,161,337,425,443]

(1). Treatment for Hodgkin's disease includes radiation therapy, chemotherapy, or a combination (treatment for children with Hodgkin's disease is more complex and is not discussed here)

(2). Several defined multimodal protocols are used in late-stage Hodgkin's disease and non-Hodgkin's lymphoma (MOPP, C-MOPP, CHOP, MACOP-B, ABVD, and so on)

(3). Often patients are referred to cancer centers for treatment of Hodgkin's disease and participation in clinical trials

(4). Cure rates of 60% to 90% are reported for localized Hodgkin's disease

(5). The first 4 years of follow-up for later-stage Hodgkin's disease is when 90% of remissions will fail

(6). Side effects of treatment

(a). The methods used to treat Hodgkin's disease often cause side effects, both short-term and permanent such as fertility problems

(b). Women's menstrual periods may stop and are more likely to return in younger women

(c). Men have impaired fertility from the disease and treatment, and younger men are more likely to regain their fertility after treatment is completed

(d). Sperm banking before treatment is an option for some men (see previous sections regarding side effects associated with radiation therapy and chemotherapy)

(e). A study of men with Hodgkin's disease 1 year after treatment reported that these patients had more generalized symptoms: fatigue, energy loss, and work impairment compared with men with testicular cancer[425]

(f). Analysis indicated that most of these differences are site specific

(g). More generalized symptoms were treatment related (stage related)

(h). Contrary to the researchers' expectations, both groups reported similar levels of infertility and erectile dysfunction[425]

(i). Cardiopulmonary impairments are also reported as a consequence of intensive radiotherapy[90,91,95,98]

b. Non-Hodgkin's lymphomas (see discussion of Hodgkin's lymphoma)

Chemotherapy for non-Hodgkin's lymphomas is usually multimodal therapy; some forms of therapy are administered orally and others by IV or intramuscular

(1). Side effects of treatment

Bone marrow transplant is a treatment option for patients who relapse. See later discussion of BMT and previous sections for side effects of radiation therapy and chemotherapy.

2. Plasmacytomas and multiple myeloma[1-3,161,337]

Plasmacytomas and multiple myeloma are difficult to cure. Patients who have a plasmacytoma receive intensive radiotherapy and often are symptom free for a long time after treatment, but multiple myeloma eventually develops in many. Treatment for those who have multiple myeloma can improve the quality of a patient's life by controlling the symptoms and complications of the disease. Patients who need treatment for multiple myeloma usually receive chemotherapy and sometimes radiation therapy. Chemotherapy using alkylating agents with or without prednisone has demonstrated little benefit. Patients who have multiple myeloma but do not have symptoms of the disease usually do not receive treatment; the risks and side effects of treatment outweigh the benefits. These patients are monitored and treatment is begun when symptoms appear.

a. Side effects of treatment: See previous sections for side effects of chemotherapy and radiation therapy

3. Leukemia

a. ALL[1-3,58,72,73,78,80,117,161,316,337,342,343,434-437]

(1). Chemotherapy. A growing number of chemotherapeutic agents are used and have been proved highly effective against ALL. Their administration either suppresses or delays the cycle of cell production, resulting in a reduction in the tumor cell load. Intensive multimodal drug therapy using vincristine, prednisone, and L-asparaginase in children and vincristine, prednisone, ara-C, and daunorubicin in adults is an important advance in treating acute leukemia. Researchers found that two or more drugs in combination had a greater ability to induce remissions than did any single-agent drug alone. More than 90% of children with ALL and 75% to 80% of adults can be expected to achieve remission. Early therapy to the CNS also is added to the regular treatment in children because of the high incidence of CNS involvement (50% to 70%) in children. Multimodal therapy is then used to maintain remission for several years, and about half the patients treated this way will still be in remission after 3 years on continuous maintenance therapy. A remission is a temporary, and potentially permanent, arrest of the leukemic process:

(a). Complete remission: There is a

complete return to a state of normal good health indicated by disappearance of symptoms, the physical findings become normal, and abnormal cells are no longer found in the bone marrow and peripheral blood

(b). Partial remission: One or more signs of leukemia may not completely disappear, and examination of the blood and bone marrow at frequent intervals enables the course of the disease to be determined and proper dosage of the appropriate chemotherapeutic drugs selected

(2). Immunotherapy. Studies have shown that most, if not all, leukemia cells have antigens distinct from those of normal cells of the patient. These tumor-specific antigens may provide a target for immune mechanisms for the patient with leukemia, which can be enhanced by BRMs. Active immunotherapy with this approach has been successful in prolonging survival in some cases, and research continues to be promising.

(3). BMT.[72–74,78,80,82,117,292,342,434–437]   BMT was initially shown to be effective in mouse leukemia and has been used in the treatment of patients with leukemia at cancer centers for more than 10 years. This technique represents an attempt to destroy the abnormal bone marrow and replace it with healthy marrow. Two primary types of transplantation are performed: autologous and allogenic. Allogenic transplant donor tissue comes from a sibling, parent or occasionally an unrelated donor. Histocompatibility is even more important in this technique than in platelet and granulocyte transfusion because the transplanted bone marrow stem cells survive and continue to divide in the patient when the graft takes. If histocompatibilities do not exist, the grafted cells may recognize the patient as "foreign" and may mount a severe immunological attack known as the graft-versus-host disease (GVHD) reaction,

which can be life threatening. Immunosuppressive drugs such as cyclosporine A and prednisone are used to control this problem, and GVHD continues to be investigated actively. Autologous transplant tissue comes from patients when they are in remission so that histocompatibility is not an issue and recovery is somewhat easier. Syngeneic transplantation is a third type of transplant in which an identical twin serves as the donor for the transplant tissue and histocompatibility is again not an issue. Both autologous and allogenic transplants are now used in a variety of hematopoietic and solid tumor cancers such as leukemia (ALL, acute myelogenous leukemia, chronic myelogenous leukemia), lymphoma (Hodgkin's and non-Hodgkin's lymphoma), multiple myeloma, lung, breast, ovarian, colon, and testicular cancer, gliomas, sarcomas, and neuroblastoma, to list a few.

b. Side effects of treatment

Other problems in treating leukemia are the result of drug side effects as well as the leukemia process itself. Chemotherapy, radiotherapy, and leukemia damage the bone marrow and impair the patient's ability to produce two important blood elements. These elements are platelets that prevent hemorrhage and white blood cells (granulocytes) that help control bacterial and fungal infections.[316] Supportive care is used to manage these side effects (see discussion of support with blood products, medical treatment).[316] Plateletpheresis (platelet transfusions) is used to reduce the occurrence of hemorrhage.

Granulocyte transfusions are used to reduce bacterial infection in some patients. Another approach to controlling infection in leukemia patients is the use of laminar airflow rooms, which are relatively germ-free environments plus decontamination procedures, to reduce the degree of contact with bacteria and thus the risk of infection. The occurrence of severe infection has been diminished significantly by the use of these isolation systems. Finally, newly developed antibiotics have been of value in the treatment of bacterial infections. Research continues to identify antibiotics more effective against certain resistant bacteria, fungi, and viruses.

Long-term follow-up of functional status and quality of life in children treated for cancer has indicated emotional and cognitive deficits and some impaired cardiopulmonary function.[56,59,62,96,97] Barr *et al.* reported on the multiple sequelae in individual patients and global morbidity burdens in survivors of ALL.[58] Overall, burdens of morbidity were greater in those who had had "high-risk" disease than in children treated less intensively for "standard-risk" ALL. Deficits in emotional and cognitive status were especially common (alone and in combination). These were more prevalent in younger patients and exhibited a close relationship to cranial irradiation.[58]

BMT also leads to many frequent side effects such as impaired cardiopulmonary, renal, or neuromuscular function or GVHD, which may impact functional status and quality of life.[73,78,80–82,85,170,171] Wingard *et al.* assessed employment status in 135 adults who survived BMT.[460] The sample was composed of 86% of eligible subjects contacted and surveyed 47 months (mean) after BMT (6 to 149 months). Sixty-nine (51%) were employed full time, 19 (14%) part time, and 43 (32%) were unemployed (there were no data for 4). Of those unemployed, 33% attended school. Of the 98 subjects employed before BMT, 71 (72%) maintained employment and 27 (28%) lost work. Of those not employed before BMT, 15 (48%) gained employment and 16 (52%) continued unemployed (there were no data for 6). Job discrimination was reported by 23%. Problems obtaining insurance were reported by 44%. Overall, illness affected job plans in 69%. Multivariate logistic regression for association with current employment and loss of employment demonstrated high social functioning and excellent health by self-report, which were positively associated with current employment and physician-rated significant illness, attending school, and perceived job discrimination as negatively

affecting work. Among those employed before BMT, GVHD and perceived job discrimination were associated with loss of work after BMT; subjects with higher social functioning and men were less likely to have lost work.[460]

References

1. American Cancer Society: *Cancer Facts and Figures, 1993.* Atlanta, GA, American Cancer Society, 1992.
2. U.S. Department of Health and Human Services: *Cancer Rates and Risks.* 3rd ed. NIH Publication No. 85-691. Washington, DC, U.S. Government Printing Office, 1985.
3. Silverberg E: Cancer in young adults (ages 15–34). *CA* 1982, 32(1):32–53.
4. Silverberg E, Lubera J: Cancer Statistics. *CA* 1986, 36:9–23.
5. Cole TM, Edgerton VR: *Report on the Task Force on Medical Rehabilitation Research.* Hunt Valley, MD, 1990.
6. American Cancer Society: *Cancer Facts and Figures for Minorities, 1986,* Atlanta, GA, American Cancer Society, 1986.
7. U.S. Department of Health and Human Services: *Healthy People 2000: National Health Promotion and Disease Prevention Objectives.* DHHS Publication No. (PHS) 91-50212. Washington, DC, U.S. Government Printing Office, 1990.
8. Update: mortality attributable to HIV infection among persons aged 25–44 years—United States, 1991 and 1992. *MMWR* 1993, 42(45):869–872.
9. O'Hare PA, Malone D, Lusk E, McCorkle R: Unmet needs of black patients with cancer posthospitalization: a descriptive study. *Oncol Nurs Forum* 1993, 20(4):659–664.
10. Jansen C, Halliburton P, Dibble S, Dodd MJ: Family problems during cancer chemotherapy. *Oncol Nurs Forum* 1993, 20(4):689–694, 694–696.
11. Goodwin JS, Hunt WC, Samet JM: Determinants of cancer therapy in elderly patients. *Cancer* 1993, 72(2):594–601.
12. Boyd-Walton J: The role of rehabilitation services in oncology. *Clin Man Phys Ther* 1985, 5(2):24–25.
13. Cammack JM. Interdisciplinary care of the patient with cancer in a community hospital. *Clin Man Phys Ther* 1984, 2(4):7–12.
14. Broadwell DC: Rehabilitation needs of the patient with cancer. *CA* 1987, 60(Suppl 3):563–568.
15. Lehman J, Engel J, Medalie J: Cancer rehabilitation: assessment of need, development and evaluation of a model of care. *Arch Phys Med Rehabil* 1978, 59:410–419.
16. Hinterbuchner C: Rehabilitation of physical disability in cancer. *NY State J Med* 1978, 78:1066–1069.
17. Cromes GF Jr: Implementation of interdisciplinary cancer rehabilitation. *Rehabil Counsel Bull* 1978, 21:230–237.
18. Lynch PD, Schaefer S, Eckert D: Cancer rehabilitation issues for occupational and physical therapists: a conference report. *Prog Clin Biol Res* 1983, 130:443–453.
19. Raven R: Future trends in rehabilitation of patients with cancerous disease. *Br J Rehabil Disabled* 1974, 91:5–11.
20. Shabashova NY, Uzunova VG, Mirotvortseva KS, *et al.*: Possibilities for rehabilitating cancer patients in old age groups. *IARC Sci Publ* 1985, 58:267–279.
21. Villaneuva R: Rehabilitation needs of cancer patients. *South Med J* 1975, 68(2):169–172.
22. Wood CA, Anderson J, Yates JW: Physical function assessment in patients with advanced cancer. *Med Pediatr Oncol* 1981, 9(2):129–132.

23. Yates JW, Chalmer B, McGengney E: Evaluation of patients with advanced cancer using the Karnofsky performance statue. *Cancer* 1980, 45:220–224.

24. Krouse JH, Krouse HJ, Fabian RL: Adaptation to surgery for head and neck cancer. *Laryngoscope* 1989, 99(8, Pt 1):789–794.

25. Hladiuk M, Huchcroft S, Temple W, Schnurr BE: Arm function after axillary dissection for breast cancer: a pilot study to provide parameter estimates. *J Surg Oncol* 1992, 50(1):47–52.

26. Bruera E, Brenneis C, Michaud M, *et al.:* Association between asthenia and nutritional status, lean body mass, anemia, psychological status, and tumor mass in patients with advanced breast cancer: *J Pain Symptom Manage* 1989, 4(2):59–63.

27. Stumm D: Considering the whole woman: rehabilitation of the breast cancer patient. *Clin Man Phys Ther* 1982, 2(1):20–22.

28. Taylor CM: The rehabilitation of persons with cancer: is this the best we can do. *J Rehabil* 1984, 50(4):60–62.

29. Oleske D, Hauck WW, Heide E: Characteristics of cancer patient referrals to home care: a regional perspective. *Am J Public Health* 1983, 73(6):678–682.

30. Ganz PA: Current issues in cancer rehabilitation. *Cancer* 1990, 65 (Suppl 3):742–751.

31. Romsaas EP, Robins HI: Early rehabilitation in cancer: a case report. *Cancer Treat Res* 1986, 30:199–203.

32. Romsaas EP, McCormick JM: Assessment and resource utilization for cancer patients, nursing and rehabilitation counseling. *Arch Phys Med Rehabil* 1986, 67(7):459–462.

33. Romsaas EP, Juliani LM: Resource utilization in an outpatient setting. Rehabilitation problems experienced by cancer patients. *Oncol Nurs Forum* 1984, 11(3):45–48.

34. Romsass EP, Juliani LM, Briggs AL, *et al.:* A method for assessing the rehabilitation needs of oncology outpatients. *Oncol Nurs Forum* 1983, 10(3):17–21.

35. Smart CR, Yates JW: Quality of life. *CA* 1987, 60(Suppl 3):620–622.

36. Campbell H, Yi P, Rothberg H, Sierocki J: Impact of cancer chemotherapy on patients and family members: a clinical study in an outpatient setting [Abstract]. *Proc Annu Meet Am Soc Clin Oncol* 1992, 11:A1342.

37. Lansky SB, List MA, Ritter-Sterr C, *et al.:* Quality of life in head and neck cancer survivors [Abstract]. *Proc Annu Meet Am Soc Clin Oncol* 1989, 8:A656.

38. Rafla S, Kowalczyk D, Weiss R: The impact of clinical stage, site and therapy on the quality of life of cancer patients [Abstract]. *Proc Annu Meet Am Soc Clin Oncol* 1991, 10:A1236.

39. Musser EH: The self-reported needs of women with breast cancer who have recently completed treatment with chemotherapy [Abstract]. *Oncol Nurs Forum* 1990, 17(Suppl 2):144.

40. Norby PA, Apte-Kakode S: Rehabilitation after conservative breast cancer surgery: management of lymphedema and limited range of motion [Abstract]. *Oncol Nurs Forum* 1990, 17(Suppl 2):209.

41. Baker CA: Factors associated with rehabilitation outcomes in head and neck cancer patients [Abstract]. *Oncol Nurs Forum* 1991, 18(2):337.

42. Fieler VK: Side effects in the patient receiving radiation therapy for prostate cancer [Abstract]. *Oncol Nurs Forum* 1991, 18(2):353.

43. Butler KM, Oakley M, Christman NJ: Symptom experience and functional status in women having radiotherapy (rt) for gynecological cancer [Abstract]. *Oncol Nurs Forum* 1991, 18(2):360.

44. Brophy LR, Sharp EJ: Physical symptoms of combination biotherapy: a quality-of-life issue. *Oncol Nurs Forum* 1991, 18(Suppl 1):25–30.

45. Dunn V: Life after mastectomy. *Com Outlook* 1988, 8:34.

46. Holmes S: Preliminary investigations of symptom distress in two cancer patient populations: evaluation of a measurement instrument. *J Adv Nurs* 1991, 16(4):439–446.

47. Satariano WA, Ragheb NE, Branch LG, Swanson GM: Difficulties in physical functioning reported by middle-aged and elderly women with breast cancer: a case-control comparison. *J Gerontol* 1990, 45(1):M3–11.

48. Guadagnoli E, Mor V: Daily living needs of cancer outpatients. *J Community Health* 1991, 16(1):37–47.

49. Houts PS, Yasko JM, Harvey HA, *et al.:* Unmet needs of persons with cancer in Pennsylvania during the period of terminal care. *Cancer* 1988, 62(3):627–634.

50. Christ G, Siegel K: Monitoring quality-of-life needs of cancer patients. *Cancer* 1990, 65(Suppl 3):760–765.

51. Schag CA, Ganz PA, Heinrich RL: Cancer Rehabilitation Evaluation System—short form (CARES-SF). A cancer specific rehabilitation and quality of life instrument. *Cancer* 1991, 68(6):1406–1413.

52. Pickard-Holley S: Fatigue in cancer patients: a descriptive study. *Cancer Nurs* 1991, 14(1):13–19.

53. Rhodes VA, Watson PM, Hanson BM: Patients' descriptions of the influence of tiredness and weakness on self-care abilities. *Cancer Nurs* 1988, 11(3):186–194.

54. Roberts DK, Thorne SE, Pearson C: The experience of dyspnea in late-stage cancer: patients' and nurses' perspectives. *Cancer Nurs* 1993, 16(4):310–320.

55. Irvine DM, Vincent L, Bubela N, *et al.:* A critical appraisal of the research literature investigating fatigue in the individual with cancer. *Cancer Nurs* 1991, 14(4):188–199.

56. Dobkin PL, Morrow GR: Long-term side effects in patients, who have been treated successfully for cancer. *J Psychosoc Oncol* 1986, 3:23.

57. Stoter G, Koopman A, Vendrik CP, *et al.:* Ten-year survival and late sequelae in testicular cancer patients treated with cisplatin, vinblastine, and bleomycin. *J Clin Oncol* 1989, 7(8):1099–1104.

58. Barr RD, Furlong W, Dawson S, *et al.:* An assessment of global health status in survivors of acute lymphoblastic leukemia in childhood. *Am J Pediatr Hematol Oncol* 1993, 15(3):284–290.

59. Byrd R: Late effects of treatment of cancer in children. *Pediatr Clin North Am* 1985, 32:835.

60. Jakacki RI, Larsen RL, Barber G, *et al.:* Comparison of cardiac function tests after anthracycline therapy in childhood: implications for screening. *Cancer* 1993, 72(9):2739–2745.

61. Groth S, Johansen H, Sorensen PG, Rossing N: The effect of thoracic irradiation for cancer of the breast on ventilation, perfusion and pulmonary permeability: a one-year follow-up. *Acta Oncol* 1989, 28(5):671–678.

62. Makipernaa A, Heino M, Laitinen LA, Siimes MA: Lung function following treatment of malignant tumors with surgery, radiotherapy, or cyclophosphamide in childhood: a follow-up study after 11 to 27 years. *Cancer* 1989, 63(4):625–630.

63. Strender LE, Lindahl J, Larsson LE: Incidence of heart disease and functional significance of changes in the electro-cardiogram 10 years after radiotherapy for breast cancer. *CA* 1986, 57(5):929–934.

64. Krakoff IH: *Cancer Chemotherapeutic Agents. American Cancer Society Professional Education Publication.* Atlanta, GA, American Cancer Society.

65. Pelletier C, Lapointe L, LeBlanc P: Effects of lung resection on pulmonary function and exercise capacity. *Thorax* 1990, 45(7):497–502.

66. Abe R: A study on the pathogenesis of postmastectomy lymphedema. *Tohoku J Exp Med* 1976, 118:163–171.

67. Viniegra M, Marchetti M, Losso M, *et al.*: Cardiovascular autonomic function in anthracycline-treated breast cancer patients. *Cancer Chemother Pharmacol* 1990, 26(3):227–231.

68. Aksoy M, Erdem S, Bakioglu I, Dincol G: Endometrial cancer due to busulfan therapy: report of 2 cases. *J Cancer Res Clin Oncol* 1984, 108(3):362–363.

69. Abeloff MD: *Complications of Cancer, Diagnosis and Management.* Baltimore, MD, Johns Hopkins University Press, 1979.

70. Beninson J: Lymphedema: pathophysiologic and clinical concepts. *Angiology* 1975, 26:661–664.

71. Van Mieghem W, Demedts M: Cardiopulmonary function after lobectomy or pneumonectomy for pulmonary neoplasm. *Respir Med* 1989, 83(3):199–206.

72. Bacigalupo A, Frassoni F, Lint van M, *et al.*: Cyclosporin A in marrow transplantation for leukemia and aplastic anemia. *Exp Hematol* 1985, 13:244–248.

73. Baello EB, Ensberg ME, Ferguson DW, *et al.*: Effect of high-dose cyclophosphamide and total-body irradiation on left ventricular function in adult patients with leukemia undergoing allogenic bone marrow transplantation. *Cancer Treat Rep* 1986, 70(10):1187–1189.

74. Batist G, Andrews JL Jr: Pulmonary toxicity of antineoplastic drugs. *JAMA* 1981, 246(13):1449–1453.

75. Bristow MR, Mason JW, Billingham ME, Daniels JR: Dose-effect and structure-function relationships in doxorubicin cardiomyopathy. *Am Heart J* 1981, 102(4):709–718.

76. Bristow MR, Minobe WA, Billingham ME, *et al.*: Anthracycline-associated cardiac and renal damage in rabbits. Evidence for medication by associative substances. *Lab Invest* 1981, 45(2):157–158.

78. Buja LM, Ferrans VJ, Graw RG: Cardiac pathologic findings in patients treated with bone marrow transplantation. *Human Pathol* 1976, 7:17–78.

79. Feingold ML, Koss LG: Effects of long-term administration of busulfan. *Arch Intern Med* 1969, 124:66–71.

80. Gluckman E, Devergie A, Lokiec F, *et al.*: Nephrotoxicity of cyclosporin A in bone marrow transplantation. *Lancet* 1981, 2:144.

81. Gottdiener JS, Appelbaum FR, Ferrans VJ, *et al.*: Cardiotoxicity associated with high-dose cyclophosphamide therapy. *Arch Intern Med* 1981, 141:758–763.

82. Keown PA, Stiller CR, Laupacis AL, *et al.*: The effects and side effects of cyclosporine: relationship to drug pharmacokinetics. *Trans Proc* 1982, 14:659–661.

83. Mills BA, Roberts RW: Cyclophosphamide-induced cardiomyopathy: a report of two cases and review of the English literature. *CA* 1979, 43:2223–2226.

84. Minow RA, Benjamin RS, Lee ET: Adriamycin cardiomyopathy: risk factors. *CA* 1977, 39:1397–1402.

85. Stern LZ, Gruener R, Kirkpatrick JB, Nemeth P: The fine structure of cortisone-induced myopathy. *Exp Neurol* 1972, 36:530–538.

86. Bernstein AE: Psychological meaning of mastectomy and surgical removal of the inner reproductive organs. *JAMA* 1985, 40:178–180.

87. Dunn EJ, Hernandez J, Bender HW, *et al.*: Alterations in pulmonary function following pneumonectomy for bronchogenic carcinoma. *Ann Thorac Surg* 1982, 34(2):176–180.

88. Quesada JR, Talpaz M, Rios A, *et al.*: Clinical toxicity of interferons in cancer patients: a review. *J Clin Oncol* 1986, 4(2):234–243.

89. Vinokur AD, Threatt BA, Caplan RD, Zimmerman BL: Physical and psychosocial functioning and adjustment to breast cancer: long-term follow-up of a screening population. *Cancer* 1989, 63(2):394–405.

90. Carmel RJ, Kaplan HS: Mantle irradiation in Hodgkin's disease: an analysis of technique, tumor irradiation and complications. *Cancer* 1976, 7:2813–2825.

91. doPico GA, Wiley AL, Dickie HA: Pulmonary reaction to upper mantle radiation therapy for Hodgkin's disease. *Chest* 1979, 75:688–692.

92. Myers CE, Kinsella TJ: Cardiac and pulmonary toxicity. In DeVita VT, Hellman S, Rosenberg SA (eds): *Cancer: Principles and Practice of Oncology.* 2nd ed. Philadelphia J. B. Lippincott Company, 1985.

93. Stover DE: Pulmonary toxicity. In DeVita VT, Hellman S, Rosenberg SA (eds): *Cancer: Principles and Practice of Oncology.* 3rd ed. Philadelphia, J. B. Lippincott Company, 1989.

94. Torti FM, Lum BL: Cardiac toxicity. In DeVita VT, Hellman S, Rosenberg SA (eds): *Cancer: Principles and Practice of Oncology.* 3rd ed. Philadelphia, J. B. Lippincott Company, 1989.

95. Watchie J, Coleman CN, Raffin TA, *et al.*: Minimal long-term cardiopulmonary dysfunction following treatment for Hodgkin's disease. *Int J Radiat Oncol Biol Phys* 1987, 13:517–524.

96. Hydzik CA: Late effects of chemotherapy. Implications for patient management and rehabilitation. *Nurs Clin North Am* 1990, 25:423–426.

97. Watchie J: Cardiopulmonary complications of cancer treatment. *Clin Man Phys Ther* 1992, 12(4):92–95.

98. Gustavsson A, Skilsson J, Landberg T, *et al.*: Late cardiac effects after mantle radiotherapy in patients with Hodgkin's disease. *Ann Oncol* 1990, 1(5):355–363.

99. Weesner KM, Bledsoe M, Chauvenet A, Wofford M: Exercise echocardiography in the detection of anthracycline cardiotoxicity. *Cancer* 1991, 68(2):435–438.

100. Silberfarb PM: Psychiatric themes in the rehabilitation of mastectomy patients. *Int J Psychiatry Med* 1977–1978, 8(2):159–167.

101. Tobin MB, Lacey HJ, Meyer L, Mortimer PS: The psychological morbidity of breast cancer-related arm swelling: psychological morbidity of lymphedema. *Cancer* 1993, 72(11):3248–3252.

102. Fox BH: A psychological measure as a predictor in cancer. In Cohen J, Martins LR (eds): *Psychosocial Aspects of Cancer.* New York, Raven Press, 1982.

103. Capovilla ED, Colotti P, Fiorentino MV: Psychological status before and after surgery for breast cancer. *Tumori* 1984, (70)3:277–279.

104. Faulkner A: Mastectomy: reclaiming a body image. *Com Outlook* 1985, May: 11–13.

105. Feather BL, Lanigan C: Looking good after your mastectomy. *Am J Nurs* 1987, 87(8):1048–1049.

106. Filiberti A, Tamburini M, Murru L, *et al.*: Psychologic effects and esthetic results of breast reconstruction after mastectomy. *Tumori* 1986, 72(6):585–588.

107. Heinrich RL, Schag CC, Ganz PA: Living with cancer: the cancer inventory of problem situations. *J Clin Psychiatry* 1984, 40(4):972–980.

108. Heinrich RL, Schag CC: Stress and activity management: group treatment for cancer patients and spouses. *J Consult Clin Psychol* 1985, 53(4):439–446.

109. Holland JC, Jacobs E: Psychiatric sequelae following surgical treatment of breast cancer. *Adv Psychosom Med* 1986, 15:109–123.

110. Schain WS: Psychological rehabilitation for breast cancer patients. *Exp Suppl* 1982, 41:352–372.

111. Scott DW: Quality of life following the diagnosis of breast cancer. *Top Clin Nurs* 1983, 4(4):20–37.

112. McLoughlin WJ, Holz S: Cancer rehabilitation is an integrated support system. *Clin Man Phys Ther* 1985, 5(6):10–12.

113. Model program explores cancer rehabilitation process. *Hosp Pract* 1984, 65(2):28–30.

114. Stumm D: Considering the whole woman: rehabilitation of the breast cancer patient. *Clin Man Phys Ther* 1982, 2(1):20–22.

115. National Cancer Institute: Coping with cancer. DHHS Publication No. 80-2080. Washington, DC, U.S. Government Print Office, 1981.

116. Viney LL, Westbrook MT: Psychological reactions to chronic illness related disability as a function of its severity and type. *J Psychosom Res* 1981, 25(6):513–523.

117. Brown H, Kelly M: Stages of bone marrow transplantation: a psychiatric perspective. *Psychiatr Med* 1976, 38:439–446.

118. Popkin MK, Stiller V, Pierce C, *et al.:* Recent life changes and outcome of prolonged competitive stress. *J Nerv Ment Dis* 1976, 163:302–306.

119. Baider L, Sarell M, Edelstein EL: Selected social-psychological characteristics of a sample of Israeli cancer patients: facts and implications. *Israel J Med Sci* 1982, 18(2):259.

120. Cohen M: Psychosocial morbidity in cancer: a clinical perspective. In Cohen J, Cullen JW, Martin LR (eds): *Psychosocial Aspects of Cancer.* New York, Raven Press, 1982.

121. Cobb B: Medical and psychological problems in the rehabilitation of the cancer patient. In Hardy RE, Cull JG (eds): *Counseling and Rehabilitating the Cancer Patient.* Springfield, IL, Charles C Thomas, 1975; pp 24–68.

122. Winick L, Robbins GF: Physical and psychologic readjustment after mastectomy: an evaluation of Memorial Hospitals' PMRG program. *CA* 1977, 39(2):478–486.

123. Jamison K, Wellisch D, Pasnau R: Psychosocial aspects of mastectomy: the woman's perspective. *Am J Psychol* 1978;135:4.

124. Meyerowitz BE, Sparks FC, Spears IK: Adjuvant chemotherapy for breast cancer: psychosocial implications. *CA* 1979, 43:1613–1618.

125. Ling MH, Perry PJ, Tswang MT: Side effects of corticosteroid therapy: psychiatric aspects. *Arch Gen Psychiatry* 1981, 38(4):471–477.

126. Weisman A: *Coping with Cancer.* New York, McGraw-Hill, 1979.

127. Derogatis LR, Akiloff MD, Melisaratos N: Psychological coping mechanisms and survival time in metastatic breast cancer. *JAMA* 1979, 242:1504.

128. Flomenhoft D: Understanding and helping people who have cancer. *Phys Ther* 1984, 64(8):1232–1234.

129. Holland JC, Jacobs E: Psychiatric sequelae following surgical treatment of breast cancer. *Adv Psychosom Med* 1986, 15:109–123.

130. Holleb AI: Human values and cancer. *Hosp Pract* 1984, 19(6):16.

131. Itano J, Tanabe P, Lum JL, *et al.:* Compliance of cancer patients to therapy. *West J Nurs Res* 1983, 5(1):5–16.

132. Schaeffer D, Garms-Homolova V: Significance of self-help groups for psychosocial rehabilitation in cancer [Translated from German]. *Rehabilitation* (Stuttg) 1986, 25(3):128–133.

133. Smith EA: *Psychosocial Aspects of Cancer Patient Care: A Self-Instructional Text.* Houston, University of Texas Health Science Center at Houston, Division of Continuing Education, 1975.

134. Snyder R: Coping: you and your patient with cancer. *Clin Man Phys Ther* 1992, 12(4):64–69.

135. Holland JC: Clinical course of cancer. In Holland JC, Rowland JH (eds): *Handbook of Psychooncology: Psychological Care of the Patient with Cancer.* New York, Oxford University Press, 1989.

136. Heber D, Byerley LO, Chi J, *et al.:* Pathophysiology of malnutrition in the adult cancer patient. *CA* 1986, 58 (Suppl 8):1867–1873.

137. Clark CM, Goodlad GAJ: Depletion of proteins of phasic and tonic muscles in tumor-bearing rats. *Eur J Cancer Clin Oncol* 1971, 7:3–9.

138. Deuster PA, Morrison SD, Ahrens RA: Endurance exercise modifies cachexia of tumor growth in rats. *Med Sci Sports Exerc* 1985, 17(3):385–392.

139. Hickson RC, Foster C, Pollock ML, *et al.:* Reduced training intensities and loss of aerobic power, endurance, and cardiac growth. *J Appl Physiol* 1985, 58:492–499.

140. Norton JA, Lowry SF, Brennan MF: Effect of work-induced hypertrophy on skeletal muscle of tumor- and non-tumor-bearing rats. *J Appl Physiol* 1979, 46:654–657.

141. Hickson RC, Davis JR: Partial prevention of glucocorticoid-induced muscle atrophy by endurance training. *Am J Physiol* 1981, 24:E226–E232.

142. Simopoulos AP: Calories and energy expenditure in carcinogenesis: conference report. *J Am Diet Assoc* 1987, 87(1):92–97.

143. Dewys WD, Begg C, Lavin PT, *et al.:* Prognostic effect of weight loss prior to chemotherapy in cancer patients. Eastern Cooperative Oncology Group. *Am J Med* 1980, 69(4):491–497.

144. Reuben DB, Mor V, Hiris J: Clinical symptoms and length of survival in patients with terminal cancer. *Arch Intern Med* 1988, 148(7):1586–1591.

145. Shizgal HM: Body composition of patients with malnutrition and cancer: summary of the methods of assessment. *CA* 1985, 55(1):250–253.

146. Dilman VM, Berstein LM, Yevtushenko TP, *et al.:* Preliminary evidence on metabolic rehabilitation of cancer patients. *Arch Geschwulstforsch* 1988, 58(3):175–183.

147. Shike M, Russell DM, Detsky AS, Harrison JE: Changes in body composition in patients with small-cell lung cancer: the effect of total parenteral nutrition as an adjunct to chemotherapy. *Ann Intern Med* 1984, 101(3):303–309.

148. Clifford C, Kramer B. Diet as risk and therapy for cancer. *Med Clin North Am* 1993, 77(4):725–744.

149. Daly JM, Hearne B, Dunaj J, *et al.:* Nutritional rehabilitation in patients with advanced head and neck cancer receiving radiation therapy. *Am J Surg* 1984, 148(4):514–520.

150. Sarna L, Lindsey AM, Dean H, *et al.:* Nutritional intake, weight change, symptom distress, and functional status over time in adults with lung cancer. *Oncol Nurs Forum* 1993, 20(3):481–489.

151. Brown JK: Gender, age, usual weight, and tobacco use as predictors of weight loss in patients with lung cancer. *Oncol Nurs Forum* 1993, 20(3):466–472.

152. Brown SC, Abraham JS, Walsh S, Sykes PA: Risk factors and operative mortality in surgery for colorectal cancer. *Ann R Coll Surg Engl* 1991, 73(5):269–272.

153. Smets EM, Garssen B, Schuster-Uitterhoeve AL, de Haes JC: Fatigue in cancer patients. *Br J Cancer* 1993, 68(2):220–224.

154. Etherington ME: Physical therapy management of the cancer patient. *Clin Man Phys Ther* 1987, 7(3):12–15.

155. Harvey RF, Jellinek HM, Habeck RV: Cancer rehabilitation: analysis of 36 program approaches. *JAMA* 1982, 247(15):2127–2131.

156. Hirschberg G, Lewis L, Vaughan P: *Rehabilitation.* 2nd ed. New York, J. B. Lippincott Company, 1976.

157. Bostwick J: Rehabilitation after mastectomy. *J Med Assoc Ga* 1987, 76(5):336–341.

158. Habeck RV, Romsaas EP, Olsen SJ: Cancer rehabilitation and continuing care: a case study. *Cancer Nurs* 1984, 7(4):315–319.

159. Kobza LL: Assessing postmastectomy care in a community hospital. *Q Rev Bull* 1983, 9(4):116–119.

160. Kudsk EG, Hoffmann GS: Rehabilitation of the cancer patient. *Prim Care* 1987, 14(2):381–390.

161. McGarvey CL: *Physical Therapy for the Cancer Patient: Clinical Physical Therapy.* New York, Churchill Livingstone, 1990.

162. Gudas SA: Directives in cancer rehabilitation. *Clin Man Phys Ther* 1992, 12(4):32–36.

163. Johnson JB, Kelly AW: A multifaceted rehabilitation program for women with cancer. *Oncol Nurs Forum* 1990, 17(5):691.

164. Toot JL: Tapestry of care. *Clin Man Phys Ther* 1992, 12(4):9–10.

165. Mellette SJ: The cancer patient at work. *CA* 1985, 35(6):360–373.

166. Anderson JL: Insurability of cancer patients: a rehabilitation barrier. *Oncol Nurs Forum* 1984, 11(2):42–45.

167. Sigel CJ: Legal recourse for the cancer patient-returnee: the Rehabilitation Act of 1973. *Am J Law Med* 1984, 10(3):309–321.

168. Winningham ML, MacVicar MG, Bondoc M, et al.: Effect of aerobic exercise on body weight and composition in patients with breast cancer on adjuvant chemotherapy. *Oncol Nurs Forum* 1989, 16(5):683–689.

169. MacVicar MG, Winningham ML, Nickel JL: Effects of aerobic interval training in cancer patients' functional capacity. *Nurs Res* 1989, 38:348–351.

170. Hicks JE: Exercise for cancer patients. In Basmajian JV, Wolf SL (eds): *Therapeutic Exercise.* 5th ed. Baltimore, Williams & Wilkins, 1990, pp 28–31.

171. Pfalzer LA: Aerobic exercise for patients with disseminated cancer. *Clin Man Phys Ther* 1988, 8(2):351–370.

172. American College of Sports Medicine: *Guidelines for Graded Exercise Testing and Exercise Training.* 4th ed. New York, Lea & Febiger, 1991.

173. Winningham ML: Walking program for people with cancer. *Cancer Nurs* 1991, 14:270–276.

174. Winningham ML, MacVicar MG: The effect of aerobic exercise on patient reports of nausea. *Oncol Nurs Forum* 1988, 15(2, Suppl):447–540.

175. Berglund G, Bolund C, Gustavsson UL, Sjoden PO: Starting again: a comparison study of a group rehabilitation program for cancer patients. *Acta Oncol* 1993, 32(1):15–21.

176. Wingate L: Efficacy of physical therapy for patients who have undergone mastectomies. *Phys Ther* 1985, 65(6):896–900.

177. Wingate L, Croghan I, Natarajan N, et al.: Rehabilitation of the mastectomy patient: a randomized, blind, prospective study. *Arch Phys Med Rehabil* 1989, 70(1):21–24.

178. Guttman H, Kersz T, Barzilai T, et al.: Achievements of physical therapy in patients after modified radical mastectomy compared with quadrantectomy, axillary dissection, and radiation for carcinoma of the breast. *Arch Surg* 1990, 125(3):389–391.

179. Swedborg I: Effectiveness of combined methods of physiotherapy for post-mastectomy lymphoedema. *Scand J Rehabil Med* 1980, 12(2):77–85.

180. Sachs SH, Davis JM, Reynolds SA, et al.: Comparative results of postmastectomy rehabilitation in a specialized and a community hospital. *CA* 1981, 48(5):1251–1255.

181. Swedborg I, Wallgren A: The effect of pre- and post-mastectomy radiotherapy on the degree of edema, shoulder joint mobility, and gripping force. *CA* 1981, 47:877–881.

182. Swedborg I: Effects of treatment with an elastic sleeve and intermittent pneumatic compression in post-mastectomy patients with lymphoedema of the arm. *Scand J Rehabil Med* 1984, 16(1):35–41.

183. van-der-Horst CM, Kenter JA, deJong MT, et al.: Shoulder function following early mobilization of the shoulder after mastectomy and axillary dissection. *Neth J Surg* 1985, 37(4):105–108.

184. Rodier JF, Gadonneix P, Dauplat J, et al.: Influence of the timing of physiotherapy upon the lymphatic complications of axillary dissection for breast cancer. *Int Surg* 1987, 72(3):166–169.

185. Petrek JA, Peters MM, Nori S, et al.: Axillary lymphadenectomy: a prospective, randomized trial of 13 factors influencing drainage, including early or delayed arm mobilization. *Arch Surg* 1990, 125(3):378–382.

186. Knobf MT: Symptoms and rehabilitation needs of patients with early stage breast cancer during primary therapy. *CA* 1990, 66(Suppl 6):1392–1401.

187. Knobf MKT: Primary breast cancer: physical consequences and rehabilitation. *Semin Oncol Nurs* 1985, 1(3):214–224.

188. Jungi WP: The prevention and management of lymphoedema after treatment for breast cancer. *Int Rehabil Med* 1981, 3(3):129–135.

189. Gaskin TA, LoBuglio A, Kelly P, et al.: STRETCH: a rehabilitative program for patients with breast cancer. *South Med J* 1989, 82(4):467–469.

190. Ganz PA, Schag CC, Polinsky ML, et al.: Rehabilitation needs and breast cancer: the first month after primary therapy. *Breast Cancer Res Treat* 1987, 10(3):243–253.

191. Ganz PA, Schag CC, Polinsky ML, et al.: Rehabilitation of patients with primary breast cancer: assessing the impact of adjuvant therapy. *Recent Results Cancer Res* 1989, 115:244–254.

192. Dawson I, Stam L, Heslinga JM, et al.: Effect of shoulder immobilization on wound seroma and shoulder dysfunction following modified radical mastectomy: a randomized prospective clinical trial. 1989, 76(3):311–312.

193. Johnson, JB, Kelly AW: A multifaceted rehabilitation program for women with cancer. *Nurs Forum* 1990, 17(5):691.

194. Scalon EF, Feldman JL: Rehabilitation of the breast cancer patient. *Semin Surg Oncol* 1988, 4(4):268–273.

195. Kobza LL: Assessing postmastectomy care in a community hospital. *Q Rev Bull* 1983, 9(4):116–119.

196. Konecne SM: Postsurgery breast cancer inpatient program. *Clin Man Phys Ther* 1992, 12(4):42–49.

197. Miller LT: Postsurgery breast cancer outpatient program. *Clin Man Phys Ther* 1992, 12(4):50–57.

198. Woods EN: Reaching out to patients with breast cancer. *Clin Man Phys Ther* 1992, 12(4):58–63.

199. Scanlon EF, Strax P: Breast cancer. In Holleb AI (ed): *The American Cancer Society Cancer Book.* New York, Doubleday & Company, 1986, pp 297–340.

200. Bostwick J: Rehabilitation after mastectomy. *J Med Assoc Ga* 1987, 76(5):336–341.

201. Danoff BF, Goodman RL, Glick JH, et al.: The effect of adjuvant chemotherapy on cosmesis and complications in patients with breast cancer treated by definitive irradiation. *Radiat Oncol Biol Phys* 1983, 9:1625–1630.

202. Dietz JH Jr: Rehabilitation of the mastectomy patient. *Breast* 1976, 2:7–11.

203. Kobza LL: Assessing postmastectomy care in a community hospital. *Q Rev Bull* 1983, 9(4):116–119.

204. Radier JF, Gadonneix P, Dauplat J, et al.: Influence of the timing of physiotherapy upon the lymphatic complications of axillary dissection for breast cancer. *Int Surg* 1987, 72(3):166–169.

205. Molinaro J, Kleinfeld M, Lebed S: Physical therapy and

dance in the surgical management of breast cancer. A clinical report. *Phys Ther* 1986, 66(6):967–969.

206. Willhite OD Jr: Pre- and post operative rehabilitation exercises for the mastectomy patient. *Home Health Nurs* 1984, 2(1):34–36, 38–39.

207. Adcock JL: Rehabilitation of the breast cancer patient. In McGarvey CL (ed): *Physical Therapy for the Cancer Patient.* New York, Churchill Livingstone, 1990, pp 67–84.

208. Snyder R: Mastectomy rehabilitation home care protocol. Special issue: Breast Cancer: Post-Mastectomy Rehabilitation. *Rehab Oncol* 1986, 4(2):9–10.

209. Walton JF: Post-mastectomy rehab protocol. Special issue: Breast Cancer: Post-Mastectomy Rehabilitation. *Rehab Oncol* 1986, 4(2):11–12.

210. Kim-Sing C, Basio V: Post mastectomy lymphedema treated with the Wright linear pump. *Can J Surg* 1987, 30:368–370.

211. Leis HP Jr: The relationship of diet to cancer, cardiovascular disease and longevity. *Int Surg* 1991, 76(1):1–5.

212. Smoking and cancer. *AAOHN J* 1986, 34(9):447–450.

213. Fernandes G, Venkatraman JT: Possible mechanisms through which dietary lipids, calorie restriction, and exercise modulate breast cancer. *Adv Exp Med Biol* 1992, 322:1–6.

214. Hegsted DM: Exercise, calories, and fat: future challenges. *Adv Exp Med Biol* 1992, 322:185–201.

215. Boyd NF, McGuire V: Evidence of association between plasma high-density lipoprotein cholesterol and risk factors for breast cancer. *J Natl Cancer Inst* 1990, 82(6):460–468.

216. Persson B, Johansson BW: The Kockum study: twenty-two-year follow-up. Coronary heart disease in a population in the south of Sweden. *Acta Med Scand* 1984, 216(5):485–493.

217. Paffenbarger RS Jr, Lee IM, Wing AL: The influence of physical activity on the incidence of site-specific cancers in college alumni. *Adv Exp Med Biol* 1992, 322:7–15.

218. Uhlenbruck G, Order U: Can endurance sports stimulate immune mechanisms against cancer and metastasis? *Int J Sports Med* 1991, 12(Suppl 1):S63–S68.

219. Zanker KS, Kroczek R: Looking along the track of the psychoneuro-immunologic axis for missing links in cancer progression. *Int J Sports Med* 1991, 12(Suppl 1):S58–S62.

220. Arraiz GA, Wigle DT, Mao Y: Risk assessment of physical activity and physical fitness in the Canada Health Survey mortality follow-up study. *J Clin Epidemiol* 1992, 45(4):419–428.

221. Lee IM, Paffenbarger RS Jr, Hsieh CC: Physical activity and risk of prostatic cancer among college alumni. *Am J Epidemiol* 1992, 135(2):169–179.

222. Thompson HJ: Effect of amount and type of exercise on experimentally induced breast cancer. *Adv Exp Med Biol* 1992, 322:61–71.

223. Cohen LA, Boylan E, Epstein M, Zang E: Voluntary exercise and experimental mammary cancer. *Adv Exp Med Biol* 1992, 322:41–59.

224. Rogers AE: Selected recent studies of exercise, energy metabolism, body weight, and blood lipids relevant to interpretation and design of studies of exercise and cancer. *Adv Exp Med Biol* 1992, 322:239–245.

225. Ballard-Barbash R, Schatzkin A, Albanes D, *et al.:* Physical activity and risk of large bowel cancer in the Framingham Study. *Cancer Res* 1990, 50(12):3610–3613.

226. Shephard RJ: Exercise in the prevention and treatment of cancer. An update. *Sports Med* 1993, 15(4):258–280.

227. Levi F, La Vecchia C, Negri E, Franceschi S: Selected physical activities and the risk of endometrial cancer. *Br J Cancer* 1993, 67(4):846–851.

228. Wannamethee G, Shaper AG, Macfarlane PW: Heart rate, physical activity, and mortality from cancer and other non-cardiovascular diseases. *Am J Epidemiol* 1993, 137(7):735–748.

229. Bernstein L, Ross RK, Lobo RA, *et al.:* The effects of moderate physical activity on menstrual cycle patterns in adolescence: implications for breast cancer prevention. *Br J Cancer* 1987, 55(6):681–685.

230. Keys A, Aravanis C, Blackburn H: Serum cholesterol and cancer mortality in the Seven Countries Study. *Am J Epidemiol* 1985, 121(6):870–883.

231. Whittemore AS, Paffenbarger RS, *et al.:* Early precursors of site-specific cancers in college men and women. *J Natl Cancer Inst* 1985, 74(1):43–51.

232. Paffenbarger RS Jr, Hyde RT, Wing AL: Physical activity and incidence of cancer in diverse populations: a preliminary report. *Am J Clin Nutr* 1987, 45(Suppl 1):312–317.

233. Vena JE, Graham S, Zielezny M, *et al.:* Occupational exercise and risk of cancer. *Am J Clin Nutr* 1987, 45(Suppl 1):318–327.

234. Wu AH, Paganini-Hill A, Ross RK, *et al.:* Alcohol, physical activity and other risk factors for colorectal cancer: a prospective study. *Br J Cancer* 1987, 55(6):687–694.

235. Shephard RJ: Exercise and malignancy. *Sports Med* 1986, 3(4):235–241.

236. Gerhardsson de Verdier M, Steineck G, Hagman U, *et al.:* Physical activity and colon cancer: a case-referent study in Stockholm. *Int J Cancer* 1990, 46(6):985–989.

237. LeMarchand L, Kolonel LN, Yoshizawa CN: Lifetime occupational physical activity and prostate cancer risk. *Am J Epidemiol* 1991, 133(2):103–111.

238. Kato I, Tominaga S, Matsuura A, *et al.:* A comparative case-control study of colorectal cancer and adenoma. *Jpn J Cancer Res* 1990, 81(11):1101–1109.

239. Nicholson WJ, Davis DL: Analyses of changes in the ratios of male-to-female cancer mortality: a hypothesis-generating exercise. *Ann NY Acad Sci* 1990, 609:290–299.

240. Trapido EJ: Age at first birth, parity, and breast cancer risk. *Cancer* 1983, 51:946–948.

241. Hamm P, Shekelle RB, Stamler J: Large fluctuations in body weight during young adulthood and twenty-five-year risk of coronary death in men. *Am J Epidemiol* 1989, 129(2):312–318.

242. Severson RK, Nomura AM, Grove JS, Stemmermann GN: A prospective analysis of physical activity and cancer. *Am J Epidemiol* 1989, 130(3):522–529.

243. Sturgeon SR, Brinton LA, Berman ML, *et al.:* Past and present physical activity and endometrial cancer risk. *Br J Cancer* 1993, 68(3):584–589.

244. Brownson RC, Zahm SH, Chang JC, Blair A: Occupational risk of colon cancer: an analysis by anatomic subsite. *Am J Epidemiol* 1989, 130(4):675–687.

245. Albanes D, Blair A, Taylor PR: Physical activity and risk of cancer in the NHANES I population. *Am J Public Health* 1989, 79(6):744–750.

246. Blair SN, Kohl HW, Gordon NF, Paffenbarger RS Jr: How much physical activity is good for health? *Annu Rev Public Health* 1992, 13:99–126.

247. Slattery ML, Schumacher MC, Smith KR, *et al.:* Physical activity, diet, and risk of colon cancer in Utah. *Am J Epidemiol* 1988, 128(5):989–999.

248. Dietz JH Jr: Rehabilitation of the cancer patient. *Med Clin North Am* 1969, 53(3):607–624.

249. Dietz J: Rehabilitation of the cancer patient: its role in the scheme of comprehensive care. *Clin Bull* 1974, 4(3):104–107.

250. Dietz JH Jr: Adaptive rehabilitation of the cancer patient. *Curr Probl Cancer* 1980, 5(5):1–56.

251. Dietz JH Jr: *Rehabilitation Oncology*. New York, John Wiley & Sons, 1981.

252. Frank-Stromborg: Health promotion behaviors in ambulatory cancer patients: facts or fiction? *Oncol Nurs Forum* 1986, 13(1):37–43.

253. Albert M: Health screening to promote health for the elderly. *Nurse Pract* 1987, 12(5):42–44, 48–51, 54–58.

254. Crosson K: Cancer patient education: what, where, and by whom? *Health Educ Q* 1984, (Suppl 10):19–29.

255. Dinning WD, Crampton J: The Krantz Health Opinion Survey: correlations with preventive health behaviors and intentions. *Psychol Rep* 1989, 64(1):59–64.

256. Havas S, Walker B Jr: Massachusetts' approach to the prevention of heart disease, cancer and stroke. *Public Health Rep* 1986, 101(1):29–39.

257. Skillrud DM: COPD: causes, treatment, and risk for lung cancer. *Compr Ther* 1986, 12(11):13–16.

258. Walter HJ, Connelly PA: Screening for risk factors as a component of a chronic disease prevention program for youth. *J Sch Health* 1985, 55(5):183–188.

259. Ross RK, Berstein L, Garabrant D, Henderson BE: Avoidable nondietary risk factors for cancer. *Am Fam Physician* 1988, 38(2):153–160.

260. Garrison J, *et al.*: Accessibility and utilization of educational materials for cancer patients. *Oncol Nurs Forum* 1983, 10(2):60–62.

261. Position of the American Dietetic Association and the Canadian Dietetic Association: nutrition for physical fitness and athletic performance for adults. *J Am Diet Assoc* 1993, 93(6):691–696.

262. U.S. Department of Health and Human Services: *Diet, Nutrition and Cancer Prevention: A guide to food choices*. NIH Publication No. 85–2711. Washington, DC, U.S. Government Printing Office.

263. Levenson FB: *The Causes and Prevention of Cancer*. New York, Stein and Day, 1984.

264. Upton AC: Principles of cancer biology: etiology and prevention of cancer. In DeVita VT, Hellman S, Rosenberg SA (eds): *Cancer: Principles & Practice of Oncology*. Philadelphia, J. B. Lippincott and Company, 1982, pp 33–58.

265. American Heart Association Scientific Council: Statement on exercise. *Circulation* 1992, 86(1):340–344.

266. U.S. dietary recommendations. Washington, DC, U.S. Government Printing Office, 1992.

267. Hamburgh RR: Principles of cancer treatment. *Clin Man Phys Ther* 1992, 12(4):37–41.

268. Pitot HC: Principles of cancer biology: chemical carcinogenesis. In DeVita VT, Hellman S, Rosenberg SA (eds): *Cancer: Principles & Practice of Oncology*. 2nd ed. Philadelphia, J. B. Lippincott Company, 1985, pp 79–100.

269. Fry RJM: Principles of cancer biology: physical carcinogenesis. In DeVita VT, Hellman S, Rosenberg SA (eds): *Cancer: Principles & Practice of Oncology*. 2nd ed. Philadelphia, J. B. Lippincott Company, 1985, pp 101–112.

270. Fidler IJ, Hart IR: Principles of cancer biology: cancer metastasis. In DeVita VT, Hellman S, Rosenberg SA (eds): *Cancer: Principles & Practice of Oncology*. 2nd ed. Philadelphia, J. B. Lippincott Company, 1985, p 112.

271. Dorr R, Fritz FW: *Chemotherapeutic Agents*. New York, Elsevier Science, 1980.

272. Prosnitz LR, Kapp DS, Weissberg JB, *et al.*: Radiotherapy: part 1. *N Engl J Med* 1983, 309(13):771–777.

273. Prosnitz LR, Kapp DS, Weissberg JB, *et al.*: Radiotherapy: part II. *N Engl J Med* 1983, 309(14):834–840.

274. Loughner JE, Carignan JR: Clinical pharmacology of antineoplastic agents. In Rosenthal S, Carignan JR, Smith B (eds): *Medical Care of the Cancer Patient*. Philadelphia, W. B. Saunders Company, 1987, pp 79–113.

275. Rubin P: Principles of radiation oncology and cancer radiotherapy. In Rubin P (ed): *Clinical Oncology: A Multidisciplinary Approach*. 6th ed. Atlanta, GA: American Cancer Society, 1983.

276. Karlberg I, Edstrom S, Ekman L, *et al.*: Metabolic host reaction to proliferation of non-malignant cells versus malignant cells in vivo. *Cancer Res* 1981, 22:597–599.

277. Foltz AT: Weight gain among stage II breast cancer patients: a study of five factors. *Oncol Nurs Forum* 1985, 12(3):21–26.

278. Huntington MO: Weight gain in patients receiving adjuvant chemotherapy for carcinoma of the breast. *Cancer* 1985, 56:472–474.

279. Lindsey AM, Dodd M, Kaempfer SH: Endocrine mechanisms and obesity: influences in breast cancer. *Oncol Nurs Forum* 1987, 14(2):47–51.

280. U.S. Department of Health and Human Services: *Clinical Practice Guideline, Acute Pain Management: Operative or Medical Procedures and Trauma*. Agency for Health Care Policy Research Publication No. 92–0032. Washington, DC, U.S. Government Printing Office, 1992.

281. Taddeini L, Rolschafer JC: Pain syndromes associated with cancer: achieving effective relief. *Postgrad Med* 1984, 75(1):1101–1018.

282. Foley KM: Cancer and pain. In Holleb AI (ed): *The American Cancer Society Cancer Book*. New York, Doubleday & Company, 1986, pp 225–237.

283. Strang P: Emotional and social aspects of cancer pain. *Acta Oncol* 1992, 31(3):323–326.

284. Strang P, Qvarner H: Cancer-related pain and its influence on quality of life. *Anticancer Res* 1990, 10(1):109–112.

285. Layzer RB: *Neuromuscular Manifestations of Systemic Disease*. Philadelphia, F. A. Davis Company, 1985.

286. Allegretta GJ, Weisman SJ, Altman AJ: Oncologic emergencies I: metabolic and space-occupying consequences of cancer and cancer treatment. *Pediatr Clin North Am* 1985, 32(3):601–611.

287. Salner AL, Botnick LE, Herzog AG, *et al.*: Reversible brachial plexography following primary radiation therapy for breast cancer. *Cancer Treat Rep* 1983, 65:797–802.

288. Minna JD, Bunn PA: Paraneoplastic syndromes. In DeVita VT, Hellman S, Rosenberg SA (eds): *Cancer: Principles & Practice of Oncology*. 2nd ed. Philadelphia, J. B. Lippincott Company, 1985, pp 1797–1842.

289. Gerber LH, McGarvey CL III: Musculoskeletal deficits and rehabilitation intervention in the cancer patient. In Wittes RE (ed): *Manual of Oncologic Therapeutics*. Philadelphia, J. B. Lippincott Company, 1989/1990.

290. Caldwell DS: Musculoskeletal syndromes associated with malignancy. In Kelly WN, Harris ED Jr, Ruddy S, Sledge CB (eds): *Textbook of Rheumatology*. 2nd ed. Philadelphia, W. B. Saunders Company, pp 1603–1619.

291. Croft PB, Wilkinson MW: The incidence of carcinomatous neuromyopathy with special reference to carcinoma of the lung and breast. In Brain WR, Norris FH Jr (eds): *The Remote Effects of Cancer on the Nervous System*. New York, Grune & Stratton, 1965, pp 45–54.

292. Pflazer L, Tutschka PJ, Harper D: Effects of interval training on muscle performance after BMT [Abstract]. *J Cardiopulm Rehab* 1989, 9(10).

293. Ganel A, Engel J, Sela M, *et al.*: Nerve entrapments associated with postmastectomy lymphedema. *CA* 1979, 44:2254–2259.

294. Shapiro WR: Tumors of the brain. In Holleb AI (ed): *The American Cancer Society Cancer Book*. New York, Doubleday & Company, 1986, pp 277–296.

295. Leestma J: Brain tumors. In Scarpelli D (ed): American Association of Pathologists, MD, 1980.

296. Levin V, Sheline G, Gutin P: Neoplasms of the central nervous system. In DeVita VT, Hellman S, Rosenberg SA (eds): *Cancer: Principles and Practice of Oncology.* 3rd ed. Philadelphia, J. B. Lippincott Company, 1989.

297. Berens M, Rutka J, Rosenblum M: Brain tumor epidemiology, growth and invasion. *Neurosurg Clin North Am* 1990, 1:1–18.

298. Black P: Brain tumors: part I. *N Engl J Med* 1991, 324:1471–1476.

299. Black P: Brain tumors: part II. *N Engl J Med* 1991, 324:1555–1564.

300. Sutton L, Packer R, Schut L: Medulloblastomas. *Neurosurg Clin North Am* 1990, 1:97–110.

301. Neatherlin J: Pineal region brain tumors. *J Neurosurg Nurs* 1985, 17:349–353.

302. Bruce J, Stein B: Pineal tumors. *Neurosurg Clin North Am* 1990, 1:123–138.

303. Allegretta, GJ, Weisman SJ, Altman AJ: Oncologic emergencies II: hematologic and infectious complications of cancer and cancer treatment. *Pediatr Clin North Am* 1985, 32(3):613–624.

304. Lindahl J, Strender LE, Larsson LE, Unsgaard A: Electrocardiographic changes after radiation therapy for carcinoma of the breast. Incidence and functional significance. *Acta Radiol* 1983, 22(6):433–440.

305. Ryttov N, Blichert-Toft M, Madsen EL, *et al.:* Influence of adjuvant irradiation on shoulder joint function after mastectomy for breast carcinoma. *Acta Radiol* 1983, 22(1):29–33.

306. Davidson G, Dean JT: Trismus after radiation therapy. *Clin Man Phys Ther* 1992, 12(4):70–76.

307. Sugarbaker PH, Lampert MH: Excision of the quadriceps muscle group. *Surgery* 1983, 93:462–466.

308. Brown H, Burns S, Kaise C: The spinal accessory nerve plexus, the trapezius muscle and shoulder stabilization after radical neck cancer surgery. *Ann Surg* 1988, 208:654–661.

309. Shone GR, Yardley MPJ: An audit into the incidence of handicap after unilateral radical neck dissection. *J Laryngol Otol* 1991, 105:760–762.

310. Schuller DE, Hamaker RC, Weidberger EC, *et al.:* Analysis of disability resulting from treatment including radical neck dissection or modified neck dissection. *Head Neck Surg* 1983, 6:551–558.

311. Leipzig B, Suen JY, English JL, *et al.:* Functional evaluation of the spinal accessory nerve after neck dissection. *Am J Surg* 1983, 146:526–530.

312. Steelman R, Sokol J: Quantification of trismus following irradiation of the temporomandibular joint. *Mo Dent J* 1986, Nov–Dec:21–23.

313. Engelmeier RL, King GE: Complications of head and neck radiation therapy and their management. *J Prosthet Dent* 1983, 49:514–522.

314. Rubin RL, Doku H: Therapeutic radiology: the modalities and their effects on oral tissues. *J Am Dent Assoc* 1976, 91:731.

315. Bodey GP: Infectious complications in the cancer patient. In Crooke ST, Prestayko AW (eds): *Cancer and chemotherapy: Vol. II.* New York, Academic Press, 1980.

316. Brody GR, Bolivar R, Farnstern V: Infectious complications in leukemia patients. *Semin Hematol* 1982, 19:193.

317. Gryfinski J: Amenorrhea-galactorrhea syndrome in the prolactin-secreting pituitary tumor: nursing implications. *J Neurosurg* 1985, 17:301–308.

318. Beals RK, Lawton GP, Snell WE: Prophylactic internal fixation of the femur in metastatic breast cancer. *Cancer* 1971, 28:1350–1354.

319. Elite JW, Bijvoet OL, Cleton FJ, *et al.:* Osteolytic bone metastases in breast carcinoma pathogenesis, morbidity and bisphosphonate treatment. *Eur J Cancer Clin Oncol* 1986, 22(4):493–500.

320. Scher HI, Yagoda A: Bone metastases: pathogenesis, treatment, and rationale for use of resorption inhibitors. *Am J Med* 1987, 82(2A):6–28.

321. Bhardwaj S, Holland JF: Chemotherapy of metastatic cancer in bone. *Clin Orthop* 1982, 169:28–35.

322. Greditzer HG III, McLead RA, Unni KK, *et al.:* Bone sarcomas in Paget disease. *Radiology* 1983, 146:327–333.

323. Kofoed H, Solgaard S: Resection alloplasty in the treatment of certain malignant bone tumors. *Cancer* 1983, 52(11):2180–2184.

324. Mankin HJ, Lange TA, Spanier SS: The hazards of biopsy in patients with malignant primary bone and soft-tissue tumors. *J Bone Joint Surg [Am]* 1982, 64(8):1121–1127.

325. Sherry AS, Levy RN, Siffert R: Metastatic disease of bone in orthopedic surgery. *Clin Orthop* 1982, 169:44–52.

326. Schajowicz F: Current trends in the diagnosis and treatment of malignant bone tumors. *Clin Orthop* 1983, 180:220–252.

327. Sherry AS, Levy RN, Siffert R: Metastatic disease of bone in orthopedic surgery. *Clin Orthop* 1982, 169:44–52.

328. Gebhart M, Roman A, Ghanem G, Lejeune F: Surgical treatment of bone metastases of the peripheral skeleton: a review of 33 cases. *Eur J Cancer Clin Oncol* 1989, 15(6):520–529.

329. Bocchi L, Lazzeroni L, Maggi M: The surgical treatment of metastases in long bones. *Ital J Orthop Traumatol* 1988, 14(2):167–173.

330. Bunting R, Lamont-Havers W, Schweon E, Kliman A: Pathologic fracture risk in rehabilitation of patients with bony metastases. *Clin Orthop* 1985, 192:222–227.

331. Friedl W: Indication, management and results of surgical therapy for pathological fractures in patients with bone metastases. *Eur J Surg Oncol* 1990, 16(4):380–396.

332. Maxon HR III, Schroder LE, Thomas SR, *et al.:* Re-186 (Sn) HEDP for treatment of painful osseous metastases: initial clinical experience in 20 patients with hormone-resistant prostate cancer. *Radiology* 1990, 176(1):155–159.

333. Poulsen HS, Nielsen OS, Klee M, Rorth M: Palliative irradiation of bone metastases. *Cancer Treat Rev* 1989, 16(1):41–48.

334. Colyer RA: Surgical stabilization of pathological neoplastic fractures. *Curr Probl Cancer* 1986, 10(3):117–168.

335. Huckstep RL: Early mobilization and rehabilitation in fractures and orthopaedic conditions. *Aust N Z J Surg* 1977, 47(3):344–353.

336. Malkawi H, Shannak A, Amr S: Surgical treatment of pathological subtrochanteric fractures due to benign lesions in children and adolescents. *J Pediatr Orthop* 1984, 4(1):63–69.

337. DeVita V, Hellman S, Rosenberg S: *Cancer Principles and Practice of Oncology.* Philadelphia, J. B. Lippincott Company, 1989.

338. Sullivan MJ, Carroll WR, Baker SR, *et al.:* The free scapular flap for head and neck reconstruction. *Am J Otolaryngol* 1990, 11(5):318–327.

339. Danoff BF, Goodman RL, Glick JH, *et al.:* The effect of adjuvant chemotherapy on cosmesis and complications in patients with breast cancer treated by definitive irradiation. *Radiat Oncol Biol Phys* 1983, 9:1625–1630.

340. Frieden RA, Ryniker D, Kenan S, Lewis MM: Assessment of patient function after limb-sparing surgery. *Arch Phys Med Rehabil* 1993, 74(1):38–43.

341. Enneking WF, Dunham W, Gebhardt MC, *et al.:* A system

for the functional evaluation of reconstructive procedures after surgical treatment of tumors of the musculoskeletal system. *Clin Orthop* 1993, 286:241–246.

342. Turner-Mcglade J, Decker W, Fehir K: Cardiopulmonary changes in bone marrow transplant patients: effects of an exercise program [Abstract]. *J Cardiopulm Rehabil* 1988, 8(10):405.

343. Sharkey AM, Carey AB, Heise CT, Barber G: Cardiac rehabilitation after cancer therapy in children and young adults. *Am J Cardiol* 1993, 71(16):1488–1490.

344. Sarna L: Women with lung cancer: impact on quality of life. *Quality Life Res* 1993, 2(1):13–22.

345. Sarna L: Fluctuations in physical function: adults with non-small cell lung cancer. *J Adv Nurs* 1993, 18(5):714–724.

346. Foote M, Sexton DL, Pawlik L: Dyspnea: a distressing sensation in lung cancer. *Oncol Nurs Forum* 1986, 13(5):25–31.

347. Lange P, Nyboe J, Appleyard M, et al.: Ventilatory function and chronic mucus hypersecretion as predictors of death from lung cancer. *Am Rev Respir Dis* 1990, 141(3):613–617.

348. Markos J, Mullan BP, Hillman DR, et al.: Preoperative assessment as a predictor of mortality and morbidity after lung resection. *Am Rev Respir Dis* 1989, 139(4):902–910.

349. Dales RE, Dionne G, Leech JA, et al.: Preoperative prediction of pulmonary complications following thoracic surgery. *Chest* 1993, 104(1):155–159.

350. Bria WF, Kanarek DJ, Kazemi H: Prediction of postoperative pulmonary function following thoracic operations. Value of ventilation-perfusion scanning. *J Thorac Cardiovasc Surg* 1983, 86(2):186–192.

351. Coleman NC, Schraufnagel DE, Rivington, et al.: Exercise testing in evaluation of patients for lung resection. *Am Rev Respir Dis* 1982, 125(5):604–606.

352. Corris PA, Ellis DA, Hawkins T, et al.: Use of radionuclide scanning in the preoperative estimation of pulmonary function after pneumonectomy. *Thorax* 1987, 42(4):285–291.

353. Bechard D, Wetstein L: Assessment of exercise oxygen consumption as preoperative criterion for lung presection. *Ann Thorac Surg* 1987, 44(4):344–349.

354. Furukawa A, Uehara H, Namima F, et al.: Postoperative care and rehabilitation of patients with lung cancer [Translated from Japanese]. *Kango Gijutsu* 1985, 31(14):1874–1878.

355. Jezek V, Ourednik A, Lichtenberg J, et al.: Cardiopulmonary function in lung resection performed for bronchogenic cancer in patients above 65 years of age. *Respiration* 1970, 21(1):42–50.

356. Juhl B, Frost N: A comparison between measured and calculated changes in the lung function after operation for pulmonary cancer. *Acta Anaesthesiol Scand* (Suppl) 1985, 57:39–45.

357. Berggren H, Ekroth R, Malmberg R, et al.: Hospital mortality and long term survival in relation to preoperative function in elderly patients with bronchogenic carcinoma. *Ann Thorac Surg* 1984, 38(6):633–636.

358. Olson GN, Weiman DS, Bolton JW, et al.: Submaximal invasive exercise testing and quantitative lung scanning in the evaluation for tolerance of lung resection. *Chest* 1989, 95(2):267–273.

359. Miyoshi S, Nakahara K, Ohno K, et al.: Exercise tolerance test in lung cancer patients: the relationship between exercise capacity and postthoracotomy hospital mortality. *Ann Thorac Surg* 1987, 44(5):487–490.

360. Sorensen PG, Groth S, Hansen SW, et al.: Patterns of perfusion and ventilation of the lungs in patients with small cell lung cancer before and after combination chemotherapy. *Clin Physiol* (Suppl) 1985, 3:99–103.

361. Sorensen PG, Osterlind K, Groth S, et al.: Effects of intensive chemotherapy on respiratory function in patients with small cell carcinoma of the lung. *Eur J Cancer Clin Oncol* 1983, 19(7):901–906.

362. Smith TP, Kinasewitz GT, Tucker WY, et al.: Exercise capacity as a predictor of post-thoracotomy morbidity. *Am Rev Respir Dis* 1984, 129(5):730–734.

363. Bagshaw MA, Kaplan ID, Cox RC: Prostate cancer. Radiation therapy for localized disease. *Cancer* 1993, 71(Suppl 3):939–952.

364. Petrovich Z, Ameye F, Baert L, et al.: New trends in the treatment of benign prostatic hyperplasia and carcinoma of the prostate. *Am J Clin Oncol* 1993, 16(3):187–200.

365. da Silva FC, Reis E, Costa T, Denis L: Quality of life in patients with prostatic cancer: a feasibility study. The members of Quality of Life Committee of the EORTC Genitourinary Group. *Cancer* 1993, 71(Suppl 3):1138–1142.

366. Schover LR: Sexual rehabilitation after treatment for prostate cancer. *Cancer* 1993, 71(Suppl 3):1024–1030.

367. Dow LP: Quality of life and rehabilitation needs following the diagnosis of prostate cancer: impact by phase of disease. *Dissertations Abstract International* [B] 1993, 53(7):3769.

368. Keith J: Testicular cancer: detection, prevention, and therapeutics. *Am Pharm* 1990, 30(7):46–51.

369. Perkins J: Gynecologic malignancies: detection, prevention, and therapeutics: part 2. Cervical and endometrial cancer. *Am Pharm* 1988, 28(12):34–37.

370. Perkins J: Gynecologic malignancies: detection, prevention, and therapeutics: part 1. Ovarian cancer. *Am Pharm* 1988, 28(11):40–43.

371. Balmer CM: Prostate cancer: detection, prevention, and therapeutics. *Am Pharm* 1988, 28(8):34–40.

372. Douglas HO Jr, Razack M, Holyoke ED: Hemipelvectomy. *Arch Surg* 1975, 110(1):82–85.

373. Blicksman AS (ed): Sarcomas of Soft Tissue and Bone in Childhood. *Natl Cancer Inst Monograph* 1981, 56:1–314.

374. Eilber FR, Eckhardt J, Morton DL: Advances in the treatment of sarcomas of the extremity: current status of limb salvage. *Cancer* 1984, 54(11):2695–2704.

375. National Institutes of Health: Limb-sparing treatment of adult soft-tissue sarcomas and osteosarcomas: Consensus development conference statement. 1984, 5(6):3–5.

376. Enzinger F, Weiss S: *Soft Tissue Tumors.* St Louis, MO, C. V. Mosby Company, 1983.

377. Maurer H, Maurer HM, Bettangadys M, Gehan EA: The intergroup rhabdomyosarcoma study: 1. A final report. *Cancer* 1988, 61(2):209–220.

378. Miser J, Pizzo P: Soft tissue sarcomas in childhood. *Pediatr Clin North Am* 1985, 31(3):779–800.

379. Pizzo P, Poplack D (eds): *Principles of Practice of Pediatric Oncology.* Philadelphia, J. B. Lippincott Company, 1989.

380. Rosenberg S: Prospective randomized trials demonstrating the efficacy of adjuvant chemotherapy in adult patients with soft tissue sarcomas. *Cancer Treat Rep* 1984, 68(9):1067–1078.

381. Suit II, Mankin HJ, Wood WC, et al.: Preoperative, intraoperative, and postoperative radiation in the treatment of primary soft tissue sarcoma. *Cancer* 1985, 55(11):2659–2667.

382. Rosenberg SA, Suit HD, Baker LH: Sarcomas of soft tissues. In DeVita VT, Hellman S, Rosenberg SA (eds): *Cancer: Principles & Practice of Oncology.* 2nd ed. Philadelphia, J. B. Lippincott Company, 1985, pp 1243–1292.

383. Kerns LL, Simon MA: Musculoskeletal sarcomas. *Surg Clin North Am* 1983, 63(3):671–695.

384. Vokes EE, Weichselbaum RR, Lippman SM: Medical progress: head and neck cancer. *N Engl J Med* 1993, 328:184–194.

385. Baker KH, Feldman JE: Cancers of the head and neck. *Cancer Nurs* 1987, 10(6):293–299.

386. Sobol S, Jensen C, Sawyer W, et al.: Objective comparison of physical dysfunction after neck dissection. *Am J Surg* 1985, 15:503–509.

387. Khafif RA, Asase DK, Attie JN: Modified radical neck dissection in cancer of the mouth, pharynx, and larynx. *Head Neck* 1990, 12:476–482.

388. Donovan E, Scheetz J, Shell B: A physical therapy program for neck dissection patients: the M.D. Anderson Cancer Center approach. *Rehabil Oncol* 1988, 6:6–8.

389. Olson ML, Shedd DP: Disability and rehabilitation in head and neck cancer patients after treatment. *Head Neck Surg* 1978, 1:52–58.

390. Barrett NV, Martin JW, Jacob RF, et al.: Physical therapy techniques in the treatment of the head and neck patient. *J Prosthet Dent* 1988, 59(3):343–346.

391. Bork B: *Head and Neck Cancer. The Physical Therapists' Role in Rehabilitation of the Shoulder Following Radical Neck Dissection: A Self-Instructional Learning Unit for the P.T.* Iowa City, IA, University of Iowa, 1980.

392. Herring D, King AI, Connelly M: New rehabilitation concepts in management of radical neck dissection syndrome: a clinical report. *Phys Ther* 1987, 67(7):1095–1099.

393. Hockenberger SJ: Fibrocystic breast disease: every woman is at risk. *Plast Surg Nurs* 1993, 13(1):37–40.

394. Bork BE: *Physical Therapy for the Post Mastectomy Patient: A Self-Instructional Learning Unit for the P.T.* Iowa City, IA, University of Iowa, 1980.

395. Fisher B, Bauer M, Wickerham D, et al.: Relation of number of positive auxillary nodes to the prognosis of patients with primary breast cancer (an NSABP update). *Cancer* 1983, 52:1551–1557.

396. Abe R: A study on the pathogenesis of postmastectomy lymphedema. *Tohoku J Exp Med* 1976, 118:163–171.

397. Beninson J: Lymphedema: pathophysiologic and clinical concepts. *Angiology* 1975, 26:661–664.

398. Lerner R, Requena R: Upper extremity lymphedema secondary to mammary cancer treatment. *Am J Clin Oncol* 1986, 9(6):481–487.

399. Bornstein BA, Zouranjian PS, Hansen JL, et al.: Local hyperthermia, radiation therapy, and chemotherapy in patients with local-regional recurrence of breast carcinoma. *Int J Radiat Oncol Biol Phys* 1993, 25(1):79–85.

400. Heuser LS, Spratt JS, Kuhns JG, et al.: The association of pathologic and mammographic characteristics of primary human breast cancers with "slow" and "fast" growth rates and with auxillary lymph nodes metastases. *Cancer* 1984, 53:96–98.

401. Brennan MJ: Lymphedema following the surgical treatment of breast cancer: a review of pathophysiology and treatment. *J Pain Symptom Man* 1992, 7(2):110–116.

402. McBride CM, Brown BW, Thompson JR, et al.: Can patients with breast cancer be cured of their disease? A sample of the M.D. Anderson Hospital experience. *Cancer* 1983, 51:938–945.

403. Winard SH: Breast cancer conservative surgery and radiation: definitions and indications. *Philadelphia Med* 1985, 85:484–486.

404. Lewis HP Jr: Selective breast carcinoma surgery. *Int Surg* 1976, 61:76–79.

405. Jones C: A case of breast disease treated by simple mastectomy and silicone breast replacement. *Natl News* 1983, 20(2):14–18.

406. Rosenblum M: General surgical principles, alternatives, and limitations. *Neurosurg Clin North Am* 1990, 1:19–36.

407. Coffey R, Lunsford LD: Stereotactic radiosurgery using the 201 cobalt-60 source gamma knife. *Neurosurg Clin North Am* 1990, 1:933–954.

408. Friedman W: LINAC radiosurgery. *Neurosurg Clin North Am* 1990, 1:991–1008.

409. Levy R, Fabrikant J, Frankel K, et al.: Charged-particle radiosurgery of the brain. *Neurosurg Clin North Am* 1990, 1:955–990.

410. Bernstein M, Laperriere N, Leung P, McKenzie S: Interstitial brachytherapy for malignant brain tumors: preliminary results. *Neurosurgery* 1990, 26:371–379.

411. Sneed P, Stauffer P, Gutin P, et al.: Interstitial irradiation and hyperthermia for treatment of recurrent malignant brain tumors. *Neurosurgery* 1991, 28:206–214.

412. Guthrie B, Laws E: Supratentorial low-grade gliomas. *Neurosurg Clin North Am* 1990, 1:37–48.

413. Daumas-Duport C, Scheithauer B, O'Fallon J, Kelly P: Grading of astrocytomas: a simple and reproducible method. *Cancer* 1988, 62:2152–2165.

414. Healey E, Barnes P, Kupsky W, et al.: The prognostic significance of postoperative residual tumor in ependymoma. *Neurosurgery* 1991, 28:666–672.

415. Lyons M, Kelly P: Posterior fossa ependymoma: report of 30 cases and review of the literature. *Neurosurgery* 1991, 28:659–665.

416. Kondziolka D, Lunsford LD: Radiosurgery of meningiomas. *Neurosurg Clin North Am* 1992, 3:219–230.

417. Dempsey P, Lunsford L: Stereotactic radiosurgery for pineal region tumors. *Neurosurg Clin North Am* 1992, 3:245–256.

418. Wilson C: Role of surgery in the management of pituitary tumors. *Neurosurg Clin North Am* 1990, 1:139–160.

419. Jackler R, Pitts L: Acoustic neuroma. *Neurosurg Clin North Am* 1990, 1:199–225.

420. Campbell C: Acoustic neuroma: Nursing implications related to surgical management. *J Neurosci Nurs* 1991, 23:50–56.

421. Wiegand D, Fickel V: *The Acoustic Neuroma Experience: Results of a Comprehensive Survey of Acoustic Neuroma Association Members.* 2nd ed., 1989.

422. Linskey M, Lunsford D, Flickinger H, Kondziolka D: Stereotactic radiosurgery for acoustic tumors. *Neurosurg Clin North Am* 1992, 3:191–206.

423. Bleehen NM, Ford JM: Radiotherapy, hyperthermia, and photodynamic therapy for central nervous system tumors. *Curr Opin Oncol* 1993, 5(3):458–463.

424. Burnham N: Bladder cancer: detection, prevention, and therapeutics. *Am Pharm* 1989, 29(6):33–38.

425. Bloom JR, Fobair P, Gritz E, et al.: Psychosocial outcomes of cancer: a comparative analysis of Hodgkin's disease and testicular cancer. *J Clin Oncol* 1993, 11(5):979–988.

426. Bergmann KA: Current concepts in clinical therapeutics: testicular cancer. *Clin Pharm* 1987, 6(9):693–706.

427. Schover LR, Fife M, Gershenson DM: Sexual dysfunction and treatment for early stage cervical cancer. *Cancer* 1989, 63(1):204–212.

428. Butler KM, Oakley M, Christman NJ: Symptom experience and functional status in women having radiotherapy (Rt) for gynecological cancer [Abstract]. *Oncol Nurs Forum* 1991, 18(2):360.

429. Dana WJ: Colorectal cancer: detection, prevention, and therapeutics. *Am Pharm* 1988, 28(6):58–62.

430. John WJ, Neefe JR, Macdonald JS, et al.: 5-fluorouracil and

interferon-alpha-2a in advanced colorectal cancer: results of two treatment schedules. *Cancer* 1993, 72(11):3191–3195.

431. Finley RS: Lung cancer: detection, prevention, and therapeutics. *Am Pharm* 1989, 29(11):39–46.

432. Peters RM, Swain JA: Management of the patient with emphysema, coronary artery disease, and lung cancer. *Am J Surg* 1982, 143(6):701–705.

433. Hays K, Rafferty DC: Care of the patient with malignant lymphoma. *Nurs Clin North Am* 1982, 17(4):677–695.

434. Clink H: Bone marrow transplantation. *Practitioner* 1984, 228:899–901.

435. Holtzman L: Physical therapy intervention in patients after bone marrow transplant [Abstract]. *Phys Ther* 1987, 67:785.

436. James MC: Physical therapy for patients after bone marrow transplantation. *Phys Ther* 1987, 67:946–952.

437. Sayre RS, Marcoux BC: Exercise and autologous bone marrow transplants. *Clin Man Phys Ther* 1992, 12(4):78–82.

438. National Cancer Institute, Office of Cancer Communications: *Radiation Therapy and You: A Guide to Self-Help During Treatment*. NIH Publication No. 88-2227. Washington, DC, U.S. Government Printing Office, 1990.

439. National Cancer Institute, Office of Cancer Communications: *Chemotherapy and You: A Guide to Self-Help During Treatment*. NIH Publication No. 88-1136. Washington, DC, U.S. Government Printing Office.

440. Ostrow S, Van Echo D, Whitacre M, et al.: Physiologic response and toxicity in patients undergoing whole-body hyperthermia for the treatment of cancer. *Cancer Treat Rep* 1981, 65(3-4):323–325.

441. Croghan MK, Shimm DS, Hynynen KH, et al.: A phase I study of the toxicity of regional hyperthermia with systemic warming. *Am J Clin Oncol* 1993, 16(4):354–358.

442. Vartak S, George KC, Singh BB: Antitumor effects of local hyperthermia on a mouse fibrosarcoma. *Anticancer Res* 1993, 13(3):727–729.

443. Baba H, Maehara Y, Takeuchi H, et al.: Optimal scheduling increases therapeutic gain of adriamycin combined with hyperthermia. *Anticancer Res* 1993, 13(3):651–654.

444. Storm FK: What happened to hyperthermia and what is its current status in cancer treatment? [Editorial]. *J Surg Oncol* 1993, 53(3):141–143.

445. Zelefsky MJ, Scher HI, Krol G, et al.: Spinal epidural tumor in patients with prostate cancer: clinical and radiographic predictors of response to radiation therapy. *Cancer* 1992, 70(9):2319–2325.

446. Stephenson RB, Kaufer H, Hankin FM: Partial pelvic resection as an alternative to hindquarter amputation for skeletal neoplasms. *Clin Orthop* 1989, 242:201–211.

447. Boman L, Bjorvell H, Cedermark B, et al.: Effects of early discharge from hospital after surgery for primary breast cancer. *Eur J Surg* 1993, 159(2):67–73.

448. Hladiuk M, Huchcroft S, Temple W, Schnurr BE: Arm function after axillary dissection for breast cancer: a pilot study to provide parameter estimates. *J Surg Oncol* 1992, 50(1):47–52.

449. Kiebert GM, de Haes JC, van de Velde CJ: The impact of breast-conserving treatment and mastectomy on the quality of life of early-stage breast cancer patients: a review. *J Clin Oncol* 1991, 9(6):1059–1070.

450. Bernstein L, Ross RK, Henderson BE: Prospects for the primary prevention of breast cancer. *Am J Epidemiol* 1992, 135(2):142–152.

451. Yokoe T, Ishida T, Tominaga S, et al.: Effect of mass screening for breast cancer from the aspect of psychosocial assessment of the quality of life. *Jpn J Cancer Res* 1993, 84(4):365–370.

452. Hacking HG, Van As HH, Lankhorst GJ: Factors related to the outcome of inpatient rehabilitation in patients with neoplastic epidural spinal cord compression. *Paraplegia* 1993, 31(6):367–374.

453. Fossa SD, Paus E, Lindegaard M, Newling DW: Prostate-specific antigen and other prognostic factors in patients with hormone-resistant prostate cancer undergoing experimental treatment. *Br J Urol* 1992, 69(2):175–179.

454. Aaronson NK: The assessment of subjective response in prostatic cancer clinical research. *Am J Clin Oncol* 1988, 11(Suppl 2):S43–S47.

455. Aaronson NK, Ahmedzai S, Bergman B, et al.: The European Organization for Research and Treatment of Cancer QLQ-C30: a quality-of-life instrument for use in international clinical trials in oncology. *J Natl Cancer Inst* 1993, 85(5):365–376.

456. Oishi K, Arai Y, Hashimura T, et al.: Quality of life of the patients with continent urinary reservoir [Published in Japanese]. *Hinyokika Kiyo* 1993, 39(1):7–14.

457. Nishimura H, Haniuda M, Morimoto M, Kubo K: Cardiopulmonary function after pulmonary lobectomy in patients with lung cancer. *Ann Thorac Surg* 1993, 55(6):1477–1484.

458. von Knorring J, Lepantalo M, Lindgren L, Lindfors O: Cardiac arrhythmias and myocardial ischemia after thoracotomy for lung cancer. *Ann Thorac Surg* 1992, 53(4):642–647.

459. Brown JK: Gender, age, usual weight, and tobacco use as predictors of weight loss in patients with lung cancer. *Oncol Nurs Forum* 1993, 20(3):466–472.

460. Wingard JR, Curbow B, Baker F, Piantadosi S: Employment of adult survivors after bone marrow transplantation (bmt) [Abstract]. *Proc Annu Meet Am Soc Clin Oncol* 1990, 9:A1180.

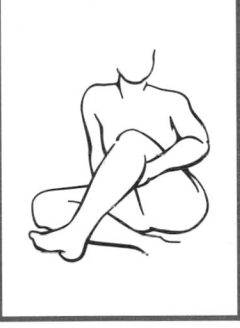

CHAPTER 5

Oncology: Examination, Diagnosis, and Treatment. Physical Therapy Considerations

Lucinda A. Pfalzer

This chapter on the physical therapy considerations of the examination and treatment of patients with cancer builds on the preceding chapter, "Oncology: Examination, Diagnosis, and Treatment. Medical and Surgical Considerations," Chapter 4.

I. Physical Therapy Examination

A. Screening

Screening is usually performed in individuals with high risk for cancer. It includes taking the patient's history, chart review, and some special tests for early detection of physical findings, signs, and symptoms implicating cancer. A systems review is used during the screening process (see Table 4–5).

B. Examination

The examination process includes the following steps (a tool for examination is shown in Figure 5–1):
1. History and chart review by system.
2. Physical examination by system and psychosocial status. The physical examination is conducted by system and (depending on the

149

SCREENING INFORMATION

NAME: _____   DATE: _____ - _____ - _____

AGE: _____ y HEIGHT: _____ cm WEIGHT: _____ kg BODY COMPOSITION (BMI, BSA, etc . . .): _____

REFERRING PHYSICIAN:_____

DIAGNOSIS AND STAGE: METASTATIC SITES:

PREVIOUS TREATMENT: CURRENT THERAPY:

MEDICATIONS (pain control, others):

MEDICAL CLEARANCE (chest x-ray; ECG; stress MUGA; PFT; blood gases; blood and platelet counts; cardiac, lung, and bone marrow biopsies; pH and electrolyte values; blood glucose tests; and kidney function tests.):

Cardiopulmonary Screen	HR(bpm)	BP(mm Hg)	RR(breaths/min)	RPE
Supine				
Sitting				
Standing				
Walking				
ADLs				

Heart Sounds (ventricular gallop, pericardial rub, etc . . .):

Chest Sounds (nonproductive cough; exertional and nocturnal dyspnea; adventitious sounds including rales, rhonchi, and wheezing):

Symptoms and Signs (chest pain, syncope, dyspnea on exertion, PND, edema, cyanosis, dizziness, nausea, etc . . .):

Musculoskeletal Screen:

Symptoms and Signs (joint pain, loss of motion, swelling, muscle weakness, tenderness, inflammation, and skin integrity):

AROM:

Flexibility:

Muscle Performance (strength and endurance):

Neurological Screen:

Symptoms and Signs (orientation, coordination, gait, muscle paralysis, tremor, paresthesia, hearing and visual disturbances, diminished or absent DTRs, sensory integration deficits, etc . . .):

Sensation (2-point discrimination, vibration, light touch, temperature):

AROM:

Muscle Performance (key muscles, DTRs, coordination, and balance):

FIGURE 5–1 Baseline information for screening a physical therapy patient. *Abbreviations:* ADLs = activities of daily living; AROM = active range of motion; BMI = body mass index; BP = blood pressure; BSA = body surface area; DTR = deep tendon reflex; DVT = deep venous thrombosis; ECG = electrocardiogram; HR = heart rate; MUGA = multiple gated acquisition; PFT = pulmonary function test; PND = paroxysmal nocturnal dyspnea; RPE = retinal pigment epithelium; RR = respiratory rate.

SCREENING INFORMATION *Continued*

Genitourinary Screen:

Symptoms and Signs (bowel and bladder continence; urinary frequency, urgency, pain, or burning; hematuria, blood in the stool; presence of stomas or appliances; problems with sexual function):

Skin Inspection and Peripheral Vascular Screen:

Symptoms and Signs (dry, thin, reddened, peeling, or blistered skin areas; diminished or absent pulses; muscle cramping, tenderness, or pain; cyanosis; nail bed changes; claudication; pulses; signs and symptoms of infection; anemia; and bleeding):

Peripheral Pulses:

Girth and Volumetric Measures (lymphedema, chords, DVTs, and emboli):

Psychosocial Screen:

Orientation (person, place, time):

Memory and Recognition (short-term and long-term memory, object recognition):

Follows Directions (one-step and multiple-step commands):

Symptoms and Signs (mental status changes, marked behavioral changes, insomnia, altered memory, depression, anxiety, nervousness, agitation, confusion, euphoria, hallucinations, etc . . .):

Other (communication; personal knowledge of health, disease, and treatment; religious beliefs; support systems; etc . . .)

Functional Status and ADLs:

Basic ADLs (Patient can perform basic ADLs):

Self-care	Yes	No (If no, specify how much assistance is needed)
Feeding		
Grooming		
Dressing		
Toileting		
Bathing		
Continence		

Mobility	Yes	No (If no, specify how much assistance is needed)
Bed mobility		
Transfers		
Ambulation and gait		
Stair climbing		

FIGURE 5–1 *Continued*

Illustration continued on following page

SCREENING INFORMATION *Continued*

Functional Status and ADLs:

Intermediate ADLs (patient can perform intermediate ADLs):

At Home	Yes	No (If no, specify how much assistance is needed)
Homemaking		
Cleaning		
Laundry		
Meal preparation		
Ability to communicate by phone or other devices		
Ability to handle finances		
Ability to use medication		
Care-giving activities for others		

Outside Home	Yes	No (If no, specify how much assistance is needed)
Shopping		
Social activities		
Employment, vocation, or avocational and recreational activities		
Ability to use car or public transportation		

PHYSICAL THERAPY PROBLEMS OR DIAGNOSES:

PHYSICAL THERAPY GOALS:

PHYSICAL THERAPY PLAN AND EXERCISE PRESCRIPTION:

Discharge Needs (*eg*, equipment, support, meals, etc . . .):

FIGURE 5–1 *Continued*

patient's goals) functional status. Objective measurement, which requires special tests such as the symptom-limited graded exercise test (SLGXT) or isokinetic tests, is used when indicated. Physical examination by system is reviewed in the chapters in this manual that discuss specific systems. Isokinetic tests and SLGXT are reviewed specific to issues related to the population with cancer.

a. SLGXT. The test is conducted to quantify and evaluate the patient's response to aerobic exercise and exercise training. Baseline data on a resting 12-lead electrocardiograph, blood chemistries, hema-tological values (see Table 4–9 and Figure 5–1), and signs and symptoms that are evident on the day that the SLGXT is administered are evaluated before the SLGXT is conducted to screen for contraindications and precautions for exercise testing. Data yielded by the SLGXT are used

- To provide baseline data on the patient's functional capacity.
- To compare results of this stress test with those of a prior test (or tests).
- To detect abnormal response to increasing exercise loads
- To determine the patient's exercise

limitations before he/she starts physical therapy treatment and exercise.

- To serve as the basis for exercise prescription for the exercise program.

(1). Testing procedures. A typical test protocol would include monitoring at the end of every stage throughout the test, at the completion of the test, and during recovery of blood pressure, heart rate and rhythm, ratings of perceived exertion (RPE), and signs and symptoms, including ratings of leg fatigue, claudication, or angina. Knowledge of how the patient is feeling during the exercise is an important complement to the physiological data that allow the therapist to better understand how subjective symptoms relate to objective measures in the limitation of functional capacity. The Borg scale or RPE (see Figure 5–2) is a simple 15-grade rating scale that has descriptive verbal anchors at every odd number (eg, 9 = very light; 17 = very hard), which indicate greater differentiation at the ends of the measurement range.[1] Numbers are selected to coincide with the individual's perceptions of the exercise intensity. The RPE is based on the assumption that a patient's percep-

Table 5–1. CRITERIA FOR TERMINATING SLGXT

1. Leg fatigue, which presents as an inability to continue pedaling an exercise bicycle at 50 cycles per minute for more than 1 minute
2. Failure of the systolic blood pressure to rise with an increasing workload, a drop of 10 mm Hg or more of systolic pressure, an increase in systolic pressure to 250 mm Hg or greater, or a rise in diastolic pressure to greater than 20 mm Hg
3. Shortness of breath
4. A complaint of nausea
5. A complaint of angina
6. A complaint of excessive generalized fatigue
7. The subject voluntarily terminating the test
8. The presence of any electrocardiogram changes and abnormalities that were consistent with the American College of Sports Medicine (1991) graded exercise test guidelines for discontinuing a test

tions of his/her physiological changes during exercise serve as potent sensory cues for perception of work intensity. A newer category-ratio scale was developed for use in rating local exertion (eg, leg fatigue) and symptoms instead of overall exertion.[2] Smutok, Skrinar, and Pandolf[3] showed that the RPE was inaccurate in predicting heart rate in patients who exercised at a low intensity; therefore the test is of limited use in clinical populations of patients with low maximal heart rates who are training at lower work intensities.[3] Sidney and Shephard[4] and Pandolf et al.[5] support this idea in relation to older subjects, whose heart rates decline with training and whose perceived exertion was unchanged. RPE levels should be used cautiously for determining and monitoring exercise intensity in older patients with cancer who have low peak exercise capacities.

(2). Criteria for terminating the SLGXT are listed in Table 5–1. Exercise heart rate responses may vary according to the patient's sex, age, and level of anxiety or anger, the nature and extent of the disease, the patient's food intake (eg, caffeine) and physical fitness, the time of day that the test is administered, and medications being taken by the patient.[6] These factors should be considered when the physical therapist

Borg's RPE-Scale		Borg CR-10 Scale	
6	No exertion at all	0	Nothing at all
7	Extremely light	0.5	Extremely weak (just noticeable)
8		1	Very weak
9	Very light	2	Weak (light)
10		3	Moderate
11	Light	4	
12		5	Strong (heavy)
13	Somewhat hard	6	
14		7	Very strong
15	Hard (heavy)	8	
16		9	
17	Very hard	10	Extremely strong (almost max)
18		•	Maximal
19	Extremely hard		
20	Maximal exertion		
© Gunnar Borg, 1985		© Gunnar Borg, 1981 and 1983	

FIGURE 5–2 Borg's rating of perceived exertion scale and CR-10 scale. (RPE scale from Borg G: *An Introduction to Borg's RPE-Scale.* Ithaca, NY, Mouvement Publications, 1985. Borg CR-10 scale from Borg G, Holmgren A, Lindblad I: Quantitative evaluation of chest pain. *Acta Med Scand Suppl* 1981, 644:43–45; Borg G: A category scale with ratio properties for intermodal and interindividual comparisons. In Geissler H-G, Petzold P (eds): *Psychophysical Judgment and the Process of Perception.* Berlin, VEB Deutscher Verlag der Wissenschaften, 1983, pp 25–34.)

interprets the patient's exercise heart rate responses to allow him/her to manage the patient's condition and to prescribe exercise appropriately, because elevated resting heart rate and blood pressure are common among cancer patients. These factors, along with the severity of the patient's deconditioning or initial fitness level, are considered when the therapist develops the exercise prescription (which includes frequency, intensity, time [duration], and type [mode] of exercise) along with flexibility and strengthening exercises.[7-10] The exercise prescription is not initially designed to increase fitness in very deconditioned patients with poor initial fitness levels; it is targeted to stimulate 40% to 60% of these patients' maximal oxygen consumption to counter the effects of inactivity.[6,11-16] Deconditioned patients can benefit from exercise even when the intensity does not lead to changes in their physical fitness.[7-10,11,12,14-17] The exercise is performed daily a couple of times a day for short periods (eg, 5 to 7 min) until the patient's exercise tolerance improves.[14,17] As the patient's endurance improves, interval exercise training may be more beneficial than continuous-load exercise because it improves the patient's strength and endurance.[17] If fatigue persists after exercise for more than 0.5 hour and the heart rate is slow to return to resting values, lower the exercise intensity during the next treatment session.

b. Isokinetic testing

(1). An isokinetic dynamometer may be used to objectively measure dynamic maximal muscle torque during concentric or eccentric muscle contraction, joint motion, peak torque in relation to joint angle, and timing between repeated contractions. Work, power, and fatigability can be calculated. Baseline data are used in determining guidelines for physical therapy treatment and exercise (strength training). Dynamometer speeds are controlled so that they range from 0 to over 300 degrees per second. Muscle contractions are performed concentrically or eccentrically with unidirectional or reciprocal contractions of antagonists. Peak values for concentric testing decrease as the speed of contraction increases because of the force-velocity relationship in skeletal muscle. Isokinetic concentric testing of the quadriceps and hamstrings muscle groups has been safely performed in patients before and after bone marrow transplantation.[17] The isokinetic testing was conducted using a protocol adapted from Lumex Corporation, Cybex Division,[18-20] and Rothstein et al.[22] for testing arthritic patients on high-dose steroids and from Greene and Strickler[23] for training and testing hemophiliacs who are at risk for joint bleeding. The protocol was designed to address the following specific concerns of this study:

- Attainment of an objective baseline measure of knee flexion/extension muscle strength to assess the effectiveness of a bicycle ergometer interval exercise program.
- Application of a form of strength assessment that would be safe in this clinical population with its increased risk of joint trauma.
- Development of a clinical method of muscle performance assessment that allows for a noninvasive estimation of Type II muscle fiber atrophy.[24-28]

(2). The velocity of movement set in the Cybex II dynamometer can be used to simulate the muscle contraction that occurs when the patient uses the bicycle ergometer and during his/her activities of daily living. Wyatt and Edwards[29] showed that rehabilitation of the knee to enable normal gait requires work ratios of between 200 and 300 degrees per second. The reliability and validity of the Cybex II have been established across a variety of age ranges. Winter et al.,[30] Fillyaw et al.,[31] Nelson and Duncan,[32] and Sapega et al.,[33] have discussed some of the problems associated with the validity and reliability of the Cybex dynamometer.

Disadvantages of the Cybex II dynamometer used in this protocol are as follow:

- Its use results in an artificial condition that does not normally occur during activity. Normal motion occurs in multiple planes around various axes at variable speed and constant resistance. The external force applied to create motion does vary throughout the joint range secondary to changes in lever arm length and the angle of pull of the muscle.
- The effect of gravity on the limb being tested produces distortion in the test results, which may cause major changes in the flexion:extension ratio.
- Torque under shoot and over shoot occurs as a result of the construction of the device and the rapid acceleration and deceleration by subjects during the initial and final phases of the range of motion (ROM) testing.
- For intersubject and intergroup comparison, age, sex, weight, and height should be considered.

(3). Testing procedures. Four aspects of strength were assessed during the test protocol to ensure repeatability; these were

- Subject positioning and stabilization.
- Test speeds.
- Reciprocal or unidirectional movement.
- Number of repetitions of contraction.

Testing of both knees was done at speeds of 90, 180, and 300 degrees per second, respectively. Additional benefits of the isokinetic test protocol were as follows:

- Isokinetic exercise is less traumatic to joints and weakened ligaments than is isotonic weight lifting for deconditioned individuals.
- The population tested has an increased risk of stress fractures and joint bleeding; therefore, testing at slow speeds was avoided, and it was not indicated for Type II fiber myopathy. If joint bleeding secondary to diminished clotting abil-

ity occurs repeatedly, it can lead to progressive joint destruction and disabling arthropathy.

- Resistive exercise is indicated for many patients, depending on the presence of pain on the stage of healing. External weight can produce traction, torsion, and compression on joints and supportive structures, and the debilitated patient may not be able to tolerate such stresses. High-speed settings on the dynamometer may be used to provide high-velocity isokinetic exercise. High-velocity exercise diminishes the maximal force generated at the joint by the contracting muscle; however, it continues to provide maximal resistance to muscle contraction throughout the ROM testing. This method of testing offers safe, early resistive strength assessment when high-load effort may be contraindicated. If pain or cramping occurs at any point during exercise testing, the subject can cease the motion, thus removing the resistance.
- Alternating reciprocal concentric muscle contractions and ROM are easily assessed objectively with the isokinetic dynamometer.

(1). The Cybex II dynamometer is calibrated before the testing session with known weights for instrument reliability. When the knee is tested, the patient is supported in a seated position at the dynamometer with the trunk and thigh being tested stabilized by Velcro straps attached to the bench. The axis of rotation of the dynamometer is aligned with the anatomical axis of the patient's knee. The lever arm is attached just proximal to the subject's ankle mortise, and ankle motion is assessed for restrictions. To enhance the reliability of the test, the patient should perform a warm-up exercise at each selected test speed to minimize a possible learning effect during testing. Other threats to the reliability and validity of the test include

- loss of instrument calibration
- variations in trunk and thigh position among subjects

- improper positioning of the lever arm axis of rotation
- learning effect from repeated trials
- improper positioning of the lever arm so that it causes interference with normal ankle motion during testing of the knee

Further research on the reliability and validity of isokinetic testing specific to the population with cancer is needed.

c. Functional or performance status.

(1). Karnofsky and Burchunel[34] developed a performance scale to assess patients' affective, physical, and functional parameters. With regard to subjective response criteria, the Karnofsky Performance Scale (KPS) and the subjective components of the World Health Organization acute and subacute toxicity scales appear to hold certain advantages over competing measurement systems. However, the available data suggest that further developmental work is needed to improve the precision of these instruments.[35,36] Mor et al.[37] examined the reliability and validity of the KPS as both a study eligibility criterion and an outcome measure in the National Hospice study. Interviewers in this study receive extensive training in the use of the tool over 4 months. The study's findings were that inter-rater reliability of 47 National Hospice Study interviewers was found to be 0.97; that the construct validity of the KPS was strongly related ($P < 0.001$) to two other independent measures of patient functioning; and that the relationship of the KPS to longevity in a population of terminal cancer patients documented its predictive validity. However, in other studies the KPS has been shown not to be uniformly reliable for testing patients whose cancer differs in site and stage.[35,36] Continued refinement of the KPS is needed to improve its reliability.

(2). Diminishing functional ability, feelings of loss of control, and changes in body image (from factors such as hair loss and weight loss) that occur as a result of cancer and its treatment may cause the patient to experience feelings of anxiety, helplessness, and futility. Baseline data can help the therapist modify the physical therapy intervention used for a patient who exhibits psychological symptoms and document the patient's functional status and quality of life. In the area of quality of life assessment, no clear choice exists among the array of available measurement tools.[38–42] Although several promising instruments for testing exist, none has had sufficient field testing to support its widespread adoption in clinical trials.[39–42] Furthermore, new tools to appropriately assess quality of life in surviving patients with cancer continue to be developed.[39–41]

(3). Other researchers have used the Eastern Cooperative Oncology Group (ECOG) Scale of Performance Status (PS) to quantify the functional status of patients with lung, head and neck, and genitourinary cancer.[40,42–44] The PS has demonstrated some ability in assisting to determine the prognosis in a number of patients with cancer.[40] The scale rates the patient's symptoms and functions with respect to his/her ambulatory status and need for care. PS O means that the patient can perform normal activity, PS 1 means that he/she has some symptoms but is still close to fully ambulatory, PS 2 means that the patient's functional level is less than 50%, PS 3 means that the patient must spend more than 50% of the day in bed, and PS 4 means that he/she is completely bedridden. Sorensen et al.[40] conducted an interobserver variability study of PS assessment to evaluate the nonchance agreement among three oncologists who rated 100 consecutive patients with cancer. They found that total unanimity was observed in 40 cases, unanimity between two observers in 53 cases, and total disagreement in 7 cases. Kappa statistics were used to evaluate nonchance agreement, and the researchers found that overall, the kappa score was 0.44 (95% confidence limits of 0.38–0.51), with the kappa scores as follow:

PS 0	0.55 (0.44–0.67)
PS 1	0.48 (0.37–0.60)
PS 2	0.31 (0.19–0.42)
PS 3	0.43 (0.32–0.55)
PS 4	0.33 (0.33–0.45)

Furthermore, it was found that when one observer gave patients scores of PS 0 to 2, another randomly selected observer placed the patients in the same category with a probability of 0.92, and when patients were scored at PS 3 to 4, the probability that the same category would be chosen was 0.82. Overall, the nonchance agreement between observers was only moderate when all ECOG PS groups were considered; however, agreement with regard to the scoring of patients at PS 0 to 2 versus 3 to 4 was high.[45] This cut-off between PS < 3 versus ≥3 is often used in clinical trials. Conhill et al.[41] assessed the relationship between the KPS and PS in 100 consecutive patients who were self-tested and tested independently by two physicians to evaluate the scales' validity and reliability. Kendall's rank correlation coefficient values were highly significant between physicians (0.76 for KPS, 0.75 for PS) and between physicians and patients (0.65 for KPS, 0.59 for PS). The authors state that patients' self-evaluation could provide a valuable and reliable assessment.[41] It appears that the patient and family self report of function or performance accurately reflects the patient's status.

(4). The European Organization for Research in Cancer Therapy QLQ-C30 has demonstrated reliable and valid measures of the quality of life of patients with cancer in multicultural clinical research settings in Europe in Phase I trials. Work is ongoing to examine the performance of the questionnaire among more heterogenous patient samples and in Phase II and Phase III clinical trials.

(5). The SCL-R-90 is a tool that is used to assess a patient's psychosocial state, symptoms, and level of functioning.[46] The SCL-R-90 is a 90-item self-report questionnaire that covers nine categories of symptoms (eg, depression, anxiety) on a five-point scale. The Brief Symptom Inventory is an abbreviated version of the SCL-R-90 that may be easier to use in clinical settings. Other available tools to assess functional status or symptoms include the Profile of Mood States, Beck's depression scale, Functional Status questionnaire, Barthel index, Katz index, Zubrod scale, Kenny Self-Care, and Pulses Profile. Each tool should include an assessment of the patient's basic and intermediate activities of daily living (see Figure 5–1) and should be carefully selected based on reliability and validity for the population being assessed (eg, ambulatory, nonhospitalized patients versus hospitalized patients). The Cancer Rehabilitation Evaluation System and its short form have been developed specifically for the assessment of patients with cancer.[47] Until objective and reliable measures of patient's quality of life and functional status can be obtained specific to cancer, the relationship between impairments, functional capacity, psychological functioning, and the qualitative level of functioning remains difficult to define. Patients with cancer who have diminished physical activity and reduced functional capacity may confuse the side effects of disease and therapy with physical and affective manifestations of inactivity (see the subsection on mental status that follows).

3. Assessment

The patient's level of function and dysfunction, and his/her special abilities, needs, problems, and diagnosis should be reviewed by system (eg, pain limiting hip flexion may impede a patient's ambulatory function). On assessment of the patient's problems, the therapist must be aware that the types of impairments and movement dysfunctions found in cancer survivors are as varied as the disease and clinical treatments and are compounded by inactivity and disuse as noted previously. Determine the patient's diagnosis and problems from an assessment of information obtained from the chart review, history, and physical examination. Decide which problems require a referral and which problems can be treated by the physical therapist.

a. Evaluate any changes in the patient's mental status, behavior, and cognitive function (see the sections on oncologic emergencies, terminal illness, neurological tumors, and clinical manifestations of cancer).

(1). Psychosocial considerations in the assessment of patients with cancer for physical therapy management. Physical therapists use a problem-centered treatment approach based on the examination, categorization, and monitoring of patient responses to initial treatment, with adjustment of the treatment plan as indicated by the responses. Cancer survivors have many impairments and dysfunctions related to the disease and its often aggressive treatments and to the resultant changes in psychosocial status, to inactivity, to disuse of the body, and to prolonged bedrest. The assessment of the patient with cancer must address the psychosocial problems that often arise.

Affective manifestations of depression, feelings of loss of control, anxiety, and severe mood swings in patients with cancer and in their family members are common. Patients also frequently experience socioemotional changes (such as fear, anger, irritability, nervousness, and denial) related to loss of insurance, loss of employment, and their physical and medical condition.[47–93] Chemotherapeutic agents, antiemetics, and corticosteroids have known effects on mood and cognition, which may confound the diagnosis of mental disorders such as depression or anxiety.[48,52,55,72,79,80,90]

- High-dose intrathecal methotrexate used in an ablative chemotherapy regimen has been reported to cause neurological alterations and delirium 10 to 13 days after administration.[71]
- The risk of high-dose corticosteroid–induced psychoses is widely known; however, changes in mood often go unrecognized.[80]
- Reported changes in mood may include agitation, insomnia, increased appetite, crying spells, and variable depression.
- Occasionally, a patient experiences difficulty when corticosteroid use is tapered.
- Improvement in mental status may be delayed for as much as 3 weeks after cessation of corticosteroid use.

Several of these affective manifestations (eg, depression, anxiety, hostility, and low morale) have been negatively associated with quality of life and survival.[34,37,40,42,46,61,72,75,82,90] An inherent interaction appears to exist between the body and the mind; this interaction affects the patient's outcomes. Weisman[81] notes that affective distress impairs the coping process and defines coping as

"the recognition of a problem from which one seeks relief; doing something about this problem; and the outcome of this action . . . coping is a process, not an isolated set of independent actions. It combines perception, performance, appraisal, and correction, followed by further activity, and directed, motivated behavior."

Many patients with cancer complain of fatigue and weakness, regardless of the stage or site of their disease—two factors that are related to diminished independence.[17,95–100] The somatic and psychic manifestations of cancer and its treatment, along with the impairment of normal socioemotional functioning, lead to a patient's inability to maintain cognitive functioning and appropriate levels of activity. As a patient's illness becomes terminal, many neuropsychiatric syndromes are common and require intervention.[101,102] When a patient is in pain, his/her functional activity is reduced. The magnitude of interaction of the physical (*eg*, fatigue) and affective factors (*eg*, pain) as they impact on the cancer patient's development of impairments, secondary disability, and dysfunction is currently being researched; quality of life and functional status are also being studied in clinical research trials.[100] The psychosocial concerns of patients and their families that may need to be explored are as follows:

(a). Effective communication and education of the patient and his/her family is a concern. Specific issues include the following:

   (i). Myths and misconceptions, *eg*, patients are *people*—not victims or a disease.

   (ii). Religious and philosophical beliefs.

   (iii). Cultural and personal attitudes.

   (iv). Reactions to a diagnosis of cancer (the degree to which a patient acknowledges the diagnosis of malignancy may be a factor in his/her initial distress level and response to treatment[103]). Related issues are
   - The patient's perceptions and feelings regarding cancer.
   - The patient's and the family's coping mechanisms. (A recent study of 40 women who acknowledged that they experienced coping difficulties in meeting the demands of everyday living as a result of their husbands' diagnosis of cancer indicated that the wives experienced a multitude of coping difficulties. Wives experienced psychological disorganization, disequilibrium, and emotional imbalance. They attempted to cope with the resultant imbalance by using their habitual problem-solving behavior patterns, and they experienced difficulty when seeking situational support. This, in turn, added to their stress. Wives also reported that their children had coping difficulties.[104])
   - The therapist should learn how to communicate with the patient and his/her family including how to discuss what he/she knows about the diagnosis.

   (v). The identification of past experiences and of potential role and relationship changes.

   (vi). The education of patients and family in how to change patterns of communication.

(b). Another concern is how to best interact with the patient and his/her family. Additional information in physical therapy interactions with patients and families is as follows:

   (i). A physical therapist may have to work with patients who are angry, aggressive, hostile, and depressed.

   (ii). A therapist may work with families and with terminally ill patients. To do so, the therapist must keep in mind society's re-

actions to death, differing cultural health beliefs, his/her own attitude toward terminally ill patients, and the stages of death, which are:
- First stage: denial and isolation.
- Second stage: anger.
- Third stage: bargaining.
- Fourth stage: depression.
- Fifth stage: acceptance.

The therapist also must be aware of neuropsychiatric syndromes in terminal illness and the choices (at home or hospice) available for the long-term care of patients.

b. Another step in assessing the patient is the detection of impaired cardiovascular function. Signs of this problem include altered peripheral pulses (such as arrhythmia) and increases in vital sign values (such as heart rate and blood pressure), angina, dyspnea on exertion, syncope, decreased O_2 saturation, and altered mental status (perfusion). See "Cardiovascular System," Chapter 6, for more information.
  (1). Impaired cardiovascular function may be disease related; the following diseases and disorders may be causes:
    (a). Paraneoplastic syndrome, electrolyte disorders, or acidosis.
    (b). Emergency situations such as superior vena cava syndrome.
    (c). Hormonal disorders or electrolyte and fluid imbalances (such as dehydration or fluid overload).
    (d). Primary tumors in the mediastinum, brain stem, head and neck, or kidney.
  (2). This problem can also be treatment related; the following types of treatment may result in cardiovascular problems:
    (a). Chemotherapy, which can cause complications such as cardiomyopathy and arrhythmia.
    (b). Irradiation to the thorax or mediastinum, which may cause cardiac fibrosis and pulmonary fibrosis.
    (c). Biological response modifiers, which can cause complications that present constitutional signs and that have system-wide side effects.
    (d). Surgical resection, which results in a loss of tissue and surgical trauma.
  (3). Inactivity and bed rest also may result in cardiovascular disorders.

c. A third step in the assessment is the evaluation of impaired pulmonary function (volumes and flow rates), demonstrated by symptoms such as abnormal breath sounds, dyspnea on exertion, increased respiratory rate, decreased chest or diaphragmatic excursion, decreased O_2 saturation, and altered mental status (ventilation). See "Cardiovascular System," Chapter 6, for more information.
  (1). Pulmonary disorders may be disease related; the following diseases and disorders may be causes:
    (a). Paraneoplastic syndrome, electrolyte disorders, or acidosis.
    (b). Emergency situations such as disseminated intravascular coagulation or pulmonary embolism.
    (c). Hormonal disorders or electrolyte and fluid imbalances (such as dehydration or fluid overload).
    (d). Primary tumors in the thorax and lungs, brain stem, or head and neck, or metastatic disease of the lungs with pathological fracture of the ribs.
  (2). Such disorders may also be treatment related; the following types of treatment may result in pulmonary disorders:
    (a). Chemotherapy, which may have complications such as pulmonary inflammation, ulceration, and fibrosis.
    (b). Irradiation to the thorax or mediastinum, which may cause cardiac fibrosis and pulmonary fibrosis.
    (c). BRMs, which may have complications, that present constitu-

tional signs and that have system-wide effects.

(d). Surgical resection, which results in a loss of tissue and surgical trauma.

(3). Inactivity and bed rest also may cause pulmonary disorders.

d. A fourth step is the examination of open wounds, skin lesions, or increased girth or volumetric measures, which may indicate the presence of lymphedema. Lymphedema, an excessive accumulation of extravascular and extracellular fluid in tissue spaces, is caused by a disturbance of the water and protein balance across capillary membranes. The lymphatic system removes plasma proteins that filter into tissue spaces. Obstruction of the lymphatic system causes retention of proteins in tissue spaces, and the increased protein concentration draws greater amounts of water into the interstitial space (increased oncotic pressure); this leads to lymphedema. Typically, obstruction of the lymphatic system occurs as a complication of treatment secondary to reduced usage and activity, of increased bed rest in conjunction with a surgical wound, of radiation fibrosis or sclerosis, of chemotherapy immunosuppression with resultant infection, of poor nutritional status and dehydration from the disease, or of all treatments that result in immunosuppression.[105–130] Other causes include the presence of varicose veins, venous stasis, leg ulcers, dermatitis, postoperative phlebitis, chronic and acute venous insufficiency, improperly fitting casts, or injury. The degree of involvement may vary from minimal (not disrupting normal functioning) to maximal (interfering with dressing and other everyday activities).

(1). Signs and symptoms of lymphatic disorders include:

(a). Lymphedema of the distal extremity, which is most often seen over the dorsum of the hand or foot.

(b). Increased weight or heaviness of the extremity.

(c). Sensory disturbances of the hand or foot.

(d). Stiffness of the fingers or toes.

(e). Tautness of the skin.

(f). Susceptibility of the skin to breakdown.

(g). Decreased resistance to infection, which can cause frequent episodes of cellulitis.

(2). Lymphedema often follows upper-quarter surgery in which lymph vessels are removed in the modified radical or radical mastectomy. Lymph nodes are also resected during axillary dissections with lumpectomy or segmental mastectomy. Lower-quarter lymphedema is common with the treatment of genitourinary cancers and lymphoma.

(3). Evaluation of lymphatic disorders should include the following:

(a). The identification of contraindications to mechanical compression therapy (such as congestive heart failure, thrombophlebitis, and pulmonary edema).

(b). Girth measurements of the extremity. McGaravey[120] described the systematic measurement of girths beginning with the initial visit. Serial circumferences are taken of both the involved and uninvolved extremities; thereafter, the involved extremity is measured at each visit, and the uninvolved periodically. To ensure consistent circumference measurement, the same therapist should measure the extremity before and after treatment, using a light indentation of the tissue if tension on the tape is appropriate.

(i). The upper extremity should be measured at the following sites: at the metacarpal phalangeal area; at the wrist; at one third of the distance between the wrist and the olecranon process, at two thirds of the distance between the wrist and the olecranon process; at the olecranon process; at one third of the distance between the olecranon process and the axilla; and at two thirds of the distance between the olecranon process and the axilla.

(ii). The lower extremity should be measured at the following sites: at the metatarsal phalangeal area; at the ankle; at one third of the distance between the ankle and the head of the fibula; at two thirds of the distance between the ankle and the head of the fibula; at the head of the fibula; at one third of the distance between the head of the fibula and the greater trochanter; and at two thirds of the distance between the head of the fibula and the greater trochanter.

(c). Volumetric measurements of the extremity. Standardized measurement is needed for measuring volumes. Commercially available volumeters allow the use of a standardized method of measurement as is described here; however, they are expensive and require storage space. The therapist measures volume based on water displacement, using a clear plastic, graduated cylinder filled with warm water into which the involved extremity will fit.

(d). Inspect both involved and uninvolved extremities for tissue quality, skin temperature, redness, tenderness, and other signs of complications. If inflammation is suspected, therapy should be withheld until the physician is consulted and the possible inflammation treated. An edematous extremity feels firm, and the skin appears stretched and shiny. With treatment, the skin should become soft and supple.

e. A fifth step in the assessment is the evaluation of pain. See the previous section on pain under clinical manifestations of cancer.

f. A sixth step in the assessment is the detection of ROM deficits.

(1). Hypermobility of a joint may be present.

(a). Loss of motor function may be the cause; this initially leads to hypermobility as the joint loses muscular stability, followed by the development over time of hypomobility. The following types of hypermobility may occur:

(i). Neurogenic, caused by central nervous system (CNS) leisons or peripheral nerve injury.

(ii). Muscular, caused by localized myasthenia.

(iii). Metastatic disease at the site of a pathological fracture.

(iv). Trauma from surgery (eg, resection of soft tissue [fascia, muscle, and nerve]) or injury.

(2). Hypomobility of a joint may occur.

(a). Loss of motor function may be the cause. The following types of hypomobility may occur:

(i). Neurogenic development over time of hypomobility with decreased active motion of joints caused by central nervous system lesions or peripheral nerve injury.

(ii). Muscular caused by local myasthenia or disuse atrophy.

(iii). Metastatic disease with resulting pain.

(iv). Segmental immobility for protection after trauma (such as surgical trauma after limb-salvage or amputation procedures, after reconstructive grafting in head and neck cancer, or after breast reconstructive surgery, or injury-related trauma after pathological fracture).

g. A seventh step in assessing a patient is

the evaluation of strength deficits and soft-tissue flexibility (*eg,* two-joint muscles).

(1). Localized weakness may be present. Various types of weakness are:

  (a). Neurogenic, caused by CNS lesions or peripheral nerve injury.

  (b). Muscular from localized myasthenia or disuse atrophy.

  (c). Segmental immobility or inactivity, such as postsurgical immobilization.

h. As an eighth step in the assessment of a patient, check for reduced endurance.

(1). Generalized weakness (common in late stage cancer) may be present, and can lead to general diminished mobility and function. See the sections on hypomobility and local weakness for more information. Various types of generalized weakness are:

  (a). Neurogenic, caused by:

  • Polyneuropathy.

  • Carcinomatous neuromyopathies and cancer-associated asthenia.

  • Ataxia.

  • Spasticity and parkinsonism.

  (b). Neuropsychiatric weakness from such disorders as depression or dementia.

  (c). Muscular from:

  • Muscular wasting (caused by malnutrition and weight loss, inactivity and disuse atrophy, or myopathy [*eg,* corticosteroid-induced]).

  • Myositis.

  • Myasthenia.

  (d). Cardiopulmonary.

  (e). Systemic conditions that diminish the patient's activity and mobility caused by:

  • Electrolyte abnormalities.

  • Endocrine disorders (*eg,* Addison's disease and panhypopituitarism, hypo- and hyperthyroidism, or hyperglycemia).

  • Anemia.

  • Dehydration.

  • Renal failure.

  • Hepatic failure.

  • Cardiopulmonary failure.

• Infection, inflammation, fever, and malnutrition.

• Deconditioning, disuse, and bed rest.

• Disease progression or metastatic spread.

• Increased intracellular destruction related to medical treatment (*eg,* chemotherapy, radiation therapy, surgery, hormonal therapy, or immunotherapy).

i. A ninth step in the assessment of a patient is the evaluation of balance and coordination deficits.

(1). If balance and coordination appear to be impaired, determine which condition exists and implement the appropriate treatment.

  (a). If the musculoskeletal system is normal, but the CNS is abnormal, check for motor output or function problems such as:

  (i). CNS lesions, caused by:

  • Polyneuropathy.

  • Carcinomatous neuromyopathies and cancer-associated asthenia.

  • Ataxia.

  • Spasticity and parkinsonism.

  • Neuropsychiatric disorders, such as depression or dementia.

  (ii). Muscular problems, caused by:

  • Muscular wasting.

  • Malnutrition and weight loss.

  • Inactivity and disuse atrophy.

  • Myopathy (*eg,* from steroid use).

  • Myositis.

  • Localized myasthenia.

  • Muscular injury.

  (iii). Peripheral nerve injury.

  (b). Motor output and function problems result in:

  (i). Impaired movement strategies.

  (ii). Impaired coordination.

  (iii). Impaired strength and endurance.

(c). Sensory input problems occur when:

   (i). Sensory feedback is impaired.

   (ii). Sensory organization is impaired.

(d). If the CNS is normal, but the musculoskeletal system is abnormal (*ie,* biomechanical problems), assess the patient for ROM deficits, strength deficits, reduced endurance, and pain, as discussed previously.

(e). If both biomechanics and CNS function are abnormal, follow the procedures discussed previously in i. (1). (a).–(c).

(2). Possible causes of balance and coordination deficits that are related to treatment are as follows:

(a). Chemotherapy and radiotherapy in patients with head and neck cancer or in children with leukemia, with resultant damage to hearing and balance.

(b). A primary tumor or metastatic tumor in the CNS or paraneoplastic syndrome.

(c). Hemorrhage in the CNS and stroke.

(d). Infection in the CNS.

(e). Distal or lower extremity loss of sensation and/or muscle weakness.

j. As a 10th step in assessing a patient, evaluate any posture deficits, impaired functional status, or mobility and ambulation problems (related to patient safety), which may be secondary to any of the above impairments and deficits discussed previously, either singly or in combination.

4. The therapist must know precautions and subsequently adapt physical therapy treatment in patients with complications (*eg,* deep venous thrombosis, embolism, cardiac arrhythmia, hypertension, metastatic disease of the lung that limits ventilation and perfusion or increases the patient's risk for rib fracture, or inappropriate response to exercise); *ie,* radiation therapy is a contraindication to the use of heat or cold in the irradiated region (see Tables 4–7 and 4–9).

a. The recognition of and appropriate action in emergency situations, including oncologic emergencies, are very important.[132-135] The physical therapist should be able to recognize signs and symptoms of:

   (1). Sepsis and tumor lysis syndrome.

   (2). Superior vena cava syndrome.

   (3). Cardiac tamponade.

   (4). Syndrome of inappropriate antidiuretic hormone.

   (5). Disseminated intravascular coagulation.

   (6). Spinal cord compression.

b. The therapist should recognize symptoms of disease and treatment-related complications (see Tables 4–7 and 4–10).

c. The therapist must be aware of contraindications to and precautions for the use of physical agents in oncology patients, *ie,* directly *over* tumor sites.

5. Physical therapy considerations for complications and side effects of surgery, radiation therapy, chemotherapy, and immunotherapy must be evaluated. See "Oncology: Examination, Diagnosis, and Treatment. Medical and Surgical Considerations, Chapter 4, Table 4–10 for more information.

6. Physical therapy planning, implementation, and management:

a. Refer to the appropriate health care providers and support systems. Communicate and document.

b. Plan for and provide information and physical therapy services.

c. Implement a treatment plan appropriate for the diagnoses and problems identified during the assessment. Monitor the patient's response. Reassess frequently.

II. Physical Therapy Treatment

A. Changes in the patient's mental status, behavior, and cognitive function

Document any changes and make appropriate referrals. Simplify commands and directions. Use memory aids when indicated.

B. Abnormal vital signs and peripheral pulses (perfusion)

If a change occurs in the patient's status, document it and make referrals; if the patient's vital signs and peripheral pulses are normal, continue physical therapy treatment.

C. Impaired pulmonary function (Also see Chapter 7.)

1. Enhance perfusion
   a. Increase cardiac output (increase oxygen supply) with:
      (1). Pharmacological management.
      (2). Exercise training.
   b. Reduce the patient's oxygen demand, decrease the amount of work that is required for him/her to breathe, increase the blood flow to poorly perfused areas of his/her lungs (improve ventilation [$\dot{V}/\dot{Q}$ shunt]).
      (1). Increase the patient's deep-breathing capacity. Decrease his/her breathing frequency (with relaxation exercises).
      (2). Position the patient to best facilitate ventilation and perfusion (use a tripod, semi-recumbent, or sidelying position, with the impaired lung positioned down to increase perfusion).
      (3). Provide supplemental oxygen, if indicated.
      (4). Clear excessive secretions from the patient's lungs (to improve $\dot{V}/\dot{Q}$ matching).
      (5). Initiate exercise training.
2. Facilitate ventilation.
   a. Initiate the following breathing exercises:
      (1). Diaphragmatic breathing.
      (2). Pursed-lip breathing.
      (3). Segmental breathing.
      (4). Low-frequency breathing.
      (5). Manual facilitation technique for inspiration or expiration.
      (6). Incentive spirometry.
   b. Position the patient ($\dot{V}/\dot{Q}$ matching).
      (1). Position the patient for bronchial drainage if secretions are excessive.
      (2). Position the patient to match ventilation and perfusion (eg, on his/her side, with the impaired lung positioned up to increase ventilation).
   c. Remove excess secretions by means of
      (1). Percussion.
      (2). Vibration or shaking.
         (a). Manual methods.
         (b). Mechanical methods.
      (3). Suctioning.
      (4). Deep-breathing techniques (discussed previously).
      (5). Bronchial drainage.
      (6). Improvement or enhancement of the patient's coughing technique.
         (a). Positioning.
         (b). Huffing.
         (c). Manual facilitation techniques.
   d. Initiate respiratory therapy; oxygen supplementation, medication for bronchial dilation, aerosol therapy, and mechanical ventilation may be used. Coordinate physical therapy treatment with the respiratory therapist.
   e. If both ventilation and perfusion are impaired, combine treatments as indicated.

D. Open wounds or skin lesions and increased girth or volumetric measures

(See Chapter 26 for more information.) If the patient has received radiation therapy to the surgical site or chemotherapy postoperatively, wound healing may be delayed.

1. Reduce lymphedema.[110-112,114-130] Successful management of edema primarily involves prevention. For cases in which edema is not preventable, four critical factors for care have been identified:
   • Early diagnosis of the underlying pathology.
   • Professional treatment.
   • Anticipation and management of complications.
   • Education of the patient with the goal of preventing recurrences.
   To increase lymphatic drainage, the hydrostatic pressure of tissues must be increased.

Lymphatic and venous return are increased by elevation of a limb or by external compression of the skin. Lymphedema caused by lymphatic disorders does not diminish as readily with elevation as does edema secondary to venous disorders.

a. It is best to prevent postoperative vascular complications. Instruct the patient:
   (1). Lower extremities.
      (a). Wear elastic support hose or an Ace wrap preoperatively.
      (b). Initiate active ROM exercises and ankle pumping.
   (2). Upper extremities.
      (a). Wear an elastic pressure-gradient sleeve or Ace wrap.
      (b). Initiate active ROM exercises to enhance blood flow (eg, arm ergometry within ROM restrictions at low work loads or low intensity).
b. Prevent or minimize postoperative lymphedema:
   (1). Elevate the involved extremity on a pillow (about 30 degrees) while the patient is lying in bed or sitting in a chair.
   (2). Wrap the involved extremity with elastic bandages or have the patient wear elastic pressure-gradient hose or an elastic sleeve.
   (3). Perform pumping exercises of the involved extremity after surgery.
   (4). Perform active ROM exercises early.
c. Decrease lymphedema if or when it develops.
   (1). A mechanical pneumatic pressure pump can be used for at least 1.5 to 2 hours a day; this is followed by having the patient don a pressure-gradient garment. The purpose of the pneumatic compression pump is to reduce edema in the extremity; the reduction is maintained by a custom-fabricated pressure-gradient garment.
      (a). Pneumatic pressure pumps vary in size, operation, style, complexity, and cost; the devices range from lightweight home models designed to treat one extremity to complex institutional models capable of treating four extremities at a time. In general, these devices function by applying high pressure for a short duration capable of applying multiple-compartment compression. The devices employ a series of overlapping compartments that apply sequential compression in a centripetal direction; they either apply single pressure, equal pressure to the entire area, or multiple or "graded" pressure to an extremity. Pressure application begins distally and then slowly spreads up the extremity to encourage the flow of lymph and venous fluids in a centripetal direction. The pneumatic sleeve is an air bladder of single-compartment or multiple-compartment design that is attached to the pump. Single-compartment sleeves inflate in a uniform or non-sequential manner, whereas multiple-compartment sleeves inflate in a sequential or distal-to-proximal direction. The intent of both of these sleeves is to promote a pneumatic massage" effect that facilitates lymphatic drainage. The external pressure in the sleeve must be greater than the internal hydrostatic pressure exerted by edematous tissues. Three variables are adjusted when a compression unit is used: the amount of pressure, duty cycle (on-to-off), and duration of treatment can all be regulated. If the patient's response to treatment is not satisfactory, it may be necessary to adjust one or more of these variables.
      (b). The patient should be made comfortable; he/she is usually placed in a supine position. Restrictive clothing and jewelry should be removed. The extremity is covered entirely with a stockinette to prevent skin abrasion and for hygienic purposes. The extremity is then elevated to enhance the return of fluid. A padded wooden wedge that has a width equal to

that of the extremity can be used to support the extremity at a 45 degree angle, with the arm and external appliance in 20 to 70 degrees of abduction. This elevated and abducted position facilitates the removal of fluid and ensures the patient's comfort. The amount of pressure used is determined by the patient's blood pressure. Gradient support pressures that are available range from 0 to 300 mm Hg. The initial setting should be 80 mm Hg or 20 mm Hg below the patient's systolic pressure. For example, if the patient's blood pressure is 120/80, the initial pressure setting is 80 mm Hg and may eventually be increased to 100 mm Hg, or 20 mm Hg less than the systolic pressure. To be effective, the amount of pressure must be equal to or greater than the patient's diastolic pressure. The pump duty cycle, if adjustable, should be set so that pressure is "on" longer than it is "off." For a 1-minute cycle, the machine should be on for 45 seconds and off for 15 seconds—a 3:1 ratio. Total treatment time per session may range from 30 minutes to 6 to 8 hours. Frequency of use depends on the nature and extent of the diagnosis and on the severity of symptoms; whereas some patients require the use of these devices for short periods (eg, weeks to months), others may require use of these devices for the duration of their disorders.

(c). A few studies have investigated the physiological effectiveness of these devices and have confirmed that their use results in the distal-to-proximal translocation of lymph.[122,123]

(d). Literature examining the effectiveness of one device compared with that of another remains scant.[110,112,118,121–130,135]

(2). Continuous elevation of the involved extremity at night and the use of an elastic sleeve or elastic hose (individually measured and fitted to the patient) during the day may help to decrease lymphedema. Further research is needed on the optimal treatment parameters and functional outcomes of this method.

(3). Manual massage from distal to proximal along the length of the extremity also may be helpful. Massage may be used to reduce hard, nonpliable edema or adhesions in the underlying tissues or to reduce excessive edema in the hand. Massage is most effective when it is used in conjunction with other forms of external compression. The massage technique most often used is effleurage or a gentle stroking in a centripetal direction. Edematous tissue must be massaged carefully to prevent stretching, scratching, or bruising of the skin.

(4). Lymphedema also may be managed with isometric and isotonic pumping exercise of the distal muscles (alternating motion of hands and feet).

(5). Avoidance of sources of increased load on the lymphatic vessels may help; these sources of increased load are as follows:

  (a). Static, dependent positioning of the limb.

  (b). Application of local heat.

  (c). Prolonged use of the muscles for even light tasks.

  (d). Hot environments.

(6). Protective skin care and the prompt administration of treatment when skin abrasions, small burns, and insect bites occur may help to prevent lymphedema.

  (a). The patient should avoid using harsh chemicals and detergents.

  (b). Moisturizers should be applied to skin frequently.

  (c). Antibiotics should be used, when appropriate, for the treatment of infection.

d. Maintain normal active ROM of the involved extremity by initiating active exercise of the involved extremity as soon as possible. When the drainage tubes have been removed, initiate daily active-assistive and active ROM exercises of the involved extremity.

e. Increase strength in the involved extremity by initiating isometric exercises of the shoulder or pelvic musculature on the first postoperative day while the patient is lying in bed. Manual isotonic resistance exercise may be initiated about 1 week postoperatively. Light resistance may be applied during exercise (approximately 2 to 3 lb with the use of such tools as weights, with TheraBands, or sand bags).

E. Treatment of pain

(See the section on the assessment of pain, I.B.3.e.) Many new patient-administered treatment systems are being used to manage cancer-related pain.[136]

1. Bone pain from cancer is not responsive to treatment by physical agents and must be managed with pharmacological therapy.
2. Cancer pain from other origins may be diminished for a short period of time with the use of physical agents.
   a. Indications for and contraindications to physical agents in patients with cancer are the same as in any other patients (*eg,* patients with acute and chronic pain). (See table in Pfalzer L: Physical agents and the patient with cancer. *Clin Management Phys Ther* 1992, 12:83–86 for general and local tumor site contraindications.[137]) Many physical agents used by physical therapists (*eg,* superficial heat, cold therapy, and ultrasound) are helpful for short-term pain relief. Application of heat modalities may be therapeutic; for example, during chemotherapy, increased blood flow to the tumor would increase drug delivery to the tumor. However, physical therapy does not deliver therapeutic deep heat at temperatures as high as those used in the treatment of tumors by hyperthermia. Heat modalities, massage, mechanical compression, and ultrasound are currently contraindicated for use directly over tumor sites. If the tumor has been irradiated, heat or cold modalities are contraindicated. The role that ultrasound may play in retarding tumor growth is being reexamined. However, a 1993 case study stated that therapeutic ultrasound is still contraindicated in patients with a history of cancer who complain of low back pain without further examination and diagnostic tests.[138]
   b. One of the first uses of transcutaneous nerve stimulation was for the treatment of pain in patients with cancer. Transcutaneous nerve stimulation can be helpful in managing acute, postoperative, and chronic pain. The transcutaneous nerve stimulation parameters are determined by the type of pain being treated (acute or chronic). Massage (including effleurage, petrissage, and myofascial trigger-point therapy), heat, cold, massage and vibration, distraction, and relaxation have been demonstrated by Rhiner and co-workers[139] and by Ferrell-Torry and Glick[140] to assist with pain relief. The authors concluded that although the exact mechanism was not known, therapeutic massage was beneficial in promoting relaxation and in alleviating the perception of pain and anxiety in hospitalized patients with cancer.[140] Massage therapy significantly reduced the subjects' level of pain perception (average = 60%) and anxiety (average = 24%) while enhancing their feelings of relaxation by an average of 58%. In addition to these subjective measures, all physiological measures (heart rate, respiratory rate, and blood pressure) tended to decrease from baseline, providing further indication of relaxation.[140]

F. ROM deficits

1. Hypermobility
   a. Management of hypermobility includes:
      (1). Internal fixation by the use of:
          (a). Medullary rods.
          (b). Plates and screws.
      (2). External fixation by the use of:
          (a). Casts and splints.
          (b). Orthoses and braces.
      (3). The initiation of strengthening exercises (usually the submaximal isometric cocontraction of agonist and antagonist muscle groups to increase stability) after appropriate internal or external stabilization.
2. Hypomobility
   a. Many patients with cancer demonstrate joint hypomobility; therefore, appropriate ROM techniques are indicated, including:
      (1). Physiological motions.
      (2). Muscle-energy techniques.
      (3). Joint-mobilization techniques.
      (4). Passive, active, and active-assistive ROM.
      (5). Continuous passive motion.

(6). Flexibility and strengthening exercises (particularly isotonic exercises with machine weights or isokinetic exercises that emphasize strengthening throughout available joint motion with isokinetic assessment of muscle weakness) may be beneficial as long as precautions are identified before treatment.

G. Strength deficits

1. Medical treatment for processes causing localized weakness and fatigue includes:
   a. The administration of corticosteroids.
   b. Nutritional support (*eg*, total parenteral nutrition).
   c. Palliative radiation, chemotherapy, or surgery.
2. Physical therapeutic management of localized weakness includes:
   a. An exercise plan (including instructions for the pacing of the exercise, for the setting of priority tasks, and for the monitoring of patients' responses).
   b. The prescription of appropriate assistive devices and orthoses or braces, as needed for stability, protection, and function of joints (for self-care and ambulation) until the muscle is sufficiently strengthened.
   c. The initiation of flexibility exercises to prevent contracture from muscle imbalance across the joint.
   d. The initiation of a strengthening program with rhythmical exercise of muscle groups assessed as being weak, with the first priorities being the strengthening of the antigravity muscles that are needed for adequate function; however, the patient must have a neurologically intact motor unit and CNS. Begin with low repetitions (five or six per set for three sets) with reasonable overload increases with each set (*eg*, the first set at 50% maximal voluntary contraction [MVC], the second set at 60% MVC, and the third set at 70% MVC). Increase the amount of overload per set over time, based on the patient's response (*eg*, the first set at 60% MVC, the second set at 70% MVC, and the third set at 80% MVC, as tolerated).[13]
   e. The observation of exercise precautions and the monitoring of the patients' response during exercise intervention to ensure the patient's safety. Review safety precautions to prevent the patient from falling if balance related to weakness is a problem.
   f. The use of functional electrical stimulation, which may be indicated if the patient's muscle is at least partially innervated, even if muscle contraction is very weak.
3. If weakness is severe, rule out motor unit problems related to disease or treatment (*eg*, peripheral neuropathy, myopathy, or muscle-tendon injury) and neuropsychiatric problems to allow for appropriate referral and treatment. If no contraindications are present, begin low-load repetitions (five or six per set for three sets) with reasonable overload increasing with each set (*eg*, the first set at 50% MVC, the second set at 60% MVC, and the third set at 70% MVC. The amount of overload increases per set, based on the patient's response (*eg*, the first set at 60% MVC, the second set at 70% MVC, and the third set at 80% MVC). If the patient's muscle is denervated, passive ROM exercise is indicated (see II.G.2.e. and f.).[13]
4. If endurance is also impaired, consider using an interval exercise training protocol to enhance both strength and endurance (*eg*, WAIT [Winnington aerobic interval training program]).[11–17]

H. Reduced endurance

1. Medical treatment for processes that cause general weakness and fatigue may include:
   a. Fluid resuscitation and electrolyte replacement.
   b. The administration of blood products.
   c. Nutritional support (*eg*, total parenteral nutrition).
   d. Administration of antibiotics and additional drugs (keeping in mind their side effects and withdrawal symptoms), including:
      (1). Antidepressant drugs.
      (2). Anticonvulsant drugs.
      (3). Corticosteroids.
      (4). Stimulants.
      (5). Antihyperglycemic drugs (such as insulin).
      (6). Analgesic agents.
      (7). Antiemetic agents.
      (8). Sedatives or antipsychotic drugs.

(9). Cardiac medications for congenital heart failure (*eg,* calcium agents or calcium channel blockers).

  e. Palliative radiation, chemotherapy, or surgery.

  f. Dialysis.

2. Physical therapy management of general fatigue and weakness (usually indicative of late-stage disease or treatment-related problems, with the patient spending most of his/her time in bed) may include the following:

  a. Encourage the patient to get out of bed to sit in a bedside chair as much as can be tolerated.

  b. Reorganize the area around the bed to put self-care items and other important personal items (*eg,* remote controls) within reach.

  c. Initiate a turning and positioning schedule and reduce the pressure over bone protuberances (*eg,* over the heels, ischial and sacral protuberances, the elbows, and the back of the head [the occiput]).

  d. Prescribe the use of assistive devices that may be needed for self-care, bed mobility, and transfers (*eg,* rails, a trapeze, a bedside tray, a bedside commode, reachers, a walker, or a wheelchair).

  e. Initiate active ROM and flexibility exercises and other exercises to maintain and improve strength and mobility (*eg,* submaximal isometric exercises of the antigravity muscle groups, deep-breathing exercises, and trunk rotation exercises).

  f. Observe exercise precautions and monitor the patient's response during physical therapy and exercise intervention to ensure the patient's safety. If balance related to weakness is a problem, review safety precautions and the patient's need for equipment to prevent falling.

  g. Set priorities for the patient's activities of daily living (*eg,* dressing, bathing, grooming, bed mobility, and ambulation).

  h. Initiate other energy-conserving techniques at an appropriate pace (*eg,* set exercise and rest intervals and the length of rest periods) and have the patient perform the most important activities first.

  i. Initiate a low-level interval exercise program for short periods of time several times a day as the patient's exercise tolerance improves, and progress to longer exercise sessions (*eg,* progress from a program of 15 to 20 minutes once a day to one of 30 to 40 minutes three times a week). (See the section on endurance exercise that follows.)

  j. Begin a strengthening program with rhythmical exercise of the large antigravity muscle groups (*ie,* the trunk, shoulder, elbow, hip, knee, and ankle extensor muscles and the trunk, shoulder, elbow, hip, knee, and ankle flexor muscles) every day at low repetitions (five or six per set for three sets) with a reasonable increase in overload with each set (*eg,* the first set at 50% MVC, the second set at 60% MVC, and the third set at 70% MVC). Increase the amount of overload per set over time, based on the patient's response (*eg,* the first set at 60% MVC, the second set at 70% MVC, and the third set at 80% MVC).

  k. Observe exercise precautions, and monitor the patient's response during exercise intervention to ensure his/her safety. Also review the safety precautions to prevent the patient from falling if balance related to weakness is a problem.

  l. Note that the exercise prescription to improve endurance contains the five aspects of activity (exercise mode, intensity, frequency, and duration and the subject's initial physical status) that are related to improving health and fitness (including cardiorespiratory endurance, muscle strength, body composition, and flexibility), as outlined by the American College of Sports Medicine,[6–17] regardless of the patient's disease state, age, or physical fitness.[6] The prescription is based on the results of a SLGXT.

    (1). Frequency. The aerobic exercise should be performed at least three times a week; patients who are hyperglycemic should be encouraged to exercise daily.

    (2). Mode. Compromised skeletal integrity may preclude weight-bearing activities. Non–weight-bearing, aerobic exercises for patients with bone and joint disease include cycling, rowing, and swimming (if the patients do not have a suppressed immune response). Additionally, patients with severe muscle weakness tolerate cycling better than ambulation.

    (3). Duration and initial fitness level. Severely debilitated patients may need to exercise twice a day for brief periods of time (*eg*, for 5 minutes). Less-debilitated patients should initially exercise for 10 to 15 minutes continuously and should progress slowly to 30 to 45 minutes, according to their tolerance.

(4). Exercise progression and intensity. The patient's exercise regimen should progress toward a program of intermittent exercise, with initial work-rest ratios of 1:1 progressing to 2:1. Such a regimen would be appropriate in severely debilitated patients. Eventual progression to 10 to 15 minutes of continuous exercise should be encouraged. Exercise intensity that is set by training heart rates may be unsafe and difficult to use with those patients who have inappropriate heart responses to exercise and who experience significant physiological changes on a day-to-day basis from disease and treatment, including changes in medications. However, exercise intensity that is set by heart rate ranges that are based on oxygen consumption or on metabolic equivalent levels has been shown to be safe, with monitoring of blood pressure and heart rate (for rhythm changes) and with Borg's ratings of perceived exertion (a score of 9–11 indicates a low exertion level, 11–12 indicates a moderate exertion level, and 13 indicates that the patient is working somewhat hard) to guide exercise intensity.

I. **Posture deficits and impaired functional status, mobility, and ambulation (patient safety)**

Treat the single deficit or combination of deficits or impairments before or contiguously with mobility training, as indicated. Reassessment may be necessary, possibly resulting in an alteration in treatment. One example that requires reassessment is when an exercise program is causing excessive fatigue (*eg*, fatigue that does not resolve within approximately 30 minutes after exercise is discontinued to a comparable pre-exercise level, or an elevated heart rate that does not return to resting values within 5 to 10 minutes in recovery); in such a case, the exercise program should be revised to a lower intensity before the next exercise session.

III. Goal Setting Specific to Physical Therapy

Goal setting relates to expected patient and family outcomes. Some examples of general and specific physical therapy goals for patients with cancer are found in Table 5–2. Examples of expected outcomes for physical therapy management of the patient and his/her family in the areas of prevention and treatment are shown in Table 5–3.

IV. Examination and Treatment for Specific Representative Cancers

A. Musculoskeletal, including bone tumors and soft-tissue tumors

1. The physical therapy examination should include the following steps:
   a. Check the patient's medical chart for results of diagnostic and laboratory tests and following surgical procedures such as limb salvage.
   b. Assess the psychosocial status of the patient, including coping mechanisms.
   c. Assess the patient's understanding of his/her condition, any physical impairments

Table 5–2. PHYSICAL THERAPY GOALS FOR PATIENTS WITH CANCER

Examples of General Physical Therapy Goals for Patients with Cancer

Prevention of deconditioning
Maximal functional skills
Prevention or treatment of cardiopulmonary impairment or dysfunction
Provision of emotional support to the patient and his/her family
Education of the patient about his/her condition, treatment options, and home exercise program
Assistance in pain and symptom control
Assistance in health promotion (*eg*, risk identification and screening for secondary prevention)

Examples of Specific Goals for Patients with Cancer

Increased strength and endurance
Diminished nervousness, irritability, and anxiety
Increased attention span and concentration
Improvement in posture
Maintenance of or improvement in ROM and flexibility
Promotion of independence in transfers, ambulation, and activities of daily living

Examples of Specific Goals for Patients with Cancer for an Endurance Exercise Program in a Comprehensive Care Plan

Ability to perform daily activities with greater efficiency
Improvements in functional capacity and health status
Participation in regulation and monitoring of exercise program; consequently, the patient learns self-care and becomes an active participant in the improvement of his/her health status
Development of a better understanding of the disease and its treatment as the patient learns about physical and affective responses to exercise, including the ways in which physical fitness may alter side effects (*eg*, the patient may feel as though he/she has more energy, he/she may feel more relaxed, he/she may have diminished anxiety and emotional stress, he/she may think more positively, and he/she may have a reduction in frustration)

and dysfunctions, and the need for physical therapy intervention.

d. Perform a musculoskeletal and neuromuscular assessment (by taking a history and by performing a physical examination) and a cardiopulmonary screen (by assessing peripheral pulses and by monitoring vital signs during postural changes and during increasing levels of activity, including activities of daily living).

e. For bone tumors, assess the patient for pain and symptoms in the involved region and assess the bone to determine the effects of the tumor (*eg*, destruction, erosion, and expansion of the bone and invasion of the soft tissue).

(1). Generally, a patient with a bone tumor has mild to constant pain that worsens at night or with activity.

(2). Pain is often an early sign of bone tumors and is often acute with fracture.

(3). Neurologic symptoms can refer from a nerve root or from plexus compression (in which case, assess the degree of nerve involvement), from entrapment, or from compartment syndromes. Neuropathic changes such as hyperesthesia, paresthesia, throbbing pain, muscle weakness, and trophic changes are common as compression or entrapment syndromes progress; perform electromyography and nerve conduction tests.

(4). Note swelling and limitation of motion and joint effusion if the tumor

Table 5–3. EXPECTED OUTCOME FOR PHYSICAL THERAPY MANAGEMENT OF THE PATIENT WITH CANCER

Expected Outcome for the Patient and His/Her Family	Specific Criteria to Achieve Desired Outcome
Should be able to manage mobility, function, self-care	Should identify the cause of the decreased mobility, inactivity, and disuse; formulate possible intervention strategies, and predict the outcomes of those interventions
	Should describe the level of mobility and ability to perform activities of daily living consistent with the patient's disease state, treatment, and functional status
	Should describe strategies to increase mobility and ability to perform activities of daily living (self-care) and to integrate the altered mobility and activities of daily living into the patient's goals and lifestyle
	Should be able to perform activities of daily living and to use self-care aids and assistive devices to improve functional abilities and mobility
	Should demonstrate methods to prevent side effects of diminished mobility, of inactivity, and of disuse

Table 5–3. EXPECTED OUTCOME FOR PHYSICAL THERAPY MANAGEMENT OF THE PATIENT WITH CANCER *(continued)*

Expected Outcome for the Patient and His/Her Family	Specific Criteria to Achieve Desired Outcome
Should be able to manage ventilation and perfusion	Should identify reasons for altered ventilation or perfusion (*eg*, anxiety, exercise, inactivity, infection, environment, reduced levels of hemoglobin, bronchospasm, inflammation, edema and effusion, airway obstruction, position, or posture) Should demonstrate methods to prevent side effects of diminished mobility and inactivity (*eg*, turning and positioning schedule and deep breathing exercises) Should describe strategies to increase ventilation or perfusion and to integrate altered ventilation or perfusion into the patient's goals and lifestyle (*eg*, positioning to increase matching of ventilation and perfusion, energy conservation techniques, performing priority tasks first, and pacing of activity with appropriate rest intervals)
Should be able to manage pain and other symptoms	Should identify the cause of pain, possible interventions, and outcomes of interventions Should report and describe level and alterations of pain Should identify strategies to modify factors that influence pain (physiological, psychosocial, and environmental) to enhance the patient's functional status Should describe strategies to reduce pain and to integrate the interventions into the patient's goals and lifestyle Should use strategies to control pain
Should be able to manage muscle weakness and fatigue	Should identify the reasons for decreased strength and endurance (*eg*, inactivity and disuse, cachexia, drug side effects) and formulate possible interventions and predict the outcomes Should report and describe the patient's level and alterations in strength and endurance Should identify strategies to modify factors that influence strength and endurance (physiological, psychosocial, and environmental) to enhance the patient's functional status Should describe strategies to reduce weakness and fatigue and should integrate the interventions into the patient's goals and lifestyle Should use strategies to control weakness and fatigue (*eg*, energy conservation techniques, performing priority activities first, and pacing activity with appropriate rest intervals)
Should be able to manage information and aid with coping	Should describe the stage of the disease and its treatment Should describe strategies for coping with predictable problems related to the disease and its treatment, such as giving postoperative care consistent with the patient's intellectual and psychosocial abilities and state Should identify personal and community resources from which to obtain information and services and then use those resources for support and to aid with coping Should communicate feelings about living with cancer and should participate in goal setting and in developing intervention strategies for mobility, self-care, ventilation, pain management, and other concerns
Should be able to manage risk identification and a prevention plan	Should identify the warning signs of cancer Should describe the risk factors for cancer Should describe and plan a risk-factor screening and self-detection strategy to maximize the patient's health status by limiting disease with early detection Should be able to perform the activities of daily living and to use self-care aids and assistive devices to improve functional status (activities of daily living and mobility) Should demonstrate methods to prevent side effects of diminished mobility, inactivity, and disuse Should screen for the patient's possible risk of falling if he/she is returning home Should assess patient and family response to physical therapy intervention and efficacy of treatment Should assess patient and family education outcomes, including assessment of prevention outcomes (*eg*, risk identification and screening for prevention, for reducing the patient's risk of falling, for enhancing physical activity

is near a joint (*eg,* the elbow or the knee); also note any deformity or changes in joint stability.

(5). Note swelling and limitation of motion and joint effusion if the tumor is near a joint (such as the knee, the shoulder, the hands, or the neck); also note any deformity.

f. For soft-tissue tumors, assess the patient for pain and symptoms in the involved region, and assess the soft tissue for the effects of the tumor (*eg,* destruction, expansion, and invasion of adjacent soft tissue and rare invasion of bone).

(1). Later in the disease, mild pain that is worse at night or with activity or constant pain that increases in severity as the tumor enlarges and compresses or stretches blood vessels, lymphatic vessels, or nerves and other neurosensitive structures is common.

(2). In patients with soft-tissue tumors, pain is acute, with nerve or vascular compression.

(3). Neurologic symptoms can refer from a nerve root or from plexus compression, or from entrapment or compartment syndromes (in which case, assess the degree of nerve involvement with electromyography and nerve conduction tests). Neuropathic changes such as hyperesthesia, paresthesia, muscle weakness, and trophic changes are common as compression or entrapment syndromes progress.

g. Physical findings may include:

(1). A palpable, tender, fixed bone mass (in patients with a bone tumor) or a fixed soft-tissue mass (in patients with a soft-tissue tumor).

(2). An increase in skin temperature over the mass.

(3). Superficial veins that are dilated and prominent.

(4). Increased girth (from tumor volume) or decreased girth (from muscle atrophy).

h. Assess the patient's strength, balance, posture, activities of daily living (*eg,* transfers, mobility and ambulation, and gait).

i. Assess the patient's endurance and exercise capacity.

2. Physical therapy diagnoses. Factors to be considered in a physical therapy diagnosis include:

a. Alterations in a patient's psychosocial status (*eg,* changes in body image related to diagnosis and treatment).

b. Alterations in a patient's ability to perform the activities of daily living, balance, posture, mobility, and ambulation as a function of the disease and its treatment.

c. Symptoms and physical impairments (neuropathic and trophic changes; decreased strength, endurance, and balance; and problems with transfers, mobility, and the activities of daily living) or pain related to a bone tumor and its treatment (*eg,* surgery, irradiation). Permanent nerve injury leads to disability.

d. Potential for injury includes the possibility of pathologic fracture related to bone tumor and immobility; of neuromuscular compromise related to the tumor and its treatment; and of vascular compromise related to the tumor and its treatment.

e. Pain related to a soft-tissue tumor, nerve and blood vessel involvement, and treatment (*eg,* surgery, irradiation). Permanent nerve injury leads to disability; for example, a patient who has undergone wide excision of the lateral vastus muscle for the removal of a sarcoma may have difficulty stabilizing the knee during the activities of daily living and ambulation, with decreased balance and abnormal gait.

f. Potential for injury also includes the possibility of neuromuscular compromise related to the soft-tissue tumor and its treatment and of vascular compromise related to the tumor and its treatment.

3. Physical therapy treatment

a. The physical therapists should provide relief of pain and treatment of neuropathic changes ("Treatment of Pain," Section II.E.) and should help the patient to avoid potential injury.

(1). Administer pain medications 0.5 hour before ambulation or other physical therapy treatment to aggressively manage pain. Many functional problems may resolve if pain is adequately controlled.

(2). Support painful extremities with positioning and elevation to reduce contracture formation but to protect the painful limb and possibly to decrease nerve compression (if it is secondary to edema).

(3). Use physical agents such as massage, cold packs, or mechanical compression for pain relief, relaxation, and the reduction of edema, as indicated; these agents are not indicated for use when pain is caused by a primary or secondary bone tumor. These agents are not to be used over a tumor site (see table in reference 137).

(4). If neuropathic or vascular changes are related to an entrapment or compartment syndrome, alleviating the compression of nerve or vein relieves the symptoms and prevents permanent tissue loss and nerve damage. Increasing mobility of the limb and stretching any adhesions may help to relieve neuropathic syndromes and to decrease edema in these cases.

(5). Prevent complications of neuropathic changes if nerve damage is permanent because neuropathic complications often lead to severe disability. Early intervention to prevent postural deficits and contractures, to enhance balance, and to protect skin integrity is needed. This can include the use of positioning techniques, instruction for skin care and protection, orthotic devices, and assistive devices and adaptive equipment (*eg,* slings, static and dynamic splints, and single-hand–use devices). To protect a neuropathic extremity support the joints when repositioning the patient, consider prescribing prophylactic orthotics, and use braces and assistive devices as necessary to guard the patient and to prevent trauma and falls; the patient and his/her family should be instructed in precautions with respect to insensate limbs. Create a hazard-free environment (*eg,* reduce the risk of falls). One method that can be used to prevent falls and to improve gait is the prescription of an ankle-foot orthosis for the management of foot drop.

b. Guard against potential injury by preventing pathological fractures (in patients with bone tumors).

(1). See Table 4–10 for appropriate therapeutic exercise regimens and for weight-bearing exercises, based on the percentage of cortical bone erosion and osteoporosis.

(2). Teach the patient to avoid trauma and falls (he/she should know activity and safety precautions) and to use braces and orthotic devices as necessary to guard against injury.

(3). Support joints when repositioning the patient and consider prescribing prophylactic orthoses.

(4). Guard the patient against injury and supply assistive devices during therapy sessions, as necessary to prevent falls.

(5). Create a hazard-free environment (*eg,* reduce the patient's risk of falling).

c. Establish maximum mobility within the limits of the patient's problems and treatment

(1). See IV.A.1. for patients with bone and soft-tissue tumors.

(2). Develop an exercise program within the patient's physical activity limits to:

(a). Encourage movement of the trunk, head, neck, and extremities.

(b). Encourage ambulation and weight bearing within the patient's physical limits when possible.

(c). Encourage increased strength and endurance for ambulation and the performance of the activities of daily living.

(d). Encourage improved balance, coordination, and gait for ambulation and the performance of the activities of daily living.

d. Strengthen the patient's coping abilities (see I.B.3.a.(1).)

(1). Create a supportive environment and educate patient and family about physical therapy intervention.

(2). Refer the patient for psychological support services, as needed.

e. Promote independence in self-care, mobility, and ambulation

(1). Encourage the patient to help himself/herself and instruct him/her in the physical therapy program with positive reinforcement.

(2). Allow sufficient time for the patient to complete tasks.

(3). Allow sufficient time between activities to prevent the patient from becoming fatigued.

(4). Assist the patient as needed in maintaining his/her independence (eg, the therapist may need to continue to increase level of support by assistive devices to help the patient to maintain his/her ability to ambulate without guarding.

(5). Enhance the patient's compliance with the therapeutic exercise program as needed, depending on his/her physical impairments and dysfunctions (eg, decreased strength, balance, and endurance).

(6). Provide appropriate preoperative and postoperative education and training in the use of assistive devices and orthoses, if indicated. The physical therapist should work to prevent complications and to minimize inactivity and bed rest. Freiden and coworkers examined the needs of 17 children undergoing limb-sparing procedures by resection and an expandable endoprosthetic replacement for the treatment of bone tumors. Each patient received postoperative inpatient and outpatient physical therapy and was followed for an average of 2.5 years. Gait training was relatively straightforward, and seven patients required neither orthoses nor ambulatory aid. The other 10 patients walked with a knee orthosis or axillary crutches, or both. Until the time came for reoperation to lengthen the implant, a shoe lift with a maximum height of 1 in was added to compensate for the limb length discrepancy. The requirements of these patients compare favorably with the more complex requirements of high proximal amputees who have external prostheses and require more involved gait training, frequent adjustments to their prostheses, and prosthetic replacements as they grow. The authors stated that children undergoing limb-sparing surgery have special needs that should be addressed, including early mobilization, gait training, adjustment to repeated brief hospitalizations for limb lengthening, and continued follow-up care to monitor their activity restriction.[141]

(7). Position the patient to reduce and prevent the development of contracture and postural deficits and the formation of pressure sores.

4. Expected outcomes
   a. The patient should achieve relief of his/her symptoms; medications or other modalities should be used to reduce pain and symptoms. Furthermore, the patient should report increased comfort.
   b. The patient should demonstrate an ability to cope with the demands of his/her condition and treatment and should participate in the decision-making process to set physical therapy goals.
   c. The patient should participate in self-care activities such as feeding himself/herself and should perform hygiene care; he/she should also be able to perform transfers and to ambulate with appropriate assistive devices.
   d. The patient should achieve wound healing at the surgical incision site.
   e. He/she should demonstrate independence in performing a home exercise regimen.
   f. The patient should be able to modify the activities of daily living as well as his/her lifestyle to accommodate functional losses related to musculoskeletal, neuromuscular, or cardiopulmonary deficits.
   g. He/she should show no signs of complications related to inactivity or bed rest.
   h. The patient should avoid potential injury (eg, neuromuscular, vascular compromise or pathological fracture); he/she should use safety precautions during activity to prevent falls and to reduce the risk of trauma and should use prophylactic orthotics appropriately.

B. Head and neck cancer

1. Physical therapy examination (see IV.A.)
   a. Perform a musculoskeletal and neuromuscular assessment (including a history

and physical examination of the head and neck and a screen of the upper quarter) and a cardiopulmonary screen by assessing peripheral pulses, ventilation, and stoma (if one is present) and by monitoring the vital signs in relation to head, neck, and shoulder girdle postural changes, increasing level of activity, and the performance of the activities of daily living.

b. As part of the neuromuscular examination, assess the patient for pain and symptoms in the involved region and for cranial nerve injury (*eg*, injury of the glossopharyngeal, auditory, facial, and trigeminal nerves, with their related functional loss, such as difficulties with chewing and swallowing). Pain in patients with head and neck tumors is acute, with nerve or vascular compression. Neuropathic changes such as hyperesthesia, paresthesia, muscle weakness, and trophic changes are common as compression or stretch injuries progress.

c. Assess the patient's strength, balance, posture, ability to perform the activities of daily living (*eg*, transfers, mobility, ambulation, and gait) and his/her cranial nerve function (*eg*, swallowing, chewing, hearing, facial expression, or balance).

d. A tool for evaluating a patient's functional status to help in the assessment of treatment outcome and in the development of successful rehabilitation for head and neck cancer has been developed.[142] The new Performance Status Scale for Head and Neck Cancer Patients assesses that the primary areas of dysfunction experienced by this population consists of three subscales: (1) understandability of speech, (2) normalcy of diet, and (3) the ability to eat in public. The researchers administered the scale to 181 patients with head and neck cancer and to a comparison group of 30 patients with breast cancer. They found that the scale is reliable across raters and sensitive to functional differences across a broad spectrum of patients with head and neck cancer.

2. Physical therapy diagnoses
   a. Evaluate the patient's symptoms and physical impairments (*eg*, neuropathic and trophic changes; decreased strength, endurance, or balance; and problems with transfers, mobility, or activities of daily living) or pain related to the tumor, to blood vessel and nerve involvement, and to treatment (*eg*, surgery or irradiation). Permanent nerve injury leads to disability; for example, one patient underwent wide excision of the mandible for the removal of a sarcoma and had subsequent difficulty with swallowing, speaking, or chewing during the activities of daily living and during ambulation because of decreased balance.

   b. Evaluate the patient's potential for injury by neuromuscular or vascular compromise related to the tumor and its treatment.

3. Physical therapy treatment (see II)
   a. Provide relief of pain and the results of neuropathic changes (see II.E.) and prevent potential injury.

      (1). Support the patient's head and neck with positioning to reduce contracture formation but to protect the head and neck from pain and possibly to decrease nerve stretch and compression (if it occurs secondary to edema).

      (2). Use transcutaneous electrical nerve stimulation or physical agents such as massage, cold packs, or mechanical compression to provide postsurgical pain relief and relaxation and to reduce edema, as indicated. These agents are not indicated for use when the pain is from a primary or secondary bone tumor and they are not indicated for use over the tumor site (see table in reference 137).

      (3). Prevent the complications of neuropathic changes if nerve damage is permanent, because these complications often lead to severe disability. Early intervention to prevent postural deficits and contractures, to enhance balance, and to protect skin integrity is needed if a stoma is present or if a tracheostomy has been performed. Intervention can include the use of positioning techniques, instruction for skin care and protection, and the use of orthotic devices. Support the patient's head and neck or shoulder girdle during repositioning and consider using prophylactic orthoses, as necessary, to guard the patient and to prevent trauma and falls (the patient and family should be educated regarding activity and balance precautions). Create a hazard-free environment (*eg*, reduce the risk of falls).

b. Establish maximum mobility within the limits of the patient's problems and treatment.

c. Strengthen the patient's coping abilities (see II.B.3.a.(1)).

d. Promote self-care activities.

e. Promote independence in self-care, mobility, and ambulation.

4. Expected outcomes

a. The patient should achieve symptom relief; medications or other modalities should be used to reduce pain and symptoms. Furthermore, the patient should report increased comfort.

b. He/she should demonstrate an ability to cope with the demands of his/her condition and treatment and to participate in the decision-making process to set physical therapy goals.

c. The patient should participate in self-care activities (*eg*, feeding himself/herself, exhibiting independence in communications, and the performance of hygiene care), and if his/her balance is impaired, he/she should be able to transfer and ambulate with the appropriate assistive devices.

d. The patient should achieve wound healing at the head and neck surgical incision site, including any sites of postsurgical reconstruction such as myocutaneous flaps.

e. He/she should demonstrate independence in performing a home exercise regimen such as the Therabite Jaw Motion Rehabilitation System (Therabite Corporation, Bryn Mawr, PA). A study compared the use of the Therabite system to the use of tongue blades as a technique for maintaining or improving mandibular ROM in patients who have undergone radiation treatment.[143] Three groups of patients were evaluated and compared; the first group performed unassisted exercise, the second performed mechanically assisted mandibular mobilization with stacked tongue depressors and unassisted exercise, and the third

used the Therabite system and unassisted exercise. No statistically significant differences between the first two groups were reported; however, the third group had a quicker and more prolonged improvement in mouth opening.

f. The patient should modify his/her activities of daily living and lifestyle to accommodate functional losses related to musculoskeletal or neuromuscular deficits.

g. He/she should show no signs of complications related to inactivity or to bed rest.

h. The patient should avoid potential injury (*eg*, neuromuscular or vascular compromise) by using safety precautions for activity and skin care to prevent falls and to reduce the risk of trauma; he/she also should use prophylactic orthoses appropriately.

C. Breast cancer

1. Physical therapy examination (see IV.A.)

a. Check the patient's medical chart for results of diagnostic and laboratory tests and surgical procedures, such as the type of resection and the potential need for breast reconstruction or implant.

b. Perform a musculoskeletal and neuromuscular assessment (including a history and physical examination for the thorax and shoulder region and a screening examination of the upper quarter region) and a cardiopulmonary screen by assessing peripheral pulses and ventilation and by monitoring vital signs in relation to postural changes, increasing level of activity, and activities of daily living.

c. For breast cancer, assess the patient for pain and symptoms in the involved region (the thorax and the upper quarter) from the effects of the tumor (*eg*, destruction, erosion, bone or lung metastases, and invasion of the soft tissue) or from treatment (*eg*, loss of shoulder motion, and lymphedema).

(1). Generally, mild to constant pain of the anterior chest wall that may refer down the arm and occasionally to the posterior thorax and is worse at night or with activity may be present.

(2). Pain is not an early sign of breast cancer; however, pain is acute when pathological fracture, nerve or vascular compression, or severe lymphedema is present.

(3). Neurological symptoms can refer from a nerve injury during a mastectomy (in which case, the therapist should assess the degree of nerve involvement) or from radiotherapy and chemotherapy. Neuropathic changes such as hyperesthesia, paresthesia, throbbing pain, muscle weakness, and trophic changes and scarring are common as a result of axillary dissection followed by radiotherapy, with compression, fibrosis, or stretching of blood vessels, lymphatics, or nerves (eg, brachial plexus and peripheral nerves) and other neurosensitive structures in the axillary region.

d. Note swelling and limitation of motion if lymphedema is present (see II.D.).

e. Assess the physical findings (see II.D.).

(1). Look for palpable, tender, chest wall adhesions; scar banding in the axilla; and soft-tissue contracture.

(2). An increase in skin temperature and dilated and prominent superficial veins are signs of lymphedema, as is increased volume or girth in the involved upper extremity.

f. Assess the patient's strength, with particular attention to the involved upper quarter region, to balance, to posture, and to the activities of daily living, such as transfers, mobility and ambulation, and gait.

g. Assess the patient's endurance and exercise capacity.

2. Physical therapy diagnoses

a. Evaluate the patient's symptoms and physical impairments (eg, lymphedema; neuropathic and trophic changes; decreased strength, endurance, and balance, and problems with transfers, mobility, or the activities of daily living) or pain related to nerve or blood vessel injury from treatment (eg, surgery or irradiation). Permanent severe lymphedema or nerve injury leads to disability; for example, one patient underwent a modified radical mastectomy, axillary dissection, and radiotherapy with involvement of the long thoracic nerve and lymphedema.

Subsequently, she experienced decreased shoulder girdle strength and stability during shoulder motion, her entire upper extremity became weakened with the loss of shoulder motion, and she had impaired ability to perform the activities of daily living that required the use of the involved upper extremity.

b. Potential for injury includes lymphedema, postsurgical pain, and immobility from disuse of the involved upper extremity; neuromuscular compromise related to the tumor or its treatment; and vascular compromise related to the tumor or its treatment.

3. Physical therapy treatment

a. Provide relief of the patient's pain and neuropathic changes (see II.E.) and prevent potential injury.

(1). Administer pain medications 0.5 hour before ambulation or other physical therapy treatment to aggressively manage pain. Many functional problems may resolve if pain is adequately controlled.

(2). Support the patient's edematous and painful extremities with positioning and elevation to reduce contracture formation but to protect the painful limbs and possibly to decrease edema and nerve compression (if it occurs secondary to edema). Also attempt to increase the patient's ROM. Treatment may include any or all of the following modalities: taping, intermittent compression, massage, exercise, and continual elevation of the involved upper extremity at night, and the use of a custom-fit gradient-support elastic sleeve or of elastic support bandaging during the day.

(3). Use physical agents such as massage, cold packs, or mechanical compression for pain relief and relaxation and to reduce edema as indicated. These agents are not indicated for use when the pain is from a primary or secondary bone tumor, and they are not indicated over the tumor site. If the axilla were irradiated, heat and cold modalities are contraindicated in this region. Stretching exercises for adhesions should

(4). If neuropathic or vascular changes are related to entrapment or to compartment syndrome (*ie*, from lymphedema), alleviating the nerve or vascular compression relieves the symptoms and prevents permanent tissue loss and nerve damage. Increase the mobility and stretch the adhesions to help relieve neuropathic syndromes and to decrease edema in these cases.

(5). Prevent complications of neuropathic changes if nerve damage is permanent because such complications often lead to severe disability. Early intervention to prevent lymphedema formation, postural deficits, and contractures; to enhance symetry in posture (especially in the thorax); and to protect skin integrity is needed. This can include the use of positioning techniques, instruction for skin care and protection, orthotic devices, assistive devices, and adaptive equipment such as slings. To protect an extremity with lymphedema and neuropathic changes, support the joints when repositioning the patient and consider using prophylactic orthotics and assistive devices as necessary to elevate the extremity and to guard the patient and to prevent trauma to the extremity (the patient and family should know the proper skin care precautions and insensate limb precautions). Create a hazard-free environment (*eg*, reduce the patient's risk of trauma, infection, sunburn, and insect bites by having him/her wear protective clothing and insect repellent when he/she is outdoors).

b. Prevent potential injury by taking precautions against lymphedema by increasing the patient's knowledge of preventing the problem. If metastatic disease is present, assess musculoskeletal system integrity and limit activity as indicated.

(1). Early presurgical and postsurgical physical therapy intervention can encourage increased use and motion of the involved upper extremity. Several studies have indicated that no increased risk of injury from early mobilization of the upper extremity exists.[144–152] It appears that some patients who have undergone mastectomies are not referred to physical therapy for postoperative rehabilitation because some physicians have doubts regarding the benefits of therapy or concerns that motion early after surgery may increase the incidence of postoperative complications such as poor wound healing. Several studies have investigated the impact of early physical therapy intervention on wound seroma and drainage and on shoulder motion and functional status.[145–152] No serious complications have been reported, and improvements in shoulder motion and functional status were found. Several studies demonstrated that the greater the amount and duration of postoperative wound drainage after lymphadenectomy, the slower the healing.[150] A greater number of positive lymph nodes and the absence of a previous surgical biopsy (as in a one-step procedure) predicted slower healing.

(2). If bone metastases are present in the spine and thorax, initiate the appropriate therapeutic exercise and weight-bearing exercise, based on the percentage of cortical bone erosion and osteoporosis that are present (see Table 4–10).

(a). The patient should avoid trauma and falls (he/she should know which activities are appropriate and how to take safety precautions) and should use braces and orthotic devices as necessary to protect cortical bone integrity.

(b). Support the patient's spine when repositioning him/her and consider prescribing prophylactic orthoses.

(c). Guard the patient and supply assistive devices, as necessary, so that he/she can avoid falls.

(d). Create a hazard-free environment (*eg*, reduce the patient's risk of falling).

c. Establish maximum mobility within the limits of the patient's problems and treatment

(1). Develop an exercise prescription within the patient's physical activity limits to:

(a). Prevent postural deformities by encouraging proper positioning and movement of the trunk, head, neck, and extremities—especially the involved extremity.

(b). Encourage ambulation and weight bearing within limits, when possible, with the use of symmetrical posture.

(c). Encourage increased strength, flexibility, and endurance for ambulation and the performance of the activities of daily living (*eg*, prescribe shoulder-shrugging and shoulder-circle exercises and active ROM exercises of the cervical spine—especially the neck extensor muscles—to encourage a relaxed upright posture). Help the patient to maintain normal ROM of the involved upper extremity and strength in the elbow, forearm, and hand musculature as soon as possible postoperatively. It is no longer necessary to delay the initiation of active-assisted and active shoulder exercises until after drainage tubes have been removed[145–152] or to limit shoulder abduction until the sutures are removed; however, do not place undue stress on the scar or cause blanching of the scar during shoulder ROM exercises. Observe the incision during exercise. These same precautions apply for ROM exercise after breast reconstruction with myocutaneous flaps. Joint mobilization techniques can be used to maintain joint play in the glenohumeral and scapulothoracic joints when

arm movement must be restricted.

(d). Maintain or increase strength in the involved shoulder with isometric pumping exercises of the shoulder musculature, initiated on the first postoperative day with the patient lying in bed. Manual isotonic resistance exercise may be initiated about 4 days postoperatively. Resistance may be applied during shoulder exercise with a light hand-held weight (approximately 2 to 3 lb).

d. Strengthen the patient's coping abilities (see II.B.3.a.(1).)

e. Promote self-care activities

f. Promote independence in self-care, mobility, and ambulation

4. Expected outcome

a. The patient should achieve symptom relief; medications or other modalities should be used to reduce pain and symptoms. Furthermore, the patient should report increased comfort.

b. He/she should demonstrate an ability to cope with the demands of his/her condition and treatment and should participate in the decision-making process to set physical therapy goals.

c. The patient should participate in self-care activities (*eg*, feeding himself/herself, performing hygiene care, and being able to perform transfers and to ambulate with appropriate assistive devices).

d. The patient should achieve wound healing at the surgical incision site and should experience a decrease in lymphedema if or when it develops.

e. He/she should demonstrate independence in performing a home exercise regimen.

f. The patient should modify his/her activities of daily living and lifestyle to accommodate functional losses related to lymphedema or musculoskeletal or neuromuscular deficits.

g. He/she should show no signs of complications related to inactivity or to bed rest.

h. If metastatic disease is present, the patient should avoid pathologic fracture and neuromuscular or vascular compromise; he/she should use precautions during activity to prevent falls and to reduce the risk of trauma. He/she also should use prophylactic orthotics appropriately.

D. CNS tumors

1. Physical therapy examination
   a. Perform a musculoskeletal and neuromuscular assessment (a history and physical examination) and monitor the patient's vital signs in relation to postural changes and to increasing level of activity and the activities of daily living.
   b. Review the patient's medical chart for the results of diagnostic and laboratory tests.
   c. Determine the patient's understanding of his/her condition, physical impairments, and dysfunctions and assess the psychosocial status of the patient for his/her coping mechanisms.
   d. Assess the patient for pain and neuromuscular symptoms related to the involved region of the brain or to the spinal cord from the effects of the tumor (*eg*, destruction, expansion and invasion of adjacent tissue, and compression secondary to elevations of intracranial pressure).
   e. Physical findings. Neurological signs and symptoms such as (1) hyperesthesia, paresthesia, and then numbness, followed by muscle weakness with paresis and then paralysis or (2) altered deep tendon refluxes, coordination, balance, posture, and gait are common as compression increases in the brain or as the tumor progresses. These signs and symptoms need to be carefully monitored and temporarily managed to retain function (*ie*, for patient safety) and to prevent impairments; however, many of these symptoms are eliminated or reduced with the effective reduction of the tumor load.
   f. Assess the patient's strength, posture, ability to perform activities of daily living (*eg*, transfers, mobility, ambulation, and gait), and overall functional status.
   g. Assess the patient's endurance level and exercise capacity.
2. Physical therapy diagnoses
   a. Assess the patient's symptoms and physical impairments (*eg*, impaired balance, coordination, and gait; problems with cranial nerve functions such as vision, hearing, speech, chewing, and swallowing; neuropathic and trophic changes; decreased strength; altered posture; and decreased endurance, mobility, and ability to perform transfers or the abilities of daily living) or pain related to the tumor, to nerve and blood vessel involvement, and to treatment (*eg*, surgery or irradiation).
   b. Potential for injury includes neuromuscular and neuropsychiatric compromise related to the tumor and to its treatment, which can result in an increased risk of falling.
   c. An alteration in the patient's psychosocial status (*ie*, changes in body image related to the disease and to its treatment from problems such as hair loss) may have occurred.
   d. An alteration in the patient's functional status, resulting in a diminished ability to perform the activities of daily living, mobility activities, and ambulation related to the disease and its treatment may have occurred.
3. Physical therapy treatment
   a. Physical therapy management is an integral part of the management of patients with neurological tumors and is similar to that for any patient with CNS compromise that results in neurological involvement; however, the natural course of disease progression varies. Many patients' problems are similar, but they may be reversed on treatment, some more rapidly than others.
   b. Patient safety during normal activities of daily living may be a concern while he/she awaits surgical or medical treatment; this issue may require the use of appropriate assistive and supportive devices and orthoses. Cranial-nerve or CNS involvement, which may alter vision or hearing or impair judgement, also needs to be addressed.
   c. Treatment of pain (see II.E.)
   d. Neuromotor and neurosensory problems
      (1). If neurosensory and neuromotor changes are related to compression, alleviating the compression by decreasing the tumor size relieves or reduces the severity of the symptoms

and prevents permanent neurological injury. Because many of these neurological symptoms and signs reverse with treatment, it is important to prevent the complications that result from a temporary loss of neuromuscular function and from sensory deficits.

(2). The usual preventive strategies for any patient who must undergo bed rest or who experiences disuse and sensory deficits need to be observed and implemented. It is important to prevent further physical impairment and loss of function related to inactivity and to bed rest as neurological function returns.

(3). Aggressively try to prevent the complications of neurological losses if brain or spinal cord damage is permanent. Rehabilitation is usually required, because these losses often lead to severe disability. Early intervention may help to prevent postural deficits and contracture; to enhance balance, coordination, and gait; or if hemiplegia or paraplegia is present, to aid in ventilation, which may be impaired. Treatment may include the use of positioning techniques, instruction for skin care and protection, the initiation of breathing exercises, or the use of orthotic devices or assistive devices and adaptive equipment (*eg*, slings, static and dynamic splints, or single-hand–use devices). To protect an insensate or paralyzed extremity, support the joints when repositioning the patient, consider prescribing prophylactic orthoses, and prescribe braces and assistive devices, as necessary, to guard the patient and to prevent trauma and falls (the patient and family should know about activity and insensate limb precautions). Create a hazard-free environment (*eg*, reduce the patient's risk of falls and increase the level of support if his/her functional status worsens).

c. Establish maximum mobility within the limits of the patient's problems and treatment

(1). Provide treatment as previously described (see IV.D.3.a.–d.).

(2). Develop an exercise prescription within the patient's physical activity limits to:

(a). Encourage movement of the trunk, head, neck, and extremities and improve ventilation.

(b). Encourage improved posture, balance, coordination, and gait for ambulation and the activities of daily living.

(c). Encourage ambulation and weight bearing within the patient's physical limits when possible; if this is not possible, prescribe assistive devices to help him/her to maintain independent mobility for as long as possible.

(d). Encourage increased strength and endurance for ambulation and the activities of daily living.

(e). Encourage breathing exercises, when indicated.

d. Strengthen the patient's coping abilities (see II.B.3.a.(1).)

(1). Create a supportive environment and educate the patient and his/her family about physical therapy intervention.

(2). Refer the patient for psychological support services, as needed.

e. Promote independence in self-care, mobility, and ambulation

(1). Encourage the patient to help himself/herself and instruct him/her in the physical therapy program with positive reinforcement.

(2). Allow sufficient time for the patient to complete tasks.

(3). Allow sufficient time between activities to prevent the patient from becoming fatigued.

(4). Assist the patient as needed to allow him/her to maintain independence; for example, the therapist may need to continue to increase the level of support by assistive devices to help the patient to maintain his/her ability to ambulate safely without guarding while he/she awaits surgical or medical treatment.

(5). Enhance the patient's compliance

with a therapeutic exercise program as needed, depending on his/her physical impairments and dysfunctions (*eg*, decreased vision, hearing, strength, balance, coordination, gait, endurance, or mobility).

(6). Provide appropriate preoperative education and training while awaiting surgical and medical treatment in the use of assistive devices and orthoses if indicated, and in the prevention of complications from inactivity and bed rest.

(7). Position the patient in such a way as to reduce and prevent contracture and pressure-sore formation and to assist in ventilation when indicated.

4. Expected outcome
   a. The patient should achieve symptom relief; medications, positioning and support, or other modalities should be used to reduce pain and symptoms. Furthermore, the patient should report increased comfort.
   b. The patient should avoid potential injury (from neuromotor or neurosensory compromise), should use safety precautions during activity to prevent falls and to reduce risk of trauma, and should use prophylactic orthoses appropriately.
   c. He/she should demonstrate an ability to cope with the demands of his/her condition and treatment and should participate in the decision-making process to set physical therapy goals.
   d. The patient should participate in self-care activities (*eg*, feeding himself/herself, performing hygiene care, and being able to perform transfers and ambulation with appropriate assistive devices or adaptive equipment such as a walker or a wheelchair).
   e. He/she should achieve wound healing at the surgical incision site.
   f. The patient should demonstrate independence in performing a home exercise regimen.
   g. He/she should modify his/her activities of daily living and lifestyle to accommodate functional losses related to neurological deficits.
   h. The patient should show no signs of complications related to inactivity or bed rest.

Clinical Decision-Making Case

At presentation, BB was a 55-year-old white woman who had been referred for physical therapy for the evaluation and treatment of 2-degree right upper-extremity lymphedema following modified radical mastectomy. Her primary complaint was pain and loss of function of her dominant hand secondary to the edema. She said that she was also concerned about the appearance of her arm.

FAMILY AND SOCIAL STATUS

BB is married and has two daughters, who are 28 and 26 years of age; both are married and live in the immediate area. She also has one 25-year-old son. She had worked full-time with the city planning department until 10 weeks before presentation. Her husband is the city mayor. They live in a three-story home in which daily housekeeping is done by a housekeeping staff. BB returned to work part time 1 month earlier and planned to return to work full time.

MEDICAL HISTORY

BB discovered a lump in her right breast 3 months previously. Her physician admitted her to the hospital for a biopsy. The biopsy results were positive, and the pathologist's report staged the cancer as stage II breast cancer. A modified radical mastectomy was performed 10 weeks before presentation for physical therapy. Other items in BB's medical history are non-contributing to her current problem, except for a long history of acute bouts of neck and upper-back pain. She complained of mild (VAS-4) pain on activity in that region. She completed a course of radiotherapy 6 weeks prior to presentation and was taking tamoxifen (as hormonal therapy) and over-the-counter pain medication. BB reported that she had never previously been treated by a physical therapist.

HISTORY OF PRESENT PROBLEM

BB reported that swelling that had become progressively worse had been present in her right arm since after the surgery; however, she only noticed it about 1 month before presentation for physical therapy. She complained that she had difficulty using her right arm and that the arm was tender to touch and aching and painful in the shoulder and hand regions. She also reported experiencing pain in her upper back and neck and some tenderness and discomfort over the mastectomy site. She was unable to perform many activities of daily living with her right arm, such as combing her hair, reaching overhead, and doing needlepoint.

INITIAL EXAMINATION

Subjective
In her medical history, BB reported tenderness and pain over the right midaxillary incision and the anterior chest wall.

Objective
BB's height was 5 ft 8 in, and she weighed 135 lb. Her heart rate was 90 beats per minute, and her blood pressure was 135/88.

Inspection
The right upper extremity was diffusely edematous; volumetric measurement indicated severe edema, as compared with her left upper extremity. Girth measures were to be taken at the following visit.

Observation
The right anterolateral surgical incision had healed, but the scar was still red in color. Atrophy was present throughout in the right upper extremity, as compared with the left, and also in the shoulder girdle—especially the right trapezius, anterior serratus, rotator cuff, and rhomboid muscles. BB's posture was asymmetrical, with the right shoulder protracted and depressed, the head in a forward posture, slight right scoliosis present, and decreased right arm swing noted on ambulation.

Sensation
BB's ability to sense a pin prick and a light touch over the right anterior chest wall was diminished; however, sensation elsewhere appeared to be intact.

Pulse
BB's right bicipital and radial pulses appeared weaker than those on the left.

Active ROM
Active ROM was within normal limits for both the lower extremities and trunk; however, neck bending and rotation to the right was more limited than that to the left, and discomfort was present in the upper back at end of the range. Active ROM also was normal in the left upper extremity and right elbow, wrist, and hand; however, a slight loss of range was present at extremes of flexion of the right versus the left upper extremity, with discomfort on overpressure at the end of the available range in the axilla and at the incision site in right shoulder external rotation, flexion, abduction, and internal rotation. Right shoulder extension and adduction appeared to be within normal limits. The right shoulder external rotation was 0 to 45 degrees, abduction was 0 to 110 degrees, flexion was 0 to 120 degrees, and internal rotation was 0 to 60 degrees.

Joint Play
The shoulder region was to be completely examined the following day; the right glenohumoral joint was restricted on distraction and on inferior glide, as compared with the left. The right scapula was abducted and upwardly rotated.

Muscle Function
Break test results were normal in the right lower extremities and in the left lower extremity. The right wrist, hand, and elbow appeared weaker than the left and ached on testing; isokinetic testing occurred the following day. The right shoulder also was weaker than the left, with aching on testing that became sharp with repetition over both the greater and lesser tubercles and over the tip of the acromion. The right grip strength was 18 lb weaker than the left, and the right lateral pinch strength was 8 lb weaker than the left.

Functional Status
Patient was independent in ambulation, transfers, and stair climbing. She required assistance in dressing, grooming, and bathing, which her daughters and husband had been providing.

DIAGNOSIS AND ASSESSMENT

Signs and symptoms consistent with the development of lymphedema and chest wall adhesions creating pain, weakness, and loss of motion in the right upper extremity were present. Signs and symptoms that indicated some loss of glenohumoral capsular flexibility secondary to inactivity, with resultant loss of coordinated motion of the shoulder and impingement of the subacromial space, also were noted.

TREATMENT PLAN

Mechanical compression was to be applied for 1.5 hours, if tolerated, and BB was to be fitted for a gradient-pressure sleeve and was to temporarily use an Ace wrap. Joint play traction was to be applied to the right glenohumoral joint, followed by active ROM and stretching exercises and light-resistance exercises (beginning with 5 lb for all motions of the right upper extremity), with special emphasis on scapular adduction and retraction exercises and postural retraining. Patient BB was instructed in skin care, in arm positioning and elevation during sitting and at night, and in a home program of stretching and resistive exercises. The patient was to be seen three times a week for therapeutic exercises and five times every 2 weeks for intermittent compression until the gradient-pressure sleeve arrived. BB tolerated initial treatment without increased pain (VAS=3 after treatment) and was asked to keep a log of her home exercises.

BB responded well to this treatment; she showed improvement in her lymphedema, pain, upper quadrant posture, active ROM, strength, and upper-extremity function. She discontinued in-office therapy at the end of 2.5 weeks when her pressure-gradient sleeve arrived, and she was able to independently don the garment and tolerate wearing it for 8 to 10 hours.

Re-evaluation

This same patient was referred for physical therapy 2 years later with a history of right neck and upper-back pain that had been present for approximately 6 weeks. On physical examination, BB's limitations were not much different from those at her last examination 2 years previously with several notable exceptions (eg, her height had become 5 ft 7 in). On physical examination with a review of her systems, BB complained of increasing dyspnea with exertion; fatigue; a slight weight loss over the previous month; and sharp pain in her right upper thoracic spine, and right posterolateral chest wall, and shoulder that increased with activity and sitting and that was a dull ache at rest and worse again at night. She also complained of headaches and that her pain would wake her at night; however, the pain could be sufficiently relieved by acetaminophen to allow her to return to sleep but was not completely relieved. Active ROM of the right shoulder was grossly within normal limits, as compared with the left; however, her symptoms reproduced in her thorax and chest wall. Palpation revealed point tenderness in both areas, with elevated skin temperature and a possible mass. Her posture was kyphotic, with anterior shifting of C7 to T1 on palpation. BB had some weakness on break testing of the T1 key intrinsic hand muscles (and grip and pinch strength), with referred pain gripping from back to front along the T1 dermatome that increased with trunk extension, flexion, sidebending, and rotation. The pain in the back was greatest on extension and sidebending to the right. Pain in the right

chest wall increased with extension, sidebending to the left, and rotation bilaterally. BB denied any other changes, signs, or symptoms. She said that she was due for her 2-year follow-up examination for her cancer 2 weeks later. The therapist's assessment was that the patient's signs and symptoms were consistent with a T1 nerve root compression with possible signs and symptoms that required the ruling out of recurrent cancer. Therefore, BB was referred to her physician. Conservative treatment for her back pain was begun (positioning, posture re-education, exercise within the painful ROM). Use of modalities was contraindicated until a definitive medical diagnosis was made. She was diagnosed with metastatic cancer of the spine, ribs, and lungs 2 weeks later.

References

1. Borg G: Perceived exertion as an indicator of somatic stress. *Scand J Rehabil Med* 1970, 2–3:92–98.
2. Noble BJ, Borg GA, Jacobs I, *et al.*: A category ratio perceived exertion scale: relationship and muscle lactate and heart rate. *Med Sci Sports Exerc* 1983, 15:523.
3. Smutok M, Skrinar G, Pandolf K: Exercise intensity: subjective regulation by perceived exertion. *Arch Phys Med Rehabil* 1980, 61:569–574.
4. Sidney KH, Shephard RJ: Perception of exertion in the elderly, effects of aging, mode of exercise and physical training. *Percept Mot Skills* 1977, 44:990–1010.
5. Pandolf KB, Burse RL, Goldman RF: Differential returns of perceived exertion during physical conditioning of older individuals using leg-weight loading. *Percept Mot Skills* 1975, 40:563.
6. American College of Sports Medicine: *Guidelines for Graded Exercise Testing and Exercise Training*, 4th ed. New York, Lea and Febiger, 1991.
7. Kottke TE, Caspersen CJ, Hill CS: Exercise in the management and rehabilitation of selected chronic diseases. *Prevent Med* 1984, 13:47–65.
8. Birrer RB: Exercise prescription: not just for cardiac patients. *Postgrad Med* 1985, 77:219–227, 230.
9. Holbrook J: Personal health maintenance for adults. *West J Med* 1984, 141:824–831.
10. Wilmore JH: *Training for Sports and Activity*. Boston, Allyn and Bacon, Inc., 1982.
11. Winningham ML, MacVicar MG, Bondoc M, *et al.*: Effect of aerobic exercise on body weight and composition in patients with breast cancer on adjuvant chemotherapy. *Oncol Nurs Forum* 1989, 16:683–689.
12. MacVicar MG, Winningham ML, Nickel JL: Effects of aerobic interval training in cancer patients' functional capacity. *Nurs Res* 1989, 38:348–351.
13. Hicks JE: Exercise for cancer patients. In JV Basmajian and SL Wolf (eds): *Therapeutic Exercise*, 5th ed. Baltimore, Williams & Wilkins, 1990.
14. Pfalzer LA: Aerobic exercise for patients with disseminated cancer. *Clin Man Phys Ther* 1988, 8:28–31.
15. Winningham ML: Walking program for people with cancer. *Cancer Nurs* 1991, 14:270–276.
16. Winningham ML, MacVicar MG: The effect of aerobic exercise on patient reports of nausea. *Oncol Nurs Forum* 1988, 15:440–447.

17. Pfalzer L, Tutschka PJ, Harper D: Effects of interval training on muscle performance after BMT [Abstract]. *J Cardiopulm Rehabil* 1989, 9.

18. Perkins J: Gynecologic malignancies: detection, prevention, and therapeutics. Part 2: Cervical and endometrial cancer. *Am Pharm* 1988, 28:34–37.

19. Perkins J: Gynecologic malignancies: detection, prevention, and therapeutics. Part 1: Ovarian cancer. *Am Pharm* 1988, 28:40–43.

20. Balmer CM: Prostate cancer: detection, prevention, and therapeutics. *Am Pharm* 1988, 28:34–40.

21. *Isolated Joint Testing: A Handbook for Using Cybex II and the UBXT.* Bay Shore, NY, Lumex, Inc., 1980.

22. Rothstein JM, Delitto A, Sinacore DR, Rose SJ: Muscle function in rheumatic disease patients treated with corticosteroids. *Muscle Nerve* 1983, 6:128–135.

23. Greene WB, Strickler EM: A modified isokinetic strengthening program for patients with severe hemophilia. *Dev Med Child Neurol* 1983, 25:189–196.

24. Barnes WS: The relationship of motor-unit activation to isokinetic muscle contraction at different contractile velocities. *Phys Ther* 1980, 60:1152–1158.

25. Coyle EF, Costill DL, Lesmes GR: Leg extension power and muscle fiber composition. *Med Sci Sports Exer* 1979, 11:12–15.

26. Ivy JL, Withers RT, Brosa G, *et al.*: Isokinetic contractile properties of the quadraceps with relation to fiber type. *Eur J Appl Physiol Occup Physiol* 1981, 47:247–255.

27. Gregor RJ, Edgerton VR, Perrine JJ, *et al.*: Torque velocity relationships and muscle fiber composition in older female athletes. *J Appl Physiol* 1979, 47:388–392.

28. Larsson L, Grimby G, Karlsson J: Muscle strength and speed of movement in relation to age and muscle morphology. *J Appl Physiol* 1979, 46:451–456.

29. Wyatt MP, Edwards AM: Comparison of quadraceps and hamstring torque values during isokinetic exercise. *J Orthoped Sports Phys Ther* 1981, 3:48–56.

30. Winter DA, Willis RP, Orr GW: Errors in the use of isokinetic dynamometers. *Eur J Appl Physiol* 1981, 46:397–408.

31. Fillyaw M, Bevins T, Fernandez L: Importance of correcting isokinetic peak torque for the effect of gravity when calculating knee flexor to extensor muscle ratios. *Phys Ther* 1986, 66:23–31.

32. Nelson SG, Duncan PW: Correction of isokinetic and isometric torque recordings for the effect of gravity. *Phys Ther* 1983, 63:674–676.

33. Sapega AA, Nicholas JA, Sokolow D, Saraniti A: The nature of torque "overshoot" in Cybex isokinetic dynamometry. *Med Sci Sports Exer* 1982, 14:368–375.

34. Karnofsky DA, Burchunel JH: The clinical evaluation of chemotherapeutic agents against cancer. In J McLeod (ed): *Evaluation of Chemotherapeutic Agents.* New York, Columbia University Press, 1949.

35. Yates JW, Chalmer B, McGengney E: Evaluation of patients with advanced cancer using the Karnofsky performance statue. *Cancer* 1980, 45:220–224.

36. Hutchinson TA, Boyd NF, Feinstein AR: Scientific problems in clinical scales, as demonstrated in the Karnofsky Index of Performance Status. *J Chronic Dis* 1979, 2:661.

37. Mor V, Laliberte L, Morris JN, Wicmann M: The Karnofsky Performance Status Scale: an examination of its reliability and validity in a research setting. *Cancer* 1984, 53:2002–2007.

38. Selby P: Measurement of the quality of life after cancer treatment. *Br J Hosp Med* 1985, 33:266–271.

39. Selby PJ, Chapman AW, Etazadi-Amoli J, *et al.*: The development of a method for assessing the quality of life of cancer patients. *Br J Cancer* 1984, 50:13–22.

40. Sorensen JB, Klee M, Palshof T, *et al.*: Performance status assessment in cancer patients: an inter-observer variability study. *Br J Cancer* 1993, 67:773–775.

41. Conhill C, Verger E, Salamero M: Performance status assessment in cancer patients. *Cancer* 1990, 65:1864–1866.

42. Bjordal K, Kaasa S: Psychometric validation of the EORTC Core Quality of Life Questionnaire, 30-item version and a diagnosis-specific module for head and neck cancer patients. *Acta Oncol* 1992, 31:311–321.

43. da Silva FC, Reis E, Costa T, Denis L: Quality of life in patients with prostatic cancer: a feasibility study. The Members of Quality of Life Committee of the EORTC Genitourinary Group. *Cancer* 1993, 71(Suppl):1138–1142.

44. Aaronson NK, Ahmedzai S, Bergman B, *et al.*: The European Organization for Research and Treatment of Cancer QLQ-C30: a quality-of-life instrument for use in international clinical trials in oncology. *J Natl Cancer Inst* 1993, 85:365–376.

45. Satariano WA, Ragheb NE, Branch LG, Swanson GM: Difficulties in physical functioning reported by middle-aged and elderly women with breast cancer: a case-control comparison. *J Gerontol* 1990, 45:M3–11.

46. Derogatis LR, Akiloff MD, Melisaratos N: Psychological coping mechanisms and survival time in metastatic breast cancer. *JAMA* 1979, 242:1504.

47. Schag CA, Ganz PA, Heinrich RL: Cancer Rehabilitation Evaluation System—short form (CARES-SF). A cancer specific rehabilitation and quality of life instrument. *Cancer* 1991, 68:1406–1413.

48. Jansen C, Halliburton P, Dibble S, Dodd MJ: Family problems during cancer chemotherapy. *Oncol Nurs Forum* 1993, 20:689–694; discussion 694–696.

49. Goodwin JS, Hunt WC, Samet JM: Determinants of cancer therapy in elderly patients. *Cancer* 1993, 72:594–601.

50. Romsaas EP, Juliani LM: Resource utilization in an outpatient setting: rehabilitation problems experienced by cancer patients. *Oncol Nurs Forum* 1984, 11:45–48.

51. Smart CR, Yates JW: Quality of life. *Cancer* 1987, 60(Suppl):620–622.

52. Campbell H, Yi P, Rothberg H, Sierocki J: Impact of cancer chemotherapy on patients and family members: a clinical study in an outpatient setting [Meeting abstract]. *Proc Annu Meet Am Soc Clin Oncol* 1992, 11:A1342.

53. Lansky SB, List MA, Ritter-Sterr C, *et al.*: Quality of life in head and neck cancer survivors [Meeting abstract]. *Proc Annu Meet Am Soc Clin Oncol* 1989, 8:A656.

54. Rafla S, Kowalczyk D, Weiss R: The impact of clinical stage, site and therapy on the quality of life of cancer patients [Meeting abstract]. *Proc Annu Meet Am Soc Clin Oncol* 1991, 10:A1236.

55. Musser EH: The self-reported needs of women with breast cancer who have recently completed treatment with chemotherapy [Meeting abstract]. *Oncol Nurs Forum* 1990, 17(Suppl):144.

56. Guadagnoli E, Mor V: Daily living needs of cancer outpatients. *J Community Health* 1991, 16:37–47.

57. Houts PS, Yasko JM, Harvey HA, *et al.*: Unmet needs of persons with cancer in Pennsylvania during the period of terminal care. *Cancer* 1988, 62:627–634.

58. Christ G, Siegel K: Monitoring quality-of-life needs of cancer patients. *Cancer* 1990, 65(Suppl):760–765.

59. Silberfarb PM: Psychiatric themes in the rehabilitation of mastectomy patients. *Int J Psychol Med* 1977–1978, 8:159–167.

60. Tobin MB, Lacey HJ, Meyer L, Mortimer PS: The psychological morbidity of breast cancer-related arm swelling: psychological morbidity of lymphoedema. *Cancer* 1993, 72:3248–3252.

61. Fox BH: A psychological measure as a predictor in cancer. In Cohen J, Martins LR (eds): *Psychosocial Aspects of Cancer*. New York, Raven Press, 1982.

62. Capovilla ED, Colotti P, Fiorentino MV: Psychological status before and after surgery for breast cancer. *Tumori* 1984, 70:277–279.

63. Heinrich RL, Schag CC: Stress and activity management: group treatment for cancer patients and spouses. *J Consult Clin Psychol* 1985, 53:439–446.

64. Holland JC, Jacobs E: Psychiatric sequelae following surgical treatment of breast cancer. *Adv Psychosom Med* 1986, 15:109–123.

65. Schain WS: Psychological rehabilitation for breast cancer patients. *Exp Suppl* 1982, 41:352–372.

66. Scott DW: Quality of life following the diagnosis of breast cancer. *Top Clin Nurs* 1983, 4:20–37.

67. McLoughlin WJ, Holz S: Cancer rehabilitation is an integrated support system. *Clin Man Phys Ther* 1985, 5:10–12.

68. Model program explores cancer rehabilitation process. *Hosp Prog* 1984, 65:28–30.

69. Stumm D: Considering the whole woman: Rehabilitation of the breast cancer patient. *Clin Man Phys Ther* 1982, 2:20–22.

70. National Cancer Institute: Coping with cancer [DHHS Publication #80-2080]. Washington, DC, U.S. Govt. Print Office, 1981.

71. Viney LL, Westbrook MT: Psychological reactions to chronic illness related disability as a function of its severity and type. *J Psychosom Res* 1981, 25:513–523.

72. Brown H, Kelly M: Stages of bone marrow transplantation: a psychiatric perspective. *Psych Med* 1976, 38:439–446.

73. Popkin MK, Stiller V, Pierce C, *et al.*: Recent life changes and outcome of prolonged competitive stress. *J Nervous Mental Dis* 1976, 163:302–306.

74. Baider L, Sarell M, Edelstein EL: Selected social-psychological characteristics of a sample of Israeli cancer patients — facts and implications. *Israel J Med Sci* 1982, 18:259.

75. Cohen M: Psychosocial morbidity in cancer: a clinical perspective. In Cohen J, Cullen JW, Martin LR (eds): *Psychosocial Aspects of Cancer*. New York, Raven Press, 1982.

76. Cobb B: Medical and psychological problems in the rehabilitation of the cancer patient. In Hardy RE, Cull JG (eds): *Counseling and Rehabilitating the Cancer Patient*. Springfield, C. C. Thomas 1975, pp. 24–68.

77. Winick L, Robbins GF: Physical and psychologic readjustment after mastectomy: an evaluation of Memorial Hospitals' PMRG program. *Cancer* 1977, 39:478–486.

78. Jamison K, Wellisch D, Pasnau R: Psychosocial aspects of mastectomy: the woman's perspective. *Am J Psychol* 1978, 135:4.

79. Meyerowitz BE, Sparks FC, Spears IK: Adjuvant chemotherapy for breast cancer: psychosocial implications. *Cancer* 1979, 43:1613–1618.

80. Ling MH, Perry PJ, Tswang MT: Side effects of corticosteriod therapy: psychiatric aspects. *Arch Gen Psychol* 1981, 38:471–477.

81. Weisman A: *Coping with Cancer*. New York, McGraw-Hill, 1979.

82. Derogatis LR, Akiloff MD, Melisaratos N: Psychological coping mechanisms and survival time in metastatic breast cancer. *JAMA* 1979, 242:1504.

83. Flomenhoft D: Understanding and helping people who have cancer. *Phys Ther* 1984, 64:1232–1234.

84. Holland JC, Jacobs E: Psychiatric sequelae following surgical treatment of breast cancer. *Adv Psychosom Med* 1986, 15:109–123.

85. Holleb AI: Human values and cancer. *Hosp Pract* 1984, 19:16.

86. Itano J, Tanabe P, Lum JL, *et al.*: Compliance of cancer patients to therapy. *West J Nurs Res* 1983, 5:5–20.

87. Schaeffer D, Garms-Homolova V: Significance of self-help groups for psychosocial rehabilitation in cancer [Translated from German]. *Rehabilitation (Stuttg)* 1986, 25:128–133.

88. Smith EA: *Psychosocial aspects of cancer patient care: A self-instructional text*. Houston, University of Texas Health Science Center at Houston, Division of Continuing Education, 1975.

89. Snyder R: Coping: you and your patient with cancer. *Clin Man Phys Ther* 1992, 12:64–69.

90. Holland JC: Clinical course of cancer. In Holland JC, Rowland JH (eds): *Handbook of Psychooncology: Psychological Care of the Patient with Cancer*. New York, Oxford University Press, 1989.

91. Heber D, Byerley LO, Chi J, *et al.*: Pathophysiology of malnutrition in the adult cancer patient. *Cancer* 1986, 58(Suppl):1867–1873.

92. Wingard JR, Curbow B, Baker F, Piantadosi S: Employment of adult survivors after bone marrow transplantation (bmt) [Meeting abstract]. *Proc Annu Meet Am Soc Clin Oncol* 1990, 9:A1180.

93. Berry DL: Return-to-work experiences of people with cancer. *Oncol Nurs Forum* 1993, 20:905–911.

94. Carmel RJ, Kaplan HS: Mantle irradiation in Hodgkin's disease: An analysis of technique, tumor irradiation and complications. *Cancer* 1976, 7:2813–2825.

95. Pickard-Holley S: Fatigue in cancer patients: a descriptive study. *Cancer Nurs* 1991, 14:13–19.

96. Rhodes VA, Watson PM, Hanson BM: Patients' descriptions of the influence of tiredness and weakness on self-care abilities. *Cancer Nurs* 1988, 11:186–194.

97. Irvine DM, Vincent L, Bubela N, *et al.*: A critical appraisal of the research literature investigating fatigue in the individual with cancer. *Cancer Nurs* 1991, 14:188–199.

98. Makipernaa A, Heino M, Laitinen LA, Siimes MA: Lung function following treatment of malignant tumors with surgery, radiotherapy, or cyclophosphamide in childhood: a follow-up study after 11 to 27 years. *Cancer* 1989, 63:625–630.

99. Smets EM, Garssen B, Schuster-Uitterhoeve AL, de Haes JC: Fatigue in cancer patients. *Br J Cancer* 1993, 68:220–224.

100. Hacking HG, Van As HH, Lankhorst GJ: Factors related to the outcome of inpatient rehabilitation in patients with neoplastic epidural spinal cord compression. *Paraplegia* 1993, 31:367–374.

101. Reuben DB, Mor V, Hiris J: Clinical symptoms and length of survival in patients with terminal cancer. *Arch Intern Med* 1988, 148:1586–1591.

102. Allegretta GJ, Weisman SJ, Altman AJ: Oncologic emergencies I: Metabolic and space-occupying consequences of cancer and cancer treatment. *Pediatr Clin North Am* 1985, 32:601–611.

103. Forester B, Kornfeld DS, Fleiss JL, Thompson S: Group psychotherapy during radiotherapy: effects on emotional and physical distress. *Am J Psychiatr* 1993, 150:1700–1706.

104. Kalayjian AS: Coping with cancer: the spouse's perspective. *Arch Psychiatr Nurs* 1989, 3:166–172.

105. Norby PA, Apte-Kakade S: Rehabilitation after conservative breast cancer surgery: management of lymphedema and

limited range of motion [Meeting abstract]. *Oncol Nurs Forum* 1990, 17(Suppl):209.

106. Abe R: A study on the pathogenesis of postmastectomy lymphedema. *Tohoku J Exp Med* 1976, 118:163–171.

107. Beninson J: Lymphedema: pathophysiologic and clinical concepts. *Angiology* 1975, 26:661–664.

108. Beninson J: Lymphedema: pathophysiologic and clinical concepts. *Angiology* 1975, 26:661–664.

109. Lerner R, Requena R: Upper extremity lymphedema secondary to mammary cancer treatment. *Am J Clin Oncol* 1986, 9:481–487.

110. Swedborg I: Effectiveness of combined methods of physiotherapy for post-mastectomy lymphoedema. *Scand J Rehabil Med* 1980, 12:77–85.

111. Swedborg I, Wallgren A: The effect of pre- and post-mastectomy radiotherapy on the degree of edema, shoulder joint mobility, and gripping force. *Cancer* 1981, 47:877–881.

112. Swedborg I: Effects of treatment with an elastic sleeve and intermittent pneumatic compression in post-mastectomy patients with lymphoedema of the arm. *Scand J Rehabil Med* 1984, 16:35–41.

113. Brennan MJ: Lymphedema following the surgical treatment of breast cancer: a review of pathophysiology and treatment. *J Pain Symptom Man* 1992, 7:110–116.

114. Beach RB: Measurement of extremity volume by water displacement. *Phys Ther* 1977, 57:286.

115. Beeby J, Broeg PE: Treatment of patients with radical mastectomies. *Phys Ther* 1979, 50:40.

116. Fell TJ: Wound drainage following radical mastectomy: the effect of restriction of shoulder movement. *Br J Surg* 1979, 66:302.

117. Hurst PAE: Venous and lymphatic disease: Assessment and treatment. In Downie PA (ed): *Cash's Textbook of Chest, Heart and Vascular Disorders for Physiotherapists*, 4th ed. Philadelphia, J. B. Lippincott Company, 1987.

118. Neel DI: Physical therapy following radical mastectomy. *Phys Ther Rev* 1960, 40:371.

119. Zeissler RH, Rose GB, Nelson PA. Postmastectomy lymphedema: late results of treatment in 385 patients. *Arch Phys Med Rehabil* 1972, 353:159.

120. McGarvey CL: Pneumatic compression devices for lymphedema. *Rehabil Oncol* 1992, 10:16–17.

121. Pekanmaki K, Kolari PJ: Sequential and graded intermittent pneumatic compression device for treatment of swollen limbs. *Biomedizinische Technik* 1987, 32:50–54.

122. Mridha M, Odman S: Fluid translocation measurement: a method to study pneumatic compression treatment of postmastectomy lymphoedema. *Scand J Rehabil Med* 1989, 21:63–69.

123. Baulieu F, Baulieu J, Vallant L, *et al.*: Factorial analysis in radionuclide lymphography assessment of the effects of sequential pneumatic compression. *Lymphology* 1982, 22:178–185.

124. Zanolla R, Monzeglio C, Balzarini A, *et al.*: Evaluation of the results of three different methods of postmastectomy lymphedema treatment. *J Surg Oncol* 1984, 26:210–213.

125. Dittmar A, Krause D: A companion of intermittent compression of single and multiple chamber systems for treatment of secondary arm lymphedema after mastectomy. *Lymphology* 1990, 14:27–31.

126. Alexander M, Wright E, Wright J, *et al.*: Lymphedema treated with a linear pump: pediatric case report. *Arch Phys Med Rehabil* 1983, 64:132–133.

127. Klein M, Alexander M, Wright J, *et al.*: Treatment of adult lower extremity lymphedema with the Wright linear

pump: statistical analysis of a clinical trial. *Arch Phys Med Rehabil* 1988, 69:202–206.

128. Zelikovski A, Haddad M, Reiss R: The "Lympa-Press" Intermittent sequential pneumatic device for the treatment of lymphedema: five years of clinical experience. *J Cardiovasc Surg* 1986, 27:288–290.

129. Richmond D, O'Donnell T, Zelikovski A: Sequential pneumatic compression for lymphedema. *Arch Surg* 1985, 120:1116–1119.

130. Yamazcki Z, Idezuki Y, Nemoto T, Togawa T: Clinical experiences using pneumatic massage therapy for edematous limbs over the last 10 years. *Angiology* 1988, 39:154–163.

131. Gudas SA: Directives in cancer rehabilitation. *Clin Man Phys Ther* 1992, 12:32–36.

132. Johnson JB, Kelly AW: A multifaceted rehabilitation program for women with cancer. *Oncol Nurs Forum* 1990, 17:691.

133. Woods EN: Reaching out to patients with breast cancer. *Clin Man Phys Ther* 1992, 12:58–63.

134. Bostwick J: Rehabilitation after mastectomy. *J Med Assoc Ga* 1987, 76:336–341.

135. Jungi WP: The prevention and management of lymphedema after treatment for breast cancer. *Int Rehabil Med* 1981, 3:129–135.

136. Abram SE: 1992 Bonica lecture: advances in chronic pain management since gate control. *Reg Anesth* 1993, 18:66–81.

137. Pfalzer L: Physical agents and the patient with cancer. *Clin Management Phys Ther* 1992, 12:83–86.

138. Sicard-Rosenbaum L, Danoff J: Cancer and ultrasound: a warning [Letter]. *Phys Ther* 1993, 73:404–406.

139. Rhiner M, Ferrell BR, Ferrell BA, Grant MM: A structured nondrug intervention program for cancer pain. *Cancer Pract* 1993, 1:137–143.

140. Ferrell-Torry AT, Glick OJ: The use of therapeutic massage as a nursing intervention to modify anxiety and the perception of cancer pain. *Cancer Nurs* 1993, 16:93–101.

141. Frieden RA, Ryniker D, Kenan S, Lewis MM: Assessment of patient function after limb-sparing surgery. *Arch Phys Med Rehabil* 1993, 74:38–43.

142. List MA, Ritter-Sterr C, Lansky SB: A performance status scale for head neck cancer patients. *Cancer* 1990, 66:564–569.

143. Buchbinder D, Currivan RB, Kaplan AJ, Urken ML: Mobilization regimens for the prevention of jaw hypomobility in the radiated patient: a comparison of three techniques. *J Oral Maxillofac Surg* 1993, 51:863–867.

144. Swedborg I: Effectiveness of combined methods of physiotherapy for post-mastectomy lymphoedema. *Scand J Rehab Med* 1980, 12:77–85.

145. Wingate L: Efficacy of physical therapy for patients who have undergone mastectomies. *Phys Ther* 1985, 65:896–900.

146. Wingate L, Croghan I, Natarajan N, *et al.*: Rehabilitation of the mastectomy patient: a randomized, blind, prospective study. *Arch Phys Med Rehabil* 1989, 70:21–24.

147. Guttman H, Kersz T, Barzilai T, Haddad M, Reiss R: Achievements of physical therapy in patients after modified radical mastectomy compared with quadrantectomy, axillary dissection, and radiation for carcinoma of the breast. *Arch Surg* 1990, 125:389–391.

148. van-der-Horst CM, Kenter JA, deJong MT, *et al.*: Shoulder function following early mobilization of the shoulder after mastectomy and axillary dissection. *Neth J Surg* 1985, 37:105–108.

149. Rodier JF, Cadonneix P, Dauplat J, *et al.*: Influence of the

timing of physiotherapy upon the lymphatic complications of axillary dissection for breast cancer. *Int Surg* 1987, 72:166–169.

150. Petrek JA, Peters MM, Nori S, *et al.*: Axillary lymphandenectomy: a prospective, randomized trial of 13 factors influencing drainage, including early or delayed arm mobilization. *Arch Surg* 1990, 125:378–382.

151. Dawson I, Stam L, Heslinga JM, Kalsbeek HL: Effect on shoulder immobilization on wound seroma and shoulder dysfunction following modified radical mastectomy: a randomized prospective clinical trial. *Br J Surg* 1989, 76:311–312.

152. Radier JF, Gadonneix P, Dauplat J, *et al.*: Influence of the timing of physiotherapy upon the lymphatic complications of axillary dissection for breast cancer. *Int Surg* 1987, 72:166–169.

PART THREE

Cardiopulmonary Systems

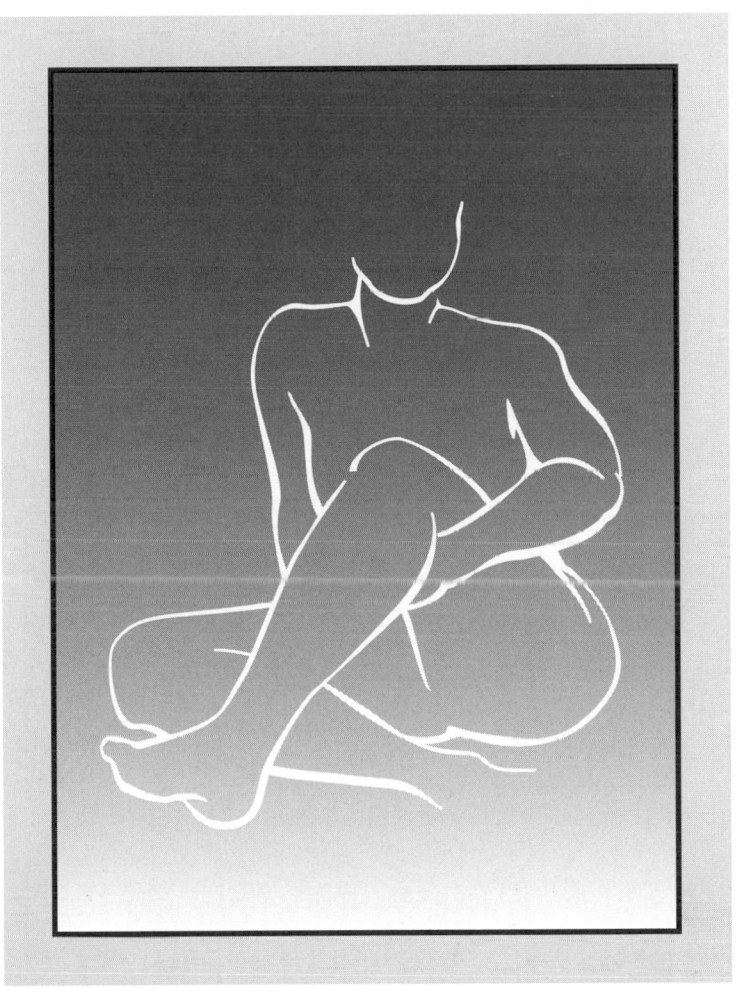

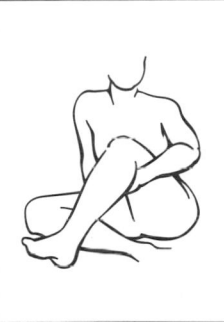

CHAPTER 6

Cardiovascular System

Catherine Certo

Over the last 20 years, cardiovascular health and disease have been the focus of attention by both the medical profession and the media. Advances in medical technology from diagnostics to surgery, pharmacological interventions, and delivery of educational services have kept the prevention and management of cardiovascular disease at the cutting edge of health care. However, despite recent encouraging reports of declines in cardiovascular

disease, it is still responsible for over half of all deaths in the United States.[1] The costs related to disease management, both directly and in terms of personal loss, are astronomical.[2]

Owing to advances in cardiovascular research, with respect to both the structure and the function of the system, the ability to evaluate cardiovascular parameters both invasively and noninvasively has grown tremendously. This has ultimately influenced the management of the disease by medical, surgical, and rehabilitative methods. To date, physical therapy intervention for cardiovascular dysfunction has encompassed acute treatment (including progressive exercise programs) of patients with medical and surgical disorders as well as more long-term outpatient, home or community-based programs designed for secondary management of cardiovascular disease. Physical therapists face the challenge of providing treatment that is responsive to current advances while dealing with a wide spectrum of issues related to cost-effectiveness, cost-containment, cultural diversity, and physical therapy shortages.

Physical therapy intervention uses exercise as a major component in the rehabilitation of patients with cardiac dysfunction. An adjunct to this may include more specific strengthening exercises to prevent or improve musculoskeletal problems. Proper patient assessment and treatment require that the physical therapist correctly obtain and accurately interpret diagnostic evaluations. Other diagnostic laboratory tests must be accurately interpreted by the physical therapist. These clinical skills, coupled with sound theoretical and factual knowledge of anatomy, physiology, and pathophysiology and the ability to develop differential diagnoses, will assist physical therapists in creating safe and effective rehabilitation programs.

It is difficult to address the multifaceted issues of the cardiovascular system without acknowledgement of the interdependence of the cardiac and pulmonary systems. Therefore, this chapter and Chapter 7 ("Pulmonary System") should be reviewed together in order to appreciate the two systems as a unit.

I. Cardiac Anatomy

A. Position

The heart is a hollow organ, positioned left of center in the chest cavity. The base of the heart is located superiorly, and the apex is directed downward and leftward and formed by the lateral tip of the left ventricle (see Figure 6–1).

B. Composition

1. The heart is encased by a fibrous protective sac called the *pericardium.*
2. The major portion of the heart is composed of muscle called *myocardium.*
3. The inner surface of the myocardium is lined with epithelial tissue called *endocardium.*
4. The fibrous membrane of the outer surface is called *epicardium* (see Figure 6–2).

C. Surfaces

The surfaces that define the heart are as follows:

1. *Sternocostal surface* (anterior), formed by the right atrium and the right ventricle.
2. *Diaphragmatic surface* (inferior), formed by the right and left ventricles.
3. *Posterior surface* (base), formed primarily by left atria (see Figure 6–3).

D. Skeleton

The heart has a skeleton composed of four fibrous rings that connect the four heart valves. Each annulus forms the foundation for a valve, linking the muscular network that comprises the four chambers.[3]

E. Function

The function of the heart is to pump oxygenated blood into the arterial system while receiving unoxygenated blood from the venous system. Thus, there is an anatomically separate right and left side, each acting as a separate pump.

F. Chambers of the heart

1. **Right and left atria.** The atria serve as reservoirs of blood and/or primer pumps that force blood into the respective ventricles. These chambers are thin walled and function under relatively low pressure.

2. **Right and left ventricles.** The ventricles serve as powerful pumps, forcing large amounts of blood either to the lung or to the systemic circulation. The walls of these chambers are much thicker and stronger than those of the atria, and they function under higher pressure to pump blood

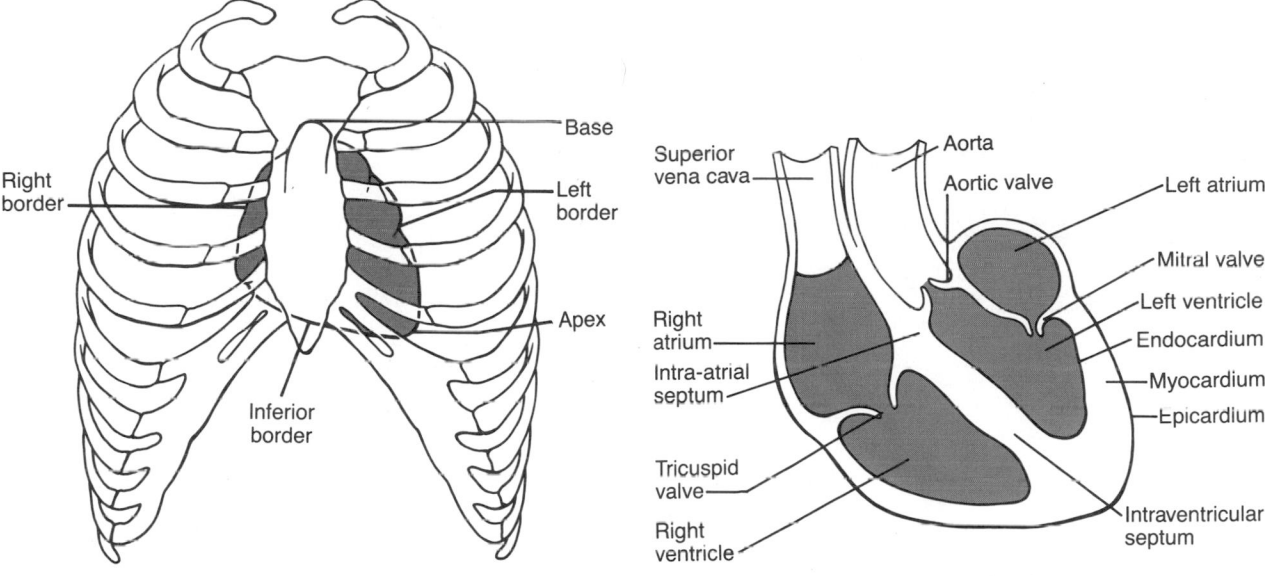

FIGURE 6–1   Anterior view of the heart.

FIGURE 6–2   The heart and its chambers.

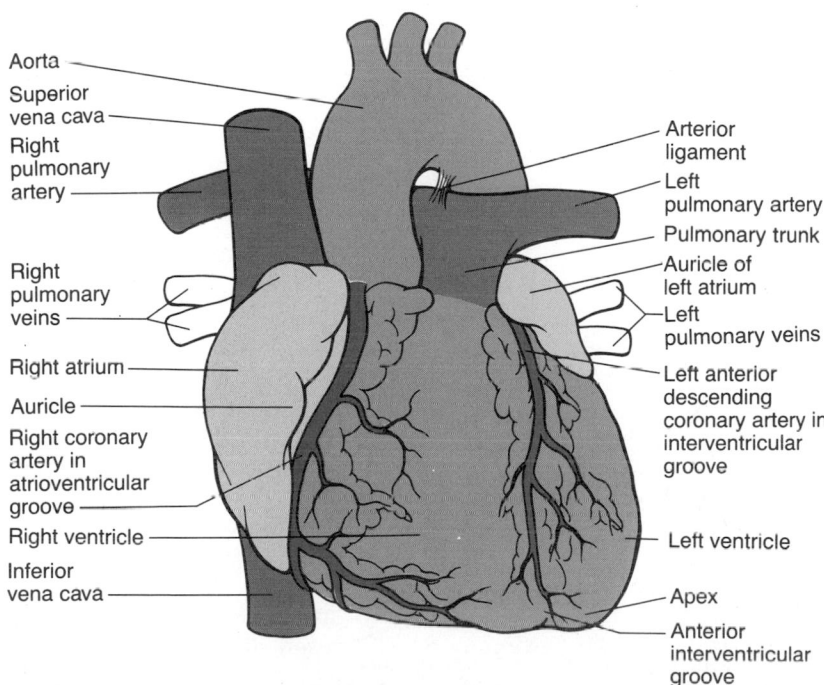

FIGURE 6–3   The sternocostal aspect of the heart.

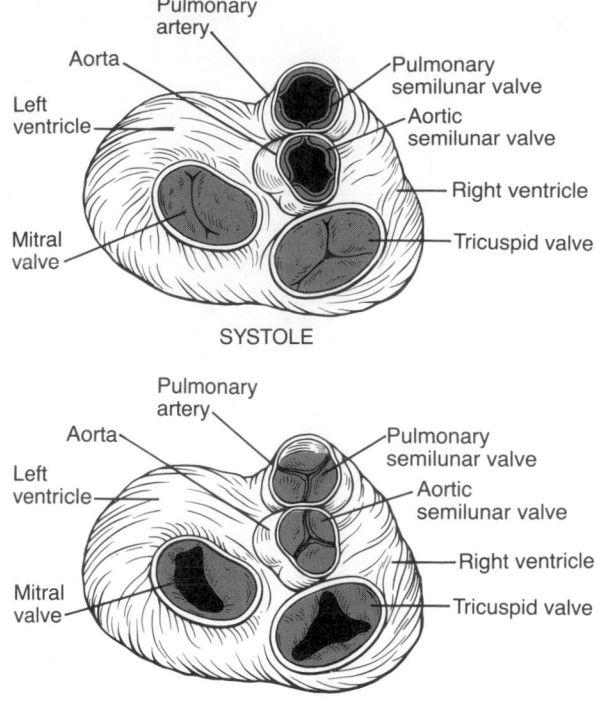

FIGURE 6–4   Valves of the heart.

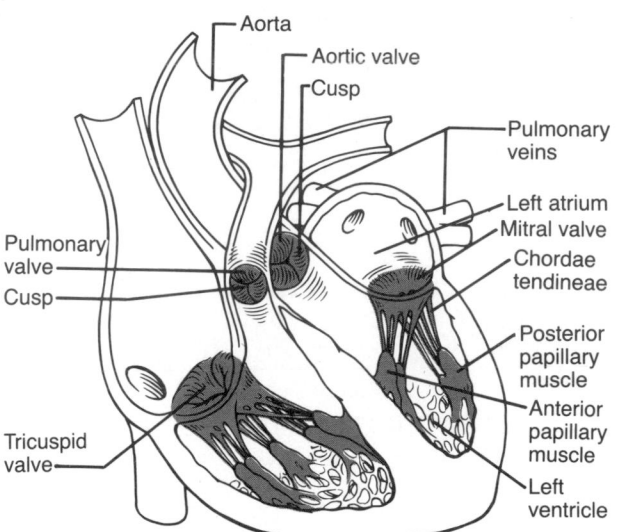

FIGURE 6–5   Structure of the mitral and aortic valves.

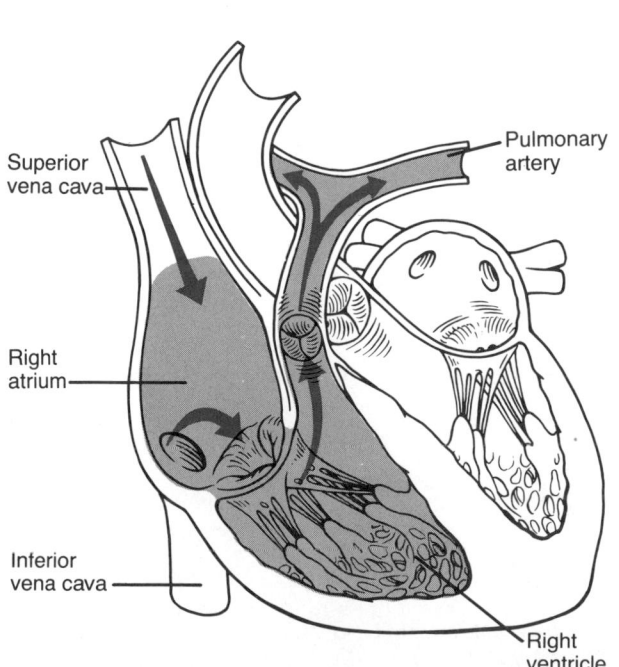

FIGURE 6–6   Blood flow from the right ventricle to the lungs.

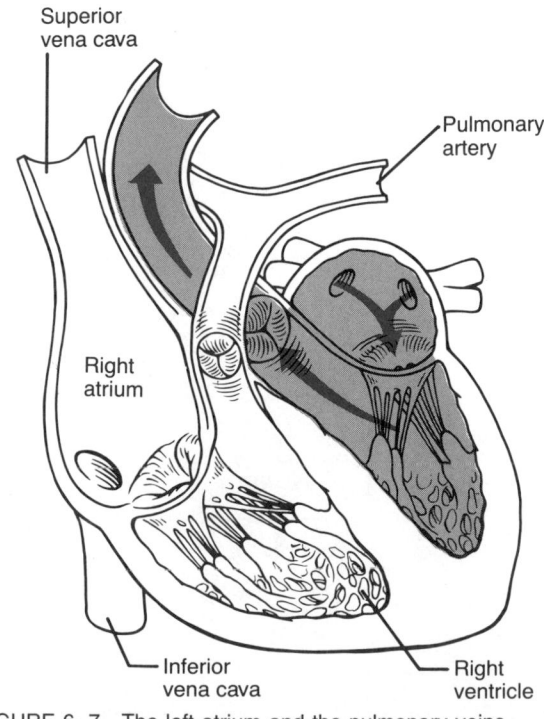

FIGURE 6–7   The left atrium and the pulmonary veins.

greater distances.[4] The walls of the left ventricle are thicker and stronger than the walls of the right because the left ventricle is responsible for pumping blood throughout the systemic circulation. It is often referred to as "the workhorse of the heart" (see Figure 6–3).

G. Valves of the heart

The four valves of the heart are all oriented so that blood never flows backward but always flows forward during contraction (see Figures 6–4 and 6–5).

1. The *tricuspid valve* controls the amount of blood between the right atrium and the right ventricle.
2. The *mitral or bicuspid valve* controls the amount of blood from the left atrium to the left ventricle. The tricuspid and mitral valves have filmlike veins that are held in place by special ligaments called *chordae tendineae,* which extend from the *papillary muscles* (see Figure 6–5).
3. The *pulmonary and aortic valves* (semilunar) prevent backward flow of blood into the right and left ventricles from the pulmonary and systemic systems. Their half-moon shaped leaflets are very strong in order to respond to the high pressure created during ventricular contraction. The probable difference between the two types of valves is that blood flows with great ease through the atrioventricular valves and is a low-pressure system, whereas the semilunar valves forcefully moving blood from the ventricles to systemic circulation and respond to a higher-pressure system (see Figures 6–4 and 6–5).

H. Systemic circulation (see Figures 6–6 and 6–7)

1. Unoxygenated blood from the venous system empties into the right atrium via the superior and inferior vena cava.
2. When a sufficient amount of blood fills the atrium, blood begins to move from the atrium through the tricuspid valve into the right ventricle.
3. When a sufficient amount of blood fills the right ventricle, the tricuspid valve closes, creating high pressure in the right ventricle. The ventricle contracts and forces blood out and through the pulmonary artery via the semilunar valve to the lung.

4. At the lung, oxygen is acquired, and oxygenated blood is transported to the left atrium via the pulmonary vein.
5. As blood fills the left atrium, blood begins to pour into the left ventricle through the mitral valve.
6. When a sufficient amount of blood builds in the left ventricle, the mitral valve closes tightly, creating strong pressure in the ventricle. The ventricle contracts and sends blood to the systemic circulation via the aorta.

I. Conduction system and the electrocardiogram (see Figure 6–8)

1. Normal cardiac impulse is initiated in the specialized pacemaker cells of the *sinoatrial (SA) node,* located at the left base of the right atrium. The impulse spreads to the left atrium and to the area of the *atrioventricular (AV) node.* This normal route occurs through specialized tracks that move the impulse quickly from the SA to the AV node. When the impulse reaches the atria, the atria depolarize electrically, producing the *P wave* on the electrocardiogram (ECG), and then they contract. Simultaneously, blood has been propelled from the atria to the ventricles.[3]
2. As the impulse reaches the AV node, conduction slows down considerably, allowing sufficient blood to flow from atria to ventricles. When the impulse leaves the AV node, conduction resumes at a rapid velocity through the common bundle or *bundle of His* and down the right and left bundle branches. This particular component is not visible on the ECG.
3. Right and left bundle branches supply the inner core of their respective ventricles through a highly myelinated network called the *Purkinje fibers.* These fibers allow for fast depolarization of the ventricles and culmination in strong ventricular contraction. When ventricular depolarization occurs, it is represented by the *QRS complex* on the ECG. At this point, large amounts of blood have been ejected from the ventricles and blood is propelled into the pulmonary artery and the aorta.[3]
4. All conduction prior to the impulse leaving the Purkinje fibers occurs between atrial and ventricular contractions, the *PR interval* on the ECG.
5. Given the complexity of the conduction sys-

tem, only the following components can be seen on the standard ECG recording (see Figure 6–8):

a. Atrial depolarization (P wave).

b. Ventricular depolarization (QRS complex).

c. Ventricular repolarization (T wave).

J. Coronary arteries (see Figure 6–9)

The function of the coronary arteries is to supply oxygenated blood to the myocardium. Oxygenated blood is supplied to the coronary arteries by the aorta.

1. **Two main coronary arteries**

    a. *Left coronary artery.* This main coronary artery bifurcates shortly after its origin, sending one branch anteriorly, the *left anterior descending* coronary artery, and one branch posteriorly, the *circumflex* coronary artery.

    (1). The left anterior descending artery supplies blood to the left anterior ventricular wall, the anterior portion of the interventricular septum, and down to the apex, where it proceeds posteriorly to anastomose with the posterior descending branch of the circumflex.

    (2). The circumflex branch of the left coronary artery passes posteriorly and to the left in the groove between the left atrium and the left ventricle. Through many branches, it supplies oxygenated blood to the posterior and lateral aspects of the left ventricle.

    b. *Right coronary artery.* The right coronary artery travels around the atrioventricular groove, and its branches supply the right ventricle. It turns to descend in the posterior interventricular groove, and its branches supply the posterior aspect of the septum and the posterior aspect of

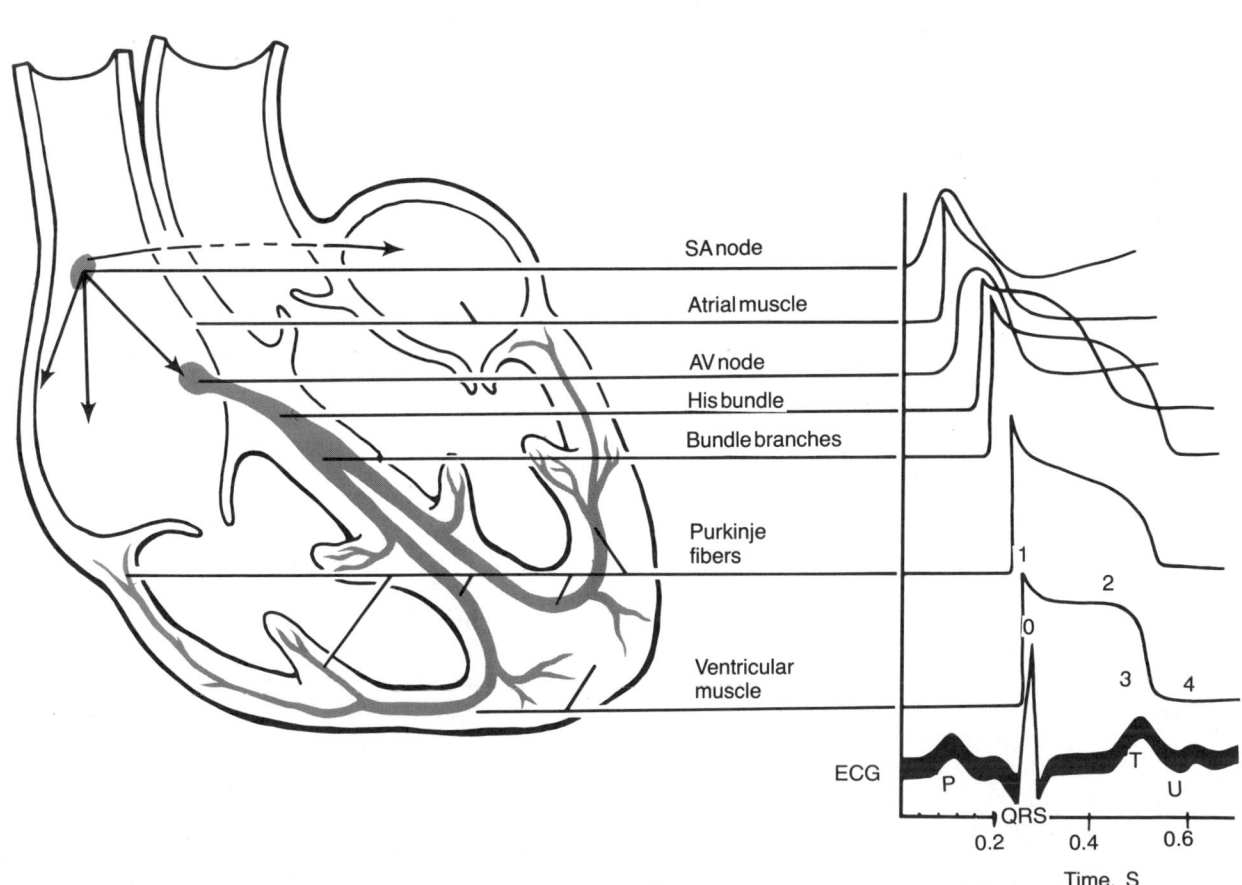

FIGURE 6–8   Conduction of the cardiac impulse and normal ECG wave configuration.

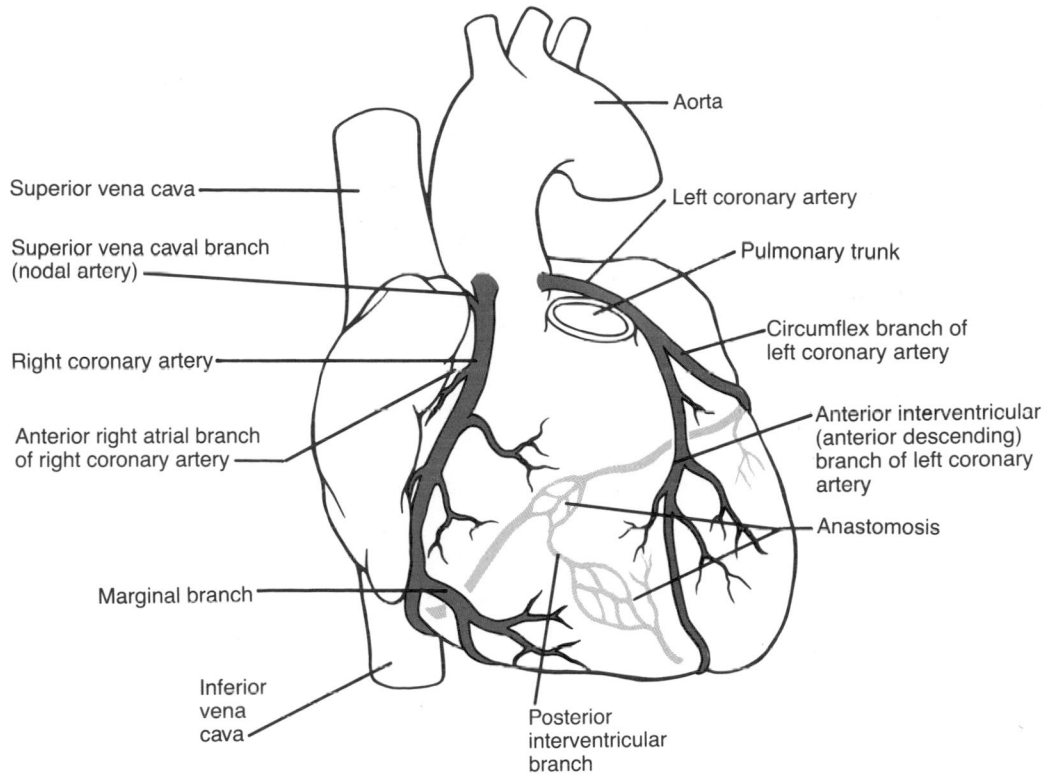

FIGURE 6–9   Coronary arteries.

the left ventricle before it anastomoses with the anterior descending branch of the coronary artery. The following are of clinical significance:

(1). The right coronary artery gives off important branches, which supply the SA node in 50% to 60% of human hearts and the AV node in 90% of human hearts.

(2). If the right coronary artery turns at the crux and supplies the posterior aspect of the left ventricle and the interventricular septum, the coronary circulation is said to be *dominant right*. About 80% to 90% of the population has a dominant right coronary circulation.

(3). When the posterior aspect of the ventricle is supplied by the left circumflex artery, coronary circulation is referred to as *dominant left*.[3,5]

■ PLEASE NOTE: The concept of dominant circulation has significant implications in the event of a myocardial infarction. The location of a myocardial infarction depends on which coronary artery is occluded and the location of the occlusion. Occlusions in large branches result in more extensive damage. Table 6–1 summarizes the areas of the heart that are supplied by the left and right coronary arteries.

Table 6–1.   COMPARISON OF RIGHT AND LEFT CORONARY DISTRIBUTION

Right Coronary Artery Supplies	Left Coronary Artery Supplies
1. SA node (55%)	1. SA node (45%)
2. AV node	2. Anterosuperior division of left bundle
3. Bundle of His (a portion)	3. Right bundle branch (major portion)
4. Posterior one third of septum	4. Anterior two thirds of septum
5. Posteroinferior division of left bundle (a portion)	5. Posteroinferior division of left bundle (a portion)
6. Inferoposterior surface of left ventricle	6. Anterolateral surface of left ventricle

(From Vinsant M, Spence M: *Commonsense Approach to Coronary Care: A Program,* 5th ed. St. Louis, C. V. Mosby Company, 1988, pp 178–210, 499, 498–500.)

(a). A left-sided coronary event usually has strong implications for systemic circulation and ultimately influences functional capacity.

(b). A right-sided coronary event, although it does not significantly influence systemic circulation, may have serious influence on arrhythmias because the right coronary artery supplies the SA node.

II. Cardiac Physiology

A. Physiological role

The physiological roles of the cardiovascular system are

1. To deliver oxygen and other substrates to the tissues of the body.
2. To remove carbon dioxide and other products of cellular metabolism.

B. Transport of nutrients through blood flow

1. Most substances carried to and from tissue are dissolved in plasma, and their transport is dependent on the volume of blood flow.[3]
2. Gases such as oxygen and carbon dioxide are transported almost entirely by red blood cells. Oxygen and carbon dioxide are transported to and from tissue depending on the blood flow and/or the metabolic needs of specific tissues or organs at any given time. For instance, during exercise, blood flow (oxygenated blood) is shunted to the exercising muscles and the skin while areas not in need of high volume at the time, eg, the kidney and stomach, experience a decrease in blood flow. Conversely, after a heavy meal, when metabolic activity of the gut is high, there is a decrease in blood flow to skeletal muscle.[3]
3. Oxygenated blood flow to the brain, however, remains nearly the same at rest or during exercise.
4. The cellular rate of metabolism is the most important determinant in the distribution of cardiac output and can be influenced or altered by age, activity, disease, trauma, and so forth.

C. Nervous regulation of cardiac function (see Figure 6–10)

1. **Role of the nervous system.** The major control system of the heart is the autonomic nervous system. It has a distinct role in the
   a. Rate of impulse formation.
   b. Speed of conduction.
   c. Strength of cardiac contraction.

2. **Divisions of the nervous system.** The two divisions of the autonomic nervous system are the *sympathetic* and *parasympathetic* systems (see Figure 6–11).
   a. The sympathetic system, known for its "fight or flight" component, is located in the medulla oblongata. Its nerve fibers supply all of the areas of the atria and the ventricles. Stimulation of its fibers elicits an increase in heart rate and in the magnitude of contraction. Norepinephrine is the primary chemical mediator, although epinephrine is also released. α- and β-Adrenergic receptors are the primary sympathetic receptors. When the α-adrenergic receptors are stimulated, they cause coronary arteriolar vasoconstriction. When the β-adrenergic receptors are stimulated, they cause coronary arteriolar vasodilation. For proper heart function, a balance between α- and β-adrenergic receptors is needed[6,7] (see Tables 6–2 and 6–3).
   b. The parasympathetic system strongly influences the heart through the vagus nerve. The center of this system is located in the medulla and is considered cardioinhibitory. Vagal nerve stimulation releases acetylcholine, which causes a decreased firing of the SA node, a decreased contractile force of the atria, and a decreased impulse conduction speed through the AV node. Vagal stimulation also causes coronary arteries to dilate, increasing coronary blood flow[6,7] (see Tables 6–2 and 6–3).

D. Additional mechanisms of control of cardiac function

In addition to the neural regulation by the autonomic nervous system, other factors can influence the heart.

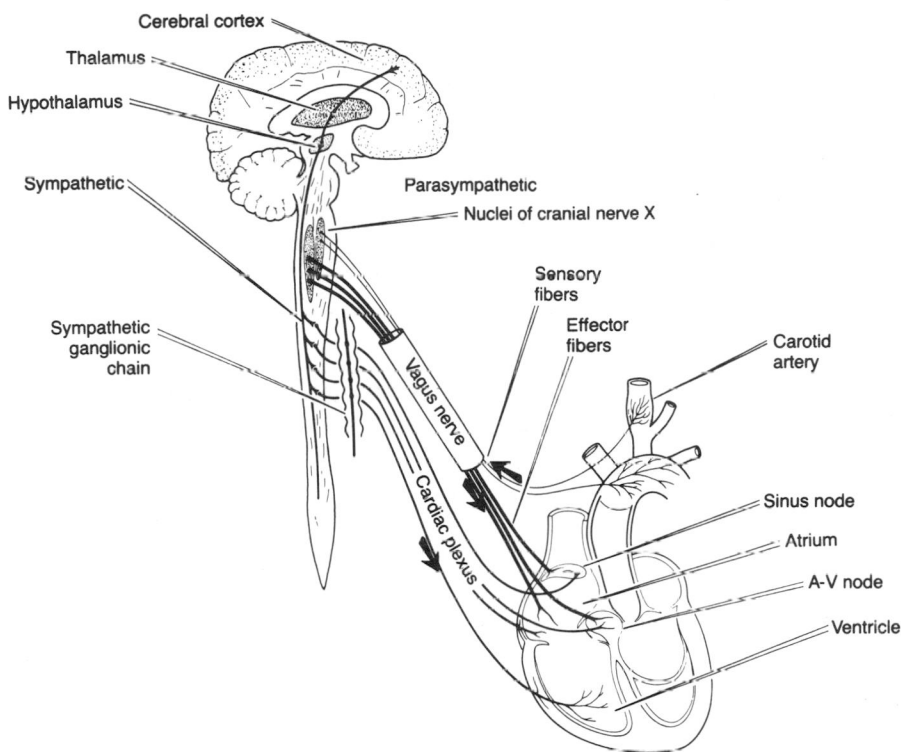

FIGURE 6–10   The innervation of cardiac muscle by the autonomic nervous system. *Abbreviation:* A-V = atrioventricular. (From Phillips E, Feeney M: *The Cardiac Rhythms,* 3rd ed. Philadelphia, W. B. Saunders Company, 1990, p 92.)

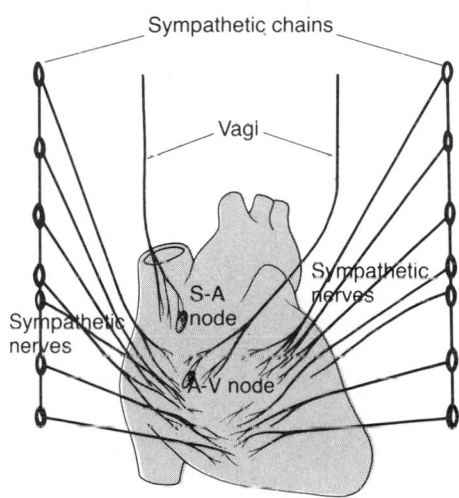

FIGURE 6–11   Innervation of the heart. *Abbreviations:* A-V = atrioventricular; S-A = sinoatrial. (From Guyton A: *Textbook of Medical Physiology,* 8th ed. Philadelphia, W. B. Saunders Company, 1991, p 107.)

Table 6–2. CARDIAC RESPONSE TO AUTONOMIC NERVOUS SYSTEM STIMULATION

Anatomy	Cholinergic Stimulation (PNS)	Adrenergic Stimulation (SNS)
Sinoatrial node	Decrease heart rate Vagal arrest	Increase heart rate
Atria	Decrease in contractility	Increase in contractility
	Increase in conduction velocity (usually)	Increase in conduction velocity
Atrioventricular node and conduction system	Decrease in conduction velocity Atrioventricular block	Increase in conduction velocity
Ventricles		Increase in contractility
		Increase in conduction velocity

(From Cohen M, Hoskins T: *Cardiopulmonary Symptoms in Physical Therapy Practice.* New York, Churchill Livingstone, 1988, p 27.)

Abbreviations: PNS = parasympathetic nervous system; SNS = sympathetic nervous system.

1. **Pressoreceptors (baroreceptors).** These are located in the arch of the aorta and the carotid sinus, and they respond to changes (elevation) in blood pressure. This stimulus sends information to stimulate the parasympathetic system, which decreases the rate

Table 6–3. BLOOD VESSEL RESPONSES TO AUTONOMIC NERVOUS SYSTEM STIMULATION

Blood Vessel	Cholinergic Impulse Response	Adrenergic Impulse Response	
		Receptor	*Type*
Coronary	Dilation	α	Constriction
		β_2	Dilation
Skin and mucosa	—	α	Constriction
Skeletal muscle	Dilation	α	Constriction
		β_2	Dilation
Cerebral	—	α	Constriction (slight)
Pulmonary	—	α	Constriction
Abdominal viscera	—	α	Constriction
		β_2	Dilation
Renal	—	α	Constriction
Salivary glands	Dilation	α	Constriction

(From Cohen M, Hoskins T: *Cardiopulmonary Symptoms in Physical Therapy Practice.* New York, Churchill Livingstone, 1988, p 30.)

and force of contraction and reduces blood pressure.[6,7]

2. **Chemoreceptors.** These are located in the carotid body and are sensitive to changes in blood chemicals such as oxygen, carbon dioxide, and lactic acid. Wide variations in chemical levels can affect heart rate.

3. **Body temperature.** Body temperature plays a role in controlling heart rate. An increase in temperature causes an increase in metabolic activity and therefore increases in heart rate. The reverse is also true.

4. **Ions and drugs.** Abnormal concentrations of certain ions and drugs in the blood have an influence on cardiac function. In particular, certain components of the ECG are influenced by increases or decreases in ions or drugs.[6,7]

5. **Autoregulation.** This is described by Starling's law (see Figure 6–12), which states that the more blood that fills the ventricle in diastole, the greater the contraction during systole. Thus, the heart automatically adapts to different levels of blood volume during filling by changing its force of contraction.

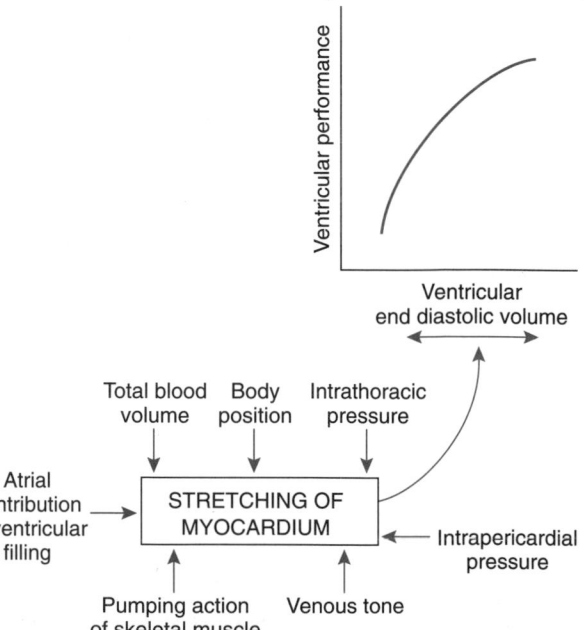

FIGURE 6–12 Relationship between ventricular and diastolic volumes and ventricular performance. (Reprinted by permission of *The New England Journal of Medicine* from Braunwald E, Ross J, Sonnenblick EH: Mechanisms of contraction of the normal and failing heart. *N Engl J Med* 1967, 277:794, Copyright 1967, Massachusetts Medical Society.)

E. Peripheral circulation

1. **Blood pressure**
   a. Blood flows when pressure in one area is higher than in another. Therefore, blood flows from areas of high pressure to areas of low pressure.
   b. Blood pressure is defined as the pressure that is exerted by the blood against the vessel walls (120/80 mm Hg is the normal value).[6,7]
   c. Blood pressure varies with age, activity, and emotional status as well as with the amount of blood in the vessel at a given time.
   d. *Systole* is the greatest pressure in the ventricles prior to contraction. *Diastole* is the lowest pressure in the ventricles prior to filling.

2. Two factors affecting blood volume and blood pressure are
   a. *Cardiac output*—the amount of blood ejected per minute, approximately (5 L). An increase in cardiac output causes an increase in arterial blood volume and blood pressure. Cardiac output is ultimately determined by heart rate or beats per minute as well as by Starling's law. Increases in cardiac output cause increases in arterial blood volume and arterial blood pressure. The reverse is also true (see Figure 6–12).
   b. *Peripheral resistance*—or resistance to blood flow—causes the volume of blood within the arteries to change and influence blood pressure. An increase in peripheral resistance causes an increase in arterial blood flow and an increase in blood pressure; the reverse is also true.[6,8] Peripheral resistance is also influenced by the viscosity of blood (determined by hematocrit) and the diameter of the vessel (determined by blood flow). Blood flows from the large arteries to the smaller arterioles; if larger amounts of blood are left in the arteries, blood volume is affected as well as arterial blood pressure.[6,8]

F. Exercise physiology

1. At rest, the body requires a steady flow of oxygen for basal metabolism.
2. Aerobic exercise requires an increased supply of oxygen to the tissue.
3. Three systems respond to the increased demand for oxygen during aerobic activity.

   a. The *pulmonary system* extracts oxygen from the environment. The pulmonary system provides oxygen from the atmosphere to the arterial blood through respiration while eliminating carbon dioxide through the venous system and back to the atmosphere. This is accomplished through diffusion at the alveolar capillary membrane. Minute ventilation (L/min) refers to the amount of air taken into the respiratory system within a minute (L/min = respiratory rate × tidal volume). When aerobic exercise is performed, more oxygen must be extracted for use in the exercising muscle, and carbon dioxide produced by the exercising muscle must be eliminated. Minute ventilation must be increased, and this is accomplished by increasing the tidal volume, increasing respiratory rate, or both.
   b. The *cardiac system* delivers oxygen to the exercising muscle. This demand for increased blood flow is accomplished by increasing cardiac output. Cardiac output refers to the amount of blood pumped per minute (cardiac output = stroke volume × heart rate). When aerobic exercise is performed, more blood must be delivered to the muscle. Cardiac output is increased by increasing heart rate, stroke volume, or both. Figure 6–13 summarizes cardiac responses to exercise.

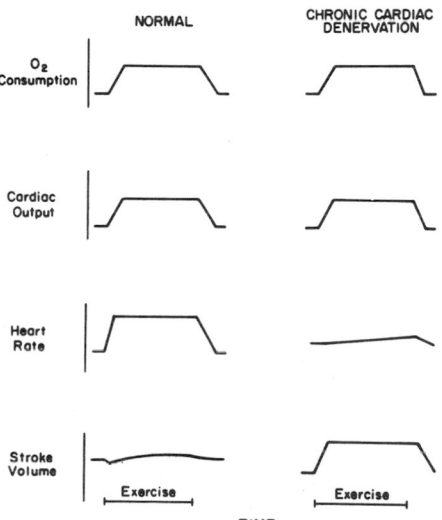

FIGURE 6–13 Cardiac responses to moderate supine exercise in humans. (Reprinted by permission of *The New England Journal of Medicine* from Kent K, Cooper T: The denervated heart. *N Engl J Med* 1974, 291:1017.)

c. *Muscle* metabolizes oxygen on delivery. Once blood has reached the muscle, the oxygen must diffuse out of the arterial blood into the mitochondria of the muscle cell, where it can be used by the exercising muscle. Carbon dioxide is diffused out of the muscle and carried away by the venous blood.

The ability of the muscles to extract and use oxygen is termed the *arteriovenous oxygen difference, ie,* the difference between the amount of oxygen delivered to the muscle by the arterial system and the amount of oxygen left in the venous system.

When exercise is performed, the muscle must extract more oxygen from the blood supply, making the arteriovenous oxygen difference greater. In order to exercise, there must be an ability to extract oxygen (lung), deliver oxygen (heart), and use oxygen efficiently at the cellular level (muscles).

◼ PLEASE NOTE: This interdependence of systems *must not* be overlooked in the exercising of any population, especially the elderly or patients with cardiac or pulmonary dysfunction.

When maximal exercise is performed, the maximal amount of oxygen is consumed by the body. This maximal level of oxygen consumption is termed $\dot{V}O_2$max. $\dot{V}O_2$max is calculated by the Fick equation:

$$\dot{V}O_2\text{max} = \text{cardiac output} \times \text{arteriovenous oxygen difference}$$

Aerobic training results in a number of physiologic adaptations[9]:
(1). Resting heart rate decreases.
(2). Resting stroke volume increases with a resultant stable cardiac output.
(3). Resting blood pressure decreases.
(4). Heart rate decreases at a given workload.
(5). $\dot{V}O_2$max increases.
(6). Myocardial oxygen consumption decreases because of an increase in efficiency.
(7). Cardiac output during maximal exercise increases.

d. In summary, cardiac output and arteriovenous oxygen difference can be increased with training, thereby improving $\dot{V}O_2$max. With aerobic training, more ex-

Table 6–4. ADAPTATION OF VARIABLES TO TRAINING AND DETRAINING

Variable	Detrained	Pretrained	Post-trained	Olympic Runner
Cardiovascular				
HR rest (beats/min)	73	68	59	38
HR peak ex (beats/min)	150	185	183	174
SV rest (mL)	55	65	80	125
SV peak ex (mL)	100	120	140	200
$\dot{Q}$ rest (L/min)	4.0	4.4	4.7	4.8
$\dot{Q}$ peak ex (L/min)	15	22.2	25.6	34.8
Heart vol (mL)	650	750	820	1200
Blood vol (L)	4.1	4.7	5.1	6.0
SBP rest (mm Hg)	140	135	130	120
SBP peak ex (mm Hg)	210	210	205	210
DBP rest (mm Hg)	80	78	76	65
DBP peak ex (mm Hg)	85	82	80	65
Metabolic				
$C(a - \bar{v})O_2$ rest	6.0	6.0	6.0	6.0
$C(a - \bar{v})O_2$ peak ex	14.0	14.5	15.0	16.0
$\dot{V}O_2$ rest (mL/kg/min)	2.4	2.6	2.8	2.9
$\dot{V}O_2$ peak ex (mL/kg/min)	21	32.2	38.4	56
Blood lactate rest	10	10	10	10
Blood lactate peak ex	100	110	125	185

(From Cohen M, Hoskin T: *Cardiopulmonary Symptoms in Physical Therapy Practice.* New York, Churchill Livingstone, 1988, p 40.)

Abbreviations: $C(a - \bar{v})O_2$ = arteriovenous oxygen difference; DBP = diastolic blood pressure; ex = exercise; HR = heart rate; $\dot{Q}$ = cardiac output; SBP = systolic blood pressure; SV = stroke volume.

ercise can be performed so that there is an improvement in functional capacity (aerobic capacity). Table 6–4 gives a comparison of variables of trained versus untrained individuals.

G. Physiological rationale for exercise

1. **Healthy population.** Exercise training in a healthy population has been shown to[10-12]
   a. Improve functional capacity.
   b. Reduce coronary risk factors.
   c. Improve quality of life.

2. **Population with cardiac and pulmonary dysfunction**
   a. *Implications.* Patients with coronary artery disease, regardless of age, have a statistically significant reduction in functional capacity ($\dot{V}O_2$max) as compared to healthy individuals. This is essentially due to poor left ventricular dysfunction and/or coronary artery disease. The physiological implications, therefore, are the following:
      (1). Impairment of left ventricular function, which
         (a). Limits the augmentation of stroke volume and, therefore,
         (b). Limits cardiac output.
      (2). Residual of the coronary artery disease, which tends to[10-12]
         (a). Lower maximal stroke volumes.
         (b). Lower maximal heart rates.
         (c). Lower peak levels of $\dot{V}O_2$max.
   b. *Considerations.* Aerobic exercise programs have been implemented as an intervention for populations with cardiac and pulmonary dysfunction. These programs have been implemented with careful consideration of

   (1). The pathophysiology of the process.
   (2). The mechanisms that limit exercise capacity.
   (3). The mechanisms that differ as a function of the underlying disease and its manifestation.

   The cardiac benefits of aerobic exercise training are listed in Table 6–5.

Table 6–5. BENEFITS OF AEROBIC TRAINING IN PATIENTS WITH CORONARY ARTERY DISEASE

Improved physical working capacity
  Able to endure at a higher exertional level for a longer period of time
  Able to perform more work at lower heart rate
  Able to perform more work at lower blood pressure
  Able to perform more work at lower rate-pressure product
Improved lactate tolerance
Improved $C(a - \bar{v})O_2$ difference, maximum and submaximum work
Higher maximum $\dot{V}O_2$
Higher resting and exercise stroke volume
Higher HDL
Higher maximum cardiac output
Higher maximum minute ventilation
Higher efficiency of breathing
Lower resting heart rate
Lower resting blood pressure
Lower percent body fat
Less neurohumoral over-reactivity
Possible benefits:
  Joie de vivre
  Increased coronary collateral circulation
  Increased diameter of coronary arteries
  Regression of coronary atherosclerosis
  Less platelet stickiness

(From Cohen M, Hoskin T: *Cardiopulmonary Symptoms in Physical Therapy Practice.* New York, Churchill Livingstone, 1988, p 83.)
Abbreviations: $C(a - \bar{v})O_2$ = arteriovenous oxygen difference; HDL = high-density lipids.

III. Cardiac Assessment

Before initiating any treatment program, a full chart review must be performed. This document usually has the most comprehensive overview of all aspects of a case.

A. Patient interview

The patient interview establishes effective communication and rapport with the patient. If necessary, the family can be consulted in order to obtain the pertinent information.

1. **Determination of chief complaint.** The underlying problem that precipitated medical attention is identified. Descriptors used to assist in problem identification are[13]
   a. Location
   b. Quality
   c. Quantity

   d. Course
   e. Setting
   f. Aggravating and alleviating factors
   g. Associated symptoms
2. **Review of patient's history**
   a. The patient's health history and current medications are evaluated. A pre-existing medical condition may influence the present evaluation and treatment plan. Frequently, patients experience symptoms of chest pain, shortness of breath, and fatigue. It is difficult to determine whether these symptoms are related to coronary disease. Tables 6–6 to 6–8 will assist the clinician in identifying the differential diagnoses of these common complaints.
   b. The patient's family history may contribute pertinent information to the assessment. Familial diseases include
      (1). Hypertension
      (2). Coronary artery disease
      (3). Rheumatic fever
      (4). Stroke
      (5). Kidney disease
      (6). Diabetes
   c. The patient's occupational history is important. From recent occupational his-

Table 6–6. DIFFERENTIAL DIAGNOSIS OF CHEST PAIN

Possible Causes	Possible Findings	Stimuli	Pathology
Myocardial ischemia	Pressure, ache, tightness, burning in midsternum, left shoulder, arm; diaphoresis; nausea; vomiting; ST-T wave changes; catheterization data show lesion	Exertion Cold air Smoking Heavy meal Fluid overload Ventricular ectopy	Coronary artery disease Coronary artery spasm
Inflammation	Auscultation of a friction rub; sharp pain, worsens with inspiration, improves with sitting	CABG Acute MI	Pericarditis
Infection	Chest tightness with breathlessness; low-grade fever; malaise; arthralgias	IV drug use Microbes	Myocarditis Endocarditis
Musculoskeletal Neck	Sharp pain with radiation to fingers; tingling; arthritic changes on x-ray	Neck motion Posture	Degenerative joint disease
Sternocostal	Improves with stretching, with heat; arthritic changes on chest x-ray	Inspiration Stretching Local pressure to produce joint motion	Degenerative joint disease
Post CABG	Feeling as if incision will separate; deep pain; sore	Cough Arm stretching	
Pulmonary	Sharp, stabbing, pain; auscultate rub of lungs on pleura	Deep breath	Pleurisy
	Hemoptysis; breathlessness; cough; increased RR; increased HR; loss of consciousness; V̇/Q̇ shows increased dead space	Prolonged bedrest Recent MI Recent surgery Fracture of long bone Atrial fibrillation	Pulmonary embolus
Vascular	Searing; severe pain; sudden onset; decreased BP	Trauma Old age Marfan's syndrome	Dissecting aneurysm
Referred pain	Burning pain; indigestion relieved by antacids	Heavy meal Spicy food	Esophageal reflux
	Belching		Hiatus hernia
Viral	Burning pain involving limited area over cutaneous distribution of nerve; skin lesions (vesicles)	Stress Immunocompromise	Herpes zoster Herpes simplex
Ventricular outflow tract obstruction	Angina pain; breathlessness; wide pulse pressure; hypertrophy of septum seen on echocardiogram; left ventricular hypertrophy on ECG	Exertion Coronary artery disease	Idiopathic hypertrophic subaortic stenosis Aortic stenosis Mitral valve prolapse

(From Cohen M, Hoskin T: *Cardiopulmonary Symptoms in Physical Therapy Practice.* New York, Churchill Livingstone, 1988, p 56.)

Abbreviations: BP = blood pressure; CABG = coronary artery bypass graft; HR = heart rate; IV = intravenous; MI = myocardial infarction; RR = respiratory rate; V̇/Q̇ = ventilation-perfusion ratio.

Table 6-7. DIFFERENTIAL DIAGNOSIS OF BREATHLESSNESS

Possible Causes	Possible Findings	Stimuli	Pathology
Increased metabolic demand for oxygen	Increased RR; increased HR; increased BP; use of accessory muscles; possible paradoxical abdominal motion	Exercise Fever	Normal Infection Hypoxia
Left ventricular dysfunction	Ventricular dilation; symmetrical rales; S_3, S_4 gallop; fatigue; decreased BP; increased HR; increased RR; poor diaphragm excursion	Chronic hypertension Exercise Chronic fluid retention	Left ventricular congestive heart failure Valve stenosis Valve incompetence
Bronchospasm	Inspiratory/expiratory wheeze; tight cough; mucoid, sparse, or copious sputum	Exercise Airborne irritants Forced expiration Bronchial irritation Drugs (beta blockers)	Asthma Allergic reaction
Hyperventilation	Increased RR disproportionate to level of exertion; pallor; diaphoresis; lightheadedness; may have loss of consciousness	Anxiety Fever Hypercapnia Hypoxia	Restrictive lung disease Metabolic or respiratory acidosis
Choking	No verbalization; ineffective breathing effort; nasal flares; rib retractions	Foreign object or tongue in airway	None
Inadequate gas exchange in lung	Resting breathlessness $Po_2 < 55$ mm Hg; accessory muscle use; increased HR; cyanosis; drowsiness; confused or unconscious; chest x-ray abnormality	Lung disease Cardiac arrest Anesthesia Hypoxia Fatigue of muscles of ventilation	Respiratory failure COPD Pneumonia Asbestosis
Lung collapse from loss of pressure gradient	Decreased movement on one side of chest; rapid onset; no pain; no cough; decreased breath sounds; increased percussion resonance	Spontaneous chest trauma Pre-existing lung disease (cystic fibrosis)	Pneumothorax
Obstruction in pulmonary circulation with interruption of blood flow	Sudden onset of breathlessness; chest pain; cough; hemoptysis; fever; loss of consciousness; increased HR; V/Q shows increased dead space; angiography shows lesion	Prolonged bed rest Recent MI Chronic CHF Atrial fibrillation Fracture of long bone Recent surgery	Pulmonary embolus

(From Cohen M, Hoskin T: *Cardiopulmonary Symptoms in Physical Therapy Practice.* New York, Churchill Livingstone, 1988, p 100.)

Abbreviations: BP = blood pressure; CHF = congestive heart failure; COPD = chronic obstructive pulmonary disease; HR = heart rate; MI = myocardial infarction; Po_2 = partial pressure of oxygen; RR = respiratory rate; V/Q = ventilation-perfusion ratio.

tory, the physical therapist can infer the patient's stress level and the physical activity level needed for his or her job. This information may include identification of other cardiac risk factors and/or need for vocational counseling.

d. Social habits, including smoking, alcohol consumption, and recreational or habitual drug use, should be documented. Each of these habits has cardiac and pulmonary implications.

e. The patient's functional and exertional activity levels should be recorded. A patient's usual activity level is important for goal setting. The expectations of the rehabilitation process will be monitored by the patient's previous activity level.

f. The patient's medication history is needed to determine potential alterations in or influence of therapeutic regimens; *ie,* a patient who is on long-term diuretics for blood pressure is at risk for electrolyte imbalance, which has further cardiovascular implications.

g. It is important to take the cough history of a patient with cardiac or pulmonary disease. Patients often minimize or dismiss cough, but it may have a cardiopulmonary association.

h. An angina pattern, if present, should be documented. Angina is referred pain, and its presentation is varied. Angina is experienced in many ways, such as left-arm pain, chest pain, right-arm pain, indigestion, or jaw pain. The onset of angina is usually consistent for each patient

Table 6–8. DIFFERENTIAL DIAGNOSIS OF FATIGUE

Possible Causes	Possible Findings	Stimuli	Pathology
Local muscle glycogen depletion	"The wall"; lack of whole body energy	Endurance exercise of long duration	None
Lactate accumulation in muscle and blood	Hyperventilation; breathlessness; loss of motivation	Deconditioning Anaerobic metabolism Organ ischemia Breath-holding activities	None
Poor motivation	Apathy; lethargy; may have pain in muscles	Overuse of muscles Depression Anxiety Drugs	Chemical imbalances in the brain (?)
Calcium ion depletion	Tetanus; muscle cramping; muscle pain	Prolonged use of muscle Electrical stimulation	None
Low cardiac output	Inotropic incompetence; low BP; increased HR; pallor; frequent ventricular ectopy	Age Deconditioning Microbes Alcoholism	Coronary artery disease Aortic valve dysfunction Cardiomyopathy Myocarditis
Anemia	General body fatigue; loss of energy; low hematocrit	Blood loss Cardiopulmonary bypass machine Dietary Deconditioning Genetic	Neoplasm Sickle cell Pernicious Iron deficiency
Dehydration	Dry mouth; general loss of energy; low BP; increased HR	Diarrhea Vomiting Heat exposure Fever Blood loss	Cholera GI bleeding Infection GI irritation
Hypothyroidism	Lethargy; dull, slow speech; slow movements	Genetic (?)	Thyroid gland dysfunction
Hypoxia	PO_2 < 55 mm Hg; O_2 saturation < 85%; cyanosis; increased RR; increased HR; pallor; breathlessness; stupor; lightheadedness	Exercise Apnea Hypoventilation	Respiratory failure Pulmonary embolus Arteriovenous shunt of heart or lungs
Hyperglycemia	Increased hemoglobin Alc; ketone breath; ketone bodies in urine; high blood sugar	High blood sugar	Diabetes mellitus with insulin deficiency

(From Cohen M, Hoskin T: *Cardiopulmonary Symptoms in Physical Therapy Practice.* New York, Churchill Livingstone, 1988, pp 132–133.)

Abbreviations: BP = blood pressure; GI = gastrointestinal; HR = heart rate; PO_2 = partial pressure of oxygen; RR = respiratory rate.

and related to increased activity. It is important for patients to recognize their particular angina pattern, realize that it is a sign of cardiac dysfunction, and understand the seriousness of its onset. Table 6–9 characterizes the differences between stable and unstable angina.

B. Physical examination

Cardiac assessment of the patient's vital signs (temperature, heart rate, respiratory rate, and blood pressure) presents a valuable statement of the systemic responses to disease or dysfunction.[13] Each of these parameters has functional significance yet alone does not have diagnostic implications. As a composite picture, each variable adds significance, and a diagnosis can

more readily be achieved. See Table 7–4 for neonatal, adult, and geriatric normal vital sign values.

1. **Temperature**
   a. Elevation above normal is common during the first few days after an acute myocardial infarction because of necrosis of cardiac muscle.
   b. Fever may be the first sign of thrombophlebitis, pericarditis, or atelectasis.
   c. An increase in temperature causes an increase in the metabolic rate of body tissues and an increase in myocardial oxygen demand. This demand places stress on an already impaired myocardium.
   d. For the patient with coronary disease, changes in skin pallor or skin temperature or excessive sweating has implica-

Table 6–9. CHARACTERISTICS OF STABLE AND UNSTABLE ANGINA PECTORIS

Characteristic	Stable	Unstable
Frequency	Regular	Increasing per week/day/hour
Onset	Consistent and predictable	More easily induced; may change from only with exertion to during rest as well
	Occurs at same RPP	Occurs at lower RPP than usual
New onset		Absent for a prolonged period and then returns
Location	Consistent	May become more variable with a spreading or changing radiation pattern
Relief	Consistent	Requires more sublingual nitroglycerin
Duration	Consistent	May take longer before relief

(From Cohen M, Hoskin T: *Cardiopulmonary Symptoms in Physical Therapy Practice.* New York, Churchill Livingstone, 1988, p 57.)

Abbreviations: RPP = rate-pressure product.

tions if associated with other symptomatology, such as pain, shortness of breath, and ECG changes.[13]

2. **Heart rate**
   a. Heart rate is one of the most accurate noninvasive methods used to determine cardiovascular efficiency.
   b. Heart rate is evaluated with respect to normal resting values and anticipated exercise responses.
   c. Heart rate normally increases in a linear manner as workloads increase. Children tend to have high heart rates at rest and with exercise.
   d. Rates of increase are affected by age, fitness, or an underlying pathological condition; *ie,* many patients with coronary artery disease and many sedentary individuals may have an abnormally high heart rate response to low-level exercise.

3. **Respiratory rate**
   a. An increase in respiratory rate is commonly related to interstitial or alveolar pulmonary edema secondary to left ventricular dysfunction or valvular impairment.
   b. A common symptom of left ventricular dysfunction is *dyspnea* (shortness of breath). Dyspnea may not be related to cardiovascular disease. Dyspnea on exertion, *eg,* may be secondary to decondi-

tioning rather than to cardiopulmonary dysfunction.
   c. Cardiac dyspnea can result when patients are lying down at rest *(orthopnea).*[13]
   d. Cardiac dyspnea may awaken a patient from sleep with a concurrent sense of suffocation *(paroxysmal dyspnea).*[13]
   e. Cardiac patients frequently have shortness of breath associated with anginal pain. This type of dyspnea may not be true dyspnea but a reaction to pain caused by ischemia.

4. **Blood pressure**
   a. Blood pressure varies with age, stress, fitness, or pathological conditions.
   b. A primary determinant of blood pressure is the volume of blood in the artery.
   c. An increase in blood volume tends to cause an increase in arterial pressure *(congestive heart failure).*
   d. Two important factors affecting blood volume and blood pressure are cardiac output and peripheral resistance, discussed earlier in this chapter.[11,12]
   e. Clinical assessment of blood pressure should be serial, with the patient at rest, sitting, standing, exercising, and after exercise.
   f. Sequential blood pressure responses are required for accurate data collection. Systolic pressure increases linearly with increasing levels of work. Diastolic pressure changes little from rest to maximum exercise in the healthy individual.
   g. Blood pressure responses to exercise may be exaggerated in patients with cardiac disease, in the elderly, and in deconditioned subjects. A patient's blood pressure response may vary from normal to hypertensive or hypotensive.
      (1). Hypertensive systolic blood pressure responses either at rest or with low-level activity are a sign of cardiovascular impairment. Systolic pressure changes greater than 20 mm Hg indicate an increase in myocardial oxygen demand and suggest potential ischemia.[14]
      (2). A blunted systolic response to increases in physical activity may be due to ventricular impairment or cardiac medications. At high levels of exercise, a blunted blood pressure response has significant implications for mortality, especially for individu-

als unable to achieve systolic pressures greater than 140 mm Hg with maximal exercise.[14]

(3). A hypotensive systolic pressure response (a decrease of > 10 to 20 mm Hg) occurring with an increase in heart rate during activity is strongly associated with ventricular dysfunction and has poor prognostic implications.

Impairment implies that ventricular contractility or the ventricular pumping mechanism is no longer capable of meeting the metabolic demands.[14]

Diastolic blood pressure reflects peripheral resistance and is a direct reflection of the driving force of blood through the coronary arteries. Diastolic pressure must be maintained to preserve adequate blood flow for perfusion of the myocardium.

C. Observation

Observation should begin with a general overview of the patient at rest and then during activity.

1. In general, but specifically for cardiac patients, observation should include[13]
   a. Facial appearance
   b. Specific skeletal abnormalities
   c. Pallor
   d. Coloration of the skin
   e. appearance of the knuckles, elbows, knees, and Achilles tendon, where swelling or deposits of cholesterol may appear
2. *Edema* can be caused by cardiac dysfunction. As the heart begins to fail, there is a slowing of the peripheral blood flow and an engorging of the capillary vessel. With the patient lying supine and with the trunk elevated about 30 degrees, jugular venous distention can be observed. Table 6–10 assists with establishing a diagnosis of edema.
3. *Peripheral edema* can be seen in gravity-

Table 6–10. DIFFERENTIAL DIAGNOSIS OF EDEMA

Possible Causes	Possible Findings	Stimuli	Pathology
Increased capillary filtration pressure (>18 mm Hg)	Vasodilation of arterioles; venular constriction; increased sodium in blood; increased BP; pedal edema; distended neck veins; ascites; weight gain; "blue bloater"; anasarca	Fluid overload (local or systemic) Increased venous pressure	Cardiac surgery Kidney dysfunction CHF of right ventricle Venous valve incompetence Venous obstruction Cardiac valve stenosis Pulmonary hypertension Cirrhosis
Prolonged elevated venous pressure in lower extremities	Frequent, indolent ulceration with pain; purple discoloration of skin; pedal edema, bilateral and pitting	Years of standing on feet (opposing gravity)	Venous stasis with venous valve incompetence
Decreased oncotic pressure	Increased urinary albumin; increased local temperature; facial puffiness	Decreased plasma protein (globulin, albumin) Accumulation of colloidal substances (active metabolites) Drugs (steroids, nifedipine)	Cirrhosis Allergic reaction Nephrosis Inflammation Infection Burns Trauma
Lymph incompetence	Massive edema confined to one location; can be painless; loss of ROM; can be postoperative (*eg,* mastectomy)	Surgery Neoplasm	Obstruction of lymph channel
Left ventricular CHF producing pulmonary edema	Frothy, pink sputum; cough; bibasilar rales; S_3 and S_4; breathlessness; increased HR; decreased BP	Exercise Ventricular ischemia	Coronary artery disease Mitral valve dysfunction Outflow tract obstruction

(From Cohen M, Hoskin T: *Cardiopulmonary Symptoms in Physical Therapy Practice.* New York, Churchill Livingstone, 1988, p 212.)
Abbreviations: BP = blood pressure; CHF = congestive heart failure; HR = heart rate; ROM = range of motion.

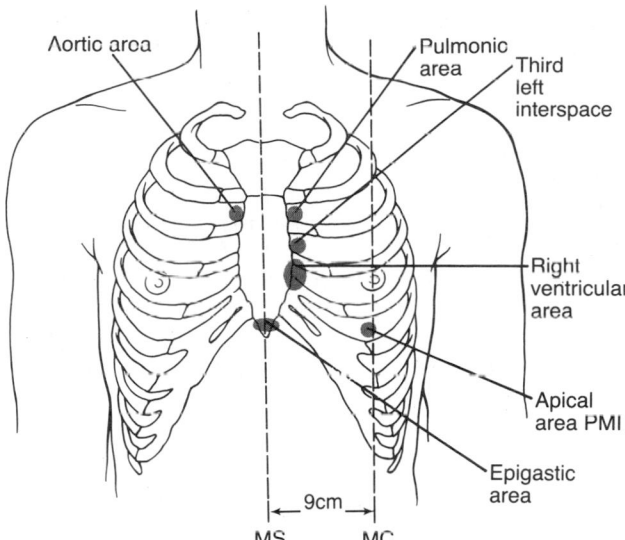

FIGURE 6–14 Palpation areas. *Abbreviations:* MC = Midclavicular; MS = Midsternal; PMI = point of maximum impulse.

dependent areas of the body (*ie,* the lower extremities, especially the ankles). Peripheral edema can also be heard within the lungs with a stethoscope.

D. Inspection and palpation

1. Universal precautions should be used when contact with a patient and/or a patient's body fluids is necessary. Certain landmarks on the anterior chest will assist the therapist in locating the heart.
   a. The base (top) of the heart is at the level of the 3rd rib.
   b. The apex (bottom) of the heart is approximately at the level of the 5th rib in the midclavicular line.
   c. The anterior surface of the thorax that overlies the heart and the aorta is the *precordium* (see Figure 6–14).

2. **Abnormal pulsations.** By observing the thorax, abnormal pulsations can be seen. Palpation of the precordium will verify observational findings.[13] With the pads of the fingers, the areas where pulsations are visible are palpated, and then the specific areas of the precordium described in Figure 6–14 are felt.
   a. The *aortic area,* the second interspace of

the right sternum, demonstrates a pulsation, thrill, or vibration during the closure of the aortic valve.
   b. The *pulmonic area,* the second and third left interspaces, are felt for abnormalities of the pulmonary artery or pulmonic valve.
   c. The *right ventricular area,* the lower left sternal border following down to the fifth intercostal space, is used to evaluate conditions associated with tricuspid valvular disease and right ventricular enlargement.
   d. The *apical area,* the fifth intercostal space, medial to midclavicular line, is palpated for the point of maximum impulse and for thrills associated with mitral valve disease.
   e. The *epigastric area,* the upper central region of the abdomen, can have visible or palpable pulsations in some normal individuals. Abnormally large pulsations of the aorta may be produced by an aneurysm of the abdominal aorta or by aortic valvular regurgitation.

E. Auscultation of the heart

Cardiac function is often evaluated by auscultation of the heart sounds. A systematic approach to cardiac auscultation is necessary so as not to miss any significant findings. Table 6–11 summarizes the major aspects of auscultation.

1. **Abnormal heart sounds**
   a. The S_3 heart sound is associated with poor ventricular compliance, large infarctions, large areas of ischemia, and even heart failure.[14]
   b. The S_4 heart sound is frequently present in patients after myocardial infarction and is commonly associated with an increase in end-diastolic pressure, which causes the atrium to contract with greater force, creating the S_4 sound.[14]
   c. The S_3 and S_4 heart sounds can occur at rest in very compromised patients or can develop as a result of exercise. Any changes or extra sounds heard during systole or diastole are called murmurs.

2. **Murmurs**
   a. Murmurs appear to be related to
      (1). High rates of flow.

Table 6–11. AUSCULTATION OF THE HEART

Regions of auscultatory interest

Aortic areas: right second intercostal space, left third inter-costal space, and cardiac apex
Pulmonic area: upper left parasternal region
Tricuspid area: lower left parasternal region
Mitral area: cardiac apex and axilla

Heart sounds

S_1: mitral and tricuspid valve closure
S_2: pulmonic and aortic valve closure
S_3: ventricular filling sounds
S_4: decreased ventricular compliance during atrial systole
Ejection click: aortic or pulmonic valve opening
Midsystolic click: mitral valve prolapse
Opening snap: opening of mitral valve in mitral stenosis

Heart murmurs

Systolic ejection murmurs
   Functional or innocent flow murmurs
   Aortic stenosis
   Pulmonic stenosis
   Idiopathic hypertrophic subaortic stenosis
   Atypical mitral regurgitation
Pansystolic or holosystolic murmurs
   Mitral regurgitation
   Tricuspid regurgitation
   Ventricular septal defect
Late systolic murmurs
   Mitral valve prolapse
Immediate diastolic decrescendo murmurs
   Aortic regurgitation
   Pulmonic regurgitation
Delayed diastolic murmurs
   Mitral stenosis
   Tricuspid stenosis
Continuous murmurs (systole and diastole)
   Patent ductus arteriosis
   Arteriovenous fistula

(From Fardy P, Yankowitz F, Wilson P: *Cardiovascular Assessment and Treatment in Cardiac Rehabilitation. Adult Fitness and Exercise Testing.* Philadelphia, Lea & Febiger, 1988.)

(2). Forward flow through a constricted or deformed valve.
(3). Backward flow through a regurgitated valve.

Table 6–11 identifies the most common heart murmurs seen clinically. Murmurs may be benign and not interfere with cardiac output, they may be transitional (as in young children), or they may be severely obstructive and compromise cardiac output.[14]

b. Murmurs are generally characterized by the following criteria:
(1). Timing—systole or diastole.
(2). Intensity—how loud.
(3). Quality—tonal characteristics.
(4). Pitch—sound frequency.
(5). Location—precordium location.
(6). Radiation—transmission across the chest.

F. Examination of the lungs

Patients with coronary disease frequently present with concomitant pulmonary complications. Therefore, a thorough examination of the lungs should occur. Evaluation should include

1. Inspection

2. Palpation

3. Percussion

4. Auscultation
Specific pulmonary evaluation tools are discussed in Chapter 7.

IV. Laboratory Studies

In addition to the specific evaluation performed by the physical therapist, laboratory studies add significantly to the documentation of coronary artery disease or to the implication of risk. None of the specific laboratory studies discussed below can be used alone to make a definitive diagnosis. It is the additive effect of each of these studies that makes a definite diagnosis. The results of many laboratory tests also have a critical influence on all aspects of intervention.

A. Chest roentgenograms

The chest x-ray is used to assess

1. The anatomical size of the heart and lungs.
2. The shape of the heart and lungs.
3. Pacemakers for lead position or lead disconnection. For patients with pacemakers that are also defibrillators, roentgenographic validation is critical.

Table 6–12. METHOD OF ELECTROCARDIOGRAPHIC INTERPRETATION

Measurements
  Heart rate (atrial and ventricular)
  PR interval (0.12 to 0.20 s)
  QRS duration (0.06 to 0.10 s)
  QT interval (heart rate–dependent)
  Frontal plane QRS axis (−30 to +90 degrees)
Rhythm diagnosis
Conduction diagnosis
Waveform description
  P waves (atrial enlargement)
  QRS complexes (ventricular hypertrophy, infarction)
  ST segment (elevation or depression)
  T waves (flattened or inverted)
  U waves (prominent or inverted)
ECG diagnosis
  Within normal limits
  Borderline abnormal
  Abnormal (list diagnoses)
Comparison with previous ECG

(From Fardy P, Yankowitz F, Wilson P: *Cardiovascular Assessment and Treatment in Cardiac Rehabilitation. Adult Fitness and Exercise Testing.* Philadelphia, Lea & Febiger, 1988.)

B. Electrocardiograms

ECGs can be of considerable value in detection of anatomical, physiological, or pathological findings. Resting and exercise ECGs are valuable clinical tools when assessing cardiac function. It is important to assess the ECG regularly, comparing resting rate with resting rate, and resting rate with exercise rate and recovery rate. Subtle changes from one ECG to the next may have pathological implications.

PLEASE NOTE: A thorough understanding of the ECG is impossible to glean from reading a text. Actual clinical practice in reading and interpreting ECGs will enhance the clinician's ability to recognize normal versus abnormal ECGs. Table 6–12 presents a method for assessing an ECG.

ECG changes occur with ischemia, myocardial infarction, arrhythmias, and conduction disturbances.

1. **Ischemia.** This is lack of oxygenated blood. If cardiac muscle becomes ischemic, ST segment or T wave changes are seen.[15,16]
   a. One millimeter of ST segment depression is considered borderline.
   b. Two millimeters of ST segment depres-

sion is considered diagnostic of coronary ischemia.
   c. ST segment alteration may be due to various causes, such as
      (1). Electrolyte imbalances
      (2). Drugs
      (3). Myocardial ischemia
      (4). Ventricular hypertrophy
      (5). Neurogenic influences
   d. ST segment depression may be observed
      (1). In the resting ECG of patients with coronary disease.
      (2). In the exercise ECG of coronary patients with increased physical activity.

Table 6–13. ECG CHANGES DURING EXERCISE*

Healthy Individual†	Individual with Coronary Artery Disease‡
1. Slight increase in amplitude of P wave	1. Appearance of a BBB at a "critical heart rate"
2. Shortening of PR interval	2. Recurrent or multifocal PVCs during exercise and/or recovery
3. Slight shift to right of QRS axis	3. VT (three or more consecutive ventricular beats)
4. ST segment depression of < 1 mm	4. Appearance of bradyarrhythmias/tachyarrhythmias—rapid rate abruptly slowing or vice versa, not related to exercise
5. Decreased amplitude of the T wave	5. ST segment depression/elevation of > 1 mm, 0.08 s after the J point
6. Single or rare PVCs during exercise and recovery	6. Bradycardia in response to exercise
7. Single or rare PJCs or PACs	7. Tachycardia that results in an HR greater than the individual's upper limit
	8. Increase in frequency or severity of any arrhythmia the individual is known to have

(From Brannon F, Foley M, Starr JA: *Cardiopulmonary Rehabilitation: Basic Theory and Application,* 2nd ed. Philadelphia, F. A. Davis Company, 1993, p 194.)
* Decreases in the resting heart rate and the submaximal heart rate are observed in both groups with physical conditioning.
† All these ECG changes are normal in response to exercise.
‡Occurrence of any one of these changes should result in cessation of exercise and thorough evaluation of the ECG change and related symptoms.
Abbreviations: BBB = bundle branch block; HR − heart rate; PAC = premature atrial contraction; PJC = premature junctional contraction; PVC = premature ventricular contraction; VT = ventricular tachycardia.

Abnormal ECG responses observed during exercise reflect an imbalance between myocardial oxygen supply and demand. Usually they are either exertional arrhythmias or alternate ST segment and T wave changes[16] (see Table 6–13).

> PLEASE NOTE: Clinicians should be aware of the danger of allowing patients to exercise with 2 mm or greater of ST segment depression. ST segment depression may increase immediately

post exercise rather than during exercise in patients with significant disease. A cool-down period that is long enough to allow a return to baseline levels is critical for these patients.

2. **Myocardial infarction.** Electrocardiographic changes that occur with myocardial infarction may include abnormalities of QRS complex and ST segment and T wave changes. In acute infarction, there is ST segment elevation in the leads over the infarction area. The eventual appearance of pathological Q waves is the ECG landmark

Table 6–14. DIFFERENTIAL DIAGNOSIS OF IRREGULAR HEART BEAT

Heart Rhythm	Possible Findings	Stimuli	Pathology
Atrial fibrillation	Irregularly irregular pulse; ventricular response rate variable	Myocardial ischemia Digitalis toxicity Atrial hypertrophy Atrial flutter	COPD CAD Mitral stenosis Aortic stenosis Cardiomyopathy
Atrial flutter	Usually rapid, regular pulse; ventricular response rate constant; atrial rate > 220 beats/min Sawtooth pattern on ECG	Myocardial ischemia Digitalis toxicity Atrial hypertrophy	COPD CAD Atrioventricular valve disease Cardiomyopathy
Paroxysmal atrial tachycardia (PAT)	Regular heart rate, 160–220 beats/min; ventricular response rate constant; spontaneous onset and cessation of "palpitations"	Caffeine High catecholamine state Anxiety	Wolf-Parkinson-White syndrome
Premature atrial contractions (PACs)	Pause in pulse can be regular or irregular, occasional or frequent May be associated with HR 60–150 beats/min	Caffeine High catecholamine state Anxiety Atrial hypertrophy Atrial ischemia	COPD Mitral valve prolapse
Premature junctional contraction (PJC), premature nodal beat (PNB)	Pause can be regular or irregular, occasional or frequent Associated with HR 40–60 beats/min Rare	AV node conduction abnormality Failure of SA node	Sick sinus syndrome
Premature ventricular contraction (PVC), ventricular premature beat (VPB)	Feel skip in pulse Pause can be regular or irregular, occasional or frequent	Conduction disturbance Drugs Spontaneous Caffeine High catecholamine state Exercise Anxiety Myocardial ischemia Failure of SA-AV nodes Low potassium	"Athlete's heart" COPD CAD Ventricular aneurysm Sick sinus syndrome
Bigeminy Couplet Ventricular tachycardia	Feel a skip every second beat Feel a longer pause Decreased blood pressure Lightheadedness	Same as above Same as above Same as above	Same as above Same as above Same as above
Pacemaker	Pause in pulse can be irregular or regular, can be rare or frequent Paced beats may be among normal beats, or all beats may be paced Pacing spike may be before or in the middle of the P wave or QRS complex	Bradycardia Acute myocardial infarction	Sick sinus syndrome Complete heart block Conduction tissue ischemia

(From Cohen M, Hoskins T: *Cardiopulmonary Symptoms in Physical Therapy Practice.* New York, Churchill Livingstone, 1988, pp 144–145.)

Abbreviations: CAD = coronary artery disease; COPD = chronic obstructive pulmonary disease; HR = heart rate.

of myocardial infarction. As the ST elevation disappears, deep T wave inversion may develop.[15,16]

3. **Arrhythmias.** These are categorized as either atrial or ventricular in origin (see Table 6–14).
   a. Most atrial arrhythmias without heart block are benign.[15,16] These are categorized from least significant to most significant:
      (1). Premature atrial contractions
      (2). Paroxysmal atrial tachycardia
      (3). Atrial fibrillation
      (4). Atrial flutter
   b. Ventricular arrhythmias are generally more lethal because their primary effect is a reduction in cardiac output.[15,16] These are categorized from least significant to critically significant:
      (1). Unifocal premature ventricular contractions (PVCs)
      (2). Multifocal PVCs
      (3). Couplets
      (4). R on T PVCs
      (5). Ventricular tachycardia
      (6). Ventricular fibrillation

4. **Conduction disturbances.** These may occur in two separate situations:
   a. Atrioventricular blocks—the result of electrical transmission interruption from the AV node to the bundle branches.
   b. Bundle branch blocks—involve the bundle of His and its branches.

C. Tests of blood lipids

1. Lipids play a serious role in the development of atherosclerosis.[17] The lipids of general importance are
   a. Cholesterol
   b. Triglycerides
   c. Free fatty acids
      Cholesterol has been more widely measured than any other lipid.

2. **Risks.** Total cholesterol levels less than or equal to 200 mg/dL are correlated with minimal risk for coronary artery disease. Total cholesterol levels greater than 200 mg/dL are associated with increased risk for developing coronary artery disease.

3. **Cholesterol and triglyceride fractionated values.** High-density lipoproteins (HDLs) carry a small portion of total cholesterol and appear to have a positive protection when they compose the greater portion of total cholesterol.[18] Recent literature suggests that the relationship between total cholesterol and risk of coronary atherosclerosis is even higher if low-density lipoprotein (LDL) levels are high. A higher ratio of HDLs to LDLs has protective value against coronary disease. High levels of LDL cholesterol can damage the endothelial lining of vessels and promote atherosclerotic lesions.[19] When clinicians assess patients' risk factors, a high lipid profile has serious implications for further management of primary and secondary risk factors.

D. Serum enzymes and MB bands

1. Serum enzymes and MB bands are used to diagnose or rule out acute myocardial infarction. Several factors play a critical role in the ultimate decision:
   a. History
   b. ECG changes
   c. Alteration in serum enzyme levels
      When there is cell death or prolonged ischemia, enzymes from the cardiac muscle leak into the bloodstream because of the increased permeability of the cell membrane. This alters the normal blood levels of the three known serum enzymes, *creatine phosphokinase* (CPK), *lactate dehydrogenase* (LDH), and *serum glutamic oxaloacetic transaminase* (SGOT).[20] The relative times and levels at which each enzyme appears in the bloodstream following infarction are shown in Figure 6–15.
      An elevated CPK level can be nonspecific for cardiac injury and can reflect either skeletal or cardiac muscle necrosis. To make a positive diagnosis of cardiac damage by the elevated CPK level, electrophoresis or radioimmunoassay is done to separate CPK into three isoenzymes. The MM isoenzyme is specific for skeletal muscle, the BB isoenzyme is unique to brain tissue, and the MB isoenzyme is a specific marker for cardiac muscle necrosis. As with CPK, LDH is fractionated into five isoenzymes. LDH is specific for myocardial damage. The third enzyme, SGOT, also is elevated after acute myocardial infarction. There is no specific isoenzyme of SGOT for myocardial tissue. SGOT alone is not diagnostic of myocardial infarction.[20]

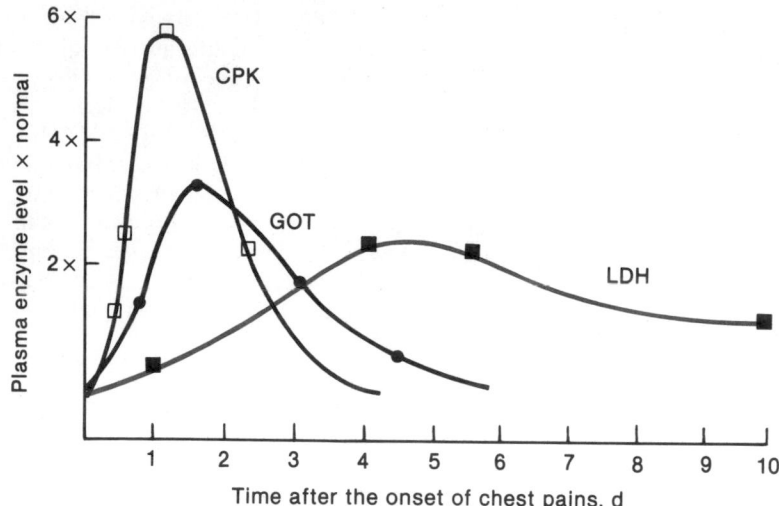

FIGURE 6–15 Typical plasma profiles. *Abbreviations:* CPK = creatine phosphokinase; GOT = glutamic oxaloacetic transaminase; LDH = lactate dehydrogenase. (Redrawn from Andreoli K, Fowkes V, Zipes D: *Comprehensive Cardiac Care,* 5th ed. St. Louis, C. V. Mosby Company, 1983.)

V. Physiological Tests

With recent advances in medical technology, specifically the new imaging techniques, cardiovascular alterations caused by coronary artery disease or dysfunction can be identified.[21]

A. Classification of tests

1. **Noninvasive** (*eg,* echocardiography and graded exercise tests)
2. **Invasive** (*eg,* radionuclide studies, cardiac catheterization, coronary arteriography, and percutaneous transluminal coronary angioplasty)

   These diagnostic tests offer information regarding the
   a. Extent of coronary atherosclerosis.
   b. Severity of coronary atherosclerosis.
   c. Location of coronary atherosclerosis.
   d. Ventricular dysfunction.
   e. Any pathology that may influence function.

   More specifically, they offer the physical therapist useful information for determining the exercise prescription for cardiac rehabilitation.

   It is impossible within this chapter to describe at length the procedural techniques, indications, and diagnostic capabilities of each of these tests. For de-

tailed information, the reader should consult additional references.

B. Echocardiography

1. Echocardiography is a noninvasive procedure that uses pulses of reflected ultrasound to evaluate the functioning heart. Because the anatomic components of the heart can be identified and their distance from the transducer measured, sizes of various chambers and vessels can be estimated with accuracy.
2. Echocardiography is performed primarily at rest, but its role in exercise studies has significantly increased.
3. Echocardiography has many important clinical applications and has surpassed the ECG in recognizing chamber enlargement, hypertrophy, and structural abnormalities. It is frequently used for differential diagnosis of heart murmurs; to provide quantitative information regarding severity of the valvular lesions; and to evaluate infectious vegetation, congenital heart disease, pericardial disease, and cardiomyopathies.

C. Graded exercise testing

Graded exercise testing is an assessment tool for evaluating functional capacity in healthy

Table 6–15.   EXERCISE TESTING FOR
              FUNCTIONAL ASSESSMENTS

Functional assessments in patients with cardiovascular disease
    Coronary heart disease
    Valvular disease
    Cardiomyopathy
    Congenital heart disease
    Peripheral vascular disease
Evaluation of patients with respiratory disease
Assessment of patients with known or suspected disabilities
Assessment for exercise training programs

(From Fardy P, Yankowitz F, Wilson P: *Cardiovascular Assessment and Treatment in Cardiac Rehabilitation. Adult Fitness and Exercise Testing.* Philadelphia, Lea & Febiger, 1988.)

individuals and in patients with cardiac disease (see Table 6–15). A graded exercise test may be used to

1. Confirm a diagnosis of coronary artery disease in a patient with suspected angina or coronary insufficiency.
2. Evaluate the functional capacity of a person with known disease for the purpose of regulating activity or treatment (see Table 6–16).
3. Assess the effects of surgery in a patient postoperatively. Several testing protocols are available. The appropriate exercise test is dependent on
   a. The patient's needs.
   b. The equipment available.
   c. The physical situation.
   d. The personnel available.

Table 6–16.   FUNCTIONAL EXERCISE
              TESTING IN CORONARY
              HEART DISEASE

Quantitation of physical working capacity for occupational and
    leisure-time activities
    Stable angina pectoris
    After myocardial infarction
    After coronary artery bypass surgery
    After coronary angioplasty
Prognostic stratification of patients into high-risk and low-risk
    subgroups
Therapeutic considerations
    Evaluating the need for surgery
    Selection of optimal therapy
    Assessing the effects of therapy
Cardiac rehabilitation
    Design of initial exercise prescription
    Determining rate of exercise progression

(From Fardy P, Yankowitz F, Wilson P: *Cardiovascular Assessment and Treatment in Cardiac Rehabilitation. Adult Fitness and Exercise Testing.* Philadelphia, Lea & Febiger, 1988.)

Table 6–17.   DATA OBTAINED FROM THE
              EXERCISE TEST TO BE USED
              IN THE DEVELOPMENT OF
              AN EXERCISE PRESCRIPTION

Subjective

Angina pectoris
Dyspnea
Fatigue—weakness
Leg discomfort
Dizziness

Objective

Physical examination
    Breath sounds
    Peripheral pulses
    Precordial examination for dyskinetic areas, murmurs, and
        gallops (before and after exercise)
    Blood pressure response
    Pulmonary function test results (before and after exercise)
    Heart rate response
    General appearance
    Oximetry/arterial blood gas results
Physical performance
    Time on treadmill/cycle
    Maximum work load (watts, kg-m/min, kp-m/min)
    Rate of perceived exertion
    Rate pressure product (heart rate × blood pressure)
Electrocardiogram
    Repolarization changes—ST segment and J point
    Rate response
    Dysrhythmias
    Conduction abnormalities—atrioventricular and ventricular
Cardiorespiratory/metabolic measurements (limited availability)
    Anaerobic threshold (AT)
    Carbon dioxide output (V_{CO_2})
    Gas exchange ratio (R)
    Minute ventilation (VE)
    Oxygen uptake (V_{O_2})
    Respiratory quotient (RQ)

(From Brannon F, Foley M, Starr JA: *Cardiopulmonary Rehabilitation: Basic Theory and Application,* 2nd ed. Philadelphia, F. A. Davis Company, 1993, p 283.)

Exercise testing is an important prerequisite for successful management of patients during cardiac rehabilitation.[9,21] The design of individual exercise programs and the rate of progression through all phases of cardiac rehabilitation depend on the results of progressive exercise testing (see Table 6–17).

Table 6–18 gives sample protocols used in the evaluation of functional capacity.

D. Radionuclide studies

Radionuclide studies of the cardiovascular system are invasive techniques accomplished

Table 6–18. SAMPLE STRESS-TESTING PROTOCOLS

Protocol	Method	Comments
Twelve-min walk*	Level walking for 12 min, distance recorded	No equipment necessary, yet correlates well with study results of more complex tests; can be used for patients who cannot accomplish either treadmill walking or bike riding because of dyspnea
Modified Naughton†	Treadmill speed constant at 2.0 mph; grade initially 0%, increased by 3.5% every 2 min	Slow speed allows patient with pulmonary impairment to be stressed without walking fast
		Intermittent-walk test for use with severely impaired patients; allows flexibility of workload assignment and establishes an accurate baseline
Balke test†	Treadmill speed constant at 3.0 mph; grade initially 0%, increased by 3.5% every 2 min	Slight increase in speed for patient with less impairment allows pulmonary and cardiovascular stress to come before leg fatigue
Bruce†	Treadmill speed initially 1.7 mph; grade initially 10%, both increased every 3 min in a specified manner	Can be used with relatively fit persons to stress accurately all systems' response to exercise; good to assess exercise-induced bronchospasm in fit persons
Bicycle test‡	Specific workload (ie, watts or kg/min); patient rides for a preset time; next workload determined by patient response	Intermittent subjective test based on patient response; requires lower extremity strength and endurance to reach high metabolic response level

* McGavin CR, Gupta SP, McHardy GJR: Twelve-minute walking test for assessing disability in chronic bronchitis. *Br Med J* 1:822–823, 1976.

† From *Physician's Handbook for Evaluation of Cardiovascular and Physical Fitness.* Nashville, Tennessee Heart Association (now called American Heart Association–Tennessee Affiliate), 1972.

‡ Ellestad NH: *Stress Testing: Principles and Practice.* Philadelphia, F. A. Davis Co, 1979.

(From Irwin S, Tecklin J: *Cardiopulmonary Physical Therapy.* St Louis, C. V. Mosby, 1985.)

through injection of a radioactive isotope. Techniques are achieved in one of two ways:

1. **Thallium perfusion imaging.** This is a diagnostic procedure for evaluating patients with suspected coronary artery disease. Positive features are

   a. Its ability to evaluate myocardial blood flow. Therefore, patients with transient, moderate, or maximal coronary perfusion deficits can be evaluated.

   b. Its effectiveness in differentiating between a true and a false-positive ST segment depression response during a graded exercise test.

   c. Its ability to assess preoperatively and postoperatively patients who have had coronary bypass surgery.

   The results of these applications of thallium scans have strong implications for the clinician involved in prescribing exercise for high-risk individuals as well as for patients with coronary artery disease.

2. **Radionuclide ventriculography.** This provides critical information regarding left ventricular dysfunction, including

   a. Wall motion.

   b. Ejection fraction.

This information is critical for clinicians to prescribe a program of exercise that is safe and effective.

E. Cardiac catheterization

Cardiac catheterization involves the introduction of catheters into the various cardiac chambers for diagnostic purposes.[21]

1. Catheterization is performed on the right and left sides of the heart to observe

   a. Chamber pressures.

   b. Pulmonary arteries.

   c. Pulmonary wedge pressure.

   d. Pressure gradients of the valves.

   e. Cardiac output in terms of ejection fraction.

   f. Oxygen content of venous and arterial blood.

PLEASE NOTE: Cardiac catheterization is considered to be one of the more life-threatening of the invasive techniques.

2. Two other special catheterization procedures have gained clinical diagnostic popularity in recent years:

   a. *Intracardiac electrophysiology studies.* These

are critical in testing drug therapy in patients who are susceptible to life-threatening arrhythmias and/or who are at great risk of sudden death.

b. *Endomyocardial biopsy.* This is a technique developed to study the rejection phenomenon in transplant patients.[21]

F. Coronary angiography

Coronary angiography is an intracardiac roentgenographic study during which radiopaque contrast medium is injected into coronary vessels and its passage is viewed as the heart beats. It provides the clinician with valuable information regarding

1. Extent of coronary artery disease.
2. Severity and location of occlusion.
3. Subsequent blood flow pattern.

Angiography has become the diagnostic tool of choice, and results are used as a baseline for all other test comparisons. One drawback of coronary angiography is that it is performed while the patient is at rest and results cannot be interpreted for performance with increased activity, *ie,* exercise.

G. Percutaneous transluminal coronary angioplasty

Percutaneous transluminal coronary angioplasty is the most recent and innovative therapy for patients with coronary artery disease. It is performed in conjunction with coronary angiography, in which the narrowed coronary artery is dilated by a special balloon-tip catheter introduced through a peripheral artery. After the balloon tip is inserted and is properly positioned within the narrowed lumen, inflation of the balloon compresses the plaque in the lumen and increases the lumen size and, therefore, increases coronary blood flow. The success rate of the procedure has reduced the need for coronary bypass surgery for many patients with coronary ischemia. Acute complications from the procedure can occur. It is necessary for the procedure to be performed in the cardiac catheterization laboratory with a back-up surgical team.

Angioplasty allows for a shorter hospitalization and a quicker return to home, work, and exercise activities. Frequently, individuals undergoing angioplasty are referred to cardiac rehabilitation post procedure.[21]

VI. Major Conditions and Special Considerations

A. Coronary artery disease

Coronary artery disease is an atherosclerotic process that manifests itself in many ways; ultimately, it reduces myocardial perfusion and therefore myocardial oxygenation.

The actual pathogenesis of atherosclerosis remains unknown. Research suggests that atherosclerosis affects any artery, with the most common sites being the aorta, the coronary, cerebral, and femoral arteries, and any other moderate to large artery.[22]

The disease is characterized by thickening of the lumen (inner layer of the blood vessel wall) caused by the accumulation of lipids. As the process continues, the wall becomes thick, the lumen narrowed, and blood flow reduced.

The Framingham heart study[14] documented the strong relationship between the presence of certain risk factors and the development of coronary artery disease. The presence of more

than one risk factor has an exponential effect on coronary disease risk.

B. Risk factors for coronary artery disease

1. **Primary risk factors**
   a. Age
   b. Gender
   c. Family history

2. **Secondary Risk Factors**
   a. Cigarette smoking
   b. High lipid profile
   c. Hypertension
   d. Physical inactivity
   e. Obesity
   f. Diabetes mellitus
   g. Certain behavioral characteristics

   Table 6–19 lists risk factors for coronary artery disease and strategies for modification. These strategies are taken

Table 6–19. RISK FACTORS FOR CORONARY ARTERY DISEASE AND STRATEGIES FOR MODIFICATION

Risk Factor	Strategy for Modification
Major	
High blood pressure	Medication
	Exercise
	Behavior modification: relaxation techniques, dietary restrictions (*eg*, salt, alcohol)
Cigarette abuse	Behavioral modification: group therapy, hypnosis, participation in community programs
	Education series: breathing techniques, benefits of quitting
High cholesterol	Diet modification (*eg*, low saturated fat, low cholesterol)
	Medication
	Exercise
Minor	
Diabetes mellitus	Diet control
	Medication
	Aerobic exercise
Sedentary lifestyle	Exercise programs: group or individual
	Increase leisure-time activities
Obesity	Weight control
	Exercise
	Behavior modification: group programs
Type A personality	Behavior modification: group programs, exercise programs
	Education: classes, literature
Nonmodifiable	
Aging	
Positive family history	
Male gender	

(From Cohen M, Hoskins T: *Cardiopulmonary Symptoms in Physical Therapy Practice.* New York, Churchill Livingstone, 1988, p 82.)

into consideration for assessment and treatment interventions.

C. Coronary artery disease manifestation

In the early stages of coronary disease, the patient is generally symptom free, meaning that he or she is able to deliver sufficient amounts of oxygenated blood to meet the demands (work) placed on the heart. As the disease progresses and significant narrowing of the vessels occurs, the demand for oxygenated blood is greater than the amount that can be supplied by the narrowed vessel (see Figure 6–16). At this point, the clinical manifestations of the disease are expressed in several progressive clinical conditions.

1. **Clinical condition: an overview**
   a. *Angina pectoris*
      (1). *Description.* Angina pectoris is pathophysiologically described as a state of transient myocardial ischemia without myocardial cell death.
      (2). *Pertinent findings.* Angina pectoris is characterized by chest discomfort and precipitated by activities that require an increase in myocardial oxygen demand. By the time angina is expressed as an overt symptom, coronary occlusion has been well established.

      Angina pain may progress from its stable state to "unstable" angina, which can occur at rest or exercise or not be associated with the usual exertional activities (see Table 6–9).

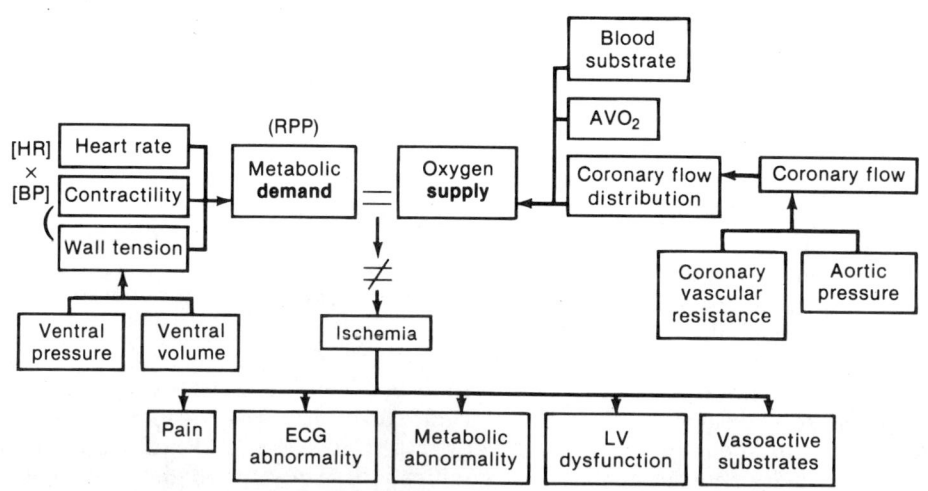

FIGURE 6–16 Myocardial oxygen supply and demand relationship. *Abbreviations:* AV = arteriovenous; BP = blood pressure; ECG = electrocardiogram; HR = heart rate; LV = left ventricular; RPP = rate-pressure product. (Adapted from Ellestad M: *Stress Testing: Principles and Practice,* 2nd ed. Philadelphia, F. A. Davis Company, 1980.)

Angina pain is classically described as crushing pain in the mid-chest with or without radiating arm pain. Nonclassical angina pain can be described as jaw pain, throat tickling, pain between the shoulder blades, radiating posterior neck pain, or even a sensation in the teeth.

(3). *Medical management.* Management is primarily pharmacological intervention, risk factor modification, and even transluminal angioplasty.

(4). *Physical therapy considerations.* These include an exercise program to improve functional capacity and delay onset of anginal pattern and patient education regarding the relationship between risk factor reduction and its influence on coronary disease, *ie*, angina.

b. *Myocardial infarction*

(1). *Description.* This is a myocardial ischemia of sufficient intensity and duration to cause cell death or necrosis of myocardial tissue.

(2). *Pertinent findings.* Common symptoms are severe and persistent chest pain, anxiety, nausea, vomiting, dyspnea, or diaphoresis. Subsequent laboratory diagnostics include ECG changes and elevated serum enzymes.

(3). *Medical management.* Initially management involves bed rest, ECG monitoring, supplemental oxygen, and pharmacological intervention. Gradually, low-level self-care measures and a progressive exercise program are implemented.

(4). *Physical therapy considerations.* These include monitoring of heart rate, blood pressure, and ECG during a gradual progressive exercise program of cardiac rehabilitation (phase 1).

c. *Heart failure*

(1). *Description.* This is the condition in which cardiac output fails to meet metabolic demands. One ventricle may fail initially, but soon the other ventricle becomes affected, leading to total decompensation.[23] Two frequent situations are left-sided failure and right-sided failure (see Table 6–20).

(a). *Left-sided failure.* This is most frequently seen post myocardial infarction. When the left ventricular pumping mechanism is altered, blood may pool in the ventricle owing to ineffective pumping. As the pressure in the ventricle increases and the volume also increases and, over time, will cause retrograde blood flow into the atrium and even into the pulmonary system and eventually cause right-sided failure. The presence of both right- and left-sided failure is critical.[23]

(b). *Right-sided failure.* This can occur unilaterally. Right-sided failure is the residual of chronic obstructive pulmonary disease (COPD) or congenital heart problems. In COPD, lung compliance decreases significantly and pulmonary vascular resistance increases significantly. The most common cause of right-sided failure is left-sided failure.[4,23,24]

(2). *Pertinent findings.* With left-sided failure, the patient is dyspneic at rest or even when sitting. As pulmonary

Table 6–20. SIGNS AND SYMPTOMS OF CARDIAC FAILURE

	Left Ventricular Failure	Right Ventricular Failure
Subjective	Dyspnea	Abdominal pain
	Orthopnea	Anorexia/nausea
	Paroxysmal nocturnal dyspnea	Bloating
		Fatigue
	Cough	Ankle swelling (bilateral)
	Fatigue	
Objective	Rales	Distended neck veins
	S$_3$ gallop	Hepatojugular reflux
	Pleural effusion	Hepatomegaly/splenomegaly
	Peripheral cyanosis	
	Increased respiratory rate	Ascites
	Cheyne-Stokes respirations	Elevated central venous pressure, right atrial pressure
	Decreased urine output	S$_4$ gallop
	Pink frothy sputum	Peripheral edema
		Decreased urine output

(From Patrick ML, *et al.* [eds]: *Medical-Surgical Nursing: Pathophysiological Concepts.* Philadelphia, J. B. Lippincott Company, 1986, p 548.)

congestion increases, the lungs become stiff and less compliant. A cough is another symptom of congestive heart failure. The cough produces frothy pink (blood) sputum, and rales are audible. If left untreated, pulmonary edema frequently becomes a medical emergency.

With right-sided failure, there is elevated central venous pressure with neck vein distention. Over time, the liver becomes engorged, the abdomen becomes distended, and there is concomitant peripheral edema of the lower limbs.

(3). *Medical management.* Congestive heart failure is treated promptly with bronchodilators, vasodilators, and diuretics.[25] Primary concern is the control of edema and adjustment of other hemodynamic problems. Treatment is directed toward decreasing circulatory load, myocardial workload, and oxygen demand while improving myocardial contractility. This is accomplished through the use of diuretics, water, and sodium restriction to reduce blood volume; cardiac glycosides (to increase myocardial contractility); and oxygen therapy.[25]

(4). *Physical therapy considerations.* Most individuals who suffer from congestive heart failure complain of fatigue and a decrease in tolerance for activity. Physical therapy treatment is directed at improving cardiac performance and cardiac output. Low-level exercises as well as energy-conservation methods are implemented in the acute stages through cardiac rehabilitation (phase I). Chest physical therapy and oxygen support are admitted as supplements to treatment when indicated.

d. *Sudden death*
(1). *Description.* Sudden death is defined as unexpected death occurring within 1 hour of the onset of symptoms.
(2). *Pertinent findings.* In patients who had no known disease, death is usually due to ventricular fibrillation.

Table 6–21. NEW YORK HEART ASSOCIATION FUNCTIONAL AND THERAPEUTIC CLASSIFICATION OF HEART DISEASE

Functional Capacity

Class I: No limitation of physical activity. Ordinary physical activity does not cause undue fatigue, palpitation, dyspnea, or anginal pain.

Class II: Slight limitation of physical activity. Comfortable at rest, but ordinary physical activity results in fatigue, palpitation, dyspnea, or anginal pain.

Class III: Marked limitation of physical activity. Comfortable at rest, but less than ordinary activity causes fatigue, palpitation, dyspnea, or anginal pain.

Class IV: Unable to carry on any physical activity without discomfort. Symptoms of cardiac insufficiency or of the anginal syndrome may be present even at rest. If any physical activity is undertaken, discomfort is increased.

Therapeutic Classification

Class A: Physical activity need not be restricted.

Class B: Ordinary physical activity need not be restricted, but unusually severe or competitive efforts should be avoided.

Class C: Ordinary physical activity should be moderately restricted, and more strenuous efforts should be discontinued.

Class D: Ordinary physical activity should be markedly restricted.

Class E: Patient should be at complete rest, confined to bed or chair.

(From Cohen M, Hoskins T: *Cardiopulmonary Symptoms in Physical Therapy Practice.* New York, Churchill Livingstone, 1988, p 84.)

PLEASE NOTE: The clinical conditions that have been mentioned here are only a sampling of the most commonly seen complications in patients with coronary artery disease. Each of these conditions is manifested differently in each patient and is dependent on the clinical course. When an individual with any of these conditions is referred for cardiac rehabilitation, he or she is often classified on the basis of personal functional capacity post graded exercise test. Table 6–21 lists the classifications identified by the New York Heart Association.

2. **Additional clinical syndromes**
   a. *Cardiomegaly*
      (1). *Description.* Cardiomegaly is an enlargement of the heart.
      (2). *Pertinent findings.* It appears that cardiomegaly is due to dilation, hypertrophy, or both. With the progression of coronary disease and

perhaps recurrent infarctions, scars form; the remaining normal tissue undergoes hypertrophy as a means of compensation. Heart size on radiograph appears enlarged. Heart dimensions measured by angiography appear increased.[23,25]

(3). *Medical management.* If the enlargement has caused some hemodynamic alteration, pharmacological agents are administered. Beta blockers may be administered to reduce myocardial workload and oxygen demand.

(4). *Physical therapy considerations.* Individuals with cardiomegaly are frequently referred to cardiac rehabilitation. Commonly, these patients may not have had a myocardial infarction and are considered at high risk for experiencing a cardiac event. In this situation, appropriate exercise prescription and careful monitoring are important while improving functional capacity. In situations in which the individual may have cardiomegaly and have had an infarction, the exercise prescription and careful monitoring are essential because many of these patients have arrhythmias.

b. *Abnormal electrocardiogram*

(1). *Description.* Changes in the ECG either at rest or with low levels of exercise strongly indicate the presence of coronary insufficiency in asymptomatic individuals.[23]

(2). *Pertinent findings.* ST segment changes are observed in the chest leads, especially V_4, V_5, and V_6, with no symptomatology. These changes include the following: 1 mm of ST segment depression that does not return to the isoelectric line within .08 seconds is considered borderline ischemia and intimates coronary disease; 2 mm of ST segment depression that does not return to the isoelectric line within .08 seconds is considered positive for coronary artery disease. Individuals with coronary disease symptoms usually display these ST segment changes.

(3). *Medical management.* To establish a diagnosis of coronary disease, an ECG is obtained during rest and exercise and into recovery. It is not uncommon for patients with angina to demonstrate similar ST segment changes as described above.

(4). *Physical therapy considerations.* Individuals may be considered high risk and may be referred to cardiac rehabilitation for improvement in functional capacity and monitoring of ECG, as well as reduction in any concurrent coronary prone risk factor.

If the individual has documented disease, a program of exercise and risk factor reduction may have positive implication for reducing coronary risk. If an individual has ECG changes but no documented disease, it is believed that the benefits of a program of exercise and risk factor reduction as primary prevention may have long-term implications for the development of coronary disease.

c. *Arrhythmias*

(1). *Description.* Abnormal conduction patterns frequently implicate coronary artery disease and may be caused by inadequate oxygenation, areas of scar formation, and even acute myocardial infarction.[23]

(2). *Pertinent findings.* Patients who have arrhythmias frequently complain of palpitations, dizziness, fatigue, or syncope.

(3). *Medical management.* Pharmacological agents are used to reduce the risk for lethal arrhythmias; a supervised exercise program is prescribed; and an assessment of risk factors for coronary disease is made.

(4). *Physical therapy considerations.* Patients are frequently referred to cardiac rehabilitation for purposes of monitoring during initial drug administration/accommodation. Establishing an appropriate exercise prescription that considers the type of arrhythmia, the functional capacity, and the heart rate associated with the onset of the arrhythmias is critical.

d. *Valvular insufficiencies*

(1). *Description.* The normal competence

of any of the valves of the heart depends on the structural and functionally intact valvular apparatus. The components of the valve, as described earlier, are the atrial walls, the leaflets, the chordae tendineae, and the papillary muscles.[23,24]

(2). *Pertinent findings.* In most situations of valvular insufficiency, the cause is related to one or many factors, including coronary artery disease, myocardial infarction, rupture of the chordae tendineae from an infarction or blow to the chest wall, and rheumatic fever.[23,24]

(3). *Medical management.* In their early stages, valvular insufficiencies are managed by careful physician observation. As the valve becomes more compromised, murmurs are generally the more overt sign of insufficiency. As these progress and the patient begins to experience severe compromise, surgical repair is indicated.

(4). *Physical therapy considerations.* Patients are referred to physical therapy for pre- and postoperative evaluation and treatment. The program is described next.

e. **Surgical intervention.** Although various philosophies and approaches exist today with respect to physical therapy treatment, it has become commonplace for all patients who are undergoing surgical intervention to be evaluated preoperatively and treated postoperatively by the physical therapist. Patients with cardiac and/or pulmonary diagnosis are at greater risk for developing postoperative complications, such as pneumonia, thrombosis, and decreased functional capacity. Programs of preoperative evaluation and assessment of both function and breathing capacity with postoperative chest physical therapy in combination with mild progressive exercise programs have been shown to reduce the risk of complications and to return the patient to normal status sooner (see Chapter 7).

(1). *Preoperative teaching and treatment*

(a). Description. At the preoperative session, the physical thera-

pist establishes a baseline of cardiopulmonary function, treats any condition that may improve the outcome of the surgical procedure, and ensures the patient's ability to perform postoperative breathing and coughing techniques.

(b). Pertinent findings. Refer to Table 7–11 for the characteristics of patients most appropriate for preoperative physical therapy evaluation and treatment.

(c). Physical therapy considerations. These are the same as those listed in Chapter 7.

(i). Introduce the patient to the therapist and the department.

(ii). Extract pertinent patient information from the medical record and physical examination.

(iii). Demonstrate techniques that may be used postoperatively.

(iv). Teach breathing exercises, splinting, and incentive spirometry.

(v). Describe the postoperative course, including treatment times, lines, tubes, discomforts, location of various rooms, and hospital guidelines for visitors.

(vi). Perform secretion removal techniques as required.

(2). *Postoperative sessions*

(a). Description. Postoperative cardiopulmonary complications are prevented by

(i). Removing any residual secretions.

(ii). Improving acration.

(iii). Gradually increasing activity (begin formal phase I progressive cardiac rehabilitation program).

(iv). Beginning formal patient education program.

(v). Returning cardiopulmonary functioning to as close to normal as quickly as possible.

(b). Pertinent physical findings. For the cardiac patient, postoperative complications could be cardiac, pulmonary, or neurologically based.

(i). Pulmonary complications are identified by an increase in temperature, increase in white blood cell count, change in breath sounds from the preoperative evaluation, shortness of breath, cough, and sputum production.

(ii). Cardiac complications are identified by an increase in temperature, increase in white blood cell count, ECG changes, unstable blood pressure, unstable hemodynamic functioning, changes in serum enzyme levels, and ventricular dysfunction or hypervolemia as a complication of the surgical procedure.

(iii). The neurological complications that occur are generally related to a complication of surgery. The most common is stroke due to an embolus or hypoxemia.

f. *Heart transplantation*

(1). *Description*

(a). This is currently the treatment of choice for end-stage myocardial dysfunction.

(b). In this procedure, a matched donor heart is used to replace the diseased heart.

(2). *Pertinent findings*

(a). Left ventricular function is less than 20%.[25]

(b). Medical therapies are ineffective.

(c). There is no expectation of recovery.

(3). *Medical management*

(a). Two major postoperative complications are infection and rejection.

(b). Immunosuppressive therapy is used to minimize rejection.

(c). Protective isolation is used to minimize the risk of infection.

(4). *Physical therapy considerations*

(a). Rehabilitation is an adjunct to medical therapy.

(b). The rehabilitation program is similar to that for a patient with coronary artery disease except for the heart's response to exercise. Heart rate cannot be used for monitoring.

(c). The response of a denervated heart is different from a normal response.

D. Common congenital anomalies affecting the cardiovascular system

The diagnoses of congenital heart defects are as diverse as the philosophies of the medical and surgical management regarding these problems.[26] The physical therapist is a member of the team working with infants and children with these anomalies.

1. **Descriptions.** A list of the more common diagnoses is given below[26]:

a. *Defects of the atrial septum and atrioventricular canal.* These involve abnormal development and structure of the atria and/or atrioventricular connections.[26]

b. *Ventricular septal defects.* These involve abnormal development and structures of the ventricle and septum.[26]

c. *Patent ductus arteriosus.* This is an open connection between the main pulmonary artery and the aorta that should have closed at birth.[26]

d. *Aortic stenosis.* This is an impedance to forward flow of blood in the aorta.[26]

e. *Coarctation of the aorta.* This is a compression or stricture in the aorta that affects blood flow.[26]

f. *Anomalies of the aortic arch.* These are embryological defects of the structure of the aorta that interfere with ejection of blood.[26]

g. *Tetralogy of Fallot.* This is a defect in the interventricular septum with stenosis of the pulmonary artery. It is the most frequent cause of cardiac cyanosis.[26]

h. *Pulmonary atresia and ventricular septal de-*

fect. This diagnosis is considered pathologically to be the severe end of the spectrum of tetralogy of Fallot. It is characterized as no direct continuity anatomically between the right ventricle and the pulmonary artery.

  i. *Pulmonary stenosis.* This is a congenital obstruction to right ventricular outflow. These anomalies are considered acyanotic with normal pulmonary blood flow, cyanotic with diminished pulmonary artery blood flow, or cyanotic with diminished pulmonary arterial flow.[26]

2. **Pertinent findings.** Depending on the extent of the disease or structural abnormality, the findings may include cyanosis, hypoxemia, poor feeding, failure to thrive, high respiratory rates, high heart rates, frequent respiratory and endocardial infections, as well as episodes of cardiac and/or pulmonary failure.[26]

3. **Physical therapy considerations.** Supportive therapy to prevent infections may be indicated. If surgical corrections are indicated, pre- and postoperative care is indicated.

   a. Chest physical therapy for medical management.
   b. Pre- and postoperative chest physical therapy for surgical intervention.
   c. Postoperative low-level range of motion program followed by a progressive exercise program. In this situation, the child's age is obviously a key factor to the rigor and duration of the treatment program.
   d. A combination of both chest physical therapy and a progressive exercise program.

VII. Physical Therapy Treatment

Cardiac rehabilitation has been shown to be successful in lowering morbidity rates in patients with cardiac disease.[27] Exercise rehabilitation programs result in improved physical, physiological, and psychological well-being of cardiac patients.[28]

A. Patient eligibility

A broad spectrum of patients are now considered eligible for cardiac rehabilitation services:

1. Patients who have had myocardial infarction.
2. Patients who have had coronary bypass surgery.
3. Patients who have had angioplasty.
4. Coronary patients with or without residual ischemia.
5. Patients with heart failure.
6. Patients with arrhythmias.
7. A variety of categories of patients with nonischemic heart disease.
8. Patients with concomitant pulmonary disease.
9. Patients who have undergone interventions such as pacemaker or cardioverter-defibrillator implantation, heart valve repair or replacement, or cardiac transplantation.
10. Elderly patients.
11. Medically complex patients.

PHYSICAL THERAPY AND CARDIAC REHABILITATION PROGRAMS

Physical therapists have been involved in planning and implementing rehabilitation programs for patients with coronary heart disease or dysfunction for several decades. By virtue of their education and training, physical therapists are experienced in exercise physiology and can combine their backgrounds in clinical pathology, postoperative management, kinesiology, and cardiopulmonary function to provide competent program management in all phases of cardiac rehabilitation.

For the patient with coronary artery disease or dysfunction, cardiac rehabilitation programs allow exercise to be performed as a treatment modality with a low risk of major complication. Contributing to the effectiveness of these programs are current guidelines of cardiac rehabilitation, which include appropriate patient selection; concurrent medical, surgical, and pharmacological therapies; patient education; careful exercise prescription, and patient monitoring.[29] Independence and self-monitoring skills are the ultimate goals of rehabilitation.

B. Phases of cardiac rehabilitation process

1. **Phase I.** The hospital inpatient period is 6 to 14 days. Phase I generally begins in the intensive care unit (ICU).
   a. *Treatment objectives.* Once a patient is medically stable after a cardiac event, the physical therapist initiates treatment with the following goals:
   (1). Preventing the deleterious effects of bed rest.
   (2). Reducing orthostatic hypotension.
   (3). Maintaining joint mobility.
   b. *Role of the physical therapist.* During the

Table 6–22. METABOLIC EQUIVALENT (MET) ACTIVITY CHART

Intensity (70-kg Person)	Endurance Promoting	Occupational	Recreational
1.5–2 METs 4–7 mL/kg/min 2–2.5 kcal/min	Too low in energy level	Desk work, driving auto, electric calculating machine operation, light housework, polishing furniture, washing clothes	Standing, strolling (1 mph), flying, motorcycling, playing cards, sewing, knitting
2–3 METs 7–11 mL/kg/min 2.5–4 kcal/min	Too low in energy level unless capacity is very low	Auto repair, radio and television repair, janitorial work, bartending, riding lawn mower, light woodworking	Level walking (2 mph), level bicycling (5 mph), billiards, bowling, skeet shooting, shuffleboard, powerboat driving, golfing with power cart, canoeing, horseback riding at a walk
3–4 METs 11–14 mL/kg/min 4–5 kcal/min	Yes, if continuous and if target heart rate is reached	Brick laying, plastering, wheelbarrow (100-lb load), machine assembly, welding (moderate load), cleaning windows, mopping floors, vacuuming, pushing light power mower	Walking (3 mph), bicycling (6 mph), horseshoe pitching, volleyball (6-person, noncompetitive), golfing (pulling bag cart), archery, sailing (handling small boat), fly fishing (standing in waders), horseback riding (trotting), badminton (social doubles)
4–5 METs 14–18 mL/kg/min	Recreational activities promote endurance; occupational activities must be continuous, lasting longer than 2 min	Painting, masonry, paperhanging, light carpentry, scrubbing floors, raking leaves, hoeing	Walking (3⅓ mph), bicycling (8 mph), table tennis, golfing (carrying clubs), dancing (foxtrot), badminton (singles), tennis (doubles), many calisthenics, ballet
5–6 METs 18–21 mL/kg/min	Yes	Digging garden, shoveling light earth	Walking (4 mph), bicycling (10 mph), canoeing (4 mph), horseback riding (posting to trotting), stream fishing (walking in light current in waders), ice or roller skating (9 mph)
6–7 METs 21–25 mL/kg/min 7–8 kcal/min	Yes	Shoveling 10 times/min (4.5 kg or 10 lb), splitting wood, snow shoveling, hand lawn mowing	Walking (5 mph), bicycling (11 mph), competitive badminton, tennis (singles), folk and square dancing, light downhill skiing, ski touring (2.5 mph), water skiing, swimming (20 yd/min)
7–8 METs 25–28 mL/kg/min 8–10 kcal/min	Yes	Digging ditches, carrying 36 kg or 80 lb, sawing hardwood	Jogging (5 mph), bicycling (12 mph), horseback riding (gallop), vigorous downhill skiing, basketball, mountain climbing, ice hockey, canoeing (5 mph), touch football, paddleball
8–9 METs 28–32 mL/kg/min 10–11 kcal/min	Yes	Shoveling 10 times/min (5.5 kg or 14 lb)	Running (5.5 mph), bicycling (13 mph), ski touring (4 mph), squash (social), handball (social), fencing, basketball (vigorous), swimming (30 yd/min), rope skipping
10+ METs 32+ mL/kg/min 11+ kcal/min	Yes	Shoveling 10 times/min (7.5 kg or 16 lb)	Running (6 mph = 10 METs, 7 mph = 11.5 METs, 8 mph = 13.5 METs, 9 mph = 15 METs, 10 mph = 17 METs), ski touring (5+ mph), handball (competitive), squash (competitive), swimming (> 40 yd/min)

(Reproduced with permission. From Fox SM, Naughton JP, Gorman PA: Physical activity and cardiovascular health: 3. The exercise prescription: Frequency and type of activity. *Mod Concepts Cardiovasc Dis,* 1972, 4:25–30. Copyright 1972 American Heart Association.)

subacute phase of cardiac care, the role of the physical therapist may be to supervise a low-level exercise program and to monitor activities of daily living while constantly evaluating heart rate, blood pressure, and the physiological response to exercise. Active exercises include assis-

tive range of motion in the supine position, progressing to sitting, standing, progressive ambulation, and finally stair climbing.

(1). *Exercise and monitoring.* During this initial critical post–cardiac event period, activities are prescribed at low

Table 6–23. INPATIENT MYOCARDIAL INFARCTION CARDIAC REHABILITATION PROGRAM

Step/Date	Cardiac Rehabilitation/ Physical Therapy	Ward Activity	Patient Education
1 1.5 METs ___/___/___	Ward Rx: Passive ROM to major joints; active ankle exercises, five repetitions; deep breathing (supine) twice a day.	1. Bed rest. 2. May feed self.	Orient to CCU. Orientation to exercise component of rehabilitation program.
2 1.5 METs ___/___/___	Ward Rx: Active-assistive ROM to major muscle groups; active ankle exercises, five repetitions; deep breathing (supine/sitting) twice a day.	1. Feeding self. 2. Partial AM care (washing hands and face, brushing teeth in bed). 3. Bedside commode.	Answer patient and family questions regarding progress, procedures, reason for activity limitation. Explain rate of perceived exertion (RPE).
3 1.5 METs ___/___/___	Ward Rx: Active ROM to major muscle groups; active ankle exercises, five repetitions; breathing (sitting) twice a day.	1. Begin sitting in chair for short periods as tolerated two times a day. 2. Bathing self. 3. Bedside commode.	
4 1.5 METs ___/___/___	Ward Rx: Active exercises—shoulder flexion, abduction; elbow flexion; hip flexion; knee extension; toe raises; ankle exercises, five repetitions; breathing (standing) twice a day.	1. Bathroom privileges. 2. Sitting in chair three times a day. 3. Up in chair for meals. 4. Bathing self, dressing, combing hair (sitting).	
5 1.5–2 METs ___/___/___	Ward Rx: Active exercises—shoulder flexion, abduction, circumduction; elbow flexion; trunk lateral flexion; hip flexion, abduction; knee extension; toe raises; ankle exercises, five repetitions (standing); twice a day. Monitored ambulation of 100–200 ft twice a day, with physician approval.	1. Bathroom privileges. 2. Up as tolerated in room. 3. Stand at sink to shave and comb hair. 4. Bathe self and dress. 5. Up in chair as tolerated.	Answer patient and family questions. Orient to ICCU phase of recovery. Present discharge booklet and other printed material (AHA). Encourage patient and family to attend group classes or do one-to-one sessions.
6 1.5–2 METs ___/___/___	Ward Rx: Standing—exercises outlined in step 5, 5–10 repetitions; once daily. Monitored ambulation for 5 min (440 ft).	1. Continue ward activity from step 5. 2. Increase ambulation up to 440 ft with assistance if appropriate, two times a day. 3. Walk short distance in hall or room.	Instruction in pulse taking and rationale. Explain value of exercise. Present T-shirt and activity log.
___/___/___	Exercise center: Transport to inpatient exercise center (IEC) for monitored ROM/strengthening exercises from step 5. Five to 10 repetitions: leg stretching (posterior thigh muscles, gastrocnemius); 10 repetitions: treadmill and/or bicycle 5 min; stair climbing (2–4 stairs) with physician approval.		
7 1.5–2.5 METs ___/___/___	Ward Rx: Standing—exercises from step 5 with 1-lb weight each extremity. Five to 10 repetitions, once daily. Monitored ambulation for 5–10 min (440–1100 ft).	1. Continue ward activity from step 6. 2. Sit up in chair most of the day. 3. Increased ambulation up to 1100 ft daily.	Begin discharge instructions with patient and family when appropriate. Encourage group class attendance or offer one-to-one sessions as needed.

levels (between 1 and 3 metabolic equivalents ["METs"]) to allow proper myocardial healing (see Table 6-22).

Another method of monitoring activity may be by using heart rate. A 20 beat/min rise above resting heart rate for myocardial infarction patients and a 30 beat/min rise for coronary bypass patients are good guidelines for exercise intensity for phase I cardiac rehabilitation. Table 6-23 outlines a progressive program in phase I for patients with

Table 6-23. INPATIENT MYOCARDIAL INFARCTION CARDIAC REHABILITATION PROGRAM *Continued*

Step/Date	Cardiac Rehabilitation/ Physical Therapy	Ward Activity	Patient Education
__/__/__	Exercise center: Transport to IEC for monitored ROM/strengthening exercises from step 6 with 1-lb weight each extremity. Five to 10 repetitions: leg stretching; 10 repetitions: treadmill and/or bicycle 5–10 min; stair climbing (4–8 stairs).		
8 1.5–2.5 METs __/__/__	Ward Rx: Standing—exercises from step 5 with 1-lb weight each extremity, 10 repetitions, once daily. Monitored ambulation for 10 min (up to 1980 ft) if appropriate.	1. Continue ward activity from step 7. 2. Increase ambulation up to 1980 ft daily.	
__/__/__	Exercise center: Ambulate to IEC for monitored ROM/strengthening exercises from step 6 with 1-lb weight each extremity. Ten repetitions: leg stretching; 10 repetitions: treadmill and/or bicycle 10–20 min; stair climbing (10–12 stairs).		
9 1.5–2.5 METs __/__/__	Ward Rx: Standing—exercises from step 5 with 2-lb weight each extremity. Ten repetitions, once daily. Monitored ambulation if appropriate.	1. Up as tolerated in room. 2. Increase ambulation up to 2640 ft daily.	Begin instruction in home exercise program. Initiate referral to phase II if appropriate. Explain predischarge graded exercise test (PDGXT) and upper-limit heart rate.
__/__/__	Exercise center: Ambulate to IEC for monitored ROM/strengthening exercises from step 6 with 2-lb weight each extremity. Ten repetitions: leg stretching; 10 repetitions: treadmill and/or bicycle 20–25 min; stair climbing (12–14 stairs).		
10 1.5–3 METs __/__/__	Ward Rx: Exercises from step 5 with 2-lb weight each extremity. Ten repetitions, once daily. Monitored ambulation if appropriate.	1. Up as tolerated in room. 2. Increase ambulation up to 3300 ft daily.	
__/__/__	Exercise center: Ambulate to IEC for monitored ROM/strengthening exercises from step 6 with 2-lb weight each extremity. Ten repetitions: leg stretching; 10 repetitions: treadmill and/or bicycle 25–30 min; stair climbing (14–15 stairs).		

(From Pollock ML, Schmidt D: *Heart Disease and Rehabilitation.* New York, John Wiley, 1986).

Abbreviations: AHA = American Heart Association; CCU = cardiac care unit; ICCU = intensive coronary care unit; ROM = range of motion.

Table 6–24. INPATIENT CARDIAC REHABILITATION PROGRAM FOR PATIENTS AFTER CORONARY ARTERY BYPASS GRAFT SURGERY

Step/Date	Cardiac Rehabilitation/ Physical Therapy	Ward Activity*	Patient Education
1 1.5 METs ___/___/___	AM Ward Rx: Sitting with feet supported—active assistive to active ROM to major muscle groups, active ankle exercises, active scapular elevation/depression, retraction/protraction. Three to five repetitions: deep breathing. Monitored ambulation of 100 ft as tolerated. PM Ward Rx: Sitting with feet supported—active ROM to major muscle groups. Five repetitions: deep breathing. Monitored ambulation 100–200 ft with assistance as tolerated.	1. Begin sitting in chair (when stable) several times a day for 10–30 min. 2. May ambulate 100–200 ft with assistance, one to two times daily.	Orient to CVICU. Reinforce purpose of physical therapy and deep-breathing exercises. Orient to exercise component or rehabilitation program. Answer patient and family questions regarding progress.
2 1.5 METs ___/___/___	Ward Rx: Sitting—repeat exercises from step 1 and increase repetitions to 5–10; deep breathing twice a day. Monitored ambulation of 200 ft with assistance as tolerated (stress correct posture) twice a day.	Continue activities from step 1.	Continue above.
3 1.5–2 METs ___/___/___	Ward Rx: Standing—begin active upper extremity and trunk exercises bilaterally without resistance (shoulder: flexion, abduction, internal/external rotation, hyperextension, circumduction backward; elbow flexion; trunk: lateral flexion, rotation); knee extension (if appropriate); ankle exercises: 5–10 repetitions, twice a day. Monitored ambulation of 300 ft twice a day.	Increase ambulation to 300 ft or approximately 3 corridor lengths at slow pace with assistance twice a day.	Begin pulse-taking instruction when appropriate and explain rate of perceived exertion (RPE) scale. Answer questions of patient and family. Reorient patient and family to ICCU. Encourage family attendance at group classes.
4 1.5–2 METs ___/___/___	Ward Rx: Standing—active exercises from step 3, 10–15 repetitions, twice a day. Monitored ambulation of 424 ft twice a day.	Increase ambulation to 500 ft at slow pace with assistance twice a day.	
5 1.2–2.5 METs ___/___/___	Ward Rx: Standing—active exercises from step 3. Fifteen repetitions, once daily. Monitored ambulation for 5–10 min (424–848 ft) as tolerated.	1. Increase ambulation up to 3 laps (up to 1320 ft) daily as tolerated. 2. Begin participating in activities of daily living (ADL) and personal care as tolerated. 3. Encourage chair sitting with legs elevated.	Orient to inpatient exercise center (IEC). Continue instruction in pulse taking and use of RPE scale. Explain value of exercise. Present T-shirt and activity log.
___/___/___	Exercise center: Walk to inpatient exercise center for monitored ROM/strengthening exercises from step 3. Fifteen repetitions: leg stretching (posterior thigh muscles, gastrocnemius). Ten repetitions: treadmill or bicycle 5–10 min (refer to treadmill/bicycle protocol) with physician approval.		
6 1.5–2.5 METs ___/___/___	Ward Rx: Standing—active exercises from step 3 with 1-lb weight each upper extremity. Fifteen repetitions, once daily. Monitored ambulation for 10–15 min (up to 1980 ft) if appropriate.	1. Increase ambulation up to 1980 ft daily. 2. Encourage independence in ADL. 3. Encourage chair sitting with legs elevated.	Give discharge booklet and general discharge instructions to patient and family. Encourage group class attendance. Individual instruction by physical therapist, nutritionist, and pharmacist.
___/___/___	Exercise center: Walk to IEC for monitored ROM/strengthening exercises from step 5 with 1-lb weight each upper extremity.		

Table 6–24. INPATIENT CARDIAC REHABILITATION PROGRAM FOR PATIENTS AFTER CORONARY ARTERY BYPASS GRAFT SURGERY *Continued*

Step/Date	Cardiac Rehabilitation/ Physical Therapy	Ward Activity*	Patient Education
7 2–3 METS ___/___/___ ___/___/___	Fifteen repetitions: leg stretching. Ten repetitions: treadmill and/or bicycle 15–20 min; stair climbing (6–12 stairs) with assistance. Ward Rx: Standing—active exercises from step 3 with 1-lb weight each upper extremity. Fifteen repetitions, once daily. Monitored ambulation for 15–20 min (up to 3300 ft) if appropriate. Exercise center: Walk to IEC for monitored ROM/strengthening exercises from step 5 with 1-lb weight each upper extremity. Fifteen repetitions: leg stretching. Ten repetitions: treadmill and/or bicycle 20–30 min; stair climbing (up to 14 stairs) with assistance.	1. Continue activities from step 6. 2. Increase ambulation up to 3300 ft daily.	Discuss referral to phase II program if appropriate.
8 2–3 METs ___/___/___ ___/___/___	Ward Rx: Standing—exercises from step 3 with 2-lb weight each upper extremity. Fifteen repetitions, once daily. Monitored ambulation if appropriate. Exercise center: Walk to IEC for monitored ROM/strengthening exercise from step 5 with 2-lb weight each upper extremity. Fifteen repetitions: leg stretching. Ten repetitions: treadmill and/or bicycle 20–30 min; stair climbing (up to 16 stairs).	1. Continue activities from step 7. 2. Increase ambulation up to 3746 ft daily.	Reinforce prior teaching. Explain predischarge graded exercise test (PDGXT) and upper-limit heart rate. Continue with possible referral to phase II.
9 2–3 METs ___/___/___ ___/___/___	Ward Rx: Standing—exercises from step 3 with 2-lb weight each upper extremity. Fifteen repetitions, once daily. Monitored ambulation if appropriate. Exercise center: Walk to IEC for monitored ROM/strengthening exercises from step 5 with 2-lb weight each upper extremity. Fifteen repetitions: leg stretching. Ten repetitions: treadmill and/or bicycle 20–30 min; stair climbing (up to 18 stairs).	1. Continue activities from step 8. 2. Increase ambulation up to 5060 ft daily.	Finalize discharge instructions. Complete referral to phase II.
10 2–3 METs ___/___/___ ___/___/___	Ward Rx: Standing—exercises from step 3 with 3-lb weight each upper extremity. Fifteen repetitions, once daily. Monitored ambulation if appropriate. Exercise center: Walk to IEC for monitored ROM/strengthening exercises from step 5 with 3-lb weight each upper extremity. Fifteen repetitions: leg stretching. Ten repetitions: treadmill and/or bicycle 20–30 min; stair climbing (up to 24 stairs). A PDGXT is recommended at this time.	1. Continue activities from step 9. 2. Increase ambulation up to 5936 ft daily.	

(From Pollock ML, Schmidt D: *Heart Disease and Rehabilitation.* New York, John Wiley, 1986.)
*Activities performed alone, with family, or with primary nurse.
Abbreviations: CVICU = cardiovascular intensive care unit; ICCU = intensive coronary care unit; ROM = range of motion.

myocardial infarction. Table 6–24 gives a phase I program for patients after bypass surgery. Table 6–25 describes a program with outcome measures.[29]

Monitoring of patients during phase I cardiac rehabilitation is usually done with the ICU's or ward's telemetry units, their hard copy of the ECG, and periodic pulse checks for changes in heart rate. Blood pressure is usually measured before and after exercise. If there is reason for concern, it can be monitored every few minutes.

(2). *Education.* Education for a healthier lifestyle is an integral part of each phase of rehabilitation, with individ-

ual instructions on identifying and modifying reversible risk factors for the prevention of further cardiac events.

(3). *Graded exercise test.* Prior to discharge, a low-level, symptom-limited graded exercise test should be performed. The purpose of this test is to evaluate the patient's functional capacity and to establish a symptom-limited heart rate to prescribe a safe and effective program for the next phase of cardiac rehabilitation.

PLEASE NOTE: Phase I cardiac rehabilitation is often coordinated by a physical therapist with the nurse and physician.

Table 6–25. DESIGN FOR PATIENT ASSESSMENT, RECOMMENDED PROGRAM, AND EXPECTED OUTCOME MEASURES

Patient Assessment and Profile	Program	Expected Outcome
Recent open chest or heart surgery (CABG, valve, AICD, pacemaker, etc.) as determined by patient medical records	Patient education program, including information on the disease process, treatment and risk factor education, activity guidelines, sexual activity, medications, and return to work	Self-care; increased understanding of surgically related concerns and improved quality of life
Recent diagnosis of CAD/MI or its treatment or sequelae, *eg,* catheterization, PTCA, arrhythmia, CHF, as determined by patient medical records	Patient education program, including information on the disease process, signs and symptoms, treatment options, risk factors, activity guidelines, sexual activity, medications, and return to work	Self-care; increased understanding of CAD-related concerns and improved quality of life
Reduced activity level, decreased functional capacity, or sedentary lifestyle as determined by a medical history or a graded exercise test, with or without oxygen-consumption measurements	Individualized exercise program based on risk stratification: • monitored • unmonitored, supervised • home exercise program and education	Increase in activity level and functional capacity, attainment of an improved level of fitness and/or regular exercise participation
Tobacco use or abuse as determined by patient or family report, CO monitoring, or isothiocyanide saliva testing	Smoking cessation program	Reduction or cessation of smoking
Any abnormality in blood lipids and/or lipoproteins as manifested by increased total cholesterol or LDL-C, and/or triglycerides, and/or reduced HDL-cholesterol as determined by fasting blood drawn (for LDL-C, triglycerides, HDL-C) and confirmed by repeat measurement	Dietary lipid/modification and medical intervention program in accordance with National Cholesterol Education Program (NCEP) guidelines: weight reduction program and/or exercise program when appropriate	Alteration toward or attainment of appropriate blood lipid and lipoprotein levels as set forth in the NCEP guidelines
Hypertension as determined by blood pressure sphygmomanometry	Hypertension management program, including medical intervention and education in accordance with the National High Blood Pressure Education Program (NHBPEP) guidelines: weight reduction, stress management, dietary modification, and/or exercise programs when appropriate	Decreased blood pressure or attainment of appropriate blood pressure as set forth in the NHBPEP guidelines, and reduction or elimination of blood pressure medication

Table 6–25. DESIGN FOR PATIENT ASSESSMENT, RECOMMENDED PROGRAM, AND EXPECTED OUTCOME MEASURES *Continued*

Patient Assessment and Profile	Program	Expected Outcome
Excess body weight or relative fatness as determined by scale, body mass index, skinfold calipers, or hydrostatic weighing	Dietary weight reduction program and/or exercise program in accordance with the American Dietetic Association guidelines	Reduction in body weight and fat stores and attainment of desirable body weight
High stress levels and/or inappropriate response to stress as determined by patient or family report, stress assessment tools, or psychological evaluation	Stress management program	Reduction in stress and/or inappropriate response to stress
Recent onset of elevated or poorly controlled blood glucose levels as determined by fasting blood draw	Diabetes education and medical intervention program in accordance with the American Diabetes Association guidelines: dietary modification, exercise, and/or weight reduction programs when appropriate	Controlled blood glucose levels
Limitation in work status due to cardiovascular medical conditions	Work hardening program and vocational rehabilitation counseling with a return to work assessment; stress management and/or exercise program when appropriate	Return to work if appropriate
Alcohol abuse as determined by patient or family report or by psychological evaluation	Alcohol abuse program, including spouse and family therapy	Appropriate alcohol use or abstinence and appropriate family interaction
Psychological disorders (anxiety, depression, phobias, aggressive behavior, etc.) as determined by patient or family report or by psychological/psychiatric evaluation	Individualized and/or group therapy	Improved psychological profile and functioning
Neuropsychological disorders (memory loss, confusion, etc.) as determined by patient or family report or by neuropsychological evaluation	Neurological or neuropsychological referral and intervention and therapy	Improved neuropsychological profile and functioning

(From *Guidelines for Cardiac Rehabilitation Programs* (p. 19, 20) by American Association of Cardiovascular and Pulmonary Rehabilitation, Champaign, IL: Human Kinetics Publishers. Copyright 1991 by American Association of Cardiovascular and Pulmonary Rehabilitation. Reprinted by permission.)

Abbreviations: AICD = automatic implantable cardioverter-defibrillator; CABG = coronary artery bypass graft; CAD = coronary artery disease; CHF = congestive heart failure; CO = cardiac output; MI = myocardial infarction; PTCA = percutaneous transluminal coronary angioplasty.

2. **Phase II.** This is the convalescent stage following hospital discharge—up to 12 weeks post cardiac event. This phase usually begins after discharge.
   a. *Treatment objectives.* The objectives of phase II cardiac rehabilitation move from recuperation to improving functional capacity, promoting early return to normal activity, and promoting positive lifestyle changes.
   b. *Role of the physical therapist.* The physical therapist's role during phase II may be to formulate a patient's exercise prescription based on graded exercise test results; monitor the patient according to level of risk (low, medium, or high) assigned (see Table 6–26); progress the

exercise prescription on the basis of physiological data; and discharge the patient from the rehabilitation program when appropriate.[29]
   c. *Treatment essentials.* Phase II cardiac rehabilitation programs emphasize the following basic essentials:
      (1). Early and repeated graded exercise tests to establish functional capacity.
      (2). Individually prescribed graded exercise programs based on the graded exercise testing procedure.
      (3). Risk factor modification programs.
      (4). Comprehensive patient education.
      (5). A multidisciplinary team approach to address the wide spectrum of patient needs.

Table 6–26. GUIDELINES FOR RISK STRATIFICATION

Risk Level	Characteristics
Low	Uncomplicated clinical course in hospital No evidence of myocardial ischemia Functional capacity ≥ 7 METs Normal left ventricular function (EF > 50%) Absence of significant ventricular ectopy
Intermediate (moderate)	ST segment depression ≥ 2 mm flat or downsloping Reversible thallium defects Moderate to good left ventricular function (EF 35%–49%) Changing pattern of or new development of angina pectoris
High	Prior myocardial infarction or infarct involving ≥ 35% of left ventricle EF < 35% at rest Fall in exercise systolic blood pressure or failure of systolic blood pressure to rise more than 10 mm Hg on exercise tolerance test Persistent or recurrent ischemic pain 24 h or more after hospital admission Functional capacity < 5 METs with hypotensive blood pressure response or ≥ 1 mm ST segment depression Congestive heart failure syndrome in hospital ≥ 2 mm ST segment depression at peak heart rate ≤ 135 beats/min High-grade ventricular ectopy

(From *Guidelines for Cardiac Rehabilitation Programs* (p. 5) by American Association of Cardiovascular and Pulmonary Rehabilitation, Champaign, IL: Human Kinetics Publishers. Copyright 1991 by American Association of Cardiovascular and Pulmonary Rehabilitation. Reprinted by permission.)
Note: 1 MET = 3.5 mL O_2/kg/min.
Abbreviation: EF = ejection fraction.

3. **Phase III.** This is an extended, supervised outpatient program, 4 to 6 months post cardiac incident.
   a. *Patient eligibility.* Phase III cardiac rehabilitation is usually a non–hospital-based community rehabilitation program. Patients in this phase may have participated in both phase I and phase II cardiac rehabilitation programs or may enter this phase with no prior involvement in an organized program. Depending on the entry requirements of the facility and the personnel involved, patients with varying levels of cardiac involvement may participate. As a rule, patients are usually 3 to 6 months post cardiac incident and have at least one of the following:
      (1). Clinically stable or decreasing angina.
      (2). Medically controlled arrhythmias during exercise.
      (3). Knowledge of signs and symptoms of cardiac disease.
      (4). An established exercise prescription.
      (5). An ability to self-regulate exercise.
      (6). A minimal functional capacity of 6 METs.
   b. *Treatment objectives.* Table 6–27 shows a 16-step walk-jog program. Objectives of this phase of cardiac rehabilitation are maintenance of function, compliance with an exercise program, and risk factor education and modification. Depending on the complexity of the patient profile, phase III may last for several months. Patients frequently remain in a program of this nature for up to 1 year to achieve initial goals and establish compliance.

Patients may be moved up and down through any level of the exercise program as the disease progresses, regresses, or remains the same. Certain "high-risk" patients will remain high risk and still achieve moderate success.[29] These supervised programs allow exercise to be performed at a low risk of major complications. Contributing to the low risk rates are the current guidelines of cardiac rehabilitation, which include appropriate patient selection for exercise programs; concurrent medical, surgical, and pharmacological therapies; patient education; careful exercise prescription; and patient monitoring.[29] Well-trained rehabilitation specialists from various disciplines with the ability to deal with cardiac emergencies quickly and skillfully have enhanced the safety of these programs.[29]

Table 6–27. SIXTEEN-STEP WALK AND WALK-JOG PROGRAM FOR CARDIAC PATIENTS IN PHASE III (COMMUNITY-BASED OR HOME) EXERCISE PROGRAM

Functional Capacity (METs)	Step	Speed* (mph)	Duration (min)	METs	METs (Average/Workout)	Energy Expenditure (kcal/min)
5 METs	1	2.5	30–60	2.5	2.5	3.0
	2	3.0	30–60	3.0	3.0	3.7
	3	3.25	30–60	3.25	3.25	4.0
5–8 METs	4	3.5	30–60	3.5	3.5	4.2
	5	3.75	30–60	4.0	4.0	4.9
	6	4.0	30–60	4.6	4.6	5.5
8 METs	7	3.75 (2 min)	30–45	4.0	4.6	4.9
		5.0 (30 s)		6.9		8.3
	8	3.75 (2 min)	30–45	4.0	5.0	4.9
		5.0 (1 min)		6.9		8.3
	9	3.75 (2 min)	30–45	4.0	5.5	4.9
		5.0 (2 min)		6.9		8.3
	10	3.75 (1 min)	30–45	4.0	6.0	4.9
		5.0 (2 min)		6.9		8.3
	11	3.75 (1 min)	30–45	4.0	6.3	4.9
		5.0 (4 min)		6.9		8.3
	12	3.75 (1 min)	30–45	4.0	6.5	4.9
		5.0 (6 min)		6.9		8.3
	13	3.75 (1 min)	30–45	4.0	6.6	4.9
		5.0 (8 min)		6.9		8.3
	14	3.75 (1 min)	30–45	4.0	6.6	4.9
		5.0 (10 min)		6.9		8.3
	15	3.75 (1 min)	30–45	4.0	7.9	4.9
		5.5 (10 min)		8.3		10.1
	16	3.75 (1 min)	30–45	4.0	8.0	4.9
		5.5 (12 min)		8.3		10.1

(From Pollock ML, Schmidt D: *Heart Disease and Rehabilitation.* New York, John Wiley, 1986.)

*Two lines denote interval training; *eg,* in step 7, the patient will alternate 2 min of walking at 3.75 mph with 30 s of jogging at 5.0 mph.

VIII. Principles of Exercise Prescription

A. Prescription

The exercise prescription is the cornerstone of any exercise program. This prescription should include[9]

1. Type of exercise
2. Intensity
3. Duration
4. Frequency
5. Progression of activity

B. Safety factors

The safety of an exercise prescription for an individual is best determined by

1. Heart rate
2. ECG
3. Blood pressure
4. Rate of perceived exertion (RPE)
5. VO_2max and METs obtained from a graded exercise test.

Table 6–28 gives examples of patient characteristics associated with exercise related to cardiovascular complications.

C. Mode of exercise

Cardiac rehabilitation programs use aerobic activity to promote the physiological adaptions of training mentioned earlier. Any rhythmical activity that uses large muscle mass for a sustained period of time is classified as aerobic. This type of exercise requires the body to provide a balance between the amount of oxygen delivered to the working muscles and the amount of oxygen used by the working muscles for a given period of time. Exercise should be chosen on the basis of

1. Patient preference.
2. Skill required for proper performance.
3. Potential for carryover at home.
4. Availability of exercise equipment.

Table 6-28. PATIENT CHARACTERISTICS
ASSOCIATED WITH
EXERCISE-RELATED
CARDIOVASCULAR
COMPLICATIONS

Category	Characteristic
Clinical status	Multiple myocardial infarctions Impaired left ventricular function (ejection fraction < 30%) Rest or unstable angina pectoris Serious arrhythmias at rest High-grade left anterior descending lesions and/or significant ($\geq$ 75% occlusion) multivessel atherosclerosis on angiography Low serum potassium
Exercise training participation	Disregard for appropriate warm-up and cooldown Consistently exceeds prescribed training heart rate
Exercise test data	Low or high exercise tolerance ($\leq$ 4 METs or $\geq$ 10 METs) Chronotropic impairment off drugs (< 120 beats/min) Inotropic impairment (decrease in systolic blood pressure with increasing workloads) Myocardial ischemia (angina and/or ST segment depression $\geq$ 0.2 mV) Serious cardiac arrhythmias (especially in patients with impaired left ventricular function)
Other	Cigarette smoker Male gender

(From *Guidelines for Cardiac Rehabilitation Programs* (p. 39) by American Association of Cardiovascular and Pulmonary Rehabilitation, Champaign, IL: Human Kinetics Publishers. Copyright 1991 by American Association of Cardiovascular and Pulmonary Rehabilitation. Reprinted by permission.)

5. Ability to increase the intensity of the activity gradually as training occurs.

ARM EXERCISE IN CARDIAC REHABILITATION

An area that has generated much controversy is the role of arm exercise in cardiac rehabilitation programs. In the past, arm exercises were prohibited because of concerns about possible adverse hemodynamic effects. Researchers have demonstrated the feasibility, safety, and effectiveness of cardiovascular training using arm ergometry in selected cardiac patients.[30] The prevalence of arrhythmias during upper extremity training is reported to be no greater than during lower extremity training. Exercise training for activities of daily living and for many preferred vocational and recreational activities that require upper extremity exercise can be safely incorporated into a cardiac rehabilitation program (see Table 6–29).

D. Exercise intensity

The most difficult aspect of designing an exercise program is the establishment of the appropriate exercise intensity. The intensity must ensure that the proper percentage of functional capacity for a given individual is achieved and maintained for the aerobic period.

The American College of Sports Medicine identifies three methods with which to establish an exercise intensity (see box).

  a. ***Exercise by METs*** The intensity of exercise may be prescribed by METs. One MET is the rate of oxygen consumed by a seated individual at rest ($\dot{V}o_2$rest) and is approximately 3.5 mL of O_2/kg/min. Average MET requirements have been calculated for a variety of common activities (see Table 6–22). It is advisable to begin an exercise program with an initial target range of 50% to 60% of maximally achieved METs on a graded exercise test.

Table 6-29. WEIGHT-TRAINING
GUIDELINES FOR LOW-RISK
CARDIAC PATIENTS

- To prevent soreness and injury, initially choose a weight that will allow the performance of 12 to 15 repetitions comfortably, corresponding to approximately 30%–50% of the maximum weight load that can be lifted in one repetition. (Note: Selected stable, aerobically trained cardiac patients may eventually use loads corresponding to a more traditional program of weight training [ie, 60%–80% of one maximum repetition])
- Perform one to three sets of each exercise.
- Avoid straining. Ratings of perceived exertion (6–20 scale) should not exceed fairly light to somewhat hard during lifting.
- Exhale (blow out) during the exertion phase of the lift. For example, exhale when pushing a weight stack overhead and inhale when lowering it.
- Increase weight loads by 5 to 10 lb when 12 to 15 repetitions can be comfortably accomplished.
- Raise weights with slow, controlled movements; emphasize complete extension of the limbs when lifting.
- Exercise large muscle groups before small muscle groups. Include devices (exercises) for the upper and lower extremities.
- Weight-train at least two to three times per week.
- Loosely hold hand grips when possible; sustained, tight gripping may evoke an excessive blood pressure response to lifting.
- Stop exercise in the event of warning signs or symptoms, especially dizziness, arrhythmias, unusual shortness of breath, and/or angina pectoris.
- Allow minimal rest periods between exercises (eg, 30–60 s) to maximize muscular endurance and aerobic training benefits.

(From *Guidelines for Cardiac Rehabilitation Programs* (p. 11) by American Association of Cardiovascular and Pulmonary Rehabilitation, Champaign, IL: Human Kinetics Publishers. Copyright 1991 by American Association of Cardiovascular and Pulmonary Rehabilitation. Reprinted by permission.)

As training effects are demonstrated, the target range can be increased to 70% of maximum MET level. The initial training intensity for elderly individuals might begin at as low as 40% of their maximum MET level.

To prescribe exercise intensity by METs, the individual may select activities for training that are known to require energy expenditures within the target range. For example, a 63-year-old man is referred to physical therapy for cardiac rehabilitation. His maximum MET level on the graded exercise test is 8 (28 mL O_2/kg/min). Because he is beginning an exercise program for the first time, we have chosen 50% to 60% of his maximum capacity for his training intensity:

$$8 \text{ METs} \times (0.50-0.60) = 4-4.8 \text{ METs}$$

A recreational activity equal to 4 to 4.8 METs might be cycling 8 mph or walking 3 mph.

b. *Exercise by Heart Rate* To prescribe exercise by heart rate, the individual's actual maximal heart rate (HRmax) must be established. The actual HRmax is the highest rate safely achieved on a graded exercise test. When exercise testing is not possible, an estimate of HRmax can be calculated. For lower extremity work, the formula is 220 − the patient's age. For upper extremity work, the formula is 220 − the patient's age − 11. This HRmax is then multiplied by a percentage (usually 70% to 85%) to determine the target heart rate range.

A 63-year-old man is referred to physical therapy for cardiac rehabilitation. No graded exercise test result is available. He has an estimated HRmax for lower extremity exercise of 220 − 63, or 157. He is to be exercising at 70% to 85% of his HRmax, so his target heart rate is calculated to be 110 to 133 beats/min.

By using a graded exercise test and acquiring an actual HRmax, the safety of the patient's exercise is certain. Predicted heart rates do not provide any information on the patient's cardiovascular response to exercise and should always be used with caution.

A second method commonly used to determine target heart rate is the Karvonen formula. In this case, the difference between the resting and the maximal heart rates is multiplied by the same percentages used to determine the target heart rate range in METs, and then resting heart rate is added:

Target HR = (maximal HR − resting HR) × (MET%) + resting HR

The same 63-year-old man, *eg*, has a resting heart rate of 70 beats/min. On a graded exercise test, he safely obtained an HRmax of 160 beats/min. Therefore,

$$\text{Target HR} = (160-70) \times (50\%-60\%) + 70 = 115-124 \text{ beats/min}$$

c. *Exercise by Rate of Perceived Exertion* Borg's RPE scale has been shown to be of benefit in evaluating a subject's response to exercise intensity.[31] This numerical scale is designed to estimate an individual's subjective response to exertion (see Table 6–30). Studies have demonstrated a linear relationship between heart rate and RPE in response to increasing intensities.[32] The RPE can be used as a means of establishing an exercise program's intensity.

The RPE selection may be more psychological than physiological. A plausible explanation is that anxiety is the patient's learned response and ultimately has a

Table 6–30. BORG'S ORIGINAL RATE OF PERCEIVED EXERTION SCALE AND REVISED SCALE

RPE		Borg CR-10 Scale	
6		0	
7	Very, very light	0.5	Very, very weak
8		1	Very weak
9	Very light	2	Weak
10		3	Moderate
11	Fairly light	4	
12		5	Strong
13	Somewhat hard	6	
14		7	Very strong
15	Hard	8	
16		9	
17	Very hard	10	
18			Maximal
19	Very, very hard		
20			
© Gunnar Borg, 1985		© Gunnar Borg, 1981, 1982	

(Left side from Borg G: An Introduction to Borg's RPE Scale. Ithaca: Mouvement Publications, 1985. Right side from Borg G, Holmgren A, Lindblad I: Quantitative evaluation of chest pain. *Acta Med Scand* 1981, 644(Suppl):45.)

negative effect on heart rate. The net result is a higher perception of exertion than the exercise intensity should produce. New patients who are not used to exercising may initially report higher RPE than predicted. With habitual exercise and continued use of the RPE scale, participants become quite accurate at predicting their exercising heart rates based on their RPE.

Although heart rate may be the most objective and accurate monitoring parameter for exercise performance, patients are forced to rely on equipment that only the rehabilitation program can offer, or they must frequently stop exercising to take their heart rate. The use of the RPE scale allows an individual to concentrate more on how a particular intensity of exercise feels yet have some assurance that he or she is within the target heart rate range. This ability to use the RPE scale makes it easier for patients to be independent in their own activity and to wean patients off external monitoring equipment.

The Borg RPE scale originally used a scale of 6 to 20. The American College of Sports Medicine recommends that a scale of 1 to 10 is more readily learned by patients in a rehabilitation program and should be instituted.[33] Table 6–30 compares the scales.

E. Exercise duration

A cardiac rehabilitation program usually begins with a warm-up period that lasts from 5 to 15 minutes. The activities are slowly progressive in intensity to prepare the individual for the more strenuous activity of the aerobic period to come. The beneficial effects of a warm-up period have been documented.[34] Proper stretching during the warm-up period reduces the incidence of musculoskeletal injuries. Slowly intensifying exercises allows the cardiovascular and musculoskeletal systems to accommodate to the increments of activity.

The period of aerobic training should begin at 15 minutes and build to 30 to 45 minutes of continuous aerobic activity. By keeping the initial exercise period under 30 minutes, the participants may be more able to avoid musculoskeletal injuries.

The aerobic training period must be imme-

diately followed by a cool-down period. Five to 15 minutes of low-level activities allows the heart rate and blood pressure to return slowly to near pre-exercise levels. If vigorous exercise is stopped abruptly, circulating blood pools in the veins of the lower extremities and causes a decrease in cardiac output, a concomitant decrease in blood pressure and coronary perfusion, and an increased potential for arrhythmias. A cool-down period of generally decreasing intensity of exercise, similar to the warm-up activities, provides a safe completion of the aerobic activity session and enhances the removal of any lactic acid (metabolic waste) that may cause muscle soreness after exercise.[34]

F. Frequency of activity

Frequency of activity refers to the number of sessions performed on a weekly basis during the exercise training period. At the onset of an exercise program, it is generally recommended that aerobic activity be performed no more than three times per week, with no more than a 2-day lapse between training sessions.[9] With an increasing frequency of exercise, participants are more likely to sustain injuries and run the long-term risk of interrupting their training schedule. For persons with low exercise intensity (ie, 3 to 5 METs), however, daily activity can be considered. If the exercise intensity is less than 3 METs, twice-daily exercise should be recommended.[34]

G. Rate of progression

Modifications in the duration and intensity level of the exercise session should occur as the individual shows physiological adaptations to exercise. For the patient with coronary artery disease, exercise progression is appropriate when the individual perceives the intensity of the exercise session to be easier, when the heart rate is lower for the same exercise intensity, and when the clinical symptoms of cardiac disease do not appear at the usual intensity or do not appear until a higher exercise intensity is achieved.

As the patient progresses, the exercise duration should first be increased by extending the amount of time in the aerobic session rather than by any change in the intensity of the activity.

As a conditioning effect occurs, adjustments of the prescription of physically active partici-

Table 6–31. EDUCATIONAL TOPICS FOR CARDIAC REHABILITATION

1. Risk factors associated with coronary artery disease.
2. Anatomy and physiology of the heart: What is a heart attack?
3. Angina: What is chest pain?
4. Relation of diet to heart disease.
5. Diet and weight control.
6. Human sexuality and coronary artery disease.
7. Stress and stress management.
8. Cigarette smoking in relation to heart disease.
9. Drugs used in the management of heart disease and their relationship to exercise.

(Reprinted from In Touch Series: *Management of Individuals with Cardiac Dysfunction.* Lesson 9. Alexandria, VA, with the permission of the American Physical Therapy Association.)

pants can be made with little fear of personal risk. Modifying an exercise prescription for sedentary; elderly; concomitant disease individuals or symptomatic individuals necessitates more caution. For these populations, the degree of risk involved in exercise is a function of the interaction of age, functional capacity, symptoms, and severity of the disease.[34] When a considerable change in the participant's ability has occurred, it is advisable to perform a new graded exercise test. These new data allow a new exercise prescription and safe progression of exercise under the most controlled guidance. If a second graded exercise test is not possible, careful monitoring of the updated exercise prescription along with patient input can provide the necessary feedback for a safe and effective program.

PLEASE NOTE: These principles of exercise apply to the development of exercise programs for persons of any age or functional capacity

in the absence or presence of disease. The major differences in prescribing exercise programs for specific populations are how the principles of frequency, intensity, duration, and rate of progression are adjusted to meet the needs of the individual.

H. Other components of the exercise program

1. **Patient education.** Education is an integral aspect of cardiac rehabilitation. To enhance compliance with exercise and behavioral changes necessary to cardiac health, the educational program instructs patients and families in all aspects of cardiac care. Table 6–31 lists topics often presented during cardiac rehabilitation.
2. **Monitoring patients during exercise.** Current cardiac rehabilitation practice allows prescribed, supervised exercise by patients to be performed at a low risk of major complications.[29] Physical therapists monitor patients during the exercise portion of the rehabilitation program to ensure safety. There is usually a check-in period before the beginning of the exercise session that includes the patient's weight, resting heart rate, blood pressure, and ECG assessment and a quick check to ensure that proper medications have been taken. During the exercise session, cardiac activity is monitored in a variety of ways. Blood pressure may be evaluated at regular intervals. ECG telemetry or hard-wired electrocardiographic equipment gives continuous feedback to the physical therapist on the status of patients in the rehabilitation group. Table 6–26 gives guidelines for risk stratification for monitoring patients. Table 6–32 lists the type of monitoring performed in cardiac rehabilitation programs.

Table 6–32. CARDIOVASCULAR COMPLICATIONS OF CARDIAC REHABILITATION PROGRAMS WITH DIFFERING EXTENTS OF ELECTROCARDIOGRAPHIC MONITORING

Type of Electrocardiographic Monitoring Used During Exercise Sessions	Programs	Patients	Patient-Hours	Cardiac Arrests	Fatalities	Myocardial Infarctions
Continuous	97	28,879	888,460	9 (10.1)*	0	4 (4.5)
Intermittent	57	12,863	1,246,111	9 (7.2)	2 (1.6)	3 (2.4)
Graduated	13	9,561	217,345	3 (13.8)	1 (4.6)	1 (4.6)
Total	167†	51,303	2,351,916	21 (8.9)	3 (1.3)	8 (3.4)
χ^2 value‡				1.13	3.12	0.77
P value				.56	.21	.68

(From Van Camp S, Peterson R: Cardiovascular complications of outpatient cardiac rehabilitation program. *JAMA* 1986; 256:1160–1163. Copyright 1986, American Medical Association.)

* Values in parentheses represent event incidence per million patient-hours.
† From 142 cardiac rehabilitation centers.
‡ Degree of freedom for all χ^2 values equals 2.

Table 6–33. CLASSIFICATION OF CARDIAC DRUGS

1. Antianginal agents
2. Antihypertensive agents
3. Digitalis glycosides and derivatives
4. Anticoagulant agents
5. Antilipidemic agents
6. Antiarrhythmic agents

(Reprinted from In Touch Series: *Management of Individuals with Cardiac Dysfunction.* Lesson 9. Alexandria, VA, with the permission of the American Physical Therapy Association.)

3. **Drug intervention.** Pharmacology plays a critical role in the medical management of all patient populations. This is especially true in the management of patients with cardiovascular disease. A wide spectrum of medications are as much a part of daily life for these patients as is exercise (see Table 6–33). Clinicians must be familiar with the commonly prescribed medications (see Table 6–34), including their indications, side effects, and hemodynamic responses at rest and with exercise. This knowledge will allow the clinician to accurately assess the patient's response to medication during functional activities and ex-

ercise (see Table 6–35). Many patients who have cardiovascular medication prescribed have other coexisting medical diagnoses that require medication. Therapists must know the influence of all medications on the hemodynamic responses as well as drug interactions.

The physical therapist must discern whether a change in a patient's exercise performance is the result of an adjustment in medication or reflective of an alteration in functional capacity. True increases in a patient's functional capacity caused by training may allow for modulation in drug dosages. In either case, the patient's exercise prescription may require an update or adjustment.

A critical component of the rehabilitation program is to educate patients about prescribed medications. This includes individual instruction and formal lectures on

- List of cardiac drugs.
- Purposes of cardiac drugs.
- Any special instructions.
- The effects on exercise.
- Any possible side effects.
- When drug issues should be reported to their physician.

Table 6–34. CARDIAC MEDICATIONS

I. Antianginal agents
  A. Nitroglycerin-related compounds
    1. Action: Smooth muscle relaxation
    2. Uses: Decrease in afterload, preload, cardiac output
    3. Side effects: Hypotension, dizziness, headaches, flushing, nausea, vomiting
    4. Drug names: Inhaled—amyl nitrate, sublingual—nitroglycerin, oral—Isordil, cutaneous—transdermal
  B. Beta blockers
    1. Action: Block beta receptors, decrease sympathetic tone
    2. Uses: Decrease heart rate, contractility, cardiac output, blood pressure
    3. Side effects: Bradycardia, heart block, congestive heart failure, pulmonary hypertension, bronchospasm
    4. Drug names: Inderal, atenolol, Lopressor, Corgard, Biocadren
  C. Calcium antagonists
    1. Action: Block influx of calcium ion concentration
    2. Uses: Vasodilate; decrease contractility, heart rate, blood pressure
    3. Side effects: Dizziness, syncope, flushing, hypotension, headache
    4. Drug names: Verapamil, nifedipine
II. Antihypertensive agents
  A. Diuretics
    1. Action: Inhibit Na^{++} and Cl^- within kidney
    2. Uses: Contraction of plasma volume, decrease blood pressure and preload
    3. Side effects: K^+ potassium ion depletion, hypovolemia
    4. Drug names: Thiazides, furosemides (Lasix), Aldactone
  B. Vasodilators
    1. Action: Smooth muscle relaxation, dilation
    2. Uses: Decrease blood pressure and afterload
    3. Side effects: Increase heart rate and contractility
    4. Drug names: Hydralazine, captopril, minoxidil
  C. Drugs interfering with sympathetic nervous system
    1. Action: Smooth muscle relaxation
    2. Uses: Decrease blood pressure, heart rate, and cardiac output
    3. Side effects: Orthostatic hypotension, dizziness
    4. Drug names: reserpine, propranolol, Aldomet, Catapres, Minipress

Table 6–34.   CARDIAC MEDICATIONS *Continued*

III. Digitalis glycosides and derivatives
 A. Action: Improve myocardial contractility
 B. Uses: Alter Ca^{++} utilization by myocardial cells
 C. Side effects: Alter ECG, arrhythmias, heart block
 D. Drug names: Digoxin, lanoxin, digitoxin
IV. Anticoagulant agents
 A. Sodium warfarin (Coumadin)
  1. Action: Inhibits synthesis of clotting factors
  2. Side effects: Takes days to maximize; bleeding
 B. Sodium heparin
  1. Action: Inactivates thrombin, prevents conversion of fibrinogen to fibrin
  2. Side effects: Bleeding
 C. Aspirin
  1. Action: Blocks production of thromboxane A2
  2. Side effects: Gastrointestinal (GI) distress, ulcers, drug interaction
 D. Persantine
  1. Action: Blocks platelet aggregation
  2. Side effects: GI distress, headache, dizziness
V. Antilipidemic agents
 A. Action: Increase excretion of bile acids
 B. Uses: Decrease in serum cholesterol
 C. Side effects: Intestinal obstruction, glucose intolerance, hyperuricemia, hepatotoxia
 D. Drug names: Cholestyramine, Lopid, niacin, Atromid-S
VI. Antiarrhythmic agents
 A. Action: Decrease Na^+ conductance and velocity of conduction
  1. Drug names: Procain, quinidine, Norpace
  2. Side effects: Fever, GI disturbance, increase in serum digitalis level
 B. Increase K^+ conductance, decrease conduction velocity
  1. Drug names: Lidocaine, Dilantin
  2. Side effects: Central nervous system; psychosis
 C. Beta blockers
  1. Drug names: Propranolol, metaprolol, atenolol
  2. Side effects: Fatigue, depression, bronchospasm, impotence
 D. Antiadrenergic
  1. Drug name: Bretylium tosylate
 E. Calcium antagonists
  1. Drug names: Verapamil, nifedipine

Table 6–35.   EFFECT OF DRUG INTERVENTIONS ON EXERCISE RESPONSES

Effect	Medication	Effect	Medication
May increase heart rate	Isoproterenol	May increase blood pressure	Bronchodilators: epinephrine, aminophylline
	Quinidine and procainamide		Nasal sprays, decongestants, Neo-Synephrine
	Bronchodilators and drugs for asthma		
	Thyroid-synthroid, thyroid USP	May increase exercise capacity	Nitrates
	Apresoline		β-Adrenergic blockers
May decrease heart rate	Propranolol and other beta-blocking agents		Digitalis: Lanoxin, digitoxin
	Reserpine	May increase cardiac contractility	Digitalis
	Some antihypertensives (*eg,* guanethidine, Aldomet)		Isoproterenol
			Aminophylline-type drugs
May decrease blood pressure	Aldomet	May decrease cardiac contractility	Propranolol and other beta blockers
	Apresoline		Procainamide and other antidysrhythmics
	Propranolol		
	Diuretics		
	Nitrates		

(From Cohen M, Hoskins T: *Cardiopulmonary Symptoms in Physical Therapy Practice.* New York, Churchill Livingstone, 1988, p 93.)

Table 6–36. SAMPLE DRUG CARD AVAILABLE FOR REHABILITATION PATIENTS

Inderal

Purpose:	Inderal is a very important drug. It acts in a way that decreases the work on the heart by causing the heart to beat at a slower, more regular rate, thus reducing the heart's requirement for oxygen. Inderal is used to a. help your heart beat regularly b. lower your blood pressure c. control angina attacks
Special instructions:	a. Inderal should be taken at regular intervals during the waking hours, preferably before each meal and at bedtime. b. While on Inderal, you should take your pulse every morning on rising and also weigh yourself every morning. c. It is important that you **do not stop, increase, or decrease** your dosage of Inderal without consulting your doctor.
Side effects to report to your doctor:	a. Nausea, vomiting b. diarrhea, constipation c. lightheadedness d. fatigue e. change in sexual functioning f. resting pulse below 50 g. unusual swelling of the ankles or unusual weight gain

(Reprinted from In Touch Series: *Management of Individuals with Cardiac Dysfunction.* Lesson 9. Alexandria, VA, with the permission of the American Physical Therapy Association.)

Table 6-37. SUGGESTED EFFICACY MEASURES FOR PROGRAM EVALUATION

Program	Efficacy Measures
Patient education program for recent heart surgery and for recent diagnosis of CAD/MI or its nonsurgical treatment	Percentage of participants completing program? Percentage of sessions attended? Percentage improvement in pre- versus post-test knowledge? Percentage answers correct on post-test? Percentage of participants returning to self-care activities at similar or improved level of performance within 1 mo? 3 mo ? 6 mo post hospital discharge? Percentage of participants returning to sexual activity at similar or improved level of performance within 1 mo? 3 mo? 6 mo post hospital discharge? Average participant score on level of understanding pre and post program? Average difference? Average participant score on level of adaptation at similar or improved level of performance within 1 mo? 3 mo? 6 mo post hospital discharge?
Individual exercise program	In hospital: Percentage of patients participating in minimum of one? three? five total exercise sessions? Percentage of patients who demonstrated functional improvements (progressed ambulation) during participation in the exercise program? Percentage of exercise sessions in which exertion-related complications required medical attention for the patient? Average number of sessions attended per patient? Average number of education sessions attended per patient? Post–hospital discharge maintenance: Percentage of participants completing program? Percentage of the total sessions attended? Percentage of participants exercising a minimum of three times per week (at home or in a structured program)? Percentage of patients increasing functional capacity after 3 mo and at 1 yr? Average change? Percentage of participants achieving a high, medium, or low fitness level based on national standards for age and gender? Percentage of patients who experienced orthopedic and/or musculoskeletal complications? Percentage of participants who withdrew from the program because of the new onset of symptoms of congestive heart failure or the worsening of baseline status in patients with congestive heart failure? Percentage of participants who experienced cardiac arrest? New or worse angina? New or worse ECG changes? Inappropriate hemodynamic responses? Percentage of participants who withdrew from program due to cardiac arrest? New or worse angina? New or worse ECG changes? Inappropriate hemodynamic responses?

Program	Efficacy Measures
	Percentage of patients who withdrew from program because of the new onset of symptoms of congestive heart failure or worsening baseline status in congestive heart failure patients?
	Percentage of participants who were successfully treated and completed program following cardiac arrest? New or worse angina? New or worse ECG changes? Inappropriate hemodynamic responses?
	Average level of behavior acceptance pre and post program? Average difference?
	Average level of behavior compliance pre and post program? Average difference?
Smoking cessation program	Percentage of participants completing program?
	Percentage of participants who dropped out at 3 mo? 6 mo? 1 yr? Percentage of participants who reduced their smoking at 3 mo? 6 mo? 1 yr? Average reduction?
	Average level of behavior acceptance preprogram to 3 mo? 6 mo? 1 yr? Average difference?
	Average level of behavior compliance preprogram to 3 mo? 6 mo? 1 yr? Average difference?
Lipid modification program	Percentage of participants who completed the program? Percentage of participants utilizing lipid-lowering medications? Frequency of adverse side effects? Percentage of participants with and without medications who reduced their lipid levels at 3 mo? 6 mo? 1 yr?
	Percentage of participants following National Cholesterol Education Program (NCEP) Step-One diet? Percentage of participants following NCEP Step-Two diet?
	Average entry total cholesterol, LDL, HDL, and triglycerides? Average exit total cholesterol, LDL, HDL, and triglycerides?
	Average change per participant at 3 mo? 6 mo? 1 yr? Percentage of participants who achieved NCEP goals at 3 mo? 6 mo? 1 yr?
	Frequency of patients experiencing adverse or limiting side effects from lipid-lowering medications?
	Average level of behavior acceptance preprogram to 3 mo? 6 mo? 1 yr? Average difference?
	Average level of behavior compliance preprogram to 3 mo? 6 mo? 1 yr? Average difference?
Hypertension management program	Percentage of participants completing the program?
	Percentage of participants who reduced medication at 3 mo? 6 mo? 1 yr? Percentage of participants who eliminated their medication at 3 mo? 6 mo? 1 yr? Percentage of participants who achieved National High Blood Pressure Education Program recommendations at 3 mo? 6 mo? 1 yr?
	Frequency of patients experiencing adverse or limiting side effects from antihypertension medications?
	Average level of behavior acceptance preprogram to 3 mo? 6 mo? 1 yr? Average difference?
Weight reduction program	Percentage of participants who completed the program? Percentage of patients maintaining initial weight loss at 3 mo? 6 mo? 1 yr?
	Percentage of participants who achieved their weight goal within 3 mo? 6 mo? 1 yr?
	Percentage of patients who have body weights $\geq$ 30% of desirable body weight?
	Average level of behavior acceptance preprogram to 3 mo? 6 mo? 1 yr? Average difference?
	Average level of behavior compliance preprogram to 3 mo? 6 mo? 1 yr? Average difference?
Stress management program	Percentage of participants completing the program?
	Percentage of participants reporting a significant reduction of stress at 3 mo? 6 mo? 1 yr?
	Average level of behavior acceptance preprogram to 3 mo? 6 mo? 1 yr? Average difference?
	Average level of behavior compliance preprogram to 3 mo? 6 mo? 1 yr? Average difference?
Diabetic program	Percentage of participants completing the program?
	Percentage of participants maintaining glucose control within American Diabetes Association (ADA) guidelines at 1 mo? 3 mo? 1 yr?
	Percentage of participants maintaining fasting blood glucose within ADA guidelines at 1 mo? 3 mo? 1 yr?
	Percentage of participants reducing medication dosage after 3 mo? 6 mo? 1 yr?
	Average level of behavior acceptance preprogram to 3 mo? 6 mo? 1 yr? Average difference?
	Average level of behavior compliance preprogram to 3 mo? 6 mo? 1 yr? Average difference?

See Table 6–36 for a sample educational drug card.

Beta blockers and calcium channel blockers are two common classifications of drugs used in the management of cardiac disease. Although the mechanisms of each of these drugs differ, the net result is a decrease in heart rate, myocardial oxygen consumption, and cardiac work. Studies have demonstrated that $\dot{V}O_2max$ is altered with the use of these drugs.[35,36] Patients taking these medications can still acquire the physiological adaptation of training with an exercise prescription based on their graded exercise test.

For patients taking medications that alter heart rate, exercise prescription based on target heart rate alone is ineffective and perhaps an inappropriate means of evaluating the level of exercise intensity performed. The use of the RPE scale to assess a person's sense of effort or feeling of exertion to a given exercise intensity may be more accurate and should be used.[33,37,38]

Finally, the Cardiac Rehabilitation Guidelines suggest that efficacy measures should be implemented at each component of the program. Table 6–37 lists the recommended efficacy measures.

IX. Special Considerations for Exercise

A. Elderly patients

It is well known that elderly individuals have decreased ventricular compliance, less total muscular mass, and musculoskeletal instability (see Table 6–38).[39,40] These individuals have a decreased aerobic capacity, and even submaximal levels of exercise are perceived as difficult and induce shortness of breath. To improve functional capacity and to ensure safety of the elderly patient, exercise based on a graded exercise test must be judiciously prescribed.

The components of an exercise session should include a warm-up phase that is considerably longer than previously discussed. For these individuals, gentle and thorough stretching to accommodate their musculoskeletal system and a slowly increasing intensity of warm-up exercises to benefit their cardiopulmonary system are advisable.

The aerobic phase of the program should include the use of large muscle groups at a prescribed intensity, frequency, and duration. Activities should be aerobic and low impact in nature. Walking, bicycling, walking-jogging, and swimming may be used for training. An adjunct to these activities might be arm ergometry to maintain upper body muscle mass (see Table 6–29).

Aerobic conditioning can occur at 50% to 85% of maximal oxygen uptake, but in the case of sedentary elderly individuals, especially those with concomitant cardiac complications, exercise intensity may be initiated as low as 30% to 40% of $\dot{V}O_2max$. By increasing the frequency, a training effect may still be achieved.[34]

Table 6–38. PHYSIOLOGICAL CHANGES DURING AGING

Structural Changes	Functional Result	Sign	Symptom
↓ Elastic tissue in vascular media	↑ Vascular stiffness	↑ Systolic blood pressure	±
Left ventricular hypertrophy ↑ myocardial connective tissue	↓ Ventricular compliance	↑ LV end diastolic pressure at rest and with exercise	Dyspnea
↓ Adrenergic responsiveness	↓ Heart rate with exercise	Orthostatic hypotension, ↓ $\dot{V}O_2max$	Postural dizziness, fatigue
	↓ Contractility with exercise ↓ Heart rate response to upright posture		
↓ Lean body mass	↓ Muscle strength	↓ Exercise time ↓ $\dot{V}O_2max$	Fatigue, weakness

(From Balady G, Weiner D: Exercise testing in healthy elderly subjects and elderly patients with cardiac disease. *J Cardiopulmonary Rehabil,* 1989, 9:36.)

The cool-down period should be slow and rhythmical. Elderly patients require an extended cool-down phase to recover to their baseline heart rate.

Modifications of any exercise program should be based on clinical signs and symptoms. For the elderly patient with cardiac disease, a supervised, telemetry-monitored program is advisable initially. Periodic updates of exercise prescriptions will keep the program safe and effective.

All of the positive effects of exercise achieved by younger individuals can be attained by the elderly population. In addition, regular exercise programs will contribute to a sense of well-being and confidence for independent living. As we look ahead to the increasing number of elderly persons and the ramifications of their health care, the need to promote wellness in this population cannot be overlooked.

B. Children and adolescents

The life span of individuals with congenital cardiac defects has greatly increased owing to the many advancements in medical, surgical, and pharmacological management. Many of these individuals now reach adulthood and live full lives, including parenthood. With present knowledge and careful medical management, many of these children and adolescents, even those at "higher risk," are able to participate in physical activity.[41] Regardless of the particular diagnosis, careful screening and an appropriate exercise prescription are the keys to successful physical activity participation.

For individuals with arrhythmias, telemetry monitoring initially is suggested.

Fatigue is a common symptom for many of these individuals regardless of the defect or diagnosis. This may or may not be reflective of ventricular dysfunction. Therefore, careful monitoring of heart rate and blood pressure, especially diastolic pressure, will give important feedback regarding the appropriateness of the exercise prescription.

For many of these diagnoses, when prophylaxis is combined with prevention practices and regular physical activity, a reduction in the number of cardiac incidences can be achieved.

As with any other group with special considerations, adherence to the principles suggested for exercise in the elderly patient, the patient with chronic ventricular failure or systemic hypertension, and even the transplant patient applies to these growing individuals. Critical to the success of this group is the individualization of the exercise prescription given the particular physical activity (mode) desired.

C. Unstable angina

Patients with unstable angina are often at great risk during exercise. There is little correlation between the adaptation of the cardiac system to exercise and their perception of angina. The usual telemetry ECG monitoring is not effective in showing the onset of ischemic cardiac changes found during exercise. For these individuals, the strict enforcement of target heart rate based on a graded exercise test is necessary. Keeping a patient's exercising heart rate below that which is known to cause ischemic changes is the safest way to exercise this patient population. Exercising during an angina attack is extremely hazardous and should be strongly discouraged.

D. Pacemakers

Patients with pacemakers are frequently paced at a fixed heart rate. Although heart rate may not change, stroke volume and, therefore, cardiac output can change to allow exercise to progress. This poses a problem for monitoring exercise performance but not for performing exercise. Using the RPE scale is an excellent means of evaluating the exercise response in patients with pacemakers.

E. Chronic ventricular failure

The potential benefits and role of exercise training in the management of patients with chronic congestive failure or cardiomyopathy are uncertain. There is no question that peripheral deconditioning and severe limitation of activity are detrimental to functional capacity. Very low levels of intermittent activity may, therefore, be prescribed for these individuals. The best monitoring tools for these individuals, aside from ECG monitoring, are blood pressure and RPE. In patients with ventricular failure, the resting systolic and diastolic blood pressure values are often increased. As these patients begin to exercise, systolic and diastolic pressures may increase further with the increased cardiac demand. If their diastolic pressure should begin to fall during exercise or the RPE rises without explanation, it is a definite sign that the failing ventricle is unable to keep up with the exercise intensity. Strict attention to a patient's signs and symptoms ensures a patient's safety during exercise.

F. Systemic hypertension

When formulating the prescription of exercise for patients with systemic hypertension, care must be taken to avoid the generation of high and potentially harmful systemic arterial pressure. Exercises that are isometric or that might cause a Valsalva maneuver should be avoided in patients with systemic hypertension.

G. Diabetes

The risk factor of glucose intolerance can be altered with exercise. This should encourage participation of patients with known coronary disease or high-risk profiles in a rehabilitation program. The clinician working with this patient population must recognize that beta blockers can mask the usual signs or symptoms of impending insulin shock. The rehabilitation team must be able to recognize the difference between an insulin reaction and a cardiac event.

H. Cardiac transplantation

Cardiac transplantation is no longer an experimental treatment for patients with severe cardiac disease. Postoperative management focuses on prevention and treatment of infection and acute rejection and early mobilization. Transplant recipients have a denervated heart,

meaning that there is no input from the autonomic nervous system. Because there is no parasympathetic influence, the resting heart rate will be elevated. With no sympathetic influence, there is an impaired chronotropic response to sudden increases in exercise. There can be an increase in cardiac output with exercise caused by an increase in stroke volume attributable to augmented preload. As exercise continues, heart rate and contractility may slowly increase because of circulating catecholamines.

Exercise for patients with cardiac transplants can and should be encouraged. Alterations must occur in their exercise program to account for their changed cardiac status. The warm-up period should be lengthened to allow the heart to accommodate increased venous return in light of the lack of possible chronotropic effects. Because of the previous severity of their illness, many patients will be fairly deconditioned. Exercise intensities must reflect their previous abilities. Monitoring these patients by heart rate and blood pressure alone is inappropriate. The RPE is a better indicator of potential abilities. The cool-down period will reflect a very slow return to baseline heart rate and blood pressure levels because catecholamines remain in the bloodstream long after exercise has ceased. With training and time, the body adapts to the denervated heart. Larger amounts of catecholamines can be produced in a shorter amount of time. A more normal heart rate response to exercise has been shown in patients 1 year post cardiac transplant.[40]

Clinical Decision-Making Cases

Case #1

LG, a 53-year-old self-employed businessman, complained of nausea and indigestion for approximately 4 hours in duration. After much procrastination, he was brought to the emergency room, where he presented with shortness of breath, chest pain, nausea, vomiting, and ECG changes. The patient had moderate hypertension (150/90) and a systolic click. A large anterolateral myocardial infarction was finally diagnosed. The patient had a hospital stay of 8 days and was dis-

charged and referred to outpatient cardiac rehabilitation.

What diagnostic testing and assessment measures will assist the physical therapist in a program that is both safe and effective for this patient?

1. Predischarge or postdischarge graded exercise stress test.
2. Any other cardiovascular diagnostic tool, *ie*, cardiac catheterization.
3. Risk factor analysis.
4. Concomitant medical problems.

5. Medication history.
6. Past and present medical history.
7. Present work status.
8. Family dynamics.
9. Time constraints.
10. Goals of the individual.

PHYSICAL EXAMINATION

Age:	53
Weight:	180 lb
Family history:	Brother obese, myocardial infarction at 47
Medical history:	Patient obese with hypertension, three previous severe angina episodes, and a systolic click; smokes 17 cigarettes/day
Medications:	Isosorbide dinitrate (Isordil), 20 mg Nitroglycerin (on occasion)
Blood chemistry:	Cholesterol: 342 mg/dL (high) HDL: 40 (poor) Cholesterol/HDL 7.5 : 1 (poor)
Resting heart rate:	59 beats/min
Resting blood pressure:	110/70

GRADED EXERCISE TEST

A treadmill graded exercise test was performed using a Balke treadmill protocol.

	Supine	Standing	Maximum	Recovery 2 min	6 min	Supine
Heart rate	59	61	170	120	115	95
Blood pressure	110/70	150/100	180/100	160/102	150/100	160/100

Total time of test: 6.15 min

Reason for test termination: Dyspnea, fatigue, 2 mm ST segment depression.

Impression: Patient performed a moderate level of exercise, limited by blood pressure and ECG responses. Patient requires an exercise prescription that takes into consideration his blood pressure and ECG responses.

CARDIAC REHABILITATION

Patient was scheduled to begin cardiac rehabilitation with the following problems:

1. Fair work capacity.
2. High coronary risk factor profile:

   • Obese
   • Cigarette smoking
   • Elevated blood pressure
   • Elevated cholesterol

3. History of coronary symptoms:

   • Angina
   • Shortness of breath

Treatment and Patient Goals

1. Improve functional capacity through progressive exercise program. Improvement will be measured by results of subsequent graded exercise test.
2. Increase knowledge of the disease within the cardiac rehabilitation program as measured by the first and subsequent test related to the education component of the program.
3. Reduction of coronary risk factors measures by a reduction in blood pressure, cholesterol values, cigarettes/day, and weight.

It is critical for the therapist to include the patient's goals in goal setting. Small, reachable goals are encouraging to the patient and reduce the overwhelming stress related to numerous lifestyle changes. Let the patient identify which of the goals is the most important to him or her. In this particular case, the patient's short-term goals were to decrease cigarette smoking and increase physical activity level. His long-term goals were to decrease cholesterol level and weight.

EXERCISE PRESCRIPTION

Intensity:	Using the Karvonen formula, the patient's target heart rate was identified: Target heart rate = 170 − 59 × (50%–60%) + 59 = 114–125
Mode:	Brisk walking at a target heart rate of 114 to 125 beats/min was prescribed. Other modalities would be added over time.
Duration:	Starting with 5 to 10 minutes of brisk walking with a rest period in between, progressing to 20 minutes with no stopping.
Frequency:	Three times per week during the regularly scheduled cardiac rehabilitation sessions and once on his own.

Exercise Session: Progression and Outcomes

The initial visit consisted of a telemetry-monitoring exercise prescription test with a check-in period, when vital signs were taken. The patient developed dyspnea at a heart rate of 105. A significant cool-down period was prescribed to bring the patient back to normal values.

At week 3, the patient was progressing, performing 8 minutes of brisk walking at a heart rate of 110. No weight loss or change in cigarette smoking was observed.

At week 5, the patient reported severe pain in both lower extremities with 9 minutes of brisk walking. He refused to exercise. The primary physician was contacted, and the patient was referred for evaluation of claudication pain. The physician validated that the pain was true claudication pain, and, with discussion between therapist, physician, and patient, a bicycling program was agreed on.

At week 8, the patient was biking for 2 to 6 minutes at 720 kpm (kilopound meters) with 2 minutes of recovery for a total of 20 minutes. Claudication pain was tolerable during exercise. The patient had quit smoking and had gained 10 lb. He reported that episodes of angina were minimal. He was frustrated by his weight gain; however, through support of the members of the team, he accepted the difficulty of dealing with multiple risk factors while attempting to improve his exercise performance.

At week 12, the patient appeared to have a change in status. He had gained 20 lb and had angina during warm-up activities. His aerobic program on the bike deteriorated and was limited to 2 minutes with substernal anginal pain, dyspnea, and leg claudication. The patient also reported an increase in the use of nitroglycerin.

At this point, the therapist contacted the cardiologist for an updated report. The cardiologist referred the patient for a follow-up graded exercise test that was positive for severe myocardial ischemia. Cardiac rehabilitation was put on hold until further diagnostic testing had been completed.

At week 17, a coronary angiogram showed abnormal coronary vasculature on the left: 70% occlusion of the left anterior descending (LAD) coronary artery, 80% occlusion of the circumflex coronary artery, and 50% occlusion of the right coronary artery. Bypass surgery was recommended.

At week 21, the patient had bypass surgery (three coronary artery bypass grafts) to the LAD, circumflex, and right coronary arteries, with no significant postoperative complications.

The patient was seen pre- and postoperatively by the physical therapy staff for chest physical therapy. On day 2, cardiac rehabilitation of the patient was begun; he ambulated and climbed one flight of stairs by discharge on postoperative day 7.

At week 27, the patient was referred for outpatient cardiac rehabilitation, having received a graded exercise test at 6 weeks post surgery. At this point, the process for the physical therapist started all over again, with consideration of the past problems and the new problems and status.

Case #2

HG is a 60-year-old black female who was brought to the emergency room and admitted with a 3-day history of increasing dyspnea at rest and with exertion. She complained of pressure in her upper chest, related to exertion. In recent days, the patient noted an increase in cough, productive of yellow-white phlegm, generalized weakness, and malaise. She stated that she had missed the last dose of her usual heart medication and admitted to an increased intake of salt in her diet, specifically corn chips. While in the rescue ambulance, the patient was treated with morphine sulfate and given lidocaine for premature ventricular contractions (PVCs). She was diuresed with furosemide (Lasix) in the emergency room and quickly became more comfortable.

WHAT SHOULD BE INCLUDED IN THE PATIENT'S DIFFERENTIAL DIAGNOSIS?

1. Myocardial infarction.
2. Pulmonary edema.
3. Hypertension.
4. Pneumonia.
5. Congestive heart failure.
6. Renal disease.
7. Chronic bronchitis.
8. Medication withdrawal.

WHAT WOULD NARROW THE DIFFERENTIAL DIAGNOSIS?

History
1. Twelve-year history of severe congestive cardiomyopathy (now end stage) with recurrent biventricular congestive heart failure and PVCs (controlled).
2. Hypertension of 5 years controlled with medication.
3. Glaucoma, taking drops.
4. Anemia.
5. Recurrent bronchitis.
6. Positive family history of heart disease.

Physical Examination
On admission, a well-developed, well-nourished black female in moderate to severe dyspnea and respiratory distress, with mild diaphoresis. Heart rate, 100; blood pressure, 120/80; respiratory rate, 22.

1. Neck: examination revealed carotid bruits, carotid distention, jugular vein distention.

2. Chest: auscultation revealed scattered rhonchi and occasional wheezes, basilar rales one third of the way up the chest.
3. Heart: examination revealed past posterior myocardial infarction, a left ventricular heave over the left precordium. Normal sinus rhythm with an S_3 gallop and a soft S_4 heard as well. Mitral valve regurgitation heard at the apex of the heart, with a systolic ejection murmur heard at the aortic area.
4. Extremities: pitting edema found bilaterally. Absent cyanosis or clubbing.

Diagnostic Tools Evaluation

1. Laboratory values: electrolytes, normal; biochemical profile, normal; serial cardiac enzymes, nonevolving and within normal limits; digitoxin levels, toxic; arterial blood gases on room air, pH 7.42, PCO_2 40, PO_2 78, bicarbonate 25; oxygen saturation 95% with mild hypoxemia present; complete blood count, normal; iron-deficient anemia was shown on bone marrow examination.
2. ECG (12 lead): revealed a left bundle branch block (LBBB), left ventricular hypertrophy, significant q waves over posterior leads, evidence of old myocardial infarction, occasional PVCs.
3. Chest x-ray: showed an unfolded aorta and massive cardiac enlargement. Some pulmonary edema and pulmonary congestion was seen.
4. Echocardiogram: showed marked dilation of the left atrium and ventricle with decreased ventricular compliance and septal motion.
5. Gaited pool study: revealed an ejection fraction of 15% and global hypokinesis.

DEFINITIVE DIAGNOSIS

Decompensated congestive heart failure secondary to congestive cardiomyopathy of unknown etiology.

The patient was admitted to the telemetry unit of the hospital (step-down unit); she was diuresed and digitized and placed on a salt-free diet. Medications subsequently included digoxin, Lasix, quinidine, tetracycline, bronchodilators, and warfarin (Coumadin). Over the course of 2 days, the patient had one episode of ventricular tachycardia resolved with lidocaine drip. PVCs continued regularly.

Subsequently, the patient was referred to physical therapy for initiation of cardiac rehabilitation program (4 days post hospital admission).

PHYSICAL THERAPY EXAMINATION

The patient's chart was reviewed, and preadmission functional status, including social status and exercise habits, was obtained during the initial interview.

Motor: Extremity strength grossly within normal limits. Active and passive range of motion within normal limits; lower extremities showed peripheral edema.

Function: Patient was independent in bed mobility; transfer ability and ambulation were not assessed.

Chest examination: Rhonchi heard with occasional wheezes. Auscultation revealed persistent S_3 gallop over apex of heart.

ECG: Patient was monitored at bedside. Occasional PVCs noted during evaluation.

On day 1, the patient was started on supine bed exercises (level II). Her heart rate was 80 to 85, within normal limits during activity; her blood pressure was 100/62 and stable during activity; and the ECG showed PVCs, LBBB, and occasional premature atrial contractions.

Interpretation of activity response: hypoadaptive heart rate with lower extremity exercise; adaptive blood pressure. ECG showed moderate ectopy and LBBB. Patient showed poor endurance and moderate dyspnea with minimal exertion.

Goals:

1. Increase strength and prevent further bed rest and deconditioning.
2. Return to independent ambulation status and activities of daily living with safe and appropriate hemodynamic responses.
3. Increase knowledge of cardiac disease and self-monitoring techniques.
4. Chest physical therapy.

On days 2 and 3, the patient continued to progress in the cardiac rehabilitation program. Exercises continued in both the supine and the sitting positions; the patient also stood at bedside with hemodynamic responses all within normal limits. Chest physical therapy was tolerated well with some sputum production.

On day 5, the patient performed exercises and began ambulation. She felt comfortable and asymptomatic; however, there was a moderate drop in systolic blood pressure. The physician consented to progression of the program. Heart rate, 68; blood pressure, 75/50; ECG, PVCs and LBBB.

On days 6 to 9, the patient continued to progress with exercises and ambulation (100 feet). She continued to have flat heart rate response and hypoadaptive blood pressure with increasing activity. She experienced no symptoms with changes in either heart rate or blood pressure.

On day 10, the patient ambulated 150 feet and climbed 4 stairs. A noticeable increase in systolic blood pressure occurred with a drop in diastolic blood pressure. ECG continued to show usual PVCs and LBBB. The physician was notified. The medication was altered in an effort to assist with the patient's abnormal hemodynamic responses to activity, which were associated with her chronic and severe cardiomyopathy, and to prevent congestive heart failure.

SUMMARY OF PROGRESSION

The patient continued a slow progression through the cardiac rehabilitation inpatient program for the duration of her hospital stay.

Her resting heart rate was variable and ran the spectrum from normal sinus rhythm (80 to 85) to irregular bradycardia (50 to 60), with occasional sinus blocks and pauses with even slower rates. Her exercise responses were flat.

Her resting systolic and diastolic blood pressures were significantly low, ranging from 80/40 to 108/50. She exhibited a consistent hypotensive blood pressure response to increasing activity, which could be expected given her compromised myocardium but which made activity difficult and proper monitoring critical.

The patient received individual instructions on a daily basis regarding coronary disease, risk factor management, and the importance of daily, low-level exercise. Attempts were made to teach the patient to take her own heart rate, emphasizing the need for self-monitoring of heart rate before, during, and after exercise in order to know the limitations to activity.

It is critical for congestive heart patients who have little symptomatology during exercise and flat heart rate and subtle changes in both systolic and diastolic pressures to self-monitor for safety during activity.

References

1. Braunwald E: The history. In Braunwald E (ed): *Heart Disease, A Textbook of Cardiovascular Medicine.* Philadelphia, W. B. Saunders Company, 1984, pp 1–13.
2. Sandler G: The importance of the history in the medical clinic and the cost of unnecessary tests. *Am Heart J* 1980, 100:928.
3. Morey M, Korsch FP: Anatomy and physiology of the heart. In Andreoli K, Fowkes V, Zipes D (eds): *Comprehensive Cardiac Care,* 5th ed. St. Louis, C. V. Mosby Company, 1983, pp 1–9.
4. Guyton A: *Textbook of Medical Physiology,* 7th ed. Philadelphia, W. B. Saunders Company, 1986, pp 160–175.
5. Braunwald E, Ross J, Sonnenblick EH: *Mechanisms of Contraction of the Normal and Failing Heart,* 2nd ed. Boston, Little, Brown and Company, 1976.
6. Brannon F, Foley M, Starr J: The heart and circulation. In Brannon F, *et al.* (eds): *Cardiopulmonary Rehabilitation: Basic Theory and Application,* 2nd ed. Philadelphia, F. A. Davis Company, 1993, pp 13–32.
7. Smith JJ, Kampine JP: *Circulation Physiology,* 3rd ed. Baltimore, Williams & Wilkins, 1990, pp 25–172.
8. West JB (ed): *Best and Taylor's Physiological Basis of Medical Practice,* 12th ed. Baltimore, Williams & Wilkins, 1991, pp 276–330.
9. American College of Sports Medicine: *Guidelines for Graded Exercise Testing and Exercise Prescription.* Philadelphia, Lea & Febiger, and London, Henry Kimpton, 1986.
10. Blessey R: The beneficial effects of aerobic exercise for patients with coronary artery disease. In Irwin S, Tecklin JS (eds): *Cardiopulmonary Physical Therapy.* St. Louis, C. V. Mosby Company, 1985, pp 137–148.
11. Skloven ZD: Hemodynamics. In Irwin S, Tecklin JS (eds): *Cardiopulmonary Physical Therapy.* St. Louis, C. V. Mosby Company, 1985, pp 23–34.
12. Hellerstein HK, Hirsch E, Cumler W, *et al.:* Reconditioning of the coronary patient: preliminary report. In LeKoft W, Moyer J (eds): *Coronary Health and Disease.* New York, Grune & Stratton, 1963.
13. Fowkes V, Andreoli K: Patient assessment: history and physical examination. In Andreoli K, Fowkes V, Zipes D (eds):

Comprehensive Cardiac Care, 5th ed. St. Louis, C. V. Mosby Company, 1983, pp 34–75.
14. Kannel W, Castelelli W, Gordon T, *et al.:* Serum cholesterol, lipoproteins and risk of coronary disease: the Framingham study. *Ann Intern Med,* 1971, 74:1–12.
15. Dubin D: *Rapid Interpretation of EKG's,* 4th ed. Tampa, FL, Cover Publishing, 1988.
16. Sivarajan ES: Exercise testing. In Underhill LS, *et al.* (eds): *Cardiac Nursing,* 2nd ed. Philadelphia, J. B. Lippincott Company, 1989.
17. Gordon T, *et al.:* High density lipoprotein as a protective factor against coronary heart disease. *Am J Med* 1977, 62:707.
18. Goldstein J, Brown M: The low-density lipoprotein pathway and its relation to atherosclerosis. *Am J Med Biochem* 1977, 46:897.
19. Freund G, Lewis JB, Reduto L: Patient assessment: laboratory studies. In Andreoli K, Fowkes V, Zipes D(eds): *Comprehensive Cardiac Care,* 5th ed. St. Louis, C. V. Mosby Company, 1983, pp 92–93.
20. Johnson M: Special diagnostic tests and procedures. *Phys Ther* 1985, 65:1856–1865.
21. Fardy P, Yankowitz F, Wilson P: *Cardiovascular Assessment and Treatment in Cardiac Rehabilitation. Adult Fitness and Exercise Testing.* Philadelphia, Lea & Febiger, 1988.
22. Cowan MJ: Pathogenesis of atherosclerosis. In SL Underhill, *et al.* (eds): *Cardiac Nursing,* 2nd ed. Philadelphia, J. B. Lippincott Company, 1989.
23. Hindle P, Wallace A: Complications of coronary artery disease. In Andreoli K, Fowkes V, Zipes D (eds): *Comprehensive Cardiac Care,* 5th ed. St. Louis, C. V. Mosby Company, 1983, pp 136–166.
24. Mechanical complications in coronary heart disease; heart failure and shock. In SL Underhill, *et al.* (eds): *Cardiac Nursing,* 2nd ed. Philadelphia, J. B. Lippincott Company, 1989.
25. Pathophysiology of coronary artery disease. In Andreoli K, Fowkes V, Zipes D (eds): *Comprehensive Cardiac Care,* 5th ed. St. Louis, C. V. Mosby Company, 1983, pp 75–97.
26. Congenital defects. In Adams F, *et al.* (eds): *Heart Disease in Infants, Children, and Adolescents,* 4th ed. Baltimore, Williams & Wilkins, 1989.

27. O'Connor GT, Buring JE, Yusuf S, *et al.:* An overview of randomized trials of rehabilitation with exercise after myocardial infection. *Circulation* 1989, 80:234–244.

28. Oldridge NB, Guyatt GH, Fischer ME, Rimm AA: Cardiac rehabilitation after myocardial infarction. Combined experience of randomized clinical trials. *JAMA* 260:945–950, 1988.

29. American Association of Cardiovascular and Pulmonary Rehabilitation: *Guidelines for Cardiac Rehabilitation Programs.* *Human Kinetics.* Champaign, IL, AACVPR, 1991.

30. Fardy PS, Webb D, Hellerstein HK: Benefits of arm exercise in cardiac rehabilitation. *The Physician and Sportsmedicine* 1977, 5:30–41.

31. Borg G: Perceived exertion: a note on history and methods. *Med Sci Sports Exerc* 1973, 5:90–93.

32. Certo C: Effects of training on heart rate speed and perceived exertion. *Am Arch Rehabil Ther* 1980, 28:8–23.

33. Gutmann M, Squires R, Pollock M, *et al.:* Perceived exertion heart rate relationship during exercise testing and training in cardiac patients. *J Cardiac Rehabil* 1981, 1:52.

34. Wolfel E, Hossack K: Guidelines for the exercise training of elderly healthy individuals and elderly patients with coronary disease. *J Cardiac Rehabil* 1989, 9:40–45.

35. Powles ACP: The effect of drugs on the cardiovascular response to exercise. *Med Sci Sports Exerc* 1981, 13:252–258.

36. Pollock ML, Foster C, Rod L, *et al.:* Effects of propranolol dosage in the response to submaximal and maximal exercise [Abstract]. *Am J Cardiol* 1982, 49.

37. Pandolf KB: Advances in the study and application of perceived exertion. *Exerc Sport Sci Rev* 1983, 2:118–158.

38. Squires R, Rod J, Pollock M: Effects of propranolol on perceived exertion soon after myocardial revascularization surgery. *Med Sci Sports Exerc* 1982, 14:276–280.

39. Bruce R, Larson E, Stratton J: Physical fitness aerobic capacity, aging, and responses to physical training in bypass surgery in coronary patients. *J Cardiac Rehabil* 1989, 9:24–34.

40. Balady G, Weiner D: Exercise testing in healthy elderly subjects and elderly patients with cardiac disease. *J Cardiopulmonary Rehabil* 1989, 9:35–39.

41. Whittemore R: Congenital heart disease in the adult. In Adams F, Emmanouilides, G, Riemenschneider T (eds): *Heart Disease in Infants, Children, and Adolescents.* Baltimore, Williams & Wilkins, 1989, pp 624–690.

Suggested Reading

American Association of Cardiovascular and Pulmonary Rehabilitation: *Guidelines for Cardiac Rehabilitation Program.* *Human Kinetics.* Champaign, IL, AACVPR, 1991.

American College of Sports Medicine. *Guidelines for Graded Exercise Testing and Exercise Prescription,* 2nd ed. Philadelphia, Lea & Febiger, 1980.

Astrand PO, Rodhahl K: *Textbook of Work Physiology.* New York, McGraw-Hill, 1970.

Atwood JA, Nielson D: Scope of cardiac rehabilitation. *Phys Ther* 1985, 65:22–29.

Borg GA: Perceived exertion: a note on history and methods. *Med Sci Sports Exerc* 1973, 5:90–93.

Braunwald E (ed): *Heart Disease: A Textbook of Cardiovascular Medicine* 2nd ed. Philadelphia, W. B. Saunders Company, 1984.

Ciccone C: *Pharmacology in Rehabilitation.* Philadelphia, F. A. Davis Company, 1990.

Cohen M, Hoskin T: *Cardiopulmonary Symptoms in Physical Therapy Practice.* New York, Churchill Livingstone, 1988.

Dubin D: *Rapid Interpretation of EKGs.* Tampa, FL, Cover Publishing Company, 1975.

Ellestad MH: *Stress Testing: Principles and Practice.* Philadelphia, F. A. Davis Company, 1975.

Fardy P, Yankowitz F, Wilson P: *Cardiac Rehabilitation: Adult Fitness and Exercise Testing,* 2nd ed. Philadelphia, Lea & Febiger, 1988.

Fardy PS, Bennett JL, Reitz NL, *et al.: Cardiac Rehabilitation Implications for the Nurse and Other Health Professionals.* St. Louis, C. V. Mosby Company, 1980.

Goldberger RL, Goldberger E: *Clinical Electrocardiography.* St. Louis, C. V. Mosby Company, 1981.

Goodman C, Snyder TEK: *Differential Diagnosis in Physical Therapy.* Philadelphia, W. B. Saunders Company, 1990.

Gutmann MC, Squires RW, Pollock ML, *et al.:* Perceived exertion heart rate relationship during exercise testing and training in cardiac patients. *J Cardiac Rehabil* 1981, 1:52.

Guyton A: *Textbook of Medical Physiology,* 7th ed. Philadelphia, W. B. Saunders Company, 1986.

Hellerstein H: Exercise Therapy in Coronary Disease. *Bull N Y Acad Med* 1968, 44:1028.

Irwin S: Clinical manifestations and assessment of ischemic heart disease. *Phys Ther* 1985, 65:1806–1811.

Irwin S, Tecklin J: *Cardiopulmonary Physical Therapy,* St. Louis, C. V. Mosby Company, 1985.

Kispert CP, Nielson D: Normal cardiopulmonary responses to acute and chronic strengthening and endurance exercise. *Phys Ther* 1985, 65:38–41.

Malone T: *Physical and Occupational Therapy: Drug Implications for Practice.* Philadelphia, J. B. Lippincott Company, 1989.

Matheson L, Selvester R, Rice H: The interdisciplinary team in cardiac rehabilitation. *Rehabil Lit* 1975, 36:366–375.

Mihevic PM: Sensory cures for perceived exertion: a review. *Med Sci Sports Exerc* 1983, 2:118–158.

Pandolf KB: Advances in the study and application of perceived exertion. *Exerc Sport Sci Rev* 1983, 2:118–158.

Weber KT, Janicki JS: *Cardiopulmonary Exercise Testing: Physiological Principles and Clinical Applications.* Philadelphia, W. B. Saunders Company, 1986.

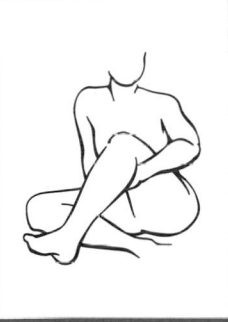

CHAPTER 7

Pulmonary System

Julie Ann Starr

Physical therapy intervention for a patient with pulmonary disease includes techniques specifically designed to improve ventilation, match ventilation to perfusion, decrease the work of breathing, and increase the functional ability of the body.

In order to tailor a treatment program for a specific patient, the clinician must be able to interpret clinical information retrieved from multiple sources: history, interview, physical examination, laboratory data, and imaging studies. The clinician's knowledge of clinical anatomy, physiology, and pathophysiology and ability to develop differential diagnoses ensures that the treatment program will comprise the most effective and efficient treatment techniques for that patient.

The therapist must appreciate the anatomical and physiological connection between the cardiac and the pulmonary systems. Any disorder in one system can and will eventually affect the other. Therefore, Chapters 6 and 7 should be studied together to appreciate this interconnection.

I. Pulmonary Anatomy

A. Thorax (see Figures 7–1 and 7–2)
1. The anterior border is the sternum: manubrium, body, and xiphoid process. The lateral borders of the trachea run perpendicularly into the suprasternal notch. The angle of Louis, the bone ridge between the manubrium and the body of the sternum, is the point of anterior attachment of the 2nd rib and of tracheal bifurcation.
2. The lateral border is the rib cage. The true ribs, 1 to 6, have a single anterior costochondral attachment; the false ribs are 7 to 12; Ribs 7 to 10 share costochondral attachments; and the floating ribs, 11 and 12, have

253

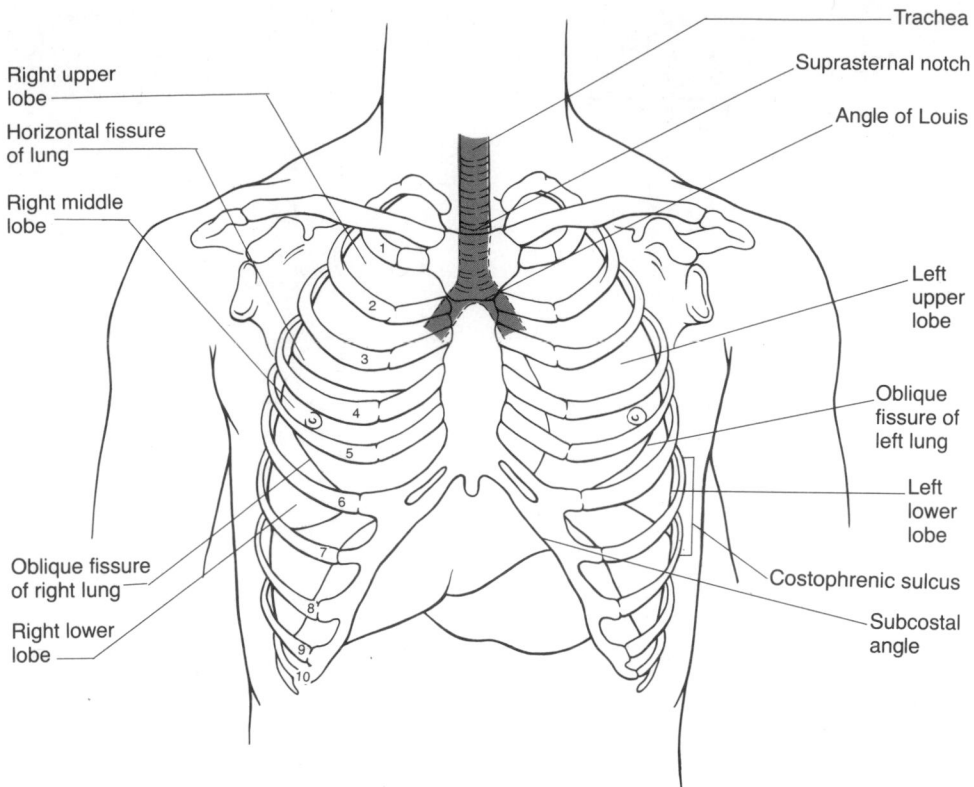

FIGURE 7–1   The bones of the thorax, anterior view.

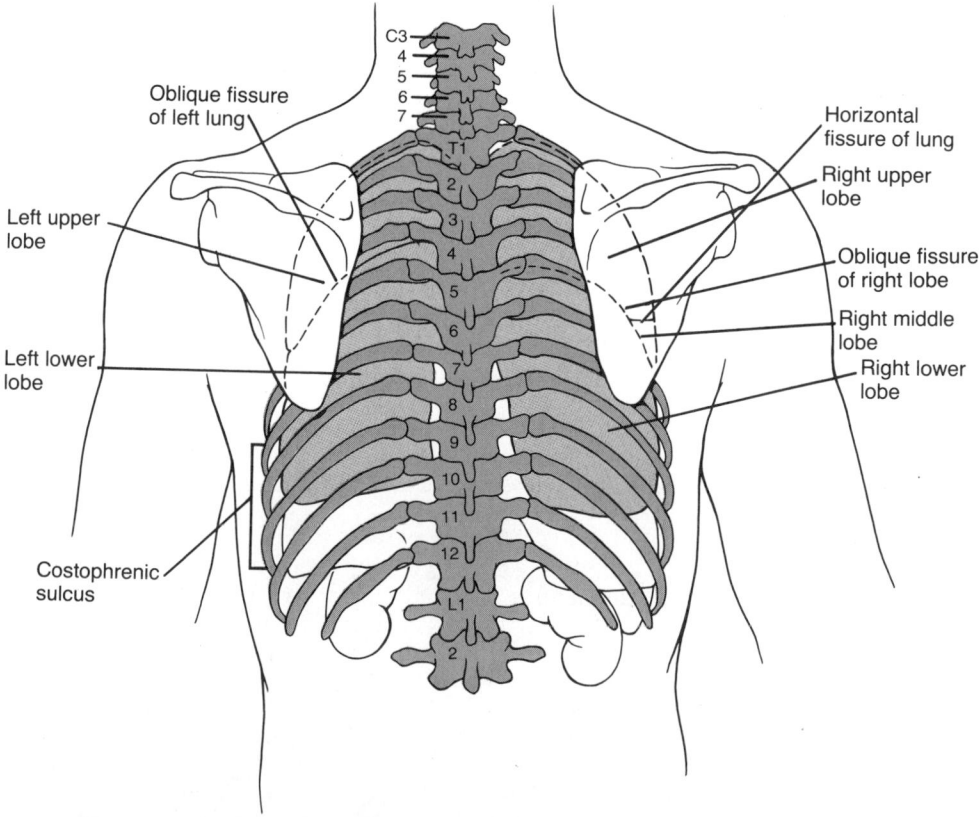

FIGURE 7–2   The bones of the thorax, posterior view.

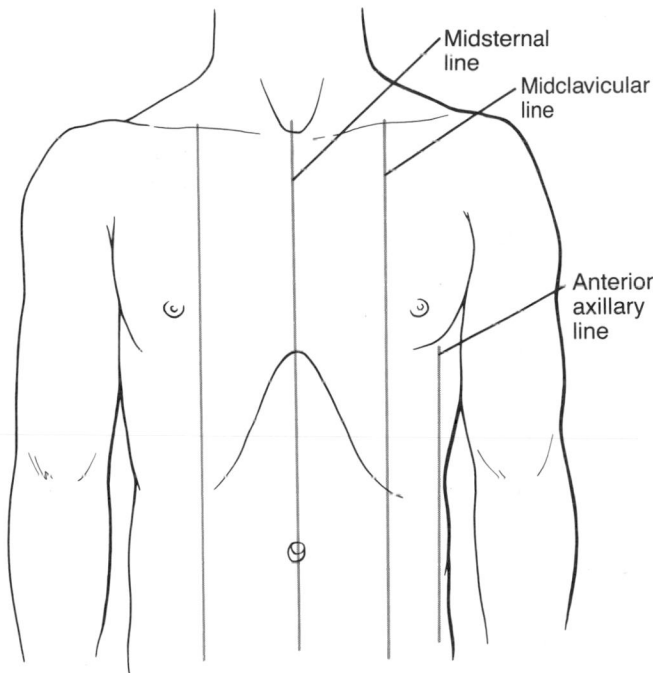

FIGURE 7–3   Surface anatomical lines, anterior view.

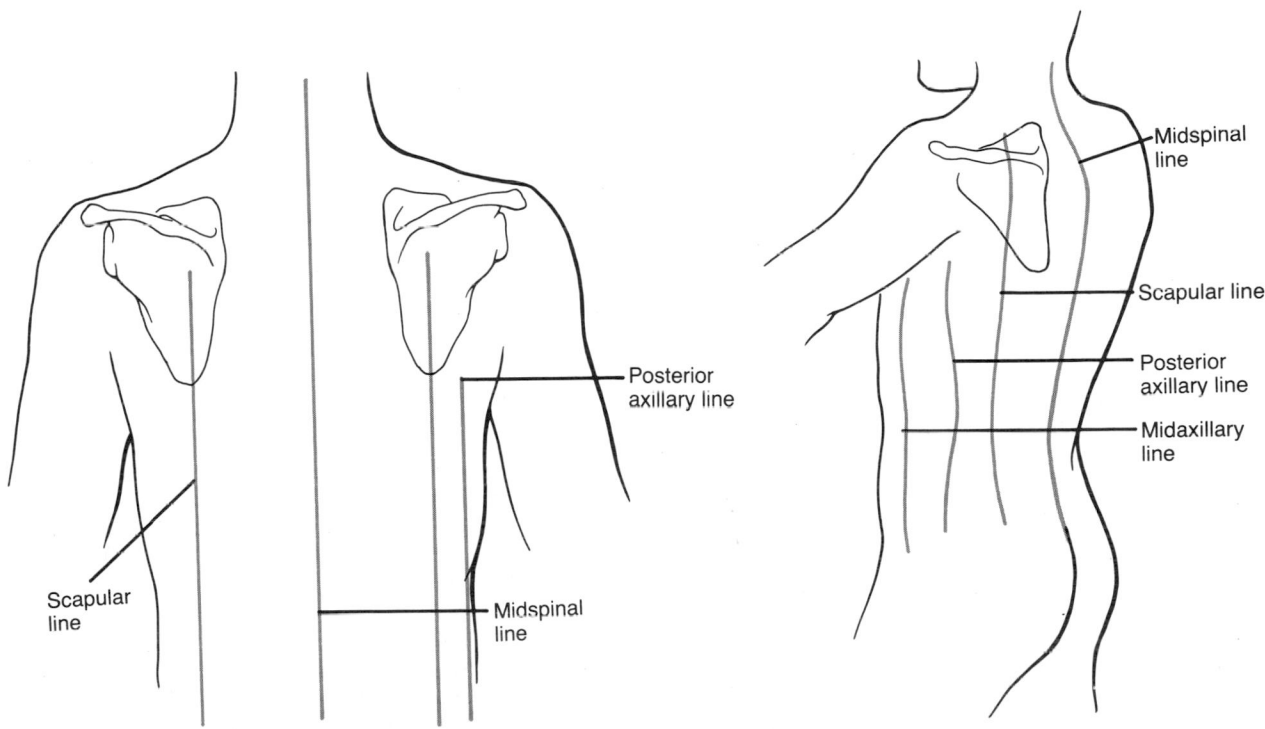

FIGURE 7–4   Surface anatomical lines, posterior view.

no anterior attachment. The subcostal angle is formed where right and left costocartilage meets the sternum. In health, this angle measures between 90 and 110 degrees.[1]

3. The posterior border is the vertebral column, T-1 through T-12. A synovial gliding joint is present between the facets of the two vertebral bodies above and below each rib and the head of the rib. Ribs 1 and 10 to 12 articulate with only one vertebral body.

4. The shoulder girdle can affect the motion of the thorax because it provides attachments to potential accessory muscles of ventilation.

B. Surface lines (See Figures 7–3 and 7–4.)

Surface anatomical lines are used as points of reference for relaying relevant patient information. For example, reporting abnormal breath sounds in a particular lung segment is imprecise because it is difficult to know exactly where within the thorax that segment is anatomically located. It is more appropriate to describe the site of abnormality by surface landmarks.

C. Internal structures

1. **Upper airways** (see Figure 7–5)
   a. The nose or mouth is the entry point into the respiratory system. The nose filters, humidifies, and warms air, but the available inspiratory flow rate is somewhat limited by the size of the nares. The mouth, able to move more air in a given amount of time, diminishes the filtration, humidification, and warming of air.
   b. The pharynx is a common area used in both the respiratory system and the digestive system.
   c. The larynx extends from the thyroid to the cricoid cartilage, connecting the pharynx to the trachea. It includes the epiglottis, which covers and protects the larynx during swallowing: solids and liquids pass into the esophagus but only air passes into the trachea. The larynx also contains the vocal cords.

2. **Lower airways**
   a. The conducting airways, trachea to terminal bronchiole, transport air only. No gas exchange occurs. C-shaped cartilaginous rings support and protect the anterior and lateral aspects of the trachea. The

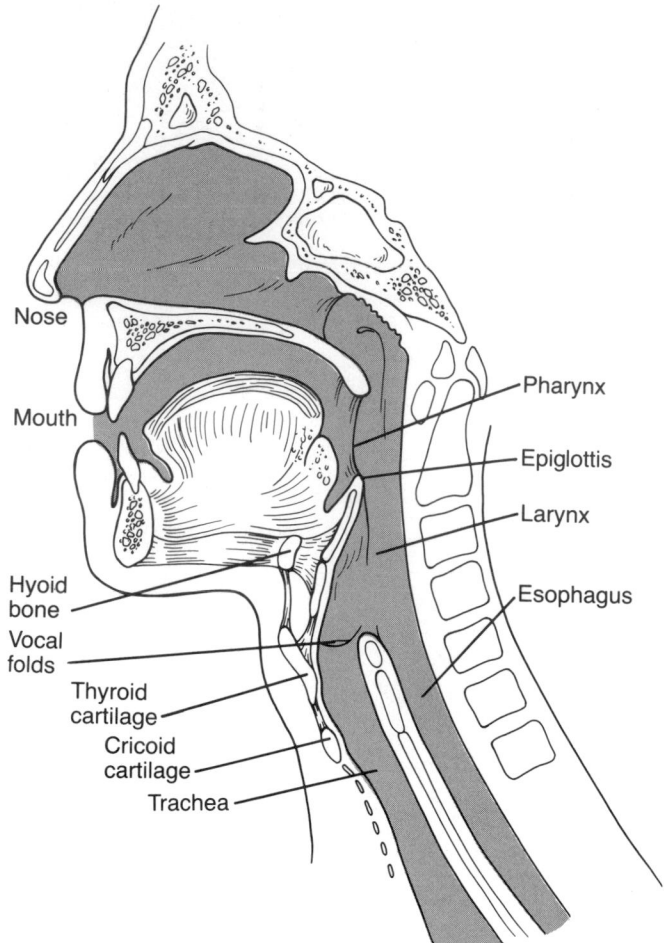

FIGURE 7–5   The upper airways.

cartilaginous support becomes more platelike and infrequent as the conducting airways branch, ceasing completely at the level of the bronchiole[2] (see Figure 7–6).
   b. The respiratory unit consists of the respiratory bronchioles, alveolar ducts, alveolar sacs, and alveoli. Gas diffusion occurs through all of these structures (see Figure 7–7).

3. **Lung structures.** Refer to Table 7–1 for approximate lung borders. Figure 7–8 shows the location of fissure lines, lung lobes, and segments.
   a. The right lung divides into three lobes by the oblique and horizontal fissure lines. Each lobe divides into 10 segments. The concave base of the right lung and the

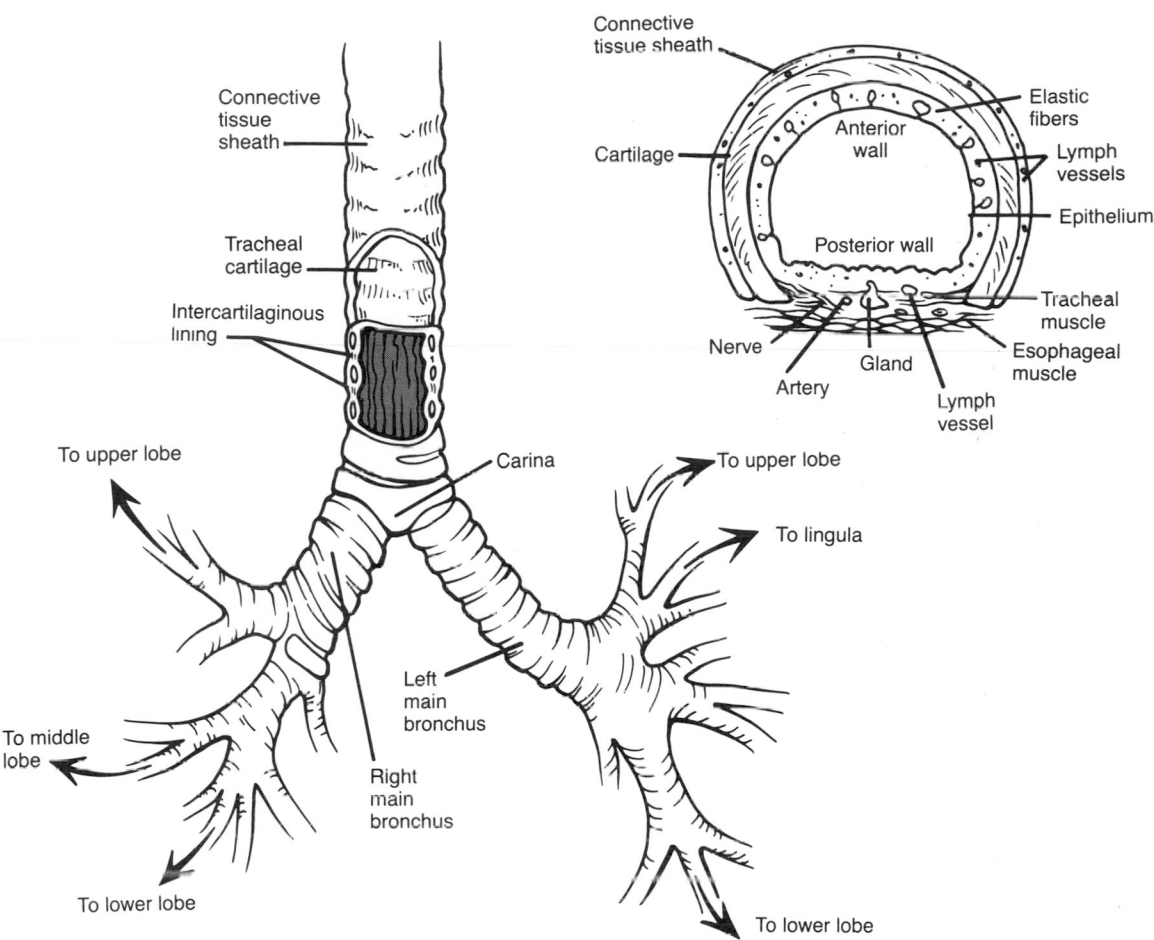

FIGURE 7–6 The lower airways. Anterior view of the trachea and primary bronchi and a cross-section through a part of the trachea that includes a C-shaped cartilaginous ring; the trachealis muscle provides the necessary support posteriorly.

right hemidiaphragm sits higher because of the liver. The right lung is somewhat shorter than the left.

b. The left lung divides into two lobes by a single oblique fissure line. Each lobe divides into eight segments. The heart, situated more within the left hemithorax, requires a larger and deeper cardiac impression in the left lung. The left lung is narrower than the right.

4. **Pleurae**
   a. Parietal pleura covers the inner surface of the thoracic cage, diaphragm, and mediastinal border of the lung.
   b. Visceral pleura wraps the outer surface of

the lung as well as covers the fissure lines that separate the lungs into lobes.

c. Intrapleural space is the potential space between the two pleurae. A small amount of serous fluid reduces friction and allows the pleurae to glide over one another during the ventilatory cycle. During inspiration, the parietal pleura moves outward with the thorax, pulling the visceral pleura with it. During exhalation, the visceral pleura moves inward, pulling the parietal pleura with it. In health, during the ventilatory cycle, a subatmospheric pressure exists between the two pleurae.

d. The costophrenic sulcus is the area be-

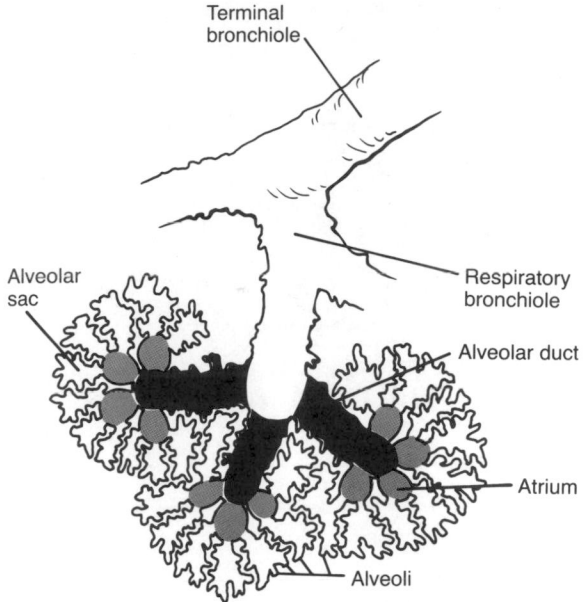

FIGURE 7–7 The respiratory unit comprises the respiratory bronchiole, alveolar ducts, alveolar sacs, and alveoli.

Table 7–1. LUNG BORDERS

Anterior apex—1.5 inches above clavicle
Anterior base—6th costicartilage
Lateral base—8th rib
Posterior apex—C-7
Posterior base—T-10

tween the bottom of the lung and the costophrenic angle (the angle created where the lateral diaphragm meets the ribs). In the upright position, this is the most gravity-dependent area of the respiratory system, where any excessive pleural fluid would be located (see Figures 7–1 and 7–2).

D. Muscles of ventilation (see Figure 7–9)

1. **Primary muscles of inspiration.** These muscles produce a normal resting tidal volume.

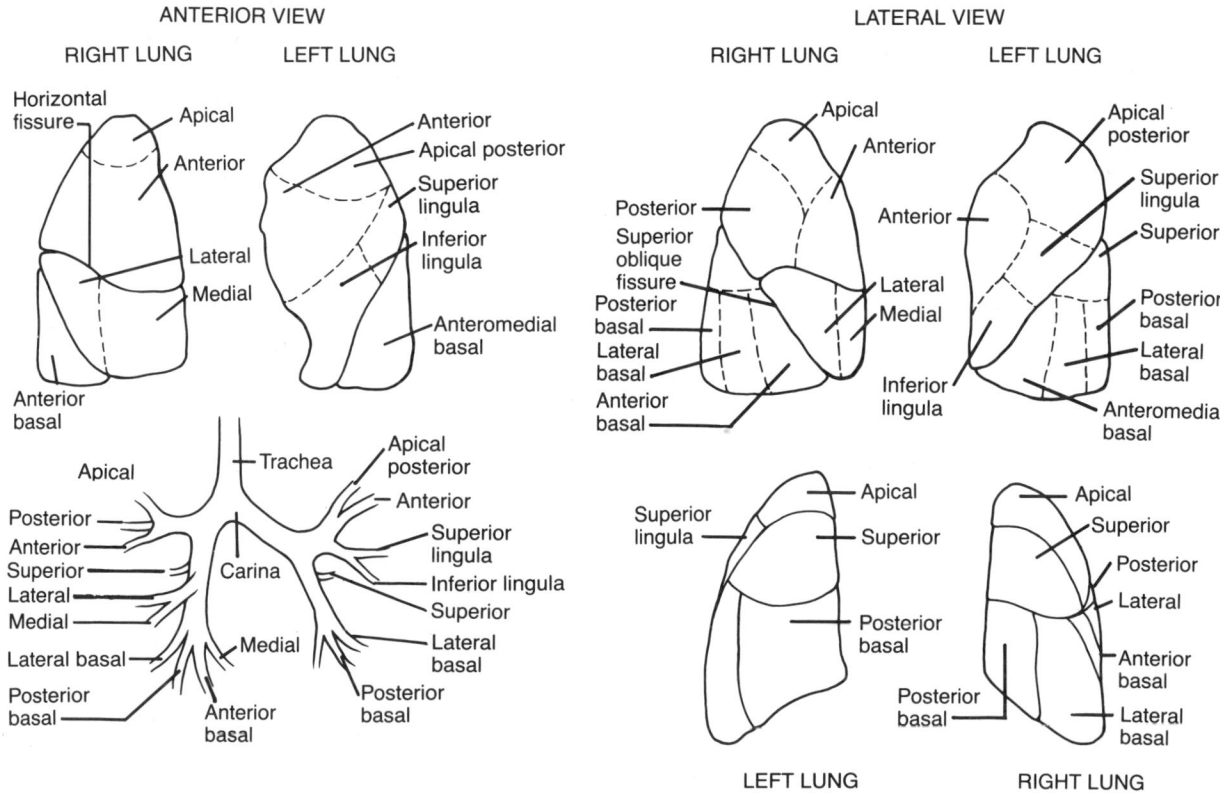

FIGURE 7–8 The segments of the lobes of the lungs. The right lung has three lobes and 10 segments. The left lung has two lobes and 8 segments.

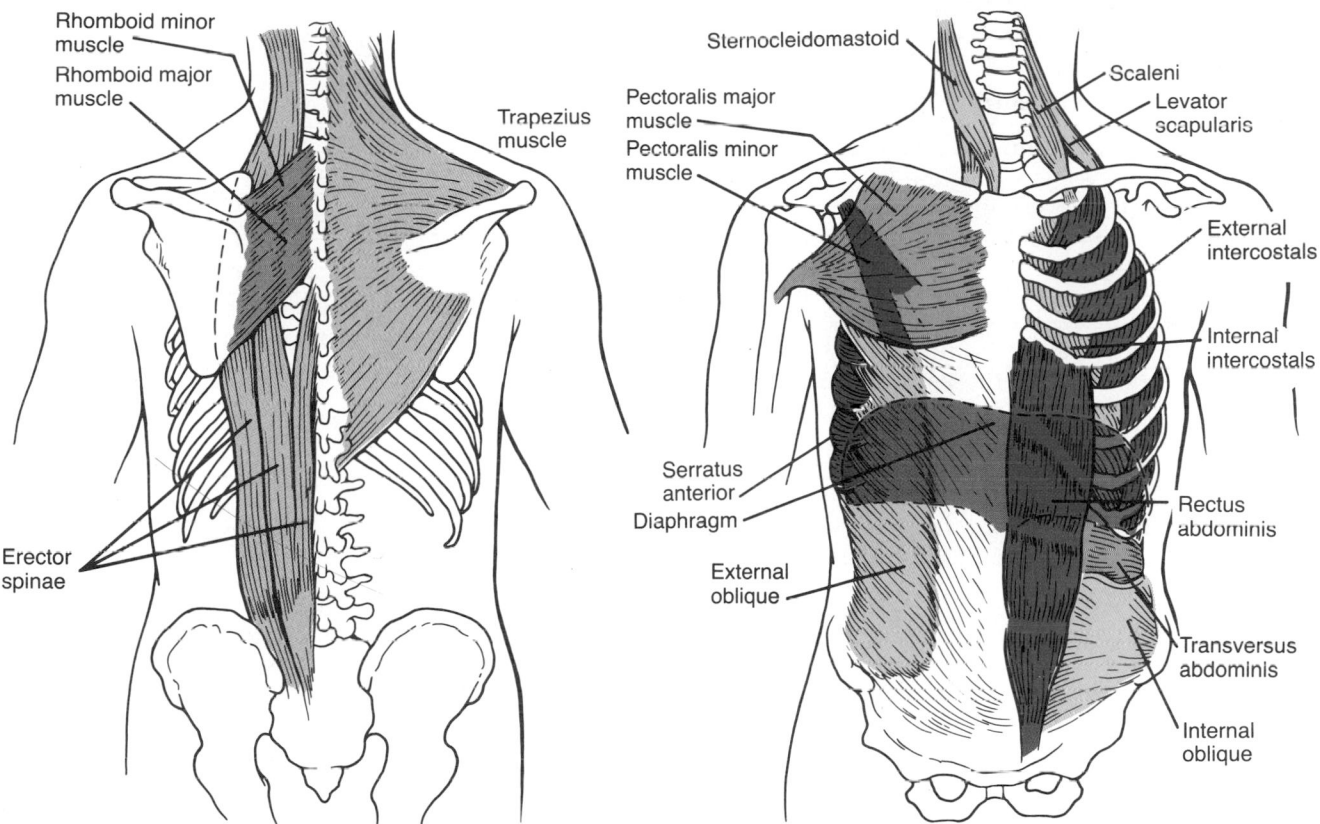

FIGURE 7–9 Muscles of ventilation, anterior and posterior views.

a. The primary muscle of inspiration is the diaphragm. Approximately 75% of fibers are fatigue-resistant (55% slow-twitch oxidative [SO] and 20% to 25% fast-twitch oxidative glycolytic [FOG]). Only about 25% are fast-twitch glycolytic.[3]

b. Additional primary muscles of inspiration are portions of the intercostals[4] (~79% SO and FOG)[3] and scalenes (~83% SO and FOG).[3]

2. **Accessory muscles of inspiration.** These muscles, used when a more rapid or deeper inhalation is required or in disease states, are the levatores costarum, sternocleidomastoid, trapezius, pectorals, serratus, and latissimus dorsi.[3]

3. **Expiratory muscles of ventilation**

a. At rest, a passive relaxation of the inspiratory muscles and the elastic recoil tendency of the lung produce expiration.

b. The expiratory muscles, used when a quicker and/or fuller expiration is desired or in disease states, are the quadratus lumborum, portions of the intercostals,[3,4] muscles of the abdomen, and the triangularis sterni.[5]

4. **Intercostals.** The action of the internal and external intercostals during ventilation is not fully understood. The internal intercostals are more active during expiration; however, the parasternal portion seems to take part in inspiration.[3,6] The external intercostals are more active during inspiration, whereas the intcrosscous intercostal contraction is expiratory in nature.[3,4] The action of both internal and external intercostals is somewhat dependent on lung volume. At low lung volumes, both intercostals help to elevate the ribs; at high lung volumes, the intercostals assist in the downward pull of the ribs.[3]

II. Pulmonary Physiology

A. Mechanics of breathing

1. **Forces acting on the rib cage** (see Figure 7–10)

   a. Elastic recoil of the lung parenchyma pulls the lungs, and therefore the visceral pleura, the parietal pleura, and eventually the bones of the thorax, into a position of exhalation, or inward pull.

   b. The bones of the thorax pull the thorax, and therefore the parietal pleura, the visceral pleura, and the lungs, into a position of inspiration, or outward pull.

   c. Muscular action makes possible both outward and inward pull, depending on which muscles are used.

   d. The intrapleural space, not a force itself, maintains the approximation of the rib cage and the lungs, allowing forces to be transmitted from one structure of the respiratory system to another.

   e. Resting end-expiratory pressure (REEP) is the point of equilibrium where these forces are balanced; it occurs at end-tidal expiration. At this point, there is no muscular action, and the thoracic outward pull is counterbalanced by the elastic recoil property of the lungs.

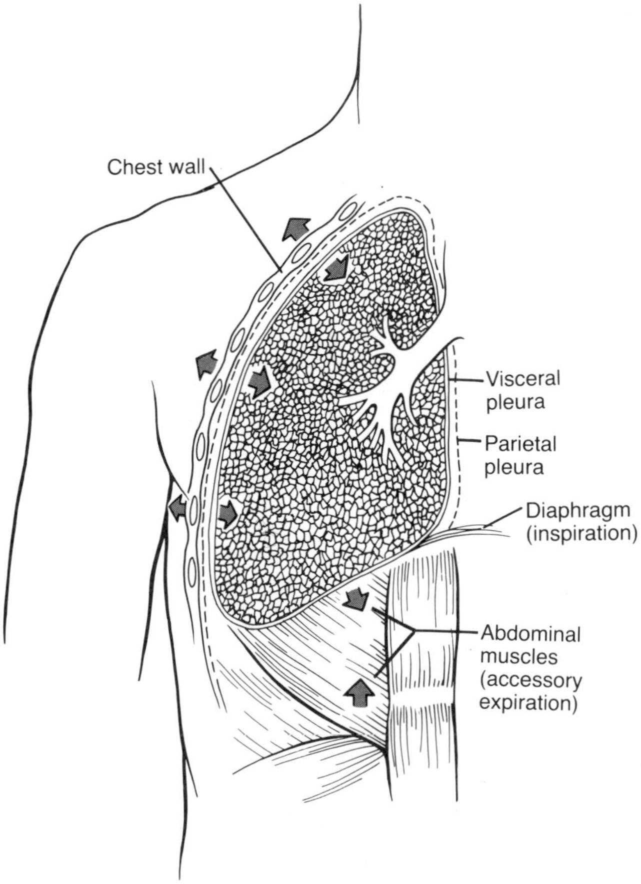

B. Ventilation

Ventilation refers to the movement of gas in and out of the pulmonary system.

1. **Volumes.** The maximum amount of gas moved by the respiratory system is divided into four volumes (see Figure 7–11).

   a. Tidal volume (TV) is the amount of gas inhaled or exhaled during a normal resting breath.

   b. Inspiratory reserve volume (IRV) is the volume of gas that can be inhaled beyond a normal resting tidal inhalation.

   c. Expiratory reserve volume (ERV) is the volume of gas that can be exhaled beyond a normal resting tidal exhalation.

   d. Residual volume (RV) is the volume of gas that, in health, remains in the lungs after ERV has been exhaled.

FIGURE 7–10 Forces acting on the rib cage: elastic recoil of the lung, outward pull of the thorax, and the muscles of ventilation.

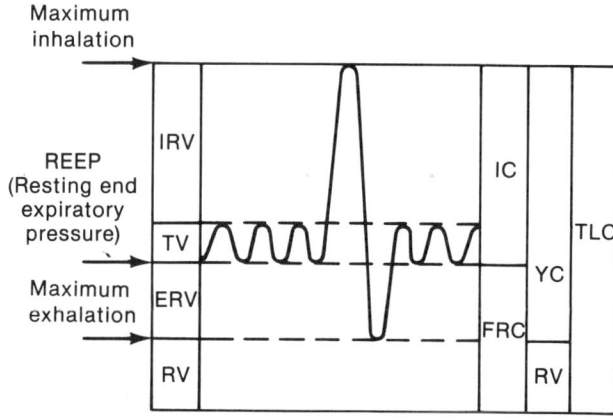

FIGURE 7–11 Lung volumes and capacities. *Abbreviations:* ERV = expiratory reserve volume; FRC = functional residual capacity; IC = inspiratory capacity; IRV = inspiratory reserve volume; RV = residual volume; TLC = total lung capacity; TV = tidal volume; VC = vital capacity.

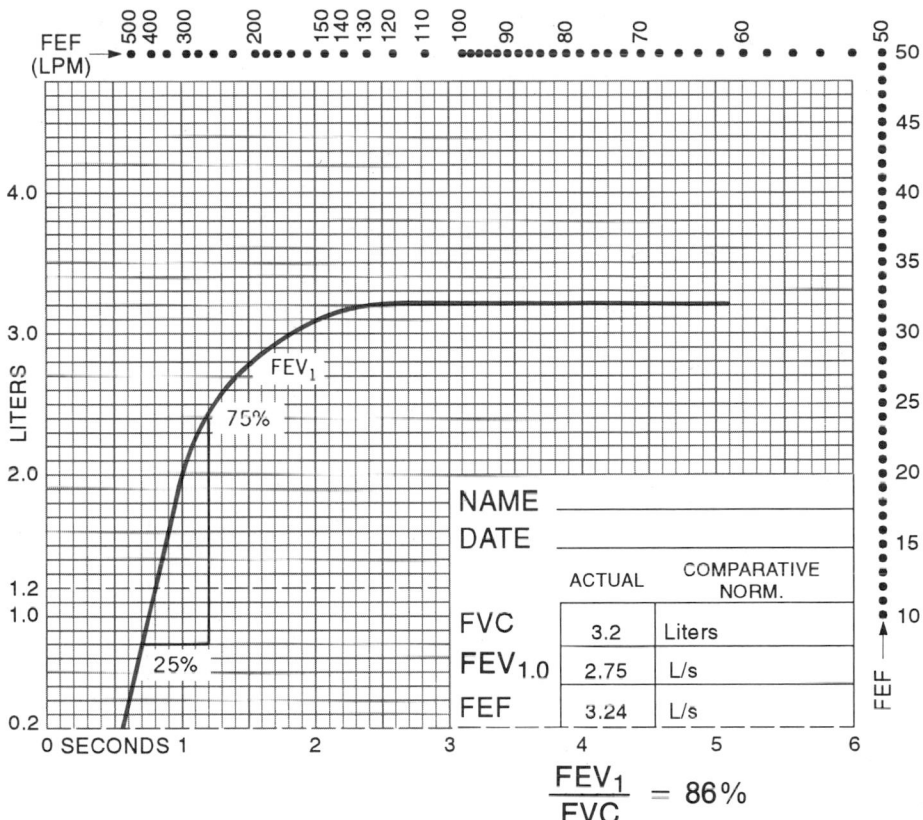

FIGURE 7–12 A forced expiratory flow rate curve. Forced vital capacity (FVC) = 3.2 L. Forced expiratory volume in 1 second (FEV₁) = 2.4 L/s. FEV₁/FVC = 75%, FEF₂₅%–₇₅% = 3.0 L/s.

$$\frac{FEV_1}{FVC} = 86\%$$

Within the figure:

FEF (LPM)→

	ACTUAL	COMPARATIVE NORM.
NAME		
DATE		
FVC	3.2	Liters
FEV₁.₀	2.75	L/s
FEF	3.24	L/s

2. **Capacities.** Two or more lung volumes added together results in a lung capacity (see Figure 7–11).
   a. Inspiratory capacity (IC = IRV + TV) is the amount of air that can be inhaled from REEP.
   b. Vital capacity (VC = IRV + TV + ERV) is the amount of air that is under volitional control, conventionally measured as a forced expiratory vital capacity. The patient is asked to breathe in as deeply as possible, then blow out all the air as hard and as fast as possible into a measuring device.
   c. Functional residual capacity (FRC = ERV + RV) is the amount of air that resides in the lungs after a normal resting tidal exhalation.
   d. Total lung capacity (TLC = IRV + TV + ERV + RV) is the total amount of air that can be housed within the thorax during a maximum inspiratory effort.

3. **Flow rates** (see Figure 7–12)
   a. FEV₁ is the amount of air exhaled during the first second of a forced expiratory vital capacity maneuver. In health, at least 75% of the forced vital capacity (FVC) is exhaled within the first second. (FEV₁/FVC × 100 > 75%.[10]) FEV₁ can predict maximum voluntary ventilation (MVV): FEV₁ × 35 = MVV.[7]
   b. FEF₂₅%–₇₅% is the slope of a line drawn between the points 25% and 75% of exhaled volume on a forced vital capacity exhalation curve. This flow rate is more specific to the smaller airways[8] and shows a more dramatic change with disease than FEV₁. However, the normal range for FEF₂₅%–₇₅% is greater than that for FEV₁, making isolated screenings difficult.[9]

C. Respiration

Respiration is the diffusion of gas (oxygen and carbon dioxide) across the alveolar-capillary membrane.

1. **Arterial oxygenation.** This is the ability of arterial blood to carry oxygen.

Table 7–2. APPROXIMATE PARTIAL PRESSURE OF AIR IN THE ATMOSPHERE AT SEA LEVEL AND AT DIFFERENT POINTS IN THE RESPIRATORY CYCLE

	Dry Atmosphere mm Hg	Moist Atmosphere	Alveolar Air	Arterial Blood
P_{O_2}	159	149	104	95
P_{CO_2}	0.3	0.3	40	40
P_{H_2O}	0.0	47	47	47
P_{N_2}	600	563	569	569

a. The fraction of oxygen in the inspired air (F_{IO_2}) is a numerical representation based on a total of 1. Room air, approximately 21% oxygen, is written as 0.21.

b. Partial pressure of oxygen in the atmosphere (P_{AO_2}) at sea level is 760 mm Hg (barometric pressure) × 21% = 159.6 mm Hg. As air travels through the conducting airways to the alveoli, water and carbon dioxide are added, displacing some of the partial pressure of oxygen.

c. The partial pressure of oxygen in the arterial blood—Pa_{O_2}—depends on the integrity of the pulmonary system, the circulatory system, and the P_{AO_2}. See Table 7–2 for the partial pressure of gases at sea level and at different points in the respiratory cycle.

d. Supplemental oxygen increases the percentage (>21%) of oxygen in the patient's atmosphere. See Table 7–3 for an approximate Pa_{O_2} in a healthy respiratory system at various F_{IO_2} concentrations.

   (1). *High flow rate devices.* All the gas that the patient breathes is drawn from a precisely controlled gas mixing system that delivers an accurate F_{IO_2} (*eg,* ventilators and Venturi masks).[10]

   (2). *Low flow rate devices.* These provide only part of the patient's minute ventilation (TV × respiratory rate) with entrained room air providing the rest. F_{IO_2} measurements can only be estimated with these devices (*eg,* nasal cannula and shovel mask).[10] See Table 7–3 for approximate F_{IO_2} delivered by some low flow rate devices.

2. **Alveolar ventilation.** This is the ability to remove carbon dioxide from the pulmonary capillary and maintain pH.

   a. pH is the negative logarithm of the concentration of free-floating hydrogen ions within the body. Normal range for pH is 7.36 to 7.44.[11] pH indirectly reflects the concentration of carbon dioxide in the blood through the equation

$$H_2O + CO_2 <=> H_2CO_3 <=> H^+ + HCO_3^-$$

   Removal or retention of carbon dioxide by the respiratory system alters the amount of free-floating hydrogen ions and therefore body pH.

   b. Pa_{CO_2}, the partial pressure of carbon dioxide within the arterial blood, is, in health, 36 to 44 mm Hg.[11]

   c. HCO_3^-, the amount of bicarbonate ion within the arterial blood, is normally 23 to 30 mEq/mL.[11] Bicarbonate is sometimes reported as base excess; *eg,* "O" base excess when pH is 7.40 and P_{CO_2} is 40. Positive base excess is a metabolic alkalosis; negative base excess is a metabolic acidosis.[12]

Table 7–3. ESTIMATED FRACTION OF INSPIRED OXYGEN (F_{IO_2}) WITH LOW FLOW RATE DEVICES

Low Flow Rate Device	Estimated F_{IO_2} (%)
Room air	21
Nasal prongs (L/min)	
1	24
3	28
3	32
4	36
5	40
6	44
Oxygen mask (L/min)	
5–6	40
6–7	50
7–8	60
Mask with reservoir bag (L/min)	
6	60
7	70
8	80
9	90
10	99 +

From Rothstein J, Roy S, Wolf S: *The Rehabilitation Specialist's Handbook.* Philadelphia, F. A. Davis Company, 1991, p. 623.

3. **Ventilation and perfusion.** Optimal respiration occurs when ventilation and perfusion are matched. Different ventilation and perfusion relationships exist.

   a. *Dead space.* This space houses gas but does not take part in respiration.

   (1). Anatomical dead space refers to the conducting airways.

   (2). Physiological dead space is additional dead space because of a perfusion abnormality, such as a pulmonary embolus. The respiratory unit is well ventilated, but, because there is no perfusion, there is no respiration[13] (see Figure 7–13).

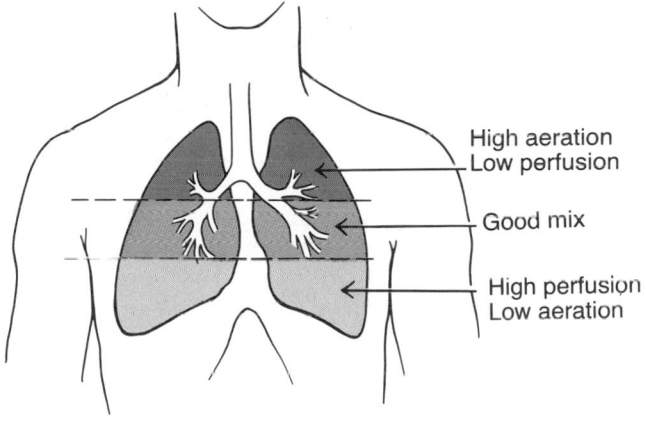

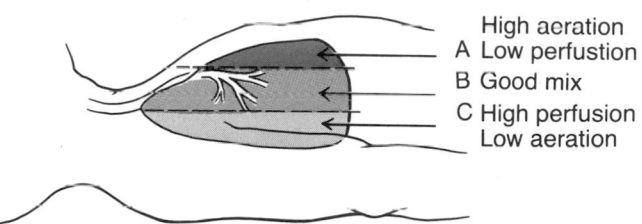

FIGURE 7–14   Relationship between ventilation and perfusion in upright sitting and supine positions. **A,** Dead space: perfusion is low, ventilation is high. **B,** Ventilation and perfusion are well matched. **C,** Shunt: ventilation is low, perfusion is high.

b. *Shunt.* With a shunt, there is no respiration because of a ventilation abnormality. For example, complete atelectasis of a respiratory unit allows the blood to travel through the pulmonary capillary without gas diffusion occurring[13] (see Figure 7–13).

c. *Body position.* For the effects of body position on the ventilation-perfusion relationship, see Figure 7–14.

   (1). *Upright position.* Gravity has the most effect on the distribution of ventilation and perfusion.

      (a). Mechanical adaptations. The anteroposterior diameter of the thorax is greater than the lateral diameter. The greatest change in dimension during the breathing cycle is in the anteroposterior direction. The muscles of inspiration are at an advantage. The intrapleural pressure is most negative at the apex of the lungs and becomes

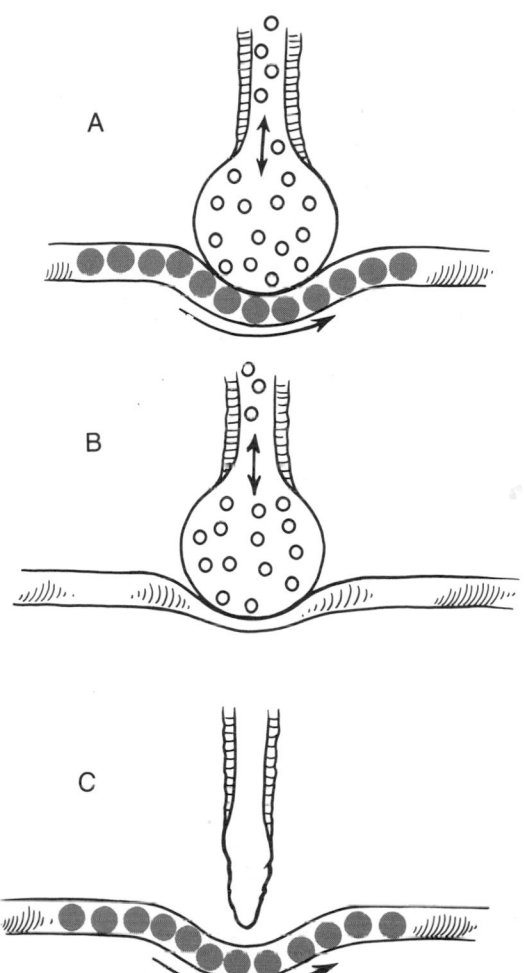

FIGURE 7–13   Relationship between ventilation and perfusion. **A,** Well-matched ventilation and perfusion. **B,** Dead space: ventilation but no perfusion. **C,** Shunt: perfusion but no ventilation.

the least negative toward the base of the lung.[14]

(b). Perfusion ($\dot{Q}$). Perfusion is gravity-dependent, meaning that in the upright position, more pulmonary blood is found at the base of the lung.[15]

(c). Ventilation ($\dot{V}$). At REEP, the alveoli in the apices are fuller than those at the base. During inspiration, more air will be delivered to the less-filled alveoli at the bases, making the greater change in ventilation ($\dot{V}_E$) at the bases.[14]

(d). Ventilation-perfusion ratio ($\dot{V}/\dot{Q}$). The apices have a low amount of perfusion to a high volume of air, resulting in an increased $\dot{V}/\dot{Q}$ ratio. The apices at rest act like dead space. In the upright position, the middle zone of the lung has the best perfusion and ventilation match. The bases have a large amount of perfusion to a small volume of air, resulting in a decreased $\dot{V}/\dot{Q}$ ratio. The bases, at rest, are similar to a shunt.

(2). *Supine position*

(a). Mechanical adaptations. The rib cage decreases in anteroposterior diameter and increases laterally.[17] The greatest change in dimension during the respiratory cycle occurs in the anteroposterior direction. The abdominal contents move the diaphragm farther into the thorax, decreasing FRC, potentially allowing airway closure.[18] This effect is especially pertinent in the geriatric patient and the diseased individual, in whom airway support is decreased.[19]

(b). Perfusion. Greater blood volume in this position is due to augmented blood return from the lower extremities and abdomen. Perfusion is more uniform in the supine than in the upright position, but gravity-dependent areas still receive more blood than gravity-independent areas.[14]

(c). Ventilation. In the supine position, $\dot{V}_E$ changes from cephalad to caudal as well as from gravity-independent to gravity-dependent.[20] In the elderly or diseased population, airway closure may occur at the lower FRC of the gravity-dependent areas, which, in the supine position, have a greater surface area. The alteration of ventilation distribution in this population may be exaggerated.[19]

(d). Results. In the elderly or diseased pulmonary system, the gravity-dependent areas of the lung in the supine position cause airway closure, resultant hypoxemia, increased perfusion, increased preload and afterload, and increased myocardial work, making the position disadvantageous.[20]

(3). *Prone position—abdomen free*

(a). Mechanical adaptations. This position is similar to the supine position for the thorax. The anteroposterior dimension of the thorax is decreased; the lateral is increased. The greatest change in dimension of the thorax occurs in the anteroposterior direction. FRC in the prone position is less than in the upright but more than in the supine.[14]

(b). Perfusion. A greater blood volume due to augmented blood return is found in the prone position as compared with the upright. Changes in cardiovascular function may be present with position change from supine to prone because of compressive forces acting on the heart in the prone position (dependent) that are not present in the supine (independent).[14]

(c). Ventilation. There is a vertical (gravity-dependent and -independent areas of the lung) as well as a cephalocaudal change in ventilation distribution.[21]

(d). Results. A greater FRC occurs in the prone position than in the supine as well as a decrease in dependent surface area; the prone position may be more advantageous than the supine in some populations but is not as optimal as the upright.

(4). *Sidelying position*

(a). Mechanical adaptations. An increase in anteroposterior dimension occurs in the sidelying compared with the supine position as well as a decrease in the lateral dimension of the thorax. The greatest change in ventilation is found laterally in the sidelying position.[14]

(b). Perfusion. A greater blood volume occurs in the sidelying compared with the upright position because of augmented blood return. There may be changes in cardiovascular function in the sidelying position, especially left sidelying, because of compressive forces acting on the heart.[22]

(c). Ventilation. The abdominal contents displace the diaphragm in a cephalad direction. The lower lung's hemidiaphragm is displaced farther than the upper lung's, resulting in a decreased FRC in the lower lung[23], making it more susceptible to airway closure, especially in the geriatric or diseased lung. The overall FRC of the sidelying position lies midway between that of the upright and supine positions.

(d). Results. The sidelying position

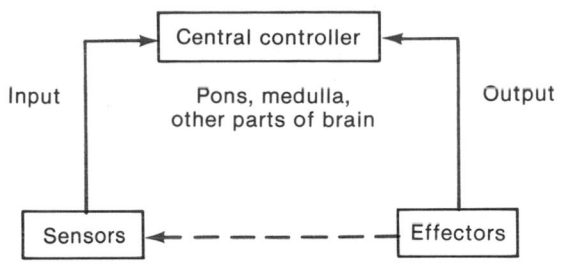

FIGURE 7–15 Schematic representation of the regulation of ventilation and respiration. (From West J: *Respiratory Physiology: The Essentials,* 2nd ed. Baltimore, Williams & Wilkins, 1979, p 115.)

is more advantageous than the supine, and, in certain populations (unilateral lung disease[24]) this position can make a difference in oxygenation.

D. Control of ventilation (see Figure 7–15)

A complex system controls the cycle of ventilation. An abbreviated discussion of the mechanisms involved in the control of ventilation follows.

1. **Receptors.** Many receptors (baroreceptors, chemoreceptors, irritant receptors, stretch receptors) within the body assist in adjusting the ventilatory cycle by sending information to the controllers.[25]

2. **Controllers.** The central control centers (cortex, pons, medulla, and autonomic nervous system) take the receptor's information, analyze the data, and send a message out to the effectors to alter the respiratory cycle in order to maintain adequate alveolar ventilation and arterial oxygenation.[25]

3. **Effectors.** Ventilatory muscles institute the changes deemed necessary by the controllers.[25]

III. Pulmonary Assessment

A. Patient interview

The patient, with the help of the patient's family, if necessary, and the medical record are consulted to obtain the following information:

1. **Chief complaint**
   a. Loss of function, such as decreased ability to perform activities of daily living.
   b. Discomfort, such as shortness of breath.

2. **Present illness**
   a. Onset of primary problem, sudden versus insidious.
   b. Initial date and sequence of events preceding current visit.
   c. Anything that worsens or improves condition, *eg*, upright sitting, rest, medications.
3. **Review of patient's history**
   a. *Occupational history*
      (1). *Past.* Some occupational exposures may cause diseases that have long latency periods, such as asbestosis, silicosis, and pneumoconiosis. Some occupations that involve potential asbestos exposure include construction worker (insulation materials) and car mechanic (brake linings). Some occupations involving risk for silicosis include stone cutter, quarry worker, and sand-blaster.[26,27] (See section on chronic restrictive pulmonary disease.)
      (2). *Present.* Antigens within the workplace can cause an episode of hypersensitivity pneumonitis within hours of exposure.[11] There is also a more chronic form of hypersensitive pneumonitis with a more insidious presentation and course. Examples are farmer's lung, caused by moldy hay, and bird-breeder's lung, caused by bird proteins.[11]
   b. *Past medical history.* Concomitant medical diagnoses and history, such as heart disease, fractured hip, or long-term steroid use, may alter physical examination or treatment plans.
   c. *Current medications.* Certain medications can mask (steroids) or exaggerate (beta blockers) symptoms.
   d. *Social habits*
      (1). Smoking in pack-years (number of packs per day × number of years smoked).[28]
      (2). Alcohol consumption.
      (3). Street-drug use.
   e. *Functional and exertional activity level.* This should be determined for periods of wellness as well as for present illness.
   f. *Cough and sputum production.* Any changes from baseline because of present illness should be recorded. All information should be checked with family members if the patient has become accustomed to his or her symptoms and is unaware of actual frequency and amounts.

   g. *Family history of pulmonary disease.* Some diseases are hereditary—eg, as cystic fibrosis, alpha$_1$-antitrypsin–deficiency, and emphysema—whereas others have familial tendencies (*eg*, a household of smokers has an increased number of upper respiratory tract infections).[29]

B. Physical examination

1. Age, gender, and vital signs are recorded. See Table 7–4 for neonatal, adult, and geriatric normal vital sign values.
   a. *Temperature.* An increase in core temperature may be a sign of infection. A decrease in skin temperature, *ie*, cold and clammy, although extremely gross in nature, may signal a decrease in cardiac output.
   b. *Heart rate.* Any medication side effects, such as increased heart rate due to sympathomimetics and methylxanthines,[30] should be accounted for.
   c. *Respiration*
      (1). Rate in breaths per minute.
      (2). Rhythm—regular or erratic.
      (3). Amplitude (volume)—shallow, deep, etc.
   d. *Blood pressure.* Any changes caused by age and current medications should be accounted for—eg, corticosteroids may increase blood pressure.[30,31]

2. The physical therapist should observe and record the following:
   a. Peripheral edema seen in gravity-dependent areas and jugular venous distention, may indicate possible heart failure. Right ventricular hypertrophy and dilation (cor pulmonale) and heart failure are common sequelae to chronic lung disease.
   b. Body positions. Stabilizing the shoulder girdle places the thorax in the inspiratory position and allows the pectorals to be

Table 7–4. EXAMPLES OF NORMAL RANGES FOR VITAL SIGNS: NEONATE, ADULT, AND GERIATRIC POPULATIONS

Vital Sign	Neonate	Adult	Geriatric
Heart rate	120–140	60–100	60–100
Respiratory rate	30–60	12–18	12–18
Blood pressure	80/46	120/80	140/85
PaO_2	40–70	95–100	$100 - 0.323$ (age)
$PaCO_2$	30–40	36–44	36–44

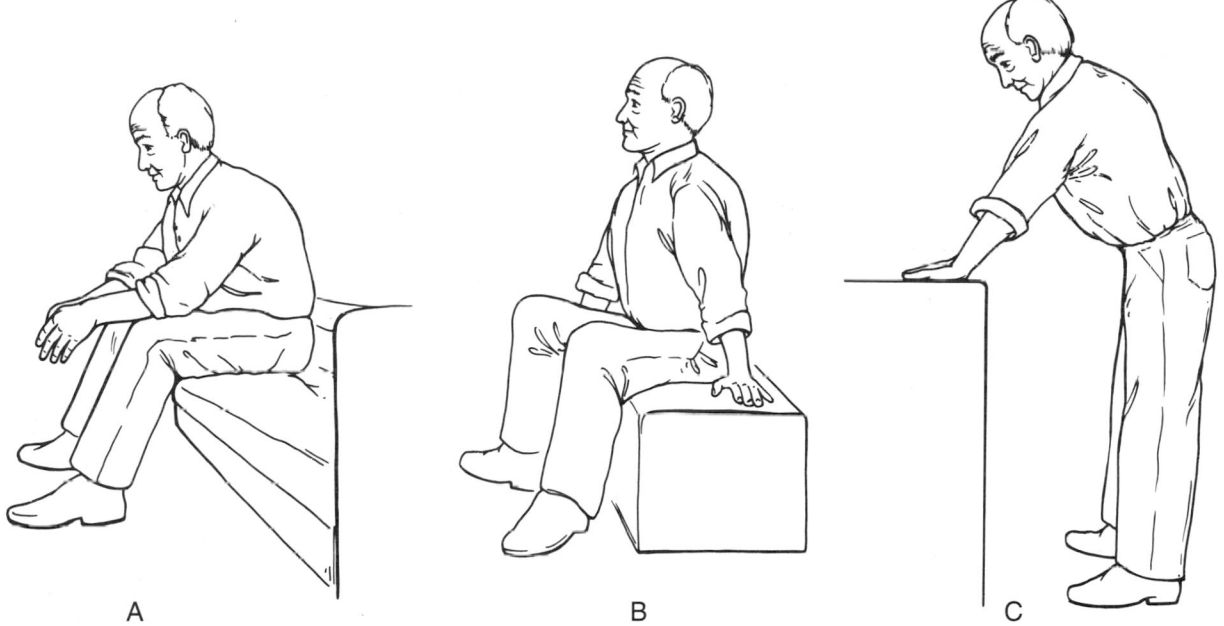

FIGURE 7–16   Postures used to assist inspiratory effort. **A,** Relaxed sitting. **B,** Upright sitting. **C,** Forward leaning.

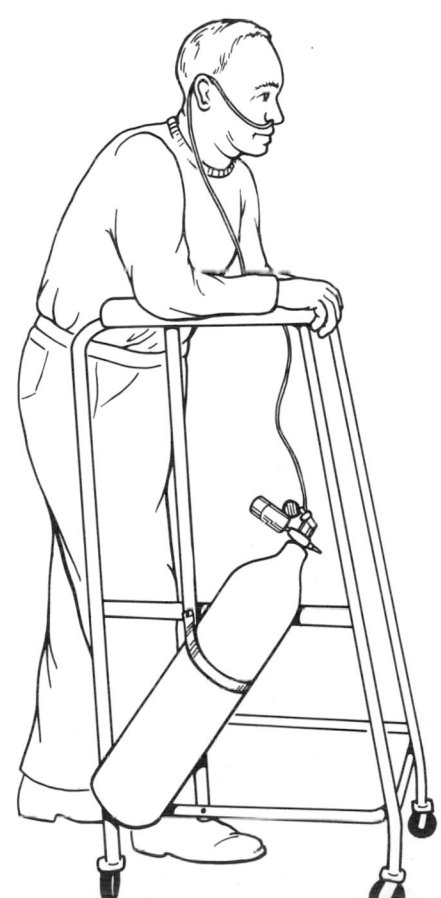

FIGURE 7–17   High-framed wheeling walker.

used as inspiratory accessory muscles.[32] See Figure 7–16 for some of these positions. Incorporation of these postures into treatment programs may assist the patient in completing a desired task (see Figure 7–17).

c. Color of the nail beds and the areas around the eyes and mouth for signs of cyanosis (hypoxemia).

d. Configuration of the distal phalanx of fingers or toes for digital clubbing (chronic hypoxemia; see Figure 7–18).

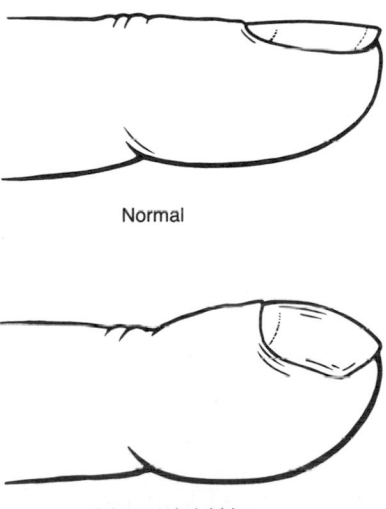

Normal

Advanced clubbing

FIGURE 7–18   Digital clubbing.

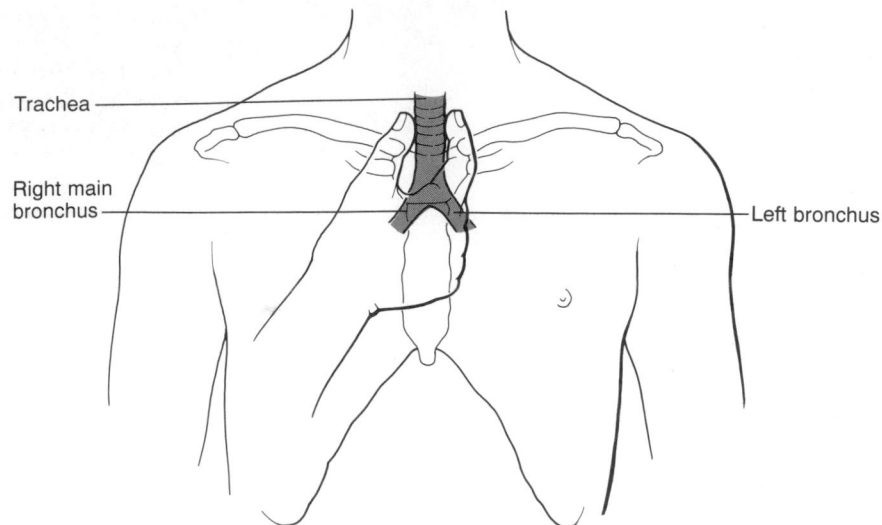

Trachea

Right main bronchus

Left bronchus

FIGURE 7–19 Palpation to assess tracheal deviation.

e. Signs of respiratory distress, especially evident in children: nasal flaring, intercostal and subcostal retractions.

3. **Inspection and palpation.** Universal precautions should be used any time the therapist can come in contact with a patient's body fluids.

a. *Neck*

(1). The trachea should run midline above the suprasternal notch (see Figure 7–19). If deviated, it is most likely because of a volume loss (deviation is toward the defect) or material in the pleural space (deviation is away from the defect)[33] (see Figure 7–20).

(2). The use of accessory muscles of ventilation should be noted.

b. *Thorax*

(1). Any changes in the bony thorax should be noted (see Figure 7–21).

(2). Anteroposterior/lateral diameter is observed. In health, there is a 2:1 ratio. With obstructive disease, this ratio can decrease because of lung tissue destruction and loss of lung recoil force, resulting in a barrel chest. If anteroposterior diameter is increased, there will also be an increase in the subcostal angle.

(3). Thoracic symmetry should be checked.

(a). Static symmetry may be altered by changes in the bony thorax (scoliosis), changes in the underlying lung and pleura (a tuberculosis patient treated with repeated pneumothoraces), or changes in the overlying skin (thoracic burn).

(b). Dynamic symmetry (see Figure 7–22) may be altered by conditions such as incisional pain, pleuritic pain, scapular immobility, or pulmonary fibrosis. Thoracic excursion in health, measured at the base of the lungs from full inspiration to full expiration, is between 2 and 3 inches.[34]

(c). Inspection is made for scars, indicating potential adhesions to underlying soft tissue or surgical removal of structures within the thorax.

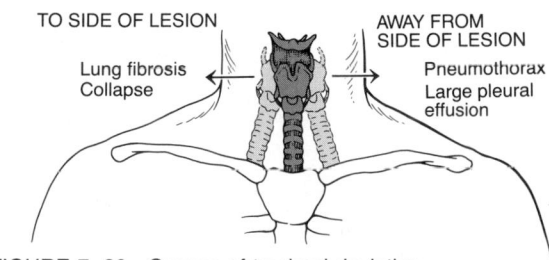

TO SIDE OF LESION

Lung fibrosis
Collapse

AWAY FROM
SIDE OF LESION

Pneumothorax
Large pleural
effusion

FIGURE 7–20 Causes of tracheal deviation.

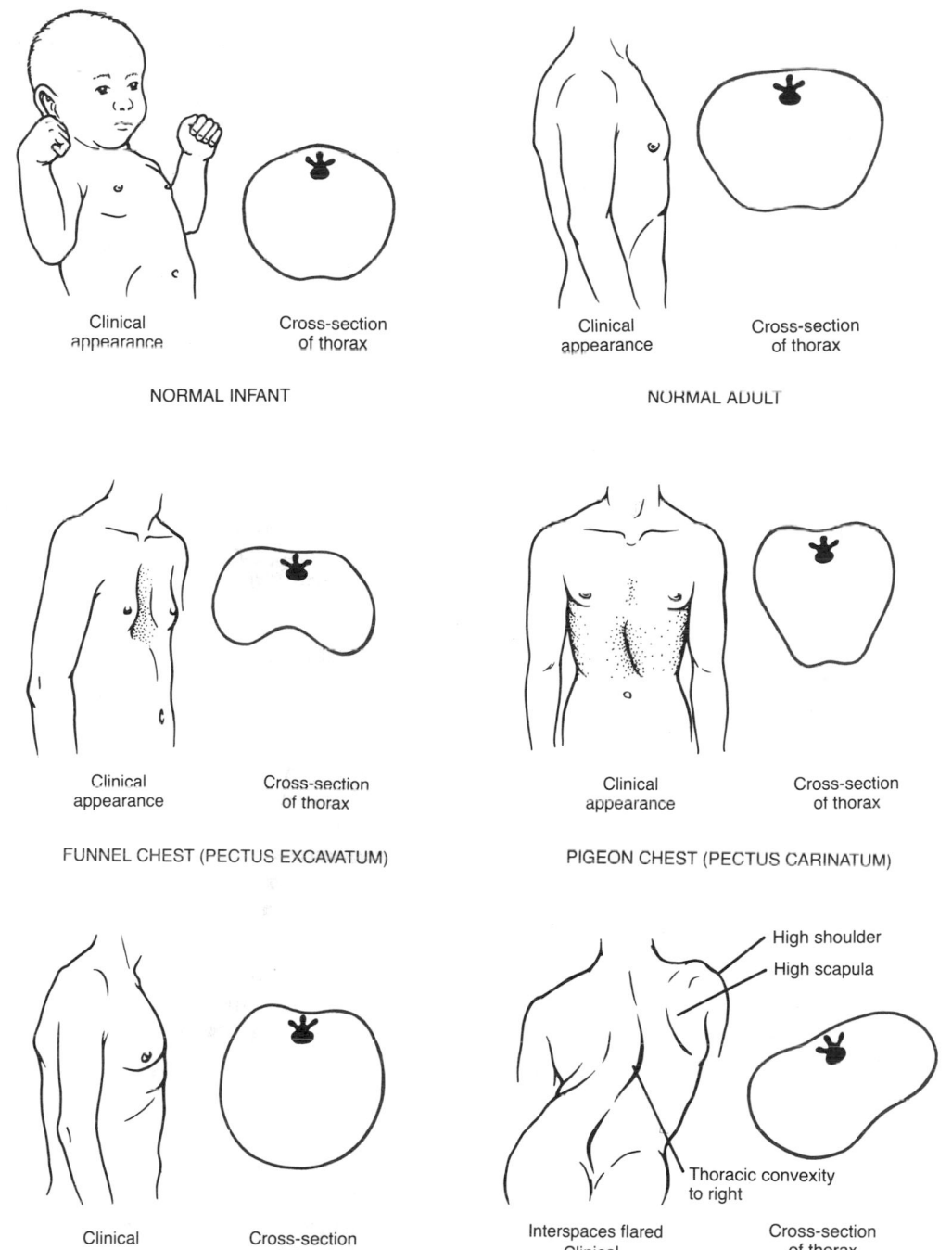

Clinical appearance   Cross-section of thorax

NORMAL INFANT

Clinical appearance   Cross-section of thorax

NORMAL ADULT

Clinical appearance   Cross-section of thorax

FUNNEL CHEST (PECTUS EXCAVATUM)

Clinical appearance   Cross-section of thorax

PIGEON CHEST (PECTUS CARINATUM)

Clinical appearance   Cross-section of thorax

BARREL CHEST

High shoulder
High scapula
Thoracic convexity to right
Interspaces flared
Clinical appearance
Cross-section of thorax

THORACIC KYPHOSCOLIOSIS

FIGURE 7–21   Normal chest configuration and thoracic deformities.

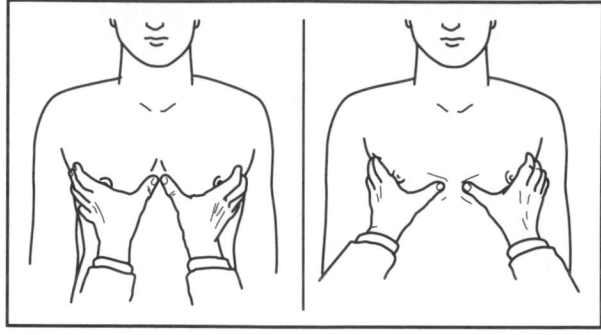

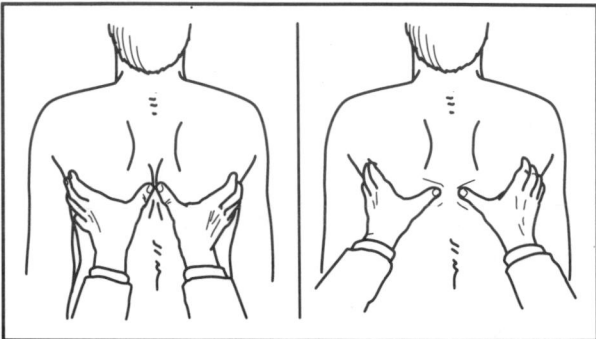

FIGURE 7–22 Assessment of dynamic symmetry, anterior (top) and posterior (bottom) views. (Redrawn from Cherniack RM, Cherniack L: *Respiration in Health and Disease,* 2nd ed. Philadelphia, W. B. Saunders Company, 1972, p 217.)

4. **Auscultation of lungs**
   a. Intensity of inspiration and expiration, when auscultated with a stethoscope, will differ over the various aspects of the thorax. The base sounds are quieter than those of the apex. Familiarity with various lung intensities is required for adequate interpretation. Figure 7–23 shows the sites generally used for auscultation.
      (1). Vesicular (normal breath sound). This is a soft, rustling sound heard throughout all of inspiration and the beginning of expiration.[35] See Figure 7–24 for sites of vesicular breath sounds in health.
      (2). Bronchial. This is a more hollow, echoing sound normally found over the right anterosuperior thorax[35] (corresponding to the area over the right mainstem bronchi) (see Figure 7–24). All of inspiration and most of expiration are heard with bronchial breath sounds.
      (3). Decreased. This is a very distant sound, allowing only some of inspiration to be heard.[35] This sound is not heard anywhere over a healthy thorax.
   b. Any adventitious (extra) sounds that are

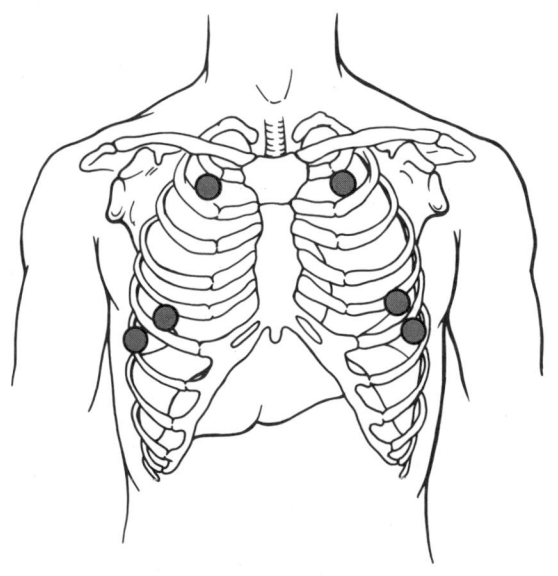

ANTERIOR VIEW

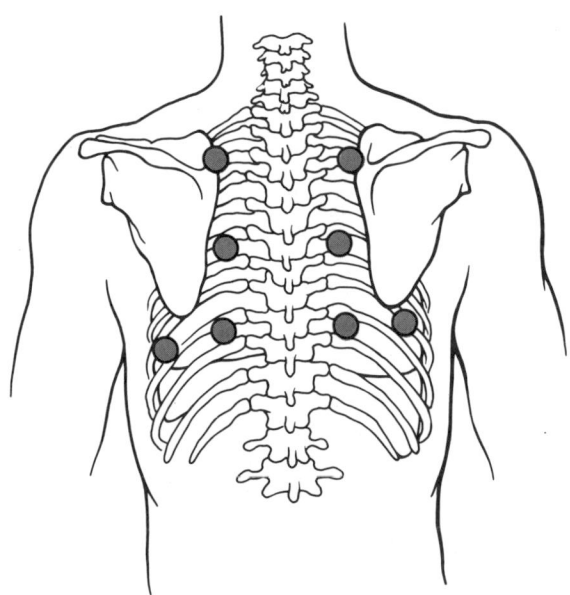

POSTERIOR VIEW

FIGURE 7–23 Anterior, lateral, and posterior auscultation sites.

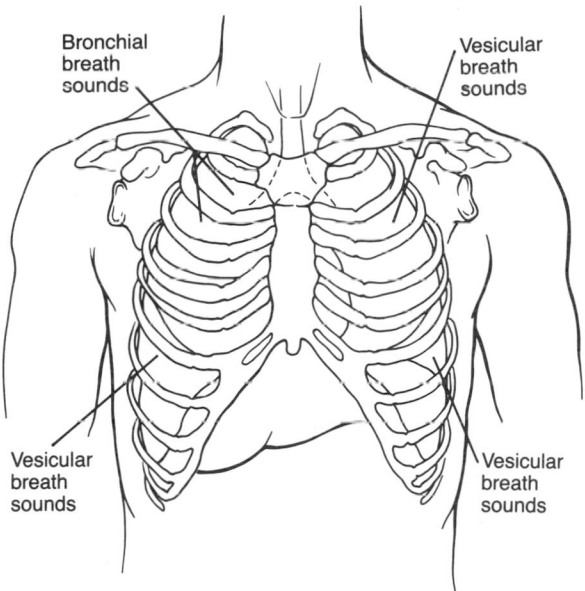

FIGURE 7–24   Normal auscultatory findings over the thorax.

heard concomitantly with intensity should be noted.

(1). *Crackles*[36]

    (a). During early inspiration, crackles may indicate airway narrowing.[37]

    (b). At the end of inspiration, crackles may indicate excessive secretions and flaccid airways, as in bronchiectasis.[37]

    (c). Throughout inspiration, crackles may indicate fibrosis.[37]

(2). *Wheezes*[36]

    (a). At the end of expiration, wheezes reflect mild airway obstruction.[34]

    (b). Throughout the expiratory phase, wheezes indicate significant airway obstruction.[34]

    (c). On both inspiration and expiration, wheezes indicate severe airway obstruction.[34]

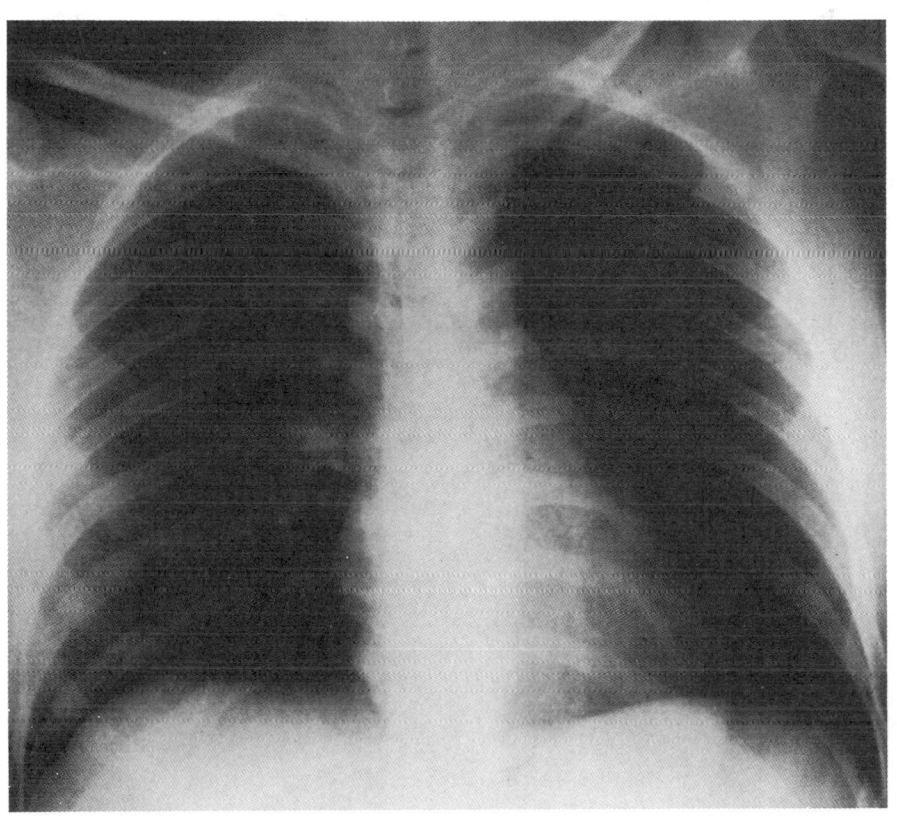

FIGURE 7–25   Normal anteroposterior chest roentgenogram. (From Hinshaw H, Murray J: *Diseases of the Chest.* 4th ed. Philadelphia, W. B. Saunders Company, 1980, p 41.)

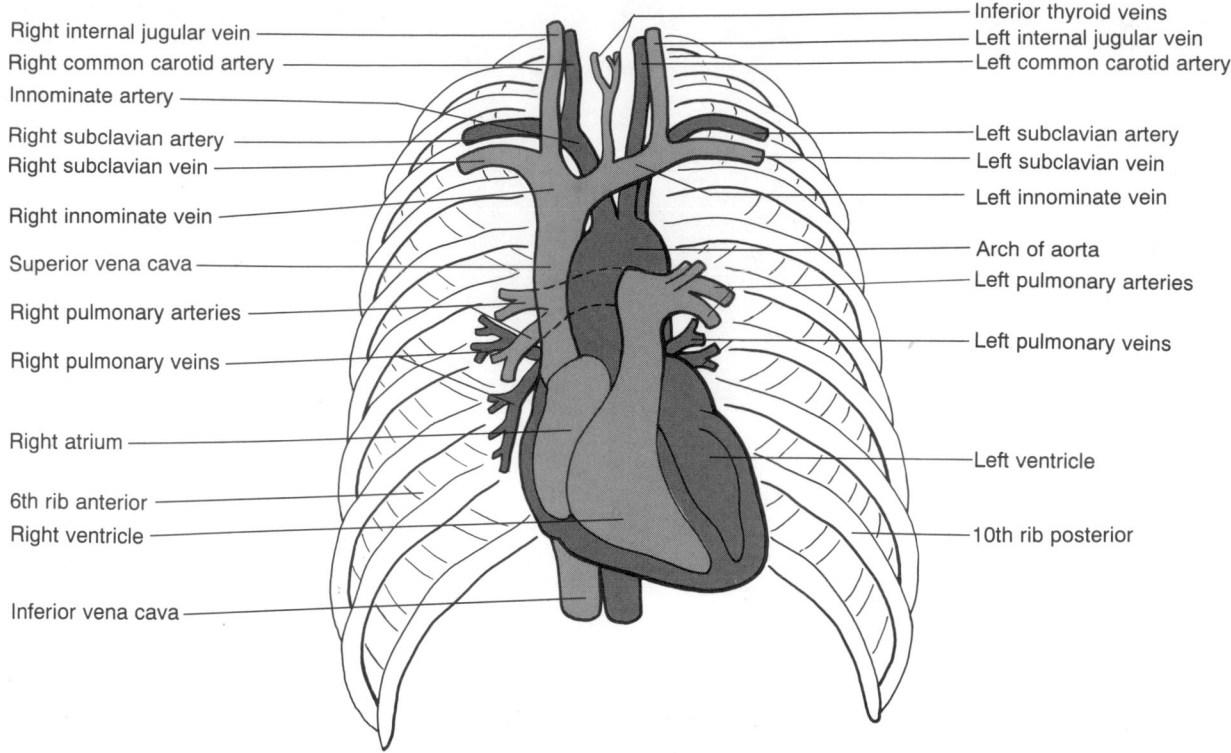

Right internal jugular vein
Right common carotid artery
Innominate artery
Right subclavian artery
Right subclavian vein
Right innominate vein
Superior vena cava
Right pulmonary arteries
Right pulmonary veins
Right atrium
6th rib anterior
Right ventricle
Inferior vena cava

Inferior thyroid veins
Left internal jugular vein
Left common carotid artery
Left subclavian artery
Left subclavian vein
Left innominate vein
Arch of aorta
Left pulmonary arteries
Left pulmonary veins
Left ventricle
10th rib posterior

FIGURE 7–26   Composite illustration showing normal relationship of the heart and great vessels to the pulmonary structures.

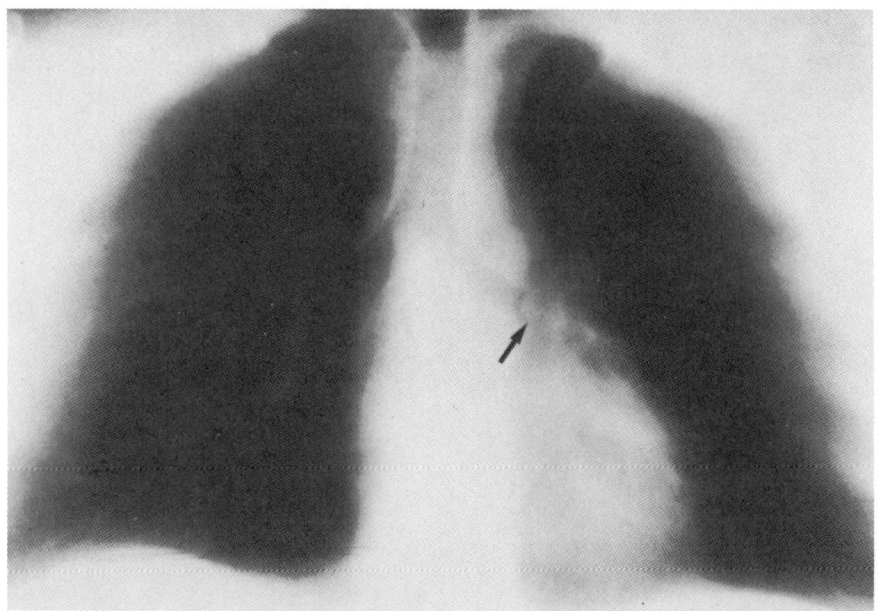

FIGURE 7–27   Lung tomogram showing oval mass (arrow) within left mainstem bronchus. In this relatively anterior section through the lung, the trachea and mainstem bronchi are well outlined. (From Weinberger S: *Principles of Pulmonary Medicine,* 2nd ed. Philadelphia, W. B. Saunders Company, 1992, p 40.)

5. **Radiographic examination**

   a. ***Chest x-ray.*** A two-dimensional radiographic film (usually lateral and postero-anterior views) detects the presence of abnormal material (exudate, blood) or a change in pulmonary parenchyma (fibrosis, collapse) (see Figures 7–25 and 7–26).[38,39]

   b. ***Tomogram.*** Tomography is a roentgenographic technique that blurs all planes except the one being studied. Identification of objects, such as tumors, and their borders may be more easily defined using the tomographic technique[11] (see Figure 7–27).

   c. ***CT (computed tomography) or CAT (computerized axial tomography scan.*** See Figure 7–28. These are computerized pictures of a cross-sectional plane of the body using the tomographic technique.[11]

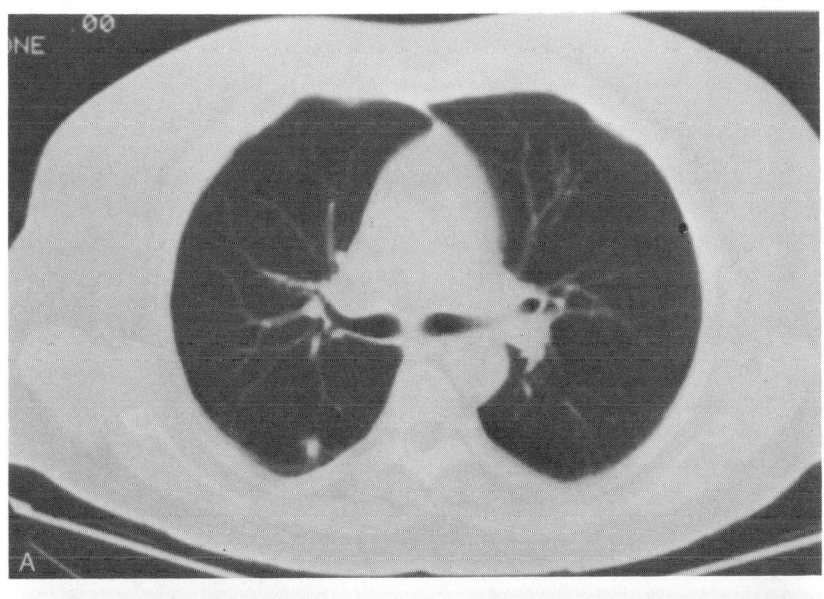

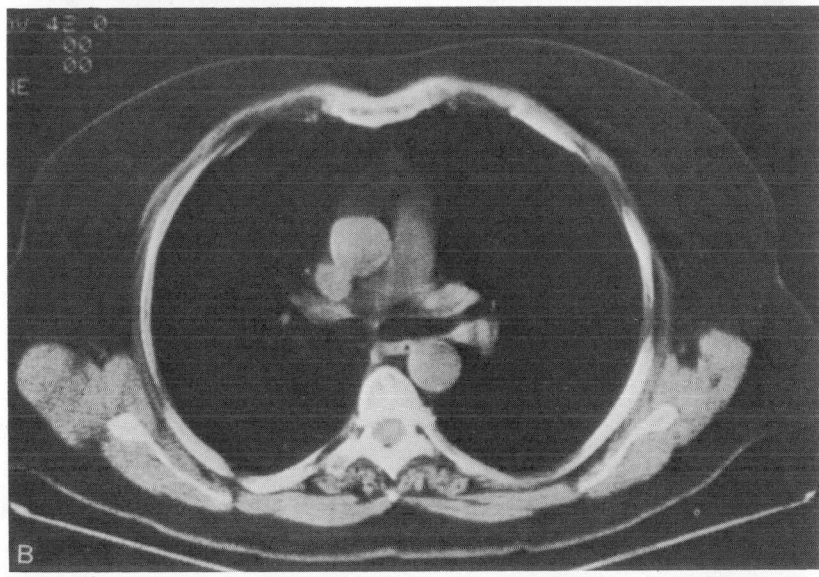

FIGURE 7–28 Cross-sectional "slice" from a computed tomographic scan performed for evaluation of solitary peripheral pulmonary nodule. Nodule can be seen in posterior portion of right lung. (From Weinberger S: *Principles of Pulmonary Medicine,* 2nd ed. Philadelphia, W. B. Saunders Company, 1992, p 41.)

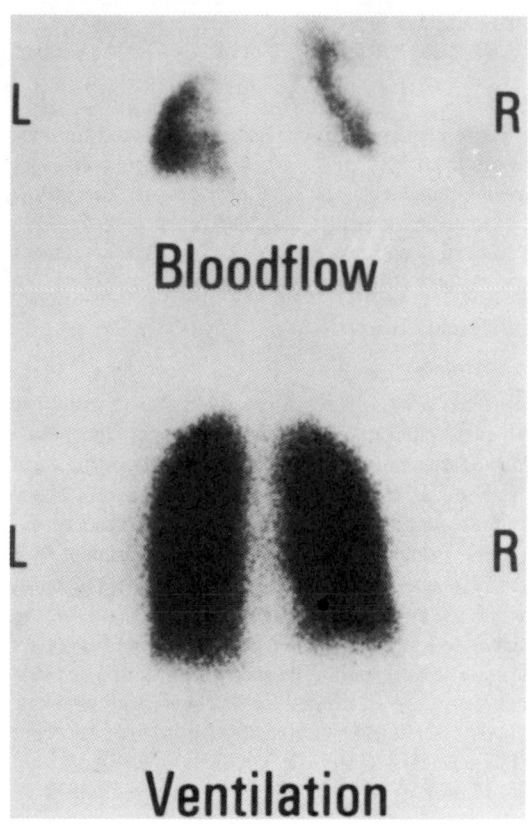

FIGURE 7–29 Lung scan in a patient with multiple pulmonary emboli. The perfusion image shows areas of absent blood flow in both lungs. The ventilation image shows a normal pattern. (From West J: *Pulmonary Pathophysiology: The Essentials,* 4th ed. Baltimore, Williams & Wilkins, 1992, p 121.)

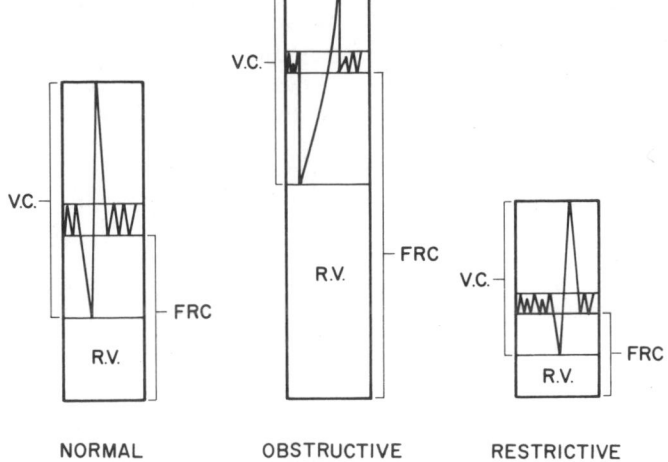

FIGURE 7–30 Total lung capacity and its subdivisions when airflow is obstructed and when distention is restricted. Note that the vital capacity (VC) is lower than expected in both patterns. In the restrictive pattern, the low VC is associated with a reduction in respiratory volume (RV), functional reserve capacity (FRC), and total lung capacity. In the obstructive pattern, the low VC is associated with an increase in RV, FRC, and total lung capacity. (From Cherniack R: *Pulmonary Function Testing,* Philadelphia, W. B. Saunders Company, 1977, p 196.)

d. *Ventilation-perfusion ($\dot{V}/\dot{Q}$) scan.* Matches the ventilation pattern of the lung to the perfusion pattern via radioisotopes. $\dot{V}/\dot{Q}$ scanning identifies the presence of pulmonary emboli[9] (see Figure 7–29).

e. *Fluoroscopy.* Examination by means of a continuous x-ray beam allows observation of movement within the body, such as diaphragmatic excursion.

6. **Laboratory tests**

a. *Arterial blood gas analysis.* This indicates the adequacy of

(1). Alveolar ventilation, by determining pH, bicarbonate ion, and partial pressure of carbon dioxide. Table 7–5 presents the five basic conditions of acid-base balance and the $Paco_2$, pH, and HCO_3^- values that accompany each condition.

(2). Arterial oxygenation, by determining

Table 7–5. INTERPRETATION OF ACID-BASE BALANCE

Condition	pH	Paco₂	HCO₃⁻	Potential Cause
Normal	7.36–7.44	36–44	23–30	
Respiratory acidosis				
No metabolic compensation	↓	↑	—	Holding breath
With metabolic compensation	↓	↑	↑	Long-term hypoventilation
Respiratory alkalosis				
No metabolic compensation	↑	↓	—	Anxiety
With metabolic compensation	↑	↓	↓	Long-term hyperventilation
Metabolic acidosis				
No respiratory compensation	↓	—	↓	Diarrhea
With respiratory compensation	↓	↓	↓	Diabetic ketoacidosis
Metabolic alkalosis				
No respiratory compensation	↑	—	↑	Vomiting
With respiratory compensation	↑	↑	↑	Adrenal disease

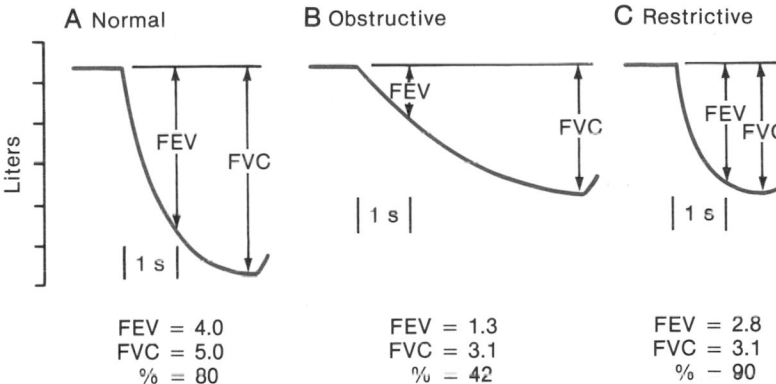

FIGURE 7–31 Normal, obstructive, and restrictive patterns of a forced expiration. (From West J: *Pulmonary Pathophysiology: The Essentials,* 4th ed. Baltimore, Williams & Wilkins, 1992, p 5.)

the partial pressure of oxygen in relation to the fraction of inspired oxygen.

b. *Electrocardiogram.* See Chapter 6 for discussion.

c. *Sputum studies*

(1). *Gram's stain.* This allows immediate identification of a type of bacteria (gram-negative or gram-positive) and its appearance (pairs, chains, etc.).

(2). *Culture and sensitivity.* This identifies the bacteria as well as the organism's susceptibility to various antibiotics. Results are available within a few days.

(3). *Cytology.* This reports the presence of cancer cells in sputum.

d. *Pulmonary function tests.* These evaluate lung volumes, capacities, and flow rates. They are used to diagnose disease, monitor progression, and determine the benefits of medical management. Figures 7–

30 and 7–31 compare normal lung values with those of obstructive and restrictive diseases.

(1). Obstructive disease shows a decreased IC and VC and an increased RV, FRC, and TLC. Flow rates decrease.[28]

(2). Restrictive disease shows a decreased IC, VC, FRC, RV, and TLC. Flow rates are variable, depending on the extent and type of restrictive disease.[7]

7. **Bronchoscopy.** An endoscope is used to view, biopsy, wash, suction, and/or brush the interior aspects of the tracheobronchial tree.

8. **Graded exercise test**

a. Evaluates an individual's cardiopulmonary response to gradually increasing exercise.[40,41] Table 7–6 lists several protocols.[42–48] Age-adjusted maximum heart rate $(220 - age)$ and MVV $(MVV = FEV_1 \times 35$ or MVV for 15 s $\times 4)$

Table 7–6. PROTOCOLS USED FOR EXERCISE TESTING FOR THE PATIENT WITH PULMONARY DISEASE

Mode	Author	Protocol
Walk tests	Cooper[42]	Ambulate as far as possible in 12 min
	Guyatt *et al.*[43]	Ambulate as far as possible in 6 min
Cycle tests	Jones[44]	Begin with 100 kpm (17 W); increase 100 kpm every min
	Carter *et al.*[45]	Begin with 25 W; 15-W increase every min
	Berman and Sutton[46]	Begin with 100 kpm/min; increase 100 kpm/min every min or 50 kpm/min every min when $FEV_1 < 1$ L/s
	Massachusetts Respiratory Hospital	Begin at 25 W; 10 W every 20 s or 5 W every 20 s when $FEV_1 < 1$ L/s
Treadmill tests	Naughton *et al.*[47]	2 mph constant 0 grade; 3.5% grade every 3 min
	Balke and Ware[48]	3.3 mph constant 0 grade; 3.5% grade every 2 min
	Massachusetts Respiratory Hospital	1.5 mph constant 0 grade; 4% grade every 2 min; 2% grade every 2 min if $FEV_1 < 1$ L/s

From Brannon F, Foley M, Starr J, *et al.: Cardiopulmonary Rehabilitation: Basic Theory and Application,* 2nd ed. Philadelphia, F. A. Davis Company, 1992, p. 269.

are calculated before initiating exercise testing to anticipate pulmonary and cardiac end points.

b. Determines the presence of exercise-induced bronchospasm by testing pulmonary function before and after testing.[49]

c. Documents the need for supplemental oxygen during an exercise program by analyzing arterial blood gas values throughout the testing.[50] These values also provide criteria for test termination. If arterial blood sampling is unavailable, pulse oximetry monitors some of the same parameters. Table 7–7 presents criteria for test termination for patients with pulmonary disease.

Table 7–7.   GRADED EXERCISE TEST TERMINATION CRITERIA

1. Maximal shortness of breath
2. A fall in PaO_2 >20 mm Hg or a PaO_2 <55 mm Hg
3. A rise in $PaCO_2$ >10 mm Hg or >65 mm Hg
4. Cardiac ischemia or arrhythmias
5. Symptoms of fatigue
6. Increase in diastolic blood pressure readings of 20 mm Hg, systolic hypertension >250 mm Hg, decrease in blood pressure with increasing workloads
7. Leg pain
8. Total fatigue
9. Signs of insufficient cardiac output
10. Reaching a ventilatory maximum

From Brannon F, Foley M, Starr J, et al.: *Cardiopulmonary Rehabilitation. Basic Theory and Application,* 2nd ed. Philadelphia, F. A. Davis Company, 1992, p. 270.

IV. Major Conditions and Special Considerations

A. Autoimmune diseases

1. **Acquired immunodeficiency syndrome.** See section on *Pneumocystis carinii* pneumonia.

2. **Goodpasture's syndrome**
   a. *Description.* Damage occurs to the basement membrane of the alveoli; associated with glomerulonephritis.
   b. *Pertinent physical findings*
      (1). Presents with pulmonary hemorrhage, hemoptysis.
      (2). Dyspnea.
      (3). Anemia.
      (4). Chest x-ray can show pulmonary infiltrate or pulmonary fibrosis.
   c. *Physical therapy considerations*
      (1). Supportive therapy if needed: supplemental oxygen, proper positioning for optimal $\dot{V}/\dot{Q}$ ratio, mechanical ventilation.
      (2). Secretion removal techniques only after exacerbation and hemorrhage resolve.

3. **Alpha₁-antitrypsin emphysema**
   a. *Description.* Alveolar destruction by trypsin because of the absence of the enzyme antitrypsin.
   b. *Pertinent physical findings*
      (1). Symptoms usually occur at younger age than emphysema from chronic obstructive pulmonary disease (COPD).
      (2). Negative smoking history may be present.
      (3). Barrel chest.
      (4). Dry cough.
      (5). Dyspnea, especially on exertion (age of onset of dypnea is earlier in a smoker [32 years] than a nonsmoker [51 years]).[50,51]
      (6). Use of accessory muscles of ventilation.
      (7). Decreased breath sounds.
      (8). Clubbing.
      (9). Cyanosis.
      (10). Arterial blood gas changes of hypoxemia and hypercapnea.
      (11). Obstructive pattern on pulmonary function tests.
      (12). Chest x-ray shows decrease in vascular markings, flattened diaphragm, hyperlucency, and cor pulmonale.
   c. *Physical therapy considerations*
      (1). Secretion removal techniques are not indicated unless there is a concomitant secretion-producing disease.
      (2). Emphasis is on breathing control with prolonged exhalation.
      (3). Improvement of functional capacity.
      (4). Inspiratory muscle training.
      (5). Energy-saving techniques.

4. **Systemic lupus erythematosus**
   a. *Description.* A systemic disease with possible pleural complications: pleuritis, pleural effusions.
   b. *Pertinent physical findings*
      (1). Shallow breathing.
      (2). Chest pain during inspiration (especially on deep breath) with pleuritis.
      (3). Effusion may be heard as decreased breath sounds over the involved area; friction rub may be present.
      (4). Chest x-ray may show fluid in the intrapleural space (effusion).
   c. *Physical therapy considerations*
      (1). Neither pleuritis nor effusion can be cleared by secretion removal techniques.
      (2). Provision of supportive therapy during exacerbation if needed: supplemental oxygen, mechanical ventilation, proper positioning for optimal $\dot{V}/\dot{Q}$ ratio.
      (3). Prevention of superinfection in affected areas by ensuring aeration with breathing exercise.
      (4). Improvement of functional capacity during remission of symptoms.

5. **Rheumatoid arthritis**
   a. *Description.* A systemic disorder with possible pulmonary manifestations of pleural effusions, pleuritis, and/or diffuse interstitial pneumonitis.
   b. *Pertinent physical findings*
      (1). Shallow breathing.
      (2). Chest pain during inspiration (especially a deep breath) with pleuritis.
      (3). Effusion auscultated as decreased breath sounds over the involved area; friction rub may be present.
      (4). Interstitial pneumonitis may produce crackles.
      (5). Chest x-ray shows increased fluid in the intrapleural space (effusion) and/or diffuse infiltrate.
   c. *Physical therapy considerations*
      (1). Neither pleuritis, pleural effusion, nor interstitial involvement can be cleared by secretion removal techniques.
      (2). Provision of supportive therapy during exacerbation if needed: proper positioning for optimal

$\dot{V}/\dot{Q}$ ratio, supplemental oxygen, mechanical ventilation.
      (3). Prevention of superinfection in affected areas by ensuring aeration with breathing exercise.
      (4). Improvement of functional capacity during remission of symptoms.

6. **Hypersensitivity pneumonitis**
   a. *Description.* Interstitial pneumonitis (acute) or fibrosis (chronic) due to the inhalation of a variety of organic dusts.
   b. *Pertinent physical findings*[52]
      (1). Correlation between pulmonary symptoms and exposure to the affecting substance.
      (2). *Acute symptoms*
         (a). Chills.
         (b). Fever.
         (c). Cough.
         (d). Dyspnea.
         (e). Chest tightness.
         (f). Tachypnea.
         (g). Cyanosis.
         (h). Crackles and/or wheezes.
         (i). Chest x-ray of diffuse patchy infiltration, reticular pattern.
      (3). *Chronic symptoms.*
         (a). Dyspnea.
         (b). Respiratory insufficiency.
         (c). Early fatigue.
         (d). Decreased functional capacity.
   c. *Physical therapy considerations.*
      (1). Identification of and removal from source of exposure.
      (2). Supportive measures and management of symptoms.
      (3). Maintenance of functional capacity.

7. **Scleroderma**
   a. *Description.* A systemic disorder characterized by diffuse fibrosis, degenerative changes, and vascular abnormalities in skin, articular structures, and other organs. Pulmonary involvement results in restrictive pattern of interstitial fibrosis, pulmonary hypertension, and cor pulmonale.[11]
   b. *Pertinent physical findings*
      (1). Early fatigue.
      (2). Tachypnea.
      (3). Crackles on auscultation.
      (4). Restricted chest wall mobility.
   c. *Physical therapy considerations.*
      (1). Supportive therapy.
      (2). Breathing exercises.

(3). Maintenance of functional capacity.

8. **Sarcoidosis**

   a. *Description.* A systemic disease, epidemiologically favoring young black women, producing noncaseating granulomas with a possibility of accompanying alveolitis. Other common manifestations of disease appear in all systems, but mainly the eyes and skin.

   b. *Pertinent physical findings*
      (1). Dyspnea, especially on exertion.
      (2). Unproductive cough.
      (3). Generalized symptoms of fever, weight loss, and anorexia.
      (4). Crackles.
      (5). Hypoxemia.
      (6). Cyanosis.
      (7). Chest x-ray of symmetrical hilar adenopathy and/or interstitial lung disease.

   c. *Physical therapy considerations.*
      (1). Maintenance of functional capacity.
      (2). Breathing exercises.
      (3). Supportive therapy if needed.

9. **Bronchiolitis obliterans with organizing pneumonia**

   a. *Description.* A disease producing connective tissue plugs in the small airways with possible pulmonary parenchymal infiltration of mononuclear cells.

   b. *Pertinent physical findings*
      (1). Dyspnea.
      (2). Wheezing.
      (3). Chest x-ray of patchy alveolar infiltrates.

   c. *Physical therapy considerations*
      (1). Maintenance of functional capacity.
      (2). Breathing exercises.
      (3). Supportive therapy if needed.

B. Trauma

1. **Rib fracture, flail chest**

   a. *Description.* Fracture of the ribs usually due to blunt trauma. Flail chest is two or more fractures in two or more adjacent ribs (see Figure 7–32).[53]

   b. **Pertinent physical findings**
      (1). Shallow breathing.
      (2). Splinting due to pain (especially with deep inspiration or cough).
      (3). Crepitation during the ventilatory cycle over fracture site.
      (4). Paradoxical movement of the flail section during the ventilatory cycle (on inspiration, the flail section is

A

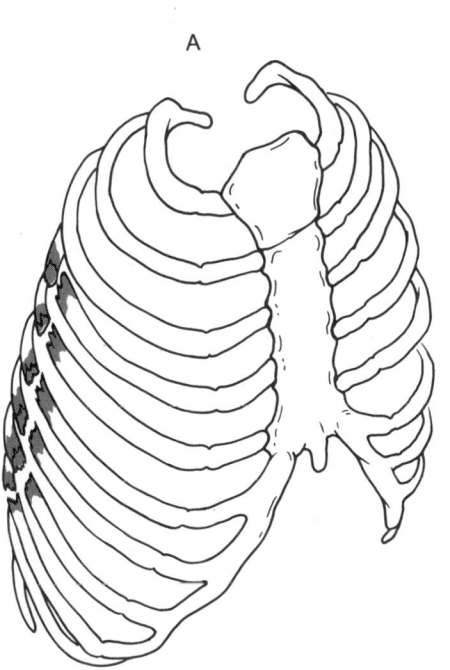

B

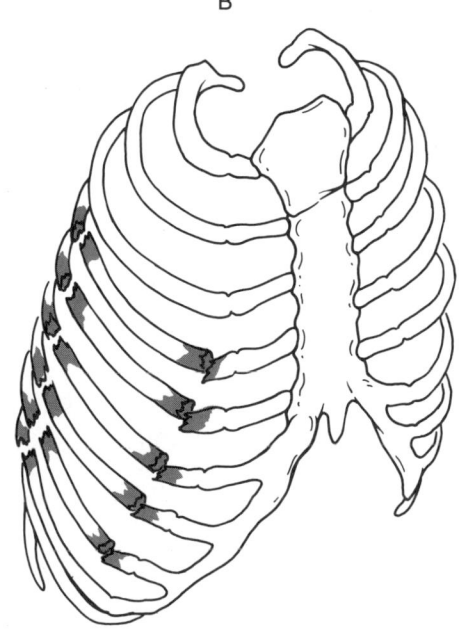

FIGURE 7–32   **A,** Rib fractures. **B,** Flail chest.

pulled inward; on exhalation, the flail moves outward).

(5). Confirmation by chest x-ray.

c. **Physical therapy considerations**

(1). Pain control may be necessary to improve ventilatory ability.

(2). Assessment for associated pleural and parenchymal complications.

(3). Prevention of pulmonary complications with breathing exercises, splinting, and appropriate positioning.

(4). If treatment of an associated parenchymal involvement is necessary, caution with, although not an absolute contraindication to, chest compressive maneuvers is recommended.[54]

2. Pleural injury

a. **Pneumothorax** (See Figure 7–33)

(1). *Description.* Air in the intrapleural space, usually through a lacerated visceral pleura from a rib fracture or ruptured bullae.

(2). *Pertinent physical findings.* All increase with the severity of injury.

(a). Chest pain.

(b). Dyspnea.

(c). Tracheal deviation away from injured side.

(d). Absent or decreased breath sounds.

(e). Cyanosis.

(f). Respiratory distress.

(g). Confirmation by chest x-ray.

(3). *Physical therapy considerations*

(a). Insertion of chest tube by medical personnel to remove the air.

(b). Assessment for associated injuries of the chest wall.

(c). Any resultant parenchymal involvement may be treated as appropriate with physical therapy techniques: segmental expansion breathing exercises, secretion removal techniques, splinting during deep breathing and coughing, and positioning for improved $\dot{V}/\dot{Q}$ ratio.

b. **Hemothorax**

(1). *Description.* Blood in the pleural space, usually from a laceration of the parietal pleura.

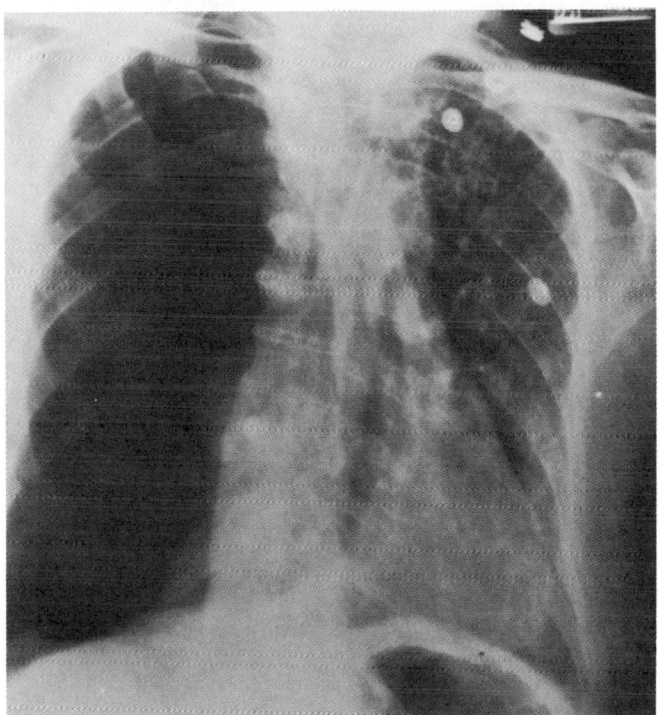

FIGURE 7–33 Chest radiograph showing right-sided tension pneumothorax. No lung markings are seen in right hemithorax, and mediastinum is shifted to left. (From Weinberger S: *Principles of Pulmonary Medicine.* 2nd ed. Philadelphia, W. B. Saunders Company, 1992, p 194.)

(2). *Pertinent physical findings.* All increase with the severity of injury.

(a). Chest pain.

(b). Dyspnea.

(c). Tracheal deviation away from side of injury.

(d). Absent or decreased breath sounds.

(e). Cyanosis.

(f). Respiratory distress.

(g). Confirmation by chest x-ray.

(h). Signs of blood loss.

(3). *Physical therapy considerations*

(a). If moderate to severe, accumulation of blood is present; thoracentesis or chest tube insertion by medical personnel may be necessary.

(b). Assessment for associated injuries of the chest wall.

(c). Any effects of parenchymal compression can be resolved with physical therapy once bleeding is resolved: breathing exercises, secretion removal techniques, splitting during deep breathing and coughing, positioning for optimal $\dot{V}/\dot{Q}$ ratio.

3. **Lung contusion**
   a. *Description.* Blood and edema within the alveoli and interstitial space due to blunt chest trauma.
   b. *Pertinent physical findings.* All increase with the severity of injury.
      (1). Cough with hemoptysis.
      (2). Dyspnea.
      (3). Decreased breath sounds and/or crackles.
      (4). Cyanosis.
      (5). Confirmation by chest x-ray of ill-defined patchy densities.

   c. *Physical therapy considerations*
      (1). Assessment of associated injuries of the chest wall.
      (2). Once bleeding is controlled, secretion removal techniques can be instituted if necessary.
      (3). Segmental expansion exercises for improved aeration.
      (4). Proper positioning for optimal $\dot{V}/\dot{Q}$ ratio.

C. Acute diseases/pulmonary infections

See Table 7–8 for comparison of various types of pneumonia.[55]

1. **Bacterial pneumonia**
   a. *Gram-positive bacteria*
      (1). *Description.* Gram-positive bacteria cause an intra-alveolar process. The

Table 7–8. DIFFERENTIATION OF PNEUMONIA RESULTING FROM INFECTIOUS AGENTS

Clinical Features	Organisms			
	Viral	*Rickettsial*	*Mycoplasmal*	*Pyogenic Bacterial*
Community history	Epidemic	Animal, bird contacts	Family illness	Not significant
Prodrome	Upper respiratory General malaise	General malaise	Upper respiratory General malaise	Occasional pharyngitis
Onset	Gradual	Gradual	Gradual	Sudden
Cough	Persistent Nonproductive	Persistent Nonproductive	Persistent Nonproductive	Persistent Purulent, bloody sputum
Chest pain	Uncommon	Uncommon	Uncommon	Common, pleuritic
Physical findings on chest examination	Minimal	Minimal	Rales, rhonchi diffuse	Localized, well defined
Roentgenogram findings	Patchy, nonspecific	Patchy, nonspecific	Patchy, lower lobes, unilateral	Localized
Leukocyte count	Normal leukopenic Mildly elevated	Normal leukopenic Mildly elevated	Normal leukopenic Mildly elevated	Polymorphonuclear leukocytosis
Sputum smear	Few leukocytes Epithelial debris	Few leukocytes Epithelial debris	Few leukocytes Occasionally leukocytes without bacteria	Numerous leukocytes Intracellular bacteria
Pleural fluid	Rare	Rare	Rare	Occasional; with empyema
Blood cultures	Negative	Negative	Negative	+10%–40%
Serology	Definitive	Definitive	Definitive	Not helpful
Response to antimicrobials	None	Good Tetracycline or chloramphenicol	Good Tetracycline or erythromycin	Good. Requires identification of organism
Secondary bacterial infection	Common	Uncommon	Uncommon	Uncommon

From Guenter C, Welch M: *Pulmonary Medicine,* 2nd ed. Philadelphia, J. B. Lippincott Company, 1982, p. 330.

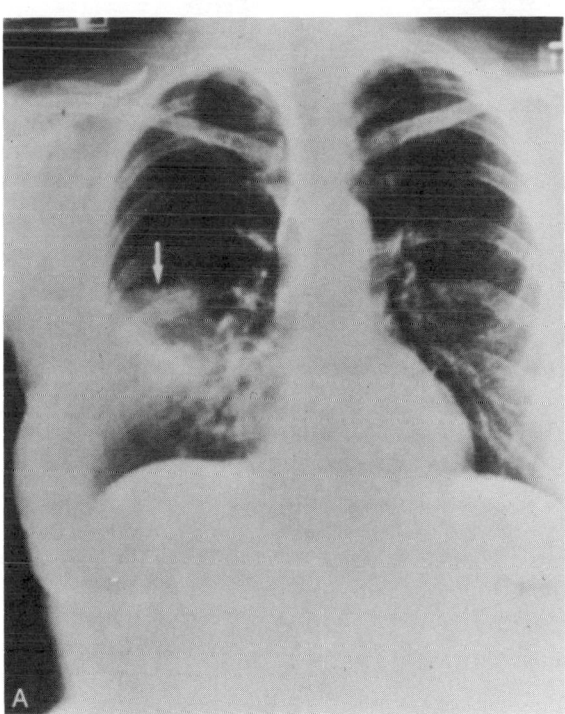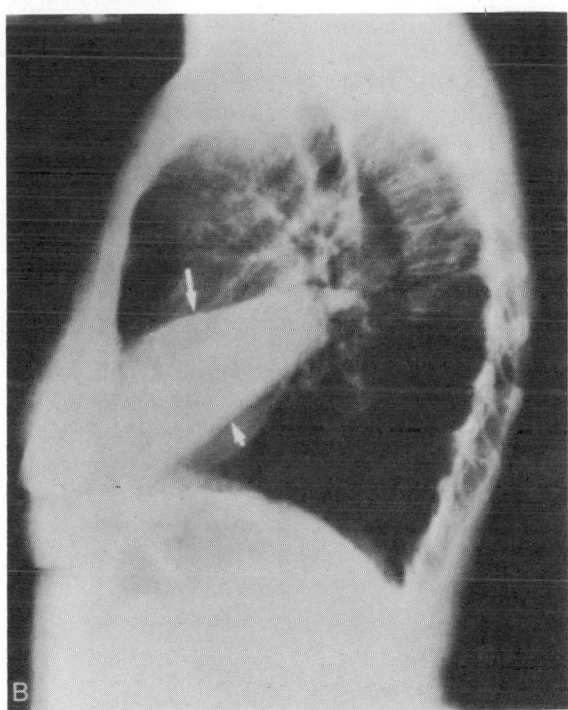

FIGURE 7–34   Posterior **(A)** and lateral **(B)** chest radiographs demonstrating lobar pneumonia (probably caused by *Streptococcus pneumoniae*) that affects the right middle lobe. In panel **A,** the arrow points to the horizontal fissure, which defines the upper border of the middle lobe. In panel **B,** the long arrow points to the horizontal fissure, and the short arrow, to the oblique fissure. (From Weinberger S: *Principles of Pulmonary Medicine.* 2nd ed. Philadelphia, W. B. Saunders Company, 1992, p 270.)

progression is from initial edema and hemorrhage (red hepatization) through phagocytosis (gray hepatization) to resolution (white hepatization). Pneumococcal pneumonia *(Streptococcus pneumoniae)* is the most common gram-positive community-acquired pulmonary infection.

(2). *Pertinent physical findings*
  (a). Shaking chills.
  (b). Fever.
  (c). Chest pain if pleuritic involvement.
  (d). Cough becoming productive of purulent blood-streaked or rusty sputum.
  (e). Decreased or bronchial breath sounds and/or crackles.
  (f). Tachypnea.
  (g). Increased white blood cell count.
  (h). Hypoxemia, hypocapnea initially, hypercapnea with increasing severity.
  (i). Chest x-ray confirmation by alveolar infiltrate and/or consolidation and air bronchogram (see Figure 7–34).

(3). *Physical therapy considerations*
  (a). Secretion removal techniques for the involved segments.
  (b). Splinting for cough and deep breathing if pleural pain is present.
  (c). Supportive therapy if needed: proper positioning for optimal ventilation-perfusion relationship, supplemental oxygen, and mechanical ventilation.

b. *Gram-negative bacteria*
  (1). *Description.* An intra-alveolar process, usually nosocomial, that results in early tissue necrosis and abcess formation. Host usually has an underlying chronic debilitating condition, severe acute illness, and/or recent antibiotic therapy. Common infecting organisms: *Klebsiella, Haemophilus influenzae, Pseudomonas aeruginosa, Proteus, Serratia.*
  (2). *Pertinent physical findings*

(a). Deterioration of general condition.

(b). Deterioration of pulmonary status.

(c). Fever.

(d). Chest pain if pleuritic involvement.

(e). Change in cough and expectoration.

(f). Decreased or bronchial breath sounds and/or crackles.

(g). Tachypnea.

(h). Increased high white blood cell count.

(i). Hypoxemia.

(j). Hypocapnea or hypercapnea, depending on the severity of illness.

(k). Chest x-ray confirmation by consolidation, cavitation, pleural effusions.

(3). *Physical therapy considerations*

(a). Secretion removal techniques for the involved segments.

(b). Splinting for cough and deep breathing if pleural pain is present.

(c). Supportive measures if necessary: positioning for optimal $\dot{V}/\dot{Q}$ ratio, supplemental oxygen, mechanical ventilation.

c. **Mycoplasmal pneumonia**

(1). *Description.* Caused by a small non-walled bacteria resulting in intersti-

tial or lobar pneumonia (usually lower lobes). *Mycoplasma* does not stain on Gram's stain.[56]

(2). *Pertinent physical findings*

(a). Typically young adults.

(b). Nonproductive or minimally productive cough.

(c). Headache.

(d). Chills.

(e). Fever.

(f). Crackles on auscultation.

(g). Sore throat and otitis often present.

(h). White blood cell normal or slightly elevated.

(i). Chest x-ray shows diffuse interstitial infiltrate (see Figure 7-35).

(3). *Physical therapy considerations*

(a). Supportive measures if necessary: proper positioning for optimal $\dot{V}/\dot{Q}$ ratio, supplemental oxygen, mechanical ventilation.

(b). Secretion removal techniques not indicated.

(c). Segmental expansion exercises for the involved lung area.

d. **Legionnaires' disease**

(1). *Description.* Pneumonia caused by inhalation of an airborne bacteria spread from contaminated source (water or soil). Although *Legionella pneumophila* is a gram-negative bac-

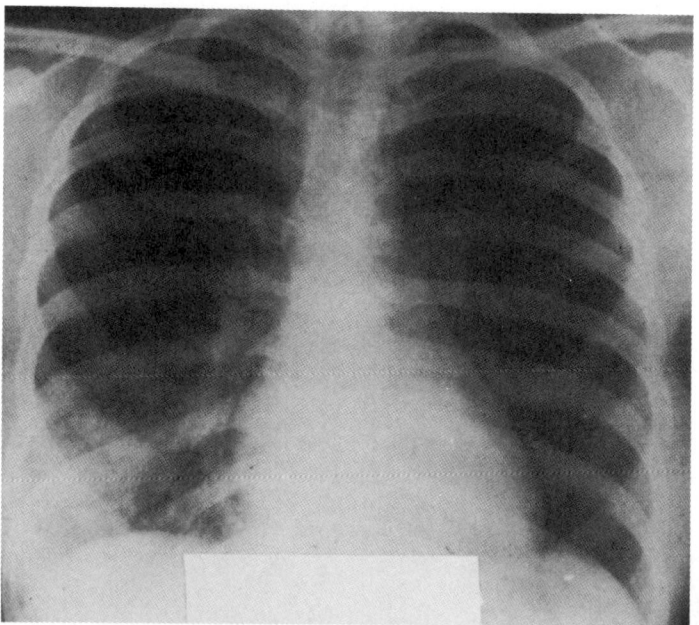

FIGURE 7–35 Pneumonia due to *Mycoplasma pneumoniae.* Young woman with mycoplasmal pneumonia demonstrating a segmental distribution and volume loss (downward displacement of horizontal fissure). (From Hinshaw H, Murray J: *Diseases of the Chest,* 4th ed. Philadelphia, W. B. Saunders Company, 1980, p 237.)

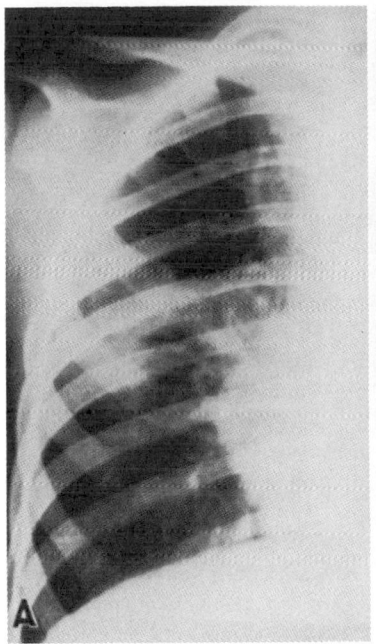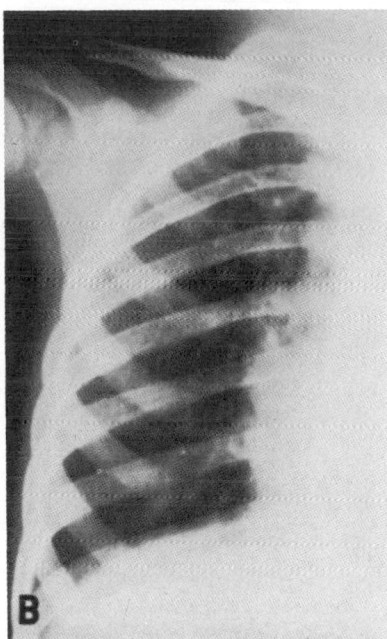

FIGURE 7–36 Viral pneumonia in a boy 11 years of age with chills, fever, cough, headache, and generalized muscle pain. **A,** Irregular infiltration in right midlung and circumscribed areas of increased translucency. **B,** One week later, almost complete resolution occurred. (From Rubin E, Rubin M: *Thoracic Diseases, Emphasizing Cardiopulmonary Relationships.* Philadelphia, W. B. Saunders Company, 1961, p 336.)

teria, it does not stain well by conventional methods and may be missed as the infecting organism.[11]

(2). *Pertinent physical findings*
   (a). Rapid onset of nonproductive or minimally productive cough.
   (b). Very high fever and chills.
   (c). Hypoxemia and hypocapnea.
   (d). White blood cell count shows leukocytosis.
   (e). Chest x-ray shows patchy infiltrates commonly in lower lobes progressing to lobar densities.

(3). *Physical therapy considerations*
   (a). Supportive measures of proper positioning for optimal $\dot{V}/\dot{Q}$ ratio, supplemental oxygen, mechanical ventilation if necessary.
   (b). Secretions are not part of the usual clinical picture of legionnaires' disease. If secretions from intubation or secondary infections are present, secretion removal techniques can be employed.

2. **Viral pneumonia**
   a. *Description.* Viral agents (influenza, adenovirus, cytomegalovirus, herpes, parainfluenza, and respiratory syncytial virus,

measles) cause interstitial and possibly alveolar edema and hemorrhage.

b. *Pertinent physical findings*
   (1). Recent history of upper respiratory infection.
   (2). Fever.
   (3). Chills.
   (4). Dry cough.
   (5). Headaches.
   (6). Decreased breath sounds and/or crackles.
   (7). Hypoxemia and hypocapnea (hypercapnea is unusual unless there is an underlying medical problem).
   (8). Normal white blood cell count.
   (9). Chest x-ray shows interstitial infiltration (see Figure 7–36).

c. *Physical therapy considerations*
   (1). Supportive therapy if necessary: proper positioning for ventilation-perfusion relationship, supplemental oxygen (although hypoxemia often remains), mechanical ventilation.
   (2). Secretion removal techniques not indicated unless a secondary bacterial superinfection arises.

3. **Aspiration pneumonia**
   a. *Description.* The aspirated material causes an acute inflammatory reaction within the lungs. Usually found in patients with an impaired swallow, impaired conscious-

ness (anesthesia), neuromuscular disease, etc. The involved areas are dependent on the body position at the time of aspiration.[33]

b. *Pertinent physical findings*

  (1). Symptoms begin shortly after aspiration event (hours).

  (2). Cough may be dry at onset, progress to producing putrid secretions.

  (3). Dyspnea.

  (4). Tachypnea.

  (5). Cyanosis.

  (6). Tachycardia.

  (7). Wheezes and crackles with decreased breath sounds.

  (8). Hypoxemia and hypocapnea; hypercapnea in severe cases.

  (9). Chest pain if inflammation extends to the pleura.

  (10). Fever.

  (11). White blood cell count shows varying degrees of leukocytosis.

  (12). Chest x-ray shows initial pneumonitis; with chronic aspiration, shows necrotizing pneumonia with cavitation.

c. *Physical therapy considerations*

  (1). Secretion removal techniques for immediate removal of aspirated contents, maintenance of patent airway, and reversal of hypoxemia, if possible.

  (2). Aspiration precautions to reduce further aspiration episodes. Positioning for optimal $\dot{V}/\dot{Q}$ ratio, if possible.

4. **Tuberculosis**

a. *Description.* An infection caused by an airborne *Mycobacterium tuberculosis* spread from an untreated infected host. Incubation period: 2 to 10 weeks. Primary disease lasts approximately 10 days to 2 weeks. Postprimary infection is reactivation of dormant tuberculous bacillus, which can occur years after the primary infection. Two weeks on appropriate antituberculin drugs renders the host noninfectious. Medication is taken for prolonged periods (6 to 12 months).[11]

b. *Pertinent physical findings*

  (1). Primary disease can be unnoticed as it causes only the following mild symptoms:

    (a). Slight nonproductive cough.

    (b). Low-grade fever.

    (c). Chest x-ray may show Ghon lesion.

  (2). Postprimary infection is characterized by the following symptoms:

    (a). Fever.

    (b). Weight loss.

    (c). Cough.

    (d). Hilar adenopathy.

    (e). Night sweats.

    (f). Crackles.

    (g). Hemoptysis.

    (h). White blood cell count showing increased lymphocytes.

    (i). Chest x-ray showing upper lobe involvement (due to the propensity for high oxygen areas) with air-space densities, cavitation, pleural involvement, and/or parenchymal fibrosis (see Figure 7–37).

c. *Physical therapy considerations*

  (1). Respiratory precautions and isolation, including masks, hand washing, and proper disposal of sputum, of suspected or newly diagnosed individuals.

  (2). If patients are unable to clear secretions independently, secretion removal techniques are indicated.

5. *Pneumocystis carinii* **pneumonia**

a. *Description.* Pneumonia caused by a protozoan in immunocompromised hosts, most often found in patients post-transplantation, neonates, or patients infected with human immunodeficiency virus.[57]

b. *Pertinent physical findings*

  (1). Insidious progressive shortness of breath.

  (2). Nonproductive cough.

  (3). Crackles.

  (4). Weakness.

  (5). Fever.

  (6). Chest x-ray shows interstitial infiltrates.

  (7). Complete blood count shows no evidence of disease.

c. *Physical therapy considerations*

  (1). Supportive measures if needed: supplemental oxygen, mechanical ventilation, and positioning for optimal $\dot{V}/\dot{Q}$ ratio.

  (2). Nebulized drug therapy (pentamidine).

  (3). Secretion removal techniques are

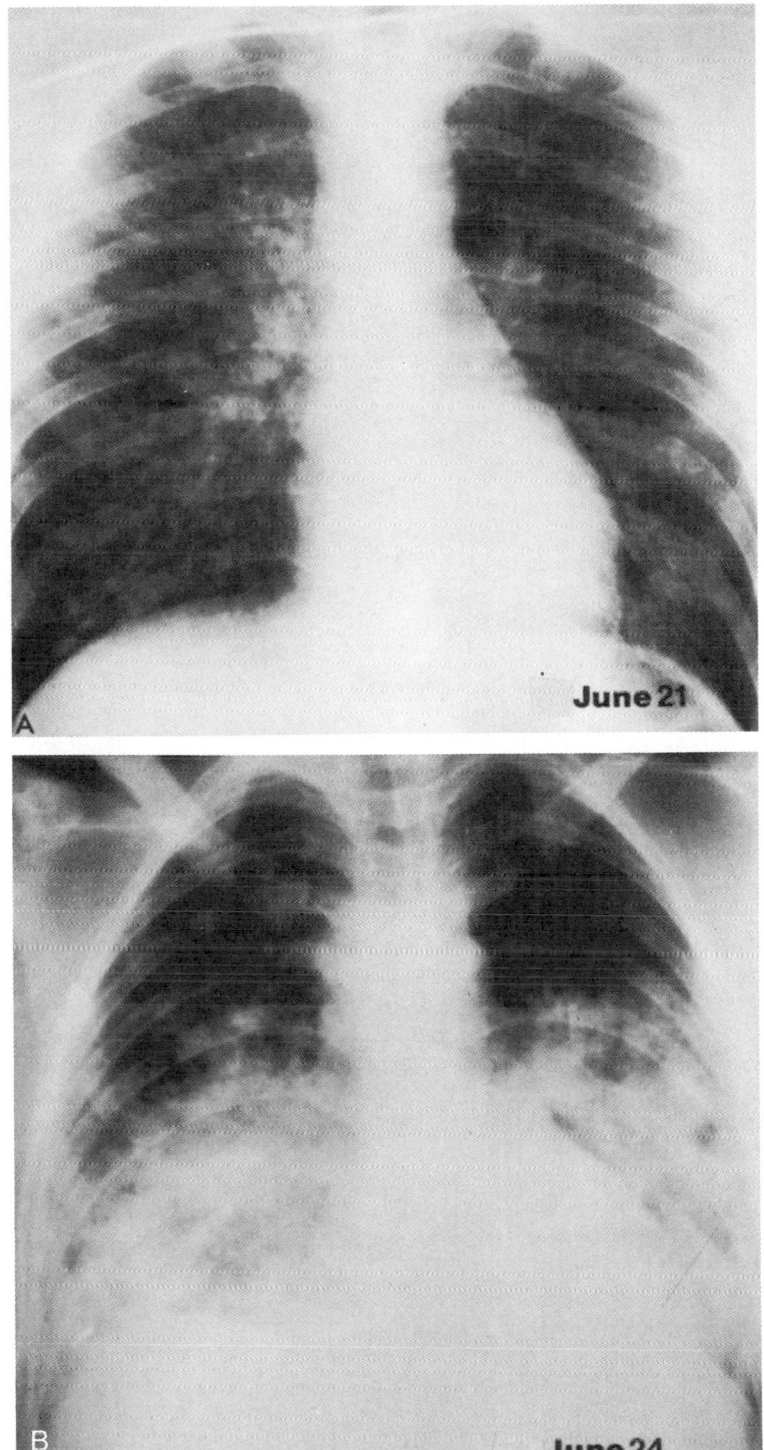

FIGURE 7–37 Cavitary tuberculosis of the right upper lobe with patchy areas of bronchogenic spread to the left lung. (From Fraser R, Paré J: *Diagnosis of Diseases of the Chest.* 2nd ed. Philadelphia, W. B. Saunders Company, 1979, p 750.)

not indicated because excessive secretions are usually not present.

(4). Segmental breathing of the involved lung segment or segments and coughing.

D. Chronic obstructive pulmonary disease

1. COPD is a disorder characterized by chronic abnormal tests of expiratory flow rates. Components of the disease include peripheral airways disease, chronic bronchitis, and emphysema.[28,58] Refer to Table 7–9 for a comparison of the results of pulmonary function tests in health and the individual disease components of COPD.

   a. *Peripheral airways disease*
      (1). *Description.* Inflammation of the distal conducting airways.
      (2). *Pertinent physical findings*
         (a). Smoking history.
         (b). Decrease in the pulmonary function tests specific to the small airways: $FEF_{25\%-75\%}$, single-breath nitrogen washout, and air and helium closing volumes.[59,60]
      (3). *Physical therapy considerations*
         (a). Smoking cessation programs.
         (b). Community health promotion programs.

   b. *Chronic bronchitis*
      (1). *Description.* Chronic inflammation of the tracheobronchial tree with cough and sputum production lasting at least 3 months for 2 consecutive years.[28]
      (2). *Pertinent physical findings*
         (a). Significant smoking history.
         (b). Cough and sputum production.
         (c). Crackles and wheezes, decreased breath sounds.
         (d). Hypoxemia, variable $PaCO_2$ levels.
         (e). Frequent respiratory infections.
         (f). Decreased functional capacity.
         (g). Cor pulmonale.
         (h). Decreased expiratory flow rates.
      (3). *Physical therapy considerations*
         (a). Smoking cessation program.
         (b). Improvement of functional capacity.

Table 7–9. STATIC LUNG VOLUMES WITH OBSTRUCTIVE DISEASES COMPARED WITH NORMALS

PFT	Chronic Bronchitis	PAD	Emphysema
TLC	—	—	↑
FRC	↑	—	↑
RV	↑	—	↑
VC	↓	—	↓
FEV_1	↓	—	↓
$FEF_{25\%-75\%}$	↓	↓	↓
FEV_1/FVC	↓	—	↓

Abbreviations: $FEF_{25\%-75\%}$ = forced expiratory flow, mid–expiratory phase; FEV_1 = forced expiratory volume in 1 second; FRC = functional residual capacity; PAD = peripheral airway disease; PFT = pulmonary function test; RV = residual volume; TLC = total lung capacity; VC = vital capacity.

      (c). Secretion removal techniques during exacerbation of the disease.

   c. *Emphysema*
      (1). *Description.* Permanent abnormal enlargement and destruction of air spaces distal to terminal bronchioles[61] (see Figure 7–38).
      (2). *Pertinent physical findings*
         (a). Significant smoking history (exception is alpha$_1$-antitrypsin deficiency [see section on autoimmune diseases]).
         (b). Barrel chest.
         (c). Dyspnea.
         (d). Hypoxemia, hypercapnea.
         (e). Obstructive pattern on pulmonary function tests.
         (f). Cough may or may not be present, depending on the severity of a concomitant chronic bronchitis.
         (g). Use of accessory muscles of ventilation.
         (h). Decreased breath sounds and/or wheezing.
         (i). Cyanosis.
         (j). Clubbing.
         (k). Cor pulmonale.
         (l). Mild weight loss.
         (m). Chest x-ray shows hyperlucency, decreased vascular markings, and flattened diaphragms (see Figure 7–39).
      (3). *Physical therapy considerations*
         (a). Breathing exercises that en-

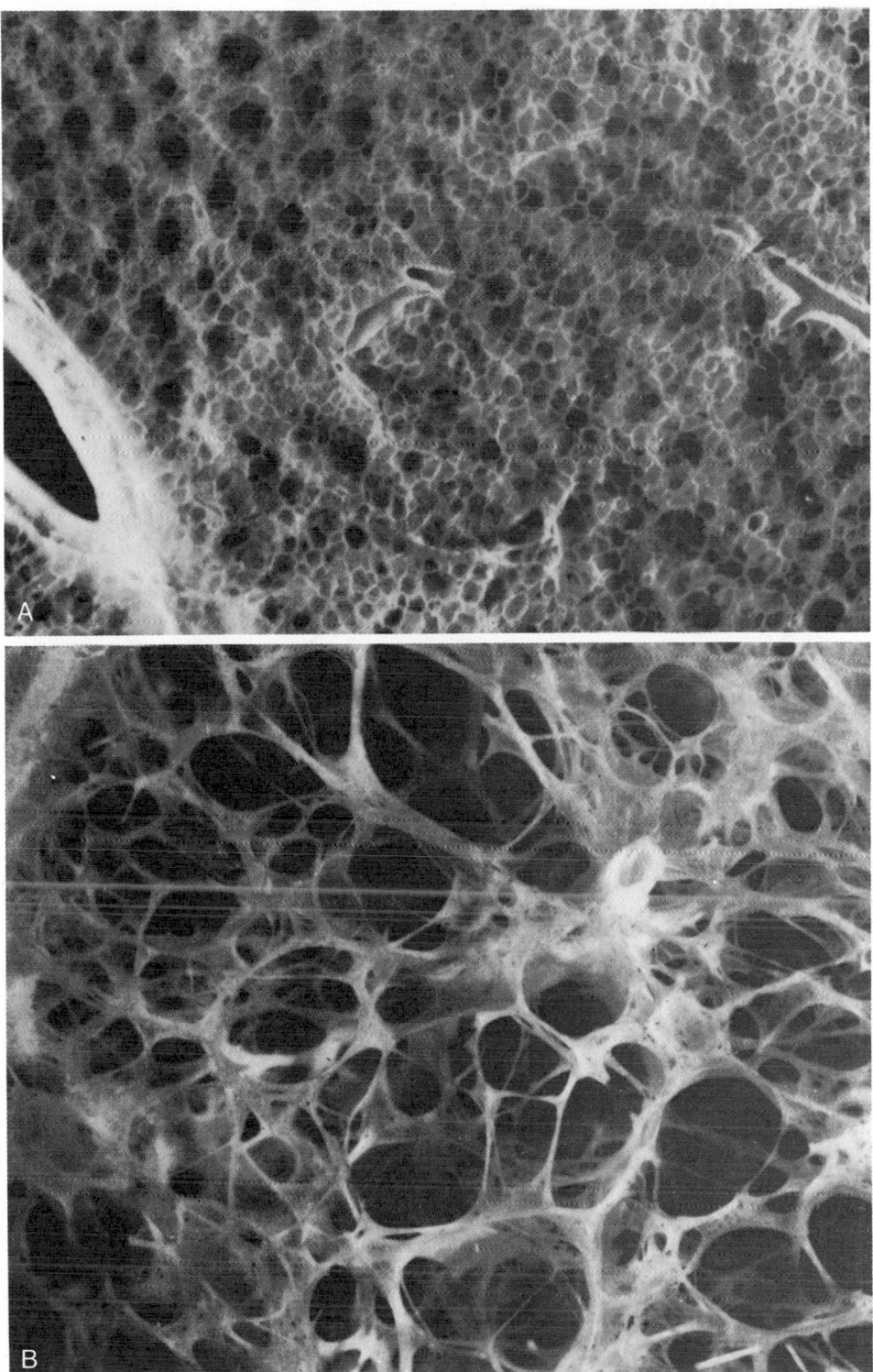

FIGURE 7-38 Appearance of slices of normal and emphysematous lung. **A,** Normal. **B,** Panacinar emphysema. (From Heard B: *Pathology of Chronic Bronchitis and Emphysema.* London, Churchill Livingstone, 1969.)

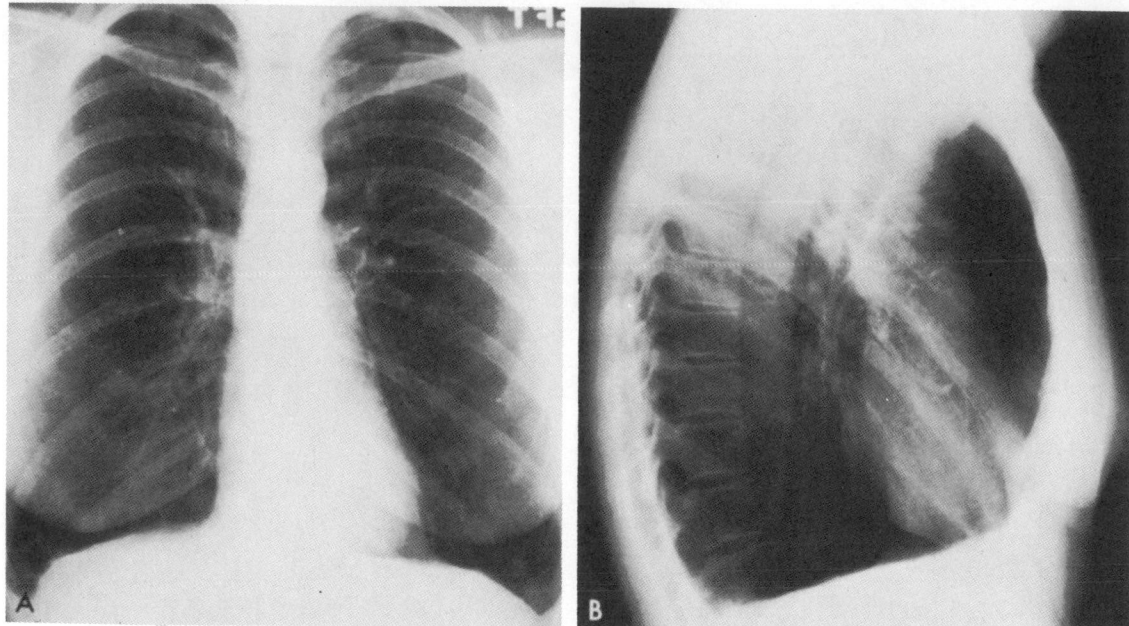

FIGURE 7–39   Posteroanterior **(A)** and lateral **(B)** chest radiographs of a 62-year-old woman with advanced chronic obstructive pulmonary disease (mainly emphysema) that show low, flattened diaphragms, large retrosternal airspace, vertically oriented heart, and hyperlucency of peripheral lung fields. (From Hinshaw H, Murray J: *Diseases of the Chest,* 4th ed. Philadelphia, W. B. Saunders Company, 1980, p 578.)

courage prolonged exhalations, such as pursed-lip breathing.

  (b). Inspiratory muscle training.

  (c). Energy-saving techniques.

  (d). Improvement of functional capacity.

  (e). Secretion removal techniques if productive cough from a concomitant bronchitis interferes with ability to perform activities of daily living or to treat exacerbation of the disease.

  (f). Smoking cessation program.

2. **Asthma**

  a. *Description.* Increased reactivity of the trachea and bronchi to various stimuli; manifests by widespread narrowing of the airways due to inflammation, smooth muscle constriction, and increased secretions. Is reversible in nature.[28]

  b. *Pertinent physical findings during exacerbation*

    (1). Wheezing, possible crackles, and/or decreased breath sounds.

    (2). Increased secretions of variable amounts.

    (3). Dyspnea.

    (4). Accessory muscle use.

    (5). Anxiety.

    (6). Tachycardia.

    (7). Tachypnea.

    (8). Hypoxemia, hypocapnea (hypercapnea in severe situations[62]).

    (9). Cyanosis.

    (10). Pulsus paradoxus.

    (11). Pulmonary function tests show impaired expiratory flow rates.

    (12). Chest x-ray shows hyperlucency and flattened diaphragms.

  c. *Physical therapy considerations*

    (1). Breathing exercises with emphasis on exhalation, such as pursed-lip breathing.

    (2). Secretion removal techniques may be used if increased secretions are problematic. Frequent assessment during treatment is necessary as bronchospasm may potentially worsen with these techniques.[63,64] Secretion removal techniques should be terminated if signs and symptoms worsen.

    (3). Maintenance of functional ability between exacerbations.

3. **Exercise-induced bronchospasm**
   a. *Description.* Bronchospasm that occurs in response to the cooling of the airways that takes place during exercise.[65–68] The following conditions promote exercise-induced bronchospasm:
      (1). Intensity of exercise at approximately 90% of predicted maximum heart rate.
      (2). Duration of exercise greater than 8 minutes.
      (3). Environment of cold, dry air with pollutants.
      (4). Running (mode of exercise most often implicated).
   b. *Pertinent physical findings*
      (1). Classically described as a decrease in pulmonary function with maximum impairment at 8 to 15 minutes post exercise.[66]
      (2). Bronchospasm at any time during exercise should be considered exercise-induced.[67]
   c. *Physical therapy considerations*
      (1). Intensity of exercise should be decreased (below 90% of predicted maximum heart rate).
      (2). Environment of exercise should be altered, such as time of day, indoors versus outdoors.
      (3). Exercise mode should be altered; swimming is an appropriate substitute as it is done in a warm, moist atmosphere, intensity is easily adapted, and breathing is controlled.
      (4). An appropriate warm-up period may be helpful.
      (5). Prescribed bronchodilator use prior to exercise is encouraged.

4. **Cystic fibrosis**[69,70]
   a. *Description.* A genetically inherited disease characterized by thickening of secretions of all exocrine glands, such as pancreatic, pulmonic, and gastrointestinal, leading to obstruction in body systems. Diagnosis is made by a positive sweat electrolyte test. Although presented here under COPD, cystic fibrosis may manifest as a restrictive disease or with both obstructive and restrictive patterns.
   b. *Clinical presentations.* The following are consistent with the diagnosis of cystic fibrosis:
      (1). Meconium ileus in a newborn.

      (2). Frequent respiratory infections, especially due to *Staphylococcus aureus* and *P. aeruginosa*.
      (3). Failure to thrive.
      (4). Inability to gain weight despite adequate caloric intake.
   c. *Pertinent physical findings*
      (1). Age of onset of symptoms variable.
      (2). Dyspnea, especially on exertion.
      (3). Productive cough.
      (4). Prolonged expiration.
      (5). Cyanosis.
      (6). Clubbing.
      (7). Use of accessory muscles.
      (8). Tachypnea.
      (9). Crackles, wheezes, and/or decreased breath sounds.
      (10). Abnormal pulmonary function tests showing an obstructive pattern, a restrictive pattern, or both.
      (11). Chest x-rays show increased markings, findings of bronchiectasis, and pneumonitis (see Figure 7–40).
   d. *Physical therapy considerations*
      (1). Secretion removal techniques performed at least twice daily.
      (2). Twenty minutes of aerobic activity can replace one session of secretion removal techniques in some children.[71,72] The increased minute ventilation that accompanies the aerobic exercise is thought to help clear the airways of excessive secretions as well as improve overall health and fitness.
      (3). Home teaching of physical therapy techniques to family members, school nurses, day-care providers, neighbors.
      (4). Maintenance of functional capacity.

5. **Bronchiectasis**
   a. *Description.* A chronic congenital or acquired disease characterized by dilation of the bronchi and excessive sputum production.[73,74]
   b. *Pertinent physical findings*
      (1). Cough and expectoration of large amounts of mucopurulent secretions.
      (2). Frequent secondary infections.
      (3). Hemoptysis.
      (4). Crackles, decreased breath sounds.
      (5). Cyanosis.
      (6). Clubbing.
      (7). Hypoxemia.

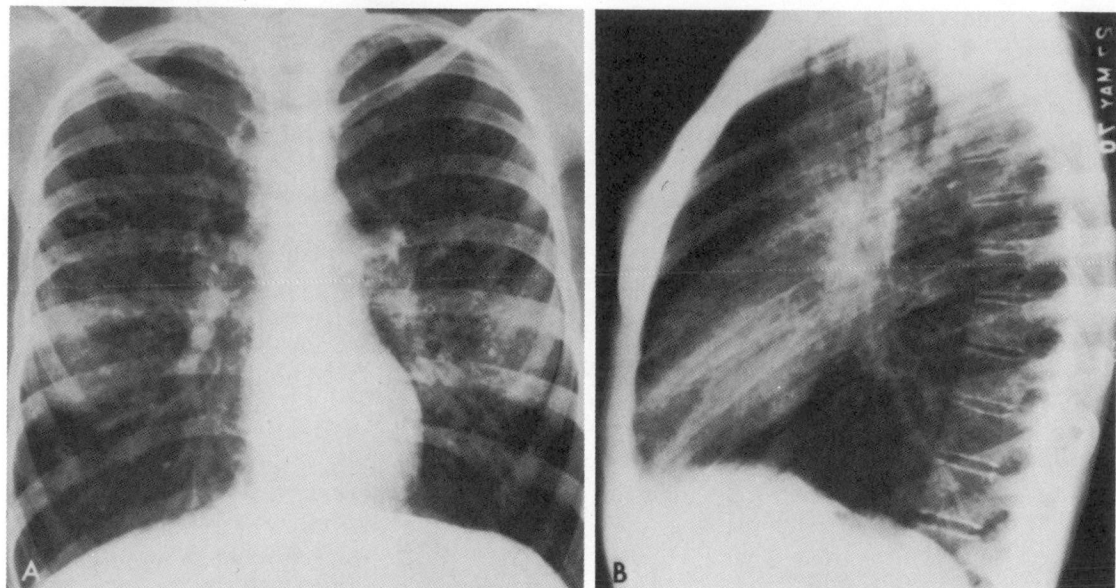

FIGURE 7–40   Posteroanterior **(A)** and lateral **(B)** chest roentgenograms of a girl 16 years of age with known cystic fibrosis, complaints of chronic cough, and moderately severe breathlessness. They show typical abnormalities of hyperinflation and diffuse mottled densities in the medial and upper lung fields. (From Hinshaw H, Murray J: *Diseases of the Chest,* 4th ed. Philadelphia, W. B. Saunders Company, 1980, p 602.)

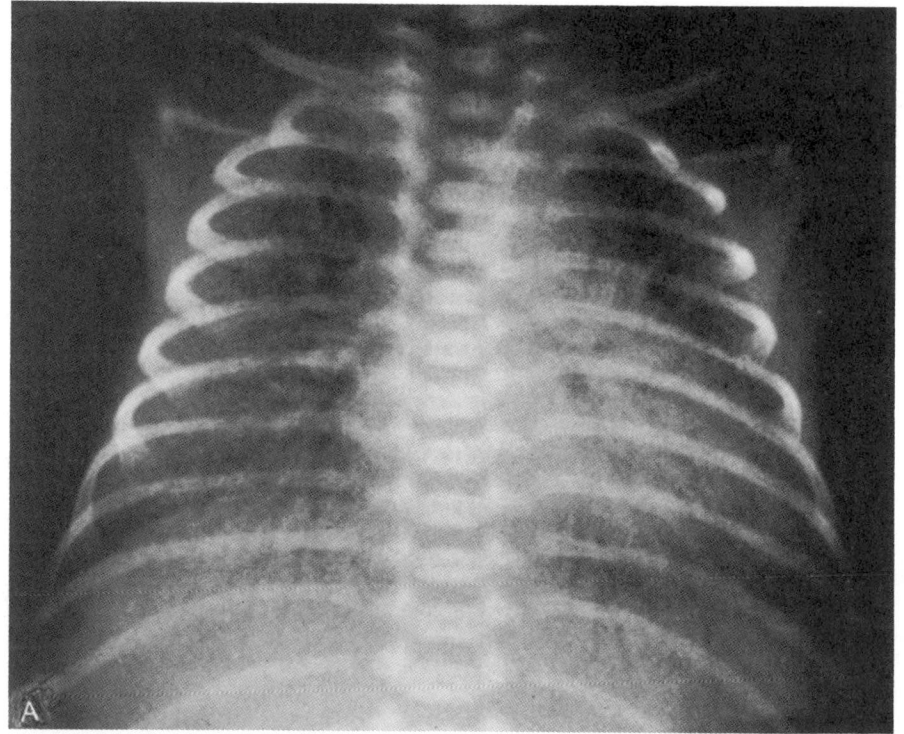

FIGURE 7–41   Chest roentgenogram of a premature neonate 2 days of age that shows finely nodular densities and striking air bronchograms. (From Hinshaw H, Murray J: *Diseases of the Chest,* 4th ed. Philadelphia, W. B. Saunders Company, 1980, p 205.)

(8). Dyspnea.

(9). Chest x-rays show increased bronchial markings with interstitial changes; bronchograms can outline bronchial dilation but are rarely needed.

c. *Physical therapy considerations*

(1). Secretion removal techniques are needed on a regular basis during periods of wellness and during exacerbations.

(2). Frank hemptosis can occur. Cessation of techniques is necessary until bleeding is under control.

6. **Hyaline membrane disease** (also called infant respiratory distress syndrome.[75]

a. *Description.* A result of lung immaturity; inadequate level of pulmonary surfactant causes alveolar collapse and respiratory distress in a premature infant.

b. *Pertinent physical findings.* The following symptoms occur within a few hours of birth:

(1). Respiratory distress.

(2). Crackles.

(3). Tachypnea.

(4). Hypoxemia.

(5). Cyanosis.

(6). Accessory muscle use.

(7). Expiratory grunting, flaring nares, retractions.

(8). Chest x-ray shows a classic granular pattern ("ground glass") caused by distended terminal airways and alveolar collapse (see Figure 7–41).

c. *Physical therapy considerations*

(1). Supportive therapy of increased F_{IO_2} and/or mechanical ventilation, proper positioning for optimal $\dot{V}/\dot{Q}$ ratio.

(2). If secretions become problematic, secretion removal techniques can be instituted. Secondary effects of therapy, such as the increased work of breathing from handling the premature infant[76] or ventricular hemorrhage,[77] must be carefully weighed against any possible benefit that physical therapy might have.

(3). Timing of pulmonary surfactant therapy via endotracheal tube should be considered when scheduling physical therapy.[78]

7. **Immotile cilia**

a. *Description.* Ciliary immotility is observed by electron microscopic studies of bronchial or nasal ciliated mucosa. Diagnosis should be suspected in children with frequent respiratory infections, otitis, and/or sinusitis.[79]

b. *Pertinent physical findings*

(1). Dyspnea, especially on exertion.

(2). Productive cough.

(3). Prolonged expiration.

(4). Cyanosis.

(5). Clubbing.

(6). Use of accessory muscles.

(7). Barrel chest.

(8). Crackles, wheezes, and/or decreased breath sounds.

(9). Pulmonary function tests show an obstructive pattern.

(10). Chest x-ray shows hyperinflation, hyperlucency, and flattened diaphragms.

c. *Physical therapy considerations*

(1). Secretion removal techniques on a regular daily basis.

(2). Maintenance of functional capacity.

8. **Bronchopulmonary dysplasia**[80]

a. *Description.* This is an obstructive pulmonary disease that is often a sequelae of premature infants with hyaline membrane disease, resulting from high pressures and/or high F_{IO_2} levels of mechanical ventilation. The lungs show areas of pulmonary immaturity and/or obstruction.

b. *Pertinent physical findings*

(1). Hypoxemia, hypercapnea.

(2). Crackles, wheezing, and/or decreased breath sounds.

(3). Increased bronchial secretions.

(4). Hyperinflation.

(5). Frequent lower respiratory infections.

(6). Delayed growth and development.

(7). Decreased pulmonary compliance.

(8). Cor pulmonale.

(9). Chest x-ray shows hyperinflation, low diaphragms, atelectasis, and/or cystic changes.

c. *Physical therapy considerations*

(1). Secretion removal techniques.

(2). Positioning to improve $\dot{V}/\dot{Q}$ ratio.

(3). Concomitant problems of oral

avoidance, developmental delay, restriction in joint range of motion, and decreased muscular strength are indications for neurodevelopmental techniques of physical therapy.[81]

E. Chronic restrictive pulmonary disease[82]

These diseases have different etiologies typified by difficulty expanding the lungs, causing a reduction in lung volumes. Table 7–10 shows the changes in pulmonary function tests due to chronic restrictive pulmonary disease.

1. **Restrictive diseases due to alterations in lung parenchyma and pleura**
   a. *Description.* These diseases involve fibrotic changes within the pulmonary parenchyma or pleura and include idiopathic pulmonary fibrosis, asbestosis, radiation pneumonitis, and oxygen toxicity.
   b. *Pertinent physical findings*
      (1). Dyspnea.
      (2). Hypoxemia, hypocapnea (hypercapnea appears with increased severity).
      (3). Crackles.
      (4). Clubbing.
      (5). Cyanosis.
      (6). Pulmonary function tests reveal a reduction in VC, FRC, and TLC.
      (7). Chest x-rays show reduced lung volumes, diffuse interstitial infiltrates, and/or pleural thickening (see Figure 7–42).
   c. *Physical therapy considerations*
      (1). Supportive therapy to reduce hypoxemia.
      (2). Maintenance of functional capacity.

Table 7–10. COMPARISON OF STATIC LUNG VOLUMES IN RESTRICTIVE DISEASE COMPARED WITH NORMALS

PFT	Restrictive Disease
TLC	↓
FRC	N to ↓
RV	N to ↓
VC	↓
Flow rates	Variable

Abbreviations: FRC = functional residual capacity; N = Normal; PFT = pulmonary function test; RV = residual volume; TLC = total lung capacity; VC = vital capacity.

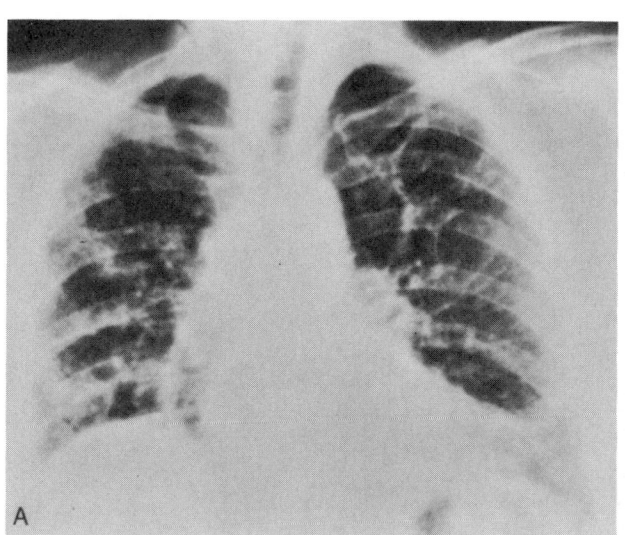
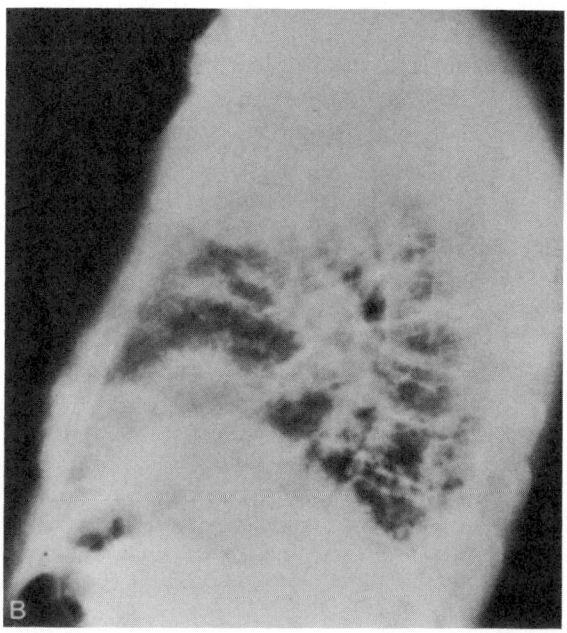

FIGURE 7–42   Posteroanterior **(A)** and lateral **(B)** chest radiographs of patient with interstitial lung disease. Reticulonodular pattern is present throughout but is most prominent in the right lung and at the base of the left lung. (From Weinberger S: *Principles of Pulmonary Medicine,* 2nd ed. Philadelphia, W. B. Saunders Company, 1992, p 39.)

Hypoxemia may worsen significantly with exercise. The need for use of supplemental oxygen with exercise is determined during the graded exercise test.

(3). Inspiratory muscle training may be beneficial.
(4). Energy-saving techniques.
(5). Breathing exercises.

2. **Restrictive diseases due to alterations in the chest wall**
   a. *Description.* These diseases involve changes of the bony thorax, restricting joint motion and therefore chest movement, and include ankylosing spondylitis, arthritis, scoliosis, pectus recurvatum, and arthrogryposis.
   b. *Pertinent physical findings*
      (1). Shallow, rapid breathing.
      (2). Dyspnea.
      (3). Hypoxemia, hypocapnea (hypercapnea with increasing severity).
      (4). Cyanosis.
      (5). Clubbing.
      (6). Crackles.
      (7). Reduced cough effectiveness.
      (8). Pulmonary function tests show reduced VC, FRC, and TLC.
      (9). Chest x-rays show reduced lung volumes and atelectasis.
   c. *Physical therapy considerations*
      (1). Maintenance of functional capacity.
      (2). Inspiratory muscle training may be beneficial.
      (3). Energy-saving techniques.
      (4). Breathing exercises.
      (5). Secretion removal techniques if indicated.

3. **Restrictive diseases due to alterations in the neuromuscular apparatus**
   a. *Description.* Decreased muscular strength results in an inability to expand the rib cage, such as in multiple sclerosis, muscular dystrophy, Werdnig-Hoffman disease, spinal cord injury, or cerebrovascular accident (CVA).
   b. *Pertinent physical findings*
      (1). Dyspnea.
      (2). Hypoxemia, hypocapnea (hypercapnea with increasing severity).
      (3). Decreased breath sounds, crackles.
      (4). Clubbing.
      (5). Cyanosis.

(6). Reduced cough effectiveness.
(7). Pulmonary function tests show reduced VC and TLC.
(8). Chest x-rays show reduced lung volumes and atelectasis.
   c. *Physical therapy considerations*
      (1). Maintenance of functional capacity.
      (2). Inspiratory muscle training, depending on the type of neuromuscular disease.
      (3). Energy-saving techniques.
      (4). Breathing exercises.
      (5). Cough assistance.
      (6). Frequent repositioning of patients who are not independent in bed mobility.
      (7). Secretion removal techniques when indicated.

F. Cancer

1. **Description.** Bronchogenic carcinoma refers to a tumor that arises from the bronchial mucosa. Smoking and occupational exposures are the most frequent causal agents. Cell types are squamous cell, adenocarcinoma, small cell anaplastic (oat cell) and large cell undifferentiated. Secondary changes due to the tumor include obstruction or compression of an airway, blood vessel, or nerve. Local metastasis is found in the pleura, chest wall, and mediastinal structures. Common distant metastases are found in lymph nodes, liver, bone, brain, and adrenals.

2. **Pertinent physical findings**
   a. Unexplained weight loss.
   b. Hemoptysis.
   c. Dyspnea.
   d. Weakness.
   e. Fatigue.
   f. Wheezing.
   g. Pneumonia with productive cough due to airway compression.
   h. Hoarseness with compression of the laryngeal nerve.
   i. Atelectasis or bacterial pneumonia with nonproductive cough due to airway obstruction.

3. **Management**
   a. Surgical resection if possible.
   b. Chemotherapy.
   c. Radiation therapy.

4. **Physical therapy considerations**
   a. Stage of the disease and potential benefits of physical therapy intervention should be determined.
   b. Secretion removal techniques in the case of retained secretions from airway compression.
   c. An obstructive pneumonia cannot be cleared with physical therapy techniques. Treatment should be held until palliative therapy reduces tumor size and relieves the obstruction.
   d. Adverse responses to therapy must be weighed carefully in treatment planning.
      (1). Possible fractures from thoracic bone metastasis with chest compressive maneuvers and coughing.
      (2). Bruising in patients with low platelets.
      (3). Fatigue that restricts other necessary activities.

G. Pre- and postsurgical teaching and treatment

1. Preoperative teaching and treatment decrease the number and severity of postoperative pulmonary complications.[83,84]
   a. *Description*
      (1). Determines baseline cardiopulmonary function.
      (2). Treats any existing condition that may alter postoperative course.
      (3). Educates patient and family regarding postoperative course and physical therapy treatment.
      (4). Enhances compliance postoperatively.
   b. *Pertinent physical findings.* Refer to Table 7–11 for the characteristics of patients most appropriate for preoperative physical therapy evaluation and treatment.

Table 7–11. PATIENT INCLUSION CRITERIA FOR PREOPERATIVE PHYSICAL THERAPY EVALUATION AND TREATMENT

Increased age	Duration of anaesthesia
Smoking history	Incision site
Concomitant disease	Poor motivation

   c. *Physical therapy considerations*
      (1). Introduction of patient to therapist and therapy department.
      (2). Extraction of pertinent patient information from medical record and physical examination.
      (3). Demonstration of secretion removal techniques used postoperatively.
      (4). Teaching of breathing exercises, splinting, incentive spirometry.
      (5). Description of postoperative course, *eg*, site of incision, monitoring and therapeutic devices, levels of discomfort, treatment times, hospital guidelines for visitors. Information should be tailored to the patient's inquiries and level of understanding.
      (6). Performance of secretion removal techniques as required.

2. Postoperative physical therapy sessions decrease the number and severity of pulmonary complications.[84,85]
   a. *Description.* Prevent postoperative pulmonary complications by
      (1). Removing any residual secretions.
      (2). Improving aeration.
      (3). Gradually increasing activity.
      (4). Returning to baseline pulmonary functioning as quickly as possible.
   b. *Pertinent physical findings.* Postoperative pulmonary complications are identified by
      (1). Increased temperature.
      (2). Increase in white blood cell count.
      (3). Change in breath sounds from the preoperative evaluation.
      (4). Abnormal chest x-ray.
      (5). Decreased expansion of the thorax.
      (6). Shortness of breath.
      (7). Change in cough and sputum production.
   c. *Physical therapy considerations*
      (1). Assessment of need for pain management.
      (2). Choosing an appropriate treatment program based on the individual patient's needs.
         (a). Secretion removal techniques.
         (b). Breathing exercises to improve aeration, incentive spirometry.
         (c). Early mobilization.

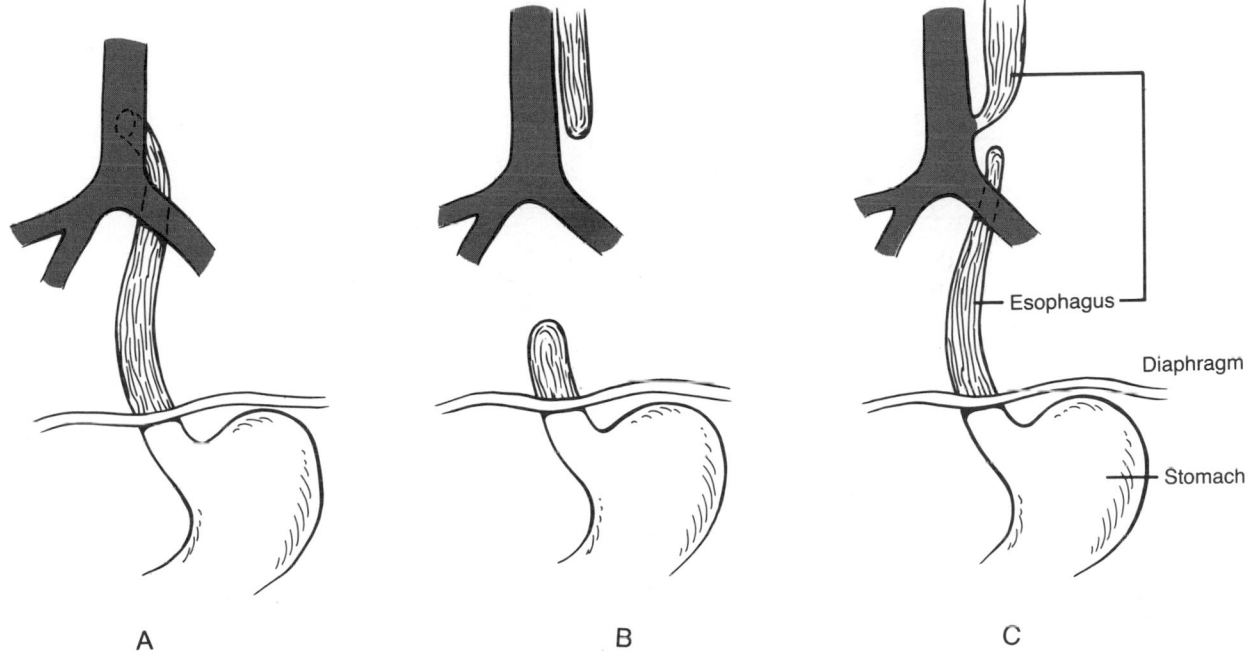

FIGURE 7–43   Three common types of tracheoesophageal (TE) fistulas and esophageal atresia. **A,** Esophageal atresia with distal TE fistula. **B,** Esophageal atresia without TE fistula. **C,** Esophageal atresia with proximal TE fistula.

H. Common congenital anomalies

1. **Tracheoesophageal fistula**[86]
   a. *Description.* An abnormal connection of the trachea and esophagus allowing esophageal contents into the trachea. Feeding gastrostomy tube, to bypass the esophagus, is necessary until surgical correction is possible (see Figure 7–43).
   b. *Pertinent physical findings.* Signs and symptoms of aspiration appear within the first few hours of life (see section on aspiration pneumonia).
   c. *Physical therapy considerations*
      (1). The patient should be positioned at all times for aspiration precautions.
      (2). Secretion removal techniques are needed if aspiration occurs. The treatment session should be scheduled just before feeding to avoid aspiration.
      (3). Postoperative care is needed when surgical correction is performed.

2. **Congenital heart defects**[87]
   a. *Cyanotic (right-to-left shunt) heart defects*
      (1). *Description.* Unoxygenated blood from the right side of the heart bypasses the lungs and is sent to the peripheral circulation, such as in tetralogy of Fallot and tricuspid atresia (see Figure 7–44).
      (2). *Pertinent physical findings.* Some or all of the following may be seen, depending on the severity of the defect:
         (a). Cyanosis.
         (b). Hypoxemia.
         (c). Poor feeding.
         (d). Failure to thrive.
         (e). High respiratory rate.
         (f). High heart rate.
         (g). Frequent respiratory and endocardial infections.
      (3). *Physical therapy considerations*
         (a). Physical therapy to prevent infections may be indicated.
         (b). Supplemental oxygen will have little to no effect on hypoxemia owing to shunt.
         (c). Pre- and postoperative care is needed when shunt is surgically corrected.

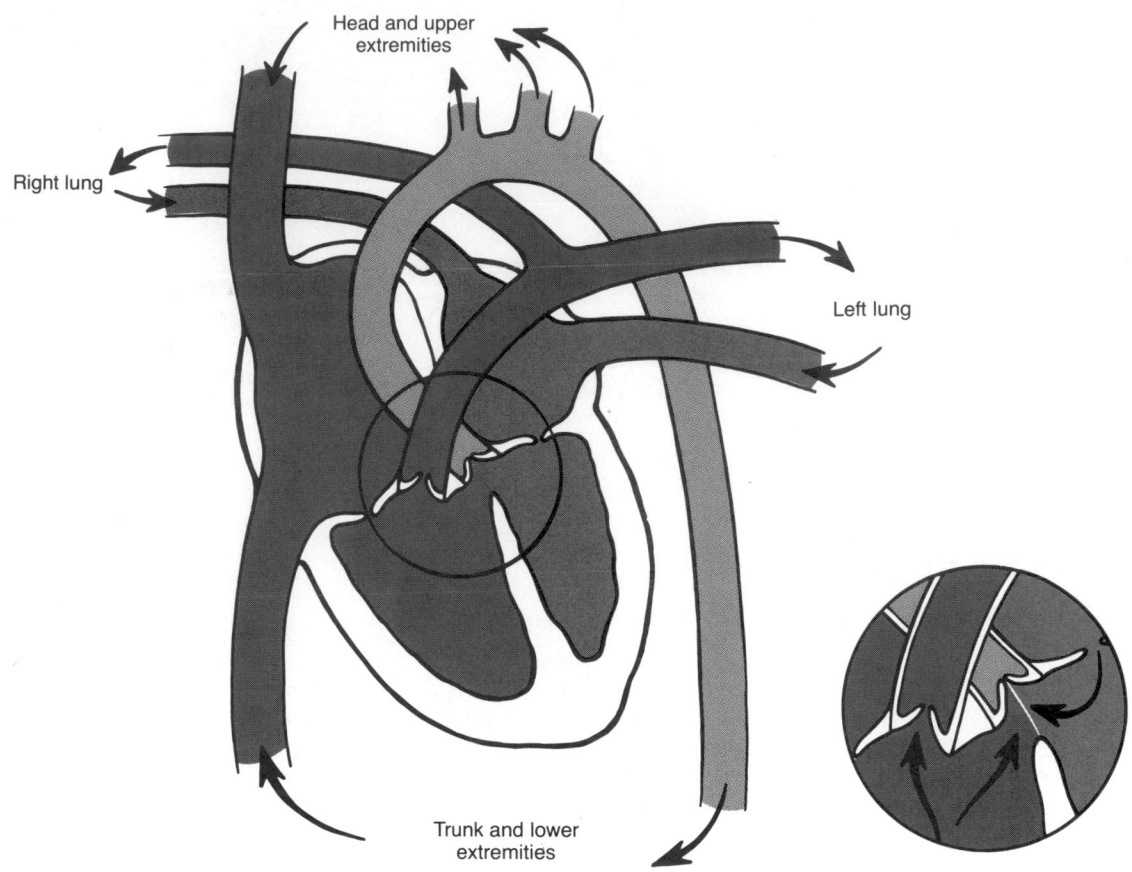

FIGURE 7–44   Tetralogy of Fallot (cyanotic heart defect).

b. **Acyanotic (left-to-right shunt) heart defects**
   (1). *Description.* Oxygenated blood from the left side of the heart is returned to the lungs, causing fluid overload of the pulmonary system, such as in ventricular septal defect and patent ductus arteriosus (see Figure 7–45).
   (2). *Pertinent physical findings.* Depending on the severity of the defect, some or all of the following may be seen:
      (a). Pulmonary edema.
      (b). Dyspnea.
      (c). High heart rate.
      (d). Failure to thrive.
      (e). Frequent respiratory and endocardial infections.
      (f). Right-sided ventricular hypertrophy.
   (3). *Physical therapy considerations*
      (a). Supportive care is indicated to decrease possible infections.
      (b). Pre- and postoperative physical therapy is needed when defect is surgically corrected.

I. Other conditions

1. **Pulmonary edema**
   a. *Description*
      (1). *Cardiogenic.* Increased pulmonary capillary pressure allows excessive seepage of fluid from the pulmonary vascular system into the interstitial space and may eventually cause alveolar edema. This is usually associated with left ventricular failure, aortic valvular disease, or mitral valvular disease.[11]
      (2). *Noncardiogenic.* This is an increased permeability of the alveolar endothelium resulting from an inhalation of toxic fumes or hypervolemia, narcotic overdose, or adult respiratory distress syndrome.[11]

b. *Pertinent physical findings*
 (1). Crackles.
 (2). Tachypnea.
 (3). Dyspnea.
 (4). Hypoxemia.
 (5). Peripheral edema if cardiogenic.
 (6). Cough with pink, frothy secretions.
 (7). Chest x-ray shows increased vascular markings, hazy opacities in gravity-dependent areas of the lung showing a typical butterfly pattern. Atelectasis is possible if the surfactant lining is removed by alveolar edema.

c. *Physical therapy considerations*
 (1). Physical therapy cannot remove the source of pulmonary edema and therefore cannot resolve the problem.
 (2). Secretion removal techniques may

be somewhat useful in the momentary decrease in some signs and symptoms.

2. **Pulmonary emboli**
 a. *Description.* A thrombus from the peripheral venous circulation that becomes embolic and lodges in the pulmonary circulation. Small emboli do not necessarily cause infarction.[12]
 b. *Pertinent physical findings without infarction*
 (1). History consistent with pulmonary emboli: deep vein thrombosis, oral contraceptives, recent abdominal or hip surgery, polycythemia, prolonged bed rest.
 (2). Sudden onset of dyspnea.
 (3). Tachycardia.
 (4). Hypoxemia.
 (5). Cyanosis.

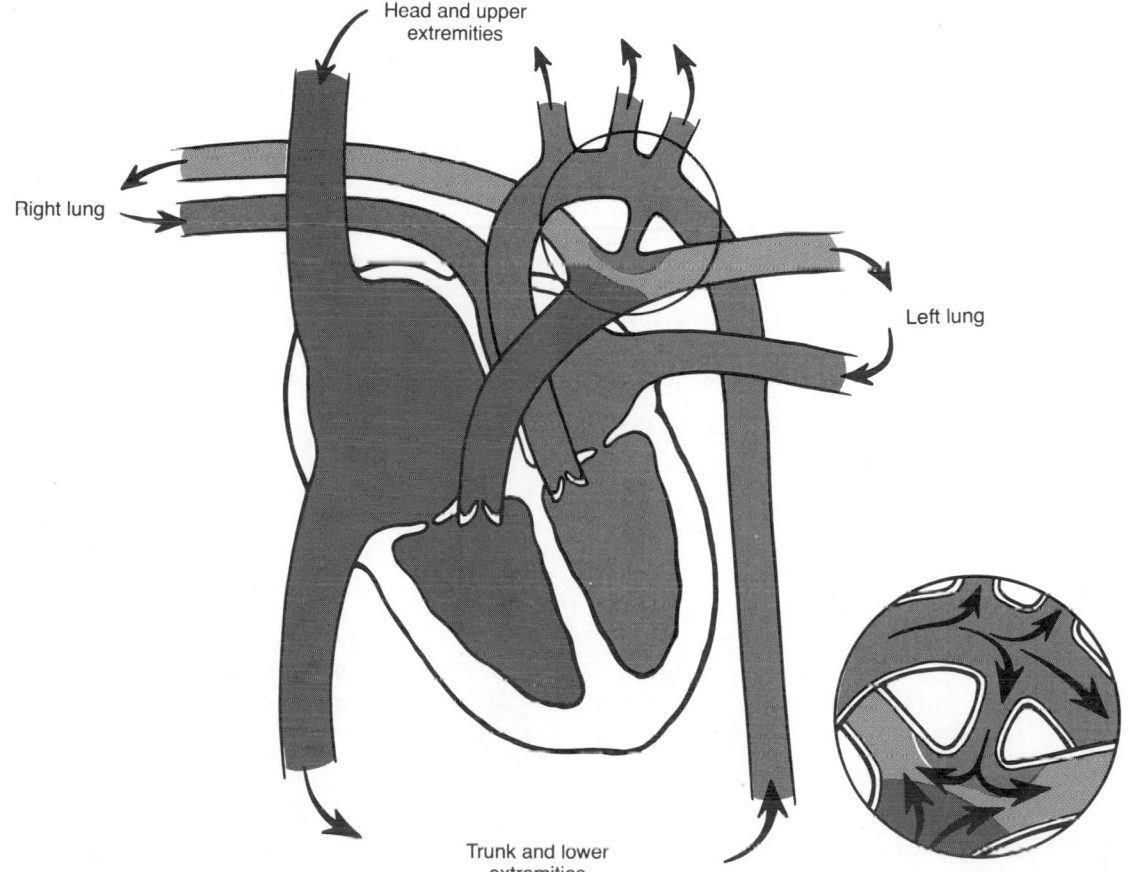

FIGURE 7–45 Patent ductus arteriosus (acyanotic heart defect).

(6). Auscultatory findings may be normal or show crackles and decreased breath sounds.

(7). $\dot{V}/\dot{Q}$ scan showing perfusion defects with concomitant normal ventilation.

c. *Additional pertinent physical findings consistent with infarction*

(1). Chest pain.

(2). Hemoptysis.

(3). Chest x-ray shows decreased vascular markings, high diaphragm, pulmonary infiltrate, and/or pleural effusion.

d. *Physical therapy considerations*

(1). Pulmonary emboli are not an indication for physical therapy techniques.

(2). Pulmonary emboli are not a contraindication to physical therapy measures if a pre-existing condition exists. Coagulation studies should be watched carefully to ensure safety.

3. **Pleural effusion**

a. *Description.* This is excessive fluid between the visceral and parietal pleura. Main causes of pleural effusion are due to[11]

(1). Increased pleural permeability to proteins from

(a). Inflammatory disease: pneumonia, rheumatoid arthritis, systemic lupus erythematosus.

(b). Neoplastic disease.

(2). Increased hydrostatic pressure within pleural space, such as congestive heart failure.

(3). Decrease in osmotic pressure, such as hypoproteinemia.

(4). Peritoneal fluid within the pleural space, such as ascites, cirrhosis.

(5). Interference of pleural reabsorption from tumor invading pleural lymphatics.

b. *Pertinent physical findings*

(1). Decreased breath sounds over effusion; bronchial breath sounds may be present around the perimeter of the effusion. Pleural friction rub may be possible with inflammatory process.

(2). Mediastinal shift away from large effusion.

(3). Breathlessness with large effusions.

(4). Chest x-ray shows fluid in the pleural space in gravity-dependent areas of the thorax if greater than 300 mL.[88]

(5). Pain and fever only if the pleural fluid is infected (empyema).

c. *Physical therapy considerations*

(1). Pleural effusions cannot be cleared with manual techniques.

(2). If the effusion is large enough to cause associated morbidity, thoracentesis or a drainage tube may be necessary.

(3). Breathing exercises and positioning can be used to reduce lung compression under the pleural effusion. Be aware of potential for $\dot{V}/\dot{Q}$ abnormalities.

4. **Atelectasis**

a. *Description.* This is a collapsed or airless alveolar unit caused by hypoventilation secondary to

(1). Pain during the ventilatory cycle, such as with pleuritis, postoperative pain, or rib fracture.

(2). Internal bronchial obstruction, such as aspiration, mucus plugging.

(3). External bronchial compression, such as tumor or enlarged lymph nodes.

(4). Low tidal volumes, such as with narcotic overdose, inappropriately low ventilator settings, or neurologic insult.

b. *Pertinent physical findings*

(1). Decreased breath sounds.

(2). Dyspnea.

(3). Tachycardia.

(4). Increased temperature.

(5). Chest x-ray with platelike streaks.

c. *Physical therapy considerations*

(1). Pain management, if appropriate.

(2). Secretion removal techniques, if atelectasis is caused by increased pulmonary secretions. Coughing alone will not be effective if air cannot be inhaled past the site of obstruction.

(3). Frequent position changes.

(4). Segmental breathing exercises to increase expansion of the thorax, especially if atelectasis is due to pain.

(5). Incentive spirometry for independent breathing exercises with emphasis on segmental expansion.

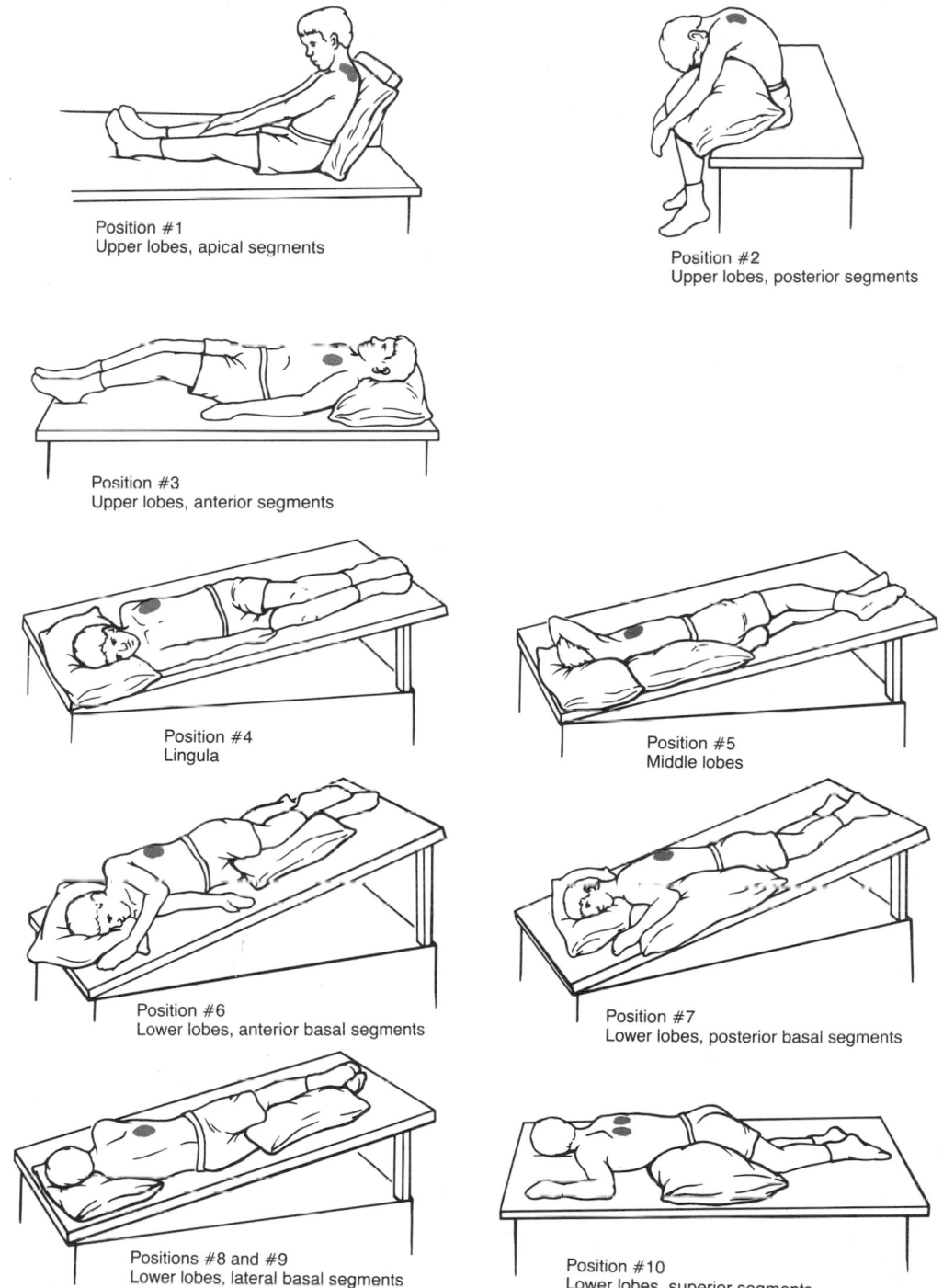

Position #1
Upper lobes, apical segments

Position #2
Upper lobes, posterior segments

Position #3
Upper lobes, anterior segments

Position #4
Lingula

Position #5
Middle lobes

Position #6
Lower lobes, anterior basal segments

Position #7
Lower lobes, posterior basal segments

Positions #8 and #9
Lower lobes, lateral basal segments

Position #10
Lower lobes, superior segments

FIGURE 7–46   Bronchial drainage positions.

V. Physical Therapy Treatment

A. Secretion removal techniques

1. **Postural drainage.** The patient should be placed in varying positions for optimal gravity drainage of secretions and increased expansion of the involved segment[89-91] (see Figure 7–46). Modification of positions may be necessary for patient tolerance.
   a. Indications for the use of postural drainage:
      (1). Increased pulmonary secretions.
      (2). Aspiration.
      (3). Atelectasis or collapse.
   b. For considerations prior to the use of the postural drainage positions, refer to Table 7–12. These considerations are not intended to imply absolute danger with the use of postural drainage positions but, rather, a possible need for position modification.
   c. *Procedure*
      (1). Explain procedure to the patient.
      (2). Place patient in the appropriate postural drainage position.
      (3). Observe for signs of intolerance.
      (4). Duration of procedure can be up to 20 minutes per postural drainage position. However, the duration typically equals the duration of the other manual techniques being used in conjunction with postural drainage.

2. **Percussion.** This is the force rhythmically applied with the therapist's cupped hands to the specific area of the chest wall that corresponds to the involved lung segment[92] (see Figure 7–47). Percussion is used to increase the amount of secretions cleared from the tracheobronchial tree.[93-95] It is usually used in conjunction with postural drainage. Modification of the technique may be necessary for patient tolerance.
   a. Indications for the use of percussion:
      (1). Excessive pulmonary secretions.
      (2). Aspiration.
      (3). Atelectasis or collapse caused by mucus plugs obstructing the airways.
   b. For considerations before the application of percussion, refer to Table 7–13. These considerations do not preclude the percussion technique; rather, they should be used to weigh possible benefits against possible detriments.
   c. *Procedure*
      (1). Explain procedure to the patient.
      (2). Place the patient in the appropriate postural drainage position.
      (3). Cover the area to be percussed with a lightweight cloth to avoid erythema.
      (4). Percuss over the area of the thorax that corresponds to the involved lung segment. The duration of percussion depends on the patient's needs and tolerance. However, 3 to

Table 7–12.   PRECAUTIONS FOR POSTURAL DRAINAGE

1. Precautions for the use of the Trendelenburg position
   a. Circulatory—pulmonary edema, congestive heart failure, hypertension
   b. Abdominal—obesity, abdominal distention, hiatal hernia, nausea, recent food consumption
   c. Shortness of breath made worse with the Trendelenburg position
2. Precautions for the use of the sidelying position
   a. Vascular—axillofemoral bypass graft
   b. Musculoskeletal—arthritis, recent rib fracture, shoulder bursitis, tendinitis making positioning uncomfortable

Reprinted from Starr J: Lesson 8. In *Touch Series.* Alexandria, VA, American Physical Therapy Association, 1990 with the permission of the American Physical Therapy Association.

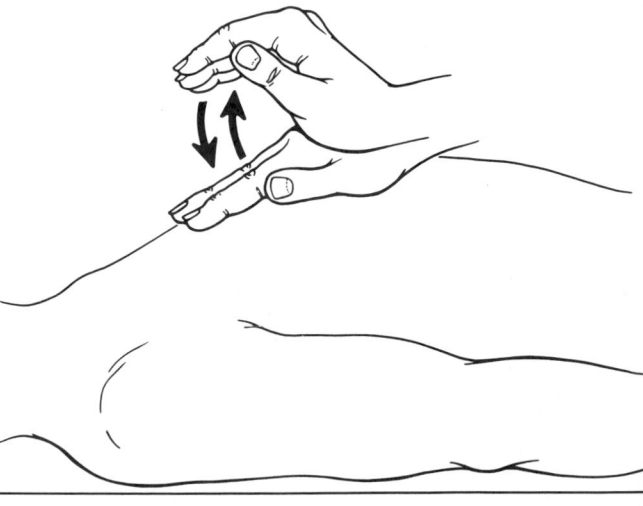

FIGURE 7–47   Percussion technique.

Table 7–13.   PRECAUTIONS FOR PERCUSSION AND SHAKING

1. Circulatory—hemoptysis, coagulation disorders (partial thromboplastin time or prothrombin time), decreased platelet count below 50,000
2. Musculoskeletal—fractured ribs, flail chest, degenerative bone disease

Reprinted from Starr J: Lesson 8. In *Touch Series*. Alexandria, VA, American Physical Therapy Association, 1990 with the permission of the American Physical Therapy Association.

5 minutes of percussion per postural drainage position with clinically assessed improvement is a guideline.

   (5). Frequency of percussion is still largely based on therapist preference rather than known efficacy. Reports of 5 to 6 Hz,[94,95] 10 to 15 Hz,[96] and 20 to 45 Hz[97] have been reported in the literature (1 Hz = 1 stroke/s).

   (6). The optimum force (intensity), according to Flower *et al.*, is that which produces voice quivering.[96]

3. **Shaking.** Following a deep inhalation, shaking is a bouncing maneuver applied to the rib cage throughout exhalation (see Figure 7–48). Shaking hastens the removal of secretions from the tracheobronchial tree.[98] It is commonly used following percussion in the appropriate postural drainage position. Modification of this technique (vibration) may be necessary for patient tolerance.

   a. Indications for the use of shaking:

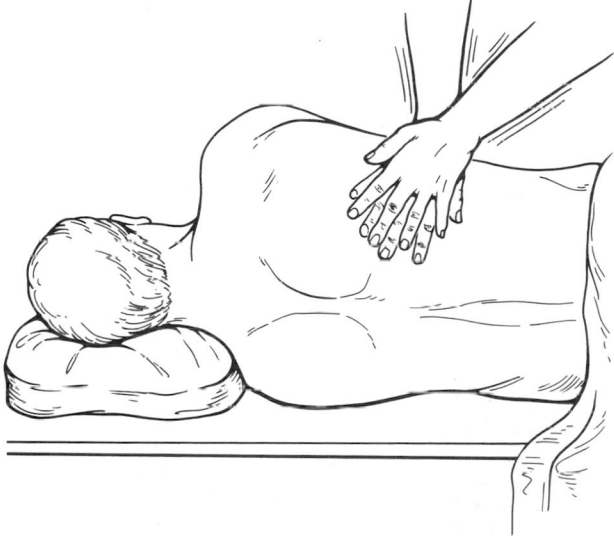

FIGURE 7–48   Shaking technique.

   (1). Excessive pulmonary secretions.
   (2). Aspiration.
   (3). Atelectasis or collapse of an airway from mucus plugging.

   b. Considerations before the application of shaking are similar to those for percussion (see Table 7–13). Again, these are not absolute contraindications to shaking but guides to its performance.

   c. *Procedure*
   (1). Explain procedure to the patient.
   (2). Place the patient in the appropriate postural drainage position.
   (3). Perform percussion, if appropriate.
   (4). As the patient inhales deeply, the therapist's hands are placed so that fingers are parallel to the ribs.
   (5). As the patient exhales, the therapist's hands provide a jarring, bouncing motion to the rib cage below.
   (6). The duration of shaking depends on the patient's needs, tolerance, and clinical improvement. Five to 10 deep inhalations with the shaking technique is generally acceptable practice. More than 10 would risk hyperventilation, and less than 5 might be ineffective.
   (7). Optimal force and frequency have not yet been qualified. It is presently based on therapist preference, patient tolerance, and clinical results.

4. **Airway clearance techniques**
   a. *Cough*
   (1). The patient should be asked to cough in the upright sitting position, if possible, after each area of lung has been treated.[99] Coughing is effective in clearing secretions from the major central airways.[100]
   (2). *Procedure.* The patient should be instructed to
      (a). Inhale deeply—cough effectiveness depends on lung volume.[101]
      (b). Close the glottis ("Close your throat" or "Hold your breath").
      (c). "Bear down" with the abdominal muscles to create a high intrathoracic pressure (up to 200 mm Hg can be created).[102]
      (d). Release the glottis and rapidly and forcefully expel the air.

b. *Huff*
   (1). The huff technique should be taught if cough is ineffective in clearing secretions. The technique is more effective in patients with collapsible airways, such as patients with chronic obstructive disease, because it prevents the high intrathoracic pressure that causes premature airway closure.[103]
   (2). *Procedure*
      (a). Ask patient to inhale deeply.
      (b). Immediately have the patient forcibly expel the air, saying "Ha."

c. *Forced expiratory technique*
   (1). *Indications.* Used to assist in the removal of the more peripheral secretions that coughing may not effect.[104]
   (2). *Procedure.* Instruct the patient to follow this sequence:
      (a). Breathe in a controlled diaphragmatic fashion.
      (b). Perform thoracic expansion exercises (with or without percussion and shaking).
      (c). Breathe as in step a.
      (d). Inhale a resting tidal volume.
      (e). Contract the abdominal muscles to produce one or two forced expiratory huffs from mid to low lung volume.
      (f). Breathe as in step a.

d. *Assisted cough (quad coughing).*[105,106] The therapist's hand (or hands or fist) becomes the force behind the patient's exhaled air. The assist to the cough must be vigorous to be effective.
   (1). *Indications*
      (a). Used when abdominal muscles cannot produce an effective cough.
      (b). Patients must lack abdominal motor control and sensation, as with spinal cord injury.
   (2). *Procedure*
      (a). Position the patient against a solid surface supine, supine in Trendelenburg's position, or sitting with wheelchair against the wall or against the therapist.
      (b). The therapist's hand is placed below the patient's subcostal

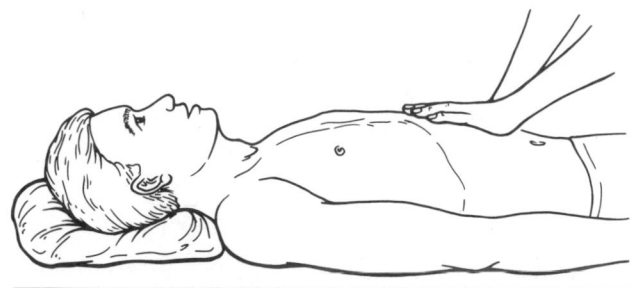

FIGURE 7–49   Assisted cough technique. In a coordinated effort, the therapist's hands become the expiratory force during the cough maneuver.

angle (similar to hand placement for the Heimlich maneuver).
      (c). The patient inhales deeply.
      (d). As the patient attempts to cough, the therapist's hand pushes inward and upward, assisting the rapid exhalation of air (see Figure 7–49).
      (e). Any secretions raised should be removed by a suction catheter if expectoration is problematic.

e. *Tracheal stimulation*
   (1). *Indications.* Used for patients with an inability to cough on command, such as infants, patients status after head trauma or stroke.
   (2). *Procedure.* The therapist's finger or thumb is placed just above the suprasternal notch, and a quick inward and downward pressure on the trachea elicits the cough reflex (see Figure 7–50).

f. *Endotracheal suctioning*
   (1). *Indications.* Suction only when the preceding airway clearance techniques fail to remove secretions adequately. Universal precautions are employed because contact with a patient's body fluid is expected.
   (2). *Procedure*[102]
      (a). Prepare suctioning apparatus, suction tubing, sterile suction catheter, a sterile glove and a clean glove, eyewear, and mask.
      (b). Explain procedure to the patient.
      (c). Preoxygenate the patient if necessary.

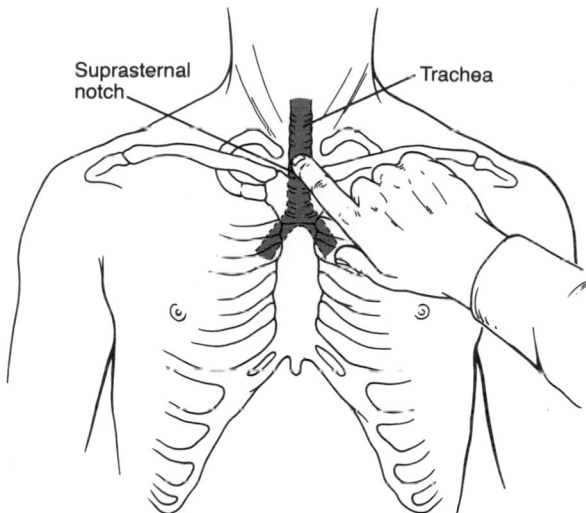

FIGURE 7–50   Tracheal stimulation to elicit the cough reflex.

(d). Wash hands, don protective eyewear and mask, the clean glove, and the sterile glove.
(e). Slide catheter out of packaging with sterile hand.
(f). Remove oxygen device with clean hand.
(g). Insert catheter through the airway to the carina, with sterile hand maintaining the suction port open. Pull back slightly.
(h). Apply suction by closing suction port with clean hand while the catheter is being rotated and removed from the airway with the sterile hand.
(i). Steps g and h combined should last for 15 seconds or less.
(j). Replace oxygenation device.
(k). Repeat steps a through j if additional passes of the catheter are necessary.
(l). Properly dispose of gloves, mask, and catheter.
(m). Wash eyewear and hands prior to leaving the patient.
(3). Complications associated with suctioning include
(a). Hypoxemia
(b). Bradycardia or tachycardia
(c). Hypotension or hypertension
(d). Increased intracranial pressure
(e). Atelectasis

(f). Tracheal damage
(g). Nosocomial infections

B. Breathing exercises

Levenson[107] divides breathing exercises into three categories.

1. The first category of exercises includes those used to increase lung volume, redistribute ventilation, restore FRC, and improve gas exchange.[107–111]
   a. ***Diaphragmatic breathing***
      (1). *Goals*
         (a). Improve ventilation/gas exchange
         (b). Decrease work of breathing
         (c). Facilitate relaxation
         (d). Maintain/improve mobility of chest wall
         (e). Prevent pulmonary compromise
      (2). *Indications*
         (a). Postoperative patients.
         (b). Posttrauma patients.
         (c). Patients with COPD with increased work of breathing and poor gas distribution.
      (3). *Procedure*
         (a). Explain procedure to patient.
         (b). Position the patient semireclined.
         (c). Place the therapist's hand gently over the subcostal angle of the patient's thorax (see Figure 7–51).
         (d). Apply gentle pressure throughout the exhalation phase of breathing.
         (e). Increase to firm pressure at the end of exhalation.
         (f). Ask the patient to inhale against the resistance of the therapist's hand.
         (g). Release pressure, allowing a full inhalation.
         (h). Progress to independence of therapist's hand during upright sitting, standing, walking, and stair climbing.
   b. ***Segmental breathing***
      (1). *Goals*
         (a). Improve ventilation to hypoventilated lung segments.
         (b). Alter regional distribution of gas.

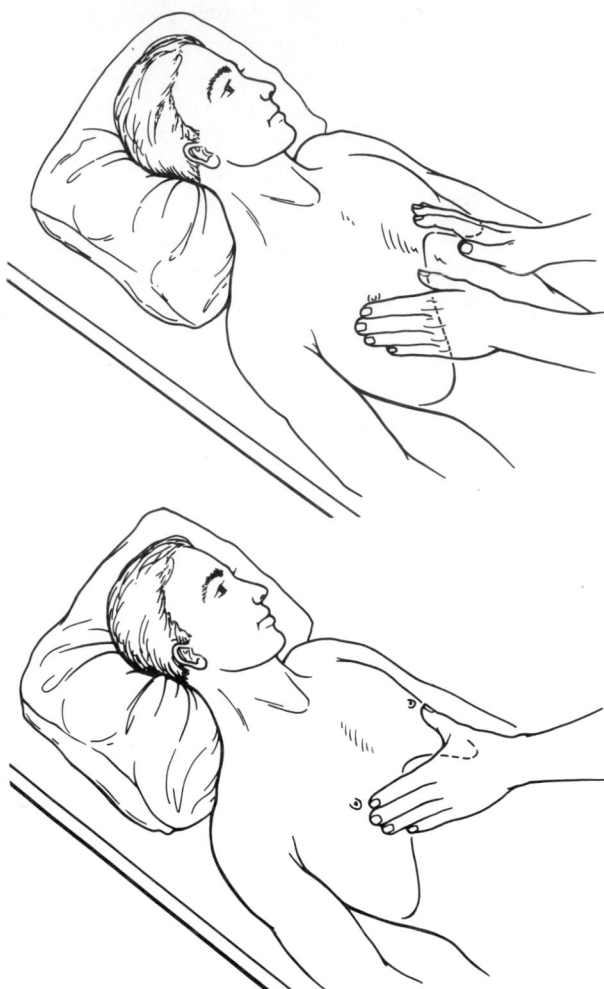

FIGURE 7-51 Placement of hand or hands for diaphragmatic breathing.

(c). Maintain or restore FRC.
(d). Maintain/improve mobility of chest wall.
(e). Prevent pulmonary compromise.
(2). *Indications.* Used with patients with the following signs and symptoms:
  (a). Pleuritic pain and splinting.
  (b). Surgical incisional pain and splinting.
  (c). Atelectasis.
  (d). Posttrauma pain and splinting.
(3). *Considerations.* Segmental breathing is inappropriate in some cases. When airway obstruction is the cause of segmental hypoventilation, segmental breathing is not effective until the cause of the obstruction is reversed (*eg,* palliative therapy used to reduce the size of a bronchogenic tumor causing external airway compression).

(4). *Procedure*
  (a). Explain procedure to the patient.
  (b). Position the patient to facilitate inhalation to a certain segment (postural drainage positions, upright sitting).
  (c). Apply gentle pressure to the thorax over the area of hypoventilation during exhalation (see Figure 7–52).
  (d). Increase to firm pressure just prior to inspiration.
  (e). Ask the patient to breath in against the resistance of the therapist's hands.
  (f). Release resistance, allowing a full inhalation.

c. *Sustained maximal inspiration (SMI)*

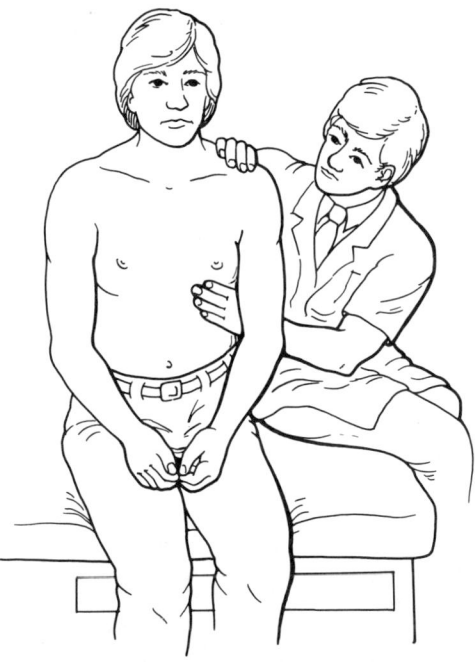

FIGURE 7-52 Unilateral (segmental) breathing emphasizing the left lower lobe. Note that the patient's shoulder must remain down, with the hands placed on the ulnar border or palm up in his/her lap. (Redrawn from Frownfelter D: *Chest Physical Therapy and Pulmonary Rehabilitation,* 2nd ed. Mosby Year Book, Chicago, 1987, p 247.)

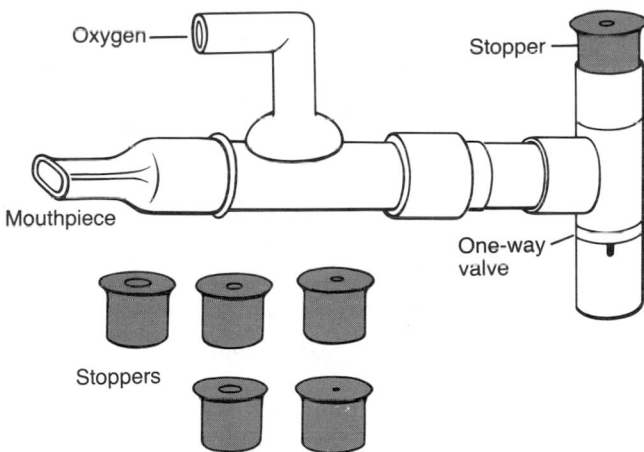

FIGURE 7–53 Duchenne's muscular dystrophy device: inspiratory muscle trainer that loads the muscles of inspiration via graded aperture openings.

(1). *Goals*
    (a). Increase inhaled volume.
    (b). Sustain/improve alveolar inflation.
    (c). Maintain/restore FRC.
(2). *Indications.* Used in acute situations for patients with
    (a). Posttrauma pain.
    (b). Postoperative pain.
    (c). Acute lobar collapse.
(3). *Procedure*
    (a). Ask the patient to inspire slowly through nose or pursed lips to maximal inspiration.
    (b). Ask the patient to hold maximal inspiration for 3 seconds.
    (c). Ask the patient to passively exhale the volume.
    (d). Incentive spirometers can assist the patient in achieving maximal inspiration with each repetition of SMI.

2. The second category of exercises includes those that improve strength, endurance, and efficiency of ventilatory muscles.[107]
  a. Inspiratory muscle trainers (IMTs) load the muscles of inspiration, as breathing is done through a series of graded aperture openings (see Figure 7–53).
    (1). *Goals.*[112–114] By increasing strength and endurance of muscles of ventilation, IMTs will
      (a). Increase efficiency of ventilatory muscles.
      (b). Decrease the work of breathing
      (c). Decrease the possibility of respiratory muscle fatigue.
      (d). Increase exercise tolerance.
    (2). *Indications.* IMTs are appropriate for patients with
      (a). Decreased compliance, such as restrictive disease.
      (b). Decreased intrathoracic volume, such as restrictive disease.
      (c). Resistance to airflow, such as obstructive pulmonary disease.
      (d). Alteration in length-tension relationship of ventilatory muscles, such as the effect of a barrel chest found in obstructive disease.
      (e). Decreased strength of the respiratory muscles, such as neuromuscular disease or long-term ventilatory use.
    (3). *Procedure*
      (a). Explain procedure to the patient, with emphasis on maintenance of respiratory rate and tidal volume during training sessions.
      (b). Determine maximum inspiratory pressure (MIP).
      (c). Choose an aperture opening that
        (i). Requires 30% to 40% of MIP (intensity).
        (ii). Allows a 15- to 30-minute training duration.
      (d). Ask patient to breathe through device while maintaining respiratory rate and tidal volume for, at least, 15 minutes.
      (e). Progression is initially focused on increasing duration to 30 minutes, then intensity is increased by the use of smaller apertures.

3. The third category of exercises includes strategies to decrease the work of breathing and facilitate relaxation.
  a. ***Pursed-lip breathing***[115,116]
    (1). *Goals*
      (a). Reduce the respiratory rate.
      (b). Increase tidal volume.
      (c). Reduce dyspnea.
      (d). Decrease mechanical disadvantage of an impaired ventilatory pump.

(e). Improve gas mixing at rest for patients with COPD.

(f). Facilitate relaxation.

(2). *Indications.* Patients primarily with obstructive disease who

(a). Experience dyspnea at rest or with minimal activity/exercise.

(b). Use an ineffective breathing pattern during activity/exercise.

(3). *Procedure*

(a). Instruct the patient to inhale slowly through nose or pursed lips.

(b). Instruct the patient to exhale passively through pursed lips.

(c). Additional hand pressure from the therapist applied to the patient's abdomen can be used to gently prolong expiration.

(d). Abdominal muscle contraction can be used judiciously to increase exhaled volume. Care must be taken not to increase intrathoracic pressure, which might produce airway collapse.

b. *Paced breathing*[107]

(1). *Goals*

(a). Accomplish a task that might otherwise be unattainable because of dyspnea.

(b). Decrease the metabolic demands of an activity over time by slowing its performance.

(2). *Indications.* Used for any patient who becomes dyspneic during the performance of an activity or exercise.

(3). *Procedure*

(a). Separate activities of daily living into manageable components.

(b). The patient inhales at rest.

(c). Upon exhalation with pursed lips, the patient completes the first component of the desired activity.

(d). The patient stops the activity and inhales at rest.

(e). Upon exhalation with pursed lips, the patient completes the next component of activity.

(f). Steps d and e are repeated until activity is accomplished in full without shortness of breath. For example, stair climbing can be done by ascending one or more stairs on the exhalation phase of breathing, ceasing activity and breathing in at rest, then climbing more stairs on exhalation, followed by another inhalation at rest, and so on.

C. Abdominal strengthening and splinting

1. Strengthening exercises can be used when abdominal muscles are too weak to provide an effective cough.

2. Patients whose abdominal muscles cannot provide the necessary support for the abdominal contents needed for passive exhalation, such as high thoracic and cervical spinal cord injuries, may find that breathing is enhanced with the use of an abdominal binder. It is important to ensure that the binder does not restrict inspiration.

D. Positioning for optimal ventilation-perfusion relationship

For each patient, there will be positions that are optional for aeration, improve perfusion, and/or maximize $\dot{V}/\dot{Q}$ ratios. Some guidelines are found in the literature, but, because each patient will have a variety of confounding variables, generalizations about optimum positioning are difficult.

1. A change in body position can shift and redistribute bronchial secretions to maintain patent airways and to facilitate secretion removal and negate their deleterious effect on oxygen transport.

a. Oxygenation improves in patients with unilateral lung disease or thoracotomy when they are placed in the sidelying position, with the affected side uppermost.[24] The worst oxygenation was found with the affected side down. In an editorial in the *New England Journal of Medicine,* Fishman[117] writes, "Down with the good lung!"

b. Patients, both pediatric and adult, with both unilateral and bilateral lung disease increased their arterial oxygenation when turned from the supine to the prone position.[118–122] (Adults should be in a prone abdomen-free position.)

c. The supine position has been found to be a disadvantage to a number of different patient populations with a variety of disease states, from healthy to chronically ill.[118–122]

2. Positioning can be used to assist in coughing. Coughing in the upright sitting position produces the highest expiratory flow rate,[99] intrapleural pressure,[123] and lung volume[124] for an effective cough.

3. Specific bronchial drainage positions use gravity to assist in the removal of secretions from a particular lung segment (see section on postural drainage).

E. Improvement or maintenance of functional capacity

1. **Interpretation of graded exercise test**

   a. Determine whether the test was terminated because of a cardiovascular or ventilatory end point. Was the maximum exercise heart rate near (within 10%) the age-adjusted predicted maximum heart rate or did the patient's $\dot{V}Emax$ (tidal volume $\times$ respiratory rate at maximum exercise) approach MVV?

   b. Determine the difference between pre- and postexercise pulmonary function tests. A decrease in 10% of FEV_1 or $FEF_{25\%-75\%}$ indicates need for bronchodilator therapy prior to the exercise regimen.[41]

   c. Determine need for supplemental oxygen. A decrease in PaO_2 of greater than 20 mm Hg or PaO_2 of less than 55 mm Hg during exercise documents the need for supplemental oxygen.[41]

2. **Prescription of exercise**

   a. *Mode.* Any sustained aerobic exercise that can be gradually increased in intensity.

   b. *Intensity.* Most therapists use a combination of target heart rate range (THRR) and rate of perceived shortness of breath.

      (1). *Heart rate reserve method.* Karvonen's formula (see Table 7–14) for THRR uses the maximum heart rate achieved on a graded exercise test and a percentage (40% to 85%) that corresponds to the patient's cardiovascular abilities, functional capacity, ventilatory maximum, and age.

         (a). If test termination occurs for

Table 7–14. KARVONEN'S FORMULA

(Maximum heart rate − resting heart rate) (40%–85%) + resting heart rate = target heart rate range

Table 7–15. SUBJECTIVE HEADINGS FOR A 10-POINT PERCEIVED SHORTNESS OF BREATH SCALE

1. Rest	Not short of breath
2. Minimal activity	Minimally short of breath
3. Very light activity	Slightly short of breath
4. Light activity	Mildly short of breath
5. Somewhat hard activity	Mildly to moderately short of breath
6. Hard activity	Moderately short of breath
7.	Moderately to severely short of breath
8. Very hard activity	Severely short of breath
9.	Breathing is not in control
10. Very, very hard activity	Maximally short of breath

Adapted from Pulmonary Rehabilitation Program, Massachusetts Respiratory Hospital, Braintree, MA.

ventilatory reasons and cardiovascular maximum was not reached, the patient can exercise at the high end of a Karvonen's calculated THRR (75% to 85%).[25]

(b). If test termination is because of reaching cardiovascular maximum with mild to moderate respiratory impairment, the patient can work in the middle of a Karvonen's calculated THRR (50% to 70%).[40]

(c). If test termination is because of cardiovascular compromise, the patient may work at the lower end of a Karvonen's calculated THRR (40% to 60%).[40]

(2). *Rate of perceived shortness of breath.* This is a variation on the Borg scale of rate of perceived exertion (RPE) that uses subjective headings to rate shortness of breath (see Table 7–15). Ratings between 4 and 6 (mildly short of breath to moderately short of breath) are appropriate.[34]

(3). *Metabolic equivalents ("METs").* Forty to 85% of maximum METs performed on a number 2 graded exercise test can be used to prescribe exercise.[40] This is probably the least accurate way to prescribe exercise for patients with pulmonary disease.

c. *Duration.* Twenty minutes of aerobic activity within the prescribed intensity is recommended.[40] If a 20-minute duration cannot be attained low duration and high frequency of exercise must be used sufficiently to allow a 20-minute duration.

d. *Frequency.* Recommended frequency is three to five times per week with a duration of 20 minutes.[40] If duration is only 10 minutes, five to seven times per week is a more appropriate frequency.

3. **Pulmonary rehabilitation session components**

a. *Check-in.* This is the time to evaluate vital signs, check for medication compliance, and check for any unusual occurrences.

b. *Warm-up.* This provides for stretching of muscles to help prevent musculoskeletal injury. Patients with chronic pulmonary disease need special attention to the head, neck, and shoulders. Light exercise is performed to increase cardiovascular responses slowly.

c. *Aerobic session.* This includes the exercise prescription of mode, intensity, and duration.

d. *Cool-down.* Light exercise is performed to reduce cardiovascular response to exercise slowly, and a stretching program is used to decrease risk of musculoskeletal injury.

e. *Education.* An education program teaches patients to become active participants in their medical management. See Table 7–16 for education session topics.

4. **Exercise progression.** Progression is first directed toward duration. Once 20 to 30 minutes' duration is achieved, intensity may be increased to maintain RPE or heart rate in target range.

5. **Adjuncts to pulmonary rehabilitation**

a. *Smoking cessation.* All types of smoking cessation programs have somewhat similar success rates[126] (see Table 7–17). If a smoking cessation program is not available within the medical facility, the American Lung Association and the American Cancer Society are good resources.

b. *Energy-saving assistive devices.* Equipment is available that allows for an activity of daily living to be accomplished with reduced energy expenditure, *eg,* a shower seat or a wheeled cart for kitchen use.

c. *Breathing exercises.* See section V.B. on breathing exercises.

Table 7–16. EDUCATION SESSION TOPICS

Anatomy and physiology of respiratory disease
Chronic obstructive pulmonary disease (COPD)
Pulmonary hygiene techniques
Effects of exercise
Nutrition and pulmonary disease
Energy-saving techniques
Stress management and relaxation
Smoking and environmental factors
Medications and oxygen therapy
Psychosocial aspects of COPD
Diagnostic techniques
General management of COPD
Community services

Adapted from Pulmonary Rehabilitation Program, Massachusetts Respiratory Hospital, Braintree, MA.

6. **Pharmacology.** Although not prescribed by the physical therapist, any clinician involved with a patient taking medications should be familiar with those medications, their effects, and their side effects. See Table 7–18 for a listing of common pharmacological agents used in the treatment of pulmonary diseases.

Table 7–17. TYPES OF SMOKING CESSATION TECHNIQUES

Propaganda	Behavior modification
Mass media messages	Self-monitoring
Posters	Stimulus control
Brochures	Contingency management
Drugs	Self-management
Lobeline	Desensitization
Dextroamphetamine	Role-playing
Imipramine	Self-punishment
Nicotine gum	Values clarification
Aversion–satiation	Sensory deprivation
Rapid smoke	Gradual reduction
Imagination	Problem solving
Smoky air in face or mouth	Others
Electric shock	Prayer
Cognitive approach	Meditation
Information	Relaxation
Books	Exercise
Articles	Acupuncture
Physician's order	
Affective approach	
Fear	
Therapy programs	
Smoking cessation clinics	
Group therapy	
Individual counseling	
Psychotherapy	
Hypnosis	

From Peters J, Lim V: Smoking cessation techniques. In Hodgkin J, Connors G, Bell CW (eds): *Pulmonary Rehabilitation: Guidelines to Success.* Boston, Butterworth Publishers, 1984, p. 94. Used by permission of J Hodgkin, MD.

Table 7–18. PULMONARY DRUGS

Use	Side Effects	Drug Names	Routes of Administration
Sympathomimetics			
Smooth muscle relaxation	Tachycardia	Isoproterenol	Inhaled
Bronchodilation	Palpitations	Epinephrine (Ephedrine)	PO
	GI distress	Isoetharine (Bronkosol)	IM
	Nervousness	Metaproterenol (Alupent)	IV
	Tremor	Terbutaline (Brethine)	
	Headache	Albuterol (Proventil, Ventolin)	
	Dizziness		
Methylxanthines			
Smooth muscle relaxation	Tachycardia	Aminophylline (Aminodur)	Inhaled
Bronchodilation	Arrhythmias	Theophylline (Elixophyllin)	PO
	GI distress	(Slo-phyllin, Theodur	IV
	Nervousness	Fleet theophylline)	PR
	Headache	Oxtriphyllin (Choladril)	
	Dizziness		
Parasympatholytic			
Blocks smooth muscle constriction	Tachycardia	Ipratropium bromide (Atrovent)	Inhaled
Maintains bronchodilation	Palpitations	Atropine sulfate	IM
	Drying of tracheal secretions		IV
	Throat irritation		Subcutaneous
	Photophobia		
	Urinary retention		
	Constipation		
Corticosteroids			
Reduces mucosal edema	Increased BP	Prednisone	Inhaled
Reduces inflammation	Sodium retention-edema	Hydrocortisone (Cortisol)	PO
Reduces immune response	Muscle wasting	Triamcinolone acetonide (Az-macort)	IM
	Osteoporosis		IV
	GI irritation	Beclamethasone (Vanceril, Beclovent)	
	Atherosclerosis		
	Hypercholesteremia		
	Increased susceptibility to infections		
Cromolyn Sodium			
Inhibits antigen-antibody response	Throat irritation	Intal	Inhaled
	Cough	Fivent	
	Bronchospasm		

From Starr J: Pulmonary rehabilitation. In Sullivan S, Schmitz T: *Physical Rehabilitation: Assessment and Treatment.* Philadelphia, F. A. Davis Company, [in press].
Abbreviations: IM = intramuscularly; IV = intravenously; PO = orally.

VI. Age-Related Considerations

A. Pediatric

Full-term neonate, 38 to 42 weeks' gestation.

1. **Anatomical and physiological differences**[86,127,128]
   a. *Airway obstruction*
      (1). High larynx contributes to the infant's propensity for nasal breathing.
      (2). The nares are smaller, reducing the flow rates available for ventilation and increasing the likelihood of obstruction.
      (3). The diameter of the airways is smaller with fewer pores of Kahn and Lambert's canals, making obstruction more likely and the resultant atelectasis more severe.

(4). Structural support of the airways is reduced, increasing the possibility for airway collapse.

b. *Increased work of breathing*

(1). The rib cage configuration is more horizontal and cartilaginous, making it a less efficient respiratory pump.

(2). Decreased lung compliance requires a greater effort to generate higher inflation pressures to maintain adequate lung volumes.

(3). Any increase in ventilation is accomplished through increased respiratory rate, not volume.

(4). The infant spends longer periods of time in rapid eye movement (REM) sleep. There is an increased work of breathing during REM sleep.

(5). Any disease process that causes nasal congestion will increase the work of breathing.

c. *Increased potential for ventilatory fatigue.* This is due to a reduced percentage of slow-twitch fatigue-resistant muscle fibers (25% in infants vs. 50% in adults) in the diaphragm of an infant.

d. *Impaired gas diffusion*

(1). The infant has a smaller number of alveoli, resulting in a smaller surface area for gas diffusion.

(2). An irregular respiratory pattern with periods of apnea impairs gas exchange.

2. **Evaluation.** Perhaps the greatest difference between the evaluation of an infant and an adult is that infants cannot answer questions; therefore, constant communication between the physical therapist and the parents and all involved medical personnel becomes essential. The following are differences in the performance and outcome of an evaluation of an infant[86,127,128]:

a. A complete history of labor and delivery is taken, including Apgar scores.

b. The mode and frequency of feeding and time of last feeding are recorded.

c. The physical examination may show the following signs of pulmonary distress that may not be seen in the adult:

(1). Retractions.

(2). Nasal flaring.

(3). Expiratory grunting.

(4). Stridor.

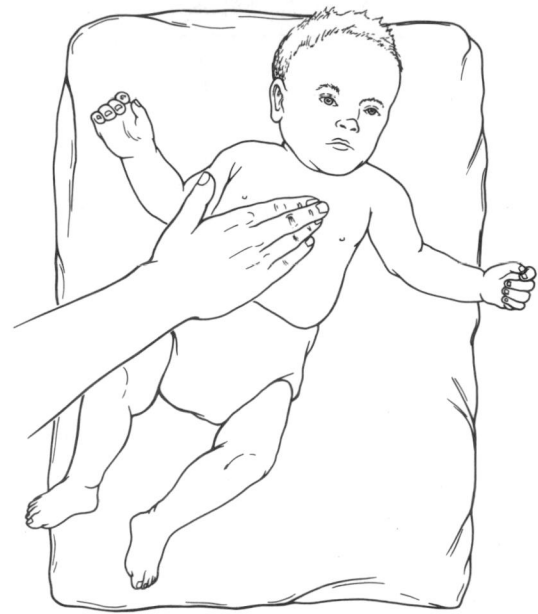

FIGURE 7–54 Tented fingers for percussion technique on small infants.

(5). Head bobbing.

(6). Bulging of the intercostal muscles.

d. Auscultation should employ a pediatric or neonatal size bell and diaphragm.

3. **Treatment differences**

a. Postural drainage of an infant can often be done on a pillow in the lap of the therapist. The most severely involved segments of the lung should be treated first. Positions of less involved segments may be combined in some cases.

b. Tented fingers may be needed on infants during the percussion technique for a better fit of the therapist's hand to the thorax (see Figure 7–54).

c. Treatment usually occurs just before the next scheduled feeding session. Risk of aspiration will be at a minimum. The child's breathing may be easier following physical therapy treatment, allowing for a better feeding session. If a child is on a continuous feeding regimen, the feeding tube should be clamped off for an acceptable amount of time prior to physical therapy care.

d. Frequency of treatment is sometimes increased, to as often as every 2 hours.

e. Suctioning and tracheal stimulation are

the only options for secretion clearance. Suction catheters must be smaller than those used for adults (5 to 6, 8, and 10 French catheters should be available).

B. Premature infant

Less than 38 weeks' gestation.[86,127,128]

1. **Anatomical and physiological differences.** All of the differences found between adults and full-term infants are of course present in the premature infant. In some instances, the difference is more exaggerated in the preterm infant.
   a. Surfactant maturity occurs at approximately 35 weeks' gestation. A decrease in pulmonary surfactant decreases lung compliance, increases the work of breathing, and causes greater respiratory muscle fatigue.
   b. The premature infant has decreased fatigue-resistant muscle fibers of the diaphragm (10% and 20% slow-twitch fatigue-resistant muscle fibers)
   c. The premature infant has decreased number of alveoli. Alveoli begin to form during the 6th gestational month, the pulmonary vascular bed is developed at approximately 26 weeks, and gas ex-

change is possible at approximately 28 weeks' gestation.
   d. Respiratory rate is more erratic in the premature infant than in the full-term infant.
   e. The premature infant has decreased or absent cough and gag reflexes.

2. **Treatment differences**
   a. Positioning the patient within the radiant warmer for treatment may necessitate altering the position of the patient, the warmer, or the sensors to maintain body temperature properly. Incubators (Isolettes), used to maintain the F_{IO_2} and temperature environment, often make therapy more difficult to perform (see Figure 7–55). If an infant can be removed from the incubator to receive physical therapy in the therapist's lap, the session will be easier. Beware of the possibility of hypothermia and hypoxemia when removing infants from their environment.
   b. The extra stimulation that holding the infant may provide may cause increased work of breathing and hypoxemia. Because handling of the infant may be contraindicated, treatment should be necessary, not routine.

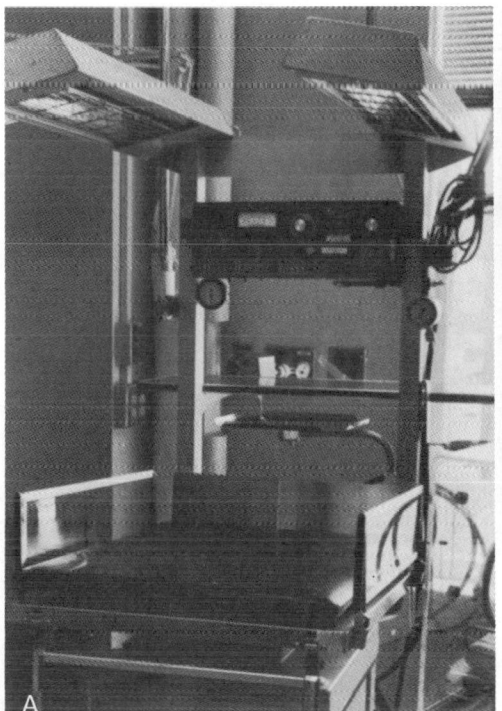
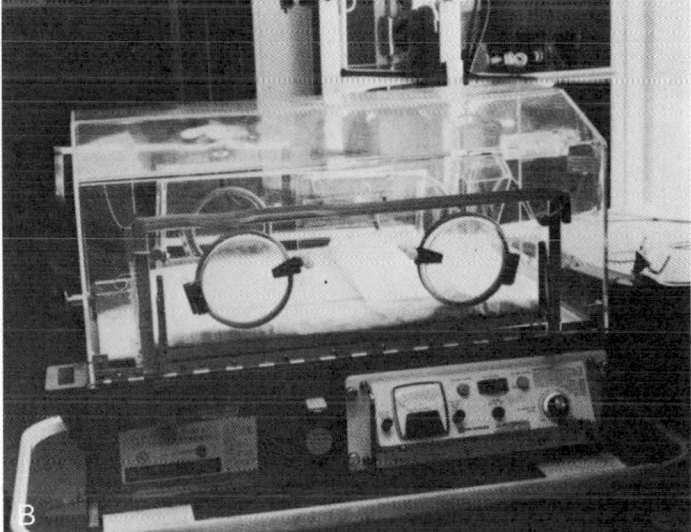

FIGURE 7–55 Examples of a radiant warmer **(A)** and an incubator **(B)** used in the care of premature infants. (From Crane L: *Physical Therapy for the Neonate with Respiratory Disease.* In Irwin S, Techklin J (eds): *Cardiopulmonary Physical Therapy,* 2nd ed. St. Louis, C. V. Mosby Company, 1990, p 397.)

C. Child

1. **Anatomical and physiological differences**
   a. As the infant grows into childhood, the respiratory system becomes more mature; respiratory rate decreases, lung volumes increase, airway size increases, resistance to airflow decreases, compliance increases, and so on.
   b. The thorax remains somewhat circular until the approximate age of 7 years, at which time it begins to elongate.
   c. Alveoli increase in both size and number until the age of 8 or 9 years, after which only an increase in size occurs.

2. **Evaluation**
   a. Constant communication between all medical personnel and parents remains essential.
   b. Age-appropriate directions are needed to obtain the desired patient response.

3. **Treatment**
   a. Age-appropriate word games, songs, and stories become necessary to keep treatment sessions successful and enjoyable.
   b. Commercially available incentive spirometers are usually designed for the adult population, making them inappropriate for pediatric patients. (The volumes needed to attain success are too great for the pediatric patient to attain.) Nonresistive expiratory maneuvers can be substituted for inspiratory devices if necessary (blowing bubbles, pinwheels, party favors, etc.).

D. Geriatric

1. **Anatomical and physiological differences**[31,129,130]
   a. *Airway obstruction*
      (1). The older patient has an increased number of mucous glands, and the mucus layer thickens.
      (2). Supportive structures of the lung decrease with age. Airways may close sooner during exhalation, trapping more air.
      (3). Loss of elastic recoil increases RV and FRC and decreases expiratory flow rates.
   b. *Increased work of breathing*
      (1). Geriatric patients have reduced mobility of the bony thorax.
      (2). Increased anteroposterior diameter of the thorax is found in older patients, negatively affecting the length-tension relationship of ventilatory muscles.
      (3). Geriatric patients have decreased strength of ventilatory muscles.
   c. *Impaired gas diffusion*
      (1). Increased time is needed for gas mixing at the alveolar level.
      (2). There is decreased arterial PO_2 via the formula $PaO_2 = 100.1 - 0.323$ (age).
   d. *Decreased exercise ability*
      (1). Geriatric patients have a decreased ability to increase minute ventilation for exercise secondary to a smaller VC.
      (2). The maximum ability to intake oxygen (VO_2 max) decreases with age.

2. **Evaluation.** Perhaps the greatest difference between the geriatric and younger adult populations is the pace at which the evaluation is completed. The process may be completed over a series of sessions, rather than in a single session. Becoming comfortable with the numerical values for geriatric pulmonary function tests, vital signs, and functional capacities will make patient assessment easier. Questions pertaining to dentition, especially if aspiration of either anaerobes or food is suspected, should be added to the evaluation.

3. **Treatment**
   a. Bones in geriatric patients are less dense; therefore, precautions, such as low-impact exercise or lighter percussion and shaking techniques, should be used.
   b. Greater cardiorespiratory response is obtained at lower work loads. Vital signs of a geriatric patient should pace the session.
   c. Fatigue at lower activity levels can be accommodated by interspersing parts of the interview or evaluation with the treatment session. These small rest periods may produce a more effective treatment session as well as make for more effective use of the therapist's time. Aerobic exercise prescription should reflect an increased frequency with a decreased intensity and duration to accommodate a patient with early fatigue.

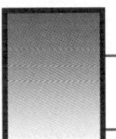

Clinical Decision-Making Cases

Case #1[131]

EPISODE I

DH is a 12-year-old female with a previously benign history of pulmonary disease. Four weeks prior to admission to this hospital, she presented to a local hospital with respiratory compromise. She was diagnosed as having a left lower lobe pneumonia and associated asthma. She was treated with intravenous antibiotics, intravenous aminophylline, and steroids. Although her wheezing never completely cleared, she was discharged on oral bronchodilators and tapering steroids.

ELEMENTS THAT SHOULD BE INCLUDED IN PATIENT'S DIFFERENTIAL DIAGNOSIS

1. Asthma.
2. Hypersensitive pneumonitis.
3. Bacterial pneumonia.
4. Viral pneumonia.
5. Atypical pneumonia.
6. Aspiration of a foreign body.
7. Cystic fibrosis (unusual for first presentation).

INFORMATION THAT WOULD HELP TO NARROW THE DIFFERENTIAL DIAGNOSIS

History

1. Inequity in caloric intake with weight gain and frequent respiratory infections (cystic fibrosis).
2. History of aspiration.
3. Recent exposure to an antigen for asthma.
4. Presentation of pulmonary compromise for insidious or abrupt symptoms of upper respiratory infection.
5. Headache, night sweats, cough, and sputum production.

Secretion Removal Techniques

These are to determine if there was a secretion problem. With asthma as a possible diagnosis, monitor continually for worsening signs and symptoms.

Sputum Studies

1. Are there secretions? (bacterial vs viral)
2. If there are secretions, what type of organism? (gram-negative vs gram-positive)
3. Presence of white blood cells?
4. Normal flora.
5. Culture and sensitivity studies.

Chest Radiograph or Other Imaging Tools (CAT Scan, Tomography, Gated Magnetic Resonance Imaging [MRI])

1. Collapse.
2. Infiltrate.
3. Hyperinflation.
4. Fibrosis.

Blood Work (Complete Blood Count)

1. Elevated white blood cell count.
2. Increase in IgE or IgG.

Blood Gas Values

A 12-year-old should be able to compensate for a small area of respiratory defect if the remainder of her lung is healthy. Is this a limited dysfunction or a more global problem?

EPISODE II

One day after discharge, DH presented to her physician with increased wheezing. She was placed on erythromycin with minimal improvement. Three days prior to admission to this hospital, she was admitted again to her local hospital for increased wheezing. There was only slight improvement with intramuscular injections of epinephrine. She was begun on intravenous aminophylline, steroids, and antibiotics. The next day, she exhibited nausea and vomiting. One day prior to transfer, her chest X-ray showed right upper lobe collapse. Arterial blood gas values were as follows:

FIO_2	pH	PaO_2	$PaCO_2$	HCO_3^-
0.21	7.48	48	29	24
0.40	7.47	68	32	24
0.70	7.43	62	30	24

DH was then transferred to this hospital for further evaluation of her respiratory status. Physical examination revealed:

History: 12 years old, 4 ft 10 inches, 85 lb well-developed, well-nourished female (WDWNF). Positive family history of asthma. No history consistent with aspiration. Decreased exercise capacity for the past month, just since pulmonary dysfunction began.

Temperature: 37.4°C
Respiratory rate: 35 breaths/min
Heart rate: 95
Blood pressure: 102/68
Review of
  systems: Within normal limits except for pulmonary system.
Lung
  examination: Diffusely decreased breath sounds over entire right lung, mild end-expiratory wheezing throughout right and left lung fields. Inspiratory to expiratory ratio was 1:1.5. No retractions evident.
Chest x-ray: Right upper lobe collapse with air bronchograms, and left upper lobe atelectasis.
Fluoroscopy: Good bilateral diaphragmatic movement.
$\dot{V}/\dot{Q}$ scan: Perfusion demonstrated that the left lung received less blood flow than the right lung. Two minor perfusion defects were noted at the left base. These defects did not have matching defects on chest x-ray. The overall ventilation was diminished, with the left lung receiving only 19% of the relative total ventilation with the major ventilatory defect at the left base.

Assessment: low possibility for pulmonary emboli. There is a surprisingly large amount of perfusion still going to atelectatic right upper lobe.

Arterial blood gases:	FIO_2	pH	PaO_2	$PaCO_2$	HCO_3^-
	0.4	7.44	58	31	20
	0.9	7.45	93	26	19
Hemoglobin:	14.8				
Hematocrit:	43.9				
White blood cell count:	8400				

Impression: The assessment was a severely hypoxemic young female with relatively normal carbon dioxide levels, minimal wheezing, and perfusion and ventilation abnormalities.

ELEMENTS THAT SHOULD BE INCLUDED IN PATIENT'S DIFFERENTIAL DIAGNOSIS

1. Asthma—although there was no air trapping on chest x-ray, no response to epinephrine, and a shortened expiratory phase rather than an elongated one.

2. Aspiration of a foreign body—although no positive history for this.
3. Pulmonary emboli—although low suspicion by $\dot{V}/\dot{Q}$ scan, and a young patient with no history to increase its likelihood (birth control pills, recent surgery, etc.).
4. Aspergillosis or other infectious agents—however, there was no eosinophilia.
5. Arteriovenous malformation—although there were no bruits along the scapula or lungs, and the right heart was not enlarged on chest x-ray.
6. Congenital heart disease well compensated until the recent pulmonary incident—although her history stated a normal exercise tolerance in the past. Also, her chest x-ray and $\dot{V}/\dot{Q}$ scan point to a pulmonary etiology.

From all of the above information and conjecture, the final assessment based on this extensive admission testing was that her respiratory difficulties were most likely caused by airway obstruction, either from an intrinsic (mucus plugging or foreign body) or extrinsic (thoracic outlet syndrome, lymphadenopathy, tumor) compression.

INFORMATION THAT WOULD HELP TO NARROW THE DIFFERENTIAL DIAGNOSIS

1. Bronchoscopy to look at the airways for signs of obstruction.
2. Chest physical therapy to identify secretions and improve aeration.

DH was admitted to the intensive care unit (ICU) and scheduled for bronchoscopy in the morning. Chest physical therapy was initiated to obtain a sputum specimen and to alleviate the collapse and atelectasis of the right and left upper lobes. Percussion and shaking were done in the appropriate postural drainage positions for the right and left upper lobes. Segmental breathing exercises were taught in the high Fowler's position, and an incentive spirometer was given to the patient for independent exercise. At this time, no sputum was produced despite a strong cough effort. Only 500 mL could be obtained on the incentive spirometer.

Re-evaluation after physical therapy prescription: No change in breath sounds, no change in respiratory rate, no change on chest x-ray. No sputum specimen was obtained. Only 500 mL on incentive spirometer shows ventilatory defect. If there are secretions, a strong cough effort with no sputum production indicates that air cannot be inhaled beyond the obstruction to remove the secretions; ie, there is either complete external compression or internal obstruction. The other possibilities include viral syndrome, atypical pneumonia with airway inflammation obstructing the airway, or aspiration with obstruction of airways. From the results of the treatment session, it was felt that breathing exercises would be more beneficial than secretion removal techniques.

On day 2, a bronchoscopy was performed. The findings were of some increased secretions in the right upper lobe but no foreign bodies, no mucus plugs, nor any external compression to the airways. Bronchial washings were sent for culture and sensitivity, and Gram's stain showed no bacteria. During right lung ventilation, only arterial blood gases on 100% showed 7.29/246/52. In the recovery room, arterial blood gases on 100% were 7.32/39/45. Chest physical therapy with secretion removal techniques was reinstituted post bronchoscopy to remove any residual fluid and/or secretions resulting from the test in order to improve DH's hypoxemia, which slowly climbed back to her baseline level.

DH was returned to the ICU. Chest physical therapy treatment was changed to breathing exercises and forced expiratory technique (FET) alone. The institution of FET was based on a supposition that secretions might be more peripheral than the bronchoscopy could detect. On re-evaluation after treatment, no change was found in breath sounds, on chest x-ray, or in sputum production.

ELEMENTS THAT SHOULD BE INCLUDED IN PATIENT'S DIFFERENTIAL DIAGNOSIS

1. Bronchoscopy findings are not consistent with asthma, bacterial pneumonia, or a foreign body aspiration.
2. A fixed right-to-left shunt from an unknown cardiac disease or an unknown pulmonary parenchymal disease seemed most likely despite the rapid onset of dysfunction and the lack of any history of disease.

INFORMATION THAT WOULD HELP TO NARROW THE DIFFERENTIAL DIAGNOSIS

1. A cardiac catheterization to look for cardiac defects.
2. An open lung biopsy for pulmonary parenchymal disease.

On day 4, a cardiac catheterization was performed. The catheterization showed no cardiac or structural pulmonary arterial or venous anomalies. All vena cavae were drained into the right atria. On room air (RA), pulmonary venous drainage from the right middle lobe was approximately normal, with a PO_2 of 114. Drainage from the right upper and lower lobes and left upper and lower lobes was found to be decreased, with essentially no increase in oxygenation during a trial of 100% oxygen ($FIO_2 = 1.0$). The PO_2 values (on RA) obtained from each segment were: right upper lobe, 29; right lower lobe, 63; left upper lobe, 58; left lower lobe, 36.

ELEMENTS THAT SHOULD BE INCLUDED IN PATIENT'S DIFFERENTIAL DIAGNOSIS

With no fixed cardiac right-to-left shunt found, no anomalies found to explain the hypoxemia, no obstruction of the major bronchial airways on bronchoscopy, and no secretions produced with any physical therapy techniques, it was postulated that the ventilation defect must be beyond the third- or fifth-generation bronchi, which were visualized by bronchoscopy and where cough is the most effective. Possibilities included pulmonary parenchymal diseases such as bronchiolitis obliterans, systemic lupus erythematosus, interstitial pneumonitis, or some process at the alveolar capillary membrane, such as Wegener's syndrome.

INFORMATION THAT WOULD HELP TO NARROW THE DIFFERENTIAL DIAGNOSIS

A lung biopsy would be needed for a definitive diagnosis. However, the patient was too ill to tolerate surgery at the time.

Still of concern was DH's continued hypoxemia and the large amount of perfusion to the atelectatic right upper lobe. On day 5, sputum cultures from the bronchoscopy were viewed by the infectious disease staff as normal flora. Antibiotic therapy was discontinued. DH's respiratory rate remained in the high 30s, and she remained afebrile. Arterial blood gases remained hypoxemic on 0.50 FIO_2 but acceptable. Breath sounds showed improvement in wheezing, and aminophylline was discontinued. There was no change on chest x-ray or in sputum production. Incentive spirometer showed an increase to 800 mL. A working diagnosis was bronchiolitis obliterans.

Chest physical therapy now included inspiratory muscle training, incentive spirometry, segmental breathing exercises, and positioning for optimal oxygenation.

On day 6, DH's chest x-ray showed an increasing opacity of the left upper lobe. However, DH was subjectively improving, and she was weaned off supplemental oxygen by day 7, with RA arterial blood gases of 7.48/64/35.

DETERMINING WHETHER EVENTS OF DAY 6 AND DAY 7 CHANGE THE DIFFERENTIAL DIAGNOSIS

DH had been on steroids for 10 days, which may have been the basis for the improvement. It was also postulated that the aminophylline may have caused vasodilation, which overcame the physiological vasoconstriction of the atelectatic, hypoxic regions. Therefore, increased perfusion through these regions (shunt) helped to decrease the overall PO_2. By discontinuing the aminophylline, a better physiological matching of ventilation and perfusion relationship occurred and improved her arterial blood gases. No change was made in her differential diagnosis.

On day 8, DH was transferred out of the ICU to the ward. Chest physical therapy continued, with the emphasis on increasing her exercise tolerance and education of her family for home physical therapy care.

On day 10, DH had pulmonary function tests performed. Her respiratory rate was now 24 to 28; she remained afebrile.

Test	Percent Predicted
FVC	41%
FEV_1	28%
$FEF_{25\%-75\%}$	12%
FEV_1/FVC	62%
TLC	47%
FRC	53%

DH was found to have a severe restrictive defect with a fixed moderate airflow obstruction. (There was no response to bronchodilators.)

DH was discharged home with home physical therapy of slowly increasing exercise duration until 20 minutes could be attained, at which time intensity would be increased. Secretion removal techniques were taught to the family in case increased secretions became present. Incentive spirometer and IMT were independently done by the patient.

DH returned to the hospital after 2 months for an open lung biopsy. At the time of her admission, chest x-ray showed continued right upper lobe collapse. The left upper lobe collapse showed a slight re-expansion of the lingular segment. A small new patch of atelectasis was present in the base of her right lung.

Three biopsy sites of the right lung were taken: posterior segment and anterior segment of right upper lobe and right middle lobe. The pathology report stated that the changes in the three biopsies were similar, although less advanced in the right middle lobe. There was a variable degree of interstitial fibrosis of the alveolar septa and a mild to moderate amount of interstitial chronic inflammatory infiltrate. The alveolar spaces contained a small number of pigment-laden macrophages, but no significant desquamation was seen. No vasculitis or viral inclusion bodies were evident.

FINAL DIAGNOSIS

Pathology findings were consistent with cellular phase of usual interstitial pneumonitis (UIP; also known as idiopathic pulmonary fibrosis). DH was discharged from the hospital on high doses of steroids for the treatment of her UIP.

Case #2

JB is an anxious 75-year-old man who presents with a chief complaint of dyspnea while performing activities of daily living (ADL). He has a past medical history of glaucoma and severe COPD. Occupational history: retired truck driver. Smoking history: 50 pack-years; he quit 3 years ago. Current medications include prednisone, a corticosteroid (Beclovent) metered dose inhaler (MDI), a bronchodilator (Atrovent) MDI, aminophylline, and antiglaucoma eye drops (Pilocar). He complains of a moderately productive cough throughout the day, which is worse in the morning. There is no family history of lung disease.

PHYSICAL EXAMINATION

Weight:	69.3 kg
Heart rate:	93
Respiratory rate:	20
Temperature:	Afebrile
Height:	178 cm
Blood pressure:	130/78

Patient was found sitting, hands grasping the edge of his seat, elbows straight, shoulder girdle elevated. Color was gray; moderate clubbing of fingers; toes not assessed. Accessory muscle use noted at rest. Barrel chest moved symmetrically with inspiration. Breath sounds were decreased throughout both lung fields; crackles heard throughout inspiration at the lower third of the left posterior thorax, which cleared with coughing. Chest x-ray was consistent with COPD: flattened diaphragm, hyperlucency, hyperinflation. Pulmonary function tests showed a FVC of 3.13 L (71% of predicted), FEV_1 of 1.14 L, and FEV_1/FVC ratio of 36%. $FEF_{25\%-75\%}$ was 17% of predicted. SaO_2 was 95%.

GRADED EXERCISE TEST

A treadmill graded exercise test was performed on room air. Results are listed in Table 7–19. JB performed a low level of exercise. Reasons for test termination were

1. Discomfort from the mouthpiece.
2. Shortness of breath.

Pulmonary function tests showed severe obstructive disease with no significant change after exercise.

Arterial blood gas studies showed significant drop in PaO_2 from 76 to 42 mm Hg. $PaCO_2$ showed an increase of 5 mm Hg.

Resting and exercise electrocardiogram (EKG) showed frequent premature ventricular contractions (PVCs), couplets twice; patient was asymptomatic. No ST-T segment changes occurred during exercise.

Table 7–19. RESULTS OF A GRADED TREADMILL EXERCISE TEST, CASE STUDY #2

Time (min)	Speed (Grade)	HR (beats/min)	TV (L)	RR (breaths/min)	VE (L/min)	BP (mm Hg)	PAO_2 (mm Hg)	pH	$PACO_2$ (mm Hg)
Rest	—	93	0.87	22	19.5	136/80	75	7.40	43
1:01	1.5/0	96	0.92	22	20.3				
2:01	1.5/0	98	1.11	19.7	21.8		52	7.40	45
3:01	1.5/4	113	1.12	23.2	26.0	168/90	44	7.38	47
4:01	1.5/4	113	1.17	30.0	35.1		42	7.36	50
4:20	1.5/4	––––––––––– Termination –––––––––––							

Reason for test termination: discomfort from mouthpiece, shortness of breath.

	Predicted	Actual
HRmax	148	113
VEmax	38.5	35.1
VO_2	1.7	0.8

Abbreviations: BP = blood pressure; HR = heart rate; RR = respiratory rate; TV = tidal volume; VE = expired volume per unit time.

VO_2max was very low; anaerobic threshold not reached.

Impression: JB performed a low level of exercise, limited by his COPD rather than by his cardiovascular system. EKG showed frequent PVCs at rest and did not change during exercise. Couplets were noted twice.

Supplemental oxygen was ordered by his physician during the exercise program (both at pulmonary rehabilitation program and at home) to begin with 2 L via nasal cannula with oximetry monitoring to keep SaO_2 above 85%.

PULMONARY REHABILITATION

JB was scheduled to begin pulmonary rehabilitation with the following problems:

1. Increased work of breathing
2. Decreased knowledge of COPD
3. Shortness of breath with minimal activity/ADL
4. Shortness of breath with stair climbing

Physical Therapy and Patient Goals

1. Decrease work of breathing within 8 weeks as measured by a decrease in accessory muscle use by teaching diaphragmatic breathing, strengthening ventilatory muscles with IMT, and pursed-lip breathing.
2. Increase knowledge of disease within 8 weeks as measured by an improved score between pre– and post–pulmonary test by attending all education sessions offered by the pulmonary rehabilitation program.
3. Decrease shortness of breath during activities within 8 weeks by improving functional capacity through aerobic exercise sessions as measured by the modified scale of perceived shortness of breath.
4. Decrease shortness of breath during stair climbing

within 1 week by teaching paced breathing technique as measured by the modified scale of perceived shortness of breath.

Exercise Prescription

Mode: JB and the therapist decided that a walking program initially would best suit his needs. Biking and arm ergometry would be added once some training had occurred.

Intensity: (maximum heart rate − resting heart rate (40% to 85%) + resting heart rate = target heart rate range; (113 − 93)(40% to 85%) + (93) = 101 to 110. JB's test was terminated due to respiratory rather than cardiac limitation; therefore, the upper end of his range was chosen as the target heart rate: 110 beats/min.

Rate of perceived shortness of breath should not exceed 6 on the modified scale of perceived shortness of breath.

Duration: An initial duration of 16 minutes of intermittent exercise was prescribed. Four bouts of 4 minutes of walking with 1 minute of rest.

Frequency: 3 times per week during regularly scheduled pulmonary rehabilitation meetings and twice weekly on his own.

Exercise Session

Pretest was given. Initial evaluation for pulmonary rehabilitation program revealed the following information: Patient lives with disabled wife in a single-story house. There are stairs to basement, where laundry facilities are located. ADL most problematic were bathing and homemaking. A 12-minute walk was performed. Total distance was 2100 ft in 7 minutes without assistive devices. Stopped due to shortness of breath. Did not continue. Heart rate from 76 to 84. Respiratory rate from 20 to 26.

It was decided that JB did not need secretion removal techniques prior to exercise. MDIs were used prior to the exercise session.

JB performed a warm-up session consisting of stretching (on exhalation) exercises and walking at a very slow pace. The aerobic portion of the exercise session was a walking program of sufficient speed to increase his heart rate to 110 beats/min. This correlated with a rate of perceived exertion of 5. He could perform four bouts of 4 minutes walking/1 minute rest. Cool-down consisted of a very slow walk for 5 minutes and a repeat of the stretching exercises. Education sessions were held once a week prior to the exercise portion of pulmonary rehabilitation.

Pacing was taught to help with home stairs to basement during his first week. (Three stairs per exhalation was found to be optimal.) The physical therapist reported that JB was able to accomplish his home stairs with a rate of perceived exertion of 3.

Progression

During the second pulmonary rehabilitation exercise session, SaO$_2$ decreased below the prescribed limits.

JB's physician was called, and 3 L of oxygen via nasal cannula was used thereafter. The prescription was changed for home oxygen as well. Within a week, the aerobic portions of the exercise sessions were performed with fewer rest periods, until, at the end of week 3, JB could perform 25 minutes of continuous walking at his target heart rate. 10 minutes of leg cycling was added to his exercise session for week 4, and 2 minutes of arm ergometry was added for week 5.

Inspiratory muscle training was begun week 4.

All education sessions were attended.

Discharge

At the end of 8 weeks of pulmonary rehabilitation, the posttest was given. A 12-minute walk showed a distance of 4500 ft with continuous walking. JB had met all goals and was discharged from pulmonary rehabilitation with a home exercise program. Referral to an outpatient maintenance group at a local mall and an invitation to return to pulmonary rehabilitation on a monthly basis were given.

References

1. Tretter S, Dueker J: Reliability of a method for measurement of the infrasternal angle [Abstract]. *Phys Ther* 1986, 66:753.
2. Martin D, Youtsey J: *Respiratory Anatomy and Physiology*. St. Louis, C. V. Mosby Company, 1988.
3. Crane L: Functional anatomy and physiology of ventilation. In Zadai C (ed): *Clinics in Physical Therapy: Pulmonary Management in Physical Therapy*. New York, Churchill Livingstone, 1992, pp 1–21.
4. De Troyer A, Kelly S, Macklem P: Mechanics of intercostal space and action of external and internal intercostal muscles. *J Clin Invest* 1985, 75:850.
5. De Troyer A, Ninane V, Gilmartin J, *et al.:* Triangularis sterni muscle used in supine humans. *J Appl Phys* 1987, 62:919.
6. De Troyer A, Sampson M: Activation of the parasternal intercostals during breathing efforts in human subjects. *J Appl Physiol* 1982, 52:524.
7. Cherniak R: *Pulmonary Function Testing*. Philadelphia, W. B. Saunders Company, 1977.
8. American Thoracic Society: Evaluation of impairment secondary to respiratory disease. *Am Rev Respir Dis* 1982, 126:945–951.
9. West J: *Pulmonary Pathophysiology: The Essentials*, 4th ed. Baltimore, Williams & Wilkins, 1992.
10. Rothstein J, Roy S, Wolf S: *The Rehabilitation Specialist's Handbook*. F. A. Davis Company, Philadelphia, 1991.
11. Weinberger, S: *Principles of Pulmonary Medicine*, 2nd ed. Philadelphia, W. B. Saunders Company, 1992.
12. Netter F: *The Ciba Collection of Medical Illustrations. Respiratory System*. vol. 7. Summit, NJ, Ciba Pharmaceutical Company, 1979.
13. Price S, Wilson L: *Pathophysiology: Clinical Concepts and Disease Processes*, 4th ed. St. Louis, C. V. Mosby Company, 1992.
14. Ross J, Dean E: Body positioning. In Zadai C (ed): *Clinics in Physical Therapy: Pulmonary Management in Physical Therapy*. New York, Churchill Livingstone, 1992.
15. Dean E, Ross J: Oxygen transportation: the basis for contemporary cardiopulmonary physical therapy and its optimization with body position and mobilization. *Phys Ther Pract* 1992, 1:34–44.
16. West J: *Ventilation/Blood Flow and Gas Exchange*, 4th ed. Oxford, Blackwell Scientific Publishers, 1985.
17. Vellody V, *et al.:* Effects of body position change on thoracoabdominal motion. *J Appl Physiol* 1978, 45:581.
18. Behrakis P, Baydur A, Jaeger M, *et al.:* Lung mechanics in sitting and horizontal body positions. *Chest* 1983, 83:643.
19. Leblanc D, Ruff F, Milic-Emili J: Effects of age and body position on airway closure in man. *J Appl Physiol* 1970, 24:448.
20. Langou R, Wolfson S, Olson E, *et al.:* Effects of orthostatic postural changes on myocardial oxygen demand. *Am J Cardiol* 1977, 39:418.
21. Amis T, Jones H, Hughes J: Effect on posture on interregional distribution of pulmonary ventilation in man. *Respir Physiol* 1984, 56:145.
22. Lange R, Katz J, McBride W, *et al.:* Effects of supine and lateral positions on cardiac output and intracardiac pressures. *Am J Cardiol* 1988, 62:330.
23. Kaneko K, Milic-Emili J, Dolovich B, *et al.:* Regional distribution of ventilation and perfusion as a function of body position. *J Appl Physiol* 1966, 21:767.
24. Zach M, Pontoppidan H, Kazemi H: The effect of lateral positions on gas exchange in pulmonary disease. *Am Rev Respir Dis* 1974, 110:49.
25. West J: *Respiratory Physiology: The Essentials*, 2nd ed. Baltimore, Williams & Wilkins, 1979.
26. American Thoracic Society: Surveillance for respiratory hazards in the occupational setting. *Am Rev Respir Dis* 1982, 126:952–956.

27. Chretien J: Pollution (atmospheric, domestic, and occupational) as a risk factor for chronic airway disease. *Chest* 1989, 96(suppl.):316S–317S.

28. American Thoracic Society: Standards for the diagnosis and care of patients with chronic obstructive pulmonary disease (COPD) and asthma. *Am Rev Respir Dis* 1987, 136:225–244.

29. Fielding J: Smoking effects and control, part I. *N Engl J Med* 1985, 313:491–498.

30. Howell S: Pharmacologic actions of bronchodilators. *Phys Ther Pract* 1992, 1:45–51.

31. Wei J: Cardiovascular anatomic and physiologic changes with age. *Top Geriatr Rehabil* 1986, 2:10–16.

32. Goss C (ed): *Gray's Anatomy of the Human Body.* Philadelphia, Lea & Febiger, 1973.

33. Burki N. *Pulmonary diseases.* Garden City, NY, Medical Examination Publishing Company, 1982.

34. Brannon F, Foley M, Starr J, *et al.: Cardiopulmonary Rehabilitation: Basic Theory and Application,* 2nd ed. Philadelphia, F. A. Davis Company, 1992.

35. Murphy R: Auscultation of the lungs: past lessons, future possibilities. *Thorax* 1981, 36:99–107.

36. Pulmonary terms and symbols. A report of the ACCP-ATS joint committee on pulmonary nomenclature. *Chest* 1975, 67:583–593.

37. Downie P (ed): *Cash's Textbook of Chest, Heart, and Vascular Disorders for Physiotherapists.* Philadelphia, J. B. Lippincott Company, 1982.

38. Hinshaw H, Murray J: *Diseases of the Chest,* 4th ed. Philadelphia, W. B. Saunders Company, 1980.

39. Rubin E, Rubin M: *Thoracic Diseases, Emphasizing Cardiopulmonary Relationships.* Philadelphia, W. B. Saunders Company, 1961.

40. American College of Sports Medicine: *Guidelines to Exercise Testing and Prescription,* 4th ed. Philadelphia, Lea & Febiger, 1991.

41. O'Ryan J, Burns D: *Pulmonary Rehabilitation from Hospital to Home.* Chicago, Yearbook Medical Publishers, 1984.

42. Cooper K: A means of assessing maximal oxygen intake: correlation between field and treadmill walking. *JAMA* 1968, 203:201–204.

43. Guyatt G, Berman I, Townsend M: Long-term outcome after respiratory rehabilitation. *Can Med Assoc J* 1987, 137:1089–1095.

44. Jones N: Exercise testing in pulmonary evaluation: rationale, methods and the normal respiratory response to exercise. *N Engl J Med* 1975, 293:541–544.

45. Carter R, *et al.:* Exercise gas exchange in patients with moderate severe to severe chronic obstructive pulmonary disease. *J Cardiopulmonary Rehabil* 1989, 9:243–248.

46. Berman L, Sutton J: Exercise for the pulmonary patient. *J Cardiopulmonary Rehabil* 1986, 6:55–59.

47. Naughton J, Balke B, Poarch R: Modified work capacity studies in individuals with and without coronary artery disease. *J Sports Med* 1964, 4:208–212.

48. Balke B, Ware R: An experimental study of physical fitness of Air Force personnel. *US Armed Forces Med J* 1959, 10:675–688.

49. Reis A: Position paper of the American Association of Cardiovascular and Pulmonary Rehabilitation: scientific basis for pulmonary rehabilitation. *J Cardiopulmonary Rehabil* 1990, 10:418–441.

50. Hutchinson D, Tobin M, Cooper D, *et al.:* Longitudinal studies in alpha$_1$ antitrypsin deficiency: a survey by the British Thoracic Society. In Taylor J, Mittman C (eds): *Pulmonary Emphysema and Proteolysis, 1986.* London, Academic Press, 1987.

51. Janis F, Phillips N, Carrel R: Smoking, alpha$_1$ antitrypsin deficiency and emphysema. In Taylor J, Mittman C (eds): *Pulmonary Emphysema and Proteolysis, 1986.* London, Academic Press, 1987.

52. Fink J: Clinical features of hypersensitivity pneumonitis. *Chest* 1986, 89:193S–195S.

53. Hood R: *Surgical Diseases of the Pleura and Chest Wall.* Philadelphia, W. B. Saunders Company, 1986.

54. Ciesla N, Rodriguez A, Anderson P, *et al.:* Incidence of extrapleural hematoma in patients with rib fractures receiving chest physical therapy [Abstract]. *Phys Ther* 1987, 67:766.

55. Guenter C, Welch M: *Pulmonary Medicine,* 2nd ed. Philadelphia, J. B. Lippincott Company, 1982.

56. Mansel J, Rosenow F, Smith T, *et al.:* Mycoplasma pneumoniae pneumonia. *Chest* 1989, 95:639–646.

57. Ranken J, Collman R, Daniele R: Acquired immune deficiency syndrome and the lung. *Chest* 1988, 94:155–164.

58. Petty T (ed): Diagnosis and treatment of chronic obstructive pulmonary disease. *Chest* 1990, 97.1S–33S.

59. Niewoehner D, Kleinerman J, Rice D: Pathologic changes in pulmonary airways of young cigarette smokers. *N Engl J Med* 1974, 291:755–758.

60. McFadden E, Kiker R, Holmes B, *et al.:* Small airway disease: an assessment of the tests of peripheral airway function. *Am J Med* 1974, 57:171–182.

61. Heard B: Pathology of chronic bronchitis and emphysema. London, Churchill Livingstone, 1969.

62. Berte J: *Critical Care: The Lungs,* 2nd ed. Norwalk, CT, Appleton-Century-Crofts, 1986.

63. Cambell A, O'Connell J, Wilson F: The effect of chest physiotherapy upon the FEV$_1$ in chronic bronchitis. *Med J Aust* 1975, 1:33.

64. Wollmer P, Ursing K, Midgren B, *et al.:* Inefficiency of chest percussion in the physical therapy of chronic bronchitis. *Eur J Respir Dis* 1985, 66:233.

65. Anderson S, Silverman M, König P, *et al.:* Exercise induced asthma: a review. *Br J Dis Chest* 1975, 69:1–39.

66. Gilbert I, Fouke J, McFadden E: Heat and water flux in the intrathoracic airways and exercise induced asthma. *J Appl Physiol* 1987, 63:1681–1691.

67. Berman B, Ross R: Exercise induced bronchospasm: is it a unique clinical entity? *Ann Allergy* 1990, 65:81–83.

68. Anderson S: Current concepts of exercise induced asthma. *Allergy* 1983, 38:289–302.

69. Murphy S: Cystic fibrosis in adults: diagnosis and management. *Clin Chest Med* 1987, 8:695.

70. Holsclaw D: Cystic fibrosis: overview and pulmonary aspects in young adults. *Clin Chest Med* 1980, 1:407–421.

71. Wolff R, Dolovich M, Obminski G, *et al.:* Effects of exercise and eucapnic hyperventilation on bronchial clearance in man. *J Appl Physiol* 1977, 43:46–50.

72. Zach M, Oberwaldner B, Hausler F: Cystic fibrosis: physical exercise versus chest physiotherapy. *Arch Dis Child* 1982, 57:587–589.

73. Daves P, Hubbard V, McCoy K, *et al.:* Familial bronchiectasis. *J Pediatr* 1983, 102:177–185.

74. Elles D, Thornley P, Wightman A, *et al.:* Present outlook in bronchiectasis: clinical and social study and review of factors influencing prognosis. *Thorax* 1981, 36:659–664.

75. Thibeault D, Gregory G: *Neonatal Pulmonary Care,* 2nd ed. Norwalk, CT, Appleton-Century-Crofts, 1986.

76. Speidel B: Adverse effects of routine procedures on preterm infants. *Lancet* 1978, 1:864–866.

77. Raval D, Yeh T, Mora H, *et al.:* Chest physiotherapy in preterm infants with respiratory distress syndrome in the first 24 hours of life. *J Perinatol* 1987, 7:301.

78. Jobe A: Pulmonary surfactant therapy. *N Engl J Med* 1993, 328:861–868.

79. Eliasson R, Mossberg B, Camner P, *et al.:* The immotile

cilia syndrome: congenital ciliary abnormality as an etiologic factor in chronic airway infections and male sterility. *N Engl J Med* 1977, 297:1–6.

80. Mayes L, Perkett E, Stahlman M: Severe bronchopulmonary dysplasia: a retrospective review. *Acta Paediatr Scand* 1983, 72:225–229.

81. Crane L: Physical therapy for neonates with respiratory diseases. In Irwin S, Tecklin J (eds): *Cardiopulmonary Physical Therapy.* St Louis, C. V. Mosby Company, 1985.

82. Petty T: *Chronic Lung Disease: A Practical Office Approach to Early Diagnosis and Management.* New York, Breon Laboratories, Inc., 1975.

83. Stein M, Cassara F: Preoperative pulmonary evaluation and therapy for surgical patients. *JAMA* 1962, 211:787–790.

84. Thoren L: Postoperative pulmonary complications: observation on their prevention by means of physiotherapy. *Acta Chir Scand* 1968, 3:193–205 (or 1954, 107:193).

85. Vraciu F, Vraciu A: Effectiveness of breathing exercises in preventing pulmonary complications following open heart surgery. *Phys Ther* 1977, 57:1367–1371.

86. Crane L: Cardiorespiratory management for the developmental therapist. In Sweeney J (ed): *The High Risk Neonate: Developmental Therapy Perspective.* New York, Hawthorn Press, 1986.

87. Guyton A: *Function of the Human Body* [In press]. Philadelphia, W. B. Saunders Company.

88. Thomas C (ed): *Taber's Cyclopedic Medical Dictionary,* 17th ed. Philadelphia, F. A. Davis Company, 1993.

89. Lorin M, Denning C: Evaluation of postural drainage by measurement of sputum volume and consistency. *Am J Phys Med* 1971, 50:215.

90. *Drainage Positions.* Cystic Fibrosis Foundation, Washington DC, 1992.

91. Rossman C, Waldes R, Sampson D, *et al.:* Effects of chest physiotherapy on the removal of mucus in patients with cystic fibrosis. *Am Rev Respir Dis* 1982, 126:131.

92. Blogett D: *Manual of Pediatric Respiratory Care Procedure.* Philadelphia, J. B. Lippincott Company, 1982.

93. Shapiro B, Harrison R, Trout C: *Clinical Application of Respiratory Care,* 2nd ed. Chicago, Yearbook Medical Publishers, 1979.

94. Bateman J, Newman S, Daunt K, *et al.:* Is cough as effective as chest physiotherapy in the removal of excessive tracheobronchial secretions? *Thorax* 1981, 36:683.

95. Mellins R: Pulmonary physiotherapy in the pediatric age group. *Am Rev Respir Dis* 1974, 110:137.

96. Flower K, Eden R, Lomax L: A new mechanical aid to physiotherapy in cystic fibrosis. *Br Med J* 1979, 2:630.

97. Denton R: Bronchial secretions in cystic fibrosis: the effects of treatment with mechanical percussion vibration. *Am Rev Respir Dis* 1962, 86:41.

98. Sutton P, Lopez-Vidriero M, Pavia D, *et al.:* Assessment of percussion, vibratory shaking and breathing exercises in chest physiotherapy. *Eur J Respir Dis* 1985, 66:147.

99. Starr J: *The Influence of Posture and Cumulative Trials on the Effectiveness of Coughing in Postoperative Cholecystectomy Patients.* Boston, Boston University, 1980. Thesis.

100. Smaldone G, Smith P: Location of flow limiting segment via airway catheters near residual volume in humans. *J Appl Physiol* 1985, 59:502.

101. Leith D: Cough. *Phys Ther* 1968, 48:439.

102. Starr J: Manual techniques of chest physical therapy and airway clearance techniques. In Zadai C: *Clinics in Physical Therapy: Pulmonary Management in Physical Therapy.* New York, Churchill Livingstone, 1992.

103. Hietpas B, Roth R, Jensen W: Huff coughing and airway patency. *Respir Care* 1979, 24:710–713.

104. Pryor J, Webber B, Hodson M, *et al.:* Evaluation of the forced expiratory technique as an adjunct to postural drainage in the treatment of cystic fibrosis. *Br Med J* 1979, 2:417–418.

105. Kocan M: Pulmonary considerations in the critical care phase. *Crit Care Nurs Clin North Am* 1990, 2:369.

106. Siebeens A, Kirby N, Puolos D: Cough following transections of spinal cord at C6. *Arch Phys Med Rehabil* 1964, 45:1.

107. Levenson C: Breathing exercises. In Zadai C: *Clinics in Physical Therapy: Pulmonary Management in Physical Therapy.* New York, Churchill Livingstone, 1992.

108. Bartlett R, Gazzaniga A, Geraghty T: Respiratory maneuvers to prevent postoperative pulmonary complications. A critical review. *JAMA* 1973, 24:1017.

109. Ward R, Danziger F, Bonica J, *et al.:* An evaluation of postoperative respiratory maneuvers. *Surg Gynecol Obstet* 1966, 123:51–54.

110. Roussos C, Fixley M, Genest J, *et al.:* Voluntary factors influencing the distribution of inspired gas. *Am Rev Respir Dis* 1977, 116:457.

111. Ravin M: Value of deep breaths in reversing postoperative hypoxemia. *N Y State J Med* 1966, 66:244.

112. Anderson J, *et al.:* Resistive breathing training in severe chronic obstructive pulmonary disease: a pilot study. *Scand J Respir Dis* 1979, 60:151.

113. Belman M, Mittman C: Ventilatory muscle testing improves exercise capacity in chronic obstructive pulmonary disease patients. *Am Rev Respir Dis* 1980, 121:273.

114. Pardy R, *et al.:* The effects of inspiratory muscle training on exercise performance in chronic airflow limitation. *Am Rev Respir Dis* 1981, 123:426.

115. Mueller RE, Petty T, Filley F: Ventilation and arterial blood gas changes induced by pursed lip breathing. *J Appl Physiol* 1970, 28:784–789.

116. Thoman R, Stoker G, Ross J: The efficacy of pursed lip breathing in patient with chronic obstructive pulmonary disease. *Am Rev Respir Dis* 1966, 93:100–106.

117. Fishman A: Down with the good lung [Editorial]. *N Engl J Med* 1981, 304:537.

118. Attiger E, Monroe R, Segal M: The mechanics of breathing in different body positions. I: In normal subjects. *J Clin Invest* 1956, 35:904–911.

119. Attiger E, Monroe R, Segal M: The mechanics of breathing in different body positions. II: In cardiopulmonary disease. *J Clin Invest* 1956, 35:912.

120. Douglas W, Rehder K, Beynen F, *et al.:* Improved oxygenation in patients with acute respiratory failure: the prone position. *Am Rev Respir Dis* 1977, 115:559.

121. Schwartz F, Fenner A, Wolfsdorf J: The influence of body position on pulmonary function in low birthweight babies. *S Afr Med J* 1975, 49:79.

122. Wagaman M, Shutack J, Moomjian A, *et al.:* Improved oxygenation and lung compliance with prone positioning of neonates. *J Pediatr* 1979, 94:787.

123. Yanazaki S, Owaga J, Shokzu A, *et al.:* Intrapleural cough pressure in patients post thoracotomy. *J Thorac Cardiovasc Surg* 1980, 80:600.

124. Curry L, Van Eeden C: The influence of posture on the effectiveness of coughing. *S Afr J Physiol* 1977, 33:8.

125. Reis A: Endurance exercise training at max targets in patients with chronic obstructive pulmonary disease. *J Cardiopulmonary Rehabil* 1987, 7:594–601.

126. Peters J, Lim V: Smoking cessation techniques. In Hodgkins J, Zorn E, Connors G (eds): *Pulmonary Rehabilitation: Guidelines to Success.* Boston, Butterworth Publishers, 1984.

127. Crane L: The neonate and child. In Frownfelter D (ed.): *Chest Physical Therapy and Pulmonary Rehabilitation: An Interdisciplinary Approach,* 2nd ed. St. Louis, C. V. Mosby Company, 1987.

128. Crane L: Physical therapy for the neonate with respiratory

disease. In Irwin S, Tecklin J (eds): *Cardiopulmonary Physical Therapy*, 2nd ed. St Louis, C. V. Mosby Company, 1990.

129. Zadai C: Pulmonary physiology of aging: the role of rehabilitation. *Top Geriatr Rehabil* 1985, 1:49–57.

130. Roy S: *Physical Activity and Aging*, 2nd ed. Rockville, MD, Aspen Publishers, 1987.

131. Starr J: Clinical case study: interstitial pneumonitis. *Cardiopulmonary Section Q* 5:5–6, 1984.

Suggested Readings

American Thoracic Society: Diagnostic standards and classification of tuberculosis. *Am Rev Respir Dis* 1990, 142:725–735.

Daniele R, Rossman M, Kern J, *et al.:* Pathogenesis of sarcoidosis: state of the art. *Chest* 1986, 89:174S–177S.

Davis G, Winn W: Legionnaire's disease: respiratory infections caused by Legionella bacteria. *Clin Chest Med* 1987, 8:419–439.

Eisenberg H: The interstitial lung diseases associated with collagen vascular disorders. *Clin Chest Med* 1982, 3:565–578.

Epler G, Colby T, McLoud T, *et al.:* Bronchiolitis obliterans organizing pneumonia. *N Engl J Med* 1985, 312:152–158.

Pepys J: Clinical and therapeutic significance of patterns of allergic reactions of the lung to extrinsic agents. *Am Rev Respir Dis* 1977, 116:573–588.

Pierce J: Antitrypsin and emphysema: perspective and prospect. *JAMA* 1988, 259:2890–2895.

Salvaggio J, de Shazo R: Pathogenesis of hypersensitivity pneumonitis. *Chest* 1986, 89:190S–193S.

PART FOUR

Neurological/ Neuromuscular System

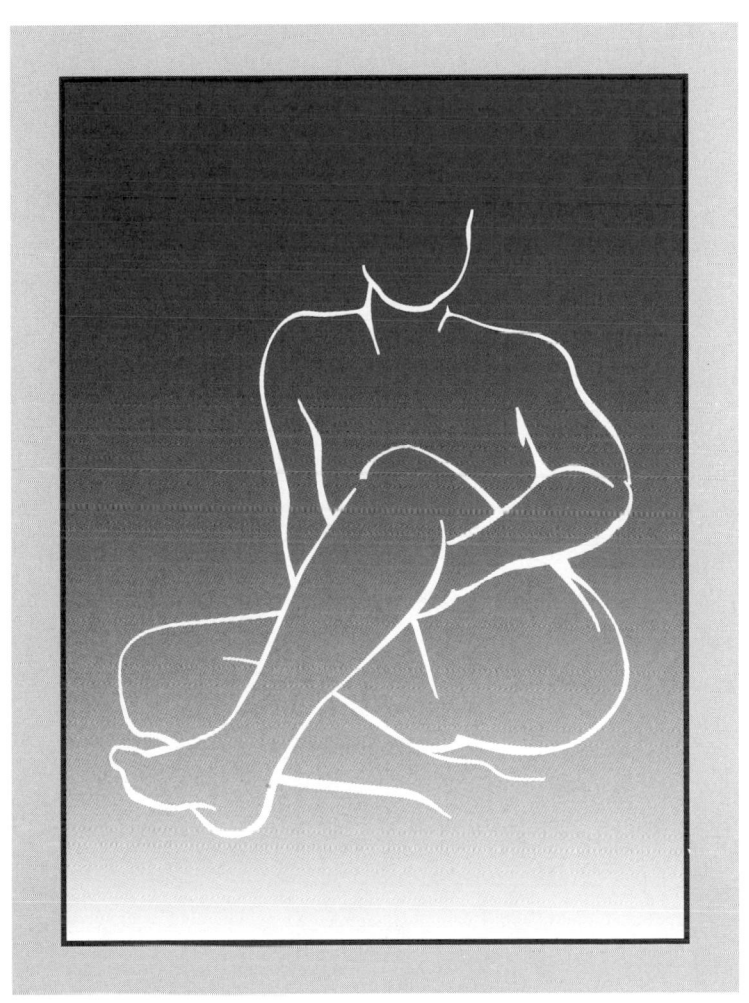

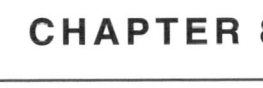

CHAPTER 8

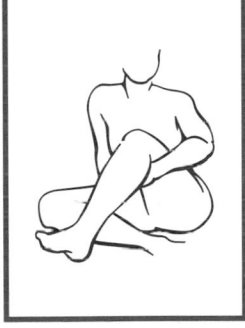

Theories and Principles of Therapeutic Intervention Based on Contemporary Models of Motor Control

Jean M. Held

The chapters in this section present a contemporary framework from which to approach the screening, evaluation, assessment, and treatment of individuals (infants, children, adults, and the elderly) with neurological damage. This chapter discusses the importance of theory to practice. In addition, it explains current models of motor control and motor learning that are influencing current practice. It provides a framework for the physiological aspect of therapeutic intervention. Chapter 9 presents three other frameworks having to do with health care that also influence physical therapy practice: the Problem Oriented System, the World Health Organization International Classification of Impairment, Disability and Handicap, and the helping/coping model.

Chapters 10, 11, and 12 discuss the processes of screening, evaluation and assessment, and treatment planning, applying the above-mentioned frameworks. The remainder of the chapters in this section comprise case studies of patients that are used to illustrate the practical application of the materials presented in Chapters 8 to 12. It is our belief that there can be no recipes for the treatment of individuals with particular problems.

Therefore, we believe that effective therapists must be aware of and must understand current theory and research and must be able to adopt a framework that will guide their practice with each individual they see. In the case studies, we have attempted to share the processes that actively practicing therapists use in their everyday practice, adhering to explicit theory and to a solid framework that keeps their practice consistent.

IMPORTANCE OF THEORY TO PRACTICE

Theory influences the way physical therapists evaluate, assess, and treat their patients. Without being aware of the theory under which therapists practice, the methods chosen for a given patient may be inconsistent or even contradictory. Additionally, using theory explicitly allows therapists to communicate to students and other health care professionals the principles and framework by which physical therapy practice is determined.[1] We therefore begin this section by presenting the theoretical framework under which physical therapists operate.

325

I. Contemporary Model of Motor Control

A. The contemporary model

The contemporary model has been referred to as the systems model, the distributed control model, or the dynamical systems model. The key elements of the contemporary model are[2]

1. **Reciprocity; multiple interconnections.** There is more than one way to route information from point A to point B. If one set of connections is interrupted, other sets are still available.

2. **Distributed control; redundancy.** Parts, units, and elements within the system may play more than one role.

3. **Emergent properties.** The output of the system is the result of cooperative interaction of all participating subsystems, as well as the interaction with the environment within which the system is operating at the time.

4. **Command by consensus.** This emerges at the point of the most relevant information. It is similar to the notion of a team. Any team member may take appropriate action at the time; no one member is in control.

B. Key concepts and theoretical assumptions of the contemporary model

1. The nervous system is organized to solve motor problems or achieve goal-directed tasks.

2. Goal-directed movement is planned in advance and emerges as a consequence of the interactions among neural subsystems, the state of the musculoskeletal components relevant to the task, and the environment within which the movement takes place.

3. The nervous system uses flexible strategies to control degrees of freedom.

   The number of degrees of freedom that must be controlled for any behavioral output is great. The nervous system finds ways to make this control simpler. These strategies have been referred to as coordinative structures, or functional synergies. Bernstein defines coordinative structures as those classes of movements that have similar kinematic characteristics, coinciding active muscle groups, and coinciding types of afferentation.[3] For each synergy there are distinctive, specific connections imposed on certain muscle groups, organizing all the muscles participating in a movement into a small number of connected groups. Most skilled movements are dependent on the assembly of complex coordinative structures. Learning, skill development, involves building synergies.

4. Input during performance is used to shape the ongoing movement (feedback mode) and to influence future movements by adjusting motor plans in advance of an anticipated disturbance (feedforward mode).

5. Apparent deficits after central nervous system damage involve a mix of positive and negative symptoms not related by cause and effect. These symptoms reflect an altered interaction among neural subsystems as well as changes at the musculoskeletal level and newly acquired compensatory strategies.[4]

   a. Negative symptoms are the loss of normal function; they result directly from damage to neural tissue. Examples of negative symptoms are weakness, loss of dexterity, and the condition of becoming easily fatigued.

   b. Positive symptoms are the result of a change in relationships as the remaining intact system attempts to function; there is a change in balance among subsystems. Examples of positive symptoms are abnormal postures, abnormal proprioceptive reflexes, disrupted autonomic control, and spasticity.

6. The damaged nervous system is both plastic and adaptive and is thus capable of recovery via various mechanisms that are probably dependent on the nature of the damage and the state of the system at the time of the damage. The reorganization of the damaged nervous system is the result of intrinsic processes that are influenced by active experience in adapting to environmental demands. Recovery is not likely to duplicate the normal developmental sequence.[5]

II. Concepts of Motor Learning and Their Application

Understanding how skill acquisition occurs naturally can provide some insight into how physical therapists can intervene to enhance skill acquisition. Gentile's framework of skill acquisition can help therapists develop guidelines for the application of motor learning theory and research to clinical practice.[6]

A. Initial stages of learning

1. **Goal setting.** The primacy of the goal.
   a. The goal must be that of the performer/patient. The therapist and patient decide mutually about the goal.
   b. The goal must be at the action level, *ie,* it must concern the accomplishment of a task, not the methods or the movements used to accomplish the task. Goal confusion should be avoided by focusing on the outcome rather than on the details of the movement. For example, when working with an individual with hemiplegia, a neurotherapeutic approach would use brushing, tapping, and/or resistance to help the person move out of flexor synergy and lift the hand to the mouth rather than supinate and flex so that the fist does not reach the ear instead. An alternative to this would be to ask the patient to lift a cup with water. The patient will need to control supination in order to prevent the water from spilling. Therefore, in a goal-directed task, the patient is better able to control the movement.
   c. The goal should be specific and challenging. The therapist should select tasks that are relevant and interesting. This will be more efficient and will enhance motivation.
   d. The patient must be confident that he/she can learn to achieve the goal. The therapist provides reassurance and support.

2. **Regulatory and nonregulatory stimuli.** Setting the goal determines which of the momentary stimuli are regulatory and which are nonregulatory.
   a. Regulatory stimuli are those that the movements must match to accomplish the task. Not until the goal is set is this determined. For example, if the goal is for the patient to walk from point A to point B in the gym prior to the arrival of other staff or patients, the regulatory stimuli will be the furniture located between points A and B, the surface of the floor, etc. If the goal is for the patient to go from point A to point B while there are several other persons in the gym, those persons whose locations and/or movement paths cross between points A and B will be additional regulatory stimuli to those encountered earlier.
   b. Nonregulatory stimuli may include announcements over the loudspeaker, the therapists working at their desks who are not near the path traversed, etc.
   c. Gentile has proposed a taxonomy of motor tasks that categorizes tasks based on the regulatory environmental conditions (see Table 8–1). In this taxonomy, Gentile considers whether the regulatory conditions are in motion or are stationary. In addition, she considers whether the conditions vary from trial to trial. Given these two dimensions, she then analyzes the demands of the task.[6] This provides physical therapists with a means of categorizing the sorts of tasks that are worked on with patients, a guide to how to structure practice, and a way to interpret the problems that a patient may display.
      (1). During the initial stages of learning, all regulatory conditions must be present. In other words, any stimuli that are normally a part of the task, and to which the movements must match, must be present. For example, when learning to play tennis, there must be a racquet (no practice of the swing without the racquet!), there must be a ball, and the ball must be traveling toward the performer in a variety of paths with varied speed. This does not mean, however, that the novice should play against the expert who uses all her

Table 8–1.   GENTILE'S TAXONOMY OF MOTOR TASKS: ENVIRONMENTAL CONTEXT

Regulatory Conditions During Performance	Intertrial Variability Absent	Intertrial Variability Present
Stationary	**Closed Tasks**	**Variable Motionless Tasks**
	1. Unlocking the front door 2. Turning on the light switch	1. Walking on different stable surfaces 2. Drinking from mugs, glasses, cups
	Self-paced* No predictive demands* Movement fixation* Reproductive mode* Monitoring decreases*	Self-paced* No predictive demands* Movement diversifies* Generative mode* Monitoring ongoing*
Motion	**Consistent-Motion Tasks**	**Open Tasks**
	1. Stepping onto an escalator 2. Stepping into an elevator	1. Sitting in a moving automobile 2. Catching a ball 3. Carrying a wiggling child
	Externally paced* Predictive demands* Movement fixation* Reproductive mode* Monitoring decreases*	Externally paced* Predictive demands* Movement diversifies* Generative mode* Monitoring ongoing*

(Reprinted from Gentile AM: Skill acquisition. In *Movement Science: Foundations for Physical Therapy in Rehabilitation* by J. H. Carr and R. B. Shepherd, (eds), p. 106, 107, with permission of Aspen Publishers, Inc., ©1987.)
* Characteristic of task.

trick shots. The complexity of the task can be reduced initially, especially when environmental conditions are moving. But, the varying, moving ball must be there.

(2). Nonregulatory stimuli can be removed or reduced initially, if necessary, to avoid distractions. In other words, patients can be treated in a quiet area without distractions.

3. **Selective attendance to stimuli.** The performer/patient must be able to attend selectively to the regulatory stimuli.
   a. The therapist determines whether the patient can recognize which features of the environment will be important to consider as he/she prepares to attempt the task.
   b. If there are some critical features that the patient has not recognized, the therapist points them out. If problems are anticipated in the identification of certain features, these can be highlighted with bright colors, stripes, etc.
   c. Distractions should be reduced initially (nonregulatory conditions).

4. **Formulation of the motor plan.** The performer/patient must develop the motor plan to accomplish the task. However, the therapist can be helpful in this process.[7]
   a. *Verbal instructions.* Verbal instructions should be global, giving only the general aspects of the intended movement and focusing on only the key features. For example, the therapist might suggest starting positions of the limbs/body in relation to significant objects/persons in the environment. Or, general strategies might be suggested. In addition, the therapist might point out how the patient can recognize his/her errors. Verbal instructions are thought to be overused. Words alone are crude descriptions of complex kinds of movements. Additionally, the learner can remember only so many instructions; this is even truer for children.
   b. *Demonstrations.* Demonstrations are best given before or between trials. The patient cannot attend to outside information during the trial without being distracted from what he/she is doing and how it feels.

Demonstrations are thought to be more effective when performed by peers during initial stages of learning. Some evidence even suggests that observing someone else learning a skill is beneficial.[8]

Demonstrations can be provided in various ways: in person or with films, videotapes, or photos. Although these methods may all seem the same, there is little experimental evidence of the effectiveness of other than in-person demonstrations.

   c. *Mental preparation.* The patient may use imagery of what he/she is going to do. The patient's state of arousal is also important; too much or too little arousal will affect performance.

5. **Response execution.** It is up to the performer/patient to respond to the execution. The therapist can observe patient performance in order to provide augmented feedback. Otherwise, the therapist should keep his/her hands off and mouth shut. This does not mean that patients should not be guarded carefully. However, the therapist should be conscious of how he/she is guarding and should not try to do anything that will change the nature of the task. For example, manual contact changes the nature of the task and talking distracts the patient from what he/she is doing; thus, the important processing of environmental stimuli and intrinsic feedback do not take place.

6. **Feedback.** There are two types of feedback:
   a. *Intrinsic feedback.* This is information related to the sensations associated with the movement itself, *eg*, the feel or the sound of the movement.[9] Intrinsic feedback comes from the sensory receptors (kinesthetic, cutaneous, vestibular, auditory, visual).
   b. *Extrinsic feedback.* This is information about the achievement of the goal that *augments* intrinsic feedback. The therapist often plays a role in providing extrinsic feedback to the patient.
      (1). The patient needs time to process and store intrinsic feedback about the performance; the therapist should delay augmented feedback to avoid interference.

      (2). The therapist should not waste time telling the performer the obvious.
      (3). Motivational feedback should be differentiated from informational feedback. For example, does "good" mean "good try" or "good performance"?
      (4). Details should be limited at this stage. The performer/patient can attend to only so much.
      (5). Feedback should be used to discourage compensatory strategies (ones that will lead to subsequent damage).

7. **Decision processes and next response**
   a. The patient should be kept motivated. The use of client goals leads to motivation.
   b. The therapist *assists* the patient in the analysis of the outcome (information feedback about outcome [IF-O] and knowledge of results [KR]) and the movement execution (information feedback about performance [IF-P] and knowledge of performance [KP]).
   c. The patient should be reminded of what has worked before (strategies, key features).
   d. Both the therapist and the patient should still be sure about the goal.
   e. If necessary, attention is refocused on regulatory stimuli in the environment.
   f. The therapist should ask the patient what he/she will do next. Patients are very good at cognitive processing related to motor learning if given the leeway to do so.

B. Later stages of learning

1. **Structuring the practice session.** More learning takes place if there are more practice trials, provided there is intent to learn and adequate feedback on performance. The problem becomes: What constitutes useful practice trials? What are the features that promote skill acquisition? Bernstein stated that "practice does not consist in repeating the means of solution of a motor problem time after time, but in the process of solving this problem again and again. Practice is a particular type of repetition without repetition."[3]

2. **Massed versus distributed practice**
   a. *Massed practice.* These are the sessions in which the amount of practice time in a trial is greater than the amount of rest between trials.
   b. *Distributed practice.* These are the sessions in which rest time equals or is greater than practice time.
   c. The best practice conditions depend on the nature of the task. In *continuous* tasks (no obvious beginning or end), limitation of rest between trials leads to systematic decrease in performance compared to distributed practice. However, following rest, there is no difference in performance. In *discrete* tasks (definite beginning and end), there is no effect of massed practice. Given limited practice time, there is an advantage to massed practice; it is more efficient.[7] However, patient endurance and motivation must also be considered.

3. **Variability in practice.** The need for variability in practice depends on the type of task. For tasks that do not vary from trial to trial, fixed (without variability) practice is better. For tasks that do vary from trial to trial, practice must vary. Research results suggest that variable practice (for variable tasks) leads to better long-term retention of the skill.[10] It is believed that variability provides practice in solving the problem, not in reproducing one solution. The skill of solving the motor problem on each occasion is what is needed in a variable task. One solution will not work for all variations of the task.

4. **Blocked versus random practice.** When a task is variable, investigators have asked whether several variations of the task practiced in blocks of each individual variation or variations practiced randomly are more effective. In other words, if the task is transfers to and from a wheelchair, is it better to practice toilet transfers 10 times, followed by bed transfers 10 times, etc., or to practice all the transfers in random order? Again, research in normal subjects has shown that blocked practice is better during the acquisition phase (initial practice phase) but that random practice is better during the retention phase (retest period at some time after the practice period).[11] Random practice requires that the patient gen-

erate each response anew rather than repeat one solution over and over again.

5. **Mental practice.** Mental practice refers to imagining performing the task without any associated overt actions. It has been found that mental practice is better than no practice but not as good as physical practice. The performer/patient must have some skill for the task in order to benefit. It may be that the patient is learning the cognitive parts of the task or is actually running off the program with decreased gain, *ie*, less electrical activity at the muscle level. This is supported by Roland's finding that mental practice causes activity in cortical areas normally associated with planning and/or execution of the movement.[12]

6. **Transfer of training.** This is the gain (or loss) in proficiency in one task as a result of practice of some other task.
   a. The amount of transfer seems to be quite small and positive unless the tasks are practically identical.
   b. Negative transfer seldom occurs.
   c. Thus, there is a great deal of specificity in gaining skill.
   d. *Part-whole transfer.* It seems logical that if therapists are attempting to aid in learning a complex motor task, it would be easier and more efficient to break the task into parts and provide practice on at least the more difficult parts before attempting the whole task. However, practice on one part in isolation may so change the motor demands/constraints for the part that it is no longer the same as it is in the context of the total skill.

      Some research has been done on this issue in the laboratory, and it appears that the effectiveness of part-whole training depends on the nature of the task. For those tasks that are serial in nature, *ie*, no overlapping parts in time, this method may help. An example of this is teaching a person with paraplegia to transfer from wheelchair to car using a sliding board. The parts are essentially serial in nature: positioning the chair, locking it, and removing the arm rest; positioning the sliding board; sliding across the board; positioning the legs inside the car; removing the sliding board.

      However, with continuous tasks, for which behavior continues more or less uninterrupted, part-whole training is less effective than practicing the whole task for the same period of time. The parts that can be isolated frequently occur at the same time as other parts and/or must be coordinated with each other. For example, we have often stated that a patient must be able to shift weight side to side prior to being able to walk. However, a recent study by Winstein *et al.*[13] demonstrated that training in lateral weight shift improved weight shift but did not improve parameters in gait in hemiplegic subjects.

7. **Feedback.** Type of feedback is task-specific.
   a. For tasks in which there is no variability from trial to trial (closed and consistent-motion tasks,[6] see Table 8–1), movement becomes fixed, consistent. Therefore, the performer/patient is acting in a reproductive mode. Consequently, the therapist needs to provide KP—feedback about the movement.
      (1). One option is for the therapist to explain to the patient verbally what the movement actually looked like and how it was or was not effective. This might be combined with a demonstration or simulation of the way the patient performed.
      (2). Another option is to videotape the patient's movements in accomplishing the task. In replaying the tape, the therapist needs to provide verbal instruction to point out important details.
   b. For tasks in which there is variability from trial to trial (open and variable motionless tasks,[6] see Table 8–1), movement becomes diversified. One movement pat-

tern will not work. Therefore, the therapist must provide KR—feedback about the outcome.
      (1). In this case, verbal feedback might include comments about environmental stimuli that the patient did not seem to notice or take into account.
      (2). One might also videotape the performer/patient within the environment, with emphasis on the environment.
      (3). The patient and the therapist need to reconsider environmental constraints and movement options.
   c. *Frequency of KR—relative versus absolute.* According to Winstein, relative frequency of KR is the proportion of practice trials for which KR is provided, whereas absolute frequency refers to the total number of trials for which KR is provided in a practice session.[9] It has been found that individuals who receive feedback less frequently actually learn the task better. It is hypothesized that dependence on feedback may decrease processing of information necessary for learning the task. With less frequent feedback, the patient may learn to detect his/her errors.
   d. *Summary KR.* Feedback is given after a number of trials rather than after each one. Again, the practice of withholding feedback and providing it after several trials leads to better long-term retention than giving feedback after each trial.
   e. *Precision of KR.* Feedback about the direction and magnitude of the error is better than either alone. The therapist can increase the detail and complexity of feedback along with the patient's skill acquisition.

III. Principles of Therapeutic Intervention Based on Contemporary Theory and Research in Motor Control and Motor Learning

A. Assessment

Assessment must be multidimensional, taking into account neurophysiology, muscle physiology, biomechanics, cognition, motor learning/motor control, and environmental constraints.

B. The therapist's role

The therapist's role is to facilitate skill, not movement patterns. This involves assisting in the selection of appropriate tasks, clarifying the goal, structuring the environment for practice, providing feedback, and helping the performer/patient with decision making.

1. Treatment is carried out in realistic, goal-directed activities.
2. The nature of the task is considered in choosing practice conditions and types of feedback to use. Skill is task-specific.
   a. Practice should be under varied conditions where appropriate.
   b. Feedback should be provided about the outcome (KR) or about the movement (KP) only when it will *augment* what the patient is able to detect on his/her own.
   c. The amount of feedback should be reduced with practice so that the patient does not become dependent on it and is able to detect errors on his/her own.
3. The patient's *active* problem solving is the key to relearning a skill. This does not mean that the patient simply actively follows directions from the therapist but, rather, actively figures out what worked and what did not so that the next try will be changed accordingly.

C. The goal of therapy

The goal of therapy is to help the patient learn to solve the motor problems that he/she will meet in everyday life.

References

1. Shepherd K: Theory: criteria, importance and impact. In Lister M (ed): *Contemporary Management of Motor Control Problems. Proceedings of the II STEP Conference.* Alexandria, VA, Foundation for Physical Therapy, 1991, pp 5–10.
2. Davis WJ: Organizational concepts in the central motor networks of invertebrates. In Herman RM, Grillner S, Stein PSG, Stuart DG (eds): *Neural Control of Locomotion.* New York, Plenum Press, 1976, pp 265–292.
3. Bernstein NA: *The Coordination and Regulation of Movements.* New York, Pergamon Press, 1967, p 127.
4. Burke D: Spasticity as an adaptation to pyramidal tract injury. In Waxman SG (ed): *Functional Recovery in Neurological Disease.* New York, Raven Press, 1988, pp 401–423.
5. Held JM: Recovery of function after brain damage: theoretical implications for therapeutic intervention. In Carr JH, Shepherd RB (eds): *Movement Science: Foundations for Physical Therapy in Rehabilitation.* Rockville, MD, Aspen Publishers, 1987, pp 155–178.
6. Gentile AM: Skill acquisition: action, movement and neuromotor processes. In Carr JH, Shepherd RB (eds): *Movement Science: Foundations for Physical Therapy in Rehabilitation.* Rockville, MD, Aspen Publishers, 1987, pp 93–154.
7. Schmidt RA: *Motor Learning and Performance: From Principles to Practice.* Champaign, IL, Human Kinetics Books, 1991.
8. McCullagh P, Weiss MR, Ross D: Modeling considerations in motor skill acquisition and performance: an integrated approach. *Exerc Sport Sci Rev,* 1989, 17:475–513.
9. Winstein CJ: Designing practice for motor learning: clinical implications. In Lister M (ed): *Contemporary Management of Motor Control Problems. Proceedings of the II STEP Conference.* Alexandria, VA, Foundation for Physical Therapy, 1991, pp 65–76.
10. McCracken HD, Stelmach GE: A test of the schema theory of discrete motor learning. *J Motor Behav,* 1977, 8:46–55.
11. Shea JB, Morgan RL: Contextual interference effects on the acquisition, retention, and transfer of a motor skill. *J Exp Psych [Hum Learn Mem],* 1979, 5:179–187.
12. Roland PE: Metabolic mapping of sensorimotor integration in the human brain. In *Motor Areas of the Cerebral Cortex* [Ciba Foundation Symposium]. New York, John Wiley, 1987.
13. Winstein CJ, Gardner ER, McNeal DR, *et al.*: Standing balance training: effect on balance and locomotion in hemiparetic adults. *Arch Phys Med Rehabil* 1989, 70:755–762.

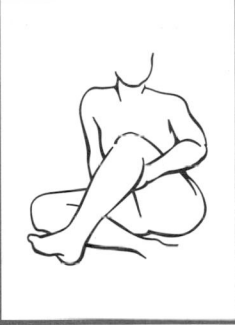

CHAPTER 9

Critical Frameworks for Evaluation, Assessment, and Treatment Planning

Lee Nelson

The most powerful of all medical and paramedical personnel is the patient—and there is one for every member of the population.[1]

I. OVERVIEW

A. Changes in physical therapy

An increased emphasis has been placed on the effectiveness and efficiency of clinical decision making in the practice of physical therapy in the past 10 to 15 years. Factors and forces that have contributed to this are numerous and reflect changes in the physical therapy profession itself as well as in the health care system at large. Changes that have occurred in physical therapy include the development and proliferation of graduate entry-level education programs (now constituting about 50% of physical therapy education programs); establishment of the

American Board of Physical Therapy Specialties, with large numbers of specialists being added to the ranks every year; increased interest in and use of clinical research; and, finally, establishment of direct access to physical therapy services without a physician referral, currently legal in greater than 50% of the states.

B. Changes in the health care system

Changes in physical therapy have happened concurrently with major shifts in the health

333

care system. These shifts have included a variety of cost-containment efforts and managed health care plans aimed at attempting to control escalating health care costs, sophisticated and costly advances in technology and medical care, a change in location in delivery of services from more acute arenas to subacute or ambulatory settings, and, most recently, more significant inquiry into and movement toward universal access to health care for every citizen.

C. The nature of problems facing physical therapists

As a result of these changes, the nature of problems physical therapists are asked to evaluate and treat are more complex, the environments within which services are rendered are changing, and the fundamental role of "treating" patients has shifted to more evaluation, consultation, and teaching. Thus, curriculum planners and faculty members throughout the United States are presented with the challenge of determining and designing meaningful curricular content and modes of delivery to prepare students to become competent practitioners.

What are the skills, attitudes, and values that future practitioners should acquire to best serve the needs of people seeking their help? What is the nature of the physical therapist's expertise and how it is acquired? Some question whether expertise is built on technical skill, application of theory or general principles, critical analysis, or deliberative action.[2] If expertise in physical therapy is not clearly defined and, therefore, not well understood, then preparing practitioners for the future, when much ambiguity will exist in the identification and provision of effective health care, becomes a major challenge.

D. Educating physical therapists

Given the recent changes, an important aspect in the education of physical therapists and other health care professionals becomes preparation for uncertainty. How are people best prepared to undertake these difficult challenges? The needs of patients in various practice environments in the next several decades will require that physical therapists possess well-honed technical and interpersonal skills as well as capabilities in ethical and clinical decision making to provide meaningful contributions to the complex situations they encounter. Instilling technical competence alone does not provide an adequate base for managing complex problems. As Weed states, "we shall always be guided more by the needs of our patients than by the power of our degree—that no matter how expert and talented we become in one part of medicine or how powerful we become in one part of society, we shall never act as if we believe that a part is greater than the whole."[1]

E. Frameworks for practice

The quest then becomes to fashion a style of practicing for each physical therapist whereby a sense of initiative, discovery, reflection, critical appraisal, technical competence, and responsibility is fostered, supported, and nurtured intrinsically and, if possible, extrinsically. In what way do these characteristics change through the course of professional education and development from novice to expert? If they are not "taught" in professional education programs, can they be "learned" when assuming the role of a practitioner? In contemplating these questions and looking at a community of practitioners with heterogeneous backgrounds who strive for excellence in clinical care and exhibit the characteristics of competent, reflective clinicians, several structures or guiding frameworks emerge. These frameworks appear to provide a backdrop against which the different yet synergistic dimensions of competence (eg, technical, ethical, decision making, affective) can interact, mature, and assist the clinician in maintaining a patient-centered focus. In this community, the following frameworks significantly contribute to the continued shaping and development of practice:

1. Problem Oriented System
2. World Health Organization International Classification of Impairment, Disability and Handicap
3. Helping/coping models

An in-depth analysis of these systems or models is not provided in this chapter, as each deserves more thorough review. Brief descriptions of the theories behind each and the manner in which each contributes to the development of a reflective practitioner who seeks excellence and maintains a patient-centered or patient primacy focus are presented.[3]

II. The Problem Oriented System

A. Originator

Larry Weed, MD, developed the Problem Oriented System (POS) of Education in the late 1960s.[4] He upset the medical community by assertively bringing forth observations about gross inadequacies in the medical care system and tracing the causes to the manner in which providers, specifically physicians, had been educated. His underlying goal in shaking up the system was to evoke better quality control programs in medicine and education. To do this, he proposed adopting new premises and tools for our health care and educational systems, the most well known being the Problem Oriented Medical Record (POMR).

B. Primary premise

One of the most important premises that Weed developed that specifically relates to professional development is that a core of behavior should be elicited from students or clinicians—not a core of knowledge taught.[5] What type of person should the clinician be? What attitudes, values, and beliefs should this person have to be able to effectively approach and manage clinical care inclusive of an increasing body of knowledge but for which uncertainty exists?

C. Development of a core of behavior

Weed proposed a system whereby a person's behavioral characteristics of thoroughness, reliability, clinical judgement/analytic sense, and efficiency are assessed from the time of being a student throughout a professional career. The rules of the process are carefully defined so that participants know what the expectations are. The behavioral characteristics are tracked via their demonstration in both audit of the medical record and observation of a treatment session. The focus and attention given to the practitioner's choices and decisions as well as to his/her actual "hands-on" management, instead of to regurgitated knowledge, support a sense of responsibility and accountability. Hence, an increased consciousness of moral obligations and rights and how individual values and attitudes affect these obligations emerges.

D. Ethical outcomes

Several ethical outcomes are possible outgrowths of this system. In a system in which behavior is monitored, truth-telling and honesty are highly rewarded. There is more room to admit error and to say "I don't know" without fear of punitive consequences. Identification and effective use of pertinent resources become important. Once a person loses fear of telling the truth, trustworthiness as evidenced through the characteristic of reliability greatly improves. The pressure to know facts is lessened or removed. This type of honesty-rearing may enable a practitioner to more effectively relate truth to a peer, patient, or family member.

E. Lifelong learning

Because much emphasis is placed on actively participating in the learning process, a healthy pattern for lifelong learning is supported. Practitioners reared in this system may be more open to peer review of the care they provide. Audit, with an educational focus, is welcomed and valued. Self-assessment skills are developed, with improved abilities to identify needed knowledge, attitudes, and/or skills as well as to take responsibility for remedying any discrepancies between the needs of patients and the skills possessed.

F. Thoroughness and reliability

In fostering development of a core of behavior rather than a core of knowledge, it is helpful to support development of the behavioral characteristics of thoroughness and reliability before focusing on efficiency. Much of the discussion of current health care changes involves an emphasis on efficiency. However, valuing and practicing efficiency when the skills of being thorough and reliable have not been developed may compromise the provision of quality services.

Thoroughness implies completion of data collection, problem identification, and formulation of goals and plans. *Reliability* addresses accuracy, reproducibility, and currency in the management of the problem. Were the plans carried out? Is there evidence of use of the most recent resources? Demonstration of thoroughness and reliability should precede demonstration of efficiency to effect comprehensive, competent care.

G. Clinical judgement

The qualities of clinical judgement or sound analytic sense and efficiency are important not only in the delivery and receipt of health care but also in terms of quality management and cost. The mystique of clinical judgement may lose some of its intrigue once patterns of logic, intuition, and critical thinking become less tacit and are able to be communicated. It is this unfolding of critical appraisal skills, through data collection, hypothesis testing, assessment formulation, and plan implementation, and a monitoring system that tracks effectiveness, that promotes sound clinical judgement.

H. Efficiency

Efficiency often implies setting priorities, and, as Weed points out, this is usually done under some sort of pressure. Efficiency cannot be attained until thoroughness is. But, if priorities are set under pressure, there may be an increased chance of being unreliable. Helping clinicians identify and learn what is being compromised and the potential consequences that may ensue and then revisiting that decision are important during these times of limited resources of varying types. In addition, the ways in which these compromises may relate to a decreased standard of quality care require our immediate attention.

I. Other measurable character traits

Although there is a timidity in identifying specific character traits that a physical therapist ought to possess, Weed's system of looking at four behavioral characteristics (thoroughness, reliability, clinical judgement and efficiency) has been helpful in learning and practicing humanistic, ethical, and scientific care. Perhaps there are other measurable character traits that we as a profession would find helpful to add.

J. Patient involvement in medical care

Another area that Weed discussed and wrote about 10 to 15 years ago was the patient's involvement in medical care.[6] Much of the movement toward patients' engagement in and responsibility for their medical care originated in the early premises of Weed. He supported empowering the patient to take an active role in understanding and managing his/her health care, including participation in goal setting and formulation of plans. His espousing of a logical and humanistic, problem-oriented, patient-centered approach to medicine has had widespread influence in our society.

As Weed described in 1978 in the introduction to his book,

. . . patients and potential patients must do their part to solve the overwhelming problems in health care—inadequate care, overutilization of care, unfair distribution of resources and uncontrolled costs. To help, the public must first develop their own point of view about health care and a system for delivering it and they must be given some tools to work with. The purpose of this book is to give them a framework in which to think and at least one useful tool with which to work.[6]

III. The World Health Organization International Classification of Impairment, Disability and Handicap (WHO-ICIDH)

A. Definitions

WHO-ICIDH has provided a sound framework for developing a perspective not only on disease and illness but also on how these affect the person and his/her functioning in society.[7] Three levels of disablement are described[7]:

1. *Impairment:* disturbances at the organ level, "concerned with abnormalities of body structure and appearance and with organ or system function, resulting from any cause."
2. *Disability:* disturbances at the level of the person, "reflecting the consequences of impairment in terms of functional performance and activity by the individual."
3. *Handicap:* disturbances at the societal level, "concerned with the disadvantages experienced by the individual as a result of impairments and disabilities; handicaps thus reflect interaction with and adaptation to the individual's surrounding."

B. WHO-ICIDH versus International Classification of Diseases

The WHO-ICIDH model presents an alternative to a previously used medical model of disease that is characterized by a pathology orientation, the International Classification of Diseases (ICD).[7] ICD is depicted symbolically as

Etiology $\longrightarrow$ pathology $\longrightarrow$ manifestation

Although this medical model provides an efficient approach to illness and disease, a consequence of this orientation is that the pathological entity is viewed as being unrelated to the person with the pathology. This is evident in our language as physical therapists, when the people we work with (the patients) are described as "the hip," "the stroke," or "the back." This is in distinct contrast to the WHO-ICIDH philosophy, which addresses the consequence of disease on everyday life, not only at the organ level, but within the context of the person and how he/she functions in society. This orientation not only supports a person-first language, *eg*, "a person with a back problem," but also better represents how physical therapists actually think and practice. Therapists pride themselves on being humanists with a functional orientation who consider "the big picture."

C. Advantages of WHO-ICIDH

1. In looking at the relationship to clinical decision making, the WHO-ICIDH fosters the practice of viewing the patient from a more comprehensive, holistic perspective and thereby supports more effective decision making, particularly about complex issues.
2. Patient contribution to and participation in goal setting, decision making, and treatment formulation are encouraged and valued.
3. The WHO-ICIDH model also brings clarity, and a more rational backdrop, to measurement of outcomes. Clinicians, better able to grasp the big picture, can more adeptly determine whether their interventions are targeted at an impairment, disability, or handicap level. Once this identification is made, measurement of effectiveness of outcomes occurs in a more focused manner, whether it be a formal clinical study or one practitioner bringing a less formal research mindset to everyday clinical care, critically appraising the intervention. Recent theories and research findings from the motor control/motor learning literature indicate the importance of goals being functional, context-specific, and owned by the patient in order to achieve expected outcomes.[8]
4. By merging the POS and WHO-ICIDH models, a richer, more meaningful encounter at the professional/patient level can emerge. Seeking a patient's contribution to goal setting, discovering what he/she wants to achieve, is a way of keying in to the person's perspective on what has happened to him/her. What does the person know about what has happened? What impact has it had on his/her life? How and what do we ask in a caring, competent way to find out what the person knows? What are the person's expectations of outcomes? What are the person's unique resources and unique constraints, and how can they be best woven into the treatment options?

IV. The Helping/Coping Model

A. Attribution of responsibility

Exploring the clinician's method of helping and the patient's manner of coping in the area of attribution of responsibility for the problem and the solution is helpful in efforts toward making this encounter the most meaningful it can be.

Examination of a helping/coping framework is helpful in trying to understand how therapists, patients, and students view responsibility for problems and solutions encountered in clinical settings:

People may not be aware of the assumptions they make about responsibility for problems and solutions. But they cannot avoid making such assumptions and the assumptions have consequences for their own behavior and for the behavior of others they influence. Each set of assumptions makes it easier to solve certain problems and harder to solve others. [9]

B. Conceptual model

Brickman *et al.* put forth a conceptual model suggesting that if behavior associated with providing help, *ie*, the therapist's behavior, and behavior associated with receiving help, *ie*, the patient's and/or student's behavior are to be understood, the two processes must be examined together.[9]

The following four models are described with varying ascriptions for responsibility for problems and solutions, as well as deficiencies found:

1. *Moral model:* a high degree of responsibility for both the problem and the solution; the individual is the only one who can effect change; loneliness is a potential outcome; typified by "est" movement.
2. *Compensatory model:* a low degree of responsibility for the problem but a high degree for the solution; exemplified by Jesse Jackson's quote, "You are not responsible for being down, but you are for getting up"; Head Start model.
3. *Enlightenment model:* a low degree of responsibility for the solution but a high degree for the problem; solution lies outside the person, and, in order to change, the person

must submit to agents of social change; Alcoholics Anonymous model.
4. *Medical model:* low degree of responsibility for both the solution and the problem; person accepts help, but the responsibility for recovery rests with the expert; sense of dependency and helplessness is fostered.

C. Implications for physical therapists

In looking at the relationship between therapist and patient, many junctures exist at which problems may occur. In considering models of helping and coping, the two parties may be out of phase with one another in attribution of responsibility for the problem and the solution. Further examination of how each party views this may be helpful in resolving possible differences.

In evaluating all four models, the models in which people are held responsible for solutions to problems, *ie*, moral and compensatory, are more likely to increase competence than models in which people are not held responsible for solutions, *ie*, medical and enlightenment.

D. Balancing responsibility

A dilemma or, at very least, a delicate balance exists in any attempt at helping. Clinician's have strong technical training and, for the most part, take pride in the "hands-on" treatment of "doing something to" a patient. A patient-centered type of decision making involves stepping back, being a good problem identifier, effectively mobilizing and incorporating the patient's own resources and desires, and collaboratively designing a plan that is meaningful to the patient. It also means that helping, in most instances, is not "doing to" or "doing for" but applying skills that enable patients to be responsible for and to participate actively in solutions to their own problems. This type of movement is evidenced in public legislation such as PL 99-457, which addresses family-centered, collaborative care whereby the person and family identify services that best meet their needs.[10]

V. Conclusions

Clinicians who can think logically, solve problems effectively and efficiently, access and utilize information appropriately, and hold onto a personal value system will be the practitioners who exhibit excellence and maintain an effective patient-centered focus despite major changes occurring in health care today. The blending of the three frameworks discussed provides a sound foundation for and is instrumental in assisting clinicians in their development as caring and competent practitioners. The importance of frameworks or systems through which physical therapists can responsibly assess progress made in lifelong learning has been highlighted. The future may bring new or modified frameworks; acknowledgement and evaluation of these will need to be made. As Weed indicates, closing the loop so that systems work to ensure quality and demand accountability in all dimensions of health care is of extreme importance today.

REFERENCES

1. Weed LL: A touchstone for medical education. *Harvard Medical Alumni Bulletin* 1974, Nov/Dec:13–18.
2. Kennedy M: Inexact sciences: professional education and the development of expertise. In Rothkopf E (ed): *Review of Research in Education.* vol. 14. Washington DC, American Educational Research Association, 1987, pp 133–168.
3. Shephard KF, Jensen GM: Physical therapist curricula for the 1990s: educating the reflective practitioner. *Phys Ther,* 1990, 9:566–577.
4. Weed LL: *Medical Records, Medical Education, and Patient Care: The Problem Oriented Record as a Basic Tool.* Cleveland, Case Western Reserve University Press, 1969.
5. Weed LL: The implications of the problem-oriented system for medical education. In Hurst JW, Walker HK (eds): *The Problem Oriented System.* New York, MEDCOM, 1972.
6. Weed LL: *Your Health Care and How to Manage It.* Essex Junction, VT, Essex Publishing Company, 1978.
7. World Health Organization: *International Classification of Impairments, Disabilities and Handicaps.* Geneva, WHO, 1980.
8. Lister M (ed): *Contemporary Management of Motor Control Problems: Proceedings of the II STEP Conference.* Alexandria, VA, Foundation for Physical Therapy, 1991.
9. Brickman P, Rabinowitz V, Karuza J: Models of helping and coping. *Am Psychol,* 1982, 37:368–384.
10. National Center for Family-Centered Care: *What Is Family-Centered Care?* Bethesda, MD, Association for the Care of Children's Health, 1990.

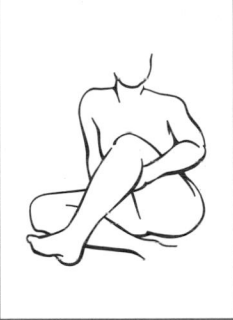

CHAPTER 10

Screening a Patient with Neurological Damage

Marianne Orest and Peggy Owen

Screening a patient, which is called cursory testing in the Problem Oriented System (POS), is performed to obtain general information about the patient in a short period of time. Screening can be useful to make quick decisions about patient care and to help determine the next steps to take. The timing of the screening can vary depending on the setting in which the patient is being seen. Data for the screening can be gathered from the patient's chart, from members of the team, and from an interview with the patient and/or family. Information should be gathered about the patient's impairments, disabilities, and handicaps.

I. Screening

A. The database

The database (see Figure 10–1) serves as a valuable guide and as the starting point for a screen. During a screen, information regarding the patient's general status background, physiological/anatomical systems, and functional motor performance can be gathered.

1. Each parameter is identified as "no problem," "problem," or "not evaluated."
   a. A "no problem" response on the database indicates that there are no pertinent data relating to the parameter that are within the consideration of physical therapy and that may contribute to a patient problem.
   b. The "problem" responses are a list of pertinent findings that may contribute to a patient problem.
   c. The "not evaluated" option is reserved for those times when examination is not feasible for reasons such as medical status or time limitations.
2. After completing the database, the screening will then proceed to an evaluation, or definitive testing as it is called in POS.

■ PLEASE NOTE: Even when using the database, it may still be difficult to separate a screen and an evaluation because, in practice, many physical therapists may naturally intertwine the two to meet the patient's needs.

The following section describes a screening for an individual with neurological damage. From this screening, an assessment can be made of the areas that need definitive evaluation.

B. Pediatric screening

Screening tools and procedures in pediatrics generally focus on the child's functional level,

Municipal Medical Center
Physical Therapy Department
*****Database*****

Doe, John
000-123-456-0

Do not thin from chart

No Problem	Problem	N/E		
			1.00	Patient profile Pt is a 62 y.o. male ō the diagnosis of ⓁCVA. Pt is retired from IBM and lives ō his wife in Essex Junction, VT. Wife is home most of the day – son and daughter live nearby. Pt was very active prior to admission. Home – one floor – 2 steps to enter ō Ⓡ rail.
				General status background
	✓		2.00	Medication Catapres, insulin, Micronase
	✓		2.10	Communication receptive aphasia
	✓		2.20	Cardiovascular HTN, atherosclerosis, ⓁCVA
	✓		2.30	Pulmonary smoking 2 ppd × 30 yrs.
	✓		2.40	Metabolic AODM
	✓		2.50	GI/GU incontinent
		✓	2.60	Vision
	✓		2.70	Behavior unable to follow simple commands
	✓		2.80	Appliances catheter, may need a w/c for use at home
✓			3.00	Pain and tenderness
				Physiological/anatomical systems data
	✓		4.00	Skin and soft tissue slight edema in Ⓡ ankle
	✓		4.10	Skeletal ↓ ROM Ⓡ shoulder and Ⓡ ankle
	✓		4.20	Neuromuscular CT scan – ⓁMCA in faret No movement noted in Ⓡ UE Ⓡ hemiparesis Limited movement noted in Ⓡ LE Decreased resistance to passive movement in Ⓡ UE
				Functional motor performance
	✓		5.00	Balance Static sitting balance – pt falls to the Ⓡ when sitting unsupported at the edge of the bed
✓			5.10	Posture
	✓		5.20	Functional mobility Bed mobility – moderate assistance needed to roll to the Ⓛ and for supine ⟶ sit Transfer – stand pivot to the Ⓛ – maximal assistance
		✓	5.30	Gait pattern

Patient aware of problem? ☐ Yes ☐ No

Therapist: _____ Date: _____ (Form #779-006, Rev.9/80)

FIGURE 10–1 Sample physical therapy database. *Abbreviations:* AODM=adult onset diabetes mellitus; CT=computed tomography; CVA=Cerebrovascular disease; GI=gastrointestinal; GU=genitourinary; HTN=hypertension; IBM=International Business Machines; L=left; LE=lower extremity; MCA=Middle cerebral artery; N/E=not evaluated; PPD=packs per day; PT=patient; R=right; ROM=range of motion; UE=upper extremity; VT=Vermont; y.o.=year old.

which is a measure at the disability and handicap levels as identified by the World Health Organization (WHO) (see Chapter 9), rather than on the child's impairment level.[1-4] If specific functional problems are identified, physical therapists may screen for impairments thought to be related to these problems.

1. Functional skills for newborns to 3-year-old children are related to motor milestones. Many texts describe motor milestones,[5,6] but whether all milestones are imperative for continued motor development needs further study. For example, many children never progress forward on their hands and knees in a quadruped position and yet they develop appropriately without difficulty. It appears that creeping on hands and knees may not be an important skill to include in a screen, but the more general skill of being able to move from one place to another to get a toy or reach a person may be important to screen.

2. Other examples of milestones thought to be important to screen are
   a. Head control in the supine and prone positions.
   b. Lifting legs up to reach for toes while in the supine position.
   c. Making a transition from one position to another on the floor.
   d. Moving from one part of the room to another to get a toy.
   e. Sitting on the floor in long sitting, on the floor in tailor-style sitting, on a bench, and with arms free.
   f. Pulling to stand.
   g. Cruising along furniture.
   h. Taking steps without assistance.
   i. Moving from the floor to stand without using arms.
   j. Squatting in play.
   k. Walking on uneven surfaces.
   l. Manipulating a toy while walking.
   m. Riding a tricycle.
   n. Playing with balls.

3. For children 3 to 7 years of age, functional skills are related to refining skills learned within the first 3 years of life. These skills include
   a. Riding a bike.
   b. Learning to hop, skip, and jump up and forward.
   c. Being able to catch a ball with hands only.
   d. Running with speed.

   e. Refining balance skills in the upright position on a variety of surfaces.

4. For children 8 years and older, functional skills are related to school environments and recreational activities.
   a. Examples of school environmental issues are
      (1). Getting from class to class safely and on time.
      (2). Participating in physical education class.
      (3). Having endurance to participate in a full day of school.
      (4). Transportation to and from school.
      (5). Positioning within the classroom.
      (6). Accessibility to all areas of the school.
      (7). Limited interaction with therapists so that the child is not thought to be "special."
   b. Examples of recreational activities include
      (1). Basketball
      (2). Baseball
      (3). Soccer
      (4). Track
      (5). Dance
      (6). Gymnastics
      (7). Skiing
      (8). Swimming
      (9). Horseback riding
      (10). Canoeing
      (11). Camping

5. Before beginning a screen with children, which occurs more frequently in the outpatient setting than in the inpatient setting, it is important to ascertain whether the child and/or family understand the reason for referral (if it is not blatant). In keeping with a family-centered approach to patient treatment, it is important to know whether the child and/or family see the need for the referral and screen and to determine what information the child and/or family would like to obtain from the screen.

C. Purpose of a screen

A screen is used to determine if problems exist that physical therapists can assist in resolving and to recommend which evaluation procedure or procedures may help determine the extent of the identified problems. Within pediatric settings, screens are used to identify children at risk for developmental dysfunction.

Screening tools are available, both standardized and nonstandardized, that assist with identifying potential problem areas and with providing an indication of "normal" or at-risk function.[1,2]

D. Setting/timing of the screening

1. **Bedside on nursing unit.** In the acute care setting, a routine screening can be done on admission to the hospital to determine if problems exist that can be managed by physical therapists. The physician can also identify problems that require further screening by the physical therapist after the medical work-up is completed. In this case, problems can be identified that are typically managed by the physical therapist or the physician may be seeking additional information from the screening. The timing of the screenings in these situations allows for early intervention by the physical therapist. A screening can also be beneficial after the patient is in the hospital for a period of time and a new problem develops necessitating physical therapy.

   Input is gathered for the screening to determine if the patient can come to the physical therapy department. At times, the patient's medical status, equipment, and/or energy level prevent her/him from coming to the department. Therefore, the screening can be performed while the patient is in bed. It can also be done while the patient is sitting in a chair if the nursing staff or the orderlies have just assisted the patient in getting out of bed or if the patient wishes to remain in the chair.

2. **Physical therapy department.** If the patient is in the rehabilitation unit, a screening can be done to better identify the major problem areas that warranted admission to the rehabilitation unit. When a patient attends therapy as an outpatient, a screening can help identify specific areas in which the patient is still having difficulty or to determine the need for physical therapy services. Screenings can also be performed in clinics that are set up for a specific patient problem, such as for children with spina bifida, or in a follow-up clinic, such as for children with at-risk function. At times, the screening can be done in the physical therapy department in the acute care setting if the chart indicates that the patient is doing well medically and is able to leave the nursing unit.

3. **Home.** Typically, problems to be addressed have been identified by the patient and/or family members. Some patients require home visits because they are unable to come to the clinic for testing because of their fragile medical status. Observing the patient performing the skills that are problematic, *ie*, observing disability level skills, will provide the information needed to assess whether a definitive evaluation is needed or whether modifications to the environment are recommended.

   The home environment is typically the most comfortable environment for screening children. Screenings performed within the home provide therapists with a more realistic view of a child's performance. When a screen is performed in the clinic, comparison of the child's performance within the clinic setting with what the family sees in the home will assist the therapist with interpreting the results of the screen.

4. **Schools and day-care settings.** A screen is often used in the school setting to help therapists address problems identified by school personnel using a minimal amount of intervention. For example, if a child is reportedly having difficulty with "sitting still" while working at the table, a brief observation of the child while she/he is working at the table would be a sufficient screen. Typically, providing the child with a supportive seat with her/his feet flat on the ground and the table at waist height is all that is necessary to remedy this problem. If the appropriate seating posture does not eliminate the identified problem, further definitive testing may be needed to determine the underlying problem of the behavior and the best plan of action to correct the problem.

E. Data Collection

1. **Patient's chart**
   a. Gathering data regarding medical stability is the primary responsibility of other members of the team to screen and evaluate. Even so, it is important to know whether or not problems in these areas exist so that the physical therapy screening can be done safely. Any problems in these areas that the therapist anticipates will have an effect on the patient's functional outcomes should be noted. General status includes medications and the

Table 10–1. GENERAL STATUS

Parameter	Example
Medications	Medications controlling intracranial pressure, spasticity, seizures, or behavior
Cardiovascular	The presence of angina or hypertension
Pulmonary	Congestive obstructive pulmonary disease or congestive heart failure
Metabolic	Diabetes
Gastrointestinal/genitourinary	Renal dialysis

cardiovascular, pulmonary, metabolic, gastrointestinal, and genitourinary systems (see Table 10–1). Information from computed tomographic (CT) scans, magnetic resonance imaging (MRI) reports, and radiographs can provide more specific information about the patient's problem as well as a clearer picture of the patient.

b. Baseline information can be gathered from the chart on communication, vision, behavior, skin/soft tissue, appliances, pain and tenderness, and skeletal, neuromuscular, and functional motor performance (including balance, posture, functional mobility, and gait pattern) (see Table 10–2). This information will also be gathered from the patient, but it is important to gather it from the chart in order to anticipate what the patient will be able to do when the screening is performed.

Table 10–2. BASELINE INFORMATION FROM THE CHART

Parameter	Example
Communication	Expressive aphasia
Vision	Homonymous hemianopsia
Behavior	Demonstration of agitated behavior
Skin/soft tissue	Open wounds or obesity
Appliances	Use of a walker prior to admission
Pain and tenderness	Increased pain with movement
Skeletal	Total hip replacement or below-knee amputation
Neuromuscular	Deficit in muscular strength or alteration in coordination
Balance	Unable to sit unsupported
Posture	Thoracic kyphosis or prolonged extensor posturing of bilateral lower extremities
Functional mobility	Deficit in ability to change positions
Gait pattern	Unable to swing left leg forward to take a step

c. Before starting the screening, the therapist should be aware of precautions for monitoring intracranial pressure, blood pressure and heart rate, seizures, and general mobility with weight-bearing status. Parameters for intracranial pressure, blood pressure, and heart rate may vary per individual depending on the patient's status and the ability to maintain control with medications. It should also be determined whether there is a need to clarify orders or precautions prior to proceeding with physical therapy. The patient's level of activity can be either bed rest or activity as tolerated. The appropriate time to begin physical therapy can be determined when the patient is medically stable, the screening can be performed within the boundaries of the precautions, and the orders are clear.

2. **Members of the team.** Members of the team may be physicians, nurses, occupational therapists, social workers, speech and language pathologists, school personnel, and day-care workers. Information can be gathered through interdisciplinary rounds and informal conversation in addition to the information from team members' notes in the chart. The information gathered may be related to medical status/changes, functional status on the nursing unit, and discharge planning.

3. **Interview with patient and/or family**
   a. The patient's goals may vary per setting. For example:
      (1). For a patient in the acute care setting, the goal may be just to get out of bed.
      (2). In the rehabilitation setting, the goal may be to walk.
      (3). At home, the goal may be to ascend and descend the basement stairs so that the patient can work on her/his projects.
      (4). As an outpatient, the goal may be orthotic trials to improve gait pattern.

PLEASE NOTE: For children, it is important to ask what their goals are when they are old enough to give realistic responses to the question.

   b. Questions about the patient's problems will provide valuable information.

(1). What does the patient feel her/his problems are?

(2). Is it a new diagnosis or a recurring problem?

(3). What are the patient's thoughts or feelings about the problem?

(4). If the problem is recurring, did the patient have physical therapy in the past?

    (a). If yes, what was the treatment and did it help?

    (b). If no, did the problem resolve on its own or what did the patient do for treatment?

c. Because patients have shorter-length hospital stays than in the past, questions in reference to discharge planning are essential.

(1). What is the home setup?

(2). Are there architectural barriers?

(3). Is there assistance available at home?

(4). Are there other discharge options?

d. For the pediatric population, a history relating to the pregnancy, delivery, and postdelivery can be taken from the child's family or caregiver. Note any problems experienced by the mother and whether she used any medications during her pregnancy. Bleeding during pregnancy may indicate that a child will be at greater risk than normal for problems postdelivery, and many drugs taken during pregnancy may affect the fetus.[6]

e. Apgar scores (measurements at 1 and 5 minutes post birth of heart rate, respiratory effort, reflex irritability, muscle tone, and color) have traditionally been an important score to gauge risk for problems in the future. Jepson *et al.* state that Apgar scores lack both sensitivity and specificity for predicting long-term neurological problems.[7] The authors recommend that Apgar scores still be used, but with caution when interpreting the level of importance. Perinatal convulsions are important to note as they could indicate future problems.[6] If a child receives oxygen post delivery, this should be noted because children receiving high doses of oxygen have had problems with lung and retinal development.

f. Other information typically collected during a history is related to the type of delivery, the length of delivery, and whether the child experienced any decel-

erations in heart rate during delivery. Whether this information is important for predicting future problems with neurological development is unclear, but it is thought to be important when looking at whether a child had an anoxic event during delivery.

g. It is also important to note the length of hospital stay post delivery; any complications such as seizures, apnea, bradycardia; and what equipment the child was discharged with from the hospital. This information is important more for safety and functional capability during the screening and evaluation rather than for prediction of neurological problems.

4. **Screening of the impairments**

a. Many times, the screening of the impairments in the adult population is done before the screening of the disabilities only so that the disabilities can be screened safely. By having a sense of what the patient is able to do at an impairment level, the physical therapist may be able to anticipate better what the patient will be able to do safely at the disability level. If, after gathering data from all sources, the physical therapist has a good sense of what the patient is able to do and does not feel that she/he or the patient would be in danger, screening may be started at the disability level rather than at the impairment level. After screening at the disability level, the physical therapist may want to go back to screening only the impairments that she/he suspects may be factors contributing to the disabilities noted. This is more desirable than starting at the impairment level and may be necessary if there are significant time constraints. Safety of the patient as well as the therapist needs to be ensured.

b. The screening of impairments consists of motor control, pain, passive range of motion, sensation, appliances, cognitive and behavior factors, vision, skin/soft tissue, posture, and communication. Cognitive and behavior factors include the level of arousal, orientation, tolerance to treatment, carryover, memory, thought process, safety, insight, and judgement. As each impairment is screened (see Table 10–3), it should be determined whether

Table 10-3. SCREENING OF THE
IMPAIRMENTS

Impairment	Action	Example
Motor control	Ask patient to move extremities within context of a goal-directed task	Patient is unable to move left extremities when attempting to roll to the right
Pain	Ask patient if she/he has any pain	Pain noted in right shoulder
Passive range of motion	Move patient's extremities through passive range of motion	Severe limitations in left ankle dorsiflexion range of motion
Sensation	Ask patient if she/he has feeling in all parts of body	Patient states that she/he has no feeling in right arm
	Ask patient if she/he can tell where arms and legs are and how they are moving	
Appliances	Ask patient if she/he used any appliances prior to admission	Patient may need wheelchair for use at home
	Ask patient if she/he has any appliances available if needed at discharge	
Cognitive and behavior factors	Observe these factors in relation to patient's participation in physical therapy	Agitation noted during screening
Vision	Note whether patient is wearing glasses	Patient seemed to ignore objects on left during physical screening process
	Ask patient if she/he is having any difficulty seeing	
Skin/soft tissue	Observe open areas/edema	Small open wound noted on patient's left heel; refer to nursing for care and monitoring
Posture	Observe patient in supine, sitting, and standing positions	Decerebrate posturing noted in supine position
Communication	Notice expressive and receptive communication	Patient had difficulty understanding directions during screening; refer to speech and language pathologist

there is "no problem" or a "problem." If there is no problem, the screening is continued. If there is a problem, definitive evaluation will need to be done.

c. For the pediatric population, special attention needs to be paid to passive range of motion/resistance to passive movement, cognitive and behavior factors, vision, posture, and auditory skills.

(1). *Passive range of motion/resistance to passive movement.* With the small child (birth to 1.5 years old), this may be done in the supine position with a quick check of hamstring length by looking at the popliteal angle. The popliteal angle test has a high specificity, to identify children who pass as being without cerebral palsy.[8] The following are checked: all hip movements to feel for a hip click, trunk flexion, trunk rotation, all arm movements, and ankle dorsiflexion with knee bent and straight. While these movements are being checked, the therapist can get a general feel for the amount of resistance to passive movement. With an older child (≥1.5 years), range of motion of arms, legs, and trunk is observed during activities, and any limitations noted require further definitive evaluation. Rather than testing resistance to passive motion, the child is observed during activities. For example, the therapist notes whether the limb is held stiff in cocontraction or whether there is limited stability in a weight-bearing joint.

(2). *Cognitive and behavior factors.* The physical therapist observes whether the child separates easily from her/his parents. The amount of assistance the child needs to stay on task is observed. If the child gets upset, how much assistance does she/he need to calm down? Is the child easily upset? What range of states does the child have and how smoothly does she/he make a transition between the states?[9] Is the child able to interact with the person doing the screen at a cognitive level that is age-appropriate? This information is important to help parents understand how much of their child's behavior is affected by central nervous system irritability rather than discipline issues and to learn ways to help the child achieve more stability in her/his behavior.

Information about the cognitive level of children is typically obtained from other sources. For example, intelligence quotient (IQ) testing is typically done in the schools and in some health department clinics. School personnel have information about the child's ability to grasp concepts taught in the classroom and whether difficulties occur in the child's learning capabilities. This information will help the therapist and family design learning and treatment opportunities that will not be frustrating for the child.

(3). *Vision.* The therapist observes the child during play to see if she/he will tilt the head sideways, turn the head to look at something with peripheral vision, or use the upper or lower quadrants of the visual field (looking with chin up or chin down) to look at toys. Does the child focus on a toy, on the therapist's face, or does she/he follow someone walking across the room? Is the child's vision linked solely to auditory cues? This information will help the parents gain better understanding of ways to engage their child in activities and to encourage development of skills in all areas.

(4). *Posture.* During spontaneous movements and static postures, the therapist notes the symmetry of right and left sides, straight spinal alignment, equal gluteal folds, and/or alignment of body parts to the head and trunk. This information is important to help rule out other orthopedic deformities.

(5). *Auditory skills.* The therapist observes whether the child reacts to loud noises (startle). Can the child locate a toy by sound without seeing where the toy is first? Does the child appear to be defensive in relation to sounds? Are there any sounds the child does not like or any sounds

that she/he shows a preference for? This information is important to determine the best environment to work in with a child, to help parents modify the home environment to allow the child to be comfortable there, and to assist the schools with possible behavior problems seen if the child is sensitive to sound. Can the child communicate her/his needs to the parents, teacher, peers, and others? This information is essential to help integrate a child into environments in which people who do not know the child well can understand the child's needs.

5. **Screening of the disabilities.** In practice, the screen can be performed according to the database until the physical therapist reaches the section on balance and functional mobility. At that point, the screen naturally turns into an evaluation. For example, if the therapist is screening the patient in the bed mobility activity of supine to sit, she/he would ask the patient to sit at the edge of the bed. Even if this activity is done only once, the therapist gains knowledge about the amount of assistance the patient needs to perform the activity. In a true screen, the therapist would acknowledge that the patient needs assistance for the activity; whereas during definitive evaluation, the actual amount of assistance required would be determined. Even though the therapist is involved in the screen at this point, it does not make sense just to document that assistance is needed when the amount of assistance that is needed is known. Therefore, it seems appropriate to perform the screening until the section on balance and functional mobility and then to switch to evaluation when using the database as a guide.

For adults, the therapist observes what the patient is able to do independently first and assists if necessary. The activities are usually done only once. Many times the screening starts at the disability level, especially if time is limited. If there is time to screen the impairments, the focus is on only those impairments that possibly limit functional activities. The activities include bed mobility, sitting balance, transfers, standing balance, and gait (see Table 10–4).

For pediatrics, observation of the child during spontaneous play will provide the

Table 10–4.   SCREENING OF THE DISABILITIES

Activity	Action	Example
Bed Mobility		
Rolling	Ask patient to roll to side	Patient needs minimal assistance to roll to the left
Supine to sit	Ask patient to sit at edge of bed	Patient needs moderate assistance for supine to sit
Sitting		
Static balance	Ask patient to sit at edge of bed unsupported	Patient falls over while sitting unsupported at edge of bed
Dynamic balance reactions	Observed through functional activities, *ie*, putting slipper/shoe on to prepare for transfers	Patient is unable to maintain balance at edge of bed while putting on slipper/shoe
Transfers		
Sit to stand	Ask patient to stand up	Patient needs maximal assistance for sit to stand
Stand pivot	Ask patient to transfer from bed to chair	Patient needs maximal assistance of two for a stand-pivot transfer
Standing		
Static balance	Ask patient to stand unsupported	Patient falls over while standing unsupported
Dynamic balance reactions	Observed through functional activities, *ie*, pulling on robe/coat while standing	Patient is unable to maintain standing balance while putting on robe/coat
Gait		
Level surfaces	Ask patient to ambulate on level surface	Patient needs supervision with ambulation while using a walker
Stairs	Ask patient to ascend and descend a flight of stairs	Patient needs contact guard to ascend stairs while using rail

greatest information. It is important to observe the child's movements without external interference so that the child's full potential can be seen. It is imperative that small children be observed without clothing or diaper to see all hip and trunk movement. To use time effectively, this observation can occur while the history is being taken from the parent. Allowing the child to engage in spontaneous play during the observation should increase the child's moti-

vation to move. To have a true measure of a child's capability, it is important to limit the amount of physical contact with the child during observation. If the child needs assistance to complete a task or to finish a movement, verbal cues should be provided. If the child is still unable to complete the task or movement with verbal cues, physical cues may be used to eliminate the child's frustration and to assist the child to learn how to finish the task or movement in the future.

a. A variety of movement patterns should be observed. Does the child move in and out of different postures (transition) using a variety of movement patterns or is she/he limited to one or two patterns? Children with cerebral palsy typically demonstrate a limited number of movement patterns.[10]

b. The speed of movement should be observed. Does the child move haltingly, ballistically, or at an appropriate speed? Slow speed of movement is typical of children with spastic cerebral palsy. Ballistic movements are seen in children with athetosis or ataxic movements.

c. The accuracy of movement should be observed. Does the child accurately reach for a toy, kick a ball, or place her/his foot during walking? Does the child over- or undershoot a toy when reaching? Does the child have tremors or shaky movements when reaching? Does the child miss the ball when trying to kick? Is the child able to place her/his foot appropriately when walking or does the child trip over her/his feet?

6. **Screening of the handicaps.** Handicaps are screened to determine the patient's ability to function at home, in school, in day care, in the community; to continue to participate in recreation and leisure activities; and to return to her/his present occupation.

F. When to stop the screening

If bed rest has been ordered for the patient, the therapist may be able to test only at the impairment level. The screening may need to be stopped when the patient is unable to perform any further activities, when the patient requires too much physical assistance to continue for the number of people available at the time, or when the patient is too fatigued to continue. If the patient (pediatric) is irritable and/or inconsolable or if the family does not feel that there is a need for the screen, the screen should not be continued.

G. Screening versus evaluation

Many times there is a need to flip back and forth between the screening and the evaluation. This is mostly because of time constraints or the need for further information immediately to make a decision. The therapist may need to interrupt screening to do more definitive testing for medical and/or safety concerns. For example, if the patient becomes dizzy after assuming sitting, the therapist may want to back up and take the patient's blood pressure before continuing. The separation between the screening and the evaluation is more readily apparent when there is no need for skilled physical therapy; essentially, the patient passes the screen and there is no need for further definitive testing.

References

1. Tecklin JS: *Pediatric Physical Therapy*. Philadelphia, J. B. Lippincott Company, 1989.
2. King-Thomas L, Hacker BJ: *A Therapist's Guide To Pediatric Assessment*. Boston, Little, Brown, 1987.
3. Campbell SK: *Pediatric Neurologic Physical Therapy*, 2nd ed. New York, Churchill Livingstone, 1991.
4. Wilhelm IJ: *Physical Therapy Assessment in Early Infancy*. New York, Churchill Livingstone, 1993.
5. Bly L: The components of normal movement during the first year of life. In Slaton D (ed): *Development of Movement in Infancy*. Chapel Hill, NC, University of North Carolina Proceedings, 1980.
6. Illingworth RS: *The Development of the Infant and Young Child*, 2nd ed. New York, Churchill Livingstone, 1980.
7. Jepson HA, Talashek ML, Tichy AM: The apgar score: evolution, limitations, and scoring guidelines. Birth, 1991, 18:83–92.
8. Johnson A, Ashurst H: Is popliteal angle measurement useful in early identification of cerebral palsy? *Dev Med Child Neurol*, 1989, 31:457–465.
9. Prechtl HFR: The behavioral states of the newborn infant: a review. *Brain Res*, 1974, 76:185–212.
10. Comparetti AM: Pattern analysis of normal and abnormal development: the fetus, the newborn, and the child. In Slaton D (ed): *Development of Movement in Infancy*. Chapel Hill, NC, University of North Carolina Proceedings, 1980.

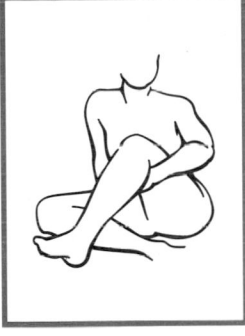

CHAPTER 11

Neurological Evaluation and Assessment

Susan Cromwell, Polly Menendez, and Peggy Owen

I. Definitions

A. Difference between evaluation and assessment

1. **Evaluation (definitive testing).** This is the collection of objective information through testing.

2. **Assessment.** This is the analysis of all the subjective and objective information that has been gathered. Assessment involves the synthesis and interpretation of the data and reflects the physical therapist's clinical judgement regarding the potential causes of a patient's problem, the significance of the problem, and what physical therapy has to offer. This leads to identifying some type of outcomes, such as goals and/or plans.

B. Traditional neurological evaluation and assessment

Traditionally, a complete and comprehensive neurological evaluation was thought to include a long list of items that were tested with every patient. Many rehabilitation hospitals created forms listing all these items and required that all areas be filled in. These evaluations often took 3 days to complete. After the evaluation was completed, the therapist would write an assessment based on data that was collected. It was assumed that all these data were necessary to understand, and thus to make an assessment about, the patient's problem.

C. Concurrent evaluation and assessment

1. We think that, in reality, physical therapists evaluate and assess their patients simultaneously. The therapist synthesizes information as it is being collected. We suggest that therapists use the information they gain from one test to guide further testing. Different types and quantities of information may lead the therapist to continue definitive testing in a few or many specific areas. This is in contrast to using an evaluation form to guide testing. The evaluation is complete when the therapist has enough information to explain the patient's problem and to plan intervention.

2. We think this circular process of evaluation and assessment is natural and reflects the process of many experienced therapists.[1]

Many therapists do not use the evaluation forms and often go back later to fill out the documentation to meet department or hospital standards. If clinicians can identify the data they need, there is no need to collect all possible data. Collecting only necessary data will make the evaluation process more efficient and thus more cost-effective. Physical therapists still need to make sure that they do not miss any key areas or that they do not evaluate only items that reflect their own interests or biases. We think that the comprehensive but brief screen combined with frequent reassessment of progress toward goals should prevent these problems.

3. To make this process of evaluation and assessment complete, we think that the order of testing procedures is important. Using the screen (see Chapter 10), the therapist quickly and grossly checks out all areas related to physical therapy. The screen should provide enough information so that the therapist can safely progress to the functional evaluation. After the functional evaluation, the therapist tests specific physical therapy impairments.

II. Evaluation Procedure

Therapists should begin all evaluations with a patient interview to gain an understanding of how the patient perceives his/her problem. The patient should be given an opportunity to state his/her goals so that the therapist can focus the evaluation on the patient's concerns. Many patients are surprised when therapists ask them about their goals and are not sure how to respond, but, with some explanation, most patients do state clear goals.

To enhance the logic of this evaluation/assessment process, we suggest two distinct cycles of data collection followed by synthesis of the information collected.

A. First cycle of data collection

1. **Objective.** During this first cycle, the therapist collects data about function.
   a. This process can include standardized functional assessment tools, such as the Barthel index (see Table 11–1), but it will also include traditional functional evaluation. The traditional functional evaluation involves watching the patient complete a number of tasks and determining the amount of assistance needed to complete the tasks. Most practice environments quantify the amount of assistance in categories such as maximal assist, moderate assist, minimal assist, contact guard, and supervision. The standardized tools are more likely to be reliable, whereas the traditional assessment allows the therapist to choose tasks based on the patient's needs. Although it is easy to criticize traditional functional testing based on current expectations of measurement, therapists must realize that their ability to show progress in key functional areas may be the foundation of their importance in health care. Documentation of functional status in the traditional format is clear and easily accessible to other health care providers.

   b. During the screen, the therapist evaluates a number of key tasks and documents the amount of assistance the patient requires to complete the tasks. The patient completes the task once during the screen. This serves as a baseline measurement and allows the therapist to make recommendations to other care providers, particularly to nursing staff.

   In an evaluation, the therapist looks at how the task is being completed. Areas to consider when evaluating a functional task include kinematics, effect of different environments, speed, efficiency, number of attempts, amount of errors, and amount of cues required. During the evaluation, the therapist observes the task several times, can suggest changes in technique, and can observe the patient's response to these changes. The amount of assistance required is likely to be different after evaluation because the therapist may have observed capabilities that were not evident initially or noted deficits that were masked during the screen.

   c. During the evaluation, the therapist looks

at more skills, and the tasks evaluated should reflect the patient's reasons for seeking physical therapy. The therapist selects tasks based on the treatment environment. In the hospital setting, the therapist selects tasks that are necessary for a safe discharge from the hospital; in the home-care setting, the therapist evaluates tasks encountered in daily life. Higher-level tasks and function in the community are evaluated in the outpatient setting. Regardless of the setting, the tasks should be evaluated in a variety of environmental contexts (see Chapter 8).

d. While observing the functional task, the therapist notes how various impairments may be contributing to the patient's difficulties. The therapist already has some idea about impairments from the screen, but, during the functional task, their possible impact on function can be observed. See Table 11–2 for suggestions on what to look for during the functional observation.

2. **Assessment.** The assessment is based on the initial interview screen and the functional evaluation.

   a. *Physical therapy impairments.* At this point, the therapist begins identifying components of the physical therapy problem. These components will include impairments such as decreased range of motion, decreased strength, or balance deficits. Through observation of function, the therapist can speculate about possible impairments and begin to develop hypotheses about how these various impairments relate to the functional problems. The therapist needs to analyze critically the list of impairments generated during the screen and to identify those impairments that are most likely to contribute to loss of function.

   b. *Plans for further testing.* Once the therapist has a theory about the probable connection between impairments and function, he/she can plan testing of impairments. We recommend limiting testing of impairments to those theorized to relate to function and thus expected to affect function.

   c. This relationship between function and impairments is an important foundation of physical therapy practice, but it is crucial to recognize that a problem can exist only in the context of the task, or, conversely, a problem can exist only when testing the impairment (out of normal context for that individual) and disappear within the context of the task. In addition, there are impairments, such as depression, that have an impact on motor function but are directly addressed by other professionals.

   d. One of the major assumptions of most of the neurofacilitation techniques was that abnormal tone (an impairment) and abnormal movement patterns (an impairment) interfered with functional capabilities. However, the therapist must be aware of the strict definition of tone (resistance to passive movement) and of spasticity (increased resistance to passive movement, which is velocity-dependent). In addition, according to Burke, "hypotonia" has never been quantitatively measured.[3] By these definitions, tone (related to passive movement), be it normal or abnormal, does not have anything to do with active movements.[3] Abnormalities of active movements may fall into either of two categories, as described in Chapter 8: positive or negative symptoms. Both categories are either the direct or the secondary result of damage to neural tissue and are not related to each other by cause and effect.

B. Second cycle of data collection

1. **Objective.** The physical therapist tests impairments that have been identified as possible contributory factors to the patient's functional problem. Standardized evaluation procedures and tests exist for some impairments (see Table 11–1). Physical therapists have a traditional set of tests for evaluating impairments that are difficult to standardize (see Table 11–3).

2. **Assessment.** In this phase, the therapist formulates specific relationships between impairments (singly or collectively) and the patient's functional problem.

   a. It is crucial that the relationship between impairments and function is clear. The

Text continued on page 358

Table 11-1. SUMMARY OF ASSESSMENTS

	Sections	Scoring	Reliability	Time (min)	Validity	Advantages	Disadvantages	Tools	Training
Fugl-Meyer Assessment (FMA) Fugl-Meyer, A.R., et al (1975) Scand. J. Rehab. Med., 7, 13–31	Jt. ROM Pain Sensation UE/LE motor Balance	0 = Cannot be performed 1 = Performed partly 2 = Performed correctly Total score is 226. Total can be scored as a fraction or a percentage. Can be scored by section.	Intratester reliability coefficients from .95–.996. Intertester reliability—significant at 0.5. Duncan et al (1983).	20–35	Concurrent validity when compared to MMAS. (Corr. between total MAS & FMA r = .92). Poole & Whitney (1988).	Includes UE & LE Reliable and valid predictor of outcome Can assess progress Can be administered in whole or in parts See Scoring	Doesn't include ADL May not be sensitive enough to identify slight improvement	Stopwatch, cotton swab, reflex hammer, tennis ball, sml cylindrical jar, pencil or pen, sml cardboard or paper	Not specifically; good idea to establish inter- & intra-rater reliability. Journal procedures & videotape are available. (Video—Duncan, P. 1986.)
Modified motor assessment scale (MMAS) Lowen, S.C. & Anderson, B.A. (1988). Phys Ther, 68(7), 1077–1081 Carr, J. & Shepherd R., et al (1985). Phys Ther, 65, 175–180	Supine to sidelying, supine to sitting, balanced sitting, sitting to standing, walking, upper-arm function, hand movements, advanced hand movements	Scores range from 0–6, a 7-point scale. 0 = Unable to perform 6 = Most difficult Total score is 48. Total scored as a fraction, can be scored by section.	Spearman rank-order correlation coefficients ranged from .83–1.00. Loewen & Anderson (1988). Inter-rater reliability ranged from .92–1.00. Poole & Whitney (1988).	15–20	MAS & FMA correlated highly (r = .92 as above). MMAS is very similar to the MAS, although a few items are different.	Includes UE & LE Assess mobility & functional hand skills Can be administered in whole or in parts Functional See Scoring	Assesses limited self-care skills (MMAS did correlate with the Barthel index) Walking & UE items may not be sensitive enough to identify slight improvement	Stopwatch, steps, styrofoam cup, 8 jellybeans or beads, 2 teacups, tennis ball, stool/bench, comb, pen & pen top, table, spoon & water, paper, sml cylindrical jar	Not specifically; good idea to establish inter- & intra-rater reliability. Journal procedures are available.

354

Assessment / Reference	Assesses	Scoring	Reliability	Time (min)	Validity	Advantages	Disadvantages	Equipment	Standardized
Rivermeade stroke assessment Lincoln, N. & Leadbitter, D. (1979). Physiotherapy, 15, 48–51	Gross function (functional movement) Arm (control & functional arm movements) Leg & trunk (control of movement)	Score 0 or 1. 0 = Unable to perform 1 = Perform activity Activities are scored in a hierarchical order. Total score is 38. Scored as a fraction. Can be scored by section.	Test-retest correlation coefficients range from .66–.93. Lincoln, N. & Leadbitter, D. (1979). Physiotherapy, 15, 48–51.	20–30	Overall reproducibility of 0.9. Lincoln & Leadbitter feel that it's a valid scale. It has not been compared to other stroke assessments tests although it is similar to the MMAS.	Easy to administer Functional Assess mobility & hand skills See Scoring	It hasn't been validated Doesn't assess ADL directly	Wheelchair, steps, beanbag, measured distances, stopwatch, large ball, tennis ball, table, paper, putty, knife & fork, plate & string	Not specifically; good idea to establish inter- & intra-rater reliability. Journal procedures are available.
Barthel index Mahoney, B.I. & Barthel, D.W. (1965). Md State Med J., 14, 61–65	Feeding, wheelchair to bed, personal toilet, on & off toilet, bathing, walking up & down steps, dressing, controlling bowels & bladder	Each item has different criteria and different point values from 0, 5, 10 & 15. Total score is 100. Scored as a fraction or by section.	Inter-rater reliability by percent agreement ranged from 71–100%. Loewen & Andersson (1988). Personal hygiene had the lower percentage agreement.	10–15	It hasn't been validated, but it has been used to predict outcome. Score of 40 or less predicts dependent mobility skills. Granger & Dewis (1979).	Well known Easy to administer Assesses ADL Used to predict outcome See Scoring	It hasn't been validated May not be sensitive enough to identify slight improvements Doesn't assess isolated movements Uses others' opinions	Feeding utensils, wheelchair, ADL supplies, clothes, steps (nursing & OT information).	Not specifically; good idea to establish inter- & intra-rater reliability. Journal procedures are available.

(Copyright reserved. Do not reproduce without permission. S. Whitney/P. Raasch-Mason, APTA Conference June 1991, Boston, MA.)
Abbreviations: ADL = activities of daily living; Corr. = correlations; Jt. ROM = joint range of motion; LE = lower extremity; MAS = motor assessment scale; OT = occupational therapy; sml = small; UE = upper extremity.

Table 11–2. OBSERVATION OF IMPAIRMENTS DURING FUNCTIONAL EVALUATION

Impairments	Impairments Noted During Evaluation of Function	Indication for Further Testing
Mental status	Note attitude toward task, ability to follow instructions, alertness, etc.	No specific physical therapy test. Relate to other disciplines (medicine, psychology, speech and language pathology, occupational therapy [OT]).
Safety awareness (part of mental status)	Note the patient's awareness of deficits. Does the patient take adequate safety precautions?	Refer to other disciplines if safety precautions are not physical in nature. If mobility is not safe, test related impairments such as balance and the ability to follow through with safety strategies.
Vision	Observe how the patient responds to the environment. Does the patient attend to the entire visual field?	Refer to OT. If OT is not available, test tracking, visual fields, and frequency of neglect.
Activity tolerance	Observe the patient's response to positional changes and complaints of dizziness and fatigue.	Problems in this area should have been identified in the screen. Vital signs should be monitored immediately when there is intolerance to change of position.
Cardiopulmonary status	Note shortness of breath and need for frequent rests. Be aware of any medical history in this area.	Monitor vital signs if the patient is short of breath or needs frequent rests.
Posture	Note major postural deviations with particular asymmetries.	
Range of motion (ROM)	Observe the quality of the movement and any potential ROM loss.	Measure only those motions that interfere with function.
Pain	Note if the patient complains of pain or makes facial expressions that indicate pain.	Measure pain if it interferes with function.
Sensation	Cannot observe this, but the patient may complain of numbness.	Gross test of sensation was part of the screen. Test more specifically only if a major problem was noted.
Tone (resistance to passive movement)	Cannot observe.	No need to test.
Reflexes/posturing	Note reflexes such as clonus, or posturing during stressful tasks.	No need for further testing. May record frequency during a task.
Balance/postural reactions	If the patient loses his/her balance, note the circumstance, the direction of balance loss, and if the patient recovers balance.	See Table 13–1.
Control of active movement Isolated movement Patterned movement MMT[2] Coordination (speed and accuracy)	Note the patient's ability to use all four extremities, head, and trunk. What parts can the patient move and what is the quality of movement.	Depending on the problem noted, MMT, standardized motor control evaluations, or a description of the movement can be completed.
Gait deviations	Note gait deviations that may be related to the patient's current problem.	Further gait evaluation is indicated if the patient has gait deviations that are a result of the current problem and are likely to be changed with treatment.

Abbreviation: MMT=manual muscle test.

Table 11–3. NONSTANDARDIZED IMPAIRMENT EVALUATION PROCEDURES

Impairment	Availability of Standard Tests	Nonstandard Procedures Commonly Used[*]

Motor control	1. Yes—see Table 11–1 for adults
	2. MMT[2,4]
	3. The Gross Motor Function Measure for children[5]
		1. If the patient moves in a synergy pattern, the therapist describes the percent of the synergy the patient is able to complete. The therapist will usually describe the position of the test. Example: patient completes about 50% of flexor synergy pattern in supine.
		2. The therapist describes the percent of isolated motion the patient can complete. Therapist often looks at all motions of all joints in position with gravity resisting and with gravity eliminated. Example: the patient completes 33% hip extension in sidelying.
		3. The therapist describes particular difficulty the patient has with movement. Examples:
		  a. The patient has difficulty initiating hip and knee flexion in supine but if therapist assists to 30 degrees, the patient can complete the motion.
		  b. The patient is able to complete the motion but with poor accuracy or control, ie, ataxia or ballistic-type movements.
		4. The therapist describes motions the patient is able to complete within functional tasks. Example: The patient is able to flex hip during rolling and gait but cannot flex hip in sitting to move leg off footrest.
		5. Observing dynamic movement patterns: Observe how the patient moves from one position to another. Note the efficiency of movement, speed of movement, and variability of movement. Example: If a patient leans backward prior to rising from sitting to standing, you would describe this as different from the normal pattern, which is to lean forward prior to standing.

Posture	No	Observe the patient in static positions that are functional for that individual. Note the ability to maintain the posture and describe significant deviations from a "neutral" posture.
Balance	Yes—see Table 11–4	See Table 13–1 for nonstandardized procedures.
Range of motion	Goniometry[6]	
Exercise tolerance/endurance	Yes—Borg scale[7]	1. Monitor vital signs in response to exercise. 2. Monitor oxygen saturation in response to exercise with finger or ear oximeter. 3. Describe tolerance to treatment, including the amount of rest needed. 4. State distances the patient ambulates and activities tolerated. 5. Particularly in the community, describe the patient's ability to function throughout his/her day.
Pain	1. Yes—for intensity of pain[8–10] 2. Fugl-Meyer—see Table 11–1	Describe the location of pain and what makes the pain better or worse. Consult the many resources in the pain and orthopedic physical therapy literature for a variety of ways to measure pain.
Sensation	Fugl-Meyer—see Table 11–1	State the modality tested and describe the pattern of sensory loss. Sensory testing is difficult when there is cognitive impairment and with young children.
Reflex/movement patterns that interfere with function	No	Describe the movement pattern and how it is interfering with function. Examples: 1. A clear example of this is clonus at the ankle set off by stretch of the plantar flexors. It interferes with function if it starts every time the patient advances his/her weight forward over the foot. 2. When one or both lower extremities pull into flexion and feet will not stay on the floor when patient attempts to bear weight, describe the movement pattern and how and when you are able to control this pattern.

Abbreviation: MMT = manual muscle test
[*]To be used when standardized testing does not provide all necessary information.

therapist should state how changes in impairment will be reflected in the patient's functional status, and this should be reflected in goal statements. For example, if a change in range of motion is expected to allow for completion of a functional task, both of these goals should be written in the same time frame.

b. At this point, the therapist may also theorize about how impairments in areas not directly related to physical therapy may influence the patient's progress toward a goal. The therapist does not treat these problems directly, but aspects of these problems may be reflected in the goal statements. For example, if a patient had impaired problem-solving skills, the learning of a physical task might take longer. Therefore, the time frames for the goals will be longer than those for a patient who does not have any cognitive impairments.

c. In the first cycle of assessment, the therapist speculates about possible impairments that may contribute to a functional problem. At this time, the impairments have been measured and it has been determined whether the impairments chosen are significant enough or likely to contribute to the functional problem. It should be recognized that if deficits are not found in the second cycle of data collection, the therapist should return to the previous assessment, speculate further about the nature of the problem, and plan further testing. This process should continue until the therapist has a reasonable theory about the patient's problem, measurable deficits, and adequate information to plan intervention.

C. Goals

Goals are the outcome of evaluation and assessment. This process began with a discussion of the patient's goals.

1. The patient's goals need to be incorporated into any goal written by the physical therapist. During the screen and evaluation, the therapist gathers data about the patient's current level of function and about impairments related to function. In the assessment, the therapist synthesizes this information in reference to functional problems. The functional problems addressed should relate to the patient's perception of the problem and thus the patient's goals.

2. Goals should address all significant problems. The therapist should write goals for function and for impairments that relate to function.

3. Measurable goals are essential for documenting progress. Some typical physical therapy goals, such as increasing range of motion by 20 degrees, are, by their nature, measurable, but therapists need to be more creative with other goals. Therapists can describe a functional skill and state how it should be completed for a functional goal. Another therapist should be able to recognize when the patient has met the goal.

4. Time frames for goals are a necessary check on the effectiveness of interventions. When the therapist commits to time frames for goals, he/she is committed to a re-evaluation schedule. If the patient meets his/her goals, the therapist needs to evaluate the need for further intervention. When patients do not meet their goals, therapists need to re-examine the premises on which the interventions were built. Physical therapy intervention is justified only when patients have achievable goals.

III. Pediatric Evaluation and Assessment

Many standardized and nonstandardized pediatric evaluation tools are available today. Therapists choose standardized or nonstandardized tools and/or procedures based on the needs of the individual client. The standardization of testing tools and its importance are described in various references focusing on pediatric evaluation.[11–14] The purpose of standardized testing is to (1) assist with determining present skill level, (2) facilitate planning of a treatment program, and (3) assist with determining the rate and trend of development when used serially.[11] Nonstandardized testing tools are typically developed by individual facilities and require careful interpretation of the results. The

Table 11–4. STANDARDIZED BALANCE TEST

Test	Sections	Scoring	Time (min)	Training	Tools	Reliability	Validity	Advantages	Disadvantages	Population
Functional Reach (FR) Duncan, Weiner, Chandler, and Studenski, J of Gerontology, 45(6): M192–197, 1990	None Subject reaches forward with hand and arm extended and parallel to a yardstick at shoulder height "Reach as far as you can without taking a step" (Weiner et al, 1992)	Scored in inches or centimeters	1–2	None required	Yardstick Small level Velcro on yardstick and Velcro on the wall	ICC across days was .81 (Duncan et al, 1990) Test-retest reliability was .89 (Weiner et al, 1992)	As reach decreases, the chance of falling increases (Duncan et al, 1992) Walking speed and FR (r = .71) Tandem walking and FR (r = .67) SLS and FR (r = .64) Mobility skills and FR (r = .65) (Weiner et al, 1992) FR and center of pressure correlated (r = .71) (Duncan et al, 1990)	Easy to perform Has documented reliability, validity, and predictive validity	Only measures one functional movement Forward is not the only direction that we move	Ages 20–87 (Duncan et al, 1990) Mean age was 78 ± 8.4 yrs (Weiner et al, 1992) 217 males (over 70 yo) were used to assess predictive validity (Duncan et al, 1992) 115 children were treated (5–15 yo) (Donahoe et al, abstract, 1993)
Berg scale Berg et al Physiother Canada, 41:304–311, 1989 Berg, Maki, et al, Arch Phy Med & Rehabil, 73:1073–1080, 1992	Items include Getting in and out of a chair Sitting unsupported Bed to chair Standing with feet together, feet apart, and EC Turning to each side and turning 360° Reaching forward Picking up object off floor Tandem and unilateral stance Dynamic weight shift	There are 14 items graded on a 5-point scale. Points are given "based on the time the position can be maintained, the distance the arm is able to 'reach forward or the time to complete the task." (Berg et al, 1992)	15	Need the Berg et al article (1989) for the scoring procedures	Ruler Watch	Intra- and interrater reliability with 10 raters and 14 subjects was .98 and .97 and the internal consistence was high (Cronbach is alpha .96), indicating that the scale is measuring one underlying concept. (Berg et al, 1989) Interobserver agreement was an ICC of .98 (Berg, 1992)	High balance scores correlated with the Barthel index (r = .67) and the timed up and go test (r = .76) plus less assistance required for ambulation (r = −.75) (Berg et al, 1992) The Berg balance scale and the balance subscale of the Tinetti test were strongly correlated (r = .91) (Berg et al, 1992)	Tests many different aspects of balance, is reliable, and also appears to be a valid measure of balance Need little equipment	Takes 15 min	31 elderly people (Berg et al, 1992)
The timed "up and go" test Podsiadlo, Richardson, JAGS, 39:142–148, 1991	Only one test	Based on time (in seconds) as measured by a stopwatch	Under 1–2	None needed	Chair with arms Space to walk 3 m Watch with a secondhand	Interrate reliability was .99 Intrarate reliability was .99 (Podsiadlo, 1991)	The Berthel index and the timed up and go log transformed score was r = .78 (Podsiadlo et al, 1991)	Requires no specialized equipment or training Can easily be included in a routine exam	Don't know if it has predictive validity	Older adults who were in the "middle portion of the spectrum of functional abilities"

Table continued on following page

Table 11–4. STANDARDIZED BALANCE TEST *Continued*

Test	Sections	Scoring	Time (min)	Training	Tools	Reliability	Validity	Advantages	Disadvantages	Population
							Gait speed and the timed up and go test log-transformed score was $r = .61$ (Podsiadlo, et al 1991) The Berg balance scale and the up and go test log-transformed scale was $r = -.81$ (Podsiadlo et al, 1991)	May be able to separate those who can be independently mobile from those who are dependent		
CTSIB (SOT) Shumway-Cook and Horak, Phys Ther, 67(12):1881–1885, 1987	Six Tests Stand on both feet, EO Stand on both feet, EC Stand on both feet, dome Stand on foam, EO Stand on foam, EC Stand on foam, dome, EO	Time it Fall or no fall Measure the amount of sway with a grid	5–7	None needed	Visual-conflict dome High-density foam	In children, only percentages by age have been reported (Dietz et al, 1991) Percentage of agreement was 68%–100% for the SOT (DiFabio and Badke, 1990) Test-retest and inter-rater reliability were $r = .99$	The Fugl-Meyer assessment and the SOT were positively correlated: sensory subscores—$p < .05$; balance subscores—$p < .01$; lower extremity score—$p < .05$ (DiFabio and Badke, 1990) Fallers had more difficulty standing on a compliant surface (Anacker & DiFabio, 1992) People with vestibular disorders were impaired compared to age-matched controls (Cohen et al, 1993)	Easy to perform Requires no specialized training	Can't compare the results from different types of foam easily	Children 6–9 yo (Dietz et al, 1991) People with hemiplegia (DiFabio and Badke, 1990) People who had fallen (Anacker and DiFabio, 1992) People with vestibular disorders (Cohen et al, 1993; Blatchly et al, 1991)

Test		Scoring	Time to administer	Standardized	Equipment	Reliability	Validity	Advantages	Disadvantages	Population
"Get up and go" (GUGT) Mathias, Nayak, and Isaacs Arch. Phy. Med. & Rehabil. 67:387–389, 1986	None—subject stands from a chair with armrests, walks a short distance, turns around, returns to the chair, and sits down.	1. Normal 2. Very slightly abnormal 3. Mildly abnormal 4. Moderately abnormal 5. Gross instability at risk for falls without support	Under 5 min depending on how fast the subject walks	Not specifically; good idea to establish inter- and intrarater reliability in your setting	Straight-backed, high-seat office chair	Not done in original article, but they looked at agreement. Kendall coefficient of concordance test was done with PTs and MDs and the agreement was higher than what would be expected by chance (p < .001). Test-retest—r = .96 (Anacker and DiFabio, 1982)	PPMC between sway (feet apart, EO, 30 s) path and the GUGT was .5/ PPMC between gait speed and the GUGT was .75 (Mathias, et al 1985) Subjects in a falls group had high GUGT scores (p < .01) and the Spearman corr. between the Sensory Organization Test (SOT) and GUGT was greater for falls (r = -.67) (Anabacker and DiFabio, 1992)	Can be done quickly Fairly well documented Need only a chair with arms Simple	Scores 2–4 are more difficult to determine Don't know if the scale is able to differentiate change in performance over time	The foam & the Equitest have a high percentage of agreement (Cass et al, in press) Older adults
Tinetti test Tinetti, JAGS, 34:119–126, 1986	Balance and gait	In original article the 0, 1, or 0, 1, 2 are not described. The scoring can be found in the PT Bulletin (Feb 10, 1993) Total balance score = 16 Total gait score = 12 Total test score = 28	Under 10	There is a manual that describes how to score the test that was obtained from Dr. Tinetti	Hard, armless chair Stopwatch or wristwatch 5-lb object 15-foot walkway	Inter-rater reliability 85%, agreement ±10%	The Tinetti balance section correlated with the Berg balance scale (r = .91) (Berg et al, 1992) Stride length correlated with mobility index (r = .62 – .68) SLS correlated with the Tinetti (r = -.59 ≥ -.64) The foam & the Equitest have a high percentage of agreement (Cass et al, in press)	Simple Easy to do Can be done quickly	May not be very sensitive The categorizations are "crude" Tinetti (1986)	Older adults

Abbreviations: EC = eyes closed; EO = eyes open; YO = years old.
(From Whitney and Borello-France: In Wilhelm IJ (ed). Physical Therapy Assessment in Early Infancy. Churchill Livingstone, New York, 1993. Do not copy without permission of the authors.)

purpose of this section is to assist pediatric therapists with making the best choice when determining which testing tools or procedures to use during an evaluation. With changes in the theoretical framework of pediatric physical therapy to include motor control and motor learning issues (see Chapter 8), evaluation tools and procedures must be reassessed on the basis of this new theoretical information to determine whether the tools and procedures provide pertinent information related to client problems.

A. Choosing an evaluation tool

1. Following a family-centered care approach, the evaluation procedure should be discussed with the caregivers to determine, jointly, the best tools and procedures to use at the time of the evaluation. The therapist should inform the caregivers about the type of information to be gained using different evaluation tools so that the caregivers can help decide which evaluation tools should be used based on the family's and child's needs.[15]

2. Evaluation tools and procedures may be chosen based on the need to predict whether a child will have significant problems in the future or to determine the best program plan for physical therapy intervention.

3. The site where an evaluation will occur may influence which evaluation tools will be used by the therapist.

   a. Public schools require age-equivalent scores to determine eligibility of children for special education services. Physical therapists have the responsibility to use testing tools that have been normed to provide this type of information to the schools.

   b. Many facilities videotape children to assist with documenting quantitative and/or qualitative change in a child's motor skills over time.[14]

   c. Within pediatric outpatient clinics, many different evaluation tools are used for many purposes. Tools should be used that help with identifying problems, assist with developing a treatment plan, and that measure change in the identified problem areas over time (see Table 11–4). Measuring change objectively over time is an essential part of physical therapy evaluation and treatment. The importance of using a standardized evaluation tool cannot be overlooked.

Table 11–5. RELATIONSHIP OF ASSESSMENT METHODOLOGY TO THE MEASUREMENT OF PHYSICAL DISABLEMENT

Methodology	Levels of Physical Disablement			
	Impairments	Functional Limitations	Disability	Handicaps
Testing of neuromotor behaviors	Loss or abnormality of a specific motor pattern component or response			
Criterion testing	Loss or abnormality of a specific prefunctional determinant of movement	Limited capability to accomplish functional/developmental motor tasks under standardized conditions		
Movement analysis	Loss or abnormality of a specific movement pattern; loss of frequency or quality of movement	Limited capability to move in a specific functional movement pattern or task		
Judgement-based assessment		Limited capability to accomplish functional motor tasks as judged by respondent	Lack of performance of functional motor activities as judged by respondent	Lack of performance of mobility-dependent social roles as judged by respondent
Observation of naturalistic movement			Lack of performance of functional motor activities observed in specific environment	Lack of performance of mobility-dependent social roles observed in specific environment

(From Wilhelm IJ: *Physical Therapy Assessment in Early Infancy.* Churchill Livingstone, New York, 1993, p 232.)

B. Necessary changes in evaluation procedures

1. Evaluations should be performed within the home whenever possible, as this environment allows the child the most comfort and provides the therapist with the most realistic view of the child's capabilities within his/her natural environment. Because this is not always possible, the therapist should verify that the performance of the child during the evaluation is consistent with the child's performance at home.

2. Ideally, evaluations should be done over a few sessions and in a variety of environments that the child typically experiences. This expanded view of the child over time and in a variety of settings provides the therapist with a true picture of the child's capabilities and needs.

3. Looking at what is evaluated, how evaluation is done, and what information is needed from evaluations may help therapists choose evaluation tools and procedures to reflect changes in the theoretical framework (see Table 11–5). According to the World Health Organization classification of the impact of an illness or disease, evaluation tools and treatment should be focused on functional tasks to evaluate and assess the disability (individual/person) level and/or the handicap (societal) level[17] (see Chapter 9) (see Table 11–5). Evaluation tools are being designed that focus on the independent movement of an infant or child without external assistance from the therapist.[5,14,16] Once a functional level is established, the therapist may want to determine what possible impairments are contributing to this level and hypothesize about the relationship between the impairments and functional level. This should direct the therapist to develop treatment plans and to develop a way to monitor change in the child's performance.

4. The purpose of an evaluation is to assist the therapist in determining the factors that are affecting an infant's or child's performance. No testing tools exist that cover all possible factors that may affect a child's overall development. Therapists should know how to refer a child and/or family to appropriate sources to gain information necessary to help the child progress as a whole toward his/her functional goals. Working as a team member is essential to be able to understand a child's problem from all angles.

5. An area typically overlooked by physical therapists is the psychological function of the children who are treated. Physical therapists typically have little formal training in dealing with psychological disorders in children with disabilities. Many authors have looked at the psychological function of children with disabilities. Rosenbaum[18] notes,

behavioral disorders such as neurosis, attention deficit, hyperactivity, misconduct, and school and adjustment problems are twice as common in chronically ill children as in healthy children of the same age. If the illness is due to brain damage or if there is an associated limitation of function the likelihood of behavioral problems may more than double.

Cadman *et al.* state that "children with both chronic illness and associated disability were at greater than threefold risk for social adjustment problems."[19] These figures are staggering, yet many therapists do not make the appropriate referrals for children experiencing mental health or social problems. Physical therapists can help with the prevention of mental health problems in children receiving physical therapy services if they will become more skilled in "the recognition of existing or incipient mental health and social problems" and refer to the appropriate resource for intervention and monitoring of progress.[20]

C. Procedure

1. The physical therapist determines the best evaluation procedures on the basis of
   a. The concerns of the parent or parents.
      (1). Clinical observations are used to evaluate specific impairments that may be related to concerns and/or problems identified by the parents.
      (2). The therapist evaluates whether the parents are interested in the child's performance in relation to peers, would like a standardized measure of performance over time, or would like to compare the child's performance over time.
   b. The information requested from the referral source.
      (1). Standardized tools should be used if a referral source wants information about a child's performance in relation to his/her peers.
      (2). Clinical observation or evaluation tools should be used to measure the

disability or handicap level skills if a referral source wants suggestions of activities to help an infant or child function within a specific environment or within the community.

c. The clinician's bias and the theoretical framework.

(1). Evaluation procedures that are non-standardized measures of impairment level skills are chosen based on the assumption that certain impairments interfere with how a child functions. For example, spasticity was once thought to be the root of all evil for children with cerebral palsy. On the basis of the hierarchical model of central nervous system function, spasticity was thought to dominate muscle function, limiting the movement patterns used by a child with cerebral palsy. Research studies looking at the effect of baclofen or dorsal rhizotomy surgery on a child's function suggest that spasticity can be reduced or eliminated with either procedure but that the overall pattern with which a child moves does not change.[3,20,21] Thus, the role of spasticity related to an adult's or child's movement patterns continues to need further study.

Table 11–5 provides information on nonstandardized evaluation procedures used with children and adults with disabilities. Nonstandardized procedures are often used to gain more information not obtained using standardized tools and to assist with measuring impairments related to disability level problems identified with standardized tools. Table 11–5 provides information about commonly used procedures and discusses factors to measure that reflect the motor control/motor learning framework. This information is provided to assist physical therapists with determining the best procedures to use during an evaluation.

(2). Determining which standardized tool (to measure functional level skills) to use during an evaluation requires knowledge of the strengths, weaknesses, limitations, and restrictions of the tests available. Using an inappropriate test could result in "inaccurate or misinterpreted information."[11] Evaluation tools should be chosen on the basis of the type of information they provide.

For example, in the case studies presented on the child with hemiplegia and the child with spastic quadriplegia (see Chapter 19), different evaluation tools were chosen on the basis of information requested by the families, the type of information gained by the evaluations, and whether the tool would be a sensitive measure of change for the children over time.

Haley *et al.* demonstrate what types of tools provide what types of information (Table 11–3).[14] Haley *et al.* provide a unique view of evaluation tools and procedures and discuss new tools not yet available for clinical use. Books by Tecklin and by King-Thomas and Hacker are wholly devoted to pediatric evaluation and assessment.[11,12] Other books devoted to general information about pediatric physical therapy also have chapters on evaluation tools and procedures. For example, the book edited by Campbell[13] has a chapter by Stengel on assessing motor development in children, and the book edited by Wilhelm[14] has a chapter by Palisano on neuromotor and developmental assessment.

Because many texts provide information about testing tools that is necessary to select the best tool to use during an evaluation, this information is not repeated in this chapter. The reader is referred to the texts listed.

(3). Measuring handicap level skills is done through therapist observation, through gaining information by informal discussion with a child and family, and through information gained by working with a recreational therapist.

Handicap level testing is being developed for adults, but no tools that specifically measure handicap level skills are available for children at this time.[17] Therapists must rely on information provided by the child and family related to extracurricular activities that the child is involved in and activities in which the child enjoys participating. The therapist should refer the child to a recreational therapist if the child and family are not involved in extracurricular activities but are interested in being involved.

Recreational therapists may play an increasing role in therapeutic intervention as the importance of having children function in society becomes more and more apparent. Therapists must be aware of how to make an appropriate referral to a recreational therapist.

No standards exist to determine whether or not a child's level of community activity is age-appropriate. The therapist must make a judgement as to whether the child's level of function in the community is appropriate to help a child develop socially.

References

1. Payton OD: Clinical reasoning process in physical therapy. *Phys Ther,* 1985, 65:924–928.
2. Kendall FP, McCreary EK, Provance PG: *Muscle Testing and Function,* 4th ed. Baltimore, Williams & Wilkins, 1993.
3. Burke D: Spasticity as an adaptation to pyramidal tract injury. In Waxman SG (ed): *Functional Recovery in Neurological Disease.* New York, Raven Press, 1988, pp 401–423.
4. Daniels L, Worthingham C: *Muscle Testing: Techniques of Manual Examination.* Philadelphia, W. B. Saunders Company, 1986.
5. Russell D, Rosenbaum P, Gowland C: *Gross Motor Function Measure Manual.* Hamilton, Ontario, McMaster University, 1990.
6. Norkin CC, White DJ: *Measurement of Joint Motion: A Guide to Goniometry.* Philadelphia, F. A. Davis Company, 1985.
7. Borg GV: Psychophysical basis of perceived exertion. *Med Sci Sports Exerc,* 1982, 14:377–387.
8. Melzack R: The McGill Pain Questionnaire: major properties and scoring methods. *Pain,* 1975, 1:277–299.
9. Huskisson EC: Measurement of pain. *Lancet,* 1974, 2:1127–1131.
10. Downie WW, *et al.*: Studies with pain rating scales. *Ann Rheum Dis,* 1978, 37:378–381.
11. Tecklin JS: *Pediatric Physical Therapy.* Philadelphia, J. B. Lippincott Company, 1989.
12. King-Thomas L, Hacker BJ: *A Therapist's Guide to Pediatric Assessment.* Boston, Little, Brown, 1987.
13. Campbell SK: *Pediatric Neurologic Physical Therapy,* 2nd ed. New York, Churchill Livingstone, 1991.
14. Wilhelm IJ: *Physical Therapy Assessment in Early Infancy.* New York, Churchill Livingstone, 1993.
15. Kolobe T: Working with families of children with disabilities. *Pediatr Phys Ther,* 1992, 4:57–63.
16. Haley SM: Assessment of motor performance in infants. In Wilhelm IJ (ed): *Advances in Neonatal Special Care.* University of North Carolina Proceedings, Chapel Hill, NC, 1986.
17. Whiteneck GG, Charlifue SW, Gerhart KA: Quantifying handicap: a new measure of long-term rehabilitation outcomes. *Arch Phys Med Rehabil,* 1992, 73:519–526.
18. Rosenbaum PL: Prevention of psychosocial problems in children with chronic illness. *Can Med Assoc J* 1988, 139:293–295.
19. Cadman D, Boyle M, Szatmari: Chronic illness, disability, and mental and social well-being: findings of the Ontario child health study. *Pediatrics,* 1987, 79:805–813.
20. Giuliani CA: Dorsal rhizotomy for children with cerebral palsy: support for concepts of motor control. *Phys Ther,* 1991, 71:249–259.
21. Katz RT, Rymer WZ: Spastic hypertonia: mechanisms and measurement. *Arch Phys Med Rehabil,* 1989, 70:144–153.

Suggested Readings

Benner P, Tanner C: Clinical judgment: how expert nurses use intuition. *Am J Nurs* 1987, 87:23–31.
Currier D (ed): Clinical measurement. *Phys Ther,* 1987, 67:1829–1897.
Jensen G, Shepherd K, Hack L: The novice versus the experienced clinician: insights into the work of the physical therapist. *Phys Ther,* 1990, 70:314–323.
O'Sullivan SB, Schmidt TJ: *Physical Rehabilitation: Assessment and Treatment,* 2nd ed. Philadelphia, F. A. Davis Company, 1988.
Rogers JC: Clinical reasoning: the ethics, science, and art. *Am J Occup Ther,* 1983, 37:601–617.
Rothstein JM (ed): *Measurement in Physical Therapy.* New York, Churchill Livingstone, 1985.
Rothstein JM, Echternach JL: Hypothesis-Oriented Algorithm for Clinicians: a method for evaluation and treatment planning. *Phys Ther,* 1986, 66:1388–1394.

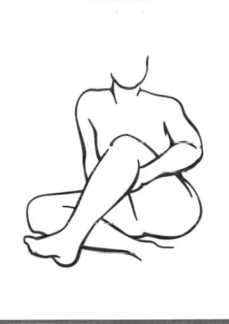

CHAPTER 12

Treatment Planning

Susan Cromwell and Peggy Owen

I. Available Treatment Approaches

The development of new theories and principles of neurological physical therapy ultimately leads to new treatment approaches and ideas. Presently, therapists use several approaches to neurological rehabilitation.[1]

A. Compensatory approach

1. This approach consists of activities that improve function rather than improving selected impairments.
2. It involves setting up the conditions of the functional task in one or two specific ways so that the patient and/or caretakers can learn how to accomplish the task in predictable and unchanging environments.

   Example: The patient in case #1 of the balance case studies (see Chapter 13) did not wish to receive ongoing physical therapy treatments. She wished to fix the problem as quickly as possible and was looking to the physical therapist for ideas on how to compensate for losing her balance while hanging out her wash. By altering the height of the clothesline and changing the position of the base of support, the therapist predicted that she would be able to hang out her wash successfully with a minimum of balance loss. If the location of the clothesline were changed, or if she started to lose her balance in another direction, the solutions the therapist suggested would probably no longer work because they were designed for one particular problem in one particular environment.

3. Therapists frequently feel that the compensatory approach perpetuates abnormal movements or limits the expression of any natural recovery process. Therefore, therapists have been reluctant to use this approach with patients unless it is requested by the patient or physical caretaker or unless a treatment approach designed to alter the impairments has failed.

B. Facilitation approaches

1. These approaches consist of activities that are designed to normalize tone, minimize

the expression of abnormal movement patterns, and facilitate normal movement patterns.[1]

2. The theoretical rationale for facilitation approaches can be found in the writings of Bobath, Brunnstrom, and Voss *et al.*[2-4]

3. Motor control is treated in isolation of functional activities. For example, the absence of hip flexion during gait may be treated by asking the patient to practice hip flexion on a powder board while in a sidelying position. The desired outcome is that hip flexion would then be exhibited within the gait cycle.

4. Skill must be gained in a sequential order based on the perceived order of difficulty or the developmental sequence. For example, gait training is often delayed until more normal movement patterns are observed in sitting and supine positions.

5. The therapist assumes the responsibility for error detection.

6. The therapist provides the patient with feedback and corrections for motor problems, often through the use of specific hands-on sensory input.

7. It is thought that abnormal tone and abnormal movement patterns interfere with the expression of normal movement; therefore, treatment is geared to normalizing tone and inhibiting abnormal patterns.

C. Motor control/motor learning (contemporary) model

1. This model consists of activities that are goal directed and functionally oriented.[1]

2. It is based on the contemporary theories of motor control and principles of motor learning as described in Chapter 8.

3. A patient practices functional activities under a variety of conditions.

4. A patient is encouraged to be an active problem solver.
   a. Verbal feedback is provided selectively by therapists to enhance skill learning and avoid overdependency.
   b. Therapists must allow the patient to experience errors.
   c. The patient must be encouraged and/or guided to use intrinsic feedback to improve future performance.
   d. The primary responsibility for error detection and problem solving is transferred to the patient. For example, rather than instructing the patient in the "best" way to ascend a flight of stairs for the first time since having a stroke, or CVA (cerebrovascular accident), the therapist allows the patient to decide on the best approach. The patient may decide to try ascending with the hemiplegic side first. Even though the therapist feels that this way may be unsuccessful, she/he allows the patient to try it that way. After the attempt (successful, partially successful, or a complete failure), the patient is asked to analyze the outcome and, if appropriate, to figure out another way that may be easier, quicker, or require less assistance. This approach does not mean that the patient is at a greater risk of falling or injury because the therapist ensures adequate safety by using aides for guarding.

II. Application of Motor Control/Motor Learning Model

For many therapists, transferring primary responsibility for error detection, problem solving, and application of solutions to motor and functional problems means a different way of practicing physical therapy. Some of these differences are reviewed, and suggestions of ways to incorporate the contemporary model into treatment plans are given.

A. Goal setting and treatment approach

1. These require the collaboration of the therapist and patient and/or family, with the patient playing a key role whenever possible.

2. The patient can be presented with available solutions to problems, but she/he must make choices. For example, the patient in

case #1 of the balance case studies (Chapter 13) desired a compensatory approach, whereas the patient in case #3 wanted to work on his disability (inability to walk on tile floors in dress shoes).

3. The therapist determines with the patient or family whether the outcome is more important than the performance details of the task. As therapists, it is difficult to determine what is most important to the patient without asking.

> **Example:** For many high-level patients, the desire to "walk more normally" is the goal because they already have the ability to walk. In these cases, it is very important to ascertain exactly what the patient means by "more normally." Does it mean faster, without an assistive device, without a limp?

> **Example:** Do the parents of a child with cerebral palsy care more about *how* their child gets to the bathroom (walk, use a wheelchair, crawl) or that the child can simply get there on her/his own?

B. Sequence of activity training

1. **Simple to difficult**
   a. Traditionally, it was thought that certain skills had to be developed before progressing to a more difficult activity. For example, independent walking should be accomplished with a walker before progressing to a cane. In the contemporary model, task difficulty is viewed differently for each patient; the traditional style of activity progression may limit the rehabilitation of some patients. Because walking with a walker is slower and inhibits stride length, some people may do better with a cane than with a walker. In addition, skill is task-specific. The task of walking with a walker is different from that of walking with a cane, and there is little evidence to suggest that training with the walker will transfer to walking with a cane. For example, balance responses are different with different assistive devices; therefore, practice should be with the assistive device most likely to be used.
   b. For difficult tasks, therapists often broke the task down into parts and had the

patient practice the parts separate from the whole. An example of this is weight shifting. Therapists frequently work on weight shifting in a standing position as a "pregait" activity. However, Winstein demonstrated no difference in gait parameters in hemiplegic patients based on their ability to shift their weight in a standing position.[5] Maybe the practice of lateral weight shifting in standing is useful for being able to wash dishes at the sink but not effective for improving lateral weight shifting during walking. If therapists feel that weight shifting during gait is a problem, one way to work on this problem during walking is by directing the patient to reach with her/his upper extremity to the right as the moment comes in gait for her/him to transfer weight forward and laterally to the right leg. By thus changing the task, the therapist may be able to elicit the weight shift within the context of the action.

2. **Developmental sequence.** It was once believed that individuals (children and adults) with central nervous system damage needed to go through the "developmental sequence" to enhance higher-level mobility activities. Using the contemporary model as a basis of treatment, developmental sequence positions and activities are used for age-appropriate or work- or recreation-related activities. For example, kneeling activities may be an important play activity for children or a work-related activity for a childcare worker. In these cases, including kneeling activities in the treatment session makes sense from a play or work perspective, but they are not done as a prerequisite to sitting, standing, or walking activities.

3. The introduction of higher level, "automatic" activities into a treatment session could enhance the movement capability of a patient with low-level (cognitive and/or motor) skills. Frequently, attempting the activity of walking with a patient with low-level skills, even if it requires using a walker and three people assisting, can produce active movement in a hemiplegic limb. For example, in a person with a head injury who is alert but unresponsive to commands, right lower extremity volitional movement is elic-

ited only when ambulating. Another example may be placing a small child with hemiplegia prone over a ball and encouraging her/him to reach for a large toy with two arms while the ball is rolled forward. This may elicit the use of the automatic two-hand reach and take advantage of the force of gravity to encourage strengthening of full arm extension on the hemiplegic side.

C. Feedback

1. Extrinsic feedback (feedback provided to the patient by outside sources, *eg*, therapists, family, other patients) should be specific.

   Example: The patient should be told "you cleared your foot 50% of the time" instead of "that was good."

2. Extrinsic feedback should be provided after the patient has had an opportunity to analyze her/his own intrinsic feedback (feedback regarding the movement from her/his own sensory organs).

   Example: Therapist to patient: "How do you think you did on that last walk?" Patient to therapist: "I felt as if I was lifting my foot off the floor more often." Therapist to patient: "You were, 50% of the time."

   With children who are old enough, or mature enough, extrinsic feedback may help them learn a task or movement; however, this technique is not used enough. Therapists tend to tell a child what happened without asking the child to describe what happened from her/his perspective. Further evaluation of a child's ability to use both intrinsic and extrinsic feedback needs to be done.

3. Extrinsic feedback should be provided only when it truly augments what the patient is able to perceive on her/his own. In addition, the frequency of feedback should be reduced over time, as the patient is better able to detect errors, analyze the problems, and alter her/his approach.

4. For small children, there are many questions about feedback. Is sensory input given by the therapist considered feedback? What type of feedback is it? Can a small child interpret the feedback, and if so, at what age? Typical types of extrinsic feedback used for children are general awards of clapping, cheering, the child gaining access to a toy, the people working with the child smiling, and/or the child receiving lots of positive attention. Often, many types of feedback can occur at the same time. Is this confusing or overwhelming for the child? And the final question is whether using feedback that is not specific (not associated with success or failure with an activity) will help a child learn to use her/his own error detection system. Does the feedback have to be discussed verbally with the child for the child to learn to detect errors? These questions are important to ask when setting up a treatment program with a child. Experimentation within the clinic may be the best way to find answers to these questions.

D. Functional-based versus impairment-based treatment

1. The summation of the impairments does not add up to the functional problem as a whole. The functional problem is a result of the interaction among the motor and the sensory impairments, biomechanical limitations, and the particular environmental constraints.

2. Treatment may be directed at the impairment if it is believed to relate directly to the functional problem.

   Example: A therapist hypothesizes that a patient walks on her toes because of range of motion limitations at the ankle. The therapist decides to work on stretching the ankle for 2 weeks. After 2 weeks, the ankle dorsiflexion has increased to a neutral position, but the patient is still walking on her toes. At this point, the therapist needs to formulate a new hypothesis of which impairments are contributing directly to the functional problem, if any, and redesign the treatment plan.

3. Treatment of impairments for children is an important issue. Children are not "little adults." They have different nervous and musculoskeletal systems from those of adults, and these systems change with the growth of the child. The combination of an impairment, *eg*, limited range of the hamstring muscles, and growth is an ever-present problem for children with any type of neuromuscular disability. Prevention of deformity with growth is a major focus of pediatric therapy. Prevention is accomplished with

a knowledge and understanding of issues related to growth and development and how to use postures, movement, play, and specific therapeutic treatments for intervention. In the case study of SM (Chapter 20), range of motion in the lower extremities was considered a major focus of intervention in the neonatal intensive care unit and for the outpatient therapist as well. Activities of play in weight-bearing positions were attempted, but direct intervention of passive stretching both manually and with splints and casts was needed to address the problem. Knowing how to balance play activities with treatment that is more focused on the impairment is important. The combination of a growing child and impairments that will change with growth leads to an impairment level focus for intervention as an important part of treatment for pediatric therapists.

4. Physical therapists need to re-examine the old assumptions regarding the relationship of impairments to functional movement patterns.

  a. *Effect of spasticity on active movement*

    (1). Spasticity is an increased resistance to passive motion that is proportional to the velocity of the motion.[6] It occurs in the presence of upper motor neuron lesions and is accompanied by other positive and negative symptoms (see Chapter 8). However, there is no research to support that spasticity is a cause of the other positive and negative symptoms.

    (2). The confusion may stem from the loose use of the term "spastic" when referring to abnormalities in active movement, such as "spastic gait."

    (3). After dorsal rhizotomy surgery, a child will no longer have spasticity, yet will continue to demonstrate movement patterns seen before surgery.

  b. *Posturing of extremities in extension or flexion and relationship to active movement*

    (1). No substantiation exists that the pattern of posturing inhibits the expression of active movement except when caused by soft-tissue contractures that result from the posturing.

    (2). Treatment of posturing has traditionally focused on inhibition and muscle stretching so that active movement would be freer to occur.

    (3). In the contemporary model of motor control, the treatment of posturing is focused on maintaining the muscle length necessary for dressing, daily hygiene tasks, and patient comfort. Treatment might include passive range of motion techniques and serial casting.

    (4). Serial casting is a valuable technique for reducing muscle contractures.[7] It can be used to prevent muscle contractures in the acute care stage in someone who is posturing severely. Serial casting is especially helpful for stretching dorsiflexors, biceps, wrist flexors, and hamstrings. It has not been shown to be helpful in permanently reducing spasticity or posturing. Children with cerebral palsy frequently require serial casting after a growth spurt to assist with decreasing the increased muscle tightness. Depending on the problem leading to muscle tightness to begin with, the response of children to this treatment is typically good.

5. A focus on impairments can be incorporated into functional activities.

  a. Ankle stretching can be accomplished through the activities of daily living task of washing dishes at the sink while standing.

  b. Hip flexion control can be accomplished by climbing stairs with the hemiplegic leg first.

  c. Upper extremity motor control can be enhanced during gait training with the cane placed in the hemiparetic upper extremity.

  d. For children, functional activities are play activities. Play activities should be chosen on the basis of the child's cognitive level, developmental level, and physical capabilities. Activities for a child who is ambulatory and approximately 4 to 5 years of age may include leg strengthening by riding a bike, balance training by playing hopscotch, or timing of muscle activity by jumping on a trampoline.

E. Environmental and training conditions

1. The environment must vary for tasks that vary from trial to trial (see Chapter 8).

  a. Transfer training can be done from

wheelchair to bed, mat, chair with arms, chair without arms, high couch, low couch, park bench, etc.

b. Gait training can be done on many surfaces. The therapist does not need to wait until proficiency is gained on an "easy" surface like linoleum before attempting gait training on grass (mowed and unmowed), thick carpet, etc.

c. Challenging a child's balance by placing her/him in the sitting position on a bench can improve the child's ability to sit in long sitting on the floor. The child may require more external support from the therapist when sitting on the bench, yet the child appears to learn to use more trunk extension in sitting. Trunk extension may be carried over to long sitting, during which the child may require no external support from the therapist.

2. The task also must vary. Changing the nature of the environment changes how the patient responds to it and so technically the task is then changed. By varying the task, the therapist provides the patient practice in problem solving. The therapist should vary

a. The direction of walking.

b. The speed of walking (frequently therapists have allowed or have even encouraged the patient to walk at one, usually nonfunctional, slow speed).

c. The patient's shoes; the patient can wear slippers, sandals, sneakers—whatever she/he might want to wear once home. If the patient is using orthotics, she/he will have fewer choices of shoes (if any), and, therefore, practice can be less varied.

d. How the task is actually performed: getting in and out of bed from both sides of the bed or by not pulling on the bed rails; walking while carrying on a conversation or stopping to admire a flower garden.

3. The therapist should also vary the structure of the practice session.

a. Randomly spaced trials of the same activity within a treatment session may result in poorer performance initially but better long-term performance than blocked trials. For example, practicing transfers to and from a wheelchair from various surfaces, such as the bed, toilet, and car, in somewhat random order may lead to greater skill over time than would be achieved by doing five identical transfers in a row under one condition.

b. Studies show that observing somebody perform the task who is also learning the task may be more beneficial than observing a skilled performer.[8] Therefore, group treatment sessions may be helpful in skill learning as well as being psychologically beneficial.

4. Therapists need to alter the treatment areas that they have worked in for so long. The typical "gym" area is foreign to most people and contains few items that people have in their homes.[9]

a. Instead of mats, "real" beds can be used, of which there are many types: futons, platform, double, single, queen, floor mattresses, even waterbeds.

b. Instead of stairs that are treaded, with rails on both sides, stairs of varying heights can be used, without rails, carpeted, and made out of concrete or stone.

c. Instead of doing all the gait training on linoleum floors and paved parking lots, it can be done on different thicknesses of carpet, old pine floors, grassy areas, gravel and dirt areas, and cracked and broken sidewalks.

d. For children, working in their familiar setting is important (eg, school, day care, home). Determining which setting is best is important.

(1). Therapy performed in the school should be educationally relevant as defined by public legislation (PL 94-142). A therapist working with a child in the school should see the child within the classroom (the consultative model) so that the teacher and/or aide can observe how to work with the child, the amount of time the child is out of the classroom is decreased, and functional problems related to the classroom are addressed. The "pull-out" model of treatment in the schools is antiquated. If a child needs direct service treatment, she/he should be seen in the clinic at a time other than during school hours.

(2). The consultative model should be used within the day-care setting also. Limiting the amount of time that an adult is in the room, possibly making the child feel that she/he is different from the other children, is important.

(3). Working with a child at home allows the therapist to see what furniture and home furnishings can be used as "therapy equipment" for the child. The therapist is also able to see what the child experiences on a day-to-day basis and is able to modify a routine activity to help the child function more independently within the home.

F. Cognitive and behavioral concerns

1. The contemporary model may seem difficult to apply to cognitively impaired adults and small children. It seems to be a formidable task to obtain their active participation in error detection, problem solving, and application of the solution to the motor and functional problem. However, in thinking this way, therapists forget the strong effect that the environmental context and intrinsic feedback can have on performance. With adults who are relearning tasks that they may have performed for 30 or more years (walking, getting out of bed), the motor plans for these activities have been in place for a long time. By providing a variety of familiar environmental contexts to the patient, therapists can provide a variety of sensory feedback that the patient can use to alter the way the activity is performed. With a few gestures or carefully constructed sentences, the therapist may be able to augment the performance with extrinsic feedback.

Pediatric therapists can provide children with feedback by encouraging them to move, allowing them to move to their fullest capability, and then augmenting the movement as much as necessary to complete the movement. In this way, the child appears to be receiving feedback about what can happen if she/he continues to move, about the way that she/he can continue to move, and about how it feels to move farther. Repetition of moving from one posture to another, but varying the movement patterns used to obtain the other posture, may be most beneficial for learning. As mentioned earlier, the amount of information available regarding feedback for children is limited and requires further study.

2. Frequently, physical therapists do not believe that they are helpful to the patient if they do not provide frequent verbal feedback. With the cognitively impaired patient or young child, it is probably enough to refrain from talking and just provide the appropriate safeguards necessary for the patient to perform the task repeatedly in as many different environments as possible. (This may also be true for cognitively intact people!)

III. Summary

Which treatment approach is better—compensatory, facilitatory, or contemporary? The answer is unknown. Many assumptions on which the compensatory and facilitatory models were founded have not been substantiated scientifically. Much research needs to be done. We can probably expect continued changes in physical therapy theories and principles in the years to come.

A. Does everything in my practice need to change?

Certainly not.

1. Be clear about why you are doing the treatment you are doing. Ask yourself if you are treating the impairments that you feel directly contribute to the patient's functional problems and goals. If you are trying to enhance skill, ask yourself if you are establishing clear goals with the patient and providing realistic environmental conditions, appropriate feedback, and optimal practice conditions.

2. Examine the techniques that you are using and be clear about the theory behind them. You will probably find that the exercises and manual techniques may not change but the reasons for doing them and when you do them may change.

    Example: Slow rocking and stretching of a posturing lower extremity may be done for the purpose of ensuring adequate range of motion for hygiene as compared with inhibiting spasticity for the improvement of motor function.

3. Evaluate the way you structure the treatment sessions and environment. You may already be enhancing the patient's problem-solving abilities more than you realize.

B. Where do I begin?

1. It can often be overwhelming and frustrating to try to change your entire practice at one time. Pick a concept (environment, feedback, practice conditions) and evaluate how you presently incorporate these items into your practice. Decide how you want to change your practice and begin with small changes.
2. Begin dialogue with colleagues. Create an environment in which discussions that challenge old and new ways of thinking can occur without defensiveness or personal affront. These discussions often bring up more questions than answers, but they can be energizing and fun.
3. For pediatric therapists, the information in "Proceedings of the Consensus Conference on the Efficacy of Physical Therapy in the Management of Cerebral Palsy"[10] may be used to initiate conversation with co-workers about ways to change practice based on new theoretical information.

References

1. Duncan PW: Stroke: physical therapy assessment and treatment. In Lister M (ed): *Contemporary Management of Motor Control Problems. Proceedings of the II STEP Conference.* Alexandria, VA, Foundation for Physical Therapy, 1991, pp 209–217.
2. Bobath B: *Adult Hemiplegia: Evaluation and Treatment.* London, William Heinemann Medical Books, 1978.
3. Brunnstrom S: *Movement Therapy in Hemiplegia.* New York, Harper & Row, 1990.
4. Voss D, Ionta M, Myers BJ: *Proprioceptive Neuromuscular Facilitation.* Philadelphia, Harper & Row, 1985.
5. Winstein C: Balance retraining: does it transfer? In Duncan P (ed): *Balance: Proceedings of the American Physical Therapy Association Forum.* Alexandria, VA, APTA, 1990, pp 95–105.
6. Burke D: Spasticity as an adaptation to pyramidal tract injury. In Waxman SG (ed): *Functional Recovery in Neurological Disease.* New York, Raven Press, 1988, pp 401–423.
7. Orest M: Casting protocol for patients with neurological dysfunction. *PT Magazine of Physical Therapy,* 1993, May:51–55.
8. McCullough P: Social psychological and learning considerations in observational learning: is correct always best? Presented at the workshop. Skill Acquisition: Implications of Research and Theory in Motor Learning for Clinical and Educational Practice, New York, Teachers College, Columbia University, April 4, 1993.
9. Behrman A: Does the rehabilitation environment need a change? *Neurol Rep,* 1993, 17:20–21.
10. Campbell SK (ed): Proceedings of the Consensus Conference on the Efficacy of Physical Therapy in the Management of Cerebral Palsy. *Pediatr Phys Ther,* 1990, 2:123–176.

Suggested Reading

Forrsberg H (ed): Treatment of children with movement disorders: theory and practice. In Hebbelink M, Shephard RJ (eds): *Medicine and Sport Science.* vol 36. Basel, Switzerland, S. Karger, 1992.

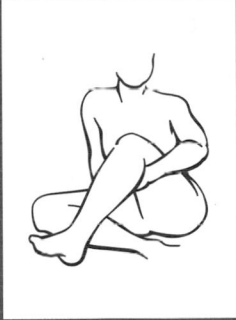

CHAPTER 13

Balance Instability

Susan Cromwell

In this chapter, three case studies are presented that involve balance problems. Each case is different with respect to age, medical history, and functional problem. Regardless of the differences, the physical therapist's thought and decision-making processes are similar. To gain a full understanding of how different impairments can be evaluated, refer to Tables 11–5 and 13–1 as you read the case studies.

I. Overview

A. Comparison of three patients

1. Patient #1 is a 75-year-old female who lives alone in a house with a yard. Her main complaint is that she consistently loses her balance when hanging clothes on a clothesline. Her doctor examined her and referred her to physical therapy. Her medical workup was negative.

2. Patient #2 is a 30-year-old female who is an inpatient in the rehabilitation unit after undergoing surgery for a malignant brain tumor. She requires assistance for all functional activities. She plans to live in her parents' home. Her parents will be the primary caretakers at discharge.

3. Patient #3 is a 40-year-old male who complains that he is unable to maintain his balance when he walks on a tile floor while wearing dress shoes. This problem has existed since his head injury 9 months previously. He states that he wishes to correct the problem and avoid compensation techniques.

B. Screening process

Traditionally, all three patients might be evaluated by using a standard format consisting of a predetermined set of impairments and functional skills. An alternative is to streamline the process by focusing the screening and evaluation process on the patient's individual problems and goals. In case #1, the primary means of obtaining information is from an interview and from evaluation of the task of hanging clothes on a clothesline. Case #2 is different because the patient has more global functional needs, and the diagnosis implies that her functional status may quickly deteriorate. The screening and evaluation are focused on gathering information that will hasten discharge from the hospital and ensure the appropriate level of care in the future. The patient in case #3 wishes to rehabilitate what he considers to be the etiology of his functional problem (poor balance). The screening and evaluation are focused on his particular functional problem using a variety of balance-specific evaluations.

375

Table 13–1. NONSTANDARDIZED CLINICAL METHODS OF EVALUATING BALANCE IMPAIRMENTS*

Parameter	Method of Evaluation	Behaviors to Observe for	Possible Interpretations of Observations	Functional Consequences of Impairment
Sway excursion	Instruct pt. to sway as far as possible in AP and lateral directions. In standing, body sway should be around the ankles (hips and knees extended). In sitting, body sway should be around the hips.	Decrease in the amount of volitional sway. Normal in standing position is 12 degrees AP and 8.5 degrees each lateral direction.[1]	If sway decreased: a. Muscle strength and/or ROM is inadequate in trunk/ankles to allow full sway excursion b. Perception of body position in space is altered	a. Difficulty in reaching items b. Altered movement patterns used for balance correction (use of a trunk flexion/extension or LE stepping for recovery of a small displacement)
Verticality	Question pt. about his/her perception of body position in space	a. Altered sense of body position b. Listing in one or more directions	Pt. has redefined, for self, where midline position is in relation to midline and vertical	a. Consistent pushing to one side or backward, which disrupts all attempts at movement b. Inability to sit or stand unsupported
Balance responses to external displacement	a. Use minimal displacement to provoke ankle pattern b. Displace pt. to edge of base of support (BOS) or by standing on short or uneven surfaces (balance beam) c. Displace outside BOS	a. No balance response b. Correctly executed response but in wrong context (eg, stepping pattern with a minimal displacement) c. Correctly chosen response, appropriate context, ineffective in balance recovery, pt. requires assistance for recovery (eg, initiates stepping pattern when displaced outside of BOS but can't complete step)	a. Lacks one or more balance responses because of physiological or biomechanical limitations (eg, solid ankle AFO biomechanically prevents use of ankle pattern) b. Slow reaction time c. Insufficient amplitude of response	a. Falls in conditions where required balance response is absent b. Attempts response but still unable to recover balance c. Needs assistive device (such as walker), which significantly reduces need for balance responses
Balance responses during volitional movements	Ask pt. to initiate and complete an activity such as reaching or bending over	a. Balance loss during initiation of activity (reaching, bending over) b. Movement patterns associated with attempts at balance recovery	a. Lacks feedback and/or feedforward capability to estimate extent of potential body displacement during activity b. Other possibilities same as listed under balance responses to external displacement	a. Unable to initiate or complete activity without losing balance b. Reduction of involvement in desired activities c. Uses assistive device
Adaptability	Repeat type of displacement (external or volitional) five to six times	Improvement in ability to recover balance	a. Improvement suggests that pt. is using feedback and feedforward mechanisms to adapt to the displacement b. Lack of improvement suggests that pt. is unable to use feedback and/or feedforward mechanisms from previous attempts to improve balance recovery	Pt.'s balance improves after the first few steps in a particular environment or during an activity, but pt. is still at risk for falling during initial contact with environmental problem (thick grass, gravel, stairs)

* Several forceplate computerized systems are commercially available to clinicians and researchers. Some include the EquiTest and Balance Master (NeuroCom International, Inc.) and the Chattecx Balance System (Chattecx Corp.). The manufacturers of these systems report the capability to measure impairments such as sensory organizational disturbances (EquiTest) and body sway excursion/verticality problems (Balance Master, Chattecx). The reliability and validity vary between researchers and patient populations. The transfer to functional abilities is questionable. We recommend a thorough investigative evaluation and trial of any system prior to purchase in your clinic.

Abbreviations: AP = anteroposterior; LE = lower extremity; Pt. = patient; ROM = range of motion.

The screening process involves the database. Each of the three patients is screened in almost the same way. If something is done differently, it is noted. The interview is a very effective way to begin completing the database. Information from the database is used to assist the therapist in formulating hypotheses about the relationship between the impairments and the functional problems.

1. **Medication.** The physical therapist notes any recent change in medications.

2. **Communication.** Any expressive or receptive language skill problems evident in general conversation are noted.

3. **Cardiovascular/pulmonary.** A history of heart disease that would be pertinent to know in an emergency or that may contribute to dizziness is noted.

4. **Metabolic.** The presence of diabetes is noted because it may be causing a peripheral neuropathy.

5. **Vision.** The therapist notes any report of balance or gait disturbances in altered light and any blindness or double vision.

6. **Behavior.** Any unusual behaviors are noted.

7. **Appliances.** The patient should be questioned about use of assistive devices in any particular environment. This question is asked even if the patient did not come to the appointment with an assistive device. The therapist should note the patient's thoughts about the use of assistive devices for mobility (*eg,* cane, wheelchair).

8. **Pain/tenderness.** These are important only if the patient experiences discomfort during a functional task that is problematic.

9. **Skin/soft tissue.** The presence of edema in legs is noted.

10. **Skeletal.** Any major limitations in range of motion, especially in the hips, trunk, and ankles, are noted. The movement behaviors used for balance correction primarily involve the trunk, hips, and ankles. In case #1, the therapist also screens for significant limitations in the shoulders that might cause the patient to use an unusual body posture when hanging clothes and thus evoke ineffective balance recovery behaviors.

11. **Neuromuscular.** The patient is questioned about any perceived asymmetry in strength in the lower extremities. The therapist checks quickly for the ability to withstand resistance in major muscle groups of the lower extremities. Any reports of sensory disturbance are noted.

12. **Balance.** This is an area to be fully explored during the definitive evaluation process. It is important to note at this time whether the patient has had or is experiencing balance problems in areas of life other than the stated problematic area.

13. **Posture.** Any severe kyphosis that places the head in a difficult position for looking and reaching upward is noted. Standing posture (wide-based stance, asymmetrical stance) also is noted.

14. **Functional mobility.** Any problem areas outside of the stated task for cases #1 and #3 are noted. For case #2, the therapist determines the level of safe mobility for functioning in the inpatient rehabilitation unit.

15. **Gait pattern.** This can be observed as the patient enters the examining area. The therapist notes any unusual pattern (limp, grossly uneven step length, reaching for walls or furniture, stumbling).

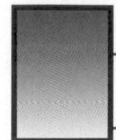

Clinical Decision-Making Cases

Case #1

SUMMARY OF SCREENING

No range of motion limitations or strength asymmetry is noted; strength is at least 3+/5. No observation of abnormal movement patterns. No cardiovascular, metabolic, skin, or neuromuscular problem. The patient is kyphotic with a forward head position. She is not using any assistive devices but has started to avoid other environmental situations, *eg*, garden and cobblestone streets, and prefers carpeting without large pile. She notices that walking in difficult environments becomes noticeably easier after 10 to 15 steps. The patient has no obvious gait deviations except slowness. She is committed to solving the present problem of hanging clothes on clothesline because she does not have a dryer and her drying rack does not hold all her clothes. She is not as concerned about her other functional limitations because she has been able to compensate for them satisfactorily.

FURTHER TESTING

Interview

The interview covers

1. The history of the problem, including whether anything helps the patient's balance.
2. Any recent alteration in home environment or manner of carrying out activities of daily living in order to enhance safety. This may indicate changes that were made that mask other existing balance problems.
3. Whether the patient has completely stopped doing any activities because of balance instability (gardening, walking across the grass).
4. Any problems with activities that require looking up (putting things in cupboards).
5. The manner in which the patient perceives that her body is trying to regain balance (does she find herself taking lots of steps, or does she sway a lot before regaining her balance).
6. Any problem with balance in low-light situations or when moving the head quickly.

Summary of Interview

The patient reports a history of balance instability when doing any activity that involves looking or reaching upward. She has been able to modify the activity by holding onto stable furniture counters. She has noticed an increase in unsteadiness in a backward direc-

tion when walking on grass, cobblestone roads, and gravel. She finds that she always loses her balance walking in a backward direction and that it takes four to five steps to correct. To date, she has not fallen.

Functional Task Evaluation

For this evaluation, the patient is asked to simulate the task of hanging clothes on a clothesline. She is asked to demonstrate how far she needs to walk from the house to the clothesline, how high she needs to lift the clothes, how she bends over and lifts the clothes to the line, and at what point she begins to feel unbalanced. She is asked to show how she loses her balance and what, if anything, she attempts to do to correct her balance.

Summary of Functional Task Evaluation

1. The clothesline is at a level 2 to 3 inches above the patient's head. Therefore, she has to lift her head to look upward and lift her arms to pin the clothes on the line.
2. As the patient lifts her head and arms, she begins to lean backward, which increases as she reaches the clothesline. When she reaches the line, she has swayed backward to a position that appears to be at the edge of her base of support. To this point, the therapist observed no attempts by the patient to correct her balance by taking any steps or flexing at the trunk or hips. The patient then appears to sway beyond her apparent base of support and takes four to five steps backward as she attempts to prevent falling. This same process happens each time the activity is repeated.

Interpretation of Interview and Functional Evaluation: Formation of Hypotheses

At this point, hypotheses are formed regarding the contribution of the impairments to the functional problem. The patient may be having difficulty with the movement behaviors usually used to recover from a balance loss. She may also be having difficulty with orientation in space when standing on altered surfaces. These hypotheses are further evaluated by impairment testing.

FURTHER IMPAIRMENT TESTING

Clinical Test for Sensory Interaction on Balance (CTSIB)

The CTSIB is a test of a person's ability to maintain balance under altered visual and somatosensory environments (see Table 11–35). Because of the patient's problem walking on uneven surfaces, the therapist wants to evaluate her ability to maintain balance under altered somatosensory and visual environments.

Balance Corrections

From the interview, the therapist hypothesizes that the patient may have a problem with the movement behaviors associated with balance correction; therefore, the therapist is interested in evaluating this impairment in an organized manner. This is an observational test of the type of body movement observed as the patient maintains her balance under different types of bodily displacements. It is not a standardized test. However, it provides descriptive information that is helpful in formulating or completing hypotheses regarding the etiology of balance problems.

First, the patient is asked to reach a minimal distance in all directions and the therapist describes the type of body movements exhibited as the patient maintains vertical (does the patient rotate around the ankles, flex/extend at the hips, bend knees, or take steps). Second, the patient is asked to stand sideways on a floor balance beam because the only way to maintain balance in this position is to flex/extend at the hips or take a step off. Third, the patient is asked to perform an activity that displaces her body outside the base of support (see Table 13–1).

Summary of Impairment Testing

The patient is able to maintain balance during all conditions of the CTSIB; however, she exhibits a large amount of body sway when standing on the foam. The patient is unable to maintain her balance when standing sideways on a balance beam. She sways, primarily in a backward direction, and at the last moment takes several steps off the beam. She does not exhibit any flexion/extension of the trunk. She appears to wait until she has almost fallen before taking any steps to regain her balance when she displaces herself close to or outside her base of support.

FINAL INTERPRETATION OF INTERVIEW, FUNCTIONAL EVALUATION, AND IMPAIRMENT TESTING

The patient is primarily using a stepping strategy for balance recovery when displaced close to the edge of her base of support. Her balance loss occurs most frequently in a backward direction; this may be accentuated by her kyphosis and forward head position,

which require a greater than normal backward lean to reach and look upward. Contributing to this problem is the high clothesline. Also, the patient uses the stepping response later than what would normally be observed and thus has to take four to five steps rather than one. She has been able to adapt her activities of daily living satisfactorily to compensate for the slow change in her balance abilities. She has not been able to adapt the manner in which she hangs her clothes.

TREATMENT GOALS

The patient will no longer lose her balance when hanging out her clothes.

APPROACH TO TREATMENT

The therapist explains to the patient that there are two approaches to the problem. The first approach involves two actions: to modify the environment by lowering the clothesline so that she does not have to reach up so high, and to place one foot in back of the other while hanging clothes so that her base of support is larger and extends backward in the direction that she most frequently loses her balance. She is informed that these two actions should significantly reduce the frequency of balance loss and that no additional physical therapy appointments are needed, merely a follow-up telephone call. The second approach would be to continue with physical therapy treatments with the goal of changing her automatic balance response so that she would react more quickly (less steps needed to regain balance) and be able to use more flexion and extension of the trunk to regain her balance (less stepping required).

The patient decides to take the first approach, which is to compensate for her problem, and to contact the therapist if the recommendations do not work. If she had chosen the second approach, the therapist would have set up a regular program of functional activities that stressed her balance and would have instructed her in using more hip flexion/extension to maintain her balance, and also to take a step sooner. This second approach assumes that consciously performed balance responses will eventually result in automatic responses. The other aspect of this approach is that the patient needs to lose her balance frequently and attempt a correction to learn to regain it. In this scenario, the therapist needs to be careful not to let the patient fall but has to restrain herself/himself from assisting the patient before she has a chance to make a response.

Case #2

SUMMARY OF SCREENING

The patient underwent cerebellar tumor removal. Residual deficits are functional limitations that require minimal assistance for transfers and moderate assistance for walking with a walker. The patient is presently using a wheelchair. No range of motion or strength deficits were noted. Inaccuracy of extremity placement was noted with functional activities. Excessive body sway was noted in the sitting and standing positions. The patient will be living in a one-story home with three entry steps; there is a railing on the right side.

FURTHER TESTING

Further testing is based on a preliminary interview and screening for impairments and functional abilities.

Interview

1. The patient is questioned more closely about the specific level of function she feels she needs to achieve before discharge.
2. She is asked to describe the environments in which she expects to be functioning.
3. She is asked how long she expects to stay at the rehabilitation center.
4. She is asked if she has any personal feelings as to how treatment ought to proceed.

Summary of Interview

The patient states that she wants to be independent with bed mobility and transfers so that she can use a bedside commode at home on her own. She states that she would like to improve her walking so that she needs only a small amount of assistance from one person. She anticipates that she will need a wheelchair for long-distance mobility and perhaps more often in the future. She would like to concentrate her treatment on getting in and out of bed and walking.

Functional Evaluation

The patient's functional mobility is evaluated for the amount of assistance that she requires and the assistive device or devices that are most useful for mobility around the house. If the patient is ambulatory, the therapist observes her walking with a standard walker, rolling walker, quadriped cane, and perhaps a straight cane. If the patient is marginally ambulatory, her ability to push a wheelchair on level surfaces, carpets, and up and down a ramp is observed.

Summary of Functional Evaluation

The patient is independent in rolling and in assuming sitting and supine positions in bed. Once sitting, she is able to sit on the edge of the bed without support. She is able to transfer to a chair with armrests if it is right next to the bed. She leans forward with one hand and holds onto the far armrest while squatting and pivoting. She requires minimal assistance to swing her hips far enough around to sit safely on the chair. The other hand remains on the side of the bed.

She is unable to stand unsupported without a moderate amount of body sway and ineffective balance responses. She is able to stand and walk with a standard walker; she needs a moderate amount of assistance for balance maintenance each time she advances the walker. With a rolling walker, she is able to walk with less assistance for balance maintenance but needs more assistance for forward deceleration. She is unable to use any type of cane for walking; each time she attempts to advance the cane, she requires moderate assistance for balance maintenance. She is able to ascend stairs with minimal assistance if she uses a railing on the right side and uses a step-to-step pattern.

Interpretation of Interview and Functional Evaluation

Although it initially appears to the therapist that the patient's balance instability is a major contributory factor to her functional instability, her balance outside of functional activities is not evaluated. The patient is most concerned about her functional status and wishes to pursue any balance retraining within the activities that need improvement for discharge. She feels that once she is home and her energy level is higher, she may want to work on her balance.

Final Interpretation of Interview, Functional Evaluation, and Balance Testing

The patient does not possess adequate skill in transferring and walking to be discharged to her home at the desired level. Given adequate opportunities for experimentation in different environments and with a variety of assistive devices, the patient should be able to solve her functional problems and be discharged to her home at the desired functional level.

TREATMENT GOALS

Independent transfers and minimal assistance for ambulation with assistive device.

APPROACH TO TREATMENT

The therapist recommends to the patient a program of functional retraining, emphasizing patient problem solving, simulating home and community environments and experimenting with different assistive devices and various methods of performing the functional tasks. She is provided with information about other resources that she may want to access in the future if her functional status changes.

Case #3

SUMMARY OF SCREENING

The patient reports that he was recently prescribed carbamazepine (Tegretol), which reduces his emotional angry outbursts but worsens his balance problem. His physician has stated that he should accommodate to the medication and that the balance problem exacerbation should diminish. The patient has no history of cardiovascular, metabolic, skin, soft-tissue, skeletal, or neuromuscular deficits. He reports a grainy texture to his vision. His posture is wide-based, and this is observed when he walks. He is independent and competent in all functional mobility activities, except he frequently slips while walking in dress shoes on a tile floor. He also reports that he feels that he avoids games with his son that require fast movement or quick turns. The patient states that he understands that he could easily compensate for the major problem of difficulty maintaining balance on a tile floor while wearing dress shoes by wearing different shoes. His goal, however, is not to compensate but to correct the problem.

FURTHER TESTING

Interview

The patient is questioned more intensely about his perception of his balance or motor problems in other activities: why he avoids fast-moving games, what happens to his body or balance when he does engage in these activities, what happens if he walks on uneven surfaces, and what his balance is like when he wears different types of shoes on different surfaces.

Summary of Interview

The patient reports that he feels unsteady during any activity that causes fast head movements or quick body turns. He has never fallen but feels as if he might. Flat, slick surfaces cause the patient more unsteadiness than uneven surfaces. The less friction he feels exists between his feet and the floor, the worse his balance is. He states that he does not feel that the problem exists if he is barefoot or wearing sneakers.

Functional Evaluation

The therapist evaluated the functional task of walking on a tile floor in dress shoes (the patient wore dress shoes and walked on the clinic's tile floor). The therapist
1. Observed the patient's natural speed of walking.
2. Observed the posture of the patient's arms, trunk, and legs.
3. Asked the patient to vary the walking speed on his own and in response to directions.
4. Observed the patient's movement behavior as he recovered his balance during walking.

5. Asked the patient to make quick turns and stops and to look over his shoulder as if someone were calling him.
6. Bumped into the patient accidentally.
7. Threw a ball to the patient.
8. Observed the patient's walking pattern on surfaces other than tile.

Summary of Functional Testing

Functionally, the patient does not appear to have any unusual patterns of movement during any functional task except while walking on a tile floor while wearing dress shoes. In this environment, he assumes a wide-based gait and shuffles his feet. He takes all turns widely and slowly and turns to look over his shoulder very carefully after his feet are planted in a wide stance. When throwing or catching a ball, he assumes a wide-based stance. When making a balance recovery on a tile floor, he shuffles his feet in many directions rather than lifting them up and planting them on the floor.

Interpretation of Interview and Functional Evaluation

The patient has a problem with balance recovery under very quick and unpredictable conditions, which is similar to the problem that many individuals have when attempting to walk on ice. He has partially compensated for his problem by altering the way he plays with his son and adjusting his posture when walking and turning. It is not certain whether the patient has a problem with movement pattern, reaction time, sensory environment, or a combination of these. Further evaluation is needed.

FURTHER IMPAIRMENT TESTING

Clinical Test for Sensory Interaction on Balance (CTSIB)

The CTSIB is chosen because the therapist wants to evaluate in a standard manner the patient's ability to maintain balance under altered sensory conditions (see Table 11–5).

Balance Corrections

This is an observational test of the type of body movement observed as the patient maintains his balance under external and internal displacements. It is not a standardized test. However, it provides descriptive information that is helpful in formulating or completing hypotheses regarding the etiology of balance problems. First, the patient is asked to reach a minimal distance in all directions and the therapist describes the type of body movements exhibited as the patient maintains vertical (does the patient rotate around the ankles, flex/extend at the hips, bend knees, or take steps). Second, the patient is asked to stand sideways on a floor balance beam because the only way to maintain balance in this position is to flex/extend at the hips or take a step off. Third, the patient is asked to perform an activity that displaces his body outside the base of support (see Table 13–1).

Reaction Time

Without electromyography or sophisticated forceplate systems, it is virtually impossible to determine if a patient is reacting quickly enough when recovering from a balance loss. The best therapists can do is to observe the patient and subjectively evaluate if a movement pattern is occurring within the time frame in which it would be expected to be effective. The value of this type of evaluation is questionable because of the lack of objectivity, reliability, and validity.

Summary of Further Balance Testing

The patient was able to maintain his balance for the specified time under all sensory conditions of the CTSIB. He maintained a wide base of support. He stated that he felt unsteady on the compliant foam and exhibited a large amount of body sway when standing on it. The patient exhibited a variety of movement patterns as he attempted to recover balance loss from external and internal displacements. He rotated around the ankles in response to minimal displacements. When displaced closer to the edge of his base of support or when standing on a narrow surface, he primarily bent his knees as he attempted to recover balance loss, although he also flexed and extended at the hips for balance correction. When responding to a large displacement of his center of gravity, he attempted to recover his balance by stepping but merely slid his feet from side to side. When this was pointed out to him, he stated that he felt he would fall if he lifted his feet off the floor. However, he did not fall when he attempted to lift his feet. He appeared to make all balance corrections in a time frame that would be effective for balance recovery.

FINAL INTERPRETATION OF INTERVIEW, FUNCTIONAL EVALUATION, AND IMPAIRMENT TESTING

The patient exhibits all of the usually observed balance recovery patterns in the appropriate contexts; however, his stepping response is ineffective because he shuffles his feet from side to side. It is unclear why his balance problem occurs primarily in fast, unpredictable, changing, and low-friction environments, except that perhaps a reaction-time problem exists that cannot be detected with the clinical or observational tools available. By avoiding challenging situations or altering the way he functions within them, the patient has lost the opportunity to "practice and sharpen" his balance responses. Theoretically, the more frequently he makes

correct and successful balance responses without compensatory habits (slow and wide turns, wide-based stance, slow speed), the better and more efficient his balance recovery system should become. The patient needs to engage in activities that challenge his balance frequently. He needs to avoid compensatory habits and use a stepping response that involves lifting his feet off the ground and stepping rather than sliding.

TREATMENT GOALS

The patient will no longer lose his balance on tile floors while wearing dress shoes, and he will feel less unsteady in fast, unpredictable, and changing environments.

TREATMENT APPROACH

The patient wishes to engage in a home program designed to rehabilitate his balance problem. The therapist's assessment of his problem and the need for him to engage in activities that challenge his balance response are explained to him. The philosophy of needing to lose one's balance in order to regain control of balance also is explained. If he understands and agrees with the approach suggested, he is instructed in the following ways to incorporate this approach into his busy life:

1. Change the wide-based stance to a normal width, especially when engaging in outdoor activities with your son or standing on a tile floor.
2. Do not make wide, slow turns on tile floors. Attempt to increase gradually the speed of these turns.
3. When walking on tile floors, stop frequently and turn to look over your shoulder as if someone were calling you.
4. Take every opportunity to walk on wet grass, slick pavement, and floors.
5. Wear dress shoes more often.
6. Eventually, run more.
7. When playing with your son, increase your body movements more by running, making quick turns, and being proactive in the game.
8. Practice standing with your feet in different positions: narrow stance, tandem stance, one-legged stance. Increase the difficulty of this activity by playing ball with your feet in those positions or by having your son try to knock you over.
9. Ongoing physical therapy treatments will be unnecessary, the therapist will follow up with you via telephone in approximately 3 weeks. With diligent attention to the program, you should notice an improvement in balance within 3 to 6 months. Goal achievement should be accomplished within 6 to 9 months.

REFERENCE

1. Nashner LM: Sensory, neuromuscular and biomechanical contributions to human balance. In Duncan P (ed): *Balance: Proceedings of the American Physical Therapy Association Forum.* Alexandria, VA, APTA, 1990, pp 5–13.

SUGGESTED READING

Woollacott MH, Shumway-Cook A (eds): *Development of Posture and Gait Across the Life Span.* Columbia, SC, University of South Carolina Press, 1989.

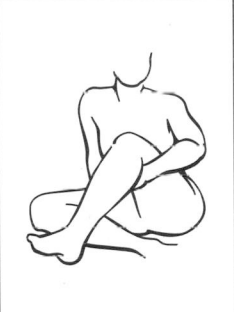

CHAPTER 14

Patients with Hemiparesis/ Hemiplegia

Marianne Orest and Polly Menendez

In the case studies presented in this chapter, the physical therapist screened, evaluated, assessed, and treated two patients who have hemiparesis/hemiplegia, with the major problem of impaired mobility. Hemiparesis/hemiplegia can result from many different causes, and each patient can present a very different picture, but these two individuals represent "typical" problems found in this patient population. The key issues addressed in these two case studies are (1) weakness and decreased motor control and (2) impaired position sense, leading to the "pusher" syndrome. These two patients are compared, looking at both the similarities and differences of the physical therapy involvement.

I. Overview

A. Introduction to two patients

1. Patient #1 is an 88-year-old female who lives alone in a trailer with a few entrance steps. She was admitted to an acute care hospital the previous day because of left-sided weakness. Her doctor examined her and referred her to physical therapy to assist with her mobility problems. She wants to be able to walk again and wishes to return to living in her trailer. Before admission, she received home health services, wore a lifeline necklace, and received Meals on Wheels.

2. Patient #2 is a 55-year-old male with a long history of diabetes with multiple complications, including bilateral below-knee amputations. He had a right cerebrovascular accident (CVA) with left hemiparesis 4 months previously. He was discharged from the acute care hospital to home at his request. The patient was followed at home by home care physical therapists and occupational therapists. He required 24-hour supervision and physical assistance with all mobility, which was provided by his partner. His

home had multiple barriers, including one step up into the bathroom and one step down into the kitchen. The home care therapists recommended admission to a rehabilitation unit because there were too many issues to work on in the home setting. The patient agreed to a 2-week stay to work on walking and left upper extremity function.

B. Screening of database items

The database is to be completed in the usual manner, with special attention to the following parameters, which are particularly important in working with a patient with hemiparesis/hemiplegia. The database assists the therapist in being aware of the patient's medical conditions, which may have an impact on the physical therapy treatment. This information can be gathered by reviewing the patient's chart, communicating with team members, and interviewing the patient.

1. **Medication.** If the patient is receiving coagulation therapy, it may affect her/his level of mobility and location of treatment. Cardiac medications may affect the patient's performance with exercise.

2. **Communication.** Any hearing deficits, aphasia, or dysarthria may affect the patient's ability to communicate her/his needs or participate in the therapy program.

3. **Cardiovascular.** The physical therapist should be aware of any cardiac conditions and/or changes that may be considered a possible etiology of hemiparesis/hemiplegia because the patient may still be at risk for additional problems. Reasons for exercise precaution, such as angina, also should be noted because they may become important during treatment.

4. **Metabolic.** Diabetes is often a consideration. The patient may have a change in her/his activity level because of the hemiparesis/hemiplegia that may affect her/his blood sugar regulation.

5. **Vision.** Visual problems such as a field cut, difficulty tracking or scanning, or a visual disregard can affect the patient's participation in physical therapy.

6. **Behavior (key area).** Cognitive and behavior problems should be noted in relation to the

patient's participation in physical therapy. Extensive testing in these areas is done by the occupational therapist, the speech and language pathologist, and the psychologist.

7. **Appliances.** The therapist should note whether the patient has previously used, or will perhaps need, any type of adaptive equipment, orthotic devices, assistive devices, splints for positioning, or wheelchair.

8. **Skin/soft tissue.** Skin abrasions or edema on the affected side may occur because the patient is not aware of the affected extremity. For example, the patient's affected arm may fall to the side when she/he is sitting in a wheelchair. The patient's hand may get caught in the spokes of the wheel, causing a skin abrasion, or may remain in a dependent position, causing edema.

9. **Skeletal.** Limitations in range of motion of the affected extremities, especially dorsiflexion and shoulder range, may affect the patient's function. For example, if dorsiflexion is limited, the patient may have difficulty during ambulation.

10. **Neuromuscular (key area).** Problems with motor control, increased resistance to passive movement, and sensation usually have an impact on functional activities in patients who have hemiparesis/hemiplegia.

11. **Balance (key area).** If the patient has a problem with static or dynamic balance, she/he should probably not be left alone for safety reasons in a sitting or standing position.

12. **Posture (key area).** If problems are noted with alignment/rotation, midline orientation, or the position of the extremities, it may indicate a weakness or a problem with the patient's perception of her/his body in space.

13. **Functional mobility (key area).** Deficits noted in bed mobility, transfers, ambulation on level surfaces, stairs, or wheelchair mobility may direct the physical therapy treatment.

14. **Gait pattern (key area).** Any deviations observed during the gait cycles should be noted. Toe clearance of the affected extremity is important to note because, if the patient is having difficulty with toe clearance, bracing may be indicated.

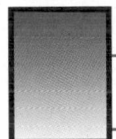

Clinical Decision-Making Cases

Case #1

SUMMARY OF SCREENING

1. Medical tests: magnetic resonance imaging report shows an infarct in the right middle cerebral artery.
2. Medication: cardiovascular, diabetic, diuretic.
3. Cardiovascular: right CVA, hypertension, coronary artery disease, peripheral vascular disease.
4. Metabolic: diabetes.
5. Gastrointestinal/genitourinary: urinary incontinence, diverticulitis, chronic renal insufficiency.
6. Vision: left homonymous hemianopsia, left neglect.
7. Skin/soft tissue: gangrene right big toe.
8. Neuromuscular: left hemiparesis, limited movement at all pivots in left extremities.
9. Balance: falls to the left when sitting at edge of bed.
10. Posture: left upper extremity hangs limply by her side.
11. Functional mobility: moderate assistance for supine to sit to the left; maximal assistance for a stand-pivot transfer to the right.

IMPAIRMENTS IDENTIFIED FROM SCREENING

The patient has decreased movement of left extremities, left upper extremity position, impaired balance, and left neglect.

IMPAIRMENTS INDICATING FURTHER EVALUATION BECAUSE OF POSSIBILITY OF CONTRIBUTING TO IMPAIRED MOBILITY

1. Motor control: Lower extremity—in sitting, the patient was able to initiate hip flexion and extend her knee through full range but had no knee flexion or dorsiflexion; in sidelying, she had half range hip extension. Upper extremity—in supine, the patient had minimal scapular elevation and protraction and slight elbow, wrist, and finger flexion.
2. Balance: The patient was unable to sit unsupported for any length of time (required continual assistance to maintain a static, unsupported position), fell to the left while trying to sit, and made no attempt to use movement in left extremities to regain balance.

ASSESSMENT

The patient needs a significant amount of physical assistance for functional activities at this time, and it is anticipated that she will need some physical assistance at discharge. She will not be able to return home alone; the patient's daughter has expressed an interest in moving in with her mother to help care for her. Admission to a rehabilitation unit may be appropriate to assist the patient in regaining as much functional independence as possible, as well as for family education.

GOALS

Goals need to be set after the initial screening to justify treatment even though the functional evaluation may not be complete. In reality, the functional evaluation is usually not completed at this time because of time constraints and patient fatigue. After the functional evaluation is complete, the goals may need to be modified.

1. Short-term goals: poor static sitting balance (occasionally able to maintain an unsupported position for less than 3 seconds, but this is inconsistent and usually depends on how she is positioned), bed mobility with minimal assistance, and transfers with moderate assistance in a time frame of 1 to 2 weeks.
2. Long-term goals: fair static sitting balance (able to maintain static, unsupported position for 3 to 30 seconds, but cannot sustain this), bed mobility with contact guarding, and transfers with minimal assistance in a time frame of 3 to 4 weeks.

FUNCTIONAL AREAS TO BE EVALUATED AFTER INITIAL SCREENING

The therapist was not able to screen the patient's ambulation during the initial screening because of time constraints and patient fatigue. Ambulation is important to evaluate because the patient wishes to walk again. Because ambulation was not screened initially, it was difficult to set a goal for ambulation because the therapist was unable to predict accurately how the patient would do. An ambulation goal was not set until ambulation was screened and evaluated.

Ambulation was screened and evaluated during a subsequent physical therapy session. The patient needed maximal assistance to ambulate approximately 10 feet. She exhibited decreased hip and knee flexion during swing and lacked heel strike.

Ambulation goals were then added to the initial set of goals. The short-term goal for 2 weeks was ambulation with maximal assistance of one and use of an assistive device, and the long-term goal for 3 to 4 weeks was moderate assistance of one and the use of an assistive device.

TREATMENT APPROACH

A functional approach of sitting at the edge of the bed for sitting balance, bed mobility training, transfer training, and gait training was used. These tasks were chosen because the patient needed to do these tasks at home. These tasks were repeated many times and in a variety of environments, allowing the patient to be an active problem solver. For example, the task of sit to stand was practiced many times from the bed, from the toilet, from various types of chairs with and without armrests, and from as many of the surfaces as possible that the patient would encounter on discharge from the hospital setting. The patient was allowed to make errors within the realm of safety and was provided the least amount of physical assistance possible. No verbal cues were provided during the task in order not to distract the patient. After the task was completed, the patient was asked how she thought the task went and what she would do differently the next time. After the patient provided her own feedback, the therapist offered additional observations regarding her performance and the outcome of the task. By making these tasks as real as possible for the patient, there is a better chance that she will be able to do them at home once she is discharged.

Use of the left extremities was incorporated into the functional activities. Movement was done within the context of goal-directed tasks to make the movement more meaningful to the patient. Increased movement may be achieved during functional activities as opposed to doing exercises on the mat with the left extremities. With shortened hospital stays, and patients spending less time in physical therapy, it may be best to spend time only on functional activities instead of on exercises.

OUTCOME

1. The treatments focused on functional mobility training, including ambulation. The patient did not do exercises to increase left extremity movements.
2. The patient's static sitting balance improved so that she was able to sit unsupported for a couple of seconds at a time, but she would still lose her balance to the left. She was beginning to use her left extremities to assist in regaining her balance.
3. Bed mobility and transfers also improved as she used her left extremities more.
4. A rolling walker was used for ambulation to keep ambulation as a spontaneous automatic activity as well as to provide support. Using the walker the therapist was able to incorporate the left upper extremity into the treatment to increase movement and work on left neglect by assisting the patient to hold onto the walker with her left hand.
5. Because of the progress the patient made and her motivation to continue improving, she was admitted to the local rehabilitation unit 1 week after physical therapy was initiated. Her acute care goals were not achieved because of her short stay in the acute care unit, but the patient was able to continue working on her goals in the rehabilitation setting.

Case #2

SUMMARY OF SCREENING

1. Discussion with patient: The patient feels that his only significant deficit is his inability to walk. He stated that he had had no difficulty walking after his amputations, saying that he walked without an assistive device on all surfaces and was able to climb ladders. He thought that he should be able to do all of these activities again. His goal for his rehabilitation stay was to walk by himself in 2 weeks.
2. Medication: cardiac and diabetic.
3. Cardiovascular: coronary artery bypass surgery 2 years previously; history of myocardial infarction and angina; recent right CVA with left hemiparesis.
4. Metabolic: brittle diabetes. Patient had his own routine for managing diabetes and did not do finger sticks. He stated that his blood sugar often drops during exercise but that he can tell when he needs to stop.
5. Vision: left homonymous hemianopsia with severe left neglect.
6. Behavior: Patient had very set ideas about what he could do and how he would accomplish his goals. He had decreased insight into the deficits because of his stroke. The patient had decreased ability to attend to tasks and was very impulsive. He frequently vented his anger at caregivers.
7. Appliances: Patient reported that he had multiple pairs of prostheses, including a pair for the shower. He had a standard wheelchair. He sat on a piece of lambswool and did not want to use a wheelchair cushion. He had a pair of crutches at home that he thought would help with his walking.
8. Skin/soft tissue: no open areas or pressure areas; some redness noted at tibial tubercle and at medial and lateral femoral condyles after walking.
9. Skeletal: bilateral below-knee amputations.
10. Neuromuscular: limited scapular movement was the only movement noted in the left upper extremity; movement at the left lower extremity dominated by the flexor synergy pattern; sensation present but impaired.
11. Balance: Patient needed intermittent assistance to maintain sitting balance on the edge of the bed

and constant assistance to maintain balance when standing.

12. Posture: Patient listed to the left in sitting and standing and resisted correction of this posture by pushing with the right arm and leg.

13. Functional mobility: Patient required moderate assistance for bed mobility and maximal assistance for transfers with bilateral prostheses. Patient stood with bilateral prostheses but was not able to take any steps with a quad cane.

ASSESSMENT OF DATABASE

When the information gathered during the screen was compared with the patient's goals, the therapist concluded that the goals were not realistic or reflective of all of the patient's needs. She was somewhat taken aback by all of the challenges put forth by the patient. The therapist had worked with many patients with hemiplegia but had minimal experience working with people after amputations. She decided to move forward, basing her judgements on previous experience with people who have had hemiplegia, and arranged for co treatment with a therapist who had had more experience working with people with amputations. The initial impressions were then discussed with the patient; further testing would be based on this discussion.

The patient continued to insist that he wanted to work only on walking but agreed that working on transfers might be helpful. Using the information from the database, the therapist decided to complete further testing of motor control of the left leg, balance, transfers, and gait.

EVALUATION PROCEDURES

Because the patient was unwilling to participate in any formal evaluation procedures, the therapist decided to base all of the testing on observations of function.

Motor Control of Left Lower Extremity

Left leg movement was observed during functional tasks, and it was noted that the patient used his right arm or leg to position his left leg for any standing or transfer activity. The patient's ability to move his left leg off his wheelchair footrest and to flex his left knee to approximately 100 degrees to prepare for standing was measured. At the initial evaluation, the patient needed complete assistance to move the left leg off the footrest. He could initiate knee flexion but needed assistance to position the foot adequately for standing.

Balance

The patient's balance was observed during a series of functional tasks (supine to sit, transfers, sit to stand, static standing, reaching and walking); he lost his sitting balance only when he was not wearing his pros-

theses. Because the patient did not want to work on sitting, sitting balance was not measured. During standing, the patient was not able to keep his center of gravity within his base of support and was always falling posteriorly and to the left. The patient reported the sensation of falling to the right, and he attempted to catch himself with a stepping response to the right. Thus, when the patient was falling, he had an incorrect interpretation of how he was falling, and his response to the fall made matters worse. Therefore, the patient's perception of his position in space and his ability to stand and walk without losing his balance were measured.

The patient's perception of his position in space was measured by asking him to describe how he was falling when he was losing his balance; his ability to maintain his balance was measured by describing how long he could stand or walk without losing his balance. At the time of the initial evaluation, the patient was not able to describe how he was falling, and he could maintain static standing without losing his balance for a few seconds.

Transfers

Bed to wheelchair transfers and sit to stand were evaluated. The techniques that the patient was using to perform these activities were inefficient and contributed to his need for more assistance. He needed maximal assistance for a stand-pivot transfer but only moderate assistance for a squat-pivot transfer. For sit to stand, which required maximal assistance, he initiated the activity by leaning backward instead of forward. These tasks were measured by documenting the amount of assistance required, but the patient's ability to use the squat-pivot transfer and whether he was leaning forward or backward before standing up also were described.

Gait

The amount of assistance the patient required for walking and the distance he could walk were measured, and gait deviations were described. The lack of reliability of observational gait analysis was recognized by the therapist,[1] but because the patient had some obvious gait deviations, a few key deviations that were thought to be limiting the patient's ability to walk without falling were documented. Temporal gait analysis was possible, but it was uncertain how the mechanics of the prosthesis (SACH foot) would affect the outcome.

Initially, the patient could not walk at all with a cane, but he could walk 10 feet in the parallel bars with his arms supported on a board across the top of the parallel bars. This required maximal assistance (two people). Significant gait deviations included increased left knee flexion in stance, excessive weight shift to the left in stance, decreased weight shift to the right in stance, decreased left foot clearance (his left foot caught on the floor most of the time), and decreased base of support (there was no space between his feet during double limb support).

ASSESSMENT

The major movement problem for the patient is his impaired sense of his position in space. He is skilled in using his prostheses, and his amputations have little effect on his current functional problems. His presentation with regard to balance and position sense is common among people who have left hemiplegia. If this patient could learn to weight shift to the right and stop pushing himself off to the left, he could learn to walk with contact guarding. This judgement was based on the therapist's past experience with patients who have had a similar postural pattern. The patient demonstrated capability for improved transfers during the evaluation, and it was felt that he could learn to transfer with supervision if he used the squat-pivot technique. It was also thought that it may be possible for him to negotiate one step with the assistance of his partner, which would make it easier for him to gain access to all areas of his house.

GOALS

The therapist wrote her goals with the patient; in the end, neither the therapist nor the patient thought the goals were reasonable, but both had compromised. Because the patient insisted on a 2-week time frame, the therapist agreed to write 2-week goals. The therapist thought that the patient needed 4 weeks to meet the goals, so it was agreed that the time frame would be reviewed near the end of the 2 weeks.

Functional Goals

1. Patient will need supervision for transfers to bed and to wheelchair.
2. Patient will walk for household distances with small-base quad cane and contact guarding from his partner.
3. Patient will be able to negotiate one step with the assistance of his partner.

In addition, four goals were written that were more reflective of improved motor control and that may relate to improved ability to walk:

1. Patient will lift left leg off the wheelchair footrest without assistance from the right leg or arm.
2. Patient will flex knee and position left foot to prepare for standing without assistance from the right leg or arm.
3. Patient will have 6 inches between his feet during double limb support.
4. When he loses his balance, patient will accurately describe how he is falling and what he needs to do to correct the problem.

TREATMENT APPROACH

Including the Patient in Active Problem Solving

Throughout all treatment activities, the therapist allowed the patient to solve his own problems. Initially, he was given some suggestions based on the therapist's understanding of his problems, and he was allowed to experiment with the suggestions. For example, it was explained that when he felt like he was falling to the right in standing, he was actually falling to the left. It was suggested that he work on this problem by shifting his weight to the right. After a strategy that worked was identified, the patient was allowed to struggle with the activity until he would remember to put all the pieces together. He sometimes did things that the therapist thought were unsafe, but he was allowed to do the activity so that he could see how it was unsafe. The therapist asked for assistance from other staff to ensure the patient's safety.

Functional Activities

The patient demanded that the therapist incorporate all of the treatment into functional tasks that had meaning to him; therefore, the patient assisted the therapist in following the principles of motor learning.[2] Most of the treatment occurred during transfers and gait, but some reaching activities in standing also were included.

Parallel bars with a board across were used to begin standing and walking activities with the patient. This setup provides a safe environment, but it also has therapeutic benefits because it promotes an upright posture and defines the limits for lateral weight shifting. The therapist had the patient reach to the right with his right arm, which subsequently forced him to weight shift onto the right leg. His right foot was blocked to prevent a stepping response to the right. This activity allowed him to experience weight shift to the right without falling to the right.

Two therapists were necessary to assist the patient in walking in the parallel bars: one therapist in front of the board, and the other therapist on a rolling stool to guard the left knee in stance and to aid with advancing the left leg in swing. Several days later, when the patient gained some control over his excessive weight shift to the left and increased knee flexion in stance, the therapist chose to use a rolling walker with a platform on the left to assist him with walking. The walker continued to define the limits of the lateral weight shift, but the patient could begin to see the ramifications of his excessive weight shift to the left because the walker would come off the floor. This is an example of having the patient attend to intrinsic feedback instead of extrinsic verbal feedback from a therapist. Because the patient could actually see what was happening, it was more effective than verbal feedback.

Within the first week, the patient walked with a small-base quad cane, which the therapist thought he would need to use for a long time. The patient wanted to try crutches, but, after one attempt, he decided it was not a good idea. The therapist particularly liked the quad cane in this case because it forced the patient to weight shift to the right and helped to correct his postural problem.

Transfer training consisted of repeated trials of transfers at a variety of times in the day. Two key components of the transfer were identified: first, that the patient should not pull on the person supervising the transfer, and, second, that he should not stand up all the way but should remain in the squat. When he attended to these issues, all the other parts of the transfer fell into place. The patient was able to do transfers with cues after 1 week.

Standing from a sitting position was a difficult challenge for this patient, and it was an area that was limited by his prostheses. Because he did not have

ankle joints, he could not lean forward enough to come to stand. This was resolved when he spread his feet farther apart and was able to come farther forward.

Directed Attention to the Left Lower Extremity

Throughout the treatment sessions, the patient was asked to complete all left leg movements with muscle power from that leg. For movements that he could not complete, such as lifting his left leg off the leg rest, he was asked to try the movement five times with his muscle before assisting with the right leg. This approach helped the patient gain some skill, but it also helped him direct attention to his left lower extremity. Throughout these activities, he had a successful experience of giving his left leg a message and eventually getting the response he was looking for.

OUTCOME

The patient agreed to stay for 4 weeks, and he met all of the goals. He did not meet his goal of walking by himself; this ability will continue to be limited because of the patient's cognitive problems, including poor judgement and limited problem-solving abilities.

II. Comparison of Patient #1 and Patient #2

A. Patient goals

Being in tune to the patient's goals is very important in providing physical therapy treatment. The goal of walking again, as was the goal of these two patients, is not uncommon for individuals with hemiparesis/hemiplegia. This is magnified by society's emphasis on walking as the accepted means of mobility. For physical therapists, it is important to listen to the patient's goals and to discuss with the patient how realistic the goals are, along with the time frame for achieving the goal. For patient #2, the time frame for achieving the ambulation goal was unrealistic. However, he did not believe the therapist until the time frame had passed and he realized that he had not achieved the goal. On the other hand, patient #1 just wanted to achieve the goal, without putting a time frame on it, but saw the ability to walk as the ticket to returning home.

For many patients, walking may not be a reasonable goal, and they may need to accept, at least for the time being, some other form of mobility. Some patients become efficient with wheelchair mobility and see this as a welcome form of independence even if they are still

working on their ambulation goal. For other patients, ambulation may not be a realistic goal, and this needs to be discussed tactfully with the individual. It is the physical therapist's responsibility to relate her/his opinion to the patient, yet therapists cannot predict the future. If the patient does have a chance to experience ambulation, there are more facts to base this decision on, and the patient may better understand the decision.

In current practice there is a shift from the physical therapist setting the goals for the patient to the patient setting the goals, with negotiation between the patient and the therapist. By understanding the patient's goals, the physical therapy treatment can be focused on working toward achieving these goals.

B. Functional approach to treatment

Because the patient's goals lead to the focus of physical therapy treatment, the functional approach to treatment seems to be the way to achieve the goals. Patient #1 had weakness in her left extremities. At the initial screening, she was able to initiate hip flexion. Her goal may be to be able to lift her leg better when she is walking, *not* to increase hip flexion movement in an isolated pattern through half of the available range against gravity. Therefore, hip flexion should be worked on within the task of ambulation rather than through exercises on the mat.[2]

Because the goal of patient #2 was very focused, he would accept only functional activities as part of his treatment. He would not even consider doing exercises because he did not see the direct relationship of the exercises to his goal. The functional approach may make the treatment more meaningful for the patient, and it gives the patient a chance to be an active problem solver during treatment.[2] The patient may be better able to do these tasks at home when she/he leaves the hospital environment because they are more real to the patient.

C. Similarities and differences between patient #1 and patient #2

1. **Impairments related to function.** In both cases, key impairments contributed to the functional problem. In patient #1, the key impairment was weakness/decreased motor control. Patient #2 also had impaired motor control, but his impaired position sense was the most limiting factor.

2. **Postural patterns.** Specific groupings of postural problems are common after a CVA.

These two patients represent two of these patterns. Patient #1 tends to list toward her involved side. She is aware that she is on the left, but she is slow to respond. Patient #2 lists forcefully to the left but perceives that he lists to the right. Patient #2 demonstrates what is commonly called "the pusher syndrome": the patient forcefully pushes himself/herself onto the involved side. The third pattern, which is not represented here, is the patient who lists to the uninvolved side and is skillful in avoiding the involved side. Forcing the patient to bear weight on the involved extremity is the therapeutic challenge in this situation.

D. Pattern recognition

The therapist treating patient #2 was unsure of her abilities to work with this patient because of her lack of experience with patients who have amputations. She used two strategies to get beyond her uncertainty. First, she recognized a pattern of movement that was familiar and worked with those problems based on previous experience.[2] Second, she consulted with someone experienced with patients who have had amputations. In the end, she was able to meet the patient's needs with minimal input from the consultant, but the consultation was important to ensure that no critical areas were overlooked.

III. Summary

Two patients who have hemiparesis/hemiplegia have been presented with a discussion of the screening, evaluation, assessment, and treatment. The principles of motor control and motor learning have been applied to these patients. These two patients represent the "typical" problems of weakness, decreased motor control, and impaired position sense. These two patients have been compared in reference to the recognition of the problem, the relationship of impairments to function, patient goals, and the functional approach to treatment. The concepts presented here are applicable to other patients who have hemiparesis/hemiplegia.

References

1. Benner P, Tanner C: How expert nurses use intuition. *Am J Nurs*, 1987, 87:23–31.
2. Gentile AM: Skill acquisition: action, movement, and neuromotor processes. In Carr J, Shepherd RB, Gordon J, *et al.* (eds): *Movement Science: Foundations for Physical Therapy in Rehabilitation.* Rockville, MD: Aspen Publishers Inc, 1987, pp. 93–154.
3. Krebs DE, Edelstein JE, Fishman S: Reliability of observational kinematic gait analysis. *Phys Ther,* 1985, 65:1027–1033.

Suggested Reading

Duncan PW: Stroke: physical therapy assessment and treatment. In Lister M (ed): *Contemporary Management of Motor Control Problems: Proceedings of the II STEP Conference.* Alexandria, VA, Foundation for Physical Therapy, 1991.
Duncan PW, Badke MB: *Stroke Rehabilitation: The Recovery of Motor Control.* Chicago, Year Book Medical Publishers, 1987.

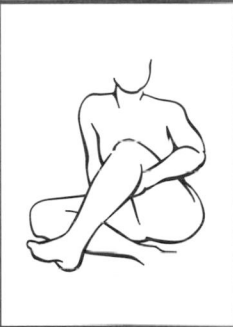

Patients with Quadriplegia

Susan Cromwell

This chapter contains three case studies about people with quadraparesis. The first case describes someone who is newly injured with a spinal cord injury. The second case decribes a person who is having new mobility problems 20 years after his spinal cord injury. The third case describes a woman with multiple sclerosis. Despite the apparent differences in diagnosis and functional history of the three people, the physical therapy process of screening, evaluating, assessing, and formulating treatment plans is very similar. This process, with minimal variations, can be applied to anyone with a quadraparesis with or without complicating factors.

I. Overview

A. Comparison of three patients

1. Patient #1 is a 20-year-old male, 3 weeks post diving accident and 2 weeks post cervical fixation for cervical subluxation. He is now wearing a Philadelphia collar whenever out of bed. He is a college student and was living with his parents for the summer. His goal is to return to his previous level of functioning.

2. Patient #2 is a 40-year-old male, 20 years post cervical spinal cord injury. He was admitted to a rehabilitation facility because of problems living independently. The patient lives alone and has personal care attendants who assist with dressing and transfers. The patient is independent in wheelchair propulsion. His goals are to be independent in transfers out of bed, to require only one person to assist with car transfers, and to be fitted with a more comfortable wheelchair.

3. Patient #3 is a 40-year old female with a 10-year history of multiple sclerosis. She experienced an exacerbation 3 weeks previously and was hospitalized for steroid treatment. She has now been admitted to a rehabilitation facility for functional mobility retraining. She lives alone in a wheelchair-accessible apartment. Before the exacerbation, she walked with forearm crutches for household distances and used a motorized scooter for community mobility. She worked as a secretary.

   Exacerbation level: quadraparesis increased, legs worse than arms. She requires assistance for bed mobility and transfers and is unable to stand or walk. She is unable to propel a manual wheelchair with her hands or legs. She is presently being weaned off steroids. She reports that there has been little improvement in her strength or function since initiation of the steroids 2 weeks previously.

B. Levels of screening

These three cases illustrate different levels of screening and evaluation based on the patients' goals, medical acuity, and potential for significant changes in medical, physical, and functional status.

1. The quadraparesis of patient #1 is very recent, and the patient is most likely still experiencing some spinal shock. Therefore, changes are anticipated in many areas, and the patient is screened for all possible and existing impairments according to guidelines suggested by the American Spinal Injury Association[1] and the Rehabilitation Institute of Chicago (RIC) guide to functional outcomes in spinal cord injury.[2] Because of anticipatory changes in motor control, respiratory function, skin integrity, sensation, and functional mobility, definitive evaluations are performed in all these areas so that an accurate baseline can be established.

2. This procedure is in contrast to what is planned for patient #2, who has had quadraparesis for 25 years. In this case, the screen is performed using the database, a functional evaluation is performed with the patient's personal care attendants, and only those impairments that are thought to have a direct relationship to the patient's bed mobility, transfers, and wheelchair seating problems are evaluated.

3. For patient #3, further significant changes are not anticipated because of the lack of response to the steroid treatment. Although it is not necessary to evaluate as many impairments as in patient #1, motor control is examined and tracked in both arms and legs in as standardized a manner as possible. Thus, a screen is performed using the database, a functional evaluation is performed, and a definitive evaluation of the patient's motor control, in addition to any other impairments that may directly contribute to her functional immobility, is done.

C. Screening process

Each patient is screened in almost the same way, and it is noted where each differs. Information from the database is used to assist in formulating hypotheses about the relationship between the impairments and the functional problem. An extensive interview with the attendants and patient #2 was conducted because

his rehabilitation admission is based on independent living problems.

1. **Medication.** The therapist notes any medications that affect alertness, resistance to passive movement, and/or reflex activity of the extremities (baclofen, dantrolene sodium).

2. **Communication.** Any speech or language problems that are noticed during normal conversation are noted, particularly the need for frequent pauses during a sentence. This could indicate respiratory dysfunction, especially in patient #1.

3. **Cardiovascular.** Any cardiac problems that would be pertinent in an emergency are documented. Patient #1 is more likely than the others to experience orthostatic hypotension, so any complaints of blurry vision and/or lightheadedness should be carefully observed. In both spinal cord cases, the patients should be questioned about any symptoms of autonomic dysreflexia.

4. **Pulmonary.** Any recent history of respiratory problems should be noted.

5. **Metabolic.** The therapist notes any metabolic disturbances.

6. **Gastrointestinal/genitourinary.** Any stomach or digestive complaints are noted. For patient #1, information on bowel and bladder continence should be noted in order to comply with the patient's schedule and to avoid embarrassment to the patient.

7. **Vision.** Visual disturbances may be most apparent in patient #3, and this should be noted.

8. **Behavior.** Any behavior that might have a negative impact on the physical therapy treatment process should be noted. The therapist should be aware that patients with new functional disabilities, as in the case of patients #1 and #3, may have mood and attitude fluctuations.

9. **Appliances.** Any assistive devices that the patients are using or that is anticipated they will need should be noted. Patients should be questioned about their attitudes regarding assistive devices. All three patients have wheelchair seating needs that will be addressed in a definitive evaluation.

10. **Pain.** Any pain should be noted.

11. **Skin/soft tissue.** Any edema should be

noted, especially in the lower extremities. Any areas of skin breakdown should be noted; key areas are the sacrum, ischial tuberosities, the greater trochanters, and the malleoli.

12. **Skeletal problem.** Any significant range of motion limitation should be noted. The presence of scoliosis or other trunk deformities should be noted because these have an impact on wheelchair seating. Any heterotopic ossification process should be noted.

13. **Neuromuscular.** Key upper extremity muscle groups to test on a screen include the shoulder flexors, abductors, elbow flexors and extensors, and wrist extensors. Motor strength greater than 3/5 in these muscle groups in anyone with quadraparesis (regardless of the etiology) indicates the potential for independent functional mobility. A quick screen can be performed for muscle activity in the major muscle groups of the legs. If any motor activity is evident below the level of the injury in the upper and lower extremities, the therapist can proceed to a definitive manual muscle testing evaluation. However, manual muscle testing has questionable use in persons exhibiting posturing and/or synergistic movement patterns.

14. **Balance.** The ability to sit and stand unsupported should be noted. Patient #3, who has been using a scooter, needs to be screened for safety in the scooter now that her motor control and mobility have deteriorated. The ability to sit supported in a wheelchair should be noted, as well as whether the wheelchair needs to be reclined. Frequently, patients with new spinal cord injuries feel most balanced when sitting slightly reclined. This is especially true if the person is wearing a halo vest or Philadelphia collar.

15. **Posture.** Sitting posture is most critical to notice in patient #2 because of the longstanding quadraparesis. For patient #3, her sitting posture on the scooter is important to note because she may wish to use the scooter rather than a wheelchair during rehabilitation.

16. **Functional mobility.** General descriptions of the amount of physical assistance that each patient needs should be communicated to the rest of the health care team so that routine care can be carried out without risk of injury to the patient or staff.

17. **Gait pattern.** This is not applicable to any of these patients.

Clinical Decision-Making Cases

Case #1

SUMMARY OF SCREENING

Patient #1 has no pertinent medical problems. There are no reports of autonomic dysreflexia. He is being started on a bowel program and has had frequent accidents. He is presently being catheterized intermittently. His skeletal injury was C5, C6 subluxation, and he underwent a posterior spinal fusion. He has slight movement in his right hand, hip, and knee as well as in shoulder musculature and elbow flexors bilaterally. Wrist extension is present in the right upper extremity. Sensation is impaired but not absent in the trunk and lower extremities. He has sat upright in a reclined wheelchair, at about 45 degrees, without experiencing orthostatic hypotension. Functionally, he requires a total lift into the reclining wheelchair. He is dependent for all self-care activities.

FUNCTIONAL EVALUATION

The functional evaluation begins with a transfer out of the wheelchair once the patient has adjusted orthostatically. He is slowly brought to a full upright position and asked to assist the therapist with his arms in any way that he can. Once sitting upright in the chair, if he has not experienced any hypotensive symptoms, a sliding board is placed under his leg and a sliding board transfer to a bed or mat is begun with the assistance of another person. Because the patient does have some movement, his ability to participate in the transfer with either of his arms or his right leg is evaluated.

Once the patient is sitting on the edge of the bed, his ability to sit unsupported with and without the support of his arms is evaluated. Evaluating this ability without the support of his arms gives the therapist an opportunity to determine whether the patient is actively using any trunk muscles.

STANDARD NEUROLOGICAL CLASSIFICATION OF SPINAL CORD INJURY

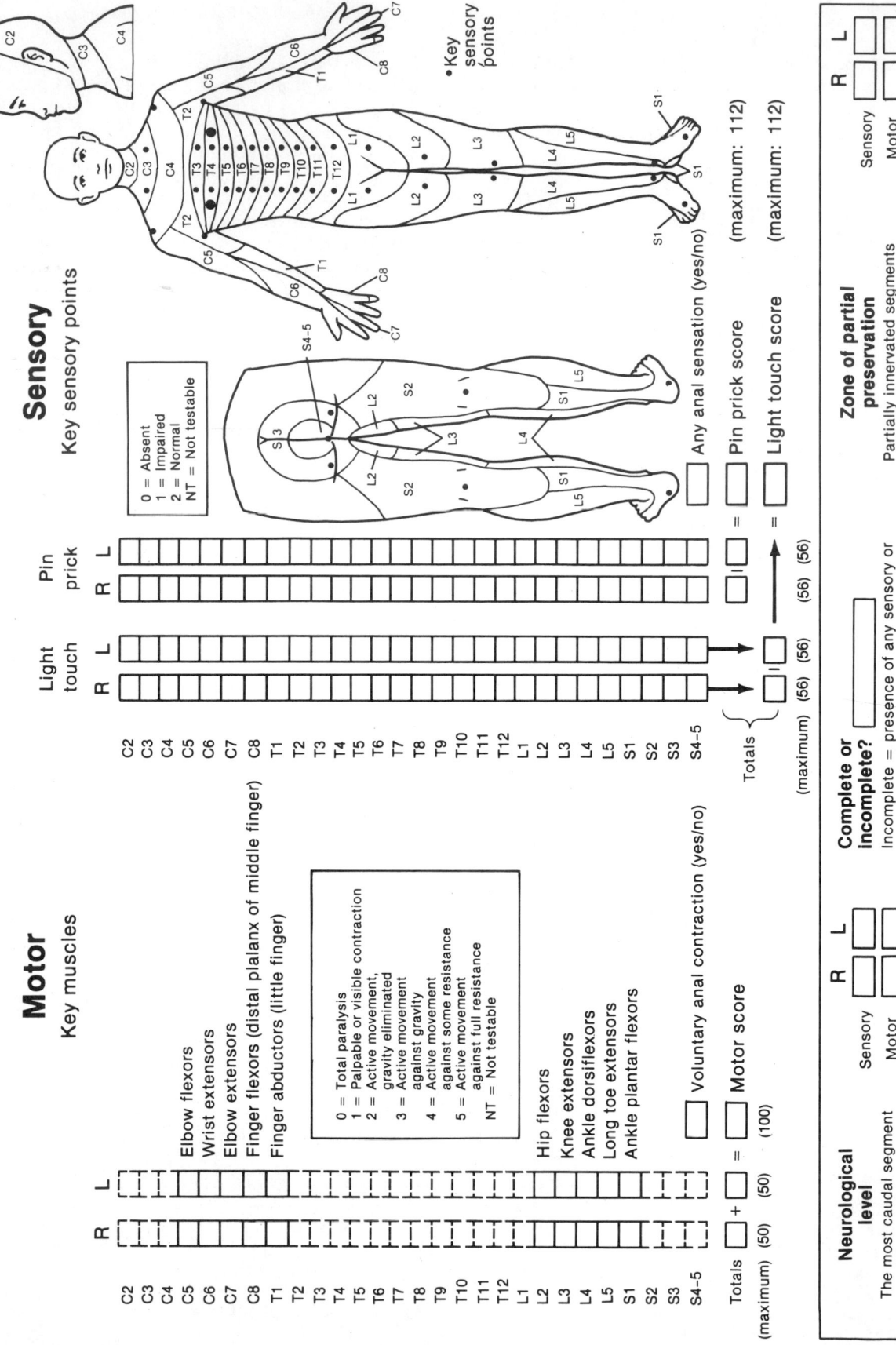

FIGURE 15–1 American Spinal Injury Association standard neurological classification of spinal cord injury form. (Courtesy of the American Spinal Injury Association.)

The patient is then assisted to a supine position, and he is again instructed to participate by using his arms and legs as much as possible. The same procedure is followed for rolling and for assuming a prone position.

For a transfer back to the wheelchair, the entire process is reversed. At that time, the patient is asked to push the wheelchair using both arms and his right leg if possible.

During the entire functional evaluation, the patient's comfort and anxiety level and his physical response to being upright are evaluated. The level of his participation is documented, as well as the movement patterns that he attempts to use during the functional activities.

Summary of Functional Evaluation

The patient participates in all activities by placing his arms in the appropriate locations. He is able to support some of his body weight with his right arm during transfers and with sitting activities. Each time he attempts to use his left arm, it slides out from under him.

The patient can push down slightly with his right leg during the transfer and also lift it off the floor about 2 to 3 inches when transitioning to a supine position. He is unable to move the left leg at all during any activity.

The patient is unable to sit unsupported without using his arms, but he can sit momentarily with his arms down on the mat, in an elbow- and wrist-extended tenodesis position.

He does not complain of any symptoms related to hypotension or dysreflexia.

The patient can place both hands on the wheelchair rim. He initiates wheel pushing with his right hand but not with his left.

Interpretation of Database and Functional Evaluation: Formation of Hypotheses

The therapist formed the following hypotheses regarding the contribution of impairments to the functional problem: This patient has significant motor loss, and this directly relates to his functional immobility. Because of his medical acuity, there is a potential for other complications to develop (pulmonary, skin, flexibility); therefore, the RIC manual will be used to assist in choosing the impairments to evaluate for use later as a baseline measure.[2] Because of the possibility that the patient's motor control could change, strength and motor recovery are evaluated carefully.

FURTHER IMPAIRMENT TESTING

The following impairments are definitively evaluated:

1. Motor strength: To evaluate the strength of any active muscle, the manual muscle testing procedure is used. The American Spinal Injury Association provides a form and standardized instructions for testing and classifying neurological and sensory impairments (see Figure 15–1).[1] Specifically, the C5, C6, C7 muscle groups and the major muscle groups of the trunk and lower extremities are tested. This procedure should be followed with every new spinal cord patient because of the high likelihood that a person may have sparing and not know it. A major muscle group in the lower extremities in someone with "complete paralysis" can be tested only to find that the person can initiate a contraction. This procedure can be performed every 1 or 2 weeks during the rehabilitation phase to keep track of any new motor recovery. However, this can be very discouraging to the patient who remains unable to produce any motor activity. With a thorough explanation, though, patients are quite appreciative of the procedure.

2. Resistance to passive movement and involuntary muscle activity: The presence or absence of resistance to passive movement is evaluated in key muscle groups: hip abductors, knee flexors, plantar flexors, shoulder adductors, elbow and wrist flexors. Severe resistance to passive movement in these areas can make hygienic care and dressing difficult tasks. The presence or absence of involuntary movements of the extremities or trunk, occurring with exertion, passive movement of a different part of the body, or sensory stimulation (foot on a foot pedal, rubbing of clothing), is also documented. Frequent involuntary movements of any extremity can interfere with functional mobility.

3. Skin integrity: This is an evaluation that requires several days or weeks to complete because the therapist is evaluating the patient's response to different wheelchairs and cushions. It is important to keep track of the length of time that a particular skin area has been under pressure, how often the area has been relieved of pressure, and what the skin looks like after the patient has been lying down or sitting on a particular wheelchair cushion.

4. Sensation: The most important sensory testing to be done is that of pressure and temperature. This is because an absence of either of these sensory experiences can mean a higher risk of skin breakdown or burns. The American Spinal Injury Association recommends light touch and pinprick sensory testing for classification purposes.[1]

5. Respiratory: The patient is asked to cough hard enough to produce sputum, if possible. This begins to tell the therapist how well the patient can handle his/her secretions. The patient is also asked to read aloud a lengthy paragraph, and the number of breaths taken are counted. Neither of these evaluative techniques has documented reliability or validity, but they provide clues to patient status that might indicate an existing problem. The other rec-

ommendations for evaluation outlined in the RIC manual are followed.[2]

6. Cardiovascular status: Blood pressure is measured and monitored, as well as symptoms for orthostatic hypotension and autonomic dysreflexia during impairment testing, but especially during the functional evaluation because that can be quite physically and emotionally stressful.

7. Wheelchair fit: The patient is provided with a wheelchair that matches his/her width, arm and leg length, and leg depth. A nonreclining wheelchair is optimal if the patient can tolerate one without becoming hypotensive or feeling as if he/she is falling forward. Otherwise, a reclining wheelchair is best to start with while gradually decreasing the recline before moving to a nonreclining chair. If the patient is unable to, or unlikely to be able to, propel a manual wheelchair (no wrist extensors), one must consider an electric chair with some type of hand-, chin-, or breath-activated controls. Several types of wheelchairs, (electric vs manual, lightweight vs active lightweight/sport) may need to be tried and evaluated during the rehabilitation admission to determine the best choice for the patient. This should be done in conjunction with an equipment specialist and reputable vendor.

Summary of Impairment Evaluation

1. Motor: Neurological injury is C5 in the left upper extremity and C7 in the right. Muscle strength in the right upper extremity is 4/5 for shoulder musculature and elbow flexors. Elbow extensors are tested at 3/5. Finger flexors are tested at 2/5. Left upper extremity has no active movement below C5 innervated muscles. Left leg has no active movement. Right leg has active hip flexion and knee extension (2/5) and plantar flexion (2/5).

2. Resistance to passive motion and involuntary muscle activity: The patient infrequently exhibits hip and knee involuntary flexion in the right leg when supine; stimulus unclear. Not observed in sitting. Mild resistance to passive movement noted in the right plantar flexors.

3. Sensation: The patient is able to detect pressure over sacrum and ischial tuberosities. He can detect the differences in ischial pressure when sitting on a wheelchair cushion and when sitting on the wheelchair upholstery alone. He is able to detect extremes of temperature.

4. Skin: The patient's skin is intact.

5. Respiratory: The patient has a weak cough. He is able to produce a little sputum with several attempts. More sputum was obtained with an assisted cough from the therapist. He is able to read a paragraph with a breath every three or four words.

6. Wheelchair fit: A 16-inch wide, nonreclining wheelchair is chosen to start with because the patient is 15 inches wide at the hips and is short, thereby requiring a chair that is lower than standard height so that he can reach the ground with his feet. Reaching the ground with his feet is important because the patient has some motor activity in his right leg, which he might be able to use for wheelchair propulsion. The patient is provided with a low-profile ROHO cushion because he has prominent ischial tuberosities and must eliminate as much pressure as possible. If he has problems with sitting balance on this cushion, which frequently occurs, he might be switched to a gel cushion.

FINAL INTERPRETATION OF DATABASE, FUNCTIONAL EVALUATION, AND IMPAIRMENT TESTING

The patient has significant motor loss, which is thought to relate directly to his functional immobility. However, he has sufficient strength in key muscle groups of the right arm and leg (elbow extensors, wrist extensors, right hand and leg function) such that even without further motor recovery his functional mobility could improve. Lack of motor activity below the level of C5 could significantly limit progress and eventual outcome. The patient does not know how to maximize and direct his existing motor strength into functional use. On the basis of this hypothesis, a treatment program is recommended that is based on compensatory muscle function and functional activity training.

TREATMENT GOALS

The patient's goals are to return to his previous level of functioning. He finds it difficult to envision himself with residual deficits. Because it is unclear what, if any, residual deficits will remain, it is suggested that his goal is kept as a long-term goal and that, in the meantime, he and the therapist work toward activities that improve his immediate living situation. For example, it is suggested that the work be aimed toward sitting up in a wheelchair, self-propelling himself, and less dependency on others for self-care and transfers. It is explained to him that standing could be a goal as soon as more pushing with the right leg during transfers is observed. He is willing to work toward these goals.

APPROACH TO TREATMENT

A program of active exercise that reverses the action of the upper extremity muscles (fixing wrist and elbows distally and moving shoulders and trunk proximally) should allow the patient to gain increased use of arm strength in a manner similar to what is needed for functional activities. Successful bed mobility and transfers for a person with this level of quadraparesis is best accomplished by placing the wrists or elbows on the bed and pushing in a multitude of directions in order to move the trunk side to side, or in and out of the vertical position. Using the muscles in this manner is foreign and requires motor re-education through exercise. Motor re-education cannot be accomplished through the traditional progressive resistive exercise programs. However, many activities of daily living require a free hand, with the proximal joint fixed. Traditional progressive resistive exercises may be helpful for these activities of daily living if done in functional movement patterns.

The psychological aspect of lifting weights is important to many people in this age group because it is an activity many individuals engage in as a route to physical fitness. Physical therapists should acknowledge the psychological benefit that traditional weight lifting may have on the overall attitude, self-esteem, and sense of community involvement of the patient during the rehabilitative process. In addition, an exercise program that emphasizes the functional use of the patient's legs will maximize the use of his right leg and provide opportunity for any motor ability of the left leg to be revealed if recovery were to continue. The bulk of the treatment activities should focus around functional activities. These activities can be very strenuous, especially if repetitively performed, and are a good mechanism for improving function as well as improving the strength in many muscles simultaneously.

Because each functional activity has its own unique characteristics, it is unlikely that the skills used in one will transfer to another. Therefore, work should be done on rolling, bed mobility, and transfers right from the beginning; the therapist should not wait for one activity to be accomplished before initiating training in another. Because of the motor activity in the patient's right leg, standing in the parallel bars is initiated as soon as both he and the therapist feel that he can push down into the floor with his right foot. It is anticipated that he will need quite a bit of support from other people, but the activity of standing will probably be psychologically therapeutic as well as therapeutic from a motor and functional standpoint.

Case #2

SUMMARY OF SCREENING

The patient has significant range of motion limitations at the hips and knees. He exhibits a moderate scoliosis with right thoracic convexity. He demonstrates incomplete quadraparesis with some minimal trunk and leg musculature. Motor control in the right arm is at a C-8 level, and at C-7 on the left. Skin integrity is good, although the patient has a history of skin breakdown on his sacrum. Functionally, he requires moderate assistance for transfers and bed mobility. He sits independently on the edge of his bed using his arms for support. In his wheelchair, he sits closer to the right armrest and has difficulty reaching the left wheel rim. His legs are windswept to the left. He presently uses a standard 18-inch wide wheelchair. He uses a 3-inch piece of T foam for a cushion. His cushion is 5 years old.

FURTHER TESTING

Interview Questions

The therapist asks the patient and his attendants

1. To explain specifically the mobility problems he is having at home and how he has attempted to fix them.
2. To describe his daily routine: what time he gets up,

how long he stays up, how often he uses his wheelchair, and how often he goes out in the car.
3. To explain what he would like in a new wheelchair.
4. To explain how well the patient feels he is able to describe to his attendants how to help him with his mobility.
5. To describe what his bed looks like, how high up off the ground it is, and the type of commode he uses.

Summary of Interview

The patient states that he used to require only minimal assistance with his legs for bed mobility and for balance during transfers. Over the past several years, his need for additional assistance has gradually increased. Home health physical therapy services have not been available in his very rural area. In terms of his daily routine, he is described as being a late riser, and he stays up in his wheelchair for about 3 hours before returning to bed. He would like to go out in his car two to three times a week but rarely has the necessary amount of assistance (two people) for car transfers. He would like a narrower wheelchair, with different footrests to prevent his feet from sliding off, and a new cushion. He feels he does not know what the best way is for his attendants to help him. He uses a hospital bed and a drop-arm commode.

Functional Task Evaluation

For this evaluation, the patient and his attendants are asked to perform the bed mobility and transfer (bed and commode) activities as if they were at home. The hospital bed in the patient's rehabilitation room is used. Car transfers are observed next. Because both of his attendants are with the patient, they are observed performing the transfer as it is done at home.

Summary of Functional Task Evaluation

1. Bed mobility: The patient rolls to both sides independently using the bed rails.
2. Supine to sit and vice versa: Before the patient attempts to come to a sitting position, the attendant places both of the patient's feet over the edge of the bed and leans over and pulls the patient up to sitting by pulling on the arms. When returning to supine position, the patient lies down on his back and the attendants lift his legs up onto the bed. In order to begin sitting up at the edge of the right side of the bed, he requires assistance to rise up on his right elbow. He then requires assistance to flex his hips and knees to a position where they fall off the edge of the bed and he can use momentum to bring his trunk up to a vertical position.
3. Bed and commode transfers: The patient is unable to maintain his balance independently while placing the sliding board. He leans backward during the transfer and needs assistance to maintain his buttocks on the sliding board. The attendants are in the habit of placing his feet on the footrests before he attempts to slide his buttocks over to the wheelchair. Once he is in the chair, he repositions his hips by alternately hooking his arms on the push handles and pulling his hips to the desired position. He requires assistance to place his feet on the footrests. When transferring to the commode, he requires assistance for positioning of his hips because there are no push handles.
4. Car transfers: During the car transfer, the attendants again first place his legs inside the car. The patient is then leaning very far backward and requires maximal assistance to come forward, grab the top of the car and slide into the driver's seat. Both attendants are assisting from the outside of the car. When he transfers out of the car, he is physically lifted by his attendants (one at the legs, and one under the arms).

Interpretation of Screening, Interview, and Functional Evaluation

It remains unclear why the patient's functional abilities have deteriorated over the last several years. It may be that his attendants changed so frequently that continuity in care was lost. Perhaps his range of motion has worsened—this is difficult to know because of a lack of baseline data. However, he has the potential to change the manner in which he performs some of his activities so that he would require less assistance. Impairments that are contributing to his mobility and seating problems are the lack of range of motion in his hips and knees and the scoliosis in his trunk. To recommend a properly fitted wheelchair, the patient's range of motion measurements at the hips, knees, and ankles are needed. It is also necessary to know how flexible the patient's scoliosis is and if he can be passively stretched to a neutral position. It is important to obtain this information because a modified wheelchair back may be necessary to support the scoliosis. Detailed muscle testing is not necessary because the patient is neurologically stable.

Further Testing

1. Range of motion measurements at the hips, knees, and ankles.
2. Flexibility of scoliosis measured by passively stretching out the patient's thoracic and lumbar area and visualizing how much of a correction can be made. This is not a reliable or valid measurement technique; no other clinical techniques that would provide the information helpful for wheelchair positioning are known.
3. Wheelchair measurements: standard measurements are seat width, seat depth, leg length, and arm length.

SUMMARY OF IMPAIRMENT TESTING

Range of motion measurements at the hips are 70 degrees on the right and 90 degrees on the left. Knee flexion is 65 degrees on the right and 100 degrees on the left. Ankle dorsiflexion is to neutral bilaterally. The patient's scoliosis is fixed. The patient's hip width is 16 inches, seat depth 19 inches, arm length 9 inches, and leg length 22 inches.

FINAL INTERPRETATION OF INTERVIEW, FUNCTIONAL EVALUATION, AND IMPAIRMENT TESTING

Significant range of motion limitations in both lower extremities and trunk definitely affect the techniques the patient can use for bed mobility and transfers. However, these limitations do not render the patient's goals unattainable. Fitting this patient in a wheelchair will involve several trials of chairs with modified cushioned backs and seat cushions. Elevating footrests may be necessary to accommodate the patient's lack of knee flexion on the right.

TREATMENT GOALS

1. The patient will be independent in bed mobility and bed/commode transfers.
2. The patient will require the assistance of only one person for a car transfer.

3. The patient will be able to procure a wheelchair that is comfortable and supports skin integrity and functional abilities.

APPROACH TO TREATMENT

A functional task relearning program is recommended to the patient and his attendants. The attendants must be involved in the process. The problem-solving process that the patient and the attendants go through, with the therapist facilitating, should make the transition to the home situation much easier and more successful over the long term. Therefore, the attendants are requested to participate actively in each treatment session (twice daily). The rehabilitation team felt very strongly that this procedure should be used in all of the patient's therapies and approached the third-party payers with the proposal. The third-party payers guaranteed continued payment for the attendants even though the patient was hospitalized.

To provide the patient with a properly fitting wheelchair, he was first given a 16-inch-wide chair with an extra-depth seat. A narrow wheelchair provides more lateral stability, prevents side-to-side movement of the pelvis, and also controls the position of the legs. The extra depth is needed because the patient sits on his sacrum owing to the lack of hip flexion. Sacral sitting gives the appearance of longer femur length, and patients generally benefit from a longer seat depth. The patient is also given a modular Jay back cushion, which allows the back foam pieces to be modified to support his scoliosis and to keep him in the middle of the wheelchair. The first seat cushion tried is a low-profile ROHO. This minimizes pressure. Because ROHO cushions are not firm, patients tend to find them slightly unstable. Other cushions exist that provide pressure relief and more stability. The patient needs to be questioned and observed as he propels the wheelchair, manages his wheelchair parts, and prepares for a transfer. An elevated leg rest may be necessary to support the right leg.

Case #3

SUMMARY OF SCREENING

The patient is being weaned from steroid treatment that she started 2 weeks previously. She has no cardiovascular, pulmonary, metabolic, or gastrointestinal/genitourinary problems. Her vision is slightly blurred. Her mood is despondent; she cries frequently and expresses resentment over her illness. She is not reporting any pain. Skin integrity is good. Range of motion is normal in both upper and lower extremities. Paresis is noted in all extremities; it is greater in the legs than in the arms. Resistance to passive motion is noted in quadriceps and plantar flexor muscles bilaterally. With exertion, lower extremities are postured in extension. The patient is able to sit unsupported on the edge of the bed if she is not engaged in an activity. When moving arms or legs, she requires assistance to prevent falling. She requires no assistance for rolling, but moderate assistance for assuming sitting and supine positions. She requires moderate to maximal assistance for stand-pivot or sliding board transfers out of bed to her wheelchair or scooter. She maintains her balance and drives her scooter in the nursing unit independently.

FURTHER TESTING

Interview Questions

The interview questions should cover

1. History of recent problem.
2. Discharge plans.
3. Goals and desired treatment focus.
4. Endurance level prior to exacerbation.
5. Physical activities enjoyed.

Summary of Interview

The patient reports that this exacerbation is the first one in 4 years. Prior to this, she had been working part-time as a secretary and swimming three to four times a week. She was able to walk around her home using forearm crutches but used her scooter in the community and at work. She is fearful that she may not return to her previous level of functioning and is making plans to live with a friend who can provide her with physical assistance. She believes that her leg strength is the key to her functional problems and would like the strength to be measured and monitored as often as possible, as she continues to hope that the steroid treatment may be effective despite physician statements to the contrary. She does not wish to consider any type of wheelchair at this time. She acknowledges that the scooter may be uncomfortable to sit in all day; however, she is hoping that her strength will increase enough that she will not need a wheelchair.

Functional Task Evaluation

The patient is asked to demonstrate the way she moves her trunk and extremities to reposition herself in bed, come to sitting and supine positions, transfer, and stand. She is asked to show or explain how she has tried to make these activities easier. The number of times she repeats the activity before she reports fatigue or until she requires more assistance is documented. Her ability to maneuver her scooter in open spaces, in tight spaces (as in a home), and outside on surfaces similar to those at her home and her friend's home is evaluated.

Summary of Functional Task Evaluation

The patient repositions herself in bed and rolls side to side independently by using the bed rails. Without the bed rails, she initiates rolling to either side but is unable to move her hips. Her legs remain in, or involuntarily move into, an extended position. She is unable to flex her trunk enough to come to a sitting position from either a sidelying or supine position. When assuming a supine position, she lies straight back and uses her arms and the bed rails to reposition herself in the bed. During a sliding board transfer, she cannot lift and push her buttocks across the board with her arms. When attempting a stand-pivot transfer, she requires moderate to maximal assistance to push up into a standing position with her legs and arms. Once standing, she remains flexed at the trunk. She is unable to pivot on her feet and requires moderate assistance to complete the transfer. She performs each activity two to three times before fatiguing. She independently maneuvers her scooter in open and tight spaces and outside on small paved hills and sidewalks.

Interpretation of Screening, Interview, and Functional Evaluation

The patient has significant motor and functional deficits resulting from the recent exacerbation of multiple sclerosis. It is hypothesized that the significant contributors to her functional problems are

1. Motor control problems (lack of active movement and extensor posturing in legs with exertion).
2. Low endurance, which contributes to her inability to tolerate trying new functional maneuvers.
3. Lack of awareness of alternative methods of carrying out functional activities.

It is hypothesized that she will not attain her previous level of functioning without significant changes in all of the above areas and that her functional abilities can improve to a minimal assistive level with an increase in awareness of alternative methods of carrying out the desired activities. The three impairments and functional abilities will be measured on a regular basis.

FURTHER IMPAIRMENT TESTING

1. Motor control: Testing of motor control is difficult to do in a case like this. Three possibilities exist: manual muscle testing, standardized testing such as the Fugl-Meyer assessment (see Table 11–1), or a description of movement behaviors during functional activities. The third choice is preferred, although it is probably less reliable and valid than the others. Describing the movement behaviors observed during

functional activities is a good choice because, in multiple sclerosis, motor behavior is frequently a function of the patient's position and the activity that the patient is trying to perform. The resistance to passive motion is not a factor in the amount of active movement or in the functional mobility of the patient, but the extensor posturing observed during exertion interferes with her ability to complete the task (see Chapter 8). Manual muscle testing reliability and validity may be compromised by her posturing. The Fugl-Meyer assessment is a possibility because it evaluates the presence of isolated and synergistic movements in all extremities in supine, sitting, and standing positions, yet not during functional movements or tasks. The Fugl-Meyer assessment was designed for people with cerebrovascular accidents, and the reliability and validity for people with multiple sclerosis cannot be assumed to be the same. For more information on these testing procedures, refer to Table 11–1.

2. Endurance: This is another area that is difficult to measure in a functionally meaningful, reliable, and valid manner. The amount of rests that the patient requests in a 45-minute treatment session in the AM and in the PM are documented. The activities (quantity and type) that take place in between each rest break also are documented. Collecting data in this manner provides the patient with useful information about structuring her days in the hospital, on therapeutic weekend passes, and at discharge. The data assist the therapist in structuring the treatment sessions so that maximal benefit can be gained.

3. Knowledge about altering the manner of carrying out functional activities: This is an area that is very difficult to measure in a reliable and valid way. The number of ways that the patient demonstrates or explains to me how she might be able to modify each of the problematic functional tasks so that they become easier are counted.

Summary of Impairment Testing

1. Motor control: The patient does not fully extend her arms from a flexed position when attempting to sit from a sidelying position or when attempting to come to a standing position with a walker. She uses elbow flexion effectively to reposition herself in bed but could not pull herself to the wheelchair during a sliding board transfer. Her legs remain in extension during rolling and when attempting to sit from supine. If her knees are passively flexed about 10 to 20 degrees, she can flex the hip and knee about another 20 degrees each. Sometimes, starting with her legs partially flexed requires less assistance for supine to sit. Her legs extend each time she pushes with her arms during a sliding board transfer; how-

ever, she is unable to fully extend her knees when assuming standing from sitting.

2. Endurance: The patient asks for five to six rest breaks of 2 to 3 minutes each during a 45-minute treatment session. In between the rest breaks, she performs several trials of rolling and assuming sitting. One transfer encompasses another part of the session. She tolerates three attempts at standing for 2 to 3 seconds each before requiring a rest break of several minutes.

3. Knowledge: This patient is unable to describe any other method or modification for carrying out any of the problematic functional activities.

FINAL INTERPRETATION OF INTERVIEW, FUNCTIONAL EVALUATION, AND IMPAIRMENT TESTING

The patient has the greatest chance at improving her functional level by learning alternative or compensatory movement strategies for performing different functional tasks. Her lack of alternative methods for these tasks and her difficulty with problem solving are limiting factors. Her endurance is probably going to limit the amount of experimentation with different movement strategies. Her reluctance to investigate wheelchair possibilities, despite the discomfort of her scooter, may promote excessive bed rest and limit the community involvement that she says she enjoys.

TREATMENT GOALS

After discussing the results of the evaluation with the patient, she described some short-term goals to work on in therapy; however, she still held onto the long-term goal to return to previous functional and motor level.

1. Minimal assistance for assuming sitting and supine positions.
2. Minimal assistance for sliding board or stand-pivot transfers.
3. Sit to stand with minimal assistance.
4. Ability to stand with a walker for 10 seconds.

APPROACH TO TREATMENT

The best approach to treatment is a functionally based treatment program, emphasizing patient problem solving and energy conservation. Caregiver training is an important component of the program because the patient is not expected to be independent by discharge. The physical therapist plans to work closely with the occupational therapist to find ways in which the patient's clothing can be modified or straps applied to her legs so that she can passively flex her hips and knees for assuming a sitting position from supine. Wheelchair evaluation is on hold at the patient's request.

References

1. *The International Standards for Neurological and Functional Classifications of Spinal Cord Injury. 1992 Edition.* Chicago, American Spinal Injury Association and the International Medical Society of Paraplegia, 1992.
2. Nixon V. *Spinal Cord Injury: A Guide to Functional Outcomes in Physical Therapy Management. Rehabilitation Institute of Chicago Procedure Manual.* Maryland, Aspen Publishers, 1985

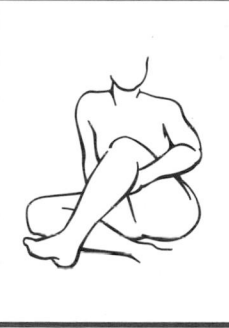

CHAPTER 16

Patients with a Low Level of Responsiveness

Marianne Orest

In the case studies presented in this chapter, the physical therapist is screening, evaluating, assessing, and treating two patients who have a low level of responsiveness, with the major problem being impaired mobility. A low level of responsiveness can result from many different causes, and each patient can present a very different picture. The cases presented here represent two patients who start at similar places yet progress differently. The treatment can be advanced depending on the progress. These two patients are compared, looking at both the similarities and differences of the physical therapy involvement.

I. Overview

A. Introduction to two patients

1. Patient #1 is a 46-year-old female who was involved in a motor vehicle accident when her car slid on ice. Cardiopulmonary resuscitation was performed at the scene of the accident. She was intubated, and a chest tube was placed at a community hospital. The patient was transferred to the regional tertiary care center because of her unresponsiveness. Four days after admission, she was referred to physical therapy. The patient is a single mother with one child still at home; she is employed as a secretary.

2. Patient #2 is a 41-year-old male who was involved in a motor vehicle accident when his car struck a tree head-on at a high speed. He was intubated at a community hospital and was posturing in the emergency room. He was transferred to the regional tertiary care center because of increased intracranial pressure (ICP). Two days after admission, he was referred to physical therapy. The patient is married with no children and is employed as a computer consultant.

B. Screening of database items

The database is to be completed in the usual manner with special attention to the following parameters, which are particularly important in working with a patient who has a low level of responsiveness. The database assists the therapist to be aware of the patient's medical conditions that may have an impact on the physical therapy treatment. This information can be gathered by reviewing the patient's chart, communicating with team members, and interviewing the patient (if possible) and/or family members.

405

1. **Medication.** Medications controlling ICP, spasticity, seizures, and behavior may affect the patient's participation in treatment.

2. **Communication.** Any hearing deficits, aphasia, or dysarthria may affect the patient's ability to communicate her/his needs or to participate in the therapy program.

3. **Behavior (key area).** Cognitive and behavior problems should be noted in relation to the patient's participation in physical therapy. Formal testing in these areas will be done by the occupational therapist and the speech and language pathologist. The patient's score on the Rancho Los Amigos levels of cognitive functioning[1] and on the Glasgow coma scale can give the therapist a sense of how the patient will be able to participate in physical therapy treatment, which may have an impact on or influence motor recovery.

4. **Appliances.** If the patient has an ICP bolt and monitor, it can be used to gauge the physical therapy treatment. The therapist should note whether the patient has previously used, or will perhaps need, any type of adaptive equipment, orthotic devices, assistive devices, splints for positioning, or wheelchair.

5. **Skin/soft tissue.** Any laceration should be noted. If an affected extremity is left in a dependent position, edema may occur.

6. **Skeletal.** Limitations in range of motion of the affected extremities, especially dorsiflexion and shoulder range, may affect the patient's function. For example, if dorsiflexion is limited, the patient may have difficulty during ambulation. The therapist lists fractures and is aware of precautions related to the fractures.

7. **Neuromuscular (key area).** Problems with motor control, increased resistance to passive movement, and sensation usually have an impact on functional activities in patients with a low level of responsiveness.

8. **Balance (key area).** If the patient has a problem with static or dynamic balance, she/he should probably not be left alone in the sitting or standing position for safety reasons.

9. **Posture (key area).** If problems are noted with alignment/rotation, midline orientation, or the position of the extremities, it may indicate a weakness or a problem with the patient's perception of her/his body in space. Any posturing of the patient's extremities should be noted.

10. **Functional mobility (key area).** Deficits noted in bed mobility, transfers, ambulation on level surfaces, stairs, wheelchair mobility, or community mobility may direct the physical therapy treatment.

11. **Gait pattern (key area).** Any deviations observed during the cycles of gait are noted. Toe clearance of the affected extremity is important to note because if the patient is having difficulty with toe clearance, bracing may be indicated.

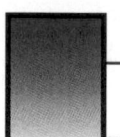

Clinical Decision-Making Cases

Cases of Patient #1 and Patient #2

SUMMARY OF SCREENING

See Table 16–1 on facing page.

IMPAIRMENTS IDENTIFIED FROM SCREENING

1. Patient #1: decreased movement, decreased responsiveness, increased posturing, decreased range of motion, impaired communication.

2. Patient #2: decreased movement, decreased responsiveness, increased resistance to passive movement, impaired communication, decreased skin integrity.

IMPAIRMENTS INDICATING FURTHER EVALUATION DUE TO POSSIBILITY OF CONTRIBUTING TO IMPAIRED MOBILITY

At this time, the patient's functional status cannot be evaluated because of the ICP bolt and the bed rest order. Therefore, the evaluation needs to stay at the impairment level.

Table 16–1. SUMMARY OF THE SCREENING

Parameter	Patient #1	Patient #2
Medical tests	MRI report shows left-sided pontine midbrain and cerebellar lesions and a right thalamic lesion	CT scan shows diffuse axonal injury and multiple punctate hemorrhages
Medication	Analgesics, diuretics, anticonvulsants, antibiotics, cardiovascular Antispasmodics	Analgesics, diuretics, anticonvulsants, antibiotics, cardiovascular
Communication	Nonverbal due to intubation	Nonverbal due to intubation
Cardiovascular	Exploratory thoracotomy with repair of epicardial tear	
Pulmonary	Intubated with full ventilator support Left upper lobe lung contusion, chest tube	Intubated with full ventilator support Pneumonia
Vision	Eyes closed throughout screening	Eyes closed throughout screening
Behavior	Unresponsive	Unresponsive Restless movement of feet and left hand
Appliances	ICP bolt, monitoring lines, ventilator	ICP bolt, monitoring lines, ventilator
Skin and soft tissue		Laceration at base of skull, ecchymotic right shoulder
Skeletal	Multiple rib fractures, limited range of motion bilateral ankle dorsiflexion	Right-sided rib fractures, right shoulder range of motion Limitations because of precautions from separation
Neuromuscular	Traumatic brain injury No movement noted	Traumatic brain injury Minimal movement noted, increased resistance to passive movement in left elbow and hip
Posture	Decerebrate on left (extension of both the upper and the lower extremity), decorticate on right (flexion of the upper extremity and extension of the lower extremity)	

Abbreviations: CT = computed tomographic; ICP = intracranial pressure; MRI = magnetic resonance imaging.

Patient #1
1. Motor control: no spontaneous movement observed.
2. Skeletal: bilateral ankle dorsiflexion range of motion to −5 degrees.
3. Behavior: unable to follow commands; Rancho Los Amigos level of cognitive functioning, II; Glasgow coma scale, 5.

Patient #2
1. Motor control: spontaneous isolated movement noted in bilateral toes and left hand through partial range.
2. Behavior: unable to follow commands; Rancho Los Amigos level of cognitive functioning, II; Glasgow coma scale, 5 to 6.

ASSESSMENT

Patient #1 has a severe traumatic brain injury. Casting may need to be considered for both ankles because of ankle range of motion limitations, possibly from prolonged posturing. The patient is at risk for losing range of motion in other joints because of prolonged posturing. She is an appropriate candidate for skilled physical therapy in order to progress her functional status and to monitor range of motion and cogni-

tive status. She will most likely benefit from a stay at a rehabilitation unit once medically stable.

Patient #2 has a severe traumatic brain injury and orthopedic injuries. He appears to have some volitional movement, left greater than right. He is an appropriate candidate for skilled physical therapy in order to progress his functional status and to monitor passive range of motion and cognitive status. He will most likely benefit from a stay at a rehabilitation unit once medically stable.

GOALS

Goals need to be set after the initial screening to justify treatment even if the functional evaluation cannot be done. In reality, the functional evaluation is usually not completed at this time because of the patient's medical status. After the functional evaluation is complete, the goals may need to be modified.

Short-Term Goals With 2- to 3-Week Time Frame
1. Patient #1: to open her eyes on command 3 out of 10 times, to increase bilateral ankle dorsiflexion to neutral (0 degrees), and to prevent loss of range of motion.

2. Patient #2: to move on command 3 out of 10 times and to prevent loss of range of motion.

Long-Term Goals

Long-term goals for both patients are deferred until the rate of progress is determined. With a patient who has a low level of responsiveness, it is difficult to anticipate how she/he will progress. Because the functional evaluation cannot be done because of the ICP bolt, it is also difficult to predict the patient's outcomes as well as the time frames in which the outcomes will be achieved.

FUNCTIONAL AREAS TO BE EVALUATED AFTER INITIAL SCREENING

The functional status of either patient could not be screened or evaluated because of the ICP bolt and the bed rest order. Functional status is important to evaluate because of the focus of the physical therapy treatment. Because functional activities were not screened during the initial screening, it was difficult to set goals for functional activities, as the therapist was unable to predict accurately how either patient would do with functional activities without the screening information. Therefore, functional goals were not set until these activities were screened and evaluated.

The functional activities to be evaluated initially include sitting at the edge of the bed for sitting balance and bed mobility. These tasks are to be evaluated because they may be familiar to the patient. The attempt is to see if the patient has the ability to respond and participate in familiar activities.

TREATMENT APPROACH

Initially, the treatment for both patients was limited because of each patient's ICP bolt and medical instability. Even so, attempts to obtain increased movement and movement on command, passive range of motion with possible serial casting to increase bilateral ankle dorsiflexion range of motion for patient #1, and passive range of motion to prevent loss of motion at all other joints can still be done.

Once each patient's ICP bolt was removed and the patients were more stable medically, the screening and the evaluation were continued. The goal at this point was for the patient to be able to tolerate functional activities without a decline in medical status.

A functional approach to treatment was taken to put the patient in different positions and to provide a greater opportunity for her/him to respond and interact with the environment. Functional activities can be incorporated into the treatment even if the patient's cognitive level is very low and even if she/he still has ventilator tubing, different monitoring lines, or other tubes.

Extra people may need to be available to ensure the safety of the patient as well as of the therapists.

A co-treatment with occupational therapy may be appropriate to meet the goals of both disciplines, to stay within the patient's tolerance to treatment, and to combine motor and cognitive skills. The patient can be put in the position of sitting at the edge of the bed using as much physical assistance as needed to see if she/he can tolerate the upright position. The physical assistance can be slightly decreased intermittently to give the patient more of a chance to try to support herself/himself in the sitting position and to control her/his head and trunk. Also in this position, familiar pictures or objects can be used to see if the patient is able to open her/his eyes on command and focus on or track the picture or object. Sitting can also be done with the patient's forearms supported on a table.

For patient #1, standing was done with the use of a standing table. Extra head support was provided, with the physical assistance slightly decreased intermittently to give the patient a chance to control her head. The standing table was also used to increase ankle dorsiflexion range of motion through weight bearing. Wheelchair seating also was done so that the patient could be out of bed in an upright position for longer periods of time throughout the day. A tilt-in-space wheelchair (keeping 90 degrees of hip and knee flexion but in a tilted position) was used with lateral supports, a head support, a lap tray, and a seatbelt in order to provide external support to keep the patient in a safe position.

For both patients, use of all extremities can be incorporated into the functional activities to promote spontaneous automatic movement and then to work toward occasionally purposeful movement. The movement was done within the context of a goal-directed task to make the movement more meaningful for the patient. For example, patient #1, who was a secretary, was assisted in reaching for the telephone after it rang to promote movement of the upper extremity in a spontaneous familiar activity as opposed to having her try to reach for an object that had no meaning to her in an unfamiliar context. Increased movement may be achieved during functional activities as opposed to doing exercises on the mat, especially with a patient who is difficult to engage. The attempt was to work toward the consistency of responses and movement on command within the functional context.

For patient #1, short leg casts were fabricated for both ankles to increase dorsiflexion. Early intervention of casting was initiated so that the patient's ankles would be in good positions for functional activities. Casting can be done in the intensive care unit, but it is usually done after the ICP bolt is removed because the effect of casting on the patient's ICP is unknown.

For patient #2, the functional program was progressed because he regained movement in his extremities. Bed mobility, transfer, and gait training, along with sitting and standing balance, were incorporated into the treatment. Because of this patient's cognitive deficits of decreased initiation, impaired motor planning, decreased attention span, increased frustration level, and impaired memory, the practice session needed to be structured. This patient became frustrated with repetition of an activity but became an active problem solver when the same activity was done in slightly different environments. For example, instead of working on transfers by moving from bed to wheelchair repetitively, transfers were practiced by moving from wheelchair to dining room chair, to seat in the car, to toilet, to seat on the stationary bicycle, to chair at the desk with the computer on it. By doing the task in a slightly different environment and keeping the context real, the patient is able to participate actively in the problem-solving process and there is a better chance of transfer of training once the patient is discharged.

For ambulation, patient #2 initially needed many people for physical assistance. He started by standing in the parallel bars, progressing to ambulation with forearm support on a rolling table, with a rolling walker, with a cane, and then with no assistive device. Stairs, running, and playing "soccer" and "basketball" also were incorporated into the treatment.

OUTCOME

Patient #1 was seen by the physical therapist during her acute care admission. At discharge from the acute care unit, the patient still had a low level of responsiveness. Her posturing continued, and she did not make many changes functionally. Most responses were seen while the patient was in the sitting position rather than supine or sidelying, and she seemed to respond appropriately with focusing and laughing. It seemed that the patient understood more than she was able to show consistently by the subtle comments she would laugh at. Because the patient is now medically stable, the therapist believes that she deserves a chance in a rehabilitation unit, where she can receive and tolerate more physical therapy to determine if more progress can be obtained.

Patient #2 was seen by the physical therapist from admission to the acute care unit until discharge from the rehabilitation unit. His present functional problems and progress with functional activities continue to be limited by his cognitive deficits and low tolerance to stress. Improvements in high-level gross motor activities will continue to occur slowly and in conjunction with greater tolerance to physical and environmental challenges. Home health physical therapy is recommended to continue to assist the patient in progressing his functional activities in the environment where the activities will be performed.

II. Comparison of Patient #1 and Patient #2

A. Screening and evaluation

Patient #1 and patient #2 both have the diagnosis of traumatic brain injury that is considered severe. The approach to the screening for the two patients was similar. The screenings were limited because the patients were on bed rest and because of the ICP monitoring. Therefore, functional activities could not be screened. Definitive evaluation was also limited initially to the key areas and then was ongoing depending on the changes the patient was making.

B. Progress

Patient #1 and patient #2 initially presented with similar motor and cognitive problems. Patient #2 made improvements in his motor control, so more functional activities could be incorporated into his treatment program. At discharge from the acute care unit, patient #2 had already begun work on bed mobility, transfers, and early gait training, whereas Patient #1 was still involved in sitting at the edge of the bed and the standing table. Patient #2 also progressed from a Rancho Los Amigos level II to a level III at discharge from the acute care unit to a level V at discharge from the rehabilitation unit. The motor ability of patient #1 seemed to plateau, and she progressed only from a Rancho Los Amigos level II to between a level II and level III at discharge from the acute care unit. If the progress of patient #1 plateaus at the rehabilitation unit and she does not make gains toward goals, skilled physical therapy cannot be continued.

C. Outcomes

Patient #1 and patient #2 are unable to return to their previous lifestyles because of the remaining motor and cognitive deficits. Patient #2 can possibly return to some previous activities and may be more limited from a cognitive standpoint than a motor standpoint. Patient #1 cannot return to any previous activities at this point.

III. Summary

Two patients with a low level of responsiveness have been presented. The screening, evaluation, assessment, and treatment information has been discussed. Treatment is based on the patient's medical stability—not the patient's cognitive level. Even if many people are needed, it is beneficial to put the patient in different positions to provide a greater opportunity for the patient to respond and interact with the environment. These two patients have been compared in reference to screening and evaluation, progress, and outcomes. The concepts presented here are applicable to other patients with a low level of responsiveness.

References

1. Malkmus D: Integrating cognitive strategies into the physical therapy setting. *Phys Ther*, 1983, 63:1952–1959.
2. Jennett B, Teasdale G: Assessment of coma and impaired consciousness. *Lancet*, 1974, 2:81–84.

Suggested Reading

Boughton A, Ciesla N: Physical therapy management of the head-injured patient in the intensive care unit. *Top Acute Care Trauma Rehabil*, 1986, 1:1–18.

Cope DM, Hall K: Head injury rehabilitation: benefits of early intervention. *Arch Phys Med Rehabil*, 1982, 63:433–437.

Cusick B: *Serial Casts: Their Use in the Management of Spasticity-Induced Foot Deformity*. Lexington, KY, Words at Work, 1987.

Heiden JS, Small R, Caton W, Weiss M, Kurze T: Severe head injury: clinical assessment and outcome. *Phys Ther*, 1983, 63:1946–1951.

Jennett B, Teasdale G: Aspects of coma after severe head injury. *Lancet*, 1977, 1:878–881.

Jennett B, Teasdale G: Assessment and prognosis of coma after head injury. *Acta Neurochir*, 1976, 34:48–55.

Lehmkuhl LD, Krawczyk L: Physical therapy management of the minimally responsive patient following traumatic brain injury: coma stimulation. *Neurol Rep*, 1993, 17:10–17.

Orest M: Casting protocol for patients with neurological dysfunction. *PT—Magazine of Physical Therapy*, 1993, 1:51–55.

Tardieu C, Lespargot A, Tabary C, Bret MD: For how long must the soleus muscle be stretched each day to prevent contracture? *Dev Med Child Neurol*, 1988, 30:3–10.

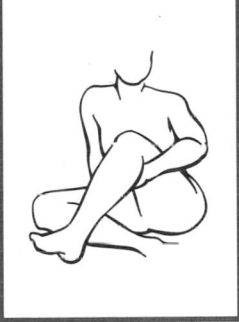

CHAPTER 17

Orthotic Management for Lower Extremity Dysfunction

Polly Menendez

In the following case studies, the physical therapist is functioning as a consultant. This is a common role for therapists who participate in brace clinics, and it allows the therapist to focus on bracing issues. However, it must be recognized that bracing can never be separated from the individual issues of the patient. The evaluation and decision-making approach (illustrated in these case studies) to bracing can aid the primary therapist in focusing on bracing, or it can help a physical therapist organize a brace clinic. The brace clinic environment usually demands quick screening and narrowly focused evaluation.

I. Overview

A. Comparison of three patients

1. Patient #1 sustained a left cerebrovascular accident with right hemiplegia 2 weeks ago. He is scheduled to go home in 5 days.
2. Patient #2 sustained a right cerebrovascular accident with left hemiplegia 4 weeks ago. He is scheduled to go home in 3 weeks.
3. Patient #3 sustained a spinal cord impingement with bilateral lower extremity paralysis from a herniated disc at L4-5. He underwent spinal fixation and spent 10 days in an acute care setting and 2 weeks in the rehabilitation unit. He was scheduled to go home in 2 weeks.

B. Screening of database items

Database items that are particularly important to consider in bracing:

1. Medication. Note medications that are antispasmodics (*eg*, baclofen), those that affect the volume of the limb (*eg*, diuretics), or those that are related to diabetes (*eg*, insulin).
2. Cardiovascular concerns. Note the presence of peripheral vascular disease.
3. Metabolic concerns. The most common metabolic problem to note is diabetes mellitus. Many disease processes exist that may be

411

relevant to bracing (*eg*, lupus erythematosus), but they are all relatively rare compared with diabetes.

4. Vision and behavior. Vision and behavior are only important to the extent that they give a therapist information about a patient's ability to use an orthosis to enhance function.

5. Appliances. Note if patient has any braces or uses any assistive devices.

6. Pain and tenderness. Note any complaint of pain or tenderness throughout screening and evaluation.

7. Balance. Although balance is often a very important area for neurological physical therapists to assess, it is only important in bracing in that it limits the function that the bracing is assisting. For example, balance could be so impaired that walking is not a possibility for a given patient.

8. Posture. Note deficits that might limit bracing or that may be improved by bracing.

9. Functional mobility. Note whether the patient can stand and walk with or without assistance.

KEY AREAS IN SCREENING

Skin and Soft Tissue Concerns

Note any open sores or red areas on the leg and foot. Note any history of skin breakdown or difficulty in healing. Also note any edema.

Skeletal Concerns

Note any limitations in range of motion (ROM) at pertinent joints. The motions that are important to examine vary according to the problem. Patients with paraplegia who want to walk with long leg braces must have a significant capacity for motion at the spine, hips, and ankles; although patients with hemiplegia also need motion in these areas, the major motion needed is ankle dorsiflexion.

Neuromuscular Concerns

Remember that this is a screen—deficits should not be measured at this time. Instead, the therapist should characterize problems. Later, the therapist chooses the deficits that are important to measure. First, list any neuromuscular disease processes from a medical standpoint. Note any deficits in motor control (strength, coordination, and patterned versus isolated motion), "posturing," or resistance to passive motion and sensation.

Gait pattern

Gait pattern is the major aspect of the bracing evaluation, and the purpose of the screening is to note whether patients have gait deviations that can be addressed through bracing.

C. Evaluation

The most important part of a bracing evaluation is the assessment of gait.

1. Based on deficits found during screening, a therapist measures specific impairments. In addition to observational gait analysis, the measurement of ankle dorsiflexion is common. Therapists often perform a manual muscle test of key muscle groups in patients with spinal cord injury or peripheral neuropathy. It is uncommon for therapists to test the ability to isolate all motions in patients with hemiplegia; however, testing a patient's ability to flex the hip, to flex and extend the knee, and to move the ankle in a sitting position gives a therapist adequate information when these test results are combined with the results of observational gait analysis.

2. Observational gait analysis.[1] A patient should be observed walking in a variety of conditions, including barefoot, with shoes, and with a variety of trial braces. The therapist should note how gait deviations change with the various conditions. The patient should walk with the same assistive device and should be provided with the same amount of assistance in all conditions to keep the focus on the issue of bracing. However, a change of assistive device sometimes provides important insight into the issue of bracing. It is important to recognize situations in which such a change is necessary. For example, if a patient with hemiplegia who uses a quad cane and an articulated ankle-foot orthosis (AFO) is not able to dorsiflex and advance his/her weight over the involved leg in late stance, a standard cane could promote forward weight shift because the patient no longer has the support of the quad cane out to the side. If the therapist had failed to look at a change in assistive device, he/she might have assumed that the patient could not use the joint of an articulated brace.

3. Observational gait analysis is not a reliable assessment tool, but it continues to be the only tool that is readily available to evaluate the impairments that are addressed in bracing.[2] Temporal gait analysis is becoming more common and may aid in evaluating changes that occur as a result of bracing.[3,4]

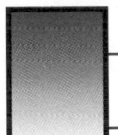

Clinical Decision-Making Cases

Case #1

FINDINGS ON SCREENING

The patient reported that he did not think he needed a brace. He had been walking on the nursing unit at the hospital with a standard cane, a posterior leaf-spring AFO, and contact guarding. He occasionally tripped over his right foot and needed assistance to regain his balance. His posture generally was flexed, and his weight was shifted to the left. He had minimal edema in his right ankle, and his ROM was limited in the same ankle. He had weakness of the right leg, and movement was influenced by synergy patterns.

FINDINGS ON EVALUATION

1. The ROM was 0 degrees of dorsiflexion on the right.
2. When motor control was evaluated, it was found that in sitting, the patient completed partial range of hip flexion, knee extension, and knee flexion, full range of plantar flexion, and no dorsiflexion.
3. The evaluation of gait deviations was completed as follows:
   a. With no brace, *in swing on the right,* foot clearance was decreased, with the foot scraping on the floor; increased plantar flexion occurred; ankle inversion increased minimally; and hip and knee flexion were decreased in early swing. *In stance on the right,* initial contact was with the forefoot, knee flexion was increased in midstance to late stance, and weight shift was decreased minimally to the right.
   b. With a posterior leaf-spring AFO (see Figure 17-1), right foot clearance improved, and the foot did not scrape on the floor. Initial contact was with the right heel, and no ankle inversion was noted.

BRACING DECISION

It was recommended that the patient use a posterior leaf-spring AFO until he had improved foot clearance.

RATIONALE FOR DECISION

The most pressing need for this patient was improved foot clearance to prevent tripping and falling. The foot clearance problem was caused by a lack of adequate hip flexion as well as by a lack of dorsiflex-ion. The posterior leaf-spring AFO worked at the ankle to prevent the foot from scraping on the floor. It also corrected the ankle inversion noted during swing; therefore, it was not necessary to pursue more aggressive bracing. The physical therapist should watch for an increase in patterned motion, which may call for a more solid orthosis; however, such an orthosis did not seem to be indicated at the time of the evaluation.

FOLLOW-UP

This patient never wore his brace after returning home, and he gained ankle dorsiflexion with good foot clearance within 2 weeks after the return home. The patient did not like wearing the brace, so he walked without the brace while his wife guarded him to prevent him from injuring himself.

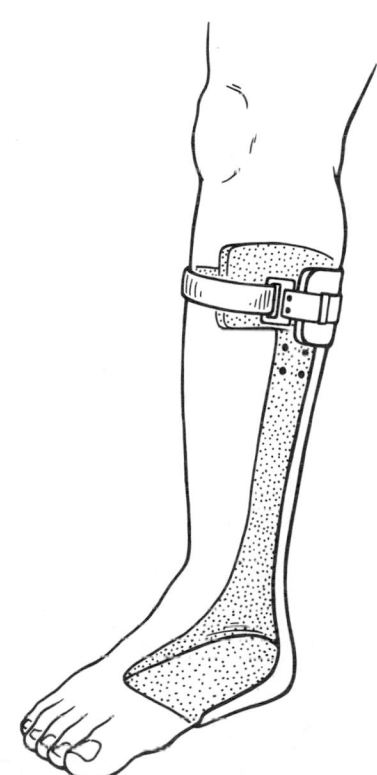

FIGURE 17–1 Custom-fitted plastic posterior leaf spring AFO.

Case #2

FINDINGS ON SCREENING

The patient reported that she would do anything to walk. She had diabetes mellitus and peripheral vascular disease, but her skin was intact. At the time of screening, the patient walked with either a cane or a rolling walker, a trial solid-ankle AFO (from the physical therapy department's stock of braces used by former patients), and minimal assistance from one person. Ankle ROM was limited, and left lower extremity movement was dominated by synergy. She lost her balance when walking, and needed assistance to regain her balance. Her posture generally was flexed, her weight was shifted to the left, and the left side of her pelvis was posterior compared with the right side.

FINDINGS ON EVALUATION

1. ROM: she lacks 5 degrees from neutral dorsiflexion.
2. When motor control was evaluated, it was found that while she was sitting, hip flexion through half of the range occurred, with ankle dorsiflexion and inversion, knee flexion and hip abduction, and lateral rotation. The patient was able to initiate knee extension.
3. On evaluation of gait deviations, the following was found:
   a. With a rolling walker and no brace, *in swing on the left,* foot clearance was decreased, ankle plantar flexion and inversion were increased, hip and knee flexion were decreased, and hip adduction was increased. *In stance on the left,* initial contact was with the forefoot, the ankle was plantar flexed and inverted, the knee remained hyperextended throughout, the left side of the pelvis was posterior compared with the right, and there was excessive lateral weight shift to the left. *In swing on the right,* a short step length was noted, and the right foot did not step beyond the left foot. *In stance on the right,* weight shift to the right decreased.
   b. With a posterior leaf-spring AFO, the only significant change was less ankle plantar flexion during swing on the left, and that initial contact on the left was with the full foot.
   c. With a solid-ankle AFO (see Figure 17–2), changes were as follows: neutral ankle position was maintained throughout, initial contact was with the heel, decreased foot clearance was still noted, but it was improved, less hip adduction in swing on the left was seen, the left knee hyperextended half of the time, and some lateral rotation of the left hip was present in stance.

BRACING DECISION

The therapist recommended increased work on gaining dorsiflexion and molding for a solid-ankle AFO with a full footplate as soon as the patient could attain neutral dorsiflexion.

RATIONALE FOR DECISION

The solid-ankle AFO is designed to hold the entire foot in a neutral position. To do this effectively, the contours of the plastic must match the contours of the foot; thus, the foot should be molded in a neutral position to maximize fit of the brace. The solid-ankle AFO prevents excessive plantar flexion and inversion by holding the ankle in a neutral position.[5] In stance, the lateral part of the brace along the tibia decreases excessive lateral weight shift to the left and promotes forward weight. In this patient, a decrease in left hip adduction in swing could result because the left leg would begin the swing from a more neutral position. This brace could aid in controlling knee hyperextension but only if the patient could progress her pelvis forward over her left foot.

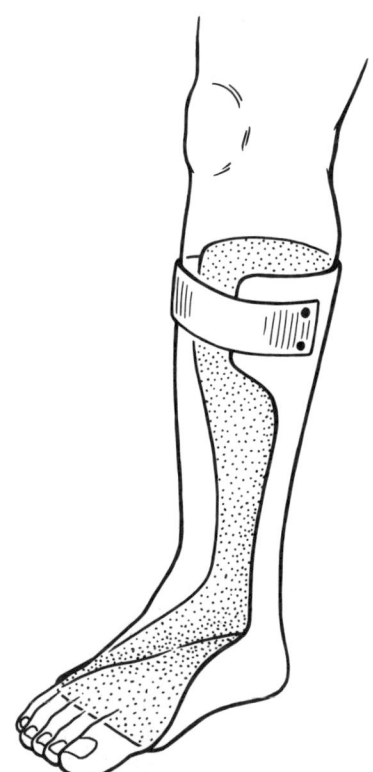

FIGURE 17–2   Custom-molded solid-ankle plastic AFO.

FOLLOW-UP

Through joint mobilization and traditional stretching, the patient gained neutral dorsiflexion in 3 days. The brace fit well, but the patient laterally rotated her left leg throughout stance. This was decreased through therapy that focused on increasing step length on the right and on increasing the gait speed. The patient did not need the full footplate because no posturing was present in the brace; thus, it was cut off just anterior to the metatarsal heads. The patient was ambulating independently for household distances at the time of discharge.

Case #3

FINDINGS ON SCREENING

The patient stated that he had a strong desire to walk and that he hoped bracing would help. He had decreased sensation on the soles of his feet, and his skin was intact. He walked with a walker, bilateral prefabricated posterior leaf-spring AFOs, and contact guarding from his therapist. He did not lose his balance when walking with the walker, but he appeared to be very careful and did not move out of his base of support. Ankle ROM was limited bilaterally. He had a steppage-type gait.

EVALUATION FINDINGS

1. The ROM was 0 degrees of dorsiflexion bilaterally.
2. When the patient's strength was tested, it was found that he was capable of active dorsiflexion to a neutral position bilaterally; however, no active plantar flexion was seen on the left, and only trace ankle plantar flexion was seen on the right.
3. On examination of gait deviations, the following was found:
   a. The patient's gait without braces showed severely increased hip and knee flexion bilaterally during swing, bilateral foot inversion and plantar flexion during swing, toe-first initial contact, and bilateral knee hyperextension throughout stance.
   b. The patient's gait with posterior leaf-spring AFOs was the same as without braces except that no ankle plantar flexion in swing was seen, and that initial contact was with flat feet.
   c. The patient's gait with a posterior leaf-spring AFO on the left and a ground-reaction AFO (see Figure 17–3) on the right (it is very unusual that a ground-reaction AFO from a previous patient would fit another patient, fortunately it did in this case) showed that a neutral ankle position was maintained throughout gait bilaterally. Initial contact was heel first bilaterally, the left knee remained hyperextended throughout stance, and in stance, the right knee remained extended but not hyperextended.

BRACING DECISION

The therapist recommended bilateral ground-reaction AFOs.

RATIONALE FOR DECISION

This patient was unable to progress forward over his feet because of a lack of strength in the plantar flexor muscles. The plantar flexor muscles act to control the forward progression of the body over the foot in late stance. This patient hyperextended his knees to gain stability during stance. The ground reaction AFOs allow

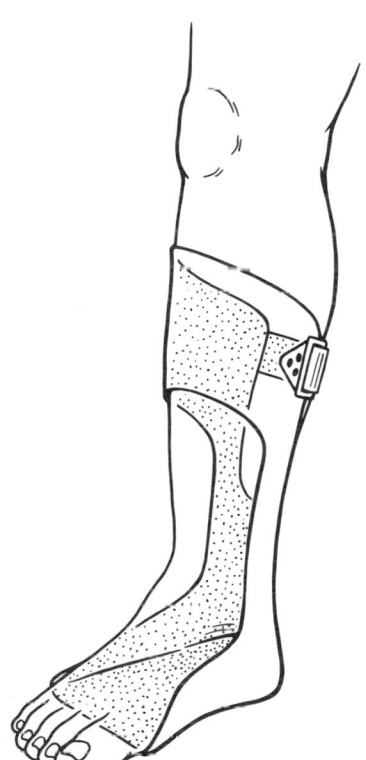

FIGURE 17–3 Custom-molded plastic ground reaction AFO. (Reprinted with permission from *The Illustrated Guide to Orthotics and Prosthetics: O & P's Guide to Medicare Codes and Reimbursements.* Alexandria, American Orthotic and Prosthetic Association, 1993.)

for some forward progression of the body, but this is limited by the anterior tibial piece. As a patient moves forward, the tibial tubercle makes contact with the brace and prevents the collapse of the tibia forward, allowing the patient to walk without knee hyperextension. The brace also prevents excessive plantar flexion by holding the foot in a neutral position.

FOLLOW-UP

The patient returned safely home, where he was able to walk independently with braces and Lofstrand crutches. He walked with less hip and knee flexion in swing (ie, less of a steppage gait). He had no knee hyperextension in stance.

II. Summary

A. Lack of adequate foot clearance

The three cases described in this chapter are similar in that all three patients lacked adequate foot clearance in swing. Foot clearance can be accomplished through hip and knee flexion in early swing and through ankle dorsiflexion in late swing. Patient #3 was able to compensate for lack of dorsiflexion by increasing hip and knee flexion. This steppage gait is common in patients with peripheral nerve lesions. In the other two patients with central nervous system damage, decreased hip and knee flexion compounded the foot clearance problem. All of the patients were fitted with AFOs that improved foot clearance. With patients #1 and #2, the therapist needs to address the problem of inadequate hip and knee flexion if the patients continue to have problems (ie, they still drag their feet on the floor).

B. Ankle inversion in swing

Patients #1 and #2 inverted their ankles in swing as they attempted to dorsiflex. This is an important deviation to correct because it leads to weight bearing on the lateral border of the foot with a varus rearfoot. In the short term, this is not a stable base for stance. A patient will feel insecure when attempting to progress his/her weight forward over this foot. In the long term, the patient will compensate for rearfoot varus through pronation of the transmetatarsal joint.[5] This allows more of the foot to come into contact with the ground, but it also may lead to other gait deviations in the hip and in the knee and to foot deformity and pain.

Ankle inversion is best controlled by a solid-ankle AFO, but other braces sometimes may be adequate. For patient #1, the posterior leaf-spring AFO was adequate to control inversion. This brace had no direct effect on inversion, but supporting the ankle in the dorsiflexed position decreased the amount of inversion due to the alignment of the bones. In addition, the anterior tibial muscle, which is often the muscle that is most active in dorsiflexion, acts more as an invertor when plantar flexion occurs. It is important to choose the type of bracing that is least invasive but that controls the problem. When such a choice is made, the therapist must watch for potential problems, such as an increase in inversion as the patient becomes more active.

It also must be recognized that it is not always possible to see what is going on inside the brace and the shoe. Therefore, it may be helpful to observe ambulation without the brace from time to time to evaluate for potential deviations or abnormal posturing.

C. Knee hyperextension

Patients #2 and #3 had knee hyperextension in stance. Patient #3 kept his knees locked because he knew that they would give out if he allowed them to flex. Patient #2 also may have hyperextended so that she could feel secure while weight bearing on that leg, but she also demonstrated a common pattern of movement seen in hemiplegia. The bracing helped to control this problem in both cases, but the approach was different in each.

For patient #3, the ground reaction brace works directly through the knee to support knee extension. The weight-bearing part of the brace at the tibial tubercle provides an extension moment by using ground-reaction forces.

The solid-ankle AFO for patient #2 decreased knee hyperextension in a more typical fashion. The ankle was maintained in dorsiflexion, creating a flexor moment at the knee. This only controlled knee hyperextension in the patient half of the time because she also rotated the left side of her pelvis backward; therefore, this patient needed to work on rotating her pelvis slightly forward while progressing her weight forward over her left foot to fully control knee hyperextension.

Traditionally, therapists have attempted to control knee hyperextension by placing the ankle in slight dorsiflexion. This is not recommended because it places the patient in an unstable crouch position. Patients usually do not tolerate this position. In double-metal uprights, patients are able to achieve plantar flexion inside the shoe, and patients often push out of the plastic braces and develop skin problems.

III. Other Considerations

A. Articulated AFOs

Recently, orthotists developed the technology for putting hinges in custom-molded braces. Generally, these braces are designed to block some plantar flexion while allowing full dorsiflexion. Some orthotists are experimenting with hinges that block dorsiflexion, but this is not a common design feature.

The combination of blocked plantar flexion and full dorsiflexion often works well in patients with hemiplegia. This allows for good foot clearance in swing and also allows forward weight shift over the foot in stance. Patients usually gain control over the stance phase prior to gaining control over the swing phase; therefore, an articulated AFO allows patients to use their strengths while supporting weaker areas.

The articulated AFO is particularly useful for patients who are very active because it makes negotiation of stairs and hills much easier. It provides benefits *different from* the solid ankle AFO and the posterior leaf-spring AFO. The posterior leaf-spring brace is flexible, allowing some of that same forward weight shift, but it does not provide comparable medial and lateral support.

In patient #2, a solid-ankle AFO was chosen over the articulated brace because of her strong tendency toward ankle inversion and her tendency to bear weight on the lateral border of the foot. The fit of the articulated AFO generally is not as intimate as that of the solid-ankle type and therefore allows some ankle inversion. The solid ankle AFO is generally indicated for patients with more serious involvement, but the choice between these two braces is always a difficult judgement call.

In this author's brace clinic, articulated AFOs have been prescribed, and in the end, the patients were unable to use the articulation. Therefore, more conservative decisions are now made about the use of articulated braces. A solid-ankle AFO is often a good choice because it can be altered as the patient gains more control—it can be gradually cut down until it becomes a custom posterior leaf-spring brace or a shoe insert.

B. No normal movement

Therapists should recognize that patients do not have normal movement when they use orthotic devices. In bracing, one abnormal component is eliminated in favor of another, more functional abnormal component. For example, with a solid-ankle AFO, increased ankle plantar flexion and inversion in swing can be controlled, but dorsiflexion cannot occur in late stance. In such a case, the patient's ability to step beyond the involved foot is limited or brings about farther gait deviations at the pelvis.

C. Evaluation of the fit

Fit evaluation is a critical issue in bracing and is one of the most difficult things for therapists to learn. Most therapists have no problems in checking for skin breakdown and in working with an orthotist to alter the brace when skin problems are present. Therapists also need to assess the way that the brace controls a patient's movement. For example, a solid-ankle AFO should maintain a neutral subtalar joint. The therapist needs to make sure that the heel fits in the brace and that no medio-lateral play, which can allow forward slippage of the foot out of the heel cup, exists. The best way to learn about fit is to work closely with an orthotist. Therapists should assist with aligning the foot for molding and spend some time in the orthotic shop to understand how braces are made.

References

1. *Observational Gait Analysis Handbook.* Downey, CA, The Patho-kinesiology Service and the Physical Therapy Department, Rancho Los Amigos Medical Center, The Professional Staff Association, 1989.
2. Krebs DE, Edelstein JE, Fishman S: Reliability of observational kinematic gait analysis. *Phys Ther* 1985, 65:1027–1033.
3. Holden MK, Gill KM, Magliozzi MR: Clinical gain assessment in neurologically impaired: reliability and meaningfulness. *Phys Ther* 1984, 64:35–40.
4. Cerny K: A clinical method of quantitative gait analysis: suggestion from the field. *Phys Ther* 1983, 63:1125–1126.
5. Ryerson S: Course Notes: the Neurological Foot. A Mechanical and Motor Control Approach [unpublished data]. Durham, NC, April 30–May 2, 1993.

Suggested Reading

American Academy of Orthopedic Surgeons: *Atlas of Orthotics: Biomechanical Principles and Applications,* 2nd ed. St. Louis, C. V. Mosby Company, 1985.
Ryerson S: The foot in CNS dysfunction. *Neurol Rep* Summer, 1989, 13:9–11.
Cusick BD: *Progressive Casting and Splinting.* Tucson, Therapy Skill Builders, 1990.

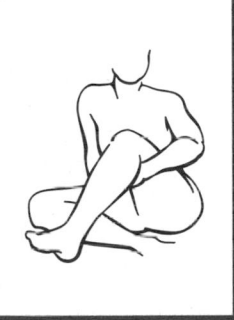

CHAPTER 18

Evaluation and Prescription for Wheelchairs and Seating

Polly Menendez

The two patients discussed in this chapter were evaluated in an inpatient rehabilitation program to determine whether they were candidates for the use of wheelchairs and seating systems. Physical therapists identify patients' needs for wheelchairs and positioning equipment in a number of settings, including acute-care hospitals, private homes, nursing homes, schools, and outpatient facilities. The best location for actually assessing a patient's seating requirements varies, depending on the services available in any particular area and the patient's needs. If a patient has complex seating needs, these can be evaluated in a wheelchair clinic or during a short hospital stay. Therapists need to make seating decisions in consultation with an equipment specialist because equipment technology is constantly changing. Equipment specialists often are vendors, but physical therapists, occupational therapists, or rehabilitation engineers also can serve in this role.

I. Overview

A. Role of the physical therapist

A physical therapist is part of a team that includes the patient and his/her family, physicians, occupational therapists, speech and language pathologists, and teachers. The physical therapist gathers information from the team to ensure that the wheelchair and seating will meet the patient's needs in all areas of his/her life. The equipment specialist is responsible for knowing what equipment is available; the therapist is responsible for understanding the patient's functional potential and positional requirements and for making sure that the equipment meets these needs. Other health care professionals may work with the physical therapist to determine which wheelchairs and seating are optimal.

B. Goals of seating

The goals of seating need to be individual to each patient, with maximal function as the major goal. Physical therapists often think about mobility when they talk about function, but function can be defined in a variety of ways. For example, tolerating sitting for longer periods aids pulmonary function. Therapists involved with seating often talk about a "functional posture."[1] In such a posture, no gross asymmetry is present; the hips, knees, and

419

ankles are at 90 degrees; the hips are in a neutral position in reference to rotation and abduction and adduction; and the shoulders are positioned over the hips. This posture is considered "functional" because patients can sit in this position for long periods without skin breakdown; this posture also may prevent some orthopedic deformities. Patients usually report being comfortable in this position.

C. Introduction to two patients

1. Patient #1 is a 42-year-old woman with a 19-year history of multiple sclerosis. She is dependent with all functional mobility, and she transfers with a Hoyer lift. She had been living at home with one full-time caregiver, and her family provided care in the evenings, at night, and on weekends. Prior to this hospital admission, she had spent all of her time in bed because she was not able to maintain her balance in the standard wheelchair that she had purchased many years ago. She and her family want her to have a chair that allows her to get out of the bedroom and to go outside. Her bedroom is on the first floor, and a threshold leading from the house onto a porch is present in the doorway. One step from the porch to the ground is present.

2. Patient #2 is a 68-year-old man who sustained a right cerebrovascular accident with a left hemiparesis 6 weeks before being examined. He was scheduled to go home 3 weeks from the time of examination. He wanted to walk, and at the time of examination, he could walk with the assistance of two people for short distances during his therapy sessions. He planned to continue working on walking but realized that he would need a wheelchair when it was time for him to return home. His family planned to take him home regardless of his care requirements. At examination, he was using a hemi-height wheelchair with a seat belt and an arm trough to support his left arm. He could wheel himself independently on the nursing unit, but he tended to slip forward as he wheeled; one time he slipped out of his chair. At home, he had pile carpet, and his family planned to build a ramp for him so he would be able to get in and out of the house.

D. Screening of database items

Most database items can have an impact on wheelchair and positioning decisions. How these items relate to seating depends on the individual patient. Following is a description of how data recorded during a physical therapist's initial screening of a patient relate to seating. Please see Table 18–1 for the database findings for patients #1 and #2.

1. Medications. Note any antispasmodics that could alter the patient's tolerance to positions and medications for seizures.
2. Communication. Augmentative communication devices may need to be mounted on the wheelchair.
3. Cardiovascular or pulmonary concerns. Cardiovascular or pulmonary disease may limit the patient's ability to propel a wheelchair or may indicate the need for a lightweight wheelchair. Peripheral vascular disease may indicate the potential for skin breakdown. If a patient needs oxygen, he/she needs a place to carry it on the wheelchair.
4. Metabolic concerns. Note the presence of any disease processes such as diabetes that may increase the potential for skin breakdown.
5. Gastrointestinal and genitourinary concerns. Note problems with bowel and bladder control that may affect the therapist's choice of cushions. If a patient has dysphagia, he/she needs to be able to attain an upright position for eating.
6. Vision. Note problems with vision that may limit wheelchair mobility. Generally, decreased visual ability limits a patient's capacity to use an electric wheelchair, and problems such as field cuts and neglect may limit the patient's ability to negotiate outdoors.
7. Behavior. A patient's behavior can affect wheelchair decisions in a variety of ways; frequently, one of the most important issues is safety awareness in reference to wheelchair use.
8. Pain and tenderness. The patient's comfort in the chair is always a primary concern because he/she often sits in the chair for most of the day.
9. Skin and soft tissue. The issues of disease processes that could increase the patient's potential for experiencing skin breakdown have already been addressed; however,

Table 18–1. SCREENING FOR WHEELCHAIR AND SEATING

Database Parameter	Patient #1	Patient #2
Medications	Baclofen	No impact on seating
Communication	Difficult to understand speech because of dysarthria; occupational therapist is evaluating ability to use a switch	No impact on seating
Cardiovascular and pulmonary concerns	History of aspiration of secretions and food; 15-y history of smoking	History of myocardial infarction 3 years before examination
Metabolic concerns	No impact on seating	No impact on seating
Vision	Limited vision; no definitive information available	Left homonymous hemianopsia with severe left neglect
Behavior	History of depression	Patient is impulsive and has poor insight into deficits
Pain and tenderness	No complaint of pain	Patient reports low back pain after sitting for several hours
Skin and soft tissue	History of sacral decubiti; no current skin breakdown or pressure areas	No pressure areas
Skeletal concerns	Limited range of motion at trunk, hip flexion, knee extension, and ankle dorsiflexion	Range of motion is limited at left hip flexion and medial (internal) rotation
Neuromuscular concerns	20-y history of multiple sclerosis; magnetic resonance imaging over the years indicated increasing involvement of the brainstem and cerebellum; has no active control of lower extremities; control of upper extremities is limited by severe ataxia; in supine and in sitting positions, right leg postures in extension, whereas left leg postures in flexion; sensation seems to be intact but is difficult to assess because of poor communication	Right cerebrovascular accident (middle cerebral artery distribution) with left hemiplegia; patient has minimal active movement at left hip and knee; sensation is intact
Balance	Patient needs maximal support to maintain static sitting position and tends to fall to the left and posteriorly	Patient can maintain static sitting on the mat but tends to list posterior and to the left
Posture	Patient sits with severe lateral trunk flexion to the left, flexing over the arm of most chairs; legs are in a "windswept" position, with both knees to the right of midline; right knee is extended, while left knee is flexed, so foot is under seating surface	In standard wheelchair, patient tends to sit with hips forward in the chair and with back hyperextended; left hip is rotated back compared with the right hip; left hip is laterally rotated
Functional mobility	Patient is dependent in all mobility, and a mechanical lift is used for transfers; she is not able to propel her manual wheelchair and is not able to manage a switch for an electric chair	Patient requires minimal to moderate assistance for bed mobility and transfers; he requires cues for management of wheelchair parts and is independent with wheelchair propulsion on smooth, level surfaces

long periods of pressure lead to skin problems in otherwise healthy skin. Note whether any areas of pressure exist, and check with the patient's nurse or his/her caregiver to determine whether he/she has seen any pressure areas.

10. Skeletal concerns. Note if the patient has scoliosis or any range of motion (ROM) limitations that prevent him/her from maintaining an optimal position in the wheelchair.

11. Neuromuscular concerns. Note weakness and posturing that alter the patient's position in the wheelchair. Lack of sensation decreases the patient's ability to detect skin breakdown.

12. Balance. Note the amount of support that the patient needs to maintain sitting balance. Sitting balance affects how much support the patient needs in his/her wheelchair.

13. Posture. First observe the patient sitting

without support (*eg*, on a mat), and then in a chair with back and arm support. Note postural deviations, including asymmetry and inability to stay within the confines of the chair. Note whether the postural deviations are fixed or flexible.

14. Functional mobility. Indicate the patient's level of mobility at the time of examination, including the type of transfer that he/she uses and the patient's ability to propel the wheelchair and to manage wheelchair parts.

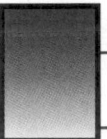

Clinical Decision-Making Cases

Case #1

EVALUATION AND ASSESSMENT

The process of fitting a patient for a wheelchair is a constant cycle of evaluation and assessment. Skin condition, posture, and functional status are evaluated with each seating system that is tried.

Measurements

Patient measurements to determine the size of the wheelchair needed should be completed before seating trials. Common measurements are as follows[1,2]:

1. Seat width (the widest part of the hips). Wheelchairs need to be 1 to 2 in wider than the patient to account for clothing and weight fluctuations.
2. Back height (the axilla to the seating surface). Back height varies, depending on the patient's trunk control or balance.
3. Arm height (the elbow to the seating surface).
4. Seat depth (the most posterior surface to the popliteal crease). The seat needs to be 1 in shorter than the patient's measurements.
5. Leg length (the popliteal crease to the floor). Leg length is used to determine the seat height; it is particularly important for a patient who propels a wheelchair with his/her feet. Consider the height of the cushion to determine the seat height.

Skin Condition

Skin condition should be monitored before and during seating trials. The areas that most frequently develop skin problems are the sacrum and ischial tuberosities; however, other areas such as the greater trochanter region and the medial surface of the knees can be a problem in a patient with asymmetrical posture. If a pressure area is seen, its size, its location, and the time it takes to disappear also should be noted. Furthermore, the length of time that the patient was sitting before the pressure area was seen should be recorded.

Posture

Most physical therapists describe sitting with the knees, hips, and ankles at 90 degrees and with the shoulders positioned over the hips as optimal.[3] Therapists evaluate their patients' ability to maintain this position comfortably. If a patient is not able to achieve this optimal position, his/her therapist must hypothesize why and measure impairments that may be contributing to the problem. Lack of ROM is often a cause of this problem. If ROM is not limited, the therapist must hypothesize further about potential causes (*eg*, weakness or excessive posturing in upright positions) and measure impairments as needed. Because the goal of seating is to provide the patient with sufficient support to maintain an adequate posture for function, the therapist evaluates the effect of various seating systems on the patient's posture, function, and comfort.

Functional Status

The evaluation of function should occur in all seating trials, and this evaluation should reflect the patient's goals. A patient's ability to propel on a variety of surfaces, as well as manage wheelchair parts, should be evaluated. How the wheelchair relates to the environment is also important. The ability of the patient to use tabletops and communication equipment, the height of the chair in reference to other people in the environment, how well the chair fits into strapping systems on public transportation, and the layout of the patient's living and working environments are some areas to consider.

SUMMARY OF EVALUATION FINDINGS AND ASSESSMENT

Measurements	Patient #1	Patient #2
Seat width	15.0 in	16.0 in
Back height	15.0 in	17.5 in
Arm height	9.0 in	9.0 in
Seat depth	22.0 in	20.0 in
Leg length	15.0 in	20.0 in

From these measurements, it can be concluded that patient #1 fits best in a chair 16 in wide, but because she has long legs, she needs a seat that is deeper than average.

A standard wheelchair measures 18 × 16 in; therefore, patient #2 can sit in a standard-width chair but needs slightly more depth. He may be able to manage in a chair with a standard back height, which is 16 in, but he may also benefit from a higher back.

Posture

Patient #1 has significant postural problems, as noted in the database. When she sat on a mat with her hips at 80 to 90 degrees and her arms supported, a therapist was able to support her trunk manually, preventing trunk rotation and lateral flexion. Significant ROM loss contributed to this patient's postural problems. ROM losses were hip flexion to 90 degrees on the right and 85 degrees on the left; 0 degrees of hip abduction on the left; and ankle plantar flexion contractures of 5 degrees.

The extended or "slumped" posture noted in patient #2 seems to have resulted from limited movement patterns. He used a total extension pattern of the leg and the trunk for all movements; this resulted in the posture described in the database. He did have some ROM losses, including 100 degrees of left hip flexion and 0 degrees of left hip medial rotation. He was able to attain an optimal sitting position on the mat but was not able to maintain this position for longer than 30 seconds.

Seating Trials and Functional Status

The functional goal for patient #1 was to allow her to tolerate sitting for longer periods and to allow her to be left unsupervised in the sitting position. The functional goal for patient #2 was to give him the capacity for independent wheelchair propulsion on a variety of surfaces without his slipping out of the chair.

For patient #1, a number of chairs and seating systems were tried. In the end, she was able to maintain a "good" sitting position for 4 hours, and she could be left alone during that time. "Good" defined the patient's ability to remain within the confines of the chair. The major issues addressed were lateral trunk flexion over the left arm of the chair, the rotation forward of the left side of the pelvis followed by the entire pelvis moving forward and out of the chair, and increased left knee flexion that resulted in the foot being under the chair. Additionally the patient was able to tolerate a near-upright position for brief periods while eating (with supervision).

During the first seating trial, a narrow reclining wheelchair (16 in wide) was tried with the ROHO cushion that the patient already owned. The recliner was evaluated at a variety of angles; however, this did not alter the patient's posture. She needed frequent read-

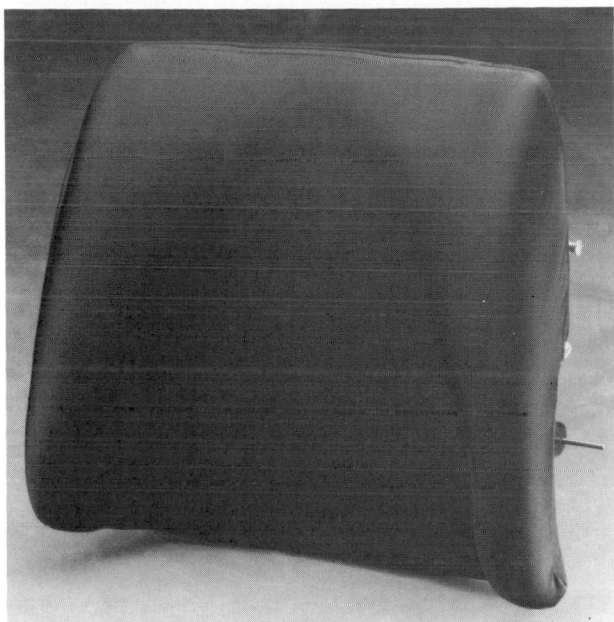

FIGURE 18–1 Avanti Personal Back. (Courtesy of Invacare Corporation, Elyria, OH.)

justments by her full-time caregiver, could not be left alone in the chair, and tolerated less than 1 hour of sitting.

During the second seating trial, various items were slowly added to the recliner; however, the therapists needed to switch the patient to an 18-in wheelchair to accommodate the seating system that was planned for the trial. First, an 18 × 18 in pommel seat with lateral padding was used; the seat was dropped in the back to create a "wedged" seat. The lateral pads on the seat were intended to prevent the "windswept" position of the legs, and the wedged seat was meant to maintain the patient's hips in the chair. The wedged seat in the recliner was intended to allow the patient's hips to be close to 90 degrees while her trunk was slightly reclined. This change did not address the lateral trunk flexion over the side of the chair, and the patient was still able to rotate her left hip forward and out of the chair.

During the third seating trial, a seat belt and the Avanti Personal Back (Invacare Corporation, Elyria, OH) with lateral supports (see Figure 18–1) were added. After this, the patient was able to maintain her hips in the chair, but she continued to laterally flex over the left armrest.

During the fourth seating trial, a large Otto Bock lateral trunk support (Otto Bock Orthopedic Industry, Minneapolis, MN) on the left did prevent the patient from laterally flexing out of the chair (see Figure 18–2).

During the fifth seating trial, the issue of the patient's

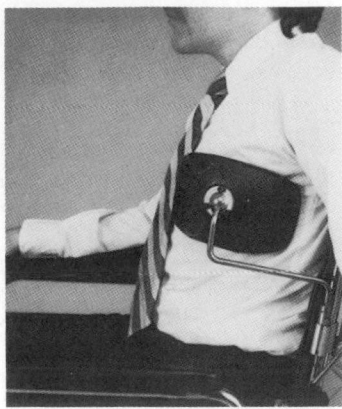

FIGURE 18–2 Otto Bock lateral support pad. (Courtesy of Otto Bock Orthopedic Industry, Minneapolis, MN.)

left leg flexing under the chair was finally addressed through the use of a foot board with several posterior straps (see Figure 18–3). The patient still sat with her right leg extended, but no solution could be found, and no significant functional problems associated with this posture were seen.

A number of seating conditions also were tried with patient #2.

During the first seating trial, the patient was initially in a hemi-height chair with a standard back height and width. He was using a prefabricated contoured foam cushion. A seat belt did not keep his hips back in the chair.

During the second seating trial, a solid dropped base was put in the chair with the back of the base slightly lowered to create a wedged seat; however, the patient still managed to slide forward in the chair.

During the third seating trial, the base was tilted more, and the patient's hips stayed back in the chair. His transfers became very difficult because he could not get out of the chair. He also had more difficulty in propelling his wheelchair because his feet barely touched the floor.

During the fourth seating trial, the extra tilt was removed from the base, and a chair with a higher back was tried to resist trunk extension pushing into extension. With this change, his transfers became easier, he was able to get his whole foot on the floor for easy propulsion, and he did not slip forward in the chair. He no longer needed a seat belt, and he was independent in wheelchair propulsion on indoor surfaces. He could not wheel independently outdoors because of his severe left neglect, not because of physical inability.

Skin Condition

Neither patient had any reddened areas in any seating arrangement. Patient #1 had no problems with skin breakdown during the seating trials, but she was at risk

in some of the earlier trials. No skin problems were seen because the patient did not tolerate the systems and went back to bed after a short time. The final system was a better measurement of skin tolerance because the patient sat in the system for 4 hours. The entire seating system contributed to skin protection because it distributed her weight over a large area, but the ROHO cushion was also an important contribution to skin protection because the patient could not shift her weight to relieve pressure on her skin.

Patient #2 also had no problems, even when he was sitting with poor posture for long periods, because he was mobile and because his frequent weight shifting prevented sustained pressure in any one area. Therefore, a foam cushion was adequate to protect his skin.

Final Wheelchair Selections

For patient #1, a standard-frame recliner wheelchair with a pommel seat 18 × 18 in with lateral padding that is dropped in the back, an Avanti Personal Back with lateral supports, a large Otto Bock lateral trunk

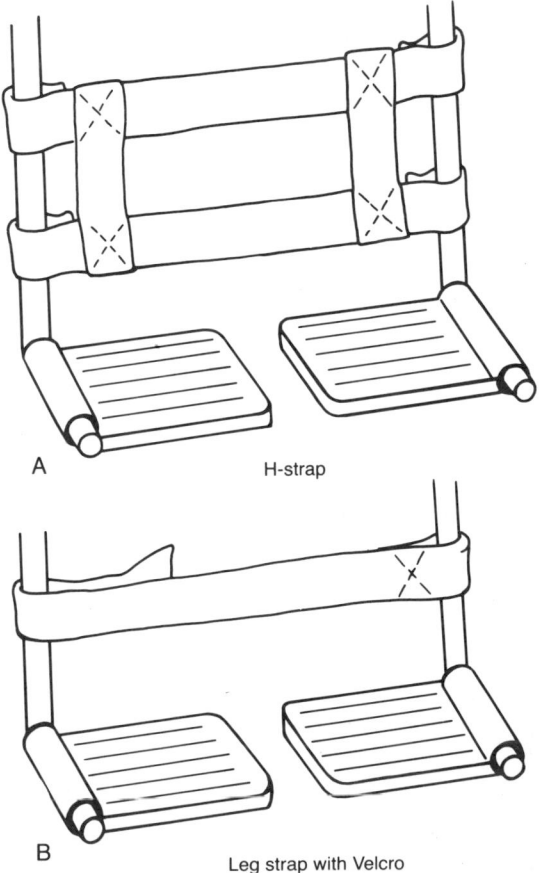

FIGURE 18–3 Posterior leg straps with Velcro hook and loop fasteners. (Courtesy of Production Research Corporation, Beltsville, MD.)

support on the left, a foot board with posterior straps, full-length armrests, a seat belt, and a low-profile ROHO cushion were selected.

For patient #2, a lightweight, 18 by 18 in hemi-height wheelchair with a tall back (18 in), a solid dropped base that is lower in the back, desk arms, a left swing-away footrest, and a prefabricated contoured foam cushion were selected.

COMPARISONS

Similarities

Both of these patients had problems with extension of the hips and the trunk that led to their sliding forward in their chairs. In each case, the therapist began addressing the problem with the use of a solid seat that was dropped in the back to create a wedge. In these cases, this did not completely resolve the problem, but in many cases, this is all that is necessary. Although this is a good solution to this common problem, care should be taken when a patient is severely tilted posteriorly at the pelvis, because pressure on the sacrum could lead to skin breakdown. Solid dropped bases make folding a wheelchair for transport more complicated, and therapists should consider less complicated approaches to this problem, such as the use of solid-back and solid-seat inserts.

Adequate back support also helps to maintain a patient's hip position, as was illustrated with both of these patients. For patient #1, the seat belt and the lateral pads on the chair also helped to keep her hips in the chair; however, for patient #2, the seat belt was not helpful.

Differences

These patients had very different seating goals, and the seating systems were recommended with these goals in mind. For example, if patient #1 had wanted to be active in the community, then the therapists would have had to consider how she was going to be transported in that chair.

Process of Wheelchair Selection

It is important to meet patients' wheelchair and seating needs with as little equipment as possible. With both of the patients discussed in this chapter, the therapist did use quite a bit of equipment but was careful to add equipment slowly and conservatively. It also is important to try simple equipment, such as seat belts, before trying more sophisticated equipment.

References

1. Wilson BA: *Wheelchairs: A Prescription Guide,* 2nd ed. New York, Demos Publications, 1992, pp 54–55.
2. Bergen AF, Colangelo C: *Positioning the Client with Central Nervous System Deficits: The Wheelchair and Other Adaptive Equipment,* 2nd ed. Valhalla, NY, Valhalla Rehabilitation Publications, 1985, pp 27–28.
3. Letts MR: *Principles of Seating the Disabled.* Boca Raton, CRC Press, 1991, pp 4–5.

Suggested Reading

Bergen AF: The prescriptive wheelchair: an orthotic device. In O'Sullivan SB, Schmitz TA (eds): *Physical Rehabilitation: Assessment and Treatment,* 2nd ed. Philadelphia, F. A. Davis Company, 1988, pp 615–628.

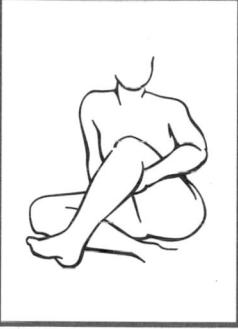

CHAPTER 19

Children with a Variety of Problems

Peggy Owen

The two children chosen for the first two cases discussed in this chapter had the problems of quadriplegia and hemiplegia, respectively. Both cases illustrate the initial physical therapy contacts with these children. The first part of the chapter discusses the screening, evaluation, assessment, and treatment-planning process for both children. At the end of this chapter, the evaluation process used for these two children is compared with the process used for two children with more complex problems to show that the evaluation process is the same for all children, regardless of the diagnosis. The specific evaluation tools and testing procedures used may vary, but the overall process of screening a patient, evaluating problems noted on screening, and assessing the case to determine the relationship between the impairments evaluated and the functional problems identified is the same for all four children discussed in these cases.

I. Overview

A. Introduction to the first two cases

1. CS is a 1-year-old (corrected age, 9 months) girl who has a diagnosis of cerebral palsy, spastic quadriplegia. CS was born prematurely at 28 weeks gestation and required ventilation assistance for only 24 hours. CS's mother thought that CS was treated with surfactant. CS was found to have periventricular leukomalasia at birth. During infancy, CS had the complications of a stomach infection and apnea, and she required a blood transfusion while she was in the intensive care nursery. CS was in the intensive care nursery for approximately 1 month before being discharged. CS was then monitored in an intensive care nursery follow-up clinic. She was referred for a physical therapy and an occupational therapy evaluation at 10 months of age (7 months, adjusted age). CS lives at home with her mother and father. She is the only child. CS's father is from the Dominican Republic and has only recently received his residency card. CS's father was in the Dominican Republic when she was born and for the first few months that CS was home. CS's parents want her to be able to sit independently, to hold her own bottle, and to reach her maximal potential.

2. PG is a 2-year-old boy with a diagnosis of cerebral palsy, spastic hemiplegia. PG's prenatal, natal, and postnatal histories were unremarkable. PG's father noticed that PG's left foot turned in when he began to walk.

PG would frequently trip while walking, so his parents decided to seek medical services. PG lives at home with his parents and two sisters, one of whom is 3.5 years old, and the other 9 months old. PG's parents are both in their early 20s. The parents' main concern is for PG's left foot to be straightened out.

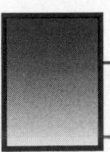

Clinical Decision-Making Cases

Case #1

SCREENING

CS was screened while her history was taken. CS was allowed to play on a mat next to her mother during the taking of the history. She was held by her mother for part of the interview so that observations of the interaction between the mother and child also could occur.

CS demonstrated no ability to get out of any position that she was placed in.

CS would swipe at toys purposefully but showed no open-handed approach to grasp a toy. She held both of her arms stiff at the elbows, with movement occurring only at the shoulders. CS had poor frequency of movement, with her arms moving more frequently than her legs.

Both legs were typically positioned in extension at the hips and knees with ankle plantar flexion. Scissoring of the legs was noted.

CS was interested in the conversation and responded to being recognized. She responded to her name by turning her head and smiling. Vocalizations were minimal. CS was able to communicate her wariness of strangers by looking to her mother and pouting and then by crying if the stranger did not retreat. CS was easily consoled by her mother.

CS reportedly was very attached to her mother to the extent that she cried when her mother left the room. CS also cried when held by her father. This was of concern to both parents.

From the information gained during screening, the following problems were identified:

- CS had a limited variety of movement patterns. Whether the limitation was related to limited range of motion or poor muscle coordination had to be determined with more specific testing.
- CS showed limited movements of her legs in the supine and supported sitting positions. Whether she would show more movement or purposeful use of her legs in the prone or supported standing position needed to be determined.
- CS showed significant delays in motor development. The tool or tools that were to be used to monitor her development and to show progress gained over time needed to be chosen.

CS showed delays in the development of both fine motor skills and in speech and language skills. She needed to be referred to an occupational therapist and a speech and language pathologist for evaluations, or if evaluations had been performed, the information needed to be reviewed, and skills that were observed during the physical therapy evaluation needed to be shared with the specialists in other disciplines.

EVALUATION OF CS

The optimal evaluating system is to perform a joint evaluation with all of the involved professionals present but with one or two professionals doing the assessment. This allows the family to decrease the number of trips that they must make to the center; it also limits the number of people calling the parents' home to schedule appointments and allows the best teaming of professionals with the child and family.

Range of Motion

Because of the limited movement demonstrated by CS, range of motion was checked to determine whether limitations were present at the time of evaluation and whether CS had any ranges that needed to be monitored to prevent joint contractures from developing in the future. No limitation in range of motion was noted.

Functional Activities

Because minimal active movement or position change was noted during screening, definitive evaluation of active movement was done to document CS's status at that time and so that a record for future reference would be available when the time came to reevaluate CS's progress.

CS was able to hold her head in midline while in a supine position.

When placed on her side, CS fell to a prone position and had difficulty getting her leading arm out from under her body.

The child's hands typically were fisted, but CS opened them to pull on the blanket covered with toys to allow her to reach the toys. Rather than reaching with her arms for the toys, CS used her mouth to get the toys and held them in her teeth. With external assistance in shifting weight to one side while she was in a prone position, she used her non–weight-bearing side to swipe at the toys.

In a prone position, CS pushed with both arms, with hands fisted, to raise her head and chest off of the floor. Her arms were not directly under her shoulder; she demonstrated shoulder flexion of approximately 120 degrees.

CS required support at the level of the axilla to maintain her head and trunk in an erect position during supported sitting. No propping with arms was noted while she was in a supported sitting position.

Head and trunk righting when the child was tilted to the side was not seen.

When CS was in a supported standing position, she maintained her knees fully locked to keep from collapsing to the floor.

Standardized Testing

CS was evaluated with the Gross Motor Function Measure (GMFM) to show the types of movement that she could actively perform, to show the amount of assistance that she needed for the completion of skills, and to provide a standardized, objective measure of change over time.[1] CS performed 20% of the lying and rolling skills; 1% of the sitting skills; and 0% of the crawling and kneeling skills, the standing skills, and the walking, running, and jumping skills.

Motor Control

According to Campbell, "Research on motor development has resulted in identification of nine different aspects of gross and fine motor development of importance in assessment of movement in the age range of 4 to 15 years. Factor analysis of items designed to test these various components of motor performance in children resulted in summary factors labeled speed, precision, strength, balance, and coordination."[2] Specific observations and testing of these factors is important for treatment planning and for monitoring the progress of treatment.

CS demonstrated movement at the shoulder for most upper-extremity skills. Her legs showed mass movement patterns, with total extension being the posture most frequently observed. Reciprocal leg movements were not seen. CS demonstrated no segmentation of her trunk during any movements.

Speed of movement was slow in the legs and ballistic in the arms when CS was swiping at toys.

Precision of reaching was poor—CS only swiped at toys. She was quite accurate, however, with her ability to reach toys with her mouth.

Strength was poor—CS was only able to maintain antigravity positions for brief periods.

Activities of Daily Living

CS required assistance to eat and drink. She continued to be spoon fed and to use a bottle for drinking most liquids. CS was able to eat soft table foods, such as ravioli. She was not drinking formula but drank milk or juice from the bottle.

CS did not assist with bathing or dressing at the time of evaluation.

This information was obtained during the screening interview. The feeding issues were to be addressed further by the occupational therapist who was to work with CS; therefore, no further testing of her feeding skills occurred at the time of evaluation.

Sensation and Skin

Sensation testing was not done because CS had limited ability to express whether she felt touch unless a noxious stimulus was used. Because the equipment that CS was using was soft, and because she spent limited amounts of time in each piece of equipment, no specific testing was needed at the time of evaluation.

Equipment

CS had an infant-sized feeder seat with a base. She used this for seating at home and also used it as an insert for positioning in her highchair and her stroller. CS used a regular child car seat.

CS had soft, bilateral thumb abduction splints.

At the time of evaluation, CS was being bathed in the sink for ease of position and holding.

Communication

CS was able to communicate her needs by crying only. She was unable to articulate words at the time of evaluation. She smiled and cooed when she was happy. Further evaluation of her speech capabilities were to be performed by a speech therapist once her parents were ready for the evaluation. CS's parents expressed a desire to wait for the speech evaluation until after physical and occupational therapeutic services had been initiated.

ASSESSMENT AND FUTURE TREATMENT PLANS

The results of CS's screening and evaluation indicated that her diagnosis of spastic quadriparesis appeared to be consistent with the findings of this evaluation. Information from the GMFM and from clinical observation showed that CS was limited in her range of movement patterns and experienced significant delay in the development of her gross motor skills when compared with other children at her adjusted age level. Motor control problems such as slow speed of movement, massed patterns of the extremities, poor movement against gravity, poor endurance, and poor precision with arm movements are important measures of skill that can be monitored over time, and their nature should direct therapeutic intervention.

The use of equipment to assist CS in becoming more functional in a variety of positions was very important. Because CS was 9 months old at the time of evaluation (adjusted age), it was important for her to work on skills in upright positions, both sitting and standing, despite the fact that she was unable to roll independently. CS was motivated to be upright. This may have been one reason that she preferred to be held; she typically was on the floor if she was not being held, and it may have been more stimulating for her to interact with the environment in a supported sitting or standing position than on the floor, where CS has limited ability to interact.

It was important to work jointly with the occupational therapist so that once CS was positioned appropriately, she could be encouraged to use her arms in a more purposeful manner to manipulate toys. Working jointly with the speech therapist also was important because CS should have been encouraged to make sounds and to communicate choice during treatment sessions when she was engaged in fun activities.

It was important to develop activities that CS's parents could do at home to work toward the joint goals of the family and the therapist. Because the parents' major goal was to have CS sit independently, therapy and the home program were to be directed toward this goal. For example, the therapist demonstrated ways to carry CS to challenge her to hold her trunk erect (as opposed to ways in which her back was always supported). Finding ways to incorporate therapeutic activities into daily activities in the home is always a challenge but may be beneficial for the child and family.

Evaluating equipment to help challenge CS to sit independently was important. A corner chair was tried. It provided some back support but minimal side support, which would encourage CS to use lateral trunk muscles and equilibrium reactions to maintain an erect sitting position. CS also was able to lean forward away from the chair to reach for toys on the table in front of her and to use active trunk extension for proper positioning.

The only form of feedback that CS gained from the therapist and parents was extrinsic feedback (see Chapter 8). CS received praise when she performed well, and holding a toy was a reward for her performing movement that would allow her to get to that toy. During a therapy session, each skill was performed in a variety of positions to encourage CS to "learn" a skill rather than to just perform the skill in one situation. For example, CS could work on sitting on her mother's lap, in the corner chair, on a bench, and on the floor in different positions.

Case #2

SCREENING

PG was screened by observation, once while he played alone and his father gave history information and once while he played with his father. Few hands-on procedures could be done because PG would not tolerate being handled by anyone other than his father. PG would use belly crawling to get from one place to another when he was in a prone position. He preferred to sit in a "W-sit" position. He reportedly never moved in a quadruped manner. PG was able to move from the floor to a standing position using a pattern of half-kneeling to standing (with the right leg forward) with one hand on the floor. Once in a standing position, PG appeared to tolerate less weight on his left foot and would keep the left side of the pelvis anterior to the right side of the pelvis. PG could walk independently, demonstrating a smaller stride on the left, limited left knee movement during the swing phase of gait, and no heel strike on the left.

From screening, the following problems that required further definitive testing were identified:

1. The static position of PG's left foot and ankle could have been related to limited range of motion or to poor muscle coordination.

2. PG's altered gait pattern could have been related to limited range of the hip muscles, a leg length difference, poor muscle coordination, or poor alignment of the pelvis.
3. The use of the "W-sit" position for sitting may have been related to PG's being more stable in this position, limited range of motion at the hips, or torsional changes at the hip.
4. Because PG showed immature social responses to the therapist, was difficult to understand, and was limited in his transition of going from the floor to a standing position with the right leg forward, developmental testing needed to be performed for gross motor skills, and a referral for a speech and language evaluation was indicated.

EVALUATION OF PG

Range of Motion

Range of motion on the left was measured because PG had limited movement at the knee and ankle. This range was compared with that on the right side, and both measures were compared with standard range of motion measures to ensure that no limitations were present on both sides. PG's range of motion was difficult to assess because he was leery of strangers and screamed when he was handled. Brief hands-on examination revealed no limitation of range at either ankle. Hip range could not be tested. When he was standing, PG had a valgus position of the left knee, questionable tibial torsion of the left leg, and midfoot pronation on the left. Measurements of leg length and pelvic alignment could not be obtained.

Functional Activities

Observation of active movement of the left side compared with that of the right was important to determine what compensations PG had learned and to see whether functional use of the left leg was occurring in all positions.

PG used both legs to belly crawl across the floor.

PG used a pattern of half-kneeling to standing when making the transition from a sitting position on the floor to a standing position. He actively did this, but only with the right leg forward. When asked to perform this task with the left leg forward, PG was able to obtain a half-kneeling position by using his hands to position his left leg; he demonstrated poor balance and poor graded control of the left leg when he pushed himself into a standing position.

PG enjoyed playing ball games with his father, and his catching and throwing skills were fair. PG had difficulty catching a large ball, and his throwing accuracy was poor.

PG was unable to run. Further definitive testing of his jumping and squatting skills was limited because of PG's being so leery of strangers. This testing was to occur over the course of the treatment sessions as PG began to feel more comfortable with the therapist.

Standardized Testing

PG was evaluated using the Peabody Developmental Motor Scales because he was very functional when he used his gross motor skills.[3] He received a total raw score of 165, which placed him within the 14th percentile for children of his age group. He received a developmental quotient of 84, which is within 1 SD of the mean. PG received an age-equivalent score of 17 months, although his chronological age was 24 months. PG had a basal level (age range where child passed the majority of skills) of 15- to 17-months and the ceiling level (age range where child passed few skills) of 24- to 29-months. PG's scores were impressive and showed that he was quite functional in gross motor skills.

Motor Control

PG showed less weight shifting to the left leg than to the right during standing and walking. Abnormal timing of the tibialis anterior with the gastrocnemius soleus muscle group on the left was suspected because PG maintained ankle plantar flexion during the swing phase of gait and because the brief measure of range of motion showed no muscle tightness. PG demon-

strated more hip and knee flexion during running than during walking, but ankle plantar flexion was not present when PG was running or walking. It appeared that PG was tripping over his left foot because his toes were dragging.

PG actively used his left arm in play when two arms were required for the activity. The quality of movement of the left arm was slightly less smooth than the quality of movement of the right arm. Overall, PG was a strong boy and was very active.

Activities of Daily Living

PG was able to feed himself without assistance. He ate table foods that were prepared for the entire family. He drank from a cup independently and demonstrated use of utensils that was appropriate for his age group.

PG bathed in the tub independently (with supervision).

PG would dress himself with some assistance. His parents had no concerns in this area; therefore, this information was obtained through questioning during the screening. No further evaluation was felt to be needed in this area.

Sensation and Skin

Because PG fell frequently, his parents were encouraged to monitor PG's environment, to limit the number of sharp objects in the house, and to provide safe areas in which PG could play. Specific sensory testing could not be performed because PG was not cooperative. While PG was being observed, he would express that he experienced pain when he fell; however, it was difficult to determine whether he could localize where he felt pain, especially on the left foot. Further monitoring of PG was to be done to assess this skill. Once his level of cooperation had improved, specific testing of whether he felt touch was to be attempted. At the time of evaluation, observation of PG when he fell and questioning of where he felt pain were used to determine whether he consistently complained of pain in a general way or if he localized a specific spot each time.

Equipment

PG had no adaptive equipment.

Communication

PG was not easily understood because he did not pronounce words; rather, he made sounds for the correct number of syllables for a word. PG became frustrated when he could not communicate his point. He was able to say no clearly.

ASSESSMENT AND FUTURE TREATMENT PLANS

PG's evaluation produced little information that was definitive because PG would not allow himself to be handled. However, the information gained through observation confirmed the parents' concerns about PG's tripping.

PG was very functional in executing his gross motor skills, as was indicated by his Peabody Developmental Motor Scale score; therefore, direct treatment for gross motor skills was not necessary.

The purpose of therapy was to determine whether intervention for ankle positioning through splinting would increase PG's function, decrease the frequency of his tripping, and assist with increasing his safety during walking. PG had not been seen by an orthopedist; therefore, he was referred to an orthopedist to have questions answered about the possible tibial torsion and to obtain the opinion of a specialist in orthopedics regarding the use of splinting for correction of the position of the left foot during walking. According to Cusick, splints cannot directly change torsional deformities in the long bones of the leg.[4] Because PG demonstrated no limitation in range of motion of the left ankle, the question of whether bracing should be used to "fix" a possible imbalanced pull of muscles around the ankle joint needed to be considered. Orthoses and splints are used primarily to maintain achievable alignment and to reduce functional deformity in children with nonparalytic neuromotor deficit.[4] Cusick stated that a well-built ankle-foot device for an equinovarus deformity assists with the goals of providing adequate toe clearance, providing a better position in stance, and preventing further deformity of the foot and the ankle. Cusick's book is a useful tool for determining whether splinting is appropriate and, if so, what the best type of splint to use would be.[4]

PG's behavior was discussed with his parents to determine whether they wanted information or guidance on ways to deal with PG so that he would not be so afraid of strangers. A referral to a social worker from the health department was given, and the special educator working with the family in the home (part of the infant and toddler project described in Part H of PL 99-457) also gave the parents some suggestions on how to deal with PG's behavior.

II. Similarities and Differences Between the Cases

The process during the screening, evaluation, assessment, and treatment planning was identical for both of the cases just discussed. The parents were questioned regarding the purpose for their seeking an evaluation. A screen was performed by observation and without hands-on intervention to gain information about each child's capabilities. Plans for what to evaluate were developed with the parents based on the parents' need for information and on the problems identified during the screenings. The definitive evaluations were performed, and the data and results were compiled to allow the therapists and the parents to jointly determine short- and long-term goals for the children and to determine the focus for future therapy, if therapy was indicated. In cases in which the child is old enough to participate in the decision-making process, he/she should assist with developing goals and with taking responsibility for the home program. It is also important for all those involved to work as a team. All professionals that evaluate a child should work together to provide information that is as comprehensive and inclusive as possible to the family. This decreases any confusion or the amount of discrepancy concerning information provided by different therapists.

A. Introduction to the second two children

1. AD is a 5-year-old boy who had a diagnosis of Lesch-Nyhan syndrome. This syndrome is progressive and results in the child demonstrating self-mutilating behaviors. Children with this diagnosis have poor motor control; however, these children may have a wide range of intellectual capabilities. AD has been followed for physical therapy services since he was approximately 2 years of age. At the time of this evaluation, AD's need for both physical therapy and occupational therapy services in his preschool was being assessed. AD was to enter kindergarten in the fall. AD lives at home with his parents and with his older brother, who had the same diagnosis. His parents were unable to transport AD for direct service treatment at the time of evaluation because AD's father was in poor health, and because his mother was unable to lift much weight owing to a back injury. AD's parents hoped that AD would continue to progress and to show developmental changes.

2. HM is a 5-year-old girl who was diagnosed

with hypothyroidism. At birth, HM was full term; there were no complications at the time of delivery. At 27 hours of age, she experienced an increase in her respiratory rate and spent a few hours in the neonatal intensive care unit. At 9 days of age, she was treated for pneumonia. She was discharged from the hospital and remained at home for 1 week. HM was readmitted to the hospital with jaundice at 2 weeks of age. Phenylketonuria test results revealed hypothyroidism. HM has taken levothyroxine sodium since she was 15 days of age. In January of 1991, HM was examined by a specialist in Boston to determine whether she had another diagnosis that would account for the

significant motor control problems that she had developed; these problems were not thought to be related to hypothyroidism. No remarkable findings were revealed. HM lives at home with her parents and a younger sister. HM has been followed in school to determine her need for physical therapy consultation and her need for direct treatment. She had been treated by a speech therapist in school and by an occupational therapist, both at school and in the clinic. HM's parents' concerns were that HM be as independent as possible and that all precautions be taken so that HM would not damage her feet, ankles, and knees.

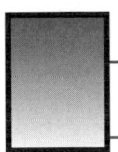

Clinical Decision-Making Cases

Case #3

EVALUATION OF AD

Range of Motion
Range of motion for all of AD's joints was full.

Motor Control
For AD, movements fluctuated from full extension to full flexion with little midrange control. His movements were ballistic. Once he extended his arms or legs, it was difficult for him to "turn off" the extensor muscles. AD's muscle tone was floppy.

Functional Activities
From a prone position, AD could move into a "W-sit" position by first pushing back into a low quadruped position. He needed arm support to maintain this position.

He rolled or "belly" crawled to get to places or to things.

AD was dependent in performing all transitions to and from equipment.

AD was being trained in maneuvering his electric wheelchair safely. He was inconsistent with his ability to stop safely. It appeared that AD had the ability to move his wheelchair straight when he was motivated to do so. AD's favorite movement in the electric wheelchair was going in circles. AD's difficulty in stopping safely appeared to be limited by his inability to release the joystick once he had obtained a fully extended arm position. AD had a better grip on the joystick and an

improved ability to release the joystick when he used it to move the chair backward rather than forward.

AD was able to push his manually operated wheelchair independently for short distances on level surfaces only.

AD's awareness of safety issues was poor.

Standardized Testing
The GMFM[1] was used to evaluate AD's skills and to examine whether any changes had occurred in his developmental level and in the amount of assistance he needed to do an activity. This was a concern of AD's parents, and it was jointly decided with the parents that the GMFM would be the best tool with which to monitor AD's developmental status over time. In 1991, AD was able to complete 96% of the lying and rolling skills; 10% of the sitting skills; 7% of the crawling and kneeling skills; 0% of the standing skills; and 4% of the walking, running, and jumping skills. In 1993, AD was able to complete 96% of the lying and rolling skills; 23% of the sitting skills; 11% of the crawling and kneeling skills; 0% of the standing skills without assistive devices; 25% of the standing skills with assistive devices; 0% of the walking, running, and jumping skills without assistive devices; and 16% of the walking, running, and jumping skills with assistive devices.

AD was evaluated using the Pediatric Evaluation Disability Inventory (PEDI)[5] in 1993 only. His functional skill score and his caregiver assistance score were greater than 4 SDs from the mean, with 2 SDs from the mean being an acceptable range. The PEDI could be used to monitor AD's progress over time; it also could be used to monitor changes in the amount of assistance that AD might need to function throughout the day.

Activities of Daily Living

AD had a modified cup with a straw for drinking. AD was able to bite food when it was brought to his mouth. He was able to lift a spoon or finger food to his mouth with guidance. AD was very messy when eating; therefore, his ability to practice independent eating at home was limited. AD worked on independent feeding at school.

AD wore a diaper at all times. His parents were not working on toilet training at the time of evaluation.

AD was totally dependent in regard to all bathing skills.

AD was dependent in regard to dressing skills. He could assist the person dressing him by pushing his arms and legs through the openings in the clothing.

Communication

AD was able to pronounce single words and had a vocabulary of approximately 10 words. He was being evaluated for an augmentative communication device. AD's language reception skills were good. AD was very social and extremely motivated to communicate with the children in his preschool class.

Sensation and Skin

Sensation was within normal limits for AD. He had no skin lesions or sensitivities. It was important to note any skin sensitivities or limitations in sensation because much of the equipment that AD used could cause irritation to sensitive skin.

Equipment

AD had both a manual and an electric wheelchair.

The electric wheelchair was chosen for AD because it was important for him to have some active control of his life, and his cognitive awareness of himself and his environment was thought to be sufficient for him to be able to learn to drive the chair. The electric wheelchair was rarely used at home because AD's parents' house had small rooms; however, AD would have the opportunity to use the electric wheelchair for independent mobility within the school.

AD also had a manual wheelchair as a backup seating system in the event that something were to happen to the electric wheelchair. The manual chair was used at home and for field trips at school.

AD used a wooden chair with arm and foot rests for activities at a table at school.

He used a ring walker for standing at the water and sand tables in class and for upright mobility within the classroom.

Impression and Future Treatment Plans

Use of the GMFM to examine AD's developmental progress showed that AD had made gains in his ability to get into a propped sitting position on the floor without external assistance. This was an important part of the evaluation because independence was one of the concerns of AD's parents.

AD was able to function independently with the assistance of many different pieces of equipment.

He continued to be dependent with all transitions to and from all pieces of equipment.

Safe, independent mobility over long distances would help AD to become mostly independent at school during the next year. Training AD to safely use the electric wheelchair was an important area to address in helping AD to become independent within the school. AD's parents had little space to use the electric wheelchair at home; thus, all of the training occurred at school.

Because AD was very small and quite light, one individual was able to lift him at school, and his father was able to lift him at home.

Communication continued to be a major limitation for AD when he tried to interact with other children in the classroom. Encouraging AD to use his independent sitting capability in school was important to increase his sitting strength and to further boost his self-esteem.

Case #4

EVALUATION OF HM

Range of Motion

Range of motion for all joints was full, with knee extension and medial and lateral ankle motions being extreme.

Motor Control

HM's movements were ataxic and athetotic. HM had no graded control of knee extension but was gaining control of mediolateral ankle movement on an inconsistent basis. A video analysis of her gait pattern was needed to provide measurable data for monitoring the changes in her ability to grade the control of her knees and ankles during walking.

Functional Activities

HM was independent with all transitions but needed stand-by guard for safety on stairs. She was able to take three to five steps without external assistance, but only with close supervision.

Standardized Testing

No standardized tests were used to evaluate HM. Because of her limited ability to jump and run, HM's score on the Peabody Developmental Motor Scales would have been extremely low. HM had good functional skills; therefore, her ability to be tested with the GMFM was limited. The PEDI was not published at the time of HM's last evaluation. Because HM's parents' concerns were related to her level of independence, the PEDI would be the best testing tool for monitoring changes in HM's independence over time. This was to be discussed with her parents to determine whether they were interested in using the PEDI at HM's next re-evaluation.

Activities of Daily Living

HM was independent with regard to eating and drinking. She was able to use a spoon and fork on her own.

HM was fully toilet trained.

HM was able to put on and take off her shirt and pants without assistance. She was able to put on her coat and to fasten one to two buttons. HM was unable to fasten zippers at the time of evaluation. She was being treated by an occupational therapist at school to assist with skills pertaining to the activities of daily living. It was important for the physical therapist to maintain communication with the occupational therapist to monitor HM's progress with regard to all areas of skill development.

Communication

HM was able to verbally communicate all of her wants and needs. She stuttered but was able to say most words if given sufficient time to speak. HM's ability to understand language was appropriate for her age level. HM was a very social, very happy girl, and she easily communicated with all people around her.

Sensation and Skin

HM had full sensation. She frequently had cuts, scrapes, and bruises on her legs from frequent falls. Documenting HM's skin integrity was important because a decrease in the number of cuts and bruises could have been another measure of increased walking skill.

Equipment

HM had a posterior walker, a manual wheelchair, and a dressing bench. HM's parents had constructed stairs and parallel bars for her. HM was independent with the use of all equipment listed. HM had had solid-ankle ankle-foot orthoses in the past but had been able to hyperextend at the knees by walking on the heels of the ankle-foot orthoses. Supramalleolar orthoses were tried to limit some mediolateral ankle movements, but no change in ankle stability was noted by HM's parents. Cusick recommends using a knee hyperextension splint for training the control of the quadriceps muscles.[4] This type of splint was to be tried for HM in the future.

IMPRESSION AND FUTURE TREATMENT PLANS

HM was independent with her mobility and with most of her skills related to the activities of daily living. HM's parents were concerned about the progress that she was making toward independence with all of her skills. The PEDI would be the best measure for following and evaluating HM's progress over time.

The other concern of HM's parents was that she not cause damage to her joints with her walking pattern. Use of a video camera to record her gait pattern, with joint markers to assist in motion analysis, would be the most objective measure of HM's ability to control her knee hyperextension and her ankle position at heel strike. These measures could be removed from the screen of the monitor using a goniometer; they would allow objective measurements of change to be seen and would allow subjective analysis of changes in the quality of HM's walking. Measurements of the frequency of falling and of the frequency of knee hyperextension also could be obtained.

Treatment for HM should be focused on increasing graded control of the knee muscles during gait by promoting a more active awareness of what movements should be avoided as well as a generalized strengthening of the muscles in both legs. Options for working on this functionally could be to strengthen HM's abilities to ride a tricycle, to climb a ladder to a slide, to go up and down stairs, and to squat during play. Monitoring the need for bracing also should continue to be a major focus of therapy.

III. Comparison of the First Two Cases and the Last Two Cases

The main similarity between these two case studies and the two case studies of the children with cerebral palsy discussed at the beginning of this chapter is that despite the variety of diagnoses, the level of involvement, and the level of independence of the children, all of the evaluations focused on the same types of concerns: those of the parents and those of school personnel. This pattern reflects the importance of the revolution of family-centered care. The families are empowered to make decisions about the type of information that they want from the evaluation and about the testing tools that will be used. The families also are able to participate in the evaluation if they so desire. The parents are then presented with the information from the evaluation, allowing the therapist and parents to formulate goals together concerning future treatments. The focus of the treatment should be directly related to the concerns of the parents or all school personnel.

References

1. Russell D, Rusenbaum P, Gowland C, *et al.: Gross Motor Function Measure Manual.* Hamilton, Ontario, McMaster University, 1990.
2. Campbell SK: Assessment of the child with CNS dysfunction. In Rothstein JM (ed): *Measurement in Physical Therapy.* New York, Churchill Livingstone, 1985.
3. Folio MR, Fewell RR: *Peabody Developmental Motor Scales.* Hingham, MA, Teaching Resources Corporation, 1983.
4. Cusick BD: *Progressive Casting and Splinting.* Tucson, Therapy Skill Builders, 1990.
5. Haley SM, Coster W, Ludlow L, *et al.: Pediatric Evaluation of Disability Inventory: Development, Standardization and Administration Manual.* Boston, PEDI Research Group, 1992.

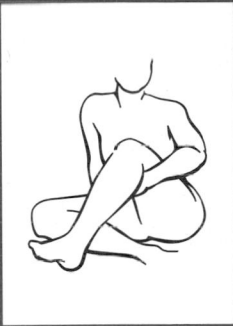

CHAPTER 20

Longitudinal Pediatric Considerations

Peggy Owen and Lee Nelson

The case study of SM is a longitudinal study that follows SM from birth through her stay in the neonatal intensive care nursery, through her initial evaluation in a rehabilitation setting within her home, and finally, to her transition from staying at home full time to starting preschool. The differences in the types of screenings, evaluations, and therapeutic intervention that were used are presented and discussed at the end of the case presentation.

I. Overview

A. Introduction to SM at birth

1. Prenatal and postnatal periods. SM is a female infant born at 34 weeks' gestation. Her mother was 28 years old and had had a history of hypothyroidism for 5 years, for which she had required Synthroid (levothyroxine sodium) therapy. The mother's pregnancy with SM was complicated by the spontaneous abortion of SM's twin during the first trimester. Congenital anomaly screenings consistently produced negative results. One month before delivery, an ultrasound examination showed placenta previa and hydramnios. SM was delivered by cesarean section secondary to complete placenta previa. Her birth weight was 1910 g, and her APGAR scores were as follows: 1 at 4 minutes, 4 at 5 minutes, and 4 at 10 minutes. At birth, SM exhibited decreased muscle tone, was without spontaneous motor activity of the arms and legs, and was without respirations, requiring ventilatory bagging and intubation ventilation. Once SM was using the ventilator, her skin color became more pink, and some movement of her arms and legs was observed. She was transferred to the neonatal intensive care unit.

2. Initial physical examination. The initial physical examination revealed the following positive signs: a low hairline; cloudy corneas bilaterally and doll's eye sign; no spontaneous respirations; hyperactive precordium without murmurs; small patent arterial ducts; contractures of both legs, with equinovarus position bilaterally at ankles; decreased movement of all extremities; hypotonic respiratory tone; elevation of the right hemidiaphragm; and normal results on cranial ultrasound (except for the presence of slightly dilated ventricles).

3. Initial findings. The initial findings sug-

gested a central nervous system cause for SM's floppy limbs and trunk and for her lack of spontaneous respiration. A discussion with SM's parents revealed that during pregnancy, SM's mother had had trouble letting go of things that she grasped and often had to shake her hands to open them. No family history of myotonic dystrophy, cataracts, or neuromuscular disease was noted. However, given the mother's history of hydramnios and SM's history of floppy limbs and trunk combined with elevated diaphragm and leg contractures, there was a strong probability of congenital myotonic dystrophy. The data from genetic and neurologic consultations, both done on SM's 3rd day of life, confirmed this diagnosis.

Clinical Decision-Making Cases

SM at Birth

SCREENING

SM was referred for physical therapy when she was 4 days old, primarily for the assessment and management of her leg contractures. A screening was performed with the database (see Chapter 10 for a description of how to use the database). This took place over the course of three sessions. Generally, it is beneficial for a physical therapist to meet with a child several times before formulating problems, goals, and treatment; it was particularly important in SM's case because of the combination of her significant musculoskeletal problems and her medical fragility. The following problems were identified on screening:

Type of Problem	Problem
Pulmonary	Ventilator-dependent
Skeletal	Congenital anomalies, including overlapping digits
Neuromuscular	Congenital myotonic dystrophy; significant contractures at the hips, knees, and ankles; paucity of volitional movement of all limbs
Postural	Extreme frog-legged position exhibited in the supine position; both legs widely abducted and externally rotated, with the lateral surfaces of the upper and lower legs resting flat on the isolette mattress

Areas such as communication and vision were not screened because SM was ventilator dependent and because her eyes remained closed. Areas such as balance, functional mobility, and gait patterns were not appropriate items to be screened for SM.

EVALUATION OF SM IN THE NEONATAL INTENSIVE CARE UNIT

Range of Motion

The one specific area that required further testing was joint mobility of the lower extremities. A complete range of motion examination was done, and the results were documented on a flowchart. The following areas were the focus of intervention:

Motion Examined	Results
Hip extension	Lacks 80 degrees to neutral bilaterally
Hip adduction	Lacks 10 degrees to neutral bilaterally
Hip internal rotation	Has 10 degrees on left and 45 degrees on right
Hip external rotation	Has 30 degrees on left and 10 degrees on right
Knee flexion	Has 115 degrees on left and 135 degrees on right
Knee extension	Lacks 30 degrees on left and 40 degrees on right
Ankle dorsiflexion	Lacks 5 degrees to neutral bilaterally

Functional Activities

No definitive testing was required.

Motor Control

No definitive testing was required.

Standardized Testing

Standardized testing was performed because the major problem identified was range of motion, which does not require the use of a standardized tool to be assessed.

ASSESSMENT

SM presented with multiple problems secondary to her diagnosis of myotonic dystrophy. Her pulmonary status was a major concern from a life-sustaining and health care maintenance point of view. The focus of physical therapy was on managing the contractures of SM's legs. Much deliberation and discussion with physicians and with SM's parents occurred regarding the safest yet potentially most effective way to accomplish this. It was decided that conservative management would be undertaken; this management would include a custom-designed, custom-fabricated soft positioning system. The primary goal was to gently but consistently reduce the contractures toward a more neutral position while carefully monitoring SM's pulmonary and medical status. Decisions regarding other developmental issues and goals were deferred because of SM's critical medical status at that time. SM's hospital course and significant events during her hospitalization included

1. A tracheostomy, which was performed when SM was 2 months old.
2. A transfer to the pediatric unit when SM was 3.5 months of age.
3. A diagnosis of myotonic dystrophy for SM's mother during SM's hospitalization.
4. A gastrostomy tube, which was placed when SM was 3 months old; SM received occupational therapy consisting of an oral-motor, prefeeding program.
5. SM's gradual learning to tolerate a ventilator schedule of 12 hours on (nocturnally) and 12 hours off; by the time she was discharged at 5 months of age, SM completely tolerated the schedule.
6. SM's growing to be a responsive infant, alert to people and her environment. At the time of her discharge from the hospital, she was able to bat at a mobile, finger small toys, bring her hands to a midline position, suck on her thumb or her hand, occupy herself by looking in a mirror, and make attempts at smiling. It was difficult to determine the degree to which facial weakness did not allow her to smile.
7. The fact that SM's parents were extremely involved and participatory in her medical and physical care.

TREATMENT

SM was treated consistently by a physical therapist throughout her hospitalization, but the sessions of this therapy varied in intensity. The soft positioning system was successfully used for approximately 1 month; it resulted in a fairly rapid reduction in hip and knee contractures to the point at which they approached normal limits. Considerable instruction in correct application of this system was given to the nursing staff and to SM's parents to ensure consistency of approach. As SM grew and as her motor activity increased in her legs, more frequent extensor patterns were observed, with strong equinovarus present at her ankles. Therefore, bilateral Aquaplast ankle-foot orthoses were fabricated, beginning when SM was 2.5 months old. It was hoped that these orthoses would help SM to maintain 90 degrees of dorsiflexion. Several more sets of orthoses were fabricated before SM was discharged from the hospital. Each set had different anchoring and strapping systems because SM's plantar flexion pattern was becoming so strong that she was able to move out of her splints.

Because of SM's diagnosis and presenting condition, she was at high risk for further contracture development and for malalignment of body segments. Initially, because of SM's medical fragility, the emphasis of therapy was on contracture reduction and on maintenance of optimal alignment. The design and initial application of this conservative, low-cost management system required intensive physical therapy services; however, the intensity decreased because the primary day-to-day responsibility for application and monitoring was assigned to the nursing staff. A minimum of weekly physical therapy monitoring and reassessment was performed to evaluate any progress or regression in SM's status. It had been uncertain whether such a simple positioning system would remediate the contractures to the degree that it did; however, because of SM's unstable medical status and the high risk that any physical intervention could have caused destabilization, this conservative plan proved to be very effective.

As SM's medical status improved, further evaluation of and treatment for improving her developmental skills and her motor activities were performed. The areas addressed were the improvement of volitional motion, prefeeding skills, increasing social interaction, and continued monitoring of joint mobility and segmental alignment. This investment in careful, consistent, and gentle efforts to promote optimal structural alignment appeared to be helpful in that it later facilitated movement and function, without causing severe musculoskeletal sequelae or medical compromise.

SM was discharged from the hospital when she was 5 months old. Her parents were trained in all aspects of her care. SM's tolerance to prolonged sitting in a car seat was tested, and her tolerance was found to be acceptable. Referrals were made for home-health physical therapy and occupational therapy, as well as for the initiation of an early intervention program.

SM at 11 Months of Age (Adjusted Age, 10 months)

SM had been referred for a physical therapy evaluation and for treatment at home. SM lives at home with her mother, father, and older sister. SM and her family had recently moved to a new home. She had received physical and occupational therapy and had been evaluated by an early intervention specialist before her family moved. Those services were to continue. Medical care conferences were held monthly to monitor SM's capabilities and to recommend alterations to her respiratory treatment programs, as needed. At the time of this evaluation, SM was off of the ventilator for 16 hours at a time each day. SM received albuterol treatments every 4 hours. Nurses assisted SM's parents for 16 hours a day. SM had a gastrostomy tube, but she was to have a button placed. Hearing and vision had not been tested, but SM's parents had no concerns about her auditory and visual abilities.

SCREENING

SM was receiving home health services from the time she was discharged from the hospital at 5 months of age until she had reached a chronological age of 11 months. SM's parents moved recently, and thus a change in service providers was required. Because SM was being transferred from services in one area of the state to services in another area of the state, the evaluation and progress notes from the first home health therapist were used as the screening.

Therapy for SM had been occurring while she was in bed. If SM was not in the bed, she was being held by her mother. SM tolerated approximately 15 to 20 minutes of therapy at a time. The main focus of therapy was to work on head control in a supported sitting position, to work on arm and leg movements against gravity, and to work on general endurance for activity. SM interacted somewhat with toys, especially with a "busy box" hanging on the side of her crib; however, further interaction was encouraged. SM's parents' concerns were that she begin performing more oral motor activities, that her feet stay straight, that she increase her head control, and that she spend more time in upright positions. From the screen, it was determined that the range of motion of SM's ankle joints needed to be evaluated, standardized testing of SM's gross motor skill level was to be performed, and the use of adaptive equipment to help SM play in upright positions was to be assessed.

EVALUATION

Range of Motion

Range of motion measurements of the hips and knees were taken because of SM's limited leg movements and because she typically had her legs positioned in hip external rotation. It was important to monitor SM's range of motion in the hips and knees so that she would not develop tightness. On evaluation, SM's range of motion was found to be full at the hips and knees.

SM had limited ankle dorsiflexion. She had a range of dorsiflexion of approximately −5 degrees when her knee was extended. With the knee flexed, the range was full, and the gastrocnemius muscle was observed to contract.

Functional Activities

SM reached purposefully and with both arms toward toys when she lay on her back. SM was motivated by the presence of toys that were in her crib.

SM spent the majority of her time in a supine position. She demonstrated the ability to kick her legs so that they barely lifted off of the bed; to raise one hip and, while keeping her shoulders on the bed, to rock her hip up and down; and to lift one shoulder to initiate a roll movement.

While in a semiprone position, SM was able to roll to the right side only to a supine position. In a prone position, she was able to lift her face and to turn her head to either side. SM was not observed to lift her head to look forward when she was supported on her elbows.

SM tolerated sitting in her tumbleform seat for 3 to 4 hours at a time. In a supported sitting position, SM demonstrated a rounded trunk and little head control.

SM was unable to support weight through her legs in a standing position at the time of evaluation.

Some functional activities were recorded, although their quality was judged subjectively. These activities will be used to evaluate SM's future progress.

Motor Control

SM's frequency of movement was high because she was constantly moving. Her movements were not considered to be writhing. She made random movements of her arms and legs. SM would flap her arms or kick one leg for brief periods. She demonstrated isolated joint movements of the ankles, knees, and hips. SM had sufficient strength to move her arms and legs against gravity, but she could only maintain these positions for brief periods. Timing the number of seconds that SM was able to hold an extremity in the air would have been one way to objectively measure changes in SM's strength and/or endurance level.

Standardized Testing

SM was evaluated using the Peabody Developmental Motor Scales (PDMS), which provided an objective measure of change in SM's gross motor status.[1] The problem with using the PDMS to measure change over time is that this tool is not very sensitive for small changes in a child's skill level. The Gross Motor Function Measure (GMFM) was not available at the time that SM was evaluated but would have been the therapist's tool of choice.[2] SM's parents were interested in having an objective measurement of their daughter's function. Before the test was administered, the limitations of the testing tool were discussed with SM's parents so that they would not be disappointed or shocked by the results. SM received a total score of 11 (which was translated into an age equivalent score of 0 months) and a developmental quotient of 65—the lowest quotient available on this test. SM's ceiling level is in the 2- to 3-month age range. Again, the PDMS can provide only limited measurement of small changes in gross motor skills.

Activities of Daily Living

Although SM was fed through her gastrostomy tube attempts were made at having her take apple juice on the end of a pacifier. SM had no active lip closure and did not show much interest in the pacifier.

Equipment

SM used a tumbleform seat, a car seat, and a stroller. None of her equipment for respiratory support was included in this section of the evaluation.

ASSESSMENT

SM showed changes in the strength of her extremities more than in that of her trunk. The size of SM's head was quite large in relation to the size of her body. It appeared that once her body grew, she would have better head control.

The standardized testing provided little specific information. The functional activity observations would be more useful for measuring change, despite the fact that these observations were subjective.

Range of motion of both ankles continued to be the concern. Fabrication of ankle-foot orthoses (AFOs) was necessary to provide the stretch needed in SM's Achilles tendons. To reduce their cost, SM's orthoses were to be fabricated from Aquaplast by the physical therapist. Aquaplast is a low-temperature plastic that is easily molded and reheated, should mistakes in molding be made. Fabricating Aquaplast AFOs is a one-

step procedure because the AFOs are molded directly to the child's sock-covered foot. This decreases the amount of time required for fabrication, resulting in a significant decrease in cost. Because SM was so small and because she was not even bearing weight at the time her AFOs were made, Aquaplast was strong enough to hold her feet in a good position.

At 10 months of age, children typically spend some time playing while in a standing posture. It was important that SM be positioned so that her legs could support some of her weight. This was important not only for bone growth but also for perceptual and social growth. It was important to work on finding equipment that would assist SM to stand and for her legs to support some of her weight.

TREATMENT

The amount of time that SM spent sitting was gradually increased over a period of 1 week until she was able to sit up 0.5 hour longer than she had the week before. SM was encouraged to work on head control while she was sitting and while she was in a prone position.

The amount of time that SM was in a prone position also was increased.

Solid-ankle AFOs were fabricated and worn for 3 to 4 hours a day. SM gradually worked up to that amount of time wearing the AFOs.

SM needed to work on active mobility. Encouraging her to do the movements she already was doing was important. She needed to be encouraged to roll to the side to reach for her "busy box." Rolling to both sides was encouraged. Work outside of the crib was limited at the time and needed to be increased.

Once the AFOs were made, it was easier for SM to work on standing. A supine stander was tried to see how SM would tolerate it. A supine stander was chosen over a prone stander because SM needed head support to maintain her head in an erect position. A prone stander also was tried to see how SM would tolerate it.

SM's parents were encouraged to first have SM perform as much of a movement as she could and to then assist her in the completion of the movement.

SM at 3 Years of Age

SM had been receiving physical and occupational therapy and early intervention services from the same facility since she was 11 months old. SM has experienced respiratory distress occasionally, but it was never bad enough for her to be hospitalized. At 3 years of age, SM was weaned from the ventilator. At first, she was able to breathe two nights consecutively without

the ventilator. She was weaned to three nights off and one night on for a few weeks; thereafter, the ventilator was discontinued for daily use to be available only on an as-needed basis. SM was starting preschool with the Early Essential Education Program in public school. SM was to be in the regular preschool classroom with other children who did not have physical disabilities. SM and her family recently moved into a new home within the same town in which they had been living since 1991. Since moving, SM appeared to be happier, possibly because the house had more space and more rooms for her to explore independently.

SCREENING

No screen was performed on SM because she had received therapy services over the 2 previous years.

SM made sounds when she was being assisted with respiration using an Ambu bag during her albuterol treatment. She was able to communicate her needs to strangers and to her parents by pointing to what she wanted or by scooting to where she wanted to go and by making sounds to get someone's attention. SM was able to shake her head to say yes and no, but she was not consistent with answering questions with this movement—she still considered it a game.

SM's parents' concerns were that SM begin taking in food orally; that she improve her general gross motor development, including getting in and out of the sitting position independently; and that she begin working on toilet training.

EVALUATION

Range of motion

SM continued to have very tight Achilles tendons. Attempts at casting were unsuccessful. SM was able to wiggle out of the casts. She also was able to wiggle out of her AFOs; therefore, they were not used. SM would not tolerate passive stretching to the Achilles tendons unless she was standing. Her tolerance of stretching while she was standing had been a recent occurrence. SM was to undergo surgery for Achilles tendon lengthening after school had started. All other range of motion measurements in both legs continued to be within normal limits.

Functional Activities

SM was able to roll from one part of the room to another.

She required moderate assistance to move from lying on the floor to a sitting position. Once in a sitting position, SM was able to scoot, either forward or backward, around the house. This was her main mode of transport at that time.

SM reportedly pulled up onto her knees when she was on the couch. She used the back of the couch to pull up with her hands and pushed with her legs so that she went from a Tailor sitting position to taking weight on her knees, while her knees were still in a Tailor sitting position.

SM was able to bear full weight standing once she was placed in that position. She was able to push with her arms and legs to move from sitting with her hips at an angle greater than 90 degrees to standing with minimal support during the push. She required support for

balance during the transition, but once she was standing, she could maintain the position for 2 to 3 seconds without external assistance.

SM was able to get off the couch, the wooden chair with arm and foot rests, or a bench independently by scooting to the edge and letting her rear end fall to the floor. She did not use her hands to slow the fall. To get off of the couch, she would lean back once she was at the edge and use her back to slow her fall to the floor.

SM was able to push a "star cart" in the house and to go from room to room. She could push the cart forward and backward, but she was stronger going backward.

Motor Control

SM had ankle clonus that was easily elicited by the stretching of her heelcords. Once she has surgery and is casted, it is hoped that the ease of initiating her clonus would be decreased.

SM's endurance for exercise during physical therapy session was increased. SM was able to tolerate a full 45-minute session, during which she performed many physical activities.

SM demonstrated accuracy of movement of both arms and legs for reaching and kicking.

SM had increased the strength in her neck extensor muscles, demonstrated by the fact that she could lean forward from a sitting position and put her head on the floor. From this position, she could lift her head and trunk by pushing with her arms to return to a sitting position. SM was able to maintain her head approximately 5 to 10 degrees in front of midline throughout this activity. She also could repeat this activity many times without fatiguing.

Increased strength was noted in all extremities, as evidenced by the amount of antigravity weight bearing that SM did with both arms and legs. SM was unable to control the position of her feet. Both feet were maintained in plantar flexion at all times. SM used both feet for weight bearing during transfers but had to stand on a wedge when she was fully upright.

Standardized Testing

SM was evaluated using the Pediatric Evaluation Disability Inventory (PEDI) and the GMFM.[2,3] The PEDI was chosen because it would measure the amount of function that SM had, the amount of caregiver assistance that was given during activities, and the number of modifications, that were needed for SM to perform activities. The functional skills measured with this tool were self-care, mobility, and social function. SM's scores indicated that she was relatively strong in regard to social skills when assistance was given by the caregiver. Mobility was SM's weakest area. SM continued to require a significant amount of caregiver assistance to perform all of the skills evaluated by the PEDI.

Because this was the first year that the PEDI had been used with SM, comparisons could not be made. (The PEDI evaluates children's abilities over time.)

SM was evaluated with the GMFM to provide objective information on her gross motor function for her parents, because this was one of their concerns. SM had been evaluated with the GMFM in the past, allowing comparisons with the earlier test results to be made. During the GMFM evaluation, SM was able to perform 45% of the lying and rolling skills, 47% of the sitting skills, 2% of the standing skills, and 0% of the crawling and walking skills. The previous year, SM had been able to complete 43% of the lying and rolling skills, 20% of the sitting skills, and 0% of the standing, crawling, and walking skills. SM was able to perform many skills independently compared with what she had been capable of the previous year.

Activities of Daily Living

SM was beginning to assist with dressing and grooming skills. She would push her arms and legs through the openings in clothing that was held for her. She would try to brush her hair and would rub her hands together while they were under water.

She continued to be fed with a tube. SM showed interest in putting toys and her feeding tube in her mouth to chew on them but had no interest in putting food in her mouth. SM preferred to feed other people. Attempts were made to put SM's feeding tube in a cup to see whether she would learn to take liquids from a cup.

SM still wore diapers, but her parents were interested in working on toilet training.

Equipment

SM had a Snug Seat wheelchair and a wooden chair with arm and foot rests, and she was to start using an electronic communication device. It was possible that SM would need some form of frame to assist her with standing once she had had her surgery and was casted. This was to be monitored.

ASSESSMENT

SM had made great gains in her overall strength, in her ability to be independently mobile in the house, and in her willingness to try new activities. SM had shown progress in gross motor function, as measured by the GMFM. She continued to require much caregiver assistance to perform most skills, but it was hoped that SM would show improvement in this area over time as she started preschool. The PEDI would be used to help monitor the changes in the area of caregiver assistance. SM was gaining strength physiologically as she was weaned from the ventilator, and she was able to tolerate 45-minute sessions of treatment. It was recommended that SM's teachers be informed that she was able to perform social skills with caregiver assistance.

TREATMENT

It was possible that the amount of treatment done in the home would change once SM had started attending preschool. SM was to be able to work on mobility and weight-bearing skills at the preschool. SM's parents had a good understanding of how to encourage her to perform skills independently; therefore, it was possible that SM would only need to be monitored on a monthly basis so that her parents could receive advice on how to work with SM during new activities.

SM was to receive physical therapy until her surgery and casting was finished and a new program for ways to work with her in the home could be prepared. Her parents would need assistance with working with SM in the casts initially. The therapy goals were to increase SM's weight bearing and her independent mobility, both at home and at preschool. With the casts on, it was possible that SM could be able to stand and walk forward in a posterior walker once she had been trained to use one. SM could use the walker at school and at home to allow her the maximal amount of training in a variety of situations.

II. Progress of SM Over Time

A. Amount and type of physical therapy intervention

SM received therapy that varied with respect to frequency and intensity in each case described. The frequency of therapy while SM was in the hospital fluctuated from daily to as tolerated, based on SM's medical status. The frequency at the 11-month and the 3-year studies remained at weekly intervention sessions. The amount of therapy while SM was in the neonatal intensive care unit was limited to short-term periods of intervention based on SM's medical status. When she was 11 months of age, SM was able to tolerate 25 to 35 minutes of intervention. Again, what determined SM's length of intervention was her physiological status; when she became fatigued, therapy was stopped or decreased to determine whether she could recover. At 3 years of age, SM was able to tolerate a full 45- to 55-minute session. SM was less fragile medically; this was reflected in her endurance level during the therapy sessions.

Intervention at all three points in time incorporated both physical and occupational therapy services. It is important for therapists providing these services to work together to help parents understand how to incorporate all of the suggestions given by each therapist; this can decrease the number of visits that a family must make to therapy settings during the week and prevent conflicting information from being given to the family resulting from the overlap of the therapists' skills.

Teamwork among the various professionals is an important part of pediatric therapy because it allows them to see a child as a whole person and to address multiple goals for the child with the child's background and circumstances in mind. The teams that worked with SM varied during her first 3 years of life, although the team at 11 months was the same as that at 3 years. The teams consisted of SM's parents, primary physician, nursing service providers, therapy service providers, and social worker. The teams at 11 months and 3 years also included insurance representatives, respite care providers, and supplies of durable medical equipment suppliers. The respective teams met monthly to discuss progress; they also met to discuss plans for SM's care based on the picture of SM as a whole person with various technical and motor problems.

B. Focus of intervention

1. The focus of SM's therapy was always driven by her medical status. Because of her fragile state at birth, much deliberation occurred regarding the splinting issues, as discussed in the beginning of the chapter. Therapeutic intervention was focused on positioning to provide comfort and to help SM to remain calm; the therapy also was intended to limit the possibility of future contractures or deformities.
2. At 11 months of age, SM was less fragile than she was at birth but continued to require monitoring of her color and respirations during activities to assess the amount of stress to her body. The focus of therapy was to provide ways to encourage more active movement while helping SM to remain calm and unstressed.

3. At 3 years of age, SM was gaining physiological strength—she was sick on an infrequent basis, and her use of the ventilator had significantly decreased. SM still was monitored for her tolerance of activities, but her endurance had improved greatly, and the number of breaks that she required had decreased significantly. Because SM was healthier and more like other children, she was, and would continue to be, challenged to perform age-appropriate activities at home and at school.

C. Amount of parent involvement

SM's parents participated in the decision-making process related to SM's care since the time of her birth. Her parents were a part of all team meetings, they chose the types of evaluation tools to be used with SM, they determined the focus of therapy throughout the time that SM received outpatient services, and they attended their first Individualized Education Program meeting so that they could prepare for when SM started school. SM's parents were to continue to have a decisive role in SM's care, using information from the team to make informed decisions.

D. Types of screenings and evaluations

Each screening and evaluation that was presented differed in the amount of information that it gathered and in how the information was gathered. The difference in screening procedures was based on the circumstances at the time of the screening.

1. SM was screened with a database while she was in the hospital so that her therapists could fully understand her physiological problems and be aware of all potential problem areas.
2. Screening information for SM at 11 months was obtained by interviewing the therapists who had been treating SM until she and her family moved, from medical information from other health care providers who had worked with SM, and by attending the final care conference for SM in her home before her family moved into its new residence.
3. No screen was performed at 3 years because SM has been treated by the same agency for the previous 2 years.
4. The types of evaluation tools used to mea-

sure SM's progress differed in each study. No standardized evaluation tool was used at SM's birth because her medical status was so fragile that the focus of intervention was on necessary procedures only. Information from a standardized assessment would not have altered the course of therapeutic intervention for SM at that time.

The PDMS[1] were chosen because the Bayley Motor Scales[4] had not yet been renormed and the GMFM[2] and the PEDI[3] were not yet available. The PDMS was the only tool that provided some information about SM. Because the PDMS does not provide information about treatment programming and is not sufficiently sensitive to measure change for a child whose status is as complex as SM's, it could be argued that no standardized measure should have been used. It was a bias on the part of the examiner that some information of a standardized measure was important to have for comparison with the results of future tests. This was a decision that was made using the parents' and the therapists' judgement. The results of the GMFM and the PEDI would be most beneficial for monitoring SM's progress over time and for developing therapeutic intervention.

III. Summary

Overall, this longitudinal case provides the reader with information on how the screening, the evaluation, and the intervention processes change as the circumstances change for the child. Physical therapy services are driven by the family and child to make the services most relevant for the family. The role of the therapist is as a teacher to the parents, the child, and the other team members. The days of having the therapist make decisions for the family are gone. The therapist must share information related to the child's diagnosis, prognosis, and possible treatment options and theories with the parents to allow them to make the best possible decision for their child. The therapist is no longer the center of the child's world. The child is the center, with therapy being only one small part of his/her world.

References

1. Folio MR, Fewell RR: *Peabody Developmental Motor Scales.* Hingham, MA, Teaching Resources Corporation, 1983.
2. Russell D, Rosenbaum P, Gowland C, *et al.: Gross Motor Function Measure Manual.* Hamilton, Ontario, McMaster University, 1990.
3. Haley SM, Coster W, Ludlow L, *et al.: Pediatric Evaluation of Disability Inventory: Development, Standardization and Administration Manual.* Boston, PEDI Research Group, 1992.
4. Bayley N: *Manual for the Bayley Scales of Infant Development.* New York, The Psychological Corporation, 1969.

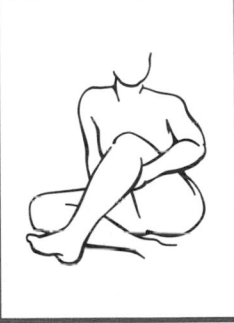

CHAPTER 21

Determining the Need for Skilled Physical Therapy

Marianne Orest and Peggy Owen

The following case studies describe the physical therapist's screening, evaluation, and assessment of three patients whose need for skilled physical therapy had to be determined. The two cases dealing with adults presented in this chapter represent the opposite ends of the spectrum in determining a patient's need for skilled physical therapy: in one case, the patient had relatively few problems, and in the other, the patient had many. The pediatric case presented in this chapter highlights the importance of taking into account all aspects of a child's life and environment to determine whether physical therapy services are needed. At the end of the chapter, these three cases are compared, to examine their similarities and differences in the type and level of physical therapy involvement that each patient required are examined.

I. Overview

A. Introduction to the two adult patients

1. Patient #1 is a 29-year-old man who was involved in a skiing accident. He had experienced a loss of consciousness at the scene and had been diagnosed as having a concussion. He was admitted to the hospital for testing and observation. He was referred for physical therapy on the day that he was admitted to the hospital. The patient was single and lived alone in a third-floor apartment but was to stay with a friend after being discharged from the hospital. He was employed as a chef and thus spent most of his work day standing.

2. Patient #2 is a 75-year-old woman who lived alone in a second-floor apartment. She had two daughters who did not live nearby. She had been admitted to an acute-care hospital 3 days before the evaluation because she had had a left cerebrovascular accident. Her doctor had examined her and referred her for physical therapy in an effort to improve her mobility. At the time of evaluation, the patient's goals were unknown because she was very lethargic and nonverbal and because her daughters were unavailable for interview.

B. Screening of database items

The database was to be completed in the usual manner. Database information can be gathered by reviewing a patient's chart, by communicating with his/her team members (i.e., the patient, his/her family, and any involved health professionals), and interviewing the patient. The database information will vary depending on the specific problems with which the patient presents (see Chapter 10).

Clinical Decision-Making Cases

Case #1

SUMMARY OF THE SCREENING RESULTS

The results of the screening for patient #1 were as follows:

Category	Results
Medical tests	Computed tomography results were negative
Medication	Antiemetic
Behavior	Glasgow Coma Scale score was 14 on admission
Pain and tenderness	Soreness throughout body—especially in the area surrounding the right knee
Skin and soft tissue	Right forehead laceration; right knee ecchymosis
Neuromuscular	Traumatic brain injury
Functional mobility training	Rail needed for ascending and descending stairs

Impairments Identified by the Screening

Increased pain and decreased skin integrity were noted.

Impairments for which Further Evaluation Was Needed Because of the Possibility of Contributing to Impaired Mobility

Further evaluation of the patient's balance and behavior was recommended because of the possibility that problems in these areas could contribute to impaired mobility.

The patient's static balance and dynamic balance were determined to be acceptable on the initial screening. However, patients with mild traumatic brain injuries frequently have problems performing more challenging balance activities; therefore, further evaluation of balance through the use of more challenging activities was recommended. The Berg Balance Scale was used to measure the patient's balance, and he obtained a perfect score (56 out of 56 possible points).

The patient's behavior was tested with the Glasgow Coma Scale. He received a score of 15.

Patient Education

The therapist discussed with the patient the possibility that he could experience balance problems as he resumed his regular routine. He was instructed to inform his physician at a follow-up visit whether he experienced any functional problems after he was discharged from the hospital.

ASSESSMENT

A physical therapy referral was made so that the patient's high-level balance could be evaluated. The patient could perform functional activities independently but required the use of a rail when he ascended or descended stairs. It was recommended to the patient that someone guard him when he used stairs that had no rail, at least initially after his discharge from the hospital. He was judged to be ready for discharge from physical therapy.

GOALS

Because the patient had no goals to work toward, there was no need for the patient to receive skilled physical therapy at that time.

Follow-up Therapy Plans

Physical therapy follow-up was not needed at that time. If problems were noted when the patient attended his follow-up appointment with his physician, follow-up physical therapy could be initiated at that time.

Impairments Identified by Screening

A lack of ability to move the right extremities, decreased strength of the left extremities, impaired balance, impaired behavioral and cognitive status, impaired ability to communicate, and impaired posture were noted.

Impairments for Which Further Evaluation Was Needed Because of the Possibility of Contributing to Impaired Mobility

Further evaluation of the patient's motor control, balance, and behavioral and cognitive status was recommended because of the possibility that problems in these areas could contribute to impaired mobility.

When the patient's motor control was evaluated, no movement was noted in the right extremities. The patient's strength in her left extremities was judged to be a grade 3 out of 5; however, it was difficult to formally test the patient's strength because of her impaired behavioral and cognitive status.

When the patient's balance was tested, it was found that she was unable to sit unsupported. She required continual assistance to maintain a static, unsupported

Case #2

SUMMARY OF THE SCREENING RESULTS

The results of the screening for patient #2 were as follows:

Category	Results
Medical tests	Computed tomography scan showed that an infarct had occurred in the left middle cerebral artery
Medication	Cardiovascular; diabetic; diuretic
Communication	Nonverbal
Cardiovascular	Left cerebrovascular accident; hypertension
Pulmonary	Smoked two packs of cigarettes a day for 30 years
Metabolic	Diabetes mellitus; obesity
Gastrointestinal/ genitourinary	Incontinence
Vision	Homonymous hemianopsia
Behavior	Very lethargic; unable to follow simple commands for performance of functional activities; apparently not oriented to people, time, or place

Category	Results
Appliances	Foley catheter
Neuromuscular	Right hemiplegia; no movement noted in right extremities; decreased strength in left extremities
Balance	Fell to the right when sitting at the edge of the bed
Posture	In a sitting position, thoracic kyphosis, forward head, rounding of the shoulders, increased weight bearing on the right; right upper extremity hung limply by her side
Functional mobility	Maximal assistance of one person needed to roll to the right; maximal assistance of one person and moderate assistance of one person needed to roll to the left; maximal assistance of two people needed to move from a supine position to a sitting position on the right side; nurses reported that patient needed the orderlies to lift her when she was transferred from the bed to a recliner lounge chair

position, she fell to the right when she tried to sit, and she made no attempt to regain her balance.

After the patient's behavioral and cognitive status was screened, she was referred to an occupational therapist and to a speech and language pathologist for a formal evaluation.

ASSESSMENT

At the time of the assessment, it was difficult to determine whether the patient would benefit from skilled physical therapy services. It was believed that her cognitive impairment would limit her ability to learn and to perform new tasks. Therefore, she was scheduled for a 1-week trial period of skilled physical therapy. If she was able to achieve the set goals, she was to receive continued skilled physical therapy. However, if she was unable to achieve the set goals, skilled physical therapy was to be discontinued, and the nursing staff was to be instructed in how to help the patient to perform activities to maintain her present status. It was anticipated that she would not be able to continue to live alone; therefore, plans to place her in a nursing home following her stay in the hospital needed to be discussed.

GOALS

The short-term goals were to be achieved within 1 week. One of the short-term goals for patient #2 was to achieve poor static sitting balance (the ability to occasionally maintain an unsupported sitting position for less than 3 seconds, but this is inconsistent and usually depends on how she is positioned. It was also hoped that the patient would learn to roll to the right with moderate assistance of one person, to roll to the left with maximal assistance of one person, and to move from a supine position to a sitting position on the right with maximal assistance of one person and moderate assistance of one person.

The determination of long-term goals for the patient was deferred until after the trial therapy period had ended, because if she did not achieve the short-term goals, physical therapy was to be discontinued.

Functional Areas to be Evaluated After the Initial Screening

The therapist was unable to screen the patient's transfers during the initial screening because of time constraints and patient's fatigue. It was important to evaluate whether the patient would be able to provide some assistance when she was being transferred or whether she would have to be lifted by the orderlies. Because transfers were not evaluated during the initial screening, it was difficult for the therapist to predict how the patient would perform in this area and to set a goal for transfers. Therefore, a goal was not set until after the transfers could be evaluated.

The patient was screened and evaluated while she performed a stand-pivot transfer during a subsequent physical therapy session. The patient required the maximal assistance of two people to perform the transfer. At that time, it was decided that it was safer for the patient and for the therapists if the patient continued to be lifted by the orderlies. Therefore, a goal was not set for transfers.

TREATMENT APPROACH

A functional approach of sitting at the edge of the bed for sitting balance and bed mobility was taken. These tasks were done because they may have been familiar to the patient. These tasks were done repeatedly to determine whether she had the ability to respond and to participate in familiar activities.

The patient's use of her right extremities was incorporated into the functional activities. Movement was performed within the context of a goal-directed task to make the movement more meaningful to the patient. For example, the therapist instructed the patient to try to reach for her glasses while she was sitting at the edge of the bed. More movement may be achieved during functional activities than during exercises of the right extremities that are done on a mat, especially when a patient is difficult to engage cognitively. Therefore, it may be best to limit physical therapy for such patients to the performance of functional activities only.

OUTCOME

Patient #2 tolerated the treatment, but she was unable to actively participate, possibly because of her lethargy and her inability to follow simple commands. The patient's functional status did not change during the trial week of treatment; therefore, she did not achieve the set goals. As outlined in the initial assessment, because the patient did not achieve the goals, skilled physical therapy was to be discontinued. Because the patient was unable to actively participate in physical therapy, she required a maintenance, or unskilled program. The nursing staff was instructed in how to help the patient to perform mobility activities that would assist in maintaining her present status. Physical therapy was to be resumed only if the patient showed significant changes in her participation level, as observed by her team members.

Case #3

GENERAL INFORMATION

Children often are referred for a physical therapy evaluation to determine whether physical therapy services are indicated. When children are clumsy and demonstrate significant delays in the development of their gross motor skills but are able to function in school, at home, or in a day-care environment, it is difficult to decide whether referrals for direct physical therapy service are appropriate. This case study focuses on a child who attended school and had significant motor deficits but was not referred for direct service treatment. This case illustrates how important it is for a physical therapist to take into account all aspects of a child's life and environment rather than just the scores on standardized testing when he/she determines whether physical therapy services are needed.

Introduction to the Pediatric Patient

Patient #3 is an 11-year-old boy who was referred for a physical therapy evaluation in his school. An observation checklist, designed by the physical therapy staff, was completed by the child's schoolteacher and was sent to the therapist at the time that the referral was made (see Figure 21–1). The problems identified on the checklist were that the child was weaker than his peers; that he tired easily; that he had difficulty hopping, skipping, jumping, and galloping; that he appeared stiff and awkward in movement; that he was clumsy; that he had difficulty sequencing motor acts; and that he had difficulty participating in his physical education class. The teacher also noted that he did not walk smoothly when he went up and down stairs and that he had difficulty adjusting his body movements to avoid obstacles in the environment. The concerns of the teacher were whether the child had significant delays in his gross motor skill development and whether he would benefit from physical therapy services, either in school or outside of school.

The child's social history was significant because he lived with his grandmother. According to the school's records, his parents were not his caregivers at the time of the evaluation. The teacher stated that the child's grandmother limited his activities significantly because she was "unable to keep up" with him. Reportedly, the grandmother thought that the child was lazy and that that was why he was unable to perform difficult tasks. The child had a younger sister who also had been evaluated regarding the possible need for physical therapy intervention. The grandmother was very limited financially and did not have access to any means of transportation.

Summary of the Screening Results

The observational checklist that was completed by the child's teacher was designed to provide screening information regarding disability level that could be used to assist in determining the type of tools needed to fully evaluate the child within the school setting. Further observation should occur when a child is walking from his/her classroom to the evaluation site. The physical therapist should observe how the child manages stairs, ramps, or uneven surfaces; how he/she negotiates doors; how he/she interacts with the teacher and the class when he/she leaves the classroom or when he/she meets peers in the hall; and how observant he/she is of his/her surroundings. In this case, patient #3 was able to guide the therapist to the room where the evaluation was to take place; however, he stopped repeatedly to peek into the windows of the classrooms along the hallway. He did not have to negotiate stairs, ramps, uneven surfaces, or doors.

The standardized testing tools chosen to evaluate the child were the Peabody Developmental Motor Scales (PDMS)[1] and the Bruininks-Oseretsky Test of Motor Proficiency (BOTMP).[2] Standardized tools were chosen for this evaluation because the teacher requested information on the child's performance in relation to the performance of his peers. Clinical observations were used in conjunction with the results of the standardized tests to determine whether physical therapy services were indicated.

The child was an amiable young boy who was distractable and required multiple cues to keep his attention focused. He demonstrated difficulty with changing from one activity to another. He needed multiple explanations of why an activity was being changed and of what the new activity would be. The child was willing to be evaluated and did not appear to mind being removed from the resource room.

SUMMARY OF THE EVALUATION

Standardized Testing

The child was initially evaluated with the short form of the BOTMP. The BOTMP is standardized tool available to measure motor function in children 7 to 14 years of age compared with that of their peers. The BOTMP also is used in making decisions about the need for therapeutic intervention.[3] Patient #3 scored within the first percentile for children in his age group. His total score was the lowest possible score that could be reported in the charts. Because the child had great difficulty performing many of the test items on the BOTMP, he was also evaluated with the PDMS.[1]

The PDMS testing was performed on a different day to determine whether the child's performance on the tests was typical of his performance at school. The PDMS is based on the capabilities of physically normal children between 0 and 8 years of age. Although patient #3 was older than the age cutoff for the PDMS, the test was used for identifying specific areas of difficulty for him. The PDMS test measures skills in five areas: reflexes, balance, nonlocomotor skills, locomotor skills, and receipt and propulsion skills.

The scores from the PDMS could not be used, but the BOTMP gave information about patient #3's performance in relation to that of his peers. The PDMS gave information regarding skill areas on which patient #3's therapy could be focused during physical education class or recess. He demonstrated difficulty with nonlocomotor strength skills and with coordination in the receipt and propulsion area.

Clinical Observations

The child was difficult to understand because he often substituted some sounds with others when he talked. For example, he said "dummer dault" instead of "somersault." He was very soft spoken; therefore, he often had to repeat phrases to make himself understood.

The child demonstrated problems that could have been caused by either motor planning deficits or by poor auditory processing skills. For example when the child was asked to stand up without having been given cues on how to do so, he could not perform the task; he lifted his feet over his head while he lay in a supine position. Furthermore, the child was not able to tie his shoes independently. When patient #3 was given a demonstration of a skill in conjunction with the command to do it, he was better able to perform.

The child's concept of body schema appeared to be poor. He was unable to consistently distinguish the right side of his body from the left side. His muscle tone was very floppy, and he appeared to be drained of energy at all times. The child's physical accuracy improved when he was given external cues on how to perform certain tasks. For example, verbal cues to "watch the ball" when he was trying to catch a ball were helpful. The child had difficulty detecting errors in his own movements. If he was questioned as to why he did not catch the ball or why he tripped, he was unable to answer. As with some of his other problems, this could be related to a possible deficit in auditory processing skills.

The child appeared to be desperate for friendship and attention. During the evaluation he would constantly ask the therapist to watch him while he tried to perform a skill. When he was praised for doing a good

OBSERVATION CHECKLIST FOR SCHOOL-AGED CHILDREN

_____ Physical therapy referral   _____ Occupational therapy referral

Student: _____

Person completing this form _____ Date _____

BASIC SENSORY FUNCTIONS

_____ 1. Dislikes being touched
_____ 2. Has trouble keeping hands to self; pokes or pushes other children
_____ 3. Excessive mouthing of objects
_____ 4. Difficulty adjusting body movements to obstacles in the environment
_____ 5. Fearful of movement (*eg,* swing, see-saw)
_____ 6. Avoids play with finger paint, "funny foam," or clay
_____ 7. Avoids crowded situations (*eg,* group story time, hallways)

MOBILITY

_____ 1. Difficulty managing adaptive device (*eg,* crutches, walker, wheelchair)
_____ 2. Difficulty getting on and off a bus
_____ 3. Unable to access the school environment (*eg,* stairs and doors present as an obstacle)
_____ 4. Unable to get in and out of a wheelchair
_____ 5. Difficulty transferring self from one position to another (*eg,* from wheelchair or walker to toilet or chair)
_____ 6. Difficulty keeping up with other children

GROSS MOTOR

_____ 1. Seems weaker than others, tires easily
_____ 2. Difficulty with hopping, skipping, jumping, galloping
_____ 3. Appears stiff and awkward in movements
_____ 4. Clumsy, difficulty with balance skills
_____ 5. Reluctant to engage in playground activities, physical education class, or both
_____ 6. Difficulty sequencing motor acts
_____ 7. Difficulty with throwing, catching, or kicking a ball

FINE MOTOR

_____ 1. Poor sitting posture (*eg,* slumps, head too close to work)
_____ 2. Difficulty with drawing, coloring, copying, cutting
_____ 3. Awkward pencil grasp
_____ 4. Switches hands often during fine motor activities; lack of an established hand dominance
_____ 5. Abnormal posturing of arms and hands
_____ 6. Tremor or shakiness in hands

VISUAL PERCEPTION/PERCEPTUAL MOTOR

_____ 1. Letter and number reversals
_____ 2. Excessive difficulty learning how to form letters and numbers
_____ 3. Difficulty copying from the board
_____ 4. Poor spacing between letters or words
_____ 5. Difficulty staying on the line when writing
_____ 6. Eye movements are not well coordinated
_____ 7. Tendency to confuse right and left (on self, others, objects)

SELF-HELP SKILLS

_____ 1. Difficulty managing fasteners
_____ 2. Difficulty with toileting
_____ 3. Difficulty placing arms or legs into clothing
_____ 4. Spillage when drinking and eating
_____ 5. Very slow eater; needs food cut up
_____ 6. Avoids certain textures of food
_____ 7. Careless when eating

continued

FIGURE 21–1 Observation checklist for school-aged children referred for physical therapy or occupational therapy evaluation.

OBSERVATION CHECKLIST FOR SCHOOL-AGED CHILDREN *(continued)*

PLAY SKILLS

_____ 1. Is a "loner" when playing
_____ 2. Unable to play purposefully during free time, flits from one thing to another
_____ 3. Selects the same play media; no interest in exploration
_____ 4. Seeks out younger children as playmates

BEHAVIOR

_____ 1. Becomes easily frustrated with motor tasks
_____ 2. Apt to be impulsive, heedless; accident-prone
_____ 3. Easier to handle in small groups or individually
_____ 4. Frequently out of seat
_____ 5. Constantly in motion
_____ 6. Needs to have instructions repeated or said slowly
_____ 7. Is very distractible

ACADEMIC

_____ 1. Written work is not commensurate with verbal skills
_____ 2. Slow worker
_____ 3. Difficulty organizing work
_____ 4. Difficulty completing work
_____ 5. Below grade level: Math ____   Spelling ____   Reading ____   Writing ____

Are there any other behavior(s) that would be important for us to know?

PLEASE RETURN TO THE CONSULTING PHYSICAL THERAPIST OR OCCUPATIONAL THERAPIST BEFORE HIS/HER VISIT.

FIGURE 21–1   *(continued)*

job or for trying hard, he smiled and repeated the praise. The child's teacher said that he did not have any close friends in his class. Because of the child's immature social behaviors and his limited language skills, it probably was difficult for the other children in his class to comfortably relate to him.

ASSESSMENT

Patient #3 is an 11-year-old boy who was found to have significant delays in his gross motor skill development when he was compared with his peers. He had demonstrated significant difficulty with motor planning, body concept, and determining when a task or skill was not performed correctly. Whether the problem was related to poor auditory processing skills needed to be evaluated further. A referral for a speech therapy evaluation was recommended if an evaluation had not been performed previously.

Determining whether the child needed physical therapy services was difficult. It was recommended that he receive physical therapy consultation in the school on a quarterly basis. It was believed that this could help the physical education teacher to determine the types of cues that would best help the child to perform well during the class. It was also hoped that therapy could

help the teacher to find ways to challenge him to use problem-solving skills to become more of a leader and less of a follower. The child performed consistently on the 2 days that he was tested, so it appeared that the test results were a good representation of his overall skill capability.

Taking into account that he had been functioning with limited motor-planning and body-concept skills for 11 years, that the age-appropriate skills he needed to practice were skills that involved group participation in sports or clubs, and that his grandmother had no transportation and did not feel that he had any problems other than laziness, direct service intervention outside of school was not feasible. The child was to be monitored by the physical therapist in school. His grandmother was given the evaluation results and suggestions for extracurricular activities that would benefit him. He was to be re-evaluated by a physical therapist at school on a yearly basis. A recommendation was to be made for the child to be evaluated by the school counselor for possible psychological problems related to his not having friends at school, his having difficulty with participating in physical education class, his having difficulty being understood when communicating verbally, and his not receiving much positive attention at home.

II. Comparison of Patient #1, Patient #2, and Patient #3

A. A skilled program versus a nonskilled or maintenance program

Physical therapists cannot continue to work with a patient if a maintenance program is being provided. Progress towards goals must be documented. The goals set by the patient need to be realistic, and the patient needs to be working toward achieving these goals.

When it is determined that a patient does not need a skilled physical therapy program, conflict may arise between the physical therapist and the patient, the family, the physician, or any other member of the patient's team. The physical therapist must be able to justify his/her decision based on the goals that wcrc set. If one treatment approach does not work, it may be worthwhile to try another treatment approach to determine whether any progress toward the goals can be made. The physical therapist must determine whether the goals identified are the patient's goals. If the goals are determined by the patient, his/her active participation in the program should improve (see Case #2 in Chapter 14).

If skilled physical therapy services are discontinued because a patient is not able or is not willing to actively participate in the program, criteria for a rereferral should be set. These criteria can include a statement such as "an additional referral for skilled physical therapy is appropriate when the patient begins to actively participate in routine daily care with the nursing staff, when a decline in the patient's functional status occurs, or when the patient consistently participates in nursing care and is willing to participate in physical therapy treatment." When criteria for an additional referral are set, the patient, the family, the physicians, and all other members of the team can feel that the physical therapist is willing to get involved again at some other time. Furthermore, fewer inappropriate additional referrals are made.

B. Use of a trial period

Sometimes on initial screening, it is obvious that a patient's level of ability is either too high or too low for him/her to benefit from skilled physical therapy, and a decision about whether to initiate services can be made. At other times, it is difficult to determine whether skilled physical therapy is needed. In such cases, a trial period of skilled physical therapy is appropriate and justified to give the patient a chance to participate in the therapy before a decision about whether he/she can benefit from it is made. If a trial period is planned, it is important to set specific goals that are to be met in a specific time frame and to discontinue physical therapy if those goals are not achieved.

C. Patient education

In cases in which a patient essentially "passes" the screening, patient education may be the role that the physical therapist should play. The therapist can discuss with the patient the findings from the screening and can call to the patient's attention any potential problems. Patients often encounter problems in their home or work environment that are impossible to simulate in a medical environment. Therefore, if the screening is not done in the place where the patient performs the activities, the patient may still encounter problems when he/she resumes his/her regular routine. The patient also can be informed by the therapist of resources related to the area of concern in the event that problems are encountered.

D. Making recommendations

It is often difficult to determine which patients would benefit from skilled physical therapy. Sometimes after making the difficult decision that physical therapy is indicated, the therapist cannot proceed with intervention because of certain problems such as a lack of transportation, the patient or the family not agreeing that physical therapy is indicated, or conflicting time schedules. In such circumstances, physical therapists may need to make recommendations to the patient or to the family regarding available resources so that the identified problems can be addressed in the patient's own environment. To monitor the patient's progress, a plan to re-evaluate him/her at specific intervals should be formulated; this allows the physical therapist to modify or update his/her recommendations. In this way, the patient has a chance to make progress without direct physical therapy intervention.

III. Summary

This chapter discussed three patients for whom the need for skilled physical therapy had to be determined. The two adult cases represent opposite ends of the spectrum in determining the need for skilled physical therapy. The pediatric case highlights the importance of taking into account all aspects of a child's life and environment to determine whether physical therapy services are needed. These three cases involve a variety of issues, including whether a skilled physical therapy program or a non-skilled maintenance program should be used, whether a trial period is needed, when patient education is necessary, and how and when various recommendations are needed. The concepts presented here can be used in the evaluation of other patients for whom the need for skilled physical therapy must be determined.

References

1. Folio MR, Fewell RR: *Peabody Developmental Motor Scales.* Hingham, MA, Teaching Resources Corporation, 1983.
2. Bruininks RH: *Bruininks-Oseretsky Test of Motor Proficiency Examiner's Manual.* Circle Pines, MN, American Guidance Service, 1978.
3. King-Thomas L, Hacker BJ: *A Therapist's Guide To Pediatric Assessment.* Boston, Little, Brown and Company, 1987.

PART FIVE

Genitourinary System

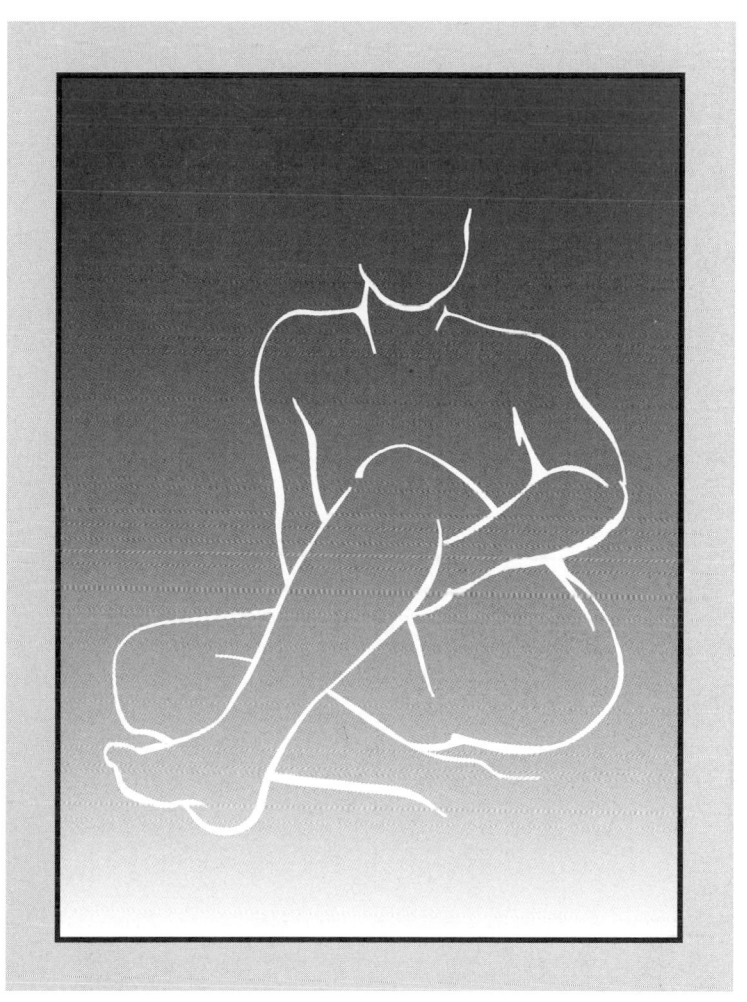

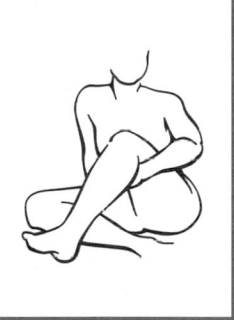

CHAPTER 22

Genitourinary System

Cara Adams and Jane Frahm

Most people take urinary continence for granted, yet incontinence is regularly experienced by as many as 1 in 4 women and 1 in 10 men. Only one third of this population seeks medical advice or assistance with the problem. Patients are sometimes referred to physical therapy expressly for the treatment of medically diagnosed urinary incontinence; however, many more patients could be helped if physical therapists were more aware of the pervasiveness of this condition and the role they could play in treating it.

It is likely that many of the patients physical therapists are now treating for the usual neuro-musculoskeletal problems also suffer silently from urinary incontinence. Simply asking patients about urine leakage will open the topic for discussion and allow patients the opportunity to learn more about this common and treatable condition.

In this chapter, the anatomy and physiology of the complex process of micturition are reviewed. Simple evaluative procedures are described, and a decision tree is provided to help the therapist design a customized intervention program for patients. Current treatments used for painful conditions of the genitourinary system are presented, and case studies of selected problems are included.

I. Anatomy[1-6]

A. Pelvic floor

The pelvic floor forms the lower border of the cylindrically shaped abdominopelvic cavity (see Figure 22–1). It is pierced by the urethra, the vagina (in the female), and the rectum and allows for parturition and daily excretory functions.

1. The main function of the pelvic floor is support of the contents of the abdominopelvic cavity during increases in intra-abdominal pressure.
2. The superior border (internally) is the peritoneum that covers the pelvic viscera and walls.

459

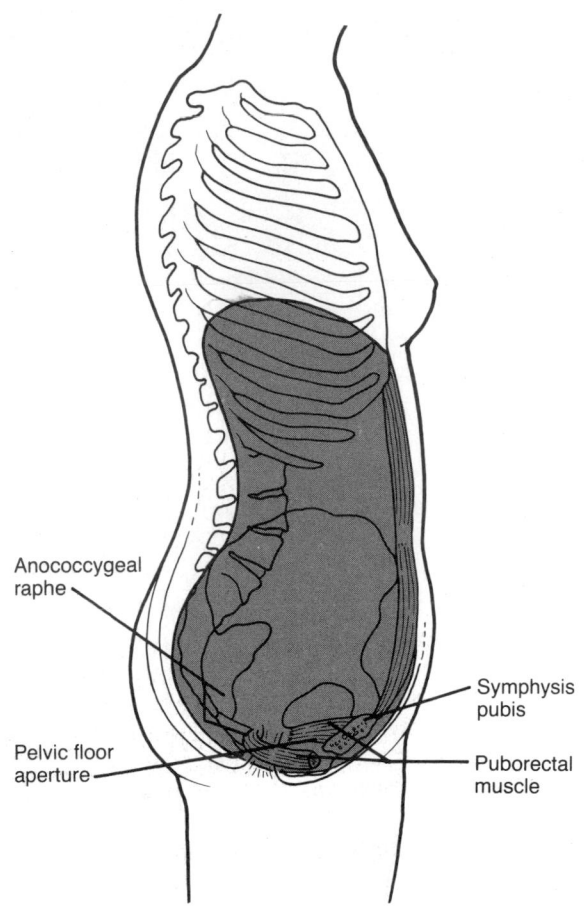

Anococcygeal
raphe

Pelvic floor
aperture

Symphysis
pubis

Puborectal
muscle

FIGURE 22–1   Abdominopelvic cavity.

3. The inferior border (externally) is the skin of the vulva, perineum, and buttocks.
4. The pelvic floor is composed of myofascial and visceral structures arranged in four general layers (see Figure 22–2).
   a. *First layer—endopelvic fascia.* The endopelvic fascia is the reflection of the superior fascia of the pelvic diaphragm on the pelvic viscera; it is one continuous body of connective tissue, surrounding and supporting the pelvic organs. Three tubes of fascia are present, encasing, respectively, the urethra and bladder, the vagina and lower part of the uterus, and the rectum. The ligaments of the pelvic organs are visceral and are a feltlike mesh of fibrous tissue containing quantities of smooth muscle. The pelvic organs are intimately positioned and dynamically supported by the endopelvic fascia. The following are significant structures in the endopelvic fascia:
      (1). The cardinal and uterosacral ligaments, which suspend the uterus within the pelvis (see Figure 22–3).
      (2). The pubocervical fascia, which supports the cervix, bladder, and vagina, and the rectovaginal fascia, which supports the rectum.
      (3). The pubourethral ligaments, which support the urethral position.

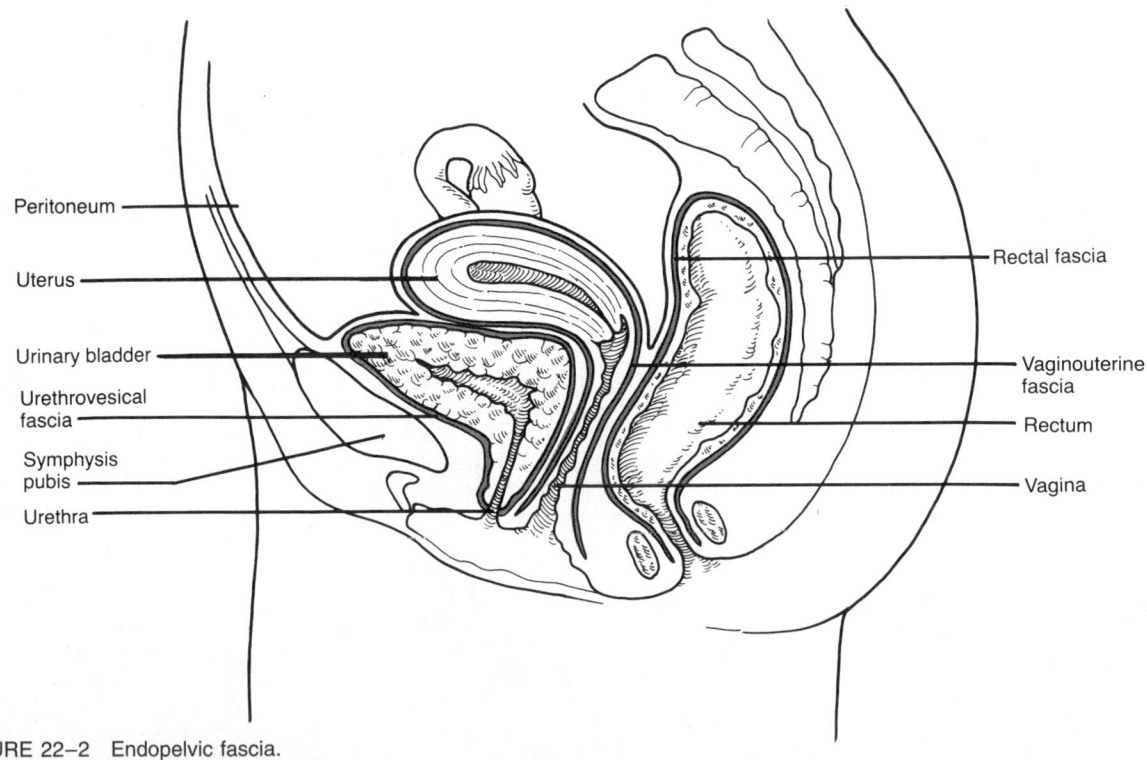

Peritoneum

Uterus

Urinary bladder

Urethrovesical
fascia

Symphysis
pubis

Urethra

Rectal fascia

Vaginouterine
fascia

Rectum

Vagina

FIGURE 22–2   Endopelvic fascia.

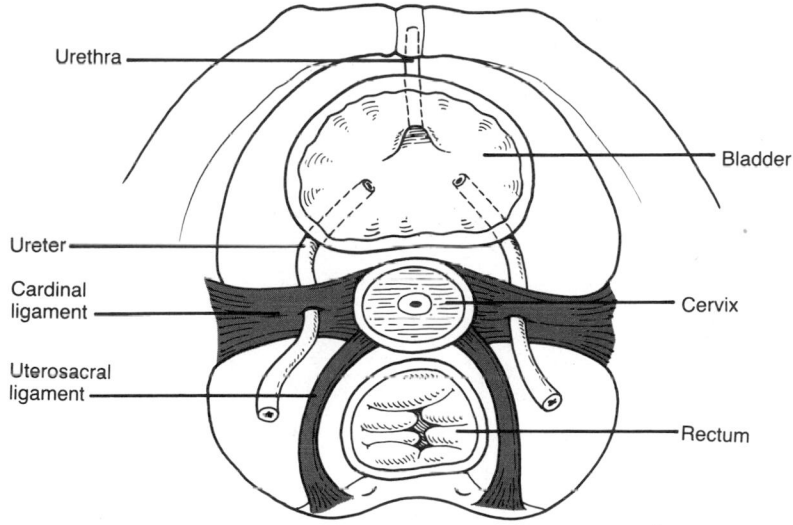

Urethra

Bladder

Ureter

Cardinal ligament

Cervix

Uterosacral ligament

Rectum

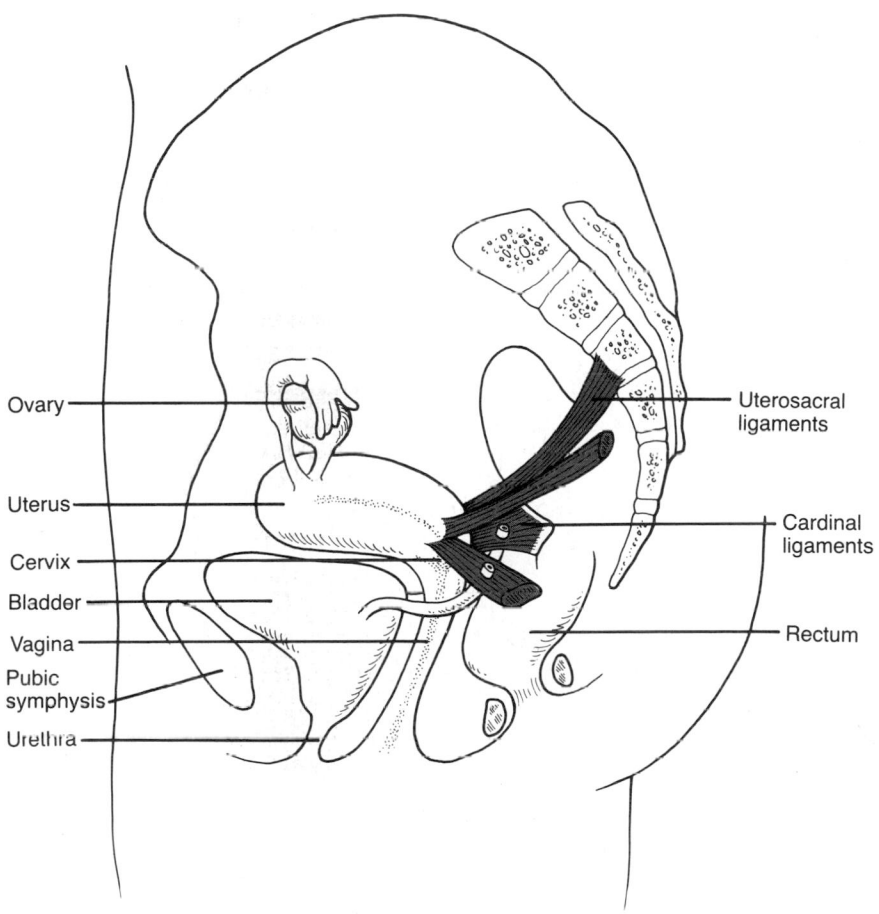

Ovary

Uterosacral ligaments

Uterus

Cervix

Cardinal ligaments

Bladder

Vagina

Rectum

Pubic symphysis

Urethra

FIGURE 22–3 Cardinal and uterosacral ligaments.

(a). The pubovesical muscle. The vesical neck is connected to the anterior and midportion of the ATFP by the pubovesical muscle—a smooth muscle offshoot of the detrusor muscle.

(b). The vaginolevator attachment. The vagina is densely attached to the levator ani muscles, just caudal to the ATFP. It is 1 cm long and 0.5 cm wide and is found at the most medial aspect of the levator ani muscle, just above the level of the urogenital diaphragm. The vaginolevator attachment lies in the region of the proximal urethra. There is no similar attachment from the levator ani to the urethra. Because of the intimate attachment of urethra and vagina, the vaginolevator attachment is in part responsible for control of urethral position and mobility. It helps elevate the urethrovesical angle during contractions of the pelvic floor muscles.

(c). Obstetrical trauma and increased intra-abdominal pres-

sure are the main reasons for the failure of the vaginal support structure.

(4). The arucus tendineus fascia pelvis (ATFP) (see Figure 22–4), which is a thickened band of the superior fascia of the levator ani muscles that attaches to the ventral end of the pubic bone, lateral to the pubic symphysis. Dorsally, it attaches to the ischial spine. Anteriorly, the ATFP lies on the medial portion of the levator ani muscles. Posteriorly, it fuses with the tendinous arch of levator ani (ATLA) muscle. It flanks the proximal urethra and vesical neck on each side.

b. *Second layer—pelvic floor muscles.* The levator ani muscles are referred to as the pelvic floor muscles (see Figure 22–5), which form a diaphragm across the pelvic cavity from the pubis to the coccyx. They are split anteriorly to allow passage of the urethra, lower vagina, and anus. The pelvic floor muscles have been shown to contain both type I and type II muscle fibers. The type I slow oxidative fibers are responsible for the resting tone of the pelvic floor muscles. The type II fast glycolitic fibers provide immediate added

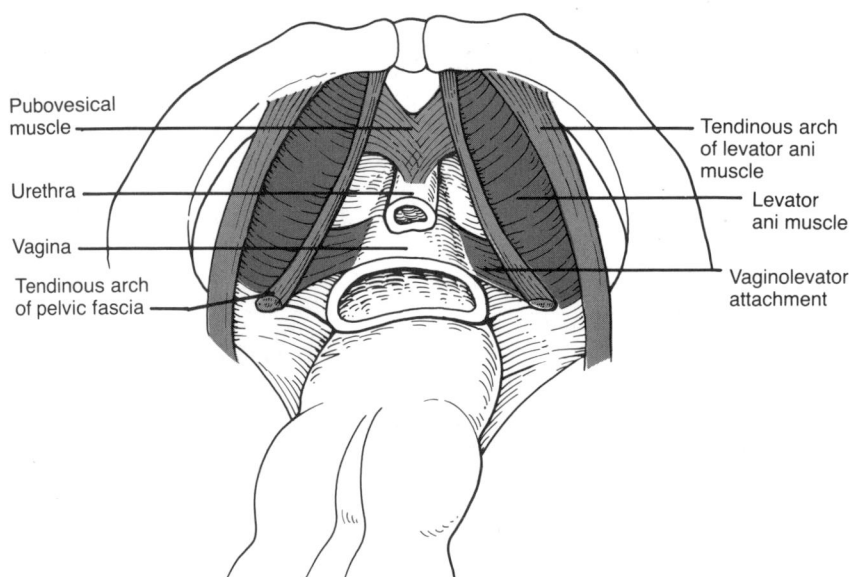

FIGURE 22–4 ATFP, pubovesical muscle, tendinous arch of levator ani muscle, vaginolevator attachment, and anterior pubourethral ligament.

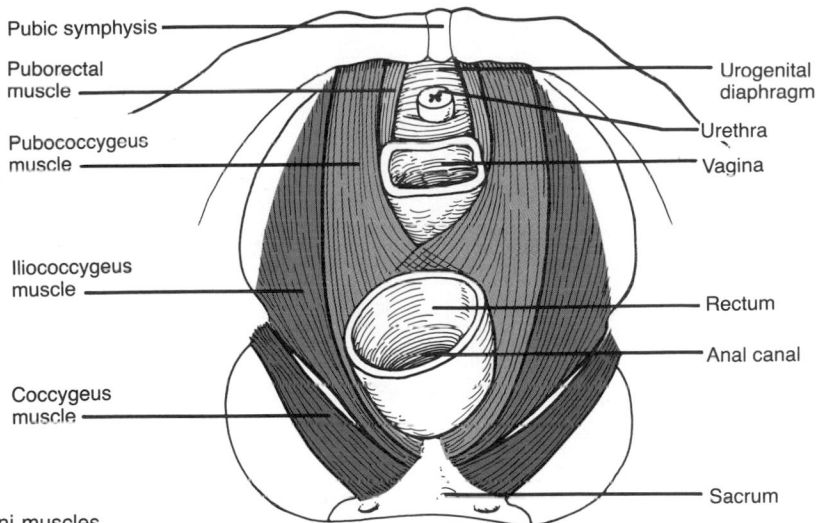

Pubic symphysis

Puborectal muscle

Pubococcygeus muscle

Iliococcygeus muscle

Coccygeus muscle

Urogenital diaphragm

Urethra

Vagina

Rectum

Anal canal

Sacrum

FIGURE 22–5   Levator ani muscles.

support in times of increased abdominal pressure, as in coughing, sneezing, lifting, or laughing. The following constitute the pelvic floor muscles[7]:

(1). *Pubococcygeus muscle*
  (a). Largest muscle of the levator ani group.
  (b). Arises from the inner aspect of the pubic bone and proximal portion of the ATLA, passes down into the anus between the internal and external sphincters, forms a sling around the dorsal aspect of the anorectal junction, and returns to the pubic bone on the other side.
  (c). Medial fibers skirt the urethra, blending with its intrinsic musculature coat; continuing fibers insert into the lateral and posterior wall of the vagina.
  (d). Fibers from both sides interdigitate between the coccyx and the rectum to form the levator plate.
  (e). Sends decussations to attach to the perineal body.
  (f). When contracted, forms a horizontal plane supporting the rectum, vagina, and urethra.
  (g). Provides support for the bladder.

(2). *Puborectalis muscle*
  (a). Lies beneath the point of origin of the pubococcygeal muscle and neighboring fascia and deep fascia of the urogenital diaphragm.
  (b). Courses along the lateral aspect of the urethra, vagina, and rectum medial and slightly inferior to the pubococcygeal muscle.
  (c). Forms a U-shaped sling encircling the posterior aspect of the rectum and returns along the opposite side of the levator hiatus to the posterior surface of the pubis (see Figure 22–6).
  (d). Affixes firmly to the vagina and to the posterior and midportions of the urethra to provide support.
  (e). Sends decussations to attach to the perineal body and provides support for the pelvic floor, vagina, and bladder neck.
  (f). Holds the rectum forward, providing continence control of the distal colon.

(3). *Iliococcygeus muscle*
  (a). Arises from a membranous insertion on the inner surface of the internal obturator muscle at the posterior portion of the ATLA.

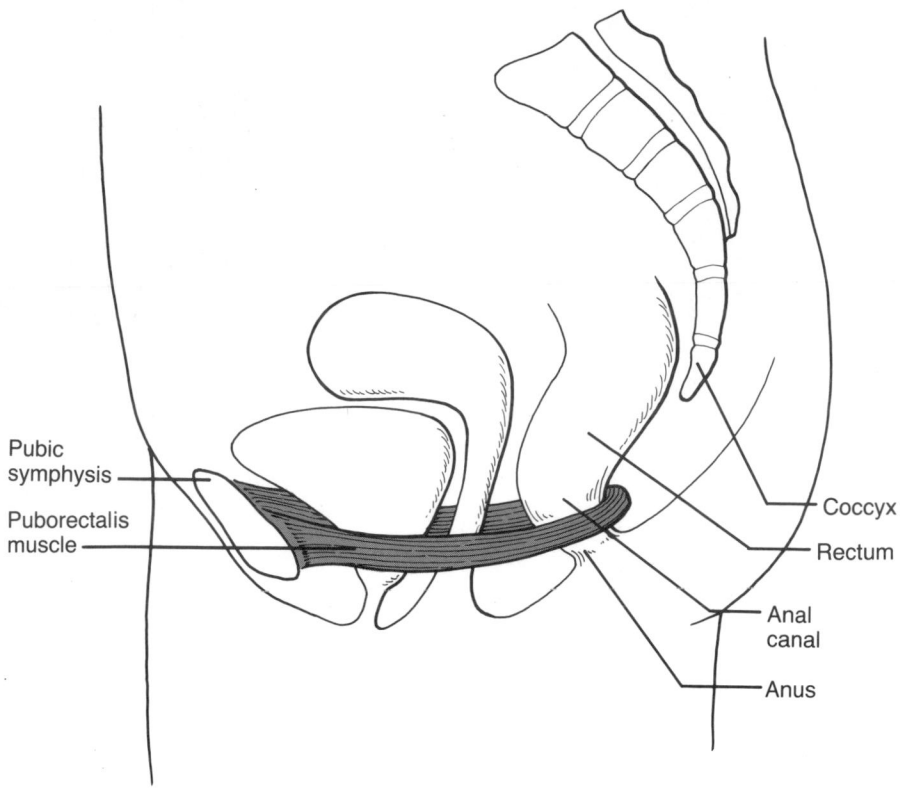

Pubic symphysis

Puborectalis muscle

Coccyx

Rectum

Anal canal

Anus

FIGURE 22–6   Action of puborectalis muscle.

(b). Inserts along the lateral margin of the coccyx and lower sacral vertebrae.

c. ***Third layer—urogenital diaphragm*** (see Figure 22–7). This is a musculomembranous partition stretched across the anterior half of the pelvic outlet, between the ischiopubic rami. It surrounds the urethral and vaginal outlets, connects the perineal body to the ischiopubic rami, and helps affix the lower urethra to these bones. It is composed of the following muscles and their enveloping fascia:

(1). Deep transverse perineal muscle.

(2). External urethral sphincter.

d. ***Fourth layer—superficial muscles at the outlets***

(1). Anteriorly: bulbospongiosus, ischiocavernous, superficial transverse perineal muscle.

(2). Posteriorly: external anal sphincter.

PLEASE NOTE: Weakness or laxity in the endopelvic fascia or other of the pelvic floor structures eventually results in partial or total prolapse of the organs it supports. The inherent sup-

portive function of the endopelvic fascia is even recognized by surgeons: "Vaginal vault prolapse, as well as recurrent cystocele, rectocele, or enterocele are disturbing complications after vaginal hysterectomy and every effort should be made to avoid them at the time of surgery." Optimal management of relaxation of the vaginal wall during vaginal hysterectomy requires clinical suspicion and precise preoperative diagnosis and therapeutic planning.[6]

See Figure 22–8 for anatomical problems caused by lack of structural support from pelvic floor structures:

• Uterine prolapse—herniation of the uterus through the pelvic floor resulting in protrusion into the vagina: first degree, the cervix remains in the vagina; second degree, the cervix appears at the perineum or protrudes on straining; third degree (procidentia), the entire uterus protrudes outside the body and there is total inversion of the vagina.

• Rectocele—protrusion of the rectum into the vagina.

• Enterocele—prolapse of a loop of the intestine usually into the pouch of Douglas, which lies

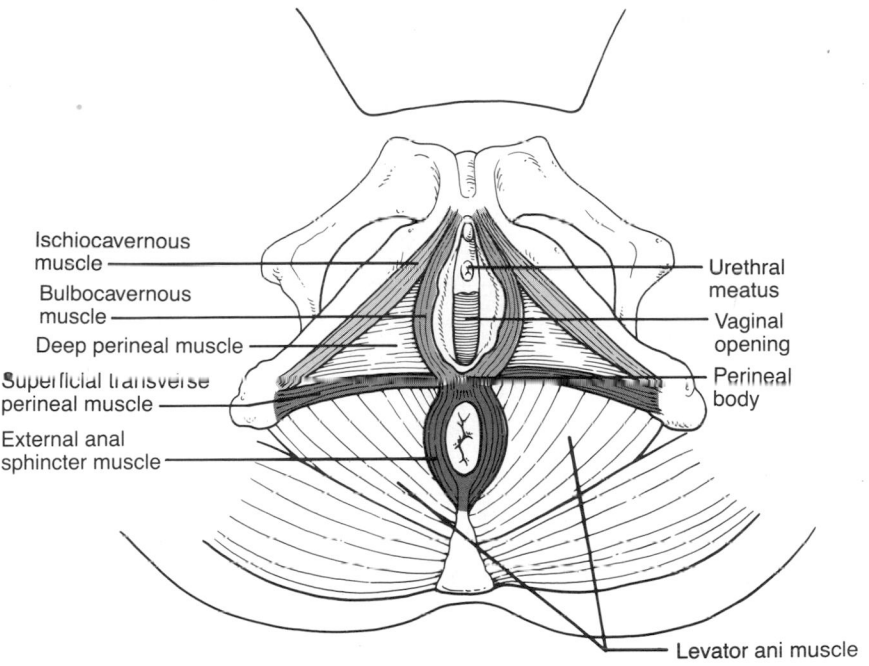

Ischiocavernous muscle

Bulbocavernous muscle

Deep perineal muscle

Superficial transverse perineal muscle

External anal sphincter muscle

Urethral meatus

Vaginal opening

Perineal body

Levator ani muscle

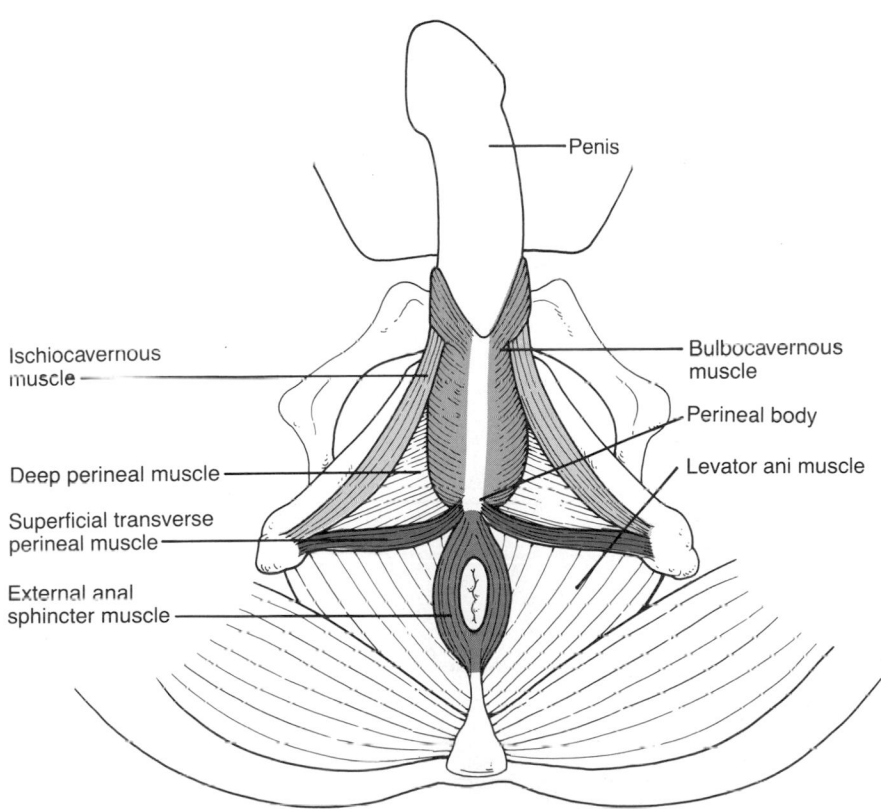

Penis

Ischiocavernous muscle

Bulbocavernous muscle

Perineal body

Deep perineal muscle

Levator ani muscle

Superficial transverse perineal muscle

External anal sphincter muscle

FIGURE 22–7   Urogenital diaphragm.

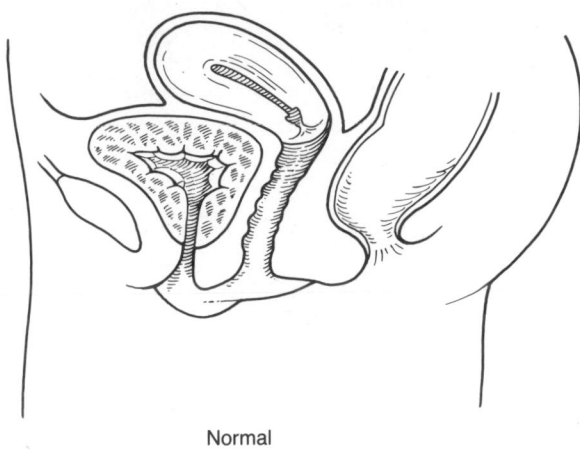

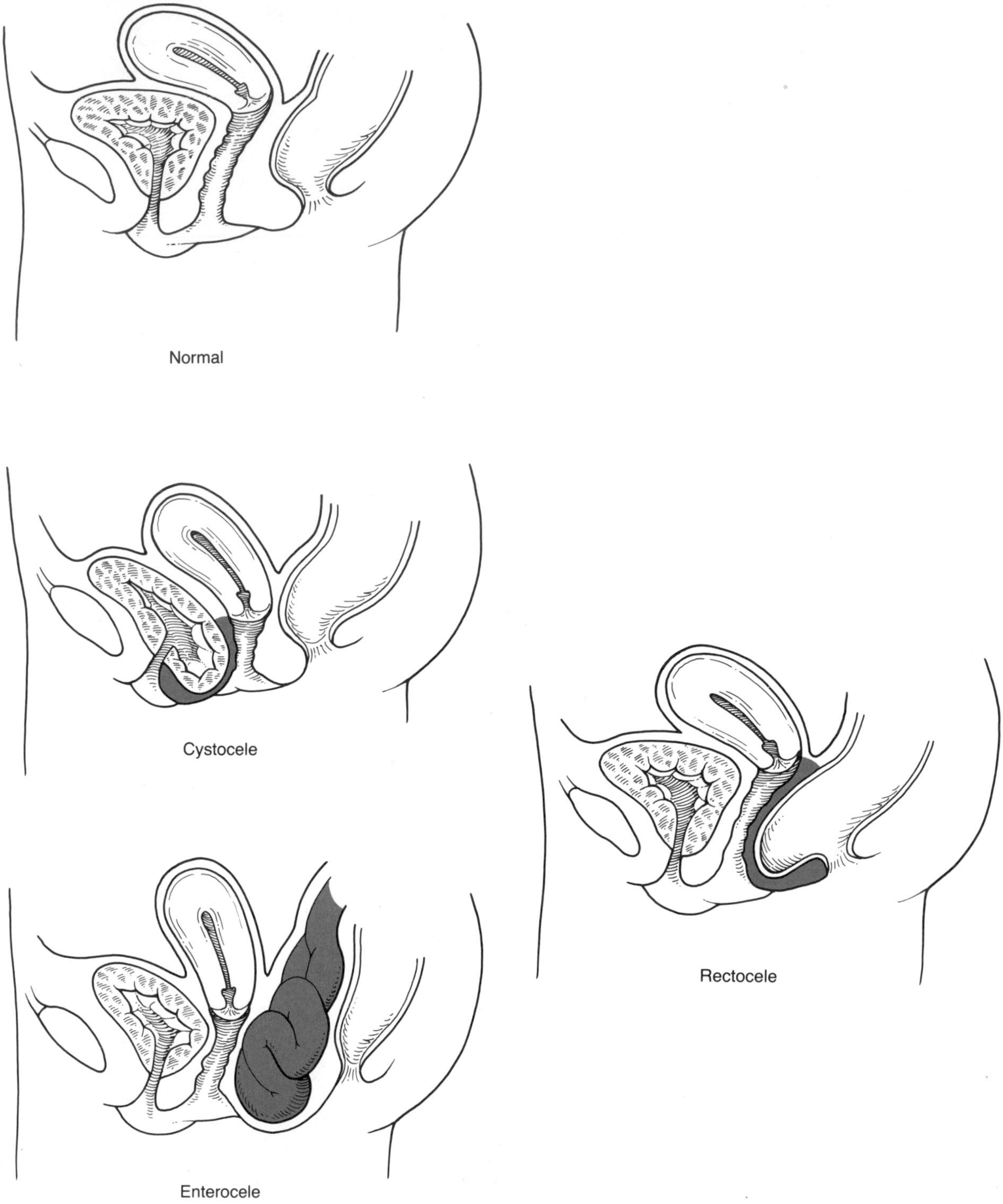

Normal

Cystocele

Rectocele

Enterocele

FIGURE 22–8   Anatomical problems caused by lack of structural support from pelvic floor structures.

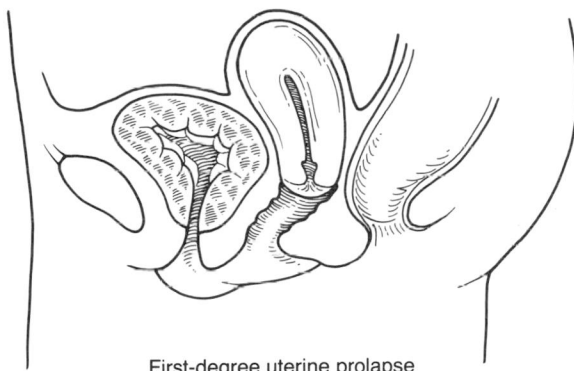

First-degree uterine prolapse

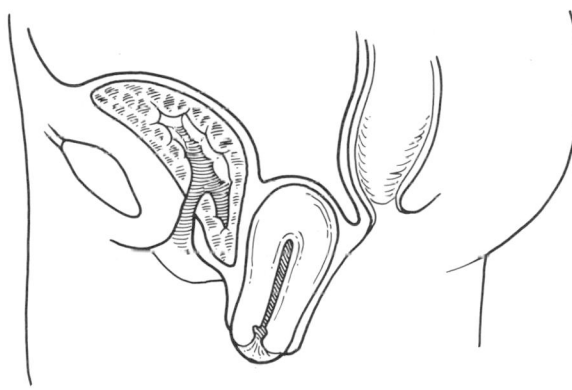

Third-degree uterine prolapse

Second-degree uterine prolapse

FIGURE 22–8   *Continued*

bctween the rectum and the vagina. It can compress the vagina and rectum and cause increased pressure on the pelvic floor.

- Cystocele—protrusion of the bladder into the vagina.
- Urethrocele—protrusion of the urethra into the vagina.

B. Perineum

The perineum is the diamond-shaped outlet of the pelvis and the soft tissues that cover it (see Figures 22–9 and 22–10). It is further defined as

1. The urogenital triangle, which is a triangular area bounded by the mons veneris anteriorly, the thighs laterally, and the buttocks posteriorly. It contains the following structures:
   a. The perineal body.

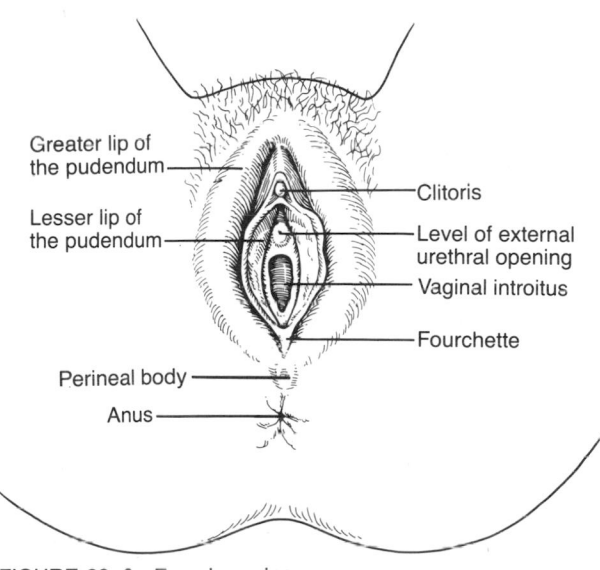

FIGURE 22–9   Female perineum.

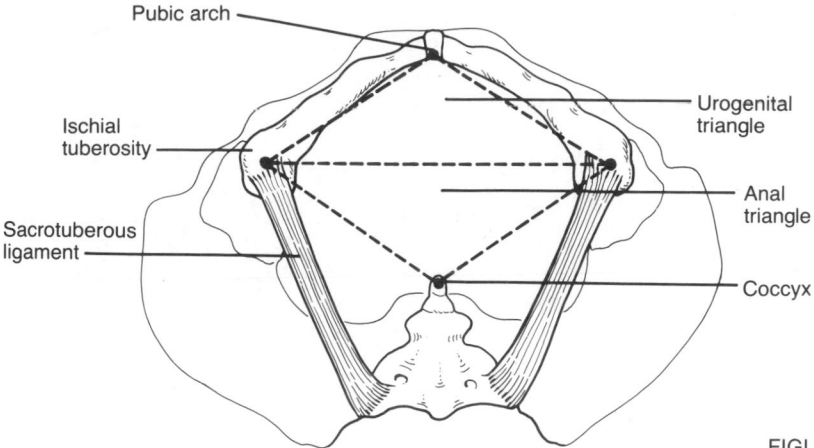

FIGURE 22–10   Divisions of the female perineum.

(1). This is the fibromuscular node between the anus and the vagina where superficial and deep musculature insert.

(2). The integrity of the perineal body lends strength to the pelvic floor; disruption leads or contributes to multiple genitourinary problems.

b. The external openings of the urethra and vagina.

PLEASE NOTE: This is the anatomical perineum. In gynecology and obstetrics, the area between the anus and the fourchette is called the perineum.

2. The anal triangle, which is bounded anteriorly by the superficial perineal muscles, laterally by the sacrotuberous ligaments and margins of the gluteus maximus, and posteriorly by the coccyx. It contains the external opening of the rectum.

C. Urinary bladder

The urinary bladder is a hollow vessel lined by a muscular coat called the detrusor muscle (see Figure 22–11).[8,9]

1. The detrusor is composed of three layers of smooth muscles: an inner longitudinal, a middle circular, and an outer longitudinal layer. Only at the outlet are these layers distinctly separate; elsewhere, muscle fibers move freely between all these layers.

2. The trigone is a muscle on the internal posterior bladder wall between the ureteral orifices and the internal urethral meatus.[8,9] It plays a role in the functional control of the vesical orifices of the ureters.

D. Urethral musculature

1. **Urethra.** The urethra is a hollow muscular tube (3 to 5 cm long in the female; 8 to 10 cm long in the male) that is approximately 6 mm in diameter. It has two muscular layers:

a. ***Inner longitudinal layer***

(1). Direct continuation of the inner longitudinal layer of the bladder.

(2). Terminates in dense collagenous tissue of the urethral wall just proximal to the external urethral meatus.

(3). Exerts a closing effect on the bladder neck.

b. ***Outer circular layer***

(1). Derived from the outer longitudinal muscle layer of the bladder.

(2). Fibers descend, loop around the urethra, and turn back again, never forming a complete ring.

(3). Fibers are thought to exert sphincteric action on the urethra.

2. **Urethral sphincteric mechanism**[8,10]

a. The internal urethral sphincter contains the following structures, which contribute to urethral closure and the maintenance of urethral resistance:

(1). Longitudinal and circular smooth muscle in urethral wall.

(2). Abundant collagenous and elastic tissue within the urethral wall.

(3). Turgor within blood vessels of submucosa contributing to the closing pressure of the urethra.

b. The external urethral sphincter is the striated voluntary muscle encircling the middle third of the female urethra and the area between the prostate and the pelvic floor muscles of the male urethra.

E. Innervation of the bladder and urethra (see Figure 22-12)

1. **Motor innervation**
   a. There is a complex triple system of control comprising parasympathetic, sympathetic, and somatic nerve supply and interconnections between the nerve networks.[8]
   b. The preganglionic parasympathetic fibers arise from S2-4 and are evenly distributed throughout the lower urinary tract musculature. They promote voiding by
      (1). Stimulation of detrusor contraction.
      (2). Inhibition of urethral contraction.
      (3). Remember: P = parasympathetic = pee.
   c. The sympathetic efferent nerves arise from T-11 to L-2 and pass via the hypogastric nerves to the bladder base and circular musculature within the proximal urethra.[11] They promote filling by
      (1). Stimulation of contraction of the bladder neck and urethra.
      (2). Inhibition of detrusor contractions.
      (3). Remember: S = sympathetic = stop.
   d. The somatic, pudendal nerves originate from S2-4 and regulate muscles of the pelvic floor.

2. **Micturition reflexes**[12,13]
   At least 12 reflexes have been identified that are important for coordinated micturition.
   a. Continence-favoring reflexes:
      (1). Sympathetic detrusor inhibiting reflex.
      (2). Sympathetic sphincter constrictor reflex.
      (3). Perineodetrusor inhibitory reflex.
      (4). Urethrosphincteric guarding reflex.

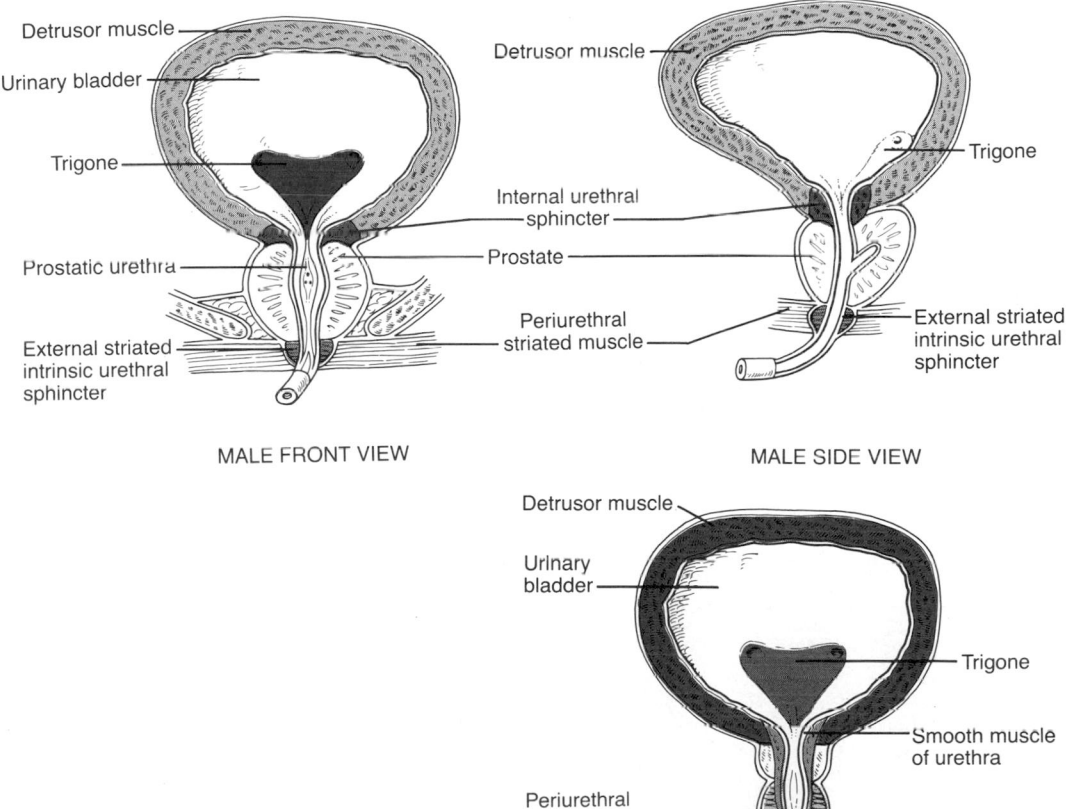

MALE FRONT VIEW

MALE SIDE VIEW

FEMALE FRONT VIEW

FIGURE 22-11 Male and female urinary tracts.

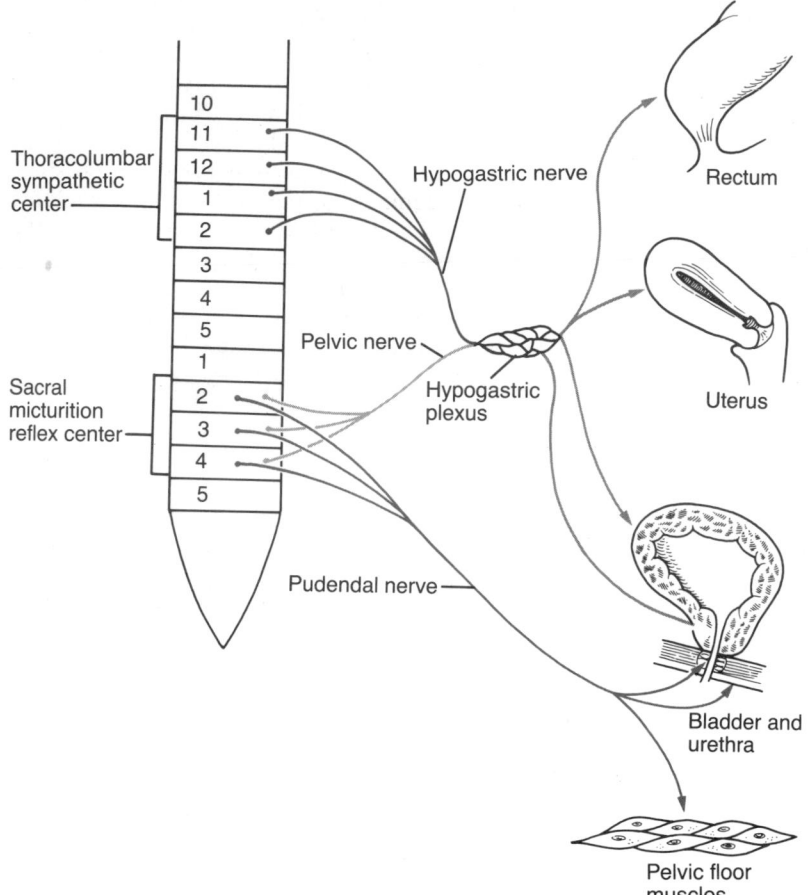

FIGURE 22–12   Innervation of the bladder, uterus, and rectum.

b. Initiation of micturition reflexes:
  (1). Perineobulbar detrusor facilitative reflex.
  (2). Detrusodetrusor facilitative reflex.
c. Intramicturition reflexes (operative during active micturition):
  (1). Detrusourethral inhibitory reflex.

  (2). Detrusosphincteric inhibitory reflex.
  (3). Urethrodetrusor facilitative reflex.
  (4). Urethrodetrusor facilitative reflex II.
  (5). Urethrosphincteric inhibitory reflex.
d. Micturition inhibitory reflex:
  (1). Perineobulbar detrusor inhibitory reflex.

II. Physiology[12,13]

Normal micturition depends on intact anatomical structures and normal nervous system control. It is a complex process dependent on the interactions of multiple neural reflexes. Any pathology that interferes with either the anatomy or the neuroanatomy of the system profoundly affects this process.

A. Mechanisms of continence
1. **Urine storage phase**
  a. The cerebral cortex exerts inhibitory control on voiding.
    (1). Modified by afferent sensations of bladder distention and pain.
    (2). Modified by knowledge of when so-

cially acceptable time and place for voiding is at hand.

b. Continence is maintained when the intraurethral pressure is higher than the existing bladder pressure.

c. Intraurethral pressure is maintained by the intrinsic and external sphincteric mechanism of the bladder neck and urethra and by the resting tone of the pelvic floor.

d. The bladder begins to fill, increasing the tension of the bladder wall.

  (1). The sympathetic detrusor inhibiting reflex inhibits the contractility of the detrusor muscle.

  (2). The sympathetic sphincter constrictor reflex stimulates the contractility of the smooth sphincter in response to the increasing tension of the detrusor muscle.

  (3). The perineodetrusor inhibitory reflex inhibits detrusor contractility in response to increasing voluntary tension in the perineal and pelvic floor muscles.

  (4). The urethrosphincteric guarding reflex stimulates contraction of the external striated portion of the urethral sphincteric mechanism in response to increasing tension in the bladder trigone or the presence of urine in the proximal urethra.

2. **Initiation of micturition**
  a. The bladder contains 300 to 400 ml of urine; socially acceptable conditions of time and place are met.

b. The pelvic floor muscles are consciously relaxed, and tension is increased in the diaphragm and abdominal wall.

  (1). The detrusourethral inhibitory reflex inhibits contraction of the bladder neck and the proximal urethra in response to increasing bladder wall tension.

  (2). The detrusosphincteric inhibitory reflex inhibits the external striated component of the urethral sphincter.

  (3). The urethrodetrusor facilitative reflexes stimulate detrusor muscle contraction in response to the presence of urine in the urethra.

c. Contractions of the detrusor in concert with relaxation of the sphincteric mechanism raise bladder pressure above intraurethral pressure and voiding begins.

d. The detrusor continues to contract, thus emptying the bladder until urine is no longer present in the urethra.

3. **Cessation of micturition.** Micturition can be halted voluntarily, before the bladder is completely emptied, under normal conditions. Voluntary contraction of the perineal and pelvic floor musculature elicits the perineobulbar detrusor inhibitory reflex, which inhibits the contraction of the detrusor muscle. This reflex facilitates the cessation of micturition and initiates the storage phase.

III. Functional Disturbances in the Urinary System

A. Urinary incontinence

Incontinence is defined as objectively demonstrated urine loss that is so severe as to cause social or hygienic problems. Urinary incontinence
1. Costs Americans $10 billion annually.
2. Is experienced by at least 10 million adults.
3. Is not a normal consequence of aging.
4. Is reported to caregivers by only about one third of the people experiencing it.
5. Is associated with depression and restricted social life.
6. Is not recognized as a significant health problem.

B. Etiology[14]

A combination of many factors may contribute to incontinence.
1. Decreased estrogen levels in menopause affect the lining of the vagina and urethra. These structures become thin and delicate owing to the decline in estrogen. Muscle contractions of the pelvic floor are not as effective in sphincteric assist as they contract around tissue that has lost much of its rich mucosal lining.
2. Childbirth and pelvic trauma can result in pudendal nerve damage of varying degree, producing weakness of pelvic floor muscles.

Table 22–1.   SOME COMMON DRUGS WITH SIDE EFFECTS
AFFECTING CONTINENCE

Broad Category	Generic Name	Brand Name	Uses	Selected Side Effects
Opioid	Morphine Hydromorphone Hydrocodone Oxycodone Codeine	MS Contin Dilaudid Vicodin Percocet, Tylox	Analgesia	Increases tone and amplitude of contractions of ureter; increases tone of detrusor muscle of bladder; increases sphincteric tone; increases urgency; increases release of antidiuretic hormone, decreasing urine output
Benzodiazepine	Flurazepam Diazepam	Dalmane Valium	Anxiety, tension Fatigue, agitation	May cause confusion and secondary incontinence, especially in the elderly
Diuretic	Furosemide Hydrochlorothiazide Bumetanide	Lasix HydroDIURIL Bumex	Congestive heart failure Cirrhosis of liver Kidney dysfunction High blood pressure	Can overwhelm bladder capacity and lead to polyuria, frequency, urgency
Calcium channel blocker	Verapamil	Calan Isoptin	Angina Hypertension Reynaud's syndrome Asthma	Can cause relaxation of bladder wall and occasionally cause urinary retention and overflow incontinence
Phenothiazine and thioxanthene	Chlorpromazine Perphenazine Prochlorperazine Thioridazine Trifluoperazine Thiothixene	Thorazine Trilafon Compazine Mellaril Stelazine Navane	Psychosis	Urinary retention overflow incontinence and may cause sedation, rigidity, and immobility
Antispasmodic	Atropine sulfate Scopolamine hydrobromide Dicyclomine hydrochloride	Donnagel-PG Transderm Scop Bentyl	Diarrhea	Urinary retention and overflow incontinence
Antiparkinsonian	Benztropine mesylate Ethopropazine hydrochloride Orphenadrine citrate Procyclidine hydrochloride Trihexyphenidyl hydrochloride	Cogentin Parsidol Norflex Kemadrin Artane	Parkinson's disease	Urinary retention associated with frequency and overflow incontinence
Antidepressant	Amitriptyline hydrochloride Doxepin hydrochloride Imipramine pamoate Nortriptyline hydrochloride	Elavil Sinequan Tofranil-PM Pamelor	Clinical depression	Urinary retention associated with frequency
Antihistaminic	Brompheniramine maleate Chlorpheniramine maleate Diphenhydramine hydrochloride	Dimetane Chlor-Trimeton Benadryl	Allergies, colds	Urinary retention associated with frequency and overflow incontinence
α-Adrenergic agonist	Pseudoephedrine	Sudafed	Decongestant Stuffy nose Broncospasm, associated with asthma	Urinary retention associated with frequency and overflow incontinence
α-Adrenergic antagonist	Prazosin hydrochloride	Minipress	Hypertension	Stress incontinence

3. Although pelvic organ prolapse may be related to parity, the underlying strength of collagen can have an impact on the continence mechanism.

4. Antihypertensive medication (α-blockers) can significantly decrease urethral pressure, and stopping the medication can alleviate the incontinence problem.

5. Obesity increases the intra-abdominal pres-

sure on the pelvic floor organs, and significant weight loss has been reported to decrease urinary leakage.[15]

6. Smoking predisposes patients to urinary incontinence and is probably related to the strength and frequency of coughing in these patients.

7. Other factors related to urinary incontinence include previous genitourinary sur-

gery, urinary tract infections, neurological disease, immobility, thyroid disease, or constipation.

C. Types and causes of urinary incontinence[16]

1. **Transient incontinence.** DIAPPERS can be used as a mnemonic for the causes of transient incontinence.
   a. Delirium: Incontinence is usually an associated symptom of delirium and will subside when the underlying cause of confusion is treated.
   b. Infection: Dysuria and urgency associated with infection will produce incontinence. Drug therapy will alleviate the problem.
   c. Atrophy: Atrophic urethritis or vaginitis may occur with menopause and can be treated by conjugated estrogen.
   d. Pharmacologic: See Table 22–1.
      (1). Sedative hypnotics (drugs or alcohol) cause confusion and impaired mobility, resulting in incontinence.
      (2). Diuretics can overwhelm bladder capacity and lead to frequency, urgency, and incontinence.
      (3). The side effects of anticholinergic agents include urinary retention with urinary frequency and overflow incontinence.
      (4). α-Adrenergic agonists (decongestants) can cause bladder relaxation with urethral tightening, leading to severe bladder distention. α-Adre-

nergic antagonists can cause relaxation of the pelvic floor muscles, leading to stress incontinence.
      (5). Calcium channel blockers can reduce smooth muscle contractility in the bladder and contribute to urinary retention and overflow incontinence.
   e. Psychological: Severe depression may occasionally be associated with incontinence.
   f. Endocrine: Excessive urine production may be due to excessive intake of liquid, endocrine imbalance, congestive heart failure, lower extremity venous insufficiency, and low albumin states.
   g. Restricted mobility: This excessively increases the time necessary to reach the toilet or complicates the process of disrobing so that urination occurs before the person is on the toilet. This is called functional incontinence.
   h. Stool impaction: The patient may have symptoms of either urge or overflow incontinence as well as fecal incontinence. Disimpaction restores continence.

2. **Stress urinary incontinence** (see Figure 22–13). This is characterized by urine loss during physical activities that increase intra-abdominal pressure (coughing, laughing, sneezing, throat clearing, nose blowing, lifting, rising from chair or bed, jogging, serving during tennis). This increased abdominal pressure causes an increase in intravesicle pressure, which exceeds urethral

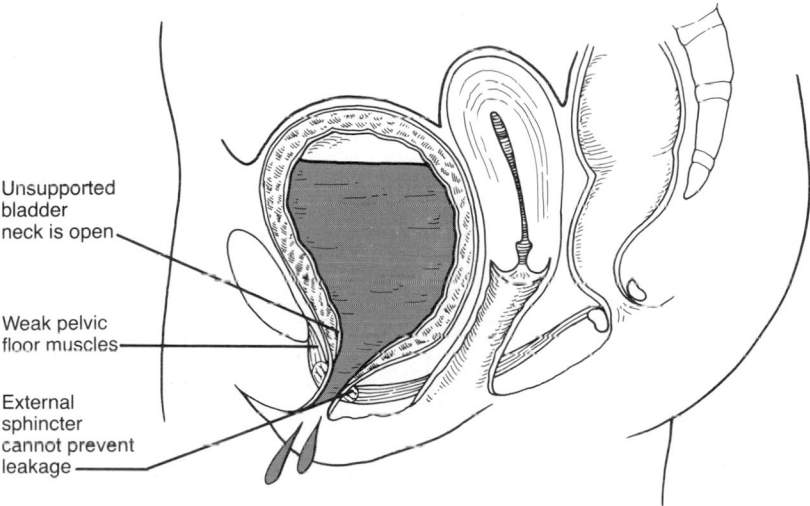

Unsupported bladder neck is open

Weak pelvic floor muscles

External sphincter cannot prevent leakage

FIGURE 22–13 Stress incontinence.

resistance, in the absence of detrusor contractions. A major factor in stress urinary incontinence is hypermobility or downward displacement of the urethra during exertion. Many times, this downward displacement is secondary to the relaxation of pelvic floor muscles during the stressful event.

   a. Associated factors in hypermobility of the bladder neck include

     (1). Perineal nerve damage, leading to weakness of the pelvic floor musculature and failure to support the bladder adequately within the abdominal cavity.[17]

       (a). Mechanical causes include

         (i). Stretching of the perineal nerve during vaginal childbirth.

         (ii). Stretching of the perineal nerve from poor bowel habits leading to frequent straining.

       (b). Traumatic causes include

         (i). Tearing of the perineum during childbirth (including extensions of episiotomy).

         (ii). Injury to the pelvic floor as a result of sexual abuse or rape.

         (iii). Injury to the pelvic floor as a result of other body trauma.

     (2). Unknown defect in the connective tissue or pelvic floor muscle or pelvic floor innervation, which leads to hypermobility of the bladder neck in some patients but not in others.

   b. Intrinsic urethral sphincter deficiency (see Figure 22–14) is due to

     (1). Congenital sphincter weakness such as myelomeningocele or epispadias (malformation of the penis in which the urethra opens on the dorsum).

     (2). Prostatectomy, trauma, radiation, or sacral cord lesion.

     (3). In women, multiple surgical anti-incontinence procedures.

   c. Neurogenic sphincter deficiency is due to neurogenic, sacral, or infrasacral lesion (myelomeningocele).

3. **Urge incontinence** (see Figure 22–14). Symptoms of urge incontinence (sometimes called instability) include the involuntary loss of moderate to large volumes of urine associated with an abrupt and strong desire to void. Patients may leak in bed at night and/or experience leakage during sexual intercourse. Four conditions lead to this problem. Patients may have urge incontinence in combination with one of the other types of incontinence.

   a. Unstable bladder (detrusor instability) with no known neurological deficits.

   b. Detrusor hyperreflexia (detrusor instability) associated with neurological lesions such as stroke, supraspinal cord lesion, multiple sclerosis.

   c. Detrusor hyperactivity with impaired bladder contractility (DHIC). Occurs in elderly patients and is usually also associated with obstructive or stress symptoms.

   d. Urethral instability (involuntary urethral

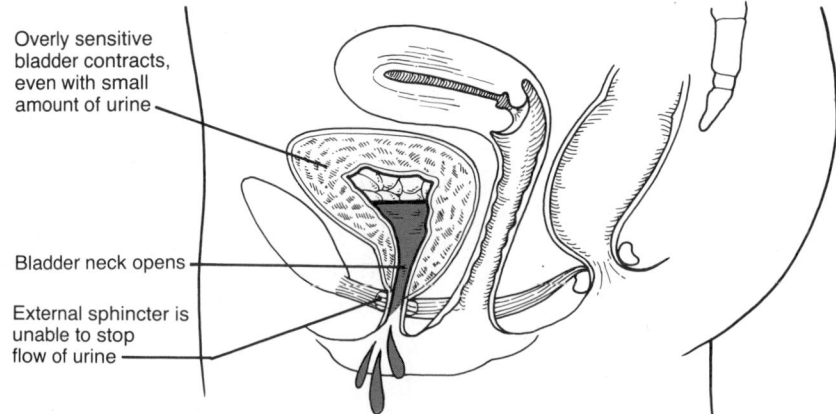

Overly sensitive bladder contracts, even with small amount of urine

Bladder neck opens

External sphincter is unable to stop flow of urine

FIGURE 22–14   Urge incontinence.

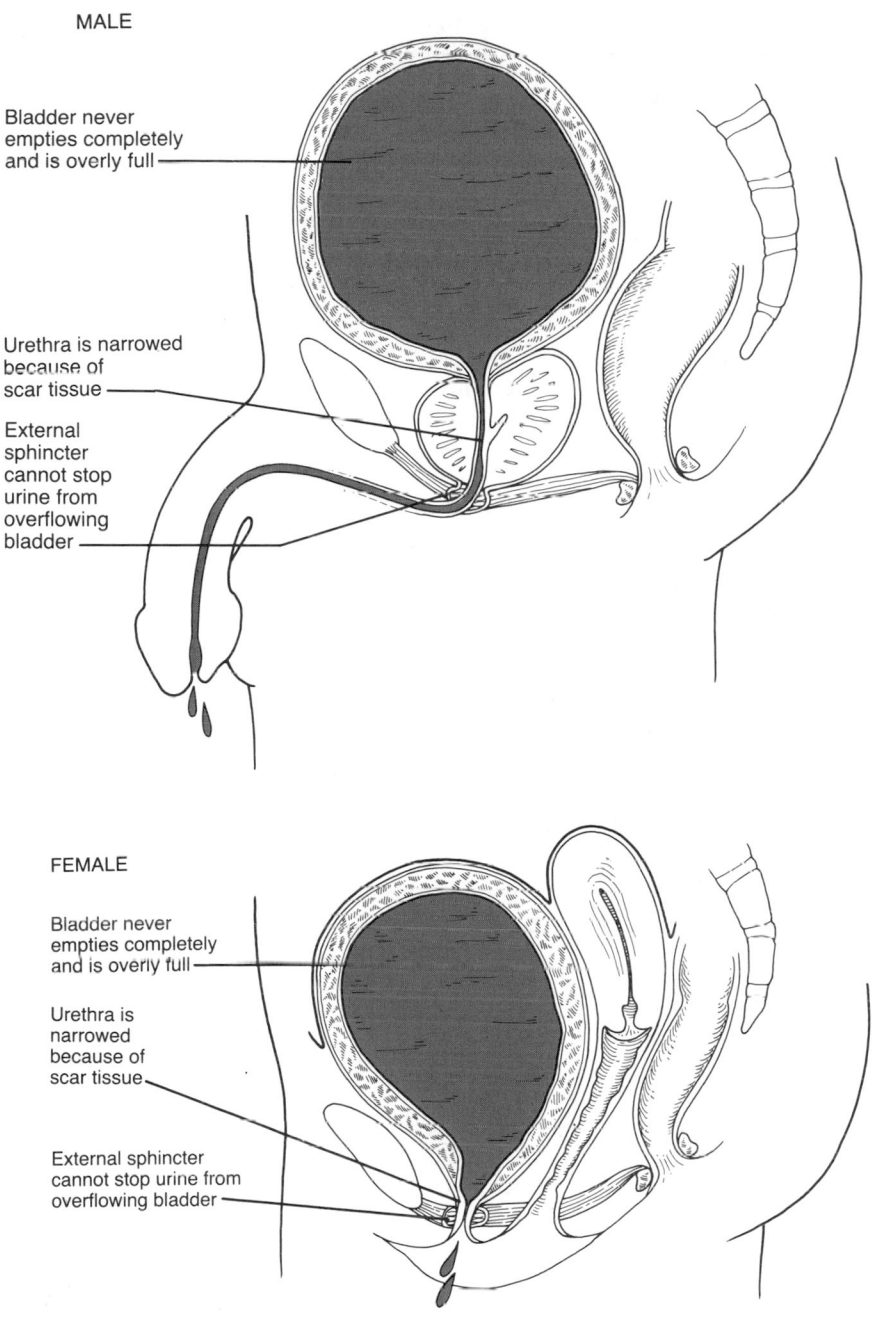

MALE

Bladder never empties completely and is overly full

Urethra is narrowed because of scar tissue

External sphincter cannot stop urine from overflowing bladder

FEMALE

Bladder never empties completely and is overly full

Urethra is narrowed because of scar tissue

External sphincter cannot stop urine from overflowing bladder

FIGURE 22–15 Overflow incontinence.

relaxation), which may occur with or without a neurological deficit.

4. **Overflow incontinence** (see Figure 22–15). Symptoms of overflow incontinence (urinary retention) include the involuntary continuous or intermittent leakage of small amounts of urine associated with overdistention of the bladder and may occur while the patient is awake or asleep. Two conditions cause this problem:

  a. Overflow from an underactive or a contractile detrusor muscle associated with outflow obstruction.

    (1). This occurs in males secondary to

      (a). Prostate gland disease

      (b). Urethral stricture

      (c). Neurogenic lesion (low spinal

cord lesion, neuropathy, post-radical pelvic surgery)

(d). Idiopathic causes

(2). This occurs in females secondary to

(a). Anti-incontinence surgery

(b). Severe pelvic prolapse, which may kink the urethra

b. Sensory neuropathy (diabetes, spinal cord injury, drugs, syphilis), which interferes with the patient's ability to recognize when the bladder is full.

5. **Mixed incontinence.** This is defined as a combination of stress and urge incontinence. Is is thought that patients with mixed incontinence may have started out with mild to moderate stress incontinence and, over the years, also developed urge incontinence.[18] The treatment of patients must be customized according to the severity of both components.

D. **Medical screening, evaluation, and assessment**[16]

1. **Urodynamic studies**

a. Uroflowmetry (flow rate) is the recording of the volume of urine passing through the urethra per unit of time (mL/s).

b. Cystometrography is the graphic recording of pressures exerted at varying phases of bladder filling. Intermittent filling of the bladder can be recorded and compared with changes in intravesical pressure. Used to test detrusor function.

c. Urethral pressure profile is a graphic recording of the pressure in the urethra at each point along its length. Gas or fluid is instilled through a catheter that is withdrawn while pressures along the urethral wall are obtained. It is used to measure the effect of exertion on the urethral closure mechanism and may help identify intrinsic sphincter deficiency.

2. **Cystourethrography.** This is roentgenographic visualization of the urethra and bladder either by retrograde injection or by voiding of contrast material. This procedure may help in identifying bladder lesions and foreign bodies as well as urethral diverticula, fistulas, strictures, or intrinsic sphincter deficiency.

3. **Videourodynamics.** This is a combination of the various urodynamic studies with simultaneous fluoroscopy. It is helpful in sorting out complex incontinence problems and can identify detrusor overactivity, detrusor sphincter dyssynergia (inappropriate contraction of the external sphincter concurrent with an involuntary contraction of the detrusor), intrinsic urethral defects, outlet obstruction, and detrusor contractility problems.

4. **Electromyography (EMG).** This is the recording and study of the intrinsic electrical properties of skeletal muscle. Fine-needle electrodes are inserted through the perineum into the periurethral or anal sphincter. Used in combination with cystometrography, it is helpful in diagnosing detrusor sphincteric dyssynergia and percentage of perineal nerve damage.

E. **Physical therapy screening, evaluation, and assessment**

Patients referred to physical therapy for the treatment of incontinence should be evaluated for the following items. The form shown in Figure 22–16 is used at the Bradford Royal Infirmary, Bradford, England, and is included as an example of a comprehensive recording form.

1. **History**

a. Age.

b. Height.

c. Weight (obesity is thought to be a contributing cause of stress incontinence).[15]

d. Occupation (include anything related to incontinence, *eg*, lifting).

e. Presenting symptoms and duration.

f. Obstetrical/gynecological/surgical history (reasons for surgery and whether there was malignancy).

g. Menopausal status (estrogen depletion during and after menopause affects the elasticity of vaginal and pelvic floor structures).

h. Date and outcome of last Pap smear. If positive, is patient undergoing treatment? (Some patients may need encouragement to follow through with treatment.)

i. Medical conditions.

(1). Cystitis.

(2). Low back pain (need to rule out

genitourinary tract structures as possible causes of referred pain).

(3). Diabetes (polyuria can produce symptoms of urgency and frequency).

(4). Respiratory diseases, including history of smoking (chronic cough associated with smoking can lead to straining and weakening of the pelvic floor).

(5). Neurological disease (multiple sclerosis, spinal cord injury can lead to various types of incontinence).

(6). Heart disease (certain medications given for treatment of heart disease can influence urine output and affect continence. See Table 22–1).

(7). Allergy (multiple coughing and sneezing episodes can contribute to pelvic floor weakness. Certain drugs can affect sphincteric mechanisms. See Table 22–1).

2. **Assessment**
   a. Activities (what enjoyable or necessary activities can the patient no longer do because of incontinence?).
   b. Drugs (including over-the-counter drugs currently being taken).
   c. Bowels—loose, normal or constipated (straining to defecate can strain and weaken the pelvic floor and possibly stretch the perineal nerve, leading to further weakness).
   d. Mobility/dexterity/orientation.
   e. Urinary symptoms.
      (1). Frequency (record the number of times the patient urinates, including leakages, in 24 hours).
      (2). Urgency (recorded as yes or no).
      (3). Stress incontinence—does the patient leak with a laugh, cough, or sneeze? (Recorded as yes or no.)

      (4). Urge incontinence—does the patient experience an uncontrollable urgency to urinate? (Recorded as yes or no.)
      (5). Nocturia (record the number of times the patient gets up during the night to urinate).
      (6). Enuresis (recorded as yes or no).
      (7). Dysuria (recorded as yes or no).
      (8). Other (eg, hesitancy).
   f. Incontinence episodes.
      (1). How often?
         (a). Almost every day.
         (b). Less than once a week.
         (c). More than once a week.
         (d). About once a month.
      (2). How severe?
         (a). A few drops.
         (b). Wets underpants.
         (c). Wets outer clothes.
         (d). Wets the floor.
   g. Attitude to incontinence (how does it affect normal activities?).
      (1). Minor inconvenience.
      (2). Slight problem.
      (3). Big problem.
      (4). Major problem.
   h. Frequency/volume chart.
      (1). Frequency during day.
      (2). Frequency during night.
      (3). Maximum volume voided.
      (4). Minimum volume voided.
      (5). Number of wet episodes.
      (6). Number of pads used.
      (7). Number of drinks (volume).
   i. Urodynamic results (from physician).
   j. Midstream urinalysis test results (from physician).
   k. Pad test (see procedure below).
   l. Stop test (used only with stress incontinence; see procedure below).
   m. Perineal examination (see procedure below).

IV. Physical Therapy Physical Evaluation Procedures

All evaluation procedures should be explained to the patient in detail before beginning the procedure, and patients should be asked to sign a consent form.

The stop test and 1 hour office pad test are used for patients with stress incontinence only.

A. Stop test or urine stream interruption test[19]

1. The patient is asked to attempt to stop urine flow voluntarily by contracting the pelvic floor muscles during midstream on the second voiding of the day. Complete cessation

1. Name _____ Hospital No. _____

Address _____ Age _____ Date _____

_____ Referral _____

_____ Tel. No. _____ Occupation _____

2. Presenting Symptoms and Duration _____

_____

_____

3. Relevant History

Obstetric: _____

Date	2nd Stage Duration	Delivery	Wt	Trauma	Exercises

Gynaecological: Surgery _____

Prolapse _____

Menopausal State _____ Smear _____

Medical			
Cysitis		Respiratory Disease	
Low Back Pain		Neurological Disease	
Diabetes		Heart Disease	
Smoking		Allergy	
Other			

Surgical: Other Pelvic Surgery _____

_____

Activities _____

4. Initial Assessment

Drugs _____

_____

Height _____ Weight _____ BMI _____

Bowels: loose/normal/constipated _____

Faecal Incontinence _____

Mobility/dexterity/orientation _____

Final Assessment   Date _____

Drugs _____

_____

Height _____ Weight _____ BMI _____

Bowels: loose/normal/constipated _____

Faecal Incontinence _____

Mobility/dexterity/orientation _____

FIGURE 22–16 Patient assessment form. *Abbreviations:* BMI = body mass index; MSU = midstream urine specimen. (Modified from lecture materials of J Laycock.)

5. Urinary Symptoms	1st	Final
Frequency		
Urgency		
Stress Incontinence		
Urge Incontinence		
Nocturia		
Enuresis		
Dysuria		
Other		
Incontinence		
How often?		
Almost every day		
More than once a week		
Less than once a week		
About once a month		
How severe?		
A few drops		
Wets underwear		
Wets outer clothes		
Wets the floor		

6. Attitude to Incontinence	1st	Final
Minor inconvenience		
Slight problem		
Big problem		
Major problem		
7. Frequency/Volume Chart		
Frequency - Day		
- Night		
Max. Vol. Voided		
Min. Vol. Voided		
No. of wet episodes		
No. of pads		
No. of drinks		
8.		
Urodynamic results		
MSU		
Pad Test		
Stop Test		

9. Perineal Examination	Initial	Final
Pelvic Floor Grading		
0 - nil		
1 - flicker		
2 - weak		
3 - moderate		
4 - good		
5 - strong		
Hold time		
No. of repetitions - slow		
- fast		
Perineometer reading		

Comments

Treatment given

FIGURE 22–16 *Continued*

or even slowing of urine flow demonstrates that the appropriate muscles are being contracted. It has been shown that the speed of stopping urine flow is positively correlated with the strength of the pelvic floor muscles.

PLEASE NOTE: This activity should not be used as an exercise as it can promote poor bladder emptying habits and may promote urinary tract infections.

B. One-hour office pad test[20,21]

1. **Purpose.** To determine an objective baseline measure of the amount of urine lost by an incontinent patient during a specified time period.

PLEASE NOTE: This test should not be done during a patient's menstrual period.

2. **Equipment**
   a. Six preweighed sanitary or incontinence pads with waterproof backing or waterproof pants for patients to wear over the pads
   b. One liter of water or juice
   c. Six plastic bags
   d. Kitchen or postal scale

3. **Procedure**
   a. *Preparatory phase*
      (1). Have the patient void before the procedure is begun.
      (2). Inform the patient what to expect.
      (3). Ask the patient to drink 1 L of water or orange juice as quickly as possible.

PLEASE NOTE: The test starts 1 hour after the patient starts to drink the fluid.

   b. *Performance phase*
      (1). Ask the patient to don one perineal pad. She will replace the pad every 10 minutes for a total of 60 minutes.
      (2). At the end of each 10 minutes, she will replace the pad, placing the used pad in a plastic bag, which will subsequently be weighed to determine any urine loss.
      (3). The patient sits quietly and rests for the first 30 minutes.
      (4). After 30 minutes, the patient begins walking and climbing stairs for a total of 15 minutes.

PLEASE NOTE: If at any time the pad becomes completely saturated before the end of the 10-minute period, it is removed and another pad is applied.

   (5). After a total of 45 minutes, the patient performs the following activities:
      (a). Sit/stand 10 times.
      (b). Cough 10 times.
      (c). Run in place for 1 minute.
      (d). Pick up objects from floor.
      (e). Wash hands.

PLEASE NOTE: The activities may need to be modified based on the patient's abilities. Variations from the norm should be noted.

   (6). After a total of 60 minutes, the last collecting device is removed. The patient voids, and the volume voided is measured.

C. *Follow-up phase*
   (1). Weigh all the pads used. Subtract the "dry" weight from the "used" weight to determine the amount of urine lost.
   (2). The findings can be interpreted as follows:

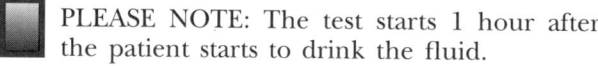

<2 g	Essentially dry
2–10 g	Slight to moderate urine loss
10–50 g	Severe urine loss
>50 g	Very severe urine loss

C. Internal evaluation of pelvic floor muscle strength[22]

1. **Purposes**
   a. To evaluate the strength of the pelvic floor muscles.
   b. To evaluate the muscle tone in the vaginal wall.

PLEASE NOTE: This test should not be done during the patient's menstrual cycle or if the patient has vaginal infection or demonstrates unusual vaginal discharge.

2. **Equipment**
   a. Perineal drape
   b. Water-soluble lubricant
   c. Gloves
   d. Gooseneck light

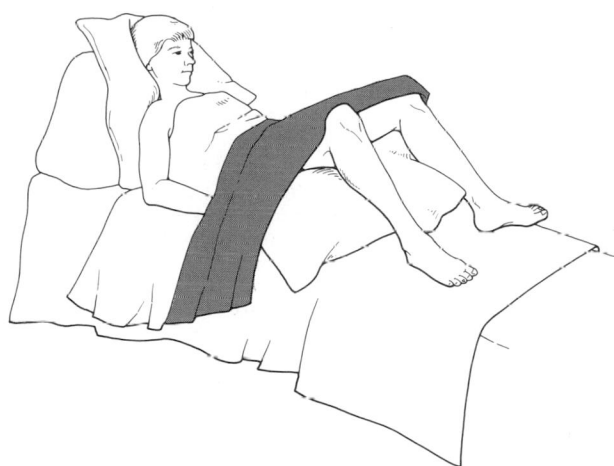

FIGURE 22–17 Patient position for internal evaluation of pelvic floor.

e. Hand mirror
f. Towel and washcloth
g. Hospital gown

3. **Procedure**
   a. *Preparatory phase*
      (1). Have the patient void before the procedure begins.
      (2). Position the patient on the examining table (underpants should be removed).
         (a). Have the patient assume the hook-lying position (see Figure 22–17).
         (b). Make the patient as comfortable as possible with pillows under her head and one under each knee.
         (c). Drape the patient to permit minimal exposure (but adequate for the examiner).
      (3). Encourage the patient to relax: tell her what you are doing and what she may feel.
      (4). Adjust the light to maximum focus.
      (5). Offer the patient the hand mirror so that she can see her perineal area if she wishes.
   b. *Performance phase*
      (1). Observe the external genitalia for any redness, swelling, drainage, lacerations or other alterations in normal anatomy such as pelvic floor laxity or bulging.
      (2). Ask the patient to contract her pelvic floor muscles. Note if the peri-

neum elevates, bulges, pulls asymmetrically, or does not move at all.
      (3). Ask the patient to cough. Note elevation or bulging or no movement. Any leakage of urine should also be noted. The bulge indicates pelvic relaxation. It may be caused by cervical prolapse (second degree) or cystocele, urethrocele, or rectocele.
      (4). Ask the patient to hold her breath and bear down. Observe as in (3).
      (5). Be gentle and take your time: don gloves; lubricate fingers. Tell the patient that she will feel the cold lubricant.
      (6). Gently separate the labia and continue visual inspection. Place one hand on the patient's thigh, maintain eye contact, and ask the patient to relax. Gently insert your middle and index fingers into the vaginal canal and turn fingerpads toward the sacrum (see Figure 22–18).
      (7). Sweep the fingertips to the left, right, and posteriorly to palpate the integrity and resting tone of the vaginal wall and pelvic floor. Be aware of any atrophy or asymmetries.
      (8). Instruct the patient to, on the count of three, squeeze the pelvic floor muscles and hold the contraction as long and as hard as she can.

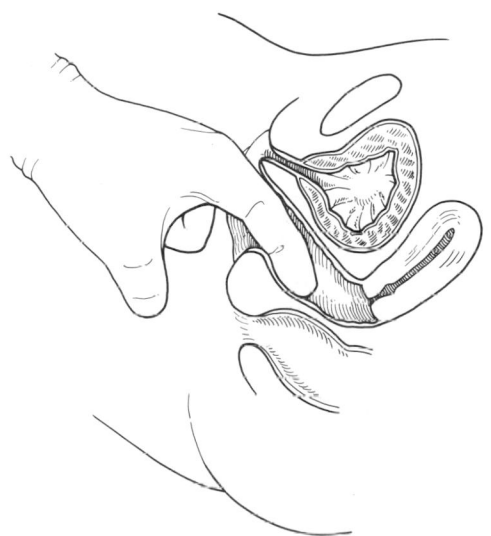

FIGURE 22–18 Palpating the pelvic floor.

If, in response to these directions, the patient tightens the gluteals, adductors, and abdominal muscles, rephrase the instructions to "Do not let me pull my fingers out" or "Tighten your muscles as if you are trying to stop urine flow or the passage of gas." This may give the desired results. Grade the muscle strength using Table 22–2 and record the duration of the contraction (duration of slow contractions is recorded in seconds). If the patient is unable to achieve any muscle contraction on the first effort, ask her to try again, this time instructing her to suck in as if using a straw while simultaneously trying to contract her pelvic floor muscles. If no contraction is felt, try to elicit a stretch reflex by pressing briskly on the puborectalis muscle. Note any muscular response.

(9). Ask the patient to repeat these held contractions for at least four repetitions or for as many as possible. Allow at least 4 seconds of rest between each contraction. Record the number of repetitions. Number of repetitions is recorded as × n.

(10). Ask the patient to contract and relax the muscles as quickly as possible with no rest period in between. Record the number of fast, 1-second contractions achieved. Number of fast (1-second) contractions is recorded following a semicolon.

(11). Surface EMG or pressure-sensing devices may be inserted at this time and appropriate assessments made (*eg*, pressure or EMG perineometers). Follow the manufacturer's recommended protocol.

C. *Follow-up phase*

(1). Assist the patient off the table.

(2). Allow the patient time and privacy to clean herself.

(3). Assist the patient in dressing if necessary. Answer any questions that she may have.

PLEASE NOTE: A possible rating might be 2/5 for 5 seconds × 3; four quick contractions. This would mean a weak contraction held for 5 seconds repeated three times followed by four

Table 22–2. PELVIC FLOOR MUSCLE GRADING SCALE

Rating	Meaning	Indication
0/5		No contraction
1/5	Trace	Contraction held less than 1 s
2/5	Weak	Contraction held for 1–3 s and/or fingers not elevated
3/5	Moderate	Contraction held for 4–6 s and fingers elevated; repeat three times
4/5	Strong	Contraction held for 7–9 s and fingers elevated; repeat three times
5/5	Unmistakably strong	Rapid contraction with elevation for >9 s; repeat four times

quick contractions. This approach allows baseline measurement for both strength and endurance of fast- and slow-twitch muscle fibers. Physical therapists wishing to gain skill in this evaluative technique are encouraged to contact the obstetrics and gynecology section of the American Physical Therapy Association regarding regional workshops and/or sites offering clinical internships.

D. Daily intake and output diary (see Figure 22–19)

Guidelines for daily diary:

1. Patients should be encouraged to drink at least 2 L of fluid per day. This is the equivalent of eight 8-oz glasses. Frequently, patients will restrict their fluid intake in hopes of preventing leakage accidents. Good hydration prevents constipation and keeps the urine diluted.

2. Urine output should be 1200 to 1500 mL.

3. The continent person voids about four to six times during the day and one to two times at night. Voiding more frequently is considered excessive.

4. The bladder needs about 300 mL of urine to empty fully. If the patient frequently voids lesser amounts, complete emptying may not be occurring.

5. Patients may wish to record the type of liquid consumed. Drinks containing caffeine (colas, coffee, tea, or chocolate) or alcohol may increase diuresis and contribute to urgency and should be taken out of the diet.

E. Urinary stress test

This is a simple test that can be used at home for active women with stress incontinence. It can help motivate patients, and it

SEVEN-DAY VOIDING LOG   Name _____

	6 AM	7 AM	8 AM	9 AM	10 AM	11 AM	12 AM	1 PM	2 PM	3 PM	4 PM	5 PM	6 PM	7 PM	8 PM	9 PM	10 PM	11 PM	12 AM	# times void at night / # pads used during day
Monday																				
Tuesday																				
Wednesday																				
Thursday																				
Friday																				
Saturday																				
Sunday																				

Instructions: Enter

E When you empty your bladder

S When you leak with cough, sneeze, exercise

U When you leak with a strong urge

FIGURE 22–19   Seven-day voiding log. (Courtesy of Frahm J. Women's Continence Program, Hutzel Hospital, Detroit MI.)

quickly and simply demonstrates improved pelvic floor function.

1. Ask the patient to empty her bladder.
2. Have the patient perform five jumping jacks.
3. Thirty minutes later, have the patient repeat the jumping jacks.
4. At the end of 1 hour, have the patient perform 10 jumping jacks while coughing during the last 5 jumps.
5. Patients who remain dry during this test are well on their way to overcoming stress incontinence.

V. Treatment

A. Treatment algorithm

1. **Mixed stress and urge incontinence** (node 6 on Fig. 22–20)
   a. *Nodes 1 and 2.* History, frequency/volume chart, pad test, stop test (see section on physical therapy evaluation, pp 477–483).
   b. *Node 3.* Discuss the patient's expectations of the physical therapy treatment. Explain the patient's role and responsibility for self-help. If the patient is committed to involvement, go to node 5. If the patient is unwilling to commit to the re-

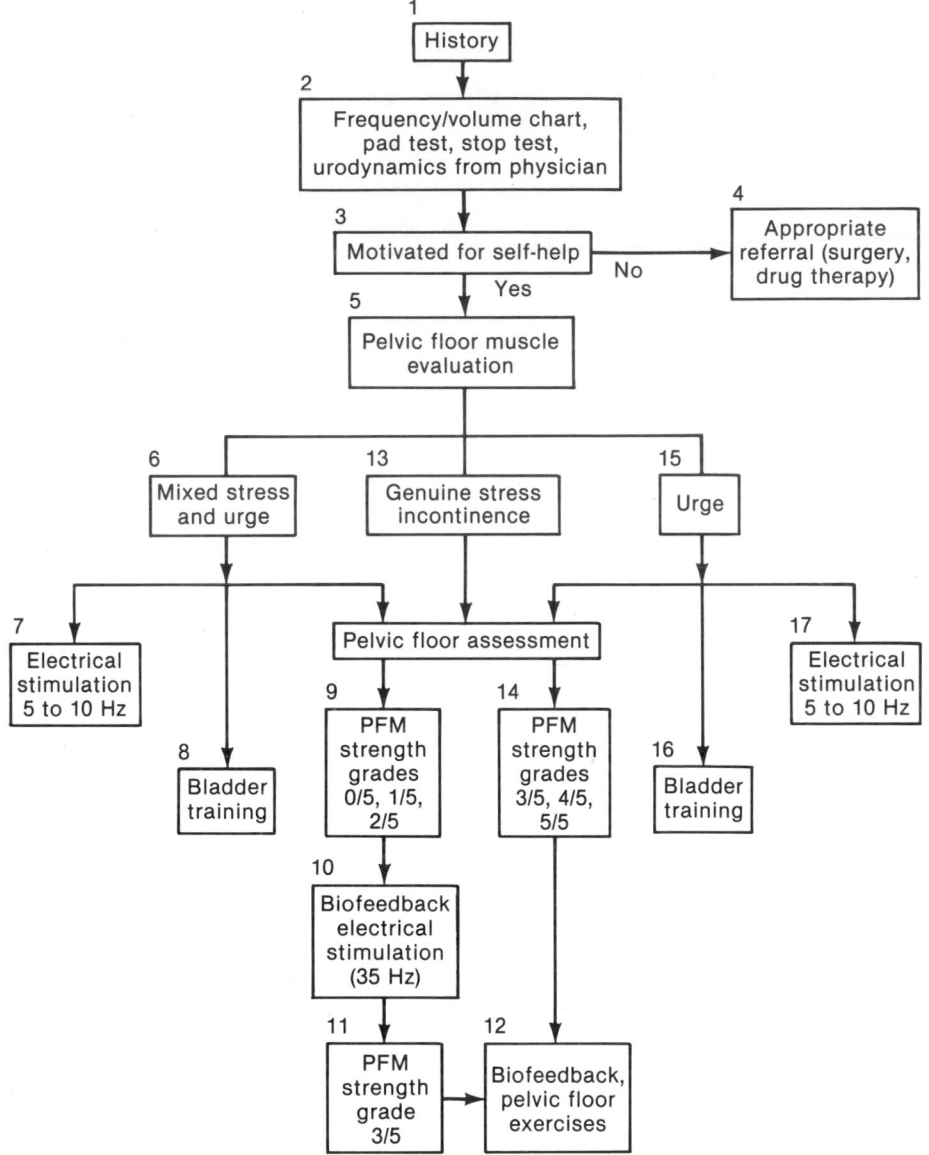

FIGURE 22–20 Protocol for physical therapy management of incontinence. (Modified from lecture materials of J Laycock.)

sponsibilities of self-help, refer the patient to the physician for alternative therapy.

c. **Node 5.** Pelvic floor muscle evaluation (see pp 480–482).

d. **Node 7.** Electrical stimulation at 5 to 10 Hz is thought to inhibit detrusor muscle contractions by influencing the sacral micturition reflex.

e. **Node 8.** Bladder training is used to help the patient break old voiding habits and increase bladder holding capacity.

f. **Nodes 9 and 10.** If the pelvic floor muscles are found to be weak (strength grades of 0/5, 1/5, or 2/5), electrical stimulation at 35 Hz will augment the voluntary muscle contractions and assist in strengthening the weakened muscles. Biofeedback will also heighten the patient's awareness of the pelvic floor muscles and their function.

g. **Nodes 11, 12 and 14.** If the pelvic floor muscles have a strength grade of 3/5, 4/5, or 5/5 (node 5), or when they attain a strength grade of 3/5, voluntary pelvic floor muscle contraction exercises will increase the strength of these muscles. Again, biofeedback is useful as a means of encouraging the patient toward greater efforts.

2. **Genuine stress incontinence** (node 13 on Fig. 22–20)
   a. *Nodes 1 through 5*. As above.
   b. *Nodes 9 and 10*. If the pelvic floor muscles are found to be weak (strength grades of 0/5, 1/5, or 2/5), electrical stimulation at 35 Hz will augment the voluntary muscle contractions and assist in strengthening the weakened muscles. Biofeedback will also heighten the patient's awareness of the pelvic floor muscles and their function.
   c. *Nodes 11, 12 and 14*. If the pelvic floor muscles have a strength grade of 3/5, 4/5, or 5/5 (node 5), or when they attain a strength grade of 3/5, voluntary pelvic floor muscle contraction exercises will increase the strength of these muscles. Again, biofeedback is useful as a means of encouraging the patient toward greater efforts.

3. **Urge incontinence** (node 15 on Fig. 22–20)
   a. *Nodes 1 through 5*. As above.
   b. *Node 17*. Electrical stimulation at 5 to 10 Hz is thought to inhibit detrusor muscle contractions by influencing the sacral micturition reflex.
   c. *Node 16*. Bladder training is used to help patient break old voiding habits and increases bladder holding capacity.
   d. *Nodes 9 and 10*. If the pelvic floor muscles are found to be weak (strength grades of 0/5, 1/5, or 2/5), electrical stimulation at 35 Hz will augment the voluntary muscle contractions and assist in strengthening the weakened muscles. Biofeedback will also heighten the patient's awareness of the pelvic floor muscles and their function.

B. **Treatment options available to physical therapists**

The following behavioral techniques are low-risk interventions that decrease the frequency of incontinent episodes in most individuals with mild or moderate symptoms. The success of all behavioral techniques depends on a patient who is attuned to self-help and a physical therapist willing to educate and provide positive reinforcement for both effort and progress.

1. **Bladder training (retraining)**[24–29]
   a. *Indications*
      (1). Best used to manage incontinence because of urgency or frequency or urge incontinence caused by detrusor instability or bladder hypersensitivity.
      (2). Very good for people who practice "just in case" toileting to avoid the possible "accident" and for those who have lost confidence in their ability to hold their urine.
      (3). Not suitable for patients with stress incontinence or overflow incontinence.
   b. *Components*
      (1). The patient is *educated* about the anatomy and pathophysiology of the lower urinary tract.
      (2). A voiding *schedule* that incorporates progressively longer periods between voiding is adopted.
      (3). The patient is taught to delay or inhibit the urge to void or to urinate only according to a timetable instead of in response to the urge to void.
      (4). Delaying is accomplished by trying to suppress the urge to urinate by
         (a). Sitting or standing still rather than rushing to the toilet.
         (b). Doing pelvic floor exercises.
         (c). Pressing on the perineum.
         (d). Performing breathing exercises to relax the abdominal muscle and diaphragm.
         (e). Performing various mental distractions such as mathematical problem solving.
      (5). The patient who practices delaying can indicate with an asterisk on a voiding log when she/he noticed the urge. The patient can then indicate by using the letters DV after the next void that this was truly a delayed void. Incidences of urges and delayed voids and interval lengths can thus be calculated, and progress is documented.
      (6). The initial interval may be as short as 1 hour while the patient is awake. A voiding schedule is not usually enforced during bedtime hours.
      (7). Patients receive positive reinforce-

ment for staying dry for longer and longer intervals. Reinforcement may be in the form of verbal praise or other, more tangible rewards.

2. **Habit training (timed voiding).**[16,19,30] Habit training is toileting on a planned schedule. The goal is to keep the patient dry by telling her/him to void at regular intervals.
   a. *Indications*
      (1). Can be useful for nursing home residents.
      (2). Unlike bladder training, there is no systematic effort to motivate the patient to delay voiding or resist the urge to void.
   b. *Components*
      (1). Determine the patient's *natural voiding pattern* over a 72-hour time span before beginning training in order to match the normal voiding interval. This can be accomplished using an electronic monitoring device.
      (2). The caretaker takes the patient to the toilet at the times matching the patient's normal intervals.

3. **Pelvic floor muscle exercises.**[25,29,31–37] These are often called Kegel exercises, named for the physician who prescribed them during the 1940s and 1950s.
   a. *Indications*
      (1). Used to treat stress urinary incontinence.
      (2). The goal is to strengthen the voluntary periurethral and pelvic floor muscles and thereby increase muscle support to the pelvic floor and improve urethral resistance.
      (3). Baseline strength measure of these muscles is important for appropriate exercise prescription. This may be done vaginally for women with an internal manual evaluation (described on pp 480–482) or by using a pneumatic or electronic perineometer. Both slow and fast contractions should be evaluated, as both are necessary to maintain continence. For men, the examiner assesses the pelvic floor muscle strength by digital examination in the rectum. The patient is sidelying, facing away from the examiner. The patient is asked to tighten the pelvic

floor muscles against the examiner's gloved and lubricated finger. Muscle strength is graded the same as noted on p 482. Patients whose muscle grades are below 3/5 need the assistance of electrical stimulation or use of biofeedback early in the course of their exercise program to ensure optimal outcome.
      (4). Patients should be seen regularly through a 6- to 8-week course of treatment. Following discharge, the patient must understand that, to be of lasting benefit, the exercise program must be done regularly for the rest of her/his life.
      (5). Training elderly patients may require a longer time.
   b. *Components*
      (1). Awareness of the pelvic floor muscles and their functions.
         (a). Diagrams of the pelvic floor can assist patients in understanding where the muscles of concern are located.
         (b). Women can be instructed to insert their own index finger into the vagina to feel when the muscle is contracting.
         (c). Have patients perform the "stop test" (described on p 477). It is recommended that this be done only once a week as a self-assessment of pelvic floor muscle strength.
         (d). Weighted vaginal cones can be used to give proprioceptive feedback and add resistance to the pelvic floor muscles (see vaginal cone retention, p 487).
         (e). A catheter, its bulb inflated with air, may be inserted into the vagina to enhance awareness of the pelvic floor muscles and add resistance to the contractions.
      (2). Using the pelvic floor muscles.[38–40] The patient should be instructed to
         (a). Sit well back on a chair with thighs and knees supported, legs slightly apart.
         (b). Lean forward with forearms on thighs.
         (c). Concentrate on the vaginal, urethral, and rectal areas.
         (d). Tighten the pelvic floor mus-

cles by drawing them in as if to stop the flow of urine or the passage of gas.

(e). Feel the tension in the pelvic floor muscles.

(f). Hold the contraction as long as possible. The goal is 10 seconds.

(g). Relax and feel the muscles softening.

(h). Tighten the muscles again. Be aware of incorrect contractions of the abdominals (*ie*, do not hold breath). A hand on the abdomen will give feedback about abdominal activity.

(i). Relax. Try to feel the difference between the contracted state and the relaxed state.

(j). Contract the muscles briefly and let go. Be certain that no other muscles are contracting.

(k). Practice this quick contraction several times.

(l). Do three repetitions to start. Weak muscles tire easily.

(m). Learn to contract the pelvic floor muscles and to maintain the contraction before and during coughing, sneezing, laughing, nose blowing, throat clearing, or lifting of heavy objects.

PLEASE NOTE: The goal is to complete a set of 10 slow contractions, holding each to the count of 10, and a set of 10 quick contractions. Six to eight exercise sets a day or hourly performance of multiple repetitions is recommended.

4. **Vaginal cone retention.**[41-44] Vaginal cones may be used in the initial or later stages of teaching pelvic floor muscle exercises (Kegel). The cones are sold in sets of five. They are equal in shape and volume but are of increasing weight, from 20 to 70 g. The cones are made of plastic and stainless steel encased in white plastic. There is a nylon string attached to the tapered end to permit easy removal (see Figure 22–21).

PLEASE NOTE: Cones should not be used while the patient is menstruating.

a. *Purposes*
(1). To increase the strength of the pelvic floor muscles.

(2). To provide direct proprioceptive feedback that the correct muscles are tightening.

b. *Equipment*
(1). Set of weighted vaginal cones. (Each patient should have her own set of cones.)

c. *Procedure* (from Femina Cones package insert)
(1). *Preparatory phase*
(a). Have the patient void before the procedure is begun.

(b). Provide the patient with an area of assured privacy.

(c). Have the patient remove her underpants.

(2). *Performance phase*
(a). Tell the patient to assume a semisquat position or to stand with one foot on a chair to facilitate insertion of the cone.

(b). Have the patient insert the lightest-weight cone into the vagina just as she would insert a tampon. It is inserted base first far enough into the vagina so that it cannot be felt protruding from the vaginal opening. The tapered end rests on the pelvic floor and the string is in the vaginal opening.

(c). Have the patient put on her underpants and walk around for 1 minute.

(d). Encourage the patient to tighten the pelvic floor muscles to hold the cone in place only if she begins to feel it sliding out.

(e). If the patient has no difficulty holding the lightest cone, repeat the process with increasingly heavy cones. (The heaviest weight retained without voluntary effort is called the passive weight and taken to represent the resting pelvic floor tone. The heaviest weight retained with voluntary pelvic floor contraction is termed the active weight.)

(f). The patient is instructed to start with the passive weight and to retain the cone for 15 minutes twice daily.

(g). Once the patient is successful

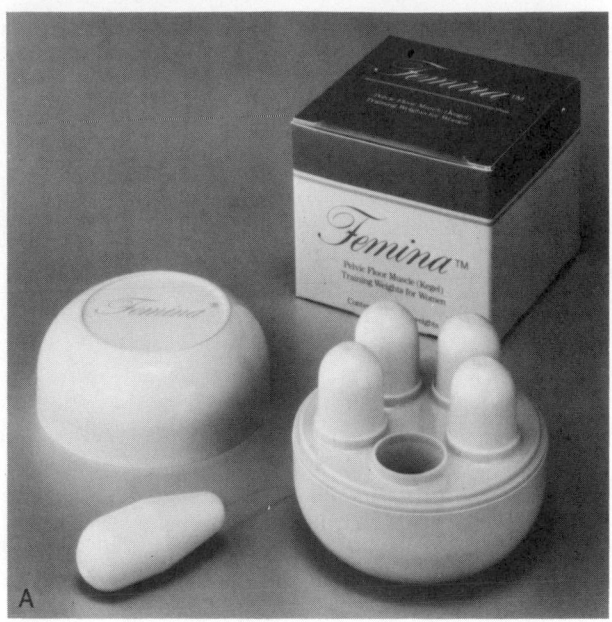

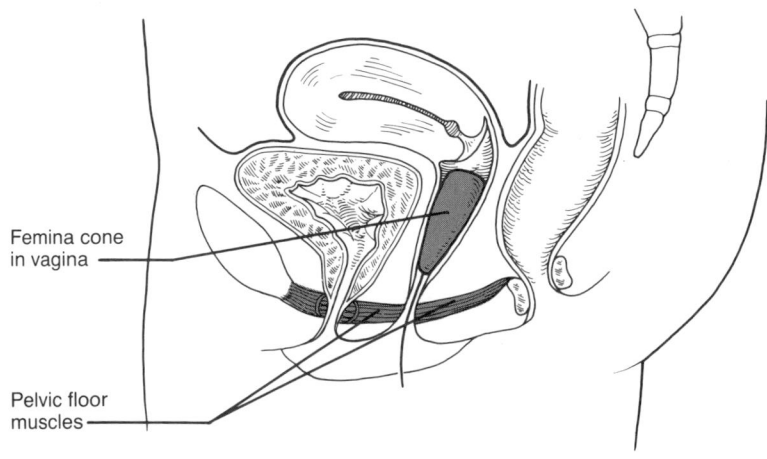

Femina cone
in vagina

Pelvic floor
muscles

B

FIGURE 22–21   **A,** Pelvic floor muscle training weights. (Courtesy of Dacomed Corp, Minneapolis, MN.) **B,** Position of Femina Cone in the vagina.

in maintaining the cone for 15 minutes on two consecutive occasions, she proceeds to the next heaviest weight.

(3). ***Follow-up phase.*** Vaginal cones should be thoroughly cleaned after each use. Rinse cone in warm water and use a soft cloth with mild soap to gently scrub cone and removal string. Rinse thoroughly and dry completely.

5. **Biofeedback.** Biofeedback uses electronic or mechanical instruments to give information to patients about their physiological activities. It was first used for urinary incontinence by Kegel, who devised an instrument called the perineometer. This was a pneumatic pressure-sensing device that, when inserted into the vagina, registered changes in the pelvic floor muscle tension, allowing the patient visual feedback about the amount of muscle force generated. Today's microchip

technology makes it possible for a portable device to provide patient feedback on both pressure changes and EMG activity during each exercise session. Some of the devices also record the outcome of each session for retrieval by the therapist when the patient returns for an office visit.

a. Used to treat patients with urge, stress, and mixed incontinence.[27,37,45–49] Patient goals are to learn voluntary inhibition of detrusor contractions, selective contraction of the pelvic floor muscles, or both.

b. Components: refer to the manufacturer's protocols.

PLEASE NOTE: The pelvic floor protocols for J & J and Verimed equipment were written by obstetrics and gynecology physical therapists Kathe Wallace and Jane Frahm, respectively.

6. **Electrical stimulation.** This can be given as faradic or interferential current.[50–60]

  a. *Indications*

   (1). Used to treat patients with stress, urge, and mixed incontinence.

  b. *Goals*

   (1). To increase strength of pelvic floor muscles.

   (2). To normalize reflex activity.[59,60]

    (a). Stimulation of afferent fibers facilitates urine storage by modifying bladder sensation.

    (b). Stimulation of efferent fibers to the detrusor muscle can induce bladder contraction.

    (c). Detrusor overactivity can be inhibited by influencing the sacral micturition reflex.

  c. *Precautions.* Electrical stimulation should not be used

   (1). During menstruation.

   (2). During pregnancy or if pregnancy is suspected.

   (3). In the presence of a known malignancy.

   (4). Over metal implants.

   (5). If the patient has a pacemaker.

  d. *Faradic current.* This may be given as acute maximal stimulation (maximal contractions two to three times per week in the clinic, or patients may use portable units that are designed to be used at home daily).

   (1). A vaginal-probe electrode containing two circuits may be used for women or a rectal-probe electrode containing two circuits for men and women. A variety of probe designs are available through distributors of stimulation equipment.

   (2). *Intensity* varies according to patient tolerance. The greater the intensity, the more motor units involved and the more effective the treatment.

   (3). The *rate* for patients with stress incontinence and pelvic floor muscle grade below 3/5 should be 35 to 50 Hz. The rate for patients with urge incontinence (unstable bladder) should be 5 to 15 Hz.

   (4). The *duty cycle* varies according to the patient's muscle grade. The rest cycle must be at least as long as the work cycle. Weaker muscles need longer rest periods. For muscles greater than grade 3/5, 2 off:1 on is an appropriate ratio. Muscles grade 0/5, 1/5, 2/5 need a 3 off:1 on cycle.

   (5). The *pulse width* for patients with stress incontinence should be 250 μs and higher to get muscle contraction similar to normal exercise. The pulse width for patients with urge incontinence should be 1 μs.

   (6). Treatment sessions are generally 20 to 30 min/d.

  e. *Chronic stimulation.*[57,58,61,62] This is thought to transform intermediate fiber types from type II (fast twitch) motor units to units with mainly type I (slow twitch), thereby increasing the resting tone of the pelvic floor muscles and resulting in a decrease in symptoms of stress incontinence. It is used for patients with stress, urge, and mixed incontinence.

   (1). Parameters are all similar to faradic stimulation except for *rate,* which should be 10 Hz, and *treatment time,* which should be 6 to 20 hr/d for a *duration* of 3 to 6 months.

   (2). The patient wears the unit while going about normal activities of daily living. Patient compliance can be a problem.

  f. *Interferential current*[53,63–65]

   (1). *Electrode placement*

(a). For four-pole application, two posterior electrodes are placed medial to the ischial tuberosities, on each side of the anus. Two anterior electrodes are placed over the obturator foramina, 1.5 to 2 cm lateral to the symphysis pubis.

(b). For bipolar application for women, a 6 × 8 cm electrode is placed directly over the anus, covering the posterior fibers of the levator ani. A 4 × 6 cm electrode is placed centrally on the anterior fibers of the pelvic floor muscle immediately inferior to the symphysis pubis.

(c). For bipolar application for men, a 6 × 8 cm electrode is placed under each of the ischial tuberosities of the seated patient so that one electrode is on each side of the gluteal cleft, anterior to the anus, and separated by about 2 cm.

(2). *Treatment protocols*
    (a). For stress incontinence:
       (i). Carrier wave = 2 kHz.
       (ii). Treatment frequency = 10 to 50 Hz ⌐.
       (iii). Intensity = maximum current tolerated.
       (iv). Duration = 15 minutes. *Followed by*
       (v). Carrier wave = 2 kHz.
       (vi). Treatment frequency = 50 Hz surged.
       (vii). Intensity = maximum current tolerated.
       (viii). Duration = 15 minutes. Total treatment time = 30 minutes.

    (b). If surged current is unavailable:
       (i). Carrier wave = 2 kHz.
       (ii). Treatment frequency = 10 to 50 Hz ⌐.
       (iii). Intensity = maximum current tolerated.
       (iv). Duration = 15 minutes. *Followed by*
       (v). Carrier wave = 2 kHz.
       (vi). Treatment frequency = 10 − 50 Hz ⌐.

(vii). Intensity = maximum current tolerated.
(viii). Duration = 15 minutes. Total treatment time = 30 minutes.

    (c). For urge incontinence:
       (i). Carrier wave = 2 kHz.
       (ii). Treatment frequency = 10 to 50 Hz ⌐.
       (iii). Intensity = maximum current tolerated.
       (iv). Duration = 30 minutes.

    (d). For mixed stress and urge incontinence:
       (i). Carrier wave = 2 kHz.
       (ii). Treatment frequency = 5 to 10 Hz ⌐.
       (iii). Intensity = maximum current tolerated.
       (iv). Duration = 10 minutes. *Followed by*
       (v). Carrier wave = 2 kHz.
       (vi). Treatment frequency = 10 to 50 Hz ⌐.
       (vii). Intensity = maximum current tolerated.
       (viii). Duration = 10 minutes. *Followed by*
       (ix). Carrier wave = 2 kHz.
       (x). Treatment frequency = 50 Hz surged.
       (xi). Intensity = maximum current tolerated.
       (xii). Duration = 10 minutes. Total treatment time = 30 minutes.

CONTENT OF SUCCESSFUL PELVIC FLOOR EXERCISE PROGRAMS[40]

1. Patient comprehension of the anatomy involved.
2. Accurate baseline measures of incontinence made for later objective demonstrations of progress.
3. Patient motivation to succeed.
4. Education and coaching provided by the therapist.
5. Some form of biofeedback.
6. A customized and regularly supervised exercise program.
7. A plan for ongoing re-evaluation both to demonstrate progress and to modify the program in response to treatment.

VI. Painful Conditions of the Genitourinary System

A. Pain originating from pelvic organs

   1. **Dysmenorrhea**[66–68]
     a. *Symptoms*
      (1). Abdominal pain and cramping.
      (2). Low back pain.
     b. *Physical therapy treatment*
      (1). Conventional transcutaneous electrical nerve stimulator (TENS) treatment has been shown to give good relief of pain of dysmenorrhea.
       (a). Electrode placement (see Figure 22–22):
        (i). Varies among patients. Some patients experience better pain relief with electrode placement posteriorly in the T-10 to L-1 segmental levels. Others have better relief with the electrodes placed on the abdomen at the most anterolateral area of pain but not higher than the umbilicus nor lower than the anterosuperior iliac spine so that the stimulation occurs in a crisscross manner.
       (b). Frequency—50 to 100 Hz.
       (c). Pulse width—40 to 75 μs.
       (d). Intensity—to produce comfortable paresthesia without muscle contraction.
       (e). Treatment time—30 minutes on, then off until pain returns, then on again for 30 minutes. Repeat as necessary.
      (2). Low-rate acupuncture, like TENS, affords pain relief but cannot be worn comfortably while performing activities of daily living.
      (3). Interferential current can also be used for pain relief.[69]
       (a). Four plate electrodes are used. Two of 100 cm² are placed anteriorly and 2 of 200 cm² are placed posteriorly (see Figure 22–23).
       (b). A rhythmical frequency of 90 to 100 Hz is used.

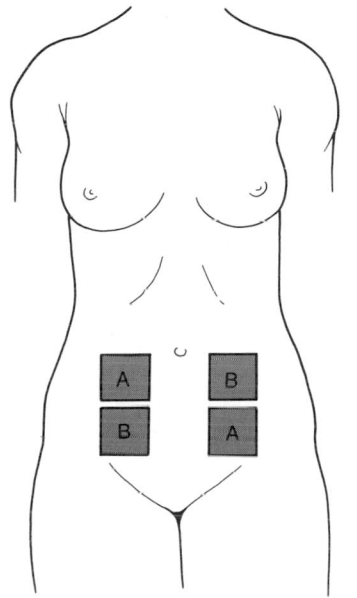
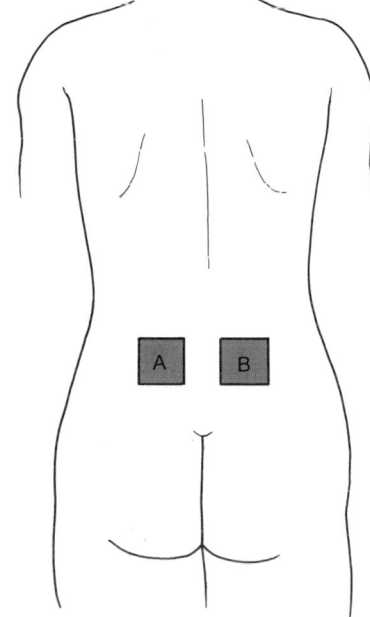

FIGURE 22–22 Electrode placement for conventional TENS for relief of abdominal and back pain of dysmenorrhea.

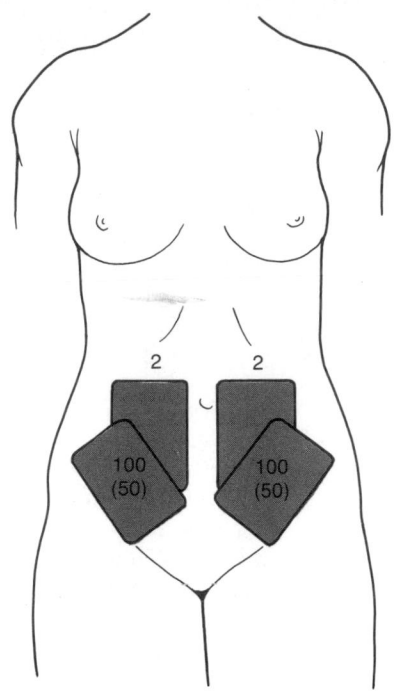

Anterior placement of 100 cm² electrodes in treating dysmenorrhea with interferential current

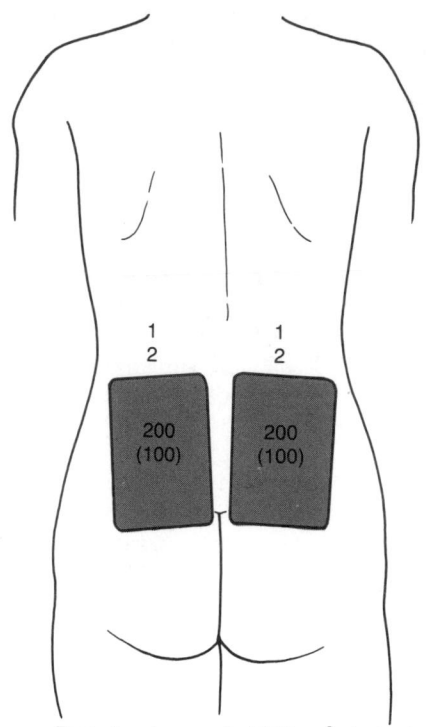

Posterior placement of 200 cm² electrodes in treating dysmenorrhea with interferential current

FIGURE 22–23   Position of electrodes in treating dysmenorrhea with interferential current.

(c). Intensity depends on patient tolerance (usually from 12 to 25 mA).

(d). Treatment time is 15 to 20 minutes daily, or every other day while pain persists.

2. **Pelvic inflammatory disease**
   a. *Symptoms*
      (1). Severe lower abdominal pain and tenderness.
      (2). Fever.
   b. *Physical therapy treatment*
      (1). Shortwave or microwave diathermy given daily or every other day, 20 minutes per treatment.[69,70]

3. **Vulvar vestibulitis syndrome**
   a. *Symptoms*
      (1). Severe focal pain of the vaginal vestibule and vulvar skin.[71]
      (2). Hypersensitivity along the labia minora.
      (3). Burning pain that occurs primarily in response to pressure and stretching.

(4). Dyspareunia.
(5). Some women experience urinary urgency, cystitis, and even interstitial cystitis (see #4).

   b. *Physical therapy treatment*
      (1). Musculoskeletal evaluation of postural problems to assess.
         (a). Spasm of inner thigh muscles.
         (b). Imbalance of hip or pelvic musculature.
      (2). Manual therapy
         (a). Joint mobilization.
         (b). Soft tissue mobilization.
         (c). Myofascial release.
         (d). Trigger point therapy.
         (e). Acupressure.
      (3). Pelvic floor muscle evaluation and treatment program to assess
         (a). Strength/weakness.
         (b). Ability to contract muscle at all.
         (c). Muscle spasm.
      (4). Electrotherapy, which may include deep heat (*eg,* diathermy or ultrasound) or TENS over sacral nerve roots for pain relief.

(5). General stretching, strengthening, or relaxation program based on evaluation.

4. **Interstitial cystitis**[65,72]
 a. *Symptoms*
  (1). Persistent, severe pelvic pain, frequent and painful urination.
  (2). Acidic, alcoholic, or carbonated beverages and coffee and tea increase pain.
 b. *Physical therapy treatment*
  (1). Bladder training (see p 485).[64]
  (2). TENS.
   (a). Electrode placement:
    (i). One set of electrodes is placed suprapubically on either side of the midline, 10 to 15 cm apart.
    (ii). A second set of electrodes may be placed at T-10 paraspinally.
   (b). Frequency—50 Hz.
   (c). Pulse width—200 μs.
   (d). Intensity—to patient maximum tolerance.
   (e). Treatment time—2 hours twice daily.
  (3). Interferential current.
   (a). Electrode placement as for treatment of incontinence.
   (b). Stimulus parameters are those for pain relief. See the manufacturer's protocol.

5. **Peyronie's disease**
 a. *Symptoms*
  (1). Severe pain on penile erection caused by fibrotic plaques on the shaft of the penis.
  (2). Deviation of the erect penis frequently preventing intromission.
 b. *Physical therapy treatment*[70,72]
  (1). Iontophoresis with 0.5% hydrocortisone cream.
   (a). Hydrocortisone cream applied to plaque.
  (b). Electrode placement:
   (i). Positive electrode wrapped around the penis.
   (ii). Negative electrode placed on patient's anterior thigh.
  (c). Intensity—5 mA continuous direct current.
  (d). Treatment time—30 minutes weekly.
  (2). Phonophoresis with 1% hydrocortisone cream.
  (3). Electrical stimulation with standard TENS unit with settings to relieve muscle spasm.
  (4). Cold laser directly on plaque for pain control.

B. Pain originating from excessive pelvic floor tension

1. Pelvic floor tension myalgia[56,73-76] is a term used to include all of the following: pyriformis syndrome, levator ani spasm, spastica pelvic diaphragm, and coccygodynia.
 a. *Symptoms*
  (1). Aching discomfort in the rectum, pelvis, or lower back, unilateral or bilateral leg pain, pain with bowel movement, coccyx pain, constipation, dyspareunia (painful intercourse).
  (2). Pain worsens on sitting and disappears on standing or lying down.
 b. *Physical therapy treatment*
  (1). Rectal diathermy. See the manufacturer's protocol for treatment parameters.
  (2). Thiele's massage[77] (see Figure 22–24).
   (a). Purposes
    (i). To evaluate the tone of the pelvic floor muscles.
    (ii). To relax the pelvic floor muscles using massage.
   (b). Equipment
    (i). Water-soluble lubricant
    (ii). Gloves
    (iii). Towel
    (iv). Washcloth
   (c). Preparatory phase
    (i). Position the patient on the examining table (underpants should be removed).

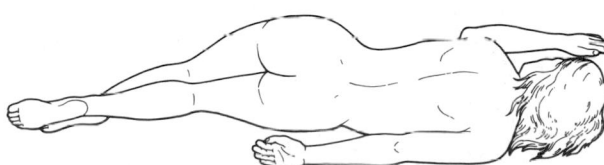

FIGURE 22–24 Position of patient for Thiele's massage.

(ii). Have the patient assume the left lateral Sims position (semiprone).

(iii). Make the patient as comfortable as possible.

(iv). Drape the patient to permit minimal exposure (but adequate for the examiner).

(v). Encourage the patient to relax; tell her what you are doing and what she may feel.

(vi). Be gentle: take your time, don gloves, lubricate your fingers, and tell the patient that she will feel the cold lubricant.

(b). Evaluation

(i). Gently insert your index finger fully into the rectum so that the finger pad is against the posterior midline. The flexor surface of your finger will lie across the fibers of the puborectalis muscle.

(ii). Place your thumb over the coccyx externally and palpate the coccyx between the thumb and the finger. Move the coccyx through its normal range of motion and note any restrictions.

(iii). Next, move the finger just lateral to the posterior midline, maintaining the flexor surface of the finger in contact with the soft tissues. The finger is now lying on the medial fibers of the gluteus maximus muscle, coccygeal, and levator ani muscles.

(iv). Keep the volar surface of your finger in contact with the underlying structures and sweep anterolaterally and ventrally to the midline of the symphysis pubis. Maintaining moderate pressure, sweep your fingers posterolat-

erally back to the coccyx. Be aware of the muscle tone palpated.

◼ PLEASE NOTE: When the entire levator ani muscle is spastic, it will feel like a firm sheet of muscle stretched tensely from its origin near the tendinous arch to its insertion into the anterior surface and lateral borders of the coccyx and lower sacrum and into the anorectum at the junction of the lower portion of the rectum with the upper part of the anal canal. Frequently, individual fascicles will stand out like tight cords, with areas of relaxed muscle between them.

(v). Ask the patient to bear down as if to pass gas or have a bowel movement. You may feel the pelvic floor muscles relax.

(c). Treatment

(i). With pressure to patient's tolerance, sweep your fingertip back and forth lengthwise along the muscle fibers from pubis to coccyx.

(ii). Repeat this movement up to 15 times on each side of the pelvis.

(d). Follow-up phase

(i). Assist the patient off the examination table.

(ii). Allow the patient time and privacy to get cleaned and dressed.

(iii). Answer any questions that the patient may have.

(3). Relaxation exercises.

(4). Hot baths daily.

(5). High-voltage pulsed current stimulation.[78]

(a). Hand-held or self-retaining rectal probe and large dispersive pad placed over lateral thigh.

(b). Pulse frequency—80 to 120 Hz.

(c). Voltage graded from 0 to patient tolerance, usually 150 to 400 V.

(d). Duration—30 to 60 minutes per session.

(e). Treatment time—every other day until symptoms resolve, usually in 5 to 10 sessions.

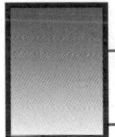

Clinical Decision-Making Cases: Incontinence

Case #1

EXAMINATION

History

HJ is a 68-year-old female; gravida 0, para 0. Her referring diagnosis is urge incontinence, unstable bladder, and dysfunctional pelvic floor muscles.

Previous medical history:	Breast cancer; bladder infections, kidney infections, arthritis, hypertension, pneumonia, thyroid disease
Current medications:	Dyazide, Myadex, tamoxifen sulfate, vitamins E and D, calcium
Previous surgical history:	Hysterectomy, mastectomy, laparoscopic cholecystectomy

HJ's chief complaints are too many urinary accidents; frequency of voiding; urine loss with coughing, sneezing, lifting, and laughing; and urge. The duration of her problem has been 7 to 12 years, and pad use is intermittent. Her initial 24-hour voiding log documents 13 voids, including 2 voids per night. She documents daily leakage. The severity of her problem (on a scale of 1 to 10) is 7/10.

Physical Examination

Evaluative data: *Observation* of perineum during contraction reveals slight elevation perivaginally and perianally; during cough, the perineum bulges. *Palpation* reveals muscle strength of 2/5. Minimal contractile activity is palpated, and there is minimal elevation of the puborectalis muscle. It is noted that in attempting contraction of the pelvic floor muscles (PFM), she uses accessory muscle assist, *ie,* abdominals and gluteals. High resting tension is palpated. *Pressure generation* (Bourne pressure perineometer measures in inches of H_2O on a scale of $\frac{1}{16}$ to $\frac{16}{16}$ inch) is $\frac{1}{16}$ inches of H_2O.

EMG data: EMG maximum is 0.937 μVs; work average is 0.657 μVs, and rest average is 0.344 μVs, which is high.

Cough assessment: With perineometer in vagina, the patient maintains a contraction of the PFM during two coughs but is unable to do so on the third.

Endurance: HJ can maintain five 10-second contractions.

ASSESSMENT/DIAGNOSIS

1. Weak, ineffective PFM (2/5).
2. High resting tension, PFM.
3. Little differentiation between work and rest on EMG or electromyogram.
4. Decreased proprioception of PFM (high resting tension).
5. Urinary frequency, 13+ voids per 24 hours.
6. Ineffective sphincter support during physical stress, *eg*, during cough, sneeze.
7. Daily urinary leakage.
8. Minimal pressure generation ($\frac{1}{16}$ inches of H_2O) on Bourne perineometer.

Note: Although the initial medical diagnosis was urge incontinence, the patient demonstrated symptoms of both urge and stress incontinence and is more accurately described as having mixed incontinence.

TREATMENT GOALS

1. Increase PFM strength to 3/5.
2. Demonstrate sphincteric support during cough on electromyogram.
3. Demonstrate increased PFM proprioception by demonstrating decreased resting tensions on electromyogram.
4. Decrease urinary frequency to five to eight voids per 24 hours.
5. Demonstrate ability to control urgency and delay voids from the time urge is felt to decrease the number of voids per 24 hours.
6. Decrease urinary leaks to less than one per day.
7. Increase pressure generation on Bourne perineometer to $\frac{3}{16}$ inches of water.

TREATMENT

1. PFM evaluation by observation, palpation, EMG, and pressure perineometry.
2. Progressive strengthening program for PFM.
3. Therapeutic exercise program of synergistic muscles to facilitate increased strength of PFM.
4. Bladder retraining, including teaching and monitoring of delayed voiding techniques.
5. On 3/4/93, electrical stimulation was assessed. After consultation with HJ's physician, electrical stimulation treatments were started in clinic three times a week for 4 weeks (start date, 3/23/93). The patient was seen a total of 15 times over a period of 3

months. Visits were on 1/13/93, 1/29/93, 2/9/93, 3/4/93, 3/23/93, 3/24/93, 3/26/93, 3/29/93, 3/31/93, 4/1/93, 4/5/93, 4/6/93, 4/9/93, 4/12/93, 4/14/93. The first four treatments were to teach PFM awareness, teach voluntary control over PFM contraction and relaxation, decrease inappropriate accessory muscle participation in PFM contractions, initiate bladder training program, teach how to keep bladder diaries, teach delayed voiding techniques. Between visits four and five, the patient saw her physician; the therapist's suggestion of electrical stimulation was agreed on, so visits 5 to 15 were for electrical stimulation in the clinic three times a week. Stimulation parameters were: phase duration, 250 μs; pulses per second, 35 (secondary to patient's muscle strength of 2/5); duty cycle, on 8 seconds/off 12 seconds; treatment time, 15 minutes. Current was applied with a vaginal electrode to right, left, and posterior vaginal walls.

TREATMENT OUTCOMES

On the second visit, the patient demonstrated $\frac{2}{16}$ inches of H_2O on Bourne perineometer, decreased leaks from three per day to three in 6 days, and ability to delay voids. On visits three and four, her voiding log documented her increased ability to delay voids (20 in 3rd week, and 23 in 4th week). Pad use decreased to one to two per day, and number of voids per 24 hours decreased to seven to eight. Perceived severity of incontinence decreased from 7/10 to 5.5/10. After 4 weeks of electrical stimulation treatments three times weekly (with a follow-up PFM functional exercise pro-

gram on a home basis), the following progress with respect to the treatment goals (p 495) was made:

1. Not met; PFM strength remains 2/5.
2. Partially met (per electromyograms).
3. Partially met; there is objective decrease in EMG activity during rest phase of functional electromyogram (work/rest mode, five repetitions of 10 seconds of work and 10 seconds of rest). Rest average decreased from 0.344 μVs to 0.190 μVs.
4. Met; frequency decreased from 13+ voids per day to 6 or 7 voids per day. Night voids decreased from two to one.
5. Patient demonstrates ability to delay voids from time of initial urge 7 to 10 times per week. Maximum time of delayed void is 4 hours, minimum time is 1 to 1.5 hours.
6. Leakage decreased to weekly, not daily.
7. Partially met; patient increased pressure generation on Bourne pressure perineometer from barely able to move the gauge to a brisk $\frac{2}{16}$ inches of H_2O.

The patient learned the exercise and bladder retraining program, which she will have to adhere to for the rest of her life.

The program was terminated because of the terms of the patient's Medicare coverage. She would have benefited from the continued use of electrical stimulation at home, but at this time the rental of an electrical stimulator is not covered for home use by Medicare. The diagnostic code used for the physical therapy program was 728.2 (muscle weakness and atrophy), and documentation of patient treatment notes was sent to Medicare for review in determining payment of claim.

Case #2

EXAMINATION

History

GC is a 75-year-old female; gravida 0, para 0. Her referring diagnosis is stress urinary incontinence. She is a retired medical technologist, referred for PFM evaluation and strengthening program.

Previous medical history: Spastic colon, prolapsed mitral valve, arthritis, ovarian cyst

Previous surgical history: Hysterectomy age 47, appendectomy

Medications: Conjugated estrogen

Allergies: Antibiotics (?)

The patient complains of urine loss with physical stress, lifting, bending, and working in garden. She has had loss of urine with laughing since childhood. She states that she wants to stop the urine loss she has

now because she does not want to be an incontinent woman in a nursing home in 10 or 15 years. She uses protective pads when out of the home. Her voiding log documents 12 voids per 24 hours and 0 voids per night. She experiences, on average, two involuntary urine leaks per day. She rates the severity of her problem as 4/10 (on a scale of 1 to 10).

Physical Examination

Evaluative data: *Observation* of perineum during contraction reveals elevation; during cough, reveals bulging. *Palpation* reveals muscle strength of 3/5. PFM contractions are easily elicited, perineal sensation is intact, but posterior contractions of puborectalis muscle are weak. At rest, her muscle tone is lax. *Pressure generation* was measured with the Milex air perineometer. Millimeters of air was measured. The gauge was calibrated from 10 to 100 mm, with no known values for norms. She made the needle rise from 12 to 14 mm of air.

EMG data: EMG maximum, 0.437 μVs; work average, 0.181 μVs; rest average, 0.072 μVs.

Cough assessment: With perineometer in vagina, the patient's PFM activity is observed to peak initially with cough but quickly relaxes during cough as documented by electromyogram.

Endurance: Although the patient can maintain a contraction for 10 seconds, her endurance (especially type I, slow-twitch fibers) is deficient, as her effort is not consistent. There is attenuation of the "hold" during this time.

ASSESSMENT/DIAGNOSIS

1. PFM strength 3/5.
2. Decreased endurance of PFM, especially against physical stress, such as change of position with increased abdominal pressure, getting out of a car, coughing, sneezing, laughing.
3. Possible excessive use of abdominal muscles, by observation and EMG activity (EMG maximum: abdominals 1.406 μVs; PFM, 0.437 μVs; 3:1 ratio).
4. Urine loss with physical stress.
5. EMG activity, low. EMG maximum, 0.437 μVs; work average, 0.181 μVs; rest average, 0.072 μVs.

TREATMENT GOALS

1. Increase PFM strength to 4/5.
2. Increase endurance to five consistently held 10-second PFM contractions.
3. Increase endurance of PFM contractions with physical stresses of coughing, as evidenced by perineal observation, clinical data, and electromyograms.
4. Decreased urine loss with stress to one per day or less.
5. Increased EMG activity of PFM to 0.500 to 0.800 μVs maximum; and work averages to 0.500 to 0.700 μVs.
6. Decreased abdominal muscle activity (per EMG data to a 1:1 ratio, or 2:1 ratio abdominal muscles to PFM).

TREATMENT

1. Teach PFM exercise for strengthening.
2. Teach abdominal muscle exercise to provide postural support for pelvis and low back.
3. Teach postural exercises, incorporating synergistic abdominal and PFM activity in patient's functional activities.
4. Teach modified cough mechanism: utilize abdominal muscles and PFM synergistically to prevent urine leakage (demonstrate PFM contraction maintenance during coughs on EMG).
5. Re-evaluate and modify program on each patient return visit.

6. Teach patient to use exercise and void logs.
7. Follow monthly for 3 months.

TREATMENT OUTCOMES

The patient was seen from March 29, 1991, through September 6, 1991, for a total of four visits. During this time, the patient maintained scrupulous exercise logs and voiding logs.

At the 2nd visit (5/15/91), leakage was about once per day, bulging of perineum was reduced with cough, maximum EMG was 0.687 μVs, work/rest averages (of five 10-second contractions) were 0.290/0.072 μVs.

At the 3rd visit (7/3/91), the perineum did not bulge with cough, maximum EMG was 0.531 μVs, with work/rest averages 0.249/0.050 μVs. Maintenance of PFM contractions with cough occurred with two out of four coughs. Abdominal muscle activity, per EMG perineometry, was at a 1:1 ratio with PFM activity, and urine loss was 1.8 leaks per day.

At the 4th and final visit, accidental urine loss was five leaks in 7 days, making loss less than once per day; PFM strength by palpation was 4/5; there was no bulge of the perineum with cough; maximum EMG was 0.609 μVs, work/rest averages were 0.405/0.084 μVs; and contractions were maintained for 10 seconds consistently for five repetitions. PFM contractions were maintained for four out of four coughs during EMG perineometry. Voids per day were reduced from 12 to 9. The patient could stop urine flow in midstream. The following progress with respect to the treatment goals was made:

1. Met.
2. Met; patient maintains five consistent 10-second contractions.
3. Met.
4. Met; patient experiencing less than one leak per day.
5. Essentially met; EMG maximum 0.609 μVs (up from 0.437 μVs initially) and work/rest averages now 0.405/0.084 μVs (initially 0.181/0.072).
6. Met; abdominal muscle to PFM ratio now about 1:1 (at onset, about 3:1).

The patient learned appropriate PFM strengthening exercises, was educated about the synergistic role that abdominal muscles play in functional activities, learned basic body mechanics, kept track of urinary activity and exercise activity, and was able to self-assess her progress in controlling urinary leakage. Increased EMG activity was significant in view of the positive subjective and objective findings of this patient. The diagnostic code used was 728.2 (muscle weakness and atrophy); Medicare reimbursed for treatments. All documentation was sent with billing.

Case #3

EXAMINATION

History

CA is a 27-year-old female; gravida 3, para 1. She was referred at 10 weeks post partum with the diagnosis of stress urinary incontinence.

Previous medical history:	Cancer-in-situ (cervix), spontaneous pneumothorax (three times), recent delivery of baby (6 lb 4 oz) over midline episiotomy
Previous surgical history:	Tonsillectomy, dilation and curettage, eye surgery
Obstetrical history:	Miscarriages (two)
Medications:	Prenatal vitamins
Allergies:	Penicillin, cephalexin
Social history:	Smokes occasionally

Physical Examination

Evaluative data: *Observation* of the perineum with contraction reveals minimal perineal elevation, noted only toward anus; major perineal bulging noted with cough. *Palpation* reveals PFM strength of 1 to 1+/5. Very weak contractions are palpated, especially on lateral walls of pubococcygeus muscle. A stretch reflex is utilized to elicit contraction of lateral walls of the pubococcygeus. The patient complains of pain over episiotomy site. Because a pressure perineometer was not available at the time of the patient's treatment, these data are not provided.

EMG data: *Note:* Because of the patient's PFM weakness, a "bridged" position was used. A pillow was placed under her buttocks while she was in the hooklying position. Work and rest averages were recorded only: work average/rest average = 0.145/0.025 μVs.

Endurance: Minimal, 3 to 5 seconds of hold.

Cough assessment: Not done with perineometry because it was felt that the patient would not be able to retain the perineometer with her limited PFM function and strength.

ASSESSMENT/DIAGNOSIS

1. Postpartum stress urinary incontinence.
2. Very weak PFM, 1+/5.
3. No endurance, holding contractions about 3 seconds.
4. Unable to maintain contraction of PFM with cough.

TREATMENT GOALS

1. Functional PFM (contract/relax at will with patient aware of same).
2. Abolish stress urinary incontinence.
3. Increase PFM strength to at least 3/5.
4. Achieve work averages of about 0.460 to 0.500 μVs for 5-second holds.
5. Long-term-goal: work average of 0.800 μVs, and 4/5 PFM strength.

TREATMENT

The patient would be followed weekly or biweekly, progressing to monthly, to monitor and modify her home program. PFM strengthening program was initiated in the first week. Arrangements were made to obtain a home biofeedback unit so that the patient could exercise and record sessions at home. She was seen for a total of nine visits from 2/27/90 through 8/23/90 at weekly, biweekly, and monthly intervals. She used a Myo 2 portable programmable biofeedback unit and performed strengthening exercises, combining them with her functional activities.

TREATMENT OUTCOMES

The visit of 3/15/90 documents 2−/5 muscle strength, with marked weakness in the right upper lateral puboccocygeal area. Maximum contraction of 0.48 μVs, with work average/rest average of 0.242/0.036 μVs. Patient says she does not have to "run" to the bathroom but still loses urine with all her athletic exercises, including walking. She does not lose urine with coughing. The Myo 2 was provided with instructions and programmed for her home exercise program.

On 3/26/90, she still lost urine with fast walking and running but denied urine loss with coughing. She is advised to temporarily stop fast walking/running and stair climber but to continue with regular speedwalking, sit-ups, leg lifts, and exercise bicycle. Palpation reveals increased PFM activity with holds for 4 seconds, 2+/5 strength, and left wall stronger than right. EMG activity in clinic for work/rest is 0.256/0.070 μVs. The patient logged 40 exercise sessions on Myo 2 unit for home program.

Visit of 4/19/90 reveals increased PFM strength to 3/5, holding 4 seconds for eight repetitions. She has had the flu with coughing. She feels more control of PFM, especially with the increased coughing during this episode of flu. Work/rest data, 0.300/0.139 μVs; 57 home exercise sessions recorded on Myo 2. Home program modified by increasing the time held for her PFM exercise.

On 5/16/90, strength is 3+/5, with only minimal stretch required to elicit a PFM contraction. With increased PFM strength, the area of weakness in the right upper pubococcygeal muscle is apparent. An air perineometer was used for the first time (millimeters of air), with ability to move air 5 to 7 mm noted. Maximum

EMG is 0.687 μVs; work/rest averages are 0.414/0.094. Evidence by EMG perineometry of maintenance of PFM contractions in two out of two coughs. Home biofeedback program increased to 8-second holds and exercise cycles of seven repetitions. Patient showing improvement in strength and function of PFM.

Assessment on 7/6/90 reveals muscle strength of 4−/5, definite elevation of perineum with contraction and quick correction of minimal bulge with cough. She moves air in the perineometer 9 to 10 mm and reports no leak episodes for about 2 weeks. She can slow urine stream and states that sexual response is much improved. She is compliant with home exercise; 45 sessions recorded on Myo 2. She also reports no urine leaks with physical activity. Cough response per EMG is positive for PFM contraction in two out of two coughs. EMG maximum is 0.609 μVs; work/rest averages (for 10-second holds) are 0.322/0.808 μVs. Noted: muscle atrophy of the right upper pubococcygeal muscle and no sensation in that area, suggestive of *pudendal nerve damage.*

There were two more visits, 7/31/90 and 8/23/90. Final data: Strength 4/5 with area of persistent weakness in right upper pubococcygeal muscle. Elevation of perineum with contraction and slight bulge with cough. Patient shows EMG evidence of PFM contraction maintenance during cough, thus enhancing the ability of the PFM to assist *sphincteric closure during physical stress.* Maximum EMG is 0.648 μVs, and work/rest averages are 0.371/0.103 μVs. The patient no longer loses urine with aerobic activities. She will continue exercising PFM, incorporating these contractions with her functional activities. Femina Cones were recommended for this patient, and she was to obtain them herself. There has been no further follow-up. The patient's function, strength, and urinary incontinence were greatly improved with a conservative exercise and monitoring program. The following progress with respect to the treatment goals (p 498) was met:

1. Met.
2. Met; abolished SUI.
3. Met; PFM strength increased from 1/5 to 4/5.
4. Partially met; patient achieved a work average of 0.371 μVs; the stated goal was 0.400 to 0.460 μVs. She achieved an increase in endurance to five consistent 8-second holds.

The patient's Blue Cross insurance was billed with the diagnostic code of 728.2 (muscle weakness and atrophy).

Case #4

EXAMINATION

History

RC is a 51-year-old female; gravida 2, para 2. Her referring diagnosis is mixed incontinence (stress and urge). She is referred for PFM evaluation and appropriate treatment measures.

Height:	5 feet 4 inches
Weight:	210 lb
Previous medical history:	Hypothyroid, irritable digestive tract
Previous surgical history:	Gallbladder, appendectomy, tubal ligation
Medications:	Levothyroxine sodium and Axid

The patient complains of stress incontinence and urgency. She states that she has had stress urinary incontinence symptoms for 10 years and urge for the past year. Urine loss is two to six times per week, occurring with sneeze, laugh, and urge. She can be sitting or standing. She usually dampens panties. She denies pad use. She perceives the severity of her problem on a 1 to 10 scale as 5/10. Her voiding log documents 9 to 12 voids per 24 hours, and she is wakened two to three times per night to void. She notices some fecal staining with irritable bowel syndrome. There is no previous Kegel exercise instruction and no history of Kegel exercise performance. She walks for exercise and states that she can partially slow urine flow with PFM contraction.

Physical Examination

Evaluative data: *Perineal observation* with contraction reveals elevation, and with cough reveals no movement. *Palpation* reveals muscle strength of 2/5 with a 3-second hold. Her PFM resting tension on palpation feels high. A measure of *pressure generation* with air perineometer demonstrates elevation of 12 mm of air.

EMG data: EMG maximum is 3.625 μVs, and work/rest averages are 1.169/0.232 μVs (resting tension is high). There is very little abdominal muscle activity noted: maximum of 0.250 and work/rest averages of 0.072/0.040 μVs.

Cough assessment: Patient elicits brief PFM contractions in two out of three coughs. Abdominal muscles are assessed as weak, and there is a 2-finger diastasis at the umbilicus.

ASSESSMENT/DIAGNOSIS

1. PFM functional, but patient lacks endurance to maintain five 10-second PFM contractions at consistent output.

2. Lack of sphincteric assist from PFM with physical activities and cough.
3. No coordination of PFM contractions (prophylactic contractions) with physical activities that cause leakage.
4. Excessive resting tension.
5. Decreased proprioception of PFM as evidenced by #4.
6. Frequency, urgency, and leakage.
7. Decreased muscular coordination in performing more than one concurrent activity.
8. Unrestricted transfer of intra-abdominal pressure onto pelvic floor with cough.
9. No abdominal pelvic floor muscle synergy.
10. Frequency, urgency.
11. Stress urinary incontinence.

TREATMENT GOALS

1. Increase endurance to five 10-second contractions at consistent output per EMG perineometry.
2. Demonstrate sphincteric assist with coughs, per EMG.
3. Increase PFM strength to 3 or 4/5.
4. Decrease resting tension to 0.090s or 0.125 μVs.
5. Decrease frequency/urgency.
6. Decrease stress urinary incontinence symptoms.
7. Increase coordination to allow PFM contractions with physical stress.

TREATMENT

Teach PFM exercises to increase strength and endurance. Initiate abdominal strengthening and awareness program. The patient will work on 6-second-hold PFM exercises and supine pelvic tilts for this treatment interval. She will be followed weekly at first, then biweekly and monthly.

Patient was seen a total of eight times from 3/30/92 to 9/25/92.

At the 4/10/92 visit, the perineum elevates with contraction and bulges with cough. Muscle strength is 2/5 with strength that attenuates quickly. EMG maximum is 1.812 μVs; work/rest averages are 0.436/0.108; very minimal abdominal activity is noted. No evidence of PFM contraction maintenance during cough evaluation on EMG. The patient reports a massive urine loss after coughing in a grocery store (3/30/92). She wore pads for a few days, then stopped. Re-evaluation: Strength still 2/5, with good initial recruitment of PFM contraction but rapid waning in 3 seconds. Palpation of PFM contraction during cough reveals strong downward mobility of urethra, bladder from intra-abdominal pressure pushing pelvic organs downward. Examiner's fingers almost pushed out of patient's vagina with this cough effort. *Note:* The patient had been issued a pessary to

help support pelvic organs and decrease incontinence. This was issued on patient's visit to physician prior to being seen by physical therapist. Much time was spent in patient education for abdominal muscles: supine pelvic tilts with head raises without breath holding and standing tummy tucks. She can perform both but demonstrates some abdominal bulging with pelvic tilts. She can maintain PFM contractions for no more than 3 seconds but is able to do this consistently for five repetitions.

Assessment of Electrical Stimulation: Tolerated AC current, 35 pulses per second, on 10/off 10, phase duration 200 μs, and intensity of 30 mA. Patient could co-contract PFM during this treatment. The physical therapist suggested that the patient possibly try girdle or support garment to lift abdomen and elevate it.

Plan: Follow in 1 week, patient to try 3-second PFM contractions every 30 minutes in sitting or lying position, plus tummy tucks. Initiate electrical stimulation in clinic and possibly obtain unit for home use by patient.

At the 4/17/92 visit, muscle contractions increased to 3/5 with ability to generate $^{8}/_{16}$ inches of H_2O pressure on Bourne perineometer (recently obtained). The week before, she generated $^{6}/_{16}$ inches of H_2O. Patient has been compliant with exercise program. The therapist can feel abdominal muscles tightening and more internal muscle activity. In addition to re-evaluation and PFM exercise, 30 minutes of electrical stimulation is done. She will increase PFM contraction "hold" time to 5 seconds. An electrical stimulation unit was obtained and proper patient education provided.

By 5/13/92, strength was 4/5, holding to 10 seconds with attenuation and maintaining PFM contraction during cough in the standing position. EMG data: maximum, 1.656 μVs; work/rest averages, 0.698/0.123 PFM and 0.226/0.085 abdominal muscles; pressure on Bourne perineometer $^{10}/_{16}$ inches of H_2O. There was progress in pressure generation and coordination of PFM during coughs. Electrical stimulation plus exercise prescribed two times a day. Three more visits ensued, 6/12/92, 7/17/92, and 9/25/92.

TREATMENT OUTCOMES

Final PFM strength was 4/5 with 10-second holds, elevation of perineum with contraction, and no movement with cough. Strong contractions elicited with palpable 7-second "hold." The patient maintained an endurance contraction for about 60 seconds. (PFM contraction of about 25% of maximum for a prolonged time period.) Severity of incontinence now 1/10. The patient reports no leaks, is maintaining $^{10}/_{16}$ inch H_2O pressure generation on Bourne perineometer. She is satisfied with her urinary control. She has been using electrical stimulation since 5/1/92 (4 months) and will continue use. She is satisfied with her progress and feels that she can continue on her own. She also enrolled in a medical weight loss program and had lost 35 lb by the time she finished her physical therapy program.

TREATMENT GOALS MET

1. Endurance: patient can hold five consistent contractions for 10 seconds each.
2. PFM with cough: there is PFM contraction before, during, and after a cough on EMG perineometry.
3. Increased PFM strength: patient achieves 4/5 with strong 7-second hold before waning of contraction.
4. Resting tension: decreased on electromyogram. Initially 0.232 μVs, on last evaluation 0.082 μVs.

5. Subjective decrease in frequency/urgency symptoms.
6. Stress urinary incontinence symptoms abolished.

Note: Electrical stimulation was used with this patient to foster awareness of PFM function, *ie*, to increase the intensity of the feeling of contracting and relaxing the PFM to help increase strength of PFM as an adjunct to her exercise program.

The diagnostic code was 728.2 (muscle weakness and atrophy). Treatment documentation was provided with billing claims.

Patients with PFM weakness who are well-motivated will show improvement in one or more areas of their presenting problems in 4 to 6 months. To expect results before this time is unrealistic.

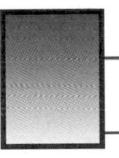

Clinical Decision-Making Cases: Interstitial Cystitis[79]

Case #1

EXAMINATION

History

YIC is a 37-year-old white female with a confirmed diagnosis of interstitial cystitis. She reports a 5- to 6-year history of urinary frequency and urgency and a 2-year history of continuous abdominal pain. Treatments have included bladder distentions, bladder instillations with silver nitrate and chlorpactin, acetaminophen with codeine, oxybutynin chloride, and propoxphene hydrochloride compound.

Chief complaint: The patient complains of frequency, urgency, and abdominal pain, which worsens approximately 1 hour after initiating physical activity. At the times of most severe pain, she needs to void up to seven times an hour and has radicular pain to her back and anterior proximal thighs.

Social history: The patient is married with three children. She cleans houses for a living but has had to reduce her workload because the activity causes an exacerbation of her symptoms. She has dropped her part-time college studies because urinary frequency prevents her from attending classes.

Physical Examination

Examination reveals an old abdominal scar from a hysterectomy. The area on either side of the scar is slightly less sensitive to touch and pinprick than the surrounding tissue. Palpation of the lower abdomen does not increase her pain. There are no other remarkable findings.

TREATMENT GOALS

1. Decrease frequency and urgency of voiding.
2. Decrease abdominal pain.

TREATMENT (TENS)

Electrode Placement

The electrodes were placed suprapubically on either side of midline, 10 to 15 cm apart. To address the patient's complaint of radicular pain to her back, the authors elected to place the other pair of electrodes at the T-10 level paraspinally.

Parameters

Stimulation was given at 50 Hz, 200 μs, with the intensity to maximum tolerance (20 to 30 mA) for 2 hours twice a day.

TREATMENT OUTCOMES

Two Weeks

The patient reported a decrease in urinary frequency, decrease in pain, ability to be active for approximately 5 hours before the onset of severe pain, and a reduction in the amount of pain medication by half. The patient had increased her wearing time from 2 hours twice a day to most of the day in order to maintain pain control.

Two Months

Because of the abdominal placement of the electrodes and the 24-hour wearing time, the patient needed to experiment with a variety of electrodes. She opted to use a combination of disposable and reusable, low-profile, low-adherence electrodes.

One Year

The patient reported using the TENS unit up to 24 hours a day for 3 days and then going without it for 1 day and still maintaining pain control. The TENS unit reduces her pain by approximately one half. She states that she has decreased her pain medication proportionately and has not had a bladder instillation in 1 year.

The patient reports an improvement in her lifestyle. Her urinary frequency has been reduced to once an hour or longer during the daytime, allowing her to resume her college studies and participate in normal daily outings. Nocturia occurs one to two times a night, enabling her to get more rest, which, she states, has improved her ability to cope with the continuing problems of interstitial cystitis.

Case #2

EXAMINATION

History

MA is a 36-year-old white female with a confirmed diagnosis of interstitial cystitis. She has had symptoms of frequency, urgency, bladder spasms, and intermittent pain for 2 years. Treatments have induced bladder distentions and bladder instillations with dimethyl sulfoxide and chlorpactin. Oxybutynin chloride is her only oral medication.

Chief complaint: The patient complained of urinary frequency (three to four times an hour during the day and two to three times during the night) with intermittent pain. She reports a higher degree of pain in the evening and when fatigued. The patient describes a continual feeling of "bladder irritability" resulting in spasms when she does not empty her bladder immediately. During her menses, the pain radiates to her back and legs.

Social history: The patient is single with one child. She works as a local administrator for a national organization. The patient does not perceive that her symptoms affect her work.

Physical Examination

There are significant physical findings. The patient has no abdominal tenderness on palpation. Sensation is intact. There are no abdominal scars or lesions.

TREATMENT (TENS)

Electrode Placement

The electrodes were placed suprapubically on either side of midline, 10 to 15 cm apart. To address the patient's complaint of radicular pain to her back, an additional pair of electrodes were placed at the T-10 level paraspinally.

Parameters

Stimulation was given at 50 Hz, 200 μs, with the intensity to maximum tolerance (15 mA) for 2 hours twice a day.

TREATMENT OUTCOMES

Two weeks

The patient stated that she was still using the unit for 2 hours twice a day. She reported some relief of symptoms but noted sacroiliac joint discomfort when using the TENS unit posteriorly. Because the patient was having only occasional radicular pain to her back, the option of discontinuing the posterior electrodes was offered. The patient felt that she might still want the option of using both electrode placements, so changes in the parameters were made. The new settings were: rate, 85 Hz; width, 75 μs; amplitude, to sensory level. After several days of using the new settings, the patient reported a decrease in pain and urinary frequency without sacroiliac symptoms.

One Year

The patient says that she is using the TENS unit for 1 to 4 hours in the morning and approximately 1 hour in the evening. If she is not having discomfort, she does not use the unit. She reports that the TENS unit relieves her pain and bladder irritability and has reduced her medication by 90%; she says there are days when she forgets she has interstitial cystitis. Frequency has been reduced to once an hour, and she sleeps through the night.

See Appendix C for more information on the genitourinary system.

References

1. Lausman HH, Robertson EG: Evolution of the pelvic floor. In Benson TJ (ed): *Female Pelvic Floor Disorders: Investigation and Management*. New York, W. W. Norton, 1992, pp. 13–18.

2. DeLancey JO, Richardson AC: Anatomy of genital support. In Benson TJ (ed): *Female Pelvic Floor Disorders: Investigation and Management*. New York, W. W. Norton, 1992, pp. 19–26.

3. DeLancey JO: Anatomy and embryology of the lower urinary tract. *Obstet Gynecol Clin North Am*, 1989, 16:18–32.

4. DeLancey JO: Functional anatomy of the female lower urinary tract and pelvic floor. *Ciba Foundation Symp*, 1990, 151:57–69.

5. DeLancey JO, Starr RA: Histology of the connection between the vagina and the levator ani muscles. *J Reprod Med*, 1988, 35:765–771.

6. Borenstein R, Elcholal U, Goldschmit R, et al.: The importance of the endopelvic fascia repair during vaginal hysterectomy. *Surg Gynecol Obstet*, 1992, 175:551–554.

7. Mattingly RF, Davis LE: Primary treatment of anatomic stress urinary incontinence. *Clin Obstet Gynecol*, 1984, 27:445–457.

8. Stanton SL: Anatomy and physiology. In *Female Urinary Incontinence*. London, Lloyd-Luke, 1977, pp 1–14.

9. Gosling JA: The structure of the bladder and urethra in relation to function. *Urol Clin North Am*, 1979, 6:31–38.

10. Bissada NK, Finkbeiner AE, Welch CT: Lower urinary tract pharmacology. *Urology*, 1977, 9:107–118.

11. Asmussen M, Miller A: Applied anatomy. In *Clinical Gynaecological Urology*. Oxford, Blackwell Scientific Publications, 1992, pp 7–19.

12. Bhatia NN: *Neurophysiology of micturition*. In Ostergard DR, Bent AE (eds): *Urogynecology and Urodynamics*, 3rd ed. Baltimore, Williams & Wilkins, 1991, pp 31–54.

13. Mahony DT, Laferte RO, Blais DJ, et al.: Integral storage and voiding reflexes. *Urology*, 1977, 9:95–106.

14. Frahm J: *Verimed Pelvic Floor Protocol*. Ft. Lauderdale, Verimed, 1993.

15. Bump R, Sugerman HL, Fantl JH, et al.: Obesity and lower urinary tract functions in women: effect of surgically induced weight loss. *Am J Obstet Gynecol*, 1992, 167:392–399.

16. *Urinary Incontinence in Adults: Clinical Practice Guideline*. Agency for Health Care Policy and Research publication 92-0038. Rockville, MD, AHCPR, US Public Health Service, 1992.

17. Snooks SJ, Badenoch RC, Tiptaft RC, Swash M: Perineal nerve damage in genuine stress urinary incontinence: an electrophysiological study. *Br J Urol*, 1985, 57:422–426.

18. Diokno AC: Practical approach to the management of urinary incontinence in the elderly. *Compr Ther*, 1983, 9:67–75.

19. Sampselle CM, DeLancey JO: The urine stream interruption test and pelvic muscle function. *Nurs Res*, 1992, 41:73–77.

20. International Continence Society: Quantification of urine loss. In *Fifth Report on the Standardization of Terminology*. Aachen, West Germany, ICS, 1983.

21. Sutherst JR, Brown MC, Richmond D: Analysis of the pattern of urine loss in women with incontinence as measured by weighing perineal pads. *Br J Urol*, 1986, 58:273–278.

22. Harrison SM: Stress incontinence and the physical therapist. *Physiotherapy*, 1983, 69:144–147.

23. Laycock J: Unpublished data, International Incontinence Seminar, Northside Hospital, Atlanta, GA, 1992.

24. McCormick KA, Burgio KL: Incontinence: an update on nursing care measures. *J Gerontol Nurs*, 1984, 10:16–19, 22–23.

25. Keating JC, Schulte EA, Miller E, et al.: Conservative care of urinary incontinence in the elderly. *J Manipulative Physiol Ther*, 1988, 11:300–308.

26. Fantl JA, Wyman JF, McLish D, et al: Efficacy of bladder training in older women with urinary incontinence. JAMA. 1991, 265(5):609–613.

27. Burgio KL, Whitehead WE, Engel BT: Urinary incontinence in the elderly: bladder-sphincter biofeedback and toileting skills training. *Ann Intern Med*, 1985, 103:507–515.

28. Burton JR, Pearce KL, Burgio KL, et al. Behavioral training for urinary incontinence in elderly ambulatory patients. *J Am Geriatr Soc*, 1988, 36:693–698.

29. Rose MA, Baigis-Smith J, Smith D, et al.: Behavioral management of urinary incontinence in homebound older adults. *Home Healthcare Nurs*, 1990, 8:10–15.

30. Schnelle JF, Newman DR, Fogarty TE, et al.: Management of patient continence in long term care nursing facilities. *Gerontol Soc Am*, 1990, 30:373–376.

31. Dougherty MC, Abrams R, McKey PL, et al.: An instrument to assess the dynamic characteristics of the circumvaginal musculature. *Nurs Res*, 1986, 35:202–206.

32. Benvenute F, Caputo GM, Bandinelli S, et al.: Reeducative treatment of female genuine stress incontinence. *Am J Phys Med*, 1987, 66:155–168.

33. Burns PA, Marecki MA, Dittmar SS, et al.: Kegel's exercises with biofeedback therapy for treatment of stress incontinence. *Nurse Pract*, 1985, Feb:28–34.

34. Kegel A: The physiologic treatment of poor tone and function of the genital muscles and of urinary stress incontinence. *Western J Surg* 1949, Nov:527–535.

35. Kegel A: Physiologic therapy for urinary stress incontinence. *JAMA*, 1950, 10:915–917.

36. Kegel A: The physiologic treatment of urinary stress incontinence. *J Urol*, 1950, 63:808–813.

37. Kegel AH: Progressive resistance exercise in the functional restoration of the perineal muscles. *Am J Obstet Gynecol*, 1948, 56:238–248.

38. Laycock J: Graded exercises for the pelvic floor muscles in the treatment of urinary incontinence. *Physiotherapy*, 1987, 73:371–377.

39. Shepherd AM: Reeducation of the muscles of the pelvic floor. In Mandelstrom D (ed): *Incontinence and Its Management*. London, Croom Helm, 1980, pp 184–195.

40. Newman DK, Smith DA: Pelvic muscle re-education as a nursing treatment for incontinence. *Urol Nurs*, 1992, 12:9–15.

41. Olah KS, Bridges N, Denning J, et al.: The conservative management of patients with symptoms of stress incontinence: a randomized, prospective study comparing weighted vaginal cones and interferential therapy. *Am J Obstet Gynecol*, 1990, 162:87–92.

42. Peattie AB, Plevnik S, Stanton SL, et al.: Vaginal cones: a conservative method of treating genuine stress incontinence. *Br J Obstet Gynaecol*, 1988, 95:1049–1053.

43. Moore D, Metcalf J: Effectiveness of vaginal cones in treatment of urinary incontinence. *Urol Nurs*, 1992, 12:69–72.

44. Peattie AB, Plevnik S: Cones versus physiotherapy as conservative management of genuine stress incontinence. *Proc Int Continence Soc*, 1988, 7.

45. Middaugh SJ, Whitehead WE, Burgio KL, et al.: Biofeedback in treatment of urinary incontinence in stroke patients. *Biofeedback Self Regul*, 1986, 15:3–19.

46. Burgio KL, Engel BT: Biofeedback assisted behavioral training for elderly men and women. *J Am Geriatr Soc*, 1990, 38:338–340.

47. Tries J: Kegel exercises enhanced by biofeedback. *J Enterostomal Ther*, 1990, 17:67–76.

48. Susset JG, Gulea G, Read L, *et al.:* Biofeedback therapy for female incontinence due to low urethral resistance. *J Urol,* 1990, 143:1205–1208.

49. Burton JR, Pearce L, Burgio KL, *et al.:* Behavioral training for urinary incontinence in elderly ambulatory patients. *J Am Geriatr Soc,* 1988, 86:693–697.

50. Fall M, Lindstrom S: Electrical stimulation: a physiologic approach to the treatment of urinary incontinence. *Urol Clin North Am,* 1991, 18:393–407.

51. Sotiropoulos A, Yeaw S, Luttimer JK, *et al.:* Management of urinary incontinence with electronic stimulation: observations and results. *J Urol,* 1976, 116:749.

52. Erikson BC, Bergman S, Elk-Nes SH, *et al.:* Maximal electrostimulation of the pelvic floor in female idiopathic detrusor instability and urge incontinence. *Neurol Urodyn,* 1989, 8:219–230.

53. Laycock J, Green GR: Interferential therapy in the treatment of incontinence. *Physiotherapy,* 1988, 74:161–168.

54. Castleden CM, Duffin HM, Asher MJ, *et al.:* Factors influencing outcome in elderly patients with urinary incontinence and detrusor instability. *Age Ageing,* 1985, 14:303–307.

55. Fall M: Electrical pelvic floor stimulation for the control of detrusor instability. *Neurol Urodyn,* 1985, 4:329–335.

56. Salvati EP: The levator syndrome and its variant. *Anorectal Disorders,* 1987, 16:71–77.

57. Erikson BC, Bergmann S, Mjolnerod OK, *et al.:* Effect of anal electrostimulation with 'Incontan' device in women with urinary incontinence. *Br J Obstet Gynaecol,* 1987, 92:147–156.

58. Lindstrom S, Fall M, Carlsson CA, *et al.:* The neurophysiological basis of bladder inhibition in response to intravaginal electrical stimulation. *J Urol,* 1983, 129:405–410.

59. Tanagho EA: Electrical stimulation. *J Am Geriatr Soc,* 1990, 38:352–355.

60. Vodusek DB, Plevnik S, Urtacnik P, *et al.:* Detrusor inhibition on selective pudendal nerve stimulation in the perineum. *Neurol Urodyn,* 1988, 6:389–393.

61. Salmons S, Vrbova G: The influence of activity on some contractile characteristics of mammalian fast and slow muscle. *J Physiol,* 1969, 201:535–549.

62. Erikson BC, Mjolnerod OK: Changes in urodynamic measurement after successful anal electrostimulation in female urinary incontinence. *Br J Urol,* 1987, 59:45–49.

63. Dougall DS: The effects of interferential therapy on incontinence and frequency of micturition. *Physiotherapy,* 1985, 71:135–136.

64. Mantle J, Versi E: Physiotherapy for stress urinary incontinence: a national survey. *Br Med J,* 1991, 302:753–755.

65. Parsons CL, Koprowski PF: Interstitital cystitis: successful management by increasing urinary voiding intervals. *Urology,* 1991, 37:207–212.

66. Lundeberg T, Bondesson L, Lundshom V, *et al.:* Relief of primary dysmenorrhea by transcutaneous electrical nerve stimulation. *Acta Obstet Gynecol Scand,* 1985, 64:491–497.

67. Gersh MR: Transcutaneous electrical nerve stimulation (TENS) for management of pain and sensory pathology. In Gersh M (ed): *Electrotherapy in Rehabilitation.* Philadelphia, F. A. Davis Company, pp 149–193.

68. Mannheimer JS, Whalen EC: The efficacy of transcutaneous electrical nerve stimulation in dysmenorrhea. *Clin J Pain,* 1985, 1:75–83.

69. Nikolova L: Gynecological diseases. In Nikolova L (ed): *Treatment with Interferential Current.* Edinburgh, Churchill Livingstone, 1987, pp 42–51.

70. Kahn J: *Electrotherapeutics.* New York, Churchill Livingstone, 1991, pp 18, 156–157.

71. Foster DC, Robinson JC, Davis KM: Urethral pressure variation in women with valvar vestibulitis syndrome. *Am J Obstet Gynecol* 1993, 169:107–112.

72. Kahn J: Use of iontophoresis in Peyronie's disease. *Phys Ther,* 1982, 62:995–996.

73. Sinaki M, Merritt JL, Stilwell GK, *et al.:* Tension myalgia of the pelvic floor. *Mayo Clin Proc,* 1977, 52:717–722.

74. Oliver GC, Rubin RJ, Salvati ED, *et al.:* Electrogalvanic stimulation in the treatment of levator syndrome. *Dis Colon Rectum,* 1985, 28:662–663.

75. Nicosia JF, Abcarian H: Levator syndrome: a treatment that works. *Dis Colon Rectum,* 1985, 28:406–408.

76. Morris L, Newton RA: Use of high voltage pulsed galvanic stimulation for patients with levator ani syndrome. *Phys Ther,* 1987, 67:1522–1525.

77. Thiele GH: Coccygodynia: cause and treatment. *Dis Colon Rectum,* 1963, 6:422–477.

78. Sohn N, Weinstein MA, Robbins RD, *et al.:* The levator syndrome and its treatment with high voltage electrogalvanic stimulation. *Am J Surg,* 1982, 144:580–582.

79. Ouelette C, Brown NN: Interstitial cystitis case studies. Presented at the American Physical Therapy Association/ Combined Sections Meeting, 1993.

Suggested Reading

Kuo HC, Chang SC, Hsa T, *et al.:* Urodynamic findings in interstitial cystitis. *J Formosan Med Assoc,* 1992, 91:694–698.

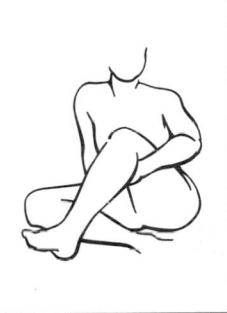

CHAPTER 23

Obstetrical Considerations

Cheryl Appel

In addition to maintaining continence, the genitourinary system of a woman plays a dramatic role in response to the considerable demands of pregnancy, childbirth, and recovery. When examining and treating women with genitourinary dysfunction, pregnancy is a condition that may either contribute to or coexist with presenting problems. Significant anatomical and physiological changes occur during pregnancy and in the immediate postpartum period. These changes are essential to accommodate the growing fetus, but they can result in stresses that the body does not otherwise experience. In this chapter, these anatomical and physiological changes are discussed, as well as conditions and complications affecting the genitourinary system during pregnancy and the postpartum period. Examination, diagnosis, evaluation, and treatment of the woman during this time, as well as essential modifications in deference to the changes her body is experiencing, are described.

I. Anatomical and Physiological Changes During Pregnancy

A. Reproductive organs[1-3]

1. **Uterus.** The muscular organ holding the fetus during pregnancy, providing nourishment to the fetus through the placenta. It is divided into the body (corpus and fundus) and the cervix (see Figure 23–1).
   a. During pregnancy, the uterus increases in weight from 60 to 1000 g. In size, it changes from 6.5 to 32 cm. In a nonpregnant state, the uterus is situated in the pelvic cavity. During pregnancy, it expands into the abdominal cavity. In addition to the growing fetus, uterine expansion is caused by an increase in connective tissue and in the size and number of blood vessels supplying the uterus (see Figure 23–2).
   b. *Ligamentous supports* (see Figure 23–3)[1-3]
      (1). Round ligaments are fibrous cords attaching to the uterus and the labia majora. During pregnancy, they become elongated and hypertrophied. They support the uterus in its move from the pelvic cavity into the abdominal cavity.
      (2). Broad ligaments are large folds of peritoneum separating the pelvis into anterior and posterior divisions. The lower portion of the ligament is known as the cardinal ligament; it

505

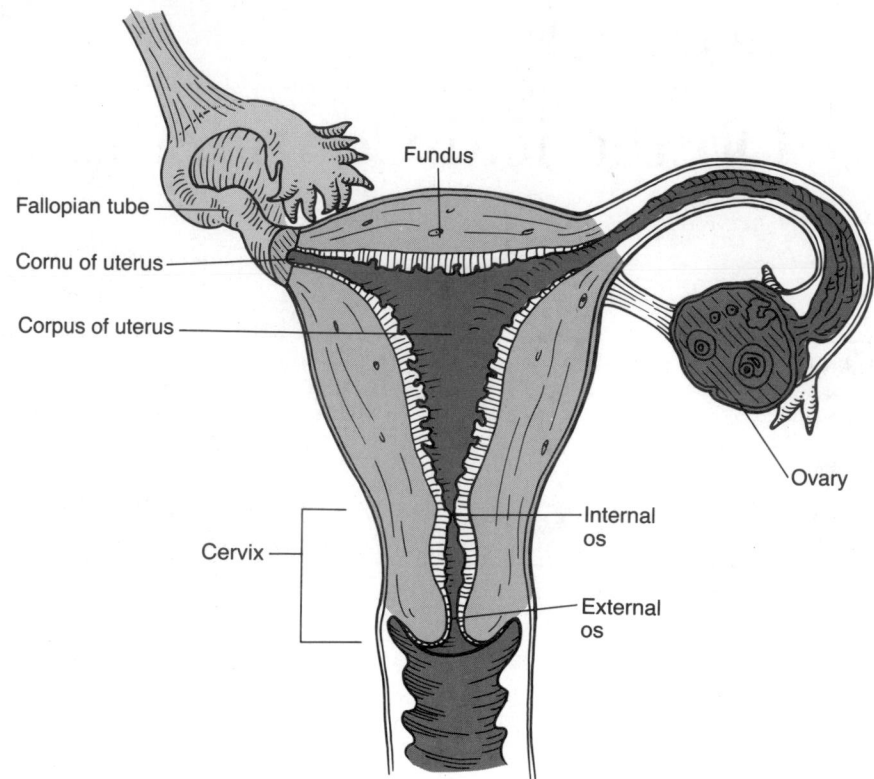

FIGURE 23–1   The female reproductive organs.

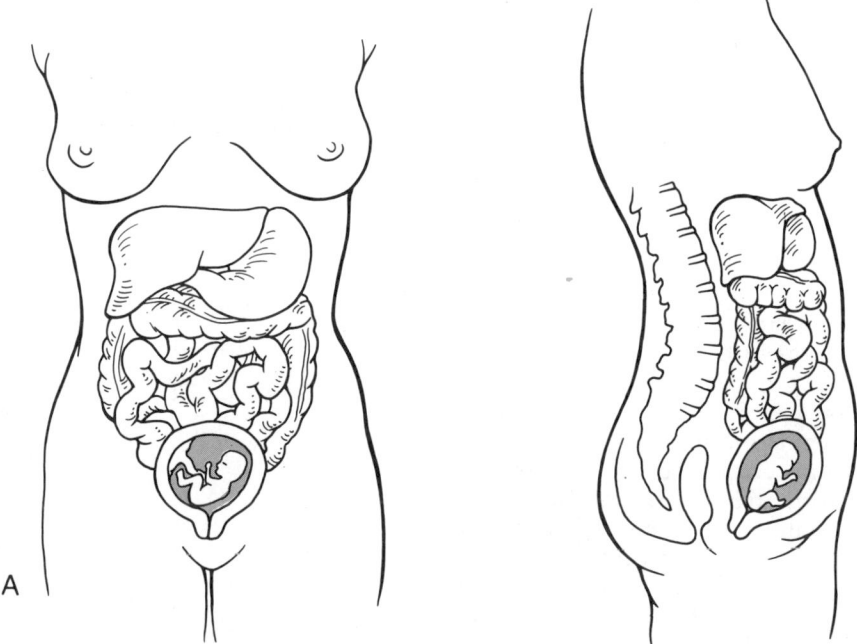

FIGURE 23–2   Changes in the size and position of the uterus during pregnancy.

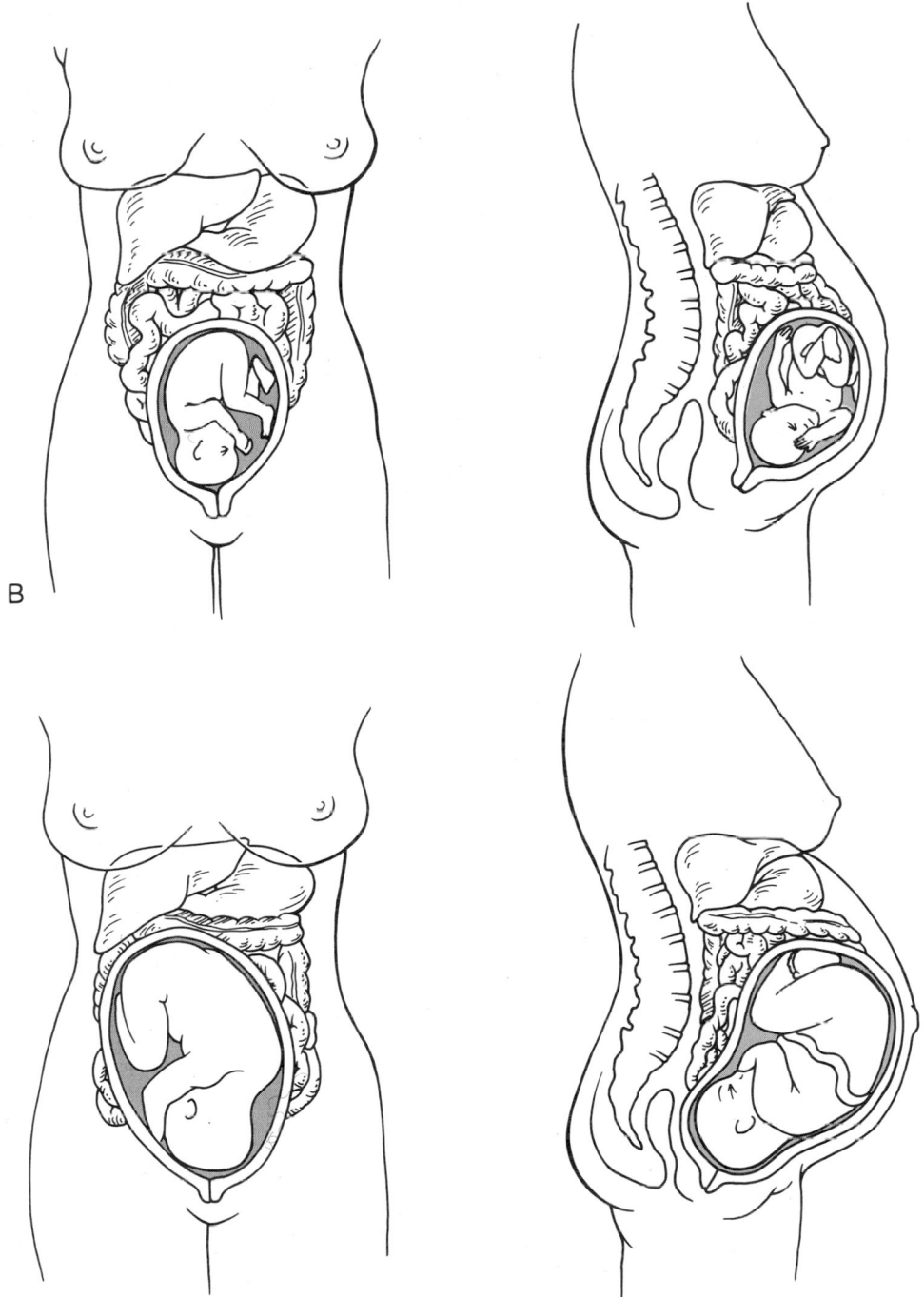

B

C

FIGURE 23–2   *(continued)*

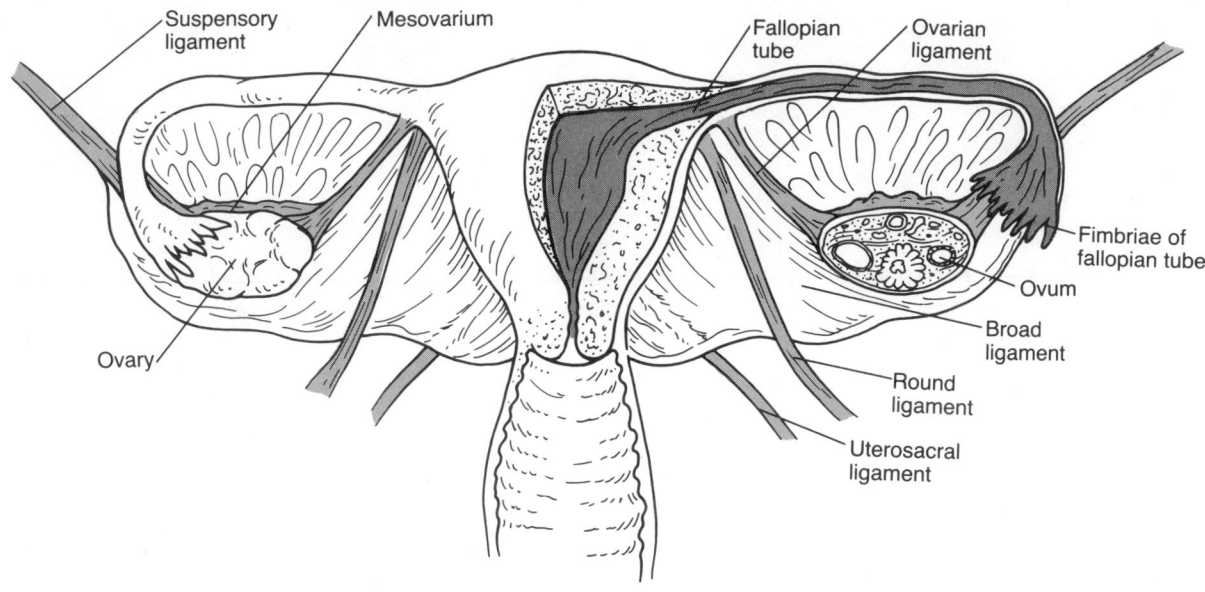

FIGURE 23–3 Ligamentous support of the uterus.

attaches the lateral aspect of the uterus to the supravaginal area of the cervix (see Figure 23–4).

(3). Uterosacral ligaments attach the sacrum to the posterior aspect of the cervix to support the cervix.

c. *Fascial and muscular supports*

(1). Other structures within the pelvic floor provide a sling to support the pelvic contents inferiorly. They are described in Chapter 22 (see Figure 23–5).

d. *Innervation*[2–4]

(1). The pudendal nerve stems from S2–4. A portion of this nerve forms the perineal nerve and innervates the lower 2.5 cm of the vagina.

(2). The uterine nerve stems from T10–12 (see Figure 23–6).

e. *Cervix.*[1,3,5] The portion of the uterus connecting the body of the uterus and the vagina (see Figure 23–7).

(1). The internal os joins the body of the uterus with the cervix.

(2). The external os opens into the vagina.

(3). During pregnancy, the cervix is closed. A mucus plug forms over the cervix, providing a protective barrier between the vagina and the uterine contents.

(4). During labor and delivery, the cervix shortens (or effaces) and widens (or dilates), effectively disappearing. A

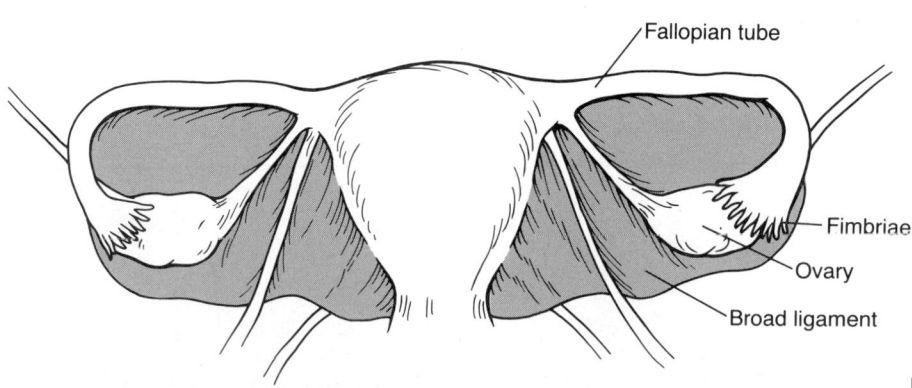

FIGURE 23–4 The broad ligament.

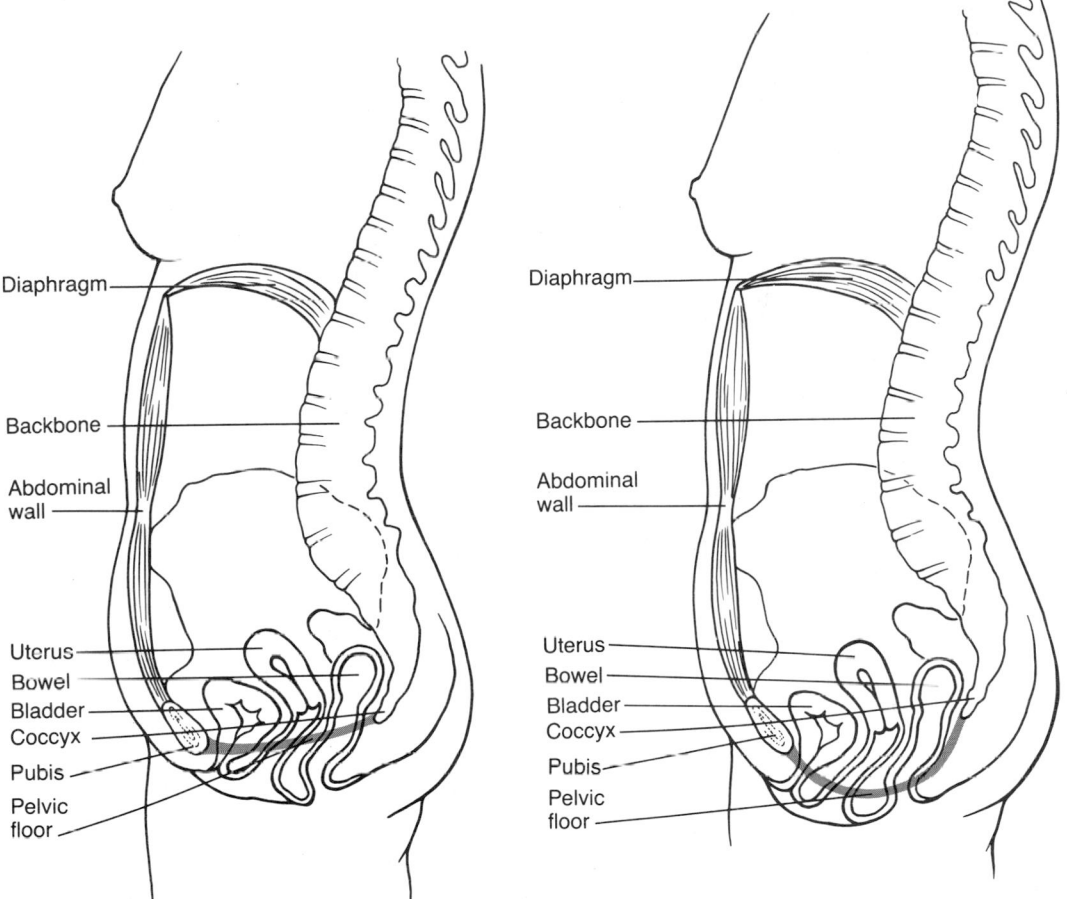

FIGURE 23-5   The pelvic floor supports the contents of the pelvis. **A,** Good pelvic floor support with a firm base and the organs in place. **B,** Inadequate support with the hammock sagging and the contents descending.

10-cm opening is left between the uterus and the vagina to allow for passage of the fetus into the birth canal (see Figure 23–8).

(5). If the cervix begins dilating prematurely, it is sometimes stitched together during the second trimester, until the fetus is mature. This procedure is known as a cerclage.

2. **Ovaries.**[1,3] The organs storing ova, or egg cells, in a primitive form. Through hormonal influence, one ovum is developed per month. It then travels into the fallopian tube and has the potential to be fertilized.
   a. One ovary is located on either side of the uterus, encased in the posterior aspect of the broad ligament.
   b. Ligamentous support is provided by the ovarian, mesovarium, and suspensory ligaments (see Figure 23–3).

3. **Fallopian tubes.**[1,2] The ducts bringing mature ova from the ovaries to the uterus via peristaltic action (see Figure 23–3).
   a. The fallopian tubes connect the uterine cavity to the abdominal cavity, near to the ovary. The opening at the abdominal site is lined with cilia to promote the peristalsis necessary to convey the ovum into the tube.
   b. They are situated in the superior margin of the broad ligament.

4. **Vagina.**[2] The connecting passage between the uterus and the perineum, serving as the birth canal.
   a. The anterior borders include the bladder and the urethra (see Figure 23–9).
   b. Laterally, the ureters and broad and round ligaments lie.
   c. Posteriorly, the peritoneum and the rectovaginal fascia surround the vagina.

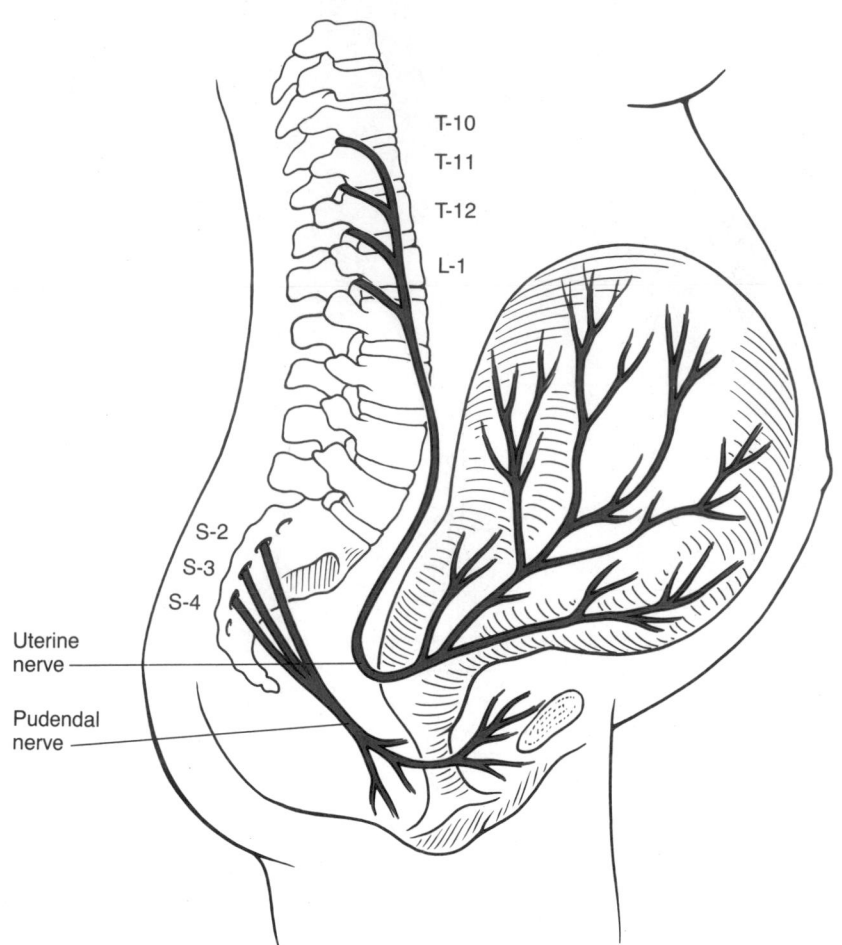

T-10

T-11

T-12

L-1

S-2
S-3
S-4

Uterine nerve

Pudendal nerve

FIGURE 23–6 The uterine and pudendal nerves.

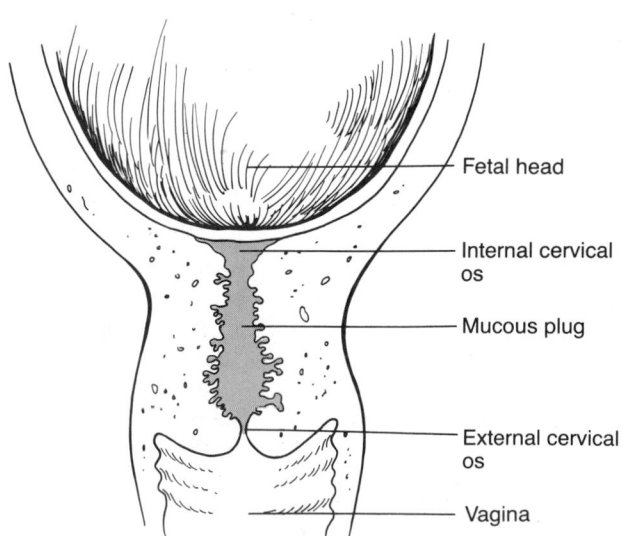

Fetal head

Internal cervical os

Mucous plug

External cervical os

Vagina

FIGURE 23–7 The cervix of a pregnant woman.

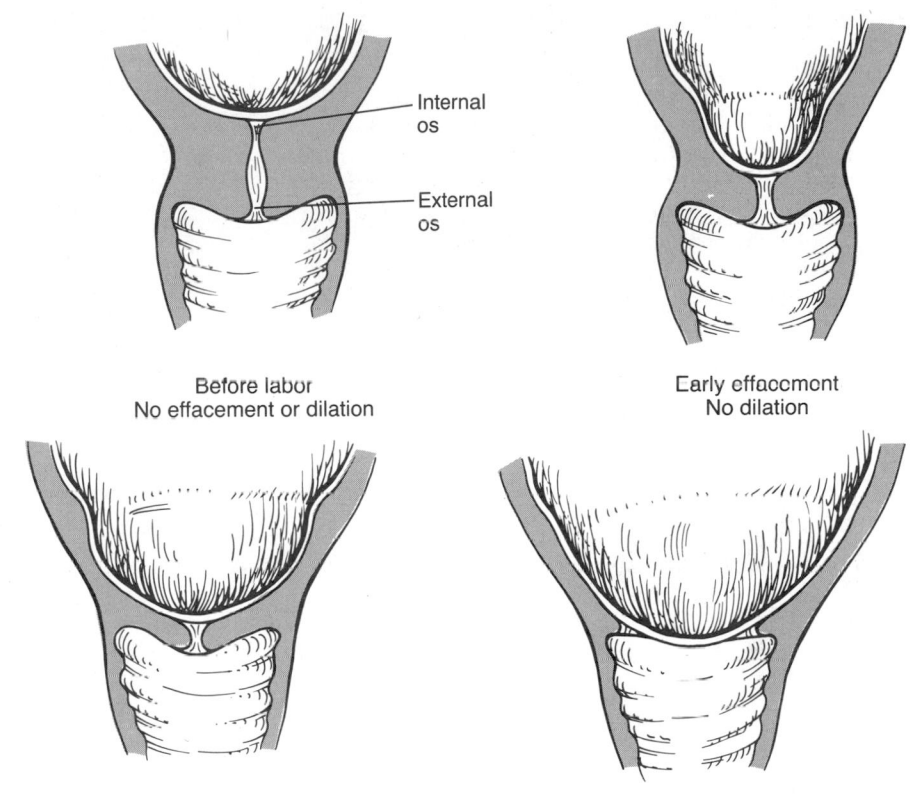

Internal
os

External
os

Before labor
No effacement or dilation

Early effacement
No dilation

Complete effacement
No dilation

Complete dilation

FIGURE 23–8   Dilation and effacement of the cervix.

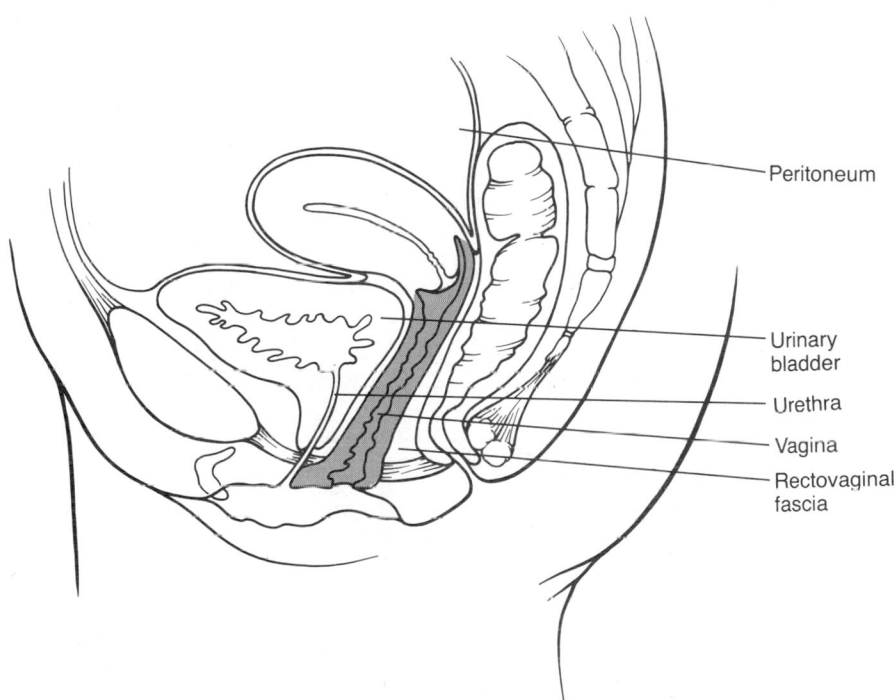

Peritoneum

Urinary
bladder

Urethra

Vagina

Rectovaginal
fascia

FIGURE 23–9   The vagina and surrounding structures.

B. Renal system[1,3,6]

1. Kidneys, bladder, and ureters expand their function and capacity in response to the demands of pregnancy (see Figure 23–10).
2. Increased urination, or polyuria, is common, occurring in 80% to 95% of pregnant women. Frequency and overall volume are both increased. This phenomenon, which primarily occurs at night, is attributed to both physiological demands and mechanical pressures.
   a. The kidney expands because of dilation of the renal pelvis and increased interstitial fluid. Additionally, glomerular filtration rate increases by 50%.
   b. Bladder compression occurs with ureter obstruction because of uterine enlargement.
3. Stress incontinence occurs in 38.5% to 85% of all pregnant women. It often increases in severity as the pregnancy progresses and drops to 5% to 14% during the postpartum period.
4. Urge incontinence is also more prevalent during pregnancy.
5. Urinary retention is common among postpartal women.
   a. A majority of women exhibit a reduction in bladder sensation and tone during the postpartum period. The result is an increase in bladder capacity from distention. Bladder distention can eventually result in atony of the muscles of the bladder. Urinary retention can result.
   b. Women who have delivered vaginally, without use of forceps, have a 9% to 14% incidence of voiding difficulties secondary to retention. With forceps delivery, the incidence rises to 38%.
6. Pregnancy increases the chance that asymptomatic bacteriuria will lead to pyelonephritis. This is associated with preterm labor and perhaps pregnancy-induced hypertension and low birth weight.

C. Cardiovascular system[1,3,5,7]

1. Heart rate increases during pregnancy, reaching a peak of 10 to 15 beats/min over nonpregnant values.
2. Blood volume increases 40% above nonpregnant values.
3. Cardiac output increases up to 30% to 50%, peaking at 28 to 32 weeks of pregnancy.

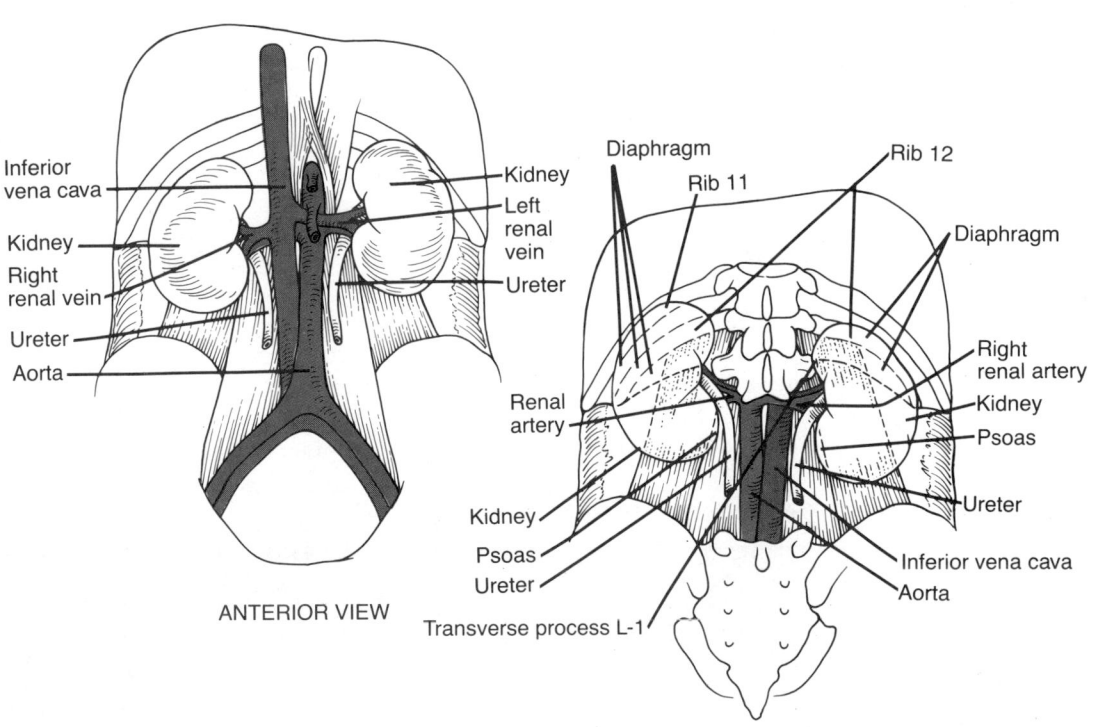

FIGURE 23–10   The renal system.

Table 23–1. HEMODYNAMIC PARAMETERS THROUGHOUT PREGNANCY

Parameter	Patient Position	First Trimester	Second Trimester	Third Trimester	Post Partum
Heart rate	L	77 ± 2	85 ± 2	88 ± 2	69 ± 2
(beats/min)	S	76 ± 2	84 ± 2	92 ± 2	70 ± 2
Stroke volume	L	75 ± 2	86 ± 4	97 ± 5	79 ± 3
(mL/min)	S	82 ± 5	85 ± 4	87 ± 5	79 ± 3
Cardiac output	L	3.53 ± 0.21	4.32 ± 0.22	4.85 ± 0.27	3.30 ± 0.17
L/min/m²	S	3.76 ± 0.24	4.19 ± 0.21	4.54 + 0.28	3.33 ± 0.21
Left ventricular ejection time	L	302 ± 2	290 ± 5	281 ± 4	310 ± 5
(ms)	S	301 ± 3	286 ± 4	260 ± 4	307 ± 5
Systolic blood pressure	L	98 ± 2	91 ± 2	95 ± 2	97 ± 2
(mm Hg)	S	106 ± 2	102 ± 2	106 ± 2	110 ± 2
Diastolic blood pressure	L	53 ± 2	49 ± 2	50 ± 2	57 ± 2
(mm Hg)	S	57 ± 2	60 ± 1	65 ± 2	65 ± 1

(From Key TC, Resnik R: In Danforth DN, Scott JR (eds): *Maternal Changes in Pregnancy in Obstetrics and Gynecology,* 5th ed. Philadelphia, J.B. Lippincott Company, 1986; adapted from Katz R, Karliner JS, Resnik R: Effects of natural volume overload state (pregnancy) on left ventricular performance in human subjects. *Circulation* 1978, 58:434, by permission of the American Heart Association, Inc.)
Abbreviations: L = lateral; S = supine

4. Arterial blood pressure decreases toward the end of the first trimester because of the reduction in systemic vascular resistance, or reduced resistance in peripheral vascular tone. It is lowest in the second trimester but remains low until the postpartum period (see Table 23–1).
   a. Maternal position has an effect on blood pressure, particularly if the uterus compresses the inferior vena cava. This occurs most often when the woman is lying supine and disappears in the left sidelying position.
      (1). This problem is known as supine hypotension or "vena cava syndrome." Profound supine hypotension affects 3% to 11% of pregnant women.
      (2). In affected women, the hemodynamic effects of vena caval occlusion are decreased venous return, decreased central venous pressure, and decreased left ventricular output. Cardiac output is reduced by 25%. Compensatory vasoconstriction typically occurs, resulting in no changes in pulse or blood pressure in most women.
      (3). Symptoms of supine hypotension include dizziness and lightheadedness. Some believe the problem can occur without obvious symptoms, however.
5. Many women have cardiac murmurs during pregnancy, particularly systolic. This is because of the increased cardiac output and the decreased viscosity of blood.
6. Mitral valve prolapse is the most common cardiac problem of pregnant women. However, complications are rare. The use of certain medications, such as prophylactic antibiotics or β-blockers, in this population remains controversial.

D. Respiratory system[3,6]

1. During pregnancy, the body is in a state of hyperventilation and respiratory alkalosis.
   a. Breathing becomes more costal than abdominal. Additionally, most women are mouth breathers during pregnancy.
   b. Anatomically, the diaphragm is progressively elevated, possibly because of expansion and elevation of the rib cage. Uterine pressure during the first and second trimesters does not appear to be a factor in this phenomenon (see Figure 23–11).
   c. Dyspnea is common, occurring in 60% to 70% of pregnant women, but is unrelated to elevation of the diaphragm. It has been hypothesized that the dyspnea is caused by either an inappropriate ventilatory response or a change in proprioceptive information transmitted to the brain. For example, a pregnant woman may feel the sensation of full inspiration or expiration at a different volume.
   d. Respiratory rate is unchanged from prepregnancy levels. However, oxygen consumption increases by 14% to 20%.
   e. Respiratory tidal volume increases during normal respiration by 200 mL, resulting in deeper breathing.

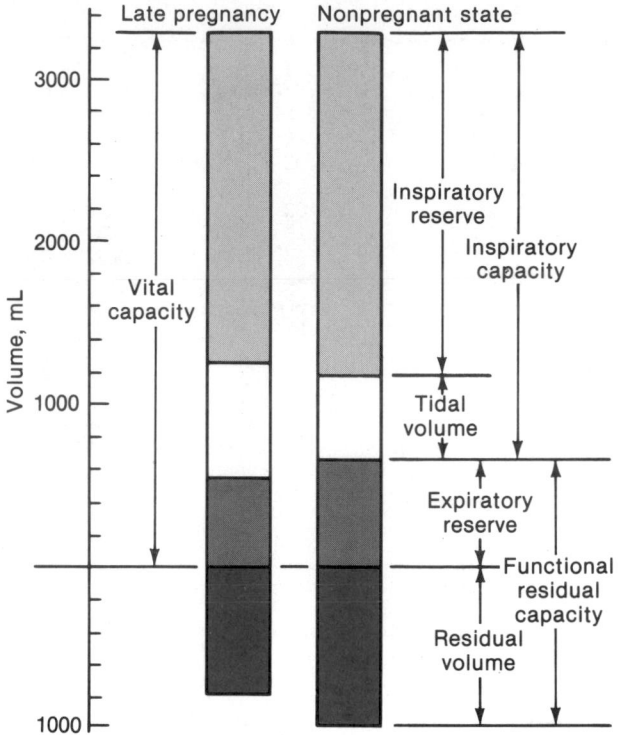

FIGURE 23–11   Respiratory parameters during pregnancy. (Redrawn from Hytten FE, Leitch I: *The Physiology of Human Pregnancy.* Oxford, Blackwell Scientific Publishers, 1964.)

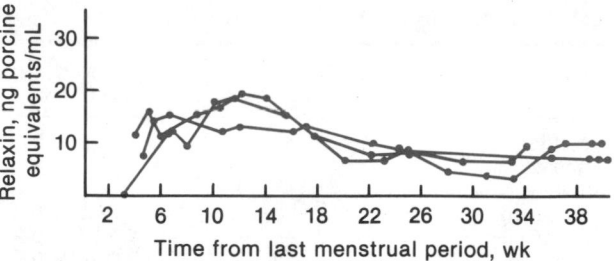

FIGURE 23–12   Relaxin levels during pregnancy and post partum. (From Quagliarello J, *et al.:* Serum immunoreactive relaxin concentrations in human pregnancy, labor and the puerperium. *Am J Ob Gyn* 1979, 135:43.)

E. Metabolic and endocrine changes[3,8–11]

1. Relaxin is a hormone secreted by the corpus luteum, the endocrine body located in the ovary, at the site of the ruptured ovarian follicle.

   a. Relaxin softens connective tissue during pregnancy in preparation for labor and delivery, when the pelvis must open to allow for the birth of the baby. Relaxin, however, is not specific to the pelvis. Other joints can also be affected.

   b. Relaxin peaks in early and late pregnancy. Women with chronic joint instability may notice an increase in symptoms during these times (see Figure 23–12).

   c. Relaxin has also been speculated to increase in the nonpregnant woman, after ovulation and throughout the menstrual period. This may cause softening of the joints and pain in affected women.

2. Other major hormones affecting a woman

f. Respiratory minute volume is elevated by 26% because of an increase in progesterone level. This is known as the "hyperventilation of pregnancy."

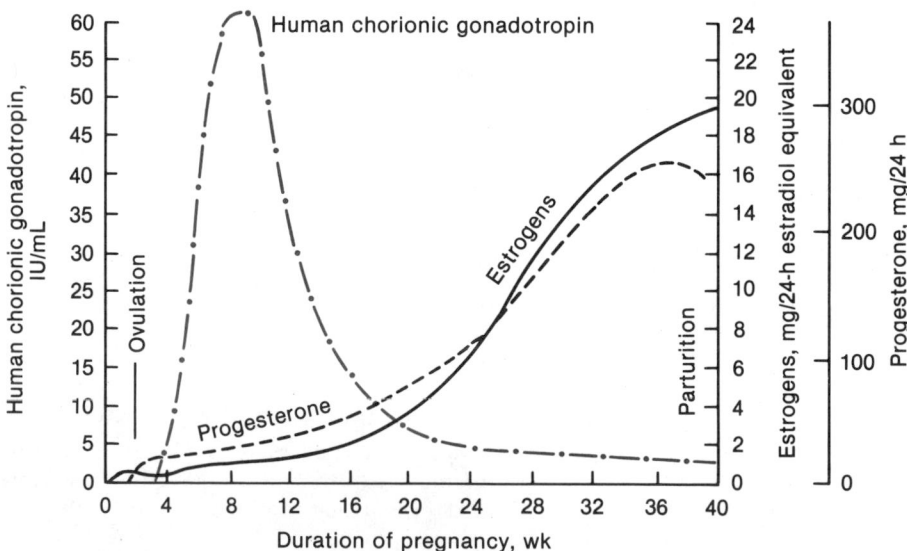

FIGURE 23–13   Rates of secretion of estrogens, progesterone, and human chorionic gonadotropin at different stages of pregnancy. (From Guyton AC: *Textbook of Medical Physiology,* 8th ed. Philadelphia, W. B. Saunders Company, 1991, p 919.)

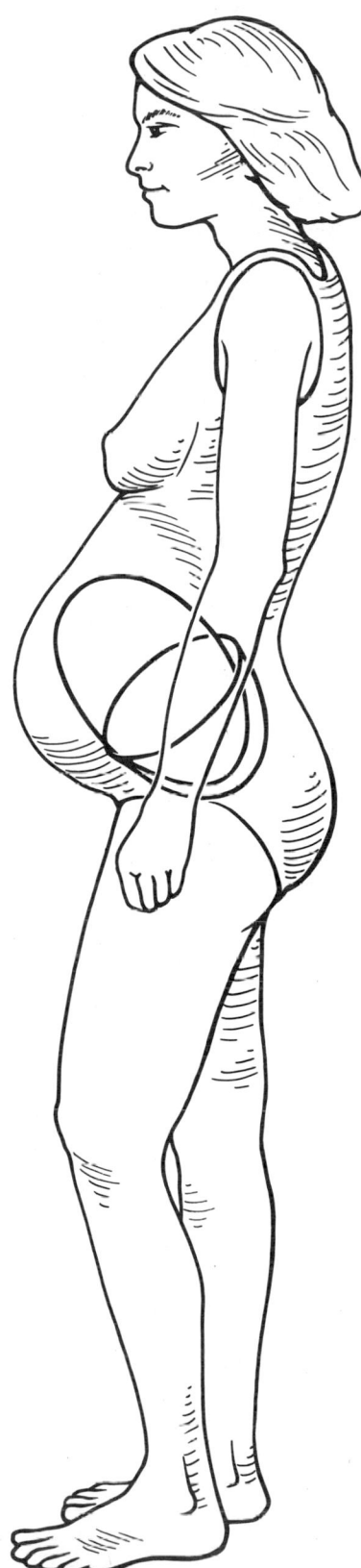

FIGURE 23–14 Postural changes during pregnancy.

during pregnancy include estrogen, progesterone, human placental lactogen, and human chorionic gonadotropin (see Figure 23–13).

3. Edema is present in the hands, feet, face and eyelids. This is due in part to sodium and water retention. Additionally, hormones circulated by the placenta, ovaries, and adrenal cortex cause increased capillary permeability, which contributes to the edema many pregnant women experience. Edema is a factor in the increased incidence of peripheral nerve entrapment syndromes experienced during pregnancy, including carpal tunnel, tarsal tunnel, thoracic outlet, and meralgia paresthetica (or lateral femoral cutaneous nerve entrapment) syndrome.

F. **Musculoskeletal system**[3,12]

1. **Postural changes.** During pregnancy, postural changes occur to accommodate for abdominal growth.
   a. These changes include forward head, rounded shoulders, increased lumbar lordosis, hyperextended knees, and pronated feet (see Figure 23–14).
   b. The center of gravity changes, resulting in changes in balance.
   c. Muscular changes are also typical. Often noted alterations include shortened hip flexors, lower back musculature, and pectorals. Abdominal muscles, neck, and upper back muscle groups elongate. This may promote stretch weakness or adaptive shortening.
   d. Extra weight is placed on the pelvic floor.

2. **Abdominal wall**[2,4] (see Figure 23–15)
   a. *Rectus abdominis*
      (1). The rectus abdominis comprises two long, narrow muscular bands connected by the linea alba; its function is to flex the trunk and to maintain the abdominal wall functions (see Figure 23–16).
      (2). The upper attachment is the 5th to 7th costal cartilage (and in some cases the 3rd and 4th ribs) and the xiphoid process and costoxiphoid ligaments.
      (3). The lower attachments are to two tendons. The lateral tendon arises from the pubic crest and tubercle. The medial tendon arises from the symphysis pubis and pubic bodies.

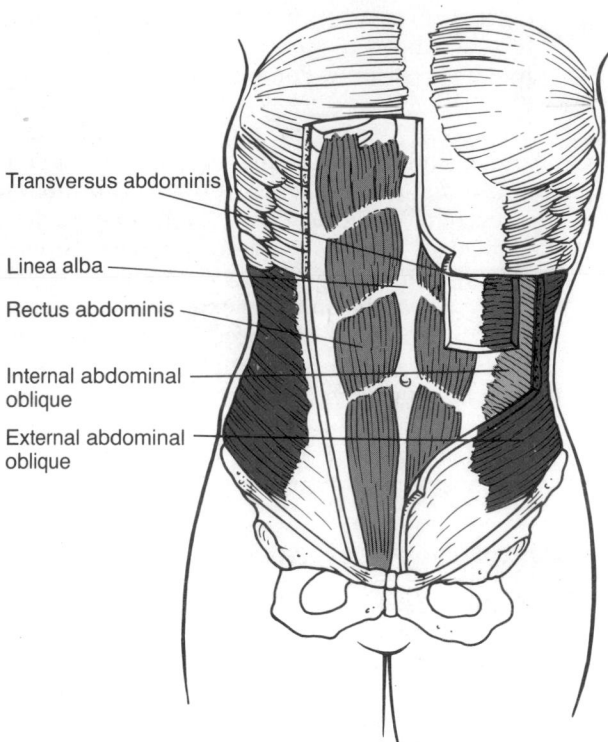

Transversus abdominis

Linea alba

Rectus abdominis

Internal abdominal oblique

External abdominal oblique

FIGURE 23–15   The abdominal wall musculature.

(4). This muscle is innervated by the spinal nerves T6–12.
b. ***External abdominal oblique***
  (1). This is the largest and most superficial of the muscles of the anterior abdominal wall. It compresses the abdomen, flexes and laterally rotates the spine, and depresses the ribs (see Figure 23–17).
  (2). The attachments are at the inferior borders and external surfaces of the lower eight ribs and the aponeurosis of the linea alba, extending from the xiphoid process to the symphysis pubis.
  (3). This muscle is innervated by the spinal nerves T6–12.
c. ***Internal abdominal oblique***
  (1). Primarily under the external oblique, this muscle also compresses the abdomen, flexes and laterally rotates the spine, and depresses the ribs (see Figure 23–18).
  (2). The attachments are at the lateral inguinal ligament, the anterior iliac crest, and the lumbar aponeurosis of the thoracolumbar fascia, leading to

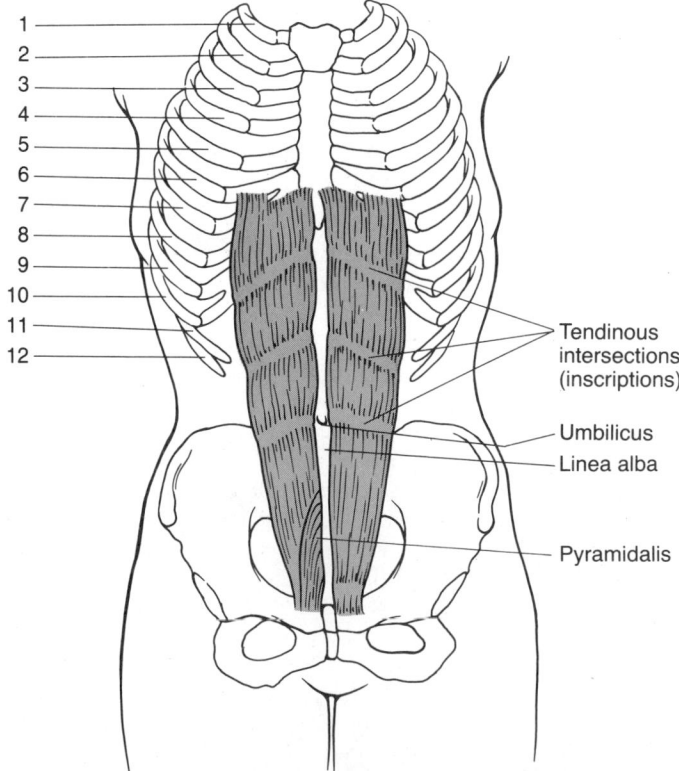

1
2
3
4
5
6
7
8
9
10
11
12

Tendinous intersections (inscriptions)

Umbilicus
Linea alba

Pyramidalis

FIGURE 23–16   The rectus abdominis muscle.

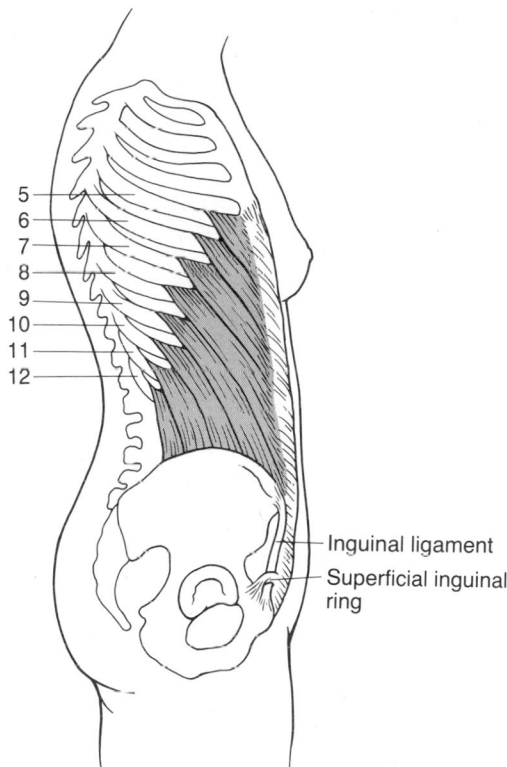

5
6
7
8
9
10
11
12

Inguinal ligament

Superficial inguinal ring

FIGURE 23–17   The external oblique muscle.

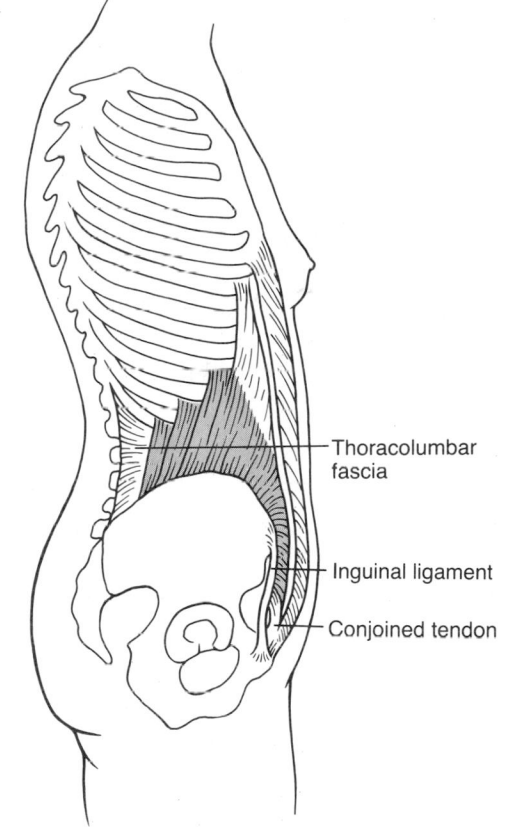

Thoracolumbar fascia

Inguinal ligament

Conjoined tendon

FIGURE 23–18   The internal oblique muscle.

the lower border of the lower four ribs, the aponeurosis of the linea alba, and the pubis and pectineal line.

(3). This muscle is innervated by T6 to L1.

d. *Transverse abdominis*

(1). The deepest of the anterior abdominal muscles, this body compresses the abdomen and depresses the ribs but has no action related to spinal movement (see Figure 23–19).

(2). The attachments are from the lateral inguinal ligament, the iliac crest, the thoracolumbar fascia, and the cartilages of the lower ribs to the aponeurosis and through to the linea alba and the pubis and pectineal line.

(3). This muscle is innervated by T6 to L1.

3. **Pelvic girdle**[1–3]

a. The pelvic girdle is composed of the hip and lower spine (see Figure 23–20).

(1). The three hip bones fusing to form

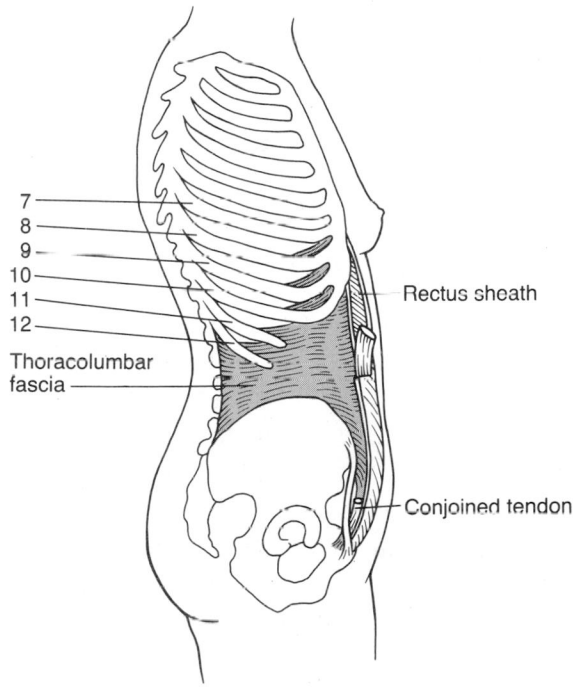

7
8
9
10
11
12

Thoracolumbar fascia

Rectus sheath

Conjoined tendon

FIGURE 23–19   The transversus abdominis muscle.

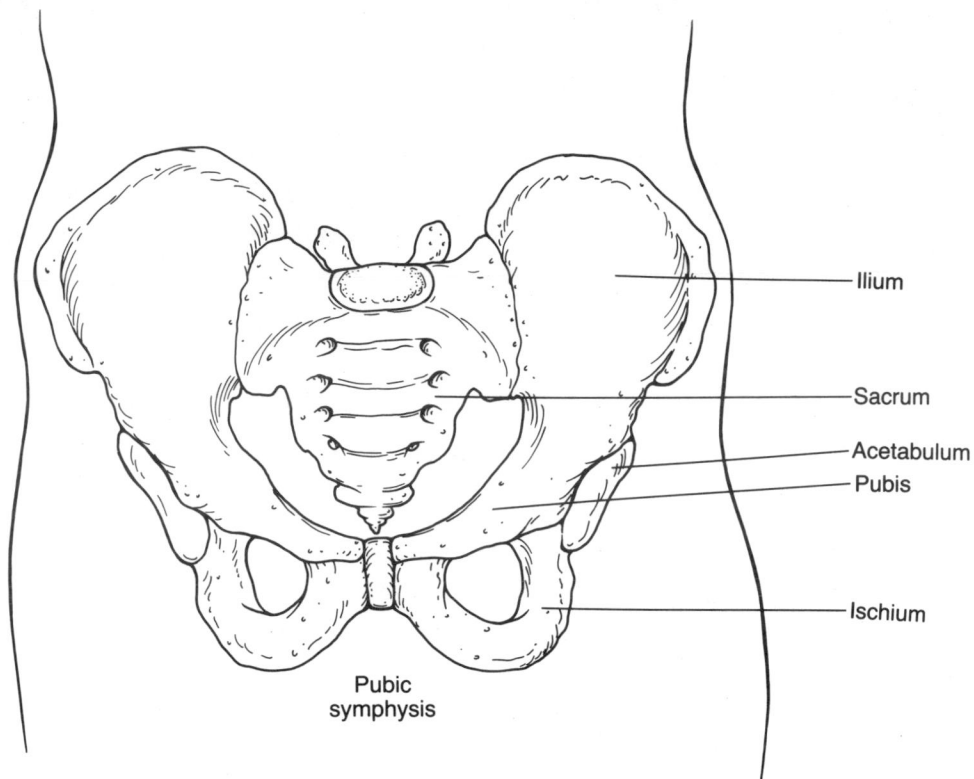

FIGURE 23–20   The bones of the pelvis.

the innominate bone include the ilium, ischium, and pubis.
   (2). The sacrum and coccyx form the central posterior aspect of the pelvic girdle.
   b. The functions of the pelvic girdle include
      (1). Transmission of body weight to the lower extremities.
      (2). Containment of a portion of the abdominopelvic organs.
   c. The pelvic inlet and the pelvic outlet surround the true (also known as lesser or minor) pelvis. The area above the pelvic inlet is the false (also known as greater or major) pelvis. During childbirth, the fetus must pass through the true pelvis (see Figure 23–21).

G. Gastrointestinal system[3,5]

1. Appetite may be increased in response to decreased serum glucose. Thirst may also be

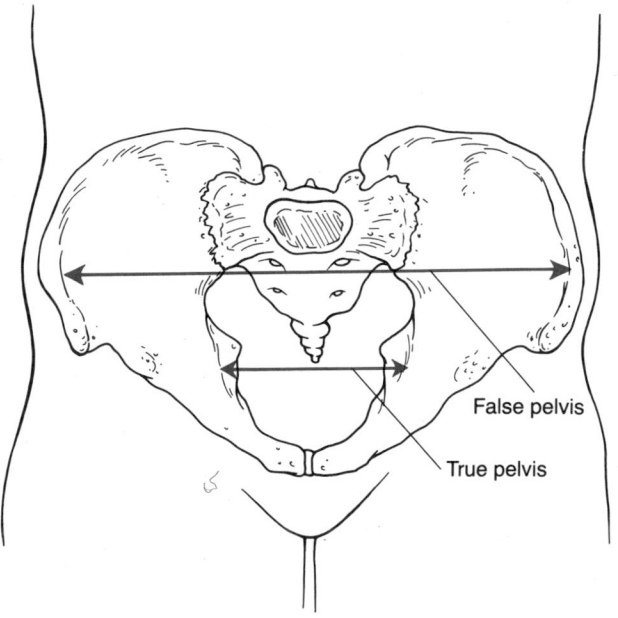

FIGURE 23–21   The true pelvis and false pelvis.

increased, partly in response to tubular reabsorption of salt and water and associated increased intake of liquids.

2. Taste threshold may be elevated, resulting in cravings.

3. Nausea or vomiting occurs in 50% to 60% of women, ranges from mild to severe, and often diminishes by 14 to 16 weeks. One suspected cause is human chorionic gonado-tropin, a hormone produced by the placenta responsible for continued production of progesterone.

4. Intestinal motility is decreased. Constipation can result.

5. Women are more predisposed to gallstones during pregnancy. Higher progesterone levels in the second and third trimesters result in decreased motility of the gallbladder.

II. Special Considerations in Physical Therapy Evaluation and Treatment

A. High-risk pregnancy[1,3,5,13,14]

1. A high-risk pregnancy is any gestation in which the prospects of optimal outcome of the mother or child are reduced.

2. High-risk pregnancies affect up to 25% of the obstetrical population.

3. High-risk diagnoses and pregnancy complications frequently encountered when working with this population include

   a. **Preterm labor.** Initiation of labor before the 37th week of a 40-week pregnancy.

   b. **Placenta previa.** A condition in which the placenta is implanted in the lower rather than the upper segment of the uterus, partially or completely obstructing the internal os of the cervix. The primary problems resulting from this are maternal bleeding and obstruction of the birth canal (see Figure 23–22).

   c. **Intrauterine growth retardation (IUGR) or fetal growth retardation.** Fetal growth below the 10th percentile for gestational age.

   d. **Placenta abruptio.** Partial or complete premature detachment of a normally situated placenta (see Figure 23–23).

   e. **Gestational diabetes.** Diabetes developing during pregnancy and resolving following delivery.

   f. **Incompetent cervix.** Inability of the cervix to retain a pregnancy due to a problem in cervical structure or function.

   g. **Preterm rupture of membranes.** Rupture of the amniotic sac prior to term.

   h. *Hypertensive disorders of pregnancy*
      (1). **Pregnancy-induced hypertension.** Blood pressure greater than 140/90 mm Hg as a consequence of pregnancy. Because normal blood pressure during pregnancy is frequently reduced, pregnancy-induced hypertension is also diagnosed if systolic blood pressure is elevated by 30 mm Hg above the patient's baseline, or if the diastolic pressure is elevated by 15 mm Hg above baseline.
      (2). **Preeclampsia.** The development of hypertension with proteinuria or edema, or both, as a result of pregnancy or the influence of a recent pregnancy.
      (3). **Eclampsia.** The occurrence of one or more grand mal seizures, not attributable to other cerebral conditions, in a patient with preeclampsia.

   i. **Disseminated intravascular coagulation.** A hemorrhagic syndrome occurring with uncontrolled activation of clotting factors and fibrinolytic enzymes in the small blood vessels. Possible consequences include thromboemboli (often affecting the kidney) and adult respiratory distress syndrome.

   j. **Multifetal gestation.** Pregnancy producing two or more infants.

   k. **Hydramnios or polyhydramnios.** Amniotic fluid volume in excess of 2000 mL, often associated with fetal malformations of the central nervous system or the gastrointestinal tract.

   l. **Oligohydramnios.** An abnormally low

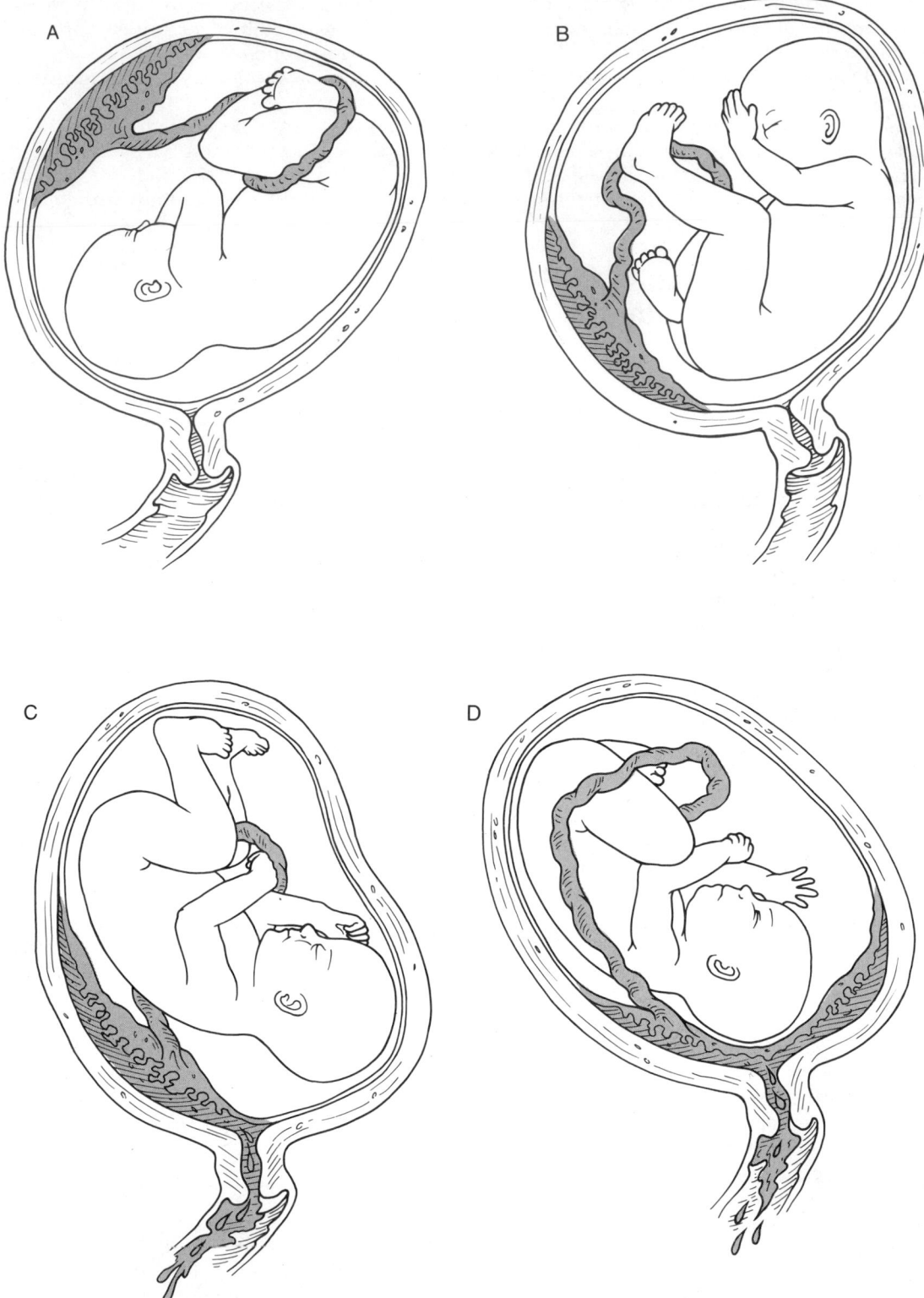

FIGURE 23–22 Placenta previa. **A,** Normal placental implantation site. **B,** Low implantation. **C,** Partial placenta previa. **D,** Complete placenta previa.

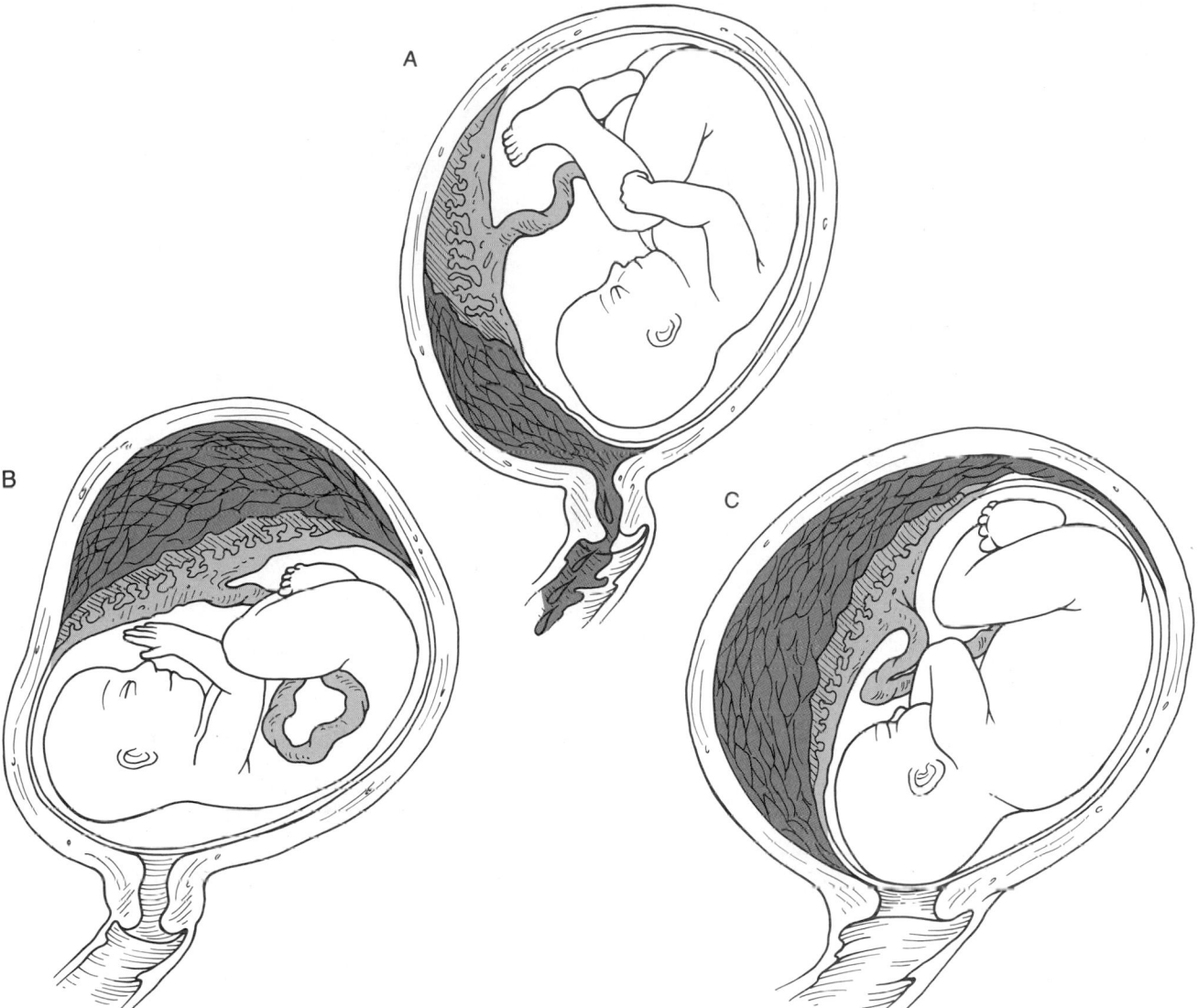

FIGURE 23–23   Placental abruption. **A,** External hemorrhage. **B,** Internal or concealed hemorrhage. **C,** Total separation.

amount of amniotic fluid, frequently caused by ruptured membranes or fetal anomaly. Primary consequences for the fetus are pulmonary hypoplasia or musculoskeletal deformities, ranging from mild contractures to congenital amputation.

4. Pre-existing conditions that can complicate a pregnancy include
   a. Diabetes
   b. Cardiac anomalies
   c. Pulmonary anomalies
   d. Systemic infection
   e. Fever
   f. High blood pressure
   g. Neoplasm
   h. Musculoskeletal conditions, *eg,* sacroiliac dysfunction or symphyseal separation
   i. Neurological conditions, *eg,* nerve entrapment syndromes or myasthenia gravis
   j. Chronic disability

5. High-risk pregnant women may have activity restrictions, ranging from light duty at

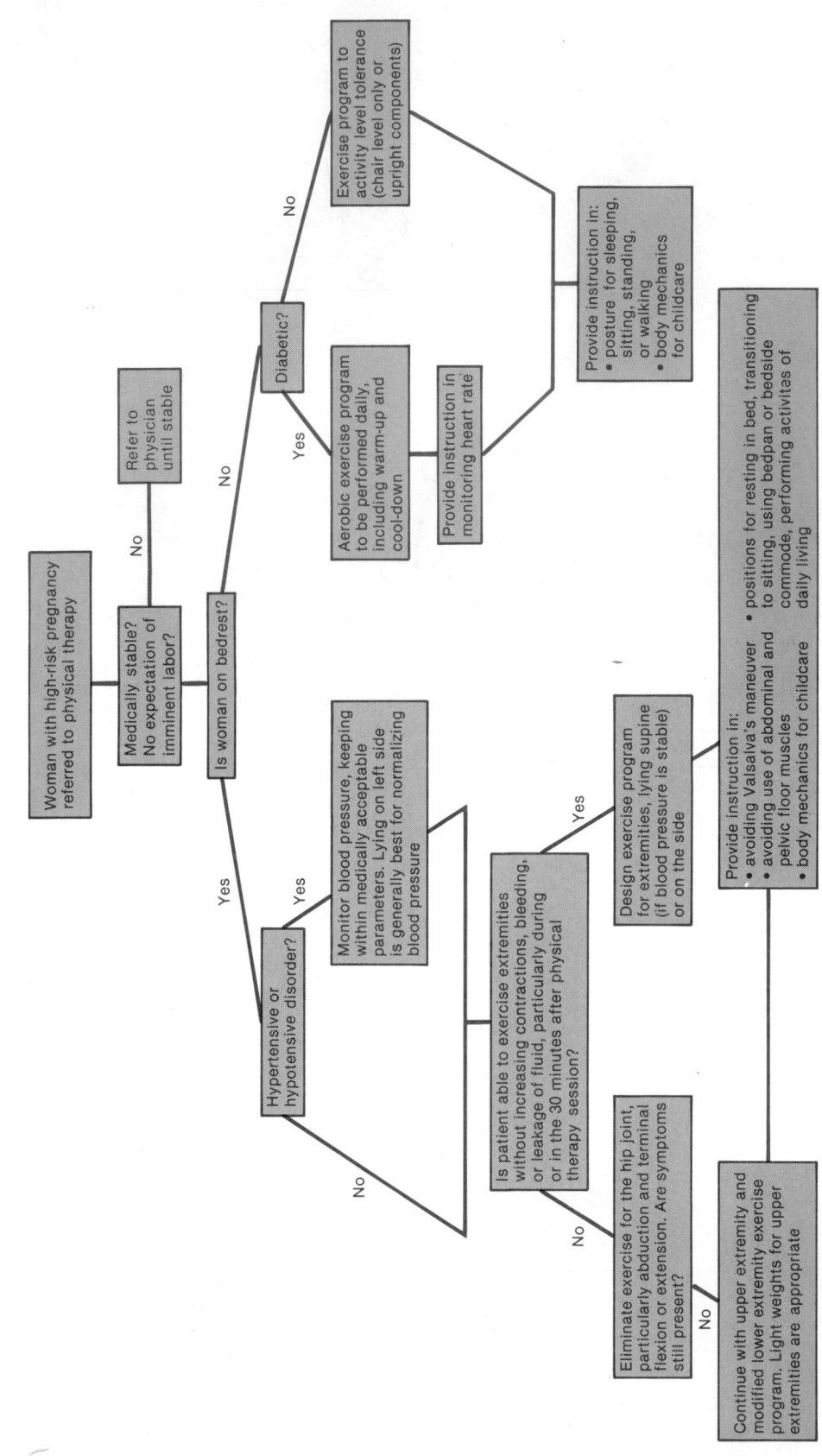

FIGURE 23–24 Physical therapy decision tree for a woman with a high-risk pregnancy.

work to bed rest. Bed rest can be intermittent or continuous. Some women are instructed to remain in specific positions, *eg*, left sidelying or Trendelenburg. Bathroom privileges may or may not be recommended. Whereas some women are hospitalized, others are on bed rest or restricted activity at home.[15,16]

6. Bed rest can be difficult psychologically for an otherwise active person who may not even feel sick. It is also difficult to go home and not be active particularly when there are young children in the home.[17]

7. **Examination of the high-risk pregnant woman** (see Figure 23–24)[15,16]
   a. History:
      (1). Present condition.
      (2). Past obstetrical history.
      (3). Past medical history.
   b. Perceived problems:
      (1). Activity related.
      (2). Pain related, including level of pain on a scale of 1 to 10, with 1 being barely noticeable and 10 being the worst pain imaginable.
   c. Current activity level.
   d. Activities that relieve or exacerbate the problem.
   e. Strength and endurance—resistive testing is not advisable.
   f. Joint range of motion—pregnancy values may vary, particularly in the trunk and hip girdle. This is a concern only when function is impaired or pain is present.
   g. Bed mobility and transfers.
   h. Gait, if ambulatory.
   i. Musculoskeletal assessment of painful or dysfunctional areas.
   j. Activities of daily living.
   k. Knowledge of energy conservation and body mechanics for pregnancy, for bed rest if indicated, and for postpartum childcare.
   l. Vital signs at rest, and with exercise, if hypertension or other relevant medical condition is a concern.

8. **Treatment goals**
   a. Maximize strength and joint range while on bed rest.
   b. Promote independence with bed mobility and activities of daily living using body mechanics that do not increase intra-ab-

dominal pressure or cause strain on the body.
   c. Counteract physiological effects of bed rest.
   d. Stimulate circulation and venous return to prevent thrombosis.
   e. Reduce stress through relaxation techniques.
   f. Increase feelings of self-control and well-being.
   g. Prevent or minimize musculoskeletal problems due to pregnancy or bed rest.
   h. If the patient is not on bed rest, maintain or improve her cardiovascular fitness with an individualized exercise program (especially diabetic patients).
   i. Promote postpartum recovery.
   j. Promote ability to care for self and infant(s) at discharge.

9. **Precautions**
   a. Avoid the Valsalva maneuver, which can increase intra-abdominal pressure. Because many patients unconsciously hold their breath during isometric exercise, isometrics should be avoided unless the patient is capable of and willing to monitor herself closely.
   b. Avoid active use or passive stretch of abdominal and pelvic floor musculature because use may cause increased contractions, exacerbation of preterm labor, or bleeding from the placenta.
   c. Check with medical or nursing staff prior to exercising with a patient who has been unstable in the recent past. Increased contractions, elevated blood pressure, bleeding, or increased leakage of fluid are reasons to consider holding treatment for the day.
   d. Other than abdominal and pelvic floor exercise, exercise that reinforces the pregnancy-related stretch weakness of certain muscles should be avoided. For example, the pectorals tighten during pregnancy and the rhomboids stretch. Circling the shoulders forward further stretches the rhomboids. Reverse shoulder circles are more appropriate because they stretch the pectorals.
   e. Isolated ankle plantar flexion may cause muscle cramps in the calves if the woman is prone to this problem.
   f. Isometric exercise and the use of Thera-Band as resistance may promote breath

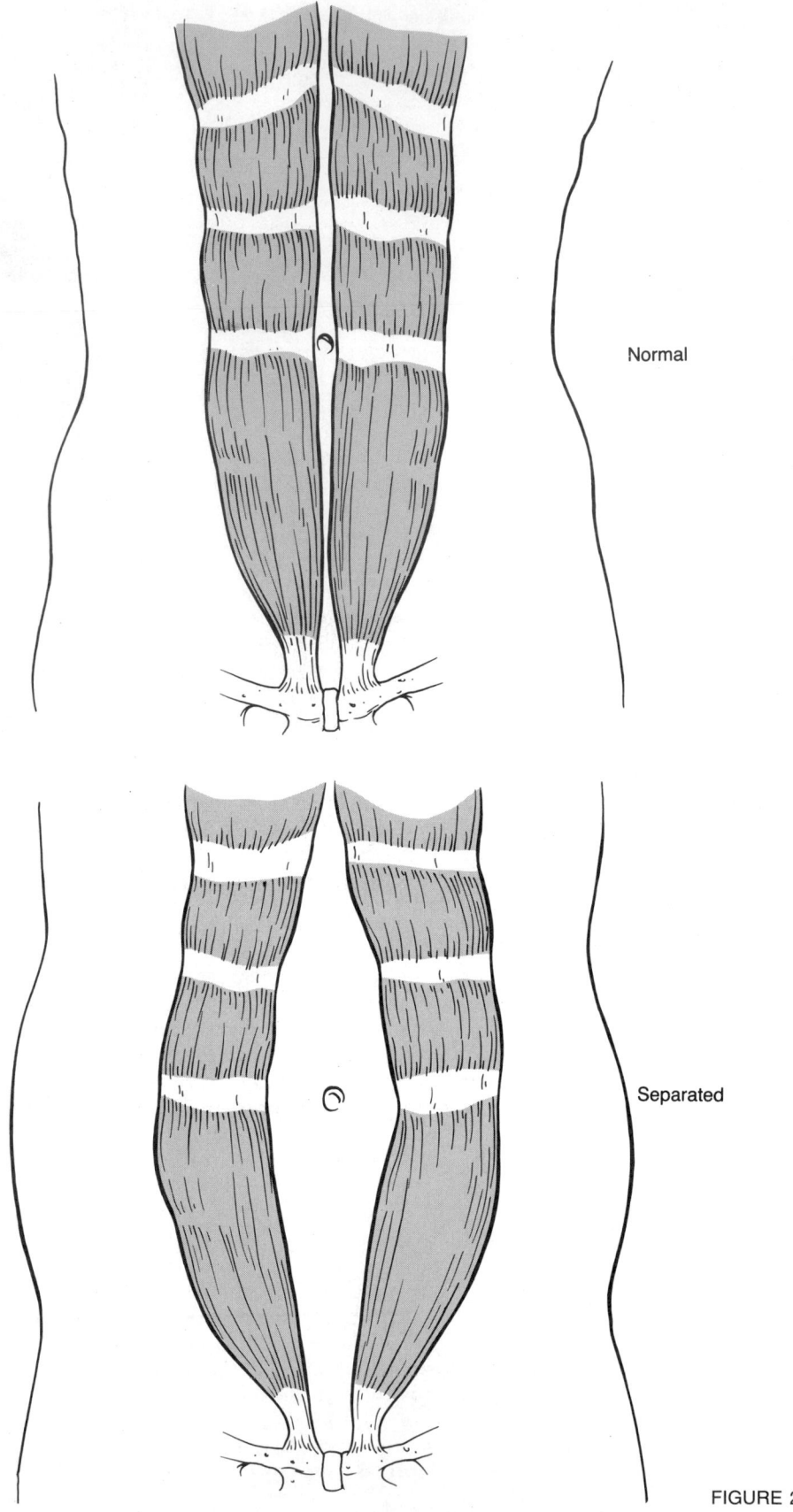

Normal

Separated

FIGURE 23–25   Diastasis recti abdominis.

holding or synergistic muscle involvement.

    g. Manual muscle testing is not advisable for the reasons cited above.

10. **Exercises**
    a. *Upper extremity*
      (1). Proprioceptive neuromuscular facilitation (PNF) diagonals (or straight-plane range of motion if the patient comprehends these exercises more easily).
      (2). Strengthening exercises to facilitate childcare during the postpartum period; for biceps, triceps, deltoids, and rotator cuff.
      (3). Light weights may be used if the woman is tolerating her exercise program without obstetrical complications and wishes to progress with weights.
    b. *Lower extremity.* Lower extremity exercise is more controversial than upper extremity exercise. Although some believe that lower extremity exercises are contraindicated with certain diagnoses, others see benefit in mild exercise. Careful assessment of patient reaction to exercise is required.
      (1). Gentle lower extremity range of motion can be performed as long as there is adherence to precautions listed previously.
      (2). If active exercise exacerbates symptoms, active assistive or passive exercise is more appropriate.
      (3). Ankle circles are important to keep blood flowing through calves because a woman on bed rest is at risk for deep vein thrombosis.
      (4). Weights and manual resistance are inappropriate with lower extremity exercise.
    c. *Neck and upper trunk.* Backward shoulder circles, chin tucks, and neck semicircles or side bending.

B. Diastasis rectus[12,18–20]

1. **Definition.** This is a condition in which the bellies of the rectus abdominis muscle, usually held close together by the linea alba, are separated. The linea alba is either thinned, completely separated, or severed altogether. Additionally, the muscle itself is stretched (see Figure 23–25).

2. **Etiology.** The most common etiology is parity. Another is surgery. Vertical abdominal incisions do not disrupt the muscle *per se* but can sever the nerve supply to the rectus. This results in paralysis, lack of union, and, finally, diastasis.

3. **Implications.** The potential exists for problems to develop during labor and delivery, *ie*, malpresentations of the fetus (such as breech or transverse) and ineffective abdominal contractions during the second stage of labor. Back pain can result. As a component of the abdominal wall, the rectus abdominis also facilitates proper posture and contributes to performance of functional activities such as coughing, defecation, urination, and vomiting. Reduced ability of the rectus to contribute to performance of these activities can result in problems in any of these areas.

4. **At-risk population.** Diastasis can occur in anyone, male or female, who has extraordinary, sustained high pressure on the abdominal wall. Examples include chronic constipation or chronic obstructive pulmonary disease.

5. **Diagnosis.** To determine if a diastasis is present, the patient is positioned in the hook-lying position. The therapist places several fingers horizontally 2 inches above the umbilicus. One fingerbreadth is estimated to be 1 cm. While lifting her head and shoulders off of the surface, the patient should exhale and reach with extended arms for her knees, as if doing an abdominal curl-up. The number of fingers placed horizontally between the muscle bellies during the curl-up (while muscle is actively contracting) indicates the degree of separation. During the later months of pregnancy, the gap may appear as a bulge. Because a diastasis may present anywhere between the sternum and the pubis, the measurement should be repeated at the level of the umbilicus and 2 inches below the umbilicus. The measurement can change throughout pregnancy, with most diastases noted in the immediate postpartum period, affecting two thirds of all women (see Figure 23–26).

6. **Treatment/precautions.** If a woman has a clinically significant diastasis (over 2 cm), she should not do full abdominal curl-ups to strengthen the rectus. Instead, she should perform a modified head lift (see Figure

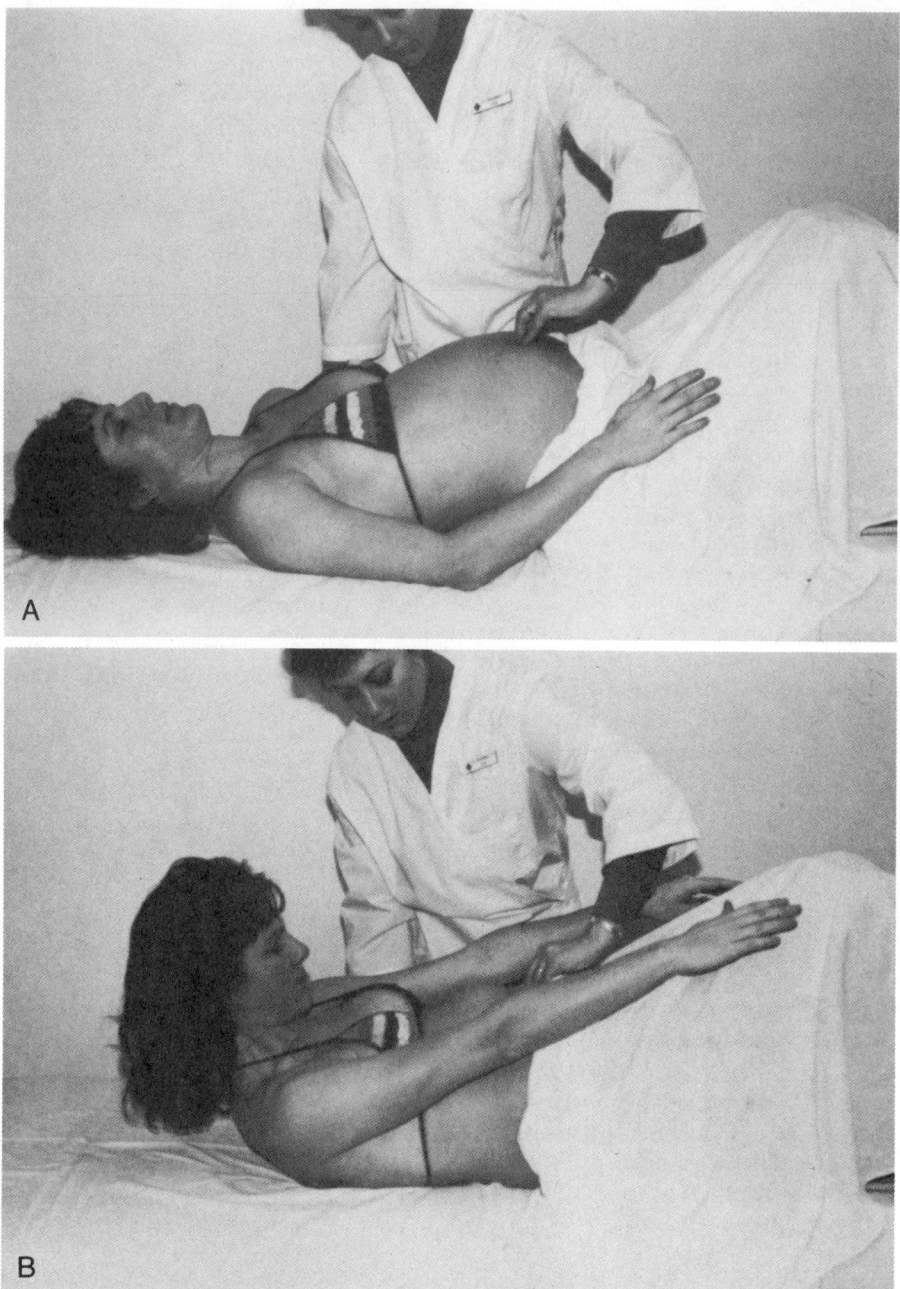

FIGURE 23–26   Assessing the abdominal wall for diastasis recti abdominis. **A,** Starting position. **B,** Final position.

23–27). This is done by starting in the hook-lying position, placing arms around the belly as shown, and exhaling while lifting the head off the surface. The woman should hold for a count of three, then slowly return to the starting position. *Note:* If the woman has supine hypotension, she may be restricted from lying on her back after the 4th month of pregnancy. Additionally, some physicians routinely discourage this position in all pregnant women after the 4th month (see Figure 23–28).

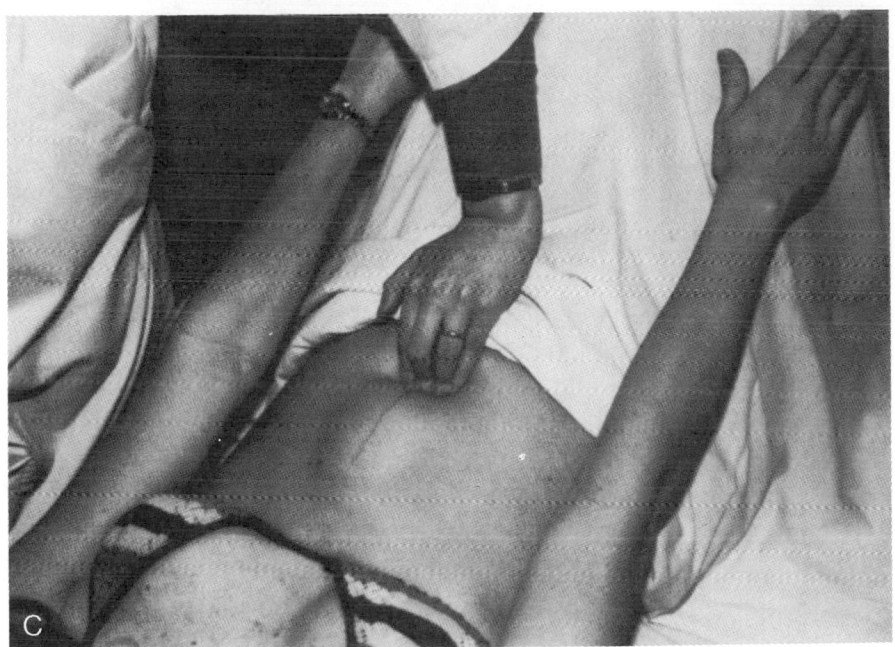

FIGURE 23–26 *(continued)* **C,** A four-finger diastasis is shown. (Panels A–C reprinted from Wilder E (ed): *Obstetric and Gynecologic Physical Therapy.* New York, Churchill Livingstone, 1988, pp 74, 75.)

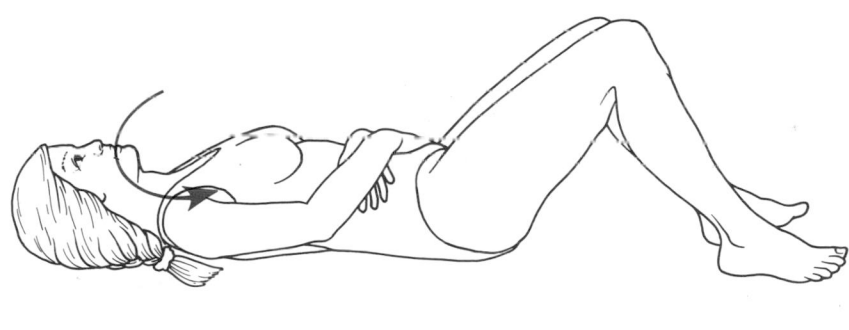

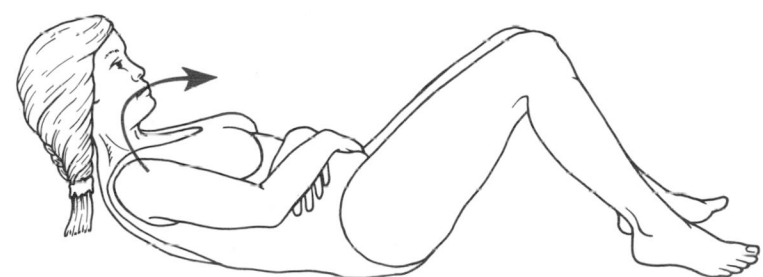

FIGURE 23–27   Modified head lift to correct diastasis recti abdominis.

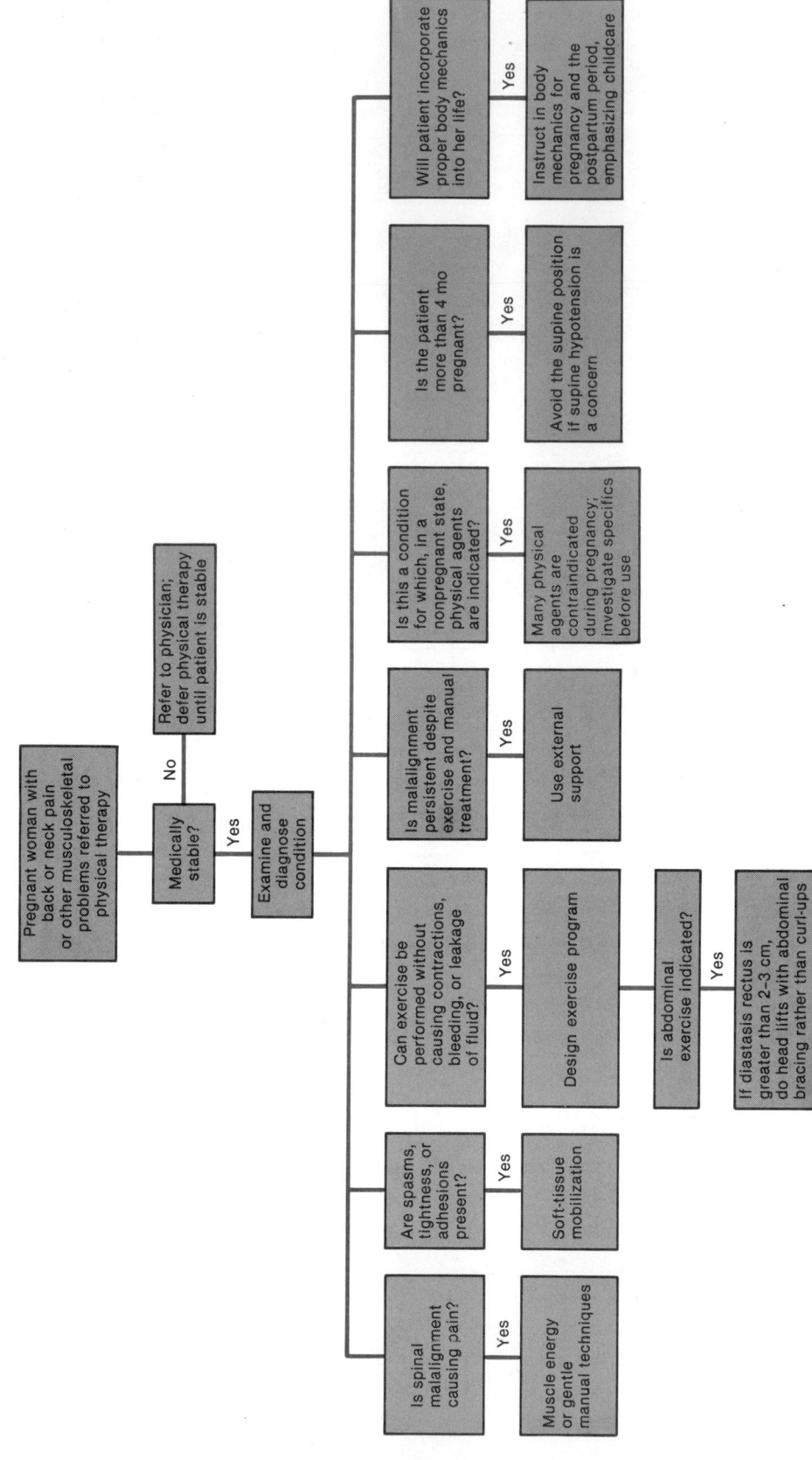

FIGURE 23–28 Decision tree for musculoskeletal conditions during pregnancy.

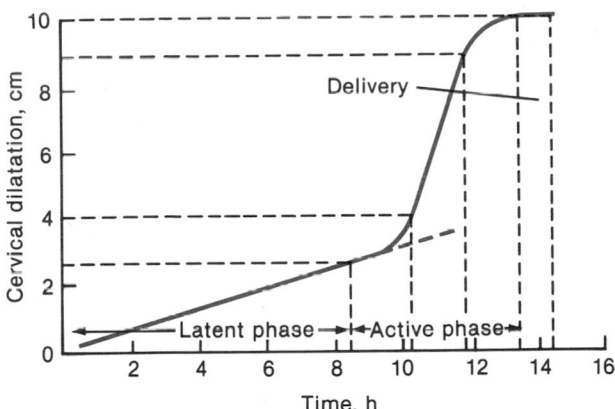

FIGURE 23–29 Labor phases and duration in the primipara. (Redrawn from Friedman EA: *Labor and Clinical Evaluation and Management,* 2nd ed. New York, Appleton-Century-Crofts, 1978, p 33.)

C. Labor and delivery

1. **Labor**[1,5]
    a. *Definition.* Labor is defined as "uterine contractions that bring about demonstrable effacement and dilatation of the cervix."[5]
    b. *Duration.* For first-time mothers, duration is 14 hours; for later births, average duration is 8 hours (see Figure 23–29).
    c. *First stage*
        (1). *Latent or prodromal labor.* Contractions begin, causing effacement and minimal cervical dilation, often to 3 to 5 cm.
        (2). *Active labor.* This occurs when the

woman's cervix dilates 1.2 to 1.5 cm/hr. It usually begins at 3 to 5 cm dilation and ends at 10 cm.

The *transitional phase* of labor, occurring during the end of the active phase, is usually when contractions are most frequent and most intense (see Figure 23–30).

2. **Vaginal birth**
    a. *Definition.* This is the second stage of labor, when the cervix is fully dilated and the fetus is being delivered.
    b. *Duration.* This phase of labor lasts an average of 50 minutes for a first-time mother and 20 minutes in the multipara (see Figure 23–30).

3. **Cesarean birth**[1,3]
    a. *Definition.* Surgical birth via an incision in the abdominal wall and the uterus. The incision is usually done in one of two ways: horizontally (transverse) or vertically (classical) (see Figure 23–31).
    b. *Indications*
        (1). *Maternal.* Maternal disease with the potential to affect the birth, including cardiac conditions, preeclampsia, infection, or diabetes; herpes; placenta previa or placenta abruptio; previous uterine surgery or cesarean delivery (particularly classical or vertical incision); and nonprogressive labor.
        (2). *Fetal.* Cephalopelvic disproportion, fetal distress, breech or transverse

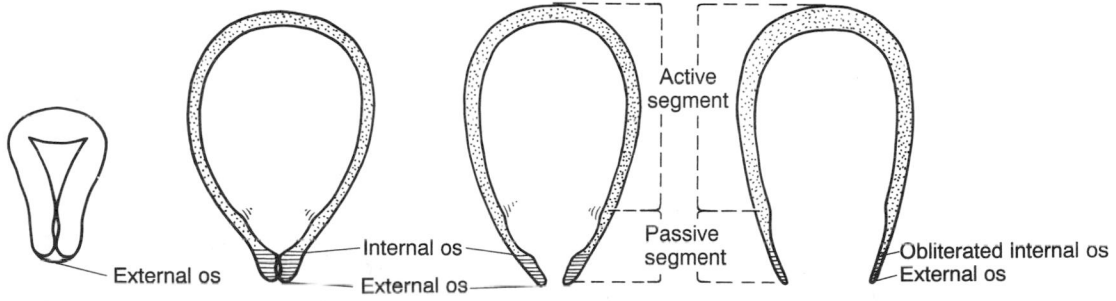

FIGURE 23–30 Comparison of uterus during phases of development. **A,** Nonpregnant. **B,** Pregnant. **C,** During labor. **D,** During delivery. (Drawing and legend for panels A–D adapted with permission from Cunningham FG, *et al.: William's Obstetrics,* 19th ed. East Norwalk, CT, Appleton and Lange, 1993, p 341.)

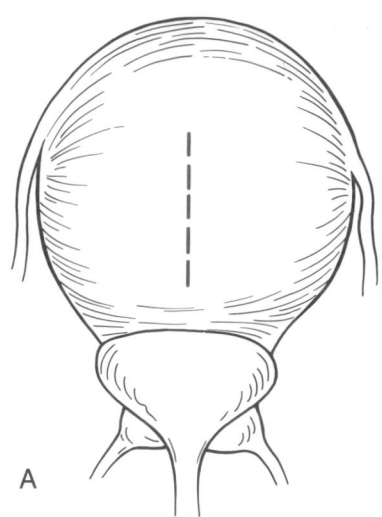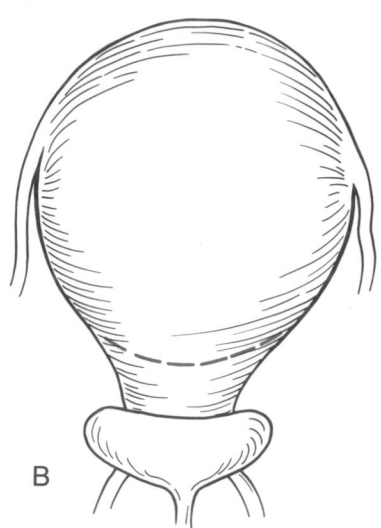

FIGURE 23–31   Uterine incisions during cesarean birth. **A,** Classical or midline. **B,** Horizontal or transverse (bladder is displaced downward).

presentation, prolapsed umbilical cord, preterm birth.

4. **Third stage of labor.** The delivery of the placenta.

5. **Transcutaneous electrical nerve stimulator (TENS) for pain control.**[21,22] TENS has been studied as a modality for pain control during labor and delivery. Subjectively, women report pain relief, particularly in the low back. Some evidence suggests that using TENS in labor and delivery reduces length of labor and decreases dependence on narcotics during and after labor. Apgar scores

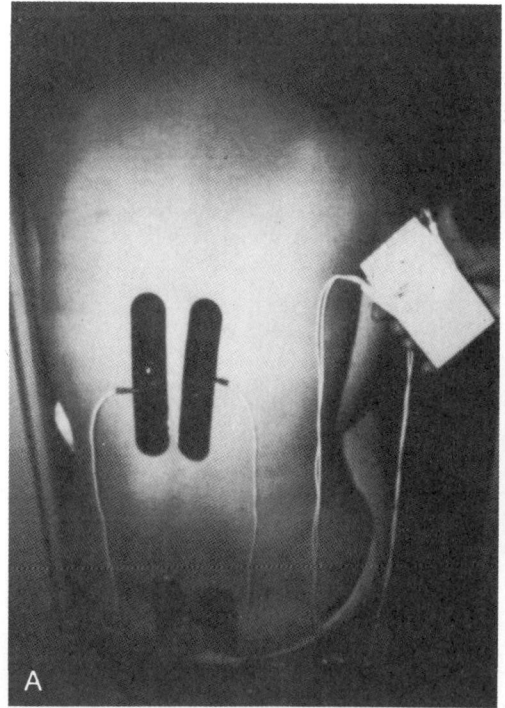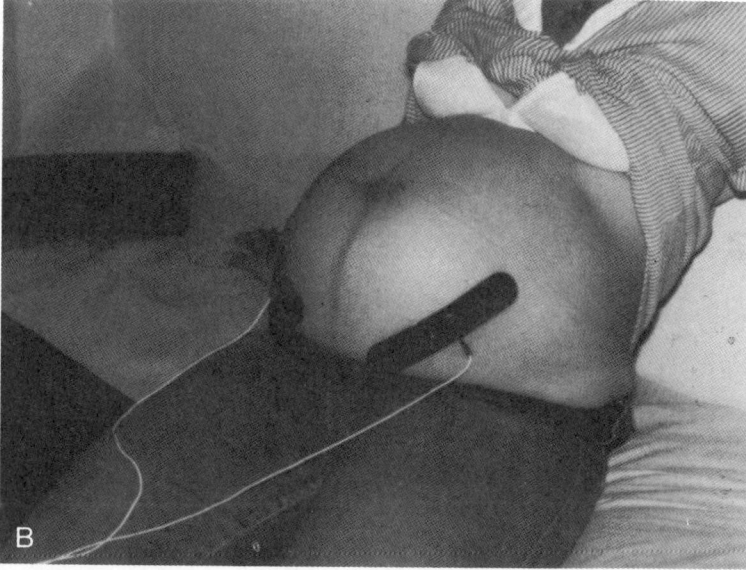

FIGURE 23–32   Electrode placement for use of TENS during labor and delivery. **A,** For uterine, back, and pelvic pain. **B,** For suprapubic pain. (Panels A and B reprinted from Wilder E (ed): *Obstetric and Gynecologic Physical Therapy.* New York, Churchill Livingstone, 1988, p 121.)

of infants whose mothers have used TENS are as high as or higher than those without.

a. ***Electrode placement*** (see Figure 23–32)

    (1). Two sets of electrodes are often used.

        (a). Electrodes are placed paraspinally T10 to L1.

        (b). Set 2 is placed paraspinally S2–S4.

        (c). For suprapubic pain or during the second stage of labor, electrodes can be placed in a V on the anterior aspect of the abdomen. This may be less effective than the spinal placements.

b. ***Parameters***

    (1). Rate—80 to 120 Hz.

    (2). Pulse width—150 μs.

    (3). Intensity—determined by the woman; can change with each contraction.

c. TENS can interfere with the fetal monitor when electrodes are placed sacrally. Filters are available to suppress the disturbance. Some women are able to be monitored intermittently and use the TENS when the monitor is not being utilized.

PLEASE NOTE: Although preliminary studies show that TENS seems beneficial, its use *during* pregnancy has not yet been sanctioned, and pregnancy remains on the list of contraindications to use of TENS. Effects of TENS on the fetus, either short term or long term, have not yet been studied sufficiently.

6. **Postpartum period.**[1,5] This is the period immediately following birth and extending until the reproductive organs have returned to their prepregnancy state.

a. ***Anatomical and physiological changes***

    (1). The uterus shrinks (or involutes), weighing 1000 g immediately after delivery, 500 g 1 week postpartum, and 100 g after 4 weeks. Uterine contractions, present especially during nursing, cause "afterpains" and assist with this process (see Figure 23–33).

    (2). The superficial layer of the endometrium is sloughed off in the lochia, or discharged from the vagina after birth. Lochia is present for 1 to 3 weeks after birth.

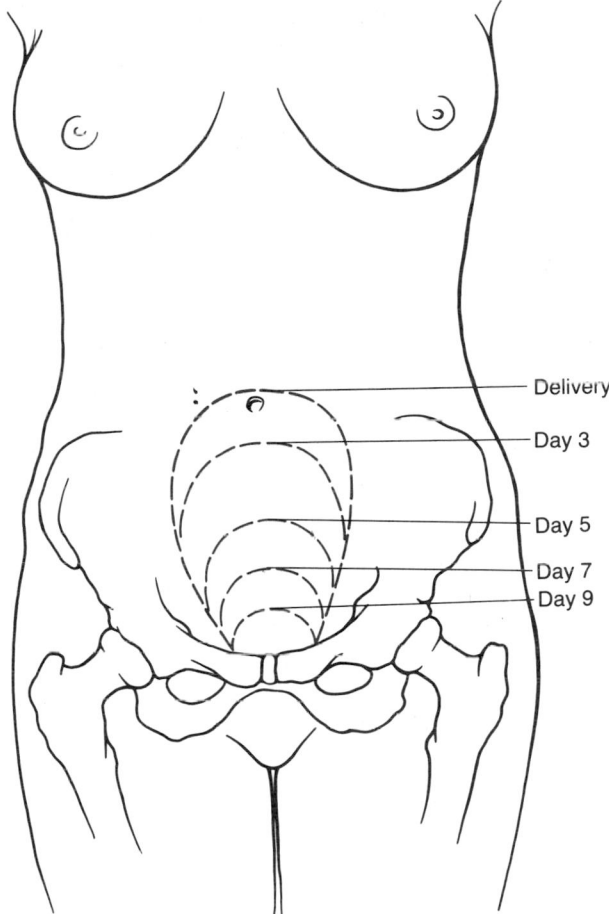

FIGURE 23–33 Uterine involution after birth.

    (3). Bladder distention is often seen, moving the uterus upward and reducing its ability to contract. This can cause uterine atony and increased bleeding. In severe cases, hemorrhage can result (see Figure 23–34).

    (4). Perineal trauma is indicated by hematoma, ecchymosis, discomfort, swelling, or erythema. Hemorrhoids also are seen at times.

    (5). Constipation is a frequent aftereffect of birth. This is caused by decreased intestinal tone, stretching of the abdomen, and a reduction in food and liquids taken in during labor and delivery. The first stool usually occurs within 2 to 3 days after delivery.

    (6). Women are at risk of developing thrombophlebitis in the early post-

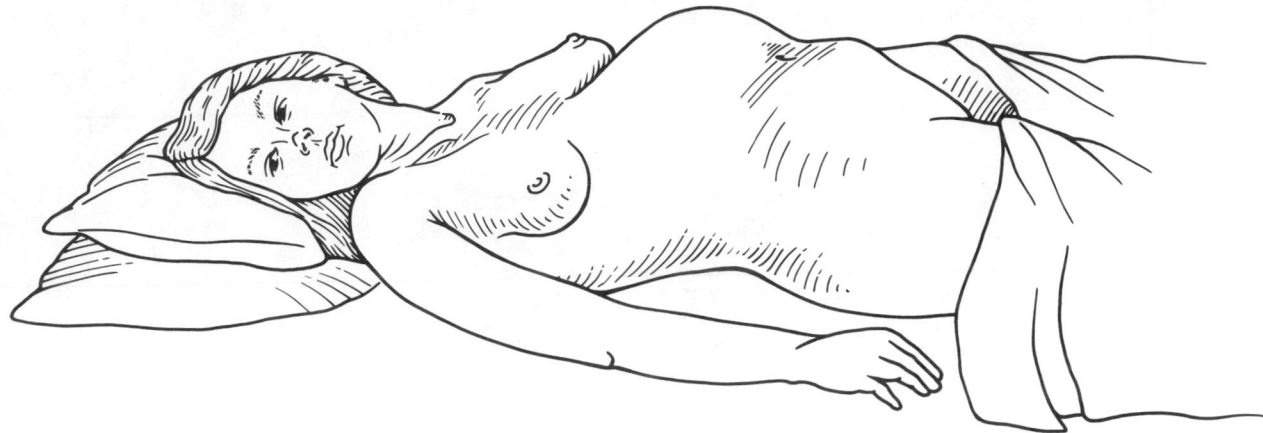

FIGURE 23–34   Full bladder displacing uterine fundus.

partum period. Decreased venous return, extended compression of blood vessels supplying the lower extremities during labor and delivery, and a tendency toward coagulation after birth predispose women to this condition.

(7). Breast engorgement occurs, causing discomfort and warmth to touch. This resolves with initiation of breast-feeding or, in the instance of bottle feeding, within a few days.

(8). *Specifics for vaginal birth*
   (a). Perineal pain is common in women who have had lacerations or episiotomies.
   (b). Early ambulation is encouraged. It has been shown to decrease the frequency of deep vein thrombosis and pulmonary emboli as well as reduce bowel and bladder complications.

(9). *Specifics for cesarean birth*[1,5]
   (a). Anesthesia increases the risk of urinary retention and decreased peristalsis as well as constipation. Ileus is often reported.
   (b). Risk of pneumonia, pulmonary embolism, and decreased oxygenation is also increased. The risk of pulmonary embolism and venous thrombosis is decreased with early ambulation.
   (c). Incisional pain.
   (d). Other potential complications include infection, bleeding from the incision, hematoma, and wound dehiscence.

7. **Postpartum examination**[12,23]
   a. Type of delivery:
      (1). Vaginal or cesarean as well as incisions (or tears) on the perineum or abdomen.
      (2). Complications of this pregnancy, birth, or postpartum period.
   b. History:
      (1). Obstetrical.
      (2). Medical.
      (3). Exercise.
   c. Current activity level.
   d. Current level of pain on a scale of 1 to 10, with 1 being barely noticeable and 10 being the worst pain imaginable.
   e. Gross muscle strength and range of motion.
   f. Bed mobility, transfers, and gait.
   g. Posture.
   h. Musculoskeletal assessment of painful or dysfunctional areas.
   i. Knowledge of postpartum body mechanics, emphasizing childcare.
   j. Diastasis rectus (not a reliable measurement until 3 days post partum owing to the rapid changes that the body is undergoing).
   k. Knowledge of pelvic floor strengthening program.

8. **Treatment goals:**
   a. Minimize pain.
   b. Independent mobility.

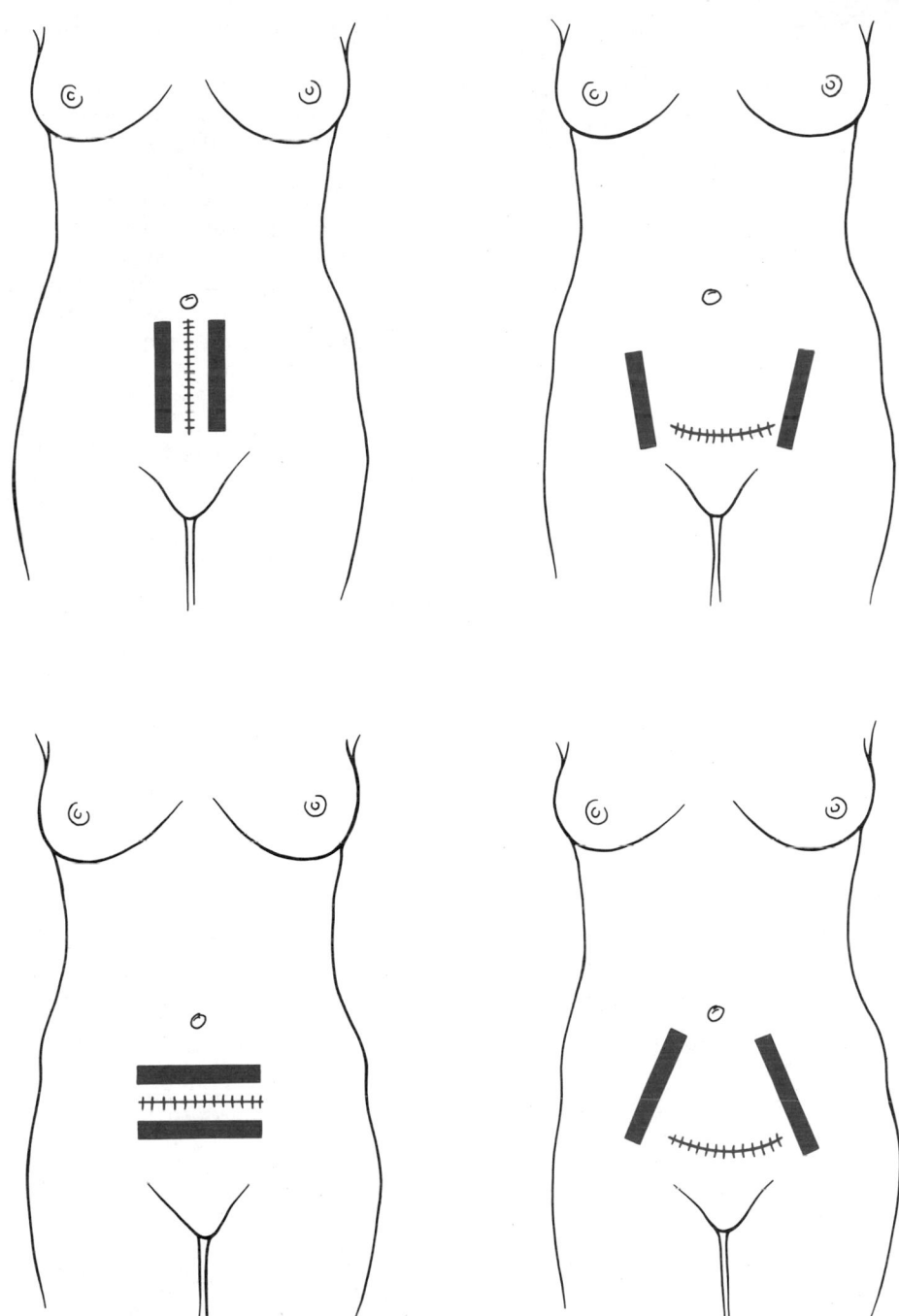

FIGURE 23–35   Electrode placements for TENS following cesarean birth.

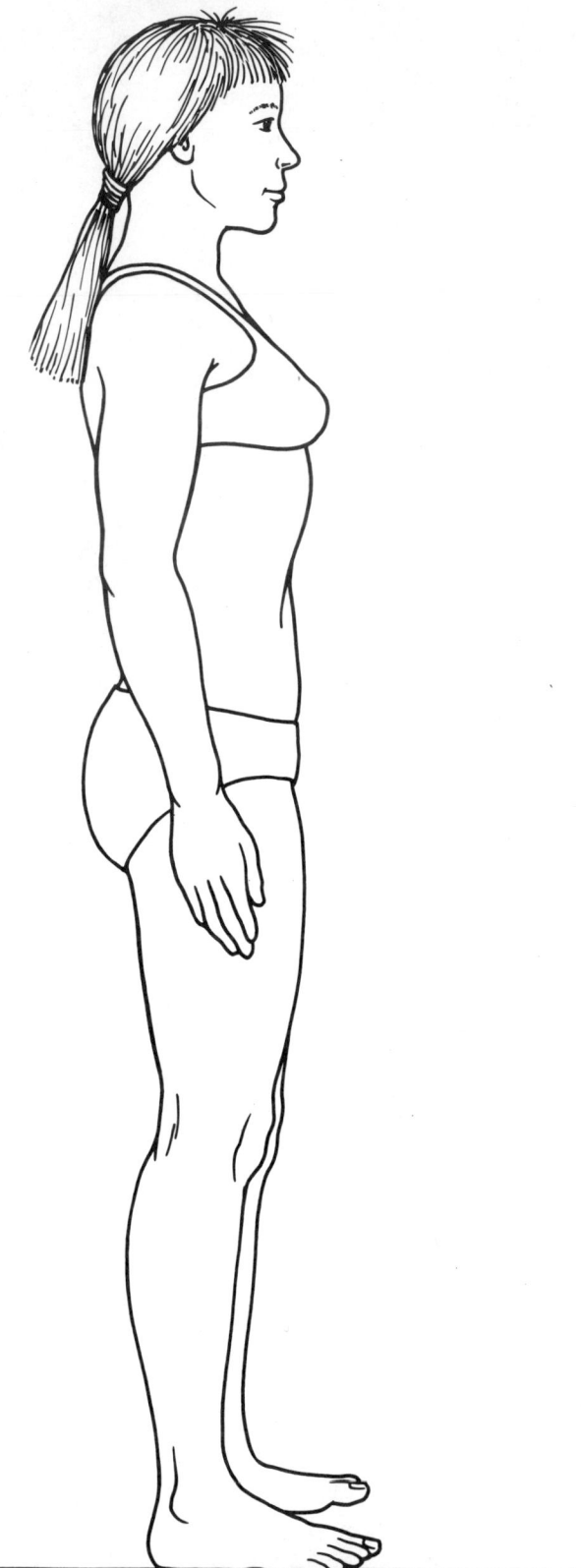

FIGURE 23–36 Good posture should be maintained after birth.

c. Prevent or correct musculoskeletal dysfunction.
d. Demonstrated knowledge of body mechanics and posture for childcare and activities of daily living.
e. Ability to monitor self for diastasis rectus.
f. Continence of bowel and bladder.
g. Independence with home exercise program.
h. Strength and endurance sufficient to care for self and infant when necessary.

9. **Treatment strategies**
   a. *Pain control*[12]
      (1). After a cesarean birth, TENS can be effective. Studies show that new mothers who use TENS require less medication for pain and have reduced nausea and vomiting. They are more alert and less depressed. They are able to ambulate earlier. They also have decreased ileus and fewer pulmonary complications than controls.
      (2). Electrodes can be placed surrounding the incision or above and below it (see Figure 23–35).
      (3). Parameters
         (a). Rate—150 pulses/s.
         (b). Pulse width—250 μs.
         (c). Intensity—determined by the patient.
   b. *Pulmonary*[24]
      (1). Abdominal breathing.
      (2). Huffing rather than coughing to clear lungs, with pillow supported against abdomen as needed for comfort.
      (3). Respiratory exercise is particularly important for those patients who have been anesthetized.
   c. *Posture and body mechanics* (see Figure 23–36)[12]
      (1). With abdominal and other musculature still stretched, postpartum women should consciously check posture when standing or walking. Abdominal muscles should be contracted to reduce lordosis. Shoulders should be over hip girdle, and head in line with trunk.
      (2). Instruction in body mechanics for the postpartum woman should include
         (a). Positioning for bottle feeding or breast-feeding.
         (b). Lifting an infant.

(c). Lifting an older child.
(d). Changing a diaper.
(e). Pushing a stroller.
(f). Bathing a baby or toddler.
(g). Placing a child in a car seat.
(h). Placing a car seat in a car.
(i). Performing household duties.
(j). Positioning for sleep.

d. *Exercises* (see Figure 23–37)
 (1). Ankle pumps and circles, for circulation.
 (2). Kegel exercises, or pelvic floor contractions.
 (3). Pelvic tilts.
 (4). Heel slides.
 (5). Abdominal exercises, according to status of abdominal wall. Diastasis should be assessed on the 3rd postpartum day.
   (a). Head lifts if diastasis is greater than 2 cm.
   (b). Curl-ups if diastasis is less than 2 cm.
   (c). Progressively, bridging, bridging with trunk rotation, diagonal curl-ups, and reverse curl-ups are added.
 (6). Upper extremity exercises.
   (a). Reverse shoulder circles.
   (b). PNF diagonals, or straight-plane range of motion, initially assisted if necessary.

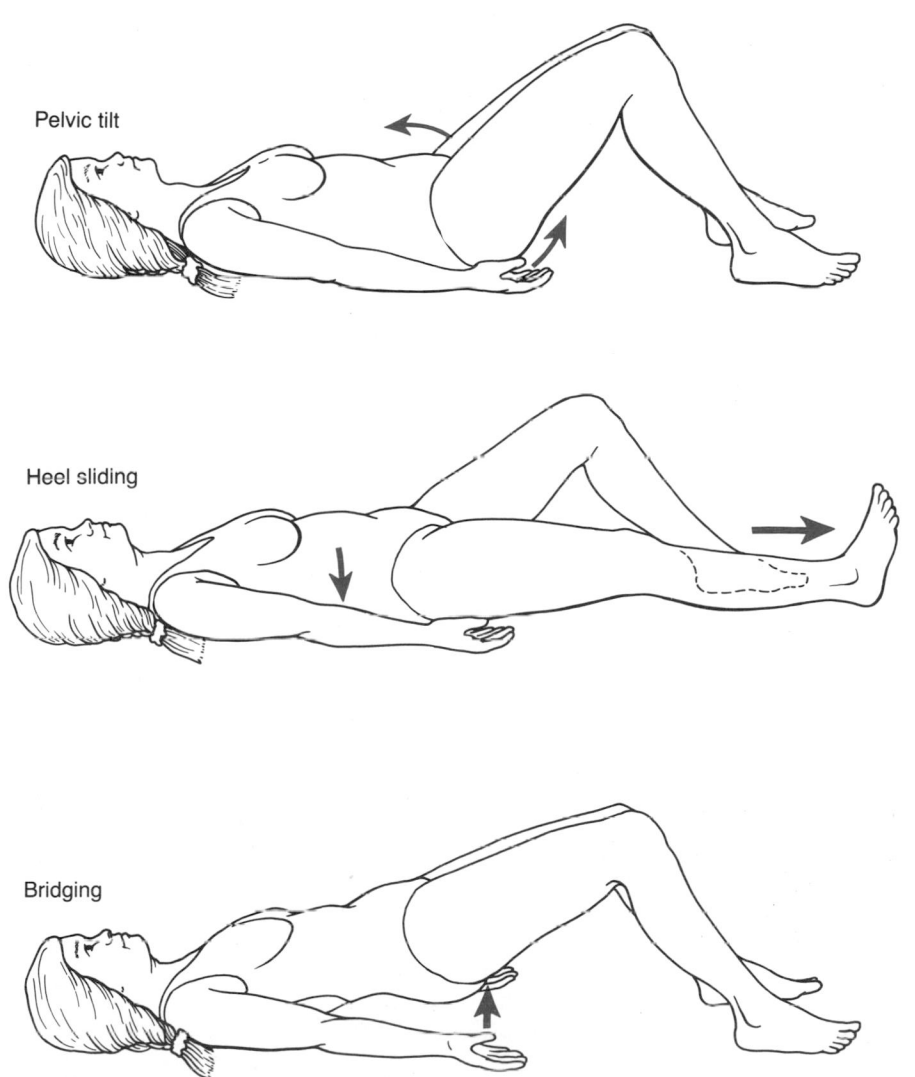

Pelvic tilt

Heel sliding

Bridging

FIGURE 23–37 Postpartum exercises.

Illustration continued on following page

Straight curl-up

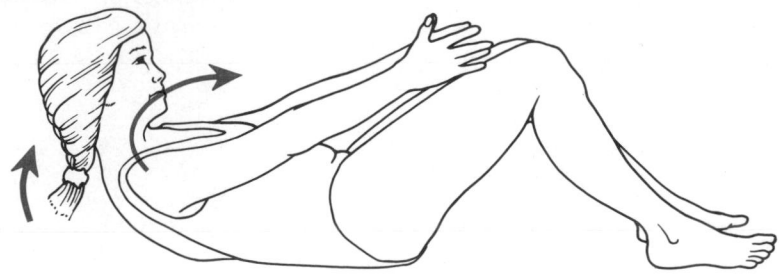

Diagonal curl-up

Heel slides

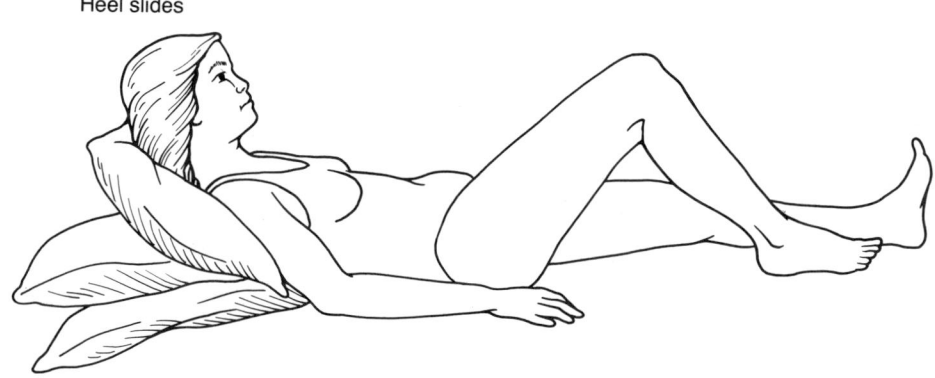

Pelvic tilt

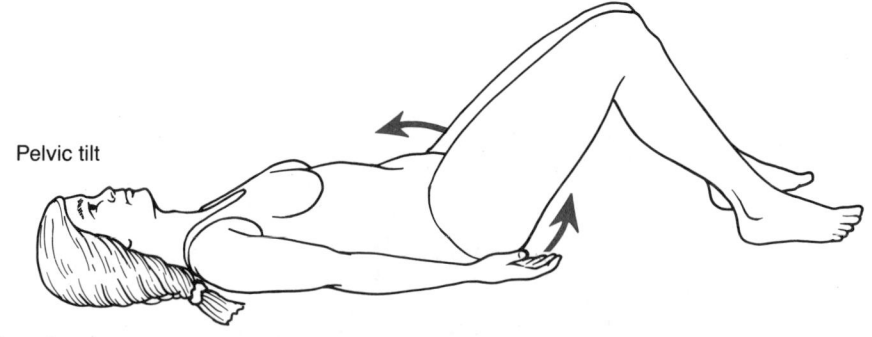

FIGURE 23–37   *(continued)*

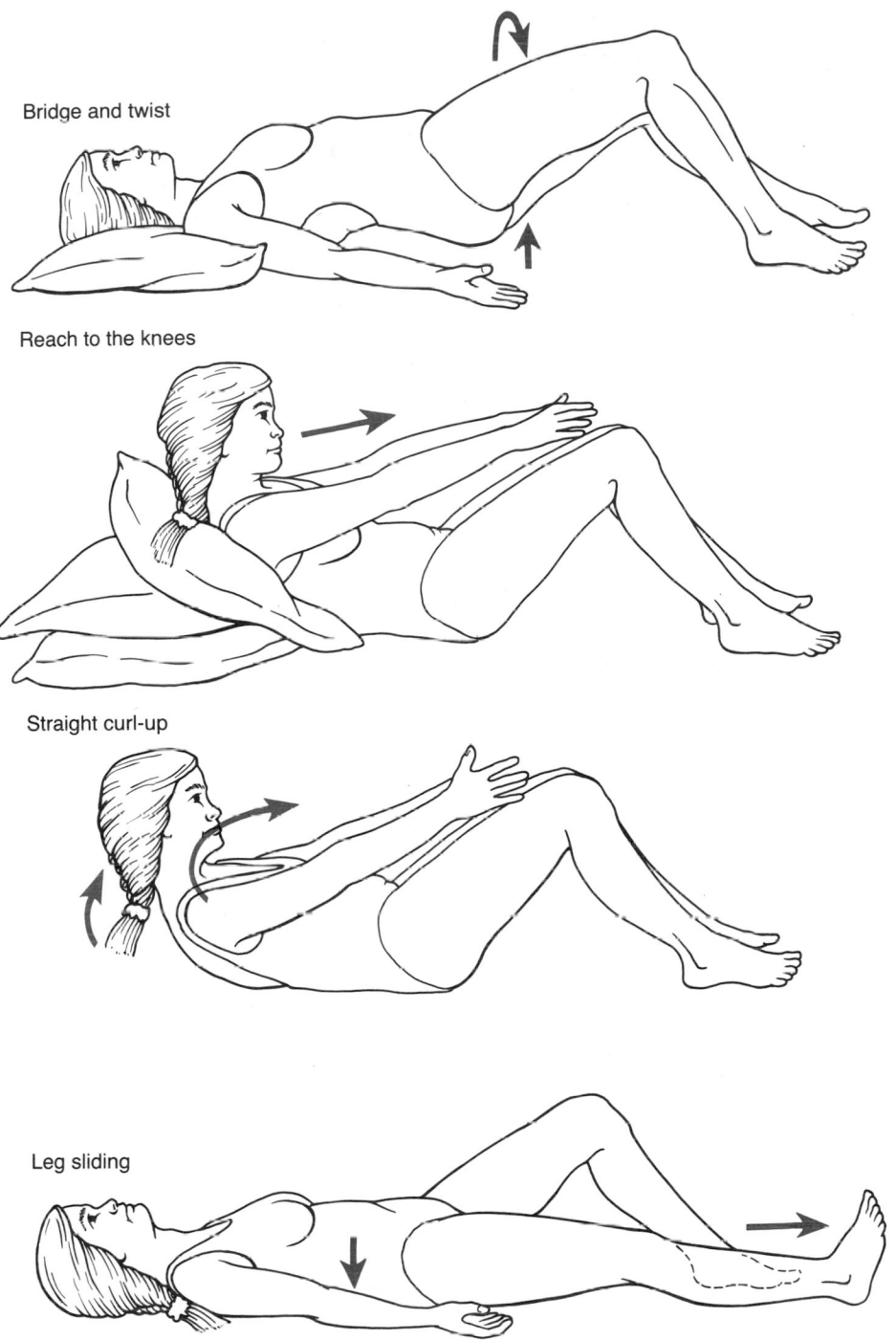

Bridge and twist

Reach to the knees

Straight curl-up

Leg sliding

FIGURE 23–37 *(continued)*

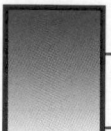

Clinical Decision-Making Cases

Case #1

EXAMINATION

History

The patient is a 30-year-old pregnant female (gravida 8, para 2) admitted to the hospital at 28⅔ weeks with preterm labor. Contractions were occurring every 2 minutes for 50 to 60 seconds.

Obstetric history: The patient has had seven previous pregnancies, resulting in one healthy full-term child, one healthy preterm child, loss of a twin pregnancy in the second trimester, and four spontaneous abortions.

Medical history: The patient has severe asthma, a mitral valve prolapse with mild mitral insufficiency, multiple sclerosis (MS) diagnosed 3 years previously, and a history of severe back pain.

Social history: The patient is married with two daughters, ages 6 and 8. She has stopped working outside the home owing to the effects of MS. She is a full-time homemaker who does a great deal of volunteer work for her church. She does not smoke, drink alcohol, or abuse recreational drugs.

Prior functional abilities: The patient ambulates with a cane "on good days," and she has also used a walker and wheelchair. Asthma and MS both limit her activity level. She has maintained her functional independence, however, and this remains one of her goals.

Medications: On admission—nortriptyline (Pamelor), prenatal vitamins, aspirin (81 g), oxycodone PRN, baclofen, flunisolide (Aerobid), ipratropium (Atrovent), terbutaline inhaler, heparin.

During hospital stay—terbutaline injections, magnesium sulfate, nifedipine, indomethacin (Indocin), furosemide (Lasix), clindamycin, gentamicin, aminophylline, methylprednisolone (Solu-Medrol), prednisone, theophylline (Theo-Dur), beclomethasone (Vanceril), and oxycodone plus acetaminophen (Percocet).

Physical Findings

Activity level: The patient is on bed rest as a treatment for her preterm labor and has been encouraged to spend as much time as possible in the left sidelying position. She is getting out of bed only to use the bedside commode.

Passive range of motion: Decreased by 25% in the lower extremities. Internal rotation of the hips at 10 degrees bilaterally.

Muscle strength/tone: 2/5 to 3/5 in both hips and knees; 1/5 to 2/5 in the ankles, with foot drop noted bilaterally. Spasticity affects both lower extremities.

Sensation: Normal for temperature; light and deep touch and sharp and dull sensation in upper extremities and left lower extremity. The right leg is reportedly numb and has reduced ability to discriminate light touch on occasion.

Mental status: Alert and oriented to person, place, and time. Able to carry on a conversation and answer questions appropriately but reports being unclear at times owing to drug interactions.

Transfers: After 1 week of bed rest, the patient required moderate assist of two for bed to commode transfer.

Gait: Not assessed owing to bed rest restrictions.

Pulmonary status: Oxygen saturation and pulse rate did not change with active assistive lower extremity exercise.

ASSESSMENT/DIAGNOSIS

The patient is a 30-year-old pregnant woman who has medical diagnoses of preterm labor, MS, and asthma. She also has mitral valve prolapse and a history of severe back pain. Physical therapy diagnoses include limitation of joint range of motion, weakness and spasticity, mildly impaired sensation, and mobility impairment secondary to MS and bed rest restrictions.

TREATMENT GOALS

1. Patient will have demonstrated knowledge of exercise program appropriate for pregnancy bed rest and will assist with this program as able.
2. Patient will have demonstrated knowledge of energy conservation and body mechanics, incorporating principles for pregnancy bed rest, asthma, and back pain.
3. Patient will have functional range of motion of the lower extremities.
4. Patient will maintain strength while on bed rest.
5. Patient will transfer bed to commode with assist of one.
6. After delivery of her child, patient will ambulate independently 25 feet with an assistive device. She will ascend and descend stairs with assist of one.
7. Within 2 months after delivery, patient will be safe

and independent with self-care, care of her infant, and ambulation with infant in a baby carrier.

OUTCOMES

After a 5-week regimen of therapeutic exercise and transfer training while on bed rest, the first five goals were met. The patient had a good understanding of her exercise program and the precautions associated with pregnancy bed rest, asthma, cardiac problem, and back pain. She was able to direct her husband in performance of her exercise program on the days therapy was not provided. Her range of motion increased to within normal limits. Strength did not further decrease. In 1 month, with instruction and practice (and a 2-week hiatus secondary to complete bed rest), she was able to transfer with assist of one.

Within 1 week of her child's birth, she was able to ambulate 30 feet using a rolling walker and wearing AFOs. She required moderate assist to ascend and descend stairs using a railing. With her child in a front pack, she was able to ambulate 5 feet with minimal to moderate assist using her assistive device.

After 2 months of twice-weekly outpatient therapy, the patient is independent in mobility on level surfaces and stairs. She has her own assistive device and custom AFOs. For long distances, she is investigating a scooter. She is able to perform self-care independently. She is caring for her infant and two other daughters. Family and friends assist with heavy household duties, as they did prior to admission. The patient is discharged from physical therapy with a home program, performing it in part independently and in part with assist of her husband.

Case #2

EXAMINATION

History

The patient is a 39-year-old female (gravida 3, para 1) pregnant with twins, admitted to the hospital at 38 weeks for induction of labor. After vaginal delivery of two healthy boys (7 lb, 8 oz and 8 lb, 3 oz, respectively), she was noted to have a large diastasis of the rectus abdominus. Referral to physical therapy was made 3 days postpartum.

Obstetric history: The patient has had a history of infertility and is now pregnant for the third time. Her first two pregnancies were achieved via in vitro fertilization, and the last via gamete intrafallopian transfer. She had one healthy full-term girl and one spontaneous abortion as a result of her first two pregnancies. This pregnancy has been uncomplicated from an obstetrical standpoint.

Medical history: The patient has no significant past medical history. She has had radiating pain to her right lower extremity during the final month of pregnancy. She was seeing a physical therapist on an outpatient basis for treatment.

Social history: The patient is married, has a 2-year-old daughter, and works full-time as a linguist. She will have part-time help at home after discharge. She does not smoke or use recreational drugs, and she did not drink alcohol during pregnancy or breastfeeding.

Prior functional status: The patient was independent in self-care and care of her daughter. Before her back became painful, she walked three times per week for aerobic exercise.

Medications: Oxytocin (Pitocin) to induce labor, and later oxycodone plus acetaminophen (Percocet) for pain.

Physical Findings

Mental status: The patient is cognitively alert and aware of her situation; she is able to carry on a conversation and assist with problem solving.

Active range of motion: Full in extremities, with the exception of hip flexion to 90 degrees bilaterally, abduction to 10 to 15 degrees, and hip rotation 10 degrees internally and 20 degrees externally. Abduction and rotation were slightly increased passively. By patient report, limitation is due to pain and not strength.

Muscle strength: Strength is grossly 4−/5 in lower extremities against midrange resistance. Upper extremities are 4/5. Trunk flexion is 2/5. She is able to perform one head lift and one pelvic tilt. Extension and rotation were not tested at this time.

Sensation: Patient reports pain at episiotomy site (which sustained a second-degree tear) and in back and leg during ambulation to the bathroom. No numbness or other sensory deficits noted. Overall, patient reports pain at a 3 to 6 level on a scale of 1 to 10.

Status of abdominal wall: Patient has a 10-cm diastasis measured 2 inches above the umbilicus and an 8-cm diastasis 2 inches below.

Bed mobility: The patient moves in bed independently but utilizes electronic bed controls and bed rails for support. She guards her trunk when shifting in bed or preparing to transfer.

Transfers/gait: The patient wears an abdominal binder when moving out of bed. She requires moderate assist to move from supine to standing. Gait is waddling and antalgic, with the patient preferring to lean on another person's arm for support. Maximal distance is 15 feet.

Child care: The patient is kyphotic during breast-feeding and is having neck pain during and after feeding her twins.

ASSESSMENT/DIAGNOSIS

The patient is a 39-year-old female with a medical diagnosis of postpartum mother, status post delivery of twins. Physical therapy diagnoses include diastasis of the rectus abdominus, impaired mobility secondary to back pain, weakness of trunk and extremities and decreased endurance, and impaired ability to breast-feed her infants secondary to neck pain.

TREATMENT GOALS

For completion during the hospital stay, the goals of treatment were:

1. Patient will be independent with home exercise program to reduce diastasis rectus and restore pelvic floor integrity.
2. Patient will have reduced back pain through positioning program and use of proper body mechanics for childcare.
3. Patient will have reduced or eliminated neck pain through exercise and use of proper body mechanics during breast-feeding.

For completion in 1 month:

4. Patient will participate in a walking program three times per week, including gentle stretching exercises to warm-up and cool-down.

OUTCOMES

The patient was seen five times during her hospital stay. She was instructed in head lifts with abdominal bracing, Kegel exercises, pelvic tilts, heel slides, and ankle circles. She was independent with these exercises and had a written copy to refer to if necessary. She was able to monitor her diastasis independently. At discharge, it had reduced to 7 cm.

A surgical consultation had been obtained the day before discharge. The surgeon noted a thinning of the linea alba but no actual herniation. He therefore felt that immediate surgery was not indicated. Recommendations included continuing to exercise, wearing a binder or a girdle for comfort and support during difficult activities, and reassessing the abdominal wall in 8 weeks.

The patient was instructed in a positioning program, including sidelying with pillow support for her back as well as using a pillow to elevate the infants when feeding them to reduce the need for flexing her neck to interact with them. She was also capable of problem solving the performance of household duties and childcare after an explanation of the principles of body mechanics. For her neck, she did chin tucks, forward neck rolls, and reverse shoulder circles. Her neck and back were feeling better, and she was transferring and ambulating independently, although her gait remained slow and slightly antalgic. Recommendations regarding beginning her walking program were made again.

After 1 month, her diastasis was reduced to 5.5 cm. She continued to exercise twice daily and was walking 30 minutes, three to four times weekly, usually wearing a girdle if her pace was rapid. Her back and neck pain were eliminated. She is pleased with her progress, and will follow up with her obstetrician and surgeon in 4 weeks.

References

1. Reeder SJ, Martin LL, Koniak D: *Maternity Nursing: Family, Newborn, and Women's Health Care,* 17th ed. Philadelphia, J. B. Lippincott Company, 1992.
2. Pansky B: *Review of Gross Anatomy,* 5th ed. New York, Macmillan, 1984.
3. O'Connor LJ, Gourley RJ: *Obstetric and Gynecologic Care in Physical Therapy.* Thorofare, NJ, Slack, Inc., 1990.
4. Williams PL, Warwick R, Dyson M: *Gray's Anatomy,* 37th ed. Edinburgh, Churchill Livingstone, 1989.
5. Cunningham FG, MacDonald PC, Grant NF: Williams Obstetrics, 19th ed. Norwalk, CT, Appleton & Lange, 1993, p 475.
6. Sand PK, Bowen LW, Ostergard DR: Urinary tract in pregnancy. In Ostergard DR (ed): *Gynecologic Urology and Urodynamics: Theory and Practice.* Baltimore, Williams & Wilkins, 1985, pp 283–298.
7. Lang RM, Borow KM: Heart disease. In Barron WM, Lindheimer MD (ed): *Medical Disorders During Pregnancy.* St. Louis, C. V. Mosby Company, 1991, pp 148–196.
8. MacLennan AH: Relaxin—a review. *Aust N Z J Obstet Gynaecol,* 1981, 21:195–202.
9. Bookhout MM, Boissonnault WG: Physical therapy management of musculoskeletal disorders during pregnancy. In Wilder E (ed): *Obstetric and Gynecologic Physical Therapy.* New York, Churchill Livingstone, 1988, pp 17–62.
10. Patterson CA, Lindsay MK: Maternal physiology in pregnancy. In Wilder E (ed): *Obstetric and Gynecologic Physical Therapy.* New York, Churchill Livingstone, 1988, pp 1–16.
11. Cartlidge, NEF: Neurologic disorders. In Barron WM, Lindheimer MD (ed): *Medical Disorders During Pregnancy.* St. Louis, C. V. Mosby Company, 1991, pp 508–533.
12. Noble E: *Essential Exercises for the Childbearing Year,* 3rd ed. Boston, Houghton Mifflin Company, 1988.
13. Duaphinee JD: Risk assessment. In Mandeville LK, Troiano NH: *High Risk Intrapartum Nursing.* Philadelphia, J. B. Lippincott Company, 1992, pp 31–39.

14. Cherry SH: The incompetent cervix. In Cherry SH, Berkowitz RL, Kase NG (eds): *Rovinsky and Guttmacher's Medical, Surgical, and Gynecologic Complications of Pregnancy*, 3rd ed. Baltimore, Williams & Wilkins, 1985, pp 702–705.

15. Pipp LM: The exercise dilemma: considerations and guidelines for treatment of the high risk obstetric patient. *J Obstet Gynecol Phys Ther*, 1989, 13:10–12.

16. Frahm J, Davis Y, Welch RA: Physical therapy management of the high risk antepartum patient: physical and occupational therapy treatment objectives and program—part III. *Clin Management Phys Ther*, 1989, 9:28–33.

17. Johnston SH, Kraut DA: *Pregnancy Bedrest: A Guide for the Pregnant Woman and Her Family*. New York, Henry Holt and Company, 1990.

18. Kotarinos RK: Diastasis recti and review of the abdominal wall. *J Obstet Gynecol Phys Ther*, 1990, 14:8–10.

19. Boissonnault JS, Kotarinos RK: Diastasis recti. In Wilder E (ed): *Obstetric and Gynecologic Physical Therapy*. New York, Churchill Livingstone, 1988, pp 63–82.

20. Boissonnault JS, Blaschak MJ: Incidence of diastasis recti abdominis during the childbearing year. *Phys Ther*, 1988, 68:1082–1086.

21. Pipp LM: Compendium of selected TENS literature. *J Obstet Gynecol Phys Ther*, 1993, 17:12.

22. Kahn J: Electrical modalities in obstetrics and gynecology. In Wilder E (ed): *Obstetric and Gynecologic Physical Therapy*. New York, Churchill Livingstone, 1988, pp 113–129.

23. Gent D, Gottlieb K: Cesarean rehabilitation. *Clin Management Phys Ther*, 1985, 5:14–19.

24. Brown G, et al.: Management of postoperative pain in obstetrical and gynecological procedures. *Obstet Gynecol*, 1983, 7:8–11.

PART SIX

Integumentary System

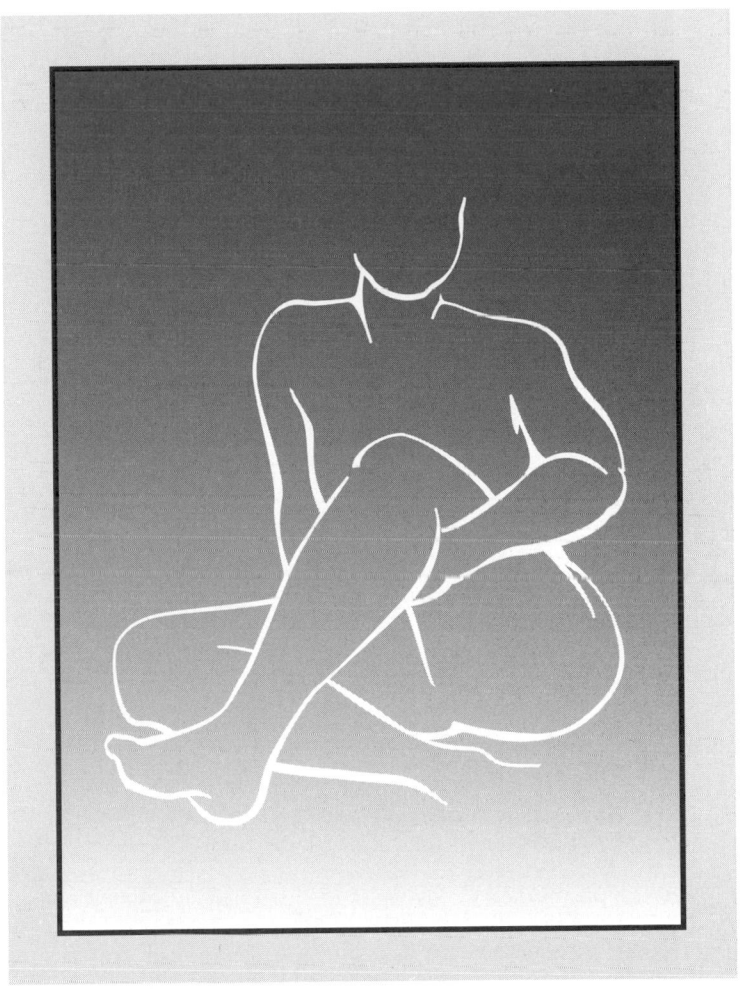

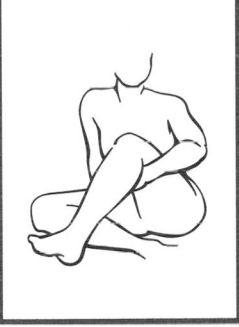

CHAPTER 24

Introduction: Anatomical and Physiological Considerations

Nancy Byl

I. Introduction

A. The skin

1. The skin is the largest organ in the body and is critical to health as it can provide insight into what may be happening in other body systems. It has many different functions.[1,2] For example, the skin
   a. Protects the underlying structures from external injury and harmful substances.
   b. Holds organs together.
   c. Contributes to fluid balance, mainly excreting fluid but also absorbing fluid.
   d. Controls temperature.
   e. Is an important organ of sensation.
   f. Absorbs ultraviolet radiation.
   g. Metabolizes vitamin D.
   h. Synthesizes epidermal lipids, which are an important protective barrier.
   i. Provides cosmesis for the body.
   j. Provides a mechanism for systemic and local drug delivery.
2. The range of disease processes that can either arise or involve the skin is large.
   a. Approximately one in every four to six patients who consults a general practitioner is likely to have a skin disorder.

b. Most patients with skin disorders can be managed as outpatients.
3. Although the physical therapist is rarely considered the primary caregiver in the management of patients with skin problems, all health care professionals should have a basic understanding of the skin and the diseases that affect it.
   a. Most commonly, therapists use the skin as a vehicle for
      (1). Facilitating motor control.
      (2). Managing pain.
      (3). Increasing extensibility.
      (4). Reducing unnecessary restrictions that might interfere with function.
      (5). Waking up the nervous system and maximizing cognitive drive.
   b. The first responsibility of the physical therapist is to be able to recognize when a serious integumentary problem exists and when a referral for care is needed.
   c. The therapist should also recognize common skin conditions that can be easily managed with common sense.
   d. The therapist should be familiar with the differences in skin at different locations

and common skin problems that occur at those sites.

e. The therapist must also understand the structure and function of the skin to be able to use the skin effectively to deliver drugs to the underlying tissues (*eg*, iontophoresis or phonophoresis).

f. The therapist must be prepared to work as part of the primary team for managing some skin problems (*eg*, nonhealing skin wounds, burns). This requires that the physical therapist be knowledgeable about the principles of healing: inflammation, repair, and remodeling.

II. Anatomical Considerations[2]

The layers of the skin are practically divided into the epidermis, dermis, and skin appendages, with the basement membrane between the dermis and the epidermis (see Figure 24–1).

A. Epidermis

The epidermis is derived from the fetal ectoderm.

1. The epidermis is the outer surface of the skin that lies on the dermis. It

a. Is thickest on the palms and soles and thinner elsewhere.
b. Is basically avascular.
c. Has a basement membrane under it, which attaches the basal cells of the epidermis to the connective tissue of the dermis.
d. Receives nutrients by diffusion of substances through the basement membrane of the underlying dermal capillaries.

2. The outermost portion of the integument is

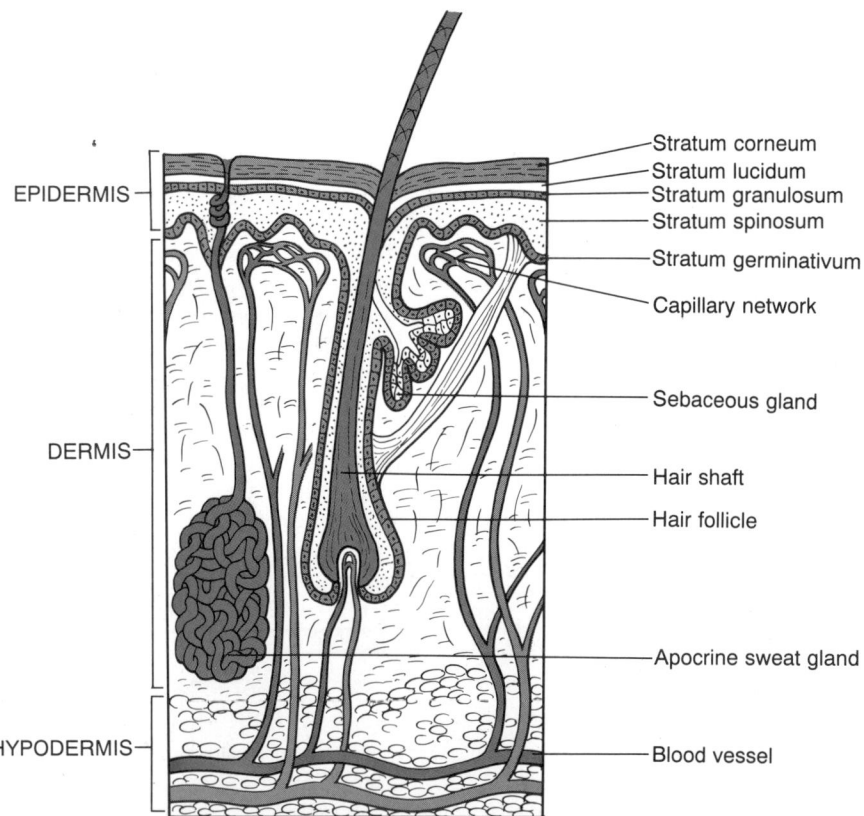

EPIDERMIS

DERMIS

HYPODERMIS

Stratum corneum
Stratum lucidum
Stratum granulosum
Stratum spinosum
Stratum germinativum
Capillary network
Sebaceous gland
Hair shaft
Hair follicle
Apocrine sweat gland
Blood vessel

FIGURE 24–1   Cross-sectional view of the human skin showing various skin tissue layers and appendages.

called the stratum corneum, the protective covering that

    a. Consists of layers of terminally differentiated keratinocytes embedded in a matrix of lipid bilayers.

    b. Serves as a barrier that prevents desiccation of the underlying tissues and excludes the entry of noxious substances from the environment.

        The production of this protective covering is the principal function of the living epidermis.

3. Four layers of the epidermis can be observed with a light microscope.

    a. The *cornified* layer is the stratum corneum, the zone where epidermal nuclei disintegrate and the production of which is the primary purpose of living epidermis.

    b. The *germinative* or *prickle cell* layer is composed of the bulk of the living epidermal keratinocytes.

    c. The *basal* layer is composed of the only keratinocytes in normal epidermis that undergo cell division.

    d. The *granular* layer is the most well protected.

4. The stratum corneum is neither continuous nor homogeneous.

    a. The fingertips, bottoms of the toes, and palmar and plantar surfaces of the hand display extensive systems of lines and ridges.

    b. Sweat pores and hairs penetrate through the stratum corneum.

    c. The cross sections of these pores are very small, and the outward movement of sweat or sebum tends to flush out substances that do not effectively penetrate the stratum corneum.

    d. Microscopically, the individual cells of the stratum corneum are roughly hexagonal and overlap at the edges with neighboring cells.

       (1). The projected area of the corneocytes varies slightly from one anatomical region to the other: least on the hands and heels and greatest in the axillary region. With age, there is an increase in the projected area of corneocytes.

       (2). The horn cells are thin and arranged in orderly stacks, with the edges of the stacked cells interdigitating.

       (3). At the dermoepidermal junction are the basal epidermal cells, which are small, vertically aligned, and roughly cuboidal.

       (4). Below the stratum corneum is the granular cell layer.

    e. Progressing from the basal layer to the stratum corneum, the cells become much flatter and wider. The stratum corneum often appears as a loosely woven and porous structure, but this is an artifact because the intact stratum corneum is a highly ordered structure.

    f. The cornification of skin varies by location.

       (1). On the inner upper arm there is a thin cornified layer and only three or four underlying layers of keratinocytes.

       (2). The keratinocyte layer of the sole of the foot is 20 to 30 cells thick.

       (3). In the younger population, cornification is usually regular, with much less evidence of the irregularity seen in older skin and on sun-exposed sites.

       (4). On chronically sun-exposed sites, chiefly the face, both the epidermis and the underlying dermis may show marked damage owing to accumulation of exposure to natural sunlight—so-called photoaging—which is seen clinically as thickened, wrinkled, furrowed skin.

       (5). Many of the alterations in the skin that we think of as aging are in fact due to ultraviolet-induced damage, and distinction should be made between photoaging, which is at least partially preventable, and chronological or biological aging.

5. Four different types of cells are in the epidermis: keratinocytes, melanocytes, Langerhans cells, and Merkel's cells.

    a. *Keratinocytes* (main cell type)

       (1). Keratins accumulate throughout epidermal differentiation and represent the major component of the stratum corneum as well as the epidermal appendages such as hair and nail.

       (2). In normal skin, keratinocyte division takes place only in the basal layer. After cell division, one daughter keratinocyte remains in the basal layer and the other moves upward through the epidermis.

(3). This cell is committed to terminal differentiation and death.

   (a). Thus, dead cells are constantly sloughed from the upper surface of the epidermis and are replaced by new cells.

   (b). The basal layer is the major source of cell renewal in the epidermis.

   (c). As a result of the proliferation of cells from the deeper layers, the cells move upward through the epidermis toward the surface, undergoing differentiation.

   (d). As differentiation proceeds, the cells become noticeably flatter; at this stage of differentiation, they are called granular cells.

(4). After a 2-week transit through the stratum corneum, corneocytes are sloughed off into the environment through the process called desquamation.

   (a). The mechanisms underlying desquamation are essentially unknown.

   (b). The factors determining the cohesion desquamation behavior of the stratum corneum are the subtle changes in the physical properties of the bilayer structure resulting from the loss of cholesteryl sulfate.

(5). Within the prickle cell layer, the keratinocytes are connected to each other by highly specialized cellular bridges or desmosomes, but there are no desmosomes between keratinocytes and melanocytes, Langerhans cells, or Merkel's cells.

(6). Hemidesmosomes are between the basal layer keratinocytes and the underlying basement membrane.

(7). Loss of function of these hemidesmosomes is important in some types of serious blistering diseases.

(8). On the granular layer, the living keratinocytes are involved in a complex series of biochemical changes during which the cell nuclei disinte-

grate, forming the granules seen in the cytoplasm.

   (a). Above this level, there is an anucleate stratum corneum.

   (b). This pattern of maturation of the epidermis is called orthokeratosis and there is an outer layer of non-nucleated cells.

   (c). In some mucosal sites, the normal maturation pattern is different and there is no granular layer.

   (d). With an outer layer of nucleated squamous cells, physiological parakeratosis occurs.

      (i). Pathological parakeratosis is seen in some diseases of the epidermis (*eg*, psoriasis).

      (ii). In this situation, the normal differentiation signals are either lacking or overridden and there is accelerated and imperfect development of the stratum corneum.

     (iii). If keratinocytes are connecting desmosomes, the outer layer is parakeratotic (as in psoriasis) rather than orthokeratotic (as in normal skin).

     (iv). It is calculated that the transit time for a daughter keratinocyte in the basal layer of normal skin to reach the outer surface is around 4 weeks. In psoriasis, this is reduced to only 4 days.

(9). The strength of the epidermis depends on the cohesion of the keratinocytes; they produce a structural protein, α-keratin, which aggregates to form tonofilaments.

   (a). These tonofilaments are continuous with the desmosomes and are easily seen with an electron microscope as large cytoplasmic bundles.

   (b). Until recently, it was believed that the major function of the epidermal keratinocyte was to produce tonofilaments.

(c). A secondary function of the tonofilament is the production of epidermal lipids, which contribute to the waterproofing function of the epidermis.

(d). The epidermal keratinocytes may produce relatively large amounts of immunological mediators.

(i). Thymus-activating factor (TAF) is structurally identical to interleukin 1. This material is synthesized in large quantities in normal keratinocytes and stored in the epidermis in a biologically inactive form.

(ii). After appropriate stimulation and release, TAF will induce synthesis of neutrophil chemotactic peptides and, therefore, may be of great importance in diseases associated with neutrophils in the epidermis, such as psoriasis and inflammatory fungal infection.

(iii). Cell adhesion also is of great current interest in understanding the interaction between cells in health and disease.

(iv). The intercellular adhesion molecule (ICAM) and the lymphocyte function antigen (LFA) act on the surfaces of two adjacent cells in a lock-and-key manner to hold the cells together.

(v). Keratinocytes in the epidermis can express ICAM, as in cutaneous, T-cell lymphoma.

(vi). In normal epidermis, the only cells that express the HLA-DR antigen are the Langerhans cells.

b. *Melanocytes* (found in basal layer)

(1). Pigment production in the skin is chiefly the function of the epidermal melanocytes, small cells with a clear halo around them.

(2). On facial skin, there may be as many as 1 melanocyte to every 5 basal layer keratinocytes; however, in the lower back skin, this ratio is usually closer to 1:20.

(3). Chronic light exposure increases the number of melanocytes relative to keratinocytes.

(4). Numbers of melanocytes are the same in equivalent body sites in white and black skin, but the rate of production of pigment and its distribution are different.

(5). Melanocytes synthesize the pigment melanin.

(a). Pigment is formed on premelanosomes catalyzed by the presence in the melanocyte of the enzymes dopa-oxidase and tyrosinase, which are not present in surrounding keratinocytes or other nonmelanocytic cells.

(b). Melanocytes are dendritic cells with an octopuslike shape: long dendritic processes stretch upward between suprabasal keratinocytes.

(c). This shape is best shown with a silver stain.

(d). Once the melanin granules are formed, they are distributed by these dendrites to surrounding keratinocytes.

(e). The combination of one pigment-producing melanocyte and several surrounding keratinocytes receiving melanin granules is termed the "epidermal melanin unit."

(f). Thus, the presence of melanin in a cell does not prove that the cell is a melanocyte.

(g). Melanocytes are found in humans in the greatest quantities in the epidermis, the hair bulb, the eye, and the brain and in very small numbers in other organs.

(i). The function of melanocytes in normal skin is thought to be to provide protection from ultraviolet radiation.

(ii). This appears to be reasonably effective in that sunlight-induced skin cancers of all types are rare in black skin but relatively common in white skin.

(6). Melanocytes are of particular interest because they give rise to the most serious type of skin cancer, malignant melanoma.

c. *Langerhans cells* (found in mid-dermis)

(1). No clearly defined function of these cells was understood when they were discovered.

(2). Today, the Langerhans cell is recognized as an important immunologically competent cell.

(3). Langerhans cells are derived from the circulating blood monocytes in the bone marrow and are found on all epidermal surfaces, usually in the mid-dermis.

(4). The bloodborne monocytes migrate into the epidermis and differentiate into Langerhans cells.

(5). The Langerhans cell is slightly larger than those around it, with a clear halo and no desmosomes.

(6). It is a dendritic cell, usually occurring in large numbers, with the dendrites of one cell in close contact with those of the next.

(7). They are the only cells to carry receptors.

(8). They are currently believed to be members of the family of immunologically important dendritic cells found in a number of body sites, including the lymph nodes and spleen.

(9). Dendritic cells capture cutaneous antigens and present them to lymphocytes in the initiation of an immune response.

(10). Their population in the epidermis is apparently constantly replenished by the bloodborne monocytes.

(11). The immunological profile of these dendritic cells suggests that they are similar to, but distinct from, macrophages and that they have the capacity to act as antigen-presenting cells.

(a). In the epidermis, which comes into contact with more foreign material than any other part of the body, this antigen-processing function is of great importance.

(b). Langerhans cells are therefore important in immunologically mediated inflammatory disease and are the cells involved in a relatively rare epidermal proliferative condition, histiocytosis X.

d. *Merkel's cells* (found mostly in basal layer)

(1). The Merkel cell appears to be an epithelial cell.

(2). A characteristic feature is the presence of many small, dense granules in their cytoplasm.

(3). Sensory nerve endings form expanded terminations in close approximation to the surface of Merkel's cells.

(4). Merkel's cells are present in relatively large numbers, particularly in sites such as the face and fingertips.

(a). They are thought to be involved with sensation and are often present in large numbers close to nerve endings.

(b). Merkel cell granules contain large quantities of catecholamines, a quality that they share with cells in other body sites.

(c). At present, the role of Merkel's cells in nonmalignant skin disease is not known.

B. The basement membrane

1. The epidermis is divided from the dermis by a complex multilayered structure called the basement membrane.

2. It has multiple layers, is not rigid, and is impervious to most substances; however, lymphocytes and Langerhans cells can traffic through it.

3. The basement membrane is important because it literally holds the skin together.

C. Dermis (mesodermal origin)

1. The three main cell types in the dermis are fibroblast, macrophage, and mast cell.
   a. Fibroblasts produce collagen.
   b. Macrophages act as general scavengers.
   c. The mast cell's exact role in normal dermal function is not yet well defined; it is an important cell in Type I immunological reactions and in interactions with the eosinophil.
2. The bulk of the dermis is composed of collagen (mainly three different types), with a fine network of elastin running through this collagen.
3. Dermal proteoglycans surround this fibrous material, and embedded within the dermis are vascular tissues, lymphatics, and nerves.
4. The outermost area of the dermis is not a flat, smooth area.
   a. It is composed of ridges and troughs with dermal papillae projecting upward and surrounded by the overlying epidermis.
   b. The papillary dermis is composed of finer collagen fibers than in the deeper area, the reticular dermis.
5. Blood supply to both the epidermis and the dermis is through a rich anastomosing superficial and deep plexus of small blood vessels.
   a. There is a large overcapacity of vessels in the dermal vasculature, normally operating only at 10% to 20% capacity.
   b. In certain physiological situations (eg, after vigorous circuit training or marathon running), heat loss via the skin is necessary and the vascular structure dilates appropriately.
   c. In a number of skin diseases, the blood supply to the skin is greatly increased, causing total body redness (erythroderma).
   d. The volume of blood flowing through the dilated dermal vessels in this situation can be so great that high-output cardiac failure results.
6. In normal skin, the lymphatic drainage system is not visible, but this also is a profuse network, running from the reticular dermis to the local lymph nodes.
7. Both free nerve endings and specialized receptors are seen in the dermis and are important for the sensation of touch, heat, cold, and proprioception.

D. The skin appendages (hair follicle, sebaceous gland, apocrine sweat gland, eccrine sweat gland)

1. The skin appendages are composed of a combination of cells derived from fetal ectoderm and mesoderm.
2. Subcutaneous fat may be involved in deeply situated skin lesions such as erythema nodosum.
3. The primary skin appendages are the pilosebaceous unit and the eccrine sweat glands.
   a. The pilosebaceous unit comprises the hair follicles, sebaceous glands, erector pili muscles, and, in some sites, the apocrine glands.
   b. On the scalp, the predominant structure is the hair follicle, with the sebaceous gland seen as a small, insignificant attachment.
   c. A small strip of smooth muscles, the erector pili, may often be seen around a lobule of sebaceous gland.
   d. In the axilla, the apocrine glands also may be seen draining into the duct leading to the surface.
4. The hair follicle is composed of a down growth of fetal ectoderm that will form the hair shaft and the hair bulb papilla, which is derived from fetal mesoderm.
   a. This papilla is vascular.
   b. The hair shaft itself is a complex multilayered structure with an outer cortex and an inner medulla.
   c. There are three recognizable types of hair: the coarse terminal hair of the scalp; the androgen-dependent terminal hair on the male chin and in the axilla and pubic region; and the fine growth of downy vellous hair on all body sites.
   d. The control of growth of scalp hair is complex.
5. Sebaceous glands are clusters of cells with a small dark nucleus and a foamy cytoplasm, which are well illustrated.
   a. These glands cluster around the hair shafts, and their secretion is formed by total destruction of the cells (holocrine secretion).
   b. The secretion drains into the hair follicle and is discharged on the surface through the hair follicle opening.
   c. Sebaceous glands are seen in large numbers on the face, chest, and upper back.

(1). They may be obvious as small, raised pearly nodules on the face of neonates when their enlargement is due to carryover of maternal hormones.

(2). They rapidly shrink and become vestigial until puberty when, in response to the individual's hormones, they become large and active, sometimes overactive, leading to the problem of acne vulgaris.

6. The apocrine sweat glands are predominately found in the axilla, with a few seen in the skin of the groin.

7. Eccrine sweat glands are seen on all body sites and are anatomically independent from the other appendages.

8. Nails could be regarded as highly modified skin appendages. The nail itself, or nail plate, grows out from the nail matrix and rests on the underlying nail bed.
   a. The pale halo at the proximal end of the nail is called the lunula, and the rim around the edge is protective cuticle.
   b. Nails often become involved in a number of skin diseases (*eg*, psoriasis and fungal infections).

E. The skin as an immune system

1. For some time, dermatologists and immunologists have suggested that there may be an epidermal equivalent of the gut-associated lymphoid tissue (GALT) found in the intestinal tract.

2. The concept of a skin immune system is much more credible.
   a. Epidermal keratinocytes can produce cytokines and other immunological mediators.
   b. Langerhans cells express immunologically relevant antigens.
   c. The above suggest that at least these two cell types have immunological capacity.
   d. Work is in progress to define the signals that activate the immunological functions of these two cell types and the skin diseases in which this aspect of the function of the epidermis is faulty.

III. Physiological Considerations

A. Electrical properties of the skin

1. Historically, people have been fascinated by the interaction of living organisms and electricity. As humans developed devices capable of measuring this current, renewed interest occurred.

2. The cellular basis of steady current has been established[3] (see Figure 24–2).
   a. Gradients are maintained across the plasma cell membrane at the expense of cellular energy.
   b. The basis of electrical excitability is the functioning of voltage-gated sodium channels.[4]
   c. The membrane potential is largely a potassium diffusion potential and leakiness to ions other than potassium compensated by various ionic pumps (*eg*, Na^+, K^+-ATPase).
   d. Virtually all cells have a negative membrane potential (the cytoplasm is electrically negative with respect to the surrounding medium), and the physiologically important ions are maintained in nonequilibrium across the plasma membrane.
      (1). The equilibrium potentials are normally tens of millivolts (mV) negative.
      (2). All cells have a measurable resting sodium permeability, allowing sodium to leak continuously into cells.
      (3). Calcium is generally further from equilibrium than sodium.
      (4). Potassium, chloride, and hydrogen ions are all out of equilibrium in the resting state of a typical cell.

3. Numerous instances of long-lasting, steady electrical currents whose polarity is associated with the morphological polarity of a developing or growing system have been reported.[5]
   a. Currents last for minutes, hours, or even days.
   b. Currents may be effectors of morphological polarity.
   c. Ion movement in and out of a cell will change the electrical state of the cell.

d. Steady currents are typically a few microamperes per centimeters squared ($\mu A/cm^2$), whereas currents during action are measured in milliamperes per centimeters squared (mA/cm^2).

e. The physiological basis of the steady currents is thought to be the regional differences in the concentration of gating substances.[6,7]

   (1). The steady current can be a result of reduced chloride conductance in the end-plate region.

   (2). Current refers to the intracellular movement of the positive charges toward the end-plate region from the flanking region in the muscle cell.

   (3). The resting membrane potential in the end-plate region is more negative than elsewhere.

   (4). Betz *et al.* and Caldwell *et al.*[6,7] estimated the steady current to be a difference of a few tenths of a millivolt on the basis of Ohm's law, and this steady current persists following denervation.

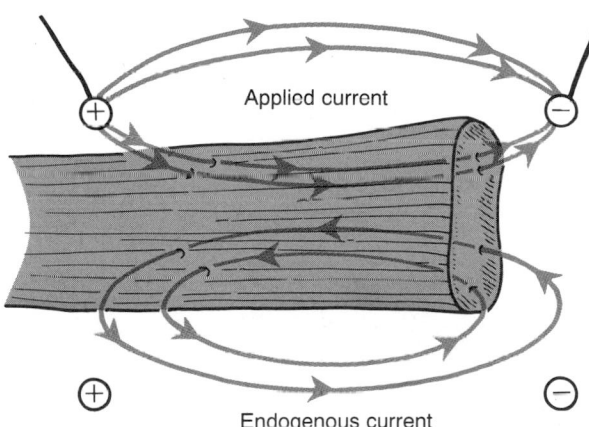

FIGURE 24-2 Polarity of endogenous and applied voltage gradients (and current flow) at the tip of a severed axon. The endogenous injury current (lower portion of the axon) shows that current enters the cut tip and flows in a distal-proximal direction inside the axon. As shown in the upper part of the drawing, an applied extracellular voltage (from a distally negative electrode pair) is of the same polarity as the extracellular component of the endogenous current; however, the applied current would penetrate the axon (because of its lowered input impedance near the cut tip), producing current flow in the reverse direction (proximal-distal) inside the axoplasm. (Redrawn from Borgens RB, Robinson KK, Vanable JW, McGinnis ME: *Electric Fields in Vertebrate Repair: Natural and Applied Voltages in Vertebrate Regeneration and Healing.* New York, Alan R. Liss, 1990, p 93, ©1990 Alan R. Liss; reprinted by permission of Wiley-Liss, a division of John Wiley and Sons, Inc.)

f. Significance of steady currents:

   (1). In salamanders, which can regenerate their limbs, the stump tip is always positive with respect to the undamaged, more proximal part of the forelimb.[5]

     (a). Potentials decline steadily after amputation over 46 days of measurement.

     (b). Distally positive surface voltages suggest that current might leave the stump end and complete its circuit by returning to the undamaged portion of the extremity.

   (2). Very weak currents were found to enter the surface of most of the proximal limb stumps (order of ~1 $\mu A/cm^2$).[8–11]

     (a). The currents are driven by the transepidermal potential (TEP).

     (b). This phenomenon was found not only in amphibians but in most vertebrates as well as humans.

     (c). Skin batteries are internally positive by about 40 to 80 mV.

       (i). Voltage is usually associated with an inwardly directed active pumping of sodium across the integument from outside to inside.

       (ii). If sodium is reduced, a proportional decrease in the potential is measured across the skin. If sodium is raised in the outside medium, the TEP is likewise increased.

   (3). Nonregenerating adult frogs drive a weak current out the end of the limb stump.

   (4). When electrical fields within the core stump tissues of the adult frog are enhanced by implanted batteries and electrodes, the measure of limb regeneration is initiated.

   (5). Steady current appears to predict the exact locus of limb-bud formation in frog and salamander larvae.

     (a). The current declines in magnitude as the bud becomes increasingly more prominent.

(b). Just prior to differentiation, the current reverses its direction.

(6). Developmental currents and fields are thought to exert their influence on nervous tissue and/or the wound epidermis (in regenerating limbs) and on migratory mesenchymal cells.

4. **Integumentary potential and wound healing**

a. The role of epidermally generated electrical potentials in the healing of vertebrate skin is not well understood.

b. The existence of wound currents has been recognized for more than 200 years.[8,12,13]

(1). In human skin immersed in saline, about 1 μA of current leaves a wound.

(2). Illingworth and Barker[13] measured

currents with densities from 10 to 30 μA/cm^2 leaving the stump surface of children's fingers whose tips had been accidentally amputated.

c. The electromotive force driving currents from wounds made in the skin is the TEP actively maintained by the epidermis.

d. Lateral fields in the vicinity of wounds:

(1). A wound in the skin creates an electrical leak that short-circuits the epidermal battery, allowing current to flow out of the wound (as long as the wound is not allowed to dry) (see Figure 24–3).

(2). The potential drop from outside the wound to inside is relatively low, but there is a steep gradient on either side of the wound.

(a). In amphibians—the epidermis

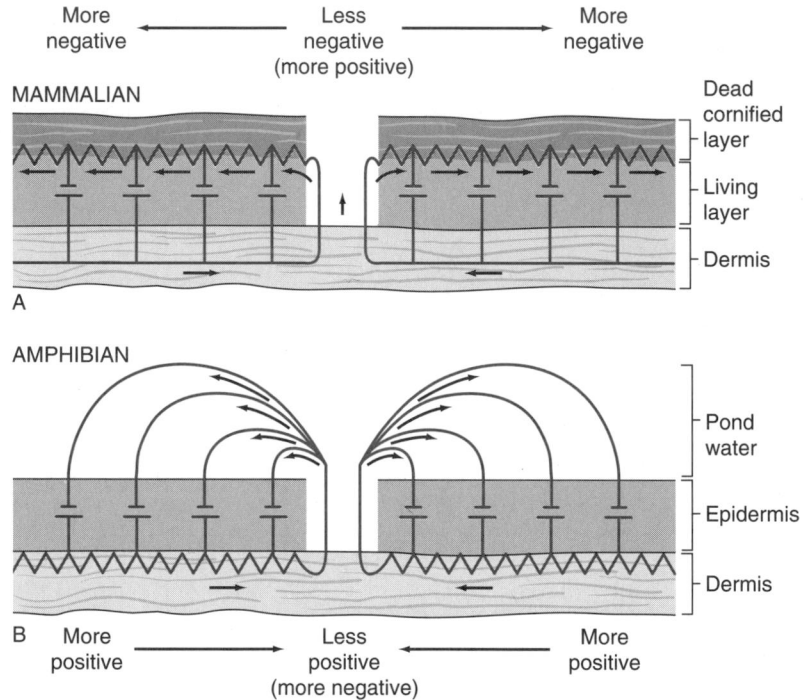

FIGURE 24–3 Comparison of the locus of the major lateral potential in mammalian and amphibian skin. **A,** Mammalian skin. A steep lateral potential develops in the high-resistance space between the living and dead cornified layers of the epidermis. This space is on the return path of the current from the wound to the epidermal battery, in which the current (positive charge) is moving, as it must, from more positive to less positive regions. In this path, then, points close to the wound are more positive than points away from the wound. **B,** Amphibian skin (and possibly mammalian cornea and oral epithelium as well as skin that is kept moist by an occlusive dressing). The dead cornified layer is thin and moist (and is ignored in the diagram) and is not a significant barrier to the movement of sodium ions into the epidermal cells. The water bathing the outer surface of the epithelium provides a low-resistance path for the return of the wound current to the epidermal battery. Here, the significant locus of lateral potential drop is subepidermal, where the current flows from the epidermal battery toward the wound, again from more positive to less positive regions. In this path, the points close to the wound are less positive (more negative) than points at a distance from the wound. (Panels A and B redrawn from Borgens RB, Robinson KK, Vanable JW, McGinnis ME: *Electric Fields in Vertebrate Repair: Natural and Applied Voltages in Vertebrate Regeneration and Healing.* New York, Alan R. Liss, 1990, p 193, ©1990 Alan R. Liss; reprinted by permission of Wiley-Liss, a division of John Wiley and Sons, Inc.)

has a lateral field, but it is opposite in polarity to that of mammalians.[14–16]

(b). In mammals—superficial epidermal cells at the edge of the wound are more negative, whereas the middle of the wound is more positive. In the deeper epidermal layer, the field is weaker and the current flows in the opposite direction (see Figure 24–3).

(3). As the distance to either side of the wound increases, the potential across the skin is found to be greater and greater until a point is reached (a few millimeters from the wound) where the potential across the skin is the full value normally found in unwounded regions of that skin.

(a). This lateral field occurs in the first 0.5 mm of skin bordering the wound.

(b). If the wound is allowed to dry, the wound resistance increases and blocks the flow of currents (eliminating the lateral potential drop at the edge of the wound).[8]

e. *In vitro* effect of electrical fields on cells:

(1). *Effect on fibroblasts*

(a). In mammalian wounds, the electrical fields exceeded 100 mV/mm.[17]

(b). Erickson and Nuccitelli[18] found that embryonic quail somite fibroblasts migrate to the cathode in fields with modest strengths.

(c). At field strengths as low as 1 mV/mm, they could just barely detect the movement.

(d). At field strengths of 50 to 100 mV/mm, the fibroblasts moved more directly toward the cathode.

(e). At field strengths of 100 to 150 mV/mm and above, the fibroblasts aligned perpendicularly to the field in addition to moving toward the cathode.

(2). *Effect on macrophages*

(a). Orida and Feldman[19] reported that macrophages migrated preferentially toward the anode after 30 minutes in *high*-strength fields.

(b). Further studies found macrophages somewhat less responsive to electrical fields than other cells.

(c). During an inflammatory reaction, the cells (probably activated macrophages in a low-strength field) aggregated preferentially to the cathode.

(3). *Effect on capillary permeability*

(a). Nannmaker *et al.*[20] reported increased capillary permeability to macromolecules and leukocytes with electrical fields.

(b). The intensity of the current needed to increase permeability may be a minimum of 5 μA.

f. Clinical trials using electrical current for wound healing:

(1). Generally, the reports on the use of electrical current to promote wound healing are positive.

(2). However, three somewhat negative reports were found in the literature on the effect of applied currents on wound healing (see Table 24–1).[21–23]

(3). The negative findings may be explained by the following:

(a). Small-needle electrodes increased the density of the current, potentially causing tissue damage rather than repair.

(b). Stainless steel and platinum wires create negative ions under the electrode, which are caustic.

(c). Open wounds are vulnerable to infection.

(4). Most of the clinical trials showed positive effects of electrical fields and wound healing (see more detailed review in Chapter 27).

(a). Most of the experiments on electrical fields and wound healing have been carried out in humans.

(b). Control subjects were evidenced in only a few studies.

(c). Studies carried out in animals were generally well controlled.

(d). Three protocols were most commonly used:

(i). The cathode was placed in the wound.

Table 24–1. SUMMARY OF CLINICAL STUDIES ON ELECTRICITY AND WOUND HEALING: NEGATIVE RESULTS

Researchers	Methods	Findings
Carey and Lepley[21]	Needle electrodes supplied 200–300 μA; treated for 2, 3, and 4 days 4-cm full-thickness wounds in rabbits	No healing at anode or cathode Anode: necrosis observed Scarcity of inflammatory cells noted where cathode implanted
Wu et al.[22]	Healing in the rectus abdominis muscle and parietal peritoneum Stainless steel wire or 30 platinum wire connecting one wound to the positive and the other to the negative terminal of a battery 40, 80, or 400 μA of current passed for 7 d	No differences in tensile strength No necrosis
Steckel et al.[23]	Full-thickness skin wounds 1.5 cm² or 2 cm² Currents of 10 or 20 μA Stainless steel electrodes Treatment—4 wk Anode threaded in wound and cathode imbedded in subcutaneous tissue in center of wound Wound not bandaged Wound cleansed every 2 d	Wounds with electrodes (with or without current) healed most slowly ES stimulated vs ES sham stimulated healed the same All wounds with electrode infected

Abbreviations: ES = electrical stimulation.

(ii). The anode was used throughout.

(iii). First the cathode and then the anode were placed in the wound.

(5). Cautions in the use of electrical currents in wounds:

(a). Avoid metallic ion contamination with the salt bridge connecting the battery to the wound.[24,25]

(b). Copper and silver ions could be deleterious to normal cell activity as ions have been measured in the skin under a silver electrode.

(c). If using a needle electrode, place it over gauze-soaked saline.

(d). The geometry and size of the electrode need to be matched to the wound.

(i). Promotion of epithelialization is not as effective with a large electrode as with a small electrode that occupies a relatively small fraction of the wound bed (in the center of a wound).

(ii). When the whole wound is covered by the electrode, the wound reaches an isopotential.[11]

(iii). A smaller electrode placed in the center of the wound produces an electrical field between the edge and the center of the wound along which the epithelial cells could migrate.

5. **Summary: electrical currents and wound healing**

a. There is much to be done before it can be said that a solid theoretical and practical understanding exists for the role of electrical fields in wound healing. Without such understanding, it is unlikely that the full potential of this approach to promoting wound healing will be achieved.

b. The epidermis of the skin acts as a battery.

(1). Sodium ions are inwardly transported to generate a TEP of about 7 mV.

(2). Wounding of the epidermis causes the TEP to provide an electromotive force to drive a steady current through the low-resistance path provided by the wound.

(3). The steady current continues as long as the wound is hydrated or until epithelialization covers the wound.

(4). In the vicinity of such wounds, steady lateral electrical fields of 100 mV/mm or more can be measured.

c. Cells in culture respond to imposed electrical fields of about 10 mV/mm or more by moving preferentially toward one pole or another.

(1). Epidermal cells and fibroblasts move to the cathode.

(2). Macrophages migrate to the anode in moderate to high electrical fields and move to the cathode in low fields or when there is an inflammatory reaction.

(3). Electrical fields imposed across capillary beds have the effect of increasing the permeability of the capillaries to macromolecules and leukocytes.

d. Lateral fields in the vicinity of mammalian wounds could affect certain aspects of wound healing if the wound is hydrated.

(1). Lateral fields promote cell migration during the inflammatory phase (leukocytes and macrophages) and fibroplasia and neoangiogenesis during epithelialization.

(2). Lateral fields could increase the permeability of local capillaries, helping to augment the supply of cells to the wound for repair.

(3). The epidermal cells closest to the lateral fields in a hydrated wound will migrate the earliest to cover the wound.

(4). Because wound contraction and collagen remodeling occur after the completion of epithelialization, they are probably not significantly affected by the electrical fields.

e. When epithelialization is delayed (as in nonsutured wounds), the strength of healing is enhanced.

f. The healing of amphibian wounds is delayed or prevented when the skin's battery is prevented from generating a TEP.

g. The healing of mammalian wounds may be promoted by the imposition of electrical fields. However, different polarities of field have been reported to be effective.

h. Further studies are needed with model systems, cell cultures, vertebrates, amphibians, and humans to clarify the parameters of current needed to facilitate wound healing.

References

1. MacKie RM: Clinical Dermatology: An Illustrated Textbook, 3rd ed. New York, Oxford University Press, 1991.
2. Murphy GF, Kwan TH, Mihm MC: The skin. In Robbins SL, Cotran RS, Jumar V (eds): Robbins Pathologic Basis of Disease, 4th ed. Philadelphia, W. B. Saunders Company, 1984, pp 1273–1301.
3. Robinson KR: Endogenous and applied electrical currents: their measurement and application. In Borgens RB, Robinson KR, Vanable JW, et al. (eds): Electric Fields in Vertebrate Repair. New York, Alan R. Liss, 1989, pp 1–23.
4. Salkoff L, Butler A, Wei A, et al.: Molecular biology of the sodium channel. Trends Neurosci 1987, 20:522–527.
5. Robinson KR: Electrical currents through full-grown and maturing Xenopus oocytes. Proc Natl Acad Sci USA 1979, 76:837–841.
6. Betz WJ, Caldwell JH, Kinnamon SC: Physiological basis of a steady endogenous current in rat lumbrical muscle. J Gen Physiol 1984, 83:175–192.
7. Caldwell J, Hand D, Betz WJ: Properties of an endogenous steady current in rat muscle. J Gen Physiol 1984, 83:157–173.
8. Barker AT, Jaffe LF, Vanable JW: The glabrous epidermis of cavies contains a powerful battery. Am J Physiol 1982, 242:R358–R366.
9. Herlitzka A: 1910 Ein Beitrag zur Physiologie der Generation. Wilhelm Roux Arch 1929, 10:126–158.
10. Kirschner LB, Kirshner LB: Electrolyte transport across the body surface of freshwater fish and amphibia. In Ussing HH, Thorn NA (eds): Transport Mechanisms in Epithelia. Copenhagen, Munksgaard, 1973, pp 447–460.
11. Vanable JW: Integumentary potentials and wound healing. In Borgens RB, Robinson KR, Vanable JW, et al. (eds): Electric Fields in Vertebrate Repair. New York, Alan R. Liss, 1989, pp 171–214.
12. Jaffe LF, Vanable JW: Electric fields and wound healing. Clin Dermatol 1984, 2:34–44.
13. Illingworth CM, Barker AT: Measurement of electrical currents emerging during the regeneration of amputated finger tips in children. Clin Phys Physiol Meas 1980, 1:87–89.
14. Becker RO: The bioelectric factors in amphibian limb regeneration. J Bone Joint Surg 1962, 43A:643–656.
15. Lassalle B: Surface potentials and the control of amphibian limb regeneration. J Embryol Exp Morphol 1979, 543:213–223.
16. Rose SM, Rose FC: Electrical studies on normally regenerating and on denervated strips of skin. Growth 1979, 38:363–380.
17. Nuccitelli R, Erickson CA: Embryonic cell motility can be guided by physiological electrical fields. Exp Cell Res 1983, 147:195–201.
18. Erickson CA, Nuccitelli R: Embryonic fibroblast motility and orientation can be influenced by physiological electric fields. J Cell Biol 1984, 98:296–307.
19. Orida N, Feldman JD: Directional protrusive pseudopodial activity and motility in macrophages induced by extracellular electric fields. Cell Motil 1982, 2:254–255.
20. Nannmaker U, Buch F, Albrektsson T: Vascular reactions during electrical stimulation. Vital microscopy of the hamster cheek pouch and the rabbit tibia. Acta Orthop Scand 1985, 56:52–56.

21. Carey LC, Lepley D Jr: Effect of continuous direct current on healing wounds. *Surg Forum* 1962, 13:33–35.

22. Wu T, Go N, Dennis C, *et al.*: Effects of electrical currents and interfacial potentials on wound healing. *J Surg Res* 1967, 7:122–128.

23. Steckel RR, Page EH, Geddes LA, Van Vleet JF: Electrical stimulation on skin wound healing in the horse: preliminary studies. *Am J Vet Res* 1984, 45:800–803.

24. Alvarez AM, Mertz DM, Smerkeck RO, Eaglston WH: The healing of superficial skin wounds is stimulated by external electric current. *Invest Dermatol* 1983, 81:144–148.

25. Berger TJ, Spadaro JA, Chapin SE, Becker RO: Electrically generated silver ions: quantitative effects on bacterial and mammalian cells. *Antimicrob Agents Chemother* 1976, 9:357–358.

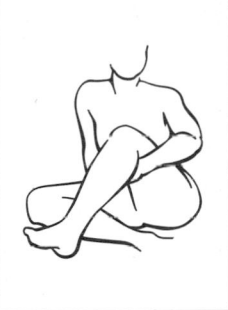

CHAPTER 25

Integumentary System Screening, Examination, and Assessment

Nancy Byl and Lucinda A. Pfalzer

I. Screening, Evaluation, and Assessment[1,2]

A. Screening for common skin lesions: age-dependent factors

1. Infants are usually brought to the physician for birthmarks, hereditary skin conditions, or infantile eczema.
2. Children are brought to the physician because of pruritic skin conditions (*eg*, atopic dermatitis) or skin infections (*eg*, warts, impetigo, scabies).
3. Teenagers go to the physician for acne vulgaris, cosmetic conditions, or skin lesions in the genital region (raising fear of venereal disease).
4. Adults most often seek medical advice when skin lesions occur on uncovered parts of the body, for unsightly lesions, if a lesion ex-

tends over one large area of the body, if a lesion is associated with severe inflammation or pruritus, or if the lesion appears to be sexually transmitted.

5. Elderly individuals have increasing problems with dry skin and adverse environmental effects (*eg*, chronic actinic skin lesions and irritant dermatitis) as well as skin tumors.

B. History and evaluation of the skin

1. The complete history and evaluation of a patient's skin should be done by a dermatologist, but the physical therapist should know some basic assessment principles when a skin problem develops in a client.

559

a. The family history may uncover heredity patterns for certain skin diseases (*eg*, atopic eczema, psoriasis).
   (1). Diabetes may predispose patients to skin conditions, (*eg*, infections such as candidosis or nonhealing wounds).
   (2). Hay fever, eczema, and allergies may be common in some families.
b. An infectious disease may have been transmitted (*eg*, lice, scabies).
c. Some skin diseases develop simultaneously in the skin and viscera (*eg*, systemic lupus erythematosus, leukemia, and scleroderma).
d. A new rash associated with a headache or a stiff neck should raise concerns about an acute infectious condition (*eg*, viral or bacterial meningitis).
e. The physical therapist should
   (1). Note the area of the lesion, when the lesion started, and the cause, including living conditions, type of work, and potential harmful agents at the workplace (*eg*, sunlight, heat, cold, cosmetics, deodorants, detergents, chemicals).
   (2). Evaluate the allergic component (*eg*, foods, animals, environmental factors in disorders such as atopic dermatitis and infectious diseases such as mycoses).
   (3). Check whether the patient has any symptoms besides the skin lesion.
   (4). Inquire about
      (a). What the rash/lesion looks like.
      (b). How it spread.
      (c). What the symptoms are (itching, burning, tingling, crawling sensation, or loss of sensation).
      (d). Systemic effects related to drugs (addictive or necessary for acute or chronic conditions) or food (tending to induce symmetrical lesions).
      (e). Seasonal factors (*eg*, certain skin disorders caused by light are more common in the spring and summer, whereas dermatoses and impaired capillary circulation are more likely to occur in the winter).
      (f). Time of month and menstrual cycle should be noted (dermatoses can develop during pregnancy).
      (g). Previous skin disorders (some infections from childhood are unlikely to occur twice and others are likely to recur; some infections may be a sign of other problems).
      (h). The duration of the current skin disorder (some diseases last for years and others are brief).
      (i). Whether the lesion causes itching.
      (j). Use of new and old drugs and how long the patient has been using the drugs.
         (i). Check past tolerances.
         (ii). Inquire about common drugs like oral contraceptives, laxatives, analgesics, and tranquilizers.

C. The physical examination

The physical examination requires inspection of the skin, including the mouth, as well as palpation of lymph nodes.
1. The entire skin should be inspected under good lighting.
2. An orderly sequence should be followed: hair, scalp, nails, buccal mucosa, skin surface.
3. General appearance is noted: temperature, moisture, dryness, skin texture.
4. The distribution and grouping of the lesions are evaluated, especially comparing the right and left side.
5. The shape, border, color, texture, and surface of the lesions are noted, and these areas are palpated.
6. The sizes of the lesions are measured.
7. If an arterial obstructive disease is suspected, the pulses are palpated.
8. Frequently, in the physical examination, other lesions will be found that the patient was not aware of (*eg*, suspicious mole or malignant melanoma).
9. When examining black skin, the physical therapist should
   a. Stretch the skin gently to decrease the reddish tone.
   b. Try to make the rash stand out from the surrounding skin.
10. Palpate for lymph nodes; take the patient's temperature; note erythema; palpate over the skin to feel the borders, skin tempera-

ture, and hardness; and observe for possible cyanosis, inspecting for a purplish-gray cast.

D. Tests and measurements

The physical examination is often accompanied by tests and specific measurements.
1. Special laboratory tests (*eg*, when suspicious of allergies; bacteriological, mycological, or virological microorganisms; autoimmune diseases; or impairments of arterial, venous, or lymphatic circulation).
2. Excising or scraping of lesions (to obtain a histological confirmation of the diagnosis, *eg*, fungus).
3. Wood's light examination (the long-wave ultraviolet light produced induces visible fluorescence in certain skin lesions).
4. Skin biopsy.
5. Patch testing (to document contact sensitivity or allergy).
6. Tzanck's smear (to evaluate blistering diseases).
7. Pustule smear.
8. Clinical photographs (to take measurements before and after treatment).
9. Depth measurements (to determine how extensive the lesion is).
10. Planimeter measurement (to measure the circumference of the wound).

E. Common skin disorders that occur by site and function

1. Different areas of the skin are subject to different disorders.
   a. The scalp is subject to specific disorders of the hair follicles.
   b. Areas rich in sebaceous glands (*ie*, face and back) are common sites for acne.
   c. The thickness of the stratum corneum and the sweat glands in the palms of the hands and the soles of the feet, which are the only sites of dyshidrosis and dyshidrosiform eruptions, can be effectively treated with galvanic stimulation.
   d. Commonly exposed areas on the extremities and areas where clothes rub another type of skin are usually responsive to physical agents, *eg*, ultraviolet light.
   e. The apocrine glands, which are in the axillae and around the areolae of the breasts, mons pubis, and perianal region, are the only areas subject to disease of the apocrine glands such as Paget's disease.

f. The transitional zones between skin and mucous membranes (*eg*, lips, genitoanal region) are at risk for herpes simplex, fixed-drug eruptions, precancerosis, and squamous cell carcinomas.
2. The difference in the function of the skin can also predispose it to certain types of problems.
   a. Acne, eczema, and skin infections are associated with seborrheic skin, whereas atopic eczema is associated with dry skin (asteatosis).
   b. In individuals with diminished peripheral circulation, dermatoses can frequently be seen, especially in the distal parts of the extremities.
   c. Decreased circulation is associated with ulcers, which are notoriously slow to heal. Patients frequently present to physical therapy for management with physical agents such as ultrasound, high-voltage galvanic stimulation, and pulsed galvanic stimulation.
   d. Where skin lies on skin (*eg*, in the umbilical, inguinal, and perianal regions or in obese patients), the evaporation of sweat and desquamation of the skin are impaired, with increased moisture and softening of the skin as a result.
      (1). This encourages the development of bacterial or mycotic infections or sensitization dermatitis.
      (2). Exposed areas of the body are also vulnerable to wounds.

F. Definition of pathological terms for the skin

1. **Macroscopic terms**
   a. **Blister.** Common term used to refer to a vesicle or bulla.
   b. **Bulla.** Fluid-filled raised area greater than 5 mm across; a large blister.
   c. **Excoriation.** Lesion that is usually a result of trauma and is characterized by breakage of the epidermis, which causes a raw, linear area (*eg*, a deep scratch).
   d. **Lichenification.** Rough, thickened area of skin characterized by prominent skin markings; this may result from repeated rubbing in people who are susceptible.
   e. **Macule.** Circumscribed area of any size characterized by its flatness. It is usually distinguished from surrounding skin by its coloration.

f. **Nodule.** Elevated solid area, like a papule, that is 5 mm or more across.

g. **Onycholysis.** Refers to the loss of the integrity of the substance of the nail.

h. **Papule.** Elevated solid area that is 5 mm or less across.

i. **Plaque.** Elevated area with a flat top, usually greater than 5 mm across.

j. **Pustule.** Pus-filled, discrete, raised area.

k. **Scale.** Platelike excrescence, horny and dry; usually the result of imperfect cornification.

l. **Vesicle.** Fluid-filled raised area 5 mm or less across.

m. **Wheal.** Transient, itchy, elevated area that can have variable blanching and erythema, formed as a result of dermal edema.

2. **Microscopic terms**

a. **Acanthosis.** Hyperplasia of the epidermal layer.

b. **Acantholysis.** Loss of the intercellular connections, which results in a loss of cohesion between keratinocytes.

c. **Dyskeratosis.** Abnormal keratinization that occurs prematurely within individual cells or groups of cells below the stratum granulosum.

d. **Erosion.** Discontinuous skin, exhibiting incomplete loss of the epidermis.

e. **Exocytosis.** Infiltration of inflammatory or circulating blood cells in the epidermis.

f. **Hyperkeratosis.** Hyperplasia of the stratum corneum, which can be associated with a qualitative abnormality of the keratin.

g. **Papillomatosis.** Hyperplasia of the papillary dermis with elongation and/or widening of the dermal papillae.

h. **Parakeratosis.** Mode of keratinization characterized by the retention of nuclei in the stratum corneum. On some membranes, like the mucous membrane, parakeratosis is normal.

i. **Spongiosis.** Where the epidermis shows intercellular edema.

j. **Ulceration.** Where the skin becomes discontinuous and exhibits a complete loss of the epidermis and portions of the dermis, including the subcutaneous fat.

k. **Vacuolization.** Refers to the formation of vacuoles adjacent to or within cells; often refers to basal cell–basement membrane.

II. Effects of the Environment and the Risks of Cancer

A. Etiology and incidence

1. Skin cancer is the most common type of cancer in the United States. Forty to 50% of Americans who live to age 65 will have skin cancer at least once. At greatest risk are individuals with blue or light-colored eyes, red or blond hair, and fair skin that freckles easily. The risk of developing skin cancer is greatest in areas with high levels of ultraviolet radiation from the sun. For example, skin cancer is more common in Texas than it is in Minnesota, where the sunlight is not as strong. Worldwide, highest rates of skin cancer are found in South Africa and Australia, areas that receive the highest amounts of ultraviolet radiation.

2. Approximately 600,000 new cases of skin cancer occur each year. Skin cancers must be diagnosed and treated early because they can invade and destroy adjacent tissues.

3. Most common skin cancers are:

a. *Basal cell carcinoma.* This accounts for more than 90% of all skin cancers. It is slow growing and seldom metastasizes.

b. *Squamous cell carcinoma.* This rarely metastasizes but does so more often than basal cell carcinoma.

c. *Melanoma.* This is less common but is increasing at the fastest rate of incidence of all cancers except for lung cancer. About 32,000 new cases were diagnosed in 1991, with 6500 deaths. In the United States, the rate of incidence is increasing at a rate of 4.3% a year; the incidence among whites from 1973 to 1988 increased approximately 75%. A positive family history increases the risk, but the cause is a lifetime exposure to ultraviolet (UV) radiation. Both UVA (320 to 400 nm) and UVB (290 to 320 nm) are implicated.

B. Diagnosis and prognosis

1. **Clinical manifestations**
   a. The most common warning sign is a change on the skin, especially a new growth or a sore that does not heal.
   b. Skin cancer does not always appear the same; it may start as a small, smooth, shiny, pale or waxy lump or as a firm red lump. Sometimes the lump bleeds or develops a crust. It can also appear as a flat, red spot that is rough, dry, or scaly. Both basal and squamous cell cancers are usually found on areas exposed to sun, such as the head, face, neck, hands, and arms. However, it can appear anywhere. Melanoma also appears in the eyes, central nervous system, anus, and esophagus. Actinic keratosis usually appears as rough, red or brown scaly patches on skin; it is a precancerous condition that sometimes develops into squamous cell cancer. It appears on sun-exposed areas, but can be found elsewhere.
   c. Changes on the skin are not sure signs of cancer but should not be overlooked. A physician should be consulted if symptoms last longer than 2 weeks.
   d. *Wounds and wound healing.* Wounds secondary to treatment of other types of cancer may present as a problem with wound healing. This may manifest as healing difficulty in a surgical site. Irradiated skin may blister, burn, or be fragile to shear stress, leading to open wounds. Because these wounds may be difficult to treat, the physical therapist is often consulted. Wounds are difficult to close because of the following:

(1). Impaired immune function and infection.
(2). Cancer cachexia with poor nutrition and dehydration with nausea and vomiting (*eg*, protein-calorie malnutrition).
(3). Poor wound healing with impaired fibroblast activity, such as decreased collagen synthesis and fibrosis (radiation therapy).
(4). Antineoplastic agents and corticosteroids commonly used in chemotherapy.
(5). Other comorbidities and advanced age (see Table 25–1).

2. **Diagnosis.** The cure rate would be 100% if all skin cancers were brought to a physician's attention before they spread.
   a. The skin should always be examined during physical examinations. The physical therapist should pay special attention to all skin areas if the patient has previously had skin cancer.
   b. The therapist should report without delay any changes (colored growths or changes in growths present).
   c. Basal cell carcinoma and squamous cell carcinoma are generally diagnosed and treated in the same way.
   d. Skin cancers are divided into two stages:
      (1). Local (affecting only the skin)
      (2). Metastatic
   e. Because nonmelanoma skin cancer rarely spreads, biopsy is often the only test needed to assess the stage. If the growth is large or present for a long time, further examination is needed, such as care-

---

Table 25–1. FACTORS DECREASING COLLAGEN SYNTHESIS AND INTRINSIC FACTORS AFFECTING WOUND HEALING

Hypoxia	Physical stress	Advanced age
Infection	Antineoplastic drugs	Trauma
Bacteria	Necrotic tissue	Foreign body
Mycobacteria	Uricemia	Chronic
Fungi or yeast	Ischemia	Factitial
Many systemic/topical antibiotics	Venous stasis	Photoaged skin
Anticoagulants	Systemic vascular disorders	Radiation injury/fibrosis
Aspirin	Atherosclerosis	Nicotine
Heparin	Anti-inflammatories	Endocrine disorders
Coumadin	NSAIDS	Diabetes
Malnutrition	Phenylbutazone	Cushing's syndrome
Trace elements (*eg*, zinc, copper)	Steroids	Ulcers
Vitamins (*eg*, A, C)	Chronic illness (*eg*, renal, cancer,	Tumor related
Protein-calorie	autoimmune, cardiovascular	Neuropathic
Starvation	hematopoietic, hepatic)	Decubitus
Emotional Stress		

Abbreviations: NSAIDS = nonsteroidal anti-inflammatory drugs.

fully checking the lymph nodes in the area.

3. **Prognosis.** Primary treatment is surgical resection.
   a. *Melanoma*
      (1). The 5-year survival rate for melanoma with early diagnosis and treatment by surgical resection is 91%.
      (2). If it has spread regionally or the cancer is being treated secondary to local invasion and spread, the 5-year survival rate is 50%.

C. Protecting the skin from the sun

1. Reducing sun exposure is the easiest and most cost-effective method to decrease risk of developing melanoma. Time of day and season affect the degree of ultraviolet exposure—60% can be eliminated by avoiding the sun between 10:00 AM and 2:00 PM (11:00 AM and 3:00 PM daylight savings time).
2. If exposure is unavoidable, the following should be used even on overcast days and especially when on or near water, snow, ice, sand, or concrete:
   a. Protective clothing.
   b. Effective sun screen (should be applied 30 minutes before exposure and at a high enough sun protection factor [SPF] rating [2 to 15] for skin color. The higher the SPF number, the greater the protection it provides in blocking ultraviolet rays). Sun screen should be reap-

Table 25–2. "IFEE" WOUND SIGNS OF INFECTION

I	Induration
F	Fever
E	Erythema
E	Edema

(From Alvarez O, Rozint J, Wiseman D: Moist environment for healing: matching the dressing to the wound. *Wounds* 1989, 1:40.)

plied after swimming or if perspiring heavily.)

3. Certain medications, such as anticancer agents, antibiotics, and antidepressants, increase a person's photosensitivity. A pharmacist or physician should be consulted.
4. Tanning lamps and booths are artificial sources of ultraviolet radiation exposure and should be avoided.

TREATMENT OF CANCER PATIENTS

Physical therapy treatment for pain and increasing functional movement is necessary if surgical resection leads to physical impairments and dysfunction. If wounds are involved, wound care is necessary to clean and close them. Wounds/excision sites should be carefully monitored for signs of infection (Table 25–2). See Table 25–1 for factors that decrease collagen synthesis and intrinsic factors affecting wound healing, and see Table 25–3 for extrinsic factors affecting wound healing. Table 25–4 includes factors that increase risk of skin injury that can be reduced or prevented, and Table 25–5 includes methods to improve wound healing.

III. Pathological Conditions of the Skin

A. Tumors[3–12]

1. The most common tumors encountered in day-to-day practice are tumors of the skin. They can be classified by their anatomical location (*eg*, the epidermis or the dermis) and by their biological behavior (benign or malignant).
   a. As a general rule, physical therapists do not treat tumors of the skin unless they

Table 25–3. EXTRINSIC FACTORS AFFECTING WOUND HEALING

Wound cleansing	Topical antimicrobials	Moist environment
Dressings	Débridement	Types of dressing (*eg*, moist vs dry)
Surgical technique	Wound/edge approximation	
Growth factors	Electrical stimulation	

Table 25–4. FACTORS INCREASING RISK OF SKIN INJURY THAT CAN BE REDUCED OR PREVENTED

Pressure	Radiation (*eg*, ultraviolet)	Poor nutrition
Friction	exposure	Emotional stress
Shear forces	Excessive moisture	Pressure gradient
Infection exposure	Trauma	Impaired mobility
Poor bowel or bladder	Mental status/level of	Inactivity
control	consciousness	Insensitive skin

are assisting in the healing process or in scar reduction after a major surgical procedure.

b. However, physical therapists should recognize potential tumors of the skin and be able to refer patients to either the patient's primary care physician or a dermatologist for appropriate care.

2. **Benign epidermal tumors**

a. *Keratinocytic tumors*

(1). This is the most common type of benign epidermal tumor.

(2). These tumors are primarily a cosmetic problem.

(3). Biopsy is required to make the diagnosis, and it can be misdiagnosed as squamous cell carcinoma.

b. *Seborrheic keratosis*

(1). This occurs most frequently after middle age and is a common benign tumor of basaloid cells.

(2). Tumors arise spontaneously, often

rapidly, and in crops. They may occur following hormonal therapy or inflammatory dermatoses.

(3). They are usually left untreated unless they cause itching or pain.

c. *Fibroepithelial polyp*

(1). This is usually called a skin tag or acrochordon and is a very common tumor.

(2). These polyps are found incidentally in middle-aged individuals, usually on the neck.

(3). They consist of squamous epithelium around a fibrovascular core and can be associated with diabetes.

(4). They do not seem to be a marker of systemic disease.

d. *Epidermal cyst*

(1). Cysts derive from the epidermis or the epithelium of the hair follicle and become filled with keratin mixed with lipid-rich debris.

(a). A pilar cyst is usually firm, well

Table 25–5. INTERVENTIONS FOR FACTORS INCREASING RISK OF SKIN INJURY THAT CAN BE REDUCED OR PREVENTED

Risk (Conduct Risk Assessment)	Intervention
Pressure	Relieve pressure, *eg*, postioning, pressure-reducing cushions and beds, or beds that mechanically turn, *eg*, rotary beds; especially relieve pressure on bony prominences, *eg*, heels
Inactivity	Turning schedule
Impaired mobility	Increase activity and mobility
Pressure gradient	Avoid pressure and improve blood flow
Insensitive skin	Do not expose to extreme heat/cold
Shear forces	Reduce shear and friction forces
Friction	Lubricate skin and do not rub red areas
Infection exposure	Provide adequate fluid intake, monitor for signs of infection, use appropriate infection-control techniques, *eg*, hand washing and skin cleansing
Poor nutrition	Assess basic diet and refer to registered dietician
Trauma	Assess area for risk of injury, slips, or falls
Excessive moisture	
Poor bowel or bladder control	Manage incontinence
Radiation (*eg*, ultraviolet) exposure	Educate about risk of skin damage from exposure
Mental status/level of consciousness	Educate family and/or primary caregiver about skin care and risk reduction program
Emotional stress	Educate about relaxation techniques and refer to psychologist as appropriate

circumscribed, and appears on the scalp. It is formed by an outer wall of keratinizing squamous epithelium without a granular layer.

(b). An epidermal inclusion cyst is also a well circumscribed, mobile, subepidermal nodule on the head, neck, or trunk. It is formed by keratinizing squamous epithelium and has a granular layer and contains keratin.

e. *Keratoacanthoma*

(1). This tumor is benign but rapid growing. It commonly appears on the face but can be seen anywhere on the head or upper extremities.

(2). It is commonly seen after middle age and begins as a round, firm, flesh-colored or red papule that grows to 1 to 2 cm or larger.

(3). There may be a temporary delay in growth and then scarring eventually ensues.

(4). It will often be excised to exclude the possibility of a squamous cell carcinoma.

(5). Clinically, they occur in older individuals as slow-growing tumors.

f. *Adenexal (appendage) tumors*

(1). These tumors originate from epithelial cells capable of pilosebaceous, eccrine, or apocrine differentiation.

(2). They are primarily benign tumors, but some malignant variants exist (sebaceous carcinoma).

(3). There are several major types of adenexal tumors:

(a). **Cylindroma.** Benign tumor of either apocrine or eccrine origin arising in early adulthood as single or multiple nodules located on the scalp.

(b). **Eccrine spiradenoma.** Benign tumor of eccrine origin arising in young adults, usually with a solitary nodule that is tender or even painful with no characteristic location.

(c). **Nevus sebaceous.** Congenital hamartoma derived from basal cells that are on the face or scalp of children.

(d). **Pilomatrixoma.** Benign tumor of hair follicle origin arising before age 20; a hard, deep nodule usually located on the face or upper extremity.

(e). **Syringocystadenoma papilliferum.** Benign tumor arising in eccrine or apocrine tissue during puberty, located on the scalp or face and usually associated with nevus sebaceous.

(f). **Syringoma.** Benign tumor in the dermis at puberty or later, usually seen in multiples of 1 to 2 mm, faintly yellow or skin colored, usually located on the face and especially the lower eyelids, abdomen, or vulva.

(g). **Trichoepithelioma.** Multiple tumors that recapitulate hair follicles, first appearing in adolescence on the face and scalp as flesh-colored papules and small nodules.

3. **Premalignant and malignant epidermal tumors**

a. *Actinic keratosis (solar keratosis)*

(1). This is a premalignant skin lesion that is usually characterized by epidermal atypia induced by chronic exposure to sunlight.

(2). It is common in fair-complexioned, middle-aged individuals with a history of high sun exposure.

b. *Basal cell carcinoma*

(1). This is a locally aggressive, common, rarely metastasizing epidermal tumor that resembles basal cells of the epidermis.

(2). This tumor rarely arises before age 40; blacks and Asians are rarely affected.

(3). It usually presents on the face and hair-bearing areas and looks pearly gray and semitranslucent with marked telangiectasis.

(4). It is uncommon on the back and forearms and common on the eyelids.

(5). When completely excised, most basal cell carcinomas are cured.

c. *Squamous cell carcinoma*

(1). This tumor has a peak incidence at 60 years and affects women more than men.

(2). The common predisposing factor is chronic sun exposure, but it may also be caused by ingestion of arsenicals; chronic ulcers or sinus tracts; prolonged contact with organic hydrocarbons; tobacco; radiation; thermal injury; xeroderma pigmentosum; and immunosuppression.

(3). Skin tumors have a low but significant potential for metastasis (less than 2% metastasize, but for those with squamous cells arising on mucosal surfaces, the metastasis rate is 20% to 50%.

(4). Complete excision is associated with cure.

4. **Tumors of the dermis**

a. *Fibrous histiocytoma*

(1). This refers to a benign dermal proliferation of fibroblasts and histiocytes, usually occurring in adults.

(2). It frequently occurs as lesions on legs of young to middle-aged women, with a history of antecedent trauma in 20%.

b. *Dermatofibrosarcoma protuberans*

(1). This is an uncommon, slow growing, and locally aggressive tumor of the dermis, with solitary or multiple nodules arising within indurated plaque; usually arises on the trunk but can be seen on the extremities, neck, scalp, and face.

(2). Along with dermatofibromas it is primarily derived from fibroblasts and the presence of variable proliferations of histiocytes.

c. *Hemangioma*

(1). These can be either benign or malignant tumors of the blood and lymphatic vessels; however, cutaneous hemangiomas are extremely common.

(2). Capillary hemangioma refers to a common benign vascular tumor that usually regresses by childhood; it is left to resolve spontaneously unless very large.

(3). Pyogenic granuloma of the skin is a benign, solitary proliferation of capillaries often associated with a history of trauma.

(4). Rarely exceeds 2 cm in diameter and is usually treated by excision.

(5). Senile hemangioma (cherry hemangioma) refers to a common, benign, tiny capillary hemangioma that usually occurs in adult life and appears as a 1- to 3-mm bright-red or purple papule that sometimes persists.

(6). Cavernous hemangioma refers to a subcutaneous or dermal vascular tumor characterized by the relatively large size of its vessels; it affects males more than females, creates irregularity in the skin, exhibits bright- to dark-red coloration, and is usually independent of systemic disorders except the following.

d. *Nevus flammeus*

(1). This is a common benign malformation of the telangiectatic vessel; it is present in more than one third of infants. It is a large, flat, pink or orange patch that changes to dark purple or even blue and may be raised.

(2). Port-wine nevus usually occurs on the face or neck and is associated with other syndromes (Sturge-Weber and Klippel-Trenaunay syndromes).

e. *Kaposi's sarcoma*

(1). This is a disease that progresses slowly but has a malignant mesenchymal neoplasm that occurs most commonly on the lower extremities of men, aged 40 to 70 years.

(2). The lesions are red-to-purple plaques containing multiple small papules and nodules on the legs.

(3). The lesions may occur anywhere on the skin; they enlarge and coalesce and form purple-red spongy tumors that are 7 cm or more in diameter.

(4). In the United States, this is a relatively uncommon disorder (0.02% of all malignant tumors), but it is more common in certain parts of Africa.

(5). This neoplasm is common in patients with HIV.

f. *Xanthoma*

(1). These tumors are characterized by collections of foamy histiocytes or granular pink cytoplasm, with cholesterol, phospholipids, and triglycerides found in the cells.

(2). They occur in all races and both sexes and may have a familial association.

(3). They may occur in association with malignancies.

(4). They may be the first indicator of high cholesterol levels.

(5). The five principal types of xanthoma are

   (a). Eruptive—usually occurring on the buttocks, posterior thighs, knees, and elbows as showers of numerous small, soft, yellow papules that come and go as plasma triglycerides and lipids wax and wane.

   (b). Tuberous—yellow nodules frequently occurring on the Achilles tendon and the extensor tendons of fingers.

   (c). Tendinous—occurring in skin folds, especially palmar creases.

   (d). Plane and xanthelasma—soft, yellow plaques occurring on the eyelids.

g. **Mastocytosis (including urticaria pigmentosa)**

(1). This refers to a group of uncommon disorders characterized by increased numbers of mast cells in the skin and other organs.

(2). It is manifested clinically by skin lesions, usually small brown papules and plaques.

(3). Urticarial lesions may develop after trauma to these sites.

(4). The release of chemical mediators from mast cell granules in these lesions is responsible for urticaria and flushing.

(5). More than 50% of patients with mastocytosis are children and infants, who develop a localized cutaneous form called urticaria pigmentosa.

(6). The disease may be localized to the skin in adults or may involve other organs (eg, liver, spleen, lymph nodes, bone).

(7). Most of the signs and symptoms are due to the effects of histamine, heparin, and other substances released by mast cells.

(8). Most patients are asymptomatic, but others have

   (a). An erythematous wheal occurring on firm rubbing of lesions.

   (b). Dermatographism, an urticaria that occurs on firm rubbing of apparently normal skin.

   (c). Pruritus and flushing triggered by hot baths, rubbing, spicy foods, cheese, alcohol, or drugs such as morphine, codeine, or aspirin.

   (d). Rhinorrhea (excessive nasal discharge).

   (e). Formation of vesicles and bullae following rubbing or minor trauma.

   (f). Melena and epistaxis (anticoagulant effect of heparin).

   (g). Bone pain due to osteoclastic and osteoblastic lesions in systemic disease.

(9). The prognosis is generally good.

(10). Ten percent of those affected experience systemic mastocytosis, and the mast cell infiltrates bone, liver, spleen, and lymph nodes as well as skin.

(11). The course of the disease is progressive, with attacks of syncope, hypotension, tachycardia, and sometimes shock; thus, the prognosis is poor for these patients.

5. **Other tumors**

a. **Mycosis fungoides**

(1). This is a T-cell lymphoproliferative disorder of the skin that sometimes evolves into generalized lymphoma.

(2). Males are more often affected than females (2:1).

(3). It may occur at any age but is most common between 40 and 60 years of age.

(4). The clinical course can be chronic (lasting up to 20 years) to rapidly progressive, with one third of the patients dying from unrelated causes.

b. **Histiocytosis X**

(1). This tumor represents an abnormal proliferation of Langerhans cells that are believed to originate in the bone marrow.

(2). The histiocytosis X cells contain Birbeck granules and express differentiation antigens that are common to both Langerhans and T cells.

c. *Metastatic carcinoma*
   (1). This occurs in 3% to 4% of all visceral malignancies.
   (2). The primary tumor can also be located in the skin, with the breast being the most common primary site in women (63%) and the lung (28%) and colon (25%) the most common in men.
   (3). Clinically, the tumors present as dermal or subcutaneous nodules that are firm and sometimes ulcerated, or they could appear as papules or plaques; they may be swollen, warm, deeply erythematous areas.
   (4). Sclerotic patches of alopecia resembling scleroderma are sometimes associated with metastatic breast carcinoma.
   (5). Most metastatic carcinoma primarily involves the dermis and spreads upward into the epidermis and downward into the subcutis.
   (6). Some tumors characteristically involve the epidermis (*eg*, Paget's disease associated with breast carcinoma).

B. Common disorders of pigmentation

1. **Freckles**
   a. This is the most common pigmented lesion of childhood in light-skinned whites.
   b. Freckles are tan to light-brown macules that vary in size from 1 to 10 mm with irregular borders.
   c. They appear early in childhood, especially after exposure to the summer sun, and usually fade in winter.
   d. The melanocytes in a freckle are larger than normal, but the number may be less than in adjacent skin.

2. **Melasma**
   a. This is a masklike hyperpigmentation often occurring in pregnant women, affecting the face as a large, flat area of blotchy light- and dark-brown pigmentation over the cheeks, temples, and forehead.
   b. Melasma results from alterations in melanocytes and leads to increased melanin production and transfer.
   c. Hyperpigmentation is bilateral.

d. It can also occur after taking agents like hydantoins.
   e. Sunlight accentuates the areas of hyperpigmentation.
   f. Melasma associated with pregnancy often resolves spontaneously.

3. **Vitiligo**
   a. This is a common disorder that affects all races but is more noticeable in dark-skinned persons.
   b. It is marked clinically by completely depigmented flat patches of bizarre and irregular configurations, with the size of depigmented areas varying considerably from inches to feet.
   c. It primarily involves the wrists, axillae, and perioral, periorbital, and anogenital skin.
   d. Histologically, there is a complete absence of melanocytes.
   e. The etiology and pathogenesis are unclear, but there is often a family history of the condition.
      (1). Most evidence supports autoimmune causation and focuses on the presence of circulating antibody against melanocytes and other melanin-producing cells.
      (2). It may be associated with other autoimmune diseases such as pernicious anemia, Addison's disease, and thyroid disease.

4. **Acanthosis nigricans**
   a. This is a clinical lesion of thickened, pigmented skin in the flexion areas (axillae, back and sides of neck, groin, and anogenital areas).
   b. It may be associated with underlying benign or malignant conditions and can be divided into
      (1). *Benign type.* This develops gradually, is not extensive, and spares distal extremities.
         (a). Common in childhood and puberty.
         (b). Represents about 80% of all cases.
         (c). Thought either to be an autosomal dominant trait or to occur in association with obesity or endocrine abnormalities, especially pituitary and pineal tumors and diabetes.

(d). Can be part of a variety of congenital syndromes.
  (2). *Malignant type*
    (a). Affects middle-aged and older individuals and is associated with adenocarcinoma. (*Note:* skin changes and tumors often present simultaneously.)

5. **Lentigo**
   a. This is a common, benign pigmented proliferation of epidermal melanocytes that occurs at all ages but often in infancy and childhood.
   b. There is no sex or racial predilection.
   c. The etiology and pathogenesis are unknown.
   d. Histologically, there is hyperplasia of the melanocytes.
   e. Lesions may involve mucous membranes as well as skin.

6. **Nevocellular nevus (pigmented nevus, mole)**
   a. "Nevus" means any congenital lesion of the skin.
   b. Nevocellular nevus specifically refers to a benign acquired or congenital tumor of neural crest–derived cells, which are modified melanocytes.
   c. Lesions are usually tan to deep brown and uniformly pigmented with well-defined, rounded borders.
   d. Some are large and contain numerous hairs, and some have a blue-black color that may be confused with certain malignancies of melanocytes.
   e. More common nevocellular nevi are acquired (noncongenital) and appear during childhood and early adulthood.
   f. Moles are very frequent, and malignant melanoma is uncommon.
   g. Between 20% and 40% of patients with malignant melanoma have histological evidence of an associated nevus.
   h. Approximately 9% to 20% of giant congenital nevocellular nevi at some point evolve into malignant melanoma.
   i. Malignant changes often occur by the age of 10 years.
   j. A large atypical mole, a dysplastic nevus, has a clear association with malignant transformation.
      (1). Moles are slightly elevated.
      (2). They are pink-brown lesions with irregular borders and a flat component, with a diameter often greater than 1 cm.

7. **Malignant melanoma**
   a. This refers to a malignant neoplasm of melanocytes.
   b. This type of lesion accounts for 1% to 3% of all cancers, with the peak incidence between 40 and 60 years of age.
   c. It occurs most often in the skin but can be found in the oral cavity, esophagus, anal canal, vagina, and leptomeninges, on conjunctivae, or within the eye.
   d. Malignant melanoma is classified into four types:
      (1). Superficial spreading melanoma
      (2). Lentigo maligna melanoma
      (3). Acral-lentiginous melanoma
      (4). Nodular melanoma
   e. Most melanomas arise *de novo*, but 20% appear to arise in association with a preexisting benign nevus.
   f. The distinction between malignant melanomas and benign nevi is that nevi usually exhibit only shades of tan to dark brown, whereas melanomas show areas of red, white, or blue in addition to brown and black.
   g. Melanomas also show irregular borders with notching and striking protrusions, whereas nevi have regular, well-circumscribed borders.
   h. The malignant melanoma is managed by surgical excision with microscopic assessment of type, level, and depth.
   i. Early detection and removal are important and can be a successful treatment.
   j. Metastases usually involve the regional rather than distal lymph nodes; however, once hematogenous metastasis occurs, the spread is to every internal organ.

C. **Inflammatory dermatoses of probable hypersensitivity origin**[13,14]

1. **Eczematous dermatitis**
   a. This is a large, common category of skin lesions characterized by severe pruritus and distinctive gross and microscopic features.
   b. One third of all patients who visit a dermatologist suffer from some type of dermatitis.
   c. The most common types are
      (1). Contact dermatitis
      (2). Atopic dermatitis
      (3). Lichen simplex chronicus
      (4). Drug-related eczematous dermatitis
      (5). Photoeczematous dermatitis

(6). One form of erythroderma

d. When the etiology is unknown, lesions are classified according to distribution, clinical appearance, and history of associated diseases.

e. Histologically, there are three categories: acute, subacute, and chronic.

f. Eczema is derived from the Greek word meaning "to boil over" and describes the clinical appearance of acute eczematous dermatitis.

g. The most obvious example of acute dermatitis is that caused by poison ivy, with pruritic, edematous, oozing erythematous plaques often showing outright blister formation.

h. Subacute dermatitis is exemplified by childhood atopic eczema with pruritic, moist, erythematous, and well-defined papules and plaques.

(1). Dermal changes include

(a). Infiltration of lymphocytes, mononuclear cells, and sometimes eosinophils.

(b). Presence of edema to some degree.

i. Chronic eczematous dermatitis has marked pruritic, dry, scaly, well-defined plaques with thickening of the skin and accentuation of skin lines.

j. The clinical effects of therapeutic agents such as topical steroids in these lesions may relate to their ability to impair the function of antigen-presenting cells and lymphocytes locally in the skin.

2. **Urticaria**

a. This refers to a common disorder of the skin characterized histologically by dermal edema and clinically by itchy pink or white wheals.

b. More than 20% of individuals experience urticaria sometime in their life.

c. There are acute and chronic types.

d. It can also be classified by etiology, but many cases are idiopathic.

e. The final common pathway is localized increases in vascular permeability with resulting dermal edema.

f. Types I and III hypersensitivity reactions as well as nonimmunological reactions can lead to increases in permeability.

(1). In Type I

(a). Immediate reactions include mast cell degranulation.

(b). Histamine is thought to be an important chemical mediator in the pathogenesis of urticaria.

(c). Antihistamines, however, fail to control the urticaria.

(2). Nonimmunological urticaria may be caused by substances that cause degranulation of mast cells.

g. All types of urticaria exhibit dermal edema, which is manifested histologically by separation of dermal collagen bundles.

h. Lymphocyte infiltrate is present and is sometimes accompanied by neutrophils and eosinophils.

i. Usually, this infiltrate is confined to the superficial dermis.

j. Occasionally, deep dermal infiltrates with nuclear debris can be observed.

k. Lesions of urticaria may occur anywhere on the body either localized or in a widely distributed pattern.

l. Lesions are transient (they characteristically last no longer than 36 hours), which distinguishes urticaria from other dermatoses.

m. If urticaria lasts less than 3 weeks, it is considered acute.

n. If lesions last more than 3 weeks, it is chronic and indicates the need for a thorough work-up to rule out an obscure etiological agent or related disease.

3. **Erythema multiforme**

a. This is a common, self-limited dermatosis that appears to be a hypersensitivity response to infections and drugs but may also be idiopathic.

b. It affects persons of any age and can commonly accompany herpesvirus and mycoplasmal infections as well as histoplasmosis, coccidioidomycosis, typhoid, leprosy, and others, the administration of drugs (sulfonamides, penicillins, barbiturates, salicylates, hydantoins, and antimalarials), or malignancies or collagen vascular diseases.

c. Lesions are multiform macules, papules, vesicles, bullae, or target lesions.

d. Erythema multiforme begins as red macules or papules that develop a pale bullous or eroded center.

e. The lesions may be distributed anywhere on the body.

f. Clinically, erythema multiforme should be classified as the minor (simplex) or major (multiplex) form.

(1). *Minor form*

(a). In the minor form, there are few or moderate numbers of skin lesions and minor mucous membrane involvement.

(b). There are no systemic symptoms, and the patient feels well.

(c). The disease is self-limited, lasting 2 to 6 weeks.

(2). *Major form*

(a). The major form is more common in children and is characterized by extensive skin and mucous membrane involvement, fever, prostration, and respiratory symptoms.

(b). Erosions and hemorrhagic crusts involve the mouth and lips and the conjunctivae, urethra, and genital and perianal areas.

(c). If the lesions become infected, the disease can be life threatening.

g. Treatment is usually symptomatic and supportive.

4. **Cutaneous necrotizing vasculitis**

a. This refers to a group of disorders characterized clinically by palpable purpura and histologically by inflammatory damage to vessel walls.

b. Immunological pathogenesis is suspected.

c. In the skin, superficial venules are involved and partially degranulated mast cells are seen, with debris-laden macrophages, endothelial cell swelling, and necrosis as well as vascular basement membrane reduplication.

d. Interendothelial cell gaps have been described.

e. IgA may be present in affected cutaneous vessels.

f. The clinical hallmark is palpable, nonblanchable purpura in crops.

g. The purpura are present on dependent areas of bedridden patients or on lower extremities of those who are ambulatory.

h. Lesions affect persons of all ages.

i. A single episode lasts 2 to 4 weeks but may recur.

j. Vasculitis may also present as chronic urticaria without purpura.

k. Fever, malaise, and arthralgia are not uncommon and may indicate the presence of vasculitis in visceral organs, kidneys, lungs, joints, gastrointestinal tract, central nervous system, and other organs.

5. **Cutaneous lupus erythematosus**

a. These cutaneous lesions consist of facial erythema and discoid plaques anywhere on the body surface, and histologically they are the only manifestations of the disease.

(1). The malar erythema is usually nonspecific, and the lesions have characteristic changes that correlate with their clinical appearance.

(2). Plaques of discoid lupus are large and well defined with scaling, erythematous surfaces.

(3). Zones of hyperpigmentation and hypopigmentation can be observed, with dilated tortuous vessels.

(4). Lesions of discoid lupus show hyperkeratosis, epidermal atrophy with loss of ridges, dyskeratosis, and vacuolization of the basal layer, a variable infiltrate of lymphocytes disposed in bandlike array along the dermoepidermal junction.

6. **Graft versus host disease**

a. This occurs following transplantation of tissue containing immunocompetent allogeneic lymphocytes to immunosuppressed individuals.

b. The lymphocytes react against a variety of sites, such as the skin, liver, and gastrointestinal tract.

c. The acute phase is several weeks after transplantation, and the chronic phase is several months to 1 year after.

d. Approximately 70% of patients receiving bone marrow transplants for leukemia or immunodeficiency states develop some form of graft versus host disease.

e. Clinically, an extensive erythematous macular eruption is seen acutely at times with scaling or bulla formation.

f. Pathogenesis of graft versus host disease is the subject of intensive investigation to study the immunofluorescence of immunoglobulins and complement at the basement membrane zone and in dermal vessels in more chronic skin lesions.

7. **Panniculitis**

a. This describes an inflammatory reaction of the subcutaneous fat that may affect the connective tissue septa separating fat lobules.

b. Erythema nodosum is the most common type and is sometimes associated with infections and drugs.

(1). The lesions are very tender, brawny, erythematous plaques and nodules (2 to 5 cm across).

(2). Most lesions often occur on the lower legs of women 20 to 30 years of age.

(3). Involution occurs in 3 to 6 weeks and leaves a bruiselike lesion, but scarring does not result.

(4). Erythema nodosum is commonly associated with β-hemolytic streptococcal infections, tuberculosis, and the administration of certain drugs, especially sulfonamides. It can also be associated with coccidioidomycosis, histoplasmosis, leprosy, use of oral contraceptives, sarcoidosis, inflammatory bowel disease, and malignancy.

c. Erythema induratum refers to a type of panniculitis characterized histologically by the presence of granulomas, vasculitis, and necrosis.

(1). It is a relatively uncommon disorder of uncertain etiology that most frequently affects adolescent and menopausal women.

(2). It may represent a tuberculoid hypersensitivity response to mycobacterial antigens.

(3). The most frequent presentation is that of either single or multiple dark-red, dusky nodules or plaques located on the calves.

(4). Ulcerations are frequent, and recurrences are common, especially in cold weather.

(5). Hypersensitivity reaction is suggested, and the disorder is usually limited to subcutaneous fat.

(6). In adults, the disease is limited to the subcutis and the prognosis is good.

(7). The disorder subsides after several months but can last up to 5 years.

(8). In children, the disease is accompanied by high fevers and can be associated with systemic life-threatening involvement.

D. Other inflammatory dermatoses not usually associated with systemic disease[15–17]

1. Acne vulgaris

a. Acne vulgaris is a chronic inflammatory disorder that is universal in the mid to late teenage years and is characterized by comedones, papules, nodules, and cysts.

b. Both males and females are affected, but males have more severe lesions.

c. It is regarded as a physiological state and may be induced or exacerbated by drugs, occupational contactants, and occlusive conditions such as heavy clothing in tropical climates.

d. Drugs that promote acne are adrenocorticotropic hormone, corticosteroids, testosterone, gonadotropins, contraceptives, trimethadone, iodides, and bromides.

e. The pathogenesis is poorly understood, but endocrine factors are implicated.

f. Fatty acids are also known to be highly irritating in the dermis, and it has been postulated that bacterial lipases break down sebum, liberating fatty acids that then cause development of the inflammatory lesions of acne.

g. Inhibition of lipase production is a rationale for administration of antibiotics to patients with inflammatory acne.

h. Lesions are divided into noninflammatory and inflammatory, characteristically distributed on the skin of the face, back, chest, and shoulders.

i. Noninflammatory lesions include open and closed comedones (blackheads and whiteheads).

j. A comedo is actually a pilosebaceous follicle filled with a keratin plug.

k. The tip of the plug is dark owing to oxidation and melanin pigment deposition.

l. An open comedo consists of a small flat or raised area with a central pore filled with impacted keratin.

m. A closed comedo pore is largely covered by epithelium; hence, it is manifested as a papule unless the skin overlying it is stretched apart.

2. Rosacea

a. *Lichen planus*

(1). Lichen planus refers to common disorders of the skin and mucous membranes.

(2). There is a distinctive gross and microscopic appearance.

(3). The lesions are itchy, violaceous, flat-topped papules highlighted by white dots or lines called Wickham's striae.

(4). The disease may present with a single lesion, but then multiple lesions arise, varying from a few to a hundred.

(5). The lesions are distributed mostly in the extremities, particularly around the wrists and elbows and occasionally the glans penis.

(6). Seventy percent of patients have oral lesions.

(7). The etiology and pathogenesis are unknown.

(8). The dermal infiltrate is composed of lymphocytes, and there is hyperplasia of Langerhans cells within the epidermis, suggesting the possibility of a delayed hypersensitivity-type response.

(9). It resolves spontaneously 1 or 2 years after onset but leaves residual postinflammatory hyperpigmentation and atrophy.

(10). Oral lesions tend to last longer, and malignant change has been described.

b. **Pityriasis rosea**

(1). Pityriasis rosea is a relatively common, self-limited dermatosis characterized by salmon-colored oval patches with a peripheral thin scale.

(2). These are distributed over the trunk in a "Christmas tree" pattern.

(3). Persons aged 10 to 35 years are most frequently affected.

(4). A viral etiology has been suspected.

(5). Eighty percent of cases begin with a herald patch, which consists of a single, sharply defined scaling red plaque, usually 2 to 6 cm across.

(6). Days or weeks later, a generalized eruption occurs usually on the trunk or extremities along the lines of the flexural cleavage.

(7). The oval patches that appear are less than 2 cm across with a collarette of fine, cigarette paper–like scale.

(8). The long axis of the oval lesion is oriented along lines of cleavage.

(9). Successive crops of lesions develop until spontaneous resolution occurs in 2 to 14 weeks.

(10). Dermal changes include a loose, focal superficial, perivascular infiltrate predominantly composed of lymphocytes.

(11). Often there is light hemorrhage in the superficial papillary dermis, which suggests the diagnosis.

(12). The herald patch is often mistaken for tinea corporis (fungus infection of the skin) and is usually not recognized until the generalized eruption blossoms (as in secondary syphilis).

(13). This rash has also been seen in patients receiving gold therapy.

3. **Psoriasis**

a. Psoriasis refers to a group of chronic disorders characterized clinically by scaly erythematous plaques and histologically by epidermal proliferation.

b. The most common type is psoriasis vulgaris, and the mean age of onset is 27 years.

c. The etiology and pathogenesis are unclear, but there is an inheritance pattern.

d. Precipitating factors include trauma, infection, and endocrine changes. It usually occurs without an identifying cause.

e. The turnover time of psoriatic skin is extremely rapid, 3 to 4 days compared with 28 days in normal skin, and thus the mitotic rate of psoriatic skin exceeds that of squamous cell carcinoma.

f. Psoriasis is sometimes associated with other organ system diseases such as psoriatic arthritis and myopathy, enteropathy, and spondylitic heart disease.

g. The clinical features are highly variable.

h. Lesions may occur anywhere, frequently on elbows, knees, scalp, lumbosacral area, intergluteal cleft, and glans penis.

i. Nails may be involved in 30% of cases.

j. Plaquelike lesions are the most common, characterized by well-demarcated pink or salmon-colored plaques surrounded by a loosely adherent silver-white scale.

k. Auspitz's sign, positive in psoriasis, consists of pinpoint bleeding sites revealed when the scale is removed.

l. Postural psoriasis is subdivided into localized (primarily on hands and feet) and generalized.

m. Psoriasis can be life threatening, with fever, leukocytosis, arthralgias, diffuse cutaneous and mucosal pustules around plaque-type lesions, and secondary infection and electrolyte disturbances.

4. **Parapsoriasis**
   a. Parapsoriasis refers to an uncommon group of chronic dermatoses that are confusing because they have no relation to psoriasis; they include several biologically unrelated disorders, and the clinical and histological appearances of the lesions are nonspecific.
   b. Guttate parapsoriasis usually affects the trunk and proximal extremities in male adolescents and young adults and is characterized by red-brown infiltrated plaques and papules 2 to 20 mm across with a thin adherent scale.
   c. Focal or diffuse parakeratosis, mild to moderate epidermal hyperplasia, and spongiosis are also common.

E. **Blistering diseases**[18-23]

1. **Pemphigus**
   a. Pemphigus refers to a group of uncommon diseases of the skin characterized clinically by vesicles and bullae and histologically by acantholysis.
   b. It is associated with serum autoantibodies. There are four types of pemphigus:
      (1). Pemphigus vulgaris
      (2). Pemphigus vegetans
      (3). Pemphigus foliaceus
      (4). Pemphigus erythematosus (most common)
   c. Acantholysis is central to the disease, referring to a loss of intercellular connections of keratinocytes, ultimately becoming round.
   d. Acantholysis occurs in other disorders, such as impetigo, herpes simplex, and herpes zoster.
   e. Autoantibodies appear to be the problem, with the patient's serum containing antibodies that react with intercellular junctions.
   f. There is a direct correlation between serum antibody titers and severity of the disease.
   g. Steroids as well as immunosuppressive drugs reverse the skin lesions and reduce the titer of autoantibodies.

2. **Bullous pemphigoid**
   a. Bullous pemphigoid is a rare form of blistering disease characterized by subepidermal bullae and is self-limited.
   b. It is more common than dermatitis herpetiformis and pemphigus, the other two major blistering disorders.
   c. Lesions can occur anywhere on the skin, but a predilection exists for the lower abdomen, groin, inner aspects of the thighs, and flexor surfaces of the forearms.
   d. The mouth is involved in 30% of patients.
   e. Typical lesions develop over 1 or more years.
   f. It appears to be caused by autoantibodies directed against some component of the lamina lucida of the basement membrane of the epidermis.

3. **Dermatitis herpetiformis**
   a. Dermatitis herpetiformis is a very rare disorder of the skin that involves itchy papulovesicular lesions and the presence of IgA at the dermoepidermal junction.
   b. It is most common in adults aged 25 to 50 years.
   c. It is plausible that the release of chemotactic agents and the influx of inflammatory cells are responsible for the damage leading to vesicle formation.
   d. There is a strong association with asymptomatic gluten-sensitive enteropathy.
   e. Clinically, it is characterized by symmetrical distribution of grouped vesicles, with the earliest sign of incipient eruption marked by pruritus and burning followed in 24 to 48 hours by erythematous urticarial lesions.
   f. Genetic factors may play a role in prolonged circulation of immune complexes.
   g. Skin lesions usually respond to oral administration of sulfonamides and a gluten-free diet.

4. **Porphyria**
   a. Porphyria refers to a group of uncommon inborn or acquired metabolic disturbances of porphyrin metabolism.
      (1). Porphyrins are pigments in hemoglobin, myoglobin, and cytochromes.
      (2). There are five major types of porphyria.
         (a). The acquired type, porphyria cutanea tarda, is the most common.
         (b). The pathogenesis is not com-

pletely understood, but it appears that cutaneous photosensitivity occurs at wavelengths of maximal absorption of ultraviolet light by the porphyrin molecule.

b. Cutaneous manifestations of hypersensitivity to light usually occur in inherited and acquired types.

c. There is edema of the papillary body, vesicle formation, and scarring around the vessels.

d. There is a dermal peg jutting into the blister cavity.

e. Sun-exposed skin exhibits deposition of eosinophilic material in the dermis, and this material is positive on periodic acid–Schiff stain and is diastase resistant.

F. Infection and infestation[24–27]

1. Normal skin is remarkably resistant to infection.
2. The most common infections of the skin are initiated by breaks in the epithelium.
3. Some superficial infections, such as folliculitis and furuncles, may be treated with local measures, whereas others, like impetigo and cellulitis, require systemic antibiotics. Deeper soft-tissue infections, such as fasciitis and myonecrosis, require surgical débridement.
4. Infections of the face and hand should be treated aggressively because of risks of intracranial spread.
5. The most common circumscribed cutaneous infections are folliculitis, furuncles, and carbuncles *(Staphylococcus aureus)*, impetigo, (group A streptococci), and ecthyma gangrenosum (gram-negative bacilli, systemic infection).
6. Vesicular or vesiculopustular lesions of the skin can also be signs of infection.
   a. ***Bacterial infections***
      (1). *Folliculitis*
         (a). Superficial infection of hair follicles.
         (b). Lesions are crops of red papules or pustules.
         (c). Hair can be seen in the center of most papules.
         (d). Staphylococci, yeast, and occasionally *Pseudomonas* sp. are responsible pathogens.
         (e). Treatment: cleansing and hot compresses are usually sufficient.

      (2). *Furuncles and carbuncles*
         (a). Subcutaneous abscesses due to *S. aureus.*
         (b). Lesions are red, tender nodules that may have a surrounding cellulitis.
         (c). Lesions occur most prominently on the face and back of the neck.
         (d). May drain spontaneously.
         (e). Furuncles may be treated with local compresses.
         (f). Larger carbuncles require incision and drainage.
         (g). Antistaphylococcal antibiotics should be given.
      (3). *Impetigo*
         (a). A common, superficial staphylococcal or streptococcal infection of the skin.
         (b). Characterized by erosive lesions covered with honey-colored crusts.
         (c). Commonly affects children and adults in poor health.
         (d). Is especially infectious in infants and usually involves exposed skin, particularly the face and hands.
         (e). A group of small red macules appear that then become pustular and break, leading to erosions (less than 2 cm across) where a drying serum forms and creates the honey-colored crust.
            (i). If crust is not removed, the process expands laterally and forms satellite lesions.
            (ii). If neglected, the lesions can have deep extensions into the full thickness of the epidermis.
   b. ***Viral infections***
      (1). *Verrucae (warts)*
         (a). Common hyperplastic epidermal lesions prevalent in children and adolescents.
         (b). Caused by papovaviruses.
         (c). Presumed mode of transmission is contact and autoinoculation.
         (d). Verruca vulgaris is the most frequent type of wart and can occur anywhere on the skin, with the hands (dorsal surface)

and periungual areas the most common.

(e). Verrucae appear as gray-white or brown and are covered with a rough, horny surface with sizes varying from 1 to 20 mm.

(f). Verruca plana, or the flat wart, is common on the face and dorsal surfaces of the hands; these are slightly elevated, flat, smooth, tan papules measuring 2 to 5 mm across.

(g). Verruca plantaris or palmaris occur on the soles on palms, and the lesions measure 3 to 25 mm across.

(2). *Molluscum contagiosum*

(a). Common viral disease of the skin.

(b). Gives rise to umbilicated papules.

(c). Most common in children and young adults, especially males.

(d). Multiple lesions (3 to 30) are seen on the skin and mucous membranes, especially the trunk and anogenital areas.

(e). Lesions appear as waxy, pink or skin-colored, firm pruritic papules with umbilicated centers that measure 2 to 4 mm in diameter but can be as big as 6 to 20 mm.

(f). Spontaneous involution of these lesions usually occurs within 2 months, but some persist.

(3). *Herpes simplex virus infection*

(a). Can occur on the hands, usually resulting from sexual contact.

(b). Virus usually creates painful erythema (usually at junction of the nail bed and skin, progressing to a vesiculopustular lesion).

(c). Resembles a paronychia (bacterial infection).

(d). When more than one digit is involved, herpes is more likely.

(e). Incision and drainage of the herpetic whitlow are contraindicated.

(f). A culture should be obtained.

(g). Treated with oral acyclovir.

(4). *Varicella-zoster virus infection*

(a). Primary infection is through a respiratory route.

(b). May also occur through contact with infected skin lesions.

(c). Viremia results in crops of papules that progress to vesicles and pustules followed by crusting.

(d). Lesions are most prominent on the trunk.

(e). Usually a disease of childhood.

(f). Systemic symptoms may precede development of rash.

(g). After primary infection, the varicella-zoster virus persists in a latent state in sensory neurons of the dorsal root ganglia.

(h). Infection may reactivate, producing syndrome of herpes zoster (shingles).

(i). Pain in the distribution of the affected nerve root precedes the rash by a few days.

(j). Dysthesia is common.

(k). In older, nonimmunocompromised patients, it is postherpetic.

(l). Neuralgia (severe, prolonged burning pain, with occasional lightning stabs in the involved dermatomes) occurs.

(m). May persist for 1 to 2 years and become disabling.

(n). Burning pain may be relieved by tricyclic antidepressants.

c. **Cutaneous mycobacterial and fungal diseases**

(1). Mycobacteria and fungi can produce cutaneous infections, manifesting generally as papules, nodules, ulcers, crusting lesions, or lesions with a combination of these features.

(2). Biopsy should be done on a chronic inflammatory nodule, crusted lesion, or nonhealing ulceration that is not readily attributed to pressure.

d. **Ulcerative lesions of the skin**

(1). *Pressure sores* (discussed in Chapter 26). These are wounds that occur at weight-bearing sites, particularly in those who cannot move.

(2). *Stasis ulcerations* (discussed in Chapter 26). Patients with lower extremity edema are at risk for infection.

(3). *Diabetic ulcerations* (discussed in Chapter 26). Particularly common in the foot.

(4). *Ecthyma gangrenosum*
  (a). Cutaneous manifestation of disseminated gram-negative rod infection (usually due to *Pseudomonas aeruginosa*) in neutropenic patients.
  (b). Initial lesion is a vesicle or papule with an erythematous halo.
  (c). Initially is small (<2 cm) but can exceed 20 cm.
  (d). The vesicle ulcerates, leaving a necrotic ulcer with surrounding erythema.
  (e). Gram's stain may reveal gram-negative rods.
  (f). Biopsy of lesion shows venous thrombosis.
  (g). Treated with aminoglycosides.

e. **Fungal infections of the skin**
  (1). Fungal infections are classified into superficial and deep types.
    (a). Superficial fungal infections are also referred to as ringworm or dermatophytosis, and the infecting organisms are limited to the cornified layer with erosion of a hair follicle and release of organisms into the dermis.
    (b). Deep fungal infections involve the epidermis, dermis, and subcutis with visceral involvement common, especially in immunosuppressed patients.
  (2). Dermatophytes grow in soil, on animals, and on humans and are responsible for superficial fungal infections. There are many different types.
    (a). *Tinea capitis* is dermatophytosis of the scalp and is common in children; symptomless, hairless patches on the scalp are associated with mild erythema, crust, and scale.
    (b). *Tinea barbae* affects the beard and is relatively uncommon (primarily occurs in men) with mild or marked inflammatory types.
    (c). *Tinea corporis* involves the trunk and extremities and affects all ages as a result of excessive heat and humidity and exposure to infected animals.
    (d). *Chronic tinea pedis* affects the feet (athlete's foot) and is common.
      (i). A papule is first seen that expands with a leading red circinate border that is elevated and scaling.
      (ii). Finally, large plaques, mounds of vesicles, and scaling patches are seen associated with red nodules.
    (e). *Tinea cruris* affects the anogenital region (jock itch).
      (i). It occurs most frequently in obese men during warm weather.
      (ii). It is also common following excessive heat, friction, and maceration.
    (f). *Tinea manus* affects the hands and almost always accompanies tinea pedis.
      (i). Common in 30% to 40% of the population, with persistent diffuse erythema and scaling, vesculobullous lesions, and macerated tissue between the toes.
      (ii). Associated with malodor, pruritus, and erythema and with onychomycosis (of the nails), which is associated with peripheral discoloration of the nail plate extending proximally.
      (iii). Associated with thickening and deformity of the nail and subungual disintegration.

f. **Arthropod bites and stings**
  (1). Arthropods can cause skin lesions, and there is wide variability in the reaction.
  (2). Some individuals suffer minimal symptoms, whereas others experience considerable discomfort, and some may die.
  (3). Lesions produced by arthropods can be caused by a direct irritant effect or by the substances excreted.
    (a). Some venoms cause specific effects (*eg*, black widow spider venom causes severe cramping and excruciating pain).

(b). There can be an immediate or delayed hypersensitivity to secretions.

(c). The arthropod can serve as a vector for bacteria, rickettsia, or parasites.

(4). A firm papule or nodule and sometimes ulceration will manifest at the site of the bite.

(5). The lesion includes dense cellular infiltrate in the dermis and underlying subcutaneous tissue composed of eosinophils, lymphocytes, and monocytes.

(6). *Scabies* is a contagious pruritic dermatosis caused by the itch mite *Sarcoptes scabiei.*

(a). The mites burrow into the interdigital skin and cause an excoriation with edema.

(b). A nonspecific chronic inflammatory infiltrate composed primarily of lymphocytes develops.

(7). *Pediculosis* is caused by the louse, and the louse or its eggs attach to hair shafts.

(a). Enlarged cervical lymph nodes are seen with pediculosis of the scalp.

(b). Pubic lice may be transmitted through sexual contact.

(c). Infection with the body louse is characterized by areas of hyperpigmentation.

g. **Diffuse lesions of the skin**

(1). *Erysipelas*

(a). An infection of the superficial layers of the skin.

(b). Usually caused by group A streptococci.

(c). Seen primarily in children and the elderly.

(d). Most commonly occurs on the face.

(e). Bright-red to violaceous raised lesions with sharply demarcated edges distinguish erysipelas from the deeper tissue infection (cellulitis).

(f). Fever commonly present, but bacteremia is uncommon.

(2). *Cellulitis*

(a). An infection of the deeper layers of the skin with a predilection for the lower extremities.

(b). Venous stasis predisposes to infection and recurrent infection.

(c). Shaking chills often occur.

(d). Linear streaks of erythema occur.

(e). Regional lymph node enlargement and tenderness common.

(f). Patches of erythema with tenderness may occur in a few.

(g). Difficult to distinguish from thrombophlebitis.

(h). Usually caused by β-hemolytic streptococci (but occasionally *Staphylococcus*).

(i). Cultures of blood from the leading edge of the wound are obtained.

(j). Most patients need to be hospitalized.

(k). Repeated attacks of cellulitis may be prevented by monthly 1-week courses of an oral antibiotic.

(3). *Soft-tissue gas*

(a). Crepitus on palpation of the skin indicates the presence of gas in the soft tissues.

(b). Subcutaneous gas can also be found after respiratory-induced barotrauma crepitus.

(c). Principles of treatment of anaerobic soft-tissue infections:

(i). Removal of necrotic tissue.

(ii). Drainage.

(iii). Appropriate antibiotics.

IV. Metabolic and Endocrine Disorders Affecting the Skin[28-34]

A. Pruritus (itching)

Pruritis is a common complaint among patients with uremia from chronic end-stage renal disease.

1. No identifiable causative factor.
2. May get relief with more frequent dialysis, parathyroidectomy, dietary phosphate restriction, and exposure to ultraviolet light.
3. Can also see a yellow discoloration due to deposition of "urochromes" and metastatic calcifications.

B. High cholesterol or disorders of lipid metabolism (including hypertriglyceridemia)

1. Xanthomas (yellow nodules or plaques of the skin composed of lipid-laden histiocytes —common around the eyes).
2. Lipid plaques, which cause thickening around the tendon.
   a. Normal low-density lipid cholesterol levels are less than 130 mg/dL.
   b. Levels of 130 to 150 mg/dL can usually be controlled with diet.
   c. Levels of 160 to 190 mg/dL necessitate diet and usually some drugs.
   d. Levels of greater than 190 mg/dL necessitate diet and drugs.

C. Scleroderma[28,29]

Scleroderma (literally, hard skin) may be classified according to the degree and extent of skin thickening and is seen most commonly in adults, whereas localized forms are commonly seen in children. It is classified according to whether it is localized, systemic, or chemically induced or according to the skin changes that mimic the disease.

1. Scleroderma-like skin changes include
   a. Raynaud's phenomenon (episodic pallor of digits following cold exposure or stress) followed by erythema, tingling, and pain (affects hands, feet, ears, nose, and tongue).
   b. Taut skin in the more proximal parts of the extremities in addition to the thorax and abdomen.
   c. Skin changes beginning on the fingers and hands.
   d. Painless pitting edema initially, followed by gradual loss of edema, leaving thick, indurated tight skin.
   e. Atrophy, which may develop at later stages of the disease, leading to laxity of the superficial dermis.
      (1). Atrophy is noted primarily over joints at the sites of flexion contractures, such as the elbow and proximal interphalangeal joints, which become prone to the development of lacerations.
      (2). Areas of hypopigmentation and hyperpigmentation are common.

D. Other scleroderma-like skin problems

1. **Eosinophilic fasciitis.** This syndrome manifests as swelling and tightness of the skin of the trunk and proximal extremities.
   a. The early stage is followed by progressive induration of the skin and subcutaneous tissue.
   b. The skin is typically shiny with an orange-peel appearance; onset frequently follows periods of physical exertion and trauma.
2. **Eosinophilic myalgia syndrome (EMS).** This syndrome has been documented in individuals who have ingested L-tryptophan and is thought to result from a contaminant in the preparation.
   a. The early phase of EMS is characterized by an acute onset of intense myalgia, skin rashes, dyspnea, fever, and weight loss.
   b. Later stages include skin induration, myopathy, and diffuse peripheral neuropathy.
3. Scleroderma-like skin changes may also occur in patients with diabetes mellitus.

E. Systemic lupus erythematosus (SLE)[30-32]

SLE is characterized by inflammation in several organ systems and production of autoantibodies that participate in immunologically mediated tissue injury.

1. General
    a. SLE usually presents with one or two symptoms, such as fatigue and arthritis, and later additional features develop.
    b. The severity of the disease varies in patients, and it is characterized by remissions and exacerbations.
2. Abnormalities of the skin, hair, or mucous membranes are the second most common manifestation of SLE (occur in 85% of patients).
3. Many different types of skin manifestations may appear.
    a. The classic malar butterfly rash is a nonpapular erythematous rash covering both cheeks and the bridge of the nose with sparing of the nasolabial folds, which may worsen with sun exposure.
    b. The second most common erythematous rash is a maculopapular rash that may be located anywhere on the body.
    c. Systemic flares of the disease are often preceded by exacerbations of skin lesions.
    d. Other skin lesions include urticaria, bullae, livedo reticularis, panniculitis, alopecia, and vasculitic lesions (manifested as livedo reticularis, tender nodules, purpuric leg ulcers, or splinter hemorrhages).
    e. Mucosal ulcers, often painless, occur on the hard and soft palate.
    f. Raynaud's phenomenon (idiopathic, paroxysmal bilateral cyanosis of the digits because of arterial and arteriolar contractions, caused by cold or emotion) may be severe.

F. Vasculitides[33]

The vasculitides represent a heterogeneous group of syndromes characterized by inflammation of the blood vessel wall (involving vessels of any size and location).

1. The inflammation may be exclusively an arteritis, exclusively a venulitis, or a combination.
2. Polyarteritis nodosa primarily involves the medium and small muscular arteries and can occur in any age group (but peak incidence is in the 5th and 6th decades of life with a male:female ratio of approximately 2.5:1).
3. Kidneys are the most commonly involved organ system (inflammation of the arcuate arteries) followed by coronary arteritis and gastrointestinal signs associated with pain, bleeding, obstruction, and perforation.
4. There are also disorders of the peripheral nervous system attributable to arteritis of the vasa nervorum and peripheral neuropathies.
5. Also, arteritis affects the integument in some form in 25% of patients.
    a. A characteristic sign is cutaneous and subcutaneous nodules (0.5 to 1 cm) that are usually movable and sometimes transient.
    b. Livedo reticularis, peripheral gangrene, and polymorphic lesions with purpura and urticaria also occur.

G. Diabetes mellitus[34-36]

1. **Characteristics**
    a. Diabetes mellitus is a common disorder, affecting 2% to 4% of the population.
    b. Complications of diabetes account for more than 25% of all new cases of end-stage renal failure and more than 50% of all lower extremity amputations. Diabetes mellitus is also the leading cause of blindness.
    c. A patient is considered to have diabetes mellitus if he/she exhibits any of the following (see Table 25–6 for more details):
        (1). Polyuria, polydipsia, ketonuria, and rapid weight loss together with gross and unequivocal elevation of plasma glucose levels.
        (2). Elevated fasting glucose concentration on more than one occasion (venous plasma glucose >140 mg/dL).
        (3). Fasting glucose concentration less than that which is diagnostic of diabetes mellitus, but sustained elevation of glucose concentration during the oral glucose tolerance test on more than one occasion. The 2-hour sample and another sample taken between the administration of the oral 75-g glucose dose should show venous plasma glucose greater than 200 mg/dL.

Table 25–6. SYMPTOMS OF DIABETES MELLITUS

Hyperglycemia	Hypoglycemia
Polyuria	Secondary to catecholamine release (adrenergic)
Polydipsia	Sweating
Polyphagia	Shakiness
Weight loss	Anxiety
Fatigue	Palpitations
Candida infections	Weakness
Blurred vision	Tremor
Vulvovaginitis	Hunger
	Faintness
	Tachycardia
	Secondary to central nervous system dysfunction
	Confusion
	Irritability
	Headaches
	Abnormal behavior
	Weakness
	Diplopia
	Inappropriate affect
	Motor incoordination
	Convulsions
	Coma
	Nocturnal hypoglycemia (due to excessive insulin)
	Morning headaches
	Lassitude
	Night sweats
	Nightmares
	Difficulty in waking
	Psychological changes
	Restlessness during sleep
	Loud respirations

2. **Classification of Diabetes Mellitus** (see Table 25–7)
   a. Type I—insulin-dependent diabetes mellitus.
   b. Type II—non–insulin-dependent diabetes mellitus.
   c. Secondary diabetes mellitus:
      (1). Pancreatic disease
      (2). Hemochromatosis
      (3). Hormonal
      (4). Drug induced
      (5). Insulin receptor abnormalities
      (6). Specific genetic syndromes
      (7). Gestational diabetes
   d. Genetic defects of the insulin receptor.

Table 25–7. CHARACTERISTICS OF DIABETES MELLITUS: TYPE I AND TYPE II

Characteristic	Type I	Type II
Age of onset	Juvenile onset usually < 30 yr	Adult onset usually > 40 yr
Ketosis	Common	Uncommon
Body weight	Not obese	Obese
Endogenous insulin secretion	Severe deficiency	Moderate deficiency
Insulin resistance	Occasional	Almost always
Islet cell antibodies	Frequent	Absent
Association with other autoimmune disease	Frequent	No
Treatment with insulin	Always necessary	Usually not required

V. Acquired Immunodeficiency Syndrome (AIDS): Skin Manifestations

A. Skin problems in patients with AIDS[37–40]

1. Human immunodeficiency virus (HIV)-infected patients may experience a variety of dermatological ailments, many of which are treatable.
2. HIV-infected individuals have higher than normal frequency of cutaneous and systemic reactions to a variety of medications, particularly sulfa-containing drugs.
   a. Severe seborrheic dermatitis often manifests as a scaly eruption between the eyebrows and the nasolabial fold.
   b. Psoriasis occurs with greater than expected frequency.
   c. Facial and genital warts also occur with increased frequency.
   d. Generalized pruritus may be a drug reaction in some cases but may also be due to dry skin or to pruritic papules (undefined etiology).
3. Many of the minor mucocutaneous problems can be readily treated, but recurrence is frequent.
   a. Thrush and candidal vaginitis usually respond initially to topical therapy.
   b. Long-term oral therapy may be required to prevent frequent relapses.
4. One of the most serious dermatological conditions in HIV-infected patients is Kaposi's sarcoma (KS).
   a. KS is recognized as a manifestation of AIDS.
   b. It occurs primarily among homosexual and bisexual men.

c. The frequency of KS has fallen from 40% at the outset of the AIDS epidemic to less than 20% in 1990.

d. The tumor may result from infection with an unidentified sexually transmissible pathogen.

e. The tumor is primarily of the skin and mucosal surface but can involve the gastrointestinal tract, lungs, and lymph nodes.

   (1). The tumor's growth is promoted by HIV-associated immunodeficiency.

   (2). The lesions may be flat or raised; may be red, brown, or blue in color; and may resemble insect bites, nevi, or cutaneous ecchymoses.

   (3). The lesions often have a firm texture when rolled between the fingers (which would not normally distinguish a benign lesion).

   (4). Symptomatic or rapidly progressive tumors must be treated.

       (a). Systemic chemotherapy can provide remissions with disseminated disease or symptomatic visceral disease.

       (b). Some patients with modest immune impairment may respond to treatment with interferon-α.

5. Another serious cutaneous presentation that is often a complication of HIV infection is non-Hodgkin's B lymphoma.

   a. Most AIDS-associated lymphomas are of small noncleaved or immunoblastic histology.

   b. Extranodal presentation is the rule.

   c. There is a high frequency of gastrointestinal or intracranial presentations.

   d. Usually, patients present with these late in the course of HIV disease, but sometimes it may be the first presenting symptom.

   e. Treatment is usually not very effective.

      (1). Chemotherapy for systemic disease or radiation therapy for central nervous system disease can provide brief clinical responses.

      (2). Few patients survive more than 6 months after diagnosis.

6. The following skin diseases are less serious but more common in patients with HIV infection:

   a. *Herpes simplex*

      (1). Clear or crusted vesicles with an erythematous base.

      (2). Ulceration common when chronic.

   (3). Location usually oral or genital mucous membranes, face, and hands.

   (4). May be treated with acyclovir; although response to initial treatment may be rapid, chronic therapy is usually required to prevent frequent relapses.

   (5). Acyclovir-resistant strains can develop, necessitating treatment with intravenous foscarnet.

   b. *Herpes zoster (shingles)*

      (1). Cluster of vesicles in a dermatomic or polydermatomic distribution.

      (2). May be preceded by unexplained pain in the involved dermatome.

      (3). May involve adjacent dermatomes or may disseminate.

      (4). Usually treated with acyclovir.

   c. *Aphthous ulcers*

      (1). Giant ulcers and esophageal ulcers are seen.

      (2). May respond to systemic corticosteroids.

      (3). Need to be cultured to be sure they are not viral in origin.

      (4). Intravenous ganciclovir or foscarnet therapy may be needed.

   d. *Staphylococcal folliculitis*

      (1). Erythematous pustules on face, trunk, and groin.

      (2). Often pruritic.

      (3). Usually treated with dicloxacillin.

   e. *Bacillary angiomatosis*

      (1). Friable vascular papules or subcutaneous nodules on skin.

      (2). May involve liver, spleen, and lymph nodes.

      (3). Treated with erythromycin.

   f. *Molluscum contagiosum*

      (1). Chronic, flesh-colored papules, often umbilicated.

      (2). Due to poxvirus infection.

      (3). Lesions on face, neck, or anogenital area.

      (4). Treated with cryotherapy and curettage.

   g. *Seborrheic dermatitis*

      (1). White scaling or erythematous patches on scalp, eyebrows, face, trunk, axilla, and groin.

      (2). Treated with hydrocortisone cream.

   h. *Psoriasis*

      (1). Scaling, marginated patches on elbows, knees, and lumbosacral areas.

(2). Treated with triamcinolone acetonide cream.
i. *Candidal rash*
(1). Urticarial scaling or erythematous patches on face, trunk, axilla, and groin.
(2). Treated with hydrocortisone or clotrimazole cream.

References

1. MacKie RM: *Clinical Dermatology: An Illustrated Textbook,* 3rd ed. New York, Oxford University Press, 1991.
2. Murphy GF, Kwan TH, Mihm MC: The skin. In Robbins SL, Cotran RS, Jumar V (eds): *Pathologic Basis of Disease,* 4th ed. Philadelphia, W. B. Saunders Company, 1990, pp 1257–1303.
3. Fisher ER, Morgan MM, Wechsler HL, *et al.:* Analysis of histopathologic and electron microscopic determinants of keratoacanthoma and squamous cell carcinoma. *Cancer* 1972, 29:1387–1397.
4. Hashimoto K, Lever WF: *Appendage Tumors of the Skin.* Springfield, IL, Charles C Thomas, 1968.
5. Gorlin RJ, Vickers RA, Keln E, Williamson JJ: The multiple basal cell nevi syndrome. *Cancer* 1965, 18:89–104.
6. Cotran RS: Metastasizing basal cell carcinoma. *Cancer* 1961, 14:1036–1040.
7. Underwood LJ, Epstein E: Squamous cell epithelioma that simulates sarcoma. *Arch Dermatol* 1951, 64:149–151.
8. Cox FH, Helwig EB: Kaposi's sarcoma. *Cancer* 1959, 12:289–298.
9. Templeton AC: Studies in Kaposi's sarcoma. *Cancer* 1972, 30:854–867.
10. Maize JC, Ahmed AR, Provost TT: Xanthoma disseminatum and multiple myeloma. *Arch Dermatol* 1974, 110:758–761.
11. Brownstein MH, Helwig EB: Metastatic tumors of the skin. *Cancer* 1972, 29:1298–1307.
12. Kopt AW: Malignant melanoma: a review. *J Dermatol Surg Oncol* 1977, 3:1–4.
13. Blaylock WK: Atopic dermatitis: diagnosis and pathobiology. *J Allergy Clin Immunol* 1976, 57:62–79.
14. Freinkel RK: Pathogenesis of acne vulgaris. *N Engl J Med* 1969, 2:1161–1163.
15. Leyden JJ: Pathogenesis of acne vulgaris. *Int J Dermatol* 1976, 25:490–496.
16. Cox AJ, Watson W: Histologic variations in lesions of psoriasis. *Arch Dermatol* 1972, 206:503–506.
17. Chowaniec O, Jablonska S, Beutner EH, *et al.:* Earliest clinical and histologic changes in psoriasis. *Dermatologica* 1961, 163:42–51.
18. Lever WF (ed): *Pemphigus and pemphigoid.* Springfield, IL, Charles C Thomas, 1965.
19. Katz SI, Strober W: The pathogenesis of dermatitis herpetiformis. *J Invest Dermatol* 1978, 170:63–75.
20. Yaoita H: Identification of IgA binding structures in skin of patients with dermatitis herpetiformis. *J Invest Dermatol* 1978, 71:213–216.
21. Ljunghall K, Schejnius A, Forsum U: Circulating reticulin autoantibodies of IgA class in dermatitis herpetiformis. *Br J Dermatol* 1979, 200:173–176.
22. Epstein JH, Williams NG, Hougston AF: Cutaneous changes in porphyrias. A microscopic study. *Arch Dermatol* 1973, 107:689–698.
23. Aimeida JD: Electron microscopic study of human warts; sites of production and nature of the inclusion bodies. *J Invest Dermatol* 1962, 38:337–345.
24. Lutzner MA: Molluscum contagiosum, verruca and zoster viruses. *Arch Dermatol* 1963, 87:436–444.
25. Finegold DS: The diagnosis and treatment of gangrenous and crepitant cellulitis. In Remington JS, Swartz MN (eds): *Current Clinical Topics in Infectious Diseases.* vol 2. New York, McGraw-Hill, 1981.
26. Gorbach SL: Diseases caused by non-spore forming anaerobic bacteria. In Wyngaarden JB, Smith LH Jr, Bennett JC (eds): *Cecil Textbook of Medicine,* 19th ed. Philadelphia, W. B. Saunders Company, 1992, pp 1685–1689.
27. Swartz, MN: Skin and soft tissue infections. In Mandell GL, Douglas RG, Bennett JE (eds): *Principles and Practice of Infectious Diseases,* 3rd ed. New York, Churchill Livingstone, pp 796–824.
28. Medsger TA: Systemic sclerosis (scleroderma), localized scleroderma, eosinophilic fasciitis, and calcinosis. In McCarty DJ (ed): *Arthritis and Allied Conditions,* 11th ed. Philadelphia, Lea & Febiger, 1989, pp 1118–1165.
29. Siebold JR: Scleroderma. In Kelley WN, Harris ED Jr, Ruddy S, Sledge CB (eds): *Textbook of Rheumatology,* 3rd ed. Philadelphia, W. B. Saunders Company, 1989, pp 1214–1244.
30. Andreoli TE, Bennett JC, Carpenter CJ, *et al.: Cecil Essentials of Medicine,* 3rd ed. Philadelphia, W. B. Saunders Company, 1993, pp 568–573.
31. Schur PHP: Clinical features of SLE. In Kelley WN, Harris ED Jr, Ruddy S, Sledge CB (eds): *Textbook of Rheumatology,* 3rd ed. Philadelphia, W. B. Saunders Company, 1989, pp 1101–1124.
32. Steinberg AD: Systemic lupus erythematosus. In Wyngaarden JB, Smith LH Jr, Bennett JC (eds): *Cecil Textbook of Medicine,* 19th ed. Philadelphia, W. B. Saunders Company, 1992, pp 1522–1530.
33. Cupps T, Fauci A: *The Vasculitides.* Philadelphia, W. B. Saunders Company, 1981.
34. Andreoli TE, Bennett JC, Carpenter CJ, *et al.: Cecil Essentials of Medicine,* 3rd ed. Philadelphia, W. B. Saunders Company, 1993, pp 513–523.
35. Brownlee M, Cerami A, Vlassara H: Advanced glycosylation end products in tissue and the biochemical basis of diabetic complications. *N Engl J Med* 1988, 318:1315.
36. Pecoraro RE: The nonhealing diabetic ulcer—a major cause for limb loss. In Barbul A, Eaglstein WH, Marshal D, *et al.* (eds): *Clinical and Experimental Approaches to Dermal and Epidermal Repair: Normal and Chronic Wounds.* New York, Wiley-Liss, 1991, pp 27–43.
37. Andreoli TE, Bennett JC, Carpenter CJ, *et al.: Cecil Essentials of Medicine,* 3rd ed. Philadelphia, W. B. Saunders Company, 1993, pp 702–719.
38. Carpenter CJ, Mayer KH, Stein MD, *et al:* Human immunodeficiency virus infection in North American women: experience with 200 cases and a review of the literature. *Medicine* 1991, 70:307–325.
39. Mann J: AIDS—the second decade: a global perspective. *J Infect Dis* 1992, 165:245–250.
40. Saag MS: HIV and associated disorders. In Wyngaarden JB, Smith LH Jr, Bennett JC (eds): *Cecil Textbook of Medicine,* 19th ed. Philadelphia, W. B. Saunders Company, 1992, p 1979.

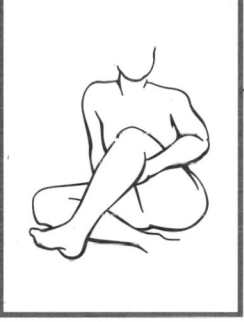

CHAPTER 26

Systemic Issues and Skin Conditions: Wound Healing, Oxygen Percutaneous Drug Delivery, Burns, and Desensitized Skin

Nancy Byl, Linda Rosenberg Zellerbach, and Lucinda A. Pfalzer

I. Principles of Wound Healing

A. Wound healing[1-21]

1. Repair and regeneration are fundamental and normal reactions to injury and occur in all organisms.[1]

   a. With increased complexity of organisms, tissue injury is healed more frequently through reconstruction of connective tissue, vasculature, and covering epithelium than through regeneration.

   b. Repair of connective tissue (collagen and proteoglycans) is essential to prolongation of life in a hostile environment.

   c. The setting for optimal repair is a healthy organism with a healthy vascular system.

585

2. General principles of repair:
  a. At the instant of injury, a complex series of events occur that proceed to repair and ultimately to scar formation.[2-4]
    (1). Some mysteries of this repair process still remain.
      (a). What in the injury stimulates repair?
      (b). How does the wound recognize that repair is no longer needed? (*ie*, Why does healing stop?)
    (2). The cascade of responses is known collectively as inflammation and repair.
  b. When tissue is disrupted, vessels are injured, cells are broken, and platelets and collagen intermingle and interact (see Figure 26–1).
    (1). The local microvasculature structure senses the injury and releases phospholipids that stimulate the intrinsic coagulation mechanisms.
    (2). The injured cells also release thromboplastin that activates the extrinsic coagulation mechanism.
    (3). The vessels nearby soon dilate, and the platelets and white blood cells begin to stick to the endothelial lining and the leukocytes migrate between the endothelial cells and into the area of injury.
    (4). Granulocytes and macrophages infiltrate within a few hours.
    (5). In the area of damaged vasculature, the tissue becomes covered with metabolic white blood cells, which will eventually be replaced by metabolizing fibroblasts.
      (a). Connective tissue has its greatest metabolic need at this time.
      (b). The circulation is least able to meet the metabolic need, and a local "energy crisis" occurs.[5-8]
        (i). However, the hypoxia and the concentrations of ascorbate and lactate that are present in wounded tissue may be critical to stimulate the fibroblasts to make collagen.
        (ii). As the cells continue to be called into the wound, anaerobic metabolism inevitably results and the extracellular P_{O_2} can fall below 10 mm Hg, a point probably below the critical or lowest optimum P_{O_2} for aerobic metabolism in both fibroblasts and leukocytes.
        (iii). Within a few days, lactate in the extracellular fluid of the central dead space of wounds is in the region of 10 to 15 mm Hg.
    (6). Within a few days, fibroblasts become visible and gradually replace the majority of white blood cells, increasing the momentum of collagen synthesis (a wound that is primarily closed begins to gain strength through collagenous links by about the 3rd day post injury) (see Figure 26–2).
    (7). Neovascularization is a constant feature of repair because the needs of inflammation and repair overwhelm the nutritional supply.

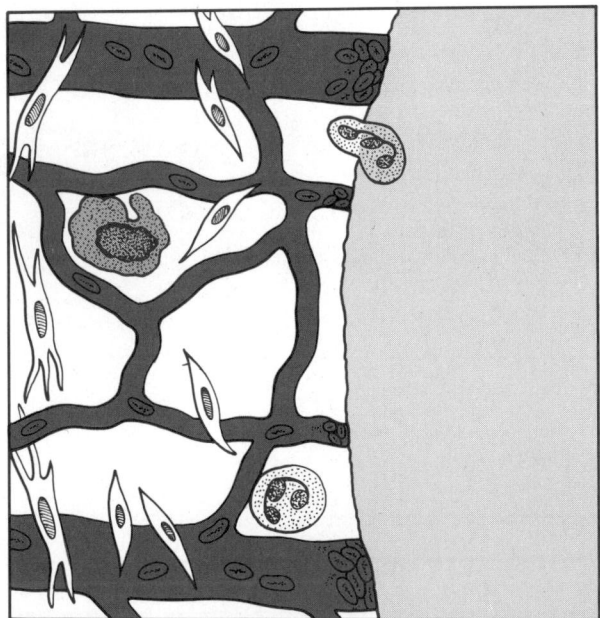

FIGURE 26–1   The edge of a wound just after injury. Vessels are thrombosed, and an inflammatory exudate, containing mostly polymorphonuclears, appears. Serum covers or fills the wound; serum contains stimulators of cell replication at least partly made by platelets.

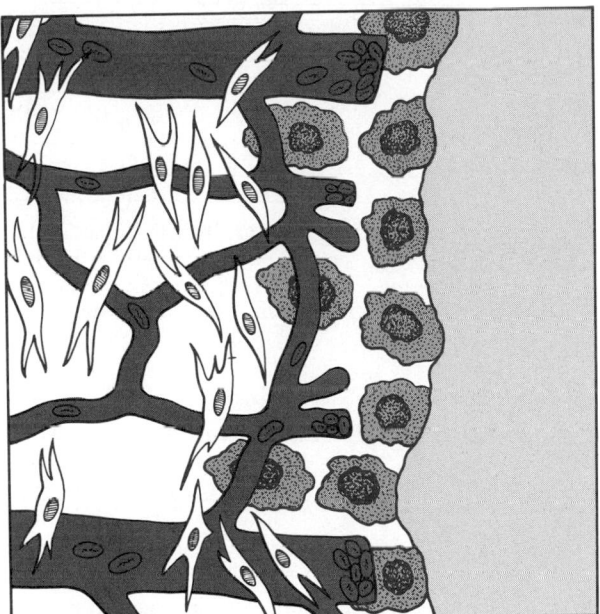

FIGURE 26–2 The developing "granulation tissue" now shows a more orderly arrangement of inflammatory response, which is predominantly macrophagic. Fibroblasts, mostly from perivascular cells, have appeared. Their mitoses are seen near the most distal functioning vessels. Endothelial capillary buds are appearing in the center of the pre-existing capillary arcade. Macrophages are now in a position to stimulate angiogenesis and fibroplasia.

(a). New circulation is seen bridging the wound space in 3 to 4 days.

(b). Aggregating platelets (eg, white blood cells) release proteolytic enzymes that amplify the distress signals of the injured tissue.

(8). Chemotactic substances accumulate and call forth the inflammatory cells.

(a). Cells follow the chemical signals to the area of injury and bind their membranes.

(b). Phagocytic cells ingest these altered substances as if to "lick the wound."

(c). Platelets and phagocytic macrophages release a substance or substances that can stimulate replication of fibroblasts.

(9). Around the 3rd day after injury, repair is well under way, with activated macrophages and granulocytes defending against bacteria.

(a). New microcirculatory loops find external support in a collagen gel secreted by the immature fibroblasts.

(b). As each new capillary loop becomes functional, more oxygen becomes available and the fibroblasts can synthesize more collagen.

(c). As the process continues, the collagen-synthesizing fibroblasts are left behind to continue the work of constructing and reconstructing the new connective tissue.

(d). A loose-knit layer of new blood vessels, macrophages, granulocytes, and fibroblasts is formed.

(e). The PO_2 in the uninjured arteriolar portion of the capillary falls to near 0 mm Hg at the surface of the macrophages and the dead spaces.

(f). The lactate, pH, and PCO_2 gradients are in the other direction: high in the dead space and lower near the functioning vessels.

(g). Scar formation occurs as a result of failed tissue regeneration.

(10). Finally, the healing is complete (see Figure 26–3).

3. The three stages of healing include
• Inflammation (1 to 10 days, with an early and a late phase).
• Granulation tissue formation (3 to 20 days).
• Matrix formation and remodeling (from day 9 on).
The three phases overlap considerably.

a. **Inflammation**

(1). Inflammation includes a vascular response, a hemostatic response, a cellular response, and an immune response.

(a). Inflammation can be caused by a variety of insults.

(b). Although the inflammatory response is the same, some insults can lead to exaggerated response in one or more events.

(2). Initially, a transient vasoconstriction of arterioles is the vascular re-

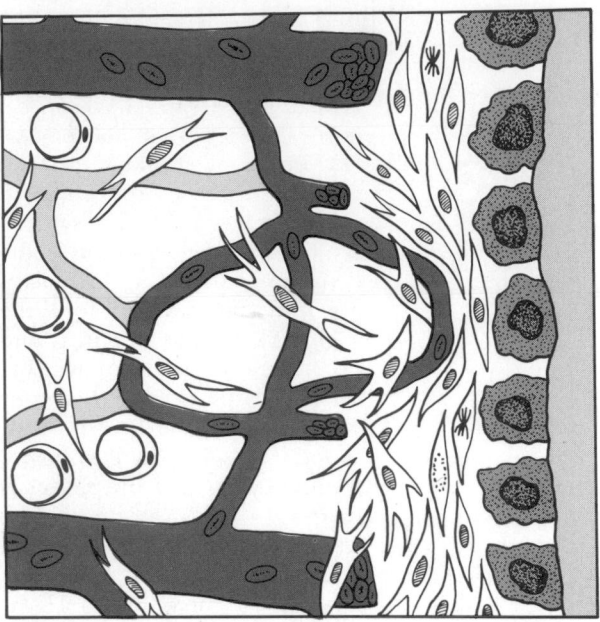

FIGURE 26–3 A new functioning capillary loop has been formed. The "wound module" is complete. Some of the old vasculature, now in an area of lessened metabolic demand, has dropped out.

sponse (usually lasting only a few minutes).[5]

(a). Capillary vessel walls (especially the postcapillary venules) become lined with white blood cells (leukocytes). This is called margination.

(b). The vasoconstriction is followed by vasodilation, which causes an increase in blood flow and a rise in vessel hydrostatic pressure.

(c). There is increased permeability of the microvessels, and this allows escape of cells, macromolecules, and fluid from the vascular system.

(d). Edema occurs because the escaping cells and macromolecules create an osmotic gradient that causes fluid to move into the interstitial spaces.

(e). The vascular response is due to local mediators released at the site of injury (histamine, bradykinin, prostaglandins, and complement fractions), each causing vasodilation and histamine release.

(f). The edema fluid is mainly water and dissolved electrolytes and is clear in appearance.

(i). As microvessel permeability increases, cells and plasma proteins escape and the fluid becomes viscous, owing to the protein, and cloudy, owing to the leukocytes.

(ii). This fluid is now called exudate (pus), and contains a large number of leukocytes.

(iii). If edema is present for long periods (especially in an area of poor circulation as in peripheral vascular disease), oxygenation is disrupted.

(g). The hemostatic response controls the blood loss when the blood vessels are ruptured.

(i). The small vessels retract and help seal themselves off.

(ii). Platelets aggregate and deposit fibrin, which traps red blood cells and creates a blood clot.

(iii). The fibrin also occludes the lymphatic channels and prevents drainage of fluid from the injured area, localizing the inflammation.

(iv). When bleeding is internal and confined to the injured area, a mass of clotted blood cell hematoma develops.

(3). During the inflammatory process, the leukocytes clear the site of microorganisms and set the stage for tissue repair. There are many different types of leukocytes—neutrophils, eosinophils, and basophils being the common polymorphonuclear cells.

(a). These different cells are predominant early and late in the process.

(b). Neutrophils characterize early inflammation, attracted by chemotactic agents released at the time of injury.

(i). They rid the site of contaminating bacteria and debris (phagocytosis).

(ii). As the neutrophils disintegrate, the enzymes perpetuate the inflammatory reaction by serving as irritants and chemotactic agents, attracting other leukocytes.

(c). During the first few days after injury, the polymorphonuclear leukocyte predominates.

(d). By about the 5th day, macrophages predominate and remain until the reparative sequence is done, retaining one or more roles throughout the life of the wound.

(e). The macrophages are phagocytic, engulfing large amounts of bacteria and cellular debris.

(f). The appearance of monocytes seems to be critical to the initiation of tissue repair.

(g). Fibroblasts are rarely far from macrophages.

(i). The tissue monocyte, the pulmonary macrophage, the peritoneal macrophage, the Kupffer cell, and other cells from the reticuloendothelial system all fit the classification of macrophages.

(ii). They are large, mobile, and well fitted for metabolism in any environment.

(h). Macrophages are probably the key cell of inflammation.

(i). They seem to act as directors, releasing chemotactic substances in order to bring in other macrophages and to release substances in order to cause multiplication of fibroblasts.

(ii). If macrophages are eliminated, repair is clearly inhibited. The injured cells and tissue are not débrided, and wound strength is poor.

(i). The macrophage débrides injured tissue, processes macromolecules to useful amino acids and sugars, attracts more macrophages, potentially signals for fibroblast formation and activation, may signal for neovascularization, and secretes lactate that stimulates collagen synthesis.

(j). Apparently, vitamin A aids the entrance of the macrophage into the wound and is vital to initiation of repair (eg, if entry of the macrophage is prevented by anti-inflammatory steroids, repair can usually be stimulated by giving the patient vitamin A).

(k). Lymphocytes are present in the later phase of inflammation. They mediate the body's immune reactions and supply antibodies for specific antigens.

(i). This immune response is both cell mediated and humorally mediated.

(ii). Besides the phagocytic activities, there is a series of enzymatic proteins that are activated by bacterial toxins or immune complexes. These enzymes increase vascular permeability and further attract leukocytes. Autoimmune diseases like rheumatoid arthritis alter the benefit of the inflammatory response because the body perceives some of its own tissues as foreign, which stimulates a chronic inflammatory response. Cortisone may inhibit repair[9]; vitamin C can accelerate repair.[10–11]

(4). Acute inflammation is complete in 2 weeks.[9]

(a). Subacute inflammation is associated with an ongoing reaction for up to a month.

(b). If it continues for months or years, it is called chronic inflammation. The predominant cells are lymphocytes, monocytes, and macrophages.

(5). In chronic inflammation, more and more fibroblasts are formed. A delicate balance between tensile strength and adequate mobility is required because the area must be strong but it must allow gliding of tissues.

b. *Tissue repair*[1]

(1). Initially in the repair phase, epithelium (the covering of the skin and the surface layer of mucous and serous membranes) and connective tissue (the cement connecting and supporting other tissues) proliferate.

(2). Some of the epithelium regenerates.

    (a). In the connective tissue, fibroplasia takes place.

    (b). Fibroblasts migrate into the inflamed area from undifferentiated mesenchymal cells and begin to synthesize scar tissue.

    (c). Endothelial buds develop from intact capillaries and supply the area. (They have a characteristic red, granular appearance.)

(3). Wound contraction also begins.

    (a). Actin-rich fibroblasts known as myofibroblasts have the ability to contract; they accumulate at the margins of the wound.

    (b). The myofibroblasts move toward the center of the wound and reduce the size of the area covered.

(4). One of the least appreciated aspects of injury repair is the regeneration of new blood vessels. The function of neovascularization or angiogenesis is to nourish tissue, supplementing the injured tissue.

    (a). New vessels always originate from existing vessels, and all new vessels begin as capillary buds.

    (b). This angiogenesis takes multiple forms, generating a whole new vascular network where a defect has to be filled.

    (c). After the initial thrombosis of the injured vessels, the wound module is assembled; and from the functioning vessels nearest the wound, sprouts of vascular cells appear from the endothelial cells.

    (d). Blood clotting does not aid neovascularization.

    (e). Initially, the basement membrane is incomplete and the new vessels are fragile and leaky.

    (f). The stimulation of new vessel formation has not been completely formulated.

       (i). It is speculated that molecular signals come from macrophages and platelets.

      (ii). Hypoxia also plays a role.[12–19]

     (iii). Circulation bridges the wound by the 2nd or 3rd day.

     (iv). This vascular regeneration is a delicate process, however; treatment modalities can interfere with it, such as chemotherapy, radiation, and steroids.

    (g). Finally, the new vessels join with unused circulation and then rejoin vessels across a primarily healing wound.

(5). Fibroblasts are prolific during this phase of healing.

    (a). Fibroblasts are rarely seen in uninjured tissue.[15]

    (b). They arise from perivascular cells and are closely tied to the vascular response.

    (c). The fibroblast is a hardy cell, but it cannot function outside a specific environment.

    (d). It needs a solid surface on which to attach and migrate.[16]

    (e). In wounds, it adheres to fibrin and collagen.

    (f). It makes collagen best in a slightly acidic environment with an oxygen tension more than about 10 to 20 mm Hg.

    (g). It needs an environment rich in ascorbate and makes more collagen if there is a high concentration of lactate.

    (h). Some fibroblasts contract and relax in response to stimuli.

    (i). They are also seen in large arteries, where they participate in arteriosclerosis.

    (j). The fibroblast has a full complement of metabolic pathways.

(i). It synthesizes proteoglycans and elastin as well as collagen.

(ii). It can also synthesize cholesterol.

(iii). Its requirements include most of the B vitamins, ascorbate, oxygen, amino acids, and trace metals such as zinc, iron, and copper.

(iv). One function of macrophages is to break down local large molecules into amino acids for fibroblast use.[15,16]

(6). Collagen is the principal structural protein of the body and the major constituent of skin, tendons, ligaments, bones, cartilage, fascia, and septa.

(a). It is the principal component of scar tissue.

(b). The term collagen actually refers to a group of glycoproteins that have

(i). Three separate linear peptide chains of equal length.

(ii). A right-handed twist to the chain so that the three chains lie parallel to each other.

(iii). Hydroxyproline and hydroxylysine are unique to collagen, and the analysis of hydroxyproline serves as a means of measuring collagen content.

(c). There are four primary types of collagen, but new types of collagen continue to be discovered.

(i). Type I is seen in bone, tendon, skin, dentin, ligament, fascia, arteries, and the uterus.

(ii). Type II is called hyaline cartilage and is seen only in cartilage.

(iii). Type III is found principally in embryonic connective tissue and in some

adult tissue in wounds, dermis, and the aorta.

(iv). Some Type III collagen is also laid down initially in dermal wounds, but, as the wound matures, it is replaced by Type I.

(v). The basement membranes are composed of Type IV.

(d). Collagen synthesis occurs similarly to other protein synthesis with some unique exceptions.

(i). RNA is not transferred for hydroxyproline or hydroxylysine.

(ii). These two amino acids cannot be directly incorporated into collagen.

(iii). Proline and lysine are included in the growing chain.

(iv). While the chain is still on the ribosome, significant numbers of each of these amino acids are hydroxylated through the action of specific enzymes, prolyl hydroxylase or lysyl hydroxylase.

(e). Rapid collagen synthesis seems to proceed at the best speed with vitamin C.

(i). The role of ascorbate is unclear.

(ii). It appears that when ascorbate is oxidized, a high-energy form of oxygen called superoxide ion (O_2^-) results.

(iii). The more O_2^- available, the more collagen synthesis is enhanced.

c. *Remodeling*

(1). This is the second phase of tissue repair.[17]

(2). Scar maturation can last for years.

(3). Fibroblasts disappear, and the collagen fibers initially laid down by fibroblasts are randomly oriented, with a fragile connective tissue matrix.

(a). With remodeling, the fibers acquire a more organized pattern, parallel to the wound surface, which creates tensile strength.

(b). At maximal strength, the scar tissue is only 70% as strong as intact tissue.

(c). It is also less vascular and creates a diffusion barrier to oxygen.

(d). Repeated injury at the same site can increase tensile strength.

(4). Remodeling is related to collagen turnover.

(a). Collagen is taken up and laid down again along strands of fibronectin.

(b). Abnormal scars develop when there is an imbalance between collagen production and uptake.

(c). A hypertrophic scar is contained within the boundaries of the original wound, whereas a keloid scar extends beyond the borders of the original wound.

(d). At first, new collagen is essentially a gel with poor wound strength.

(i). In order to continue resynthesis, amino acid must be brought in from elsewhere.

(ii). Collagenase is the primary extracellular enzyme involved in collagen lysis. This is produced by inflammatory cells, including polymorphonuclear leukocytes and macrophages, and by regenerating epidermis. Lysis can be accelerated by starvation or specific protein deficiency. It is also seen in patients with scurvy, burns, sepsis, or shock.

(e). Wound strength is a balance between lysis of the old collagen and new collagen (see Figures 26–4 and 26–5).

(i). New collagen must be adequately cross-linked before it is strong.

(ii). The balance of collagen synthesis and collagen lysis represents the well-being of the wound.

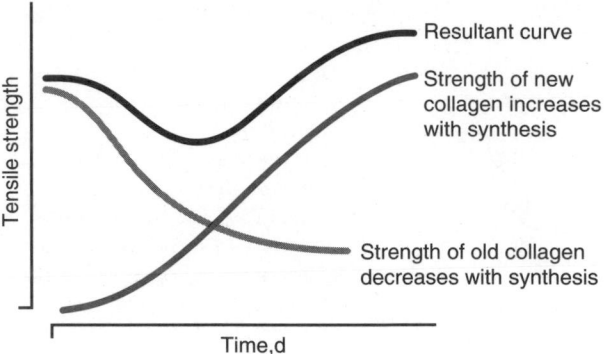

FIGURE 26–4   Concept of wound strength that is expressed as a balance between lysis of the old collagen, which holds the sutures and the new collagen, which welds the wound edges. Any deficit of synthesis or exaggeration of lysis makes the wound's weak point even weaker for a longer time. (Redrawn from Hunt TK, Dunphy JE: *Fundamentals of Wound Management.* New York, Appleton-Century-Crofts, 1979, p 33.)

(iii). The peak rate of collagen synthesis in a primarily healing wound is reached at about 5 to 7 days, and this corresponds with the most rapid rate of increase of tensile strength.

(iv). By about the 3rd week, the primarily healing wound has about the greatest mass it will have, and the strength of the wound increases during this time.

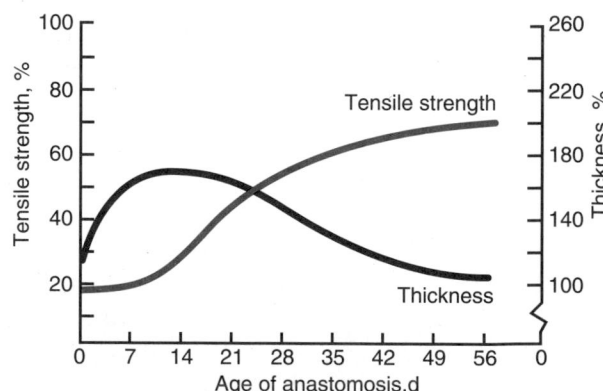

FIGURE 26–5   Tensile strength development in the wound. Note the rapid increase of strength after the initial "lag phase." The initial peak in thickness is clinically defined as the *healing ridge.* The late, slow increase in strength despite loss of thickness reflects collagen turnover and remodeling. (Redrawn from Lange Medical Publications In Dunphy JE, Way LW [eds]: *Current Surgical Diagnosis and Treatment,* 3rd ed. New York, Appleton-Century-Crofts, 1977, p 113.)

(f). As collagen in the maturing wound is turned over, its synthesis and deposition probably follow different rules.

  (i). The vascular system is not complete. The wound has continuity, and stresses and strains on the tissue are again normal.

  (ii). The electrical charges produced by the stresses probably result in an alignment of the proteoglycans and collagen fibers.

  (iii). Movement encourages wounds to heal faster.

  (iv). Fibroblasts and collagen tend to line up along lines of tension.

  (v). Normal tension associated with normal movement is an important stimulus.

B. Factors that modify Inflammation and repair[18–21]

1. Age, nutrition, anemia, peripheral vascular problems, and especially systemic disease such as diabetes mellitus can alter healing.

2. Some drugs can inhibit inflammation, like corticosteroids, but interfere with collagen deposition.

3. Some drugs used for chronic inflammatory conditions stabilize cell membranes and inhibit production of prostaglandins and related thromboxanes and leukotrienes.

4. Nonsteroidal anti-inflammatory drugs (NSAIDS) such as aspirin and ibuprofen also inhibit inflammation by interrupting production of prostaglandins.

5. Prolonged immobilization promotes the development of adhesions and limited motion.

   a. Remobilization is critical to recovery of function after the inflammation.

   b. Remobilization is also critical to repair (which is one reason why continuous passive motion devices are often employed early after injury).

   c. Soft-tissue techniques modify the lines of stress and release adhesions.

   d. Controlled exercise and weight bearing change the lines of stress.

6. Effect of thermal agents on inflammation and repair:

   a. Inflammation and repair are natural and desirable.

   b. Selection of physical agents used to modify inflammation and repair depends on

      (1). Type of lesion (eg, open full-thickness wounds, nonhealing decubitus surgical incisions, abrasions?)

      (2). Stage of injury (acute inflammatory conditions, eg, sprains/strains; chronic inflammatory conditions, eg, rheumatoid arthritis?)

      (3). Problems secondary to healing, such as peripheral vascular problems, edema, limited joint mobility, or contractures?

   c. The modalities frequently used to facilitate healing include heat (deep and superficial), cold, light (laser and sunlight or ultraviolet light), and electrical current.

   d. Intervention with physical agents should be designed to facilitate or accelerate the process or control the undesirable side effects (eg, excessive swelling, pain, immobilization, and infection).

   e. Acute injuries must be managed differently than chronic conditions.

      (1). As a general rule, treat the acute problem with cold, compression wrap, elevation, and rest. The goal in the early treatment is to prevent edema, minimize pain, and take the stress off the tissues.

         (a). In the case of early-onset inflammation, cold minimizes acute edema and hemorrhage and provides a good analgesic effect.

         (b). Cold decreases the effects of histamine on capillary permeability and lowers leukocyte counts; it reduces muscle spasm and soreness.

      (2). In acute inflammation also

         (a). Consider continuous passive motion to maintain mobility without damaging tissue.

         (b). Protect the injured area.

         (c). Consider the benefit of therapeutic modalities listed below that can be used to facilitate healing for both acute as well as chronic conditions.

            (i). Diathermy (pulsating) at a low intensity can be used in the acute phase.

            (ii). Low-intensity ultrasound

(0.5 W/cm²) delivered in a pulsating mode can facilitate healing (*eg*, collagen deposition) without increasing heat.

(iii). Neuromuscular stimulation to muscle contraction may keep the muscles active without joint movement.

(iv). Transcutaneous electrical stimulation may be given to control pain.

(v). Galvanic current, high-volt pulsed current, or pulsed direct currents can be used to facilitate healing, including assistance with wound cleaning.

f. For subacute and chronic conditions, heat is recommended to
   (1). Inhibit inflammation.
   (2). Alter the viscoelastic properties of connective tissue and make it more extensible.
   (3). Increase blood flow and thereby increase oxygen and increase collagen deposition.
   (4). Assist in the reabsorption of late inflammatory exudate and debris.
   (5). The deeper the lesion, the more beneficial the modalities of ultrasound or diathermy.
   (6). Heat can
      (a). Localize the inflammation.
      (b). Accelerate abscess formation so that the abscess can be drained.
   (7). Heat should not be used within the first 24 hours after injury because it could
      (a). Exacerbate hemorrhage and edema.
      (b). Increase blood flow and increase microvascular hydrostatic pressure.
   (8). Caution must be executed in the application of modalities during the treatment of patients with rheumatoid arthritis.

(a). Patients with rheumatoid arthritis are often referred for moist heat during a flare.

(b). Heat during the acute phase could be harmful.

(c). It has been reported that temperature increases of 5° were found to degrade cartilage by fourfold.[22]
   (i). This may have been because of an elevated metabolic rate of the macrophages.
   (ii). Increased destructive enzymes are associated with this autoimmune disease.

(d). Others actually recommend superficial heat (*ie*, hot packs) and claim that it has not been associated with cartilage destruction in patients with rheumatoid arthritis.
   (i). This may be due to the fact that joint temperature actually falls in response to hot packs.
   (ii). There may be a reflex shunting of blood flow away from the joint to the more superficial tissues.

(e). More research is needed to clarify whether heat (superficial or deep) or cold is the best treatment for an acute exacerbation of pain and inflammation for a patient with rheumatoid arthritis.

7. In summary, healing and repair are complex tasks. Although we do not have all the answers, it is clear that physical therapists have a role to play to facilitate the healing process. The physical therapist must
   a. Consider what is desired at each point along the healing continuum.
   b. Critically analyze the problem and apply logical problem solving to determine the most appropriate treatment.
   c. Carefully evaluate the response to treatment and determine whether it is necessary to modify the treatment.

II. Postsurgical Management and Infections: The Role of Oxygen[23–52]

A. Introduction

1. Healing of wounds that are well perfused, noninfected, and otherwise healthy proceeds in an orderly and predictable sequence.
2. Healing can be compromised by host or environmental factors such as diabetes mellitus, trauma, infection, proliferative endarteritis following therapeutic irradiation, peripheral vascular disease, steroids, foreign bodies, nutritional disorders, hypovolemia, or anemia.
3. Infections are most likely to start in injured and poorly vascularized tissues, where a decrease in the delivery of oxygen, leukocytes, and other immune substances, which inhibit the removal of carbon dioxide occurs.
4. An inevitable result of tissue injury is hypoxia.[23–25]
   a. Hypoxia is a stimulus to repair but also imposes vulnerability to infection.
   b. Oxygen delivery changes with tissue injury and repair.
   c. The question is whether the clinical administration of oxygen can be used to prevent and treat infection.

B. Tissue response to injury

1. Injury elicits inflammation, fibroblast proliferation, angiogenesis, connective tissue synthesis, and epithelialization.
2. Surgery and trauma also disrupt tissue architecture and lead to hemorrhage.
3. Injury disrupts vessels, which fill with blood and clot.
   a. Blood is exposed to collagen, and this activates Hageman's factor and causes degranulation of platelets.
   b. Four major biochemical amplification systems result from the activation of Hageman's factor and the tissue injury:
      (1). The complement cascade.
      (2). The intrinsic coagulation mechanism.
      (3). The kinin cascade, which causes vessels to dilate.
      (4). The fibrinolytic system.
   c. Each biochemical reaction amplifies the original signal and produces mitogens and chemoattractants.
4. Repair is heavily populated by polymorphonuclear neutrophils and lymphocytes (phagocytic leukocytes). Phagocytic leukocytes are the most important line of defense against infection, but killing of granulocytes is normal only to the degree oxygen is available. Whereas some healing occurs automatically, oxidative killing is more effective and efficient and white blood cells increase their respiration.[26–30]
   a. The degranulating platelets release substances (eg, serotonin) that further amplify the coagulation mechanisms and ensure complete activation of the complement and kinin cascades.
   b. Kinins activated by Hageman's factor cause surrounding vessels to dilate.
   c. Many small infarcts cause surrounding vessels to dilate.
   d. Small infarcts result from blockage of the main outflow of vessels.
   e. Intravascular thromboses result from blockage of the main outflow of vessels.
      (1). Intravascular thromboses accumulate back to the point where blocked vessels connect to vessels with free flow.
      (2). Circulation that was once adequate to meet the needs of uninjured tissue is diminished, and the demands made on circulation are increased.
      (3). The wound becomes an energy sink.[6–12]
         (a). This mismatch leads to tissue hypoxia, local acidosis, and lactate accumulation.
         (b). The environment is then ready for microorganisms to proliferate and invade the tissue.

C. Normal tissue oxygen tension

1. Inspired oxygen pressure, pulmonary function, cardiac output, intravascular volume, tissue perfusion, oxygen-carrying capacity of blood, and local oxygen consumption affect the amount of oxygen transported to tissues.
2. No single value can be specified as "normal oxygen tension," but a series of gradients whose steepness varies is known.
3. Molecular oxygen must be present to accommodate basic metabolic cell needs.

a. About 90% of the molecular oxygen consumed by tissues is involved in the creation of adenosine triphosphate (ATP).

b. Nine percent is used to remove hydrogen from amino acids and amines (oxidation).

c. One percent is incorporated into complex organic molecules like biogenic amines and hormones (oxygenation).

4. Tissue oxygen also varies with type of sensor, which measures the mean value over a region of tissue.[25,31–34]

a. Under conditions of air breathing at 1 atmosphere absolute pressure (ATA), a 100-μm membrane-covered electrode draws oxygen from a region of tissue about 450 μm in diameter and records a Po_2 of 25 to 35 mm Hg near the surface of healing wounds and a Po_2 of 5 to 10 mm Hg in nonhealing wounds.

b. It has been reported that cells can live with oxygen tension as low as 2 mm Hg, but oxygen tension of approximately 30 mm Hg is required for active cell division and normal wound healing.

5. The optimum dose of oxygen has not yet been established.[45,46]

a. It is clear that most individuals with wounds require no additional oxygen, whereas others require a very high dose of hyperbaric oxygen to achieve healing.

b. A specific dose for each individual probably exists, but a great deal of work is still needed in this area.

6. Knighton et al.[30] isolated an angiogenesis factor that is produced by hypoxic macrophages and appears to signal proliferation of capillaries.

a. This was initially thought to hypothesize that hyperoxia inhibited repair.

b. Because hyperoxia does not inhibit repair, further studies suggested that lactate also stimulates macrophages to produce the angiogenesis factor.

c. Macrophages also secrete lactate, even under aerobic conditions.

d. Hyperoxia reduces wound lactate only slightly; thus, it does not shut down angiogenesis until high oxygen tension is maintained for a prolonged period.

7. In hyperbaric exposure, a patient's skin oxygen tensions are elevated for approximately 30 minutes[40] to 4 hours.[36,37]

a. A sufficient time is needed for macrophages to resume a hypoxic status and trigger production of the angiogenesis factor prior to the next hyperbaric oxygen exposure.

b. It is also likely that fibroblast proliferation and collagen production are stimulated by the wound oxygenation and provide a structural support for capillary angiogenesis.

8. Measurements of oxygen following breathing of oxygen show different responses in chronic nonhealing wounds compared with those in acute wounds.

a. Baseline wound oxygen tension is 20 mm Hg in the chronic wound as compared to 27 mm Hg in the acute wound (while air breathing).

b. Acute wounds immediately respond to increases in oxygen, but chronic wounds do not.

c. Also, with increased breathing of 100% oxygen, acute wounds show a sharp increase of oxygen whereas chronic wounds show a gradual but slight increase in oxygen, rising to a lower level than in normal wounds.

9. Transcutaneous (Tc) oxygen measurements have been used to predict healing. For example:

a. In a series of 288 diabetic patients with peripheral vascular disease, those with leg/foot $TcPo_2$ values below 20 mm Hg were significantly more likely to have ulcers and rest pain and to require amputation of the limb compared with those with leg/foot $TcPo_2$ values above 20 mm Hg.[50,51]

b. Peripheral vascular disease patients requiring below-knee amputations were observed to heal spontaneously if preoperative below-knee $TcPo_2$ values were above 35 to 40 mm Hg and to fail if the values were below 35 mm Hg.[51]

c. In a series of 11 patients, diabetics with below-knee $TcPo_2$ values less than 20 mm Hg were shown to heal during a course of hyperbaric oxygen treatment if a $TcPo_2$ value of 900 to 1100 mm Hg could be achieved on initial exposure to 100% oxygen breathing at 2.4 ATA. Conversely, if the wound response to hyperbaric oxygen failed to achieve those $TcPo_2$ values during initial treatments, healing did not occur.[52]

d. In another study, successful healing cases were above 30 mm Hg and unsuccessful, nonhealing cases declined below 30 mm Hg.[53]

D. Host defense mechanisms

1. The most important line of defense against infection in injured tissue is phagocytic leukocytes.
2. The killing capacity of granulocytes is normal only to the degree to which oxygen is available to them. This is probably the basis for the observation that local immunity is proportional to blood supply.
3. Normally, leukocytes move and ingest bacteria equally well by using anaerobically or aerobically derived energy.[53]
   a. The capacity of leukocytes to kill bacteria depends on molecular oxygen.[39–42,48]
   b. Bacterial killing usually comprises two major mechanisms.
      (1). The first mechanism is degranulation. Ingested bacteria are exposed within the phagosome to various antimicrobial compounds derived from leukocyte granules. These "packages" of enzymes are carried by leukocytes from bone marrow to the site of phagocytosis.
      (2). The second mechanism is "oxidative killing." This depends on the molecular oxygen that is captured by leukocytes and converted to high-energy radicals such as superoxide, hydroxyl radical, peroxides, aldehydes, and hypochloride, which are toxic to bacteria in varying degrees. The rate of production of toxic radicals, and hence the adequacy of oxidative bacterial killing, is directly proportional to local oxygen tension.
4. The first evidence of the oxidative killing mechanism came to light 50 years ago; it was noted that white blood cells increased their respiration as much as 25-fold in a short burst immediately after phagocytosis.
   a. The "respiratory burst" was related to a primary oxidase located in white blood cell membrane and activated by phagocytosis.
   b. Energy requirements were furnished largely by the hexose monophosphate shunt, which rapidly consumes molecular oxygen by converting it to superoxide (the first step in the respiratory burst).
   c. Understanding that leukocytes failed to mount a respiratory burst led to the discovery that the respiratory burst coincides with bacterial killing.
   d. Oxygen radicals are produced by leukocytes and contribute to microbactericidal mechanisms.[42]
   e. Absence of primary oxidase is equivalent to anoxia.
      (1). Normal leukocytes lose approximately half of their maximum killing capacity when oxygen tension is reduced to near zero.
      (2). Major loss of killing capacity occurred when local P_{O_2} fell below about 30 mm Hg.
      (3). Oxygen tensions below this level are commonly reached in injured animal and human tissues.[55,56]
   f. Some bacteria are susceptible and others are resistant to oxygen radicals.
      (1). Bacteria that can quench or detoxify these radicals seem more resistant than others.
      (2). It is unclear whether all of the subspecies within a given bacterial strain behave the same in this respect.
      (3). Organisms affected by the oxidative pathway are those involved in abscesses and wound infections.
   g. In studies designed to test the importance of oxygen relative to infection, bacteria were implanted in a variety of animal studies and exposed to different conditions of oxygen. Again and again it was found that
      (1). The clearance of bacteria was directly proportional to tissue oxygen supply.
      (2). Increasing oxygen in the breathing mixture decreased both the incidence and the extent of necrosis.[27,44]
         (a). Compared with breathing 12% oxygen, exposure to 21% oxygen reduced lesion size by 50% and reduced the number of lesions by 30%.
         (b). Exposure to 45% oxygen, compared with 12% oxygen, resulted in a 63% reduction in lesion diameter and a 57% reduction in the number of necrotic lesions.
         (3). Hyperoxia and antibiotics were additive so that only rarely was evidence of infection seen in animals treated

with both, whereas every injection site became infected in hypoxic animals receiving no antibiotics.[27,46]

(a). Resistance to clinically important wound pathogens is proportional to the oxygenation of the tissue surrounding the area of inoculation.

(b). Increasing oxygen delivery even 12 hours after inoculation diminishes lesion size, whereas antibiotics lose their effectiveness if given more than 3 hours later.

(4). Experiments suggest that the effects of oxygen are as important as those of antibiotics in many infections.

h. Experiments designed to test the effect of blood perfusion on oxygen found that[47–49]

(1). Oxygen tension measured in the distal aspect of random, poorly perfused skin flaps was approximately 20 mm Hg, whereas the P_{O_2} in their proximal portion was approximately 40 mm Hg.

(2). Tissue oxygen tension in the normal (undisturbed) tissue and in both the proximal and the distal levels of the musculocutaneous (well-perfused) flaps was approximately 50 mm Hg.

(3). When the flaps were inoculated with *Staphylococcus aureus* and lesion size was measured at 24 and 48 hours after inoculation:[47]

(a). Infection of the distal (hypoxic) area of the poorly perfused flaps resulted in confluent infectious gangrene.

(b). The poorly perfused flaps showed many white blood cells, some bacteria, no containment of infection by abscess formation, and considerable intravascular thrombosis.

(c). Lesions in the well-perfused flaps and control tissues were far smaller than those in the poorly perfused flaps.

(d). In the poorly perfused flaps, the infection spread rapidly until it met better oxygenated tissue.

(e). Greater numbers of radioactive leukocytes were in the poorly perfused flaps than in the well-perfused flaps, confirming that access of leukocytes was adequate in the hypoxic tissue but that the white blood cells that did arrive became inefficient in the hypoxic environment.[55]

(f). These studies prove only that ischemia decreases local immunity in a pattern that corresponds to oxygen tension and that infection thrived only in tissue whose P_{O_2} was below 30 to 40 mm Hg, potentially defining the "critical" zone.[47]

i. To determine if oxygen was actually the critical factor, other experiments were done that found that[47]

(1). Tissue oxygen tension at the tip of poorly perfused flaps was about 15 mm Hg and could be raised only slightly by breathing additional oxygen; whereas up on the flaps was a zone in which tissue P_{O_2} could be raised from 30 to over 40 mm Hg by having the patient breathe supplemental oxygen.[55]

(2). The area of infection necrosis was found to be inversely proportional to the content of oxygen in the breathing mixture and corresponded quite precisely to the tissue P_{O_2} in the area of inoculations.

(3). Tissue whose P_{O_2} could be raised above about 40 mm Hg was protected against invasive infection.

(4). When leukocytes and their enzymes of the respiratory burst are activated, the rate of production of superoxide is limited by oxygen supply.

(a). As the supply rises, the added oxygen will be consumed, which leads to a steeper gradient but that only marginally elevates the P_{O_2} around the activated leukocytes.

(b). The net result is a steeper oxygen gradient and increased superoxide production.

E. Oxygen and collagen

1. Oxygen is used in the hydroxylation of proline and lysine. This is a necessary step for the release of collagen from cells and its incorporation into fibers.

a. Hunt and Pai[8] measured arterial and wound-space oxygen tension and showed that the amount of hydroxyproline more than doubled when arterial oxygen tension increased from 40 to 200 mm Hg. Wound-space Po_2 also increased but by far less, showing that the added oxygen was used for collagen synthesis.

b. Niinikoski[7] reported that rats in a 70% oxygen experimental group with subcutaneous cellulose sponge implants developed almost twice as much hydroxyproline as did those in the 18% oxygen control group.

c. In studies of patients with chronic, indolent soft-tissue wounds, all of the nonhealing wounds were hypoxic with Po_2 values ranging from 5 to 20 mm Hg, as compared to control tissue values of 30 to 50 mm Hg.[31]

2. Cells live and divide normally in a broad range of oxygen tensions (24, 49, and 137 mm Hg), but cellular growth and proliferation are retarded when oxygen tension is insufficient.

3. Cell growth and proliferation are also retarded when oxygen is continuously excessive.[49]

a. Although a daily high dose of oxygen is needed to correct hypoxic environments of fibroblasts in the problem wound, oxygen must be delivered on an intermittent schedule to avoid possible "toxic" effects on the cells.

b. Because the cell cycle for human fibroblasts is approximately 24 hours and mitosis occurs in a period of about 1 hour, an oxygen dose of about 1 to 2 hours every 24 hours is probably appropriate.

c. The optimum Po_2 for constant exposure seems to be about 50 to 100 mm Hg.

d. The implication is that normal wounds of any magnitude are hypoxic and that the rate at which they heal is oxygen dependent.

F. Clinical studies

1. Postoperative tissue oxygen tensions in the range of 25 to 40 mm Hg that are unresponsive to breathing increased oxygen mixtures have frequently been found.[42,49]

2. No clinical means exist to accurately predict tissue Po_2 in clinical circumstances.

3. Simple dehydration can depress tissue Po_2 into the critical range.[42]

4. Dehydrated patients are excessively susceptible to infection.

a. Patients undergoing hemodialysis will experience a drop in Po_2 as they lose weight and fluid.

b. The Po_2 remains low in these patients even at the completion of the dialysis run.

5. Rabkin and Hunt[51] demonstrated that local heat (ie, the traditional hot pack) raises tissue oxygen tension.

a. The effectiveness of local heat in treating wound infection may be due to change in tissue Po_2, change in perfusion, or most likely both.

b. Keeping patients warm both generally and peripherally could help to maintain good perfusion and good oxygen supply.

c. In conclusion, pathogens are more efficiently killed with well-oxygenated leukocytes.

6. Hyperbaric oxygen studies have shown that

a. Well-oxygenated leukocytes are far more efficient than hypoxic leukocytes as killers of some major pathogens

b. Degrees of hypoxia that are often reached in human and animal tissues under common physiological conditions can seriously inhibit leukocyte function.

c. Bacterial killing can be increased with oxygen to a degree that is of the same order of magnitude achieved by antibiotics.

d. The increased killing achieved by oxygen is additive to that of antibiotics.

(1). It is important to emphasize that oxygen can be delivered only by an intact and functioning vascular system.

G. Therapeutic guidelines for oxygen use

1. Simply having a patient breathe oxygen under normal or hyperbaric pressure does not guarantee delivery of oxygen to tissue.

2. Current clinical skills are not able to determine the extent to which oxygen reaches tissue.

3. The ultimate utilization of the oxidative killing mechanism of leukocytes awaits the development of a generally useful means to measure tissue oxygen tension in patients.

4. Meanwhile, the best way to ensure that oxygen is delivered is to use good clinical assessment.

a. Increase arterial P_{O_2}.

b. Give fluids aggressively enough to keep capillary return normal, peripheral skin warm, eyeball turgor normal, and mucous membranes moist, and ensure that no changes in vital signs occur when the patient assumes an erect posture.

c. Thirst is often a sign of dehydration.

d. Urine output is misleading.

   (1). Low urine output warrants fluid volume expansion.

   (2). However, normal or even high urine output carries no guarantee of good peripheral perfusion.

e. Delivery of oxygen to the infected subcutaneous and connective tissues is important.

f. Infected tissues are extremely vulnerable to vasoconstrictive influences, such as sympathetic discharge that occurs during hypovolemia.

   (1). Infected tissues can be poorly perfused and hypoxic while brain, liver, kidney, and heart are well perfused.

   (2). Subcutaneous tissue can be made hyperoxic with the patient breathing oxygen; all other tissues whose vascular anatomy is normal can probably be hyperoxygenated as well.

g. Many patients (30% to 80%) leaving the recovery room after major abdominal surgery have "tissue hypoxia."

h. This hypoxia is almost always correctable by more aggressive fluid administration and increased oxygen in the breathing mixture.

i. A role for oxygen in the treatment of infection has been established; all patients at high risk for serious infection who are undergoing operations or who are in the acute recovery phase after injury should receive oxygen.

   (1). When should oxygen be given?

   (2). When should perfusion be supported?(

   (3). When should hyperbaric treatment be elected?

   (4). How long should treatment last?

   (5). What percentage of time should oxygen be breathed?

j. If acute infection is established, the use of hyperbaric oxygen may be indicated by existing criteria.

   (1). The fact that causative organisms are aerobic does not remove hyperbaric oxygen from therapeutic consideration.

   (2). In making these decisions, assessment of tissue perfusion is critical.

   (3). If ischemic tissue is present, it must be surgically removed.

   (4). Alternatively, the presence of marginally ischemic tissue may be used as an indication for hyperbaric oxygen therapy provided that some evidence exists that the added oxygen will reach its intended goal.

   (5). Hyperbaric oxygen is recommended as adjunctive therapy for refractory osteomyelitis and other soft-tissue infections.[32,52]

k. What is the evidence that hyperbaric oxygen actually gets to the tissue?[31,32,37,41,52]

   (1). Hyperbaric oxygen therapy is delivered either with the patient inside a pressurized hyperbaric chamber filled with pure oxygen or by an oxygen mask or oxygen hood delivery system.

   (2). These procedures increase the partial pressure of oxygen in the lung and increase plasma oxygen, increasing tissue oxygen tension.

   (3). This results in an increase in the oxygen diffusion distance from functioning capillaries into zones of hypoxic tissue.

   (4). Breathing 100% oxygen at sea level increases dissolved oxygen by 1% to 2%.

l. The oxygen transport rate is dependent on the number and distribution of capillaries and the permeability of capillary walls and tissue.

   (1). Diffusion distance varies directly with the oxygen tension along the length of the capillary.

   (2). In several different studies, a dramatic increase in tissue oxygen tension has been demonstrated after exposure to hyperbaric oxygen at 2 ATA.

      (a). Values were increased from 50 mm Hg to over 4000 mm Hg during a 1-hour exposure.

      (b). In a series of 20 patients, oxygen tension in chronic, indolent soft-tissue wounds was monitored by implanted polygraphic oxygen electrodes before hyperbaric oxygen treatment.

(c). The wounds were all hypoxic during ground-level air breathing, but wound PO_2 increased during the several days of hyperbaric oxygen treatment.

(d). Even wounds with severely compromised microcirculation or infected wounds with high oxygen consumption showed markedly increased benefit with hyperbaric oxygen compared with ground-level oxygen inhalation.

(e). In most cases, wound PO_2 values decreased to 30 to 50 mm Hg within 30 minutes following the hyperbaric oxygen.

(f). Wound response to oxygen appeared to increase as healing occurred, with week-to-week variability in approximately 6-week cycles.

(g). There also appeared to be a relationship between changes in wound size (healing) and wound PO_2 values of the previous week.

(h). Wound oxygen values were highly variable (5 to 20 mm Hg during air breathing at 2 ATA, 100 mm Hg or higher during 100% oxygen breathing at 1 ATA, and 1000 mm Hg during 100% oxygen breathing at 2.3 ATA).[31]

(i). Hyperbaric oxygen therapy cannot overcome poor blood flow.

m. Whenever hyperbaric oxygen therapy is considered, the possibility that surgical therapy may be preferable also must be considered.

n. The principles of transplanting a blood supply is now well developed in surgery.

o. Hyperbaric oxygen may remain a valuable adjunct to débridement.

p. It is becoming clear that if one can bring either enough blood or more oxygen within an existing vascular supply to a localized infection, one can probably cure it.

5. The length of oxygen treatment is dictated by considerations of toxicity.

a. How often oxygen treatment should be repeated is an open question.

b. One hour a day of oxygen exposure does not seem to be too little to produce a clinically noticeable effect.

c. The addition of 1% to 2% volume of dissolved oxygen to the blood, brought about by breathing 100% oxygen at sea level, may effect little or no change in wound PO_2 because of the rapid consumption of oxygen in wounded, infected tissue.

(1). Addition of 4% to 5% of oxygen to the blood, by raising arterial oxygen tension (PaO_2) above 1000 to 1200 mm Hg under hyperbaric conditions, may well bring tissue PO_2 into the range of effective bacterial killing.

(2). Hyperbaric oxygen cannot easily overcome the obstacles of poor blood flow.

(3). It is imperative that blood flow be maximized whenever any form of oxygen therapy is needed.

6. Infections of various sorts have been treated with hyperbaric oxygen.

a. Specifically, hyperbaric oxygen therapy is currently recommended as adjunctive therapy in refractory osteomyelitis and soft-tissue infections, including extensive necrotizing fasciitis and gas gangrene.

b. The use of hyperbaric oxygen therapy in several other areas is undergoing further evaluation, such as in burns, intra-abdominal abscesses, empyema, refractory actinomycosis, and selected mycobacteria.

H. Local oxygen therapy

1. Some clinicians have administered oxygen at either normobaric or hyperbaric pressures directly over wounded or infected tissue.

2. This is as an alternative approach to increasing inspired oxygen concentration as a means of increasing oxygen tension in tissue.

a. This theoretically circumvents the impaired vascular supply.

b. However, oxygen penetrates the skin poorly or by diffusion only. Approximately 70 μm of penetration is all that can be expected, even under maximum tolerable hyperbaric oxygen pressures.[40]

c. Directly applied hyperbaric oxygen elevates tissue PO_2 only in the superficial dermis (little systemic absorption of the oxygen occurs).[40]

d. Local hyperpressure may discourage local blood flow but may promote both epithelialization and clearing of superficial infections.

I. Summary

1. Hypoxia is a characteristic of wounded tissue.
   a. Normal leukocytes kill bacteria poorly in hypoxic conditions.
   b. Measurement of oxygen tension reveals that wounds are often hypoxic to a degree that compromises leukocyte function.
   c. Tissue oxygen measurements have confirmed hypoxia in chronic, indolent human wounds and have demonstrated elevation of wound oxygen tension with hyperbaric oxygen treatment.

d. It is usually possible to raise wound tissue PO_2 out of the critical zone by using aggressive fluid resuscitation or normobaric and hyperbaric oxygen administration.
e. The immunological benefits of raising tissue PO_2 out of the critical zone are roughly equivalent to the effects of antibiotic administration. The effects of oxygen and antibiotics are additive.
f. Local measurements of mean tissue PO_2 will likely resolve the question about exact essential levels of PO_2.
g. It appears that chronic, intractable infections due to *S. aureus, Escherichia coli, Proteus* sp., *Salmonella* sp., *Klebsiella* sp., etc., are likely to respond to oxygen therapy.
h. Tissue oxygen measurements are becoming a valuable tool in the medical decision-making process for nonhealing soft-tissue wounds.

III. Percutaneous Drug Delivery: Mechanical and Barrier Properties of the Skin

A. General issues[53–56]

1. Delivering drugs through the skin is referred to as transdermal drug delivery or percutaneous drug delivery.
2. Transdermal drug application is a method of systemic drug delivery.
3. Advantages of transdermal drug delivery:
   a. The drug goes immediately into the bloodstream and eliminates the absorption required by the gastrointestinal tract (see Figure 26–6).
   b. The drug is easy to apply, and it can be applied at a specific site.
   c. The drug bypasses the liver and avoids first-pass metabolism.
      (1). Drug molecules follow the path of least diffusional resistance.
      (2). This path is determined by the physicochemical nature of the membrane (including thickness, molecular mobility, and membrane capacity), the viscosities, the extent of cross-linking, and the packing of polymetric matter.
4. The stratum corneum is the primary limiting barrier layer to the permeation of drugs.[53] It is necessary to
   a. Predict the rate at which materials penetrate the skin.

b. Assess potential toxicological hazards.
c. Identify enhancers to improve topical administration.
5. One major difficulty in generating a good percutaneous model is the inherent biological variation of the skin.[56]

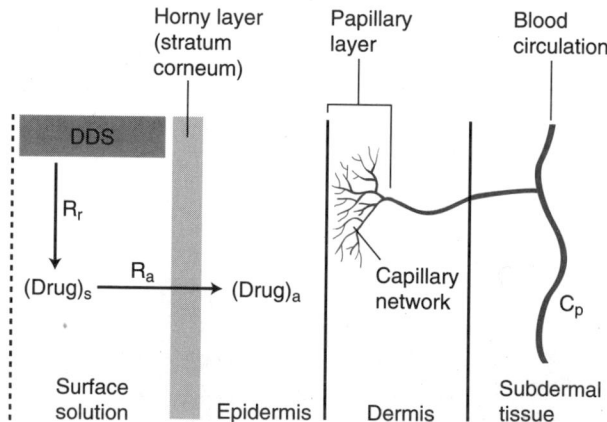

FIGURE 26–6   Relationship between the rate of drug release (R_r) from a transdermal drug delivery system (DDS) and the rate of drug absorption (R_a) by the skin. (Redrawn from Chien Y: *Transdermal Controlled Systemic Medication.* Marcel Dekker, Inc., N.Y. 1987, p 28 by courtesy of Marcel Dekker, Inc.)

a. Diseased or damaged skin often presents less resistance.

b. Regional variations in the permeability are noted in the stratum corneum.

6. Compounds are thought to transfer through the skin by a passive diffusion mechanism.[53-56]

a. Fick's laws of diffusion can be applied to determine drug levels in the skin, blood, and urine after topical administration (see Table 26-1).

b. The stratum corneum is a very impermeable barrier, and a long time is required to establish steady-state conditions.

c. Each skin layer has different properties, which must be calculated into the model.

7. Absorption can be enhanced with high concentrations of[53-56]

a. Solvents (eg, chloroform and benzene).

b. Dimethyl sulfoxide (DMSO).

8. Enhancers promoting drug absorption break down the stratum corneum lipids, denature the stratum corneum structural keratin proteins, or delaminate the horny layer.

a. Burning the skin may or may not alter diffusion.

(1). If skin temperature is lower than 75°C, it retains its essential barrier properties until some time passes and the devitalized tissue is digested and sloughed.

(2). If burns are inflicted at temperatures of 85°C or higher, the permeability of skin is immediately altered regardless of the depth of the tissue damage.

(3). Although burning initially melts the lipids, the lipids actually recrystallize quickly on cooling.

(4). Phenol at 5% to 6% (aqueous)

creates instantaneous and complete destruction of the horny element and makes the permeability similar to that of skin membranes that are stripped of the stratum corneum, opening the intracellular structure similarly to high temperatures.

b. Surfactants alter the protein conformations and enhance polar pathway transport.

c. Solvents can swell the stratum corneum and may also be able to solubilize lipids.

d. Physical approaches for skin penetration enhancement have been evaluated, such as stripping the stratum corneum, thermal energy, iontophoresis, and ultrasound.

9. In summary, over the last few years, intensified interest has been devoted to novel routes of drug administration such as transdermal drug delivery.

a. Despite major research, development efforts, and the many advantages, only a few transdermal delivery systems are clinically available: clonidine, estradiol, scopolamine, and nitroglycerin.

b. A major limitation to transdermal drug delivery is the impermeability of human skin and its biological variability.

c. It is well accepted that the stratum corneum is the major rate-limiting barrier to molecular diffusion.

d. Because most drugs do not permeate the skin in therapeutic amounts, chemical and physical approaches have been examined to lower the skin barrier properties and enhance transdermal permeation.

B. Transdermal drug delivery in physical therapy[57]

1. Drugs are frequently incorporated into physical therapy treatments.[57]

a. Anesthetics, counterirritants, and anti-inflammatories are most commonly used (see Table 26-2).

b. The goal of treatment is to get the drug inside the target cells.

c. Corticosteroids are most frequently used by physical therapists, with either ultrasound or electrical current as an enhancer.[9,58-61]

(1). With corticosteroids, the glucocorticoid binds to the high-affinity cytoplasmic receptor.

Table 26-1. FICK'S FIRST LAW OF DIFFUSION*

$$d = \frac{dQ}{dt} - \frac{DK_pc}{h_s}$$

* From this formula, one can see that the partitioning behavior is important as well as the diffusion of the drug through the skin, the driving force for diffusion, and the concentration of the dissolved drug.

Abbreviations: c = concentration of drug in vehicle (equation is valid only if it is assured that the concentration of drug in receptor phase is zero); d = diffusion; D = effective diffusion coefficient of drug in stratum corneum; dQ/dt = rate of skin penetration; h_s = effective diffusion path length through the skin barrier; K_p = partition coefficient of drug between skin and vehicle.

Table 26–2. DRUGS FREQUENTLY USED BY PHYSICAL THERAPISTS IN PHONOPHORESIS OR IONTOPHORESIS

Anesthetics—substances blocking pain receptors by creating numbness (*eg*, lidocaine or menthol).

Counterirritants—substances that cause inflammation of the skin for purposes of relieving pain from stimulation rather than depression of cutaneous sensory receptors (*eg*, methyl salicylates).

Anti-inflammatories—medications such as adrenal cortical steroids (*eg*, hormones, including glucocorticoids, dexamethasone, and hydrocortisone). Of these corticosteroids are clearly the most common.

---

(2). This activated hormone-receptor complex is then translocated into the nucleus, where it interacts with nuclear chromatin acceptor sites (glucocorticoid regulatory elements).
  (a). This interaction results in the expression of specific genes followed by transcription of mRNA.
  (b). Subsequent translation of mRNA produces proteins that may be either inhibitory or stimulatory, depending on the tissue type.
(3). During an inflammatory response, glucocorticoids influence the cells involved in the inflammatory reaction by
  (a). Increasing the number of circulating neutrophils, accompanied by a demargination and migration.
  (b). Decreasing the neutrophils at sites of inflammation.
  (c). Inhibiting the phagocytosis by neutrophils and monocytes, the release of degradative enzymes, and the production of inflammatory cytokines (lymphokines and monokines).
(4). The effects of corticosteroid penetration are usually measured clinically by[22,70–73]
  (a). A decrease in pain.
  (b). A decrease in swelling.
  (c). A decrease in redness of the involved tissue.
  (d). The extravasation of plasma proteins.

(e). Reduction in fluid accumulation.
(f). Reduction in local heat or change in polymorphonuclear cells and/or mononuclear phagocytes at the site of the lesion.
(g). Biochemical analyses of exudate, including chemotactic and chemokinetic activities of inflammatory tissue.
(h). Retardation of collagen deposition.
(i). The corticosteroids interfere with fibroblast division when the concentration exceeds the normal physiological level, particularly when the steroid reaches the tissue shortly after an injury or when long-term administration of anti-inflammatory steroids is seen.

C. Ultrasound and transcutaneous drug delivery: phonophoresis (sonophoresis)[62–81]

1. The use of ultrasound to increase drug diffusion is called phonophoresis (the movement of drugs through living intact skin and soft tissue under the influence of ultrasonic perturbation).[62–65]
   a. Physical therapists must obtain a prescription from a physician for each specific patient who is to be treated with a steroid mixed into the ultrasound gel.
   b. Therapeutic ultrasound is approved by the US Food and Drug Administration but there is no specific approval for "phonophoresis." Thus, this treatment should be documented as the use of ultrasound with corticosteroid either applied to the skin or mixed with the sonic gel.[57]
2. As a longitudinal sound wave with variable amplitude and a frequency above audible sound ($>20,000$ Hz), the ultrasound can be directed toward the target, and both heating and mechanical effects are produced.
   a. As sound waves move through body tissues, particles have periodic oscillations about their resting positions, with displacement of a particle proportional to the intensity of the beam and the number of oscillations proportional to the frequency of the ultrasound waves.

b. Sound waves create compression and expansion of the cells, creating a piezoelectrical effect (negative and positive charges).

c. Sound waves also undergo reflection, refraction, and/or absorption, depending on the properties of the encountered medium.

d. Attenuation of ultrasound is measured in terms of energy loss.

e. As energy is lost to the tissue, heat is created.

f. Waves are mechanical and create a localized shear stress of the wave, potentially causing structural alterations that can increase the permeability of the tissue.

3. Ultrasound enhances drug absorption by[65–70]

a. Creating a radiation pressure from the ultrasound beam and potentially forcing the medication away from the target tissue.

b. Heating the tissue and increasing the kinetic energy of the molecules, enabling greater diffusion.

c. Sonic streaming, which changes cell permeability, enhancing tissue diffusion.

d. Depolymerizing proteins.

e. Exciting calcium bound to proteins.

f. Decreasing the viscosity of the intracellular and extracellular colloidal substances.

4. Pharmaceutical research provides evidence for ultrasound as an enhancer, based on both the kinetic energy theory and the cell permeability theory as the most likely explanations, with the pressure theory the least likely explanation.

5. When selecting a drug for phonophoresis, one must first determine whether[57,71,72]

a. The drug transmits or blocks the ultrasound.

b. The energy from the ultrasound must reach the tissue.

(1). In recent studies, it was determined that hydrocortisone blocked the sound waves, potentially causing the ultrasound machine to turn off as if the sound head has lost contact.

(2). With hydrocortisone, no ultrasound reaches the target tissue.

6. Guidelines exist for the use of ultrasound in clinical practice, but clinical studies usually provide only subjective measures of patient improvement with phonophoresis.[73–76]

a. Griffin et al.[76] found that

(1). Patients receiving hydrocortisone

phonophoresis had a significantly greater reduction in pain compared with controls.

(2). Patients receiving ultrasound had a 68.1% reduction in pain after 4.5 treatments with 1.5 W/cm², 1 MHz for 8 minutes per treatment, compared with a 27.7% improvement in the control group.

b. Newman et al.[77] found that patients with subdeltoid bursitis made significant gains in pain relief and function when treated with ultrasound and either intra-articular injections of hydrocortisone or hydrocortisone hypospray compared with ultrasound alone.

c. Others[78–81] have demonstrated reduction in muscle soreness, enhanced cutaneous blood flow, and anesthesia by the administration of drugs other than steroids.

7. Animal studies have traced the diffusion of steroid down to the subcutaneous tissue and nerve tissue but not to levels of muscles, tendons, or joints.[53,80–82]

a. Using a swine model, following 5 minutes of ultrasound (1 to 3 W/cm², continuous, 1 MHz, using a stationary sound head), Griffin and Touchstone[74,75] demonstrated that hydrocortisone penetrated around nerve and subcutaneous tissue but not around muscle. Some tissue burning was described at this intensity.

b. Davick and associates[83] documented that a single application of hydrocortisone with ultrasound for 8 minutes (1.5 W/cm², continuous, 1 MHz)

(1). Diffused through the stratum corneum and was traced to the subcutaneous tissue in dogs.

(2). Did not penetrate beyond the epidermis.

c. In a controlled study with greyhound dogs carried out by Muir et al.[82]

(1). No significant differences in intra-articular hydrocortisone levels were found between the phonophoresed and skin-rubbed knee joints.

(2). The intra-articular steroid level in the injected knees was significantly higher than both the control and the skin-rubbed joints.

d. Using a swine model, one recent controlled study by Byl et al.[72] measured the effects of corticosteroid (dexamethasone and hydrocortisone) on the deposition of collagen when rubbed into the skin, injected, sonated, or sham sonated.

(1). Collagen deposition was estimated based on hydroxyproline measurements calculated from subcutaneously implanted polytetrafluoroethylene (ePTFE) tubing (commercially called Impra or Gore-Tex).

(2). One treatment was provided.

(3). After 1 week of healing, hydroxyproline and DNA were measured through laboratory analysis of the ePTFE.

(4). A total of 1.1 mg of hydrocortisone and 0.065 mg of dexamethasone were applied to each pig.

(5). These researchers found that

   (a). The injected ePTFE tubes (hydrocortisone and dexamethasone) and the phonophoresed dexamethasone tubes each had about one half the collagen that was measured in the controls.

   (b). There were no significant differences between the skin-rubbed ePTFE tubes and the controls.

   (c). The ePTFE sonated with hydrocortisone had the same level of hydroxyproline as the controls.

   (d). Interestingly, in the swine, the levels of hydroxyproline in the control wounds was half that measured in previous studies with swine.

   (e). This raised some questions about potentially systemic effects of the steroids rather than just local effects.

   (f). A total of 1.1 mg of hydrocortisone and 0.065 mg of dexamethasone had been applied in all the wounds in this study.

   (g). Also, interestingly, the DNA was monitored and found to be high in all of the measurements, suggesting that there had been no effect of the steroids on reducing the inflammation.

e. Novak[78] demonstrated ultrasound-facilitated diffusion of lidocaine into both skin and muscle in human subjects.

f. Ciccone et al.[79] measured a significant decrease in muscle soreness and muscle stiffness (as measured by range of motion) following sonation of trolamine salicylate with 1.5 W/cm², continuous, 1 MHz, for 3 days.

(1). Another group was similarly treated, but the ultrasound was not turned on.

(2). D-mannitol, inulin, and physostigmine were used as the model drugs because they are totally and rapidly eliminated and therefore appear completely in the urine.

(3). The radioactivity of the collected urine was measured by liquid scintillation counting.

(4). There was a significant effect of ultrasound on mannitol permeability.

(5). By chromatography, there was no decomposition of the mannitol by the ultrasonic energy.

(6). Histological evaluation of exposed skin samples showed no damage.

(7). The amount of drug measured in the urine was five times greater in the sonated rats than in the controls.

(8). The amount of drug measured increased within the 1st hour, and the maximum difference was measured 5 hours later.

(9). When mannitol was placed on the skin alone (no ultrasound), there was a slight increase in mannitol measured in the urine beginning at 3 hours post application.

g. *Summary*

(1). The majority of phonophoresis studies have used the continuous mode of ultrasound.

(2). Frequency was either 1 or 2 MHz with an intensity of 1 to 3 W/cm².

(3). Most of the researchers validated that the target drug transmitted ultrasound before carrying out the study.

(4). None of the studies found intra-articular penetration, and only one validated intramuscular penetration.

(5). Some of the studies were not well controlled, and the outcomes were not objectively documented or were not measured with sensitive instruments.

h. In the clinics, physical therapists should objectively evaluate when phonophoresis may be helpful.

(1). If ultrasound is applied with a continuously moving sound head in the therapeutic range of 1 to 3 W/cm² for 5 to 7 minutes, no harm is expected.

(2). A contact medium is required when applying ultrasound, and it is important that this medium be degassed.

(3). When using ultrasound to treat open, nonhealing wounds, lower doses are suggested (eg, 0.5 W/cm²).

(4). In pharmaceutical research on percutaneous (transcutaneous) drug delivery, drug patches are usually left on for several hours.

(5). The pulsating mode will minimize the heating effects.

(6). When treating over bony surfaces, it is suggested that ultrasound be applied in water.

(7). If phonophoresis does enable a drug to penetrate directly into the vascular system, therapists must carefully evaluate if there is any contraindication for using a steroid with a given patient.[105,110]

(8). If the sound head is stationary or if the wattage begins to approach 10 W/cm², structural damage can occur.

(9). The precise parameters of ultrasound to select for transdermal drug delivery are not well defined, but both the high and the low doses have been associated with improvement.

(a). Research in pharmaceutical chemistry suggests that the frequency needs to be very high (≥10 Hz) in order to penetrate the stratum corneum.

(b). Studies reporting the greatest penetration use continuous, stationary ultrasound, which is contraindicated in patients because of burning.

(c). An intensity of 1.5 W/cm², continuous 1 MHz, has been associated with increased steroid in the tissue.

(d). The heating effects of the ultrasound could assist in drug penetration, suggesting that the lower doses may not adequately heat the tissues to enable successful drug diffusion.

(10). Ultrasound might be an answer to two major problems facing the field of transdermal drug delivery: lag time and low drug penetration. It is relatively easy to use and has minimal side effects when used in the therapeutic range.

(11). Ultrasound may be an enhancer of transcutaneous drugs, but, to achieve these eventual objectives, some critical studies will be needed to examine[67,111]

(a). The effect of the frequency of ultrasound and intensity on enhancement.

(b). The effect and compatibility of ultrasound on "transdermal patches."

(c). Whether there are morphological and chemical changes in the skin when it is exposed to ultrasound and the reversibility and kinetics of the ultrasound.

(d). The effect of ultrasound relative to drug properties: size, polarity, charge.

(12). When phonophoresis is used, it should be billed as ultrasound with documentation of the specific drug mixed with the conductive medium.

D. Iontophoresis in physical therapy[86–113]

1. Iontophoresis (ion transfer) is the introduction of topically applied ions into the skin using direct current.[86–88]

a. Electrically charged electrodes will repel an ion that is similarly charged.

(1). Ions with a positive charge can be introduced into the body with a positive electrode.

(2). Ions with a negative charge can be introduced into the body with a negative electrode.

(3). Table 26–2 summarizes the drugs that are commonly used by physical therapists for iontophoresis.

b. Iontophoresis has long been used in the practice of medicine and is not unique to physical therapy. It is also a more established method of transcutaneous drug delivery than phonophoresis.[89]

2. Iontophoresis is most commonly used to treat problems of
   a. Edema.[90,91]
   b. Skin ulcers.[92]
   c. Hyperhidrosis.[93–98]
   d. Fungus infections.[99]
   e. Arthritis (particularly gout).[100,101]
   f. Tendinitis.[102]
   g. Musculoskeletal inflammatory conditions.[103,104]
   h. Local anesthesia.[105–111]
   i. Plantar wart scar-tissue modification.[111,112]
   j. Wound healing.[113]

3. Iontophoresis requires the use of direct, galvanic current.
   a. Low doses of current are used (microamperage intensity is the most comfortable, but it takes longer to apply; often up to 5 mA is used if the patient can tolerate it).
   b. The drug can be applied simply by placing it on a cotton sponge and placing the treatment electrode over the gauze over the target area.[76]
   c. The drug can be delivered using special phoressor devices that are sold for purposes of enhancing drug delivery into the skin.
      (1). These units have some analgesic in the electrode to decrease the pain, and then the treatment drug is added.
      (2). These units provide specific guidelines for drug administration, which is often more comfortable than when applied with a traditional galvanic machine; however, they are expensive.
   d. Usually about 1 mL of a drug is placed in or on an electrode.
   e. The time required to administer the drug will vary by the amount of current.

4. Physical therapists must have a prescription from a physician to deliver a controlled drug into the tissue; however, some therapists are using over-the-counter drugs (eg, Flexall, DMSO).

5. Effectiveness of iontophoresis:
   a. Many studies have reported the positive effects of iontophoresis.[90–113]
   b. Most report effectiveness, but often good controls are lacking.
      (1). Magistro[91] used hyaluronidase to reduce edema in a study of 100 patients (with hyaluronidase enhancing fluid absorption).
         (a). Total edema reduction ranged from 0.6 to 1.9 cm.
         (b). Time of edema reduction was not noted.
         (c). No controls were used.
      (2). Harris[104] administered xylocaine and dexamethasone for problems of musculoskeletal inflammation three times a week for 1 week using a phoressor and a current of 1 mA increased to 5 mA for 15 minutes.
         (a). Excellent pain relief for 38 of 50 patients; 5 reported no long-term relief.
         (b). No control subjects were used.
      (3). Russo et al.[106] used local anesthetics (lidocaine and a placebo).
         (a). Lidocaine produced local anesthesia for longer duration than topically applied lidocaine.
         (b). Lidocaine iontophoresis anesthesia was shorter than the anesthesia produced by injection.
         (c). Average anesthesia was 5 minutes with iontophoresis.

6. Many patients do not like iontophoresis because
   a. They are afraid of the current.
   b. The galvanic current is uncomfortable.
   c. The results may not be very long lasting.
   d. The skin may feel burned under the electrode.

7. Many therapists are hesitant to use iontophoresis because
   a. They are uncomfortable using galvanic current.
   b. They do not have a special unit.
   c. They do not have a close working relationship with a physician to obtain a prescription.
   d. They are not convinced that it is effective.
   e. It takes too much time.

8. Electrical current can be an enhancer for assisting the absorption of drugs into the tissues; however, if used:

a. The physical therapist must be knowledgeable about the polarity of the drug.
b. The skin must be watched carefully to prevent burning.
c. A prescription must be obtained.
d. The treatment should be only one aspect of the management of the problem.
e. The therapist should carefully screen the patient for potential drug allergies or other contraindications for the drug selected.

IV. Burns[114–122]

A. General

1. Because the experience of a burn is so devastating to the patient, it is impossible to treat him/her in any way other than as a whole person.
2. The losses may include loved ones, a home, and all possessions, but most distressing may be the loss of personal appearance.
3. Burn rehabilitation must be done by a team, and the participation of the patient and his/her family and friends is important to ensure a successful outcome.
4. Teaching begins immediately because the best results are anticipated by preventing problems rather than by repairing them.
5. Physical therapy evaluation begins on admission, if possible, or within 24 hours of admission, as practical. The following information is included in the initial assessment.

B. Etiology

1. **Mechanism of injury**
   a. *Thermal*
      (1). May include flame, steam, hot liquids, hot tar, hot metals, extreme cold.
      (2). Severity is related to temperature and duration of contact of the agent that caused the burn.
   b. *Electrical*
      (1). Injury due to contact with electrical current depends on voltage, type of current, duration of contact, pathway of current.
      (2). Body tissues and fluids conduct electricity, with heat produced as a function of voltage drop and current density.
         (a). High-tension electrical injury therefore results in more frequent severe injuries to the digits and extremities than to the trunk.
         (b). After current flow has stopped, the superficial tissues cool faster than the deeper ones, with deeper tissues at risk for more severe injury.
         (c). A small surface wound may be misleading as there may be extensive deep tissue damage.
      (3). Current may arc across flexor surfaces of joints and char skin.
      (4). Associated flame burns may also be caused by arcing of current.
      (5). Entrance and exit wounds are characteristic.
      (6). Cardiac arrest or cardiac arrhythmias are frequent sequelae.
      (7). Neurological deficits may be a result of nerve destruction by the current. Their onset may be immediate or delayed.
      (8). Children are at risk for mouth injuries caused by contact with electrical cords or sockets.
   c. *Chemical*
      (1). Strong acids, such as sulfuric, nitrous, or hydrochloric.
      (2). Strong alkalis, such as lime or ammonia.
      (3). Contact burns with agents such as gasoline.
   d. *Inhalation injury*
      (1). Patients with inhalation injuries may

present with or without a visible surface burn.

(2). Inhalation injury is suspected if the burn occurred in an enclosed space. Physical clues include facial or neck burns with singed facial hair, hoarseness, or productive cough with carbonaceous sputum.

(3). Bronchoscopy assists with diagnosis when clinical signs are vague.

e. Other skin-loss syndromes may require wound care and follow-up similar to treatment of burns.

(1). Toxic epidermal necrolysis syndrome, also known as Stevens-Johnson syndrome, is characterized by an initial rash progressing to loss of skin.

(a). The etiology is not fully understood, but it is suggestive of an autoimmune or allergic process.

(b). Medications are implicated in the majority of cases.

(c). The patient may be referred to a burn center when the skin rash begins to slough.

(d). Epidermal separation exposes a viable dermis that should heal within 14 days without scarring if there is no infection.

(e). If wounds progress from partial to full thickness, the course becomes much more complex, with medical and rehabilitative complications.

(f). Eyes and mouth can be affected, as well as the esophagus and urethra.

(g). Treatment includes wound care techniques such as hydrotherapy, débridement, and use of topical antibiotic dressings and biological dressings.

(h). If lesions become infected, these disorders can be life threatening because of systemic response to generalized sepsis.

(i). Protective isolation techniques are used to help combat the increased risk of septic complications.

(2). Erythema multiforme in the major or complex form may be the initial

diagnosis in the early stages of these diseases.

(3). Psoriatic arthritis can also progress to a serious skin-loss disorder.

C. Extent of injury

1. Total body surface area (TBSA) of the injury can be calculated by using the "rule of nines."

   a. The body is divided into anatomical regions that represent 9% (or a multiple of nine) of the total body surface.

   (1). Head and neck: 9%.

   (2). Upper extremity (each): 9%.

   (3). Lower extremity (each): 18%.

   (4). Anterior trunk: 18%.

   (5). Posterior trunk: 18%.

   b. The size of the patient's palm represents about 1% of TBSA.

   c. The ratios are different in infants and in children, whose heads are larger in relationship to their bodies.

   d. Duration of hospitalization is frequently estimated to be 1.5 days per percentage of body surface area burned.

D. Location of burns

1. If the burned area includes face, hands, feet, or perineum, hospitalization in a burn center is recommended.

2. If joint surfaces are crossed by the burn, intervention by the physical therapist is crucial to the functional outcome.

E. Depth or degree of burn

1. **First-degree burn**

   a. May be caused by sunburn or minor flash injury.

   b. Epidermis is only layer affected.

   c. Dry, very painful, may range from pink to bright red.

   d. Tends to heal by itself within 1 week. These burns do not scar.

   e. When the TBSA is calculated, these burns are not included.

2. **Second-degree burn (partial-thickness burn)**

   a. *Superficial*

   (1). May be caused by flash injury, scald caused by a spill.

(2). The outer portion of the dermis is affected.

(3). Characterized by blisters, with exudate.

(4). Red, may be mottled, very painful.

(5). Can heal with good wound care (no infection) within 10 to 14 days.

(6). Not likely to scar, but scar maturation should be monitored.

(7). Change in pigmentation of this area may occur.

b. *Deep*

(1). May be caused by scald of longer duration (or central area of spill), brief exposure to flame, brief contact with hot material such as tar.

(2). More of the dermis is compromised, with some alteration in the sweat glands, hair follicles, etc.

(3). May be red with white or yellow areas.

(4). If these wounds are not grafted, they will take several weeks to heal.

(5). The quality of the healed skin is fragile, inelastic, and abrades easily.

(6). These burns are most likely to scar when they are allowed to heal spontaneously.

(7). Skin grafting is usually done if there is adequate unburned skin available for donor sites, especially if burns are on the hands or cross a joint surface.

(a). The exception to this is facial burns.

(b). The cosmetic appearance of healed deep dermal burns is usually better than when skin is grafted.

c. **Third-degree burn (full-thickness burn)**

(1). May be caused by flame, immersion scalds of sufficient duration, strong chemicals, electricity, prolonged contact with hot objects.

(2). Can be gray or white, may be charred in appearance.

(3). Eschar, a leathery, inelastic layer of tissue, must be removed in order for healing to occur either by wound contraction and epithelialization or by skin grafting.

(4). Because the entire dermis has been destroyed, this wound has no sensation.

(5). Skin grafting must be done for a full-thickness burn greater than 2 inches in circumference.

(6). Scarring is expected.

d. **Fourth-degree burn**

(1). May be caused by prolonged contact with flames, electricity.

(2). This term may be used to describe burns that include subcutaneous tissue, including muscle, tendon, and bone.

(3). Surgical treatment may be more extensive than split-thickness skin grafting, possibly including such techniques as use of tissue flaps.

(4). Scarring is expected with some degree of changes in contour.

F. Medical history

1. Includes significant prior illnesses or surgeries, prior level of function, and psychological and social history.

a. *Psychological/social profile*

(1). Burn patients are frequently individuals who have history of drug and/or alcohol abuse.

(2). May have documented psychiatric history.

(3). May be homeless or transient.

(4). May be victims of abuse.

(a). Health care professionals must fulfill their obligation to report any suspected child or elder abuse.

(5). Compliance with inpatient and follow-up outpatient program is difficult with these patients.

G. Morbidity and mortality

1. **Criteria for admission to a burn center**

a. Burn wound greater than 15% TBSA in an adult.

b. Burn wound greater than 10% TBSA in a child.

c. Patient with greater than 2% full-thickness burn.

d. Smoke inhalation injury.

e. Burns of the hands, feet, face, or perineum.

f. Associated illnesses or injuries.

g. Electrical injuries.

h. Child abuse.

2. **Infection control**

a. The skin's function of providing a protective barrier is disrupted.

b. The patient is at risk for altered homeostasis and immune competence and for infection.

　(1). *Wound infection*

　　(a). Colonization begins at time of injury.

　　(b). By the 4th day, gram-negative organisms such as *Pseudomonas aeruginosa* may replace normal bacterial flora.

　　(c). Status of wound is monitored by wound cultures and biopsies.

　　(d). Choice of topical antibiotic may change depending on test results.

　　(e). Methicillin-resistant *Staphylococcus aureus* requires strict infection control.

　　(f). Infection can cause a burn to convert to a deeper wound, requiring more aggressive care.

　(2). *Systemic infection*

　　(a). Severe wound infections can become systemic infections.

　　(b). Intravenous antibiotics are chosen based on blood cultures.

　　(c). Septic shock is a cardiovascular response to bacterial invasion.

　　(d). Altered mental status is frequently the first clinical sign.

　　(e). Other symptoms include decreased urine output, tachypnea, hypotension, hypothermia, coma.

　　(f). Condition is potentially life threatening.

　　(g). Patients with inhalation injuries are at high risk for sepsis.

c. Infection control procedures are essential to prevent cross-contamination of patients.

　(1). Hand washing is the mainstay.

　(2). Universal precautions are observed when handling body fluids.

　(3). Protective devices include gloves, masks, and eye shields (such as glasses or goggles); hats, gowns, and shoe covers are worn.

H. Burns: outpatient treatment

1. Many burns occur that do not meet the above criteria.

2. Whenever possible, outpatient status will be maintained with visits to a clinic as needed.

3. Most frequently, small burns are inspected and dressings changed once a day by staff, with second treatment to be done by family member or other available caregiver.

4. If problems arise, status may change to inpatient for more aggressive treatment of burns, particularly surgery or control of infection.

5. The focus of rehabilitation in this patient population is the prevention of contractures and maintenance of function and cosmesis.

I. Phases of treatment

1. **Emergent (or shock) phase.** This phase is 0 to 72 hours from the time of injury.

a. *Fluid resuscitation*

　(1). Because of increased permeability of blood vessels, fluid leaks out of the cells into the extracellular space, resulting in intravascular hypovolemia.

　(2). Calculations are made in order to infuse the patient with sufficient volume to maintain adequate organ perfusion.

　　(a). There are many formulas, including the Parkland or the Brooke, that use information such as degree and depth of injury to determine the amount and rate of infusion.

　　(b). Urine output is monitored closely to ensure adequate resuscitation.

b. *Implications for physical therapy*

　(1). The patient may become grossly edematous during the emergent phase.

　(2). Positioning and exercise focus on edema control.

2. **Acute (or healing) phase.** This phase is from the end of the emergent phase until the majority of the burn wounds are healed.

a. *Wound care objectives*

　(1). To prevent infection.

　(2). To cleanse and débride as quickly as possible.

　(3). To prepare for healing and grafting.

(4). To reduce scarring and contracture formation.

(5). To protect injured tissue.

(6). To protect granulation tissue and new grafts.

b. Physical therapists are frequently required to assist in wound care following whirlpool applications to the upper or lower extremity.

(1). During a whirlpool, mechanical débridement may be appropriate.

(2). This may be accomplished with a sponge, washcloth, or gloved fingertip and antibacterial soap or other cleansing agent.

(3). A chemical agent, such as povidone-iodine (Betadine), may be used in the whirlpool.

(a). The choice of a chemical agent may depend on which topical agent has been chosen.

(b). Povidone-iodine is not appropriate for use with some chemical débriding agents.

(c). Bleach may be used with hydrochloric acid to balance the pH.

(4). Use of an agitator may be appropriate for smaller burns but may be too painful early in the acute phase.

(5). Treatment time is limited to 20 minutes.

c. **Guidelines for débridement.** Débridement is the removal of nonviable tissue.

(1). *Mechanical*

(a). The preferred and safest method of learning wound débridement is by observation, return demonstration, and practice with supervision.

(b). Eschar is painless and bloodless, but exposed tissue underneath is painful.

(c). Débridement should not cause bleeding, as bleeding indicates that viable tissue has been reached.

(d). Pus under eschar is an indication for débridement.

(e). Forceps can be used to pick up eschar; scissors should be held parallel to the wound.

(f). Sharp débridement of the face should be done using dressings

or by a surgeon in the operating room.

(g). Fat should not be débrided unless it is necrotic.

(h). Débridement over exposed tendons is usually done with dressing changes. Moist dressings are necessary to help maintain the viability of an exposed tendon.

(i). The peroneal nerve is superficial, and therefore caution should be used lateral to the knee.

(2). *Chemical*

(a). Proteolytic enzymes may be used to digest dead tissue.

(b). Physical therapy treatment should be done prior to the application of these dressings, which may be painful once applied.

(3). *Surgical*

(a). The current trend is early surgical débridement to achieve the earliest possible total wound closure.

(b). Skin grafting is the definitive choice for coverage after débridement.

(c). If the granulation bed is not yet ready to accept skin grafts, other wound coverage may be necessary.

d. **Wound coverage**

(1). *Topical agents*

(a). These are used for prevention of infection and to assist with mechanical débridement.

(b). Choice of agent is determined by a physician; however, input from entire team can be helpful in decision making.

(c). It is important to be able to determine whether the wound care regimen is effective or not.

(d). Application of dressings should enable the patient to perform at maximal functional level.

(e). Individual dressings for digits of hands and feet help prevent webbing as well as promote greater independence in activities of daily living.

(f). Silver sulfadiazine cream (Silvadene) is the mainstay of topical antibiotics used in the treatment of burn wounds.

  (i). It is a soothing white cream, used prophylactically in the early treatment of burns.

  (ii). It penetrates eschar sufficiently.

  (iii). It is changed at least once a day, usually twice or three times per day.

(g). Other topical agents include solutions such as Dakin's, mafenide acetate (Sulfamylon), silver nitrate, povidone-iodine, neomycin/polymyxin B sulfate (Neosporin).

(2). *Biological dressings*

(a). Help decrease heat loss.

(b). Reduce water and protein loss by acting as a temporary physical barrier.

(c). Prevent contamination of the wound with environmental microorganisms.

(d). Decrease pain.

(e). Prepare wound for grafting by promoting granulation.

(f). Serve as a test to ascertain the readiness of the wound for autografting.

(g). Provide immediate coverage of partial-thickness burns.

(h). Protect exposed vital structures.

(i). Provide mechanical débridement of wounds after eschar separation.

(j). Provide coverage of granulated tissue between autografts.

(k). Provide immediate wound coverage after excision.

(3). *Types of biological dressings*

(a). Xenograft (heterograft)

  (i). The most common animal skin used is porcine (pigskin).

  (ii). It is readily available in split-thickness fresh or frozen preparations, meshed or unmeshed.

(b). Homograft (allograft)—uses cadaver skin taken as split thickness.

(c). Human amniotic membrane—obtained from placenta.

(d). Semisynthetic materials—may consist of nylon, Silastic, and collagen derivative.

(e). Synthetic materials.

(f). Artificial skin—collagen dermis covered by Silastic epidermis.

e. *Nutrition*

(1). The metabolic rate during healing is accelerated.

(2). It is difficult for the acutely ill patient to keep up with caloric requirements.

(3). Caloric requirements are calculated based on the patient's TBSA and weight.

(4). The patient's weight and daily calorie and protein intake are monitored.

(5). The dietician is an important member of the burn team.

(6). Insertion of a nasogastric tube is frequently required.

(7). Intravenous hyperalimentation also is used if tube feedings are inadequate or not tolerated.

f. *Surgical management*

(1). *Débridement*

(a). Escharotomy/fasciotomy

  (i). A full-thickness burn can constrict.

  (ii). Because of the pressure from the massive fluid shift, a tourniquet effect can cause loss of viability of tissue distal to this constriction.

  (iii). Escharotomy or fasciotomy may be necessary for circumferential injuries of the neck, trunk, or extremities.

  (iv). These procedures are used to prevent circulatory occlusion and to relieve respiratory distress.

  (v). Incisions are made with care to avoid tendons and nerves.

  (vi). General anaesthesia is not required because full-thickness burns are insensate.

(b). Excision of eschar

  (i). Tangential (or sequential)

excision is used in deep dermal burns. Eschar is shaved in layers to the level of profuse and uniform capillary bleeding.

(ii). Fascial excision is used in full-thickness burns. The entire dermal layer and subcutaneous tissue down to the level of fascia are excised.

(2). *Skin grafting*

(a). The only kind of graft that will be able to remain in place permanently is an autograft, *ie,* skin from the burned person grafted to himself/herself.

(b). Autograft is obtained from patient during the surgical procedure.

(c). Usually a "split-thickness" graft is used, *ie,* a layer of skin that includes part of the dermis.

(i). Meshed grafts help enlarge the available skin to cover a larger area. A surgical instrument puts tiny holes into the skin after it has been harvested. The holes vary in size to allow more stretch as needed to cover then excised area.

(ii). Sheet grafts cover an area equal to that of the donor site from which the skin was removed. Sheet grafts are used for faces, hands, and over joint surfaces when possible. The use of a sheet graft gives a better cosmetic and functional result.

(iii). Frequently, a combination of both types of split-thickness skin grafting is used.

(iv). Split-thickness coverage may not be the best choice to cover bone or tendon.

(v). A skin flap that includes subcutaneous tissues may be used to increase the ability of skin to glide over tendon or bone and to decrease the risk of abrasions over these surfaces.

(d). A donor site is the area from which the skin graft is obtained.

(i). The site is treated essentially as a "manmade" partial-thickness burn, requiring 10 to 14 days to heal.

(ii). The location of the donor site depends on the availability of unburned skin.

(iii). When possible, skin grafts for the face are taken from donor sites above the nipple line, known as the "blush area."

(iv). The scalp is a frequent choice. It heals quickly. Hair growth will conceal any scar from the donor site.

(v). Donor sites can be reused after they have healed. The best skin is available from the first harvest. The first use of donor skin is usually used for face, hands, and joint surfaces.

(vi) A mild change in pigmentation may remain after the scarring process is complete.

(e). Cultured epithelial autograft

(i). This is used when burns are so extensive that there is not enough available donor site to cover burn wounds.

(ii). Human epidermal cells from a small skin biopsy can be cultured to produce epithelial sheets for wound coverage.

(iii). A specimen of 2 cm^2 can be expanded by a factor of 10,000 in 3 to 4 weeks.

(iv). Physical therapy implications with use of cultured epithelium: Skin is much more fragile than autografts, which have support from at least part of the dermis. Extreme care must be taken during routine therapy procedures, such as splinting or exercise.

g. *Complications*
(1). *Amputations*
(a). With full-thickness injury, digits of hands and feet are the most common sites for amputation.
(b). More extensive amputations of limbs occur with electrical injuries.
(c). Patients with high risk for amputations with burns include those with pre-existing medical conditions such as peripheral vascular disease or diabetes.
(2). *Heterotopic ossification*
(a). Excessive calcium is deposited in joints.
(b). This is frequently seen in elbows and knees.
(c). Treatment is somewhat controversial.
(d). Consensus seems to be that active range of motion should be encouraged to maximize functional range.
(e). Immobilization may cause decreased motion.
(f). Surgery may be performed when the process is no longer active, if there is severe pain, and/or there is loss of mobility.
(3). *Peripheral neuropathies*
(a). Peroneal nerve and brachial plexus injuries may occur.
(b). The type of neuropathy varies with location of the burn.
(4). Children under 5 and adults over 50 have greater rate of complications.
(a). The skin of an infant may be less than half as thick as that of an adult.
(b). Dermal atrophy begins in patients over 50 years of age, with resulting thinning of the skin in elderly patients.
(c). Scald burns can be particularly deceptive in this population

and are frequently underestimated in extent and depth.

3. **Rehabilitation phase**
a. *General considerations*
(1). The patient is medically stable, with few open areas requiring wound care.
(2). Acute surgical intervention is no longer required; however, reconstructive procedures may be done during this phase.
(3). Discharge planning is the focus, with all team members involved.
b. Rehabilitation of the burn patient requires a team effort, including the physician, psychologist and/or psychiatrist, physical and occupational therapists, nurse, social worker, dietician, art and play therapist, vocational counselor, clinical pharmacist, and, most important, the patient, family, and friends.
(1). Psychological support should be provided by all members of the team.
(2). Team conferences help to identify a patient's variable needs.
(3). Children are routinely seen by an art and play therapist.
(4). A patient's response to the injury may be influenced by his/her perception of how it occurred.
(a). A burn may be self-inflicted; the patient may be an innocent bystander or a victim of his/her own carelessness.
(b). The patient may respond with corresponding feelings of guilt, anger, vulnerability, and embarrassment.
(5). Acceptance of an altered body image may require a great deal of time and effort.
(6). Families and significant others may benefit from individual meetings with social workers.
(7). Patients and/or families may benefit from support groups offered during and after the hospitalization.
(8). Psychiatrists are especially helpful when premorbid status includes a pertinent history.
(9). Pain control is an important element in the patient's tolerance of the experience.

(10). Hypnotism has been used in addition to pain medications.

(11). Psychological and social rehabilitation is an ongoing process that may take years.

c. *Reconstructive procedures*

(1). The focus of rehabilitation is to prevent or minimize the need for reconstructive surgery.

(2). Common techniques to correct burn scar contracture include Z-plasty and scar excision with primary closure or grafting.

(3). Tissue expansion can be used to extend available healthy skin in place of scars. This is often used for increased hair coverage on the scalp.

(4). Reconstructive procedures are usually not done until the burn scar has matured.

(5). Exceptions to this include correction of functional deficits such as eyelid and lip ectropion or severe joint contractures.

d. *Long-term sequelae*

(1). Hypertrophic scars can be stiff, dry, itchy, painful, thick, hypersensitive, and hyposensitive. (More on this process is found in the section on burn care, in Chapter 27.)

(2). Hair loss is possible with deep partial- or full-thickness injury.

(3). Sweat gland disruption causes decreased sweating in burned areas, with increased sweating in unburned areas.

(4). Disruption of sebaceous glands requires long-term external lubrication.

(5). Skin is more fragile after burns have healed, with resulting open areas from minor trauma such as bumping into an object.

(6). Patients with poor peripheral circulation before burn are at risk for chronic ulcers when burn is in a dependent area.

(7). Joint pain and stiffness may occur because of the constant force of the scarring process.

(8). There may be orthopedic asymmetry in children.

(a). Inelastic scar bands may not allow bones to grow to optimal length.

(b). Pressure garments may inhibit growth; *eg*, a chin strap may affect the growing temporomandibular joint.

V. Special Problems of Desensitized Skin[123-129]

A. General issues

1. Healthy skin has an inherent protection against injury but is easily repaired and healed following injury.

2. Denervated skin is more at risk for injury.

a. Unnecessary decubitus (pressure ulcers) can lead to amputations.

b. Pressure sores can interfere with successful rehabilitation of the elderly and patients with spinal cord injuries.

c. Pressure sores increase the number of hospital days and lost time from rehabilitation and lead to poor staff and patient morale.[123]

3. Adequate blood flow to the tissue is critical for healthy skin.

a. Blood brings oxygen and other nutrients to the cell.

b. Blood removes carbon dioxide and metabolic waste products.

c. If blood flow is disrupted, tissue function will be compromised.

d. Compression (pressure) is the primary risk factor for tissue damage, creating ischemia and altering normal cell metabolism.

e. Normal capillary pressures have been measured at 32 mm Hg at the arteriole end and 15 mm Hg at the venule end.

(1). Any pressure greater than this internal pressure will cause capillary obstruction and ischemia, leading to increased capillary permeability and extravasation.[124]

(2). One to 2 hours of pressure at 60 to 70 mm Hg on innervated or denervated tissue causes pathological changes.

(3). Pressure of 40 to 100 mm Hg over a 4-hour period results in cellular ischemia.[125]

4. Loss or diminished mobility or sensory function, autonomic and sympathetic dysfunction, metabolic disturbances, nutritional deficiencies, loss of bowel and bladder control, spasms, hemoglobinemia, and emotional depression further increase the risk of developing pressure sores.

5. External risk factors such as friction, shearing forces, moisture (especially from incontinence), fever, and infection further heighten the risk.

6. If the patient is compromised by severe trauma and must be immobilized for healing, a planned program of skin care must be implemented to prevent the development of ulcers.

   a. Different areas of the body are more sensitive than others to ischemia.

      (1). Skin over body prominences is likely to be more susceptible to tissue damage.

      (2). Skin can withstand high pressures for short periods of time when there are brief intervals of relief.

   b. Without conscientiousness, normal individuals change positions frequently to relieve and redistribute pressure.

   c. Those without sensations of pressure must assume cognitive control of changing positions because pressure receptors will not provide the information that they are overloaded.

7. Body weight usually exceeds 100 mm Hg.

   a. Patients sitting in a chair most of the day will create irreversible damage in 4 hours or less, especially over the ischial tuberosity.[123]

   b. Pressure sores usually develop more rapidly with far less pressure than 100 mm Hg.

   c. Elderly patients are at the greatest risk of skin breakdown.

      (1). Pressure is confounded by metabolic problems.

      (2). The major challenge is to keep patients active to prevent unnecessary pressure.

      (3). The elderly often require constant attention by nurses, aids, and family members to change positions to prevent bed sores.

      (4). Ideally, patients should be kept ambulatory or at least standing so that they can assume some responsibility to maintain mobility.

   d. Risk of decubitus in patients with spinal cord injuries is related to the level and completeness of the injury.

      (1). Of patients with complete quadriplegia, 43% to 57% developed pressure sores during their initial hospitalization.[126,127]

      (2). Risk for skin breakdown is the greatest during the early phase of hospitalization, when the metabolic disturbances are the greatest. Patients remain vulnerable for pressure sores for the rest of their lives.

8. Patients, health care providers, and families need to recognize abnormal skin responses so that they can identify problems early.

   a. *Blanching*

      (1). A normal response to pressure; the instant change in color that occurs following compression.

      (2). May not be visible in dark-skinned patients.

      (3). Is easy to demonstrate by applying pressure on a nail bed.

   b. *Pressure mark*

      (1). Following temporary ischemia, a normal compensatory response occurs: bright skin flush that occurs within seconds (reactive hyperemia).

      (2). Fades within 1 hour when pressure is removed.

      (3). There is no tissue damage.

   c. *Pressure area*

      (1). Refers to an abnormal color change that does not fade and may or may not blanch.

      (2). Characterized by elevated local temperature ("hot spot").

      (3). Edematous swelling or lumps and blisters or pimples may be common.

      (4). May take several days to heal and may be the start of a Grade I pressure sore.

   d. *Pressure sore*

      (1). Abnormal area of ulceration characterized by exudate from open areas.

(2). Dark or necrotic tissue is in the middle of the sore.

(3). May take up to 1 year to heal and may require surgery.

(4). Can be life threatening.

9. Grading the severity of pressure sores.[128]

a. Pressure sores are graded from I to IV, with Grade IV potentially life threatening and Grade I clearly a reversible lesion that should be immediately treated.

(1). *Grade I.* These sores involve both the epidermis and the dermis and may or may not have some shallow skin breakdown.

  (a). Blister formation may be present, but no blanching (reactive hyperemic response).

  (b). Usually there is some heat, swelling, induration, and redness.

  (c). Usually takes 10 to 14 days to re-epithelialize.

(2). *Grade II.* Involves the epidermis, dermis, and subcutaneous fat.

  (a). Looks like an irregular, full-thickness ulcer with increased inflammation and fibrotic involvement.

  (b). The surrounding area may have redness, heat, and swelling.

  (c). May take 3 weeks to 3 months to heal; re-epithelialization contains collagen that is poorly keratinized and results in scar tissue.

  (d). This is a reversible lesion.

(3). *Grade III.* These sores involve the adipose tissue and the muscle in addition to the epidermis, dermis, and subcutaneous tissue.

  (a). There is extensive undermining; the sore has thick, rolled edges, and infection is usually present.

  (b). Extensive loss of fluid and protein occur.

  (c). Bone can respond to the local inflammation, and subperiosteal new bone and local osteoporosis can develop.

  (d). Joints may develop capsular swelling and synovial effusion and begin to restrict motion.

  (e). Wound must be débrided of necrotic tissue to allow healing.

  (f). Healing time depends on whether infection is present and whether surgery is needed.

  (g). These sores can be life threatening.

(4). *Grade IV.* These sores involve soft-tissue necrosis down to the bone and joint structures.

  (a). Anemia, infection, fluid, and protein are extensive.

  (b). There is extensive undermining of the tissue.

  (c). Osteomyelitis, septic arthritis, subluxations, and dislocations can occur.

  (d). Radiographs are needed to indicate the extent of the involvement and the osteomyelitis.

  (e). Surgical scraping or removal of necrotic bone must occur before healing is possible.

  (f). These sores can be life threatening.

b. Pressure grades are used to assess and document the level of tissue involvement.

c. The patient's and physical therapist's early recognition of skin changes and knowledge of what to look for and how to visually and tactilely inspect the skin are essential elements for successful healing.[129]

d. The parameters to monitor for skin dysfunction include

(1). Color (pale, redness, jaundice, hyperemia, rashes).

(2). Elasticity (skin turgor, signs of dehydration, dryness).

(3). Moisture (presence of perspiration, urine, drainage).

(4). Cleanliness (odor, dirt, crumbs).

(5). Dryness (presence of cracks, fissures, flakiness).

(6). Temperature changes should be palpated ("hot spots," "cold spots," or fever).

(7). Edema should be noted (swelling, tightness, spongy soft tissue).

10. Inspection of the skin by the patient should occur before going to bed at night, getting up in the morning, during and after bathing, and during and after toileting, transfers, and other activities.

a. Visual inspection includes major pressure points as well as stress points resulting from clothes, casts, or braces.

    b. Mirrors can assist in visualizing areas that are difficult to see and reach (*eg*, sacrum, trochanter, ischia, and heels).

    c. The dorsum of the hand can also be used to feel body surfaces that can be felt but not seen (good for picking up any underlying lesions that have not yet caused a change in the skin appearance [*eg*, a hidden Grade II]).

11. In summary, skin breakdown in patients with insensitive skin must be prevented.

    a. With diligence and concern on the part of the patient, the family, and all caregivers, it is possible to prevent these problems.

    b. When skin breakdown does occur, all of the concepts of positioning, turning, relieving pressure, and basic wound care techniques must be implemented.

References

1. Hunt TK, Van Winkle W: Normal repair. In Hunt TK, Dunphy JE (eds): *Fundamentals of Wound Management*. New York, Appleton-Century-Crofts, 1979, pp 4–68.
2. Davis JC, Hunt TK: *Problem Wounds: The Role of Oxygen*. New York, Elsevier, 1988, pp 1–242.
3. McLean AEM, Ahmed K, Judah JD: Cellular permeability and the reaction to injury. *Ann N Y Acad Sci* 1964, 116:986–989.
4. Schoefl GI: Studies on inflammation. III. Growing capillaries; their structure and permeability. *Virchows Arch [A]* 1963, 337:99.
5. Im MJC, Hoopes JE: Energy metabolism in healing skin wounds. *J Surg Res* 1970, 10:459.
6. Niinikoski J, Hunt TK, Dunphy JE: Oxygen supply in healing tissue. *Am J Surg* 1972, 123:247–252.
7. Niinikoski J: Oxygen and wound healing. *Clin Plast Surg* 1977, 4:361–374.
8. Hunt TK, Pai MP: Effect of varying ambient oxygen tensions on wound metabolism and collagen synthesis. *Surg Gynecol Obstet* 1972, 135:561–567.
9. Ehrlich HP, Hunt TK: Effects of cortisone and Vitamin A on wound healing. *Ann Surg* 1968, 167:324–328.
10. Gould BS: Ascorbic acid–independent and ascorbic acid–dependent collagen-forming mechanisms. *Ann N Y Acad Sci* 1961, 92:168–174.
11. Barnes MUJ: Function of ascorbic acid in collagen metabolism. *Ann N Y Acad Sci* 1975, 258:264–277.
12. Babior BM: Oxygen-dependent microbial killing by phagocytes. *N Engl J Med* 1978, 298:659–668, 721–725.
13. Remensnyder JP, Majno G: Oxygen gradients in healing wounds. *Am J Pathol* 1968, 52:301–304.
14. Levene CI, Bates CJ: The effect of hypoxia on collagen synthesis in cultured 3T6 fibroblasts and its relationship to the mode of action of ascorbate. *Biochim Biophys Acta* 1976, 444:446–452.
15. Nimni ME: Collagen: its structure and function in normal and pathologic connective tissues. *Semin Arthritis Rheum* 1974, 4:95.
16. Tanzer ML: Crosslinking of collagen. *Science* 1973, 180:561.
17. Gay S, Miller EJ, Fischer G: *Collagen in the Physiology and Pathology of Connective Tissue*. New York, Springer-Verlag, 1978.
18. Hunt TK: Disorders of repair and their management. In Hunt TK, Dunphy JE (eds): *Fundamentals of Wound Management*. New York, Appleton-Century-Crofts, 1979, pp 68–149.
19. Moserova J, Houskova E: *The Healing and Treatment of Skin Defects*. New York, Karger, 1989, pp 1–62.
20. Ehrlich RF, Rodeheaver G, Thacker JG, et al.: Technical factors in wound management. In Hunt TK, Dunphy JE (eds): *Fundamentals of Wound Management*. New York, Appleton-Century-Crofts, 1979, pp 408–483.
21. Davis JC: Local Management of Problem Wounds. In Davis JC, Hunt TK (eds): *Problem Wounds, The Role of Oxygen*. New York, Elsevier, 1988, pp 211–223.
22. Michlovitz SL: *Thermal Agents in Rehabilitation*. Philadelphia, FA Davis Company, 1986, pp 99–115.
23. Erlich HP, Grislis G, Hunt TK: Metabolic and circulatory contributions to oxygen gradients in wounds. *Surgery* 1972, 72:578–583.
24. Hunt TK, Twomey P, Zederfeldt B, et al.: Respiratory gas tensions and pH in healing wounds. *Am J Surg* 1967, 114:203–208.
25. Silver IA: Cellular microenvironment in healing and non-healing wounds. In Hunt TK, Heppenstall RB, Pines E, et al. (eds): *Soft and Hard Tissue Repair*. New York, Praeger, 1984, pp 50–66.
26. Beaman I, Beaman BL: The role of oxygen and its derivatives in microbial pathogenesis and host defense. *Annu Rev Microbiol* 1984, 38:27–48.
27. Hohn DC: Oxygen and leukocyte microbial killing. In Davis JC, Hunt TK (eds): *Hyperbaric Oxygen Therapy*. Bethesda, Undersea Medical Society, 1977, pp 101–110.
28. Hunt TK, Halliday B, Knighton DR, et al.: Impairment of microbial function in wounds: correction with oxydation. In Hunt TK, Heppenstall RB, Pines E, et al. (eds): *Soft and Hard Tissue Repair, Biological and Clinical Aspects*. New York, Praeger, 1984, pp 455–468.
29. Klebanoff S: Oxygen metabolism and the toxic properties of phagocytes. *Ann Intern Med* 1980, 93:480–489.
30. Knighton DR, Halliday B, Hunt TK: Oxygen as an antibiotic: a comparison of inspired oxygen concentration and antibiotic administration on in vivo bacterial clearance. *Arch Surg* 1986, 121:191–195.
31. Wallyn RJ, Gumbiner SH, Goldfien S, et al.: Treatment of anaerobic infections with hyperbaric oxygen. *Surg Clin North Am* 1964, 44:107–112.
32. Mader JT, Hulet WA, Reinarz JA: Potential value of hyperbaric oxygen in inoperable pelvic and intraabdominal sepsis [abstract 630]. 20th Interscience Conference on Antimicrobial Agents and Chemotherapy, 1980.
33. Kellog EW III, Fridovich I: Liposome oxidation and erythrocyte lysis by enzymatically generated superoxide and hydrogen peroxide. *J Biol Chem* 1977, 252:6721–6728.
34. McRipley RJ, Sbarra AJ: Role of the phagocyte in host-parasite interactions. Relationship between stimulated oxidative metabolism and hydrogen peroxide formation and intracellular killing. *J Bacteriol* 1967, 94:1417–1424.
35. Knighton DR, Halliday B, Hunt TK: Oxygen as an antibiotic: the effect of inspired oxygen on infection. *Arch Surg* 1984, 119:199–204.
36. Sheffield PJ: Tissue oxygen measurements with respect to soft tissue wound healing with normobaric and hyperbaric oxygen. *Hyperb Oxyg Rev* 1982, 6:18–46.
37. Wells CH, Goodpasture JE, Horrigan DJ, et al.: Tissue gas measurements during hyperbaric oxygen exposure. In Smith G (ed): *Proceedings of the Sixth International Con-*

gress on Hyperbaric Medicine. Aberdeen, Aberdeen University Press, 1977, pp 118–124.

38. Wyss CA, Matsen FA III, Simmons CW, et al.: Transcutaneous oxygen tension measurements on limbs of diabetic and nondiabetic patients with peripheral vascular disease. *Surgery* 1984, 95:339–345.

39. Gottlieb SF, Solosky JA, Aubrey R, et al.: Synergistic action of increase oxygen tensions and sodium sulfisoxazole on some gram negative bacteria. In Trapp WG, Banister EW, Davison AJ, et al. (eds): *Fifth International Hyperbaric Conference Proceedings.* Vancouver, Simon Fraser University Press, 1974, pp 577–583.

40. Selvaraj RJ, Sbarra AF: Relationship of glycolytic and oxidative metabolism to particle entry and destruction in phagocytosing cells. *Nature* 1966, 211:1272–1276.

41. Sheffield PJ, Workman WT: Noninvasive tissue oxygen measurements in patients administered normobaric and hyperbaric oxygen by mask. *Hyperb Oxyg Rev* 1985, 6:47–62.

42. Chang N, Goodson WH III, Gottrup F, et al.: Direct measurement of wound and tissue oxygen tension in postoperative patients. *Ann Surg* 1983, 197:470–478.

43. Gottrup F, Firmin R, Hunt TK, et al.: Dynamic properties of tissue oxygen in healing flaps. *Surgery* 1983, 95:532–536.

44. Gregory EM, Fridovich I: Induction of superoxide dismutase by molecular oxygen. *J Bacteriol* 1973, 144:543–548.

45. Hunt TK, Halliday B, Knighton DR, et al.: Impairment of microbicidal function in wounds: correction with oxygenation. In Hunt TK, Heppenstall RB, Pines E, et al. (eds): *Soft and Hard Tissue Repair, Biological and Clinical Aspects.* New York, Praeger, 1984, pp 455–468.

46. Chang N, Mathes SJ: Comparison of the effect of bacterial inoculation in musculocutaneous and random-pattern flaps. *Plast Reconstr Surg* 1982, 70:1–10.

47. Jonsson K, Hunt TK, Mathes SJ: Effect of environmental oxygen on bacterial-induced tissue necrosis in flaps. *Surg Forum* 1984, 35:589–591.

48. Hohn DC, MacKay RD, Halliday B, et al.: The effect of O_2 tension on the microbicidal function of leukocytes in wounds and in vitro. *Surg Forum* 1976, 27:18–20.

49. Feng LJ, Price D, Hohn D, et al.: Blood flow changes and leukocyte mobilization in infection: a comparison between ischemia and well-perfused skin. *Surg Forum* 1983, 34:603–605.

50. Goodson WH III, Andrews WS, Thakral KK, et al.: Wound oxygen tension of large vs small wounds in man. *Surg Forum* 1979, 30:93–95.

51. Rabkin J, Hunt TK: Local heat increases blood flow and oxygen tension in wounds. *Arch Surg* 1987, 122:221–222.

52. Mader JT: Update: HBO and infections. In Hart GB, Strauss MB (eds): *Proceedings of the Eighth Annual Conference for the Clinical Application of Hyperbaric Oxygen.* Long Beach, CA, Memorial Hospital, 1983, p 39.

53. McNeill SC, Potts RO, Francoeur ML: Local enhanced topical delivery (LETD) of drugs: does it truly exist. *Pharm Res* 1992, 9:1422–1427.

54. Webster RC, Maibach HI: Individual and regional variation with in vitro percutaneous absorption. In Bronaugh RL, Maibach HI (eds): *In Vitro Percutaneous Absorption: Principles, Fundamentals, and Applications.* Boston, CRC Press, 1991, pp 26–30.

55. Guy RH, Hadgraft J: The effect of penetration enhancers on the kinetics of percutaneous absorption. *J Control Rel* 1987, 5:43–51.

56. Bucks D, Guy R, Maibach H: Effects of occlusion. In Bronaugh RL, Maibach HI (eds): *In Vitro Percutaneous Absorption: Principles, Fundamentals, and Applications.* Boston, CRC Press, 1991, pp 85–114.

57. Henley EJ: Iontophoresis and phonophoresis transcutaneous drug delivery. Presented at the 65th Annual Conference of the American Physical Therapy Association, Santa Ana, CA, June 24, 1990.

58. Munck A, Guyre PM: Glucocorticoid physiology and homeostasis in relation to healing. In Schleimer RP, Claman HN, Oronsky AL (eds): *Anti-inflammatory Steroid Action: Basic and Clinical Aspects,* San Diego, Academic Press, pp 30–48.

59. Tsurufuji S, Sugio K: Molecular mechanism in the manifestation of antiinflammatory activity of glucocorticoids. *Eur J Rheumatol Inflamm* 1978, 1:226–231.

60. Tsurufuji S, Ohuchi K: In vivo models of inflammation: a review with special reference to the mechanisms of action of glucocorticoids. In Schleimer RP, Claman HN, Oronsky AL (eds): *Anti-inflammatory Steroid Action: Basic and Clinical Aspects.* San Diego, Academic Press, 1989, chapter 11.

61. Harvey W, Grahame R, Panayi GS: Effects of steroid hormones on human fibroblasts in vitro. I. Glucocorticoid action on cell growth and collagen synthesis. *Ann Rheum Dis* 1974, 33:437–441.

62. Lehmann JF (ed): *Therapeutic Heat and Cold. Rehabilitation Medicine Library.* Baltimore, Williams & Wilkins, 1990.

63. Ziskin MC, McDiarmid T, Michlovitz SL: Therapeutic ultrasound. In: Michlovitz SL (ed): *Thermal Agents in Rehabilitation,* 2nd ed. Philadelphia, F. A. Davis Company, 1990, pp 134–169.

64. Hayes KW: *Manual for Physical Agents.* Norwalk, CT, Appleton & Lange, 1993, p 169.

65. Tyle P, Agravala P: Drug delivery by phonophoresis. *Pharm Res* 1989, 6:355–361.

66. Scott RC: In vitro absorption through damaged skin. In Bronaugh RL, Maibach HI (eds): *In Vitro Percutaneous Absorption: Principles, Fundamentals, and Applications.* Boston, CRC Press, 1991, pp 129–135.

67. Dinno MA, Crum LA, Wu J: The effect of therapeutic ultrasound on electrophysiological parameters of frog skin. *Ultrasound Med Biol* 1989, 15:461–470.

68. Dinno MA, Dyson M, Young SR, et al.: The significance of membrane changes in the safe and effective use of therapeutic and diagnostic ultrasound. *Ultrasound Med Biol* 1989, 34:1543–1552.

69. Bommannan D, Okuyama H, Stauffer P, Guy RH: Sonophoresis I. The use of high-frequency ultrasound to enhance transdermal drug delivery. *Pharm Res* 1992, 9:559–564.

70. Bommannan D, Menon GK, Okuyama H, et al.: Sonophoresis II. Examination of the mechanism(s) of ultrasound-enhanced transdermal drug delivery. *Pharm Res* 1992, 9:1043–1047.

71. Cameron MH, Monroe LG: Relative transmission of ultrasound by media customarily used for phonophoresis. *Phys Ther* 1992, 72:142–148.

72. Byl N, McKenzie A, West J, et al.: Low-dose ultrasound effects on wound healing: a controlled study with Yucatan pigs. *Arch Phys Med* 1992, 73:565–664.

73. Antich TJ: Phonophoresis: the principles of ultrasonic driving force and efficacy in treatment of common orthopedic diagnoses. *J Orthop Sports Phys Ther* 1982, 4:99–102.

74. Griffin J, Touchstone JC: Ultrasonic movement of cortisol into pig tissues: I. Movement into skeletal muscle. *Am J Phys Med* 1963, 42:77–85.

75. Griffin J, Touchstone JC: Ultrasonic movement of cortisol into pig tissues: II. Movement into peripheral nerve. *Am J Phys Med* 1965, 44:20–25.

76. Griffin, JE, Echternach JL, Price RE, Touchstone JC: Patients treated with ultrasonic drive hydrocortisone and ultrasound alone. *Phys Ther* 1967, 47:595–601.

77. Newman MK, Kill M, Frampton G: Effects of ultrasound alone and combined with hydrocortisone injections by needle or hypospray. *Am J Phys Med* 1958, 37:206–209.

78. Novak EJ: Experimental transmission of lidocaine through intact skin by ultrasound. *Arch Phys Med Rehabil* 1964, 45:231–232.

79. Ciccone CD, Leggin BG, Callamaro J: Effects of ultrasound and trolamine salicylate phonophoresis on delayed-onset muscle soreness. *Phys Ther* 1991, 71:666–678.

80. Benson HA, McElnay JC, Harland R: Use of ultrasound to enhance percutaneous absorption of benzydamine. *Phys Ther* 1989, 69:113–116.

81. Hong CZ, Shellock FG: Effects of a topically applied counterirritant (Eucalyptamint) on cutaneous blood flow and on skin and muscle temperatures. A placebo-controlled study. *Am J Phys Med Rehabil* 1991, 70:29–33.

82. Muir WS, Magee EP, Longo JA, et al.: Comparison of ultrasonically applied vs intra-articular injected hydrocortisone levels in canine knees. *Orthop Rev* 1990, 29:351–356.

83. Davick JP, Martin RK, Albright JP: Distribution and deposition of tritiated cortisol using phonophoresis. *Phys Ther* 1988, 68:1672–1675.

84. Williams AR: Phonophoresis: an in vivo evaluation using three topical anaesthetic preparations. *Ultrasonics* 1990, 28:137–141.

85. Kost J, Levy D, Langer R: Ultrasound as a transdermal enhancer. In Bronaugh RL, Maibach HI (eds): *Percutaneous Absorption: Mechanisms-Methodology-Drug Delivery,* 2nd ed. New York, Marcel Dekker, 1989, pp 595–601.

86. Eli Glick, ES Snyder-Mackler L: Iontophoresis. In Snyder-Mackler L, Robinson AJ (eds): *Clinical Electrophysiology: Electrotherapy and Electrophysiologic Testing, Rehabilitation Practice Series.* Baltimore, Williams & Wilkins, 1989, pp 247–260.

87. Cummings J: Iontophoresis. In Nelson RM, Currier DP (eds): *Clinical Electrotherapy,* 2nd ed. San Mateo, CA, Appleton & Lange, 1991, pp 317–329.

88. Gersh MR: *Electrotherapy in Rehabilitation.* Philadelphia, F. A. Davis Company, 1992, pp 337–342.

89. Behl, C, Jumar, S, Malick AW, et al.: Iontophoretic drug delivery: effects of physicochemical factors on the skin uptake of drugs. In Bronaugh RL, Maibach HI (eds): *Percutaneous Absorption: Mechanisms-Methodology-Drug Delivery,* 2nd ed. Marcel Dekker, 1989, pp 603–631.

90. Schwartz MS: The use of hyaluronidase by iontophoresis in the treatment of lymphedema. *Arch Intern Med* 1955, 95:662–668.

91. Magistro CM: Hyaluronidase by iontophoresis in the treatment of edema. A preliminary clinical report. *Phys Ther* 1964, 44:169–179.

92. Cornwall MW: Zinc iontophoresis to treat ischemic skin ulcers. *Phys Ther* 1981, 61:339–340.

93. Akins DL, Meisenheimer JL, Dobson RL: Efficacy of the Drionic unit in the treatment of hyperhidrosis. *J Am Acad Dermatol* 1987, 26:828–832.

94. Hill BHR: Poldine iontophoresis in the treatment of palmar and plantar hyperhidrosis. *Aust J Dermatol* 1976, 27:92–93.

95. Stolman LP: Treatment of excess sweating of the palms of iontophoresis. *Arch Dermatol* 1987, 123:893–896.

96. Grice K, Sattar H, Baker K: Treatment of idiopathic hyperhidrosis with iontophoresis of tap water and poldine methylsulphate. *Br J Dermatol* 1972, 86:72–78.

97. Shrivastava SN, Sing G: Tap water iontophoresis in palm and plantar hyperhidrosis. *Br J Dermatol* 1977, 96:189–195.

98. Abdell E, Morgan K: Treatment of idiopathic hyperhidrosis of glycopyrronium bromide and tap water iontophoresis. *Br J Dermatol* 1974, 87:87–91.

99. Haggard HW, Strauss MJ, Greenberg LA: Fungous infections of hand and feet treated by copper iontophoresis. *JAMA* 1939, 223:1229.

100. Psaki CE, Moss S, Carroll JF: Acetic acid ionization: a study to determine the absorptive effects upon calcific tendonitis of the shoulder. *Phys Ther Rev* 1955, 35:84.

101. Kahn J: A case report: lithium iontophoresis for gouty arthritis. *J Orthop Sports Phys Ther* 1982, 4:113.

102. Bertolucci LE: Introduction of antiinflammatory drugs by iontophoresis: double blind study. *J Orthop Sports Phys Ther* 1982, 4:203.

103. Glass JM, Stephen RL, Jacobsen SC: The quantity and distribution of radiolabeled dexamethasone delivered to tissues by iontophoresis. *Int J Dermatol* 1980, 19:519–525.

104. Harris PR: Iontophoresis: clinical research in musculoskeletal inflammatory conditions. *J Orthop Sports Phys Ther* 1982, 4:109.

105. Brunnett A, Corneau M: Local anesthesia of the tympanic membrane by iontophoresis. *Trans Am Acad Otolaryngol* 1974, 78:453.

106. Russo J, Lipman AG, Comstock TJ, et al.: Lidocaine anesthesia: comparison of iontophoresis injection and swabbing. *Am J Hosp Pharm* 1980, 37:843–847.

107. Gangarosa LP: Iontophoresis for surface local anesthesia. *J Am Dent Assoc* 1974, 88:125.

108. Chantraine A, Lundy JP, Berger D. Is cortisone iontophoresis possible? *Arch Phys Med Rehabil* 1986, 67:38–40.

109. Garzione JE: Salicylate iontophoresis as an alternative treatment for persistent thigh pain following hip surgery. *Phys Ther* 1978, 58:570–571.

110. Brunnett A, Corneau M: Local anesthesia of the tympanic membrane by iontophoresis. *Trans Am Acad Otolaryngol* 1974, 78:453.

111. Gordon AH, et al.: Sodium salicylate iontophoresis in the treatment of plantar warts. *Phys Ther Rev* 1969, 49:869–870.

112. Tannenbaum M: Iodine iontophoresis in reduction of scar tissue. *Phys Ther* 1980, 60:792.

113. Falcone AE, Spadaro JA: Inhibitory effects of electrically activated silver material on cutaneous wound bacteria. *Plast Reconstr Surg* 1986, 77:455–458.

114. Alsbjörn BF: Biologic wound coverings in burn treatment. *World J Surg* 1992, 16:43–46.

115. Depew CL: Toxic epidermal necrolysis. *J Crit Care Nursing Clin North Am* 1991, 3:255–267.

116. Dyer C: Burn wound management: an update. *Plast Surg Nurs* 1988, Spring.

117. Gallico GG, O'Connor NE, Compton CC, et al.: Permanent coverage of large burn wounds with autologous cultured human epithelium. *N Engl J Med* 1984, 311:448–451.

118. Heimbach D, Engrav L, Grube B, Marvin J: Burn depth: a review. *World J Surg* 1992, 16:10–15.

119. McDonald K, Johnson B, Prasad JK, Thomson PD: Rehabilitative considerations for patients with severe Stevens-Johnson syndrome or toxic epidermal necrolysis: a case report. *J Burn Care Rehabil* 1989, 10:167–171.

120. Nolan WB: Acute management of thermal injury. *Ann Plast Surg* 1981, 7:3.

121. Robson MC, Barnett RA, Leitch IOW, Hayward PG: Prevention and treatment of postburn scars and contracture. *World J Surg* 1992, 16:87–96.

122. Salisbury RE, Newman NM, Dingeldein GP: *Manual of Burn Therapeutics.* Boston, Little, Brown and Company, 1983.

123. Kosiak M: Etiology of decubitus ulcers. *Arch Phys Med Rehabil* 1961, 42:19–29.

124. Berecek K: Etiology of decubitus ulcers. *Nurs Clin North Am* 1975, 20:157–170.

125. Constantian MD: *Pressure Ulcers: Principles and Techniques of Management.* Boston, Little, Brown and Company, 1980.

126. Young J, *et al.:* Pressure sores and spinal cord injured. In *Spinal Cord Injury Statistics: Experience of the Regional Spinal Cord Injury System, Part I.* Phoenix, Good Samaritan Hospital, 1982, p 108.

127. *Regional Spinal Cord Injury Care System of Southern California.* Final Report. Downey, CA, Rancho Los Amigos Hospital, 1982.

128. Shea JD. Pressure sores: classification and management. *Clin Orthop* 1975, 223:89–100.

129. Enis JE, Sarmiento A: The physiology and management of pressure sores. *Orthop Rev* 2:25–27, 1973.

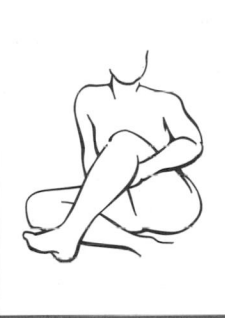

Treatment and Prevention: Goals and Objectives

Nancy Byl, Michelle Cameron, Luther C. Kloth, and Linda Rosenberg Zellerbach

I. Decisions: Goals and Objectives of Treatment

A. Goals

1. Six primary goals should be addressed when treating patients with problems of the integumentary system:
   a. Prevention of unnecessary trauma to the skin.
   b. Relief of underlying biomechanical causes of integumentary problems.
   c. Reduction of pain and edema.
   d. Facilitation of healing and repair.
   e. Maintenance and restoration of function.
   f. Maintenance of overall fitness and health.
2. Some goals address specific integumentary problems, and several goals pertain to several problems.
3. Individual goals must be outlined for each patient and supplemented with specific ob-

jectives that are objectively and functionally measurable.

B. Objectives

1. Goal: To prevent unnecessary trauma to the skin. The patient should be instructed to
   a. Avoid unnecessary skin pressures.
   b. Provide pressure relief at regular intervals.
   c. Maintain clean, well-lubricated skin.
   d. Examine the skin on a regular basis to identify lesions early.
   e. Minimize skin shearing and rubbing forces.
   f. Protect exposed skin areas from the sun (*eg*, use sun block).

625

g. Protect exposed skin from harmful substances (*eg*, wear gloves or protective clothing).

h. Ask for help in examining the skin in inaccessible places (*eg*, the back, the bottom of the foot).

2. Goal: To relieve underlying biomechanical causes of integumentary problems. The physical therapist should

a. Make sure the patient's clothing is loose and comfortable with no pressure spots.

b. Instruct the patient to incorporate activity or weight shifting into a schedule that will keep pressure off vulnerable areas.

c. Evaluate the patient's workplace and determine whether less dangerous materials can be used and/or better protective clothing is available.

d. Perform an environmental survey for potential allergic contributions to skin conditions (*eg*, grasses, animals, dust).

e. Educate the patient about careful drying to prevent constant moisture against the skin (as from sweating or post showering).

f. Teach the patient how to identify early pressure points.

g. Educate the patient about potentially worrisome lesions.

h. Evaluate the patient's skin condition before physical therapy, referring the patient to a dermatologist or other physician if potential cancerous lesions are noted and protecting self from skin conditions that may be infectious.

3. Goal: To reduce pain and edema.

a. Immediately after injury, unnecessary edema and bleeding should be prevented with compression, elevation, and ice.

b. Modalities used to reduce edema:
 (1). Intermittent pressure.
 (2). Electrical stimulation (microcurrent or less than muscle contraction).
 (3). Pulsating ultrasound.
 (4). Phonophoresis or iontophoresis.
 (5). Continuous passive range of motion.

c. Physical agents used to relieve pain:
 (1). Cryotherapy.
 (2). Superficial heat (heating pad, hot pack, whirlpool).
 (3). Transcutaneous neuromuscular stimulation.

 (4). Low-intensity, pulsating diathermy.

4. Goal: To facilitate healing and repair. The physical therapist should

a. Enhance the inflammatory process.
 (1). Débride necrotic tissue.
 (2). Enhance macrophages and leukocytes with cathodal stimulation (pulsed direct or try high voltage).

b. Minimize infection.
 (1). Topical and systemic antibiotics might be recommended.
 (2). Use ultraviolet treatment when appropriate (*eg*, for psoriasis).

c. Maintain good blood flow to the area.

d. Keep the involved and surrounding areas clean.

e. Maintain hydration (*eg*, have the patient drink lots of water).

f. Keep open areas moist, preferably covered to prevent drying and the formation of a scab.

g. Increase oxygen to the wound (*eg*, have the patient drink lots of water; possibly have patient breath oxygen-enriched air; heat the area; free up the soft tissue; and involve patient in general exercise).

h. Identify the stage of healing and apply the modality or procedure that could facilitate appropriate cellular activities (*eg*, increasing leukocytes, macrophages, fibroblasts, collagen deposition, collagen remodeling).

i. Encourage the patient to maintain a well-balanced diet that is potentially high in proteins and vitamins, especially vitamins B, C, and E.

j. Enhance the wound injury current with electrical stimulation (*eg*, cathodal treatment electrode for bone healing and positive electrode for soft-tissue repair, unless one wants to temporarily increase clean-up with negative electrode on the wound site for the first 3 days followed by anodal stimulation).

k. Do soft-tissue mobilization around the edge of an open wound to maintain tissue mobility and facilitate collagen deposition.

l. Prevent unnecessary wound pressure.

m. Avoid wound compression unless trying to control edema.

n. Keep the wound covered (be careful not to put adhesive tape on the skin).

o. Débride dead tissue.

p. Maintain active movement of the involved extremity, at least at the proximal joint.

q. Instruct the patient to stay generally active.

5. Goal: To maintain and restore function

a. If immobilization is needed, put the extremity in a position of function with the joint in an open position but ligaments taut (to avoid shortening) and consider dynamic rather than static splinting.

b. Keep mobile parts moving.

c. Begin active movement as soon as possible.

d. Progress activities consistent with the stage of healing and repair.

e. Use soft-tissue and joint mobilization techniques to release underlying adhesions and scars.

f. Use therapeutic modalities to relieve pain and inhibit muscle spasm to free up for functionally necessary motions.

g. Evaluate the need for assistive devices to support the area and enable independent function ambulation.

h. Protect the area from further trauma (eg, splint, change in performance criteria, more frequent rests).

i. Assess other medical problems that may be interfering with restoration of func-

tion and make an appropriate referral if necessary.

j. Assess psychosocial problems that could interfere with recovery and refer for treatment.

k. Assess and develop a mechanism for monitoring pain.

6. Goal: To maintain overall fitness and health. The patient should be instructed to

a. Follow a regular exercise program developed by the therapist.

(1). Exercise three times a week.

(2). Energy output should average 60% to 70% of maximum heart rate (for elderly and those with chronic disease) to 80% to 85% of maximum heart rate (for those who are healthy and <35 years of age, with this capacity approved by a physician when the patient is >35). Maximum heart rate is 220 beats per minute.

b. Eat well-balanced meals.

c. Be conscientious of maintaining good hydration.

d. Get reasonable rest (minimum of 6 hours a night).

e. Make time for relaxation.

f. Reduce stress.

II. Prevention

A. Prevention of ulcers in patients with desensitized skin[1-3]

1. Decubitus should be prevented.

a. If decubitus begins to develop, the goal is to make an early diagnosis and estimate severity.

b. Prevention as well as treatment must include pressure relief and avoidance of shearing and friction forces on the skin.

2. An ischial pressure relief program must be carefully and clearly outlined.

a. In some cases, mechanical devices may be helpful (eg, foam egg-crate mattresses, air-fluidized beds, mechanical beds such as the circle-electric bed and Stryker-frames).

b. Wheelchair cushions may decrease pressures (but none provide a panacea or allow unrelieved sitting).

c. Capillary pressure must be monitored, and relief achieved by pushups and weight shifting at least every 15 to 30 minutes.

3. In the acute phase, pressure relief and skin care must address the needs of patients confined to bed or wheelchairs.

a. Range of motion exercises are critical and should be started immediately.

b. A turning program must be initiated within 24 hours for all patients who are bedridden, specifically for those with a spinal cord injury (with turning at least every 2 hours).

(1). Skin should be examined every time the patient is turned.

(2). All sides of the patient should be used, and each turn should be 15 to 30 degrees.

(3). Turning intervals can be increased if patient tolerance improves.

(4). Pillows and soft rolls should be used to relieve pressure over bony prominences or reddened areas, especially under heels.

(5). Patients with increased tone may need to have extra supervision to maintain position.

(6). Local massage to pressure points may be helpful to maintain circulation, especially if the patient cannot be turned.

(7). Avoid pulling or sliding patients across the sheets or rough surfaces.

(8). Bedsheets need to be tight and free of wrinkles.

(9). Pillows may be needed to keep patients in neutral position and to reduce tone.

(10). Stimuli that increase tone should be avoided.

c. In chairs and in beds:

(1). The patient's weight should be kept evenly distributed.

(2). Shear and friction forces should be avoided.

(3). Wheelchair-bound patients should raise their buttocks every 15 minutes for 15 seconds (more often for paraplegic patients).

(4). If the patient needs assistance, he/she should be raised every hour for 1 minute.

(5). Pants and pocket stitching should not be tight over the ischia.

(6). Pushups on forearms should be performed in the chair in all possible positions (lifting on the chair arms, leaning backward, sideways, or forward, and reclining backward).

(7). The patient's body should be well aligned in the chair, and the foot rests properly positioned.

4. Hygiene is critical to prevention as well as healing.

a. Daily bathing can help to decrease the bacterial population of the skin.

b. Skin that is moist from perspiration, urine, vaginal secretions, or feces has decreased resistance; bacteria localize in moist, warm, and ischemic tissues.

c. Patients should be instructed in at-home self-care measures as follows:

(1). Take a daily bath or shower (including more than one a day) followed by careful inspection of the skin.

(2). Avoid soaps, alcohol, and powders.

(3). Use lotion that lubricates and preserves the skin.

(4). Perform perineal hygiene daily, including soap and water wipes if there is incontinence.

(5). Avoid tightly fitting external catheters.

(6). Wear cotton or natural-fiber clothing to absorb moisture and decrease perspiration.

(7). Avoid adhesive tape on skin.

(a). Use paper, plastic, or silk tape if necessary.

(b). Try to anchor bandaging on other bandaging rather than directly on the skin.

5. Good nutrition is essential for healing.

a. Weight must be regulated along with diet.

b. Good hydration is critical to circulation and perfusion of oxygen (*eg*, up to 300 mL of fluids in 24 hours is encouraged).

c. Diet should be high in protein, vitamins, and fiber, with sufficient calories to maintain weight and, when necessary, to replace protein that is lost as a result of an injury.

d. For those who cannot eat normally, food supplements may be advised.

e. Excessive fats and excessive calories should be avoided.

f. Diet drinks may help keep weight down but are dehydrating.

6. Psychological variables must be considered.

a. Patients who have sustained a significant injury or disease as well as the elderly may be hopeless and depressed.

b. Emotional issues complicate problems of decubitus.

c. Health care professionals need to work with the patient's family on these issues; in some cases, professional help from a psychologist or a social worker can be helpful.

7. Patients must be educated about the basic mechanisms of skin breakdown.

a. Patients and families should be taught how to

(1). Inspect the skin.

(2). Keep the skin clean.

(3). Relieve pressure with weight shifting.

(4). Maintain mobility.

(5). Maintain a normal diet.

(6). Recognize vulnerable areas.

    (a). Fatty tissue and thick muscle layers are at risk.

    (b). Bony areas are at greatest risk.

b. The physical therapist should give positive reinforcement and feedback to patients and families when they are successful in preventing decubitus.

c. All individuals who work with elderly patients, diabetic patients, and those with spinal cord injuries or other conditions that are associated with loss of sensation of the skin need to be knowledgeable about skin care (nurses, aides, physical therapists, family members, and the patients themselves).

B. General principles of preventive and management of skin complications for patients with diabetes mellitus

1. General management of diabetes

  a. Eliminate symptoms.

  b. Prevent long-term complications of diabetes.

    (1). Try to normalize blood glucose levels.

    (2). Prevent end-stage liver or kidney disease, adrenalin insufficiency, autonomic insufficiency, ethanol abuse, and psychiatric disturbances.

    (3). Establish good metabolic control.

      (a). Maintain consistency in the timing of eating and caloric content of meals, particularly reducing high cholesterol and other risks for vascular disease.

      (b). Balance food intake with insulin.

      (c). Incorporate high-fiber content into diet.

      (d). Pay attention to sugar and complex carbohydrates in diet.

      (e). Keep weight under control.

      (f). Tailor the insulin regimen for each patient (type of insulin—rapid, intermediate, or long acting—and timing of insulin).

      (g). Regulate oral medications when diet is insufficient to regulate blood sugar.

      (h). No smoking.

2. Establish a balanced physical therapy program to address general fitness and specific wound care.

  a. Outline a general program of fitness and a home program.

  b. Instruct the patient in skin care, particularly of the feet:

    (1). Keep feet clean and dry carefully.

    (2). Examine feet carefully.

    (3). Have others examine feet if you cannot get a good look.

  c. Recommend good shoes that incorporate good biomechanics and weight bearing.

  d. Evaluate the need for foot orthotics.

  e. Develop an early wound care program at the first signs of skin redness or a break in the epidermis.

    (1). Relieve the pressure off the area.

    (2). Soak in warm water/whirlpool to keep it clean.

    (3). Administer ultrasound to increase cell permeability and collagen deposition.

    (4). Give high-volt transcutaneous electrical nerve stimulator (TENS) treatment.

    (5). Try a low-volt microcurrent stimulation negative treatment electrode initially to clean wound; positive treatment electrode to increase collagen deposition with treatment 8 to 24 h/d.

    (6). Consider low-intensity or pulsating diathermy or electromagnetic fields.

C. Complications

1. Microvascular disease, which affects the small blood vessels and is manifested by eye and kidney disease.

2. Macrovascular disease, which involves the large blood vessels and is manifested by coronary, cerebral, and peripheral vascular disease.

3. Neuropathy, which can affect the motor, sensory, cranial, and autonomic nervous system.

4. Foot ulcers and other skin lesions, usually resulting from large-vessel atherosclerosis, microangiopathy, neuropathy, or a combination.

  a. Ulcers on the tips of the toes are usually secondary to large-vessel disease.

  b. Ulcers due to neuropathy occur in areas

of weight bearing and pressure (plantar surface).

5. Once an ulcer has developed, the patient should be instructed to
   a. Keep the area clean.
   b. Keep active but take the load off feet.
   c. Elevate feet above the level of the heart.
   d. Débride with whirlpool and disinfectant.
   e. If there is evidence of infection: anaerobic cultures should be obtained; antibiotics need to be effective against gram-positive, gram-negative, and anaerobic bacteria.
   f. Exercises should be done with feet elevated to assist circulation.
   g. Oxygen therapy may be provided either by breathing oxygen-enriched air or by hyperbaric treatments.
   h. Recent research points to the possible

link between nonhealing decubitus and lack of inportant growth factors.

6. Amputations: rehabilitation
   a. Most amputations today result from diabetes and not from trauma.
   b. Special care must be given to healing the residual limb and being sure that the prosthesis does not cause unusual pressure in any one area.
   c. Emphasis is on education of the patient regarding care of the residual limb and early weight bearing.
   d. Teaching regular skin inspection is important because the patient often has no feeling in the residual limb.
   e. Follow traditional rehabilitation protocols for care of prosthesis and ambulation training.

III. Use of Therapeutic Agents to Facilitate Wound Repair

A. Ultrasound for tissue healing

1. **History.** Ultrasound is acoustic energy of a frequency beyond the audible range, greater than 20 kHz. Frequencies between 0.7 and 3 MHz are usually used for therapeutic purposes. It is a condensation rarefaction wave requiring a viscoelastic medium for propagation. Methods to generate and detect ultrasound first became available in the 19th century and were first used on a large scale during World War II, when sonar (sound navigation and ranging) was used to detect submarines. Ultrasound was introduced into medical practice in the 1930s for deep heating, and more recently it has also been employed for its nonthermal therapeutic effects. For the past 50 years or more, ultrasound has been widely used as an effective physical therapy treatment. Robinson and Snyder-Mackler reported that 91% of physical therapists used ultrasound and that 94% had an ultrasound unit available to them.[4]

2. **Effects at the cellular level.** Ultrasound affects biological processes by heat, cavitation (stable or unstable), and/or acoustic streaming. The following cellular level effects have been experimentally demonstrated:
   a. Increased cell membrane permeability and cell diffusion.
   b. Increased intracellular calcium.
      (1). Mortimer and Dyson applied ultrasound at 0.25 to 1.5 W/cm^2, pulsed 1:5, 1 MHz, for 1 to 20 minutes to chick fibroblasts.[5] They found significantly increased intracellular calcium at 0.5 to 0.75 W/cm^2 for 5 minutes. Further increases were observed with increased time. This effect was reversed within 20 minutes after treatment. Cell damage and lysis were observed at 1.5 W/cm^2.
      (2). Dinno *et al.* applied ultrasound at 0.60 to 2.4 W/cm^2, continuous or pulsed 1:5, 1 MHz, for 12 minutes at 22°C or 12°C to abdominal frog skin.[6] They found decreased transepithelial potential and resistance (5% to 50%) and increased ionic conductance (20% to 250%). Pulsed ultrasound caused a significantly greater effect than continuous, and the effect was reversible. The changes were attributed to nonther-

mal mechanisms because they were much greater than the effects of temperature alone.

c. Mast cell degranulation.[7]
d. Histamine and chemotactic factor release.[7]
e. Increased rate of protein synthesis.[8]
f. Fibroblast stimulation, with increased collagen synthesis and strength.[8]
g. Changes in electrical activity of nerves.[9]
h. Increased enzyme activity.
i. Increased angiogenesis.[10]

  (1). Young and Dyson studied the effects of ultrasound at 0.5 W/cm², pulsed 1:5, 0.75 or 3 MHz, for 5 minutes on full-thickness surgical skin lesions in rats.[10] At 5 days post surgery, there was greater angiogenesis in the 0.75 MHz group than in the controls. By 7 days, there was no significant difference between the groups. This suggests that ultrasound affects angiogenesis during the early phase of healing. The authors propose that this is due to ultrasound stimulating macrophages to activate angiogenesis.

3. **Healing of specific tissues: research and mechanisms.** The thermal and nonthermal effects of ultrasound may all facilitate tissue healing. Animal and human studies on the effects of ultrasound on the healing of dermal ulcers, incisional wounds, tendon lesions, bone fractures, and nerve injuries have been carried out, attempting to delineate the optimal treatment parameters for these pathologies.

a. *Dermal ulcers*

  (1). Dyson and Suckling studied 25 patients with lower extremity varicose ulcers.[11] The ulcers were treated with ultrasound at 1 W/cm², pulsed 1:5, 3 MHz, for 5 to 10 minutes, three times a week for 4 or more weeks. Ultrasound was applied around the edges of the ulcers. At 28 days, the treated ulcers were significantly more reduced in area than the placebo-treated ulcers (see Figures 27–1 to 27–3).

  (2). McDiarmid *et al.* studied 40 patients with pressure sores.[12] They used ultrasound at 0.8 W/cm², pulsed 1:5, 3 MHz, for 5 minutes, three times a week. Overall, the treated sores healed more quickly, but this was not statistically significant. However, infected sores healed significantly more quickly with ultrasound treatment than with placebo treatment.

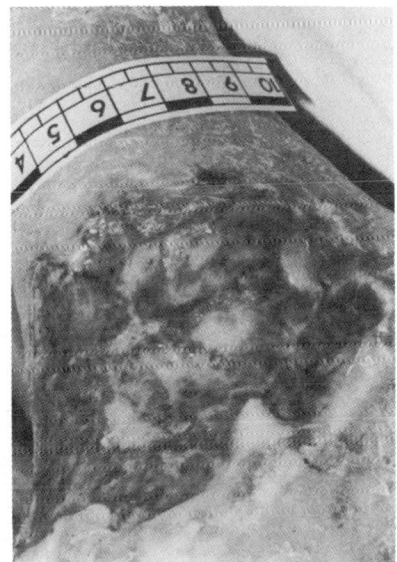

FIGURE 27–1 Ulcer before treatment with ultrasound. (From Kloth LC, *et al.* (eds): *Wound Healing: Alternatives in Management.* Philadelphia, FA Davis Company, 1990, p 269.)

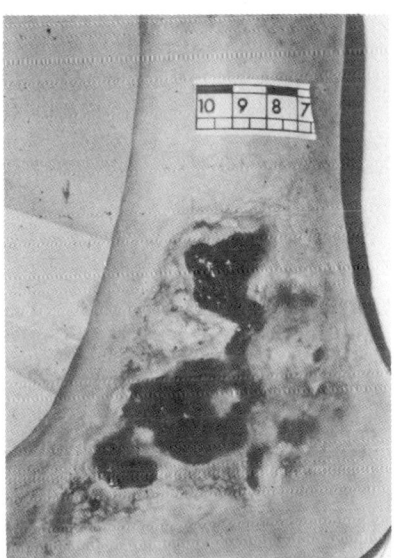

FIGURE 27–2 Ulcer after 17 treatments with ultrasound. The epithelium is extending over well-vascularized granulation tissue. (From Kloth LC, *et al.* (eds): *Wound Healing: Alternatives in Management.* Philadelphia, FA Davis Company, 1990, p 270.)

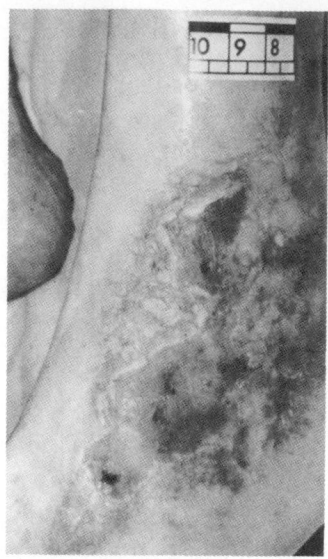

FIGURE 27–3 Ulcer after four more treatments with ultrasound. Epithelialization is virtually complete. (From Kloth LC, *et al.* (eds): *Wound Healing: Alternatives in Management.* Philadelphia, FA Davis Company, 1990, p 271.)

(3). Lundeberg *et al.* and Eriksson *et al.* both treated patients with venous ulcers with ultrasound.[13,14] Lundeberg *et al.* used 0.5 W/cm^2, pulsed 1:9, 1 MHz, for 10 minutes, on 22 patients with 22 controls, three times a week for 4 weeks, then once a week for the following 4 weeks. Eriksson *et al.* used 1 W/cm^2, 1 MHz, for 10 minutes, on 19 patients with 19 controls, twice a week for 8 weeks. Both reported no significant difference in the percentage of healed ulcers. Eriksson *et al.* also reported no significant difference in ulcer size.

■ PLEASE NOTE: It is proposed that ultrasound facilitates wound healing by the nonthermal effects of acoustic streaming and stable cavitation, resulting in wound contraction and protein synthesis. Studies using 3 MHz have been more successful in demonstrating improved healing; however, there are no studies directly comparing 1 MHz and 3 MHz for ulcer treatment. The study by McDiarmid *et al.*[12] indicates that ultrasound may be most beneficial for treatment of infected dermal ulcers.

b. *Wound healing*
   (1). Byl *et al.* have carried out a series of

studies on the effects of ultrasound on surgical wounds in pigs.[15,16] They have found that ultrasound increases wound healing strength, collagen deposition, and mast cell degranulation and decreases wound size. A low dose of 0.5 W/cm^2, pulsed 1:5, 1 MHz, or a high dose of 1.5 W/cm^2, continuous, was effective for the first week of treatment, whereas only the low dose was effective for 2 weeks or longer.

c. *Tendons*
   (1). Stevenson *et al.* cut and sutured the flexor profundus tendons of 77 hens and treated them with ultrasound at 0.75 W/cm^2, 3 MHz, for 5 minutes daily for 20 days, starting after 4 weeks of immobilization.[17] They found that the functional recovery, in terms of toe flexion range of motion, was significantly greater for the treated group than for the placebo group from 3 weeks of treatment on. This study demonstrates that ultrasound improves tendon healing and does not result in excess scar-tissue formation.
   (2). Enwemeka *et al.* have studied the effects of ultrasound on tendon healing.[18,19] They treated cut and sutured Achilles tendon lesions in rabbits with 1 MHz ultrasound at 1 W/cm^2 (1989) and 0.5 W/cm^2 (1990) for 5 minutes daily for 9 days, starting 1 day post surgery. The strength of the treated tendons was significantly greater than the untreated controls at day 10 in both studies, and the strength of those treated at 0.5 W/cm^2 was greater than those treated at 1 W/cm^2.

■ PLEASE NOTE: Ultrasound enhances tendon healing by increasing the strength of individual collagen fibers and the amount of collagen synthesized.

d. *Bone fractures*
   (1). Duarte treated osteotomized fibulas and femurs of 45 rabbits with ultrasound using two different transducers, one with 4.93 MHz frequency and the other with 1.65 MHz frequency, both at approximately 10

W/cm² pulsed 1:200 to produce a spatial average temporal average (SATA) intensity of 50 mW/cm².[20] This is equivalent to 0.25 W/cm² pulsed at 1:5. Duarte treated for 15 minutes daily, starting 1 day post surgery. Callus formation was greater in the treated bones, with most effect in the first 10 to 12 days. No temperature increase occurred in either the ultrasound- or placebo-treated bones.

(2). Pilla *et al.* studied 139 rabbits with bilateral fibular osteotomies (see Figure 27–4).[21] They treated with ultrasound at 1.5 MHz pulsed to produce a SATA intensity of 30 mW/cm². This is equivalent to 0.15 W/cm² pulsed at 1:5. Pilla *et al.* treated for 20 minutes daily, starting 1 day post surgery. Maximum strength increases of 40% to 85% were found in the treated group from postoperative day 14 to 23. The treated fractures were as strong as intact bone from postoperative day 17 to 28, whereas the control fractures did not reach this strength until day 28. Biomechanical healing was accelerated by a factor of 1.7.

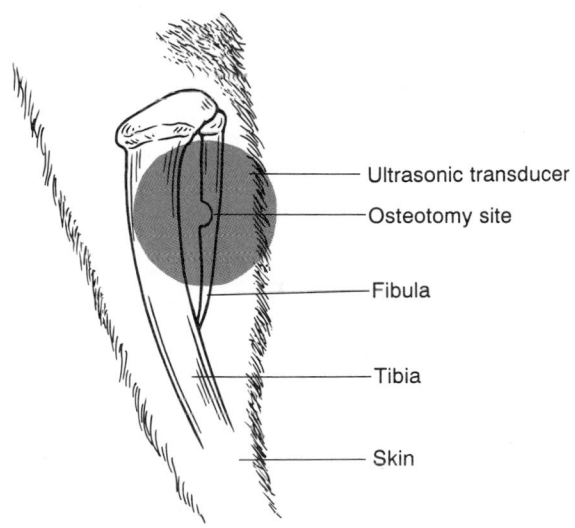

RABBIT HIND LEG

FIGURE 27–4 The lateral view of the tibia and osteotomized fibula. The osteotomy is made in a C shape to provide bone contact and to maintain a relatively stable healing curve. Note that the ultrasound transducer completely encompasses the osteotomy site. (Redrawn from Pilla AA, Mont MA, Nasser PR, et al.: Non-invasive low-intensity pulsed ultrasound accelerates bone healing in the rabbit. *J Orthop Trauma* 1990, 4:246–253.)

PLEASE NOTE: Proposed mechanisms for the effect of ultrasound on bone healing include cell membrane ionic permeability changes and the piezoelectric effect. The piezoelectric effect is the generation of electrical currents in response to physical deformation; it was discovered by Pierre Curie and first described in bone by Fukada and Yasuda.[22]

e. *Nerves*

(1). Farmer found that ultrasound at 0.5 W/cm² or 3 W/cm² increased nerve conduction velocity (NCV) of motor axons in humans, whereas at 1 to 2 W/cm² it decreased NCV.[23]

(2). Kramer and Halle *et al.* also studied the effect of ultrasound on nerves in humans.[24,25] They found that ultrasound increased NCV and decreased conduction latencies. Halle *et al.* determined that this change was due to a thermal effect.

(3). Hong *et al.* studied the effects of ultrasound on mechanically induced peripheral nerve compression injuries in rats.[26] They found that NCV and amplitude of the evoked compound muscle action potential (ACMAP) recovered significantly faster in those treated with 0.5 W/cm² than in controls. However, the ACMAP recovered more slowly with treatment at 1 W/cm² than in controls. Although the authors propose that these changes are caused by increased local blood flow, facilitation of hematoma clearance, and increased temperature, no explanation was proposed for the difference in effects at 0.5 and 1 W/cm².

(4). Hong treated patients with lower extremity polyneuropathy and control subjects with ultrasound for 2 minutes at 0.5, 1, and 1.5 W/cm².[9] He found a decreased ACMAP amplitude and increased proximal latency during treatment for patients treated at 1 and 1.5 W/cm² and no significant effects at 0.5 W/cm². The treatment effect was reversed within 5 minutes.

PLEASE NOTE: Research on the effects of ultrasound on nerve conduction has so far yielded contradictory results. Some studies report increased conduction velocity, and others report decreased conduction velocity. It appears that the effects of ultrasound on nerve conduction may be dependent on intensity and temperature. At this time, the research supports the use of low-dose ultrasound for facilitation of nerve healing after compression injury.

4. **Adverse effects**

   a. *Blood cell stasis and endothelial cell damage.* Blood cell stasis has been demonstrated in the vessels of chick embryos exposed to ultrasound of 1 to 5 MHz frequency.[27] This occurs with both continuous and pulsed ultrasound with intensity as low as 0.5 W/cm^2 with as short as 0.1-second exposure. This is thought to be due to standing wave formation as may occur when a stationary technique is used. The process is reversible but may cause damage to the endothelial cell lining of blood vessels. This effect can be avoided by moving the sound head at all times.

5. **Guidelines for clinical application: general**

   a. A medium should be used between the sound head and the treatment area that excludes air and transmits ultrasound.

      (1). For areas where the skin is intact, such as over a bone or tendon, a gel or lotion made specifically for ultrasound transmission should be used.

      (2). For areas where the skin is not intact, such as dermal ulcers, gel should be applied directly on the wound or, to avoid wetting the wound, applied to the wound perimeter, or hydroscan sheets should be used.

      (3). More contoured areas should be treated in water. The body part to be treated and the ultrasound transducer are placed in a plastic container filled with water. The transducer should be kept approximately 1 cm from the skin surface. The therapist's hand should not be placed in the water.

   b. Frequency is selected according to depth of penetration.

      (1). 1 MHz for 0.5 to 5 cm.

      (2). 3 MHz for 0.5 to 2 cm.

   c. Intensity is selected according to desired temperature or by research recommendations for nonthermal effects. The lowest intensity necessary to achieve the desired therapeutic effect should be used. Higher intensities are not necessarily more effective. Lower intensities are used close to bone or for tissues with a high protein content (*eg,* tendon, ligament). Higher intensities are used to reach deeper lesions.

   d. Duty cycle is selected according to desired thermal or nonthermal effect. The maximum thermal effect will be achieved with continuous ultrasound. A moderate thermal effect occurs with a 1:2 duty cycle. No thermal effect occurs with a 1:5 duty cycle. Nonthermal mechanical effects occur with all duty cycles.

   e. Treatment time is selected according to the size of the treatment area. Treatment time is 5 minutes for twice the effective radiating area (ERA; *eg,* with an ERA of 5 cm^2 and a treatment area of 20 cm^2, treatment is for 10 minutes).

6. **Guidelines for clinical application: tissue specific**

   a. *Dermal ulcers.* These are treated with 3 MHz, 0.8 to 1 W/cm^2, pulsed 1:5, 5 to 10 minutes, three times a week. This is more likely to be effective with infected ulcers.

   b. *Incisional wounds.* These are treated with 1 MHz, 0.5 W/cm^2, pulsed 1:5, or 1.5 W/cm^2, continuous, for 1 week; 0.5 W/cm^2, pulsed 1:5, for 2 weeks or longer.

   c. *Tendons.* Frequency is selected according to depth, 0.5 W/cm^2, continuous. Should be started as early as 1 day post injury if possible.

   d. *Bones.* Frequency is selected according to depth, 0.15 to 0.25 W/cm^2, pulsed 1:5, for 15 to 20 minutes, daily. Start 1 day post fracture. Greatest effect is likely in the first 2 weeks.

   e. *Nerves.* Treatment with 0.5 W/cm^2 may facilitate recovery from nerve compression injury.

7. **Contraindications/precautions**

   a. The sound head must be moved to avoid hot spots, unstable cavitation, blood cell stasis, or blood vessel damage.

   b. Ultrasound should not be applied over

      (1). Growing epiphyses.

      (2). Methyl methacrylate cement, as used for prosthetic joints. Although ultrasound does not penetrate through the bone to the cement of most total hip or knee replacements, its use is still not recommended with cemented prostheses.[28]

    (3). The abdomen or low back at any time during pregnancy.[29]

    (4). A limb or body part with a malignant tumor. Although ultrasound is used for tumor treatment, only a narrow temperature window, 42°C to 43°C, is effective. Other temperatures may enhance tumor growth or damage healthy tissue.

    (5). The chest of a patient with a pacemaker.

    (6). The eye.[30]

c. Although there are no research data documenting adverse consequences with these applications, it is also recommended that ultrasound not be applied over the following areas.[31,32]

    (1). Central nervous tissue, as may be exposed in the postlaminectomy spine or at the base of the skull.

    (2). Ovaries or testes.

    (3). Areas of thrombophlebitis or recently repaired blood vessels.

    (4). Areas of infected bone. This could spread infection.

    (5). Cervical ganglia, stellate ganglia, vagus nerve, or thorax near the heart in patients with coronary artery disease. This may cause arterial constriction.

d. Caution should be used when applying ultrasound over the following areas.[32]

    (1). Areas of decreased or absent sensation.

    (2). Directly over a nerve (eg, deep peroneal nerve at the lateral knee, ulnar nerve at the elbow).

e. Ultrasound may be safely employed over metal (eg, screws, plates, or uncemented prostheses).[33]

f. Because ultrasound is poorly transmitted through air, a person applying ultrasound is unlikely to receive accidental exposure. During underwater application, the therapist's hand should be kept out of the water to avoid exposure.

B. Electricity in wound healing

Therapeutic electricity has been used successfully to promote healing of chronic dermal ulcerations for decades.

1. The clinical use of this modality for wound healing is based on evidence that a bioelectrical system exists in skin and subcutaneous tissues and that exogenously applied doses of electricity enhance the healing rate of nonhealing or slow-healing skin lesions, especially pressure ulcers.

2. Clinical studies have reported using two types of therapeutic current:
   a. Direct current
   b. Pulsed current

3. Clinical research findings for direct current:
   a. Wolcott et al.[34] delivered 200 to 800 μA to 75 dermal ulcers for 6 hours a day for an average of 7.7 weeks. All wounds were initially treated with the cathode for 3 days or until infected wounds were aseptic. When subsequent anodal treatment resulted in a cessation of ulcer healing, treatment electrode polarity was reversed until healing recurred. This alternation of polarity was repeated during the study period each time a cessation of healing was observed. Wolcott et al. reported that 45% of the ulcers healed completely in an average of 9.6 weeks at a healing rate of 18.4% a week, whereas 55% of the ulcers healed incompletely to an average volume decrease of 64.7% in 7.2 weeks at a healing rate of 9.3% a week. Overall, they reported that during an average of 7.7 weeks, electrical stimulation produced an 81.8% decrease in wound volume at a healing rate of 13.4% a week for the 75 treated ulcers. In comparison, eight control ulcers healed at a rate of 5% a week.

   b. Gault and Gatens[35] replicated the Wolcott et al. study protocol on 100 ischemic ulcers. They reported that over a mean treatment period of 4.7 weeks, 100 ulcers treated with microamperage direct current healed at an average rate of 28.4% a week, compared with an average healing rate of 14.7% a week over a mean period of 4 weeks for 6 control ulcers. After a mean treatment time of 4.7 weeks, 48 of the 100 treated ulcers healed completely, whereas none of the 6 control ulcers had healed completely over a mean time of 4 weeks.

   c. In 1985, Carley and Wainapel[36] reported that 15 indolent skin ulcers treated with 300 to 700 μA of cathodal followed by anodal direct current, 5 days a week for 5 weeks, healed from 1.5 to 2.5 times faster than 15 control ulcers that received either wet-to-dry dressings or hydrotherapy. In addition, treated ulcers had stronger scar tissue, were less painful, and required less débridement than control wounds.

4. Clinical research findings for pulsed current:
   a. Other studies have applied pulsed current from high-voltage pulsed current devices that are capable of delivering average current to treatment electrodes in the same microamperage range as delivered from microamperage direct current devices. Kloth and Feedar[37] found the following:
      (1). Ulcers of nine patients in a treatment group healed at a rate of 45% a week and healed completely in 7.3 weeks.
      (2). Ulcers of seven patients in a sham-treated (control) group increased in size a mean of 29% during 7.4 weeks.
      (3). After ulcers of three patients in the control group were crossed over to the treatment group, their wounds, which had increased in area by 1.2%, healed at an average rate of 38% a week and were completely healed in an average of 8.3 weeks.
   b. Griffin et al.[38] used high-voltage pulsed current to treat pressure ulcers in spinal cord injury patients. A treatment group (N = 8) received 500 μA of average cathodal current to their ulcers for 60 minutes a day for 20 consecutive days. A placebo group (N = 9) received 60 minutes of sham stimulation to their ulcers for the same period of time. They found that ulcers in the treatment group had significantly greater percentage-of-change decreases in surface area at 5, 15, and 20 days after treatment compared with mean pretreatment ulcer size.
   c. Pulsed current delivered at milliamperage levels has also produced favorable results toward healing of chronic wounds. From a multicenter study on 50 ulcers having various etiologies, Feedar et al.[39] reported that 30 minutes of pulsed cathodal or anodal stimulation at an amplitude of 29.2 mA twice a day applied to 26 Stages III and IV chronic ulcers for 4

weeks resulted in a 56% decrease in size of treated wounds compared with a 33% decrease in size of 24 control wounds. Treated ulcers healed at a rate of 14% a week compared with 8.25% a week for control ulcers.
   d. Using the same stimulator device and protocol used in the Feedar et al. study, Gentzkow et al.[40] assigned 19 ulcers to sham-treatment groups and 21 ulcers to active stimulation groups. After 4 weeks, stimulated ulcers healed an average of 49.8% a week compared with sham-treated ulcers which healed an average of 23.4% a week. Healing rates per week were 12.5% and 5.8% for stimulated and sham groups, respectively. At the end of 4 weeks, 15 patients whose ulcers had healed an average of 13.4% while in the sham group were crossed over to the treatment group and, after 4 weeks of active stimulation, their wounds had healed an average of 47.9%.

5. Many other studies in which either direct current or pulsed current was used on induced wounds in animals or cell cultures at microamperage current levels have reported a number of findings that have significance to wound healing augmentation with electrical stimulation, including
   a. Increased re-epithelialization and collagen synthesis.[41]
   b. Greater tensile strength of scar tissue.[42]
   c. Enhanced wound closure.[43]
   d. Solubilization of clotted blood.[44,45]
   e. Increased skin protein synthesis and adenosine triphosphate concentration.[46,47]
   f. Migration of fibroblasts toward the cathode.[48]
   g. Increased protein and DNA synthesis.[49]
   h. Epidermal cell migration toward the cathode.[50]
   i. Bactericidal or bacteriostatic effects.[51,52]
   j. Migration of macrophages toward the anode.[53]
   k. Migration of neutrophils toward the anode and cathode.[54]

6. Based on clinical studies reported in the literature, the wounds most frequently treated with electrical current have been pressure ulcers. The following is a guideline for treating a pressure ulcer with pulsed current:
   a. Thoroughly evaluate the patient and ulcer.

(1). Exclude the use of electrical stimulation to treat a patient's wound if
  (a). Osteomyelitis is present in bone deep in the ulcer.
  (b). The patient is severely cardiac compromised.
  (c). Wound tissues contain neoplastic cells.
  (d). Ions from Mercurochrome or povidone-iodine are present in the wound tissue.
  (e). The patient has a demand-type cardiac pacemaker.
  (f). The patient's skin is very friable or is easily irritated by electrical current.
  (g). The wound volume is more than 25% necrotic tissue.

(2). Use precautionary measures when using electrical stimulation to treat a patient's wound if
  (a). The patient's skin is insensate or anesthetic as it may be in those with spinal cord injury.
  (b). The location of the wound would require placing electrodes tangential to the heart.

(3). When evaluating the wound before treatment
  (a). Record its dimensions by measuring its length, width, and depth in centimeters, or trace its area on plastic wrap superimposed over sterile, exposed radiographic film.
  (b). Describe the characteristics of any wound drainage in terms of color, viscosity, quantity, and odor.
  (c). Determine percentages of necrotic and viable tissue.
  (d). Repeat steps a to c at weekly intervals for comparison against pretreatment baseline values.
  (e). Decide whether to use electrical stimulation as a treatment for the ulcer by determining from patient records and prior treatments given whether the ulcer has been progressing toward healing, showing no change, or increasing in size. Electrical stimulation is most appropriate for the latter two

conditions. Also, base your decision on the exclusions previously presented.

7. If electrical stimulation is selected as the therapeutic intervention, the following may be used as a guideline for treatment:
  a. Select an electrical stimulation device that delivers either pulsed current in the microamperage or low milliamperage range or continuous direct current in the microamperage range.
    (1). A high-voltage pulsed current stimulator is an appropriate choice of a device that has been reported to accelerate healing of chronic dermal ulcers.[37,38]
    (2). The guidelines for treatment are as follows:
      (a). If the ulcer contains necrotic tissue, débride it first.
      (b). Position the patient comfortably for treatment.
      (c). Clean, beefy-red ulcers or ulcers with small amounts of necrotic tissue should be irrigated with sterile water or sterile 0.9% saline.
      (d). Using appropriate infection-control procedures, moisten 2×2 or 4×4 sterile gauze and fill the Stage III or IV ulcer crater with this gauze to promote electrical conductivity to the wound tissues.
      (e). Create a treatment electrode made of heavy-duty aluminum foil by folding the foil three to four times and cutting the folded foil so that its dimensions are 1 cm smaller than the gauze in the wound.
      (f). Place the foil electrode on the gauze and secure it in place so that the foil does not make contact with any tissues.
      (g). Connect an insulated lead wire with an alligator clip to the foil so that the metal in the alligator clip does not contact tissues.
      (h). Connect the opposite end of the lead wire from the treatment electrode to the cathode of the high-voltage stimulator device.

(i). Moisten the sponge of a commercial nontreatment electrode (that is two to five times larger than the foil treatment electrode) with tap water and secure it to the patient's intact skin, avoiding electrode applications that would allow current to pass through the left thoracic region and the heart.

(j). Connect the opposite end of the lead wire from the nontreatment electrode to the anode of the high-voltage stimulator device.

(k). Set the electrical stimulation parameters as follows:

  (i). Pulse frequency: 100 per second.

  (ii). Polarity of treatment electrode: negative.

  (iii). Stimulation amplitude: submotor; tingling paresthesia.

  (iv). Treatment time: 60 minutes a day, 5 days a week.

(l). Following each electrical stimulation treatment, check the ulcer for any undesirable changes, such as development of periulcer inflammation, foul odor, change in appearance and/or quantity of drainage, development of undermining or tunneling, and increase or no change in wound dimensions.

8. **Clinical decision making.** Certain clinical decisions related to electrotherapy treatment may have to be made when undesirable changes are observed in the ulcer or when concerns related to the patient's medical diagnosis arise.

  a. *Inflammation.* In the presence of inflammation, the cathode should be the treatment electrode because a few studies have reported that negative polarity causes neutrophils to move toward the cathode via a "galvanotaxic effect."[54–56]

  b. *Débridement of necrotic tissue.* If the ulcer contains necrotic tissue consisting of coalesced blood elements, the cathode may be used to solubilize clotted blood as shown by Sawyer.[45,57,58]

  c. *Wound edema.* In the presence of wound edema, studies have shown that the cathode repels albumen, the main colloidal protein in blood, and in so doing causes fluid shifts that may facilitate edema reduction.[50,59–61]

  d. *Infected ulcers.* There is a lack of agreement on which polarity to use for an antibacterial effect. Some *in vitro* and animal studies have reported bacteriostasis[51] or bacterial killing with the cathode.[52] In another study, positive polarity produced a bactericidal effect on intact human skin.[62]

C. **Transcutaneous drug delivery**

1. **Phonophoresis**[15,63–69]

  a. Phonophoresis is used to increase the diffusion of topically applied drugs mixed with ultrasound gel.[63,64]

  b. Analgesics, anti-inflammatories, and anesthetic drugs can be mixed with the ultrasound gel.[65]

    (1). Mixtures of these types of drugs in ultrasound gel can be purchased from a pharmacy or mixed by the physical therapist. In either case, the mixture must be free of air.

    (2). Dexamethasone is more appropriate to use than hydrocortisone because it transmits 99% of the sound waves.[66]

      (a). Steroids equivalent to 5% to 10% are commonly used.

      (b). Some therapists have used over-the-counter topical steroids, which are only 1%.

    (3). Over-the-counter analgesics also can be used (*eg*, BenGay, Flexall, but there is no evidence that ultrasound assists in the diffusion of these particular drugs.

  c. *Indications*

    (1). To reduce inflammation.

    (2). To decrease pain.

    (3). To decrease exercise-induced muscle soreness.

    (4). To decrease cdcma.

  d. *Precautions and contraindications*[67]

    (1). The physical therapist should

      (a). Be sure that a prescription has

been obtained from a physician for prescription drugs.

    (b). Check the patient for allergies to topical agents.

    (c). Check whether patients have had negative effects to any common analgesic, anti-inflammatory, or anesthetic drug because topically applied drugs are systemic.

    (d). Be careful using phonophoresis in patients with desensitized skin.

    (e). Be careful using phonophoresis around metallic objects (although there is currently no evidence that this is contraindicated) and around joint replacements where the intensity of the ultrasound is high enough to "thin" the glue.

    (f). Get approval from a physician for using ultrasound over artificial joints (there is concern about the ultrasound creating too much heat for the glue.)

    (g). Use lower-intensity ultrasound in patients with compromised vascular systems.

(2). The physical therapist should *not*

    (a). Apply medications to open wounds, in general.

    (b). Apply ultrasound directly over nerves, around the vitreous humor of the eyes, or over pacemakers, in general.

e. ***Duration of treatment.*** Five to 7 minutes.

f. ***Intensity of ultrasound***[67]

(1). The intensity most commonly used in physical therapy has been 1 to 1.5 W/cm^2, continuous, 1 MHz.

(2). No studies have been found that study the differences between continuous and pulsating or between high- and low-intensity ultrasound.

    (a). Pulsating ultrasound produces less heat.

    (b). Pulsating ultrasound may have increased mechanical effects.

g. ***Frequency of ultrasound***

(1). Ultrasound between 800,000 Hz and 3 MHz is approved for therapeutic use.

(2). No studies have been done comparing the use of 1 MHz and 3 MHz.

(3). Most studies have used 1 MHz for phonophoresis.

(4). Pharmaceutical research suggests that 10 MHz is more effective than 1 MHz, but high-frequency ultrasound is not approved by the US Food and Drug Administration, and this frequency is associated with partial destruction of the cells in the stratum corneum.[68,69]

h. ***Length of treatment***

(1). No studies have been found on the required frequency (number of times per week) and duration (number of weeks) that ultrasound should be used to maximize drug delivery.

(2). Most animal studies have focused on a single application of the ultrasound with the transcutaneous drug.

(3). Clinical studies have measured subjective responses following phonophoresis two to three times a week for several weeks.

(4). The provider must equate phonophoresis with other drug prescription practices.

(5). Studies with ultrasound alone have shown increases in healing by 30% after 1 week of therapy.[15]

    (a). If phonophoresis is equated with injection, only one treatment should be needed.

    (b). If ultrasound is suggested to be less effective than injection, several treatments with phonophoresis may be needed in a short period of time (*eg*, three times a week for a week) to be equivalent to an injection.

    (c). If phonophoresis is equated with a short dose of steroids, the treatment should be given daily for 1 to 2 weeks.

i. ***Preparation of the drug for use with ultrasound***

(1). Some therapists apply the drug to the skin and put ultrasound gel over the top and then administer the ultrasound.

(2). Some pharmacies will premix the drug in the ultrasound gel.

(3). It is important to minimize gas bubbles in the medium with or without a prescription drug.

2. **Iontophoresis**[70–84]

a. Iontophoresis is the introduction of topically applied active ions into the epidermis by the use of continuous direct current.[70,71]

(1). The force of the electrical current needed to move an ion through the body depends on the strength of the current and the impedance of the tissue.

  (a). The strength of the current can be enhanced by increasing the amplitude or increasing the density of the current.

  (b). Normal intact skin will not tolerate more than approximately 1 mA/cm^2.

(2). The electrodes have a predictable effect on the tissues.[70,71]

  (a). The anode produces an acidic reaction (creating hardening and mild heating).

  (b). The cathode produces an alkaline reaction in the underlying skin and has a softening effect (and produces mild heating).

    (i). The alkaline effect is very caustic and can cause burning.

    (ii). Usually, a large electrode is used for the cathode to minimize the risk of burning (twice the size of the anode).

    (iii). The difference in electrode size should be followed whether the cathode is the treatment or the control electrode.

  (c). Continuous unidirectional current has an anesthetic effect, and the patient may not be aware of burning.

    (i). A mild hyperemia is expected under both electrodes.

    (ii). The therapist should check under the electrodes every 3 to 5 minutes; sometimes it is help-ful to give a trial dose of the current before topical drugs are added.

b. Iontophoresis is usually used to decrease pain, decrease inflammation, or create an anesthetic area.[70,71]

(1). The therapist must determine the purpose of the treatment.

(2). The therapist must select the drug of choice:

  (a). Acetate (negative)—breaks up calcium deposits.

  (b). Chloride (negative)—softens scars and adhesions.

  (c). Copper (positive)—decreases fungus infections.

  (d). Dexamethasone (positive)—decreases inflammation.

  (e). Hyaluronidase (positive)—decreases edema.

  (f). Magnesium (positive)—muscle relaxant.

  (g). Salicylate (positive)—decreases edema.

  (h). Tap water (alternating polarity)—improves hyperhidrosis.

  (i). Xylocaine (positive)—decreases inflammation.

  (j). Zinc (positive)—improves healing.

(3). The therapist must discuss the treatment with a physician.

  (a). A prescription is needed from a physician for a prescription drug.

  (b). If there is an open lesion, this should also be discussed.

(4). *Contraindications*[70,71]

  (a). Iontophoresis should not be used on anesthetic skin or on newly scarred areas.

  (b). The therapist must make sure that the patient is not allergic to any topical agent or ions intended for use.

  (c). If metal electrodes are used, they must not be in contact with the skin.

  (d). The electrodes must be well soaked in water or the ionic solution, or special electrodes may be used that allow the therapist to inject the drug into a pouch on an electrode.

(5). *Precautions*

(a). The electrodes should not be removed without turning off the current first.

(b). The therapist must make sure that the electrodes make good contact with the skin and keep constant pressure.

(c). The therapist must carefully explain the procedure to the patient.

(d). The patient must be instructed to report any signs of pain or burning immediately.

(e). A reliable machine should be used so that the current density can be calculated under the electrodes.

(f). The current should always be started on the slow side, and the intensity slowly turned up.

(6). *Administration*[70,71]

(a). The skin should be carefully cleaned with alcohol.

(b). The skin should be evaluated carefully, especially for sensation.

(c). The drug needed and the polarity of the ions should be identified.

(d). The therapist should check to be sure that the patient is not allergic to the drug.

(e). The machine is selected to deliver the direct current.

(f). The patient is informed about procedures.

(g). The solution containing the ion is applied to the skin by massaging it into the tissue or by injecting the solution into a special electrode.

(i). A towel moistened with warm tap water or with saline solution is placed over the skin.

(ii). The therapist should be careful to avoid wrinkling the towel.

(iii). The toweling must be larger than the electrode.

(iv). The electrode is placed over the towel with good contact with the towel, but the electrode does not touch the patient.

(v). The ground electrode is placed approximately 18 inches away; this ground is larger and is placed over toweling that is moist but does not have the drug on it.

(vi). The electrodes are secured in place with a rubber strap.

(vii). The machine may be turned on and the intensity adjusted to 0.1 to 0.5 mA/cm^2 of the active electrode surface. The patient is again warned to call if the skin begins to feel as if it is being burned.

(viii). The current is administered for 10 to 15 minutes, but the patient should be checked every 3 minutes.

(ix). If alternating polarity is to be used, the current should be alternated approximately once per minute. The machine must be turned off to alternate the current.

(x). The current may have to be turned down as treatment progresses.

(xi). At the end of treatment, the machine is turned down slowly and then the electrodes are removed.

(xii). The skin should be carefully inspected.

(xiii). The therapist should pay attention to irritation and note any redness that is seen in the chart.

(xiv). The therapist should massage an astringent into the tissues to help minimize the burning.

(7). Iontophoresis with certain types of

drugs has been shown to be effective.

(a). Lidocaine can produce a local anesthesia for about 2 minutes.[72]

(b). Magistro found a reduction in tissue volume of 0.6 to 1.9 cm after 20 to 40 minutes of electrical stimulation with 250 mL of 0.1 M acetate buffer solution with a pH of 5.4.[73]

(c). Schwartz measured significant reduction of edema with hyaluronidase.[74]

(d). Glass *et al.* found that dexamethasone sodium phosphate could be iontophoresed into the tendon.[75]

(e). Harris reported high reduction in pain relief following delivery of 1-mL solution containing 4 mg of dexamethasone sodium phosphate along with 2 mL or 4 mL of 4% lidocaine with an increasing current from 1 mA/cm² to 4 mA/cm² for 30 minutes.[76]

(f). Patients younger than 45 years of age respond more favorably than older people to iontophoresis with anti-inflammatory drugs.[77,78]

(g). Kahn,[79] Levit,[80] and others[81,83] reported success in treating hyperhidrosis (range of treatment, 15 to 29 mA for 10 to 15 minutes two to three times a week).

(h). Falcone and Spadaro[84] demonstrated bacterial-free areas on tissues treated with silver-coated fabric.

1. Hydrotherapy is frequently used in rehabilitation for purposes of heating tissues by conduction and convection.[85–88]
   a. The water is hotter than the skin, and heat moves to the skin.
   b. The body moves in the heated water, and, as the body moves, heat is also achieved by convection.
   c. Increases in temperature are associated with other benefits, such as increase in metabolism, local perspiration, local vasodilation, initial vasoconstriction of deeper tissues, muscle relaxation, sedation of nerve endings, general increase in respiratory and pulse rates and decreased blood pressure, and increased capillary pressure and cell permeability.

2. Agitated water provides mechanical effects such as buoyancy (making movement easier) and massage.[85–88]
   a. Agitation of the water is usually created by a turbine.
   b. Water and air are mixed to create increased turbulence with increased aeration.
   c. The turbine is usually mounted on a column and has spring-type action to allow height adjustment (be careful to keep face away from the top of the turbine in case the spring releases the turbine too quickly).
      (4). There is usually more agitation near the surface than deeper.
      (5). The turbine should be angled toward the involved area.

3. **Indications**
   a. Hydrotherapy is most often used to relieve pain, decrease muscle spasm, and relieve stiffness.[89,90]
   b. Hydrotherapy with appropriate medications in the water can be used for cleansing, sterilizing, débriding, and promoting wound healing (*eg*, for ulcers and burns).[91–94]
   c. Hydrotherapy can promote mobility by use of buoyancy.
   d. Hydrotherapy can also be used to increase hydrostatic pressure, which can increase circulation.[95–98]
   e. Frequently, hydrotherapy is recommended for patients with rheumatoid arthritis,[99–101] joint injuries or replacements,[102] paraplegia, or poliomyelitis and polyneuritis.[103]
   f. Hydrotherapy can be used to increase exercise tolerance and strength by increased speed of movement, increased depth of water, or with the use of paddles which increase density and resistance.[102,104]

4. *Contraindications*[105–107]
   a. Fever that already exists.
   b. Infectious conditions that may spread.
   c. Heat intolerance because of cardiac instability, hypertension, or respiratory instability.
   d. Malignancies that may be subject to metastasis with high heat.
   e. Active bleeding conditions increased by heat.
   f. Mental confusion and disorientation.
   g. Areas of skin with loss of sensation.

5. *Precautions*[105–107]
   a. The therapist must be sure that the skin can tolerate the increased temperature and turbulence (both the area involved and the surrounding tissue).
   b. Patients should not be incontinent, but can be catheterized.
   c. Caution must be used with patients who could be negatively affected by heat (*eg,* upper respiratory infection, uncontrolled blood pressure, febrile conditions, severe mental disorders, uncontrolled epilepsy, cardiac or pulmonary conditions with a vital capacity less than 1500 mL, and multiple sclerosis with heat sensitivity).
   d. Caution should be used with patients who fear water.
   e. Debilitated patients must be watched carefully.
   f. When the body temperature equals the environmental temperature, heat is lost from evaporation.
      (1). If a large proportion of the patient is immersed, the remaining skin surface may not be sufficient to lose heat adequately, and faintness or fever may develop.
      (2). The patient should be provided cold compresses to the head and cool drinks of water.

6. **Temperature ranges used for heat and cold**[105,106]
   a. Temperature ranges for warmth include:
      (1). Warm: 96°F to 98°F or 35.5°C to 36.5°C.
      (2). Hot: 98°F to 104°F or 36.5°C to 40°C.
      (3). Very hot: 104°C to 115°F or 40°C to 60°C.

   b. Temperature ranges for cold include:
      (1). Very cold: 35°F to 55°F or 1°C to 13°C.
      (2). Cold: 55°F to 65°F or 13°C to 18°C.
      (3). Cool: 65°F to 80°F or 18°C to 27°C.
      (4). Tepid: 80°F to 92°F or 17°C to 33.5°C.

7. **Types of hydrotherapy units**[108]
   a. Hydrotherapy can be provided in an extremity tank (upper extremity, lower extremity) or in a Hubbard tank (which is large enough for the whole body, and also allows an individual to begin walking).
   b. A regular pool can also be considered a form of hydrotherapy.
   c. Hot tubs are often used for the benefits of hydrotherapy, particularly at home.
      (1). Hot tubs should be used for closed lesions only.
      (2). Hot tubs should not be used if the patient has consumed alcohol.
   d. Hydrotherapy units can be movable or fixed (or an agitator motor can be purchased for the bathtub at home).
   e. Contrast bath temperatures are also considered hydrotherapy.[109]
      (1). A whirlpool at 38°C to 44°C and another container with water at 10°C to 18°C can be used.
      (2). The extremity is placed into the warm water for 10 minutes and then into the cold water for 1 minute and then back into the warm water for 4 minutes.
      (3). This cycle is repeated for 30 minutes, with the last immersion in the warm water.
      (4). The general hot:cold ratio is 3:1 or 4:1.
      (5). Contraindications include small-vessel disease because of diabetes, arteriosclerotic endarteritis, or Buerger's disease.
      (6). Caution should be exercised with patients with peripheral vascular disease with water hotter than 40°C.
      (7). It is used for patients with arthritis or peripheral joints, joint sprains, muscular tenderness strains and some peripheral vascular diseases.

8. **Treatment procedures**[105,106]
   a. Keep the area for hydrotherapy warm.

b. Fill the tank with water.
c. Select the proper temperature based on the medical condition and treatment objectives (see previous discussion for heat and cold and contrast bath temperatures).
   (1). Temperatures of 36.5°C to 40.5°C are acceptable for heat except in the case of peripheral vascular disease, sensory loss, or full body immersion, where it may be necessary to use 1°C above skin temperature to a maximum body temperature.
   (2). In the presence of cardiovascular or pulmonary disease, the temperature should not exceed 38°C (mild warmth).
   (3). Patients with painful conditions may receive hot to very hot baths.
   (4). Patients in the whirlpool for exercise should receive tepid baths.
   (5). Generally, do not exceed 110°F.
d. Inspect the part to be treated for temperature, edema, open lesions, color, muscle spasm, sensation, and other systemic problems.
e. Make sure that agitation is gentle for painful lesions (eg, ischemic ulcers or burns).
f. Adjust agitation toward the body area that needs to be treated or needs to avoid the agitation.
g. Use a disinfectant when treating open wounds (eg, povidone-iodine or sodium hypochlorite).
h. Place the patient in a comfortable position.
i. Treat for 10 to 30 minutes.
   (1). Twenty minutes is usually indicated to get the maximum benefit of the heat (increasing temperature).
   (2). For débridement, the duration is 5 to 20 minutes, depending on the patient's medical status.
   (3). Have the patient supine or sitting for 5 to 10 minutes before standing.
j. Do not leave the patient unattended.
   (1). If the patient is unstable, secure him/her with a strap.
   (2). Give the patient a bell if attending several patients simultaneously.
   (3). Elderly or confused patients should not be treated unless carefully watched.

k. Inspect the wound area when removed from the water.
l. Redress wounds and keep them covered to prevent drying.
m. Treat patients with acute conditions twice a day; once a day or several times a week may be adequate for patients with chronic conditions.

9. **Care of whirlpool: safety precautions**[110–120]
a. The tank should be properly grounded.
b. The tank and turbines should be cleaned after each use.
   (1). The inside is scrubbed with commercial disinfectant that will not cause corrosion, rinsed thoroughly with clean water, and dryed.
   (2). Disinfect with chlorine at 200 ppm to get rid of common forms of bacteria.
   (3). Glutaraldehydes, formatin alcohol, ethylene oxide, and β-propriolactone are used for spore-forming bacteria.
   (4). Chloramine-T (100 to 200 ppm) is effective in reducing gram-negative organisms and *Pseudomonas* and can be used to disinfect after wound treatment.
c. Culture samples are obtained from the tank in accordance with guidelines determined by the hospital infection-control department.
d. For protection from human immunodeficiency virus (HIV), the physical therapist should[119,120]
   (1). Check with the Centers for Disease Control and Prevention for changes in standards.
   (2). Always wear gloves.
   (3). Avoid contact with blood, bloody fluid, body fluids containing visible blood, tissues, cerebrospinal fluid, synovial fluid, pleural fluid, peritoneal fluid, pericardial fluid, and amniotic fluid.
   (4). Wear masks, gown, and goggles when treating large wounds, especially in a patient who has infections in addition to HIV.
   (5). Wear gloves and protection when cleaning the tank.
   (6). Use sodium hypochlorite at 500 to 5000 ppm to inactivate the HIV rap-

idly, and sterilize as described above for other infections.

E. Use of intermittent compression for vascular insufficiency

1. **Definition.** Pneumatic units (compression pumps) are designed to reduce edema by giving controlled, usually alternating external pressure.
   a. Intermittent compression reduces edema by moving excess interstitial fluid to sites of normal lymphatic or venous drainage.
   b. Pressure needs to be higher distally and lower proximally.
   c. Pressure may decrease pain and improve range of motion (secondarily by decreasing swelling).

2. **Indications**
   a. Traumatic edema.[121–126]
   b. Venous insufficiency.[127,128]
   c. Lymphedema post mastectomy.[129–132]
   d. Amputations.[131]

3. **Contraindications**[132,133]
   a. Presence of thrombi that could become mobile.
   b. Edema related to cardiac dysfunction or from renal/kidney dysfunction.
   c. Infections (where there is risk of moving the bacteria into the lymphatic or venous drainage system).
   d. Arterial insufficiency and increased peripheral resistance.
   e. Obstructed lymphatic drainage.
   f. Cancer where it may be possible to promote metastasis.
   g. Patients who are obtunded and cannot tell when the pressure is excessive or painful.

4. **Procedures**[133]
   a. Instruct the patient in the procedures.
   b. Evaluate and inspect the skin carefully and take circumference measurements. Repeat after treatment.[134]
   c. Place the patient in a comfortable position.
   d. Place a stocking/stockinette over the area with all wrinkles smooth.
   e. Apply the appliance and attach the rubber tubing to the source of air.
   f. Increase the pressure but do not exceed the diastolic blood pressure.
   g. Apply the pressure for 45 to 90 seconds and release for 15 to 30 seconds (3:1 ratio).
   h. Have the patient keep the extremity moving.
   i. Treat for a minimum of 2 hours out of every 24 hours (even better done twice a day).
   j. Remove appliance and check skin hourly.
   k. Recheck the skin and blood pressure when done.
   l. Wrap the extremity with an Ace bandage to keep the pressure and integrate elevation and exercise.

5. **Frequency**
   a. The pump should be used twice daily if possible.
   b. It usually takes 3 to 4 weeks to achieve the desired effect.
   c. The patient should consider renting a unit for home use.

F. Use of ultraviolet treatment in the management of skin problems

1. Ultraviolet treatment has been used in physical therapy primarily to treat disorders of the skin. Usually, the goal is to cause an erythema response. Today, ultraviolet treatment is rarely used in physical therapy clinics; instead, it is administered by dermatologists or their assistants.

2. Ultraviolet lamps manufactured in the United States have a broad spectrum.
   a. An ultraviolet (UV) lamp is housed in a cabinet with a single bulb or multiple bulbs that have different spectrums:[135,136]
      (1). UVB (250 to 320 nm)
      (2). UVA (320 to 400 nm)
      (3). UVB narrow band (311 to 312 nm)
   b. Newer equipment usually includes multiple lamps.

3. The purpose of ultraviolet treatment is to cause an erythema response.[135]
   a. The response should be seen in 2 to 4 hours.
   b. The peak response is usually about 12 hours post treatment.
   c. The earliest the response is seen is 1 hour post exposure.

4. The dosimetry of ultraviolet treatment:
   a. Dosimetry is based on two laws: the inverse square law and the cosine law.[137]
      (1). The inverse square law states that the intensity of illumination varies with the square of the distance from the source.
      (2). The cosine law states that the energy of illumination varies proportionally to the cosine of the degrees of deviation from the perpendicular (thus, the dose increases as the area being irradiated becomes more oblique).
   b. The goal is to create a desired erythema dose: suberythema dose, minimal erythema dose (MED), or first-, second-, or third-degree erythema dose.[138]
      (1). These doses not only relate to time of exposure and distance, but also to age, skin color, and other factors, such as sensitivity to the sun.
      (2). Each person must be tested for sensitivity and to set the MED.[139]
         (a). Testing is usually done on the forearm.
         (b). Four window squares (1 or 2 cm^2) are cut in a piece of cardboard.
         (c). These windows are used to determine the MED.
         (d). The area around the windows is draped so that no skin is exposed.
         (e). The lamp is set up so that it is 60 to 80 cm away and the light is penetrating in a perpendicular direction (or the machine's specific instructions for distance should be followed).
         (f). The first window is exposed for 120 seconds.
         (g). The second window is opened and exposed for 60 seconds (while the first window continues to be exposed).
         (h). The third window is opened and exposed along with the other two for 30 seconds.
         (i). Finally, the fourth window is opened and exposed for 30 seconds along with the others.
         (j). The patient must then wait 8 hours to determine which exposure shows mild reddening of the skin, which should disappear in 24 hours, and this most commonly is the treatment dose.
            (i). A first-degree erythema appears after 6 hours and may last several days.
            (ii). A second-degree erythema occurs after 2 hours or less and is like a severe sunburn, with the skin hot, tender, and maybe even swollen.
            (iii). The patient should check the area in bright light every 2 hours when awake and record which marks have appeared and faded (a form should be provided for this purpose, and the patient can return the form at the next visit).
         (k). Over time, the skin builds up a tolerance for the exposure; thus, to maintain the MED, either the time of exposure must be increased or the distance from the bulb must be decreased.
            (i). This increase may need to be 35% each day.
            (ii). For first-degree burns, exposure would have to be increased 50% each day.
            (iii). Maximum exposure is 5 minutes.
            (iv). If more than 5 minutes is needed, the distance must be decreased.
   c. *Other treatment procedures*
      (1). Have the room comfortably warm and private.
      (2). Have the patient properly draped and positioned for
         (a). Local exposure.
         (b). Total body exposure (four-quadrant method).
      (3). Have good circulation in the room (to get rid of the ozone).
      (4). Warm up the machine for about 5 minutes before use.

(5). Wash the area prior to exposure (area should be free of dirt, oil, makeup, or exudate).

d. *Indications*[139-148]

(1). *Psoriasis*

(a). First-degree erythema level should be used.

(b). Treatment is once or twice a day (until the plaques disappear).

(c). The exposure may vary by the other type of treatment being administered and skin sensitivity.

(2). *Acne*

(a). Second-degree erythema level is usually used.

(b). The goal is to dry out skin and promote peeling.

(c). Usually other medications are given.

e. *Precautions*[150,151]

(1). A patient's sensitivity to sunburn should be carefully evaluated.

(2). Ultraviolet treatment should not be administered around the eyes without lenses over the eyes of the patient to prevent burning.

(3). The therapist should carefully evaluate whether this is the proper modality when patients have had known problems with skin cancer.

(4). Areas of the skin not usually exposed to the sun should be treated with one third to one half the dose of the rest of the body.

(5). The therapist should wear polarized goggles to protect against the ultraviolet light.

(6). The skin should always be carefully examined before and after treatment.

(7). The therapist should be sure that the patient is not on medications that cause photosensitivity (*eg*, sulfonamides, tetracyclines, and quinolones [for bacterial infections], psoralens [for psoriasis], gold salts [for rheumatoid arthritis], amiodarone hydrochloride and quinidines [for cardiac arrhythmias], and phenothiazines [for anxiety]).

(8). Patients with syphilis should not be treated with ultraviolet light.

(9). Patients who are substance abusers are not appropriate candidates for ultraviolet treatment.

(10). The patient should not be heated before treatment.[151]

(11). Caution should be used when patients have eaten strawberries, eggs, or shellfish.

(12). Women on estrogen may also have an increased sensitivity to ultraviolet light.

f. *Frequency and duration of treatment*[150]

(1). Each application of ultraviolet radiation must be given after the effects of the previous dose have disappeared.

(2). The exposure is increased by 25% with each treatment.

(3). If a treatment is missed, the next exposure should be decreased by 25% of the previous dose.

(4). Duration of treatment is determined by the patient's response to treatment and the effect of other therapy and is negotiated with the physician.

1. This is performed during admission procedures or as soon as feasible, within 24 hours of admission.

a. Active range of motion, passive range of motion, strength, sensation, coordination, mental status, functional skills, including activities of daily living, transfer, and gait, if appropriate, are evaluated.

b. Resistive tests are appropriate only to unburned areas, as local pressure to a burned area can cause further damage because of microtrauma.

c. Patients with inhalation injuries benefit

from cardiopulmonary physical therapy considerations when appropriate.

2. **Education**
   a. Essential for successful outcome.
   b. Long-term recovery depends most on the patient's understanding and compliance with the program, especially after discharge from inpatient care.
   c. Patients and family members should become "experts" in burn care.
   d. Education begins during the first meeting of therapist and patient and/or family or other significant visitors.
   e. Family and/or friends are usually anxious to be helpful. (Individuals who would like to be physically involved can assist with positioning.)
   f. The family is often fearful of touching the patient at all. Because the touch of a loved one is extremely therapeutic, teaching the family how to touch the patient can be included in this process.

B. **Positioning (see Color Plates 1 to 4)**

1. **General principle**
   a. Maintaining length in the area with a burn wound as it heals, with or without skin grafting procedures.
   b. Splints or other positioning devices may need to be fabricated to assist with positioning.

2. **Positioning in emergent phase**
   a. Elevation is a critical element in positioning, especially during this period of fluid resuscitation.
   b. May be for prolonged periods because of priority of medical monitoring and procedures.

3. **Positioning in the acute phase**
   a. The activity tolerance of the patient determines whether the positioning is constant or intermittent.
   b. As the patient becomes medically more stable, positioning becomes more important when the patient is at rest, especially overnight.
   c. Splint-wearing schedule is re-evaluated daily.
      (1). Depends on the patient's functional abilities, depth of injury, and mental status.
      (2). For example, if the patient is able to ambulate to the bathroom, ankle

splinting is not likely to be necessary.
      (3). If the patient is on bed rest, an ankle-foot orthosis may be needed to keep length in the gastrocnemius.
   d. Pressure areas are prevented.
      (1). With elderly patients, monitoring for decubitus is standard.
      (2). Even a relatively young patient is at risk for decubitus if the burn is severe and narcotics are used for pain control.
      (3). Pressure on a burned area can result in a burn of greater depth.
      (4). Special beds are available to assist with positioning, including beds using air pressure, silicone beads, and other materials.
   e. The position of comfort is the position of contracture.
   f. Elevation of burned extremities is required from the onset of the burn until pressure bandages or garments have been fitted to the patient.
   g. Examples of commonly used positions and accompanying assistive devices:
      (1). *Head*
         (a). Mouth
            (i). To maintain horizontal opening, a microstomia prevention device, or "mouth-spreader," may be used.
            (ii). To monitor vertical opening, a simple device of tongue depressors stacked and counted cannot only stretch the mouth opening but also can serve as an objective measure.
         (b). Ears
            (i). Ears can be fragile when burned, with second-degree burns converting to third-degree burns (partial thickness to full thickness).
            (ii). Because of its cartilaginous base, the ear is at risk for desiccation.
            (iii). Ear protectors may be made in the form of

foam "donuts" or thermoplastic mesh cages for longer-term patients on ventilators.

(c). Elevation of the head is achieved using head-of-bed control in conjunction with regular pillows if there is a posterior neck burn or no neck involvement.

(d). If the anterior neck is involved, a very small, firm "pillow" may be used, but neck extension should be maintained.

(2). *Neck, anterior surface*

(a). The tendency is for neck flexion contracture, with scar bands.

(b). To prevent this, initial positioning requires *no pillow*.

(c). Support under shoulders in supine position may be required to keep neck in slight extension or at least neutral extension.

(d). A soft collar made of 1 inch of foam covered with stockinette may be used very early to assist with positioning.

  (i). Plastic wrap helps to keep exudate from invading the foam cells.

  (ii). Both the stockinette and the dressing can be changed at the same time.

(e). A hard collar (made of a low-temperature thermoplastic material) is often used after more healing has occurred.

  (i). It can assist with providing pressure to this area when sufficient healing has occurred, as well as keep the neck in extension.

  (ii). Disadvantages to using a hard collar include difficulty eating, inability to drive secondary to limited rotation, and sweating.

(3). *Neck, posterior surface*

(a). Burns here are less common but should be kept in an elongated position.

(b). Use of pillow is allowed.

(4). *Neck, circumferential*

(a). Principles for prevention of neck flexion contracture take priority.

(b). The patient may be on a ventilator, which may require additional precautions.

(5). *Axilla*

(a). If the axilla itself or the anterior or posterior axillary fold is involved in the burn, diligent reinforcement of the positioning program is essential to prevent adduction and flexion contractures.

(b). Shoulder abduction should be kept at 90 degrees, as tolerated.

(c). Sensation must be carefully monitored, as this position may cause stress to the brachial plexus.

(d). Abduction (or airplane) splints may be fabricated to assist with this positioning, especially when immobilization is needed after skin grafting.

(6). *Elbow, antecubital surface*

(a). Elbow extension is the preferred position.

(b). Hyperextension should be avoided.

(7). *Elbow, posterior surface*

(a). Slight flexion of the elbow is desired, as elbow flexion is needed for functional activities.

(b). Splints are rarely necessary for these burns.

(8). *Wrist*

(a). Neutral to 30 degrees of extension is appropriate.

(b). The wrist should be in neutral deviation.

(9). *Hands, dorsal*

(a). Most burns occur on the dorsum of the hand because of the natural tendency to cover the face with the palms for protection.

(b). The burned hand will naturally assume a position of wrist flexion and radial deviation, thumb adduction, metacarpolphalangeal (MP) joint hyperextension, and interphalangeal (IP) joint flexion.

(c). To prevent contractures in these positions, splints are fabricated in a functional position.

  (i). The wrist should be positioned as noted above.

  (ii). The thumb should be in functional abduction.

  (iii). MP joints should be in 45 to 70 degrees of flexion.

  (iv). IP joints should be in extension.

(d). If dorsal burns have already caused extensive damage over the proximal interphalangeal (PIP) joints and reconstruction is not feasible, the IP joints may be positioned in partial flexion so that fusion may occur in a position for function. (If fusion is desired, a surgical pinning may be appropriate.)

(10). *Hands, palmar*

(a). Because the skin on the palm is thicker than on the dorsum, palmar burns tend to be less deep.

(b). If burns are on the palm only, a more open position is appropriate, with the wrist in neutral.

(11). *Hands, circumferential*

(a). The desired position closely resembles that for the dorsal burn, with more thumb extension and flexion of the MP joints less extreme.

(b). Dressings must be applied to digits individually for individual functional use as well as to prevent distal migration of web spaces.

(12). *Hips*

(a). Because of the need to elevate burned lower extremities, a bedridden patient may be at risk for hip flexion contractures.

(b). They are usually avoided as activity level permits increased exercise and/or gait.

(c). Prone positioning may be indicated when medical status permits. (This may be contraindi-

cated if a nasogastric tube is present because of aspiration precautions.)

(13). *Knees*

(a). The knees are usually kept extended, as the tendency of bedridden patients is for knee flexion contracture.

(b). If the popliteal area is spared, slight flexion is preferred over hyperextension.

(14). *Ankles*

(a). Neutral dorsiflexion may be difficult to maintain using pillows or footboards.

(b). Ankles are at risk for skin and joint contractures as well as nerve damage from prolonged positioning.

(c). Ankle-foot orthoses may be indicated for a patient without ankle or foot burns who is on prolonged bed rest or has difficulty achieving neutral dorsiflexion for any other reason.

(15). *Feet*

(a). The dorsum of the foot is more commonly injured than the plantar surface.

  (i). The skin on the dorsum is thinner.

  (ii). The mechanism of injury frequently involves a spill onto this area.

(16). *Toes*

(a). Because the dorsum of the toes is more likely to be injured than the plantar surface, the tendency for contracture is for toe dorsiflexion.

(b). When sufficient healing has occurred, the pressure program should work to counteract this tendency.

(c). Dressings must be applied to individual toes to counteract the tendency for web spaces to migrate distally.

h. Splinting has been mentioned earlier as an aid to positioning.

(1). An important principle when using splints to assist with protective positioning is to make efforts to splint appropriately.

(2). Oversplinting can contribute to increased stiffness of joints and increased feelings of dependence due to inability to perform activities of daily living.

(3). Increased use of splints may be necessary if the patient is unable to achieve a range of motion goal in an appropriate length of time during treatment.

(4). Night splinting is especially helpful to maintain motion gained during function and exercise during the daily routine.

C. Complications of improper positioning

1. **Peroneal nerve stretch**

   a. The "frog leg" position, with hips abducted and externally rotated, knees flexed, ankles inverted and plantar flexed, can result in dorsiflexor weakness.

   b. Although this may be a well-known position to avoid with lower extremity burns, it may be the position the burn team has chosen for a patient with burns in the groin area.

   c. If chosen as a primary position for healing, appropriate alternatives should be used during the day to avoid peroneal nerve stretch.

   d. The peroneal nerve can also be injured by dressings too tightly applied at the fibular head.

2. **Brachial plexus compromise**

   a. If a position of greater than 90 degrees of shoulder abduction is used over a prolonged period, the patient may report pain or paresthesias in the distal upper extremities because the brachial plexus is stretched.

   b. Pressure should also be avoided in this area.

3. **Cubital tunnel syndrome**

   a. This may be caused by pressure from dressings or bed positioning on the ulnar nerve at the elbow.

   b. Prolonged positions of ulnar nerve stretch are also to be avoided.

4. **Tendon rupture**

   a. Any exposed tendon may be at risk for damage by prolonged stretch.

   b. Tendons should be kept in a "slack" position until there is adequate wound closure over the tendon.

c. Protective positioning for this problem usually requires splinting.

d. In the hand, boutonnière deformity may occur if the central slip of an extensor tendon ruptures. The extensor may move from the dorsal surface to the lateral surface, assisting flexion of the digit instead of extension.

D. Exercise

1. Active range of motion exercises begin as early as tolerated by the patient, within 24 hours of admission if possible.

2. If the patient is unable to participate, passive range of motion exercises should be done unless contraindicated by damaged tendons, fractures, or other complications.

3. Exercise is often done during the daily hydrotherapy treatment.

   a. During this time, the patient may have the maximum allowable dosage of pain medications.

   b. It may be easier to achieve the range of motion goals without the friction of sometimes bulky dressings.

   c. Buoyancy in water may allow the patient greater success in active exercises.

   d. Wound inspection allows hand placements that avoid the more painful areas of an open wound.

4. **General principles for exercise**

   a. Potential problem areas are noted in the initial evaluation, during which a comprehensive plan for positioning, splinting, and exercise is established.

   b. Whenever possible, it is most helpful to have the patient personally involved in all aspects of his/her care.

   c. It is always easier to prevent problems rather than to repair them.

      (1). Patients often do not understand that timing is crucial.

      (2). If exercise is deferred until all wounds are healed, the patient may develop functional deficits that reconstructive surgery cannot correct.

   d. Frequent short exercise sessions are better than one long session.

   e. Active motion is always more desirable than passive motion.

   f. Maintaining length of the skin during healing is of primary concern. Adequate length of the skin at the end-range of joint range of motion is the goal.

g. Skin loses its elastic properties when it has been burned.

h. Skin shrinks as it heals.

i. Granulation tissue contracts and hypertrophies.

j. Joints contract across flexor creases.

k. Each patient's pain threshold varies and must be considered.

   (1). Pain medicine may be coordinated with exercise sessions.

   (2). Relaxation and imagery may help with tolerance.

   (3). Giving the patient some control over the process often helps with compliance and success; *eg*, the patient may choose when the session occurs or the sequence of exercises.

l. Hand contact with burned surfaces should be minimized.

m. Observing the skin during exercise is helpful to determine the type and amount of exercise needed.

   (1). Blanching of the skin is a good indication that stress is being applied to the area.

   (2). Sustained stretch is frequently used.

n. Passive exercise may be indicated if the patient is unable to assist with exercises because of

   (1). Medical instability.

   (2). Heavy sedation.

   (3). Perceived pain of great intensity.

   (4). Neuropathies or spinal cord or head injuries.

   (5). Fractures or other neuromuscular or musculoskeletal disorders.

5. **Appropriate exercise during different phases of burn care**

  a. *Day of admission*

    (1). Evaluation; gentle active, assisted, and passive exercises.

    (2). Passive exercise is not done when burn depth is unclear and deeper structures may be compromised, such as the extensor tendons in the hand.

    (3). Rapport building and introduction to the role of the therapist.

    (4). Education begins as the rationale for exercise is explained to the patient and the family.

  b. *Emergent phase*

    (1). Few repetitions needed, positioning monitored.

    (2). Medical status requires close monitoring and takes priority over exercise program.

  c. *Acute phase*

    (1). Wound is débrided, wound care is vigorous.

    (2). During this phase, exercise becomes more a focus for the patient because the wound contracts during healing.

    (3). Functional exercise is stressed, as the patient's self-esteem benefits greatly from increased independence in activities of daily living.

     (a). Patient should be encouraged to feed self as soon as possible to reinforce the importance of nutrition in the healing process.

     (b). Equipment may be adapted to increase function by increased circumference or length of eating utensils or other items such as a toothbrush.

     (c). Referral to an occupational therapist may be indicated and treatment coordinated between the physical therapist and the occupational therapist.

      (i). Role delineation between physical therapists and occupational therapists differs in each facility.

      (ii). Good communication is essential for the best treatment planning and implementation.

    (4). Before skin grafting, maximimal range of motion is the goal in preparation for immobilization of the grafted area.

    (5). During surgery, a physical therapist may perform passive range of motion while the patient is under anesthesia to evaluate joint mobility in a pain-free environment (see Color Plates 5 and 6).

     (a). The end-range can be safely achieved using guidelines

from joint mobilization techniques.

(b). Close observation of the skin for maximal stretch without tearing tissue is essential.

(c). Once joint mobility and skin length have been assessed, the goals of treatment can be more clearly defined post surgery.

(6). After skin grafting, exercise is usually deferred for 3 to 7 days to wait for good adherence of the skin graft to the vascular bed.

(a). Active range of motion exercises begin without dressings so the effects of exercise on the new graft can be observed.

(b). When there is adequate adherence of the autografts to the granulation tissue, passive and resistive exercises may be added to the program to increase range of motion and strength.

(c). Fluid may accumulate under sheet grafts, which can undermine adherence. A cotton swab may be used to "roll" this fluid to the edge of the graft, where it can be removed.

6. **Postoperative splinting**
   a. Splints are used during this phase for immobilization and to promote healing.
   b. Splints that maintain a position of maximal skin length and joint function may be fabricated by the physical therapist before the skin grafting procedures.
   c. Because the patient will be wearing these devices for a prolonged period, a good fit is essential.
   d. Splints may also be fabricated in the operating room by physical therapists or surgeons.

7. **Guidelines for hand exercises** (see Color Plates 7 and 8)
   a. *First-degree (superficial) and mild second-degree (partial-thickness) burns*
      (1). Active functional use is encouraged.
      (2). Active range of motion is moni-

tored, but formal exercise or splinting program is usually not indicated.

(3). Mild second-degree burns may require splinting during the emergent phase if the patient is unable to maintain good position.

b. *Second-degree (partial thickness) burns*
   (1). Hands are splinted in the functional position already described, except during supervised exercise or activities of daily living sessions.
   (2). For deeper partial-thickness burns, precautions in the exercise program should be observed. Range of motion exercises include
      (a). Wrist motions, with focus on extension.
      (b). Stretching of whole hand, including palmar stretch and abduction of all digits.
      (c). Thumb MP joint motions, including abduction, extension, circumduction, with focus on stretching the first web space.
      (d). MP joint flexion: passive assist may be required to achieve full range.
      (e). IP joint exercises include active and passive extension.
      (f). Full fist making should be avoided during this stage.
         (i). Because the depth of burn is not always clearly defined during the earliest stages of burn care, extensor tendons of the digits should be protected.
         (ii). To achieve flexion, MP and IP joint flexion exercises should be done independently. (MP joint flexion with PIP joints extended. PIP and distal interphalangeal [DIP] joint active flexion with MP joints stabilized in neutral.)
         (iii). *No* passive PIP joint flexion.
   (3). Splints may be removed during the day when sufficient healing warrants. Criteria for making this decision include

(a). Healed skin coverage over PIP joints.

(b). Demonstration by patient that positioning can be maintained and that precautions are understood.

(4). Activities of daily living must be done in a way that prevents excessive stretch of the extensors.

c. *Third-degree (full-thickness) burns*

(1). Extensor tendon precautions are followed, with the patient resting in splints continuously except during supervised exercise sessions.

(2). Skin grafting is scheduled as early as feasible for the patients, and exercise is resumed 3 to 7 days after surgery, depending on the graft "take."

(3). Once there is healed skin coverage over the PIP joint primarily and MP joint secondarily, fist making can be resumed as an exercise.

(a). The exercise program becomes more aggressive, with increased frequency and independence.

(b). More hand exercise equipment can be introduced to encourage coordination, strength, desensitization, and independence in activities of daily living.

8. **Exercise after cultured epithelial autograft**

a. These grafts are more fragile than split-thickness skin grafts and require a longer period of immobilization after application in surgery.

b. After 7 to 10 days, exercise may begin with no dressings in order to visualize the grafts.

9. **Exercise during rehabilitation phase** (see Fig. 27–5)

a. When most areas are healed, it is appropriate to use any exercise technique that is effective for the patient, as long as stated precautions are observed.

b. Exercises may include active, passive, assistive, or resistive exercises in functional or diagonal patterns, open or closed chain, aquatic, and isokinetic, etc.

c. Continuous passive motion machines are being used for inpatients as well as outpatients who need the additional support of these devices.

d. Function remains a priority, and the patient may need individual treatment for stretching of healed burns as well as joint mobilization.

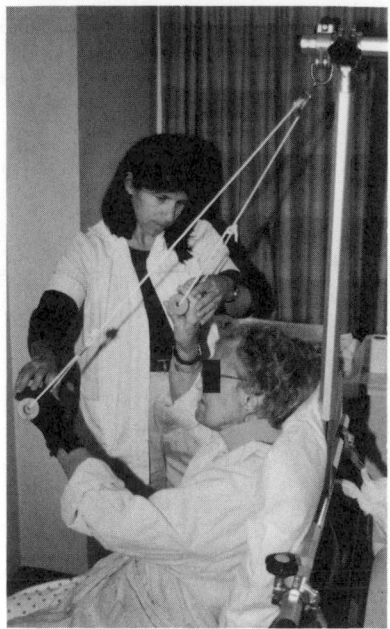

FIGURE 27–5 Equipment may be installed in a patient's room to encourage frequent and independent exercise sessions.

e. Isolated movements must be combined to achieve full functional mobility. For example, wrist and elbow extensions are more difficult when they are done simultaneously, but they are frequently combined in functional activities.

10. **Conditioning program**

a. Conditioning exercise is usually a necessary part of the rehabilitation phase because of the prolonged hospitalization required for wound healing.

b. The program may include use of a stationary bicycle, treadmill, stair-climbing machine, free weights, or any equipment found in a physical therapy gym or available at a fitness center.

11. **Serial splinting or casting to assist with range of motion** (see Color Plate 9)

a. Splints may also be used in conjunction with exercise programs to increase the range of motion of a joint.

b. A splint can be fabricated to fit while the joint is in the position of maximum stretch.

c. If kept in an elongated position, the tissue should adapt and lengthen. The splint can then be remolded to accommodate any changes.

d. Plaster casts are often used for this purpose, especially with children.

12. **Dynamic splinting**
   a. This may be appropriate during this phase as an adjunct to intensive exercise.
   b. Tension may be adjusted using elastic, springs, or wires to assist motion or to provide resistance for strengthening.

E. Ambulation

1. **General considerations**
   a. To help prevent problems associated with prolonged bed rest patients are encouraged to ambulate as soon as tolerated.
   b. Early ambulation helps to
      (1). Prevent thrombophlebitis and pneumonia.
      (2). Prevent lower extremity contractures.
      (3). Maintain skeletal mass.
      (4). Maintain strength and endurance.
      (5). Prevent decline of mental status by increasing orientation and reducing anxiety.
   c. **Contraindications**
      (1). Burns on the soles of the feet if on weight-bearing surfaces (see Color Plate 10).
      (2). Cellulitis.
      (3). Burn wounds too severe.
      (4). Fractures.
      (5). Tendon damage.
      (6). Thrombophlebitis.
      (7). Low hemoglobin.
      (8). Unstable medical status.
   d. If a patient has lower extremity burns, dressings need to be applied and then elastic support must be provided to
      (1). Prevent edema.
      (2). Support the capillary bed in new granulation tissue.
      (3). Prevent conversion of a burn to a deeper degree.
         For example, if a patient were to ambulate with deep dermal (partial thickness) burns on the lower extremities with no vascular support, the wound could convert from a partial- to a full-thickness wound, which would require skin grafting for healing to occur instead of healing spontaneously with good wound care.
   e. Ace bandages should be used if
      (1). Donor sites do not exhibit sufficient healing, especially on the lower legs.

(2). Lower extremities are edematous.
(3). The patient was on prolonged bed rest, even if there are no burns on the lower extremities. This will help counteract hypotensive response.
(4). The patient is elderly.
(5). There is known vascular insufficiency.
   f. Guidelines for Ace bandage wrapping for ambulation:
      (1). The figure-of-8 wrap is most effective for promoting vascular return.
      (2). Wrapping should always be done distal to proximal, from base of toes to groin.
      (3). The heel should be included in the wrap to prevent ballooning of edema.
      (4). The toes should be included in the wrap if they are burned.
      (5). When standing a patient for the first time, a second layer may be appropriate.
      (6). A second layer is recommended for the first time ambulating after lower extremity skin grafting.
   g. Assistive devices are used only if absolutely necessary.
      (1). This encourages the patient to bear full weight on the lower extremities.
      (2). Postural adjustments of the trunk are facilitated as well.
      (3). If independent ambulation was the patient's prior level of function, the progression is usually fairly rapid from the initial gait pattern of gross flexion and antalgia to ambulation with a more natural gait, using standard gait-training techniques.
   h. A tilt table may be useful if burn wounds are severe or if there are medical problems such as postural hypotension.
   i. Foam pads may be necessary to cushion the plantar surface of the foot if this area was burned.
   j. Ambulation after skin grafting:
      (1). The number of days that the patient is kept from ambulating depends on the area of the burn and the condition of the graft.
      (2). Ambulation may begin as early as 1 day post surgery with Unna's boot (a zinc oxide–calamine-gelatin bandage) applied for support.
      (3). If there is grafting of the lower leg, such as the ankle or foot,

the surgeon may choose to wait up to 10 days before initiating gait training.

F. Discharge rounds

1. The burn team should meet regularly with a focus on discharge plans. This weekly meeting should begin during the first week of admission.
2. Included is the disposition planned, the support system available to the patient, the insurance coverage, and current patient care plans of all of the participating disciplines.
3. Plans are made for the coming treatment period, including any recommended referrals.

G. Scar management (see Color Plate 11)

1. **General considerations**
   a. Patient education is critical for the best outcome for scar control.
   b. Because the scarring process accelerates in the 1 or 2 months after discharge, the patient and family must be well versed in the care of the burn scar before discharge.
   c. If a burn wound heals without a skin graft within 2 weeks, scarring is unlikely, and pressure therapy for this area is not necessary.
   d. If the wound heals within 3 weeks, close monitoring is indicated if the patient
      (1). Is a child.
      (2). Has a positive scar history.
      (3). Is dark skinned or highly pigmented.
      (4). Has lower extremities requiring vascular support.
      (5). Has lower extremity donor sites.
   e. If the patient has skin grafting or still has not achieved wound closure within this 3-week period, there is a likelihood of scar formation.
   f. Most burn wounds have a satisfactory, flat appearance on the patient's discharge from the hospital; however, it is somewhat deceiving to the patient who has not been prepared for the process of scar maturation.
      (1). The healing burn wound is characterized by a marked increase in vascularity.
      (2). A scar that remains hyperemic after 2 months and becomes firmer is likely to become hypertrophic.
         (a). There is also a marked increase in fibroblasts, myofibroblasts, collagen, and interstitial material.
         (b). The contractile properties of the myofibroblasts can distort features and cause joint contractures.
         (c). If unopposed, the burn wound will continue to shrink.
         (d). The collagen fibers fuse together and become piled up in whorls and nodules in a random configuration.
         (e). Scar contractures usually consist of a firm mass of collagen covered by a thin layer of epithelium.
      (3). The early hypertrophic scar is readily influenced by mechanical forces (see Figures 27–6 to 27–8 and Color Plate 12).
         (a). Because the bonds in the collagen linkages are not as stable in early scars, they respond well to pressure devices.
         (b). The best results are seen with the earliest intervention.
      (4). Scar hypertrophy is characterized by a red or inflamed appearance, raised above the level of the normal skin, with a stiff, firm texture.
      (5). Surgical correction is usually not done during the phase of active scar-

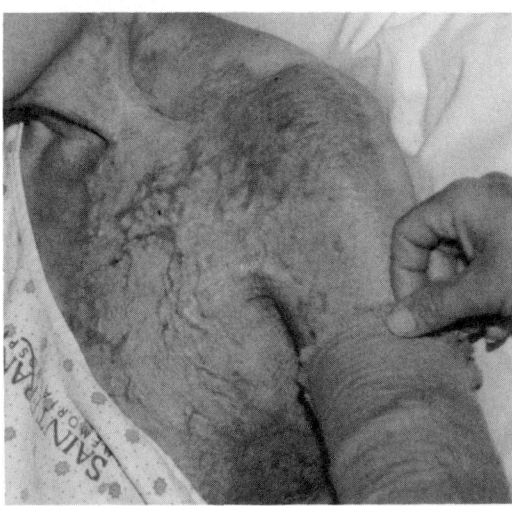

FIGURE 27–6 Early hypertrophic scarring on the neck and axilla in the presence of a pressure sleeve.

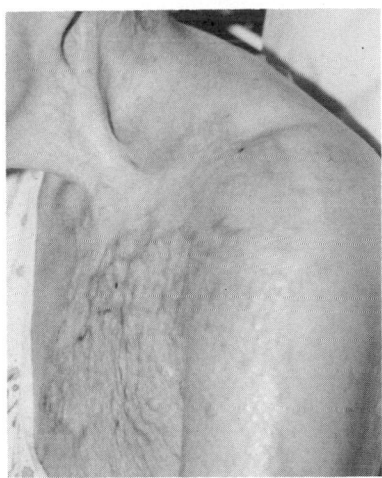

FIGURE 27–7 Early hypertrophic scarring on the neck and axilla in the absence of a pressure sleeve.

ring because the additional trauma can cause more scarring.

2. **Pressure therapy**
   a. Pressure therapy can begin as soon as open wounds are no larger than approximately 5 cm in diameter.
   b. Elastic bandages of all sizes can be used as the first pressure devices.
   c. The first methods of applying pressure should be relatively easy to apply and remove, as the skin is quite sensitive and may require light dressings.
   (1). Self-adhering elastic bandages are particularly useful for fingers and hands, toes and feet.
      (a). For example, a 7-month-old infant with a scald burn that healed within 4 weeks without surgery showed the beginning signs of hypertrophic scarring.
      (b). Because of the rate of an infant's growth, it would be very difficult and expensive to try to keep the patient in custom-made garments that provided sufficient pressure.
      (c). A 1-inch-wide self-adhering elastic bandage was wrapped into a glove that was changed daily by the parents.
      (d). The parents were able to demonstrate good technique with pressure wrap and home exercise program.
      (e). An excellent result was achieved.
   (2). Tubular elastic pressure devices can provide good interim pressure for extremities.
   (3). Elastic gloves and stockings are available.
   (4). Bicycle shorts or girdles offer good vascular support of donor sites on the proximal thigh and buttock.
   (5). Interim garments for all parts of the body are available in a variety of standard sizes for use until adequate healing has occurred or edema has subsided.
   (6). Caution should also be used if the open wound is on a joint surface, as friction from the garment over the wound should be minimized.
   d. *Custom garments* (see Figure 27–9)
   (1). Many companies now offer custom-made pressure garments.
   (2). Garments are available in colors from some vendors, which may help improve the self-image of the wearer.
   (3). The ideal pressure for scar control is about 25 mm Hg, which is close to capillary level.
   (4). Measurement for the garments is done according to the instructions of the individual vendor.

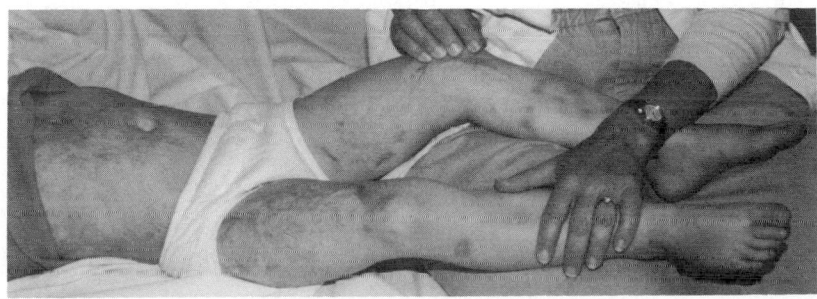

FIGURE 27–8 Burn scars 1 year after discharge. Inflammation is barely visible; burn scars are almost mature.

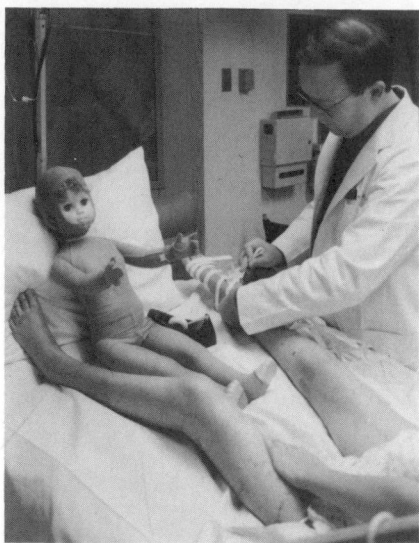

FIGURE 27–9 Measurements for custom garments are taken. (The doll dressed in garments is used for education.)

(a). Circumferential measurements are taken about every 1.5 inch on the extremities.

(b). Various vertical, horizontal, and circumferential measurements are taken of the head, neck, and torso.

(5). Fitting is done by an experienced individual because the fit must be tight enough, but not too tight.

(6). Instructions for wear, care, and replacement are issued to the patient and family.

(a). Garments should be worn at all times except when the patient is bathing.

(b). Usually two of each garment are ordered so that one can be washed while the other is worn.

(c). Because of constant use and frequent laundering, the garments need to be replaced every 2 or 3 months.

e. *Adjuncts to elastic garments*

(1). Low-temperature thermoplastic splints may be made to conform closely to the healed burned area to provide additional pressure.

(2). Body areas with concavities, such as the face, neck, axilla, chest, and hands, often require additional inserts for adequate pressure.

(a). A variety of materials are avail-able for fabrication of inserts for wear with splints or pressure garments.

(b). Materials include flexible Silastic elastomer, many types of foam, neoprene, silicone gel sheets, and sheepskin.

(c). Shoes should have closed toes and be made of firm materials. High-tops may apply additional pressure to ankles.

(3). Transparent face masks are preferable to opaque garments (see Color Plate 13)

(a). Compliance with opaque garments can be extremely difficult.

(b). Although the transparent face mask is still noticeable, it is accepted by the patient better because it is more acceptable to others.

(c). Soft face masks do not conform sufficiently to the features of the face. The obvious need for functional holes causes decreased pressure, especially in the center of the face.

(d). Opaque masks conceal the personality and identity of the individual and, in fact, can present a frightening substitute, causing the patient to resemble a masked criminal.

(4). Fabrication of transparent face masks:

(a). They are custom-made of molded high-temperature plastic, such as Uvex.

(b). Because this material cannot be molded directly onto a patient's face, a plaster mold of the patient's face must be fabricated.

(c). The heated plastic can then be pulled over the plaster mold.

(d). Proper fit is essential for good results, and regular follow-up is necessary.

H. Discharge conference

1. The transition from inpatient to outpatient can be very difficult after a prolonged hospitalization.

2. Patients may require continued rehabilita-

tion in an inpatient acute rehabilitation unit or a skilled nursing facility.

3. Once the final skin graft is stable, the patient is usually ready for discharge within a few days.

4. The team approach continues, with the patient and family or significant others present.

5. A written home program for skin care and exercise is standard.

6. A videotape of the procedures may be the best method of providing clear discharge instructions, including

    a. Bathing

        (1). The patient should have a tub bath or shower daily, using antibacterial bar soap.

        (2). The patient should then air dry for about 15 to 30 minutes to facilitate healing of any small open areas.

    b. Skin care

        (1). Lubrication

            (a). This is needed because of damage to sebaceous glands in full-thickness injury.

            (b). Application of lotion may be required to skin-grafted areas for years.

        (2). Massage

            (a). Friction should be avoided over the surface of the burn scar, as the superficial layer can be fragile.

            (b). With firm contact on the surface, underlying soft tissue can be manipulated to help restore elasticity.

            (c). A "scar massager," a small commercially available device, can help with this technique.

        (3). Treatment of open areas

            (a). The patient and caregivers review verbally and manually the procedure for dressing applications.

            (b). Review of characteristics of wound healing assists with choice of dressing materials.

        (4). Exercise program

            (a). Priorities in specific exercises for problem areas are stressed.

            (b). General guidelines for conditioning are included.

        (5). Use of adaptive equipment may be included.

        (6). Pressure garments and splints: wear-

ing schedules, how to care for them, and plans for replacement are included in the discharge plan.

I. Outpatient rehabilitation

1. Home physical therapy visits may be the first intervention, with focus on safety and functional ambulation on stairs in order to progress from "homebound" to outpatient status.

2. Outpatient physical therapy may include

    a. Range of motion exercises and strengthening:

        (1). Treatment may be very time-consuming and must be prioritized.

        (2). Therapy time should focus on the management of the patient's problem areas, those that cannot be managed by the patient and family in a home program.

        (3). Home programs are essential for maintaining the gains made in therapy sessions.

    b. Splinting may be used as an adjunct to the pressure program as well as to maintain or increase range of motion and strength.

    c. Modalities:

        (1). Paraffin may be applied to the scar tissue while in a lengthened position to help soften and release the scar as well as to decrease joint stiffness.

        (2). The temperature may need to be lower than usual because healed burn tissue can be hypersensitive.

    d. Edema control.

    e. Prosthetic training.

    f. Gait training.

    g. Treatment of associated injuries, such as fractures, sprains, back injuries, and joint problems.

    h. Conditioning:

        (1). Patients frequently continue their conditioning programs on their own, with more distant supervision as their progress permits.

        (2). Movement classes (aerobics, yoga, step, stretch, tai chi, karate, jazz, ballroom dancing, Feldenkrais) can be an excellent way for individuals to stay excited and involved in their exercise programs.

        (3). The social aspects of classes are beneficial as well.

3. Return to work:

    a. Specific training should be provided when

patients plan to return to their prior occupation or to a new one.

b. Work tolerance screening and job analysis may be included, as well as vocational evaluation and workplace modification.

c. Functional status before burn injury helps establish goals.

d. Specific work hardening programs may be helpful.

4. Common complaints encountered in outpatient physical therapy:

a. Itching

(1). Frequent lubrication is helpful.

(2). Lotions that include anesthetic medications may be used.

(3). Medication such as diphenhydramine (Benadryl) is often prescribed.

(4). Itching may be exacerbated at night, possibly due to decreased external stimulation or distractions.

(5). Scratching can cause new open areas in recently healed burns and is to be avoided.

b. Pain and stiffness of skin and joints, with accompanying fear of movement.

c. Hypersensitivity to heat and cold.

d. Decreased or altered sensation, including burning, tingling, numbness.

e. Folliculitis due to ingrown hairs, particularly in the beard areas on men with facial burns.

f. Local areas of infection under healed grafts.

g. Swelling.

h. Depression.

J. Outpatient visits: follow-up burn clinic

1. Scar maturation continues for 1 to 2 years after the open burn wound has healed.

2. Continued assessment of the wound, functional status, psychological status, and general progress of the patient is necessary.

3. Comprehensive follow-up may be arranged through a burn clinic, during which the patient may be seen by the physician(s), physical and occupational therapist, art and play therapist, social worker, dietician, and pharmacologist.

4. Referrals can be made for further evaluation of any problem reported or observed.

5. Recommendations may be made to a cosmetologist for assistance with camouflage makeup.

6. The patient is followed in the clinic until the burn scar has matured.

7. Burn scar maturation is achieved when the scar has faded and there is no longer any appearance of inflammation.

8. Pressure garments can be discontinued at this time.

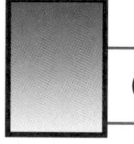

Clinical Decision-Making Case

EXAMINATION

History

The patient is a 50-year-old white male who sustained 22% total body surface area full-thickness flame burns to the left side of face, left side of neck, left upper extremity, left chest, abdomen, and right lower extremity. He was burned in a house fire that may have been caused by a smoldering cigarette.

The patient also sustained an inhalation injury.

Medical history is significant for alcohol abuse, chronic smoking, atrial fibrillation, alcoholic liver disease, diabetes mellitus, an unnamed psychiatric disorder, and lumbar laminectomy.

Physical

The patient was intubated and had escharotomies to the left upper extremity in a local hospital before transfer to the burn center. Wounds were covered with silver sulfadiazene (Silvadene).

Preparations for surgery were made, including cardiovascular, respiratory, and nutritional support (including hyperalimentation and insulin drip to control blood sugar).

The patient was noted to be a large man, about 6 feet tall and weighing 200 lb.

Surgical Procedures

On the 6th day after burn, the patient's wounds were débrided and covered with xenograft. Systemic antibiotics were begun at this time.

On the 9th day, the xenograft was débrided and an autograft was placed.

The grafts were examined on the 14th day after burn, with good graft take. The palmar surface of the left hand required continued dressing changes for healing to be complete.

Mental Status

The patient became less responsive to stimulation, and, on the 13th day post burn, neurological consultation was performed. The patient's coma was determined to be reversible. He was seen by a psychiatrist as well, and appropriate medications were prescribed.

The patient continued to require persistent respiratory support, with improvement of his mental status and diabetic control.

His sister began to visit and provided a great deal of emotional support and motivation.

Extubation occurred 4 weeks after burn.

Antibiotic therapy was stopped after 2 weeks but was resumed 10 days later when *Pseudomonas* was found in his sputum.

Local wound care continued. The patient had sufficient wound healing to allow a transfer to the skilled nursing unit 2 months after the burn occurred.

ASSESSMENT/DIAGNOSIS

During the initial physical therapy evaluation, the patient was restless and combative, thrashing around in bed. He was positioned on an air bed during this phase. Wrist restraints were required to preserve intubation.

The left upper extremity was evaluated during hydrotherapy. Full-thickness injury was apparent, with escharotomies already performed. The anterior axillary fold was included in the burned area. The patient presented with risks for decreased function of entire left upper extremity as well as hypertrophic scarring.

Because of the inhalation injury, the patient was also at risk for multiple medical problems, not only directly from this injury but also from the period of prolonged bed rest that would be required to recover.

TREATMENT GOALS

1. Independent transfers and ambulation.
2. Independent self-care activities with full use of left upper extremity.
3. Independent home exercise program with maintenance of range of motion and functional strength.
4. Independent home pressure program with adequate control of hypertrophic scarring.
5. Demonstration of knowledge of skin care post burn.

TREATMENT

Treatment was begun at the time of evaluation with exercises performed following hand protocol to protect extensor tendons. A left hand splint was fabricated in the functional position, and the left upper extremity was positioned in elevation, elbow extension, with shoulder abducted to 90 degrees.

Exercises to all extremities and neck also continued daily until skin grafts were applied. Range of motion in unburned extremities was limited by therapist when arterial lines were present.

After autografting, positioning was monitored until postoperative day (POD) 6, when passive range of motion exercises to all extremities except left upper extremity were begun. The patient was generally resistant to movement throughout.

On POD 7, passive range of motion exercises for the left upper extremity were begun, with full range easily achieved in the shoulder and elbow. Left wrist flexion and extension were limited to 20 degrees each, radial and ulnar deviation to 5 degrees each. Hand exercises continued with extensor tendon precautions, with 90 degrees of passive MP joint flexion available in the digits.

This program of exercise continued, with the patient resisting movement in general. Muscle tone was generally increased throughout. By POD 13, the patient had full passive range of motion to left hand and wrist but supination was limited to 50%. The facial and neck burns healed.

During the next phase of functional mobility retraining, exercise and functional use of the left upper extremity continued daily as tolerated.

POD 15: The patient was transferred from supine to sitting position on the edge of the bed with maximal assist of two therapists (and three other staff assisting with endotracheal tube, cables from monitors, and intravenous lines.) Two layers of elastic bandages were applied from toes to groin before this activity.

POD 16: The patient was extubated. Continuing with Ace wraps as above, the patient was lifted (by four people) to recliner chair for upright sitting for 10 minutes, then was reclined after blood pressure began to fall.

POD 17: Increased conversation and level of alertness noted. The patient was oriented to person and year, not to place. Four-person transfer made from bed to tilt table. He tolerated tilting to 45 degrees, with chief difficulty being shortness of breath.

POD 18: Tilt table toleration continued, to 60 degrees. Increased tolerance to sitting up in chair, to 3 hours. Four-person assist needed for stand-pivot transfer back to bed from chair.

POD 21: Complaints about low back pain began. Bed exercises began with focus on relief of back pain. The patient was unable to tolerate other bed mobility work or transfer training.

POD 22: Resumed tilt table, but back pain limited tolerance to activity.

POD 23: Began use of battery-powered standing frame with increased ability to maintain upright posture.

POD 26: Able to work on transfer from sit to stand with bed height raised, with two persons assisting.

POD 27: Sit to stand transfer practiced with walker. The patient refused all left hand and wrist exercises at this time.

POD 29: The patient cooperated with left hand and wrist exercises, with 50% wrist motions and only 10% flexion of digits.

POD 30: Began work on wheelchair mobility using right hand and both feet for steering.

POD 33: Left elbow extension splint fabricated for use at night, as it was very difficult for patient to stretch into extension each morning.

POD 34: Use of self-adhering elastic pressure wrap began on left hand over light dressings, then Ace wrap from hand to axilla. Patient able to propel self in wheelchair. Patient continued to ramble in and out of appropriate verbal communication.

POD 37: Patient was able to ambulate 8 feet with contact guard.

POD 39: Occupational therapy began with activities of daily living assessment and treatment.

POD 40: The patient was able to ambulate 100 feet with close supervision.

POD 41: He was able to ambulate 200 feet.

POD 44: Back pain again limited rehabilitation. Transcutaneous electrical nerve stimulation (TENS) trial used for back pain.

POD 45: Back pain became more tolerable with TENS and new medication. The patient was able to tolerate more independence in exercise program, using foam ball and other equipment. He was able to tolerate manual resistive exercises to left shoulder and elbow musculature.

POD 46: Left hand soaks used as a medium for exercise.

POD 47: Back pain again limited functional mobility; however, the patient has become much more cooperative for hand therapy and activities of daily living.

About 2 months after the burn injury, the patient was transferred to the skilled nursing unit for continued rehabilitation.

A schedule of activities, including treatments twice a day for both physical and occupational therapy, was developed during a team conference attended by social services, nursing, the activities director, and physical and occupational therapists.

The patient was measured for and fit with custom pressure garments, including gloves for left hand, vest with sleeves, and waist-high garment to support both legs (in place of elastic wraps).

Included in the patient's activities of daily living program were skin care and lubrication.

During this period of aggressive physical and occupational therapy, the patient resumed cigarette smoking. He was also treated for urinary retention with a surgical procedure.

After 2 weeks on the unit, the patient was discharged to a board and care facility. He required assistance to apply his pressure garments, and meals were provided. Otherwise, he was independent in activities of daily living.

After 1 week of physical therapy and occupational therapy home care, the patient began outpatient treatment at the hand therapy clinic. During the month of hand therapy, he was treated two or three times a week. The patient appeared for one scheduled appointment with alcohol on his breath.

The patient then moved to his sister's home in the country. He has not returned for follow-up visits since.

OUTCOMES

1. The patient achieved the goals of independent transfers and ambulation.
2. He achieved independence in activities of daily living by the end of his course of therapy. This included care of healed burns and skin grafts.
3. He was able to wear his pressure garments. He did not always wear the support to his lower extremities. (Because these areas were primarily healed donor sites and not deep burns or skin grafts, he was not symptomatic when he did not wear them.)
4. His left upper extremity was fully functional, although continued work by the patient was required to maintain full range of motion and to regain full strength.

References

1. Constantian MB: *Pressure Ulcers: Principles and Techniques of Management.* Boston, Little Brown and Company, 1980.
2. Shea JD: Pressure sores: classification and management. *Clin Orthop* 1975, 223:89–100.
3. Enis JE, Sarmiento A: The physiology and management of pressure sores. *Orthop Rev* 1973, 2:25–27.
4. Robinson AJ, Snyder-Mackler L: Clinical application of electrotherapeutic modalities. *Phys Ther* 1988, 68:1235–1238.
5. Mortimer AJ, Dyson M: The effect of therapeutic ultrasound on calcium uptake in fibroblasts. *Ultrasound Med Biol* 1988, 14:499–506.
6. Dinno MA, Crum LA, Wu J: The effect of ultrasound on electrophysiological parameters of frog skin. *Ultrasound Med Biol* 1989, 15:461–470.
7. Dyson M, Luke DA: Induction of mast cell degranulation in skin by ultrasound. *IEEE Trans and Ultrasonics, Ferroelectrics, and Frequency Control (UFFC)* 1986, 33:194.
8. Harvey W, Dyson M, Pond JB, Grahame R: The stimulation of protein synthesis in human fibroblasts by therapeutic ultrasound. *Rheumatol Rehabil* 1975, 14:237.
9. Hong CZ: Reversible nerve conduction block in patients

with polyneuropathy after ultrasound thermotherapy at therapeutic dosage. *Arch Phys Med Rehabil* 1991, 72:132–137.

10. Young SR, Dyson M: The effect of therapeutic ultrasound on angiogenesis. *Ultrasound Med Biol* 1990, 16:261–269.

11. Dyson M, Suckling J: Stimulation of tissue repair by ultrasound: survey of mechanisms involved. *Physiotherapy* 1978, 63:105–108.

12. McDiarmid T, Burns PN, Lewith GT, Machin D: Ultrasound and the treatment of pressure sores. *Physiotherapy* 1985, 71:66–70.

13. Lundeberg T, Nordstrom F, Brodda-Jansen G, *et al.:* Pulsed ultrasound does not improve healing of venous ulcers. *Scand J Rehabil Med* 1990, 22:195–197.

14. Eriksson SV, Lundeberg T, Malm M: A placebo controlled trial of ultrasound therapy in chronic leg ulceration. *Scand J Rehabil Med* 1991, 23:211–213.

15. Byl NN, McKenzie AL, West JM, *et al.:* Low-dose ultrasound effect on wound healing: a controlled study with Yucatan pigs. *Arch Phys Med Rehabil* 1992, 73:656–664.

16. Byl NN, McKenzie A, Wong T, *et al.:* Incisional wound healing: a controlled study of low and high dose ultrasound. *J Orthop Sport Phys Ther* 1993, 18:619–628.

17. Stevenson JH, Pang CY, Lindsay WK, Zuker RM: Functional, mechanical and biochemical assessment of ultrasound therapy on tendon healing in the chicken toe. *Plast Reconstr Surg* 1986, 77:965–970.

18. Enwemeka CS: The effects of therapeutic ultrasound on tendon healing. *Am J Phys Med Rehabil* 1989, 68:283–287.

19. Enwemeka CS, Rodriguez O, Mendosa S: The biomechanical effects of low intensity ultrasound on healing tendons. *Ultrasound Med Biol* 1990, 16:801–807.

20. Duarte LR: The stimulation of bone growth by ultrasound. *Arch Orthop Trauma Surg* 1983, 101:153–159.

21. Pilla AA, Mont MA, Nassen PR, *et al.:* Non-invasive low-intensity pulsed ultrasound accelerates bone healing in the rabbit. *J Orthop Trauma* 1990, 4:246–253.

22. Fukada E, Yasuda I: On the piezoelectric effect of bone. *J Phys Soc Jap* 1957, 12:10.

23. Farmer WC: Effect of intensity of ultrasound on conduction of motor axons. *Phys Ther* 1968, 48:1233–1237.

24. Kramer JF: Effect of therapeutic ultrasound intensity on subcutaneous tissue temperature and ulnar nerve conduction velocity. *Am J Phys Med* 1985, 64:1–9.

25. Halle JS, Scoville CR, Greathouse DG: Ultrasound's effect on the conduction latency of the superficial radial nerve in man. *Phys Ther* 1981, 61:345–350.

26. Hong CZ, Liu HH, Yu J: Ultrasound thermotherapy effect on the recovery of nerve conduction in experimental compression neuropathy. *Arch Phys Med Rehabil* 1988, 69:410–414.

27. Dyson M, Pond JB, Woodward B, Broadbent J: The production of blood cell stasis and endothelial damage in blood vessels of chick embryos treated with ultrasound in a stationary wave field. *Ultrasound Med Biol* 1974, 1:133.

28. Normand H, Darlas Y, Solasso IA, *et al.:* Etude experimental de l'effet thermique des ultrasons sur le materiel prothetique. *An Readaptation Med Phys* 1989, 32:193–201.

29. McLeod DR, Fowlow SB: Multiple malformations and exposure to therapeutic ultrasound during organogenesis. *Am J Med Genet* 1989, 34:317–319.

30. Sokoliu A: Destructive effect of ultrasound on ocular tissues. In Reid JM, Sikiov MR (eds): *Interaction of Ultrasound and Biological Tissues.* Washington DC, Department of Health, Education and Welfare, Food and Drug Administration Publication 73-8008, 1972.

31. Oakley EM: Dangers and contra-indications of therapeutic ultrasound. *Physiotherapy* 1978, 64:173–174.

32. *Biological Effects of Ultrasound: Mechanisms and Clinical Implications.* NCRP Report No. 74, Bethesda, MD, 1983, pp 196–198.

33. Skoubo-Kristensen E, Sommer J: Ultrasound influence on internal fixation with rigid plate in dogs. *Arch Phys Med Rehabil* 1982, 63:371–373.

34. Wolcott LE, Wheeler PC, Hardwicke HM, *et al.:* Accelerated healing of skin ulcers by electrotherapy: preliminary clinical results. *South Med J* 1969, 62:795–801.

35. Gault W, Gatens P: Use of low intensity direct current in management of ischemic skin ulcers. *Phys Ther* 1976, 56:265–269.

36. Carley P, Wainapel S: Electrotherapy for acceleration of wound healing: low intensity direct current. *Arch Phys Med Rehabil* 1985, 66:443–446.

37. Kloth L, Feedar J: Acceleration of wound healing with high voltage, monophasic, pulsed current. *Phys Ther* 1988, 68:503–508.

38. Griffin JW, Tooms RE, Mendens JK, *et al.:* Efficacy of high voltage pulsed current for healing of pressure ulcers in patients with spinal cord injury. *Phys Ther* 1991, 71:433–442.

39. Feedar J, Kloth L, Gentzkow G: Chronic dermal ulcer healing enhanced with monophasic pulsed electrical stimulation. *Phys Ther* 1991, 71:639–649.

40. Gentzkow GD, Feeder J, Kloth L, *et al.:* Improved healing of pressure ulcers using Dermapulse, a new electrical stimulation device. *Wounds* 1991, 3:158–170.

41. Alvarez OM, Mertz DM, Smorkeck RO, *et al.:* The healing of superficial skin wounds is stimulated by external electrical current. *J Invest Dermatol* 1983, 81:144–148.

42. Assimacopoulos D: Low intensity negative electric current in the treatment of ulcers of the leg due to chronic venous insufficiency. *Am J Surg* 1968, 115:683–687.

43. Brown M, McDonnell M, Menton D: Polarity effects on wound healing using electric stimulation in rabbits. *Arch Phys Med Rehabil* 1989, 70:624–627.

44. Sawyer P, Wesolowski S: Studies on direct current coagulation. *Surgery* 1961, 49:486–489.

45. Sawyer RN: Bioelectric phenomena and intravascular thrombosis: the first 12 years. *Surgery* 1964, 56:1020–1026.

46. Cheng N, Van Hoof H, Bock E, *et al.:* The effects of electric currents on ATP generation, protein synthesis and membrane transport in rat skin. *Clin Orthop* 1982, 171:264–272.

47. Kaziro Y: The role of guanosine-5'-triphosphate in polypeptide chain elongation. *Biochim Biophys Acta* 1978, 505:95–99.

48. Erickson E, Nuccitelli R: Embryonic fibroblast motility and orientation can be influenced by physiological electric fields. *J Cell Biol* 1984, 98:296–307.

49. Bourguignon GJ, Bourguignon LYW: Electric stimulation of protein and DNA synthesis in human fibroblasts. *FASEB J* 1987, 1:398–402.

50. Cooper M, Schliwa M: Electrical and ionic control of tissue cell locomotion in DC electric field. *J Neurosci Res* 1985, 13:223–244.

51. Rowley BA: Electrical current effects on *E. coli* growth rates. *Proc Soc Exp Biol Med* 1972, 139:929–934.

52. Kincaid C, Lavoie K: Inhibition of bacterial growth with high voltage, monophasic pulsed current. *Phys Ther* 1989, 69:651–655.

53. Orida N, Feldman J: Directional protrusive pseudopodial activity and motility in macrophages induced by extracellular electric fields. *Cell Motil* 1982, 2:243–255.

54. Fukushima L, Senda N, Incii H, *et al.:* Studies on galvano-taxis of leukocytes. *Med J Osaka Univ* 1953, 4:195–208.

55. Dineur E: Note sur la sensibilité des leucocytes à l'électricité. *Bull Seances Soc Belge Microscopic (Bruxelles)* 1891, 18:113–118.

56. Monguio J: Über die polare wirkung des galvanischen stromes auf leukozyten. *Z Biol* 1933, 93:553–559.

57. Sawyer P, Deutch B: The experimental use of oriented electric fields to delay and prevent intravascular thrombosis. *Surg Forum* 1955, 5:173–178.

58. Sawyer P, Deutch B: Use of electrical currents to delay intravascular thrombosis in experimental animals. *Am J Physiol* 1956, 187:473–478.

59. Blank M: Recent developments in the theory of ion flow across membranes under imposed electric fields. In Marino A (ed): *Modern Bioelectricity.* New York, Marcel Dekker, 1988.

60. Newton R: High voltage pulsed galvanic stimulation: theoretical bases and clinical applications. In Currier DP, Nelson RM (eds): *Clinical Electrotherapy.* Norwalk, CT, Appleton-Century-Crofts, 1987, pp 201–220.

61. Pethig R: Electrical properties of biological tissue. In Marino A (ed): *Modern Bioelectricity.* New York, Marcel Dekker, 1988.

62. Bolton L, Foleno B, Means B: The effects of direct current stimulation on microorganisms in repairing wounds. *Bioelectricity Repair Growth Soc Proc* 1981, 1:70.

63. Ziskin MC, McDiarmid T, Michlovitz SL: Therapeutic ultrasound. In S Micholovitz SL (ed): *Thermal Agents in Rehabilitation.* Philadelphia, F. A. Davis Company, 1990, pp 153–154.

64. Tyle P, Agravala P: Drug delivery by phonophoresis. *Pharm Res* 1989, 6:355–362.

65. Antich TJ: Phonophoresis: the principles of ultrasonic driving force and efficacy in treatment of common orthopedic diagnoses. *J Orthop Sports Phys Ther* 1982, 4:99–102.

66. Cameron MH, Monroe LG: Relative transmission of ultrasound by media customarily used for phonophoresis. *Phys Ther* 1992, 72:142–148.

67. Lehmann JF (ed): *Therapeutic Heat and Cold,* 3rd ed. Baltimore, Williams & Wilkins, 1990.

68. Bommannan D, Okuyama H, Stauffer P, Guy RH: Sonophoresis I. The use of high-frequency ultrasound to enhance transdermal drug delivery. *Pharm Res* 1992, 9:559–564.

69. Bommannan D, Menon GK, Kouyama H, *et al.:* Sonophoresis II. Examination of the mechanism(s) of ultrasound-enhanced transdermal drug delivery. *Pharm Res* 1992, 9:1043–1047.

70. Cumming J: Iontophoresis. In Nelson RM, Currier DP (eds): *Clinical Electrotherapy,* 2nd ed. San Mateo, CA, Appleton & Lange, 1991, pp 317–330.

71. Harris R: Iontophoresis. In Licht S (ed): *Therapeutic Electricity and Ultraviolet Radiation.* Baltimore, Waverly, 1967.

72. Russo J, Lipman AG, Comstock TJ, *et al.:* Lidocaine anesthesia: comparison of iontophoresis injection and swabbing. *Am J Hosp Pharm* 1980, 37:843–847.

73. Magistro CM: Hyaluronidase by iontophoresis. *Phys Ther* 1964, 44:169–175.

74. Schwartz MS: The use of hyaluronidase by iontophoresis in the treatment of lymphedema. *Arch Intern Med* 95:662–668, 1955.

75. Glass JM, Stephen RL, Jacobsen SC: The quantity and distribution of radiolabeled dexamethasone delivered to tissues by iontophoresis. *Int J Dermatol* 1980, 19:519–525.

76. Harris PR: Iontophoresis: clinical research in musculoskeletal inflammatory condlitions. *J Orthop Sports Phys Ther* 1982, 4:109–112.

77. Bertolucci LE: Introduction of antiinflammatory drugs by iontophoresis. Double blind study. *J Orthop Sports Phys Ther* 1982, 4:203–205.

78. Psaki C, Carol J: Acetic acid ionization. A study to determine the absorptive effects upon calcified tendinitis of the shoulder. *Phys Ther Rev* 1955, 35:84–87.

79. Kahn J: *Clinical Electrotherapy.* Syosset, NY, Joseph Kahn, 1973.

80. Levit F: Simple device for treatment of hyperhidrosis by iontophoresis. *Arch Dermatol* 1968, 198:505–507.

81. Abdell E, Morgan K: Treatment of idiopathic hyperhydrosis by glycopyrronium bromide and tap water iontophoresis. *Br J Dermatol* 1974, 92:87–91.

82. Akins DL, Meisenheimer JL, Dobson RL: Efficacy of the Drionic unit in the treatment of hyperhidrosis. *J Am Acad Dermatol* 1987, 16:828–832.

83. Hill BHR: Poldine iontophoresis in the treatment of palmar and plantar hyperhidrosis. *Australas J Dermatol* 1976, 17:92–93.

84. Falcone AE, Spadara JA: Inhibitory effects of electrically activated silver material on cutaneous wound bacteria. *Plast Reconstr Surg* 1986, 77:455–458.

85. Holmes G: Hydrotherapy as a means of rehabilitation. *Br J Phys Med* 1942, 5:93–95.

86. Scott PM: *Clayton's Electrotherapy and Actinotherapy* 7th ed. Baltimore, Williams & Wilkins, 1975.

87. Cohen A, Martin G, Wakim K: The effect of whirlpool bath with and without agitation on the circulation in normal and diseased extremities. *Arch Phys Med Rehabil* 1949, 39:212–219.

88. Lehmann JF, DeLateur BJ: Therapeutic heat. In Lehmann JF (ed): *Therapeutic Heat and Cold.* 3rd ed. Baltimore, Williams & Wilkins, 1982, pp 417–581.

89. Abraham E, McMaster WC, Kriiger M, Waught TR: Whirlpool therapy for treatment of soft tissue wounds complicated by extremity fractures. *J Trauma* 1974, 4:222–226.

90. Hoyrup G, Kjorvel L: Comparison of whirlpool and wax treatments for hand therapy. *Physiother Can* 1986, 38:79–82.

91. Headley B, Robson MC, Krizek TJ: Methods of reducing environmental stress for the acute burn patient. *Phys Ther* 1975, 55:5–9.

92. Richard RL, Finley RK, Miller SF: Effect of hydrotherapy on burn wound bacteria [Abstract]. *Phys Ther* 1984, 64:746.

93. Koepke G: The role of physical medicine in the treatment of burns. *Surg Clin North Am* 1970, 150:1385–1390.

94. Steve L, Goodhart P, Alexander J: Hydrotherapy burn treatment: use of chloramine-T against resistant micro-organisms. *Arch Phys Med Rehabil* 1979, 60:301–303.

95. Abramson D: Physiologic basis for the use of physical agents in peripheral vascular disorders. *Arch Phys Med Rehabil* 1965, 46:216–244.

96. Abramson D, Brunnet C, Bell Y, *et al:* Changes in blood flow, oxygen, uptake and tissue temperatures produced by a topical application of wet heat. *Arch Phys Med Rehabil* 1961, 42:305–318.

97. Borrell R, Parker R, Henley EJ, *et al.:* Comparison of in vivo temperatures produced by hydrotherapy, paraffin wax treatment, and Fluidotherapy. *Phys Ther* 1980, 60:1273–1276.

98. Hellerbrand T, Holutz S, Eubank I: Measurement of whirlpool temperature, pressure and turbulence. *Arch Phys Med Rehabil* 1950, 32:17–26.

99. Fricke FJ, Gersten JW: Effect of contrast baths on the vasomotor response of rheumatoid arthritis patients. *Arch Phys Med* 1952, 33:210–216.

100. Hollander JL, Horvath SM: The influence of physical ther-

apy procedures on the intra-articular temperature of normal and arthritic subjects. *Am J Med Sci* 1957, 218:543–548.

101. Harrison RA: Tolerance of pool therapy by ankylosing spondylitis patients with low vital capacity. *Physiotherapy* 1981, 167:296–297.

102. Roberts P: Hydrotherapy: its history, theory and practice. *Occup Health Saf* 1982, 235:5.

103. Stewart JB, Basmajian JF: Exercises in water. In Basmajian JV (ed): *Therapeutic Exercise* 3rd ed. Baltimore, Williams & Wilkins, 1978, pp 303–308.

104. Downey JA, Darling RC, Miller JM: The effects of heat, cold, and exercise on peripheral circulation. *Arch Phys Med Rehabil* 1968, 49:309–313.

105. Walsh MT: Hydrotherapy. In Michovitz S (ed): *Thermal Agents in Rehabilitation*. Philadelphia, F. A. Davis Company, 1993, pp 109–133.

106. Hayes K: Hydrotherapy. In Hayes K (ed): *Manual for Physical Agents*, 4th ed. Norwalk CT, Appleton & Lange, 1993, pp 16, 17.

107. Gieck J: Precautions for hydrotherapeutic devices. *Clin Management* 1983, 3:44.

108. Whitehall hydrotherapy equipment catalog no. 680. Hackensack, NJ.

109. Woodmansey A, Collins DH, Ernst MM: Vascular reactions to the contrast bath in health and in rheumatoid arthritis. *Lancet* 1938, 2:1350–1353.

110. Miller JK, LeForest NT, Hedberg M, *et al.:* Surveillance and control of Hubbard tank bacterial contaminants. *Phys Ther* 1970, 50:1482–1487.

111. McMillan J, Hargess C, Nource A, *et al.:* Procedure for decontamination of hydrotherapy equipment. *Phys Ther* 1976, 56:567–570.

112. Simonetti A, Miller R, Gristin J: Efficacy of povidone-iodine in the disinfection of whirlpool baths and Hubbard tanks. *Phys Ther* 1972, 52:1277–1282.

113. Ziegenfus RW: Povidone iodine as bactericide in hydrotherapy equipment. *Phys Ther* 1969, 49:582–585.

114. McGukin M, Thorpe R, Abrutyn E: Hydrotherapy: an outbreak of *Pseudomonas aeruginosa* wound infections related to Hubbard tank treatments. *Arch Phys Med Rehabil* 1981, 62:283–285.

115. McMillan J, Hargiss C, Nourse A, Williams O: Procedure for decontamination of hydrotherapy equipment. *Phys Ther* 1976, 56:567–570.

116. Miller JK, LeForest NT, Hedberg M, Chapman V: Surveillance and control of Hubbard tank contaminants. *Phys Ther* 1970, 50:1482–1487.

117. Nelson RM, Reed JR, Kenton DM: Microbiological evaluation of decontamination procedures for hydrotherapy tanks. *Phys Ther* 1972, 52:919–923.

118. Sykes JH: Calcium hypochlorite for disinfection of hydrotherapy equipment. *Phys Ther* 1963, 43:345–347.

119. Centers for Disease Control: Update: universal precaution for prevention of transmission of human immunodeficiency virus, hepatitis B virus and other bloodborne pathogens in health care setting. 1988, *MMWR* 37:388.

120. Microbiologic Control Branch Bacterial Disease Division, Bureau of Epidemiology. Centers for Disease Control, Atlanta, GA, 1977 (contact for current standards).

121. Matsen FA, Krugmire RB: The effect of externally applied pressure on post fracture swelling. *J Bone Joint Surg* 1974, 56-A:1586–1591.

122. Quillen WS, Roullier LH: Initial management of acute ankle sprains with rapid pulsed pneumatic compression and cold. *J Orthop Sports Phys Ther* 1982, 4:39–43.

123. Kolb P, Denegar C: Traumatic edema and the lymphatic system. *Athletic Training* 1983, 17:339–341.

124. Airaksinen O, Kolari PJ, Herve R, Holopainen R: Treat-

ment of post-traumatic oedema in lower legs using intermittent pneumatic compression. *Scand J Rehabil Med* 1988, 20:25–28.

125. Murphy K: The combination of ice and intermittent compression system in the treatment of soft tissue injuries. *Physiotherapy* 1988, 74:42.

126. Wilkerson J: Contrast baths and pressure treatment for ankle sprains. *Physician Sportsmed* 1979, 7:143.

127. McCulloch JM: Intermittent compression for the treatment of a chronic stasis ulceration. *Phys Ther* 1981, 61:1452–1453.

128. Nelson PA: Recent advances in treatment of lymphedema of the extremities. *Geriatrics* 1966, 21:162–173.

129. Jungi WF: The prevention and management of lymphoedema after treatment for breast cancer. *Int Rehabil Med* 1981, 3:129–134.

130. Leis HP, Bowers WF, Dursi J: Postmastectomy edema of the arm. *N Y State J Med* 1966, 66:618–624.

131. Sanderson RG, Fletcher WS: Conservative management of primary lymphedema. *Northwest Med* 1965, 64:584–588.

132. Swedborg I: Effects of treatment with an elastic sleeve and intermittent pneumatic compression in post-mastectomy patients with lymphoedema of the arm. *Scand J Rehabil Med* 1984, 26:35–41.

133. Hayes KW: Intermittent compression pump. In Hayes KW (ed): *Manual for Physical Agents*, 4th ed. Norwalk, CT, Appleton & Lange, 1993, pp 71–73.

134. Swedborg I: Voluminometric estimation of the degree of lymphedema and its therapy by pneumatic compression. *Scand J Rehabil Med* 1977, 9:131–135.

135. Scott BO: Ultraviolet application. In Stillwell K (ed): *Therapeutic Electricity and Ultraviolet Radiation*, 3rd ed. Baltimore, Williams & Wilkins, 1983, pp 228–262.

136. Shriber WJ: *A Manual of Electrotherapy*, 4th ed. Philadelphia, Lea & Febiger, 1973.

137. Goats GC: Appropriate use of the inverse square law. *Physiotherapy* 1988, 74:8.

138. Low J: Quantifying the erythema due to UVR. *Physiotherapy* 1986, 72:60–64.

139. Tromovitch TA, Thompson LR, Jacobs PH: Testing for photosensitivity. *J Am Phys Ther Assoc* 1963, 143:348–349.

140. Haarber LC, Bickers DR: *Photosensitivity Diseases: Principles of Diagnosis and Treatment*, 2nd ed. Toronto, B. C. Decker, 1989.

141. Fitch DH, Soderstrom RM, Kinzie S: PUVA therapy in the treatment of psoriasis. *Clin Management* 1987, 7:24, 26–27.

142. Fusco RJ, Jordon PA, Kelly A, Samuel M: PUVA treatment for psoriasis. *Physiotherapy* 1980, 66:39–40.

143. Gorham H: Treatment of psoriatic arthropathy by PUVA. *Physiotherapy* 1980, 66:40.

144. Klaber MR: Ultra-violet light for psoriasis. *Physiotherapy* 1980, 66:36–38.

145. Shurr DG, Zuehlke RL: Photochemotherapy treatment for psoriasis. *Phys Ther* 1981, 62:33–36.

146. Solomon WM, Netherton EW, Nelson PA, Zeiter WJ: Treatment of psoriasis with the Goeckerman technique. *Arch Phys Med Rehabil* 1955, 36:74–77.

147. Taylor RB: Clinical study of ultraviolet in various skin conditions. *Phys Ther* 1972, 53:279–282.

148. Van Scott EJ: Therapy of psoriasis. 1975. *JAMA* 1976, 235:197–198.

149. Snyder-Mackler L, Seitz L: Therapeutic uses of light in rehabilitation. In Michlovitz S (ed): *Thermal Agents in Rehabilitation*. Philadelphia, F. A. Davis Company, 1990, pp 214–217.

150. Hayes K: Ultraviolet radiation. In Hayes K (ed): *Manual for Physical Agents*, 4th ed. Norwalk, CT, Appleton & Lange, 1993, pp 61–69.

151. Montgomery PC: The compounding effects of infrared and ultraviolet irradiation upon normal human skin. *Phys Ther* 1973, 53:489–496.

152. Ahn ST, Monafo WW, Mustoe T: Topical silicone gel for the prevention and treatment of hypertrophic scar. *Arch Surg* 1991, 126:499–504.

153. American Burn Association: Rehabilitation and reconstruction of the burned patient (Unpublished). Salt Lake City.

154. Chan SC, Pedretti LW: Burns. In Pedretti LW, Zoltan B (eds): *Occupational Therapy Practice Skills for Physical Dysfunction*, 3rd ed. St Louis, C.V. Mosby Company, 1990, pp 445–457.

155. Harnar T, Engrav L, Marvin J, *et al.:* Dr. Paul Unna's boot and early ambulation after skin grafting the leg. *Plast Reconstr Surg* 1982, 69:359–360.

156. Malick MH, Carr JA: Flexible elastomere molds in burn scar control. *Am J Occup Ther* 1980, 3:603–608.

157. McGough CE: Introduction to CPM. *J Burn Care Rehabil* 1988, 9:494–495.

158. O'Donnell LK: Bothin Burn Center rehabilitation therapy procedure manual (Unpublished). San Francisco, St. Francis Memorial Hospital.

159. Rivers EA, Strate RG, Solem LD: The transparent face mask. *Am J Occup Ther* 1979, 33:108–113.

160. Tanigawa MC, O'Donnell LK, Graham PL: The burned hand: a physical therapy protocol. *Phys Ther* 1974, 54:696–700.

161. Whitmore J, Burt M, Fowler R, *et al.:* Bandaging the lower extremity to control swelling: figure 8 vs spiral technique. *Arch Phys Med* 1972, 53:487–490.

162. Reich J, *et al.:* Different polarity electrical stimulation can manipulate the number of mast cells during the healing of superficial wounds. *J Invest Dermatol* 1991, 96:574.

163. Weiss D, Eaglstein, Falanga V: Exogenous electric current can reduce the formation of hypertrophic scars. *J Dermatol Surg Oncol* 1989, 15:1272–1275.

PART SEVEN

Musculoskeletal System

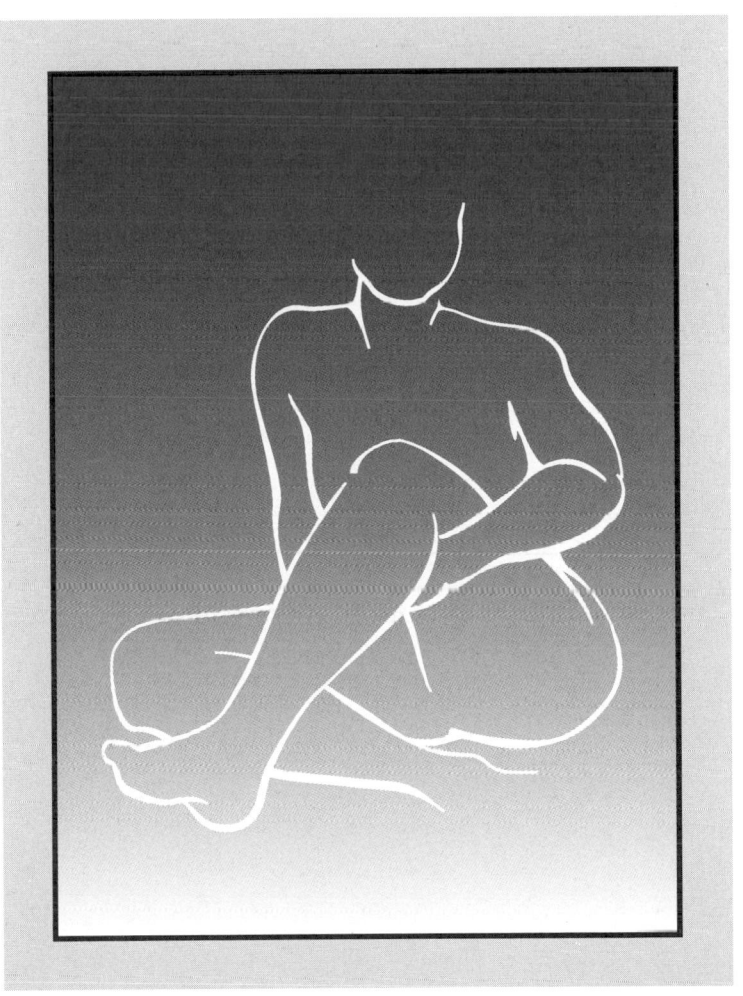

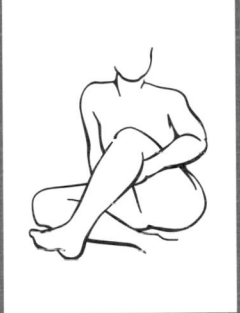

CHAPTER 28

Craniomandibular Examination and Treatment

Barbara Bourbon

The study of occlusion and of head position and its relationship to how the masticatory system functions has gained wide interest and popularity in the profession of physical therapy since the early 1980s. Tremendous interest in this area accompanied by a lack of complete knowledge has stimulated those in the field to propose numerous concepts, theories, and treatment methods. Although the level of knowledge today is greater than ever before, there is still much to learn. Competent clinicians must establish their treatment methods based on both their present knowledge and their constant evaluation of the information that they receive from the extensive amount of continuous research.

The purpose of this chapter is to present the basic framework of the craniomandibular system in a logical and practical manner and to examine the concepts used for the evaluation and treatment of problems related to this multifaceted system.

This chapter is divided into six main sections that cover four major subject areas: anatomical and physiological features, screening and evaluation techniques, temporomandibular joint (TMJ) disorders, and treatment methods. The first four sections discuss the normal anatomical and physiological features of the craniomandibular complex. Knowledge of the normal relationship of the head and neck and their interdependence with masticatory function is essential to the understanding of dysfunction within the system. The fifth section describes screening evaluation techniques that physical therapists use to diagnose specific signs and symptoms of craniomandibular disorders. The sixth section is similar to the fifth section but more succinctly addresses TMJ disorders and gives the

669

rationale for and sequence of appropriate treatment techniques. The case study format is used to emphasize the appropriateness of treatment choices and to illustrate how clinical decisions are made.

I. Functional Anatomy and Biomechanics of the Craniomandibular System

A. Dentition and supportive structures

1. Dentition
   a. The human dentition is made up of 32 permanent teeth, and each tooth can be divided into two basic parts: the crown, which is visible above the gingival tissue, and the root, which is submerged in and surrounded by alveolar bone.
   b. The 32 permanent teeth are distributed equally in the alveolar bone of the maxillary and mandibular arches Sixteen maxillary teeth are aligned in the alveolar process of the maxilla, which is fixed to the lower anterior portion of the skull. The remaining 16 teeth are aligned in the alveolar process of the mandible, which is the movable jaw.
   c. The maxillary arch is slightly longer than the mandibular arch; this causes the maxillary teeth to overlap the mandibular teeth both vertically and horizontally when they are in occlusion.
   d. A discrepancy in size of each tooth can result from either greater maxillary arch width or greater facial angulation of the maxillary arch, which creates horizontal and vertical overlapping of the two arches.
   e. The teeth can be classified according to crown morphology.
      (1). Incisors. The anterior teeth are incisors. They have a characteristic shovel-like shape. The four maxillary incisors, which overlap the four mandibular incisors, are larger than the mandibular incisors. The function of incisors is to cut food during mastication.
      (2). Canines. The canine teeth are distal to the incisors, have a single cusp and root, and are the longest of the permanent teeth. Humans have two maxillary and two mandibular canine teeth. Their function is to cut or tear food.

   (3). Premolars. Premolars are next in the arch. They are also called bicuspids because they generally have two cusps. Humans have four maxillary and four mandibular premolars. Their function is to crush food to begin effective breakdown for digestion.
   (4). Molars. Molars are posterior to premolars. Their crown has either four or five cusps. The function of the six maxillary and six mandibular molars is to crush and grind food, primarily in the later stages of chewing.
2. Periodontal ligament
   a. The periodontal ligament is made of connective tissue that spans from the cementum of the roots of the teeth to the alveolar bone.
   b. Its fibers run obliquely from the cementum in a cervical direction to the bone.
   c. It attaches each tooth firmly to a bone socket and helps to dissipate forces applied to the bone when the teeth functionally contact each other, *ie,* it acts as a "natural shock absorber" (see Figure 28–1).

B. Skeletal components

1. Maxilla
   a. The maxilla is actually two bones that are fused at the midpalatal suture (see Figure 28–2).
   b. Superiorly, the maxilla forms the floor of the nasal cavity and the floor of the eye sockets.
   c. Inferiorly, it forms the palate and alveolar ridges, which support the teeth.
   d. The maxillary teeth are considered to be a fixed part of the skull; they make up the stationary component of the masticatory system.
2. Mandible
   a. The mandible is a U-shaped bone that

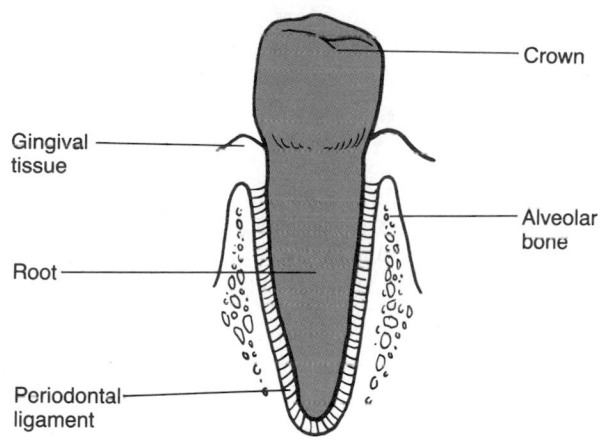

FIGURE 28–1   The tooth and its periodontal supportive structures.

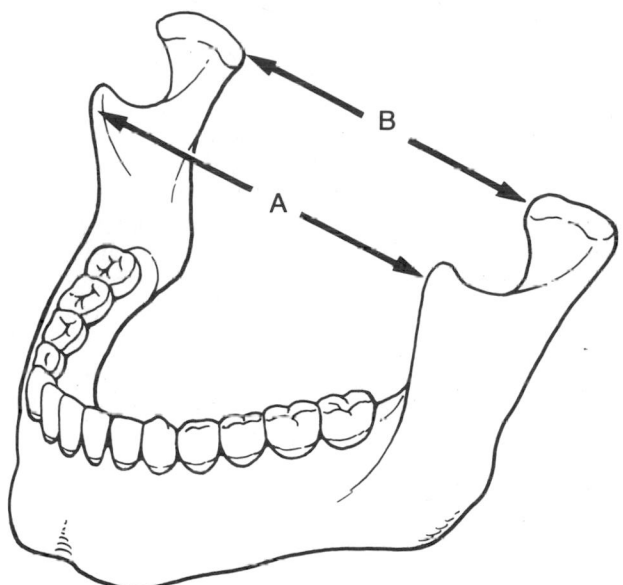

FIGURE 28–3   The ascending ramus extends upward to form the coronoid process **(A)** and the condyle **(B)**.

supports the lower teeth and makes up the lower facial skeleton.

b. No bone structure attaches it to the skull.

c. It is suspended below the maxilla by muscles and ligaments.

d. The superior aspect of the arch-shaped mandible consists of the alveolar process and the teeth.

e. The mandible extends posteroinferiorly to form the mandibular angle and posterosuperiorly to form the ascending ramus.

f. The ascending ramus is formed by a vertical plate of bone that extends upward as two processes: the coronoid process (anteriorly) and the condyle (posteriorly) (see Figure 28–3).

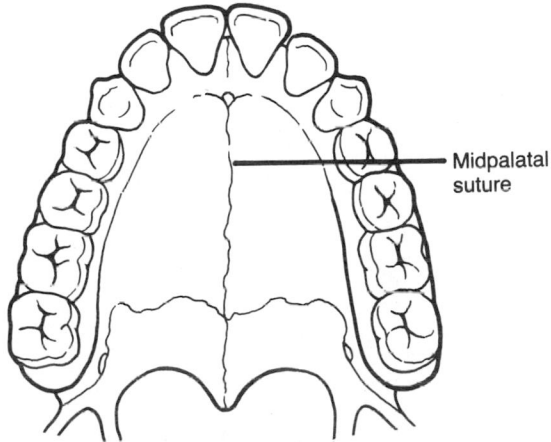

FIGURE 28–2   The midpalatal suture results from fusion of the two maxillary bones during development.

g. Condyle

(1). The condyle is the portion of mandible that articulates with the cranium. Movement occurs around the condyle.

(2). From the anterior view, it has medical and lateral projections called *poles.*

(3). The mediolateral length of the condyle is 15 to 20 mm; the anteroposterior width is between 8 and 10 mm.

(4). The articulating surface of the condyle extends both anteriorly and posteriorly to the superior aspect of the condyle.

(5). Its posterior articulating surface is greater than its anterior surface.

(6). The articulating surface of the condyle is quite convex anteroposteriorly and only slightly convex mediolaterally.

3. Temporal bone

a. Squamous portion

(1). This portion of the temporal bone is made up of the concave mandibular fossa (also known as the articular or glenoid fossa), in which the condyle is situated when it is at rest.

(2). It articulates at the base of the cranium with the mandibular condyle.

(3). Immediately anterior to the fossa is

a convex prominence of bone called the *articular eminence.*

(4). The degree of convexity of the articular eminence is highly variable; however, its steepness dictates the pathway of the condyle when the mandible is positioned anteriorly.

(5). The posterior roof of the mandibular fossa is quite thin, indicating that this area of the temporal bone is not designed to sustain heavy forces.

(6). The articular eminence consists of thick, dense bone covered by a fibrocartilaginous lamina able to tolerate heavy forces.

C. Temporomandibular joint (TMJ)

1. The TMJ is a ginglymoarthrodial joint that provides a hingelike movement in one plane, referred to as *rotation,* and a gliding movement in the opposite plane, known as *translation.*

2. Components of the TMJ
   a. The mandibular condyle. This component fits into the mandibular fossa of the temporal bone.
   b. The disc
      (1). The disc is interposted between the mandibular condyle and the temporal bone.
      (2). It is attached to the capsular ligament anteroposteriorly; mediolaterally the disc divides the joint into two distinct cavities.
      (3). The disc is composed of dense fibrous connective tissue that is devoid of blood vessels and nerve fibers.
      (4). It is sagittally divided into three regions, according to thickness:

- The anterior border, which is thicker than the central area.
- The central area (intermediate zone), which is the thinnest region.
- The posterior border, which is the thickest area.

(5). Anteriorly the disc is attached to the capsule of the joint and the superior belly of the lateral pterygoid muscle.

(6). Posteriorly the disc is attached to highly vascular and neural loose connective tissue, known as *retrodiscal tissue.*

(7). Retrodiscal tissue (see Figure 28–4)
   (a). One part of the retrodiscal tissue is the superior retrodiscal lamina, which contains many elastic fibers. It attaches the articular disc posteriorly to the tympanic plate.
   (b). Another part of the retrodiscal tissue is the inferior retrodiscal lamina, which is composed of collagenous fibers. This section attaches the inferior border of the posterior edge of the disc to the posterior margin of the articular surface of the condyle.
   (c). The remainder of the retrodiscal tissue is attached to a large venous plexus that fills with blood as the condyle moves forward.

3. Joint capsule (see Figure 28–5)
   a. Attachments. Superiorly the joint capsule is attached to the temporal bone along the borders of the articular surfaces of the mandibular fossa and the articular eminence; inferomedially it is attached to

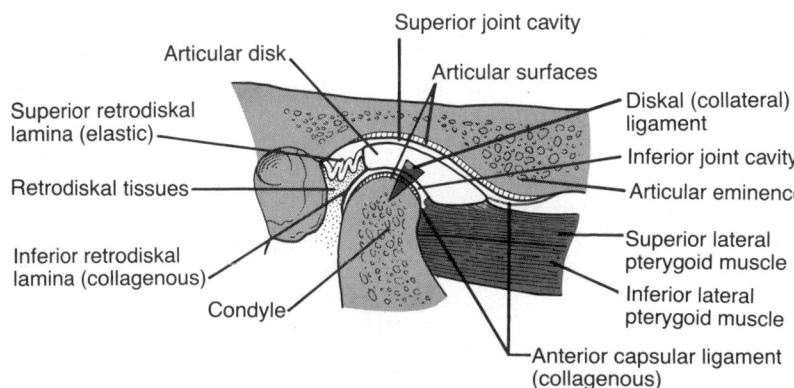

Superior joint cavity

Articular disk

Articular surfaces

Superior retrodiskal lamina (elastic)

Diskal (collateral) ligament

Retrodiskal tissues

Inferior joint cavity

Articular eminence

Inferior retrodiskal lamina (collagenous)

Superior lateral pterygoid muscle

Inferior lateral pterygoid muscle

Condyle

Anterior capsular ligament (collagenous)

FIGURE 28–4 Anatomic components of the TMJ.

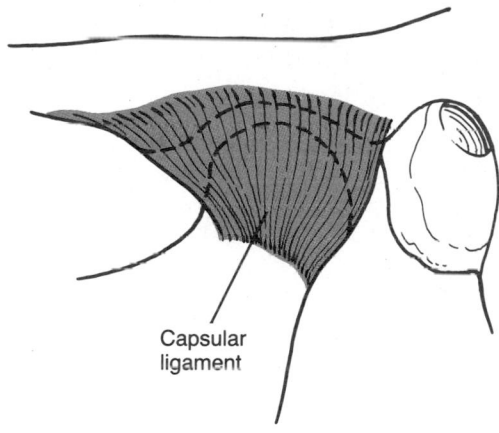

FIGURE 28–5 Capsular ligament (lateral view). Note that it extends anterior to include the articular eminence and encompass the entire articular surface of the joint.

the neck of the condyle, and inferolaterally to the disc.
b. Function. The joint capsule encompasses the TMJ, thus retaining the synovial fluid.
c. Innervation. The capsule is well innervated by the auriculotemporal nerve and provides proprioceptive feedback to the brain regarding the position and movement of the joint.
4. Synovium
a. The synovium covers the superior cavity bordered by the mandibular fossa and the superior surface of the disc.
b. It also covers the inferior cavity bordered by the mandibular condyle and the inferior surface of the disc.
c. The synovium is made up of specialized endothelial cells.
d. This lining, along with a specialized synovial fringe located at the anterior border of the retrodiscal tissues, produces synovial fluid.
e. Synovial fluid provides nonvascular articular joint surfaces with their metabolic requirements.
f. Synovial fluid serves as a lubricant between the articular surfaces during function.
g. Synovial fluid lubricates by two mechanisms.
(1). Boundary lubrication. When the joint is moved, fluid is forced from one area of the cavity to another.

(2). Weeping lubrication. The ability of the articular surfaces to absorb a small amount of synovial fluid helps to eliminate friction in the compressed but nonmoving joint.
5. Temporomandibular ligament (see Figure 28–6)
a. The temporomandibular ligament comprises tight fibers of the capsular ligament that reinforce the joint laterally.
b. It is composed of two parts.
(1). The outer oblique portion. This extends from the outer surface of the articular tubercle and the zygomatic process posteroinferiorly to the outer surface of the condylar neck. Its function is to limit rotational opening.
(2). The inner horizontal portion. This extends from the outer surface of the articular tubercle and the zygomatic process posteriorly and horizontally to the lateral pole of the condyle and to the posterior part of the articular disc. Its function is to limit posterior movement of the condyle and disc, thereby restricting excessive retrusion. It also protects the retrodiscal tissues from possible damage caused by the posterior displacement of the condyle, and it protects the lateral pterygoid muscle from excessive lengthening.

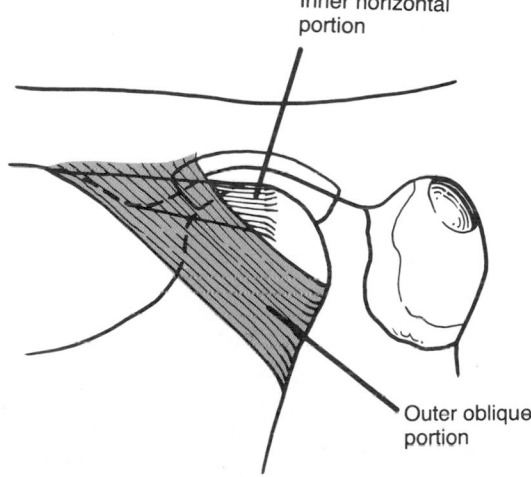

FIGURE 28–6 Temporomandibular ligament (lateral view). Note that there are two distinct parts: the outer oblique portion and the inner horizontal portion. The outer oblique portion limits normal rotational opening movement and the inner horizontal portion, posterior movement of the condyle and disc.

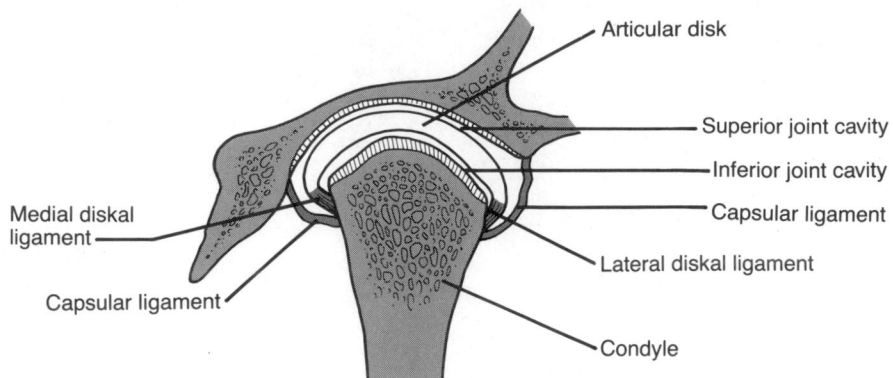

FIGURE 28-7   Anterior view of TMJ.

6. Collateral (discal) ligaments (see Figure 28-7)
   a. Collateral ligaments attach the medial and lateral borders of the articular disc to the medial and lateral poles of the condyle.
   b. They are responsible for dividing the TMJ mediolaterally into the superior and inferior joint cavities.
   c. Their function is to restrict the movement of the disc away from the condyle, which causes the disc to move passively with the condyle as it glides anteriorly and posteriorly.
   d. These ligaments are vasculated and innervated.
   e. The nerves to these ligaments provide information to the brain regarding joint position and movement.
7. Sphenomandibular ligament (see Figure 28-8)
   a. This ligament extends from the spine of the sphenoid bone downward to the medial surface of the inferior ramus (lingula).
   b. The sphenomandibular ligament imposes no specific limitations on the mandible.
8. Stylomandibular ligament (see Figure 28-8)
   a. The stylomandibular ligament extends from the styloid process downward and forward to the angle and posterior border of the mandibular ramus.
   b. Its function is to limit any excessive protrusive movements of the mandible.

D. Muscles of mastication

1. Masseter (see Figure 28-9)
   a. The masseter is a rectangular muscle that originates from the zygomatic arch and extends downward to the lower border of the mandibular ramus. This muscle inserts onto the inferior-posterior border of the angle of the mandible.
   b. It is made up of two heads: the *superficial portion,* which contains fibers that run downward and slightly backward, and the *deep portion,* which contains fibers that predominantly run vertically.
   c. The masseter is a powerful multipenniform muscle that functions as a mandibular elevator. Its superficial fibers aid in protrusion, and its deep fibers stabilize the condyle against the articular eminence.

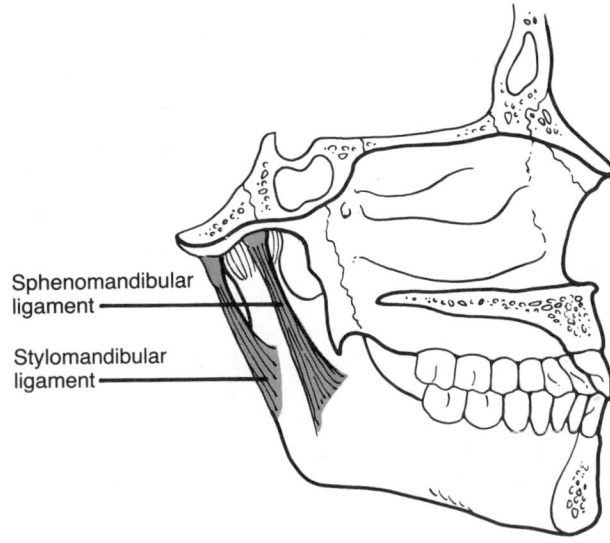

FIGURE 28-8   Mandible, TMJ, and accessory ligaments.

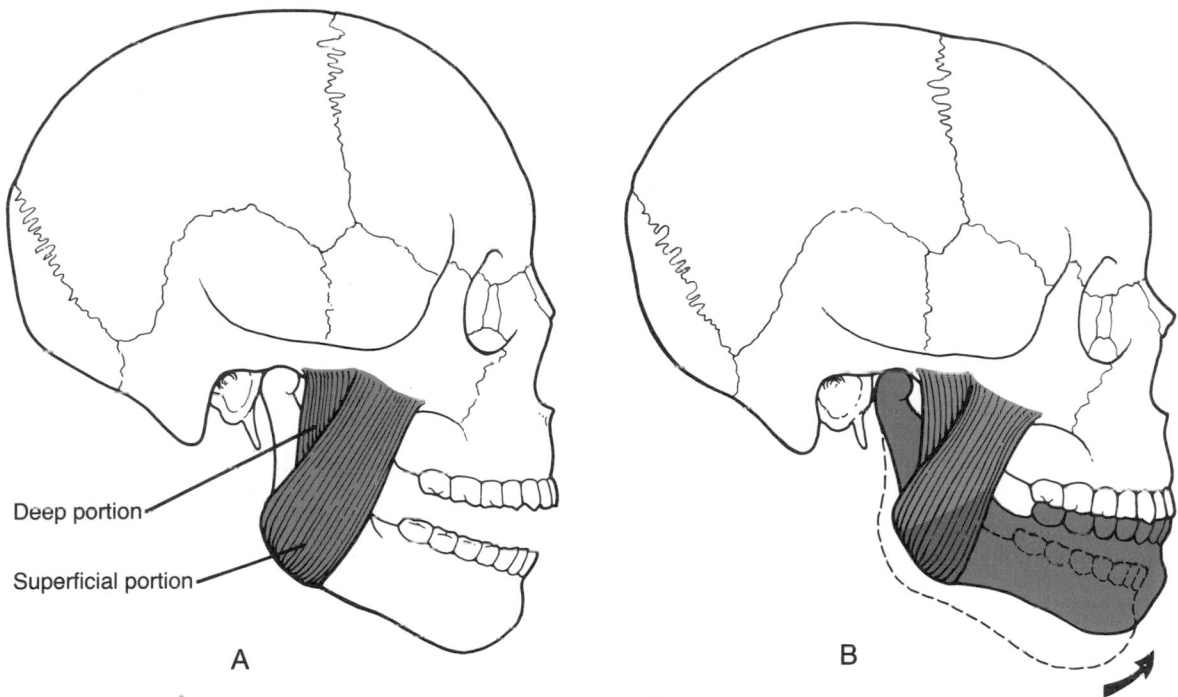

Deep portion

Superficial portion

A

B

FIGURE 28-9 **A,** Masseter muscle. **B,** This muscle elevates the mandible.

2. Temporal muscle (see Figure 28-10)
   a. The temporal muscle is a fan-shaped muscle that originates from the temporal fossa of the parietal bone. Its fibers converge as they extend downward between the zygomatic arch and the lateral surface of skull to form a tendon that inserts onto the coronoid process and the anterior border of the ascending ramus.
   b. It is subdivided into three distinct areas according to fiber direction and ultimate function: the anterior vertical fibers, which raise the mandible vertically; the middle oblique fibers, which elevate and retrude the mandible; and the posterior horizontal fibers, which retrude the mandible. Collectively, the components of this muscle exert significant positioning force on the mandible.
3. Medial pterygoid muscle (see Figure 28-11)
   a. This muscle originates from the medial lip of the lateral pterygoid plate and extends downward, backward, and outward to insert along the medial surface of the mandibular angle.
   b. Along with the masseter, it forms a muscular sling that supports the mandible at the mandibular angle.

   c. Its function is to elevate the mandible. This muscle is also active in protruding the mandible. Unilateral contraction of the medial pterygoid muscle causes a mediotrusive movement of the mandible.
4. Lateral pterygoid muscle (see Figure 28-12)
   a. Inferior lateral pterygoid muscle
      (1). This muscle originates at the lateral lip of the lateral pterygoid plate and extends back, up, and out to attach to the neck of the condyle.
      (2). The muscle performs two functions: bilaterally, it pulls the condyles downward and forward; unilaterally it creates a mediotrusive movement on the condyle that causes a lateral movement of the mandible to the opposite side.
   b. Superior lateral pterygoid muscle
      (1). This muscle is considerably smaller than the inferior lateral pterygoid. It originates at the infratemporal surface of the greater sphenoid wing and extends horizontally backward and downward to attach to the articular capsule, the disc, and the neck of the condyle.
      (2). This muscle is active during the clo-

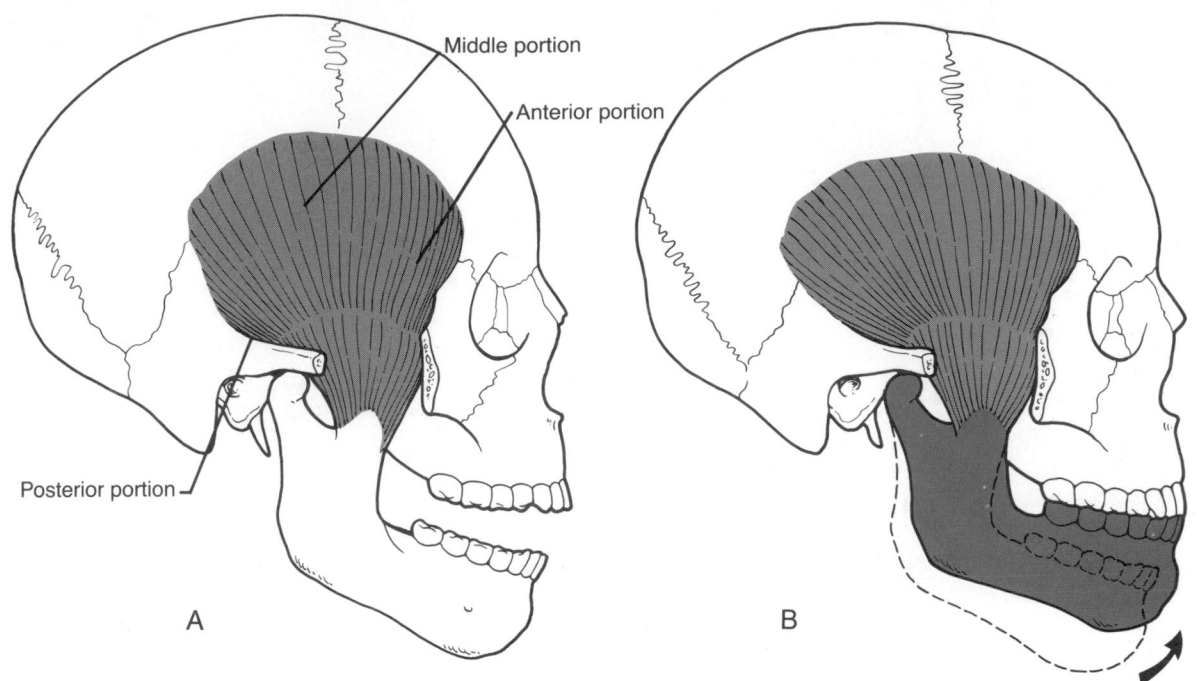

FIGURE 28–10   **A,** Temporalis muscle. **B,** This muscle elevates the mandible. The exact movement is determined by the location of the fibers being activated.

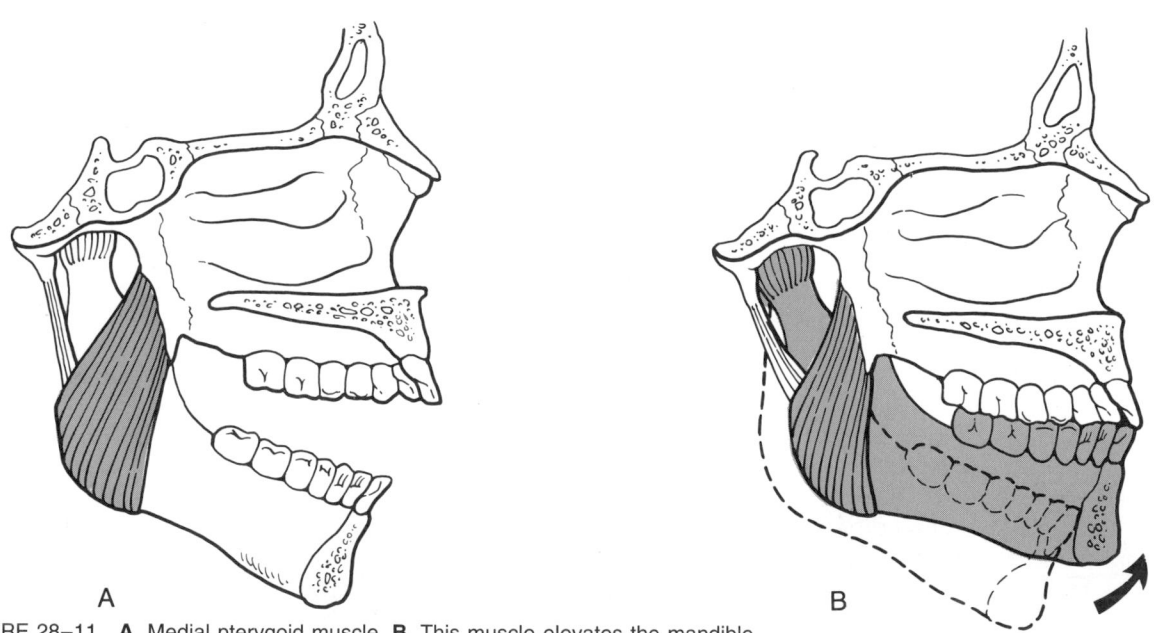

FIGURE 28–11   **A,** Medial pterygoid muscle. **B,** This muscle elevates the mandible.

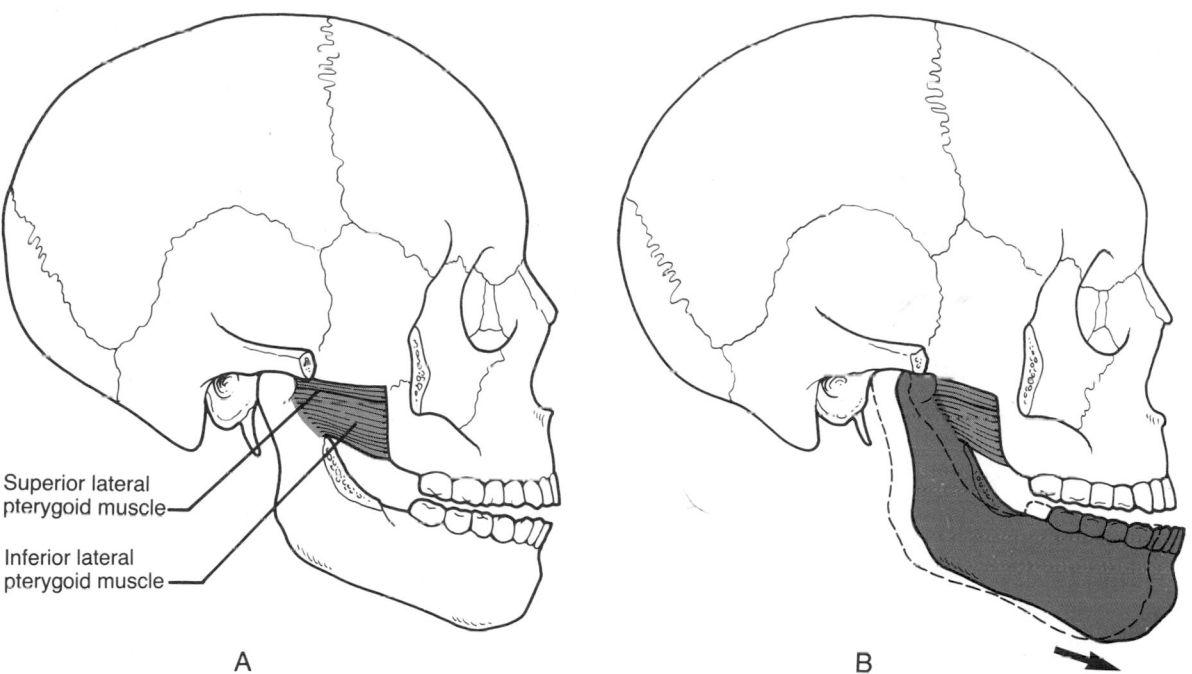

FIGURE 28–12 A, Inferior and superior lateral pterygoid muscles. **B,** The inferior lateral pterygoids cause protrusion of the mandible.

sure of the mandible against forms of resistance such as chewing and clenching of the teeth.

c. Lateral pterygoid muscles
   (1). These two muscles exert influence on the disc and the condyle in a significantly medial direction.
   (2). When the mouth is wide open, the direction of the muscle pull is almost entirely medial.

5. Digastric muscles (see Figure 28–13)
   a. Posterior belly
      (1). This muscle originates from the mastoid notch, just medial to the mastoid process. Its fibers run forward, downward, and inward to the intermediate tendinous attachment to the hyoid bone.
      (2). When bilateral contraction of the posterior belly occurs, the mandible is depressed and pulled back, and the teeth are brought out of contact.
      (3). This muscle assists in mandibular stabilization during swallowing.
   b. Anterior belly
      (1). The anterior belly originates at a fossa on the lingual surface of the mandible close to midline. Its fibers extend downward and backward to

attach to the same intermediate tendon as the posterior belly.
      (2). Bilateral contraction of this muscle tends to elevate the hyoid bone.

6. Buccinator muscle (see Figure 28–14)
   a. This muscle is thin, flat, and rectangular and is attached laterally to the alveolar processes of the maxilla and the mandible, opposite the molar teeth and the pterygomandibular raphe. Medially, its fibers blend with those of the orbicular muscle of the mouth.
   b. This muscle aids in mastication and swallowing by pressing the cheeks against the molar teeth during chewing; this action pushes the food against the occlusal surfaces of the teeth. The buccinator muscle is also used during whistling and sucking, *ie,* it forces the cheeks against the teeth.

E. Biomechanics of the TMJ

1. The TMJ is a compound joint.
   a. The TMJ is made up of bilateral joints that can simultaneously act separately; however, each joint cannot act without some influence from the other.
2. The TMJ comprises two distinct units.
   a. One unit is that of the condyle and the

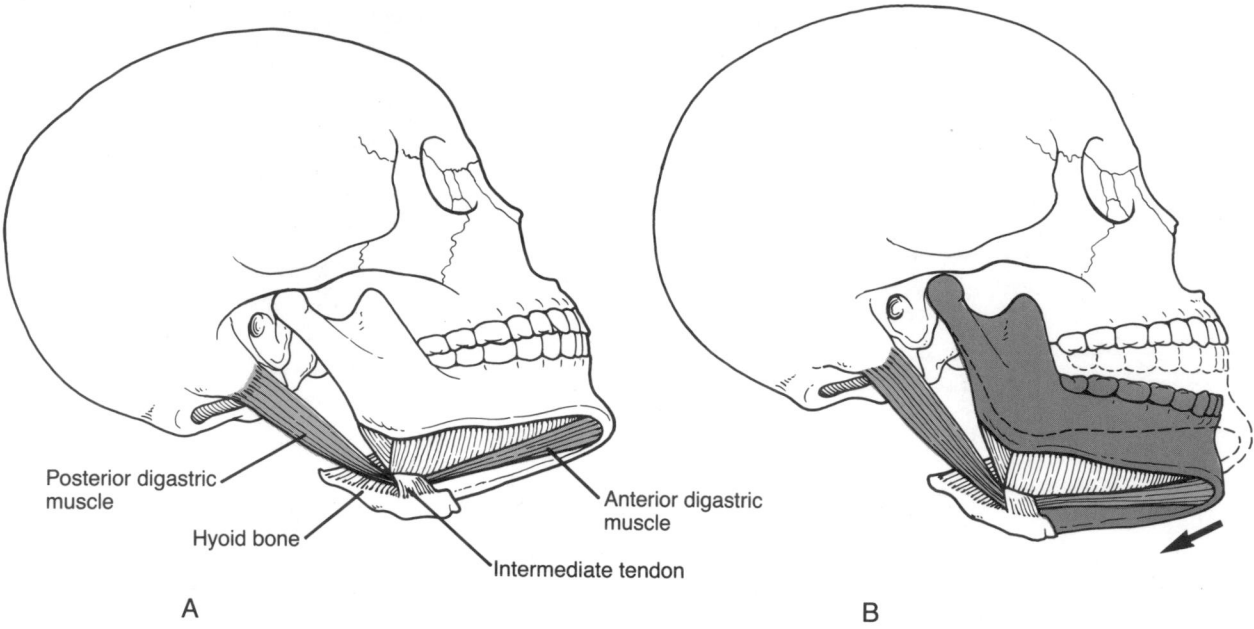

FIGURE 28–13 A, Digastric muscle. **B,** This muscle depresses the mandible.

articular disc (the space between them is the inferior synovial cavity). The disc is tightly bound to the condyle by the medial and lateral disc ligaments; the only physiologic movement that can occur is *rotation* of the disc on the articular surface of the condyle.

b. The other unit comprises the condyle-

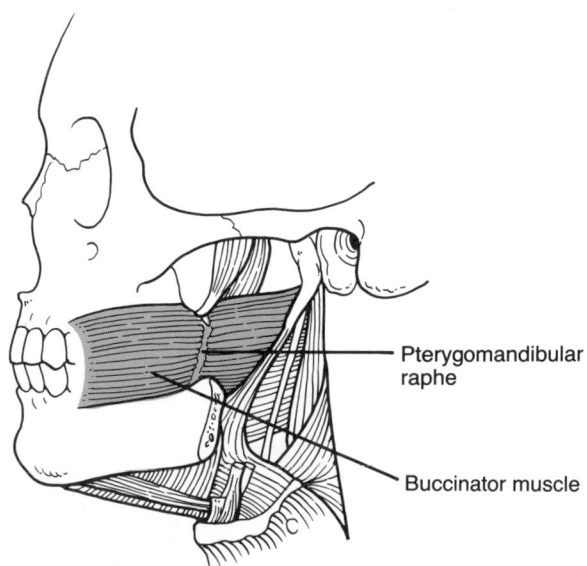

FIGURE 28–14 Buccinator muscle. This muscle positions boluses of food onto dentition.

disc complex, which is adjacent to the temporal bone (the space between these elements is the superior synovial cavity). The movement that occurs is the sliding of the joint between these surfaces; this motion is referred to as *translation*.

3. Disc
   a. When interarticular pressure is low, as in the closed resting position, disc space widens; when the pressure is high, as during clenching of the teeth, the disc space narrows. The contour and movement of the disc permit constant contact of the articular surfaces of the joint.
   b. As interarticular pressure increases, the condyle seats itself on the thinner, intermediate zone of the disc.
   c. When pressure is decreased and the disc space widens, a thicker portion of the disc is rotated to fill the space.
   d. The direction of disc rotation is determined by the superior bilaminar zone and the superior lateral pterygoid muscle.
   e. As the mandible moves into a full forward position and during its return to its resting position, the retraction force of the superior retrodiscal lamina holds the disc rotated as far posteriorly on the condyle as the width of the articular disc allows.

f. The disc is maintained with the translating condyle because of its discal attachments, its morphology, and the interarticular pressure.

g. At rest when the mouth is closed, the condyle normally is in contact with the intermediate and posterior zones of the disc.

h. The superior retrodiscal lamina is the only structure capable of retracting the disc posteriorly onto the condyle.

4. Condyle
   a. As the mandible moves into a full forward position and during its return to its resting position, the retraction force of the superior retrodiscal lamina holds the disc rotated as far posteriorly on the condyle as the width of the articular disc space allows.
   b. During translation, the combination of disc morphology and interarticular pressure maintains the condyle on the intermediate zone, and the disc is forced to translate forward with the condyle; only when the morphology of the disc has been altered does the ligamentous attachment of the disc affect joint function.
   c. During rotation, the condyle-disc complex is pulled downward and forward by the digastric muscles and the inferior lateral pterygoid muscle.
   d. As soon as the condyle has moved sufficiently forward to cause the retractive force of the superior retrodiscal lamina to be greater than the muscle tonus force of the superior lateral pterygoid muscle, the disc will be rotated posteriorly to the extent permitted by the width of the articular disc space.
   e. When the condyle is returned to the resting closed-joint position, the superior lateral pterygoid muscle becomes the predominant force, and the disc is repositioned forward as far as the disc space permits.

5. Function (see Figure 28–15)
   a. When resistance is met during mandibular closure, such as when the teeth bite down on hard food, the interarticular pressure on the biting side is decreased; this occurs because the force of closure is applied not to the joint but to the food.
   b. With the condyle moved forward and the disc space increased, the tension of the superior retrodiscal lamina tends to retract the disc from the functional position, which results in separation of the articular surfaces, resulting in dislocation.
   c. To avoid this, the superior lateral pterygoid muscle becomes active during the power stroke, rotating the disc forward onto the condyle so that the thicker posterior border of the disc maintains articular contact; this stabilizes the joint during the power stroke of chewing.
   d. As the teeth chew the food and approach intercuspation, the interarticular pressure is increased; as the pressure increases, the disc space decreases, with the disc mechanically rotated posteriorly so that the thinner intermediate zone fills the space.
   e. When the force of closure is discontinued, the resting joint position is once again assumed.

6. Orthopedic principles
   a. The ligaments do not actively participate in TMJ function—they restrict joint movements both mechanically and through neuromuscular reflex activity.
   b. The ligaments do not stretch; once ligaments have been elongated, joint function usually is compromised.
   c. The articular surfaces of the TMJ must be maintained in constant contact. This contact is produced by mandibular elevators (the masseter, temporalis, and medial pterygoid muscles).

II. Functional Neuroanatomy of the Masticatory System

A highly refined neurologic control system regulates and coordinates activities of the entire masticatory system. It consists primarily of nerves and muscles, hence, the term neuromuscular system.

A. Muscles
1. Motor unit
   a. Many muscle fibers are innervated by one motor neuron. This allows them to perform only one function—contraction.

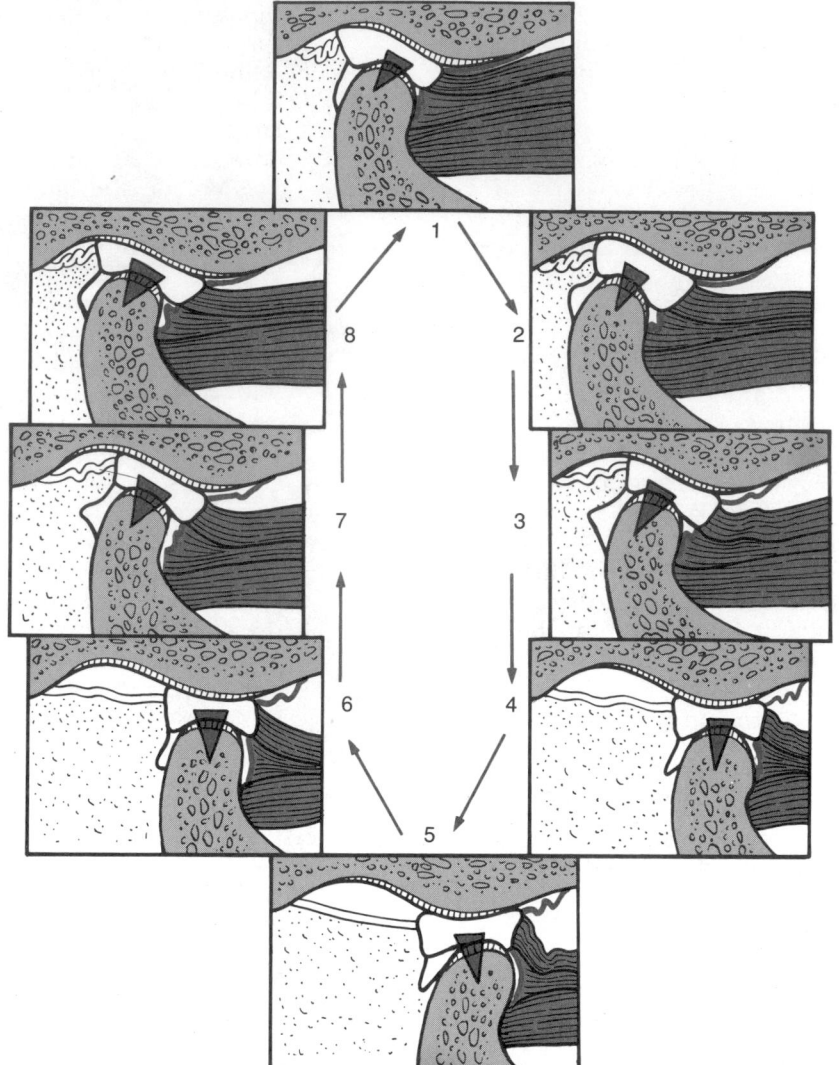

FIGURE 28–15   Normal functional movement of the condyle and disc during the full range of opening and closing. Note that the disc is rotated posteriorly on the condyle as the condyle is translated out of the fossa. The closing movement is the exact opposite of the opening movement.

b. The fewer the muscle fibers per motor neuron, the more precise the movement (*eg*, the lateral pterygoid muscle). Muscles with fewer fibers are capable of the fine adjustments in length needed to adapt the horizontal changes in the mandibular position.

c. The greater the number of muscle fibers per motor neuron, the more forceful the movement (*eg*, the masseter muscle). Muscles with more fibers are capable of providing the force necessary during chewing.

2. Function
   a. The muscles of the masticatory system have three potential functions:
      • Isotonic contraction. This function involves the shortening of a muscle under a constant load. The masseter muscle performs this function when the mandible is elevated.

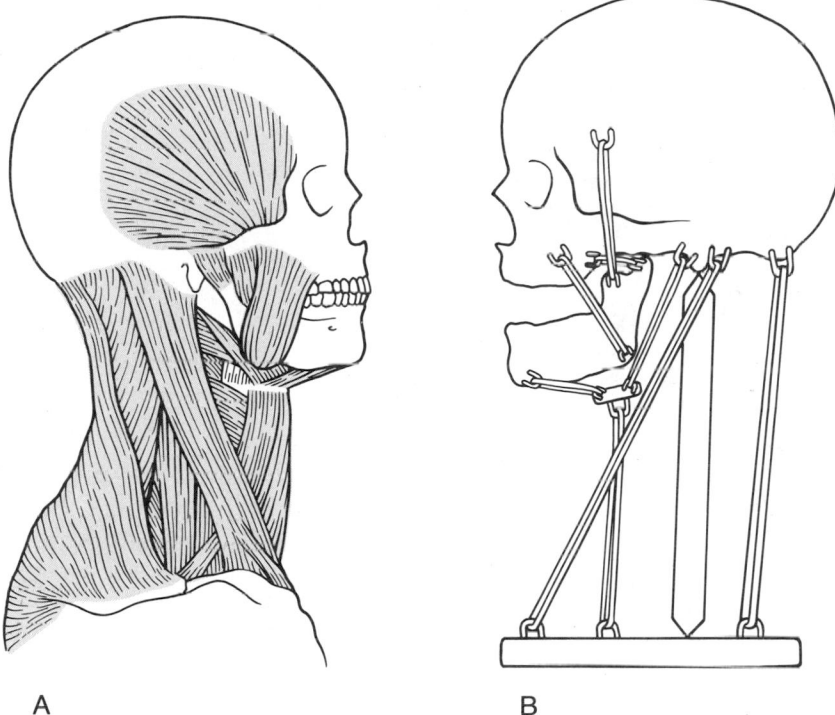

A   B

FIGURE 28–16   Precise and complex balance of the head and neck muscles must exist if proper head position and function are to be maintained. **A,** The muscle system. **B,** Each of the major muscles acts like an elastic band. The tension provided must precisely contribute to the balance that maintains the desired head position. If one elastic band breaks, the balance of the entire system is disrupted and the head position is altered. (Panels **A** and **B** from Okeson JP: *Management of Temporomandibular Disorders and Occlusion,* 3rd ed. St. Louis, Mosby Year Book, 1993, p 30.)

- Isometric contraction. This function entails muscle contraction without shortening. The masseter muscle performs this function when an object is held between the teeth.
- Eccentric contraction. This function involves the lengthening of a muscle. The masseter performs this function when the mouth opens to accept more food during mastication.
  b. If the head is turned to the right, certain muscles must shorten (isotonic contraction), others must relax (controlled eccentric relaxation), and still others must stabilize or maintain certain relationships (isometric contraction) (see Figure 28–16).

B. Neurologic structures

1. Sensory receptors
   a. **Muscle spindles.** These are specialized re-

ceptor organs that are found in muscle tissue; they monitor tension within the skeletal muscle and consist of contractile extrafusal fibers. These spindles make up the bulk of the masticatory muscle. Their cell bodies are located in the trigeminal motor nucleus.
   b. **Golgi tendon organs.** These receptors monitor tension and are located in the muscle tendon between the muscle fibers and their attachment to the bone.
   c. **Pacinian corpuscles.** These corpuscles monitor the perception of movement and firm pressure. They are found in the tendons, joints, periosteum, tendinous insertions, fascia, and subcutaneous tissue.
   d. **Nociceptors.** Nociceptors monitor the condition, position, and movement of the tissues in the masticatory system; some respond to noxious mechanical and ther-

FIGURE 28–17 The nociceptive reflex is activated by unexpected biting on a hard object. The noxious stimulus is initiated by stress directed toward the tooth and periodontal ligament. Afferent nerve fibers carry the impulse to the interneurons in the trigeminal motor nucleus. The afferent neurons stimulate both excitatory and inhibitory interneurons. The interneurons synapse with the efferent neurons in the trigeminal spinal tract nucleus. Inhibitory interneurons synapse with efferent fibers that lead to the elevator muscles. The message carried is to discontinue contraction. The excitatory interneurons synapse with the efferent neurons that innervate the jaw-depressing muscles. The message is to initiate contraction, which brings the teeth away from the noxious stimulus. (Redrawn from Sessle BJ: In Roth GI, Calmes R [eds]: *Oral Biology.* St. Louis, C. V. Mosby Company, 1981, p 61.)

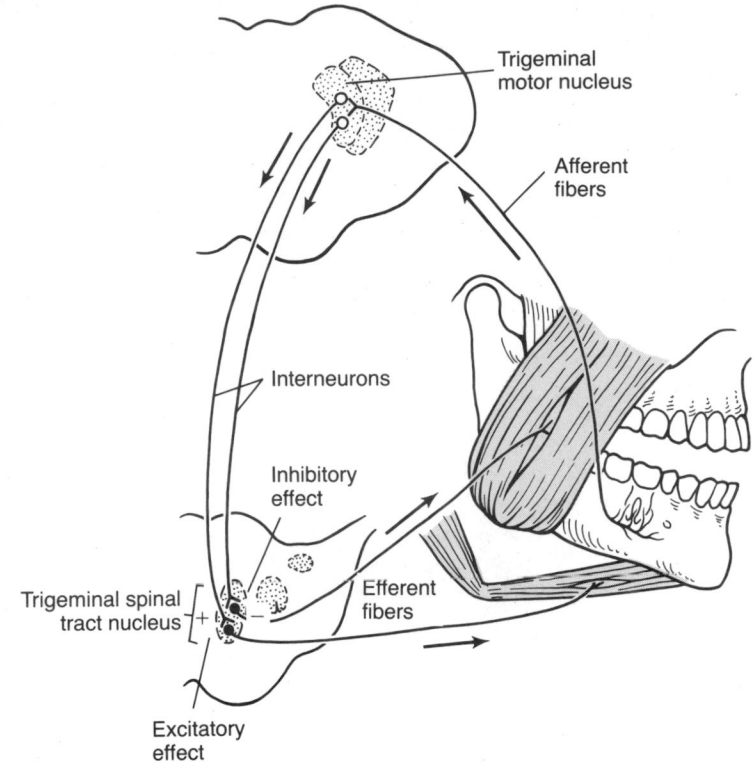

mal stimuli, others to noxious injury. Still others are low-threshold receptors for light touch, pressure, or facial hair movement. (The third type of receptor is also known as a *mechanoreceptor.*)

2. Function
   a. One function of the neurologic structures of the masticatory muscles is myotatic reflex. This is the only monosynaptic jaw reflex; a sudden downward tap on the chin causes the jaw to be reflexly elevated and the masseter to contract, resulting in tooth contact, which can be used to determine the resting position of the jaw.
   b. Another function of the muscles is nociceptive (flexor) reflex (see Figure 28–17). This is a polysynaptic reflex to noxious stimuli that is considered to be protective. This reflex occurs when a hard object is suddenly encountered during mastication; it protects the teeth and supportive structures from the damage that could occur from the sudden and unusually heavy functional forces that result.

C. Pain

1. Primary
   a. Primary pain occurs when the site and the source of the pain are in same location (*eg,* toothache).
2. Heterotrophic
   a. Central heterotrophic pain occurs in situations such as when a tumor is present in the central nervous system (CNS); the pain is often felt in the peripheral structures (*ie,* the neck, shoulders, or arms).
   b. Projected (radiating) heterotrophic pain occurs in situations such as when a nerve

is trapped in the cervical region; the pain is felt radiating down the arm to the hand.

c. Referred heterotrophic pain occurs in situations such as when myocardial infarct pain is felt in the neck and mandible.

Referred pain occurs within a single nerve root; can be felt outside the nerve responsible for it; moves cephalad; and occurs in the trigeminal area—referred pain never crosses the midline.

III. Functional Physiology of the Masticatory System

There are three major functions of the masticatory system: mastication, swallowing, and speech. Sensory input from the structures of the masticatory system is received and integrated with existing reflex actions and learned muscle activity to achieve a desired functional activity.

A. Mastication

1. Chewing stroke
   a. Each opening and closing of the mandible represents a chewing stroke.
   b. The complete chewing stroke has a movement that is described as being "tear shaped"[1] (see Figure 28–18). It can be divided into the closing phase and the opening phase.
      (1). Closing phase
         (a). Crushing is the first action that occurs during the closing phase; during crushing, the food is trapped between the teeth.
         (b). Grinding is the second action that occurs during the closing phase; during grinding, the bolus is trapped and the mandible is guided by the occlusal surfaces of the teeth back to the intercuspal position, which causes the cuspal inclines of the teeth to pass across each other. This motion permits the teeth to shear and grind the bolus of food.[2]
      (2). Opening phase
         (a). Gliding contact occurs as the cuspal inclines pass by each other during opening of the mouth and grinding. The mean percentage of gliding contacts during chewing is 60% during grinding and 56% during the opening phase.[3]
         (b). The molars move slightly forward during the opening phase.
2. Tooth contact
   a. In the final stages of mastication just before swallowing occurs, contacts occur during every stroke.[4]

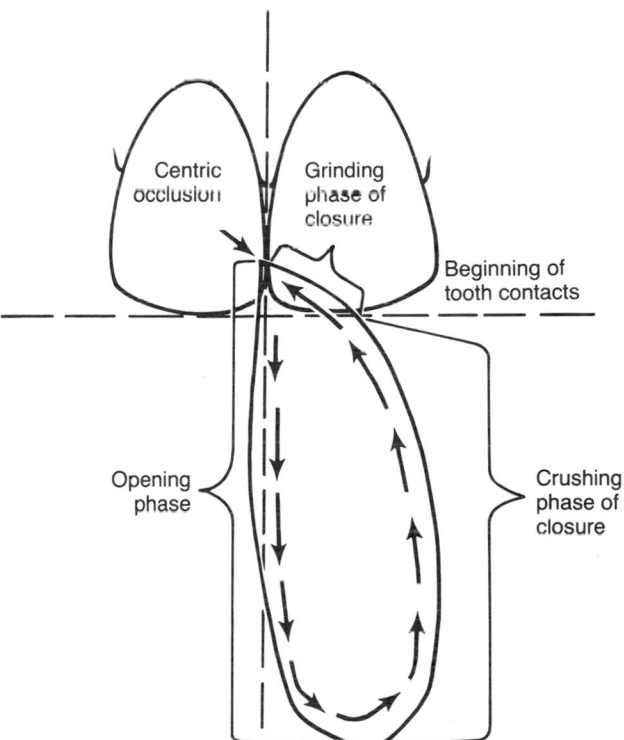

FIGURE 28–18 Frontal view of the chewing stroke. (From Okeson JP: *Management of Temporomandibular Disorders and Occlusion,* 3rd ed. St. Louis, Mosby Year Book, 1993, p 51.)

b. The average length of time for tooth contact during mastication is 194 milliseconds.[3]

c. During mastication, the quality and quantity of tooth contacts constantly relay information back to the CNS. This feedback system allows the chewing stroke to be altered according to the particular food being chewed.

d. Tall cusps and deep fossae promote a vertical chewing stroke, whereas flattened or worn teeth encourage a broader chewing stroke.

e. Normal chewing strokes are well rounded with definite limits and are repeated less frequently. TMJ dysfunction results in shorter and slower strokes with irregular pathways and more repetitive patterns; these irregular movements appear to be related to the altered functional movement of the condyle around which disorder is centered.[5]

3. Forces

a. Women have a maximum biting load that ranges from 79 to 99 lbs; men have a maximum biting load that varies from 118 to 142 lbs. The highest recorded maximum biting force is 975 lbs.[6]

b. The average range of maximum force applied to the first molar is 91 to 198 lbs, whereas the average maximum force applied to the central incisor is 29 to 51 lbs.[7]

c. Increased biting strength appears to be attributable to facial skeletal relationships.[8]

d. During chewing, the greatest amount of force is placed on the first molar.[9]

4. Soft tissue

a. The lips guide and control the intake of food and liquids and seal off the oral cavity.

b. The tongue maneuvers food in the oral cavity to promote efficient chewing; initiates the process of food breakdown by pressing it against the hard palate; pushes food onto the occlusal surfaces of the teeth; repositions partially crushed food onto the teeth for further breakdown; and sweeps the teeth to remove any food residue that is trapped in the oral cavity.

c. The buccinator muscle positions and repositions boluses of food onto the occlu-

sal surfaces of the teeth from the buccal sides of the mouth.

B. Swallowing (deglutition)

1. Stages (see Figure 28–19)

a. First stage. During the first stage, voluntary lip closure occurs, and the teeth are brought into maximum intercuspal position to stabilize the mandible (somatic swallowing). Infantile swallowing (visceral swallowing) occurs when the mandible is braced by the tongue as it is placed forward between the dental arches or gum pads; over-retention of the habit of infantile swallowing can result in the lateral displacement of the anterior teeth, which may cause an anterior open bite.

b. Second stage. This stage is involuntary; once the bolus of food has reached the pharynx, a peristaltic wave caused by the contraction of the pharyngeal constrictor muscles carries it down the esophagus. The soft palate rises to touch the posterior pharyngeal wall, sealing off the nasal passage, and the epiglottis blocks the pharyngeal airway to the trachea and keeps the food in the esophagus. These first two stages of swallowing last about 1 second.

c. Third stage. During the third stage, reflex muscular activity occurs, allowing the bolus to pass through the length of the esophagus into the stomach via peristaltic waves; this takes about 6 to 7 seconds. Studies have documented that the swallowing cycle occurs approximately 590 times during a 24-hour period: 146 cycles during eating, 394 cycles between meals during the waking hours, and 50 cycles during sleep. (Lower levels of saliva during sleep result in a decreased need for swallowing.)[10]

C. Speech

1. Articulation of sound

a. The relationship of the lips and tongue to the palate and teeth varies.

b. The controlled contraction and relaxation of the vocal cords or bands of the larynx create a sound with a desired pitch.[11]

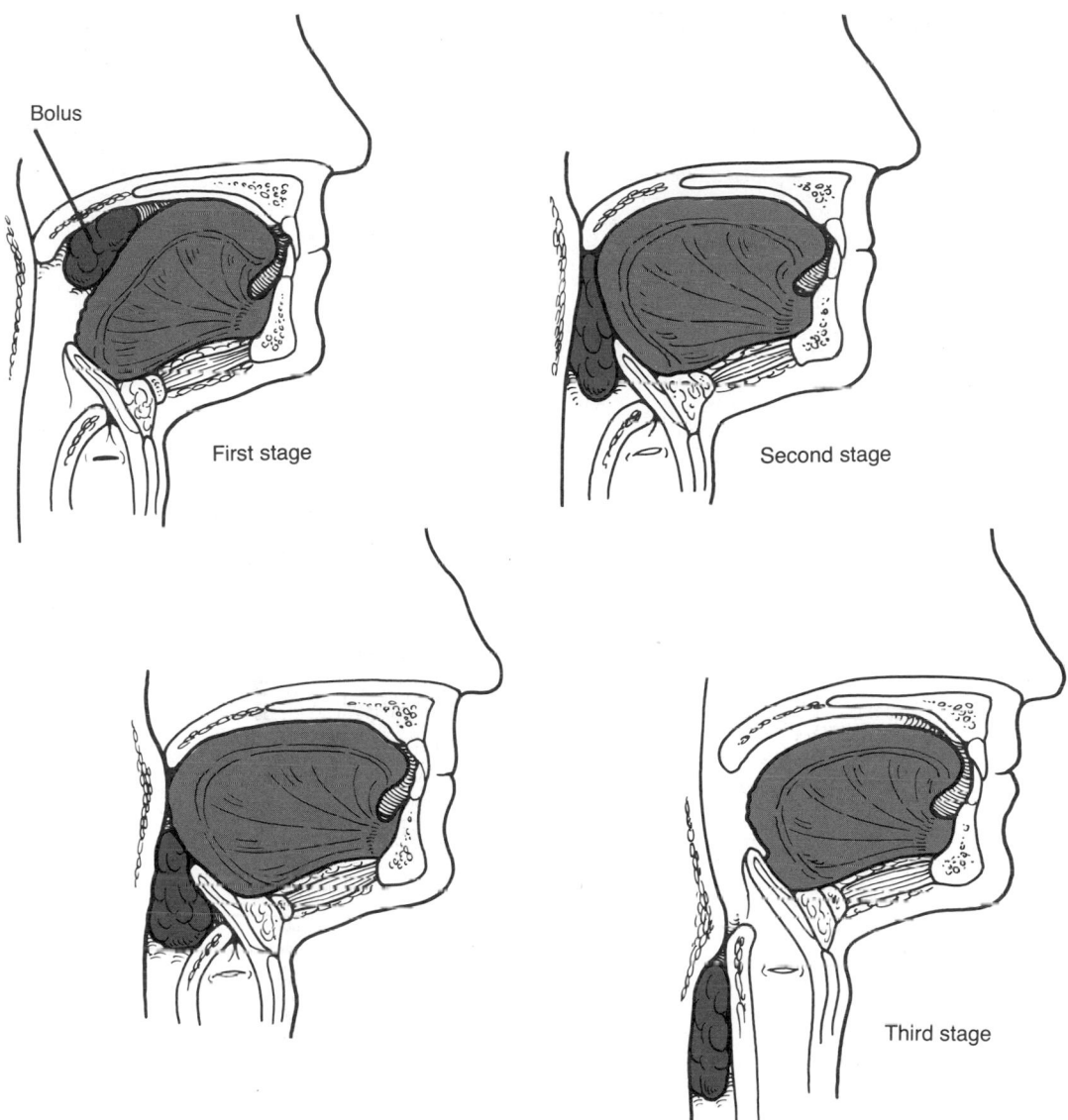

Bolus

First stage

Second stage

Third stage

FIGURE 28–19   The three stages of swallowing.

c. The sounds for *m*, *b*, and *p* are formed by the lips as they come together and touch.

d. The sound for *s* is made when the incisal edges of the maxillary and mandibular teeth approximate one another and air is passed between the teeth.

e. The sound for *d* is articulated when the tip of the tongue reaches up to touch the palate directly behind the incisors.

f. When the sound of *th* is made, the tongue touches the maxillary incisors.

g. The sounds for *f* and *v* are formed when the lower lip touches the incisal edges of the maxillary teeth.

h. The sounds for *k* and *g* are articulated when the posterior portion of the tongue rises to touch the soft palate.

2. As a learned reflex. Once speech becomes a pattern of reflexive response, it becomes controlled unconsciously by the neuromuscular system.

IV. Mechanics of Mandibular Movement

Mandibular movement occurs as the result of a complex series of inter-related three-dimensional rotational and translational activities determined by the combined and simultaneous activities of both TMJs.

A. Types of movement

1. Rotation
    a. Rotation occurs when the mouth opens and closes around a fixed point (axis) within the condyles.
    b. It occurs as a movement within the inferior cavity of the joint between the superior surface of the condyle and the inferior surface of the articular disk.
    c. Rotation can occur in all three reference planes: horizontal, frontal, and sagittal.
        (1). In the horizontal axis, rotation occurs as an opening and closing motion that is referred to as the *hinge axis* (see Figure 28–20).
        (2). In the frontal (vertical) axis, rotation occurs when one condyle moves anteriorly out of the terminal hinge position and the vertical axis of the opposite condyle remains in the terminal hinge position (see Figure 28–21).

        (3). In the sagittal axis, rotation occurs when one condyle moves inferiorly while the other remains in the terminal position (see Figure 28–22).
2. Translation (see Figure 28–23)
    a. Translation occurs when the mandible moves forward.

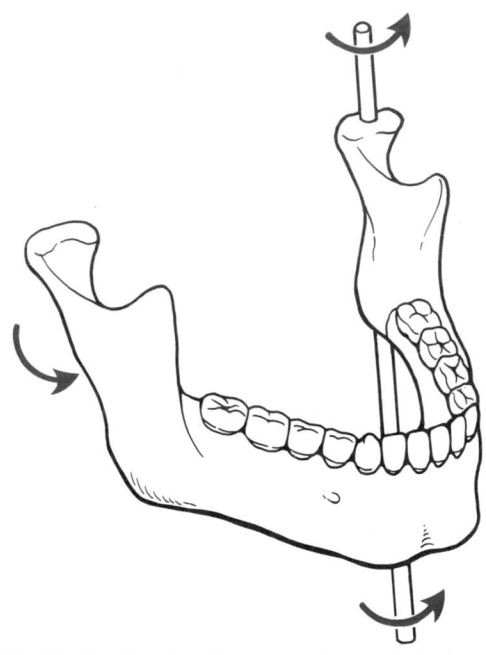

FIGURE 28–21   Rotational movement around the frontal (vertical) axis.

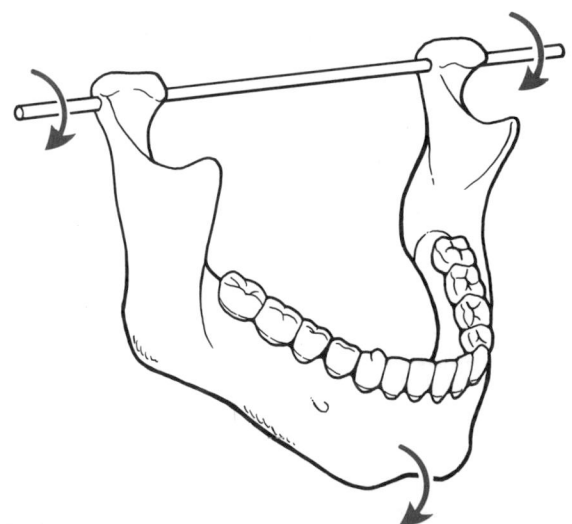

FIGURE 28–20   Rotational movement around the horizontal axis.

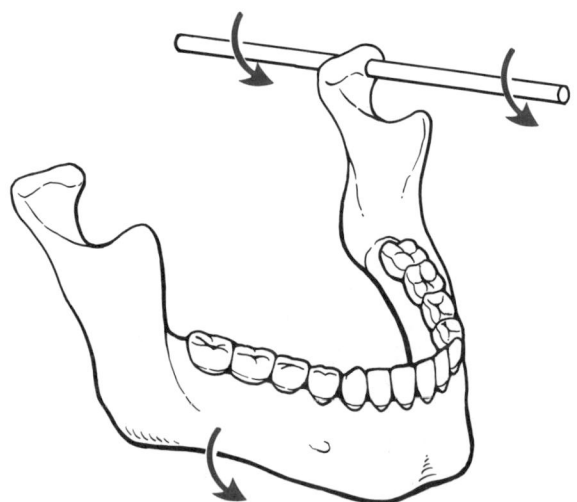

FIGURE 28–22   Rotational movement around the sagittal axis.

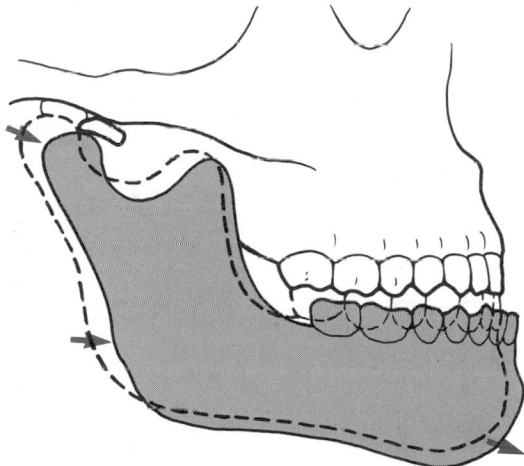

FIGURE 28–23   Translational movement of the mandible.

b. The teeth, condyles, and rami all move in the same direction and to the same degree.

c. Translation occurs within the superior cavity of the joint between the superior surface of the articular disc and the inferior surface of the articular fossa (*ie*, between the disc-condyle complex and the articular fossa).

B. Border movements

1. Sagittal plane

   a. Posterior opening border movements occur as two-stage hinging movements. During the first stage, pure rotational opening can occur until the anterior teeth are 20 to 25 mm apart; during the second stage, the condyle is translated down the articular eminence as the mouth rotates open in the range of 40 to 60 mm.

   b. Anterior opening border movements occur when the mandible is maximally opened. Closure is accompanied by contraction of the inferior lateral pterygoid muscles, which keep the condyles positioned anteriorly.

   c. Superior contact border movements are determined by the characteristics of the occluding surfaces of the teeth. The precise delineation of these movements depends on

      • the amount of variation between the centric relation and the centric occlusion.

• the steepness of the cuspal inclines of the posterior teeth.
• the amounts of vertical and horizontal overlap of the anterior teeth.
• the lingual morphology of the maxillary anterior teeth.
• the general interarch relationships of the teeth.

2. Horizontal plane

   a. Mandibular movements in this plane are measured with a Gothic arch tracer (a recording plate attached to the maxillary teeth and a recording stylus attached to the mandibular teeth).

   b. As the mandible moves, the stylus attached to the mandibular teeth generates a pathway on the recording plate attached to the maxillary teeth.

   c. A rhomboid-shaped pattern that has four distinct movement components can be seen. These components are
      • left lateral border.
      • continued left lateral border with protrusion.
      • right lateral border.
      • continued right lateral border with protrusion.[12]

3. Frontal plane

   a. A shield-shaped pattern with four distinct movement components can be seen (see Figure 28–24). These components are
      • left lateral superior border (see Figure 28–25).

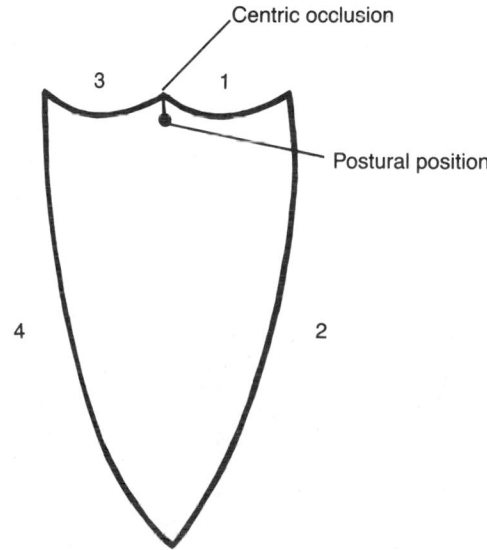

FIGURE 28–24   Mandibular border movements in the frontal plane. 1, left lateral superior; 2, left lateral opening; 3, right lateral superior; 4, right lateral opening.

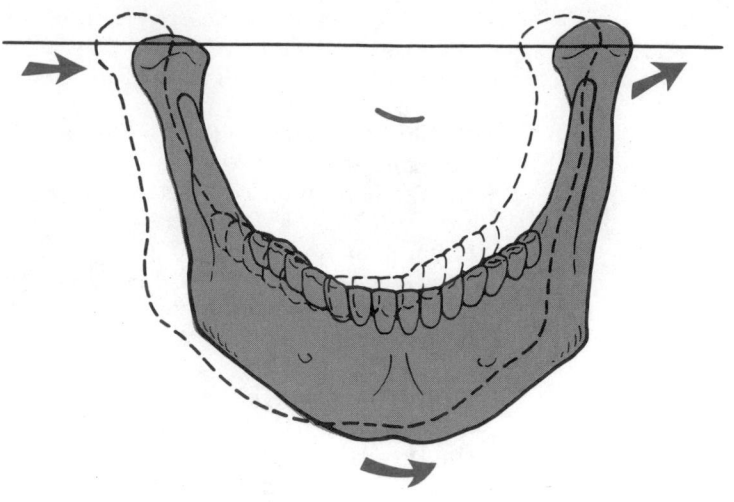

FIGURE 28–25 Left lateral superior border movement recorded in the frontal plane.

• left lateral opening border (see Figure 28–26).
• right lateral superior border (see Figure 28–27).
• right lateral opening border (see Figure 28–28).

C. Functional movements

1. Sagittal plane
   a. At rest, the mandible is open 2 to 4 mm and it is in a position below centric occlusion; this is the clinical rest position.
   b. In this position, the teeth can quickly and effectively be brought together for immediate function.
   c. With the head upright, the teeth are elevated directly into centric occlusion from the postural position.
   d. With the head posteriorly angled 45 degrees, the postural position of the mandible becomes more posterior—this is the drinking posture.[13]
   e. With the head angled forward 30 degrees (this is the alert feeding position), the mandible becomes more anterior.
2. Horizontal plane
   a. The horizontal plane most often occurs near the centric occlusion position.
   b. The range of jaw movements begins at a

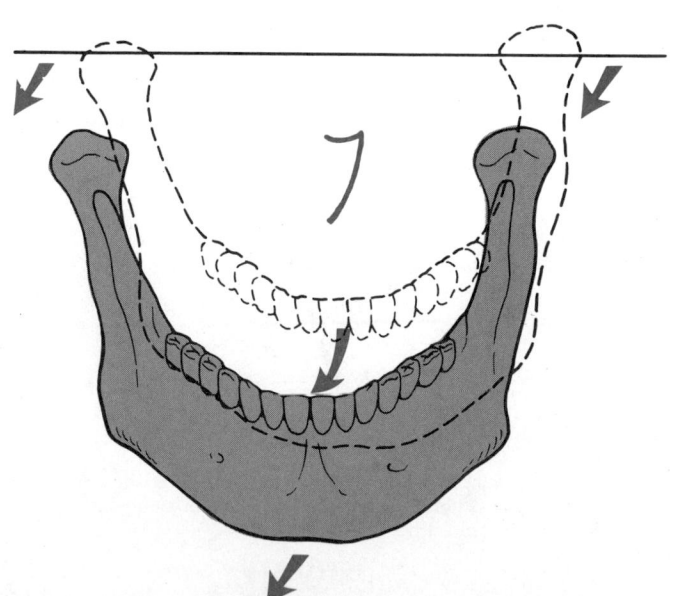

FIGURE 28–26 Left lateral opening border movement recorded in the frontal plane.

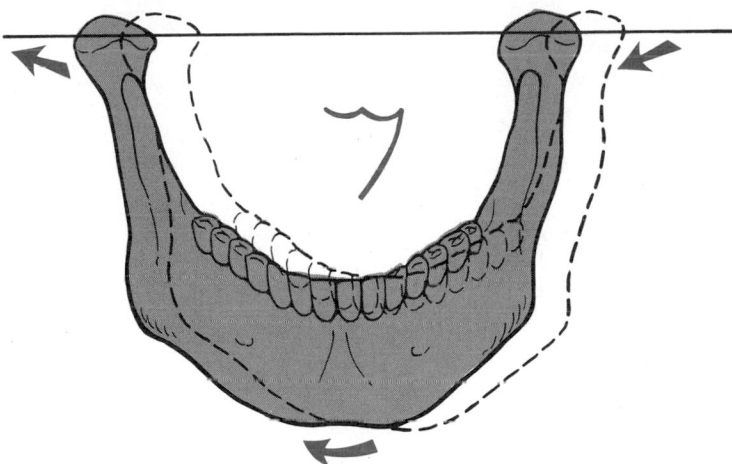

FIGURE 28–27 Right lateral superior border movement recorded in the frontal plane.

moderate distance from centric occlusion; as food is broken down, the jaw position moves closer and closer to centric occlusion.

3. Frontal (vertical) plane
   a. The frontal plane begins and ends at the centric occlusion position.
   b. During chewing, the mandible drops inferiorly until the desired opening is achieved; it then shifts to the side of the bolus and rises up.
   c. As the mandible approaches centric occlusion, the bolus is broken down between the opposing teeth.
   d. During the final millimeters of closure,

the mandible quickly shifts back to a position of centric occlusion.

D. Three-dimensional movement

1. An example of three-dimensional movement is right lateral excursion.
   a. The mandible moves to the right, and the left condyle is propelled out of its centric relation position.
   b. The left condyle orbits anteriorly around the frontal axis of the right condyle.
   c. The left condyle encounters a posterior slope or an articular eminence; this causes an inferior movement of the con-

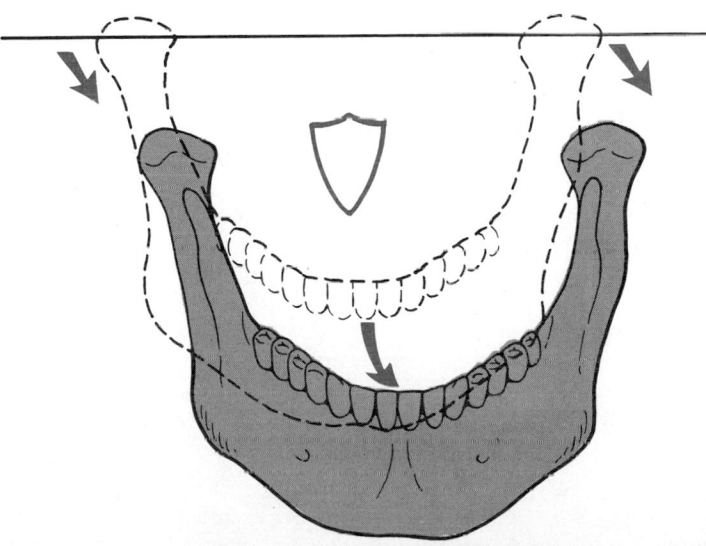

FIGURE 28–28 Right lateral opening border movement recorded in the frontal plane.

dyle around the sagittal axis, resulting in tilting of the frontal axis.

   d. Because the left condyle is moving anteriorly and inferiorly, the horizontal axis also is shifting anteriorly and inferiorly.

   e. During this simple lateral movement, motion occurs around each of the three axes; simultaneously, each axis tilts to accommodate the movement occurring around the other axes.

   f. The mechanism is intricately controlled by the neuromuscular system.

V. Craniomandibular Disorders

A. Etiology of functional disturbances in the masticatory system

During functional activities of the masticatory system, neuromuscular reflexes actively protect the teeth and other structures from damage. Often, an interruption of this protection occurs, leading to functional disturbances.

1. Malocclusion
   a. Functional malocclusion is influenced by alteration of the occlusal condition.
   b. Parafunctional malocclusion is provoked by abnormal tooth contact.
      (1). The following abnormal oral habits can be a factor:
      - cheek and tongue biting.
      - finger and thumb sucking.
      - unusual postural habits.
      - biting of pencils, pins, or fingernails.
      (2). Bruxism also can be a factor and includes excessive and unwarranted clenching and grinding of the teeth.
2. Stress
   a. Emotional stress refers to the degree of psychologic stress experienced by a patient.
   b. Physiologic tolerance is influenced by diet, general body health, and fatigue.
   c. Structural tolerance relates to the point at which physical breakdown begins (*eg*, with the unilateral loss of the posterior teeth, the force of parafunctional activity to the joint on the unsupported side is much greater than that on the contralateral side).
3. Cyclic effect of emotional stress. Malocclusion can lead to emotional stress, which can cause an increase in muscle hyperactivity. This may result in physical breakdown that causes pain and dysfunction, which in turn may lead to increased emotional stress and further malocclusion.
4. Trauma
5. Systemic diseases
6. Developmental disorders

B. Signs and symptoms of craniomandibular disorders

Each of the major sites of potential physical breakdown is discussed in this section. These include the muscles, the TMJs, and the dentition. The associated etiologic factors that either cause or contribute to each disorder also are discussed.

1. Muscles
   a. Muscle splinting
      (1). Splinting is an involuntary CNS-induced hypertonic condition.
      (2). It is caused by an alteration in sensory or proprioceptive input to the CNS.[14]
      (3). Splinting is a normal attempt by the musculoskeletal system to stabilize and protect a part of itself from damage.
      (4). Two major factors in the etiology of splinting are changes in the oral condition and stress.
         (a). Splinting can result from any change in the oral condition, such as the mouth's opening too wide during a long dental examination.
         (b). Increased emotional stress also can cause splinting through the mechanisms of muscle hyperactivity (*eg*, bruxism).

(5). The clinical symptoms of splinting are myalgia and muscle weakness.

b. Myospasms

(1). Myospasms are involuntary CNS-induced continual muscular contractions.[14]

(2). They result in clinical shortening of the muscles.

(3). The three major causes are splinting, increased emotional stress, and constant deep pain.

(4). The clinical symptoms of myospasms are as follow:
- Pain increases during use of the muscles.
- Structural dysfunction of the muscles is present.
- A reduction of muscle length occurs.
- A reduction of mandibular movement is seen.
- The symptoms are usually present for more than 2 to 3 days.
- The symptoms may come and go with changes in a patient's stress level.

c. Myositis

(1). Myositis is an inflammatory condition of the muscle tissue.

(2). The two major causes of myositis are protracted myospasms and spreading infection.

(3). The main clinical symptom is constant pain.

d. Myofascial trigger point pain

(1). This type of pain arises from hypersensitive areas in the muscles called trigger points.

(2). A very circumscribed region is involved, and relatively few motor units contract.

(3). Palpation of the taut bands elicits pain.

(4). Certain nerve endings in the muscle tissues may become sensitized by algogenic substances that create a localized zone of hypersensitivity.[15]

(5). This is a source of deep, chronic pain.

(6). The major causes of myofascial trigger point pain are muscle stress, increased emotional stress, and the spontaneous development of the symptoms.

(7). The clinical symptoms of this type of pain are as follows:
- Palpable tenderness.
- Referred pain (*eg*, trigger point pain in the trapezius muscle refers "headache" pain to the temporal region) (see Figure 28–29).
- Trigger points in the shoulder or cervical muscles produce spasms in the masticatory muscles.[16]

2. TMJ derangement of the condyle-disc complex

(1). A single click (see Figure 28–30) is a sign that the disc could stick or be bunched slightly, causing an abrupt movement of the condyle over the disc into a normal condyle-disc relationship.

(2). A reciprocal click (see Figure 28–31) occurs:
- During mandibular opening, the click that is heard indicates that the condyle is moving across the posterior border of the disc to its normal position on the intermediate zone.

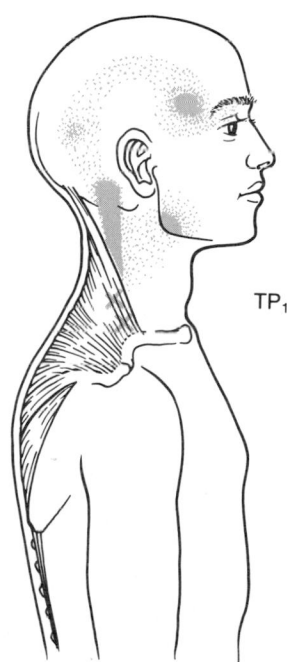

FIGURE 28–29 Note how trigger points (TP₁) located in the trapezius muscle (marked with X) refer pain to behind the ear, the temple, and the angle of the jaw. (Redrawn from Travell JG, Simons DG: *Myofascial Pain and Dysfunction: the Trigger Point Manual.* Baltimore, Williams & Wilkins, 1983, p 184.)

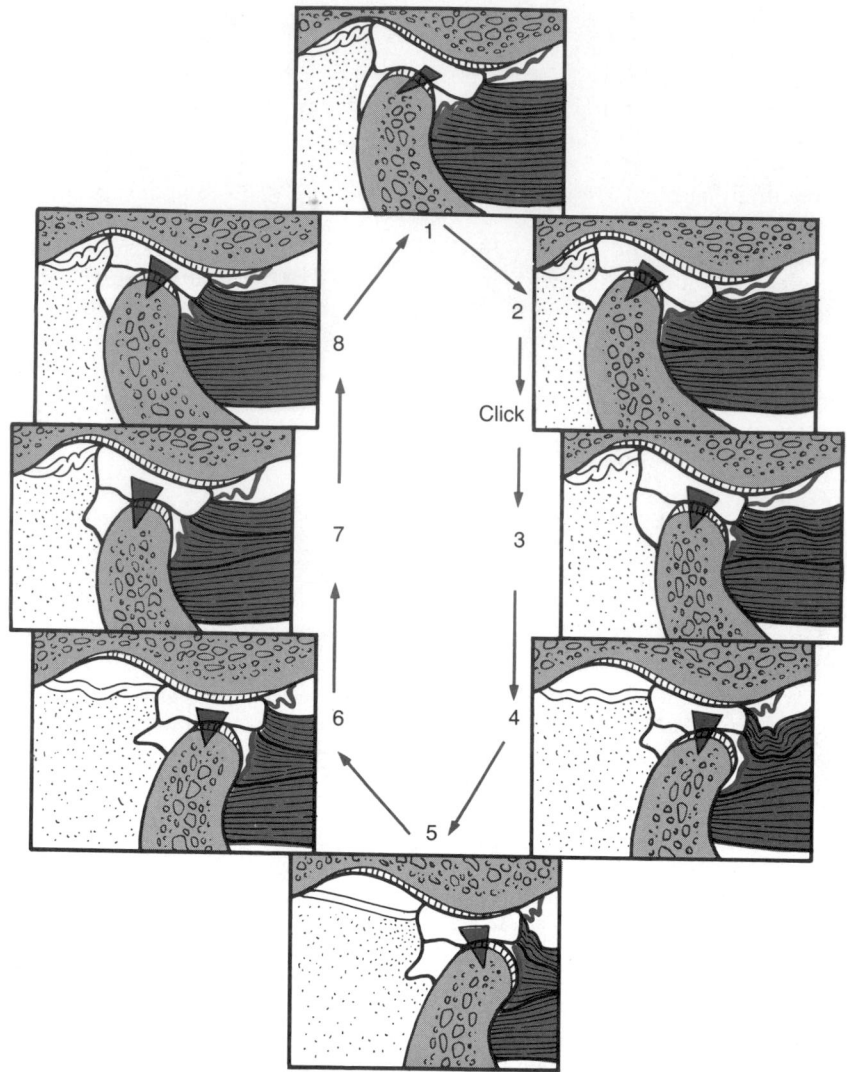

FIGURE 28–30   Single click. Between positions 2 and 3, a click is felt as the condyle moves across the posterior border into the intermediate zone of the disc. Normal condyle-disc function occurs during the remaining opening and closing movement. In the closed joint position (1), the disc is again displaced forward (and medially) by activity of the superior lateral pterygoid muscle.

• During closing, the normal disc position is maintained until the condyle returns to very near the closed joint position.

• As the closed joint position is approached, the posterior pull of the superior retrodiscal lamina is decreased.

• The combination of the disc morphology and the pull of the superior lateral pterygoid muscle allows the disc to slip back into a more anterior position; this final movement of the condyle across the posterior border of the disc creates a second clicking sound (a *reciprocal* click).

(3). Functional dislocation of the disc with reduction (see Figure 28–32) has the following features:

• Limitation of opening.

• Anteromedial positioning of the disc.

• No joint sounds.

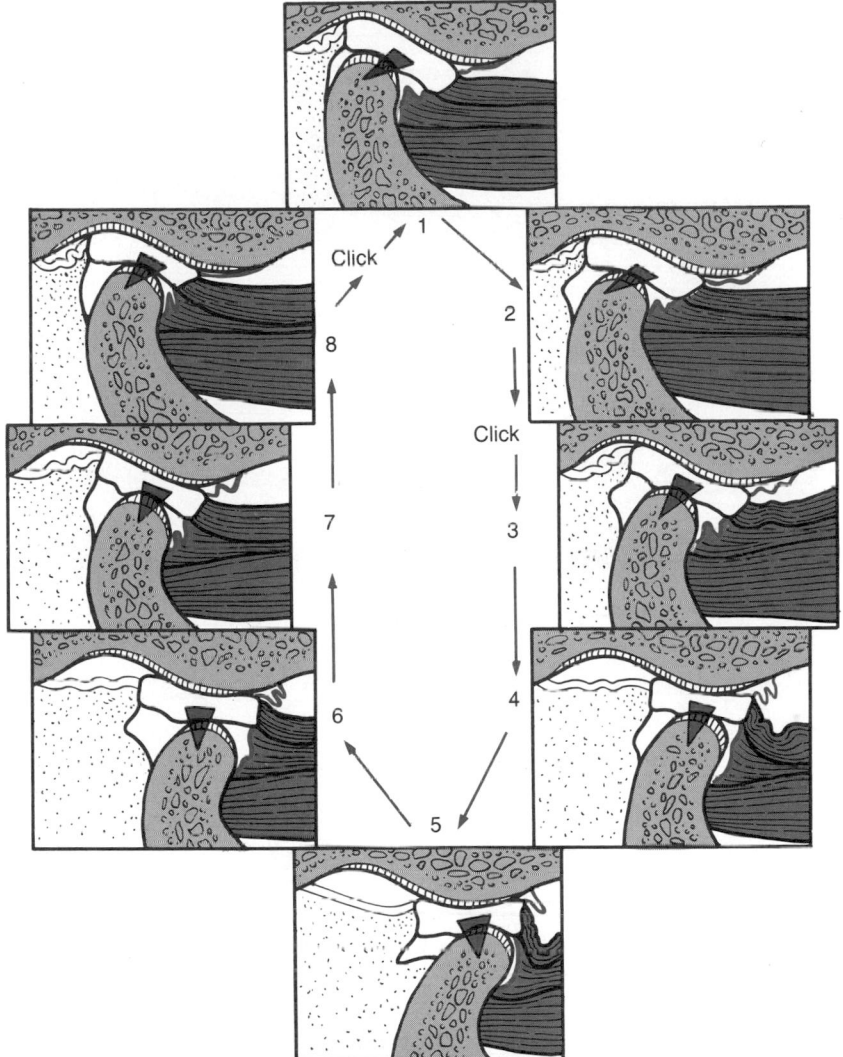

FIGURE 28–31   Reciprocal click. Between positions 2 and 3, a click is felt as the condyle moves across the posterior border of the disc. Normal condyle-disc function occurs during the remaining opening and closing movement until the closed joint position is approached. A second click is heard as the condyle once again moves from the intermediate zone to the posterior border of the disc (between positions 8 and 1).

- Occasional locking.
- The ability of the patient to resolve with no assistance.
- The patient's jaw "catching."
- Arthralgic pain associated with elongation of the joint ligaments.

(1). Functional dislocation of the disc without reduction (see Figure 28–33) is defined as follows:
- The limitation of opening is 25 mm interincisally.
- The midline of the mandible is deflected to the affected side.
- Lateral movement to the unaffected side is restricted.

b. Another type of craniomandibular dysfunction is the structural incompatibility of articular surfaces.
(1). Weeping lubrication of synovial fluid can exhaust the joint's required supply of lubrication, resulting in the sticking of articular surfaces.
(2). Static loading of the joint occurs commonly with muscle hyperactivity (clenching).
(3). Clicks caused by adhesions can be

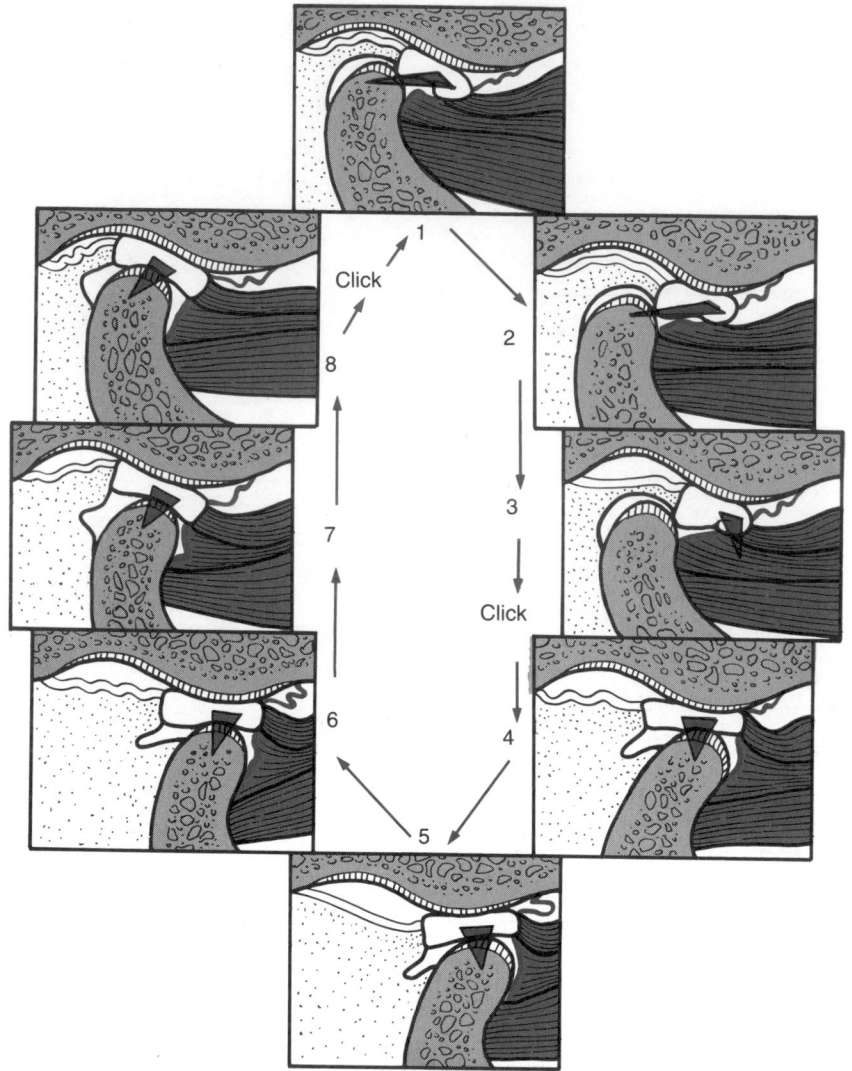

FIGURE 28–32   Functional dislocation of the disc with reduction. Note that during opening, the condyle passes over the posterior border of the disc onto the intermediate area of the disc, thus reducing the dislocated disc.

differentiated from clicks associated with disc displacements because they occur only once following a period of static loading.

(4). *Adhesions* can occur between the disc and the condyle, as well as between the disc and fossa.

  (a). When adhesions occur in the inferior joint space, rotation is limited—this condition is similar to closed lock.

  (b). When adhesions occur in the superior joint space, translation is limited—this condition is similar to closed lock.

(5). Subluxation may occur.

  (a). The articular eminence has a short, steep posterior slope and a longer, flatter anterior slope.

  (b). The anterior slope is more superior than the crest of the eminence.

  (c). The maximum rotational movement of the disc is reached before the maximum translation of the condyle.

  (d). The last portion of the translatory movement occurs with a bodily shift of the condyle and the disc as a unit.

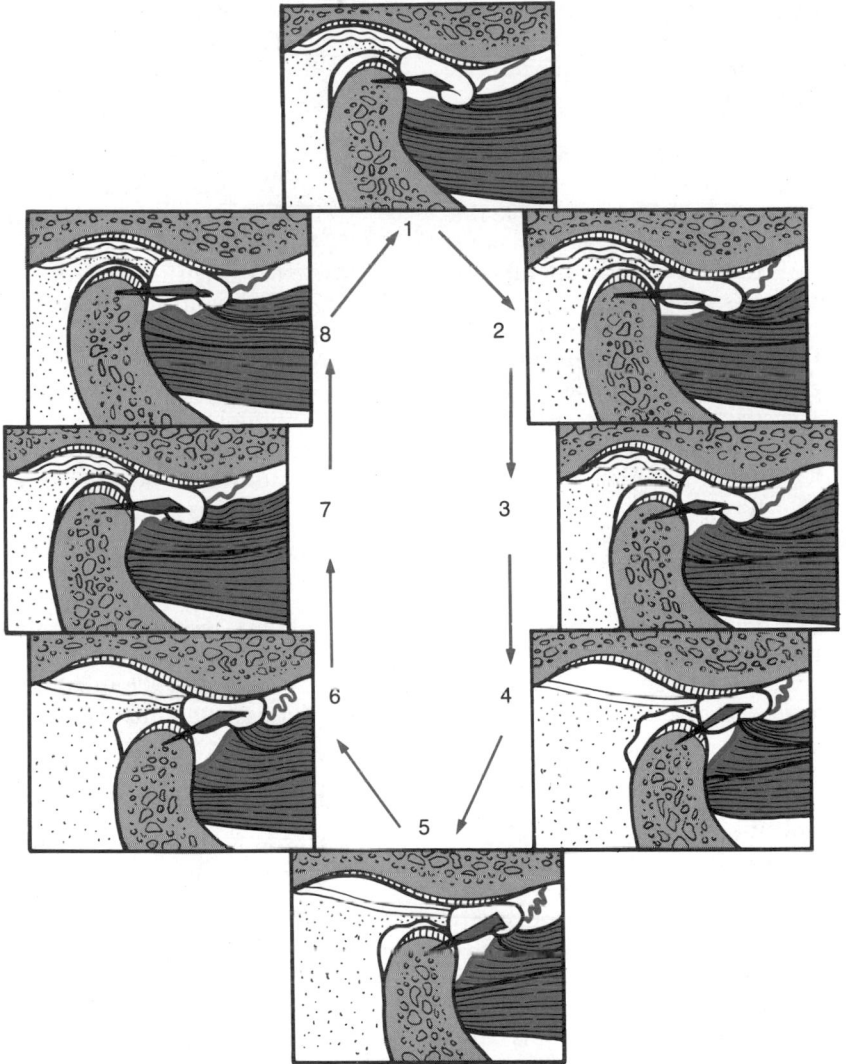

FIGURE 28–33 Closed lock. Note that the condyle never assumes a normal relationship on the disc but instead causes the disc to move forward ahead of it. This condition limits the distance it can translate forward.

(e). This creates a quick forward leap and a thud of the condyle-disc complex.[17]

(6). Spontaneous dislocation may be present.

 (a). "Open lock" is a condition in which the mouth is opened beyond its normal limits and the mandible locks open.

 (b). The patient cannot close his/her mouth.

 (c). The anterior slope of the articular eminence is more superior than the crest; therefore, the locking is mechanical in the open-mouth position.

c. Factors that predispose a patient to disc-interference disorders.

 (1). The degree of steepness of the articular eminence may contribute to the severity of disc-interference disorders.

 (a). A flat eminence results in a minimal amount of posterior rotation of the disc on the condyle during opening.

 (b). A steep eminence causes significant posterior rotation of the disc on the condyle during opening; this results in a high incidence of disc-interference disorders.

(2). The morphology of the condyle and the temporal bone is another contributing factor.

(a). A flat condyle or a gable-like condyle that articulates against inverted V-shaped temporal components seems to have an increased incidence of disc-interference disorders and degenerative joint disease.

(b). A steep articular eminence seems to have a relationship to a higher incidence of disc-interference disorders.

(3). Joint laxity is a factor in these disorders. Women typically display greater ligamentous laxity than men.[18,19]

(4). Variations of superior lateral pterygoid muscle attachment may contribute to the severity of these disorders.

d. Inflammatory disorders are another type of craniomandibular disorder.

(1). One specific inflammatory disorder is capsulitis. The symptoms are tenderness at the lateral pole of the condyle and pain during the opening of the mouth.

(2). Retrodiscitis, a constant dull aching pain that is increased by clenching, is another inflammatory disorder.

(3). A third disorder is degenerative joint disease. The symptoms are pain that is accentuated by jaw movement and, commonly, crepitation. This disorder can occur anytime the joint is overloaded; this causes surfaces to erode and flatten.[20]

(4). Inflammatory arthritis is another inflammatory disorder, which results in true inflammation caused by trauma or infection; it may also develop as a result of systemic conditions.

3. Functional disorders of the dentition

a. Mobility. Increased mobility of the dentition may be caused by a loss of bone support secondary to periodontal disease or unusually heavy occlusal forces.

b. Pulpitis

(1). Alterations in the blood supply to the pulp may cause pulpitis. If the blood supply is severely altered or if lateral forces are great enough to completely block or sever the artery that passes into the apical foramen, pulpal neurosis may occur.[21]

(2). Caries may progress to pulpitis.

(3). Sensitivity to heat or cold may be a sign of pulpitis.

(4). Pain of short duration also may signify pulpitis.

c. Tooth wear is a sequella to parafunctional activity.

4. Other symptoms associated with temporomandibular disorders (see Figure 28–34)

a. Tinnitus (ringing in the ears)

b. Vertigo, or dizziness

c. Headache

d. Secondary hyperalgesia

e. Cervicospinal pain that creates masticatory myospasms

f. Central excitatory symptoms (*eg*, eye, nose, or sinus symptoms)

C. Examination for craniomandibular disorders

The purpose of recording patient history and performing physical examination is to identify any area or structure of the craniomandibular system that shows breakdown or pathologic changes. Breakdown in the system is generally signified by pain and/or dysfunction.

1. Screening history

a. Administering a written questionnaire is the first step in the screening history. The following questions should be asked:

• Do you have difficulty opening your mouth?

• Do you hear noises emanating from your jaw joints?

• Do you have frequent headaches?

• Does your jaw get ''stuck'' or ''locked?'' Does it ''go out?''

• Do you have pain in or about your ears or cheeks?

• Do you have pain when you chew or yawn?

• Does your bite feel uncomfortable or unusual?

• Have you had a recent injury to your head or neck?

• Do you have arthritis?

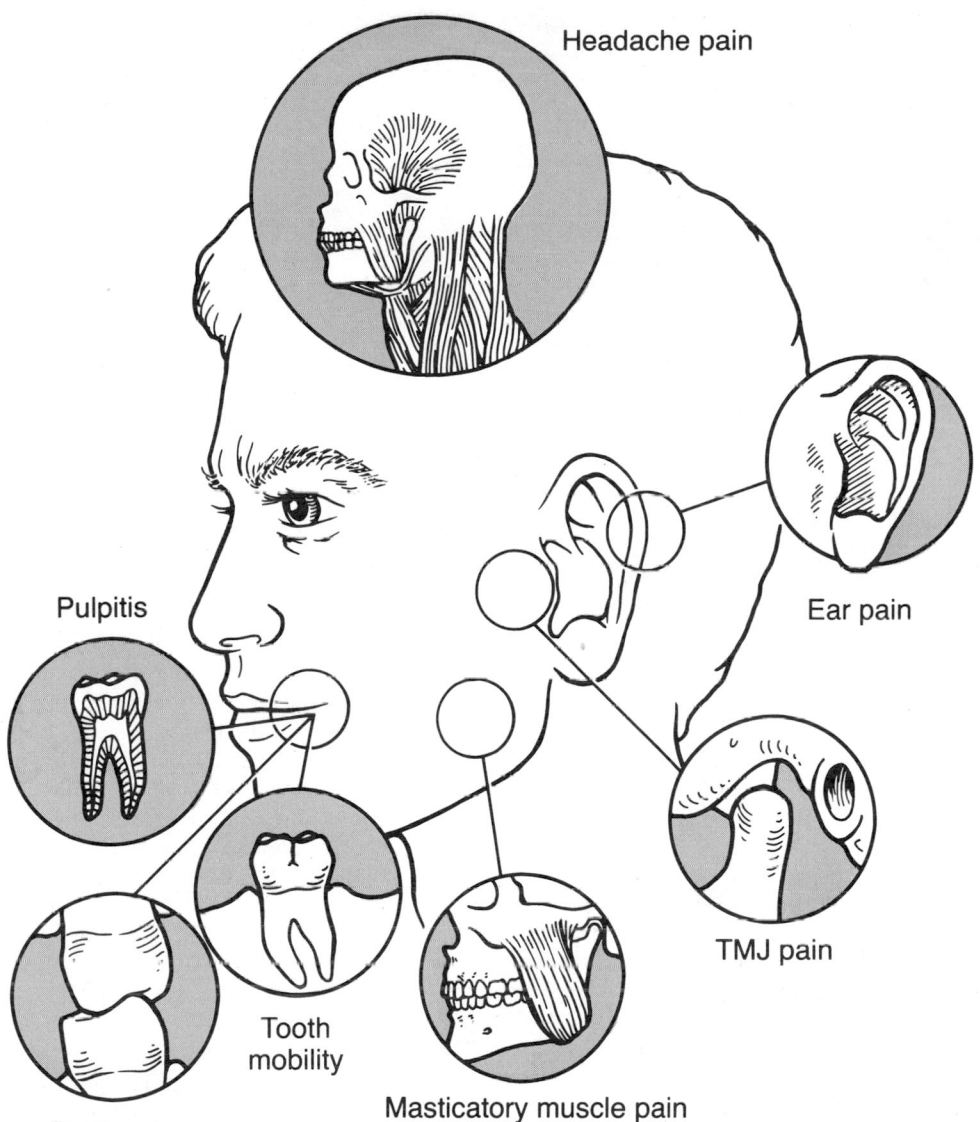

FIGURE 28–34 When parafunctional activity of the masticatory system increases, various structures can break down, causing symptoms. Some of the more common are (1) pulpitis, (2) tooth wear, (3) tooth mobility, (4) masticatory muscle pain, (5) TMJ pain, (6) ear pain, and (7) headache pain. (Redrawn from Okeson JP: *Management of Temporomandibular Disorders and Occlusion,* 3rd ed. St. Louis, Mosby Year Book, 1989, p 158.)

- Do you have any muscle or joint problems?
- Have you ever been treated for TMJ disorders?

b. The screening should include questions eliciting a history of pain.

(1). The *location* of the pain should be noted. Pain may be localized in a specific area, or it may be present in a large, ill-defined region. The area of pain may be constant or spreading.

(2). The *characteristics* of the pain should also be noted. It should be determined whether the pain occurred just once or whether it is recurrent. Whether the pain is constant or intermittent and whether it is relieved by movement or by heat or cold should be noted.

(3). The *quality* of the pain is important to determine. It may be sharp (stimulating) or dull (depressing). "Pain" may be expressed more as an itching sensation, which is a subthreshold pain or as a "prickling feeling," such as the sensation that is felt when one's limb "goes to sleep." A "burning" pain may be felt—this is pain combined with a feeling of warmth. The patient may complain of an "aching" pain, a constant level of "annoying" pain, or a throbbing or "pulsatile" pain, which occurs in time with increased systolic pressure provided by the rhythmic heartbeat.

(4). The *duration* of the pain refers to how long the episode lasts (days, weeks, months) and to how long the pain lasts during each episode.

(5). It is difficult to measure the *degree* of pain; the pain scale is a helpful tool, but it is not reliable for comparing the pain levels among different patients.

c. Dysfunction should be noted on screening. The following questions should be asked:
- Are your jaw movements limited?
- Are joint sounds being experienced?
- Have any changes occurred in your biting position?
- Have there been any alterations in the effectiveness and comfort of functional activities?

d. On screening, the onset of a patient's problems should be determined.

(1). The time of onset should be noted to establish whether a problem is acute or chronic.

(2). The circumstances of the onset of a problem should be noted. Note the history or occasion of the following:
- Trauma (*eg*, a blow to the face).
- Microtrauma (*eg*, yawning or a long dental procedure).
- Parafunctional activity (*eg*, holding a pencil or a pipe between the teeth).
- Bruxism, grinding, or chronic clenching of teeth.
- Extraoral habits (*eg*, holding a telephone between the chin and shoulder, resting the mandible in the hands while sitting at a table, or playing a violin or another similar instrument).

e. A patient's history of previous treatment should be noted, including the type and outcome of prior treatment as well as any medications that were prescribed and their effectiveness.

f. On screening, associated symptoms should be determined.

(1). If the patient has headache pain, determine the following:
- Its frequency.
- Its location.
- Its quality.
- Its duration.
- Its intensity.

(2). If ear pain is the patient's complaint, note whether he/she has ringing, a feeling of fullness in the ear, or a loss of hearing.

(3). If cervical disorders (such as complications resulting from whiplash injury) are noted, ask the patient whether he/she has pain, stiffness, a reduction of movement, or numbness in the head, neck, shoulder, or arm.

2. Clinical examination

a. Cranial nerves

(1). The *olfactory* (I) *nerve* is tested by asking the patient to detect differences between the odors of peppermint, vanilla, and chocolate.

(2). Test the *optic* (II) *nerve* by having the patient cover one eye and read a few one-line sentences 10 feet away.

(3). The *oculomotor* (III), *trochlear* (IV), and *abducens* (VI) *nerves* are tested by having the patient follow a finger as it moves to form an X shape; both eyes should move slowly and similarly as they follow the finger. The pupils should be rounded and equal in size, and they should react to light by constricting.

(4). Test the *trigeminal* (V) *nerve's* sensory input by lightly stroking the face with a cotton swab bilaterally in three regions: the forehead, the cheek, and the lower jaw. Gross motor input is tested by having the patient clench his/her jaw while the masseter muscle and the temporalis and medial pterygoid muscles are palpated.

(5). The sensory input of the *facial* (VII) *nerve* is tested by asking the patient to distinguish between sugar and salt using the tip of his/her tongue. This nerve's motor component is tested by asking the patient to raise both eyebrows, smile, and show his/her lower teeth.

(6). The *acoustic* (VIII) *nerve's* association to hearing can be evaluated by rubbing a strand of hair between the first finger and thumb near the patient's ear and by noting any difference between the sensitivity of the right and left ears. If a question of balance exists, ask the patient to walk heel-to-toe along a straight line.

(7). The *glossopharyngeal* (IX) and *vagus* (X) *nerves* are tested together because they both are located at the back of the throat; the patient should be asked to say "ah," while the soft palate is observed for symmetric elevations.

(8). The *accessory* (XI) *nerve* can be tested by asking the patient to shrug against resistance and by having him/her look first to the right and then to the left against resistance.

(9). Test the *hypoglossal* (XII) *nerve* by asking the patient to protrude his/her tongue; note any uncontrolled or consistent lateral deviation.

b. Muscle palpation

(1). For the *temporalis muscle*, each area should be independently palpated, including the anterior region above the zygomatic arch, the middle region directly above the TMJ and superior to the zygomatic arch, and the posterior region above and behind the ear. The tendon of the temporalis muscle can be palpated by placing a finger of one hand intraorally on the anterior border of the ramus and a finger of the other hand extraorally on the same area.

(2). Palpate the *masseter muscle* bilaterally at its superior and inferior attachments.

(3). Palpate the *medial pterygoid muscle* intraorally along the ramus.

(4). The *sternocleidomastoid muscle* should be palpated bilaterally near its insertion on the outer surface of the mastoid process, behind the ear, and through the entire length of muscle down to its origin on the clavicle.

The trigger points in this muscle are frequent sources of referred pain to the temporal muscle and the circumferential region of the temporomandibular joint.

(5). The *splenius muscles* of the head and neck and the *trapezius muscle* should be tested; the trapezius commonly has trigger points that refer pain to the face.

c. Functional manipulation of the muscles. Each muscle is contracted and then stretched. If the muscle is the true source of the patient's pain, both activities increase the pain.

(1). The *inferior lateral pterygoid muscle* should be checked. Have the patient protrude the muscle against resistance provided by the examiner; this activity increases pain if this muscle is the source of the pain. When the teeth are clenched, pain increases if this is the source; biting on a separator does not increase the pain and may even decrease it.

(2). Test the *superior lateral pterygoid muscle*; clenching increases the pain. Stretching of the muscle occurs at maximum intercuspation; therefore, stretching and contraction of this muscle occur during clenching.

(3). The *medial pterygoid muscle* should be examined; clenching increases the pain. This muscle is stretched when the mouth is opened wide; therefore, opening the mouth wide increases the pain if the medial pterygoid muscle is the source.

d. TMJ

(1). Any pain, which can be determined by digitally palpating the joints during static and dynamic movement, should be noted.

(2). Determine whether any dysfunction is present.

(a). Joint sounds such as a click or crepitation are a sign of dysfunction.

(b). Joint restrictions also signify dysfunction.

(3). Evaluate the TMJ with one or more of the following four basic radiographic diagnostic procedures:
• Panoramic radiography.
• Lateral transcranial radiography.

- Transpharyngeal radiography.
- Transmaxillary radiography.

(4). Tomography can be used to evaluate the TMJ. Tomograms can be obtained at very precise sagittal intervals so that true sections of the joint are seen; this type of image is more accurate than panoramic or transcranial radiographs for identifying abnormalities or changes of the bones. The disadvantages are high cost, lack of convenience, and exposure of the patient to inordinately high levels of radiation.

(5). The TMJ can be examined by arthrography; a contrast medium is injected into the joint spaces to outline important soft tissue structures. With arthrography, it is possible to ascertain the position and condition of the articular disc, and dynamic movements of the disc and the condyle can be visualized. The disadvantages include high cost, invasiveness, and exposure of the patient to high levels of radiation.

(6). Computed tomography scanning can be used to produce digital data that reflect the extent of x-ray transmission through various tissues; these data may be transformed into a density scale and used to generate or reconstruct a visual image. The technique's main advantage is that it images both hard and soft tissue; therefore, the disc-condyle relationship can be observed and evaluated without disturbing the existing anatomic relationships. The disadvantages are high cost, the fact that it is time consuming, and exposure of the patient to high doses of radiation.

(7). Magnetic resonance imaging uses a strong magnetic field to create changes in the energy level of soft tissue. These molecular changes can be used to create a computer image. The main advantage of this technique is that it introduces no radiation that might produce tissue damage. The disadvantages are high cost and limited availability.

e. Dental examination

(1). Check for tooth mobility, which can result from a loss of the supporting bone (periodontal disease) or unusually heavy occlusal forces (traumatic occlusion). Three signs that indicate that heavy occlusal force may have occurred are a widened periodontal space, condensing osteitis (osteosclerosis), and hypercementosis.

(2). Examine the patient for pulpitis. Tooth sensitivity is a sign of pulpitis, and it may be induced by dental caries, heavy occlusal forces, a crack in a tooth, or referred pain from trigger zones in the temporalis muscle, masseter, or anterior belly of the digastric muscle.

(3). Check for tooth wear, which may be the result of parafunctional activity. Tooth wear is determined by the examination of wear facets on the teeth. Furthermore, the patient should be questioned regarding any oral habits that he/she may have such as biting on a pencil or a pipe.

f. Occlusal examination

(1). Check the centric relation position. The condyles should be positioned most superoanteriorly in the mandibular fossa and braced against the posterior slopes of the articular eminences, with the disc properly interposed. From this position, the mandible can be rotated in either an open or a closed position approximately 25 mm interincisally while the condyles remain in their centric position.

(2). Examine the centric occlusion position. Check the relationship of the teeth in their maximum intercuspation; if the mandible moves laterally from this position, then the noncentric cusps come into contact and guide it. If the mouth is opened and then closed, then the noncentric cusps help to guide the mandible back to centric occlusion.

(3). Compare *centric occlusion stability and joint stability.* Small discrepancies (1 to 2 mm) commonly exist between centric relation and centric occlusion; if a significant shift occurs in the mandibular position from light tooth contact to the clenched position, a lack of stability between joint and tooth positions should be suspected. A lack of stability between intercuspation and joint position can be a major contributing factor to disc-interference disorders.

(4). Check the arch integrity; any loss of arch integrity (resulting from tooth loss or carious loss of tooth structure) should be noted. Record any drifting, tipping, or supereruption of the teeth.

(5). The vertical dimension of occlusion represents the distance between the maxillary and mandibular arches when the teeth are in occlusion. This position can be affected by loss of teeth, caries, drifting, or occlusal wear; posterior bite collapse is a cause of a loss of vertical dimension.

(6). Evaluate eccentric occlusal contacts. The superior eccentric border movements of the mandible are dictated by the occlusal surfaces of the teeth; when anterior teeth occlude during eccentric mandibular movement, they provide guidance for the remainder of the dentition. In some instances, they do not come into contact with each other in centric occlusion (anterior open bite), and eccentric guidance is provided by the posterior teeth.

(7). Examine the patient's *protrusive contacts.* Ask the patient to move his/her mandible from centric occlusion into a protrusive position; occlusal contacts should be observed until the mandibular incisors have passed over the maxillary incisors (~8 to 10 mm). Place blue paper between the teeth and ask the patient to close and protrude several times. Next, place red paper and ask the patient to close again and tap in centric occlusion; the red marks denote centric occlusal contacts, and the blue marks denote protrusive contacts.

(8). Test the patient's *laterotrusive contacts.* Ask the patient to move his/her mandible laterally until the canines pass beyond an end-to-end relationship or 8 to 10 mm, whichever comes first.

(9). Evaluate the *mediotrusive contacts.* Place articulating paper between the posterior teeth and instruct the patient to clench while a constant pulling force is maintained on the paper. The patient moves in a mediotrusive direction; if the mandible moves less than 1 mm and the paper becomes disengaged, no mediotrusive contact exists. It has been suggested that mediotrusive contacts contribute significantly to functional disturbances.[22,23]

D. Diagnosing craniomandibular disorders

Separating masticatory disorders into common groups of symptoms and etiologies is necessary before an appropriate diagnosis can be ascertained. A diagnosis is achieved by careful evaluation of the information obtained during the recording of the history and the examination procedures.

1. Masticatory muscle disorders
   a. A diagnosis of muscle splinting—an involuntary CNS-induced hypertonic state of a muscle—can be made as follows.
      (1). The history findings may indicate a recent event that altered the structures of masticatory system (*eg,* a new restoration or dental injection). Splinting is an immediate response to altered input that lasts only a few days and is associated with muscle weakness.
      (2). The examination findings may show symptoms of pain with muscle use but little or no pain when the muscles are at rest. This is not associated with dysfunction; therefore, normal range of motion can be achieved.
   b. Myospasms. Myospasms are involuntary CNS-induced contractions of a muscle that arise from muscle splinting that is not resolved within several days (*eg,* such as when increased levels of emotional stress lead to muscle hyperactivity).
      (1). The history findings may indicate a myalgia following an event that has altered the structure (*eg,* overuse of jaw muscles). Pain may be associated with increased emotional stress.
      (2). The examination findings may indicate increased myalgia with muscle

use. The pain often diminishes or disappears with rest; structural dysfunction with limitation of mouth opening may exist, and the point of restriction, characterized by a "soft-end" feel, may be at any degree of opening.

   c. Myositis. This disorder is characterized by local inflammation of muscle tissue resulting from protracted myospasms or a spreading infection.

     (1). The history findings may show that myositis creates myalgia even when the jaw is at rest, and jaw use accentuates the pain. Dysfunction is present secondary to constant pain and local tissue changes.

     (2). On examination, it may be noted that the muscles are extremely painful to palpation and that pain lingers long after palpation.

   d. Myofascial trigger points. Trigger points arise from hypersensitive areas in muscle tissues that tend to refer pain to distant sites by central excitatory effects.

     (1). The history findings may indicate that the most common complaint for this disorder is headache (referred) pain.

     (2). The examination findings may show that pressure applied to the active trigger points increases the pain at the referred site. A patient complaining of temporal headaches referred from trigger points in the sternocleidomastoid muscle might have some discomfort when turning his/her head (indicating dysfunction of the sternocleidomastoid muscle but no problem in the temporal muscle, *ie*, no pain on palpation and

no limitation of function). Four conditions are likely:

- Constant deep pain, which may create trigger points not only at the source but also far away from them (satellite trigger points).
- Increased levels of emotional stress, which can activate trigger points.
- Muscle strain or overload (as from a sudden stretch during a motor vehicle accident).
- Spontaneous trigger points (*eg*, from vitamin B deficiency).

2. Disc-interference disorders

   a. Disc displacement (see Figure 28–35). The inferior retrodiscal lamina is elongated, with discal collateral ligaments causing thinning of the posterior border of the disc. This condition allows the disc to be displaced more anteriorly.

     (1). It is common for the history findings to indicate trauma to be associated with onset of joint sounds; accompanying pain may or may not be present. If pain is present, it is intracapsular with a concomitant dysfunctional "click."

     (2). The examination findings may show that joint sounds are audible during opening and closing. Disc displacement is characterized by a normal range of motion of the jaw during opening; any limitation of motion is due to pain and not a structural dysfunction. When reciprocal clicking is present, two clicks usually occur at different degrees of opening, with the closing click occurring very near the intercuspal position.

   b. Disc dislocation with reduction (see Fig-

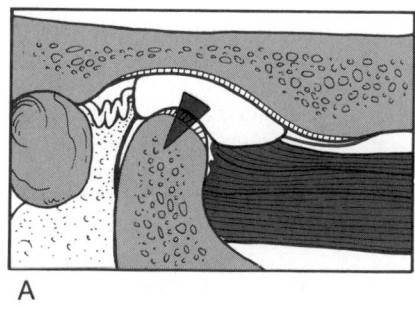
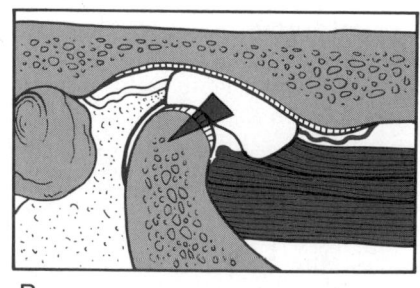

A   B

FIGURE 28–35 Functional displacement of the disc. **A,** Normal condyle-disc relationship in the resting closed joint. **B,** Anterior functional displacement of the disc. The posterior discal border has been thinned, and the discal and inferior retrodiscal lamina are elongated sufficiently to allow the superior lateral pterygoid muscle to displace the disc anteromedially.

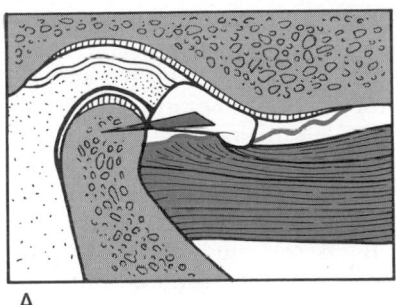 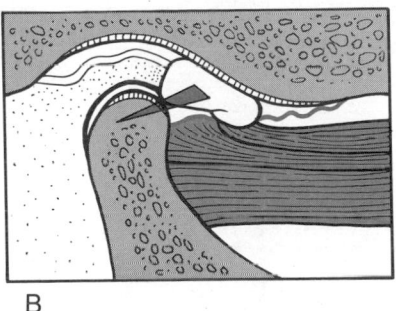 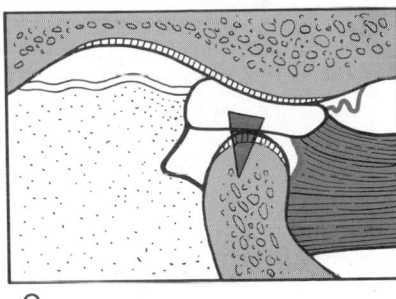

A   B   C

FIGURE 28–36 Anteriorly dislocated disc with reduction. **A,** Resting closed-joint position. **B,** During the early stages of translation, the condyle moves up onto the posterior border of the disc. This can be accompanied by a clicking sound. **C,** Remainder of opening. The condyle assumes a more normal position on the intermediate zone of the disc as the disc is rotating posteriorly on the condyle. During closure, the exact opposite occurs. In the final closure, the disc is again pulled forward by the superior lateral pterygoid muscle and the dislocation is re-established. Sometimes this is accompanied by a second (reciprocal) click.

ure 28–36). If the inferior retrodiscal lamina and discal collateral ligaments become further elongated and the posterior border of the disc becomes thinner, the disc can be pulled completely through the discal space. Because the disc and condyle no longer articulate, a dislocation occurs. If the patient can reposition the condyle onto the posterior border of the disc; then the disc is reduced.

(1). The history findings may show a long history of clicking with a more recent catching sensation. The patient may report that when the joint catches and gets stuck, he/she can move his/her jaw a little and get it functioning again; the catching may or may not be painful.

(2). The examination findings may indicate that the patient presents with a limited range of opening. When opening reduces the disc, associated deviation in the opening pathway occurs; often a sudden loud "pop" is heard during the recapturing of the disc. Following reduction, a normal range of mandibular movement is present. Often, having the patient keep his/her mouth in a slightly protruded position following recapture of the disc eliminates the catching sensation, even during opening and closing.

c. Dislocation without reduction (see Figure 28–37). As elasticity of the superior retrodiscal lamina is broken down, recapturing of the disc becomes more difficult; when the disc is not reduced, forward translation of the condyle forces the disc in front of the condyle.

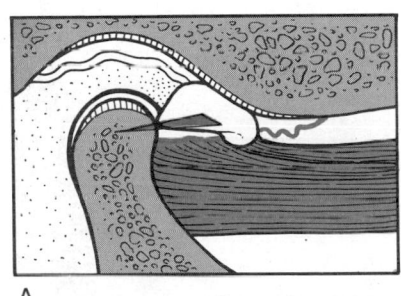 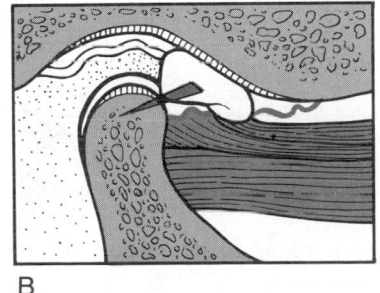 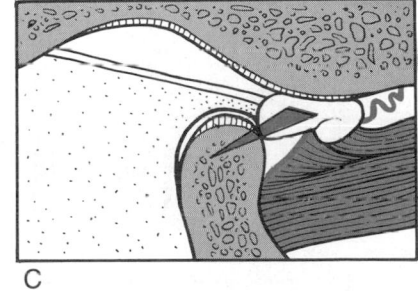

A   B   C

FIGURE 28–37 Anteriorly dislocated disc without reduction. **A,** Resting closed-joint position. **B,** During the early stages of translation, the condyle does not move onto the disc but instead pushes the disc forward. **C,** The disc becomes jammed forward in the joint, preventing the normal range of condylar translatory movement. This condition is referred to clinically as a closed lock.

(1). The history findings usually show that the patient is acutely aware of when the dislocation occurred (*eg*, when he/she bit into an apple or had his/her mouth open for a prolonged period). The patient may report that his/her jaw is locked in the closed position; pain is a common sequela, and when it is present, it accompanies attempts to open the mouth beyond the joint restriction. The history may reveal that the clicking occurred before the disc dislocation was resolved.

(2). The examination findings may indicate that the active range of motion is 25 to 30 mm and that the mandible deflects to the involved joint. The maximum point of opening may reveal a "hard-end" feel; eccentric movements may be relatively normal to the ipsilateral side but restricted to the contralateral side. Loading the joint with bilateral manual manipulation is often painful because the condyle is seated on retrodiscal tissue.

3. Structural incompatibilities of the articular surfaces
   a. Adhesions (see Figure 28–38) represent a sticking of the articular surfaces and may occur between the condyle and the disc (inferior joint space) or between the disc and the fossa (superior joint space). Adhesions can be diagnosed as follows.
      (1). The history findings often show that a patient underwent a long period during which the joint was loaded (such as when clenching occurs during sleep). It may be found that as

the patient tried to open his/her mouth, a single click was felt and normal range of motion returned. Adhesions occur because static loading of the joint exhausts weeping lubrication; when adhesion is broken, boundary lubrication takes over, and sticking does not recur unless static loading is repeated. Patients usually report morning stiffness until the joint is "popped" and normal movement is restored. If pain is a symptom, it is normally associated with attempts to increase opening, such as yawning, which elongates the ligaments.

(2). The examination findings indicating adhesions in the superior joint space may be as follows. Normal translation of the condyle-disc is inhibited; therefore, the movement of the condyle is limited to rotation. The patient presents with 25 to 30 mm of jaw opening. If adhesions are longstanding, discal collateral and anterior capsular ligaments can become elongated; the condyle begins to translate forward, leaving the disc behind; this leads to posterior dislocation of the disc. (Most posterior disc displacements are associated with adhesion problems.)[24] These posterior dislocations are characterized by the patient's inability to get the teeth back into occlusion.[25] Adhesions in the inferior joint space can be diagnosed as follows. Sticking occurs between the condyle and the disc with a loss of normal rotational movement. The patient can open

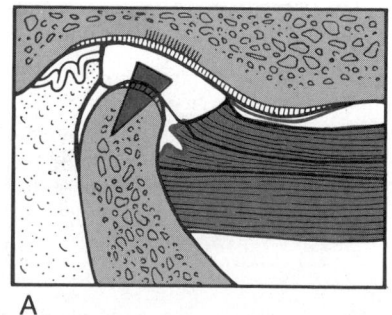 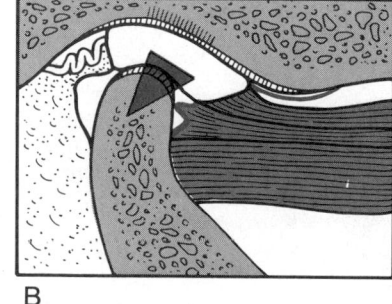 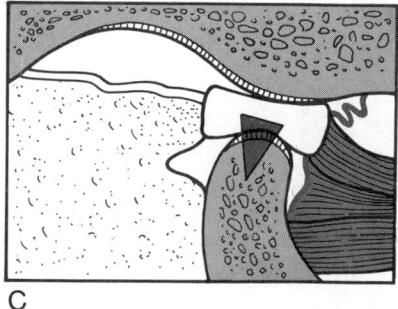

A   B   C

FIGURE 28–38   **A,** Adhesion in the superior joint space. **B,** The presence of the adhesion limits the joint to only rotation. **C,** If the adhesion is freed, normal translation can occur.

his/her mouth but experiences a "catching" or "jumping" sensation while he/she attempts maximum opening. Translation between the disc and the fossa is normal.

b. Alterations in form are caused by actual changes in the shape of the articular surfaces. These changes include thinning of both the borders and the perforations. They can be diagnosed as follows.

   (1). The history findings may indicate long-term dysfunction with or without pain; often, the patient has learned a pattern of mandibular movement that avoids the alteration in form.

   (2). The examination findings may show that dysfunction is observable at the same point of opening. During closing, the dysfunction is observed at the same degree of mandibular separation as during opening. The speed and force of opening do not alter the point of alteration.

c. Subluxations represent a sudden forward movement of the condyle during the latter phase of mouth opening. This represents normal joint movement as a result of certain anatomic features and is characterized by having a TMJ whose articular eminence has a steep, short posterior slope articulating with a longer anterior slope of the abutting condyle.

   (1). The history findings may indicate that the patient reports that his/her jaw "goes out" anytime he/she opens wide; the joint sound is best described as a "thud."

   (2). During the examination, the patient should open wide; at the latter slope of opening, the condyle jumps forward, leaving a small depression. The midline pathway seems to deviate and return as the condyle moves over the eminence. Usually, no pain is associated with this movement.

d. Spontaneous dislocation occurs when the TMJ hyperextends, leading to anterior dislocation of the disc; the resultant condition fixes the joint in the open position, preventing any translocation. This problem occurs most often in a TMJ with anatomic features that produce subluxation and can be diagnosed as follows.

   (1). The history findings may show that the problem is associated with wide-open mouth procedures, such as a long dental examination. The patient may report that he/she cannot close his/her mouth. Pain is associated with stretching of the capsular and discal ligaments.

   (2). The examination findings may indicate that the patient cannot verbalize the problem because his/her jaw is locked open; this augments the distress and pain that the patient feels.

4. Inflammatory joint disorders. These disorders are characterized by continuous deep pain that is influenced by function. The symptoms usually are referred pain, excessive sensitivity to touch (hyperalgesia), or an increase in myospasm frequency.

a. Synovitis or capsulitis

   (1). The history findings often include an incident of trauma or abuse. Continuous pain usually originates in the joint area, and any movement that elongates the capsule increases pain, which is characterized as a deep, constant pain.

   (2). The examination findings may indicate palpable pain over the lateral pole of the condyle and limitation of opening due to myospasms secondary to pain with a "soft-end" feel. If edema is present, the condyle may be displaced inferiorly; this creates a disocclusion of the ipsilateral posterior teeth.

b. Retrodiscitis

   (1). The history findings may indicate an incident of trauma or chronic grinding (bruxing). Pain is constant, it originates in the joint area, and it is aggravated by jaw movements.

   (2). The examination findings may show that a "soft-end" feel is present unless the inflammation is associated with a disc dislocation. Edema may force the condyle forward and down the eminence; this creates an acute malocclusion with disocclusion of the ipsilateral posterior teeth and heavy contact of the contralateral anterior teeth.

c. Degenerative joint disease. This is actually a noninflammatory condition in which the articular surfaces and underlying bone deteriorate.

(1). The history findings may indicate that the patient reports unilateral pain that is aggravated by mandibular movement, with the pain usually worsening during the day.

(2). The examination findings may find limited mandibular opening with a "soft-end" feel. Crepitation can usually be felt. The diagnosis may be confirmed with TMJ radiographs that reveal structural changes of the condyle or the fossa (*eg*, flattening, osteophytes, or erosions).

d. Inflammatory arthritis

(1). For traumatic arthritis, a positive history of macrotrauma may be present. The patient may report constant arthralgia aggravated by movement, limited mandibular opening secondary to pain, and a "soft-end" feel. Acute malocclusion may exist if swelling is present.

(2). Infectious arthritis, which is a nonsterile inflammatory reaction of the articular surfaces, can be associated with systemic disease, bacterial invasion, or immunologic response. The history findings may reveal a local infection of adjacent tissues or a penetrating wound to the joint. Constant pain is present and is aggravated by movement. Joint swelling and elevated tissue temperature are present. The study of the patient's blood as well as his/her fluid aspirated from the joint may assist in diagnosis. Blood cultures are positive indicators of systemic joint disease in approximately 50% of patients. The leukocyte count of the synovial fluid may be greater than 110,000 per microliter, with 90% or more of the cells being polymorphonuclear. Synovial fluid sugar is usually low, and a Gram's stain of the synovial fluid has positive results in 75% of staphylococcal infections and in 50% of gram-negative infections.[26]

(3). Rheumatoid arthritis is characterized by inflammation of the synovial membranes that extend into the surrounding connective tissues and articular surfaces, which become thickened and tender. This disorder is associated with a history of joint complaints. The diagnosis may be confirmed by blood studies during both the acute and chronic phases. The erythrocyte sedimentation rate, the level of gamma globulins (immunoglobulins M and G), and the platelet count are typically elevated, whereas the white cell count is typically normal.[24]

(4). Hyperuricemia (gout) occurs when high levels of serum uric acid persist, causing urates to be precipitated in the synovial fluid of the TMJs. Symptoms of pain and swelling commonly recur in both joints. This disorder is usually seen in elderly patients.

5. Chronic mandibular hypomobility

a. Muscle contracture

(1). Myostatic contracture occurs when a muscle is restrained from fully relaxing (stretching) for prolonged periods of time.

(2). Myofibrotic contracture occurs as a result of excessive tissue adhesions within the muscles. This commonly follows trauma to the muscle. The restriction of movement is not painful.

b. Capsular fibrosis

(1). The history findings often indicate that a patient reports a previous injury or capsulitis. Trauma may be due to surgical intervention in the joint.

(2). The examination findings may show that movement is restricted in all positions. If fibrosis is unilateral, midline pathway deflection occurs to the involved side during opening.

c. Coronoid impedance

(1). The history findings may show that painless restriction of opening exists.

(2). The examination findings may reveal that limitation is evident in all movements—especially in protrusion. In the case of unilateral coronoid involvement, opening deflects the mandible to the affected side.

d. Ankylosis

(1). The history findings may show that intracapsular surfaces of the joint develop adhesions that prohibit normal movement. This condition results from a fibrous union between sliding surfaces. The patient usually has had sustained trauma or a joint infection.

(2). On examination, it may be determined that mandibular movement is restricted in all planes. Clinically, the patient has neither pain nor acute malocclusion.

6. Growth disorders
   a. Hypoplasia is incomplete development or underdevelopment.
   b. Hyperplasia is overdevelopment.
   c. Neoplasia, which is rare, involves the formation of a neoplasm (eg, a rare, metastatic adenocarcinoma).

V. Treatment

A. Treatment of functional disturbances of the masticatory system

At least 28 treatment modalities that have been recognized as appropriate therapy for craniomandibular disorders have been identified in the literature.[27] Each produces varying degrees of success; this fact has contributed to the vast amount of confusion surrounding the treatment of these disorders.

1. Supportive therapy. Over-the-counter drugs suggested by a physical therapist or prescription drugs recommended by a physician in conjunction with appropriate physical therapy treatment offer a comprehensive approach to the treatment of many masticatory disorders. Care must be taken in regard to the type of drugs prescribed and the manner in which they are to be used. Because many disorders present symptoms that are periodic or cyclic, there is a tendency to prescribe drugs on a "take-as-needed" basis, which may encourage drug abuse; the drugs most commonly abused are narcotic analgesics and tranquilizers.
   a. Pharmacologic therapy
      (1). Analgesics may be prescribed in regular doses over a short period of time. These include aspirin, acetaminophen, ibuprofen, and codeine combined with salicylate or acetaminophen.
      (2). Tranquilizing agents are used to alter the patient's perception or reaction to stress and include diazepam (Valium) and amitriptyline.
      (3). Local anesthetics include lidocaine and mepivacaine (Carbocaine).
      (4). Anti-inflammatory agents include aspirin, naproxen, ibuprofen, and hydrocortisone (by injection).
   b. Physical therapy offers supportive treatments that often are instituted in conjunction with dental interventions.
      (1). Thermotherapy by moist heat or ultrasound is based on the premise that heat increases circulation to the applied area.
      (2). Coolant therapy involves the use of ice or a vapor spray, such as fluoromethane.
      (3). Electrical stimulation may be used. Two varieties are electrogalvanic and transcutaneous electric nerve stimulation.
      (4). Acupuncture point stimulation, which works by stimulating endorphins for pain modulation, may be used.
      (5). A therapist may try soft-tissue manipulation through massage, passive muscle stretching, or the mobilization of a joint (accomplished by placing the thumb in the patient's mouth over the lower second molar area on the side to be distracted; this does not require translation but merely unloading in the closed-joint position).
2. Exercise protocols and instructional paradigms help to establish normal mandibular function
   a. Restrictive use of affected joints or muscles
      (1). The patient should be instructed to function within a painless range ("if it hurts, don't do it").
      (2). The patient's diet should be altered to include softer foods, and he/she should be told to take small bites and to chew slowly.
      (3). The patient should attempt to discontinue parafunctional habits.

(4). He/she should learn to control clenching and bruxing.

(5). Appliance therapy may be indicated by a dentist to control nocturnal bruxing.

b. Passive exercise

(1). These exercises should be performed within a painless range of movement.

(2). They aid in maintaining the normal function of blood flow to the muscles.

(3). They help to train a patient to do certain movements that will help him/her to overcome dysfunction.

c. Active exercises

(1). Assisted stretching exercises are used when a need to regain muscle length is noted; they should be performed with gentle intermittent force that is gradually increased. Patients often can perform stretching on their own because they are not likely to overstretch or traumatize the involved tissue. The reduction in symptoms that is associated with the use of fluoromethane spray is enhanced when stretching is accomplished immediately after the overlying area has been sprayed.

(2). Resistive exercises are based on the concept of reciprocal inhibition; when the patient opens his/her mouth, the mandibular depressors are active and the elevator muscles relax slowly, keeping the mandible from dropping suddenly. If the depressor muscles meet resistance, the neurologic message sent to the antagonistic muscle (elevators) is to relax more fully. These exercises are repeated 10 times each session five times a day.

(3). Isometric exercises (see Figure 28–39) are based on the concept of reflex relaxation to provide an increase in the mandibular opening. The patient is instructed to open his/her mouth against the resistance of a fist; this promotes relaxation of the elevator muscles, thus allowing increased mandibular opening.

B. Treatment of masticatory muscle disorders

The predominant complaint of patients with masticatory muscle disorders is myalgia, which

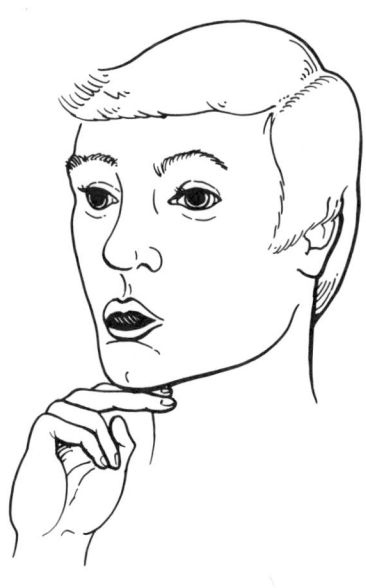
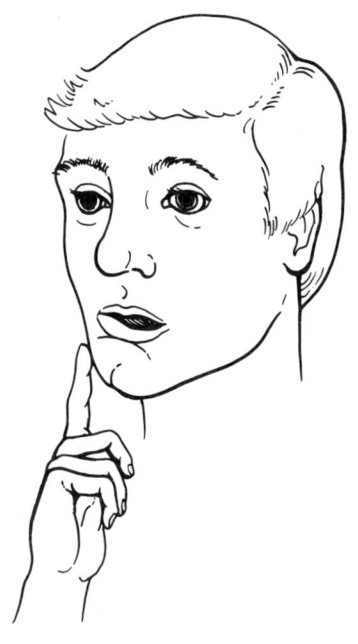

A   B

FIGURE 28–39   Gentle isometric jaw exercises are helpful for increasing the strength of hypotrophic muscles. **A,** The objective is to resist movement. **B,** The patient moves the jaw laterally while resisting the movement with the fingers. This is done for 3 to 5 seconds in a protrusive as well as a right and left lateral movement. The exercises are repeated throughout the day.

often is reported as having a sudden onset and as being recurrent. The treatment of the four subclassifications of masticatory muscle disorders is discussed in this section.

1. Muscle splinting
   a. Etiologic considerations
      (1). Splinting is the initial reaction of muscles to altered sensory or to proprioceptive input or injury.
      (2). Patients commonly report symptoms of short duration (several days) and often associate a particular event with the onset of a problem.
      (3). The causative event or factor may have been trauma (such as that from prolonged open-mouth dental or surgical [intubation] procedures), an alteration in the patient's occlusion, or soreness surrounding a recent injection site.
      (4). Patients often report myogenic pain during functioning but have no restriction in mandibular movement.
      (5). Muscle weakness is a common complaint.
   b. Definitive treatment
      (1). If the splinting was caused by trauma, definitive treatment is not indicated because the causative factor is no longer present.
      (2). If the trauma resulted from poorly fitting restorations, the treatment consists of altering the restorations to harmonize with existing occlusion; however, alteration of the occlusal condition is directed only at the offending restoration and not at the entire dentition. Once the offending restoration is eliminated, the occlusal condition is returned to its pre-existing state; this should resolve the symptoms.
   c. Supportive therapy
      (1). If the cause is trauma, supportive therapy (eg, ice) is the most effective type of treatment.
      (2). A soft diet is recommended until the patient's pain has subsided.
      (3). Short-term pain medication may be indicated.
      (4). Gentle mandibular active range of motion exercises should be performed by the patient in all planes to maintain joint integrity.

2. Myospasms
   a. Etiologic considerations
      (1). Protracted muscle splinting that lasts more than 2 to 3 days may cause myospasms.
      (2). Increased emotional stress may not be associated with a distinct clinical event but may be related to a prolonged course of rising and falling symptoms.
      (3). Constant deep pain can create central excitatory effects, referring myospasms to the muscles of mastication.
   b. Definitive treatment
      (1). Mandibular use should be restricted to within painless limits, and a soft diet, along with recommendations to take smaller bites and to chew more slowly, is encouraged.
      (2). Painless contraction and relaxation of a muscle seem to reduce myospasms, but the muscle must never be overworked.
      (3). The patient should disengage the teeth; this reduces input and assists in muscle relaxation. The patient should be instructed to keep his/her lips together and his/her teeth apart. An occlusal appliance may be required for a nocturnal bruxer. A muscle relaxation centric relation appliance provides even occlusal contacts when the condyles are in their anterosuperior position resting on the articular discs against the posterior slopes of the articular eminences.
      (4). The pain cycle should be interrupted through the use of analgesic medication, anesthetic injections, or muscle relaxation procedures.
   c. Supportive therapy
      (1). Moist heat applications can be used.
      (2). A coolant spray (fluoromethane) may help.
      (3). Ice massage can be useful.
      (4). Therapy with high-voltage pulsed current can help.
      (5). Continuous ultrasound can be used.
      (6). Transcutaneous electrical nerve stimulation can help.

3. Myositis
   a. Etiologic considerations
      (1). An inflammation of the muscle tis-

sue resulting from either protracted myospasms or spreading infection may be the cause.

(2). The patient may be experiencing an advanced stage of myospasms.

(3). Protracted muscle hyperactivity may be present.

b. Definitive treatment

(1). Restrict mandibular use to within painless limits. The patient should keep his/her jaw as immobile as possible. A soft diet should be initiated, along with recommendations to chew more slowly and to take smaller bites.

(2). The patient should disengage the teeth. A muscle relaxation centric appliance can be used in the same manner as for the treatment of myospasms.

(3). Anti-inflammatory medication such as nonsteroidal ibuprofen may be recommended and should be taken on a regular basis (600 mg four times a day) for 3 weeks so that blood levels are sufficiently elevated to achieve a clinical effect. Ibuprofen is another analgesic that can help to reduce the cyclic effect of myospasms that lead to myositis.

c. Supportive therapy

(1). Gentle isometric jaw exercises to increase the use and strength of the involved muscles should be performed.

(2). Passive stretching to regain the original length of the elevators should be used.

(3). Moist heat and ultrasound may be helpful.

(4). The patient should be progressed slowly with exercise and other treatment modalities because too aggressive a treatment may worsen symptoms.

4. Myofascial trigger point pain

a. Etiologic considerations

(1). Myofascial trigger point pain originates from local hypersensitive areas within the muscle tissues.

(2). These trigger points can arise from any source of constant deep pain, from strain or overload of the muscles, or from increased levels of emotional stress.

(3). Trigger points can develop spontaneously.

(4). Trigger points may be activated by upper respiratory tract or viral infections.

b. Definitive treatment. Listed here are a variety of techniques to be used either independently or in combination to achieve the desired results. The spray and stretch technique works particularly well in the treatment of trigger point pain.

(1). The spray and stretch technique consists of using a coolant spray (eg, fluoromethane) on the tissue overlying the muscle that has a trigger point and then stretching the muscle. The muscle is stretched to its full length, and the vapocoolant applied from a distance of 18 in toward the site of the referred symptoms (the precise technique for each muscle has been described by Travell and Simons).[28]

(2). Pressure and massage can be used. Pressure should be increased to approximately 20 points and maintained for 30 to 60 seconds.

(3). Ultrasound provides deep heat to the area of the trigger point; this allows for local muscle relaxation.

(4). High-voltage pulsed current rhythmically pulsates the muscle to a level of fatigue; this causes the muscle to relax.

c. Supportive therapy

(1). Vitamin supplements should be given because hypovitaminosis appears to be a common finding in people with this disorder; deficiencies of the B-complex vitamins are especially common.

(2). Hypoglycemia and hypothyroid conditions must be addressed medically.

(3). The patient should get adequate amounts of sleep because a lack of sleep seems to be a contributing factor.

(4). Poor posture should be corrected; muscles that are maintained in a shortened length tend to develop trigger points. Daily stretching of the muscles to full length can help to reduce pain. Regular exercise also should be encouraged.

C. Treatment of disc-interference disorders

Disc-interference disorders are characterized by intracapsular symptoms that result from dysfunction of the condyle-disc complex against the mandibular fossa. Common clinical features range from joint sounds and sticking to jamming or irregular catching of the joint. This section addresses the four common categories of disc-interference disorders: derangement of the condyle-disc complex, structural incompatibility, subluxations, and spontaneous dislocations.

1. Derangement of the condyle-disc complex
   a. Treatment for displacements and dislocations with reduction
      (1). An anterior repositioning appliance, which causes the mandible to be positioned slightly anterior to centric occlusion, can be used; use of this appliance causes the mandible to be retruded only slightly (see Figure 28–40).
      (2). The appliance must be worn for 2 to 4 months 24 hours a day; if it is removed, the posterior teeth come together and the condyle slips behind the disc and re-establishes the pathologic condition.
      (3). An anterior repositioning appliance does not heal the TMJ; it merely provides a favorable joint position that allows the tissue maximum opportunity for repair.
      (4). The length and success of appliance therapy depend on three factors: the acuteness of the injury, the extent of the injury, and the age and health of the patient.
   b. Treatment for dislocation without reduction
      (1). Initial treatment should include an attempt to reduce or recapture the disc by manipulation.
      (2). Success of reduction depends on the following factors:
         • Relaxation of the superior lateral pterygoid muscle.
         • An increase in disc space (so that the disc can be repositioned on the condyle).
         • Maximum forward positioning of the condyle (translatory condyle).
      (3). The patient should attempt to reduce the dislocation by effecting side-to-side mandibular excursions without assistance until the mandible reaches the maximum protrusive position.
      (4). Manipulation may be needed (see Figure 28–41). If it is, the thumb should be placed intraorally over the mandibular second molar on the affected side; the fingers should be placed on the inferior border of the mandible anterior to the thumb's position. Firm but controlled downward force should then be exerted on the molar as upward force is placed by the fingers. While the joint is being distracted, the condyle should be brought downward and forward; this motion translates the

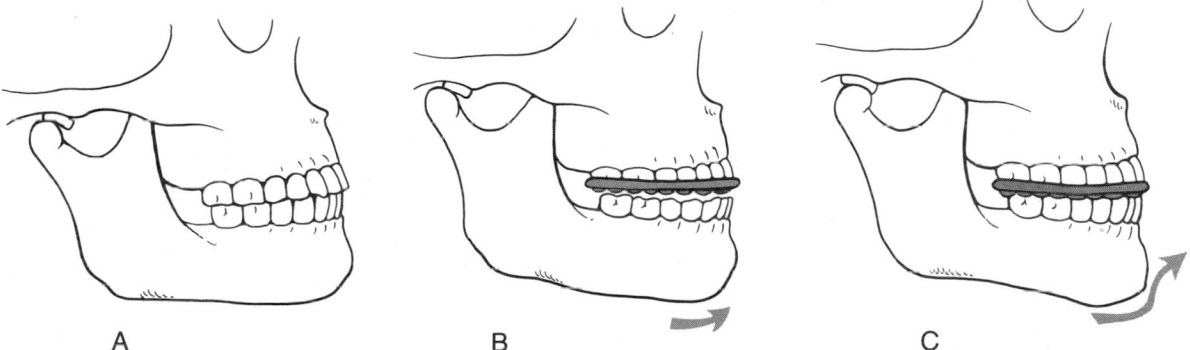

A   B   C

FIGURE 28–40 **A,** In the resting closed-joint position, the disc has been anteriorly displaced from the condyle. **B,** A maxillary occlusal appliance has been fabricated and creates an occlusal condition that requires the mandible to shift slightly forward. **C,** Note that when the appliance is in place and the teeth are occluding, the condyle is repositioned on the disc in a more normal condyle-disc relationship. It is for this reason that this device is called an *anterior repositioning appliance.*

condyle out of the fossa. An anterior re-positioning appliance should immediately be placed to prevent occlusion of the posterior teeth, which would redislocate the disc.

c. Supportive therapy
  (1). Therapy should be directed at managing the patient's pain and secondary myospasms.
  (2). When pain is a factor, analgesics may be indicated.
  (3). Ultrasound, high-voltage pulsed current, moist heat, and phonophoresis over the joint area may be helpful in reducing the pain.

d. Surgical consideration for condyle-disc derangement disorders
  (1). The goal of surgery is to return the disc to a normal functional relationship with the condyle.
  (2). Surgery should be considered only when conservative therapy fails to resolve the symptoms.
  (3). When a disc is displaced or dislocated, the surgical procedure of choice is plication.
  (4). Plication involves removal of a portion of the retrodiscal tissue and the inferior lamina; the disc is then retracted posteriorly and secured with sutures.

  (5). Removal of the disc (discectomy) also has been considered.
  (6). Discal implants such as Silastic implants have been used.
  (7). Dermal grafts may be needed.

2. Structural incompatibilities
  a. Treatment of adhesions
    (1). A muscle relaxation appliance is indicated to minimize muscle hyperactivity.
    (2). A referral for arthroscopic surgery to break down fibrous attachments may be necessary.
    (3). Passive stretching with ultrasound should be used.
    (4). Distraction of the joint may be helpful.
    (5). The patient should be instructed to adopt appropriate patterns of movement that do not aggravate the adhesions.
  b. Treatment of subluxations
    (1). Refer a patient with subluxations to an oral surgeon for surgical alteration of the joint. An eminectomy reduces the steepness of the articular eminence and decreases the amount of posterior rotation of the disc and condyle during full translation.
    (2). Educate the patient to restrict open-

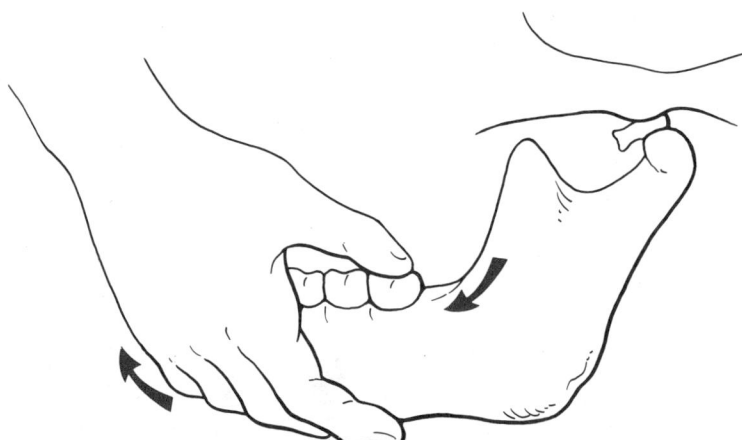

FIGURE 28–41 Manual disc reduction technique description (steps A–F). A, The patient presents with an acute disc dislocation without reduction in the left TMJ (closed lock). There is a maximum opening of only 23 mm. B, The clinician's right thumb is placed intraorally over the patient's left mandibular second molar, and the mandible is grasped. With the left hand stabilizing the cranium, gentle but firm force is applied downward on the molar and upward on the chin to distract the joint. C, Arrows depict the proper force vectors for effective joint distraction. D, Once the joint is distracted, the mandible is brought forward and to the right, enabling the condyle to move into the area of the dislocated disc. When this position is achieved, constant distractive force is applied for 30 to 40 seconds while the patient relaxes. E, After the distraction, the thumb is removed and the patient is asked to close on the anterior teeth, maintaining the jaw in a slightly protrusive position. F, When the patient has rested a moment, he/she is instructed to open maximally. If the disc has been reduced, a normal range of movement (48 mm) is possible.

ing so as not to reach the point of translation that initiates the interference.

(3). Recommend that an intraoral device be worn for 2 months; use of such a device causes the development of myostatic contracture of the elevator muscles, thus limiting opening to the point of subluxation.

c. Spontaneous dislocations

(1). The goal of treatment is to increase the disc space; this increase allows the superior retrodiscal lamina to retract the disc.

(2). The patient should be instructed to open wide as in yawning; this activates the mandibular depressors and inhibits the elevators as slight posterior pressure is simultaneously applied to the chin.

(3). If dislocation remains resistant to this method, then both of the therapist's thumbs should be placed on the mandibular molars and downward pressure should be exerted as the patient yawns; this will usually provide enough space to recapture the disc.

(4). If dislocation is still not reduced, it is likely that the inferior lateral pterygoid muscle is in myospasm, preventing posterior repositioning of the condyles. If this is the case, it is appropriate to refer the patient to a dentist for local anesthetic injection into the lateral pterygoid muscle in an attempt to break up the myospasm and promote relaxation.

(5). If the elevator muscles appear to be in myospasm, local anesthetic may be helpful.

(6). When supportive therapy fails to eliminate or reduce the problem to an acceptable level, the patient should be referred to an oral surgeon for surgical consultation.

D. Treatment of inflammatory disorders of the temporomandibular joint

Inflammatory disorders of the TMJ are generally characterized by continuous pain in the joint area that is often aggravated by function. Inflammatory conditions of the joint structures often occur simultaneously with or secondary to other inflammatory disorders. The four catego-

ries to be covered in this section are capsulitis and synovitis, retrodiscitis, degenerative joint disease, and inflammatory arthritis.

1. Traumatic capsulitis and synovitis
   a. Restrict all mandibular movement to within painless limits.
   b. A soft diet combined with slow movements and small bites is recommended.
   c. Analgesics may be needed to relieve pain.
   d. The application of moist heat for 15 minutes four or five times a day may help.
   e. The application of cold packs for 15 minutes four or five times a day[29] may be alternated with the application of moist heat; approximately 2 hours should lapse between alternating treatments.
   f. Ultrasound application may be used for 6 minutes three times a week.[30]
   g. When a single traumatic injury has been experienced, a single injection by the dentist of a corticosteroid to the capsular tissue may be helpful.
2. Secondary inflammatory capsulitis or synovitis
   a. When the inflammatory condition arises secondary to an adjacent structural infection, appropriate antibiotic therapy and medical care are recommended, and the patient should be referred to a dentist or physician.
   b. If the capsulitis is a direct result of an arthritic condition, the arthritis should be treated.
   c. When the capsulitis appears to be secondary to a disc-interference disorder, the disorder should be treated.
3. Retrodiscitis from extrinsic trauma. When trauma such as a blow to the chin is received, the condyles are likely to be forced posteriorly into the retrodiscal tissues.
   a. Careful observation of the occlusal condition should be made.
   b. If no evidence of acute malocclusion is noted, the patient may be given analgesics by a dentist for pain, may be instructed to restrict movements to within painless limits, and may begin a soft diet.
   c. To decrease the likelihood of ankylosis, some movement is encouraged.
   d. Ultrasound and moist heat may be helpful in reducing pain.

e. A muscle relaxation appliance should be fabricated by a dentist to stabilize the occlusal condition; the appliance must be regularly adjusted as the retrodiscal tissues return to normal.

f. As soon as the proper occlusal condition is re-established, the fixation can be discontinued.

4. Retrodiscitis from intrinsic trauma. As the disc becomes more anteriorly positioned, the condyle assumes a position on the posterior border of the disc as well as on the retrodiscal tissue.

a. When retrodiscitis is the result of an anteriorly displaced or dislocated disc, treatment is directed toward establishing a proper condyle-disc relationship.

b. An anterior repositioning appliance may be used to reposition the condyle off the retrodiscal tissues and onto the disc.

c. After the symptoms have resolved, the appliance is slowly reduced, returning the mandible to the normal condylar position.

d. The motion of the mandible is restricted to within painless limits.

e. Analgesics may be prescribed for pain.

f. Ultrasound applications three to four times a week may be helpful in controlling symptoms.

g. Applications of moist heat or ice to a painful joint may be used as needed.

5. Degenerative joint disease. Mechanical overloading is associated with compromise of the articular structures.

a. An anterior repositioning appliance may be used to correct the condyle-disc relationship.

b. A muscle relaxation appliance may help to decrease the loading force; it should be worn as much as possible—especially at night.

c. Pain medication and anti-inflammatory agents may be used to decrease the general inflammatory response.

d. The patient should restrict movements to within painless limits.

e. A soft diet is recommended.

f. Ultrasound and moist heat applications may be beneficial.

g. Gentle active range of motion exercises within painless limits may help to lessen the likelihood of myostatic or myofibrotic contractures as well as to maintain joint function.

6. Traumatic arthritis

a. If trauma is anticipated as a result of a sports-related injury, a mouth protector may be recommended.

b. Jaw use should be decreased.

c. A soft diet is recommended, along with taking small bites and chewing more slowly.

d. Nonsteroidal anti-inflammatory medications are often recommended by dentists to reduce inflammation.

e. Moist heat may be applied as needed.

f. If symptoms persist beyond 7 to 10 days, ultrasound treatment may be indicated.

7. Infectious arthritis

a. The dentist initiates appropriate antibiotic medication to eliminate the invading organism.

b. Active range of motion exercises to maintain normal range of motion and to avoid postinfection fibrosis or adhesions may be necessary.

c. Ultrasound and moist heat should be used.

8. Rheumatoid arthritis

a. A muscle relaxation appliance may be used to decrease pain.

b. Moist heat may help.

c. Ultrasound also may be used.

d. Gentle active range of motion exercises to maintain mandibular range can be useful.

9. Temporal tendonitis (chronic hyperactivity of the temporal muscle)

a. A muscle relaxation appliance may help to rest the temporalis muscle.

b. Analgesics may be recommended.

c. Anti-inflammatory medications may be prescribed by a dentist or physician.

d. The intraoral application of ice may be helpful.

e. Ultrasound also can be used.

10. Stylomandibular ligament inflammation (pain at the angle of the mandible radiating to the TMJ and ear)[31]

a. Resting the jaw is recommended.

b. Analgesics and anti-inflammatory medications may help.

c. The intraoral application of ice may be useful.

11. Suboccipital neuralgia

a. Exercise may be used to correct forward head position.

b. Moist heat may be helpful.

c. Ultrasound also can be used.

d. A gentle myofascial release technique that is designed to liberate the restricted soft tissue surrounding the suboccipital muscles may help.

e. Ice may be applied to the affected muscles.

f. Re-education exercises to correct postural deficiencies are recommended.

g. Potential ergonomic contributory factors should be assessed. These may include harmful postures on the job or harmful sitting positions in the car, at home, or at work.

E. Treatment of chronic mandibular hypomobility

Chronic mandibular hypomobility is rarely accompanied by painful symptoms or progressive changes; however, when pain is a factor, it usually originates from an inflammatory reaction secondary to movement beyond the patient's restriction.

1. Contracture of the elevator muscles

   a. Myostatic contracture. The treatment goal is to re-establish the original resting length of the mandibular elevators. The resting length of the muscles can be re-established by two types of exercises: passive stretching exercises (see Figure 28–42), which are to be performed gently over a reasonable length of time, and resistant opening exercises (see Figure 28–39), which utilize reciprocal inhibition and thus initiates mild contraction of the antagonistic muscle groups (reflex relaxation). Pain implies that too much treatment has been given too soon; when pain occurs, the patient and the physical therapist should decrease the force and number of repetitions used. Supportive therapy should include the use of moist heat and ultrasound.

   b. Myofibrotic contracture. The treatment goal is to liberate the muscle tissues and sheath that have become bound by fibrous connective tissue. The connective tissue develops as a scar resulting from inflammation. Elongation of the muscle can be accomplished by continuous elastic traction. Surgical detachment and reattachment of the muscle involved may be necessary.

2. Ankylosis. Ankylosis occurs when the disc

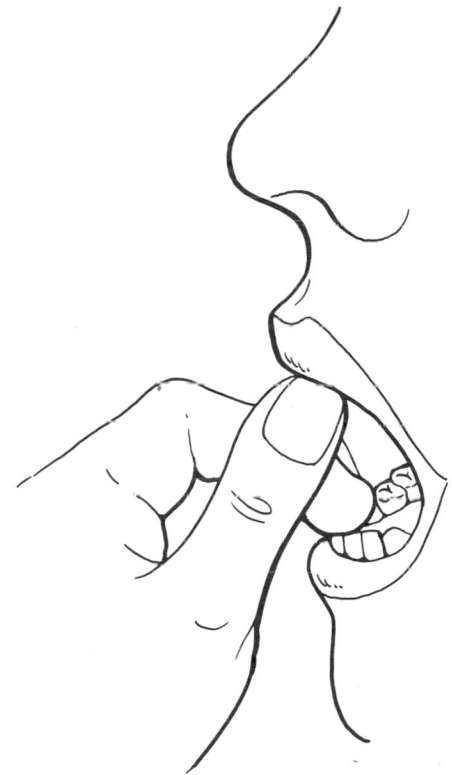

FIGURE 28–42 Passive stretching exercise. With the mandible opened to the point of restriction, the fingers are placed between the teeth. Momentary gentle force is applied to stretch the elevator muscle. The exercise should not elicit pain.

adheres to the articular fossa. Treatment should include a referral for arthroscopic surgery, prescription of analgesics, and the restriction of movements to within painless limits.

F. Occlusal appliance therapy

An occlusal appliance (splint) is a removable device, usually made of hard acrylic, that fits over the occlusal and incisal surfaces of the teeth in one arch, creating precise occlusal contact with the teeth of the opposing arch. This appliance is commonly referred to as a *bite guard, interocclusal appliance, night guard,* or *orthopedic appliance.*[32] These appliances are most commonly fabricated by a dentist; however, physical therapists are receiving more education and training in the fabrication of these appliances.

1. **Muscle relaxation (centric relation) appliance.** This appliance is used to decrease muscle hyperactivity.

a. A description of the appliance is as follows.
  (1). It is fabricated for the maxillary arch and provides an occlusal relationship that is considered optimal for the patient.
  (2). When the appliance is used, the condyles are in their most stable musculoskeletal position at the time of tooth contact.
b. Treatment goals
  (1). Muscle hyperactivity should be decreased.
  (2). The parafunctional activity that often accompanies stress should be decreased.
  (3). Symptoms associated with myospasms and myositis should be reduced.
  (4). Bruxing should be reduced.
c. Criteria for the use of the muscle relaxation appliance
  (1). It must accurately fit the maxillary teeth and provide total stability and retention when it comes into contact with the mandibular teeth.
  (2). In centric relation, all posterior mandibular buccal cusps must contact the flat surfaces of the appliance with even force.
  (3). During protrusive movements, the mandibular canines must contact the muscle relaxation appliance with even force.
  (4). In any lateral movement, only the mandibular canine teeth should exhibit laterotrusive contact on the appliance.
  (5). Mandibular posterior teeth must contact the muscle relaxation appliance only in centric relation closure.
  (6). In the feeding position, the posterior teeth must contact the muscle relaxation appliance more prominently than the anterior teeth.
  (7). The occlusal surface of the appliance should be as flat as possible with no imprints for mandibular cusps.
  (8). The occlusal appliance should be polished so that it does not irritate any adjacent soft tissue.
d. Instructions
  (1). The patient is to wear the muscle relaxation appliance at all times except during meals and when brushing or flossing teeth.
  (2). If wearing the appliance causes pain,

the patient should discontinue its use and report the problem to the dentist or physical therapist immediately so that it can be evaluated and corrected.
  (3). The patient may experience an increase in saliva production, which resolves in a few days.
  (4). The patient may have difficulty speaking; this resolves as soon as the tongue adapts to the thickness of the resin.
  (5). The appliance should be brushed immediately after being taken out of the mouth to prevent buildup of plaque and calculus.
  (6). Adjustments in the muscle relaxation appliance should be made as a more superoanterior position of the condyle is assumed.

2. **Anterior (orthopedic) repositioning appliance**
  a. Description
    (1). It is an interocclusal device that encourages the mandible to assume a position that is more anterior than centric occlusion.
    (2). The appliance is a full-arch hard acrylic appliance that can be used in either arch.
  b. Treatment goals
    (1). The appliance should provide a better condyle-disc relationship in the fossae so that normal function can be re-established.
    (2). It should eliminate the signs and symptoms associated with disc-interference disorders.
    (3). It does not permanently alter a mandibular position but does change the position temporarily while normal condyle-disc complex function returns (see Figure 28–43).
  c. Criteria for the anterior repositioning appliance
    (1). It should accurately fit the maxillary teeth with total stability and retention when it is in contact with the mandibular teeth.
    (2). In the established forward position, all of the mandibular teeth should come into contact with it with even force.
    (3). In the established forward position, the joint symptoms during opening and closing should be eliminated.

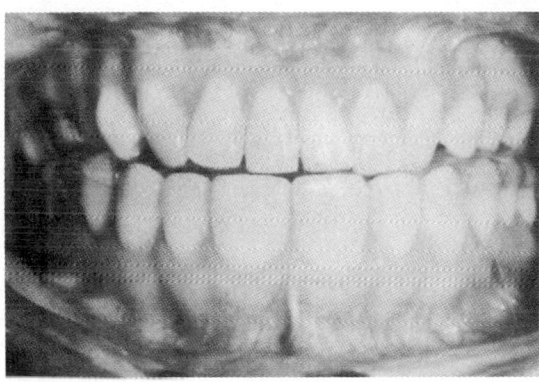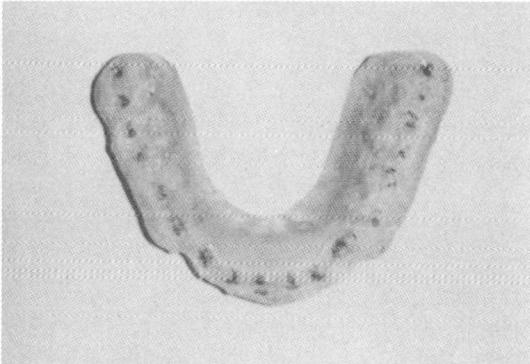

FIGURE 28–43   *Left panel,* Maxillary anterior repositioning appliance. Note the contact of all the teeth and the prominent retrusive guidance ramp. *Right panel,* Esthetics have been improved by removal of the acrylic, labial to the maxillary anterior teeth. (Left and right panels from Okeson JP: *Management of Temporomandibular Disorders and Occlusion,* 3rd ed. St. Louis, Mosby Year Book, 1993, p 483.)

(4). In the retruded range of movement, the lingual retrusive guidance ramp should contact the appliance, and on closure direct the mandible into the established forward position.

(5). The appliance should be smoothly polished and compatible with adjacent soft tissue.

d. Instructions

(1). It is to be worn at all times, even during eating.

(2). Problems with chewing and speech may occur initially.

(3). The patient must be instructed to maintain the forward position if a mandibular appliance is worn.

(4). The maxillary appliance is prescribed for wear during sleep.

(5). The length of time for use is determined by the type, extent, and chronicity of the disorder.

3. **Anterior bite plane**

a. Description

(1). It is a hard acrylic appliance worn over the maxillary teeth; it provides contact with only the mandibular anterior teeth (see Figure 28–44).

b. The treatment goals and use of the appliance are listed here.

(1). The appliance should disengage the posterior teeth and thus eliminate their influence on the function of the masticatory system.

(2). It can be used for the treatment of muscle disorders, especially myospasms that originate from an occlusal treatment.

(3). It is useful for the treatment of para-

functional activity associated with unfavorable posterior tooth contacts.

(4). Its use should be closely monitored, and it should only be used for short periods.

4. **Posterior bite plane**

a. Description. This hard acrylic appliance is worn over the mandibular teeth and is connected by a cast metal lingual bar.

b. The treatment goals with this appliance are to achieve major alterations in vertical dimension and to achieve mandibular repositioning.

c. Indications

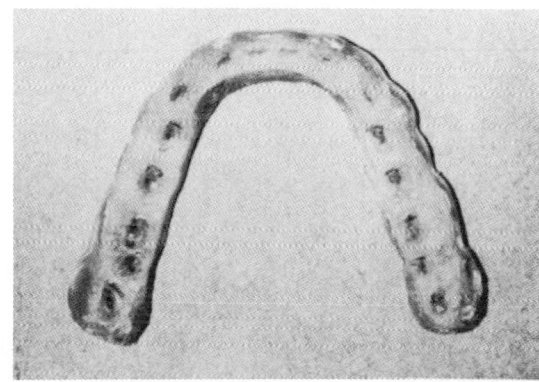

FIGURE 28–44   Mandibular anterior repositioning appliance. Unlike the centric relation appliance, each centric cusp on this appliance fits into a small depression or fossa that dictates the desired forward position. This appliance is used only during the day and is replaced with the maxillary repositioning appliance for nighttime use. (From Okeson JP: *Management of Temporomandibular Disorders and Occlusion,* 3rd ed. St. Louis, Mosby Year Book, 1993, p 485.)

(1). It can be used to restore severe loss of vertical dimension.

(2). It is useful for making major changes in anterior repositioning of the mandible.

(3). It can be used for certain disc-interference disorders.

(4). Its constant and long-term use should be discouraged.

5. **Treatment considerations for appliance therapy**

Much research suggests that occlusal appliance therapy can successfully reduce the symptoms of TMJ disorders.[31] The greatest contribution of this type of therapy appears to be the reduction of muscle activity, which, in turn, decreases myogenic pain. The reduction of muscle activity also reduces the forces imposed on the TMJs.[32] Six general features that may contribute to the decrease in muscle activity are common to all appliances; they are as follows.

a. Alteration of the occlusal condition. A change toward a more stable condition decreases muscle activity and eliminates symptoms.

b. Alteration of condylar position. A change may occur that moves the condyle to a more stable musculoskeletal position or a more structurally compatible and functional position.

c. Increase in vertical dimension. This results in a decrease in muscle activity and symptoms.

d. Cognitive awareness. The appliance acts as a reminder to the patient to alter activities that may affect the disorder.

e. Placebo effect. The appliance may cause a placebo effect because of the competent and reassuring manner in which therapy is provided.

f. Increased peripheral input to the CNS. Changes at the peripheral input level seem to have an inhibitory effect on CNS activity, *eg*, when an occlusal appliance is placed between the teeth, it provides a change in peripheral input and thereby decreases CNS-induced bruxism.

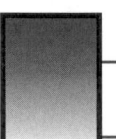

Clinical Decision-Making Cases

Case #1

HISTORY

The patient, a 35-year-old secretary, complained to the physical therapist that she had pain in her right masseter and temporal muscles that had been present for 2 days and had begun shortly after an amalgam restoration was placed.

EXAMINATION AND ASSESSMENT

The neuromuscular examination revealed tenderness in the right temporal muscle and pain in the right masseter muscle. The maximum comfortable interincisal opening was 32 mm, with a maximum opening of 52 mm. The TMJ examination revealed pain and tenderness in the belly of the right masseter and temporal muscles. A click in the right jaw was noted at 24 mm of opening. It was asymptomatic, and the patient reported that it had been present for 15 years. The occlusal examination revealed a complete, natural dentition that was in a good state of repair.

DIAGNOSIS

Muscle splinting secondary to placement of a high restoration.

TREATMENT

The amalgam restoration was adjusted by the dentist to contact evenly and simultaneously with the adjacent and surrounding teeth. The physical therapist instructed the patient to limit movement to within painless ranges until the pain subsided. She also was instructed to apply ice as needed.

OUTCOME

When the patient returned to the physical therapist in 5 days, the pain had subsided and no symptoms were present.

Case #2

HISTORY

A 20-year-old male college student reported to an outpatient physical therapy facility complaining of a generalized muscle soreness on the left side of his face. The pain was aggravated by chewing. It had been present for approximately 1 week. In discussing the problem, the patient revealed that this type of pain had been present on three other occasions 2, 6, and 8 months earlier, respectively. He did not report any noticeable change in his occlusion but felt that the pain did limit his mandibular opening. Further questioning revealed that each of the three previous episodes of pain, as well as the present episode, accompanied his college examinations.

EXAMINATION AND ASSESSMENT

The neuromuscular examination revealed tenderness of the right and left masseters and the left temporal muscle. The patient's comfortable interincisal opening was measured at 22 mm. The TMJ examination revealed no pain or sounds. There were no other significant findings in the history or clinical examination.

DIAGNOSIS

Myospasms secondary to increased emotional stress associated with college examinations.

TREATMENT AND GOALS

The patient was made aware of the relationship between emotional stress, parafunctional activity, and the symptoms that he was experiencing. Active range of motion exercises were outlined for him, and a series of six ultrasound applications were administered to the affected muscles. In addition, spray and stretch techniques were used to increase the extensibility of the mandibular elevators. The patient was also instructed to restrict movement to within painless limits and, when possible, to control parafunctional activity.

OUTCOME

At the termination of the sixth ultrasound application, all symptoms had resolved.

Case #3

HISTORY

A 38-year-old homemaker complained of a 3-week history of fairly constant pain originating in the muscles on the right side of her face. She reported that she had had recurrent episodes of similar pain but that it had never been so bad or lasted so long. The history revealed no trauma, but the symptoms were related to stresses associated with raising her two young children.

EXAMINATION AND ASSESSMENT

The neuromuscular examination revealed generalized tenderness to palpation of the right temporal and sternocleidomastoid muscles and severe pain in the right masseter muscle. The maximum comfortable mandibular opening was 18 mm. The TMJ examination failed to disclose any pain or dysfunction. During the occlusal examination, it was noted that both mandibular first molars had been extracted and that the second molars had drifted into the existing space, causing a lateral shifting of the mandible from centric relation to centric occlusion. There were no other significant findings in the history or clinical examination.

DIAGNOSIS

Myositis secondary to protracted myospasms and related to parafunctional activity, probably associated with both emotional stress and malocclusion.

TREATMENT AND GOALS

The patient was made aware of the relationship among her occlusion, stress, parafunctional activity, and symptoms. A muscle relaxation appliance was fabricated by her dentist, and she was instructed to wear it at all times (except during meals). Progressive relaxation techniques were outlined, and she received ultrasound treatments three times a week for 3 weeks.

OUTCOME

After 2 weeks, the symptoms were approximately 50% resolved. By the 3rd week, active exercises were instituted to regain maximum comfortable mandibular opening. By the 4th week, almost all of the symptoms had resolved, and assisted stretching exercises were added to aid in regaining a normal range of movement. After 6 weeks, the patient was completely free of symptoms. Passive and assisted stretching exercises were continued for an additional 3 weeks until a normal range of opening was achieved.

Case #4

HISTORY

A 41-year-old secretary was referred by her dentist to the physical therapy office because of her complaint of tightness in her jaw muscles and a constant headache. The headache had been present for 4 months and appeared to be worse in the late afternoon after she had been typing all day. The tightness in the jaw muscles was aggravated by chewing.

EXAMINATION AND ASSESSMENT

Examination revealed a comfortable mandibular opening of 24 mm, with a maximum opening of 39 mm. A normal range of eccentric movements also was present. No joint pain or sound was noted. Bilateral masseter tenderness was present. Although the headache was felt in the temporal regions, the temporal muscles were not tender to palpation. Palpation of the posterior neck and trapezius muscles revealed multiple trigger points. Pressure applied to the trigger zones in the trapezius aggravated the headache in the temporal area. There were no other significant findings in the history or the clinical examination.

DIAGNOSIS

Myofascial trigger point pain in the posterior cervical and trapezius muscles with referred pain to the temporalis muscles.

TREATMENT AND GOALS

Trigger points in the trapezius and posterior cervical muscles were sprayed and stretched. An explanation was given to the patient regarding myofascial trigger point pain and the common etiologic factors. The patient was also told about emotional stress and the possible effect of incorrect posture during typing. She was then told to follow a home treatment program that included moist heat and passive stretching of the neck and shoulder muscles. In addition, correct postural attitudes were outlined for the patient, with the suggestion that a lumbar support be used to facilitate correct head and neck alignment during her prolonged periods of sitting.

OUTCOME

She returned 2 weeks later with significantly reduced headache pain. Comfortable mandibular opening had reached 35 mm, with a maximum range of 44 mm.

Case #5

HISTORY

A 44-year-old computer analyst complained of right TMJ tenderness and sounds. He also reported generalized facial muscle tightness with occasional tenderness. The current joint problems had been present for 4 days and had been recurring approximately every 2 months for the past year. The history revealed no trauma or previous treatment for the prior episodes. It appeared that a relationship existed between the recurrence of joint symptoms and a heavy workload associated with alternate monthly deadlines.

EXAMINATION AND ASSESSMENT

Examination revealed a single click in the right TMJ at 3 mm of opening. The joint was tender to palpation. The left joint was asymptomatic. Transcranial radiographs revealed normal TMJ function and bone surfaces. The neuromuscular examination revealed that the left and right temporal muscles and the right masseter were tender. On palpation, the left masseter, left sternocleidomastoid, and posterior cervical muscles were painful for the patient. The right lateral pterygoid muscle also was painful to palpation. The occlusal examination disclosed a generally healthy dentition with moderate wear on the canines and posterior teeth. No missing teeth, caries, or significant periodontal disease was present. Also, no other significant findings could be found in the history or clinical examination.

DIAGNOSIS

The primary diagnosis was disc displacement; the secondary was myospasms. Both of these diagnoses were related to parafunctional activity associated with increases in emotional stress.

TREATMENT AND GOALS

A muscle relaxation appliance was fabricated by the patient's dentist. The patient was instructed to wear the appliance all day, taking it out only when eating and performing oral hygiene activities. To control nocturnal parafunctional activities, he was also to wear it during sleep. The relationship among heavy workload, emotional stress, parafunctional activity, and the patient's symptoms was discussed with him. Alternate work patterns were suggested to lighten peak workloads. Progressive relaxation training was begun, and the patient was instructed to spend at least 20 minutes a day developing relaxation skills. Mandibular active range of motion exercises were initiated using reflex inhibition techniques.

OUTCOME

After 1 week, the patient reported a reduction of symptoms of approximately 50%. After 2 weeks, the symptoms were almost completely reduced, and 1 week after that, all symptoms were eliminated. The patient then discontinued appliance therapy but continued with the exercise program. During a routine 6-month follow-up appointment, the patient reported that he had experienced two recurring episodes, which he managed successfully with exercise and relaxation techniques.

Case #6

HISTORY

A 36-year-old homemaker reported that her jaw kept locking. She stated that on the previous day, after she had repeatedly clenched her jaw, she had been unable to open her mouth completely. For the past 2.5 months, her right TMJ had been making sounds, and on occasion, she had felt as if it were going to get "stuck." This was the first time that her jaw had actually become locked, and the sounds had ceased to be present in the joint.

EXAMINATION AND ASSESSMENT

Examination revealed tenderness of the right TMJ and no symptoms associated with the left joint. No joint sounds were heard. The patient's maximum interincisal opening was 26 mm. She had a normal range of lateral movement to the right side (8 mm), but left lateral movement was limited to 4 mm and elicited pain. Transcranial radiographs revealed a restricted pattern of movement in the right TMJ. The articular surfaces of both joints looked normal. The neuromuscular examination produced negative results, with the exception that tenderness was observed in the right masseter muscle. All dentition was present and in a good state of repair. Although the occlusal condition looked clinically nor-

mal, the patient complained that "the back teeth didn't seem to bite right." There were no other significant findings in the history or clinical examination.

DIAGNOSIS

Disc dislocation secondary to parafunctional activity.

TREATMENT AND GOALS

The mandible was manipulated in an attempt to reduce the dislocated disc. This was successful, but shortly after closing, the dislocation recurred. An anterior repositioning appliance was fabricated. The mandible was once again manipulated, and the disc was successfully reduced. The appliance was immediately placed, and the patient closed in the forward position as determined by the appliance. Repeated opening and closing in this position failed to cause dislocation of the disc.

OUTCOME

The patient wore the appliance constantly for 3 months, after which time she wore it only at night. After 4 months, the TMJ range returned to normal pain-free function.

Case #7

HISTORY

Immediately after a dental procedure during which three extensive amalgam restorations were completed, the 31-year-old male patient, an executive, could not close his mouth. Occlusal examination revealed that the posterior teeth were relatively close to their occluding teeth, but that the anterior teeth were not. The patient repeatedly attempted to close and with each failure became increasingly uncomfortable and frustrated.

He had earlier related that when he opened his mouth wide, the joint would commonly hesitate and jump forward, but no pain was associated with this movement or any history of previous locking.

DIAGNOSIS

Spontaneous dislocation secondary to a long dental procedure.

TREATMENT AND GOALS

The therapist's thumb was placed on the patient's chin, and slight posterior force was applied. At the same time, the patient was asked to open wide as if yawning. The mandible immediately reduced itself, and the occlusion was re-established. The patient was reassured with an explanation of the problem. Because he had reported a history of subluxation, he was instructed to maintain normal function within the range so as not to provoke this condition. Whenever possible, any procedures requiring a wide-open mouth were discouraged. It was suggested that he eat his food cut into small pieces so that minimal opening would be required until the symptoms had completely resolved.

OUTCOME

No recurrence was reported.

Case #8

HISTORY

A 27-year-old male graduate student reported to the physical therapy office with severe pain in his left TMJ. He had been in a car accident 4 days earlier, and his head had hit the dashboard. He had received several cuts around the cheek, eye, and chin. He had been treated in a hospital emergency room for these cuts and released. On the day after the accident, his left TMJ was tender, and it became progressively more painful each day thereafter. He had had no symptoms in this joint prior to the accident.

EXAMINATION AND ASSESSMENT

Examination revealed an extremely painful left joint. The right joint was asymptomatic. No joint sound or noticeable swelling was present in the joint area. Pain was constant and was aggravated by mandibular movement. The patient could open only 22 mm interincisally without pain. Maximum opening was 35 mm. Transcranial radiographs revealed no obvious bone involvement. Panoramic and anteroposterior radiographs failed to identify any evidence of condylar fracture. The neuromuscular examination disclosed tenderness in the left masseter muscle and in the right and left temporal muscles. The clinical examination revealed a complete and healthy complement of teeth with no obvious dental disease. No evidence of trauma to any teeth was seen. The occlusal condition was within normal limits, and the patient reported that he could bite on his posterior teeth without eliciting pain. No other significant findings were noted in either the history or the clinical examination.

DIAGNOSIS

Capsulitis secondary to extrinsic trauma.

TREATMENT AND GOALS

The patient was instructed to restrict all mandibular movement to within painless limits and to eat only a soft diet. Analgesics were prescribed to control pain. It was suggested that he apply moist heat to the painful joint area for 10 to 15 minutes four to six times a day. After 4 days, ultrasound was applied three times a week for 2 weeks.

OUTCOME

During the 1st week, the patient reported that most of the pain had resolved. After 1 additional week of the therapy, he was no longer experiencing pain and was able to resume normal function. Follow-up visits revealed no recurrence of symptoms.

Case #9

HISTORY

A 12-year-old female junior high school student reported that she had been feeling severe pain in her right TMJ for 2 days after she had fallen off her bike and hit her chin on the sidewalk. She had had no previous history of any type of pain in this joint.

EXAMINATION AND ASSESSMENT

Examination revealed pain in the right TMJ and no tenderness in the left. No noticeable sounds were present in either joint. The maximum comfortable interincisal opening was 17 mm, and the maximum opening 41 mm. Transcranial radiographs revealed normal function and subarticular surfaces. Panoramic and anteroposterior radiographs did not reveal any evidence of fracture of the condyle. The neuromuscular examination showed some tenderness of the right temporal muscle. The occlusal examination revealed a relatively normal healthy dentition in a good state of repair. No teeth were missing, and posterior support appeared to be sound; however, the patient reported that the pain increased when she clenched on her posterior teeth. With a tongue depressor placed between the posterior teeth, clenching did not elicit pain. There were no other significant findings in the history or clinical examination.

DIAGNOSIS

Retrodiscitis secondary to extrinsic trauma.

TREATMENT AND GOALS

The patient was instructed to restrict all mandibular movement to within painless limits and to begin a soft diet. Analgesics were recommended to control the pain. Moist heat was applied at home four to six times a day. The patient returned in 5 days and reported that the pain was still present and was most severe on awakening in the morning. Neuromuscular examination revealed that other muscles (the left and right mas-

seters, the right temporalis, the occipitalis, and the right sternocleidomastoid muscles) had become tender to palpation. The physical therapist thought that parafunctional activity could be a coexistent factor that was influencing the outcome of the retrodiscitis. An occlusal appliance was fabricated to produce a comfortable mandibular position, and the patient was instructed to wear the appliance during sleep or anytime that clenching or bruxing was noticed. Exercise therapy for muscle relaxation was also initiated.

OUTCOME

The patient returned after 1 week and reported a 50% reduction in the symptoms. The same therapy was continued, and in 1 week she had no symptoms. She was encouraged to continue wearing the appliance at night for 4 more weeks to promote complete healing of the retrodiscal tissues. At that time, appliance therapy was discontinued.

Case #10

HISTORY

A 46-year-old housepainter came to the physical therapy office with pain in his right TMJ. He reported that this joint had become "locked" 2 months earlier but had only recently been painful.

OBJECTIVE

TMJ examination revealed a maximum comfortable interincisal opening of 25 mm and a maximum opening of 27 mm. The patient was able to move his mandible normally in a right lateral direction but was severely restricted in the left lateral movement. Transcranial radiographs revealed limited movement in the right joint. The subarticular surfaces of both joints appeared normal. The neuromuscular examination revealed tenderness in the right and left temporalis and right and left masseter muscles. The occlusal examination showed several missing posterior teeth and considerable drifting of the remaining molars and premolars. The anterior teeth exhibited signs of heavy occlusal contact. When the patient was asked to clench on his remaining posterior teeth, pain was elicited. Biting on a separator did not accentuate the pain but in fact relieved it. There were no other significant findings in the history or clinical examination.

DIAGNOSIS

Retrodiscitis secondary to intrinsic trauma from an anteriorly dislocated disc.

TREATMENT AND GOALS

This patient was referred to a dentist who fabricated an anterior repositioning appliance that moved the condyle off the retrodiscal tissues onto the disc. After 8 weeks of continuous appliance therapy the appliance was gradually thinned in an attempt to reduce the anterior positioning of the disc. After the second adjustment, the pain returned. The symptom-free position of the mandible was then re-established on the appliance. Over the next 4 weeks, repeated attempts were made to thin the appliance, but the symptoms always returned. Treatment options were presented to the patient, and surgery to repair the protracted and dislocated disc was selected. The surgical procedure revealed that the disc was anteriorly and medially dislocated but in good repair, and that it was successfully repositioned on the condyle. A postsurgical occlusal evaluation revealed residual postoperative pain and joint restriction. The patient was referred to physical therapy for exercises designed to stretch the restricted elevators and joint capsule; modality intervention accompanied the stretching techniques, and a home exercise program was designed.

OUTCOME

After 6 weeks of physical therapy, the patient regained a pain-free functional mandibular range of 39 mm.

Case #11

HISTORY

A 50-year-old female college professor came to the dental office complaining of chronic right TMJ pain. She was able to locate it by placing her finger over the distal aspect of the right condyle. The pain had been present for 6 weeks and seemed to be getting worse. The pain was always present, but it was less in the morning, and it became worse as the day progressed. She was aware of a grinding sound in her right TMJ. Movement aggravated the pain. On questioning the patient, the therapist learned that the right TMJ had "locked" 9 to 10 months previously and that she had only recently begun to regain a normal opening range. She commented that her wide opening was still limited compared with what it had been 1 year ago.

EXAMINATION AND ASSESSMENT

Examination revealed pain in the right TMJ that was aggravated by movement. The left joint was only slightly tender to palpation during function. The patient experienced pain at 20 mm of interincisal opening but could open to 36 mm maximally. During opening, a deflection of the midline to the right side occurred. Definite crepitation in the right TMJ was noted. Transcranial radiographs revealed alteration in the subarticular surfaces in the right condyle consistent with degenerative joint disease. The neuromuscular examination revealed tenderness of the left and right masseter muscles, the left and right temporalis muscles, and the left sternocleidomastoid muscle.

DIAGNOSIS

The primary diagnosis was degenerative joint disease secondary to functional anterior dislocation of the disc; the secondary diagnosis was muscle splinting and myospasms secondary to chronic joint pain.

TREATMENT AND GOALS

The patient was informed of the causes and prognosis of degenerative joint disease. She was told that the disease is often self-limiting but that the course of the symptoms might last 8 to 12 months. It was emphasized that conservative therapy usually is successful in controlling pain and helps to limit the inflammatory process. The patient was also to restrict jaw movement to within painless limits and to begin a soft diet. Analgesic and anti-inflammatory medications were recommended on a regular basis for 4 weeks. Moist heat was to be applied several times each day at home.

OUTCOME

The patient returned in 1 week and reported a considerable decrease in pain. The same therapy was continued, and she began passive exercises within painless limits to maintain a normal range of movement. The patient complained that she had a very limited range of painless movement. The therapy continued for 1 month, at which time the pain had greatly diminished.

References

1. Hilderbrand GY: *Studies in the Masticatory Movements of the Lower Jaw.* Berlin, Walter De Gruyter, 1931.
2. Hilderbrand GY: A further contribution to mandibular kinetics. *J Dent Res* 1937, 16:551.
3. Suit SR, Gibbs CH, Benz ST: Study of gliding tooth contacts during mastication. *J Periodontol* 1975, 47:331–334.
4. Adams SH, Zander HA: Functional tooth contacts in lateral and centric occlusion. *J Am Dent Assoc* 1964, 69:465.
5. Mongini F, Tempia-Valenta G: A graphic and statistical analysis of the chewing movements in function and dysfunction. *J Craniomandibular Pract* 1984, 2:125.
6. Gibbs CH, Mahan PE, Manderli A, *et al.*: Limits of human bite strength. *J Prosthet Dent* 1986, 56:226–229.
7. Howell AH, Manly RS: An electronic strain gauge for measuring oral forces. *J Dent Res* 1948, 27:705.
8. Waugh LM: Dental observations among Eskimos. *J Dent Res* 1937, 16:355.
9. Howell AH, Brudevald F: Vertical forces used during chewing of food. *J Dent Res* 1950, 29:133.
10. Schneyer LH, Pigman W, Hanahan L, Gilmore RW: Rate of flow of human parotid sublingual and submaxillary secretions during sleep. *J Dent Res* 1956, 35:109–114.
11. Jenkins GN: *The Physiology of the Mouth,* 3rd ed. Philadelphia, F. A. Davis Company, 1966, pp 461–476.
12. Preiskel HW: Some observations on the postural position of the mandible. *J Prosthet Dent* 1965, 15:625.
13. Mohl ND: Head posture and its rate in occlusion. *N Y State Dent J* 1976, 42:17.
14. Bell WE: *Temporomandibular Disorders,* 2nd ed. Chicago, Year Book Medical Publishers, Inc, 1986, pp 66–67.
15. Friction JR, Kroening R, Haley D, Siegert R: Myofascial pain syndrome of the head and neck: a review of clinical characteristics of 164 patients. *Oral Surg Oral Med Oral Pathol* 1985, 60:615–623.
16. Travell JG, Simons DG: *Myofascial Pain and Dysfunction: The Trigger Point Manual.* Baltimore, Williams & Wilkins, 1983.
17. Bell WE: *Temporomandibular Disorders,* 2nd ed. Chicago, Year Book Medical Publishers, 1986, pp 194–195.
18. Pullinger A: Sex Differences in TMJ Laxity and Jaw Opening. *J Dent Res* 1985, 64:269.

19. Bates RE Jr, Stewart CM, Atkinson WB: The relationship between internal derangements of the temporomandibular joint and systemic joint laxity. *J Am Dent Assoc* 1984, 109:446–447.
20. de Bont LG, Boering G, Liem RS, *et al.:* Osteoarthritis and internal derangement of the temporomandibular joint: a light microscopic study. *J Oral Maxillofac Surg* 1986, 44:634–643.
21. Ramfjord SP, Ash M: *Occlusion*, 3rd ed. Philadelphia, W. B. Saunders Company, 1983, pp 313–314.
22. Ramfjord SP: Bruxism, a clinical and electromyographic study. *J Am Dent Assoc* 1961, 52:21–44.
23. Williamson EH, Lundquist DO: Anterior guidance: its effects on electromyographic activity of the temporal and masseter muscles. *J Prosthet Dent* 1983, 49:816–823.
24. Blankestyn J, Boering G: Posterior dislocation of the temporomandibular disc. *Int J Oral Surg* 1985, 14:437.
25. Gallagher D: Posterior dislocation of the temporomandibular joint meniscus. *J Am Dent Assoc* 1986, 113:411.
26. Schroeder SA: *Medical Diagnosis and Treatment*. Norwalk, CT, Appleton & Lange, 1993.
27. Okeson JP: Conservative management of masticatory disorders. *Proceedings of the American Equilibration Society's 32nd Annual Meeting*. Chicago, February 11–12, 1987.
28. Travell JG, Simons DG: *Myofascial Pain and Dysfunction. The Trigger Point Manual*. Baltimore, Williams & Wilkins, 1983.
29. Zarb GA, Speck JE: The treatment of mandibular dysfunction. In Zarb GA, Carlsson GE (eds): *Temporomandibular Joint Function and Dysfunction*. St. Louis, C. V. Mosby Company, 1979, p 382.
30. Krentziger KL, Mahan PE: Temporomandibular joint degenerative joint disease. *J Oral Surg Oral Med Oral Pathol* 1975, 40:12.
31. Shankland WE: Ernst syndrome as a consequence of stylomandibular ligament injury: a report of 68 patients. *J Prosthet Dent* 1987, 57:502.
32. Okeson JP: *Management of Temporomandibular Disorders and Occlusion*. Philadelphia, C. V. Mosby Company, 1989.
33. Clark GT: Occlusal therapy: occlusal appliances. In *The President's Conference on the Examination, Diagnosis, and Management of Temporomandibular Disorders*. Chicago, American Dental Association, 1987, p 137.
34. Sheikholeslam A, Holmgren K, Riise C: A clinical and electromyographic study of the long-term effects of an occlusal splint on the temporal and masseter muscles in patients with functional disorders and nocturnal bruxism. *J Oral Rehabil* 1986, 13:137–145.

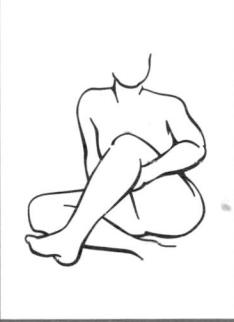

CHAPTER 29

Cervical Spine

Margaret Anderson, Barbara Stevens, Jan Richards, and Gail Jensen

THE MAITLAND APPROACH AND CLINICAL DECISION MAKING: OVERVIEW

The Maitland approach focuses on assessment, examination, and treatment and provides a conceptual framework to assist clinicians in their decision-making process by linking theoretical knowledge with clinical evidence. Several other approaches to musculoskeletal evaluation and treatment are frequently used by physical therapists (eg, osteopathic, Kaltenborn, Cyriax, Mennell, McKenzie). These approaches emphasize different "philosophical bases." For example, the Kaltenborn approach has a strong biomechanical component and the emphasis is on biomechanical assessment of joint movements. These various approaches also have many similarities, such as the type of interview and physical examination data the clinician collects.[1] We believe that the Maitland approach provides an excellent framework for collecting and analyzing clinical data. The framework is one that is detailed, logical, and requires the clinician to generate clinical working hypotheses as the basis for planning and modifying treatment.

The following two sections provide definitions of key terms and an introduction to the basic components of the Maitland approach, the overall philosophy of treatment, and an introduction to the major concepts in the evaluation process.

I. Definition of Key Terms

Active physiological movements. Movements that the patient can perform, eg, flexion, abduction, extension, rotation.

Asterisks. These are used to highlight the main subjective complaints and the objective signs comparable to the patient's problems against which change or the patient's progress can be monitored. The objective signs must be measurable.

Clear. The term used when no clinical signs are present. If no signs are present, a joint will have full range and painless movement with overpressure.

PLEASE NOTE: A joint may be painlessly stiff and not give rise to symptoms, ie, normal for that person. Such a stiff, painless joint may be considered a "normal abnormal" joint for that person. A joint cannot be considered clear unless firm overpressure is applied with no more discomfort than the normal joint on the opposite side.

Comparable sign. A finding on examination that reproduces the pain or demonstrates the abnormality comparable to the complaint for which the patient is seeking treatment.

End-feel. The therapist's assessment of the sensation that is perceived when a joint is moved passively to the end of range of movement. Cyriax described five types of end-feel (bone to bone [hard], springy block, muscle spasm, soft-tissue approximation, and empty).[2] Others, eg, Kaltenborn,[3] advocate just three—soft, firm, and hard.

Manipulation. A passive movement technique that is

1. Performed at the limit of the available passive range at such a speed that it is beyond the patient's control.
2. Performed as a slow, sustained stretch at the end of the passive range with the intent of increasing range by tearing the limiting structures.

Mobilization. A passive movement technique performed by the physical therapist in a manner and at a speed that are within the ability of the patient to control the movement.

Overpressure. Oscillatory movement that is applied passively to a joint at the limit of the range of motion. The therapist gets a sense of the end-feel of the joint when applying overpressure.

Passive accessory movements. Movements available in a joint that are performed passively by the examiner but which the patient cannot perform actively. These include the translatory movements between articular surfaces (eg, slide, roll, spin, which are performed as treatment movements such as posteroanterior movements).

Passive physiological movements. Movements that are performed by the therapist, not the patient.

Sign. A finding on physical examination that is measurable (objective examination). It may be anything within a joint/structure that interferes with movement (eg, stiffness, palpable soft-tissue changes, pain).

II. Basic Components and Philosophy of the Maitland Approach[4]

A. Process of problem solving

All good clinicians use some process of problem solving, which allows them to do the following:
1. Collect data through examination of the patient.
2. Interpret the data.
3. Reach a decision based on that interpretation regarding what and how to treat.
4. Act on the basis of that interpretation and carry out the treatment program.
5. Observe, evaluate, and respond to changes in the patient's condition during the course of treatment.

B. Process of systematic examination

The process of examination-assessment-treatment is the foundation of the Maitland approach.

1. **Role of clinical evidence versus pathology.** The Maitland approach is not based on biomechanical or pathoanatomical theory; rather, it is an approach to problem solving that is focused on *clinical evidence.* This includes
   a. *Symptoms.* These constitute the patient's complaint. Many types of symptoms can occur, including pain, paresthesia, stiffness, weakness, giving way, or specific functional loss.
   b. *Signs.* Any abnormalities of tissue, movement, or function

2. **Role of two-compartment thinking.** Two-compartment thinking is used to separate the theoretical framework and clinical assessment and is aided by the concept of the brick wall (see Figure 29–1). As seen in the figure, "the theoretical concepts influence examination and treatment while examination and treatment leads one back to a reconsideration of theoretical premise."[4]

3. **Role of the permeable brick wall.** The brick wall should actually be thought of as permeable, that is, theory should help illuminate the clinical evidence, and clinical evidence should assist with the recognition of clinical

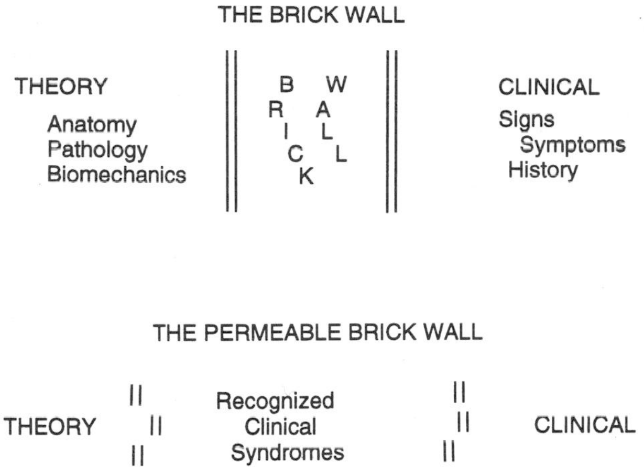

FIGURE 29–1 Theoretical framework. (From Maitland GD: *Vertebral Manipulation*, 5th ed. Churchill Livingstone, New York.)

syndromes. This type of thinking frees the clinician from prejudice and restraints that are imposed by a "diagnosis" and assists the clinician in
   a. Speculating and formulating a working hypothesis that remains responsive to emerging data.
   b. Treating safely and effectively without knowing a precise diagnosis.
   c. Creating evaluation and treatment techniques to meet the needs of a given clinical situation, unhindered by theory.
   d. Speculating, treating, and monitoring the patient's response.

C. Process of assessment

The process of assessment is the cornerstone of the Maitland approach. If the assessment is to be accurate and relevant, the examination and treatment must necessarily be performed with skill and accuracy. Assessment is detailed in a later section.

D. Process of examination

The examination process in the Maitland concept is divided into the subjective and objective phases.

1. The subjective examination
   a. Provides the basis for understanding and interpreting the patient's symptoms as they will relate to the physical examination findings; demonstrates the therapist's ability to listen to the patient and understand the problem from the patient's perspective.
   b. Requires the development of a high level of communication skills, particularly the ability to listen to the patient.
   c. Seeks to establish the following:
      (1). Precise area of all symptoms, including depth, character, and an indication of the worst area.
      (2). Whether one area of symptoms is present or multiple areas.
      (3). The behavior of each area of symptoms related to the time of day or in response to movement or body position.
      (4). The chronological history of the disorder.
      (5). The presence of any contraindications to examination or treatment.
   d. Provides the basis for assessment that may be used in planning the objective examination and treatment. This may include
      (1). The cause of the symptoms.
      (2). The manner in which the disorder is presenting, ie, the
         (a). Severity.
         (b). Irritability.
         (c). Nature.
         (d). Stage and stability.
      (3). The characteristics of the patient as a person.
      (4). A baseline level of function against which progress may be assessed.

2. The objective examination purpose:
   a. To interpret the patient's concept of disability in terms of structures and movement by
      (1). Producing the symptoms that the patient is complaining of.
      (2). Finding comparable signs (and abnormality of movement of function) in appropriate structures.
      (3). Determining the nature and extent of abnormalities of movement or function.
   b. To determine physical factors that may have predisposed the patient to the onset of the disorder.
   c. To be a specific exploration of the patient's complaint and to be guided by the assessments made following the subjective examination. Every examination will vary in
      (1). Content and emphasis.
      (2). Extent and detail.
      (3). Vigor.
   d. To explore movement through various ways of movement testing.
      (1). These movements or combinations of movements are important for producing the appropriate symptomatic response.
      (2). The importance of the following should be noted:
         (a). Relating the change in symptoms to the test movements.
         (b). The detail of the palpation of soft tissue and the use of accessory movements.
         (c). Using principles of differentiation when possible.
         (d). Making appropriate use of compression.

III. Anatomy of the Cervical Spine

The cervical vertebrae represent the most mobile segments of the vertebral column. They bear the least amount of weight and are relatively small and thin with respect to the size and shape of their vertebral arch and vertebral foramen.[5,6] The diameter of a cervical vertebra is greater transversely than in the anteroposterior direction. In addition, they are easily identifiable by their transverse processes, which are perforated by a foramen, the foramen transversarium, that transmits the cervical arteries and vessels.[5-7]

Of the seven cervical vertebrae, the 1st and 2nd (C1–C2) present special features that necessitate a separate description. C3–C7 conform to a fairly typical type of vertebra and are covered by a common description.

A. Vertebrae C3–C7

Vertebrae C3–C7 are each composed of a body, vertebral arch, spinous process, and two transverse processes. Posterior to the body is the vertebral arch, consisting of two pedicles and two laminae. The pedicles project back from the body and form the two sides of the intervertebral arch. On the inferior aspect of each pedicle is a deep vertebral notch, and on the superior aspect a shallow notch. The two adjacent notches, along with the intervertebral body and disc, form the intervertebral foramen for the exit of the spinal nerve. The two laminae are oriented posteriorly and medially to join in the midline with the spinous process.

Projecting from the arch are the two transverse processes and a single spinous process. The transverse processes have two projections, the anterior and posterior tubercles. These two tubercles serve as origins for the cervical muscles. Between the anterior and the posterior tubercles of the transverse process is a sulcus for the exiting spinal nerve (see Figure 29–2).

The spinous process of each vertebra projects posteriorly from the junction of the laminae. They are typically short at the C3–C6 levels and are usually bifid.

The 7th cervical vertebra is considered transitional and is somewhat modified from the other typical vertebrae. The inferior aspect of the C7 vertebral body is larger than the superior aspect. The C7 spinous process is larger than the spinous processes of the other cervical vertebrae and therefore more easily palpable[5–7] (see Figure 29–3).

1. **Intervertebral discs.** The intervertebral disc consists of an inner core of fibrogelatinous material, the nucleus pulposus, surrounded by an outer laminated ring of fibrocartilage, the annulus fibrosus.

The intervertebral disc binds adjacent vertebral bodies together, functioning as a shock absorber and stabilizer throughout the vertebral column from the sacrum to the axis.

The cervical intervertebral discs differ in many respects from the intervertebral discs of the lumbar spine. The vertical height of the cervical intervertebral disc is two times greater anteriorly than posteriorly. In the lumbar spine, the disc height is only slightly greater anteriorly.[8] This increased anterior height contributes to the curve of the cervical spine. In the erect standing position, the cervical intervertebral disc and facet joints bear equal vertical compressive forces, whereas the lumbar intervertebral disc bears approximately 85% of the vertical compressive force; the facets bear the remaining 15%.[7,9,10]

Horizontal fissuring of the annulus fibrosus of the intervertebral disc begins around the end of the first decade of life and is increasingly prevalent in the later adult years.[7] As a result, there is an overall loss of disc height. This process is associated with a

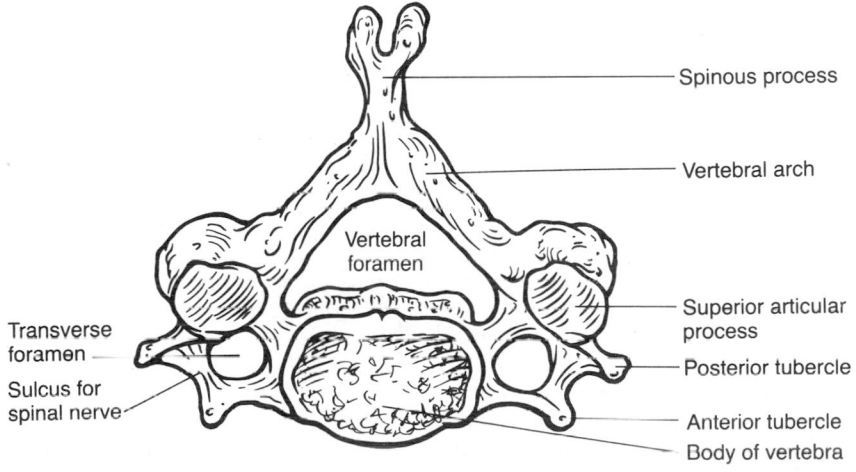

FIGURE 29–2 Fifth cervical vertebra.

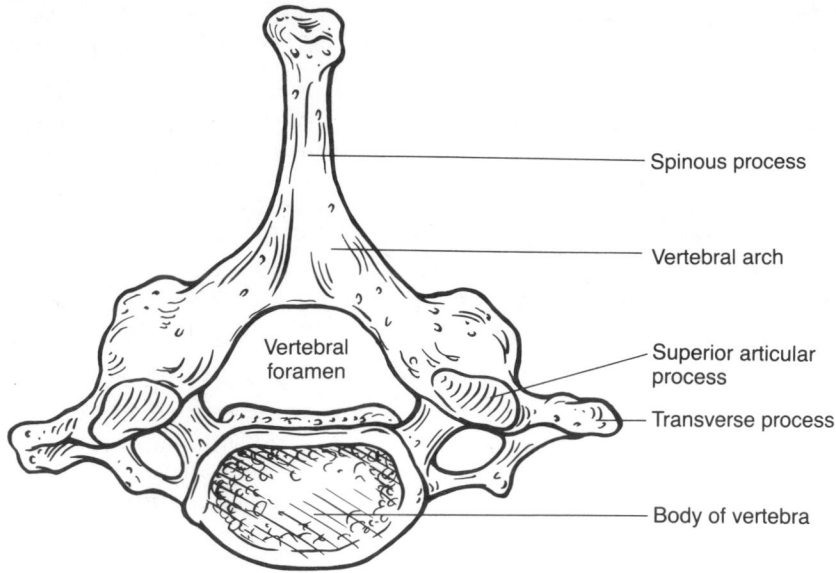

Spinous process

Vertebral arch

Superior articular process

Transverse process

Body of vertebra

Vertebral foramen

FIGURE 29–3   Seventh cervical vertebra.

gradual loss of nuclear material through the posterior and lateral fissures.[7] In the adult spine, the nucleus pulposus of the cervical intervertebral disc is typically absent.[7] If any nuclear material remains in adult years, it is more likely to herniate backward into the spinal canal than laterally into the intervertebral foramen.[7]

2. **Zygapophyseal joint or facet joint.** The articular facets from adjacent vertebrae join to form a small-plane synovial joint referred to as the zygapophyseal or facet joint. Facet joints in the cervical spine are designed to allow free movement in all planes of motion. The structure and orientation of the articular facet determine the available intervertebral movement.

In the cervical spine, the articular surfaces of the facet joints are oriented 45 degrees to the transverse plane, with a range of 30 to 60 degrees, and are parallel to the frontal plane and at a right angle to the sagittal plane.[10] The superior facets are oriented upward and posteriorly, and the inferior facets are oriented downward and anteriorly. Movement occurs in a coupling fashion, meaning each type of motion is always accompanied by another. For example, axial rotation is always coupled with lateral flexion during movement of the cervical spine[9–13] (see Figure 29–4).

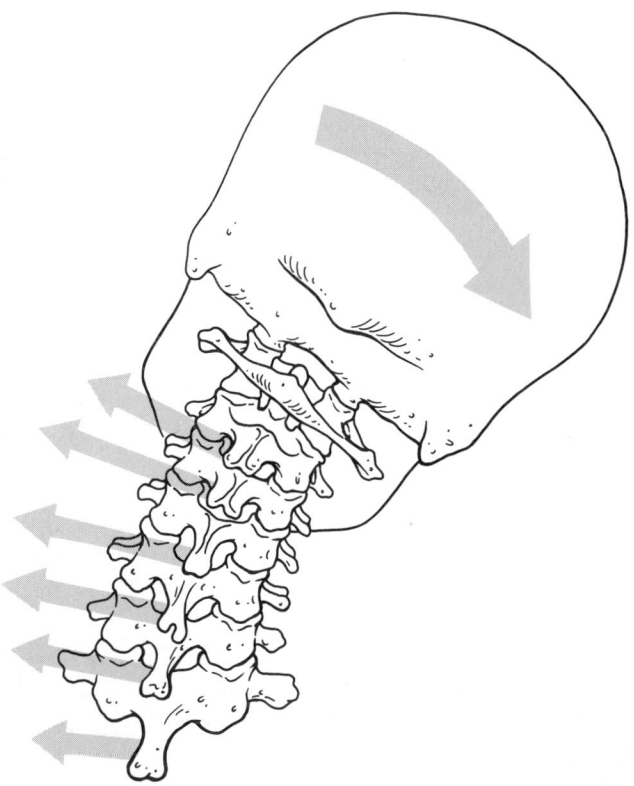

RIGHT LATERAL BENDING

FIGURE 29–4   Coupling movements in the cervical spine.

Approximately 45 degrees of axial rotation and 49 degrees of lateral flexion occur to each side of neutral at levels C3–C7.[10] During flexion and extension, there is a total range of approximately 64 degrees, with 24 degrees of extension and 40 degrees of flexion.[9] However, there is a wide variation in the amount of motion contributed by each individual vertebral segment.[9–13]

3. **Uncovertebral joints.** The uncovertebral joints (or joints of von Luschka) are formed between the uncinate processes, the lateral vertebral margin of the upper surface of the inferior vertebral body, and the lower body of the vertebral body above.

It is believed that degenerative changes in the uncovertebral joints are twice those in the facet joints.[6] Degenerative change is most likely related to excessive stress placed on the uncovertebral joints because of

a. Additional uncovertebral joint loading associated with increased disc fissuring and loss of disc height.
b. Shear forces on the joint during cervical spine movement, leading to osteophytic spurring around the spinal canal, exiting nerve roots, and vertebral artery.[7,11,14,15]

4. **Nerve supply.** Structures in the cervical spine that are posterior to the intervertebral foramen and cervical nerve roots, defined as posterior elements, receive their nerve supply from the dorsal rami of the cervical spinal nerves.[16] The anterior elements, or structures that lie anterior to the cervical nerve roots, which include the intervertebral disc and the anterior and posterior longitudinal ligaments, receive their innervation from the ventral rami of C1–C6.[16–21] Superficial posterior neck muscles are innervated by the lateral branches of the cervical dorsal rami, whereas the medial branches of the cervical dorsal rami supply the deeper muscles of the neck.[16–21] In addition, these nerves provide innervation to the cervical facet joints.[15]

B. Upper cervical spine (C1–C2) atlanto-occipital and atlantoaxial joints

The 1st and 2nd cervical vertebrae differ from the other vertebrae in size, shape, and function. The upper cervical area also differs from the remainder of the vertebral column because of the absence of intervertebral discs. This unique area of the upper cervical spine forms a complex articular system that primarily permits nodding and rotational movements of the head.

The 1st cervical vertebra, C1, or the atlas, is atypical in that it lacks a body and consists primarily of an anterior and posterior arch. The atlas has paired lateral masses in which the upper surfaces have concave articular facets for the articulation of the occipital condyles.[5,6,22] On the lower surface of the atlas are inferior articular facets for the articulation with C2 (axis).

Along the upper edge of the posterior arch is a groove in which the vertebral artery runs posteriorly and medially, entering the skull at the foramen magnum. The posterior tubercle of the posterior arch is a rudiment of a spinous process and is often difficult to palpate because of its deep position under the occiput (see Figure 29–5).

The 2nd cervical vertebra, C2, or the axis, is distinctive primarily for its odontoid process, or dens. The dens is an articular process that projects superiorly from the vertebral body and articulates with the anterior arch of C1[5,6,22] (see Figure 29–6).

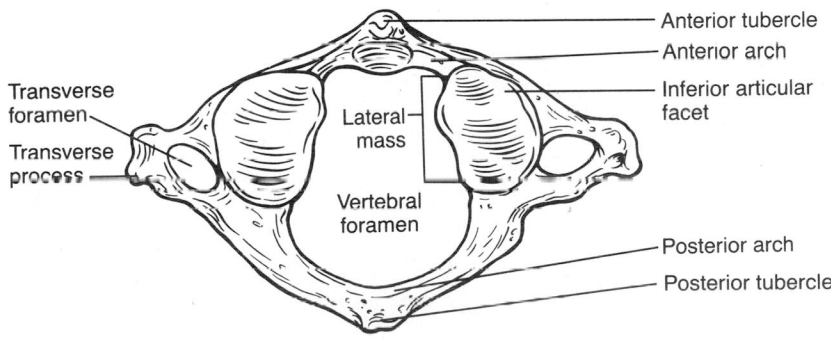

FIGURE 29–5 Atlas.

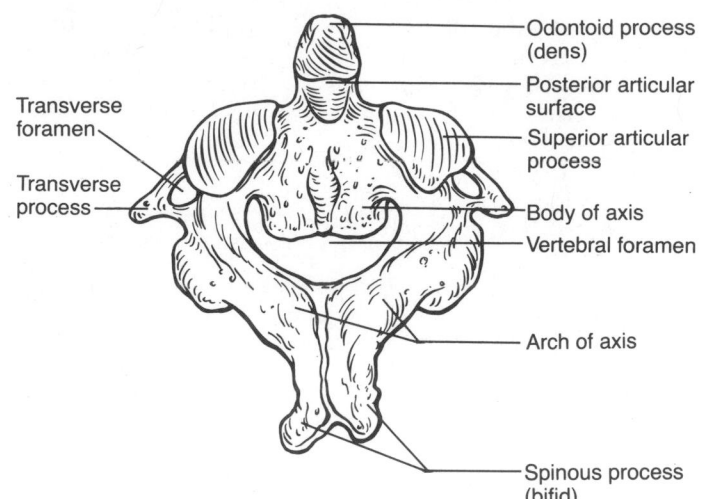

FIGURE 29–6   Axis.

The ligamentous structures of the upper cervical spine are the primary stabilizer for this region. The atlanto-occipital joint is surrounded by strong, loose fibrous capsules. The atlantoaxial joint capsules are reinforced by accessory ligaments. Between the occiput and the anterior arch of the atlas is a broad, thick membrane, the anterior atlanto-occipital membrane, a continuation of the anterior longitudinal ligament.[6] Posteriorly, the paired ligamenta flava are represented by a somewhat thinner membrane, the posterior atlanto-occipital membrane. These membranes provide additional support for this region[6] (see Figure 29–7).

Each lateral mass of the atlas has a tubercle for the attachment of the strong transverse ligament (see Figure 29–8). The transverse ligament passes behind the dens, stabilizing the dens in contact with the anterior arch of the atlas, controlling anteroposterior movement at the atlantoaxial joint. Atlanto-occipital stability is provided by the alar ligaments that extend from the superior and lateral aspect of the dens to the lateral margins of the foramen magnum. The thin apical ligament extends from the tip of the dens to the anterior margins of the foramen magnum, also providing stability for the atlanto-occipital region[5,6,22,23] (see Figure 29–9).

Motion at the atlanto-occipital region consists of 10 to 15 degrees of flexion and extension and 8 degrees of lateral flexion.[10,12]

During flexion, the head moves forward while the convex occipital condyles slide posteriorly on the concave superior facet joints of the atlas. This movement is coupled with a relative anterior and superior translation of the

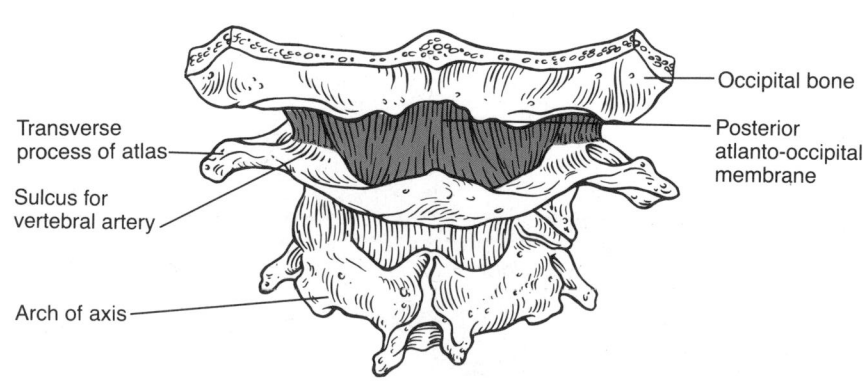

FIGURE 29–7   Posterior atlanto-occipital membrane.

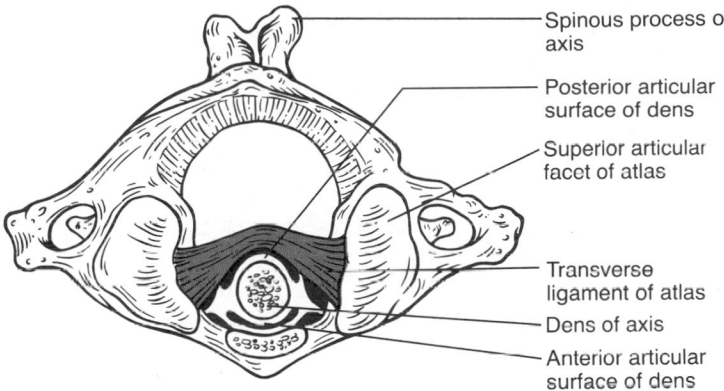

Spinous process of
axis

Posterior articular
surface of dens

Superior articular
facet of atlas

Transverse
ligament of atlas

Dens of axis

Anterior articular
surface of dens

FIGURE 29–8   Transverse ligament.

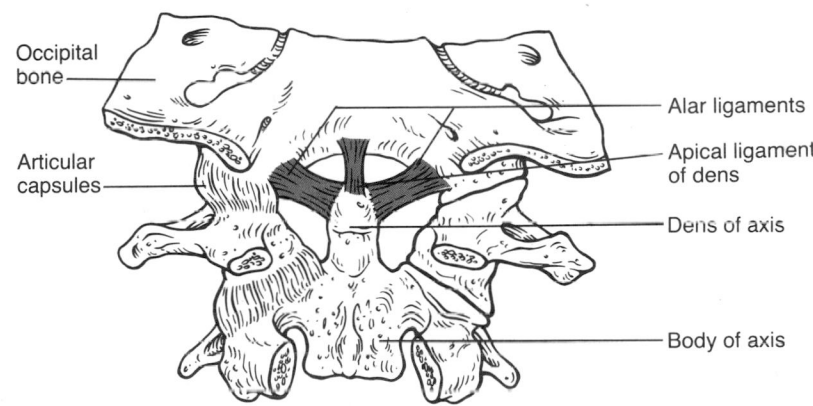

Occipital
bone

Articular
capsules

Alar ligaments

Apical ligament
of dens

Dens of axis

Body of axis

FIGURE 29–9   Alar and apical ligament.

atlas. The alar ligaments restrict flexion at the atlanto-occipital joint by tightening as the occipital condyles slide posteriorly and superiorly.

During extension, the head moves backward while the convex occipital condyles slide anteriorly on the atlas. The primary restraint during extension of the head is the increase in tension of the membrane and the anterior capsular fibers of the atlanto-occipital joints.

Little to no axial rotation occurs at the atlantoaxial joint. Any rotational force on the head is transformed into movement at the atlantoaxial joint.[10]

The primary movement of the atlantoaxial joint is axial rotation. This rotational movement has been measured between 38 and 47 degrees and represents 50% to 60% of the total axial rotation available in the cervical spine.[10] Approximately 10 degrees of flexion and extension occurs at the atlantoaxial joint, with minimal to no lateral flexion occurring at this region.[10,12]

1. **Nerve supply.** The suboccipital muscles of the cervical spine receive their innervation from the C1 and C2 dorsal rami.[15] The C1 and C2 ventral rami provide the innervation for the atlanto-occipital and atlantoaxial joints.[16–21]

IV. Subjective Examination of the Cervical Spine

A. Primary objectives

1. To ascertain the kind of disorder with regard to
   a. **Severity**—the clinician's assessment of the intensity of the patient's symptoms as they relate to a functional activity.

      Example: A patient avoids turning his head quickly to the right because of a sharp stabbing pain in the midcervical area; the pain is severe. This type of pain tends to be sharp, stabbing, and intense but does not last a long time; it subsides immediately after the provoking activity is stopped.

   b. **Irritability**—the clinician's assessment based on relating the amount of activity needed to bring on the patient's symptoms and the amount of time before the symptoms return to a resting or a nonaggravated level.

      Example: When the patient described above turns his head to the right and experiences sharp midcervical pain. The pain now radiates into his shoulder and takes up to 2 hours to begin decreasing. This means that the patient's condition is extremely irritable (little activity brings on considerable pain that lasts for a long period of time).

   c. **Nature**—The clinician's assessment of
      (1). The pathology or structure of the primary complaint.
      (2). Other pathology (*eg*, rheumatoid arthritis, diabetes, osteoporosis, general poor health that limits examination and treatment and prevents a good recovery).
   d. **Stage and stability**—the clinician's assessment of the progression of symptoms and the stability of the condition.

      Example: The patient described above, 1 week later, now complains that the pain spreads into the shoulder and arm. It is keeping him from doing his work. This would indicate that the pathological condition may be worsening and that the patient is not "stable."

2. To determine the characteristics of the patient (the clinician's assessment of the patient's pain tolerance, including consideration of cultural differences).
3. To determine the present level of function as a baseline against which progress may be assessed.

B. Major elements of the examination

- Patient profile.
- Kind of disorder.
- Area of symptoms.
- Behavior of symptoms.
- Special questions.
- History.
- Medical history.

1. **Patient profile.** This provides the background for the interpretation of the patient's complaint and is necessary if the therapist is to establish an accurate prognosis and set realistic goals for treatment. Some items should be asked directly, whereas others must be pieced together from other areas of the interview. The profile may include
   a. Biographical data (*eg*, age, gender).
   b. Occupation, including the physical demands, ergonomic situation, time constraints.
   c. Recreational activity, including frequency and intensity.
   d. Present level of activity (*eg*, work, recreation, rest).
   e. Psychobehavioral factors.
   f. Socioeconomic factors.
   g. Insurance, compensation, litigation status.

2. **Kind of disorder.** The therapist ascertains the patient's priorities and/or reasons for seeking treatment. The initial question should encourage spontaneous comment: What is your main problem? Pain is the most common reason for seeking treatment, but other reasons include
   a. Stiffness.
   b. Giving way.
   c. Instability.
   d. Weakness.
   e. Loss of function.
   f. Recurrent episodes.
   g. Trauma, accident, surgery, hospitalization.

3. **Area of symptoms.** This may be the single most important part of the subjective examination. It forms the basis for the remainder of the examination, with possible implications for the following:
   - Structures involved.
   - Severity of the disorder.
   - Area to receive major emphasis.

 PLEASE NOTE: Figure 29–10 provides an example of a body chart.

   a. *Hints*
      (1). The patient should be adequately undressed.
      (2). The therapist should observe gestures and the manner in which the patient uses his/her hands; in par-

ticular, the patient's first movements should be noted.
      (3). The therapist may place his/her hands on the patient to save time and to assist in clarification of where the symptoms are located; the therapist should use his/her hands in the same manner as the patient.
   b. *Recording on the body chart.* Accuracy is critical in determining the following:
      (1). The extent of the symptoms.
      (2). The depth of the symptoms.
      (3). The character/quality of the symptoms.
      (4). Paresthesia/anesthesia.
      (5). The worst area.
   c. *Areas to routinely question the patient about for the cervical spine*
      (1). Central over the spine.

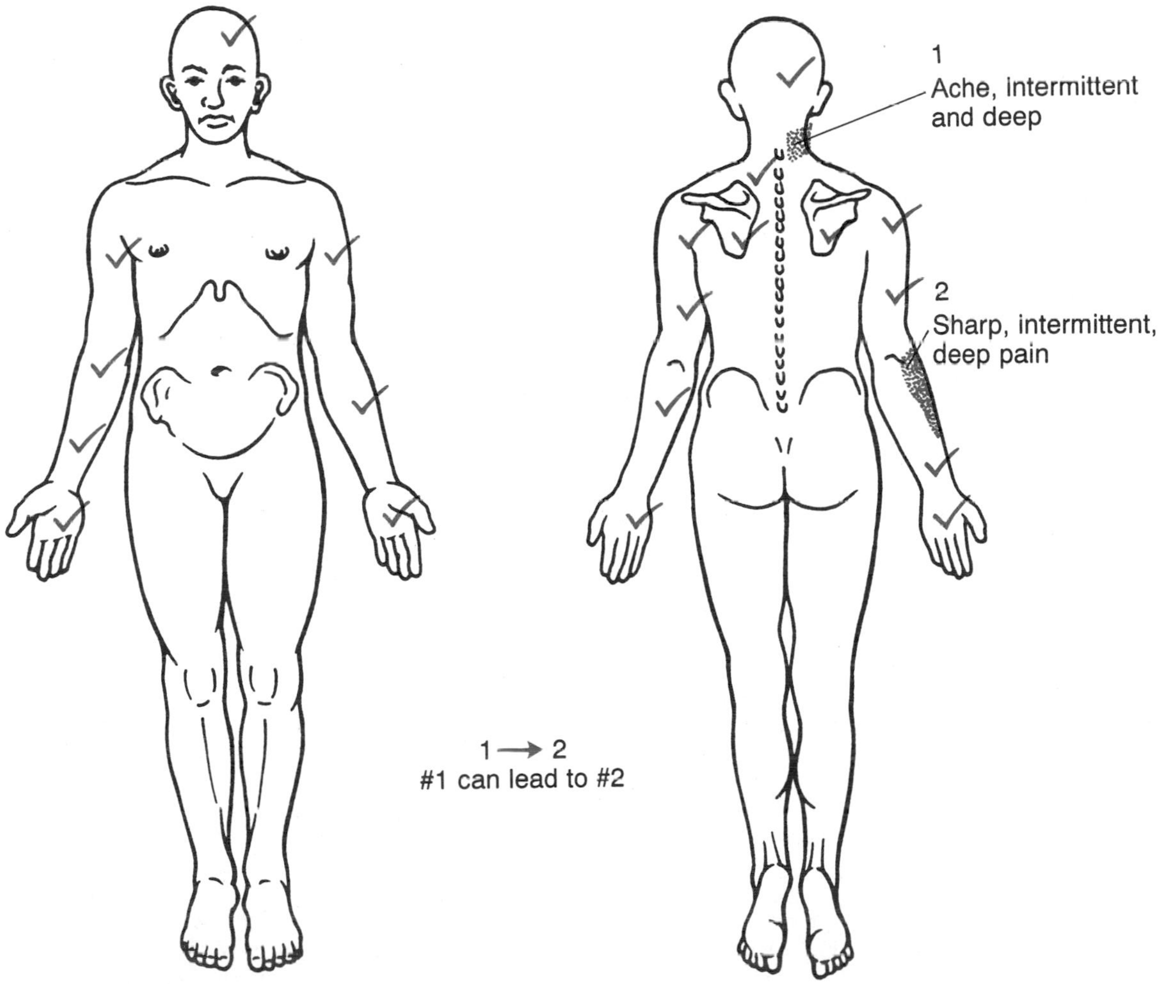

1
Ache, intermittent and deep

2
Sharp, intermittent, deep pain

1 → 2
#1 can lead to #2

FIGURE 29–10   Example of a body chart.

(2). Pain referred into the extremity.

(3). Pain on the opposite side of the spine or referred into the opposite extremity.

(4). Pain referred to the medial border of the scapula.

(5). Headaches.

(6). Shoulder pain.

(7). Paresthesia/anesthesia.

4. **Behavior of symptoms.** The therapist questions the patient about the pattern of the symptoms throughout the day (*ie*, behavior of the symptoms). The therapist does the following:

a. Establishes and explores the mechanical nature of the problem.

b. Assesses the irritability of the condition. In assessing irritability, the therapist must consider the following three components:

(1). The amount of activity required to bring on the symptoms.

(2). The severity of the symptoms produced.

(3). The time required for symptoms to subside or recover to the previous level.

c. Establishes a baseline level of function against which progress can be measured.

d. Other considerations for establishing behavior of the symptoms include:

(1). Whether the symptoms are constant or intermittent (*eg*, vary with time of day, activity, posture, or position).

(2). Aggravating factors (the positions or movements/activities that bring on the symptoms are identified).

(3). Easing factors (the positions or movements/activities that ease the symptoms are identified; the effect of rest is determined).

(4). Symptom behavior over a 24-hour period.

PLEASE NOTE: For each subjective complaint, the therapist should establish objective parameters (*eg*, patient self-report of what changes the symptoms). These can be used as a baseline against which progress can be measured, giving the therapist a more accurate impression of the impact of the problem on the patient's life.

5. **Special questions.** These are asked in an attempt to reveal conditions that may require caution or may contraindicate treatment. The patient is questioned about

a. General health.

b. Relevant weight changes.

c. Use of steroids and anticoagulants.

d. Radiographs and other diagnostic tests.

e. Medications for this or any other condition (*eg*, analgesics, anti-inflammatory drugs).

f. Possible spinal cord symptoms:

(1). Bilateral numbness and tingling in the feet.

(2). Disturbance of gait.

6. **History.** The history of the present episode must describe the circumstances/manner of onset, the development of the episode, and the present stage and stability of the disorder.

a. When did it start?

b. Manner of onset:

(1). *Sudden*

(a). A specific incident (the therapist attempts to understand the mechanics of the forces involved).

(b). A spontaneous injury:

(i). Did the patient wake with the symptoms?

(ii). When did the patient first notice it or what was the patient doing when it was first noticed?

(iii). What were the predisposing factors?

(c). The therapist attempts to relate

(i). The nature of the incident.

(ii). The severity of the symptoms.

(iii). The patient's ability to continue work.

(iv). The severity of symptoms the next morning.

(2). *Gradual*

(a). When did the patient first notice symptoms?

(b). What were the predisposing or precipitating activities?

c. Progress of the symptoms since the onset:

(1). Changes in area and severity of symptoms.

(2). Spread in the extremities; development of paresthesias or anesthesias.

(3). Development of new symptoms.

(4). Rate and direction change: are symptoms static, worsening, or improving? If symptoms are static, for what period of time?

d. Treatment given.

e. Diagnostic studies.

7. **Previous history**

a. Description of first episode in detail: cause, duration, treatment, level of recovery.

b. Successive bouts: frequency, ease of provocation, severity, time to recover, treatment and its effect, level of recovery.

c. How does this episode compare to others?

8. **Medical history.** The therapist looks for

a. Previous surgeries that may not be related to the presenting problem (eg, total hip replacement).

b. History of other diseases (eg, diabetes, hypertension, malignancy, heart disease, rheumatological conditions).

c. Recent fracture.

PLEASE NOTE: The medical history may set limits on how much vigor the therapist can use in examination and is important for predicting prognosis and planning for patient management.

V. Planning the Objective Examination for the Cervical Spine

After collecting the subjective data, the clinician should be able to fill out a planning sheet according to the following outline either on paper or in the head (see case study #1, p 767).

A. Structures at fault

Which structures must be examined as a possible cause of the patient's symptoms?

1. Which joints lie under the area of symptoms?

PLEASE NOTE: Joints lying under the area of symptoms need to be checked so that possible secondary joint problems are not overlooked. *The clinician should not fall victim to the error of omission.*

2. Which joints may refer into the area of symptoms?

3. Which contractile structures are under the area of symptoms (eg, rotator cuff, forearm muscles)?

4. Which other structures need to be examined (eg, thoracic outlet, carpal tunnel)?

5. Which of these structures is most likely to cause the patient's symptoms? (Consider all of the possible and most probable structures.)

6. Will a neurological examination be needed? (Yes, if the symptoms go below the acromio-clavicular joint or are in the scapula or thoracic area.)

B. Influence of symptoms on the examination

1. **Severity.** Are the symptoms minimal, moderate, or severe?

2. **Irritability.** Are the symptoms irritable? Give an example of

a. Activity causing the symptoms.

b. Severity of the symptoms.

c. Time for the symptoms to subside.

3. **Nature.** Does the nature of the disorder indicate caution? Is specific testing required?

4. **Stage.** Does the stage of the disorder guide or limit the examination?

5. Are there any contraindications to the examination or treatment?

C. Kind of examination

1. Will you be gentle or vigorous with the examination? Why?

2. Will you

a. Move to the first report of pain (P1)?

b. Move to the limit (L)?

c. Add overpressure?

d. Use sustained, repeated, or combined movements?

3. Which symptoms will you reproduce?

4. Do you expect a comparable sign to be easy or hard to find?

D. Associated examination

Are there other factors that must be examined as reasons why the affected structure has become painful or why the disorder may recur (*eg*, lifestyle, posture, physical fitness)?

E. Prognosis

Begin to estimate the patient's expected level of recovery.

VI. Objective Examination for the Cervical Spine: Introduction

The objective examination either substantiates or negates information obtained from the subjective examination. The examination also provides data to assist the therapist in decision making, in treatment selection, and in determining the prognosis. The pattern of the patient's level of function is also obtained as the clinician marks with an asterisk objective signs that can be monitored throughout the course of the treatment.

A. Examination goals

1. To find the joints and/or muscles at fault.
2. To reproduce the patient's symptoms or to find comparable signs at an appropriate joint.
3. To look for deviation in movement patterns that confirm the patient's complaints.

B. Physical examination tests

1. Intervertebral joints:
   a. Active physiological movements.
   b. Passive accessory intervertebral movements.
   c. Passive physiological intervertebral movements.
2. Muscles.
3. Pain-sensitive structures in the vertebral canal and intervertebral foramen.
4. Neurological function:
   a. Upper motor neuron lesions, spinal cord.
   b. Lower motor neuron lesions, nerve root or peripheral nerve impairment.
5. Peripheral joints underlying the area of pain.
6. Other special tests:
   a. Vertebral basilar artery insufficiency.
   b. Thoracic outlet syndrome.

C. Limits of the objective examination

1. **Relevant testing.** All tests are not appropriate and will not necessarily be performed on the first visit. One always works systematically when examining tissue from which pain and other symptoms may arise. Some tests are routine, whereas selection of the most pertinent will improve with clinical experience.
2. **Pain reproduction.** During the examination, the clinician decides which category the patient falls into—irritable or nonirritable—and then considers the following criteria:
   a. *Severe/irritable symptoms.* The examination is limited to
      (1). One or two movements because
         (a). The patient has to be treated in the first session and their symptoms relieved.
         (b). A comparable sign will be easy to find.
         (c). Details of the objective examination can be obtained during subsequent visits.
      (2). Movements just to the onset of pain (called P1) or just beyond so that the behavior can be noted.
   b. *Nonirritable symptoms.* It is not necessary to limit the examination. The patient can move to the limit of his/her range (called L).
      (1). Active physiological movements are used, then oscillatory overpressure, increasing from gentle to vigorous; range, behavior of symptoms, and end-feel are noted.
      (2). Repeated/quick movements, sustained movements, combined move-

ments, and functional tests may be necessary to reproduce symptoms.

3. **Alterations during movement testing.** Changes are made when
   a. Emerging information indicates that the patient's symptoms are more irritable/severe than estimated in the subjective examination or vice versa.
   b. The nature of the presenting problem indicates more or less caution; there is latency in symptoms.
   c. The subjective examination indicates that it is unlikely to reproduce symptoms, and the objective examination indicates that information will not be obtained by a more detailed or vigorous examination. (The therapist proceeds to palpation for a comparable sign or uses treatment to bring about change.)
   d. Adequate data are collected from the objective examination, and further information will not change treatment selection (*eg*, in cases of cervical spondylosis).

REMEMBER: Knowledge of clinical presentation tells the therapist what to expect; when something atypical arises, *caution* is required, *ie*, rethink your hypothesis.

VII. Objective Examination Sequence for the Cervical Spine

A. Observation

The patient is observed for
1. General appearance, affect, visual cues of symptoms.
2. Willingness to move, undressing.
3. Body structure, somotype, level of fitness.
4. Posture.
5. Changes of body contour suggestive of atrophy, swelling, spasm.
6. Scarring, thickening, edema.

B. Sitting

1. Functional quick tests (these are the patient's demonstration of movements that aggravate the problem).
2. Active cervical movements.
   a. Flexion.
   b. Extension.
   c. Rotation, right and left.
   d. Lateral flexion, right and left.
   e. Quadrant, right and left (combined movement) (see Figure 29–11).
3. When indicated, the therapist does the following:
   a. Corrects the deformity where it occurs.
   b. Applies overpressure.
   c. Differentiates between upper and lower cervical spine.
   d. Performs repeated movements.
   e. Performs sustained movements.
   f. Uses compression or distraction.
   g. Performs vertebral artery testing.

C. Standing

1. Shoulder tests to clear the joint:
   a. Abduction.
   b. Hand behind back test (see Figure 29–12).
   c. Static (resisted) tests for the rotator cuff muscles.

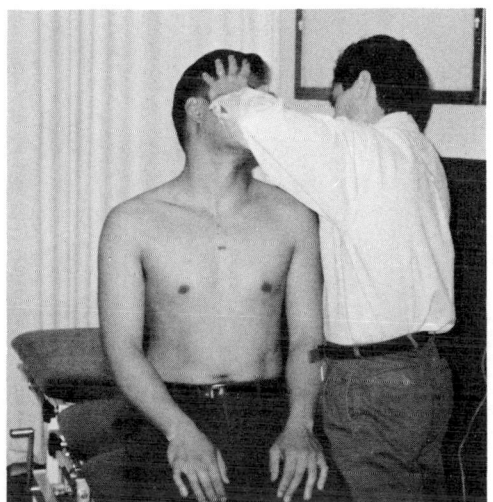

FIGURE 29–11 Cervical spine quadrant test.

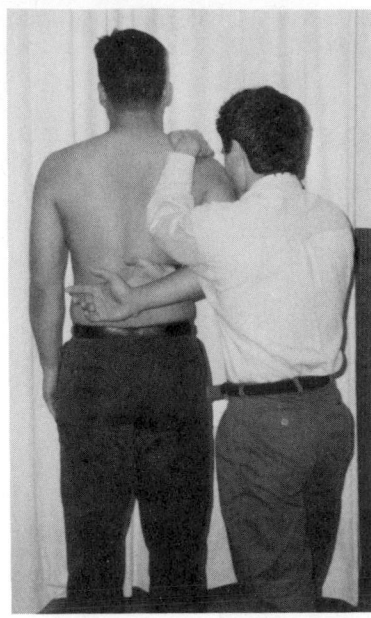

FIGURE 29–12   Hand behind back test.

D. Supine

1. Neurological tests (see following section on neurological examination for the cervical spine).

2. Passive peripheral joint tests.
3. Passive physiological intervertebral movements.
4. Further vertebral artery testing.
5. Elbow and wrist tests to clear the joints.
   a. Elbow:
      (1). Flexion.
      (2). Extension.
      (3). Extension and adduction.
      (4). Extension and abduction.
   b. Wrist:
      (1). Flexion.
      (2). Extension.
      (3). Radial and ulnar deviation.

E. Prone

1. Palpation:
   a. Temperature and swelling.
   b. Soft tissue.
   c. Position and alignment.
   d. Passive accessory intervertebral movements.

VIII. Neurological Examination for the Cervical Spine

A. Lower motor neuron lesions

1. Nerve roots:
   a. Loss of power in myotome.
   b. Loss of sensation in dermatome.
   c. Loss of reflex.
2. Peripheral nerves:
   a. Loss of power in muscles supplied.
   b. Loss of sensation in skin supplied.

B. Upper motor neuron lesions

1. Spinal cord:
   a. Hyperreflexia.
   b. Babinski's sign.
   c. Clonus.

C. Indications for neurological examination for cervical spine at initial visit

1. Complaint of pain/symptoms referred into extremity that may be referred from the spine:
   a. Pain or burning into the scapular area.
   b. Pain below the acromioclavicular joint.
2. Any complaints of weakness or paresthesia/anesthesia.
3. Any symptoms suggestive of upper motor neuron lesions of spinal cord compression:
   a. Bilateral numbness and tingling in the hands and feet.

b. Incoordination or disturbance of gait suggestive of spasticity.
4. Previous history of referred symptoms.

D. Indications for repeating neurological examination

1. At first follow-up visit when any neurological deficit was found at initial visit.
   a. Only abnormal findings need to be rechecked unless there has been a change in the patient's symptoms.
2. Any worsening of the patient's condition characterized by
   a. A marked change in severity or area of symptoms.
   b. Spread of local symptoms into the extremity.
   c. New complaints of weakness, giving way, paresthesia.
   d. Development of symptoms suggestive of cord or cauda equina compression.
3. Complete and dramatic relief of pain suggesting the possibility of a complete conduction loss.
4. When a neurological deficit is present, it should be checked frequently, if not at every visit.
   a. Useful to monitor recovery.
   b. Essential to monitor if patient's condition is worsening.

E. Content of Neurological Examination for Cervical Spine

1. **Muscle strength**
   a. Key muscles are tested at each nerve root level:
      (1). C5: deltoid.
      (2). C6: biceps.
      (3). C7: triceps.
      (4). C8: flexor digitorum longus and the extensor digitorum longus.
      (5). T1: interossei.
   b. Testing may be done only on the affected side; however, if there is a finding of weakness:
      (1). Comparison with opposite side should be made.
      (2). Testing should be done in a midrange.

c. Testing should build to a maximum isometric contraction.
d. Testing may be inconclusive in the presence of pain.

2. **Reflexes**
   a. The following are tested:
      (1). C6: biceps.
      (2). C7: triceps.
      (3). C8 flexor digitorum longus.
   b. The test should always be performed six times, looking for fatigue in the reflex.
   c. The reflex is graded as follows:
      (1). Equal bilaterally.
      (2). Diminished.
      (3). Absent.
      (4). Fatigues (the number of repetitions noted).
   d. Reinforcement:
      (1). Gritting teeth to raise general level of tonicity reinforces all reflexes.
      (2). When reinforcement is required, it must be used bilaterally and recorded.

3. **Sensation**
   a. Testing required only when the patient complains of paresthesia/anesthesia.
   b. Pinprick test:
      (1). Each dermatome of the affected side should be compared with the normal side.
      (2). Performed around the extremity.
   c. If there is a deficit, the area should be mapped.

4. **Babinski's sign and clonus**
   a. Tested if there is any suggestion of upper motor neuron lesion (eg, head trauma, cardiovascular accident, cord compression).
5. Most common levels of nerve root involvement and sensory loss associated with compression. Upper limb:
   a. C4: supraclavicular area.
   b. C5: radial aspect of wrist.
   c. C6: pad of thumb.
   d. C7: pad of index finger.
   e. C8: hyperthenar eminence.
   f. T1: ulnar aspect of wrist.

IX. Dizziness Testing and Cervical Spine Treatment

A. Anatomy of vertebrobasilar complex (see Figure 29–13)

1. Arises from subclavian vessels and runs through the foramina transversaria of the six upper cervical vertebrae.
2. Pierces the posterior atlanto-occipital membrane and enters the foramen magnum.
3. Unites in front of the brain stem to form the basilar artery and then divides into two posterior cerebral arteries.
4. Supplies the spinal cord, meninges, nerve root plexuses, muscles and joints of the neck, medulla, cerebellum, and vestibular nucleus.

B. Incidents

1. Between 1947 and 1988, 58 cases of patients who were injured by physical treatment to the cervical spine because of the injury to the vertebrobasilar complex were documented in the literature; 44 of these cases were from chiropractic manipulations.[24] These patients
   a. Were young adults (mean age, 37 years).
   b. Underwent multiple manipulations in one session.
   c. Did not have warnings of vertebral basilar complex symptoms before manipulation.
   d. Had early onset of neurogenic symptoms within minutes of manipulations.
   e. Underwent rotation manipulations.
2. The dominant level of insult was the atlantoaxial joints of the vertebral basilar complex.

C. Predisposing factors

1. Anomalies in the atlantoaxial region:
   a. Subject to stretching when larger rotation occurs at C1 and C2.

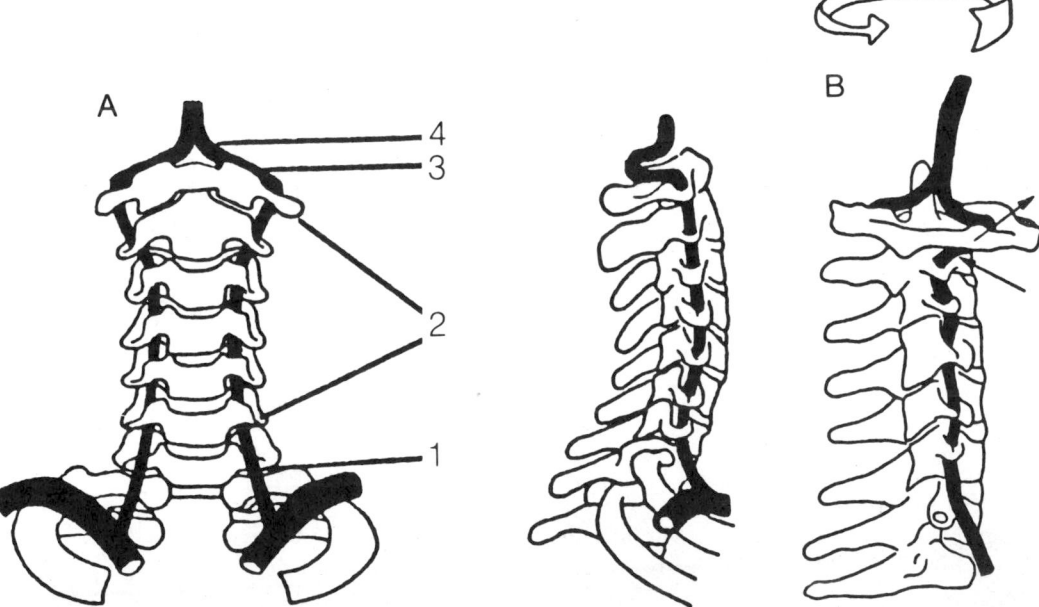

FIGURE 29–13 **A,** Anterior and lateral views of the vertebral artery. The course of the vertebral artery may be described in four parts: (1) the first part extends from the subclavian artery to the C6 foramen transversarium; (2) the second part runs vertically through the foramina transversaria of the upper six cervical vertebrae; (3) the third part passes through the foramen transversarium of the C1 vertebra and turns horizontally across it; (4) the fourth part enters the foramen magnum to join the opposite artery to form the basilar artery. **B,** A sketch of the right vertebral artery demonstrates how the atlantoaxial segment (arrow) is stretched forward by left rotation of the atlas. (Panels **A** and **B** from Bogduk N: Dizziness and the vertebral artery. In *The Cervical Spine and Headache Symposium.* Brisbane, Australia, Manipulative Therapists Association of Australia, 1981, pp 113, 116.)

b. Artery is relatively immobile at the C1 and C2 foramina transversaria.
c. Injury: subintimal tears and hematoma, perivascular hemorrhage, thrombosis, embolism, and spasm.
2. Bony changes compromising the artery throughout its course.
3. Muscle bands.
4. Stretching.

D. Symptoms: The Five "Ds"

1. Dizziness.
2. Diplopia.
3. Drop attacks.
4. Dysarthria.
5. Dysphagia.

PLEASE NOTE: Dizziness is the most common symptom. Dizziness as an unaccompanied symptom may be difficult to differentiate from distortion of normal afferents (cervical vertigo) and labyrinth of the inner ear.

E. Clinical evaluation

1. **Subjective examination.** In every patient presenting with upper quadrant dysfunction, questioning is specifically directed to elicit the presence of dizziness.
   a. Type, degree, frequency, and duration of dizziness.
   b. The occurrence or aggravation of dizziness by head movements or sustained positions of the head and neck, particularly rotation, extension, or a combination of these movements, or any other posture volunteered by the patient.
   c. The nature and type of any symptoms associated with dizziness.
   d. The history of the dizziness vis à vis the history of the neck, headache, or other symptoms.
   e. The status of dizziness.
   f. Previous treatment.
2. **Objective examination**
   a. Sustained extension.
   b. Sustained rotation, left and right.
   c. Sustained rotation with extension, left and right.
   d. Quick rotation.
   e. Standing: head held still, sustained trunk rotation, left then right.
   f. Supine: sustained extension and rotation; sustained position held for 10 seconds.

X. Assessment

Assessment is the cornerstone of the Maitland concept. It is a skill that must be used at the initial evaluation and continuously throughout the course of treatment, as it forms the foundation of a methodical approach to the evaluation and treatment of musculoskeletal disorders. The term assessment is used with two meanings:

• Analytical assessment: making sense out of what the patient is able to say and demonstrate about the disorder.
• Assessment during the course of treatment: proving the value of each technique that is used.

A. Assessment at the initial evaluation

1. Related to diagnosis:
   a. From the subjective examination, the clinician assesses how the disorder presents: severity, irritability, pathology, and stage of the condition.
   b. From the subjective and objective examination, the clinician interprets findings to
      (1). Recognize clinical syndromes.
      (2). Develop a prognosis.
      (3). Plan treatment.
2. The location, nature, and extent of the movement abnormality are determined.
   a. Range of movement.
   b. What limits movement, eg, pain, resistance, spasm.
   c. Quality of movement through range and its end-feel.
   d. Relationship of the factors of pain, resistance, and spasm.
   e. Behavior of each factor with movement.
3. The patient is assessed as a person.
   a. Psychological effect.
   b. Socioeconomic effect.
   c. Reliability as a witness.
   d. Pain tolerance.

B. Assessment during the course of treatment

This requires that the clinician

- Think.
- Plan.
- Prove.

1. **Think**
   a. Signs and symptoms plus a chronological history guide the development of a working hypothesis, including
      (1). Structures involved.
      (2). Presentation of the disorder (severity, irritability, nature, and stage and stability of the condition).
      (3). Characteristics of the patient.
      (4). Recognizable clinical syndromes.
   b. The therapist determines expectations:
      (1). What do you expect to change?
      (2). How much change can you expect?
      (3). At what rate?
      (4). When more than one problem or area is involved, what do you intend to change first?

2. **Plan**
   a. What you will do during the
      (1). Examination.
      (2). Treatment.
   b. What the patient will do:
      (1). Home exercise.
      (2). Rest, medication.
      (3). Work, recreation, activities of daily living.
   c. What will occur with the passage of time:
      (1). Healing.
      (2). Natural progression of the disorder.

3. **Prove**
   a. Your thoughts on
      (1). The working hypothesis.
      (2). The prognosis.
   b. The value of each technique.

C. Assessment of technique

The ability to assess the effect of the technique depends on the therapist's

- Ability to detect change.
- Ability to determine why the change has occurred.

1. What has changed? The clinician considers
   a. Range:
      (1). Quantity.
      (2). Quality.
   b. Pain:
      (1). Area.
      (2). Quality.
      (3). Severity.
      (4). Irritability.
      (5). Behavior with movement.
   c. Spasm:
      (1). Portion of the range.
      (2). Ease with which it is provoked.
      (3). Extent to which it limits movement.
   d. Function.
2. How much change has occurred?
   a. The clinician must be able to detect and measure the difference.
   b. Measurement should be quick, accurate, and reproducible.
3. Is the change sufficient? The clinician considers
   a. The rate and extent of change.
      (1). For this treatment session.
      (2). At the conclusion of a course of treatment.
   b. The goals and prognosis. Is the intent to
      (1). Clear the joint?
      (2). Make the patient symptom free? (Signs may persist at a level that is normal for that person.)
      (3). Prevent or reduce recurrence?

D. Assessment and comparison

1. Before each treatment session:
   a. The clinician determines the effect of the last treatment. There are three times that are of particular importance to question the patient about:
      (1). Immediately following the last treatment.
      (2). That evening.
      (3). The next morning.
   b. The therapist clarifies what is better or worse. For example
      (1). What is better?
      (2). Better than what?
   c. The clinician reassesses the subjective and objective examination items that are marked with an asterisk.
2. During each treatment session:
   a. As each technique is performed, the therapist "talks to the joint" by[25]
      (1). Questioning the patient.
      (2). Observing closely.
      (3). Palpating.
   b. After each technique, the clinician
      (1). Assesses the subjective and objective

examination items that are marked with an asterisk.

  (a). Assessment must be accurate relative to

    (i). Patient position.

    (ii). Order of tests.

    (iii). Manner in which tests are performed.

  (2). Attempts to elicit spontaneous comments.

  (3). Decides to

    (a). Repeat.

    (b). Modify.

    (c). Add.

    (d). Discard.

c. At the conclusion of a treatment session, the clinician assesses the overall changes in the patient's condition.

3. A progressive assessment is made every three of four sessions.

4. A retrospective assessment is made at the conclusion of a course of treatment.

5. A final analytical assessment is made with respect to

  a. The possibility of recurrence.

  b. Prophylactic measures.

  c. Suggestions for medical measures.

  d. The remaining disability.

REMEMBER: If assessment is to be accurate and relevant, the examination and treatment must be performed with accuracy and skill.

XI. Treatment Planning

A. Major elements

- Problem(s) identification leading to a working hypothesis and prognosis.
- Formulation of treatment goals.
- Priorities for implementation.
- Technique selection and prescription.

1. **Problem identification**

  a. Each problem requires an assessment of

    (1). Joint/structure to be treated.

    (2). Presentation (severity, irritability, nature, and stage and stability). An assessment of these components must be made to ascertain the amount of treatment given.

    (3). Pathology:

      (a). Nature of the pathology affecting the joint or structure to be treated.

      (b). Coexisting musculoskeletal conditions of medical problems that will affect treatment/management of the condition.

    (4). Limitation of motion:

      (a). Directions (eg, cervical extension limited more than left rotation and flexion).

      (b). Extent of the limitation (measured objectively in degrees).

      (c). Nature of the limiting factor:

        (i). Pain.

        (ii). Stiffness/resistance.

        (iii). Spasm.

        (iv). Weakness.

        (v). Incoordination.

      (d). Relationships of the factors of pain, resistance, spasm.

      (e). Response of each factor to movement.

    (5). Relevant psychosocial factors.

    (6). Associated factors:

      (a). Reasons why the joint/structure has become painful.

      (b). Underlying or related condition/biomechanical factors.

  b. Identification of the problems leads to a prognosis.

    (1) The prognosis is a prediction of the rate and level of recovery following treatment and may be modified throughout the course of treatment.

    (2). Numerous factors influence the prognosis.

      (a). Age and physical condition of the patient.

      (b). General health and concurrent medical/musculoskeletal problems.

      (c). Nature of the pathology.

      (d). Severity and irritability of the condition.

      (e). Underlying pathology.

      (f). Altered mechanics or loss of structural integrity.

2. **Formulation of treatment goals**

  a. Correction of existing problems and attainment of optimum function.

    (1). Relief of symptoms.

    (2). Normalizing of tissues (free of signs).

(3). Full recovery of function (mobility, strength, coordination, endurance).

b. Compensation for problems that cannot be fully corrected.

   (1). Control of symptoms.

   (2). Improved condition of the tissues (some signs will persist).

   (3). Improved level of function.

c. Prophylaxis.

   (1). Risk factors are identified that may limit full recovery or make progression of the pathology/recurrence more likely.

   (2). Certain treatment goals must be targeted to minimize or control risk factors.

3. **Priorities for implementation.** Once goals are established, it is useful to establish priorities for implementation. Many factors may be considered.

  a. Importance to the patient.

  b. Relative severity.

  c. Relative importance of the problem (primary, secondary, contributing).

  d. Relative ease or anticipated change.

  e. Structural, pathological, or biomechanical considerations.

4. **Technique selection**

  a. Every technique has parameters that should be considered:

   (1). Type of movement (physiological, accessory, combined).

   (2). Direction of movement.

   (3). Amplitude.

   (4). Position in range.

   (5). Force.

   (6). Speed.

   (7). Rhythm.

  b. Every technique should have a specific intent.

  c. If symptoms will be provoked, a conscious decision should be made with respect to their nature and intensity.

5. **Other factors influencing spinal technique selection**

  a. *Area of symptoms*

   (1). Symmetrical: a technique should be selected that affects both sides of the joint in a symmetrical manner (*eg*, central posteroanterior pressure, traction, flexion/extension).

   (2). Asymmetrical: a technique should be selected that affects the joint in an asymmetrical manner (*eg*, unilateral posteroanterior, rotations, transverse pressures).

  b. *Effectiveness of technique.* With the following, the initial application of the technique is performed as indicated to produce an opening in the joint:

   (1). ⤵ Away from the side of pain.

   (2). ⤵ On the side of pain.

   (3). ⟶ Toward the side of pain.

  c. *Intervertebral level from which symptoms arise*

   (1). Upper cervical spine (C1–C3).

   (2). Lower cervical spine (C4–C7).

  d. *Pathology*

   (1). Spondylosis: treatment requires movement through range with many different techniques.

   (2). Acute/severe nerve root pain: gentle traction.

   (3). Chronic nerve root:

    (a). Mobilization of joint signs.

    (b). Treatment of tension signs.

   (4). Discogenic problems: selection depends on presence of deformity, severity, irritability, and stability of condition.

    (a). Traction in line with the deformity.

    (b). Central and/or unilateral posterior anterior pressures at the affected level.

  e. *Grade of technique*

   (1). Selection of grade may depend on the intention to treat pain or resistance.

    (a). Pain: Grades I, II.

    (b). Resistance: Grades III, IV.

   (2). Selection of grade may be influenced by pathology.

    (a). Nerve root: subacute, chronic.

    (b). Discogenic problems.

  f. *How technique is performed*

   (1). *Speed*

    (a). Speed may be used to amplify force.

    (b). Where spasm is present, slow movement is essential.

   (2). *Rhythm*

    (a). Where pain predominates or spasm is a factor, an even rhythm is required.

    (b). Staccato rhythm is useful for amplification of force of catching pain.

(c). Sustained techniques may be used with spasm, where a prolonged stretch is required, or in the treatment of disorders in which symptoms develop as a result of sustained positions.

B. Treatment plan

1. At the initial evaluation and treatment, the physical therapist should
   a. Expect a certain change in the patient's pain response and movement patterns.
   b. Consider unfavorable response.
   c. Instruct patient in home care/exercises as applicable.
2. At subsequent visits, the following actions are taken based on the patient's status:
   a. If improved: repeat, may increase vigor.
   b. If status quo: repeat, increase vigor if pain permits.
   c. If no change: consider whether the vigor of the treatment was adequate or whether the correct area was treated.
   d. If worse: assess carefully to determine the cause (*eg*, treatment, home exercises, patient activity).
      (1). If exercises: discontinue at this time.
      (2). If treatment: repeat more gently or change.
3. Order of addition/progression will depend on the signs and symptoms.

C. General treatment guidelines

1. If the spine is the primary problem, or a large component of a peripheral problem, the spine is treated first.
2. If more than one area of the spine is involved, the spinal areas are treated in order of severity.
3. If the peripheral joint is clearly the problem (as determined by history, area, behavior, and physical findings), it is important to treat the peripheral problem first.
4. When the working hypothesis implicates a tension sign, the general treatment plan should be:
   a. Treatment of the cervical signs.
      (1). Central and unilateral posteroanterior pressures at varying angles.
      (2). Traction.
      (3). Rotation away.
      (4). Lateral flexion away.
      (5). Stretching all related muscle groups:
         (a). Trapezii.
         (b). Levator scapulae.
         (c). Scalenes.
      (6). Treatment of the shoulder.
      (7). Treatment of the soft tissues of the upper extremity at any interface that may influence the tension sign.
      (8). Mobilizing the tension sign.

XII. Recording and Documentation

A. Characteristics

1. Establishes a baseline at the time of the initial examination of the patient.
2. Determines whether changes have been made subjectively and/or objectively by providing detailed information regarding the quality, quantity, and symptomatic response of each movement.
3. Serves as a justification in performing a specific technique, changing a technique, or adding or deleting a technique.
4. Allows the therapist to follow a methodical approach to examination and treatment and provides a critical assessment of the effect of the treatment and treatment progression.

B. Method of recording

When recording a joint or structure that is found to have full painless movement with overpressure, two check marks (✔✔) can be used. (The first check mark indicates the range of motion with overpressure applied at the limit of the range. The second check mark indicates the symptomatic response the patient reports.)

Example 1: A patient performs left cervical spine rotation to full range of motion with overpressure applied at the limit of the range. The patient has full range of motion and is painless with that specific movement.
Recording: Cervical spine rotation left: ✔✔

Example 2: A patient has a symptomatic response during a movement.
Recording: Cervical spine rotation left: 75 degrees P1 (pain onset), left lower cervical spine pain.

PLEASE NOTE: P1 refers to the point at which pain is first encountered. The location of the symptoms produced during the movement is also recorded.

C. Recording treatment

1. The following is a format of documentation that is clear, concise, and easy to follow:

   S/E: subjective examination
   O/E: objective examination
   PP: present pain
   Rx: treatment
   Plan: Plan

   a. **S/E.** The subjective examination refers to the patient's complaints. The main subjective complaints, designated by asterisks, are reassessed on a basis by which change or progress can be monitored.
   b. **O/E.** The objective examination typically includes objective signs, designated by asterisks, to reassess before treatment. Objective reassessment is important to establish a baseline before the treatment session. Objective reassessment also provides information regarding the effect of the previous treatment performed.
   c. **PP.** Resting symptoms should be assessed before and after the treatment to determine whether any change has occurred.
   d. **Rx.** The following is a format for recording treatment:

Rx	Effect of Rx
a) Technique used/ level	a) Subjective response
b) Position for technique	b) Objective reassessment
c) Grade of movement	
d) Duration/number of times performed	
e) Effect of technique during performance of treatment	

   e. **Plan.** The plan comprises what action will be taken during the next treatment session.

   ### Example of Rx

   PP: complaint of mild left lower cervical spine area pain

Rx: posteroanterior pressure C6 Grade IV ($\downarrow$ C6 IV)
60 seconds × 1
Slight discomfort while performing the technique

   Assessment

   S/E: "neck feels looser"
   O/E: cervical spine rotation ✔✔

D. Symbols of mobilization: vertebral column

1. Physiological movements:
   F: flexion
   E: extension
   ↷ :   rotation to the right
   ↗ :   lateral flexion to the right
2. Accessory movements:
   ↓ :   central posteroanterior (PA) pressures.
   ↱ :   unilateral PA pressures to the left.
   ↰ :   unilateral anteroposterior (AP) pressures to the left.
   ← :   transverse pressure to the left.
   ↔ :   longitudinal movement.
3. Commonly used abbreviations for specific tests/movements:
   ULTT: Upper limb tension test
   PPIVM: Passive physiological intervertebral movements
   PAIVM: Passive accessory intervertebral movements
   OP: Overpressure

E. Grades of movement

Grades of movement are applied to both physiological and accessory movements. Grades are numbered from I to IV according to the point in the range at which the movement is performed, and the amplitude of the movement.

Grade I.   Small amplitude of movement within the resistance-free range.
Grade II.   Large amplitude of movement within the resistance-free range.
Grade III.   Large amplitude of movement into resistance.
Grade IV.   Small amplitude of movement into resistance.

XIII. Prognosis, Recovery, and Discharge Planning

A. Prognosis

Prognosis is a prediction of the level and rate of recovery in the patient's condition. It is important to formulate the prognosis early so that the following can be adequately planned:

1. The treatment plan:
   a. Selection of technique.
   b. Frequency and duration of application.
2. Treatment progression:
   a. Optimum rate.
3. The discharge plan:
   a. Treatment goals must be realistic and consistent with the patient's goals.
4. Patient education related to self-care and prevention of recurrence.

B. Formulation of a realistic prognosis

The therapist must consider
1. The working hypotheses.
2. The natural history of the disorder.
3. The patient's physical condition.
4. The extent and rate of functional change.

C. Expected outcome

The prognosis should express the expected outcome. The therapist must consider:

1. The optimal level of recovery (both the patient's and the therapist's).
2. Limitations to the attainment of optimal function.
3. The anticipated level of recovery.
4. The rate of recovery.
5. The likelihood of recurrence.
   a. The natural history of the disorder.
   b. Factors contributing to the likelihood of recurrence: age, physical condition, motivation, related medical conditions, occupation.

D. Level of recovery

The therapist may
1. Clear the joint (ie, free of symptoms and signs).
2. Make the patient symptom free (signs may persist with specific movements).
3. Improve the present level of function (signs and symptoms may persist, but the patient returns to higher level of function).
4. Prevent or reduce the level of recurrence.

E. Factors influencing level of recovery

1. Age, general health, and fitness level of the patient.
2. Patient's motivation.
3. Underlying pathology (eg, rheumatoid arthritis).
4. Altered mechanics:
   a. Fracture.
   b. Malunion.
   c. Ligamentous instability.
   d. Spondylolisthesis.
5. Deformity or structural anomalies:
   a. Scoliosis.
   b. Congenital fusions.
6. Joints that were limited in range of motion before the current episode:
   a. Dysfunction from previous episodes.
   b. Degenerative joint changes.
7. Multiple levels of dysfunction.
8. Factors present in the history.

F. Factors influencing rate of recovery

1. Fast (one to four treatments)
   a. Area of pain, local or near the source of the problem.
   b. Nonirritable patient, few aggravating factors.
   c. Sudden onset, without great progression of symptoms.
   d. Low severity.
   e. Getting better.
   f. Improved quickly in the past with treatment.
2. Intermediate (five to nine treatments)
   a. Moderately irritable.
   b. Symptoms suggestive of an inflammatory process; ie, wakes at night, symptoms not because of a specific posture or position, has difficulty falling asleep.
   c. Insidious onset over a period of a few weeks or months.
   d. Getting worse, especially in upper or lower extremity.
   e. Similar episode in the past that took a period of time to resolve.
   f. Poor response to therapeutic passive movement in the past.
   g. Joints restricted in all directions.
3. Slow (10 + treatments)
   a. All of the above.

b. Movements limited in all directions that reproduce sharp, shooting-type pains.
c. C8 nerve root lesions.
d. Long-standing tilts, shifts, deformities.
e. Previous surgeries, especially fusions.
f. Positive ULLT.
g. Clinically significant findings on magnetic resonance imaging or computed tomography.
h. Distal pain greater than proximal pain.
i. Bilateral upper extremity symptoms of equal severity.
j. Symptoms suggestive of two nerve root lesions.
k. Neurological signs that are getting progressively worse.
l. Multiple areas of pain persisting over a long time.

PLEASE NOTE: Response to treatment may modify the prognosis or alter the working hypothesis.

XIV. Adverse Mechanical Tension in the Upper Limb

A. History

In 1978, Elvey devised the brachial plexus tension test (now the ULLT) for a selection of patients who were referred to him with the diagnosis of frozen shoulder.[26–28] As these patients did not respond to traditional treatment, he decided that it was necessary to differentiate between intrinsic shoulder pain and shoulder pain of cervical origin.

Although it has been recognized in the literature for some time that shoulder and cervical problems coexist, the cervical component was not easily identified with standard tests taught in physical therapy programs. No test existed to document the selective stressing of cervical nerves, so Elvey studied cadavers to demonstrate movement of the cervical nerve roots with movement of the arm and neck.[26–28] He found that the largest excursion occurred at the C5, C6 roots, with less movement at the C7 root. No movement was observed at the C8, T1 roots.

Today, with new information on adverse mechanical tension in the nervous system, clinicians must look at musculoskeletal problems in a much broader perspective. ULTTs should be incorporated in the examination.

The musculoskeletal system must still be examined, and the therapist should continue to assess the effects of treatment. As with some musculoskeletal presentations, the results of treating neural tissue are less likely to be immediate.

Butler, after reviewing the literature, adopted the concept of considering the nervous system as an organ with a continuous tract containing chemical properties and interfacing with other tissue.[29–31] The nervous system mechanically adapts to a wide variety of ranges, speeds, and combinations of movement without interrupting the normal flow of impulses.[32,33] It also limits some combinations of movement. If regarded as a continuum, the therapist is free to examine anywhere along the tract for relevant signs.

B. Tests for the upper limb

In our opinion, the nervous system is far too complex to use tests for individual nerves. ULTTs may show a bias for one nerve rather than another.

The use of one traditional tension test is not enough. Upper limb tension testing is a concept of testing. In treatment, the therapist should use the base tests (asterisks) for assessment and treat in other ways to effect change.

1. **Hints**
   a. Check the unaffected limb first: know what to expect before testing.
   b. Know details of all symptoms before testing.
   c. Know resting symptoms.
   d. Monitor symptoms throughout:
      (1). Communicate with the patient.
      (2). Make patients aware of their pain.
   e. Pay attention to resistance and its relationship to pain.
   f. Take component to onset of symptoms or resistance in tissue, release slightly, then add next component to produce the symptoms again.

g. Start with the neck in midposition; do not fixate because it becomes the escape valve for unexpected responses.

2. **Mechanism.** It is postulated that:
   a. Glenohumeral abduction causes an axial stretch on nerve roots of the brachial plexus, particularly C5–C7.[33]
   b. Glenohumeral lateral rotation causes a wraparound effect of the musculocutaneous nerve and medial nerve in the upper arm that further increases brachial plexus tension.
   c. Elbow extension stretches all nerves in the arm except the ulnar nerve.
   d. Forearm supination causes a wraparound effect of the ulnar nerve.
   e. Wrist and finger extension causes a maximal distal movement of the medial nerve to further increase tension.[34]
   f. Cervical movements alter the position of the cord and nerve roots within the canal.
   g. Lateral flexion causes nerve roots on the convex side to be drawn up into the canal and stretched taut; therefore, cervical lateral flexion away increases tension and cervical lateral flexion toward decreases tension. Therefore
      (1). If the addition of cervical movements changes the symptoms, it implicates tension in the nerve root, not joint or soft-tissue stretch.
      (2). If the addition of wrist and finger extension causes a change in the proximal symptoms, it implicates tension in nerve roots.
   h. If symptoms produced in the ULTT are not reproduced by tests of individual structures (*eg,* joints), this implicates tension in the neural system.
   i. Any cervical pathology or anatomical anomaly further increases vulnerability of cervical nerve root.

3. **Normal responses for ULTT base test**[35]
   a. Deep stretch sensation in the cubital fossa (99%) and in the palm of the hand (80%).
   b. Tingling sensation anterior/radial aspect of forearm, thumb and/or middle three fingers (77%).
   c. Anterior shoulder stretch (10%).
   d. Responses were altered most (94%) with lateral flexion.

4. **Positive responses for ULTT**
   a. Reproduction of the patient's symptoms.
   b. Asymmetrical elbow/wrist extension: *ie,* resistance or symptoms are different from what is known to be normal or in comparison with the opposite side.
   c. Symptoms must change with neck movement (this is a more positive response than alteration of symptoms when a component is released, *eg,* wrist or elbow extension).
   d. Most common pattern of symptoms occurs in the C5–C6 dermatome.

5. **ULTT 1 (base test)** (see Figure 29–14)
   a. Patient supine with shoulder near table edge and arm at side.
   b. Shoulder depression blocked with fist on table.
   c. Humerus just behind coronal plane.
   d. Wrist held in neutral.
   e. Shoulder abduction to about 90 to 100 degrees.
   f. Lateral rotation of arm.
   g. Forearm supination.
   h. Wrist extension.
   i. Elbow extension.
   j. Cervical lateral flexion, left and right.

6. **ULTT 2**
   a. *Comments*
      (1). Shoulder depression is unavoidably lost in ULTT 1.
      (2). Shoulder depression is highly sensitive in terms of imparting tension and is the main component of ULTT 2's bias.
      (3). Used in patients with restricted glenohumeral motion.
   b. *Median nerve bias—ULTT 2M* (see Figure 29–15)
      (1). The therapist performs the test by standing on the patient's left, facing the patient's feet.
      (2). The patient is supine, lying diagonally, so that the scapula is off the table edge.
      (3). Shoulder depression is achieved with the therapist's thigh on the superior aspect of the patient's shoulder.
      (4). The therapist's left hand is on the patient's wrist, and right hand under elbow.
      (5). Elbow extension, maintaining shoulder depression.
      (6). Lateral rotation/supination.

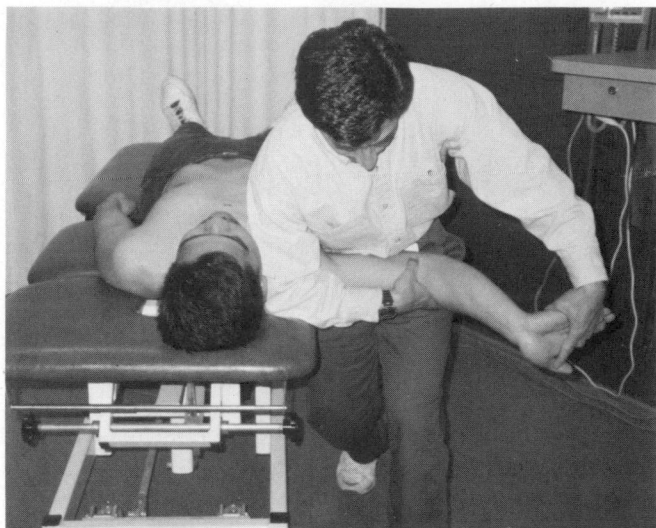

FIGURE 29–14   ULTT 1.

(7). Wrist/finger extension.
(8). Shoulder depression is released with distal symptoms.
(9). Wrist extension is released with proximal symptoms.
(10). Further progression is made by abduction as needed, taking care with this movement.
(11). Sensitization may occur with shoulder protraction/retraction.

c. *Radial nerve bias—ULTT 2R*
  (1). The therapist's position is as just described.

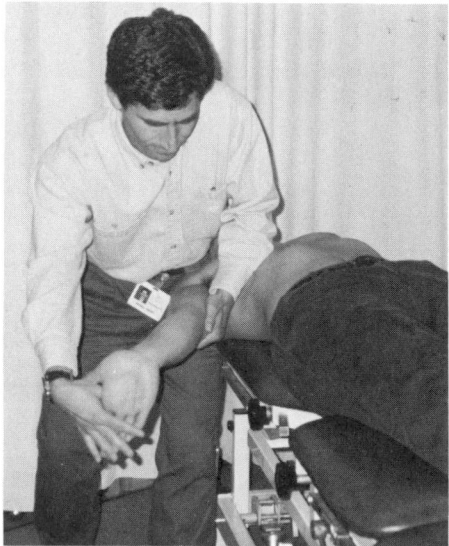

FIGURE 29–15   ULTT 2.

(2). Shoulder depression.
(3). Elbow extension.
(4). Forearm pronation and shoulder medial rotation simultaneously.
(5). Wrist flexion (may be added before elbow extension).
(6). Further sensitization with thumb flexion (for the superficial radial nerve; may be added before elbow extension).
(7). Abduction.
(8). Shoulder depression is increased if symptoms are not already reproduced.

7. **ULTT 3: ulnar nerve bias**
  a. The patient's and therapist's positions are the same as for ULTT 1.
  b. The therapist starts with the patient's elbow just below the anterosuperior illiac spine (ASIS).
  c. Wrist/finger extension.
  d. Supination.
  e. Elbow flexion.
  f. Lateral rotation of shoulder.
  g. Shoulder depression is blocked with fist on table.
  h. Arm is walked up into abduction.

C. Treatment

1. Skill in treatment by nervous system mobilization requires time to develop. This treatment is potentially dangerous because
  a. It is easy to be overly vigorous.
  b. Sensitivity of the patient's nervous system is heightened in the presence of a pathological process.
  c. It is difficult to estimate irritability.
  d. It is difficult to visualize the complex anatomy and mechanisms of the nervous system compared with those of the joints.
2. Pathoanatomical involvement:
  a. Joints underlying the symptoms.
  b. Muscles and soft tissue.
  c. Neural tissue.
  d. The safest way to start is to treat underlying joints, muscles, and soft tissue first and continually reassess each component that has an asterisk.
3. Presentation (severity, irritability, nature, stage, and stability)[36]:
  a. Irritable:
    (1). Treatment is short of pain, progressing into pain.
    (2). Grades I and II are used with slow, rhythmic movements.
    (3). Indirect component (*ie*, the therapist

should consider treating away from the site of symptoms).

    (4). Latency.

b. Nonirritable:

    (1). Treatment is into resistance.

    (2). Grades III and IV are used.

    (3). Sustained techniques should be considered.

    (4). Direct component (*ie*, treatment closer to the source of symptoms).

    (5). Combined tension movements and positions are used.

    (6). The therapist should consider axial versus transverse tension.

c. Mechanical—through range versus end of range problems:

    (1). *Extraneural*

      (a). Through range: Grades II and III are used.

    (2). *Intraneural*

      (a). End of range: Grade IV is used.

d. Functional:

    (1). *Direct*

      (a). Tension component in the patient's functional aggravating position is treated.

    (2). *Indirect*

      (a). Prophylaxis is used (posture, ergonomic design of furniture and equipment).

XV. Differentiation of Cervical Spine and Shoulder Problems

A. Basic principles

Given the following:

1. Shoulder pain may arise from the cervical spine, glenohumeral joint, viscera, or neural structures.

2. Cervical and shoulder problems frequently coexist.

3. Patients may present with glenohumeral complaints that originate from the cervical spine. They may

  a. Deny cervical pain or stiffness on presentation or in the recent past.

  b. Demonstrate restricted glenohumeral mobility and pain.

4. Subjective and objective examinations may not differentiate between shoulder pain arising from the cervical spine and/or the shoulder joint.

5. The hypothesis must be formulated early and continually reviewed in accordance with the emerging data as treatment and assessment are undertaken.

6. Treatment and accurate reassessment are required to differentiate the primary cause of the problem.

7. Three basic categories are considered here:

  a. Clear cervical problem with referred pain to the shoulder and doubtful shoulder joint involvement.

  b. Clear shoulder problem with doubtful contribution from the cervical spine.

  c. Combined cervical and shoulder involvement.

8. Sometimes these presentations will appear to have other peripheral joint or peripheral nerve involvement (*eg*, repetitive strain injuries). Thus, the concept of adverse mechanical tension in the neural structures of the upper limb (ULTTs) must be considered.

9. Given this clinical phenomena:

  a. The subjective and objective examinations must be consciously focused to disclose the primary cause of the problem.

  b. A working hypothesis must be developed and continually reviewed.

  c. A plan of treatment must aim to support or disprove the working hypothesis.

REMEMBER: Accurate interpretation of findings requires that the therapist make everything fit: *think, plan, prove.*

10. When interpreting data, the therapist must be careful not to

  a. Overemphasize findings that support an existing hypothesis.

  b. Misinterpret noncontributory information as confirming an existing hypothesis.

c. Ignore findings that do not support a favored hypothesis.
d. Obtain redundant information.

11. Goals for the first visit:
   a. Detailed examination of the primary area of concern.
   b. Clear or establish reliable signs in the secondary area of concern.

B. Clearly cervical problem with doubtful shoulder involvement

1. **Subjective examination**
   a. *Area*
      (1). Primarily and characteristically cervical:
         (a). Cervical pain and/or stiffness, usually greater on the side of referred symptoms.
         (b). Pain referred into the medial border of scapula.
         (c). Pain in the supraspinous fossa.
         (d). Dermatomal pain in the C4, C5, C6 nerve roots may be patchy or throughout the entire dermatome.
         (e). In acute nerve root pain, the pain and/or numbness may be worse in the distal extent of the dermatome.
      (2). Pain not classic glenohumeral joint pain, *ie*:
         (a). Anterior glenohumeral joint pain.
         (b). Pain at the deltoid insertion.
         (c). Pain in a band around the upper one third of the humerus.
   b. *Behavior of symptoms*
      (1). Symptoms are aggravated by activities involving movement or sustained positions of the cervical spine.
      (2). The patient may or may not deny difficulty using the arm; therefore, the therapist must clarify significant negatives (*eg*, hand behind back).
      (3). When the patient experiences difficulty using the arm, what position is the neck in?
      (4). The ULTT positions should be considered in relation to cervical and arm movements.
      (5). Patient position at night for cervical spine problems is usually lying on the affected side and is unable to tolerate long periods on the opposite side. The therapist must ask about this specifically if the patient does not volunteer the information.

 PLEASE NOTE: Differentiation often involves the clarification of significant negatives.

   c. *History*
      (1). Characteristics of the cervical spine should be considered in terms of
         (a). Area of onset.
         (b). Gradual spread from the cervical spine to shoulder or no central pain.
         (c). Onset of cervical stiffness or loss of movement before pain.
      (2). Insidious onset for no apparent reason is common in spinal problems.
      (3). Sudden onset is common in cervical spine problems and is often associated with quick movements of the head.
      (4). Previous history of cervical pain/stiffness/trauma.
      (5). Previous treatment (*eg*, cortisone injection into the glenohumeral joint) of no benefit.

2. **Plan for the objective examination**
   a. Detailed examination of the cervical spine.
      (1). Attempt to reproduce the distal symptoms from the neck if severity and irritability allow. Sometimes this is not feasible, and one has to rely on palpation and response to treatment to prove the hypothesis.
      (2). Palpate the cervical spine.
      (3). Reassess subjective and objective movement signs (asterisks) selected during the examination to see whether change has occurred.
   b. Clear or implicate the shoulder.
      (1). Active movements with overpressures:
         (a). Flexion.
         (b). Abduction.
         (c). Hand behind back.
      (2). Passive test: quadrant.
      (3). Resisted static tests.
   c. Neurological tests.
   d. Screen for positive ULLTs.

3. **Objective examination findings**
   a. If the patient has a cervical problem, the objective examination findings should support the working hypothesis; *ie*, signs will be most comparable and reproduced with cervical procedures.
   b. Shoulder signs will be minimal and less comparable (it is not uncommon to have pain or limitation of motion with quadrant or static resisted tests).

4. **Initial treatment.** The therapist should
   a. Treat the most comparable/significant cervical sign first: it will produce more change in the cervical spine and give clearcut data more quickly.
   b. Reassess:
      (1). Cervical asterisks that show movement abnormalities.
      (2). Shoulder asterisks that demonstrate clearly abnormal glenohumeral movement signs, *eg*, the quadrant.

5. **Confirmation of working hypothesis.** This requires
   a. Improvement of cervical symptoms and signs with parallel improvement in glenohumeral symptoms and signs; *ie*, as the cervical spine improves, so should the shoulder.
   b. Conversely, if the cervical spine improves and clears with no change in the shoulder, the working hypothesis has been disproved and treatment of the shoulder may be commenced.

C. **Clearly shoulder problem with doubtful cervical involvement**

1. **Subjective examination**
   a. *Area*
      (1). Classic for the glenohumeral joint.
      (2). Pain throughout the C5 dermatome.
      (3). Pain referred to the deltoid tubercle or a band of pain around the arm with no pain over the glenohumeral joint, anterior shoulder joint line pain.
      (4). The patient denies pain of symptoms in classic neck areas, including ipsilateral neck, supraspinous fossa, medial border of scapula. Symptom-free areas should be checked.
      (5). Patient denies cervical stiffness or loss of movement.
   b. *Behavior*
      (1). Symptoms aggravated by activities involving the glenohumeral joint, including hand behind head or hand behind back.
      (2). The patient presently has or previously had difficulty lying on the affected side.
      (3). The patient denies pain or limitation of motion of the neck, particularly turning, looking overhead, or sustained cervical flexion.
   c. *History*
      (1). Onset of symptoms in the area of the glenohumeral joint and not an

area of symptoms referable to the cervical spine.
      (2). Onset related to overuse or incident involving the shoulder, such as repetitive throwing or reaching over to the back seat of the car.
      (3). Onset is rarely insidious, for no apparent reason.

PLEASE NOTE: Patients in the 35- to 45-year-old age range may experience the onset of symptoms from a very minimal incident because of predisposing, age-related wear and tear.

      (4). The patient denies previous history of neck pain or stiffness.

2. **Plan for the objective examination**
   a. Examine the shoulder in detail.
   b. Eliminate the cervical spine as a source of symptoms.

REMEMBER: In the older age group there will be secondary changes in the neck, so the therapist will be unable to eliminate the neck as clear; therefore, comparability on palpation becomes important.

      (1). Extension, rotation toward, sustained.
      (2). Low cervical quadrant test.
      (3). Occasionally: flexion or lateral flexion away.
      (4). *Palpate the cervical spine:* finesse is required here. Need to distinguish between new and old changes in levels that are comparable to the shoulder.
      (5). Neurological tests.

3. **Objective examination findings**
   a. Significant limitations in shoulder movements (shoulder asterisks).
   b. The cervical spine has no abnormalities in movement and on palpation.

PLEASE NOTE: This means the therapist should clear centrally at different angles on the spinous process and unilaterally over the facets.

   c. Age-related, asymptomatic palpation findings may be present in the cervical spine.

4. **Initial treatment.** The clinician should
   a. Always reassess the glenohumeral asterisks after cervical palpation.
   b. If there are no symptoms referred from

the cervical spine and no signs, proceed with treatment of the shoulder.

  c. If there are cervical signs, or when the signs are those found on palpation (thickening, stiffness and local pain at a comparable level):

    (1). Treat the cervical spine.

    (2). Reassess the strongest shoulder findings (asterisks).

    (3). Before a conclusion is reached, the cervical signs must be clearly altered. When the only signs are palpation findings, they must change during the course of treatment (continuous assessment).

    (4). To prove that the cervical spine is not contributing to the shoulder, treat several comparable levels (centrally and unilaterally) at varying grades to change the signs.

5. **Confirmation of the working hypothesis.** This requires

  a. Alteration of cervical signs with no change in the shoulder signs; *ie*, effective treatment of the cervical spine does not affect the shoulder joint.

  b. Shoulder joint signs improve with treatment of the shoulder joint.

6. When irritability, severity, or pathology clearly implicates the shoulder, it is perfectly acceptable to treat the shoulder on day 1 without palpating the neck. This can be done at subsequent treatments when the shoulder improves (*eg*, fractured neck of humerus).

D. Combined shoulder joint and cervical involvement

1. **Subjective examination**

  a. *Area*

    (1). Combines cervical and shoulder areas.

    (2). If there are any cervical areas, the cervical spine must be at least partially involved.

    (3). The extent of shoulder involvement can be determined only by the history.

      (a). The history will confirm the initial hypothesis made from reviewing the body chart.

      (b). The history of onset will help the therapist rank the areas in order of importance.

REMEMBER: The longer the history, the greater the secondary changes and the more confusing the picture may become: *ie*, chronic tension signs will be present.

The objective examination will result in asterisks (movement signs) for each area, and sometimes there is confusion.

The response to treatment is often the only way the therapist can obtain more data to support a hypothesis or sort out what is relevant to the patient's presenting problems.

    (4). If the area is dermatomal, the therapist must prove that there is no nerve root involvement.

  b. *Behavior*

    (1). Aggravating activities are a combination of the shoulder, cervical spine, and sometimes ULTT positions.

    (2). The therapist must obtain one to two significant asterisks for each area.

  c. *History*

    (1). Often unclear, possibilities must be considered.

    (2). Particular care is required to ascertain the initial area of onset and the chronological development of symptoms thereafter.

    (3). Past history must include detailed questioning about shoulder and cervical problems: this may help the therapist to rank problems in order (*eg*, shoulder trauma superimposed on chronic neck problems, or past history of whiplash, cervical trauma).

2. **Planning for the objective examination**

  a. The objective examination is dependent on the history, but generally

    (1). A detailed examination of the shoulder and cervical spine is required. If time is limited, the therapist should be prepared to examine the cervical spine and clear/implicate the shoulder on day 1. The examination of the shoulder must be completed on day 2.

    (2). In some cases if it is clear that both areas are intimately involved, it is acceptable to screen both areas, obtain asterisks, including ULTTs, and then obtain more data during treatment so that the problems can be ranked in order more clearly.

(3). Neurological tests must be performed.

(4). Palpation of the cervical spine and shoulder are critical. Asterisks documented for the shoulder and cervical spine should be reassessed after the palpation.

(5). Examination must aim to reveal clear, comparable signs in the cervical spine and shoulder. The therapist should plan to pursue tests until a clear diagnosis is obtained.

3. **Objective examination findings**
   a. Findings are highly variable.
   b. The therapist should obtain at least two significant asterisks for the cervical spine and two for the shoulder, preferably in two planes of movement.

 PLEASE NOTE: The more significant the asterisk, the better the assessment.

4. **Initial treatment**
   a. The therapist should always begin with the cervical spine. The cervical, shoulder, and ULTT asterisks are reassessed after each technique.
   b. The cervical symptoms and signs must change to reach a clear conclusion about the shoulder.
   c. Meticulous assessment and the ability to detect change are critical skills.

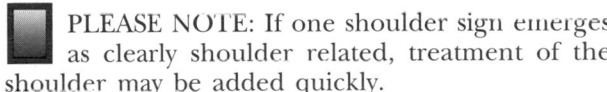 REMEMBER: Different techniques will change different components of the patient's problem.

   d. Treatment of the cervical spine is continued until change in the progress of the shoulder signs plateaus or becomes insignificant. At this point, shoulder treatment may be initiated.

PLEASE NOTE: If one shoulder sign emerges as clearly shoulder related, treatment of the shoulder may be added quickly.

XVI. Exercise and Home Program

The prescription of exercise relies on the same principles of evaluation, treatment, and assessment that guide the application of other forms of manual therapy. Effective exercise programs must be based on the specific evaluation of each patient. The results of the physical therapist's assessment will determine the goals of the exercise program and guide the selection and application of specific exercises. Continuous assessment of the patient's exercise program in relation to performance, emerging data, changes in the symptoms and signs, and changes in the condition must guide the application, modification, or progression of the program.[36,37]

Although it is beyond the scope of this chapter to discuss every type of exercise that might be used in the treatment of the cervical spine, consideration of each of the components of the physical therapy assessment in relation to specific examples are provided to illustrate the decision-making process as it relates to the application of exercise.

A. Physical therapy assessment

The physical therapy assessment requires the therapist to interpret the presenting symptoms and signs in relation to

1. Structures that will require treatment.
2. The presentation of the condition in terms of severity, irritability, nature, and stage and stability.
3. The mechanical assessment of the postures, positions, movements, and stresses that aggravate or ease the symptoms and their relation to function.
4. The cause of the patient's functional restrictions as they relate to mobility, strength, endurance, and coordination.[38]
5. Psychosocial/personal characteristics of the patient that may influence the attitude toward and compliance with the exercise program.
6. The physical or ergonomic factors that may have caused the problem to occur or be perpetuated.

B. Factors influencing ability to exercise

In addition to the assessment of the condition to be treated, the therapist must be alert to other factors that will influence the patient's ability to exercise, such as age, general fitness level, and coordination or athletic ability. The patient may present with constraints related to other medical conditions, such as cardiovascular disease, musculoskeletal problems in related areas, or postural deformities.

C. Goal setting

Based on the results of a comprehensive assessment, specific goals can be set by the therapist. Morgan and Stevens[39] stress that the goals should reflect whether treatment is directed to correct the problem, compensate for problems that cannot be fully corrected, or prevent a problem. The treatment plan must reflect the specific work, recreation, and activity level to which the patient will return.

D. Exercise prescription

Each exercise should be prescribed for a specific purpose that is clearly understood by the patient. Exercises may be prescribed to relieve or prevent the onset of symptoms; to improve mobility of joints, muscles, or neural elements; to improve strength, endurance, or aerobic capacity; or to improve coordination or patterns of movement. The specific tissue to be treated, the intention of the exercise, and the presentation of the condition will determine the specific prescription or dosage of the exercise. Important parameters in exercise prescription may include

1. Position of the patient.
2. Direction of the movement.
3. Position in range.
4. Amplitude of the motion.
5. Forces involved.
6. Speed or rhythm.
7. Time (duration).
8. Repetition.
9. Frequency or timing of the exercise sessions.

PLEASE NOTE: The integration and application of these principles might be best illustrated with respect to the clinical syndromes previously discussed.

E. Exercise and posture

Clinically, the role of posture is important in the treatment of most cervical spine syndromes. The posture syndrome has been defined by McKenzie[40] and Stevens and McKenzie.[41] They believe that the pain associated with poor posture is caused by mechanical deformation when the soft tissues (joint capsule, ligaments, and muscle) adjacent to the vertebral segment are subjected to prolonged, uninterrupted stress at the limit of the available range of motion. Poor posture is characterized by the forward head position (see Figure 29–16), which places the upper cervical spine at end-range extension and the lower cervical spine in flexion. In relaxed, unsupported sitting, the thoracic and lumbar regions are also fully flexed. Other characteristics of the syndrome include the following:

1. The patient is typically under the age of 30 with a sedentary occupation and a general lack of fitness.
2. The patient complains of a symmetrical area of symptoms near the midline and denies referral to the medial border of the scapula or into the extremities. Patients may complain of secondary areas of symptoms in the midthoracic and low lumbar regions.
3. Symptoms are never characterized as severe or irritable. They are aggravated only when particular postures or postions are adopted

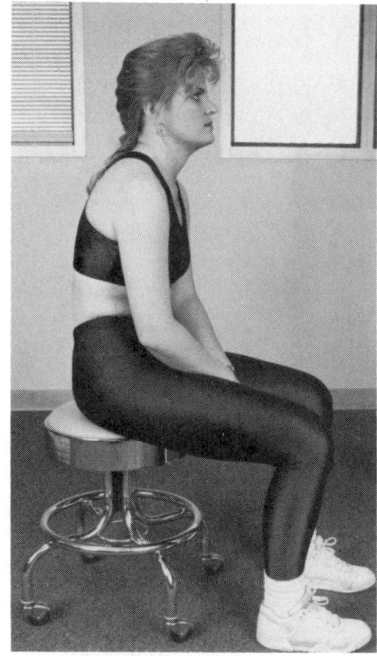

FIGURE 29–16   Poor postural position: forward head.

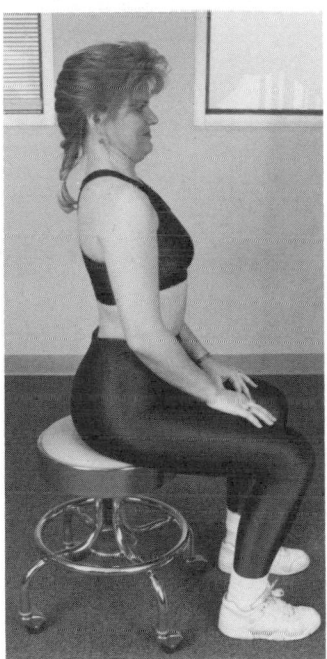

FIGURE 29-17   Slouch-overcorrect exercise.

for prolonged periods. The symptoms are relieved immediately with movement or a change of position.

4. On examination, there are no signs of abnormal movement. Range of motion is not limited, and pain is not reproduced with the addition of overpressure or the use of repeated motion. The symptoms can be reproduced only when the patient is placed in the position purported to reproduce the symptoms for a period of time.

a. *Focus of exercise program.* The exercise program for this type of patient focuses on several important elements and uses the training principles outlined by Morgan *et al.*[42]:

(1). The relationship between poor posture and symptoms is established. Verbal admonishments are rarely sufficient. Patients learn by doing and must be taught that maintenance of the spine in a functional position alleviates symptoms.

(2). The kinesthetic awareness necessary to control spinal postures and movement is developed. Exercise provides the repetitive movement experiences that are essential in establishing safer, more functional patterns of movement. Correct posture must become habitual.

(3). Strength and endurance are improved so that the positions can be maintained in static situations and during normal activity.

b. *Slouch-overcorrect exercise.* The patient may be taught the slouch-overcorrect exercise (see Figure 29–17). Patients with habitual poor posture often have difficulty coordinating the appropriate movements of head on neck and neck on trunk. The upper cervical region is flexed as the lower cervical region is retracted. The important contributions of lumbar and thoracic movement to the functional positioning of cervical spine become readily apparent.

c. *Lumbar support.* The patient may use a lumbar support to assist with the maintenance of lumbar lordosis while practicing the cervical retraction movement (see Figure 29–18). Both exercises may be progressed to a gymnastic ball to introduce a less stable surface (see Figure 29–19). The ball also facilitates training in a variety of positions, which is an essential element of the training sequence. With movement away from the vertical, strengthening against gravity is introduced. Figure 29–20 illustrates the retraction exercise in the supported quadruped position. Figure 29–21 illustrates a partially recumbent position.

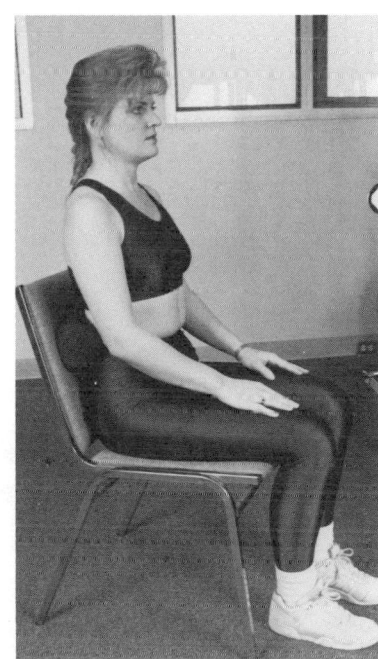

FIGURE 29–18   Cervical retraction movement.

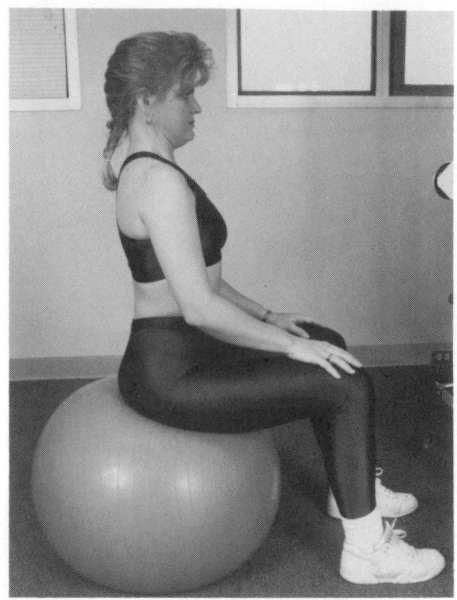

FIGURE 29–19   Gymnastics ball: unstable surface.

d. ***Upper extremity exercises.*** When the patient can produce coordinated motion and maintain the functional neutral position in the seated, partially recumbent, and supported quadruped positions, a variety of upper extremity exercises may be added.

(1). Scapular retraction in the seated po-

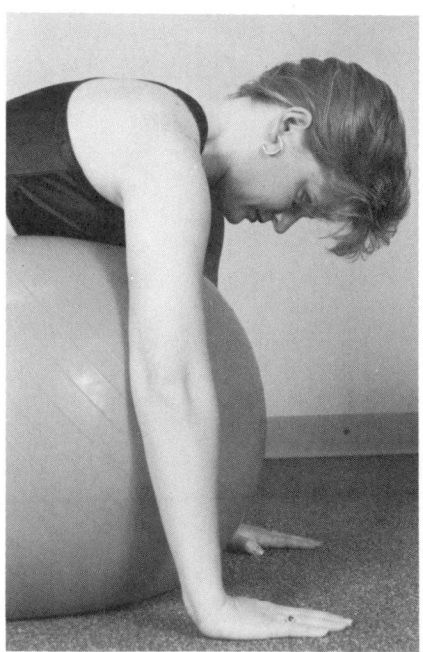

FIGURE 29–20   Retraction exercise in quadriped position.

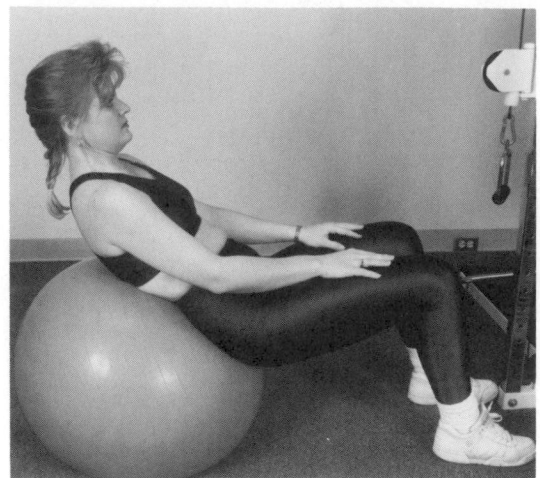

FIGURE 29–21   Partially recumbent position.

sition on the gymnastic ball (see Figure 29–22).

(2). Supported quadruped: cervical retraction with scapular retraction (see Figure 29–23).

(3). Supported quadruped: cervical retraction with upper extremity flexion (see Figure 29–24).

(4). Supported quadruped: cervical retraction with horizontal abduction (see Figure 29–25).

(5). Partially recumbent: cervical retraction with upper extremity flexion (see Figure 29–26).

(6). Partially recumbent: cervical retraction with horizontal abduction (see Figure 29–27).

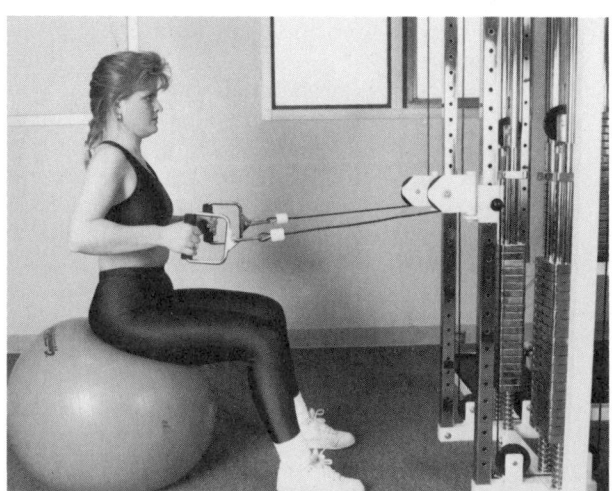

FIGURE 29–22   Scapular retraction in seated position.

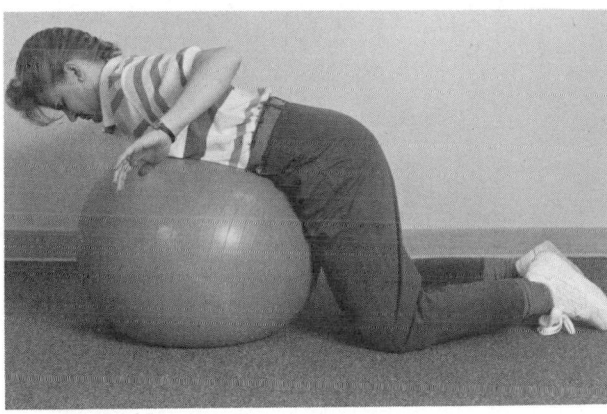

FIGURE 29–23   Supported quadriped: scapular retraction.

■ PLEASE NOTE: Maintaining the functional position of the cervical spine during upper extremity activities is difficult for most patients and requires training the trunk extensors and retractors of the scapula as well as the cervical extensors.

   e. *Addition of weight.* Weight may be added to all exercises, but it is critical that the emphasis remains on the quality of movement. Repetitions are increased before weight, and weight should be increased gradually as the patient is able to perform the correct movement repeatedly. The exercise is terminated when the patient can no longer effectively control the position of the spine in a smooth and coordinated fashion.

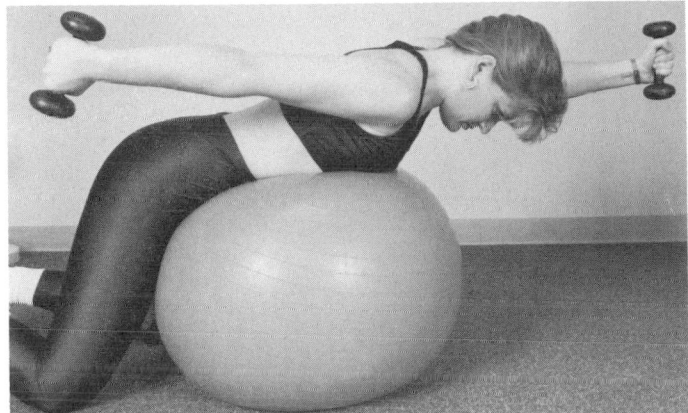

FIGURE 29–24   Supported quadriped: upper extremity flexion.

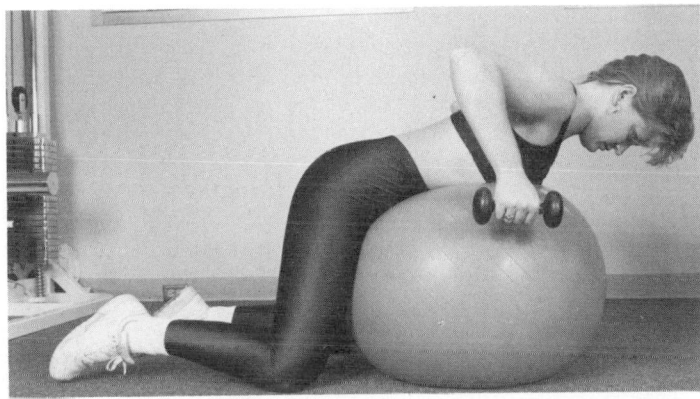

FIGURE 29–25   Supported quadriped: horizontal abduction.

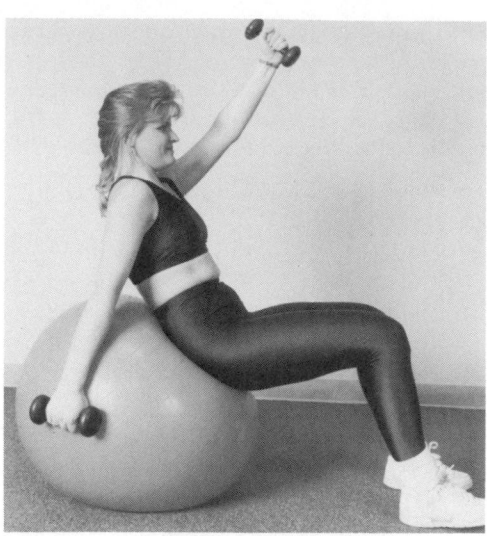

FIGURE 29–26   Partially recumbent: upper extremity flexion.

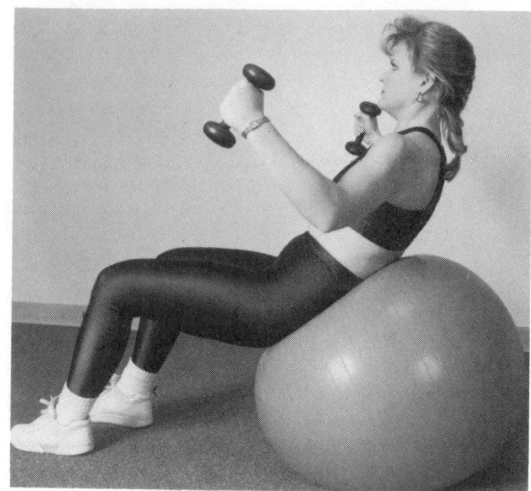

FIGURE 29–27   Partially recumbent: horizontal abduction.

F. Cervical spondylosis: application of the principles

Clinically, these patients present with pain and limited motion that is multisegmental and multifactorial: involving limited motion of the joints, tightness of the cervical musculature, as well as signs of adverse mechanical tension. Jull and Janda[39] stress the importance of considering the basic interdependence of all structures involved in the production and control of motion. It is important to conceptualize this integrated and interdependent neuromusculararticular system correctly when assessing the cause and effect of disability in patients with low back pain. Dysfunction in any component of this system can affect the activity of muscles and thus the control of the motor response.[43]

1. The goals and components of the physical therapy assessment can be used in the development of the program. The exercise program for these patients is directed toward compensation because full correction is not likely. When the history reveals a pattern of recurrent episodes, prophylaxis should receive considerable attention. Treatment may be directed at increasing range of motion or improving the pain-free range of motion. Increased strength and endurance may contribute to an improved level of function.

2. Treatment is often directed toward a specific structure, with the understanding that multiple structures may be affected. The therapist must continually assess the patient's response to exercise and remain alert to the stresses any exercise may place on the structures in the region. Stretching the neck in full rotation with a sustained overpressure may be effective for improving joint mobility; however, in some patients this may compromise the vertebral artery. Patients with spondylosis usually require treatment directed at multiple joints and muscles.

   a. Treatment of limited joint motion should be addressed before muscle stretching begins.

   b. Jull and Janda have described common patterns of muscle imbalance.[43] In the cervical region, the hypertrophic muscles commonly include the cervical erector spinal, the upper trapezius, the levator scapulae, the scalenes, and the sternocleidomastoid. Muscles prone to weakness in this region include the short cervical flexors and the stabilizers of the scapula, the serratus, the rhomboids, and the lower portions of the trapezius. Jull and Janda believe that the emphasis of the program should initially be placed on regaining the normal length of the tight muscles.[43] After an effective stretching program, exercises may be directed toward facilitating and strengthening weak muscles and improving the patterns of movement. A comprehensive text on stretching has been completed by Evjenth and Hamburg.[44] An example is illustrated in Figure 29–28. With stretching directed at muscles, proprioceptive neuromuscular facilitation techniques, such as contract relax or hold relax, are extremely useful.

3. The severity and irritability of the condition vary considerably and are important factors in determining the focus of the exercise program and the manner in which it is initi-

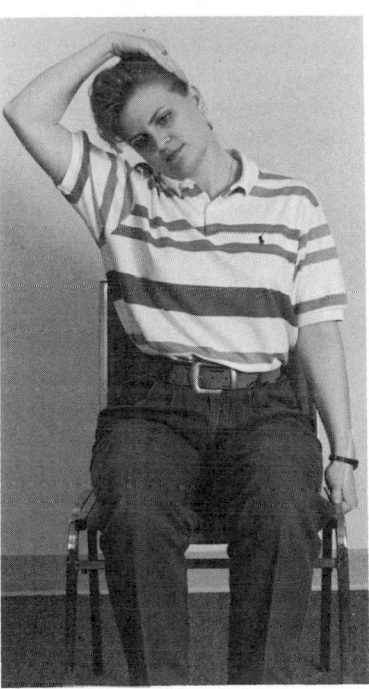

FIGURE 29–28   Stretching.

ated and progressed. In an irritable condition, the focus of the program is on relief of symptoms and exercises to maintain or improve motion. Strength training may be deferred or limited to isometric exercises. Several modifications may be necessary.

a. The patient may be positioned supine to alleviate the compressive forces of gravity. The neck and upper thoracic region may be supported on pillows or wedges in a neutral or midrange position (see Figure 29–29).

b. The direction on movement should be away from pain and resistance. As the irritability decreases, the patient may progress to movements in the painful directions, gradually stretching into the resistance.

c. The patient should be instructed to move as far as possible in the pain-free range. As the pain and irritability decrease, the patient may increase the amplitude of the motion and begin to stretch into a controlled amount of discomfort.

d. The movement should be slow.

e. The number of repetitions should be low, corresponding to the irritability. It may be advantageous at this stage for the therapist to ask the patient to perform several brief sessions of exercise followed by a period of rest. With irritable conditions, rest is an important factor in the recovery process. As the irritability decreases, the number of exercises in each session is increased.

f. For many patients, time of the day may influence their compliance with the exercise program. Some patients have great difficulty with exercise immediately on waking. They may benefit from heat and a period of time to move about before commencing exercise.

4. The mechanical presentation in spondylosis is one of motion limited by pain and stiffness in all directions. Grieve[45] lists the segments most commonly affected by cervical spondylosis as C5 C6, C6 C7, C4 C5, and C7 T1. Spondylosis is also associated with arthrotic changes in the facet joints. He also notes the importance of the cervical thoracic junction as a region where the most mobile region of the vertebral column is physically interdependent with a region of very limited movement. Also, a number of connective tissue structures and muscles cross the C7 T1 segment.

5. Stretching of the thoracic region and mobilization of the cervical thoracic junction facilitate the recovery of motion in the lower cervical spine. The exercise ball is useful in promoting thoracic extension and may be used in a variety of ways depending on the capability of the patient. Examples are illustrated in Figures 29–30 and 29–31. Attempts to recover extension may be limited by structural deformities such as scoliosis or accentuated thoracic kyphosis. The age of the patient must also be considered.

6. The retraction exercises in the section on exercise and posture may be implemented.

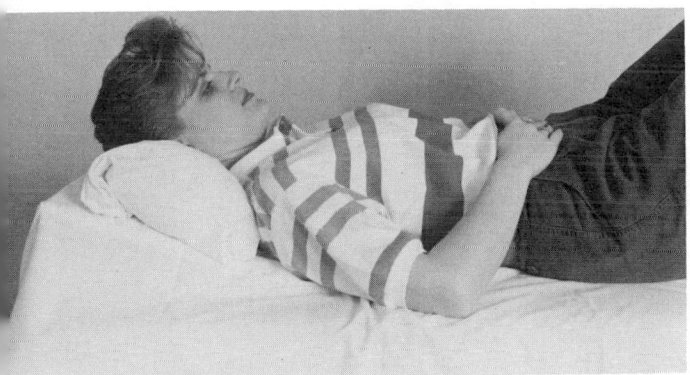

FIGURE 29–29   Positioning techniques.

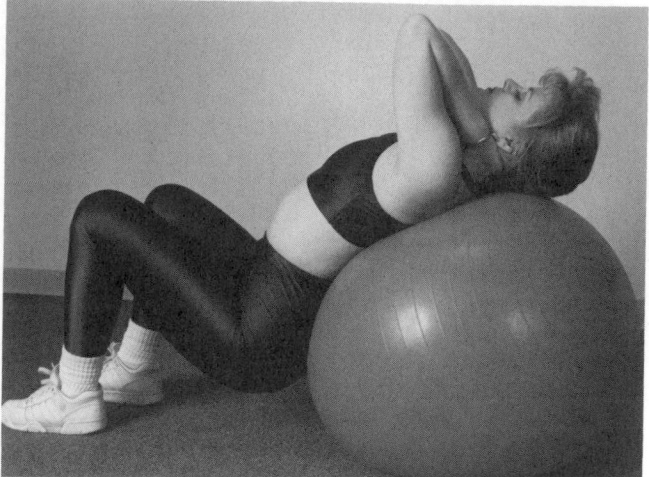

FIGURE 29–30 Ball exercise: thoracic extension.

Most patients will need range of motion exercises in all directions. Overpressure may be added where more vigorous stretching is appropriate (see Figure 29–32). With spondylosis, there is potential for narrowing of the intervertebral foramen, particularly with extension. Exercising in extension should be approached carefully, and the patient is instructed to avoid those motions that produce symptoms referred into the upper extremity. Because these patients are often aggravated by sustained positions at the limit of the range, the stretching should be intermittent in nature.

7. The forward head posture commonly adopted by patients maintains the upper cervical spine in extension, promoting tightness of the suboccipital musculature and restriction of flexion in the upper cervical joints. Retraction in sitting will influence motion in this area. When a specific stretch is desired, the exercise may be done in supine (see Figure 29–33).

8. The assessment of the patient's functional restrictions in relation to mobility, strength, endurance, and coordination usually reveals deficits in all areas. The improvement of strength and endurance should be approached carefully. In general, patients must exercise with the neck maintained in a midrange or functional neutral position, taking care to avoid the extremes of range. Exercise for cervical patients is complicated by the difficulties of maintaining the correct position of head on neck and neck on trunk. Like lumbar patients, they benefit from repetitive movement experiences aimed at improving kinesthetic awareness and patterns of movement. Clinically, errors with exercise are more likely to provoke exacerbations in cervical patients.

9. Upper extremity exercises used for cervical patients should be assessed carefully, with consideration of the effect of the arm position on the cervical and thoracic regions. For example, raising the shoulders forward to the limit of range increases thoracic extension and encourages protrusion of the head forward. Patients must be taught to maintain the correct position of the cervical spine when moving the upper extremities, just as lumbar patients are taught to maintain a functional position of the spine during activities. It is frequently necessary to limit the excursion of the upper extremities to avoid losing the functional position.

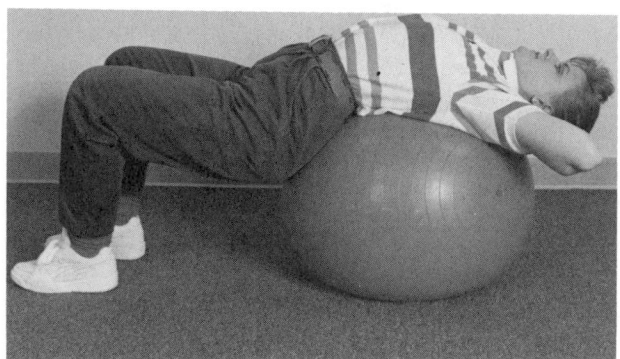

FIGURE 29–31 Ball exercise: thoracic extension.

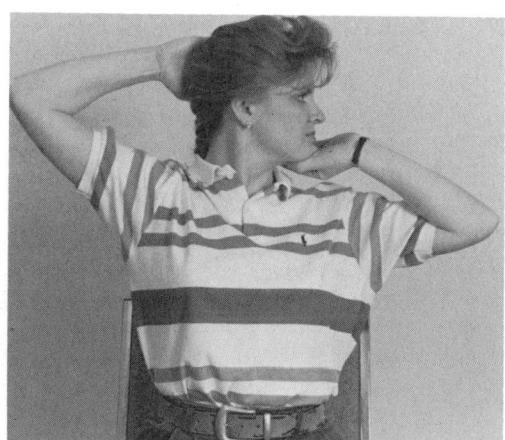

FIGURE 29–32 Overpressure added to stretching exercise.

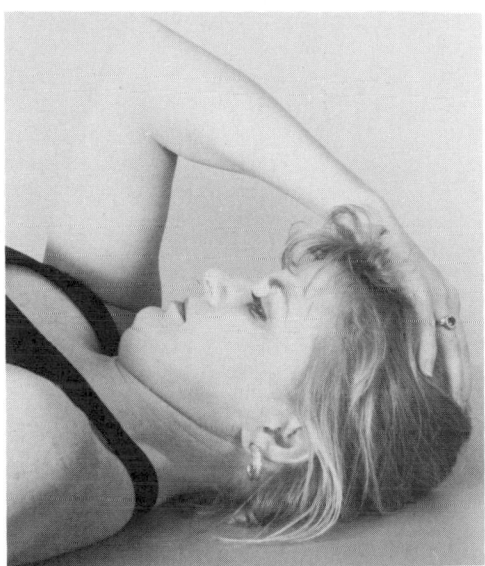

FIGURE 29–33 Supine position for stretching exercise.

cated.[31] The therapist must determine if through range movement or end of range stretching is indicated. Other forms of exercise may require evaluation with respect to the effects on the nervous system. The trapezius stretch will also influence the nervous system, and the doorway stretch, commonly used to stretch the pectoral muscles, will strongly stretch the glenohumeral joint and the nervous system. Exercises aimed at other structures may be modified slightly to more effectively include the nervous system.

G. Conclusion

Exercise is an important part of the treatment plan for patients with musculoskeletal problems. There is no protocol for an exercise program that is suited to all patients.

Remember: to be effective, an exercise program must be

1. Designed for the individual.
2. Based on a comprehensive evaluation of the patient that focuses on the presenting symptoms and signs, the mechanical behavior of the spine, and the relationship of these to the patient's functional restrictions.
3. Monitored carefully for correct performance.
4. Assessed in relation to the changes it produces in the patient's condition.

Training of the musculature that stabilizes the scapula is emphasized.

10. Particular care is required when exercising the upper extremities in the presence of an upper limb tension sign. The patient may be given specific exercise to mobilize the tension sign when stretching is indi-

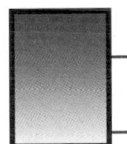

Clinical Decision-Making Cases

Case #1: Planning Objective Examination for Cervical Spine

SUBJECTIVE EXAMINATION

Patient Profile
1. 55-year-old female, secretary.
2. Working full time at new job.
3. Recreation includes reading and needlework.

Area of Symptoms (see Figure 29–34)
1. Constant vague, deep ache in right occipital area radiating to right trapezius muscle and to right shoulder and arm as far as deltoid tubercle.
2. Intermittent sharp, severe pain right midcervical.
3. Constant deep pain in central C7 area.
4. Constant deep ache medial border right scapula and intermittent vague numbness right hand.
5. Occasional dizziness with sustained looking overhead to place things on a high shelf.

Aggravating Factors
1. Sustained flexion for 15 minutes increases neck, arm, and scapula ache; to settle, raises head and moves about for 5 minutes.
2. Right cervical rotation to reverse her automobile produces sharp pain; stops immediately, but a dull ache persists for 15 minutes.
3. Quick movement right produces severe right neck pain and locking; takes 30 minutes to settle.
4. Dizziness looking overhead 1 to 2 minutes; settles quickly.

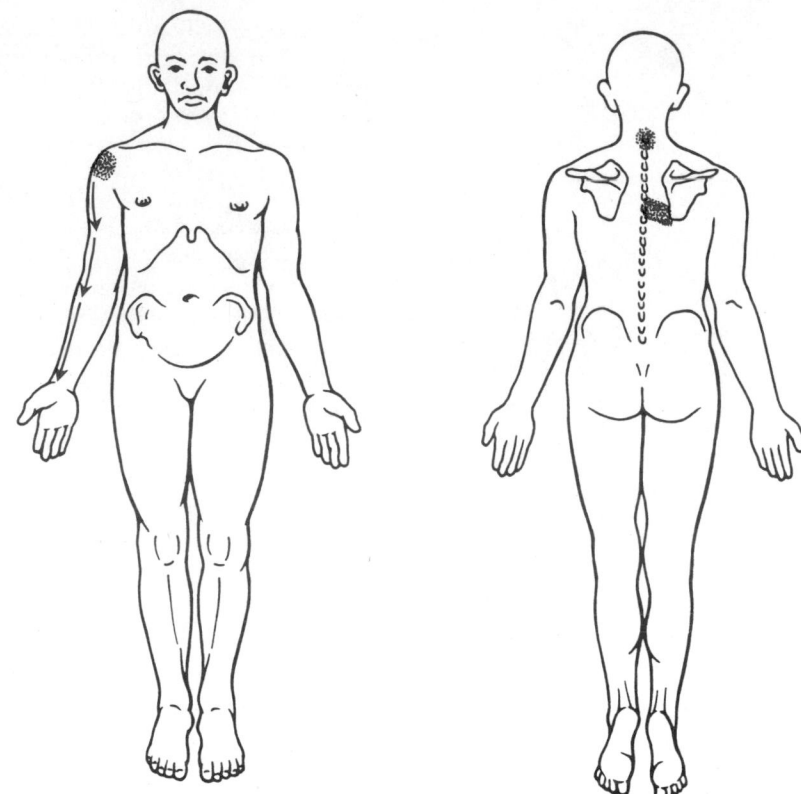

FIGURE 29–34   Body chart: shoulder and cervical pain, 55-year-old female.

5. Numbness/tingling in hand only during night or on waking in morning; up to move, settles quickly.

Easing Factors
1. Rest.
2. Avoiding movement.
3. Medication as listed below.

24-Hour Behavior
1. Night: wakes occasionally with numbness; settles quickly with getting up to move.
2. Day: all areas worse, spreads to arm by midday. Severe pain dependent on activity.

Special Questions
1. Vertebral artery: dizziness related to neck position (*ie,* when looking up).
2. Cord: negative.
3. Cauda equina: negative.
4. Medications: ibuprofen, four times a day.
5. Weight loss/gain: stable.
6. General health: history of rheumatoid arthritis.
7. Steroids: 10 years ago, required prednisone, 20 mg/d, for rheumatoid arthritis, which is now in remission.
8. Tests: 6 months ago, radiographs showed degener-

ative changes at C4–C5, C5–C6 without evidence of foraminal encroachment.

History
Gradual onset of right neck stiffness led to pain 6 weeks ago, after beginning new job as typist. Three weeks ago, pain spread to scapula and right shoulder. Hand symptoms are worse since onset of neck pain; now worsening. Sharp pain with turning developed 1 week ago. No treatment.

Past History
Motor vehicle accident occurred 10 years ago, severe bilateral neck and arm pain for 6 weeks. Recovered 90%. Intermittent episodes of right neck pain with exertion or sleeping in the wrong position. Usually lasts 1 to 2 weeks and recovers without treatment. This is first episode of scapula pain and the first recurrence of arm pain since the accident. Five-year history of carpal tunnel syndrome.

OBJECTIVE EXAMINATION

After collecting the subjective data, the clinician should be able to fill out a planning sheet as outlined below, either on paper for a less experienced clinician or mentally for a more skilled practitioner.

Structures at Fault

1. Which structures must be examined as a possible cause of the patient's symptoms?
   a. Although one may place great emphasis on particular aspects of the examination, no one test will give all the answers; therefore, the puzzle must be pieced together by considering all structures.
   b. One is not going to examine all areas. However, if all options are not considered, the obvious may be overlooked (error of omission).
   c. One must examine all areas under the symptoms.
   d. If the patient is not improving in one aspect of the problem, this provides a reference of structures to be examined further.
2. Which joints lie under the area of symptoms?
   a. C0–C7 apophyseal joints; later focus will be directed at the right.
   b. C4–C5 or C5–C6 joints because these are where sharp pain occurs.
   c. C6–C7 or C7–T1 intervertebral joints.
   d. T7 costotransverse joint or costovertebral joint.
   e. Glenohumeral, acromioclavicular, wrist, thumb, hand, finger joints.
3. Which joints may refer into the area of symptoms?
   a. The cervical spine may refer symptoms into the glenohumeral, acromioclavicular, wrist, and hand joints.
   b. The thoracic spine may refer symptoms into the wrist and hand area.
4. Which contractile structures are under the area of symptoms (eg, rotator cuff, forearm extensors)?
   a. Upper cervical musculature.
   b. Right trapezius muscle.
   c. Right erector spinae muscles.
   d. Deltoid muscle.
   e. Rhomboid muscles.
   f. Muscles of the hand.
5. Which other structures need to be examined?
   a. Thoracic outlet tests.
   b. ULTTs.
   c. Median nerve: carpal tunnel syndrome tests for median nerve compression at the wrist.
6. Which of these structures are *most likely* to cause the patient's symptoms? That is, from the above structures, which ones may be possible causes for the patient's presentation? The focus needs to be narrowed to the most probable causes, hence helping to narrow the focus of the objective examination.
   a. C6–C7, C7–T1 discogenic.
   b. C4–C5 apophyseal joint.

c. Carpal tunnel syndrome.
d. Vertebrobasilar insufficiency.
7. At this stage, what is the *hypothesis*?
   a. Spondylitic neck with C4–C5 apophyseal joint impingement, with C6–C7 discogenic problems superimposed.
9. Will a neurological examination be needed?
   a. It is necessary to undertake neurological tests for the upper extremity because the patient has symptoms radiating beyond the acromion and numbness and tingling into her hand.

Influence of Symptoms on the Examination

1. Severity: are the symptoms minimal, moderate, or severe? This is a judgment call on the part of the therapist. All symptoms should be considered because examination of one area may need to be limited while other areas can be examined with vigor.

Local	Referred	Symptoms
Cervical sharp pain—yes	Medial scapula—no	Dizziness—no
Cervical deep ache—no		Numbness or tingling—no

2. Irritability:
   a. Are the symptoms irritable?
   b. Give an example.
   c. Activity causing the symptoms.
   d. Severity of the symptoms.
   e. Time to subside.

Local	Referred	Symptoms
Cervical sharp pain—yes. Pain on quick turning, which locks for 30 min	Medial scapula pain and all pain increases at end of the day + is activity dependent	Dizziness, numbness, or tingling—no

3. Nature, ie, fragility of the problem (eg, recent fracture, osteoporosis, and pathology of the presentation):
   a. Nature limits vigor used for some movements and procedures (eg, a history of recurrent dislocations in the shoulder would indicate that care is needed with abduction/external rotation tests).
   b. Does the nature of the disorder indicate caution?
   c. Care should be taken with upper cervical testing (history of rheumatoid arthritis).
   d. Dizziness testing not possible or ineffective; therefore, care should be taken with techniques that may compromise the vertebral artery.

4. Is specific testing required?
   a. Local tests for carpal tunnel syndrome.
   b. Later, ULTTs need to be performed.
5. Stage and stability of the condition (do these guide or limit the examination?):
   a. This episode is worsening because symptoms are spreading to other areas and involving other structures.
   b. The present episode is acute and is superimposed on long-standing chronic conditions.
6. Are there any *contraindications* to the examination or treatment?
   a. No manipulation or end-range techniques in the upper cervical spine because of the patient's age (55 years old, possibility of osteoporosis). Also, there is a history of rheumatoid arthritis and steroid medication.

KIND OF EXAMINATION

1. Will you be gentle or vigorous with your examination? Why?
2. Will you examine structures to
   a. P1? (Onset of pain and beyond or increase of symptoms.)
   b. L? (Limit of patient's active movements.)
   c. Add overpressure?
   d. Use sustained, repeated, combined movements?

Symptoms: Local	Referred	Other
P1 for right cervical rotation. Add overpressure for flexion, extension, and left rotation	Limited by severity and irritability of local symptoms	Test cervical movements to onset of patient's dizziness within limits of local and referred

5. Which symptoms are you prepared to reproduce?

Symptoms: Local	Referred	Other
P1 of sharp pain	Unable to get because of limitations in local symptoms and dizziness	Dizziness

6. Circle the appropriate. Do you expect
   a. A comparable sign? (Movements or other tests that reproduce the patient's symptoms will be easy or hard to find?)
   b. To be treating pain, resistance, pain and resistance, or spasm?

ASSOCIATED EXAMINATION

Other factors must be examined to determine why the affected structure has become painful or why the disorder may recur. These include upper trapezius and upper cervical spine muscle length and posture.

SECOND HYPOTHESIS

1. Do you wish to modify the first hypothesis?
2. To the first hypothesis under "Structures at Fault" (7.a.), one would add carpal tunnel syndrome as a contributing factor.

PROGNOSIS

The prognosis is a prediction of the rate and level of recovery the patient is expected to achieve. Early formation of a prognosis is necessary to guide the therapist in further examination and treatment selection. As further information becomes available, the prognosis may need to be modified.

This patient's prognosis is good. The therapist can expect significant relief of symptoms (*ie*, elimination of the sharp right cervical pain and general right ache); however, she will always have residual signs (*ie*, limitation of cervical movement and stiffness on palpation of the cervical spine).

It may be difficult to change the symptoms of carpal tunnel syndrome if they are directly caused by compression of the median nerve at the wrist. If these symptoms are referred from the cervical spine, one would expect an improvement.

Generally, in a clinical situation in which the therapist sees an acute injury on chronic problems, the prognosis is poorer.

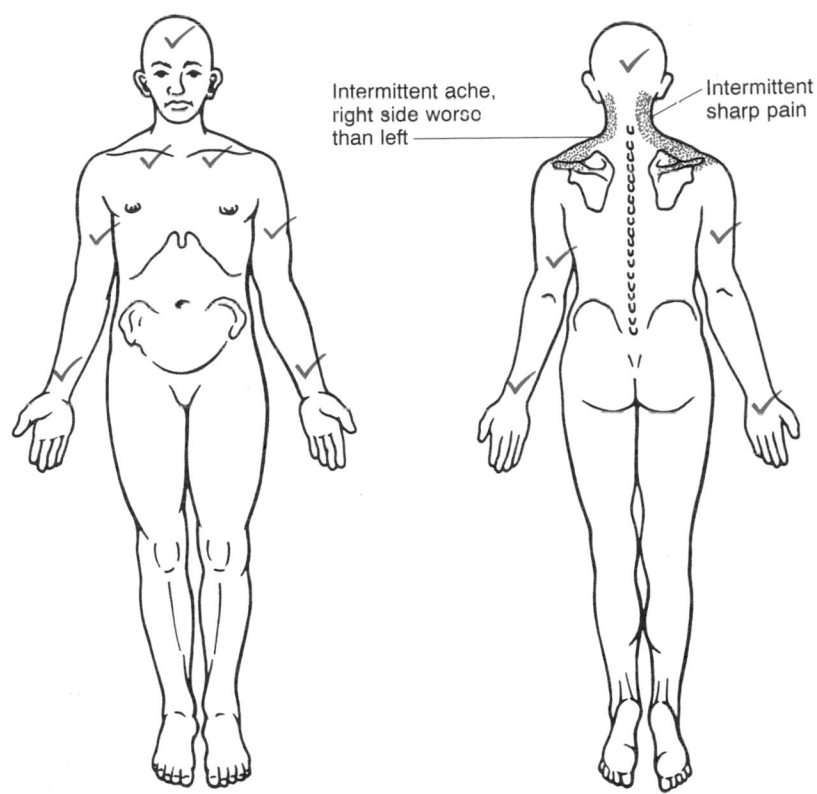

Intermittent ache, right side worse than left

Intermittent sharp pain

FIGURE 29–35 Body chart: cervical spondylosis, 55-year-old female.

Case #2: Cervical Spondylosis

INTRODUCTION

Cervical spondylosis is the product of cervical disc degeneration. It results as part of the aging process and may be aggravated by stresses of daily living and trauma. The common finding is narrowing of the intervertebral disc, which contributes to apophyseal joint arthropathy and narrowing of the intervertebral foramina, which in turn may lead to nerve root compression.

SUBJECTIVE EXAMINATION

Patient Profile

1. 55-year-old female, unloads boxes from a conveyor belt.
2. She has to constantly turn her head to the right, which she is able to do with care or by rotating her body.
3. She likes to sew patchwork quilts and watch television in the evening; this is difficult to do because of neck ache.

Area of Symptoms

1. Bilateral, intermittent cervical ache, right greater than left; when symptoms are aggravated, they radiate into supraspinous fossa.
2. Intermittent sharp pain midcervical on right (see Figure 29–35).

Aggravating Factors

1. Ache increases with driving for more than 1 hour or sitting to sew for 1 hour; she is able to continue activity, but ache intensifies if she persists with activity. She also feels stiff.
2. Quick turning to the right results in sharp pain, eases after a few seconds. She avoids this movement at work by moving with care or rotating whole body.

Easing Factors

1. Rest, heating pad.
2. Moving neck around, massage.
3. Ibuprofen, as needed.

24-Hour Behavior

1. Sleeps right sidelying throughout the night, wakes with sharp pain if turns, returns to sleep immediately.
2. Morning: stiff in all directions, eases in half an hour with hot shower.

3. End of day: stiff and painful, especially after a work-day; she avoids sewing in the evening.

Special Questions

✓✓, except radiographs show diffuse degenerative joint disease at C3–C4, and C5–C6.

History

1. Always had neck pain but worsened over the last year or so.
2. Sharp pain began 2 weeks ago, after a plane trip cross-country to visit sick relatives.
3. Had car accident about 20 years ago but does not remember neck being a problem.

OBJECTIVE EXAMINATION

Posture

Sits with a poking chin posture, tight upper cervical musculature, and slight increase in the thoracic kyphosis.

Active Physiological Movements

1. Flexion: half range, unable to get chin on chest or to reverse cervical lordosis, hinges into flexion at C7.
2. Extension: midcervical movement, C7 area pain, stiff with overpressure.
3. Axial extension (ie, dorsal glide): unable to get to neutral, low cervical pain.
4. Left rotation: 45 degrees, left cervical pain, very stiff end-feel (stiff + +) with overpressure.
5. Right rotation: 30 degrees, right pain, very stiff end-feel with onset of sharp pain on overpressure.
6. Left lateral flexion: stiff upper cervical movement.
7. Right lateral flexion: stiff upper cervical movement.

Palpation

1. Tight upper trapezius and upper cervical muscles, local tenderness over right midcervical area.
   a. Central posteroanterior pressure (PAs↓) on the spinous processes of C4, C5.
   b. Left unilateral posteroanterior pressures (↓↦) on apophyseal joints of C4–C6.
   c. Right unilateral posteroanterior pressures (↦↓) on apophyseal joints of C3, C4 at Grade IV reproduce sharp pain and stiffness.

Passive Physiological Intervertebral Movements

1. Rotation:
   a. Left, no opening.
   b. Right, no closing.
   c. Stiff + + at C3–C4.

Reassessment After Objective Examination

1. Flexion: slight increase in half range.
2. Extension: range same, slight decrease in stiffness with overpressure.
3. Right rotation: 40 degrees, onset of sharp pain with overpressure.

4. Physical therapist's assessment: patient no worse; in fact, slight improvement in range with no exacerbation of pain. Patient requires movement as treatment.

ASSESSMENT AT CONCLUSION OF OBJECTIVE EXAMINATION

Diagnosis

1. Radiographically documented multilevel degenerative changes.
2. Locked joint on right midcervical level.

Presentation

1. Severity: sharp pain on right midcervical area severe, other areas not.
2. Irritability: because the patient is able to work, the condition is not irritable with the exception of quick right rotation, which locks for 30 minutes.
3. Stage: chronic with one acute level superimposed.
4. Stability: deteriorating over time.
5. Mechanical: all active movements limited.
6. Functional:
   a. Right rotation limited by pain and stiffness.
   b. Sustained postures.

Further Assessment

1. Psychosocial factors: happily married with good health insurance coverage, planning for retirement.
2. Contraindication to treatment: age may limit vigor.
3. Possible causes: age-related changes, repetitive neck movement at work, airplane flight.

Prognosis

1. Natural history of the disorder: progressively worsening over patient's lifetime, may have nerve root disorders later.
2. Level of recovery (goals):
   a. Eliminate sharp right-sided pain.
   b. Reduce generalized ache to pain-free periods.
   c. Improve range of movement.
   d. Increase sustained pain-free periods.
3. Rate: slow.
4. Factors that may limit full recovery:
   a. Age.
   b. Documented pathology on radiograph.
5. Likelihood of recurrence: characteristics of the pathology are episodic.

TREATMENT

Spondylosis is a multijoint degenerative disease and requires movement through range with many different treatment techniques.

Day 1

1. Apply unilateral posteroanterior pressures on C3, C4 with Grade IV − short of pain: addresses the most severe level first, where the therapist will expect the most change.

a. Reassess right rotation: 40 degrees, decreases sharp pain.
b. Continue technique, increasing to a Grade IV, reproducing pain and addressing stiffness.
c. Reassess right rotation: 60 degrees, decreases sharp pain with overpressure.

2. Address other restricted levels by adding left unilateral posteroanterior pressures.
a. Start gently at Grades IV − and III −.
b. Assess if improvement or no exacerbation; continue with more vigorous Grades IV and III.

Day 2

1. Reassess if maintained gains from previous treatment session. Repeat.
2. Consider increasing vigor by medially directing the posteroanterior pressures.
3. Consider adding other techniques:
a. Cervical rotation.
b. Cervical traction.
4. Commence addressing other factors:
a. Muscle tightness.
b. Posture.
c. Work situation.

Case #3: Cervical Headaches

Introduction

Headaches may occur for many reasons. Physical therapists are often able to help in cases that occur from disorders in the articular, muscular, or soft-tissue structures of the upper cervical spine. Through the convergence of cervical and trigeminal afferents on common neurones in the trigeminocervical nucleus, any structure innervated by any of the upper three cervical nerves may refer pain to the head and face.

Common areas of head pain recorded for cervical headache sufferers are frontal, orbital, temporal, and occipital and are shown in the body chart (see Figure 29–36). Headaches are commonly unilateral but can be bilateral; headaches of cervical origin do not typically change sides, as can occur in migraines.

The pain may be an ache, may be a deep boring pain, or, less commonly, may have a throbbing quality. Patients may also complain of tenderness over the occipital muscles and a feeling of local swelling. Superficial, shooting or lancinating pain is typical of true neuralgia.

Neurogenic symptoms in benign cervical musculoskeletal headaches are rare. Headache is a referred pain rather than irritation or compression of cervical

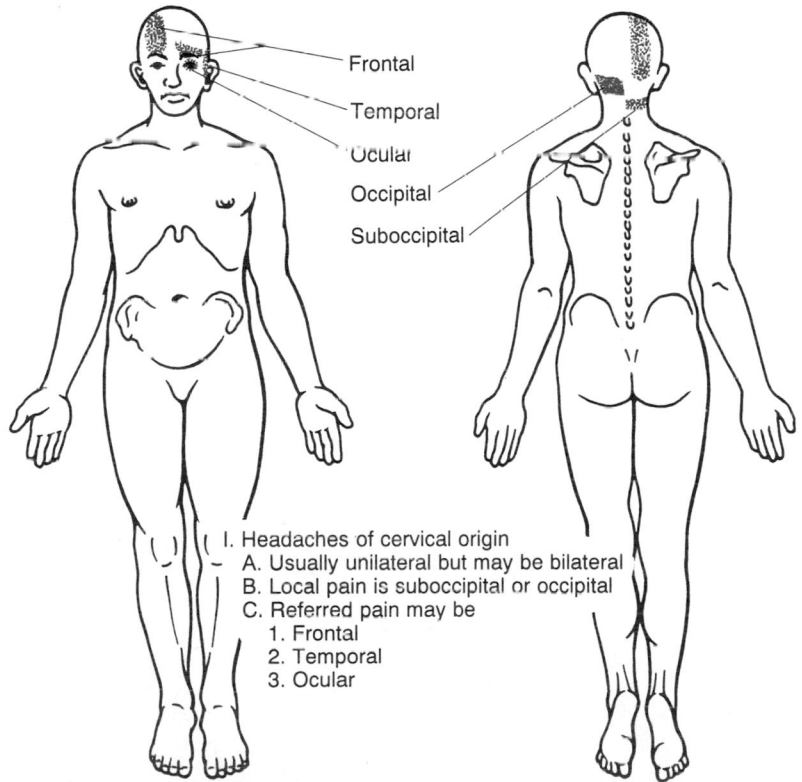

Frontal

Temporal

Ocular

Occipital

Suboccipital

I. Headaches of cervical origin
   A. Usually unilateral but may be bilateral
   B. Local pain is suboccipital or occipital
   C. Referred pain may be
      1. Frontal
      2. Temporal
      3. Ocular

FIGURE 29–36   Common areas of head pain/cervical headache.

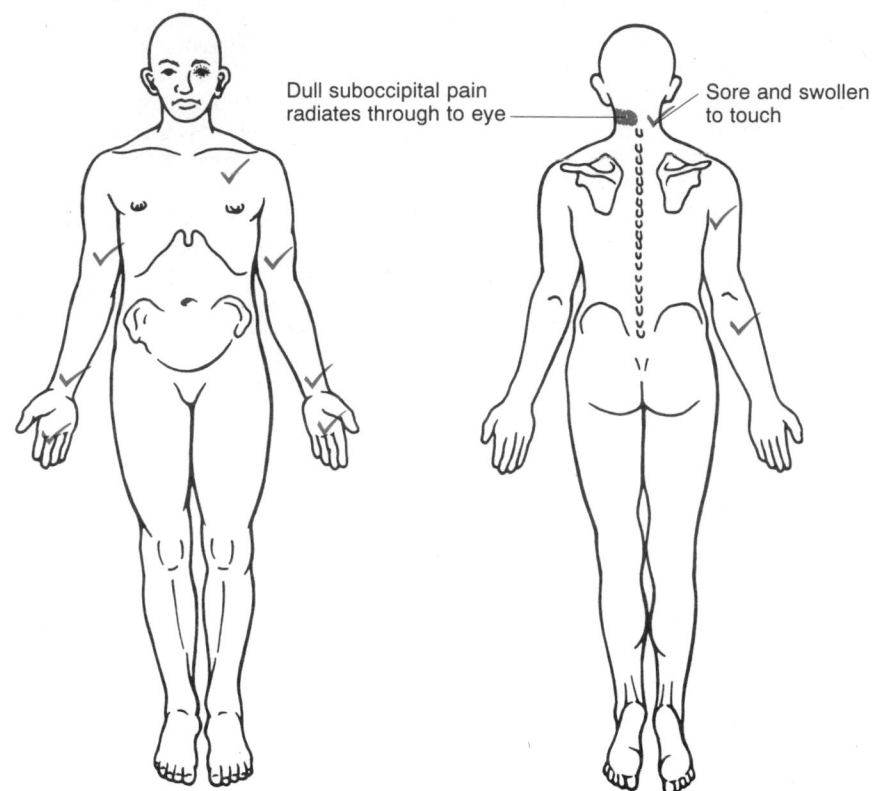

Dull suboccipital pain radiates through to eye

Sore and swollen to touch

FIGURE 29–37   Body chart: cervical headaches, 65-year-old female.

nerve root, but the therapist must always question the patient about sensory changes in the scalp.

Classic areas for specific cervical segment involvement are now proving tenuous but are still helpful to the therapist when trying to establish the level at fault from the body chart in the subjective examination.

1. C0–C1
   a. Occipital, not suboccipital.
   b. Can give pain to the ear.
2. C1–C2
   a. Suboccipital.
   b. Posterior head to the forehead.
   c. Into and behind the eye.
   d. Temporal pain.
3. C2–C3
   a. May irritate C2 or C3 nerve root.
   b. Pain as for C1–C2 and anterior neck pain.

SUBJECTIVE EXAMINATION

Patient Profile
1. 65-year-old female.
2. She looks after her grandchildren, works on various charitable committees.
3. She is always busy.

Area of Symptoms
1. Left-sided dull suboccipital pain that radiates behind left eye.
2. Suboccipital area sore to touch and feels swollen.
3. She denies right-sided pain, pain radiating into the upper extremity, or any numbness and tingling (see Figure 29–37).

Aggravating Factors
1. The patient says that her headaches come on for no apparent reason. The only pattern that she is aware of is that she typically wakes at midnight following a busy day or at 4 AM if she was not busy during the day.
2. The pattern of headaches often differs from the typical mechanical behavior of other musculoskeletal problems. The pattern is often not one of immediate cause and effect as in an impingement syndrome in the shoulder. Therefore, the therapist should ask about the following:
   a. The pattern of occurrence and duration (eg, sometimes headaches will occur daily, two or three times a week, or once a month).
   b. The initiating factors (these may include stress, premenstruation, or postural components).

c. Aggravating factors once the headache is present (*eg*, turning the head, looking up, reading).

d. Associated symptoms. These will give a clue as to the severity of the headaches or whether they are coming from other sources, such as vascular or instability problems. Therefore, the patient should always be asked about nausea and vomiting, eye symptoms (blurring, double vision, spots), and ear symptoms (pain/ache, ringing, buzzing).

e. Activities that provoke upper cervical symptoms. These often involve sustained upper cervical extension; therefore, ask about activities such as driving (poking chin), reading with chin in hand, and sleeping position. Also, ask whether there is difficulty with swallowing, as this can indicate anterior cervical swelling in trauma or a C3 discogenic problem.

Easing Factors

1. The patient said that she took acetaminophen when her headache was severe, after which she could return to sleep.

2. In addition, the therapist should ask about the effect of rest when the headache is present. Is the pain eased if the patient lies down or sits quietly? Also, medications should be identified.

PLEASE NOTE: Because the behavior of headaches differs from the usual musculoskeletal patterns, irritability is often difficult to establish.

24-Hour Behavior

1. The typical pattern for headaches over a 24-hour period may be waking with the headache because of poor sleeping position or a busy previous day. Cervical stiffness may occur in the morning, ease with activity, and then intensify by the end of the day. This would be consistent with an arthritic condition.

2. In this case, the patient said that she always woke with a headache, which eased within 1 hour, and that she was unaware of any cervical stiffness.

3. During the day, she was fine and never had a headache.

Special Questions

The patient took acetaminophen as needed. She had never taken steroids or anticoagulants. Her general health was good, her weight was stable, and she had no dizziness or gait disturbance. The physician had not taken radiographs of her neck.

History

1. Because patients will present with headaches of weeks', months', or, more often, several years' duration, the therapist has to be careful with a differential diagnosis. A headache can be a symptom of a disease or disorder of many origins, including neurological, vascular, ophthalmological, otolaryngological, dental, psychiatric, and musculoskeletal.

2. Many patients relate the onset of cervical headaches to an injury or have a past history of head or neck trauma.

3. A common cause of perpetual strain to the upper cervical joints can be poor posture, poor postural habits, or poor sensory motor performance.

4. The insidious onset of headaches may be in direct response to the onset of degenerative joint disease.

5. In this case, the patient's headaches began when her husband was seriously ill 6 months previously, and she thought they were because of stress. Her husband recovered, but her headaches did not clear. They now remain in the unchanging pattern described previously. In the past, she had neck pain about 7 years ago. It was an insidious onset and was treated successfully with manipulation.

OBJECTIVE EXAMINATION

Observation

Poking chin posture, unable to correct. Tight upper cervical muscles and tight upper trapezius muscle.

Active Movements

1. Flexion: poor unrolling of upper cervical, no pain with overpressure.

2. Left rotation: 85 degrees, stiff end-feel, no pain.

3. Right rotation: 70 degrees, tight, left suboccipital, no pain.

Passive Physiological Intervertebral Movements

1. C2–C3 blocked to opening movement and closing in rotation and lateral flexion.

Palpation

1. Tight upper cervical musculature, left greater than right.

2. Unilateral posteroanterior pressure on left C2–C3 apophyseal joint at Grade IV is thickened—stiff and reproduces pain greater than on the right ($\llcorner$⌐ C2–C3 thickened, stiff local pain IV ≫ ⌐$\lrcorner$).

3. Unilateral posteroanterior pressure on left apophyseal joint at C1–C2 reveals spasm, no pain at Grade IV ($\llcorner$⌐ C1 C2 spasm ✔IV).

ASSESSMENT AT CONCLUSION OF OBJECTIVE EXAMINATION

Diagnosis

1. Headache of C1–C2, C2–C3 origin.

2. Secondary/chronic muscle shortening and spasm.

Presentation

1. Severe when headache occurs because it wakes patient from sleep.
2. Irritable.
3. Stage: chronic.
4. Stability:
   a. Not changing, very stable pattern.
   b. This indicates that the physical therapist may have difficulty changing the pattern of headaches and eventually may have to treat vigorously to have an effect.

Mechanical

1. Active cervical ranges of movement are not markedly restricted, but C2–C3 restricted to lateral flexion and rotation passive physiological intervertebral movements.
2. Adaptive muscular tightness predominates.

Functional

1. The patient is not limited in activity during the day, but the time of onset of the headache at night appears to be dependent on the activity during the day.

Further Assessment

1. Psychosocial: well-adjusted elderly woman.
2. Contraindication to treatment: none, but care should be taken with vigorous techniques because of age.
3. Possible causes:
   a. Age and posture changes resulting in adaptive shortening in muscles and stiffness in the upper cervical joints.
   b. Stress of husband's recent illness.

Prognosis

1. Natural history of the disorder: chronic problem, flared after long symptom-free period, may tend to worsen as posture and muscles tighten.
2. Level of recovery:
   a. If tissue responds well in the first few treatments, patient should be symptom free for prolonged periods.

   b. If secondary changes are set, one would expect only to decrease the intensity of the headaches and perhaps enable the patient to sleep longer before being awakened.
3. Rate: depends on initial response to treatment, so would expect six visits.
4. Factor limiting full recovery: age.
5. Likelihood of recurrence: will recur but should be minimized with an effective home program of stretching and appropriate sleeping positions.

TREATMENT

1. Treatment should focus on three aspects of the patient's problem: stiff upper cervical joints, tender and shortened musculature, and adaptive postural changes.
2. The physical therapist's primary goal will be to mobilize the stiff upper cervical joints; however, because the musculature is tender and shortened, the joint mobilization will not be effective until the musculature is looser.
   a. Aim to mobilize the stiff upper cervical joints.
   b. This may be difficult as a first choice of treatment because of the muscular tenderness complained of in the subjective examination.
3. In this case, the physical therapist may choose to commence treatment by stretching the upper cervical musculature and the upper trapezius muscle.
4. Mobilization of the upper cervical joints may then be added.
5. To alleviate upper cervical tenderness, soft-tissue massage could be added.
6. After several treatments, when the patient is responding to the above treatment, the therapist may wish to teach the patient home stretching exercises to maintain the treatment gains.

   PLEASE NOTE: Cervical traction for the upper cervical spine tends to exacerbate headaches emanating from this area and is usually avoided as a treatment choice.

Case #4: Acute Nerve Root

INTRODUCTION

Acute nerve root lesions occur when the nere root is compressed or irritated by another structure; generally, they occur because the cervical disc has herniated and is compressing the nerve as it exits the intervertebral foramen. The presence of osteophytes may also compromise the nerve. In the acute phase, an inflammatory process is usually involved in the pathology.

SUBJECTIVE EXAMINATION

Patient Profile

1. 38-year-old female, department store buyer.
2. Travels monthly from San Francisco to New York.
3. Exercised on Nautilus equipment twice a week for the last month.

Area of Symptoms

1. Constant severe, deep right arm pain; worse in dorsum of forearm.

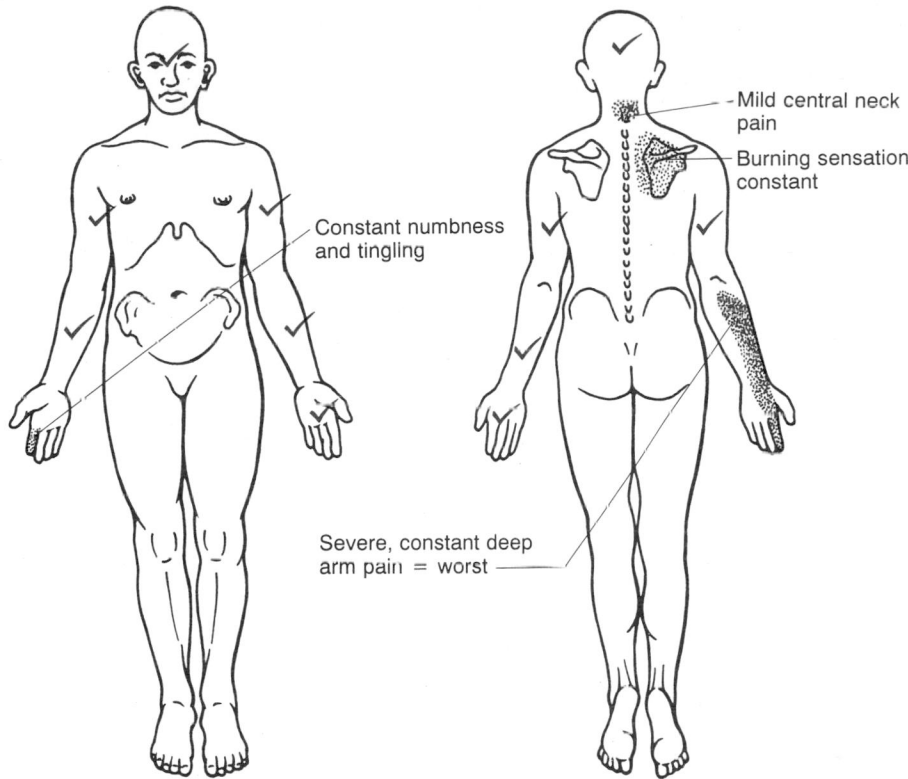

FIGURE 29–38   Body chart: acute nerve root.

2. Constant numbness/tingling tip of index finger.
3. Burning medial border and across the scapula.
4. Mild central neck pain.
5. This is a classic picture for an acute C7 nerve root irritation: the pain is severe and in a dermatomal pattern. It is worse distally, and paresthesia is present in the distal part of the C7 dermatome (see Figure 29–38).

Aggravating Factors

1. Any movement, particularly right rotation or extension, gives flash of forearm pain that takes 15 minutes to settle and leaves a deep ache; increased numbness persists for 30 minutes.
2. Unable to lie supine, prone, or on right side.
3. Sustained flexion 5 minutes gives scapula pain, takes 1 hour to settle.
4. Cough gives forearm pain.
5. Pain limits the patient's movement, and in this situation it is the distal symptoms that are produced with a small amount of movement. The most provocative movements are those that narrow the intervertebral foramen, eg, rotation toward the side of pain and extension.

Easing Factors

1. Never free of symptoms; best position is lying in a recliner with neck carefully supported, arm resting across chest. Because of the constant severe symptoms, the patient's daily activities are significantly restricted.

24-Hour Behavior

1. Night: wakes every 2 to 3 hours with deep burning in forearm, gets up for medications, then tries to return to sleep. This indicates an inflammatory process and also shows that slight movement throughout the night aggravates the condition.
2. Morning: better if able to maintain resting position; denies stiffness.
3. Day: progressively worse when out of recliner for 2 to 3 hours.

Special Questions

1. Vertebral artery/dizziness: negative.
2. Cord signs: negative because the patient denies bilateral numbness and tingling in a glove distribution in hands and feet; also, she does not have any gait disturbances.
3. No history of steroid use.

4. General health is good.
5. Weight is stable.
6. Medication: ibuprofen 2 days, 30% relief (now able to sleep briefly).
7. Tests: radiographs show diffuse degenerative changes at C4–C5, C5–C6, and C6–C7 with mild foraminal encroachment at C6–C7.

History

1. Present:
   a. Woke 3 days ago with neck stiffness and scapular pain after returning from New York, exercised on Nautilus that day, scapular pain became more severe and spread to forearm.
   b. Next morning woke with numbness in finger and severe pain in arm.
   c. Slight decrease in neck stiffness and medial border of scapula pain with medications, but distal symptoms continued to worsen.
   d. Visited physician, who diagnosed C7 nerve root irritation of discogenic origin and prescribed ibuprofen, 600 mg, four times a day, and physical therapy.
2. Past:
   a. The patient said that she tends to have many accidents, as she has had numerous falls down stairs while at work and a motor vehicle accident 10 years ago for which no prolonged treatment was given.
   b. Always has a stiff neck after a plane flight and carrying heavy luggage; it resolves within a few days.
   c. Began weight training program 1 month ago; some neck stiffness after pulling the latissimus dorsi bar down behind her neck, but usually resolved in a day.

OBJECTIVE EXAMINATION

Observation

1. Healthy-looking female.
2. Sits uncomfortably in pain, with head in slight flexion and right rotation, cradles arm across chest.

Active Movements

1. Extension: 10 degrees, increases forearm pain, increases numbness and tingling in the index finger for 15 seconds, which takes 1 minute to subside.
2. Rotation right: 30 degrees, increases forearm pain.

Neurological Findings

1. Right triceps reflex has decreased.
2. Decreased sensation to pinprick in the right index finger and anterior forearm.
3. Triceps 3+/5, pain in arm (needs retesting when less severe).

Manual Traction in Semireclined Position

1. Eases arm pain.

ASSESSMENT AT CONCLUSION OF OBJECTIVE EXAMINATION

Diagnosis

1. C7 nerve root irritation/compression of discogenic origin.

Presentation

1. Severe.
2. Irritable.
3. Stage: acute.
4. Stability:
   a. This episode is improving with ibuprofen, but recent onset does not indicate whether the condition will deteriorate.
   b. Previous episodes of cervical stiffness have worsened to serious pathology.
5. Mechanical: all movements limited by severe distal pain and numbness.
6. Functional:
   a. Severely limited, can barely tolerate being up out of a recliner for more than 2 to 3 hours.
   b. Cervical movements markedly restricted, position of rest limited to head supported in a reclining chair.

Further Assessment

1. Psychosocial factors:
   a. High-achieving female executive who has supportive husband.
   b. Good insurance coverage.
   c. Able to take time from work to facilitate recovery.
2. Contraindications:
   a. Gentle treatment required because of severity of pathology.
   b. Condition may deteriorate without intervention, and physical therapy treatment must not be seen as the reason for the decline.
3. Possible causes:
   a. Documented degenerative changes in the cervical spine, indicating that there has been long-standing pathology in the area.
   b. Overwork and poor positions.
   c. Fatigue.
   d. New exercise activity (Nautilus) may have exacerbated dormant problems.

Prognosis

1. Natural history of the disorder:
   a. Chronic problem deteriorating over time.
   b. Now a full-blown herniation with nerve root involvement.

c. Unsure whether this episode will deteriorate further, resulting in surgical intervention.
2. Level of recovery:
   a. Depends on size of herniation and whether nerve root is fully compromised, may not be able to affect numbness in hand.
   b. At best, try to return patient to former functional level, ie, episodes of stiffness.
3. Rate: will be slow. Expect to treat patient for approximately 3 months.
4. Factors limiting full recovery:
   a. Documented degenerative changes in cervical spine with foraminal encroachment.
   b. Size of herniation.
   c. Inability of patient to tolerate pain during recovery, may elect surgery.
   d. Length of time able to take off work for recovery.
5. Likelihood of recurrence: May live with recurrent episodes, which, if well managed, will be less severe than this one.

TREATMENT

1. Aim to relieve distal symptoms.
2. Instruct the patient in posture and support, which may include a soft collar.
3. Traction is generally the treatment of choice because it affects the joint indirectly, is clinically known to help, and, in this case, relieved symptoms when tested in the objective examination.
4. Rotation away from the side of pain with Grade IV −

may be considered as an alternative treatment choice.
   a. Perform manually in a pain-easing position.
   b. Begin gently without provoking symptoms or fully relieving distal symptoms.
   c. Progress time before weight.
   d. Rest after treatment or between rounds of traction.
5. Mobilization added:
   a. When severity and irritability are decreased.
   b. Able to move neck beyond P1.
   c. Mobilize in a manner that does not provoke symptoms with movement; ie, use slow, small, gentle-amplitude oscillations.
   d. Rotation away is usually the first choice (Grade IV −).
   e. Add thumbs only when the pain is not severe or latent.
6. Repeat neurological examination at each visit to monitor whether patient is maintaining or deteriorating.
7. In early stages:
   a. Time is the therapist's best ally because the inflammation needs time to settle and neural tissue recovery has recognized recovery periods.
   b. Response to treatment will be slow: expect small objective changes in the patient's condition before she reports favorable subjective changes.
   c. Consider the advantages of bringing the patient into the clinic versus rest at home with sound advice.

Case #5: Chronic Cervical Nerve Root

INTRODUCTION

A chronic cervical nerve root may be the result of a past acute cervical radiculopathy that has not completely resolved. Clinically, the symptoms are often described as an intermittent aching pain throughout a patchy dermatomal pattern.

SUBJECTIVE EXAMINATION

Patient Profile

1. 35-year-old female, executive secretary. She continues to work but is limited in the amount of time that she can spend at her desk typing.
2. Mother of two children, ages 10 and 6 years.
3. Activities include StairMaster/stationary bike 30 minutes, four times a week. She has been able to continue with these activities.

Area of Symptoms

1. Left intermittent cervical spine pain. She describes the pain as an ache that can be sharp at times.
2. She also reports a left intermittent forearm ache and intermittent numbness/tingling in the left thumb (see Figure 29–39).

Aggravating Factors

1. *Typing for greater than 30 minutes, with her neck in positions of sustained flexion, will increase her cervical spine pain. Symptoms ease in 5 minutes when she is out of the typing position. If she continues typing for greater than 60 minutes, she will notice increased numbness/tingling in the thumb and an increase in the forearm ache. Symptoms settle in 2 to 3 minutes when she gets up from her desk. Once symptoms settle, she is able to resume typing.
2. *Backing up car, turning her head to the left, increases her neck pain. Symptoms settle immediately when out of position and looking straight ahead.

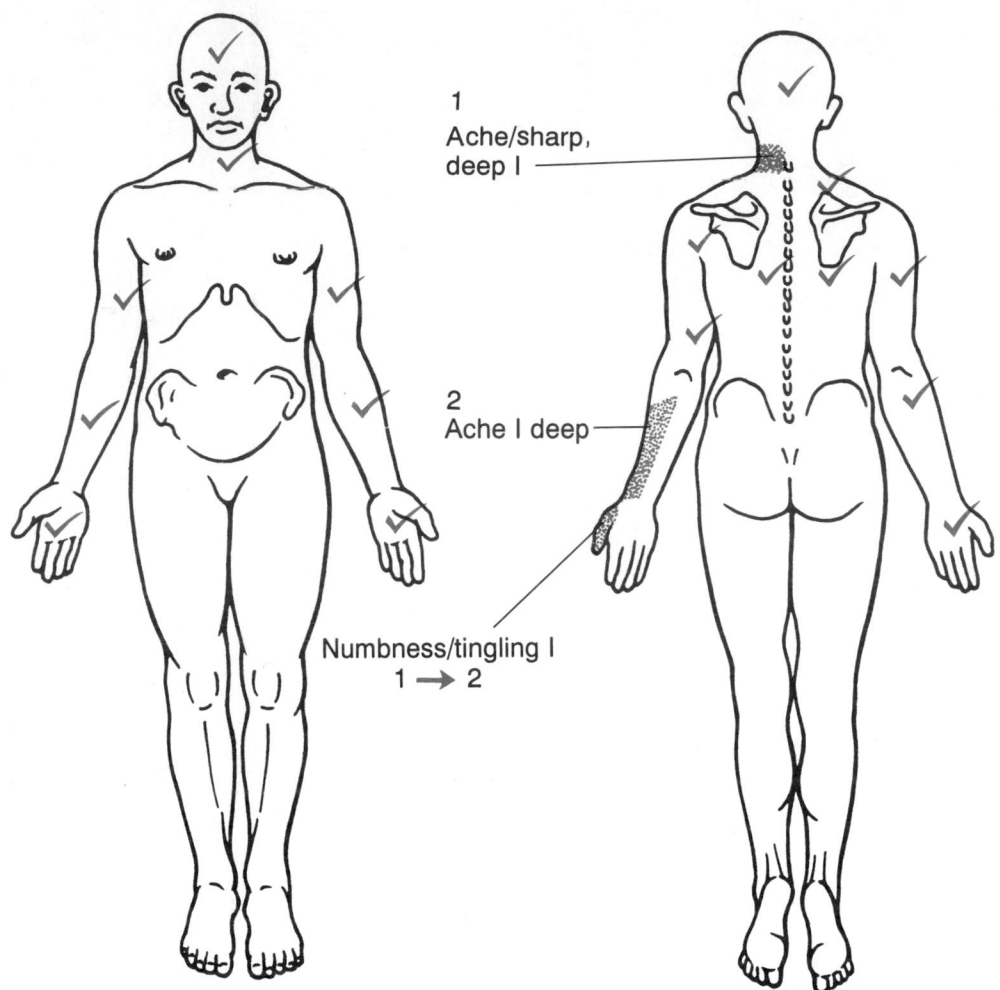

FIGURE 29–39   Body chart: chronic cervical nerve root.

1
Ache/sharp,
deep I

2
Ache I deep

Numbness/tingling I
1 → 2

Easing Factors
1. Avoiding typing for extended periods of time.
2. Exercising; walking.

24-Hour Behavior
1. *Night: occasionally wakes in left sidelying with forearm pain and thumb numbness. Settles immediately with change of position.
2. *Morning: stiffness in cervical spine. Settles in 5 to 10 minutes with shower.
3. End of day: worse when working. Better on weekends when she is able to avoid prolonged sitting at her desk.

Special Questions
1. General health: good.
2. Medications: none.

3. Vertebral artery: no complaints of vertebral artery symptoms.
4. Anticoagulants/steroids: none.
5. Weight loss/weight gain: stable.
6. Cord: no complaints of spinal cord symptoms.
7. Tests: none.

History
Nine months ago, the patient noticed gradual increase in neck pain. There was no apparent reason for onset. Seven months ago, she began to experience left forearm pain and left thumb numbness and tingling. Cervical spine symptoms were more constant and intense at that time. She saw a physician, who prescribed a soft collar and ibuprofen, 600 mg. She was also referred to the physical therapist for traction and exercise. The patient felt her progress had reached a

plateau after 2 months of therapy. Result: 70% relief but unable to function at 100% for an 8-hour day. Symptoms have remained unchanged for the past several months.

OBJECTIVE EXAMINATION

Observation
Forward head, slouched sitting posture. When sitting posture is corrected, the forward head position is reduced.

Shoulder Clearing
1. Flexion: full range of motion and painless with overpressure.
2. Abduction: full range of motion and painless with overpressure.
3. Hand behind back: full range of motion and painless with overpressure.

Rotator Cuff
1. Resisted tests: strong and painless with resisted movement.

Cervical
1. Flexion: full motion, complaint of pulling in the left cervical area with overpressure.
2. Extension: 75 degrees, complaint of left neck pain, overpressure increases the pain.
3. *Left rotation: 75 degrees, increase in left neck pain, overpressure increases the pain.
4. Right rotation: full range of motion and painless with overpressure.
5. Left lateral flexion: complaint of left neck pain.
6. Right lateral flexion: complaint of pulling in the left cervical spine.
7. *Left quadrant: increase in left cervical spine pain. On return to neutral, slight increase in forearm ache.
8. Right quadrant: full range of motion and painless with overpressure.

Neurological Findings
1. *Strength: slight weakness of the left biceps.
2. Reflexes: bicep jerk, equal bilaterally; tricep jerk, equal bilaterally.
3. Sensation: intact; normal sensation, although the patient has complaints of numbness/tingling in the thumb.

ULTT 2
1. *Left upper limb: increase in forearm ache and numbness in thumb with full shoulder depression, external rotation, forearm supination, wrist/finger extension to 20 degrees. Lateral flexion of the cervical spine to the right increases the symptoms (see Figure 29–39).

2. Right upper limb: forearm stretch at 50 degrees wrist/finger extension.

Palpation
1. C5–C6 Grade IV: central posteroanterior pressure at level C5 and level C6 causes an increase in local pain.
2. C5–C6 Grade IV: left unilateral posteroanterior at level C5–C6 increases local pain with a spread of pain to the supraspinous fossa.

Reassessment After Objective Examination
1. Cervical rotation left: slightly better movement, less increase in cervical pain with overpressure.
2. Neurological findings: same.
3. ULTT 2 left: wrist/finger extension to 30 degrees with increase in same symptoms.

ASSESSMENT AT CONCLUSION OF OBJECTIVE EXAMINATION

Diagnosis
1. Chronic cervical nerve root disorder, clinical findings:
   a. Area of symptoms: cervical spine, distal forearm and thumb (C6 distribution).
   b. Manner of onset 9 months ago: beginning in the cervical spine and progressing into the left upper extremity.
   c. Chronic and stable symptoms at present.
   d. Restricted and painful movements of the cervical spine and on the ULTT.

Presentation
1. Severity: not severe. The patient continues to work but is limited in her typing activities. She is able to continue her normal level of exercise.
2. Irritability: not irritable. Typing increases her symptoms, yet all symptoms settle within a few minutes with a change of position. Turning her head increases her neck symptoms, and symptoms settle immediately when she is out of that position.
3. Stage: chronic.
4. Stability: stable at this time; symptoms have been the same for the past several months.
5. Mechanical:
   a. Restricted and painful cervical spine movements.
   b. Restricted and painful movement on the ULTT.
   c. Restricted and painful passive accessory movements in the cervical spine at the C5–C6 intervertebral level.
6. Functional: limited in work activities, specifically sustained postures at the computer terminal.
7. Further assessment:
   a. Psychosocial: active, motivated woman.
   b. Contraindications to treatment: none; however, care is needed with possible nerve root involvement.

c. Possible causes: sustained postures at the computer terminal.

Prognosis

1. Natural history of the disorder: episodic, may have recurring symptoms if she continues with her unmodified lifestyle.
2. Level of recovery (goals):
   a. Return to full work activities.
   b. Free of symptoms; signs may persist with certain movements.
3. Rate: moderate.
4. Factors limiting full recovery:
   a. Sustained postures at work.
   b. Length of current episode.
5. Likelihood of recurrence: possible, especially if patient remains in sustained postures throughout her workday.

TREATMENT

Initial treatment will be directed to the C5–C6 level. The initial selection of technique will be a left unilateral posteroanterior pressure at the C5–C6 intervertebral level. Consider:

1. The most comparable joint sign found during the palpation examination was a left unilateral posteroanterior pressure at the C5–C6 intervertebral level.
2. There was a positive response to palpation, with an increase in cervical rotation; therefore, a palpation technique was chosen (left unilateral posteroanterior pressure) as the initial form of treatment over a technique such as cervical spine rotations.
3. Traction was not chosen as the initial technique because the patient had received traction in the past and she felt that she had reached a plateau. At this time, mobilization techniques will probably be more effective in making changes in her signs and symptoms.

Treatment 1

1. Left unilateral posteroanterior pressure at the C5–C6 Grade IV, short of pain reproduction.

2. Reassess objective asterisks (*):
   a. Left rotation: slightly better range, less increase in pain.
   b. Left quadrant: return to neutral, no increase in forearm symptoms.
   c. ULTT 2: same.
3. Advice/patient education:
   a. Avoid sustained flexion (change positions frequently).
   b. In sitting, maintain an appropriate lumbar spine position to avoid accentuating the forward head position.
   c. Work station/ergonomics: address early on in the treatment of this patient to assist in maintaining gains.

Treatment 2

1. Reassess if gains have been maintained from the initial treatment.
   a. Subjectively, the patient reports that she is able to type for a longer period of time before the neck pain begins. She reports no change in the numbness/tingling in the thumb and the forearm ache. Symptoms continue to increase after 60 minutes of typing.
   b. She maintained the gains in cervical spine movements from the initial treatment.
   c. ULLT: same.
2. Repeat the left unilateral posteroanterior pressure at C5–C6. Progress the grade of movement as pain and resistance move farther into the range.
3. Progression: additional techniques can be quickly added in the treatment of this patient owing to the low severity and irritability of her condition:
   a. Central posteroanterior pressures.
   b. Rotations.
   c. Traction.
4. With a chronic cervical nerve root condition, it is often necessary to use the ULTT as a form of treatment. For example, if there is no change in the ULTT following treatment to the intervertebral joint, one may choose to begin treatment of the neural tension sign using a technique such as the ULTT.

Case #6: Discogenic Pain

INTRODUCTION

Discogenic pain typically occurs in individuals in the 20- to 55-year-old range. Symptoms often develop as a result of sustained postures, such as prolonged sitting at a computer terminal or heavy lifting activity within the past 24 hours. The area of symptoms may include pain and stiffness in the cervical spine, medial border of the scapula, and supraspinous fossa. A cervical spine postural deformity may be present.

SUBJECTIVE EXAMINATION

Patient Profile

1. 40-year-old male, certified public accountant, currently working 8 to 10 hours a day.
2. Symptoms of scapular pain force him to stop work several times a day.

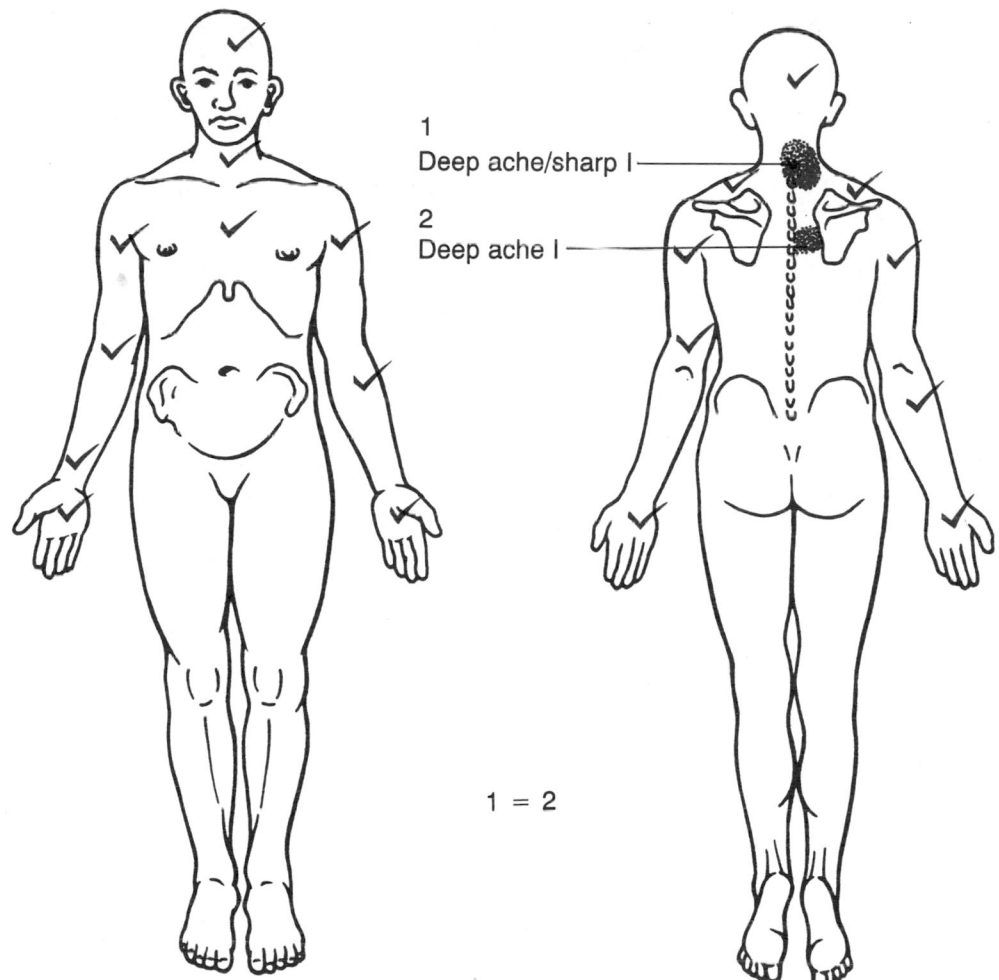

1
Deep ache/sharp I
2
Deep ache I

1 = 2

FIGURE 29–40   Body chart: discogenic.

3. Symptoms are eased with movement and change of position.
4. Recreational activities include running and cycling four times a week. He has been unable to run or cycle since the beginning of this episode owing to the increase in neck and scapular pain.

Area of Symptoms
1. Intermittent neck pain radiating to the supraspinous fossa and the medial border of the right scapula. The patient describes the symptoms as deep and aching in character and states that the worst pain is the scapular pain. He denies symptoms referred to the right upper extremity or numbness and tingling (see Figure 29–40).

Aggravating Factors
1. *Working at his computer terminal with the neck in positions of sustained flexion for more than 30 minutes increases neck and scapular pain. Symptoms resolve in 10 minutes when he changes positions or moves about.
2. *Shaving with the neck in the extended position produces an immediate increase in right cervical pain, which subsides with return to the erect position.
3. *Reading the newspaper, with the neck in the flexed position, upper extremities unsupported, for greater than 20 minutes increases neck and scapular pain. Symptoms settle in a few minutes with a change of positions.

Easing Factors
1. Hot tub.
2. Ice.

24-Hour Behavior
1. *Night: wakes occasionally with change of positions. Returns to sleep easily.
2. *Morning: neck stiffness. Eases with movement in 15 to 20 minutes.

3. Day: symptoms vary depending on activities. He can be asymptomatic if he avoids all aggravating factors.

Special Questions

1. General health: good.
2. Medications: naproxen, 500 mg, twice a day.
3. Tests: radiographs show mild narrowing of C5–C6 disc.
4. Weight loss/weight gain: stable.
5. Steroids/anticoagulants: none.
6. Vertebral artery: denies any vertebral artery symptoms.
7. Cord: denies any unsteadiness of gait, bilateral numbness/tingling in hands or feet.

History

One week ago, the patient woke with a stiff and painful neck. Pain was also present in the right scapula region. He was unable to extend or rotate right. He denies specific trauma but reports marked increase in desk and computer terminal work in past month preparing for tax season. Severe pain felt in the neck and scapula area persisted for 2 days. Feeling slightly better at this time, with increased mobility and decreased pain.

Past History

Experienced similar symptoms three times in the past 5 years. In all cases, it has cleared without treatment in 2 to 3 days. He occasionally experiences neck, right supraspinous fossa aching, especially if he is at the computer terminal for long periods. He reports that this is the worst episode, with increased intensity and duration of symptoms.

OBJECTIVE EXAMINATION

Observation

Forward head posture. Retraction of forward head position increases sharp cervical spine pain and scapula area pain.

Shoulder Clearing

1. Flexion: full range and painless with overpressure.
2. Abduction: full range and painless with overpressure.
3. Hand behind back: full range and painless with overpressure.

Cervical

1. *Flexion: two fingers, pulls in cervical spine and scapula area.
2. *Extension: 25 degrees, sharp increase in cervical, scapula area pain.
3. *Right rotation: 50 degrees, increases in right cervical area pain.
4. Left rotation: 75 degrees, increase in cervical area pain.

5. Right lateral flexion: 25 degrees, increase in right cervical pain.
6. Left lateral flexion: 50 degrees, increase in cervical area pain.

Neurological Findings

1. Strength: within normal limits.
2. Reflexes: biceps jerk, equal bilaterally; triceps jerk, equal bilaterally.
3. Sensation: intact.

Palpation

1. Central posteroanterior pressure at C5 and C6 levels at Grade IV increases local pain and scapular area pain ($\downarrow$C5, C6 IV); stiffness at C5 greater than at C6.
2. Right unilateral posteroanterior pressure at the C5–C6 level at Grade IV increases local pain with a slight spread to the scapular region; restricted movement at C5–C6 ($\longleftarrow\downarrow$C5–C6 IV).

Reassessment After Objective Examination

1. Cervical flexion: same.
2. Cervical extension: slight increase in motion to 40 degrees.
3. Cervical rotation right: same.

ASSESSMENT AT END OF OBJECTIVE EXAMINATION

Diagnosis

1. Discogenic C5–C6: clinical findings:
   a. Area of the symptoms: lower cervical spine and medial border of the scapula.
   b. Manner of onset: prolonged periods of sustained postures at computer terminal, woke with stiffness and pain.
   c. Patterns of cervical spine movement restrictions.

Presentation

1. Severity:
   a. Minimal: limited at work but able to continue working an 8- to 10-hour day. Unable to perform normal recreational activities.
2. Irritability:
   a. Mild: working at computer terminal greater than 30 minutes will increase symptoms, which take 10 minutes to settle when out of this position.
3. Stage: subacute.
4. Stability: improving.
5. Mechanical:
   a. Active cervical spine movements are restricted and painful.
   b. Passive accessory movements are restricted at the C5–C6 level.
6. Functional:
   a. Limited in sustained postures.
   b. Limited in recreational activities.

7. Further assessment:
   a. Psychosocial: motivated, athletic.
   b. Contraindications to treatment: none.
   c. Possible causes: sustained postures, increased work hours.

Prognosis

1. Natural history of the disorder:
   a. Worsening over time; with this episode, more intense and of longer duration.
   b. Recurrent episodes.
   c. May progress over time to involve cervical nerve root.
2. Level of recovery (goals):
   a. Free of symptoms.
   b. Improved mobility (signs may still persist with certain movements).
   c. Reduced level of recurrences.
3. Rate of recovery:
   a. Fast, symptoms have cleared quickly in the past.
   b. He is improving at this time.
4. Factors limiting full recovery:
   a. Occupation, sustained postures.
   b. Recurrent episodes
5. Likelihood of recurrence:
   a. History of disorder: this is fourth episode of similar symptoms.
   b. Occupation, sustained postures.
   c. Degenerative changes: present at C5–C6 level.
   d. Age: patient is at prime age for discogenic problems.

TREATMENT

1. Initial treatment will be directed to the C5–C6 level using a central posteroanterior pressure. Consider:
   a. C5–C6 was the most comparable and restricted level; therefore, progress will be easy to detect.
   b. There was a positive response to palpation, with increased cervical spine extension following the palpation examination.
   c. Clinical experience has taught us that central posteroanterior pressures are very effective in the lower cervical spine, even when the symptoms are primarily unilateral.

Treatment 1

1. Central posteroanteriors at C5–C6 Grade IV: short of pain reproduction.
2. Reassess objective asterisks (*):

a. Retraction: correction of forward head posture.
b. Cervical flexion: one finger, increase in pulling pain.
c. Cervical extension: 50 degrees, increase in cervical area pain.
d. Cervical rotation: 70 degrees, increase in cervical area pain.

3. Progress grades of movement as the onset of pain and resistance at the C5–C6 level move farther into the range.
4. Advice/patient education (in a subacute condition, the therapist must immediately instruct the patient in the activities to avoid; otherwise, the patient is unlikely to maintain the gains produced with treatment):
   a. Avoid sustained flexion.
   b. Interrupt position before onset of symptoms.
   c. Maintain correct posture (explain the importance of this).

Treatment 2

1. Reassess if gains have been maintained from previous treatment:
   a. Subjectively, the patient reports that he has been sleeping well through the night and waking with less morning stiffness and that he has been conscious of his posture and avoiding sustained flexion at his computer terminal.
   b. Objectively, the patient maintained the gains in cervical mobility from the initial treatment.
   c. Palpation findings revealed better movement at the C5–C6 level, with onset of pain farther into the range.
   d. The treatment was repeated at C5–C6, progressing farther into range.
2. Patient education:
   a. Ergonomics/work station: modifications must be introduced early in treatment for progress to be ensured. Without these modifications, the patient may be faced with a pattern of exacerbation and remission.
   b. Exercise: incorporate appropriate exercise for the stage of the patient's condition.

Progression

1. Adding other techniques:
   a. Rotations.
   b. Traction.
   c. Unilateral posteroanterior pressures.
2. Changing the vigor/grade of the techniques.

References

1. Farrell JP, Jensen GM: Manual therapy: a critical assessment of role in the profession. *Phys Ther* 1992, 72:843–852.
2. Cyriax J, Cyriax P: *Illustrated Manual of Orthopedic Medicine.* Boston, Butterworth Publishers, 1983.
3. Kaltenborn FM: *Manual Mobilization of the Extremity Joints,* 4th ed. Oslo, Olaf Norlis Bokhandel, 1989.
4. Maitland GD: *Vertebral Manipulation,* 5th ed. London, Butterworth Publishers, 1986, pp 1–13.
5. Warwick R, Williams PL: *Gray's Anatomy,* 36th ed. Edinburgh, Longmans, 1980.
6. Hollinshead WH, Rosse C: *Textbook of Anatomy,* 4th ed. Philadelphia, Harper & Row, 1985.
7. Twomey LT, Taylor JR: Joints of the middle and lower cervical spine: age changes and pathology. In *Proceedings of the Manipulative Therapists Association of Australia. Biennial Conference.* Adelaide, Australia, Manipulative Therapist's Association of Australia (MTAA), 1989, pp 215–220.
8. Grant JC: *An Atlas of Anatomy,* 5th ed. Baltimore, Williams & Wilkins, 1962.
9. Kapandji I: *The Physiology of Joints, The Trunk and Vertebral Column,* 2nd ed. vol 3. Edinburgh, Churchill Livingstone, 1974.
10. Nordin M, Frankel VH: *Basic Biomechanics of the Musculoskeletal System,* 2nd ed. Philadelphia, Lea & Febiger, 1989.
11. Penning L: Differences in anatomy, motion, development, and aging of the upper and lower cervical disc segments. *Clin Biomechanics* 1988, 3:37–47.
12. Penning L: Normal movements of the cervical spine. *Am J Roentgenol* 1978, 130:317.
13. Schneider G, Pardoe M: Translation of the facets during coupled motion in the cervical spine: a pilot study. *Aust J Physiother* 1985, 31:39.
14. Hayashi K, Yabuki T: Origins of the uncus and Luschka's Joint in the cervical spine. *J Bone Joint Surg* 1985, 67A:788–791.
15. MacNab I: Cervical spondylosis. *Clin Orthop* 1975, 109:69–74.
16. Bogduk N: Innervation and pain patterns of the cervical spine. *Clin Phys Ther* 1988, 17:1–13.
17. Bogduk N: Innervation of the vertebral column. *Aust J Physiother* 1985, 31:89.
18. Windsor M, Inglis A, Bogduk N: The innervation of the cervical intervertebral discs. *J Anat* 1985, 142:218.
19. Aprill C, Bogduk N: The prevalence of cervical zygapophyseal joint pain. A first approximation. *Spine* 1992, 17:744–747.
20. Dory MA: Arthrography of the facet joints. *Radiology* 1983, 148:379.
21. Bogduk N: The clinical anatomy of the cervical dorsal rami. *Spine* 1982; 7:319.
22. Rothman RH, Simeone FA: *The Spine.* vol 1. Philadelphia, W. B. Saunders Company, 1975.
23. Saldinger P, Dvorak J, Rahn BA, Perren SM: Histology of the alar and transverse ligaments. *Spine* 1990, 15:257–261.
24. Grant R: Dizziness testing and manipulation of the cervical spine. *Clin Phys Ther* 1988, 17.
25. Maitland GD: *Peripheral Manipulation,* 3rd ed. London, Butterworth-Heinemann Publishers, 1991, pp 64–106.
26. Elvey RL: Brachial plexus tension signs and the pathoanatomical origin of arm pain. In Glasgow EF, Twomey LT, Scull ER (eds): *Aspects of Manipulative Therapy.* New York, Churchill Livingstone, 1985.
27. Elvey RL: The investigation of arm pain. In Grieve GP (ed): *Modern Manual Therapy of the Vertebral Column.* New York, Churchill Livingstone, 1986, pp 530–535.
28. Elvey RL: *Brachial Plexus Tension and the Pathoanatomical Origin of Arm Pain. Aspects of Manipulative Therapy.* Carlton, Australia, Lincoln Institute of Health Sciences, 1980, pp 105–110.
29. Butler DS: Adverse mechanical tension of the nervous system: a model for assessment and treatment. *Aust J Physiother* 1989, 35:227–238.
30. Butler DS, Gifford L: The concept of adverse mechanical tension in the nervous system. Part 1: Testing for dural tension. *Physiotherapy* 1989, 75:622–636.
31. Butler DS: *Mobilisation of the Nervous System.* Edinburgh, Churchill Livingstone, 1991.
32. Brieg A: *Adverse Mechanical Tension in the Central Nervous System.* Stockholm, Almquist and Wiksell, 1978.
33. Sunderland S: *Nerve Injuries and Their Repair.* Melbourne, Churchill Livingstone, 1991.
34. McLellan DL, Swash M: Longitudinal sliding of the median nerve during hand movements: a contributory factor in entrapment neuropathy. *Lancet* 1975, 1:633–634.
35. Kenneally M, Rubenach H, Elvey RL: The upper limb tension test: the SLR of the arm. *Clin Phys Ther* 1988, 17:167–194.
36. Maitland GD: *Vertebral Manipulation,* 5th ed. London, Butterworth Publishers, 1986.
37. Morgan DM: The industrial back patient: a physical therapist's perspective. *Top Acute Care Trauma Rehabil* 1988, 2:38–46.
38. Morgan DM: Concepts in the functional training and postural stabilization for the low back injured. *Top Acute Care Trauma Rehabil* 1988, 2:8–17.
39. Morgan DM, Stevens B: Evaluation and treatment of the cervical spine. Personal communication, Marin Orthopedic Rehabilitation, Mill Valley, CA, 1989.
40. McKenzie RA: Mechanical diagnosis and treatment of the lumbar spine. Course notes. 1989.
41. Stevens BJ, McKenzie RA: Mechanical diagnosis and treatment of the cervical spine. *Clin Phys Ther* 1988, 17:271–289.
42. Morgan DM, *et al.:* Training the patient with low back dysfunction. Course notes, Folsom Physical Therapy, 1987.
43. Jull JA, Janda V: Muscles and motor control in low back pain: assessment and management. *Clin Phys Ther* 1988, 13:253–278.
44. Evjenth O, Hamburg J: *Autostretching: The complete manual of specific stretching. Auta Rehabil Forlag* 1989.
45. Grieve GP: *Common Vertebral Joint Problems,* 2nd ed. Edinburgh, Churchill Livingstone, 1988, pp 254, 259.

Suggested Reading

Aprill C, Dwyer A, Bogduk N: Cervical zygapophyseal joint pain patterns. II: A clinical evaluation. *Spine* 1990, 15:458–461.
Bland JH, Booushey DR: Anatomy and physiology of the cervical spine. *Arthritis Rheum* 1990, 20:1–20.
Bogduk N: Cervical causes of headache and dizziness. In Grieve G (ed): *Modern Manual Therapy of the Vertebral Column.* Edinburgh, Churchill Livingstone, 1986, p 289.
Bogduk N: The clinical anatomy of the cervical dorsal rami. *Spine* 1982, 7:319.
Bogduk N: The rationale for patterns of neck and back pain. *Patient Management* 1984, 13:17.
Bogduk N, Lambert G, Duckworth JW: The anatomy and physiology of the vertebral nerve in relation to cervical migraine. *Cephalalgia* 1981, 1:11.
Bogduk N, Marshall A: Third occipital headache. *Cephalalgia* 1985, 5(supp 3):310.
Brieg A: *Adverse Mechanical Tension in the Central Nervous System.* New York, John Wiley & Sons, 1978.

Chester JB: Whiplash, postural control, and the inner ear. *Spine* 1991, 16:716–720.

Cloward RB: Cervical discography. *Ann Surg* 1959, 150:1052.

Dalton PA, Jull GA: The distribution and characteristics of neck-arm pain in patients with and without a neurological deficit. *Aust J Physiother* 1989, 35:3–8.

Dillin W, Booth R, Cuckler J, *et al.*: Cervical radiculopathy, a review. *Spine* 1987, 11:988–991.

Dwyer A, Aprill C, Bogduk N: Cervical zygapophyseal joint pain patterns. I: A study in normal volunteers. *Spine* 1990, 15:453–457.

Edwards BC: Combined movements of the cervical spine (C2–C7). Their value in examination and technique choice. *Aust J Physiother* 1980, 26:165.

Elvey RL: The investigation of arm pain. In Grieve GP (ed): *Modern Manual Therapy of the Vertebral Column.* Edinburgh, Churchill Livingstone, 1986, p 530.

Grant R (ed): Physical therapy of the cervical and thoracic spine. *Clin Phys Ther* 1988, 17:111–124.

Grieve GP: *Common Vertebral Joint Problems.* Edinburgh, Churchill Livingstone, 1981.

Holt S, Yates PO: Cervical spondylosis and nerve root lesions. *J Bone Joint Surg* 1966, 48B:407–423.

Kikuchi S, Macnab I, Moreau P: Localization of the level of symptomatic cervical disc degeneration. *J Bone Joint Surg* 1981, 63B:272–277.

Macnab I: Cervical spondylosis. *Clin Orthop* 1975, 109:74.

Macnab I: The whiplash syndrome. *Orthop Clin North Am* 1971, 2:389–403.

Magarey ME: Examination of the cervical spine. In Grieve GP

(ed): *Modern Manual Therapy of the Vertebral Column.* Edinburgh, Churchill Livingstone, 1986, p 503.

Maitland GD: Palpation examination of the posterior cervical spine: the ideal, average and abnormal. *Aust J Physiother* 1982, 28:3–12.

Maitland GD: *Vertebral Manipulation,* 5th ed. London, Butterworth Publishers, 1986.

McLellan DL, Swash M: Longitudinal sliding of the median nerve during movements of the upper limb. *J Neurol Neurosurg Psychiatry* 1976, 39:566.

Murphy RW: Nerve roots and spinal nerves in degenerative disc disease. *Clin Orthop* 1977, 129:46.

Norris SH, Watt I: The prognosis of neck injuries resulting from rear-end vehicle collisions. *J Bone Joint Surg* 1983, 65B(5):608–611.

Penning L: Differences in anatomy, motion, development and aging of the upper and lower cervical disc segments. *Clin Biomechanics* 1988, 3:37–47.

Penning L: Normal movement of the cervical spine. *Am J Roentgenol* 1978, 130:317–326.

Wells P: Cervical dysfunction and shoulder problems. *Physiotherapy* 1982, 68:71.

White AA, Southwick WO, Panjabi MM: Clinical instability in the lower cervical spine: a review of past and current concepts. *Spine* 1976, 1:15–27.

Windsor M, Inglis A, Bogduk N: The innervation of the cervical intervertebral discs. *J Anat* 1985, 142:218.

Wyke B: Neurology of the cervical spinal joints. *Physiotherapy* 1979, 65:72–76.

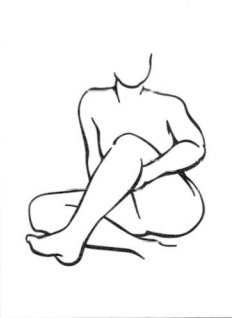

CHAPTER 30

Upper Extremity: Shoulder

Wayne Diamond

The shoulder region is anatomically complex, consisting of several articulations: the glenohumeral, acromioclavicular, sternoclavicular, and pseudoscapulothoracic joints. The relationship of the subacromial space and its space-occupying structures makes the shoulder somewhat perplexing because of the many different structures that can become dysfunctional, leading to pain. The most proximal joint of the shoulder girdle, the cervical-thoracic region, can refer pain to the shoulder without having pain itself.

The glenohumeral joint was considered by Cyriax and Cyriax[1] to be "the best joint" and by Maitland[2] to be one of the most interesting joints to treat by passive movement. Many therapists, however, do not concur with these thoughts because of the difficulty and poor success rate with passive treatment. The difficulty or success with treatment lies with accurate assessment of the joint and the ability to apply an appropriate technique for the problem. Far too often the therapist does not apply the principles of assess-

ment in determining the treatment (which treatment, how much, when to perform, etc.). When the patient does not respond to treatment, the technique is abandoned because it is thought to be of no value. However, the technique may have been appropriate for the patient, but the performance of the technique may have been too vigorous. The other possibility is that the technique was used too early in the treatment plan. If an adequate subjective examination is performed, followed by a well-planned objective examination, the involved structure can be localized, and then it can be determined whether any treatment would be sufficient for the patient at that point in time. According to Maitland,[2] certain types of patients respond to passive techniques:

1. Patients unable to move a shoulder properly because of stiffness more than pain.
2. Patients who have a painful shoulder in which pain is the limiting factor.

789

3. Patients who have a component of stiffness and pain.
4. Patients who have a momentary catch type of pain and can reproduce the pain only with certain activities.

The options available to the therapist for treatment are many. The focus of passive treatment relies on physiological and accessory movements in the pain-free, slightly into pain, and/or into stiffness ranges.[2] The goal of the therapist is to assess subjectively, to plan accordingly, and to perform the objective examination. From the information gathered, the therapist makes a working assessment of the problem, modifying it as needed but committing to a clinical decision. The outcome of this decision will in essence prove or refute the hypothesis or physical therapy diagnosis.[3,4]

The exercise or active portion of any treatment approach should be functional as well as an adjunct or complement to the treatment plan. The exercise needs to be appropriate for the problem that the patient presents based on signs and symptoms. For example, the patient with secondary impingement (see operational terms and definitions, p 792) because of instability of the scapula will reap little benefit from conventional rotator cuff strengthening exercises. The exercises need to be taught and evaluated in the same critical fashion as the passive treatment approach. The Maitland concept of the patient's condition (see subsequent discussion)—the Severity, Irritability, Nature, Stability, and Stage of the disorder (SINS; see operational terms and definitions)—governs the evaluation and treatment of the patient.

THE MAITLAND CONCEPT IN THE ASSESSMENT OF THE SHOULDER COMPLEX

In examining the shoulder, passive and active approaches are applied using the Australian or Maitland concept. Maitland[5] stated, "The Maitland concept requires open-mindness, mental agility, and mental discipline linked with a logical and methodical process of assessing cause and effect. The central theme demands a positive personal commitment (empathy) to understand what the person (patient) is enduring. The Maitland concept is the basis of this chapter because it relies heavily on clinical decision making, on which expert clinicians base their treatment.

Clinical decision making has become a major focus for the advanced clinician. Myers and Rose[6] and a committee edited an entire issue of the journal *Physical Therapy* devoted to articles based on presentations made at the 1988 Conference of Clinical Decision Making in Physical Therapy because of the exciting changes that this focus brings to the scope of physical therapy practice. With the advent of direct-access practice, the competency of physical therapists to formulate a physical therapy diagnosis and treatment plan became an issue. More important, the physical therapist had to develop advanced clinical skills to identify problems beyond the current scope of physical therapy practice that require follow-up visits by another specialist. In a special issue of *Physical Therapy* on manual therapy, Farrell and Jensen[3] discuss the role of the physical therapist's ability to assess pain and function. From this assessment, the physical therapist must implement a treatment program and establish real functional goals related to the patient's problem.[3]

"Clinical reasoning" is a thought process involving many steps—from decisions made from the moment the patient is greeted on initial treatment until eventual discharge.[3,4,7,8,19] It is the same process that is used in the medical community known as "hypothetico-deductive" reasoning: the process of collecting data and analyzing the information for hypothesis generation. From the hypothesis, which is continually changing with the patient's signs and symptoms, the treatment is designed.[4,7]

A working hypothesis is developed based on the source of the symptoms, which is determined from subjective and objective segments of the evaluation.[9-11] The information is then evaluated and a hypothesis is formulated. A common pitfall for novice clinicians is deductive reasoning. Jones states, "reasoning that is deductive is at a level on which conclusions are made logically from the presented data."[4] The expert clinician, however, takes this process one step further by applying inductive reasoning: looking at all possibilities as multiple sources or structures that can lead to dysfunction and pain. The expert clinician has the knowledge base or database of previous patients to draw from, which the novice has yet to acquire.[12-18] These past clinical treatments and outcomes become patterns for the expert clinician, allowing a more complete approach to patient management. Jones[4] and others[8,13,14] have noted that the expert clinician is superior in organizational skills, using the knowledge base, clinical patterns, and hypothetico-deductive reasoning. The expert will give more thought to several possible hypotheses and options for treatment. The novice will often take another approach, arriving at a conclusion of one simple hypothesis or problem, and will not thor-

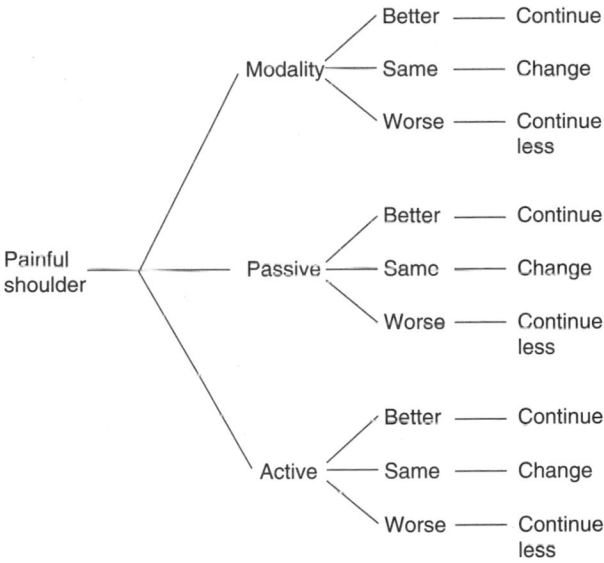

FIGURE 30–1   Decision tree. (Reprinted from *Physical Therapy* with the permission of the American Physical Therapy Association; adapted from Watts NT: Clinical decision analysis. *Phys Ther* 1989, 69:569–576.)

oughly examine other possible structures for provocation of pain and dysfunction.

The reason so much emphasis has been placed on the Maitland concept is because it parallels the clinical decision making process. "The permeable brick wall" that Maitland speaks of divides theory/diagnosis on one side from signs and symptoms on the other.[15–17] "Making the features fit" with the information gathered from the evaluation is an attempt to bring theory and signs and symptoms together.[5,19] The emphasis of this approach is the continual assessment, not the use of techniques, in determining the SINS. The Maitland concept uses the subjective and objective portions of the evaluation to determine factors such as how the patient will tolerate the examination and what might be expected on follow-up visits.[19]

Rothstein[20] and Gonnella[21] have provided the basis on which to study this approach through case reports and single-case designs.[20,21] These case reports are clinically relevant and document what was observed. Observation is subjective and thereby may be biased in interpretation by the observer. Controversy exists concerning subjective assessment in the evaluation.[9–11] When we document information that the patient reports to us, how accurate is that information? The accuracy of the subjective data rests on the clinician and how the questions are asked. If the question asked is open ended, less observer bias will be added, allowing

the patient the opportunity to offer his/her interpretation of the symptoms. As long as the therapist is consistent in asking the questions, the information will be consistent. Maitland[19] stresses the importance of continual assessment: not just of the patient but also of the therapist. If therapists are critical and consistent in the manner in which they seek information, whether subjectively or objectively, reliability may increase. Multiple authors have found good intrarater reliability in measurement, more so than inter-rater reliability.[11,20,22]

The Maitland concept of analytical assessment is a validation of every step of the evaluation process: the need to prove or disprove the hypothesis by inductive reasoning.[3,5,23] There are many ways of performing this analytical assessment, *eg*, by using models such as clinical decision trees,[24] hypothesis-oriented algorithms,[25] and cognitive mapping[18] (see Figures 30–1 and 30–2). These models are similar in that they involve collecting data and making an initial hypothesis or assessment from the information. The treatment plan is then implemented based on the information but is assessed as it is performed. Subjective and objective

History and evaluation

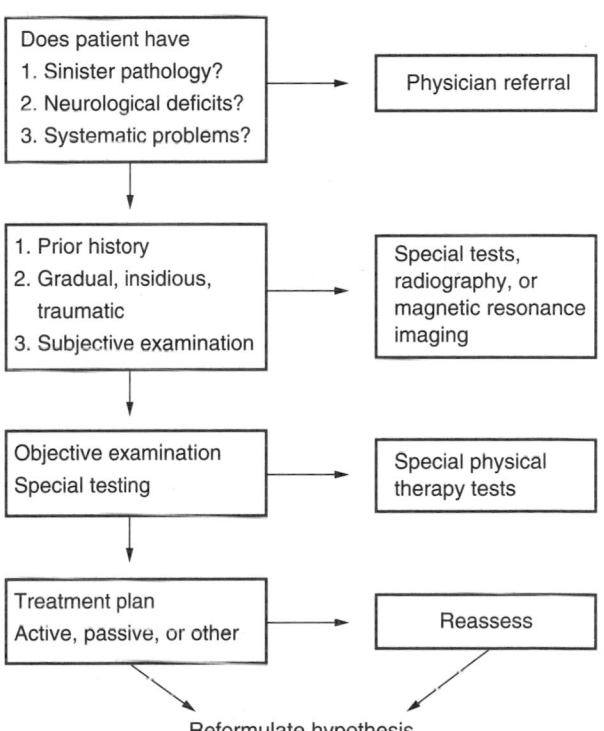

FIGURE 30–2   Shoulder pain algorithm. (Courtesy of Physical Therapy Department, Roger M. Nelson, PhD, PT, U.S. Public Health Service Hospital, San Francisco, CA.)

data are reassessed at follow-up visits, and the efficacy of the treatment plan is determined at that stage. If it is not effective, re-evaluation and interpretation of signs and symptoms are needed with insight into the problem. The primary aspect of this approach or concept is continual assessment in search of the correct answer.

This chapter follows the Maitland concept because we as clinicians need to validate and justify what we do in our treatments.[4] This approach uses clinical decision making and critically assesses all evaluative processes. The reassessment process justifies whether or not to continue a treatment approach for that particular patient problem. Each patient is a single-case design or report requiring continual critical assessment for changes in signs and symptoms. If clinicians are critical of themselves as well as their patients, more accurate data can be obtained. This data can then be used with future patients for more cost-effective treatment approaches that resolve symptoms more quickly. However, it must be stressed that objectivity and an open mind will allow the expert clinician to avoid false assumptions and to treat patients methodically.[23]

OPERATIONAL TERMS AND DEFINITIONS

Terms that are commonly used in the literature and throughout this chapter are defined below.

Active movement. Any movement of a mobile segment produced under a patient's own muscular control.

Aggravating factor. An activity performed on a regular basis by the patient that makes the complaints or symptoms worse.

Assessment. Findings of the examination that provide the therapist with necessary information to make a diagnosis. Also used for changes that take place as a result of the use of a technique to prove/disprove the effect of a technique. Analytically used during or at the conclusion of a treatment.[3,5,19,23,26]

Asterisk signs. Outstanding signs used for quick assessment and reassessment of the patient's progress. They can be subjective or objective. The main objective is to highlight those elements deemed important.[5,19,26]

Bankart lesions. The humerus translates forward during dislocation, and the glenoid labrum avulses from the anterior part of the periosteum, stripping the capsule. These lesions are suggestive of recurrent subluxations or dislocations of the humeral head.[27,28]

Capsular pattern. Typical pattern of limitation at a joint examined by passive movement, constrained by pain and/or resistance. The capsular pattern varies by joint and is determined by a proportion of the limitation, not the total amount. For example, the capsular pattern for the shoulder is as follows: medial rotation is most limited, followed by abduction, and then by lateral rotation, which is the least restricted.[1]

Clear. Area is free from signs or symptoms when movement is performed actively and/or passively with overpressure applied. The affected joint should be similar to the unaffected side.[2,4]

Comparable sign. A combination of pain, stiffness, and/or spasm that the therapist finds on examination and considers to be comparable to the patient's symptoms.[3,5,19]

Easing factor. Anything that will make the complaints or symptoms of the patient less significant.[5,19,26]

End-feel. What the therapist feels when performing passive movement to a joint, normally at the extremes of range of that joint.[1,5,19]

Hill-Sachs lesion. A radiological finding thought to be a compression fracture of the posterior humeral head. It is caused by traumatic translation of the posterior humeral head over the sharp anterior lip of the glenoid rim.[28–32]

Hypermobility. Excessive range of movement, if there is complete muscular control, to provide for stability.[27,33]

Impingement syndrome. Variety of shoulder disorders generally leading to shoulder pain with overhead activities. Structures in the subacromial space are compromised to the point of pain and pathology. These disorders can have two different etiologies, either primary or secondary impingement.[27,34–41]

Primary impingement involves the rotator cuff being mechanically impinged underneath the coracoacromial arch. Degenerative changes to the rotator cuff, most often the supraspinatus muscle, lead to tendinopathies, tear, and rupture. It is often present in those over 35 years of age. Surgery is performed when conservative treatment fails. Neer[37] considers primary impingement in three stages:

- Stage I—edema and hemorrhage.
- Stage II—fibrosis and tendinitis.
- Stage III—tears of the rotator cuff, biceps ruptures, and bone changes.

Secondary impingement is also mechanical in nature and involves glenohumeral or functional scapular instability. It generally occurs in a younger group of individuals (<35 years of age) involved with throwing- or racquet-type sports. The nonoperative approach is more often used with these individuals. Jobe, as cited in Silliman and Hawkins,[27] classified anterior shoulder pain patients into four groups:

- Group I—Athletes who demonstrate pure impingement.
- Group II—Athletes who have instability secondary to anterior ligament and labral injury with secondary impingement.
- Group III—Athletes who have instability due to hyperelasticity and secondary impingement.
- Group IV—Athletes who have pure anterior instability.[27,38–41]

Instability. Excessive displacement anteriorly or posteriorly of the humeral head in relationship to the glenoid tested *clinically*. Lack of anterior or posterior static and dynamic stabilizers of the shoulder determine the condition and direction. There are two common types of instability:[33,42]

1. TUBS—Traumatic Unidirectional Anterior Instability with Bankart lesion requiring Surgery.[43]
2. AMBRII—Atraumatic Multidirectional Bilateral laxity Rehabilitation Inferior Capsule and Rotator Interval. TUBS lesions often require surgery for repair, whereas AMBRII lesions require more of a rehabilitation approach. Surgery is not as successful but can be performed if necessary.[43]

Irritability. Irritability is assessed by three factors:

1. How easily the symptoms are brought on with various activities.
2. How severe the symptoms become.
3. How long these symptoms persist after the activity has stopped.

Irritability can be assessed as: nonirritable, minimal, moderate, or severe.[5,19]

Joint. *Intra-articular* refers to the structures (1) from subchondral bone through to subchondral bone of adjacent joint surfaces, and (2) everything within the joint space, including the inner capsule. *Periarticular* refers to structures outside the joint adjacent to and including the outer capsule.

Laxity. The ability of the humeral head to be translated anteriorly, inferiorly, and/or posteriorly *passively* in the glenoid fossa.[33]

Nature of a disorder. The therapist's interpretation and assessment of the structure and its pathology in regard to the patient's complaints. All areas of the subjective examination play a role in determining the nature of the disorder.[5,19,26]

Overpressure. A passive movement applied by the therapist, from gentle to moderate to vigorous, applied at the limit of the available range. This procedure needs to be performed in individuals considered to have full range of motion and to be painless. The joint is considered normal if overpressure is applied and is compared with the contralateral side.[5,19,26]

Painful arc. Pain elicited in the range of 60 to 120 degrees of shoulder elevation. Pain is often worse on lowering in this range, which is more indicative of a rotator cuff problem due to eccentric control of tendon(s).[1,35]

Passive movement. Any movement of a mobile segment that is produced by any means other than that under the patient's muscular control.

1. Physiological: movements performed by the examiner, although they can be performed actively.
2. Accessory: movements available in a joint performed passively by the examiner. These cannot be performed actively.

Scaption. Elevation of the arm in the plane of the scapula.[44–56]

Sign. An objective finding; anything within a joint or structure regarding its movement that is found to be abnormal.[5,19,26]

Stability of a disorder. Present area or symptoms as compared to area during initial onset of symptoms. For example, a stable disorder is one that is in the same area as during initial onset of condition. A condition with a worsening progression of symptoms is shoulder pain that was local in the past but that is currently referring distally to the forearm and hand.[5,19,26]

Stage of a disorder. The stage of the condition as it relates to the chronicity of the disorder, but this is not the only factor in its determination. An acute condition can overshadow a chronic underlying condition. A classic example is that of a frozen shoulder; severe pain with full range of motion progresses to decreased pain with increased stiffness and finally to stiffness presenting as the dominant factor with minimal pain.[2–4]

Subluxation. Partial loss of joint congruency, which can normally be controlled with dynamic stabilizers. Affected by a certain amount of normal translation within the glenohumeral joint.[27,42]

Sulcus sign. On observation, an indentation of the skin distal to the acromion indicating possibly inferior laxity of the glenohumeral joint. Often present in individuals with multidirectional instability.[43]

Superior Labrum Anterior Posterior Lesions (SLAP). Superior labral avulsion at the biceps insertion.[27,57,58]

Symptom. Something the patient complains of, *eg*, pain, stiffness, numbness.

I. Functional Anatomy

Anatomy gives a view of one structure as it relates to another from a static point of observation. The clinical examination of structures by palpation, stretch, contraction, and/or compression appears to be a logical progression through which methodical testing can assist in determining the structure's integrity. The shoulder, because of its large degree of mobility, can possess multiple-structure pathology. This inter-relationship of many different structures emphasizes the need for assessing the shoulder in many different positions during movement or examination. The shoulder can be difficult to evaluate when it is examined statically because often it is the dynamics of the shoulder that are dysfunctional. Therefore, shoulder anatomy must also be assessed dynamically for a more realistic picture of the patient's problem.

This section provides an update on the functional anatomy of the shoulder. Certain tests are mentioned as they relate to specific anatomy and pathology. More details are given in the section on special tests. The shoulder is explored based on its joint structure and related components. Figure 30–3 illustrates the five joints of the shoulder complex: glenohumeral, coracoacromial, acromio-

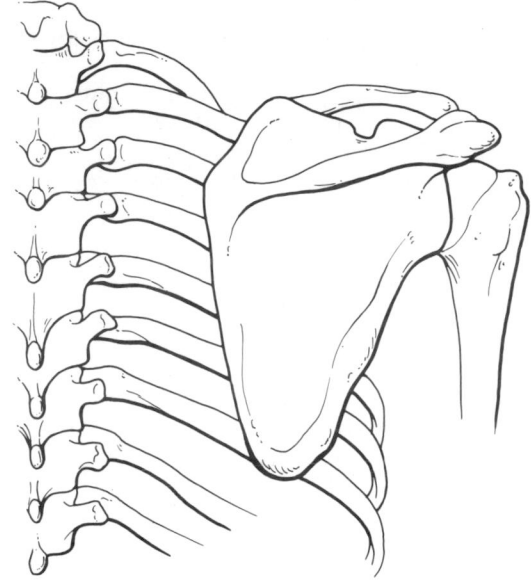

FIGURE 30–4 Relationship of the scapula to the thoracic cage.

humeral (more of a space than a joint), sternoclavicular, and scapulothoracic (more of an articulation than a joint). This section focuses on the glenohumeral and coracoacromial joints and their related structures, as these play the most important roles in function and dysfunction.

A. Glenohumeral joint

The glenohumeral joint has a true ball-and-socket relationship in regard to its strict bony articulation. The articular surface of the humeral head is markedly larger than the female proximal surface of the glenoid facing superiorly, medially, and posteriorly. The axis of the head and the longitudinal axis of the shaft of the humerus may vary from an angle of 130 degrees to 150 degrees in the frontal plane.[59] In a transverse plane, the axis of the humeral condyles is 30 degrees posterior or retroverted to the elbow.[60,61] The clinical significance of the retroversion of the humeral head is that it hides the joint from palpation by placing the greater tuberosity more anteriorly.[60] Therefore, for the therapist to attempt to palpate the rotator cuff tendon, specifically the supraspinatus, the humerus would have to be placed in internal rotation and slightly adducted.

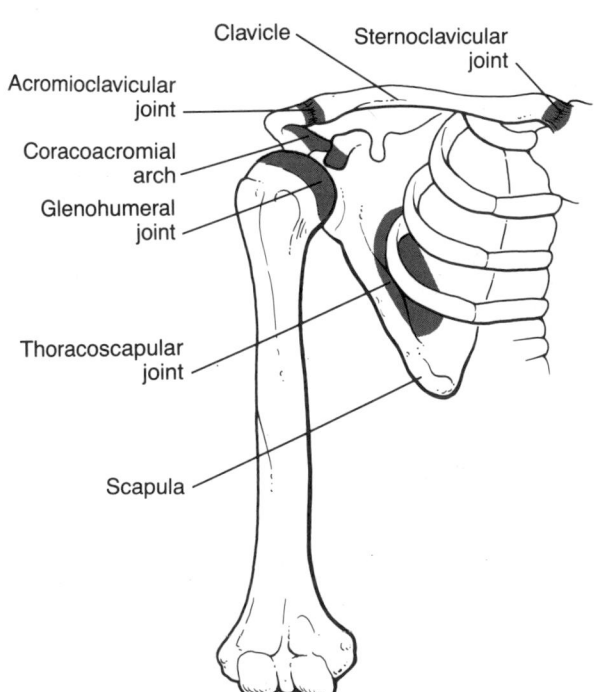

FIGURE 30–3 Shoulder complex and its five related joints.

The glenoid fossa of the scapula faces superiorly and anteriorly at rest. When the arm is held at the side in a dependent position, the fossa tilts 5 degrees downward and faces posteriorly 7 degrees. Figure 30–4 demonstrates the relationship of the scapula to the thorax as it lies at a 30- to 45-degree angle to the coronal plane.[52,54] Thus, elevation in the path of least resistance would be along the same plane as the scapula, 30 to 45 degrees to the coronal plane, known as scaption.[39,55] The glenoid fossa surface contact is one third to one quarter the size of the humeral head, leading to increased mobility at the expense of stability.[61,62]

B. Acromiohumeral joint

The acromiohumeral joint or subacromial region is a specific space described by its bony and ligamentous borders.[59] The borders of this joint are the superior aspect of the humerus inferiorly, the acromion and spine of the scapula superiorly and posteriorly, the coracoacromial ligament superiorly, and the coracoid process superiorly and anteriorly.

Structures within the acromiohumeral space are discussed from inferior to superior. Most inferior is the synovium and joint capsule of the glenohumeral joint, with a sliding intra-articular biceps tendon encased within this structure. Above the superior glenohumeral and coracohumeral ligaments are the rotator cuff muscles (supraspinatus, infraspinatus, and teres minor), attaching to the greater tuberosity. The subscapularis attaches to the lesser tuberosity below the coracoid process and coracoacromial ligament.[59,61]

The most superior structure in the acromiohumeral joint is the subacromial or subdeltoid bursa. These bursae are collectively referred to as the subacromial bursa because they are often continuous in nature and considered to be the most important of the bursae. The subacromial bursa is located between the coracoacromial ligament and acromion above and the rotator cuff (primarily supraspinatus) below, extending beneath the deltoid muscle and coracoid process. It adheres to the coracoacromial ligament and supraspinatus muscle below. The bursae communicate with the joint in cases of pathology such as a ruptured rotator cuff muscle.[60,62,63] Diagnostically, leakage of dye during arthrography would be indicative of a rotator cuff tear. The major function of the bursae is to aid in shoulder mechanics where motion between adjacent structures can cause friction. The subacromial bursa prevents friction between the humerus and the supraspinatus tendon but can cause pain independently or concurrently when the supraspinatus no longer functions properly.[48]

The subscapular bursa lying between the subscapularis muscle tendon and the anterior neck of the scapula protects the tendon as it passes under the coracoid process. The subscapular bursa and the subacromial bursa do not communicate with the joint cavity except in the case of a rotator cuff tear.

The coracoacromial arch (see Figure 30–5), a bony ligamentous arch, is made up of the undersurfaces of the acromion and coracoid processes and the coracoacromial ligament placed posteriorly to the glenoid.[64] This arch forms a secondary restraining socket for the humeral head, protecting the joint from trauma above and dislocation of the humeral head superiorly.[64] Beneath this arch lies the acromiohumeral space occupied by the rotator cuff and its bursa. A narrowing of this space, *ie*, humeral head migration, can predispose a person to an impingement syndrome of any of the above space-occupying structures, including its bony borders. The coracoacromial arch can be modified arthroscopically by cutting the coracoacromial ligament or by acromioplasty in cases of impingement.[10,60,64]

The acromion, which represents the roof of the subacromial space, has received much at-

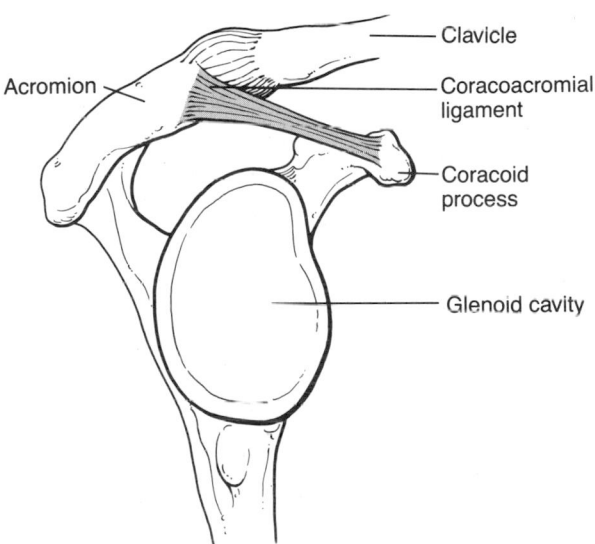

FIGURE 30–5   Coracoacromial arch.

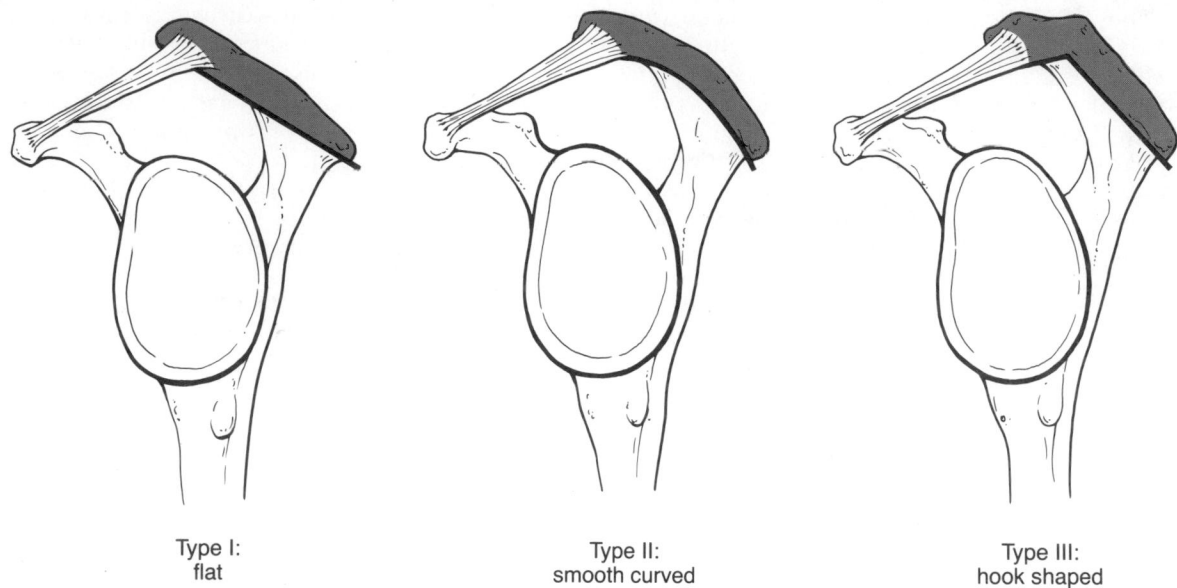

Type I:
flat

Type II:
smooth curved

Type III:
hook shaped

FIGURE 30–6   Three types of acromions: flat, smooth-curved, and hook-shaped.

tention in the past few years. The shape of this bony structure has been implicated as a major factor in rotator cuff pathology.[65,66] Bigliani *et. al.*[65] described variations in acromion shape correlated with tears of the rotator cuff. Acromion shapes (see Figure 30–6) were classified as Type I, flat; Type II, smooth curved; and Type III, hooked. The hooked acromion had a higher frequency of complete rotator cuff tears. This information may be of value in reviewing radiological films of patients with impingement-type complaints leading to a potential rotator cuff tear.[35,65,66]

C. Joint capsule

The joint capsule attaches to the glenoid rim and the anatomical neck of the humerus, allowing considerable laxity for large, unresisted arcs of motion. The capsule is loose anteriorly and inferiorly but tight superiorly. This slack of the capsule allows for normal distraction of the humeral head from the glenoid fossa of approximately 1 inch. A sulcus sign,[42] an indication of inferior instability, would be evident at the lateral border of the acromiohumeral space if displacement was greater than 1 inch. The capsule also acts as a stabilizer in extremes, winding back on itself. With immobilization of the shoulder, periarticular changes can occur, leading to pain and significant decrease in mobility at the joint.[67-72] The typical capsular pattern, as described by Cyriax and Cyriax,[1] is one of marked limitation of medial rotation, followed by abduction, and then by lateral rotation. If these restrictions are not in these proportions, it might be appropriate to examine the cervical spine for referral of pain leading to restriction at the shoulder.[67,73-75]

The capsule can also act as a stabilizer, improving stability anteriorly. At the same time, if restricted, it can limit flexion and external rotation.[33] If the capsule has slack instability, frank dislocation can occur in a dependent position of the humerus. However, for patients with shoulders unchanged through conservative treatment, a release of the capsule may afford more mobility.[33,42,71]

D. Glenoid labrum

The glenoid labrum provides additional stability to the glenohumeral joint by deepening the articular surface of the glenoid. Its main function is to deepen and provide the necessary stability for function.[57,60] Therefore, trauma or pathology to this structure can lead to instability of the joint, which would require stability testing. The glenoid labrum, made of fibrous connective tissue that is ligamentous in nature, has a small band of fibrocartilage in the transition zone, with articular cartilage covering the joint surface (see Figure 30–7). The inner surface of the labrum is covered with

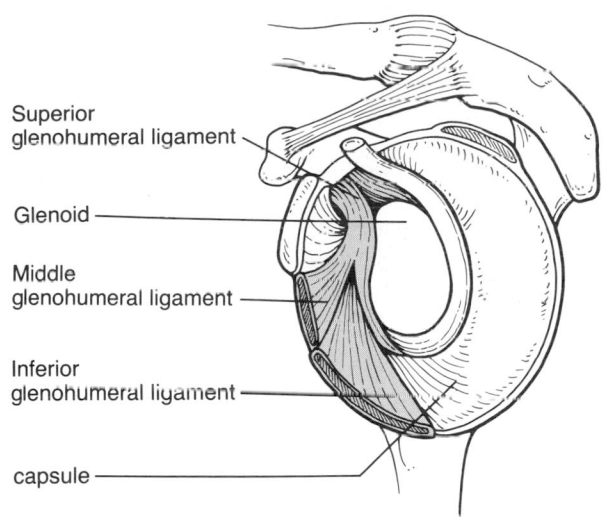

Superior
glenohumeral ligament

Glenoid

Middle
glenohumeral ligament

Inferior
glenohumeral ligament

capsule

FIGURE 30–7   Glenohumeral ligaments of the shoulder.

synovium, and the outer surface is continuous with the periosteum of the scapular neck.[76,77] The superior part of the labrum inserts directly into the biceps tendon, which may explain the tenderness often experienced during palpation over the bicipital groove.[77] The inferior glenohumeral ligament blends the anterior portion of the labrum and the anterior glenoid rim. Most labral detachments in this area commonly result in a catching or popping sound during overhead and external rotation activities. The patient may have a sensation of the arm going "dead." The direction of the injury will determine which part of the labrum is torn. For example, an anterior dislocation will possibly tear the anterior labrum, resulting in anterior instability. Most labral tears occur in the anterosuperior quadrant of the glenoid. Flap tears are most common in this region, possibly related to a traction injury to the biceps tendon on the labrum. These are often referred to as SLAP lesions affecting the labrum.[27,58] The shoulder quadrant test would be an excellent way to stress this area in relation to the anterior instability tests for provocation of symptoms. (See the section on special tests for more details on the quadrant test.)

E. Coracohumeral ligament

The coracohumeral ligament is a broad band that strengthens the superior anterior aspect of the capsule. It runs from the base and lateral border of the coracoid process and passes obliquely downward and laterally to the front of the greater tuberosity, blending with the supraspinatus muscle and the capsule.[62,76] This ligament, along with the superior capsule, acts in the stability of the dependent arm. Because of its anterior orientation to the axis of rotation, it also checks lateral rotation and extension.[59] This could be a factor leading to restriction similar to the capsular pattern of the shoulder.[33,71] If this is the case, perhaps mobilization of this ligament would assist in improving range of motion and in decreasing (certain types of shoulder) pain.

F. Glenohumeral ligaments

These ligaments are closely related to the capsule and attach to the upper and middle part of the medial margin of the glenoid cavity, blending with the labrum.[78] The superior ligament descends and parallels the bicipital tendon, attaching to a small depression above the lesser tuberosity of the humerus and the base of the coracoid process. This ligament may prevent inferior dislocation but is primarily a static stabilizer during the dependent position of the arm. The sulcus sign might imply that the integrity of this ligament could be compromised.

The middle glenohumeral ligament extends from the superior glenohumeral ligament and part of the glenoid rim, attaching to the anterior aspect of the anatomical neck of the humerus lying underneath the tendon of the subscapularis muscle. This ligament limits external rotation in the ranges of 0 to approximately 45 degrees of abduction. As the humerus exceeds that range of abduction, approaching 90 degrees of external rotation, protection is no longer afforded by this ligament.[79] Stability testing, eg, the anterior drawer test from 0 to 45 degrees, will test for the middle glenohumeral ligament, but not at greater ranges of abduction.[80–82]

The inferior glenohumeral ligament is considered the most important static stabilizer and is the thickest of all three ligaments. Attached to the anterior, inferior, and posterior margins of the glenoid labrum and the inferior aspect of the humeral neck is the thickest part of the capsule. This ligament can be divided into two bands, superior and inferior, referred to as the axillary pouch of the inferior glenohumeral ligament. This ligament provides most of the anterior stability of the shoulder in ranges of 45 to 90 degrees of abduction with external rotation.[82] In performing the anterior drawer test, at greater than 45 to 90 degrees of abduction, the inferior glenohumeral ligament would check that motion, providing a firm end-feel.[33,79]

In examining the shoulder, many positions and ranges need to be explored because no one structure is primarily responsible for stability. As summarized by Turkel *et al.,*[80] all three ligaments affect stability at different positions. In the dependent position, the support of the superior glenohumeral and coracohumeral ligaments provides stability. In middle ranges of abduction, the middle glenohumeral ligament and the superior band of the inferior glenohumeral ligament are stabilizers. Upper ranges of abduction are checked by the axillary pouch of the inferior glenohumeral ligament, thus preventing anterior subluxation or dislocation.[79,80] (See the section on special tests for more information about stability tests.)

G. Rotator cuff

The rotator cuff comprises the supraspinatus, infraspinatus, teres minor, and subscapularis muscles. They are referred to as a rotator cuff because they blend with the capsule, acting as dynamic reinforcement. They cause individual as well as component motion of rotation of the humerus in the glenoid. This causes some compression of the humerus into the glenoid, which promotes the dynamic stability necessary for function and skilled activities.[48] Testing for intra-articular pathology may be indicated and, if painful, could implicate the rotator cuff in adding compression to the glenoid. The focus of this section is on the supraspinatus, as this muscle leads to most of the pathologies of the shoulder. The shoulder complex muscles are discussed in the section on biomechanics of the shoulder.

1. Supraspinatus

This muscle has probably had the most written on it in regard to the impingement syndrome and related shoulder pathology. The supraspinatus muscle in the shoulder can be affected by trauma but also undergoes underlying chronic degenerative change leading to tendinopathies and rupture. Tears have been classified as small, moderate, and large. This classification relates to the number of tendons involved, *ie*, the more rotator cuff tendons, the larger the

classification.[83] The anatomy of the cuff has been shown to be a mesh or combining of the tendons as they insert into the capsule and the greater tuberosity of the humerus. Thus, if the tear is small or minor, the supraspinatus is probably the only tendon involved. This may be related to a long chronic history of shoulder symptoms, no trauma, and symptomatic impingement processes.[37,38] When trauma is added to the history of an older patient with some chronic changes, this might implicate more of a moderate to large tear involving the infraspinatus along with the supraspinatus tendon. Also, the amount of external rotation loss would implicate the infraspinatus tendon.[83–86]

Pathological changes of the cuff can be divided into intrinsic and extrinsic factors. Intrinsic factors are those directly related to the tendons themselves. The degenerative nature of the tendon and its diminished blood supply, especially with age, lead to pathological changes. Most tears of the cuff begin on the articular surface; thus, in these cases, other factors are secondary to the primary factor of pathology to the cuff itself.[85]

Extrinsic causes affecting the cuff are the secondary changes from outside the tendon. This would relate to the impingement syndrome involving structures such as the acromion and the coracoacromial arch and allowing enough space for clearance during shoulder elevation. If the space narrows or degenerative changes occur, the rotator cuff bears additional wear, leading to early tendinitis and eventual tears. Also, secondary impingement from glenohumeral instability can cause functional changes in rotator cuff action and result in overuse and additional wear of the tendons.

The cuff plays an important role in stability and function of the shoulder. (This area is discussed further in the section on biomechanics of the shoulder.) Examination of the shoulder by history, palpation, functional movement, and resistive testing can implicate cuff pathology. Special tests, such as magnetic resonance imaging and arthrography, can be confirming and of value if a decision needs to be made concerning operative repair.[30,35,83] With arthroscopic procedures, tendinitis, an area of hyperemia in the tendon's undersurface, can be seen. Degeneration or a partial tear can be diagnosed by fraying and fibrillation of the tendon. Magnetic resonance imaging can relate the size of the cuff tear to atrophy of the muscle. This testing is helpful in a differential diagnosis of a complete or partial-thickness tear of the cuff, tendinitis, or normal tendons. The significance of this testing is that there is a high correlation between the diagnostic testing and cuff pathology.[30] Although diagnostic testing is helpful in determining the severity of the lesion, this testing will not play a major role in treatment if surgical repair is not chosen by the patient. The therapist needs to treat signs and symptoms (the Maitland concept), advancing the rehabilitation program as the patient progresses.[19]

2. Subscapularis tendon

The subscapularis tendon acts as a passive and active stabilizer, although its role decreases with increased abduction. At 0 degrees of abduction, the subscapularis is loose but tightens as the humerus approaches 45 degrees of abduction. The external rotation that accompanies abduction is the reason for the tightening of this muscle. As abduction increases to 90 degrees, the muscle tightens. As more external rotation occurs, the muscle moves superiorly over the humeral head and no longer covers the inferior portion of the humeral head, losing its static role.[60,80]

H. Bicipital tendon sheath

The long head of the biceps arises from the superior glenoid tubercle and crosses the head of the humerus down the bicipital groove. It doubles back on itself to ensheath the tendon. This provides a gliding surface by using the synovial lining of the capsule and decreases stress in its articular course.[59,60] The long head of the biceps tendon is probably related to some lesions affecting the labrum. The biceps plays an important role once pathology is present. It then acts as an elevator as well as control for superior migration of the humeral head.

II. Biomechanics of the Shoulder

The shoulder, with its many different articulations and functional components, links the hand to the trunk. The shoulder is actually a complex of joints working in coordination with each other, producing the largest range of motion in the body. This amount of motion provides great mobility, but at the expense of stability. This section describes the kinematics of the four articulations of the shoulder complex—the glenohumeral, acromioclavicular, sternoclavicular, and scapulothoracic joints—and their significance to the orthopedic examination. Abnormal structure or function might indicate abnormal mechanics and function. The concept of scapulohumeral rhythm is relevant as it relates to normal scapulothoracic range of the shoulder. If shoulder range is abnormal between two joints, the body will compensate and substitute with other joints. Then, abnormal firing patterns and substitution of muscle function occur. The relevance of this is in the ability to evaluate a joint and its related structures passively and dynamically, comparing one side to the other. This is the only true way to identify "normal" for an individual patient.

Shoulder elevation can be defined as movement of the humerus away from the body. The movement can be in any plane of motion. Forward flexion in the sagittal plane, abduction in the frontal plane, or elevation in the scapular plane can be evaluated in their respective planes for smooth, coordinated movement with normal range as compared to that of the contralateral shoulder. Although all movements need to be evaluated, elevation in the scapular plane[54] and in the plane that the patient complains of during the subjective and objective sections of the evaluation needs to be performed. The scapular plane is considered by many authors to be the most functional form of elevation because the glenohumeral capsule inferiorly is not twisted, allowing for the greatest amount of elevation.[47,54] The plane of the scapula lies midway between the frontal and the sagittal planes secured along the thoracic cage. If winging or lateral slide of the scapula were noted during elevation, this would be significant as it relates to the plane of the scapula and glenohumeral motion.[31] A change in scapulohumeral rhythm should be noted at the point in the range when it occurs during the objective evaluation for clinical relevance. Dynamic stability plays a major role in scapulohumeral rhythm and is discussed in detail in the section on scapulothoracic evaluation.

During examination of the shoulder, the passive structures, such as the capsule, glenohumeral ligaments, and labrum, need detailed attention. For example, anatomical studies have demonstrated the influence of the translation of the humeral head in the glenoid during different movements in controlling motion. In flexion movements beyond midrange, the humeral head translated anteriorly. In extension, the humeral head translated posteriorly. Translation was not significant during internal and external rotation movements. Harryman et al.[42] observed that during glenohumeral flexion, anterosuperior translation occurred; during extension and external rotation, the humeral head translated posteriorly; and during internal rotation and horizontal adduction movements, the humeral head underwent anterior translation. The shoulder lock and quadrant tests (see the section on special tests for an explanation of these tests) could be of value in determining which part of the passive structures could be implicated as possible sources of pathology.[87,88] On cadaver dissection, Slade[88] found that parts of the capsule were lax or taut during different degrees of abduction. Between 105 and 120 degrees, the humeral head bulged anteriorly, which might be of clinical significance if the capsule is especially taut during the quadrant test.[88] This test could then be used as treatment for the offending structure. Following the Maitland concept, examination techniques can be incorporated into the treatment techniques or plan.

A. Scapulohumeral rhythm

The scapulothoracic joint works in conjunction with glenohumeral movement. The humerus moving on the glenoid fossa in relation to the scapula's position on the thoracic cage is significant to how the dynamic stabilizers will function for coordinated movement. There has been much discussion as to how much scapular-to-humeral movement exists during elevation. Poppen and Walker[52] found, overall, a 2:1 ratio of glenohumeral motion to scapulothoracic motion. During the initial phase of elevation, 30 to 60 degrees, the scapula attempts to set itself for stability during humeral motion.[89] This scapulohumeral rhythm is primarily dependent on the sternoclavicular and acromioclavicular joints. A "force couple" de-

velops between the trapezius and serratus anterior muscles, upwardly rotating the scapula.[48]

The following is the sequence of events, as described by Norkin and Levangie,[48] that occurs during elevation of the shoulder:

1. **Phase one.** The upper and lower portions of the trapezius muscles force couple with the upper and lower portions of the serratus anterior muscles, producing an upward rotational force on the scapula. As this movement continues, force is placed on the clavicle, producing elevation to approximately 90 to 100 degrees. The scapula maintains contact with the rib cage because of checking of the coracoclavicular ligaments.

2. **Phase two.** The trapezius and serratus muscles continue to pull, generating an upward rotational force on the scapula. Rotation is taken up by the clavicle, which is rotational around its axis. This rotation is possible because of the freedom of the sternoclavicular and acromioclavicular joints to move in an unrestricted manner. Inman et al.[89] found that total clavicular elevation at the acromioclavicular joint was 20 degrees, occurring in the first 30 and the last 45 degrees of shoulder elevation. At the sternoclavicular joint, range of elevation was approximately 40 degrees, occurring in the first 90 degrees of elevation. Reciprocal motion at the acromioclavicular joint will affect the sternoclavicular joint. Clinically, this would make it necessary to clear both joints to rule them out as sources of pathology.[56]

B. Rotator cuff

The supraspinatus, infraspinatus, teres minor, and subscapularis muscles, also known as the rotator cuff, contribute significantly to dynamic stability of the glenohumeral joint. The rotator cuff not only provides a rotational force at the humerus, it also adds compression to the glenoid fossa and results in stability (see Figure 30–8). The cuff offsets the translational pull of the deltoid muscle, reducing shear forces during elevation of the humerus. Actually, there is a force couple that develops between the deltoid muscle and the combined action of the infraspinatus, teres minor, and subscapularis muscles. This force couple produces pure rotation within its instantaneous axis of rotation if dynamically stable.[48,52] If one notes that the supraspinatus is not as strongly involved in this

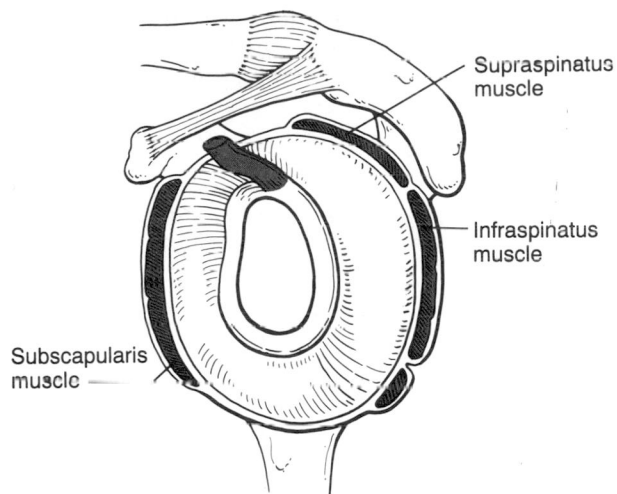

FIGURE 30–8 Glenoid surrounded by the rotator cuff and capsule.

C. Scapula stabilizers

There are two force couples present in the shoulder: the upper trapezius and upper serratus anterior muscles and the lower trapezius and lower serratus anterior muscles. The upper force couple elevates the arm with upward rotation of the scapula. The lower force couple acts as a synergist, controlling winging and allowing for the distal segment of the scapula to remain in contact with the thoracic cage (see Figure 30–9). The trapezius is more critical for abduction, and the serratus functions more in flexion. Both muscles act as stabilizers for the deltoid, allowing the arm to elevate on the scapula, the fixed segment. Along these same lines, the middle trapezius and rhomboid muscles are critical to stabilizing the scapula through eccentric control.[48] The latissimus dorsi and pectoral muscles, by attachment to the humerus, will fix the scapula to the thoracic cage, providing stability for arm movement. Actions such as shoulder depression, especially if the hands are fixed in weight bearing, will assist greatly in scapula stability.[48,59]

D. Clinical relevance

If therapists give home exercise programs to increase muscular strength and to decrease pain and dysfunction, it is imperative to evaluate which muscles are functioning and, more

stability, more attention must be paid to the other cuff muscles. The supraspinatus provides dynamic stability but can also function as a primary abductor, a major problem with overhead activities and impingement of the shoulder.

The infraspinatus and teres minor muscles are important, in addition to their stabilizing function, for providing external rotation of the humerus and thereby clearing the greater tuberosity from butting up against the acromion and decreasing the chance of impingement. The clinical significance of this is in patients with "painful arcs" and impingement. The supraspinatus may be the primary structure being impinged. The subscapularis provides the same function of dynamic stability as the infraspinatus and teres minor muscles but also has a very important function for preventing anterior shoulder dislocation by medially rotating the humeral elevation. Performing special tests for anterior stability is static in nature. To evaluate the dynamic stability, the therapist needs to observe the joint for smooth, coordinated muscular function.

The deltoid muscle, although not part of the cuff, acts as the counterbalance by increasing joint compression force and helping with stabilization dynamically. Deltoid weakness is rarely a problem, unless possibly with nerve involvement, abnormal firing pattern leading to early humeral head elevation, and impingement.

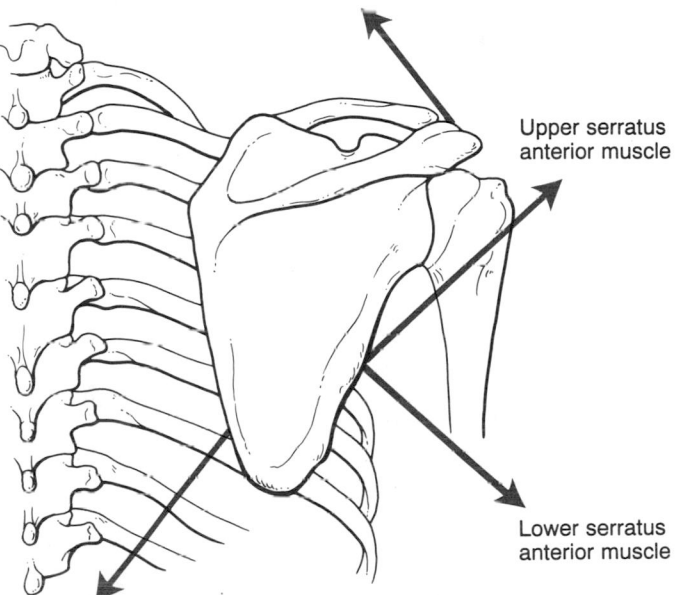

FIGURE 30–9 Force couple of the scapula.

important, their normal timing and firing patterns.[90] This process of evaluation is not static but dynamic, as is the exercise program. The exercises need to be directly related to what is or is not functioning for the patient. Scapula dynamic stability is pivotal if success is to be obtained in patients demonstrating glenohumeral instability and impingement problems.[50] The scapulothoracic evaluation sections on evaluating muscle passively and actively, treatment, and home exercise programs address these issues.

III. Subjective Examination

The primary objective of the subjective examination is to ascertain the disorder involved, *ie*, pain, stiffness, weakness, or loss of function. From this information, the severity, irritability, nature, stability, and stage (SINS) of the problem can be determined as well as how the patient is affected by the disorder in his/her occupation. Handedness can be important in determining whether the patient can work and function in the activities of daily living. The concerns of the patient as they relate to precautions and contraindications to certain procedures and possibly to referral to a specialist, can be highlighted in a special questions section.[90,91] The subjective examination is the key to these determinations and much more. The reader is referred to Chapter 29 for greater detail on the content of the subjective examination.

A. Body chart

The body chart, a symptomatic representation of a patient's complaints, is considered to be one of the most important elements of the subjective examination and will guide both the subjective and the objective examinations.

1. The chart shows possible structure(s) involved that can be inferred as the pathological source of pain or symptoms. The chart is used to document for analysis
   a. Type and severity of the pain or symptoms.
   b. Depth of the pain or symptoms.
   c. Constancy of the pain or symptoms.
   d. Relationships of the pain or symptoms (are one or more structures involved?).

■ PLEASE NOTE: Figures 30–10 to 30–19 are body charts illustrating various areas (1 to 10) of pain and symptoms. Below, possible structures in each area that may be implicated in the pain or symptoms are listed along with the procedures that the therapist can perform to determine the involvement of the structure in the provocation of the pain or symptoms.[92–94]

2. **Sites of shoulder pain for differentiation**
   a. *Area 1* (see Figure 30–10)
      (1). *Sternoclavicular joint/first rib.* The shoulder should be placed in the pain-provoking position and accessory movements performed on the sternoclavicular joint and the 1st rib. If symptoms change, this joint may be the source of the patient's complaint.
      (2). *C3 Vertebral segmental referral.* Physiological movements of the cervical spine should be performed in stretch or compressed positions that reproduce the pain or local neck

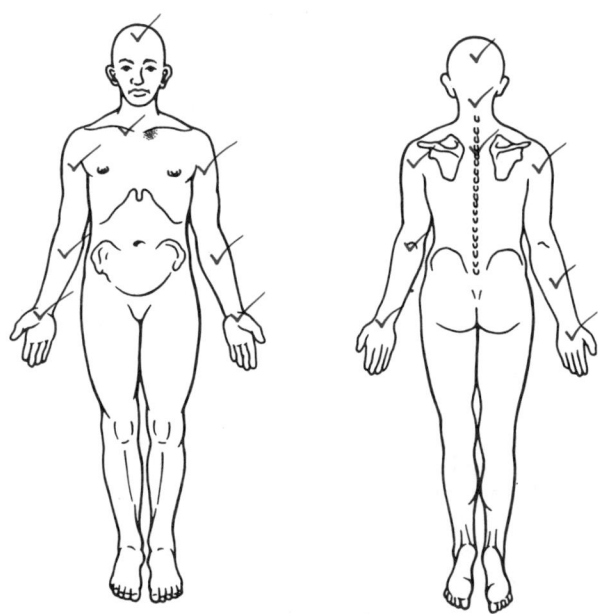

FIGURE 30–10   Body chart of area 1.

pain. Passive accessory intervertebral testing of the C3–C4 vertebral level might be implicated in hypomobility of the ipsilateral joint.

(3). *Soft-tissue structures* (*eg*, sternocleidomastoid muscle). Any attachment of soft tissue can be implicated by resisted testing for muscular tissue. Stretching can implicate inert tissues as well as muscular tissue. Palpation can assist in localizing subtle differences of thickening, tenderness, or tightness.

(4). *First sternocostal articulation*. Passive accessory motion of the 1st rib should be performed, reproducing signs and symptoms. The rib should be palpated for thickening, tenderness, or, most important, hypomobility as compared to the other side.

b. *Area 2* (see Figure 30–11)

(1). *Acromioclavicular joint*. The shoulder should be placed in the pain-provoking position and accessory movements of the acromioclavicular joint performed. If symptoms change, this may be the source of the patient's complaint. Compression should be added to the maneuver, and palpation repeated. The joint should be palpated for thickening, tenderness, or abnormal mobility.

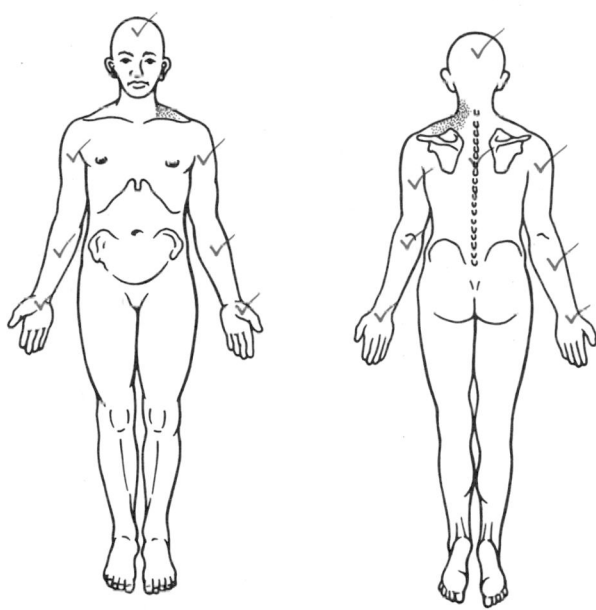

FIGURE 30–12   Body chart of area 3.

(2). *C3–C4 Vertebral segmental referral*. Physiological movements of the cervical spine should be performed in stretch or compressed positions that reproduce the pain or local neck pain. Passive intervertebral testing of the C3–C4 and C4–C5 vertebral levels might be implicated with hypomobility of the ipsilateral joint(s).

(3). *Soft-tissue structures* (*eg*, deltoid muscle). Any attachment of soft tissue can be implicated by muscle testing for inert versus contractile structures. Stretching can implicate inert tissues as well as muscular tissue. Palpation can assist in localizing subtle differences of thickening, tenderness, or tightness.

c. *Area 3* (see Figure 30–12)

(1). *Soft-tissue structures* (*eg*, levator scapula, trapezius, or supraspinatus). Any attachment of soft tissue can be implicated by resisted testing for muscular tissue. Stretching can implicate inert tissues as well as muscular tissue. Palpation can assist in localizing subtle differences of thickening, tenderness, or tightness.

(2). *C3–C6 Vertebral segmental referral*. Physiological movements of the cervical spine should be performed in

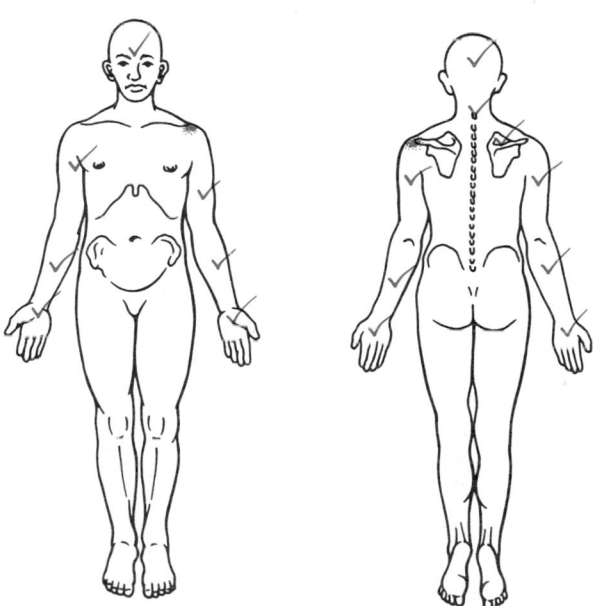

FIGURE 30–11   Body chart of area 2.

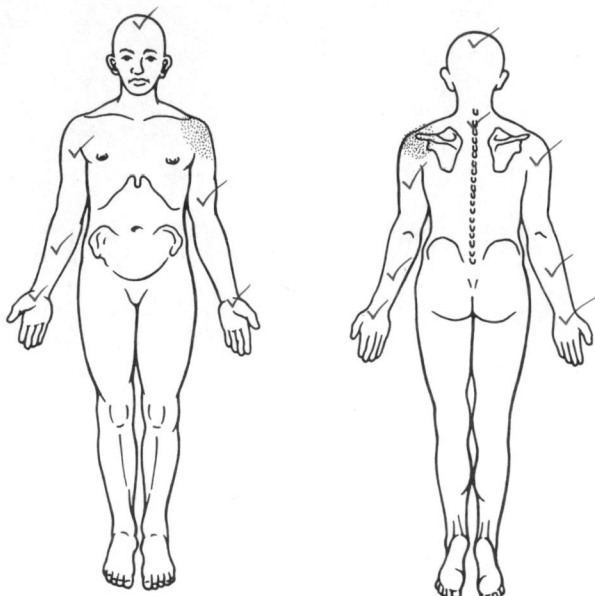

FIGURE 30–13   Body chart of area 4.

stretch or compressed positions that reproduce the pain or local neck pain. Passive intervertebral testing of the C3–C4, C4–C5, and C5–C6 vertebral levels might be implicated with hypomobility of the ipsilateral joint(s). Also, there may be referred discogenic pain, as described by Cloward.[95]

d. **Area 4** (see Figure 30–13)

(1). *Glenohumeral joint.* The shoulder should be placed in the pain-provoking position and accessory movements performed on the glenohumeral joint. If symptoms change, this may be the source of the patient's pain or symptoms. The joint should be compressed or distracted while performing this maneuver to determine whether an intra-articular or a periarticular structure is the source of the condition.

(2). *Subacromial joint.* The shoulder should be placed in the pain-provoking position and accessory movements of the subacromial joint area performed. If symptoms change, this may be the source of the patient's complaint. The joint should be compressed or distracted while performing this maneuver to determine

whether an intra-articular, a periarticular, or a soft-tissue structure (*eg,* cuff or bursa) is the origin.

(3). *C4–C6 Vertebral segmental referral.* Physiological movements of the cervical spine should be performed in stretch or compressed positions that reproduce the shoulder symptoms or local neck pain. Passive accessory intervertebral testing of the C4–C5 and C5–C6 vertebral levels might be implicated with hypomobility of the ipsilateral joint(s). This level needs to be compared with the area of pain.

(4). *Adverse neural tension.* The shoulder should be placed in the pain-provoking position and the position changed by performing one of the following: shoulder depression; elbow extension; wrist, thumb, and finger extension; or side flexion of the head away from the affected shoulder. Any changes in signs or symptoms, as compared with the other side, can implicate a structure as dysfunctional.[96]

e. **Area 5** (see Figure 30–14)

(1). *Glenohumeral joint.* See Area 4.

(2). *Subacromial joint.* See Area 4.

f. **Area 6** (see Figure 30–15)

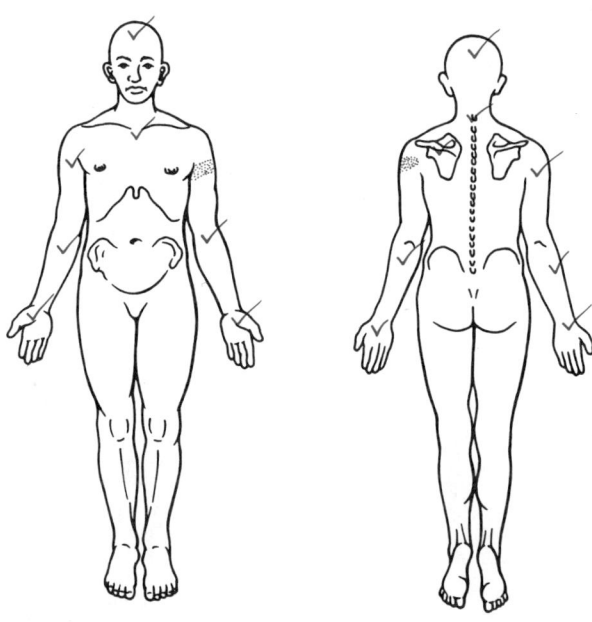

FIGURE 30–14   Body chart of area 5.

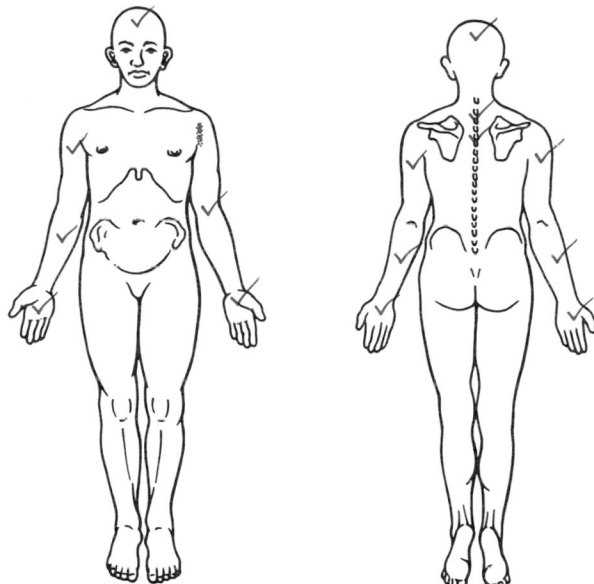

FIGURE 30–15   Body chart of area 6.

(1). *Soft-tissue structures* (*eg*, biceps). Any attachment of soft tissue can be implicated by resisted testing for muscular tissue. Stretching can implicate inert tissues as well as muscular tissue. Palpation can assist in localizing subtle differences of thickening, tenderness, or tightness.

    (2). *Glenohumeral joint.* See Area 4.
    (3). *Subacromial joint.* See Area 4.
g. **Area 7** (see Figure 30–16)
    (1). *Soft-tissue structures* (*eg*, subscapularis). Any attachment of soft tissue can be implicated by resisted testing for muscular tissue. Stretching can implicate inert tissues as well as muscular tissue. Palpation can assist in localizing subtle differences of thickening, tenderness, or tightness.
    (2). *T1–T2 Vertebral segmental referral.* Physiological movements of the lower cervical spine should be performed in stretch or compressed positions that reproduce the pain or local neck pain. Passive accessory intervertebral testing of the C7 to T1 and T1–T2 vertebral levels might be implicated with hypomobility of the ipsilateral joint(s). This level needs to be comparable with the area of pain.
h. **Area 8** (see Figure 30–17)
    (1). *Soft-tissue structures* (*eg*, infraspinatus). Any attachment of soft tissue can be implicated by resisted testing for muscular tissue. Stretching can implicate inert tissues as well as muscular tissue. Palpation can assist in localizing subtle differences of thickening, tenderness, or tightness.

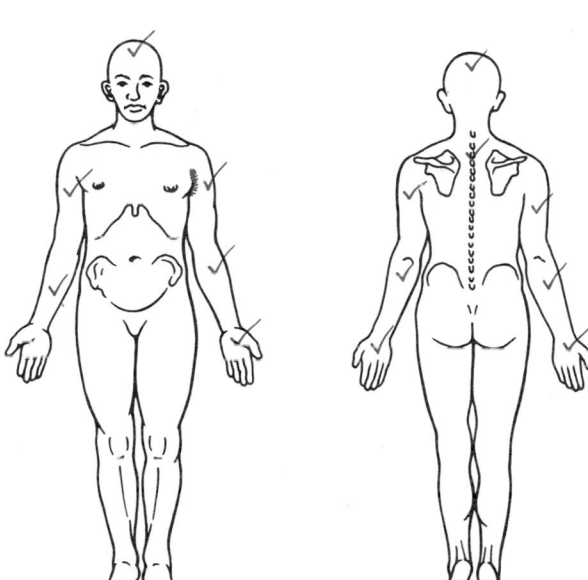

FIGURE 30–16   Body chart of area 7.

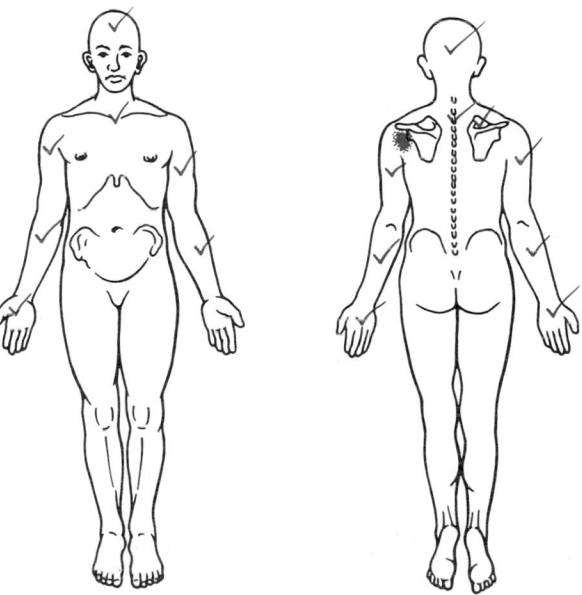

FIGURE 30–17   Body chart of area 8.

(2). *C6–C8 Vertebral segmental referral.* Physiological movements of the lower cervical spine should be performed in stretch or compressed positions that reproduce the pain or local neck pain. Passive accessory intervertebral testing of the C5–C6, C6–C7, and C7 to T1 vertebral levels might be implicated with hypomobility of the ipsilateral joint(s). This level needs to be comparable with the area of pain.

i. *Area 9* (see Figure 30–18)

(1). *Glenohumeral joint.* See Area 4.

(2). *Subacromial joint.* See Area 4.

(3). *C5–C6 Vertebral segmental referral.* Physiological movements of the mid/lower cervical spine are performed in stretch or compressed positions that reproduce the pain or local neck pain. Passive accessory intervertebral testing of the C5–C6 and C6–C7 vertebral levels might be implicated with hypomobility of the ipsilateral joint(s). This level needs to be comparable with the area of pain. Look for noncapsular patterns; *ie,* shoulder flexion and abduction are limited secondary to pain, but lateral rotation and hand behind back are nearly full range.[1,67]

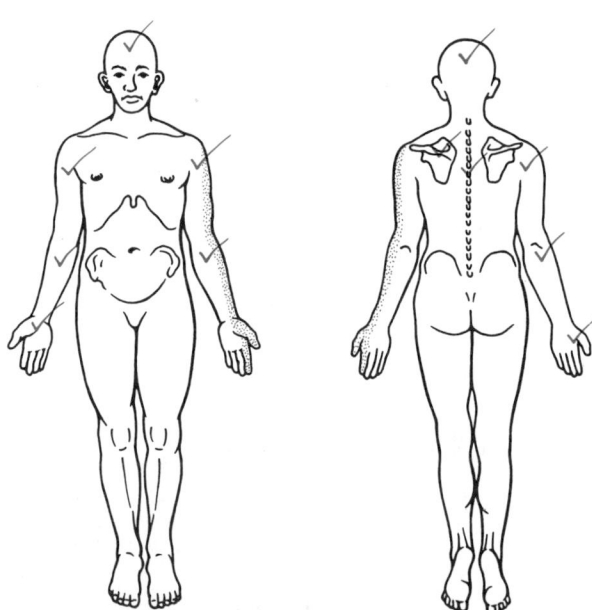

FIGURE 30–18   Body chart of area 9.

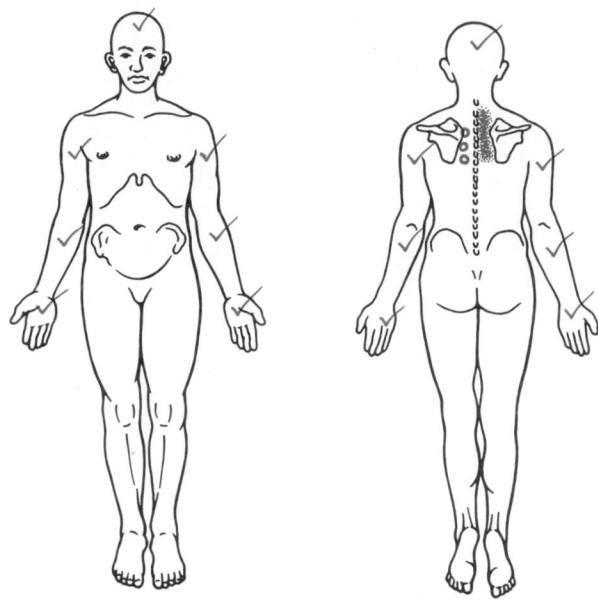

FIGURE 30–19   Body chart of area 10.

(4). *C5–C6 Nerve root pain.* The therapist should look for neurological differences as compared with the other side. The therapist checks myotomes for strength, checks dermatomes for sensation, and checks for diminished reflexes.

(5). *Adverse neural tension.* The shoulder should be placed in the pain-provoking position and the position changed to one of the following: shoulder depression; elbow extension; wrist, thumb, and finger extension; or side flexion of the head away from the affected shoulder. Any changes in signs or symptoms, as compared with the other side, can implicate a structure as dysfunctional. Mechanical tension is stressed on nerve roots C5–C7 and/or the brachial plexus.[96]

j. *Area 10* (see Figure 30–19)

(1). *Soft-tissue structures* (*eg,* rhomboids). Any attachment of soft tissue can be implicated by resisted testing for muscular tissue. Stretching can implicate inert tissues as well as muscular tissue. Palpation can assist in localizing subtle differences of thickening, tenderness, or tightness.

(2). *C6 to T5 Vertebral segmental referral.* Physiological movements of the lower cervical and thoracic areas of the spine should be performed in stretch or compressed positions that reproduce the pain or local neck pain. Passive accessory intervertebral testing of C6–C7 to T4–T5 vertebral levels might be implicated with hypomobility of the ipsilateral joint(s). This level needs to be comparable with the area of pain.

(3). *C3–C7 Discogenic referral.* Mid/lower cervical extension of cervical spine can cause irritation in an inflamed disk and cause referred pain into the interscapular area.[95]

B. Behavior of symptoms[91–94]

1. **Aggravating factors.** These are the mechanical movements or positions that elicit pain or dysfunction. Below are listed specific aggravating factors and the physiological and accessory movements that might be related that would be examined by the therapist.
   a. Reaching into forward elevation as in placing an object on a shelf.
      (1). Physiological movements of the glenohumeral joint:
         (a). Flexion.
         (b). Abduction.
         (c). External rotation.
      (2). Accessory movements of the glenohumeral joint:
         (a). Anterior/posterior pressures.
         (b). Posterior/anterior pressures.
         (c). Caudal glides.
   b. Hand behind back as in tucking in a shirt or reaching for a wallet.
      (1). Physiological movements of the glenohumeral joint:
         (a). Hand behind back (combination of extension/internal rotation).
         (b). Internal rotation.
         (c). Forward flexion.
      (2). Accessory movements of the glenohumeral joint:
         (a). Anterior/posterior pressures.
         (b). Lateral glides.
         (c). Caudal glides.
   c. Reaching across the chest as in reaching for a seat belt.
      (1). Physiological movement of the glenohumeral joint:
         (a). Horizontal flexion.

         (b). Internal rotation.
         (c). Forward flexion.
      (2). Accessory movements of the glenohumeral joint:
         (a). Anterior/posterior pressures.
         (b). Lateral glides.
         (c). Caudal glides.
      (3). Accessory movements of the acromioclavicular joint:
         (a). Anterior/posterior pressures.
         (b). Posterior/anterior pressures.
         (c). Caudal glides.
   d. Performing simultaneous abduction and external rotation as in pitching a baseball.
      (1). Physiological movement of the glenohumeral joint:
         (a). Abduction.
         (b). External rotation.
         (c). Flexion.
         (d). Shoulder quadrant (see the section on special tests).
      (2). Accessory movements of the glenohumeral joint:
         (a). Anterior/posterior pressures.
         (b). Posterior/anterior pressures.
         (c). Caudal glides.
      (3). Testing for shoulder stability (see the section on special tests):
         (a). Anterior drawer.
         (b). Posterior drawer.
         (c). Inferior glide.

PLEASE NOTE: All accessory movements should be performed in the physiological position that is most comparable to the signs and symptoms that are elicited.

2. **Easing factors.** These are the movements or positions that might decrease signs or symptoms, indicating a pathophysiological condition. Below are listed possible positions that the therapist can use to ease symptoms or can suggest to the patient for self-treatment.
   a. Supporting arm across chest.
      (1). Treat in position of ease with accessory movement of glenohumeral joint short of pain:
         (a). Posterior/anterior pressures.
         (b). Caudal glide.
      (2). Treatment modality (see the section on treatment):
         (a). Ice.
         (b). Electrostimulation.
         (c). Ultrasound.

(d). Sling or tape for support.
(e). Medication (preferably nonster-oidal anti-inflammatory drugs).

3. **24-Hour behavior**
   a. *Morning*
      (1). Pain/stiffness:
         (a). Duration greater than 30 min-utes. (Think possibly inflamma-tory.)
         (b). Duration less than 30 minutes. (Think arthritic condition.)
   b. *Night*
      (1). Can patient sleep on shoulder? (Think compressive structures, *ie*, intra-articular structures.)
      (2). Shoulder hanging in a dependent position awakens patient. (Think periarticular structures.)
      (3). Constant pain much worse at night. (Think serious pathology, *eg*, cancer, Pancoast's tumor.)
      (4). Patient awakens with tingling in hands during sleep hours. (Think neural tension or thoracic outlet pa-thology.)
   c. *Day*
      (1). Morning worse than afternoon. (Think inflammatory.)
      (2). Afternoon worse than morning. (Think overuse, postural, etc.)
      (3). Time of day not a factor. (Think more activity specific.)

4. **History.** The following scenarios necessitate examination of specific structures.
   a. Sudden insidious onset without trauma:
      (1). Capsule.
      (2). Glenohumeral joint.
      (3). Cervical spine.
   b. Sudden onset with trauma:
      (1). Capsule/labrum/ligaments.
      (2). Rotator cuff.
   c. Gradual onset:
      (1). Overuse, *eg*, rotator cuff.
      (2). Degenerative pathology.
      (3). Glenohumeral joint.
      (4). Other related structures.

5. **Past history**[71]
   a. Shoulder versus contralateral shoulder.
   b. Past treatment and its effect.
   c. Past trauma or dislocations.

6. **Special questions**[91,92]
   a. *General health:*
      (1). Current or past history of cancer.
      (2). Diabetes.[96]
      (3). Surgeries that required arm in ab-ducted and externally rotated posi-tion.
   b. *Weight:*[91,99]
      (1). Loss/gain from serious pathology.
   c. *Steroids:*
      (1). Past injections to shoulder.
         (a). How many?
         (b). Where?
         (c). Pain relief?
   d. *Special tests:*[29-32]
      (1). Arthrography.
      (2). Magnetic nuclear imaging.
      (3). Radiography.
   e. Other relevant questions as stated in Chapter 29.

IV. Objective Composite Examination

The objective composite examination is a com-prehensive examination of the patient who is con-sidered to be nonirritable to mildly irritable. Also included is the patient who on subjective examina-tion indicates pain(s) or symptom(s) that might be difficult to reproduce with simple procedures. The therapist conducts the examination taking into consideration factors such as severity, irritability, nature, stability and stage of the disorder (SINS). Directions are given to the patient before any movement is actually performed.

Therapist's responsibilities:

• Establish baseline symptoms before performing the movement.
• Note where the symptoms are reproduced in the range and whether they subside once out of that position.
• Are the symptoms of the same type and quality as those originally stated?
• Do the symptoms abate before performing the next movement?

Please see Chapter 29 for more detail about these examination principles and planning the objective examination.

A. Standing

1. **Observation**
   a. Muscle atrophy (neurologically related vs because of pain and disuse).
   b. Hypertrophy (substitution patterns or dominant hand).
   c. Structural deformities (*eg*, hooked acromion[65,66] or uneven acromioclavicular joint due to separation).
   d. Abnormal movement patterns (observe during undressing).
   e. Scapular positioning on thoracic cage.[50,98]

2. **Shoulder: active physiological movements.** The baseline for pain and/or symptoms must be established. Where in the range are the symptoms reproduced? If reproduced, are they of the same type and quality as described? Correct for deviation of movement during the test and note whether the response is different with correction. If correction does not affect pain or symptoms, the deviation may not be related to the condition. Overpressure needs to be applied and compared to the contralateral shoulder for pain, range, and end-feel responses. If different, this should be noted and reassessed after treatment for possible changes.
   a. Functional movement, *ie*, the movement that reproduces the patient's complaint.
   b. Flexion.
   c. Abduction.
   d. External rotation.
   e. Horizontal flexion.
   f. Hand behind back.

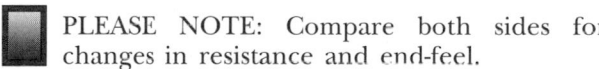 PLEASE NOTE: The therapist may need to modify movement by changing the direction, speed, or number of repetitions of the movement to reproduce the patient's complaints or symptoms.

3. **Rotator cuff resistive tests.** These tests should be performed with a slow buildup in resistance during contraction. The therapist looks for the quality of the contraction and possible substitution of other muscles. Scapula elevation is a common substitution in a painful or weak rotator cuff.
   a. Abduction.
   b. External rotation.
   c. Internal rotation.
   d. Elbow flexion.

B. Sitting

1. **Shoulder palpation.** Both sides must be compared for tenderness. The therapist looks for swelling, discoloration, warmth, or thickened areas.
   a. Acromion (hooked acromion increases propensity for cuff pathology).[65,66]
   b. Bursa.[1]
   c. Supraspinatus.[1]
   d. Biceps.[1]
   e. Infraspinatus.[1]
   f. Rib[1] (important to rule out thoracic outlet types of complaints[91,97]).

2. **Cervical spine clearing test.** Determine whether there is cervical spine involvement.[19]
   a. Rotation left and right.
   b. Extension.
   c. Lower cervical quadrant.

3. See Chapter 29 for more details on these movements.

C. Supine

1. **Neurological examination** (see Chapter 29)

2. **Passive physiological movements[5]**
   a. Flexion.
   b. Abduction.
   c. External rotation.
   d. Internal rotation.
   e. Horizontal flexion.

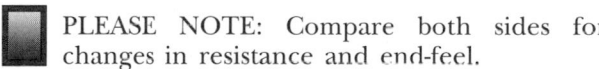 PLEASE NOTE: Compare both sides for changes in resistance and end-feel.

3. **Special tests**[2,5,27,35–41,50,57,58,80,87,89,93,94,101–103]
   a. Instability tests:
      (1). Anterior drawer.
      (2). Posterior drawer.
      (3). Inferior glide.
      (4). Jobe three-part relocation.
   b. Lock test
   c. Shoulder quadrant test
   d. Differentiation tests:
      (1). Glenohumeral structures:
         (a). Intra-articular.
         (b). Periarticular.

(2). Subacromial structures:
   (a). Contractile.
   (b). Intra-articular.
   (c). Inert.
e. Neural tension tests:
   (1). Upper limb tension test (see Chapter 29).

4. Shoulder: passive accessory movements
a. *Glenohumeral joint*
   (1). Neutral:
      (a). Anterior/posterior pressures.
      (b). Posterior/anterior pressures.
      (c). Caudal glide.
      (d). Lateral glide.
   (2). In shoulder flexion:
      (a). Anterior/posterior pressures.
      (b). Posterior/anterior pressures.
      (c). Caudal glide.
   (3). In abduction:
      (a). Anterior/posterior pressures.
      (b). Posterior/anterior pressures.
      (c). Caudal glide.
   (4). In horizontal flexion:
      (a). Posterior/anterior pressures.
      (b). Caudal glide.
      (c). Lateral glide.
b. *First rib*
   (1). Caudal glide.
c. *Cervical spine palpation*
   (1). Anterior/posterior unilateral pressures.[19,75]

D. Prone

1. Shoulder: passive accessory movements
a. *Glenohumeral joint*
   (1). In hand behind back:
      (a). Performed on the scapula.
         (i). Posterior/anterior pressures.
         (ii). Lateral glide.

2. Cervicothoracic spine palpation/clearing (see Chapter 29)
a. Central pressure.
b. Unilateral pressure.

E. Sidelying

1. Scapulothoracic joint. Evaluation of the scapulothoracic joint involves proprioceptive neuromuscular facilitation patterns of the scapula (see the section on scapulothoracic evaluation).

a. Muscle length by technique of rhythmical initiation.[90,99–101]
b. Dynamic evaluation of muscle.[90]
   (1). Smooth, coordinated movement.
   (2). Contraction is smooth and strong throughout the range.
   (3). Strength from initiation of the movement to the conclusion of the movement.
c. Scapula patterns:
   (1). Anterior elevation.
   (2). Posterior depression.
   (3). Anterior depression.
   (4). Posterior elevation.

F. Passive physiological movements for the shoulder

It is assumed that all movements are performed from the patient's right side.

1. Flexion (see Figure 30–20)
a. Patient position: supine with glenohumeral joint close to edge.
b. Therapist position:
   (1). Walk-stand.
   (2). Right hand stabilizes patient's scapula in supraspinatus fossa.
   (3). Left hand holds proximal humerus, controlling rotation.
   (4). Humerus taken to available end range dependent on SINS.

2. Abduction (see Figure 30–21)
a. Patient position: supine with glenohumeral joint close to edge.
b. Therapist position:
   (1). Facing patient.
   (2). Left hand stabilizes patient's scapula over acromion process.
   (3). Right hand holds humerus at elbow in neutral rotation.
   (4). Humerus taken to available end range dependent on SINS.

3. External rotation (see Figure 30–22)
a. Patient position: supine with arm abducted to approximately 45 degrees.
b. Therapist position:
   (1). Walk-stand, supporting patient's arm on thigh.
   (2). Right elbow stabilizes patient's scapula over the anterior glenohumeral joint (see Fig. 30–22*B*).
   (3). Left hand holds patient's wrist.
   (4). Patient's wrist taken to available end range dependent on SINS.

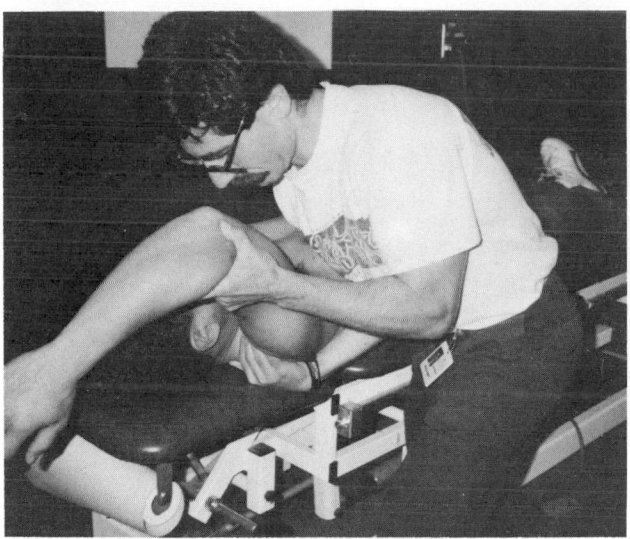

FIGURE 30–20   Passive physiological shoulder flexion.

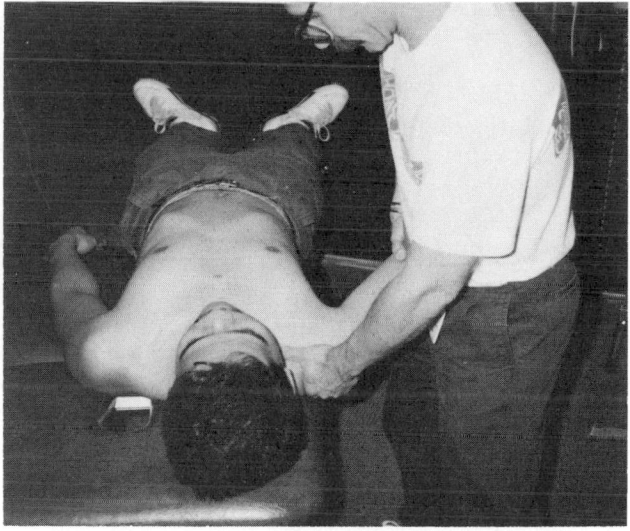

FIGURE 30–21   Passive physiological shoulder abduction.

4. **Internal rotation** (see Figure 30–23)
   a. Patient position: supine with arm abducted to approximately 45 degrees.
   b. Therapist position:

   (1). Walk-stand, facing patient's feet and supporting patient's arm on thigh.
   (2). Left elbow over patient's anterior glenohumeral joint.

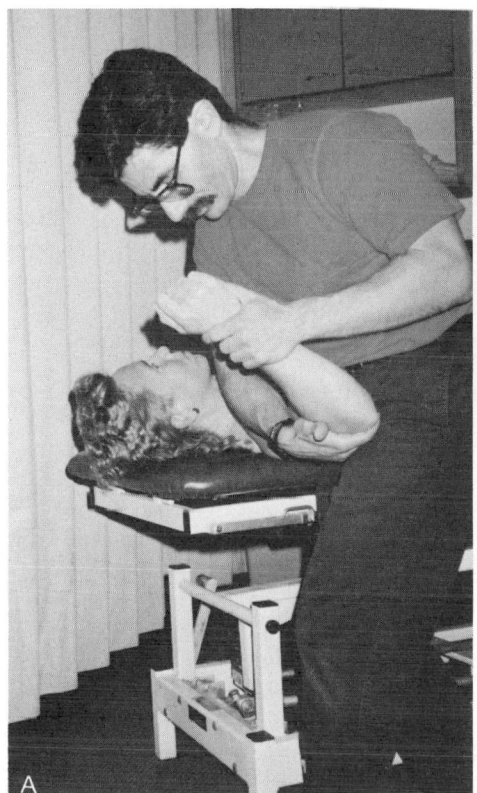

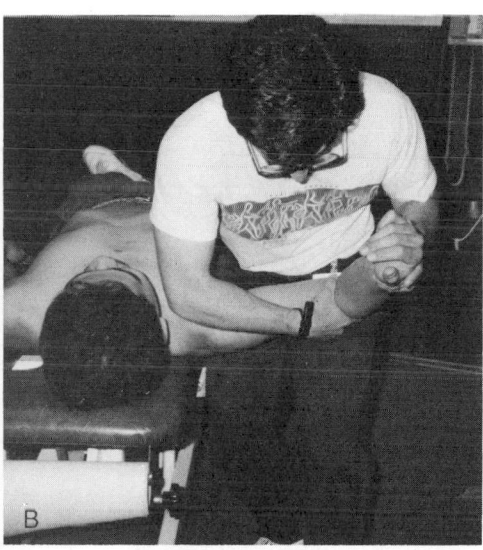

FIGURE 30–22   Passive physiological shoulder external rotation.

(3). Right hand holds patient's wrist.
(4). Patient's wrist taken to available end range dependent on SINS.

5. **Horizontal flexion** (see Figure 30–24)
   a. Patient position:
      (1). Supine with scapula close to edge.
      (2). Arm held at 90 degrees of flexion, 0 degrees adduction, neutral rotation.
   b. Therapist position:
      (1). Facing patient.
      (2). Right hand stabilizes at lateral border of patient's scapula.
      (3). Left hand holds humerus at elbow in neutral rotation.
      (4). Humerus taken to available end range dependent on SINS.

G. Special tests

These tests are done when the therapist needs to differentiate the structure causing the symptoms. For each test, it is assumed that the patient's right shoulder is being evaluated and treated.

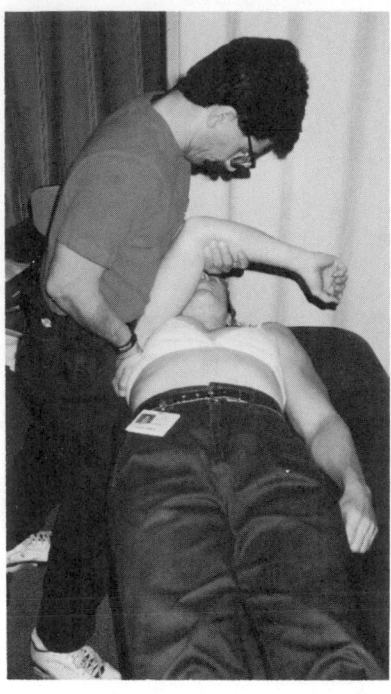

FIGURE 30–24 Passive physiological shoulder horizontal flexion.

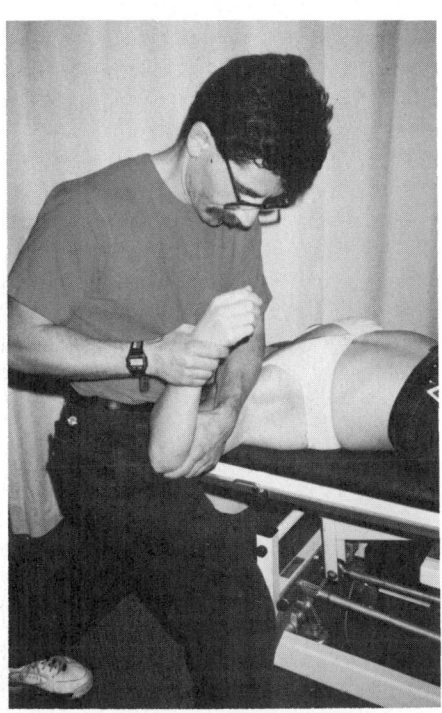

FIGURE 30–23 Passive physiological shoulder internal rotation.

1. **Indications**
   a. Clinical signs minimal.
   b. Momentary catch pain with certain activities.
   c. Normal examination does not reproduce symptoms.
   d. To rule out possibility of instability.

2. **Tests**
   a. Lock test
   b. Quadrant test
   c. Impingement tests
   d. Stability tests:
      (1). Inferior glide.
      (2). Anterior drawer.
      (3). Posterior drawer.
      (4). Jobe three-part relocation.
   e. Differentiation tests

3. **Lock test**[5,87]
   a. *Indications*
      (1). Pain localized to shoulder region.
      (2). Pain or restriction on movement of hand behind back.
      (3). Catch type of pain.

b. *Patient position*
   (1). Supine with right shoulder at edge of table.
   (2). Right shoulder in 45 degrees abduction and 30 degrees medial rotation, and elbow 10 degrees posterior to frontal plane.

c. *Therapist position*
   (1). Standing perpendicular to patient.
   (2). Walk-stand, with outside leg ahead of inside leg.
   (3). Right hand under scapula with fingertips stabilizing trapezius and with thumb on vertebral border of scapula.
   (4). Left hand on patient's left elbow.
   (5). Patient's right hand resting on right shoulder of therapist.

d. *Method*
   (1). *Start position* (see Figure 30–25)
      (a). Above position maintained; assess for resting symptoms.
      (b). Slowly glide patient's elbow forward by weight shift to front leg.
      (c). Note location of onset of resistance and/or pain in available range.
   (2). *End position* (see Figure 30–26)
      (a). Patient's right shoulder in maximal humeral abduction with overpressure.
      (b). Neither patient nor therapist can externally rotate arm while at this end range.

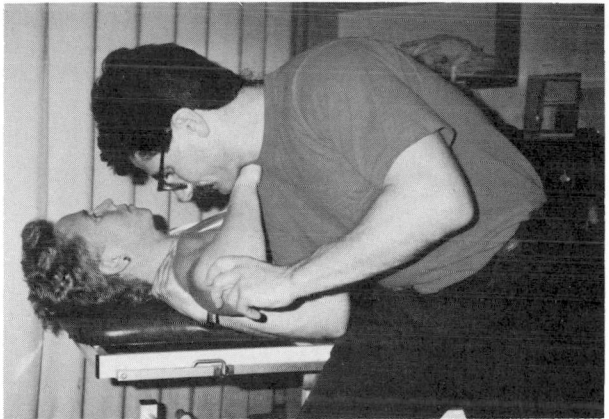

FIGURE 30–26   End position for lock test.

e. *Positive/significant findings*
   (1). Patient's symptoms reproduced.
   (2). Affected shoulder more painful than unaffected shoulder.
   (3). Range of motion restricted as compared to contralateral side.

f. *Treatment*
   (1). Same position as for testing.
   (2). If pain is severe, Grade IV (small oscillatory techniques just into resistance.[15,19]
   (3). Reassess asterisk signs:
      (a). Better: continue with same treatment and reassess.
      (b). Same: increase grade slightly or increase vigor and reassess.
      (c). Worse: continue with same treatment at lesser grade.
   (4). Once technique completed, perform abduction (large amplitude, short of resistance) to ease treatment soreness.

4. **Quadrant test**[5,87,88]
   a. *Indications*
      (1). Pain localized to shoulder region.
      (2). Pain with horizontal flexion and/or extension type of movements.
      (3). Catch type of pain.
      (4). Restricted flexion, abduction, and/or external rotation movements.
   b. *Patient position* (see Figure 30–27)
      (1). Supine with right shoulder at edge of table.
      (2). Right shoulder in abducted position with forearm parallel to floor.

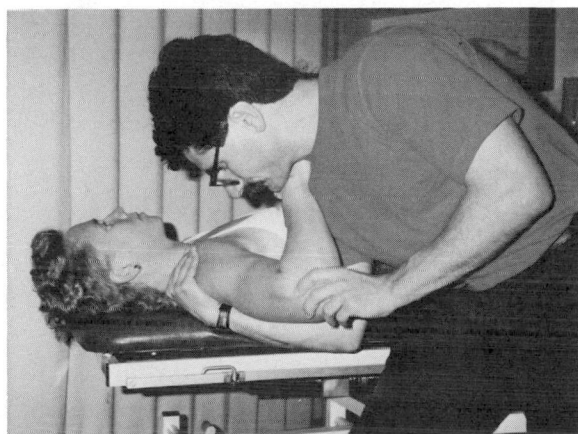

FIGURE 30–25   Start position for lock test.

(3). Right arm in approximately 90 degrees of external rotation (this is considered the "top of the hill" or the "hump").

c. *Therapist position*
(1). Standing perpendicular to patient.
(2). Walk-stand, with outside leg ahead of inside leg.
(3). Right hand under scapula with fingertips stabilizing trapezius and with thumb on vertebral border of scapula.
(4). Left hand on patient's right elbow.

d. *Method*
(1). *Start position*
(a). Assess for resting symptoms.
(b). Slowly glide patient's elbow toward floor in an anteroposterior direction.
(c). Note location of onset of resistance and/or pain in the available range.
(2). *Next position*
(a). Position as above, placing patient's forearm in various degrees of internal and external rotation (see Figures 30–28 and 30–29).
(b). Apply anteroposterior pressure perpendicular to forearm, not the floor.
(c). Each time, note onset of pain and resistance.

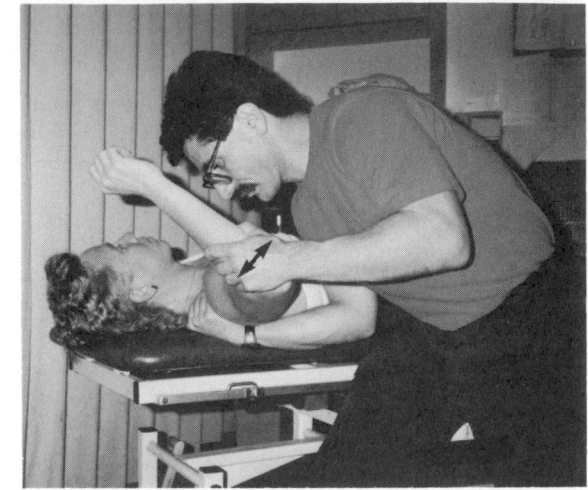

FIGURE 30–28   Assessing right shoulder quadrant below hill.

(d). Compare with opposite or unaffected shoulder.

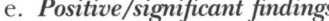 PLEASE NOTE: Release anteroposterior pressure before assessing other positions.

e. *Positive/significant findings*
(1). Patient's symptoms reproduced.
(2). Affected shoulder more painful than unaffected shoulder.
(3). Range of motion restricted compared with opposite side.

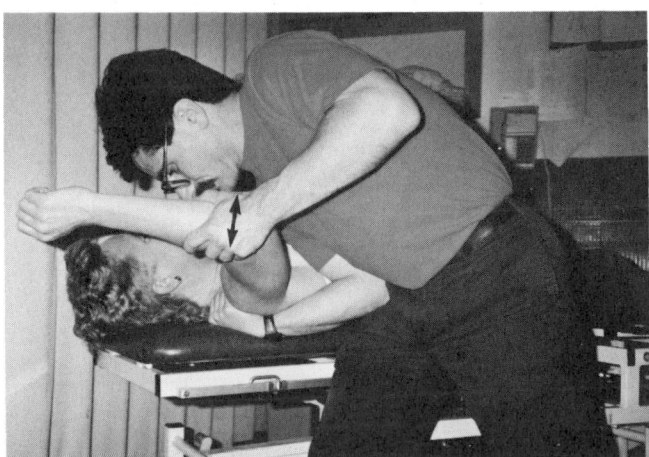

FIGURE 30–27   Assessing right shoulder quadrant at top of hill.

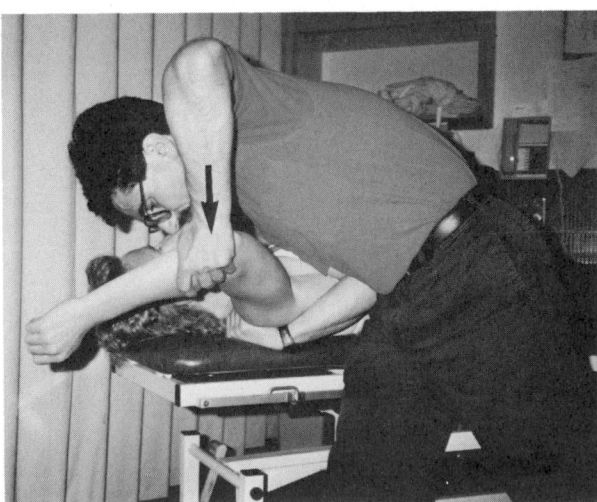

FIGURE 30–29   Assessing right shoulder quadrant above top of hill.

f. *Treatment*
(1). Same position as for testing.
(2). If pain is severe, Grade IV (small oscillatory techniques just into resistance).
(3). Reassess asterisk signs:
   (a). Better: continue with same treatment and reassess.
   (b). Same: increase grade slightly or increase vigor and reassess.
   (c). Worse: continue with same treatment at lesser grade.
(4). Once repetitions of technique completed, perform flexion/abduction (large amplitude, short of resistance) to ease treatment soreness.

5. **Impingement tests 1 and 2**[27,34–41,98,102]
a. *Indications*
(1). Arc of pain or catch pain.
(2). Crepitus.
(3). Weakness as related to muscle or pain, not neurological.
b. *Impingement test 1*
(1). *Patient position* (see Figure 30–30)
   (a). Standing, with right shoulder into flexion/abduction position.
(2). *Therapist position*

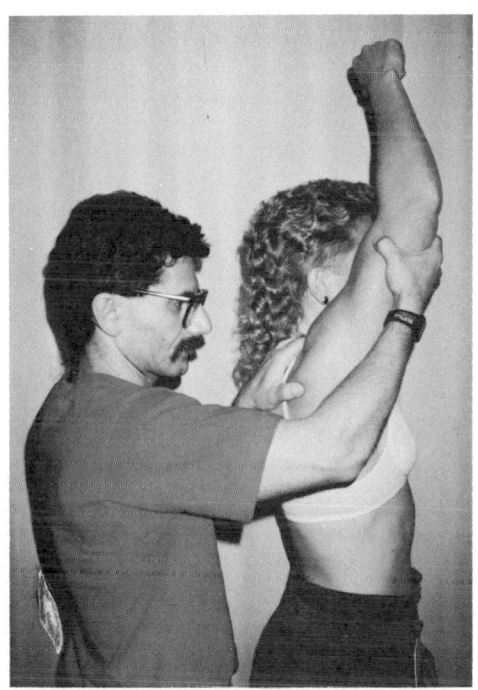

FIGURE 30–30   Impingement test 1.

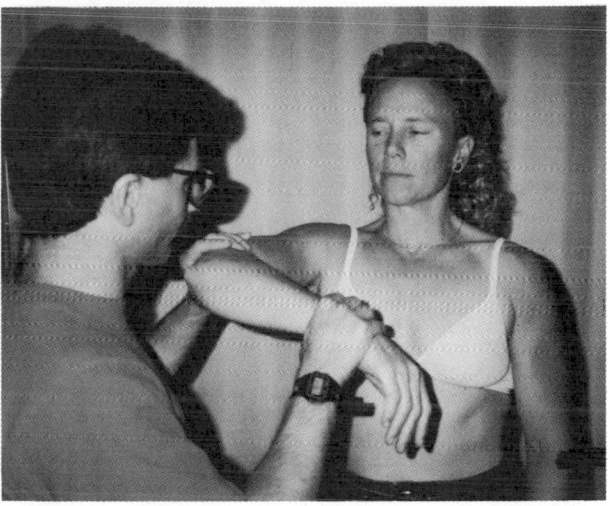

FIGURE 30–31   Impingement test 2.

   (a). Standing parallel to right side of patient.
   (b). Stabilize patient's right scapula with therapist's right hand at joint.
   (c). Therapist's left hand proximal to joint on forearm.
(3). *Method*
   (a). Start position
      (i). As above; patient actively flexes and abducts arm.
      (ii). Apply overpressure to active movement; note response.
      (iii). Note location of onset of resistance and/or pain in available range.
      (iv). Compare with opposite or unaffected shoulder.
c. *Impingement test 2*
(1). *Patient position* (see Figure 30–31)
   (a). Sitting, with right arm in 90 degrees of flexion and 90 degrees medial rotation.
(2). *Therapist position*
   (a). Standing, facing patient.
   (b). Therapist's left hand on patient's right elbow, and right hand on right wrist.
(3). *Method*
   (a). Start position
      (i). As above; patient actively flexes arm to 90 degrees and medially rotates arm.

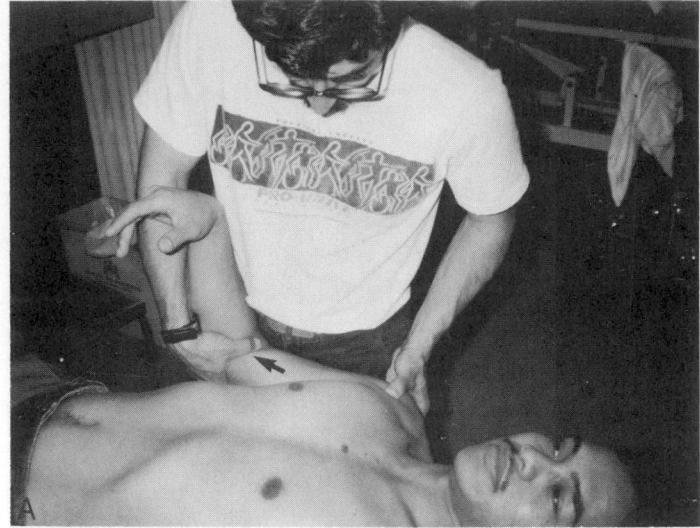
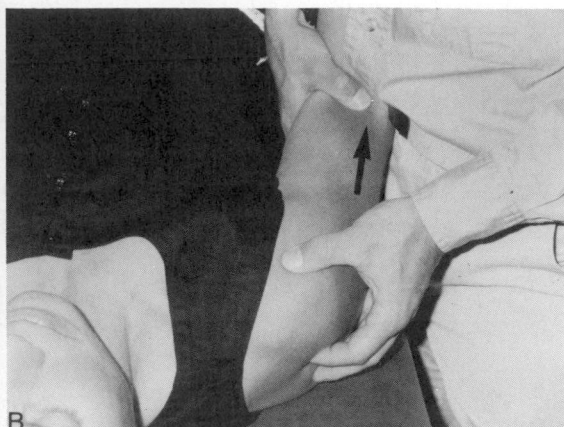

FIGURE 30–32   Inferior glide test.

(ii). Apply overpressure to medial rotation; note response.
(iii). Compare with opposite or unaffected shoulder.
(4). *Positive/significant findings*
    (a). Patient's symptoms reproduced.
    (b). Affected shoulder more painful than unaffected shoulder.
    (c). Range of motion restricted as compared to opposite side.

6. **Stability tests**[83,102,103]
  a. *Indications*
    (1). History of trauma to shoulder.
    (2). Shoulders of athletes, especially those involved in throwing or overhead activities.
    (3). Signs and symptoms of subacromial impingement.
    (4). Younger than 35 years of age.
  b. *Inferior glide test* (see Figure 30–32)
    (1). *Patient position*
      (a). Supine with right shoulder at edge of table.
      (b). Right shoulder at side.
    (2). *Therapist position*
      (a). Standing, facing patient's right shoulder.
      (b). Therapist's left thumb and forefinger palpate anterior acromion and subadjacent humeral

head as right middle finger palpates posterior aspect of subacromial space.
      (c). Patient's elbow and forearm tucked between therapist's right arm and thorax.
      (d). Therapist's right hand cups anteromedial aspect of patient's arm.
    (3). *Method*
      (a). Start position
        (i). Above position is maintained; assess for resting symptoms.
        (ii). Slowly perform longitudinal caudal glide of humerus toward feet until scapula moves.
        (iii). Note location of onset of resistance, end-feel, and/or pain in range.
        (iv). Compare with opposite or unaffected shoulder.
  c. *Anterior drawer test* (see Figure 30–33)
    (1). *Patient position*
      (a). Supine with right shoulder abducted to 70 or 120 degrees.
      (b). Right arm cradled in neutrally rotated position.
    (2). *Therapist position*
      (a). Therapist's right hand cups patient's right shoulder.

(b). Therapist's right thumb pad on patient's coracoid process, and index finger on spine of scapula.

(c). Therapist's left hand grasps midshaft of patient's right humerus.

(3). *Method* (can be done at 70 and 120 degrees of abduction)

(a). Perform a quick flick of patient's right humerus in a posteroanterior direction.

(b). Stabilize scapula with right hand.

d. **Posterior drawer test** (see Figure 30–34)

(1). *Patient position*

(a). Supine.

(b). Right arm in 90 degrees of flexion and 0 degrees of abduction.

(2). *Therapist position*

(a). Facing patient.

(b). Therapist's right hand supports undersurface of patient's right forearm.

(c). Therapist's left thumb pad on anterior surface of humeral head.

(3). *Method*

(a). Perform horizontal flexion and internal rotation with patient's right forearm.

(b). With left thumb, simultaneously perform an anteroposterior

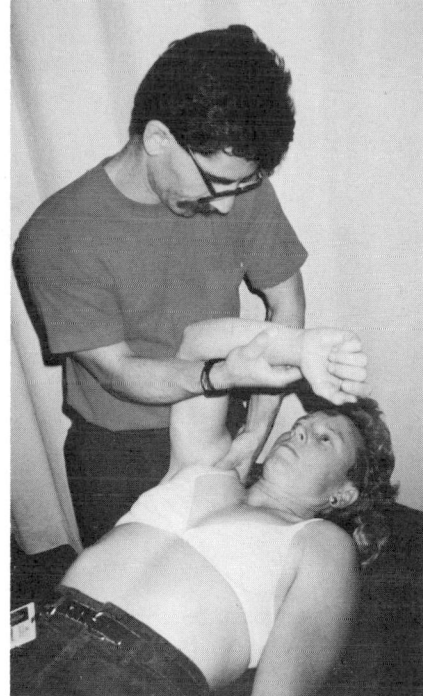

FIGURE 30–34   Posterior drawer test.

pressure through the humeral head.

(4). *Results of test*

(a). Grading of range of movement.

(b). Pain and resistance to movement.

(c). End-feel.

(d). Click or apprehension.

e. **Jobe three-part relocation test**[87]

(1). *Indications*

(a). Similar to above tests for instability.

(b). History of subluxations and not dislocations.

(2). *Patient position*

(a). Supine with right shoulder abducted to 90 degrees, and externally rotate to 90 degrees.

(3). *Therapist position*

(a). Standing, facing patient.

(b). Therapist's abdominal area supports patient's right elbow.

(4). *Method*

(a). Start position

(i). Pain is present in the above position or position of apprehension.

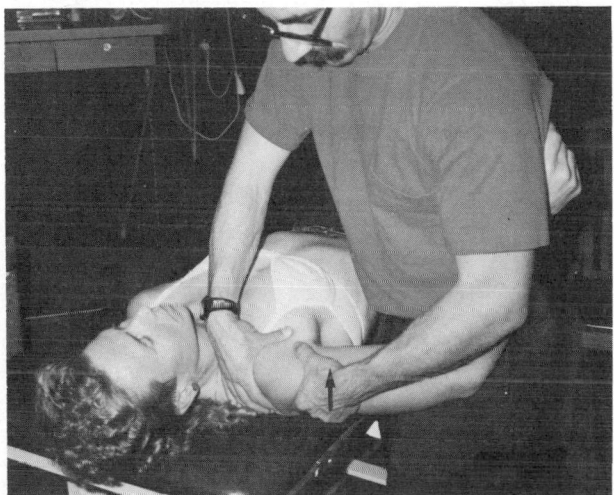

FIGURE 30–33   Anterior drawer test.

(ii). While patient is in this position, perform a posteroanterior pressure on humeral head. What is response?

(iii). While patient is in this position, perform an anteroposterior pressure on humeral head. What is response?

(5). *Positive/significant findings*

(a). Pain or apprehension of shoulder in external rotation/abduction.

(b). Increased pain when a posteroanterior pressure is performed.

(c). Decreased pain when an anteroposterior pressure is performed.

7. **Differentiation tests**[5,92–94]

a. *Indications*

(1). To determine which pathological structure(s) is (are) responsible for signs and symptoms.

(2). To determine appropriate treatment for area and structure related.

b. *Principle.* Find the position or movement to implicate one specific pain-provoking structure. Repeat the same position or movement and alter one structure. The one structure that is altered can be the offending structure and is implicated as the pathological problem. Also, adding compression to a joint can implicate the articular surface of the joint.

c. *Differentiation of intrinsic disorders of rotator cuff from shoulder impingement*

(1). *Patient position*

(a). Supine with right shoulder at edge of table.

(b). Right shoulder in 30 degrees of abduction.

(2). *Therapist position*

(a). Standing, facing patient.

(b). Therapist's two arms support patient's right arm.

(3). *Method*

(a). Patient actively contracts in abduction against resistance.

(b). Note pain response and location.

■ PLEASE NOTE: A positive (painful) response may indicate supraspinatus tendinitis and/or impingement. The next test differentiates between impingement and involvement.

(c). Perform same test as above but with slight distraction of the humerus from the glenoid and acromiohumeral space.

(4). *Findings*

(a). Pain reproduced only with first test: could be either tendinitis or impingement.

(b). Pain reproduced with both tests: supraspinatus tendinitis implicated as source of pain.

d. *Differentiation of supraspinatus tendinitis from impingement of acromiohumeral space.* Intra-articular: glenohumeral joint versus acromiohumeral space.

(1). *Indications*

(a). Localized pain to glenohumeral joint and acromiohumeral space.

(b). Subjective complaint of pain deep in joint.

(2). *Patient position*

(a). Supine with right shoulder at edge of table.

(b). Right shoulder in range from 0 to 90 degrees of abduction.

(3). *Therapist position*

(a). Standing, facing patient.

(b). Left arm at head of humerus for glenohumeral joint.

(c). Left arm on top of acromion for acromiohumeral joint.

(d). Right arm supporting elbow.

(4). *Method*

(a). Passively abduct patient's arm in range where patient complains of painful arc.

(b). Add compression with left hand through humeral head for glenohumeral joint.

(i). Positive finding. Pain provocation indicative of pathology in the glenohumeral intra-articular surface (see Figure 30–35).

(c). Repeat above procedure but add compression with left hand through acromion and shaft of the humerus.

(i). Positive finding. Pain provocation. Indicative of pathology in the acromiohumeral space (see Figure 30–36).

e. Testing of intra-articular compressive force on glenohumeral and acromiohumeral joints

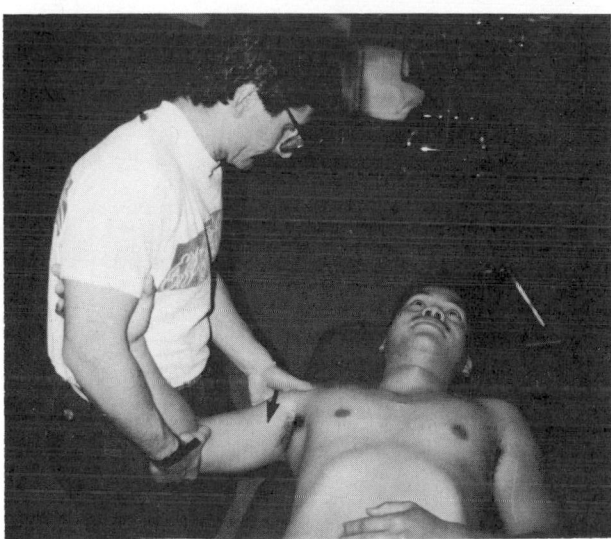

FIGURE 30–35   Glenohumeral intra-articular lesion.

(1). *Indications*
   (a). Pain with lying on shoulder or weight bearing through shoulder joint.
   (b). To identify pathology of glenoid, versus acromion, versus humerus.

(2). *Patient position*
   (a). Supine with right shoulder at edge of table.
   (b). Right shoulder in quadrant position that represents pain position.

(3). *Therapist position*
   (a). Standing, facing patient.
   (b). Both hands supporting proximal humerus from below.
   (c). Therapist's abdomen supports patient's elbow.

(4). *Method*
   (a). Place shoulder in quadrant position.
   (b). Bring elbow down to point of onset of pain.
   (c). Lift humerus in posteroanterior direction with both hands.
      (i). Positive findings. Symptoms increase: possibly a periarticular problem. Symptoms decrease: possibly an acromiohumeral space problem.
   (d). Perform an anteroposterior pressure on humerus.
      (i). Positive findings. Symptoms increase: an acromiohumeral space problem. Symptoms decrease: a periarticular problem.

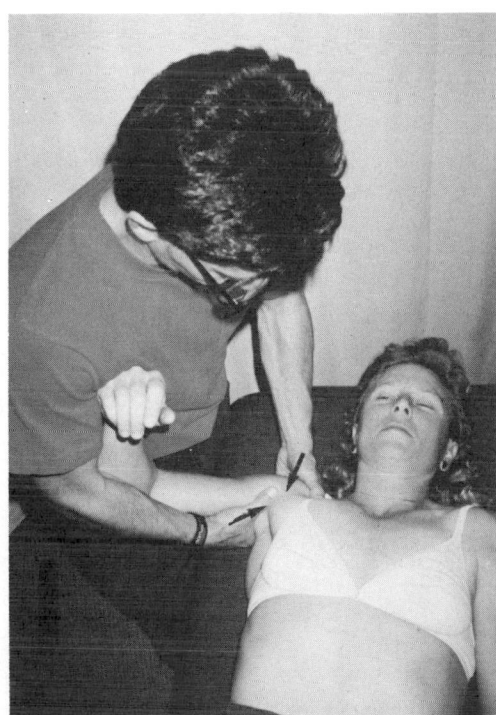

FIGURE 30–36   Acromiohumeral space lesion.

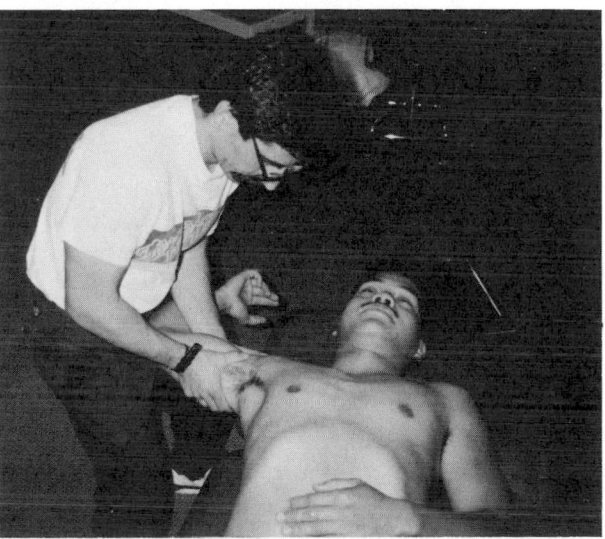

FIGURE 30–37   Differentiating periarticular structures of the glenohumeral joint.

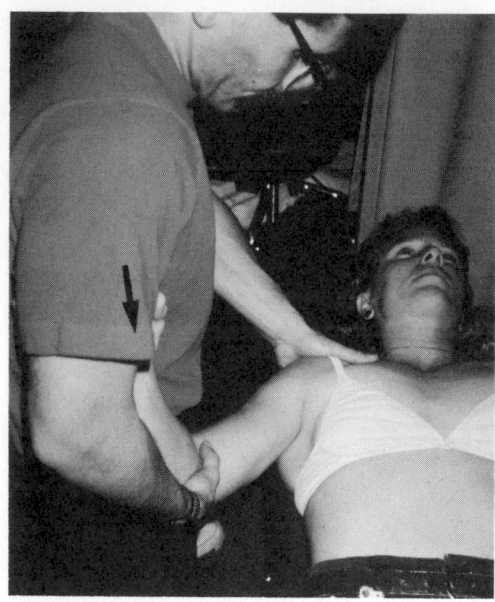

FIGURE 30–38   Differentiating acromiohumeral structures.

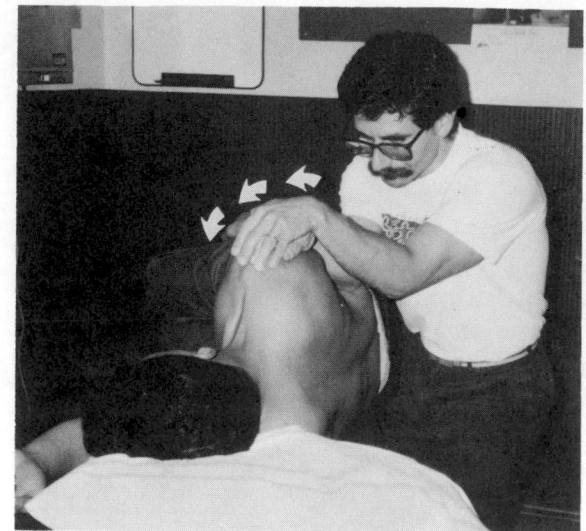

FIGURE 30–40   Start position for anterior elevation.

(e). In quadrant position, apply posteroanterior pressure on humerus, placing stress on periarticular structures (see Figure 30–37).

(f). In quadrant position, apply cephalad pressure on humerus and caudad pressure on acromion, placing slack on periar-

ticular structures (see Figure 30–38).

(g). Place anteroposterior pressure on anterior tubercles of transverse processes or cervical vertebrae at levels comparable to level of shoulder symptoms (see Figure 30–39).[73–75,95,96]

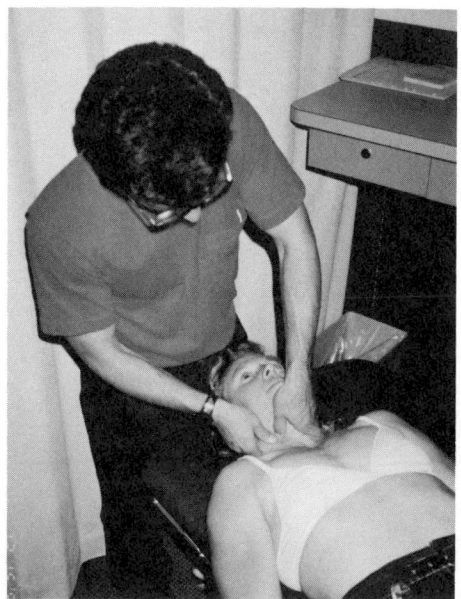

FIGURE 30–39   Anterior palpation of the cervical spine.

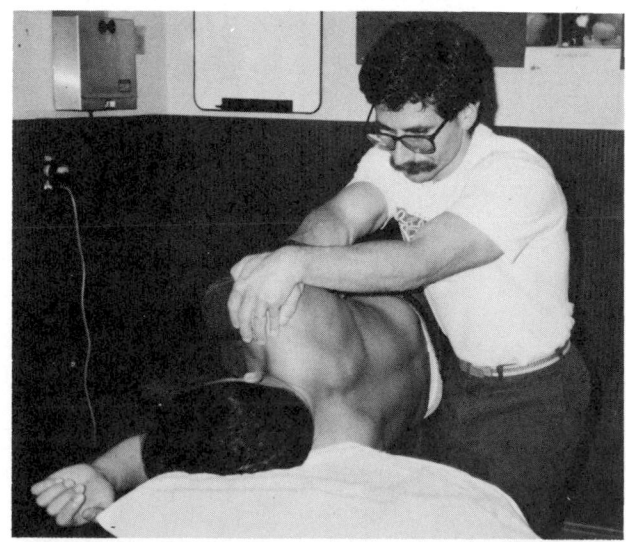

FIGURE 30–41   End position for anterior elevation.

H. Scapulothoracic evaluation

1. **Proprioceptive neuromuscular facilitation patterns**[90,100,101]
   a. In performing this evaluation, the following need to be considered:
      (1). Muscle length.
      (2). Muscle strength throughout range.
      (3). Muscle contraction (smooth, coordinated vs ballistic movement).
      (4). Most important, comparison of affected with unaffected side.
   b. The following steps should be performed for optimal performance of the techniques:
      (1). *Patient position*
         (a). Sidelying, affected side up.
         (b). Hips and knees between 70 and 90 degrees of flexion with spine in a neutral position.
         (c). Head and neck also in a neutral position with assist of pillows.
      (2). *Therapist position*
         (a). Posterior to the patient.
         (b). Hand placement specifically on surface to be facilitated.
         (c). Hips facing in line of diagonal.

2. **Scapula patterns**
   a. *Anterior elevation.* Place hands overlapped on superolateral surface of acromion process (see Figures 30–40 and 30–41).

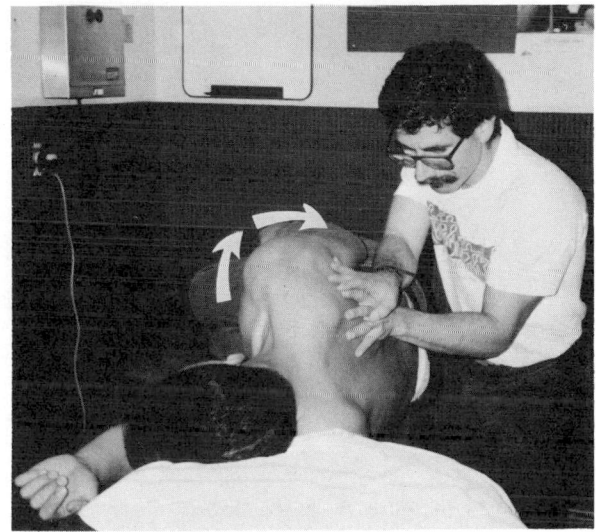

FIGURE 30–43   End position for posterior depression.

   b. *Posterior depression.* Place hands on inferior angle of scapula (see Figures 30–42 and 30–43).
   c. *Anterior depression.* Place hands on anterior and posterior surfaces of axilla (see Figures 30–44 and 30–45).
   d. *Posterior elevation.* Place hands on superior portion of acromion process (see Figures 30–46 and 30–47).

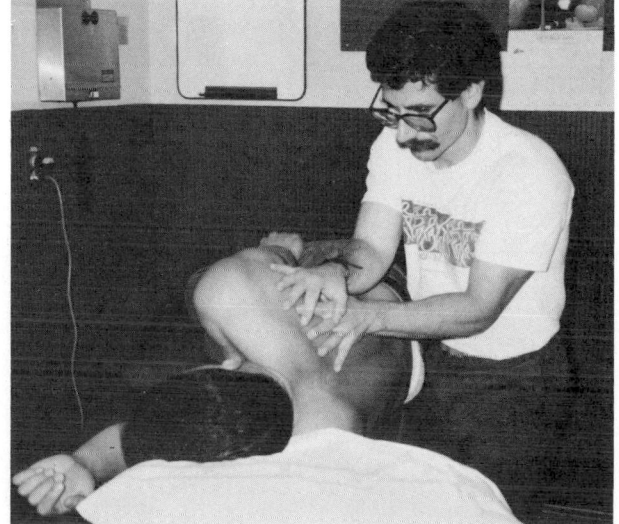

FIGURE 30–42   Start position for posterior depression.

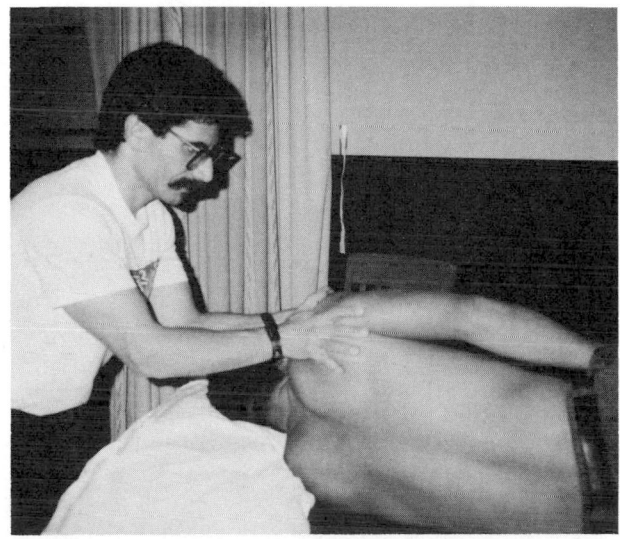

FIGURE 30–44   Start position for anterior depression.

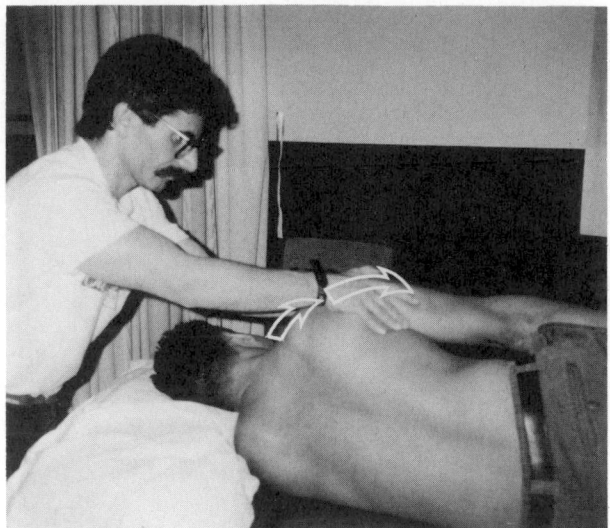

FIGURE 30–45   End position for anterior depression.

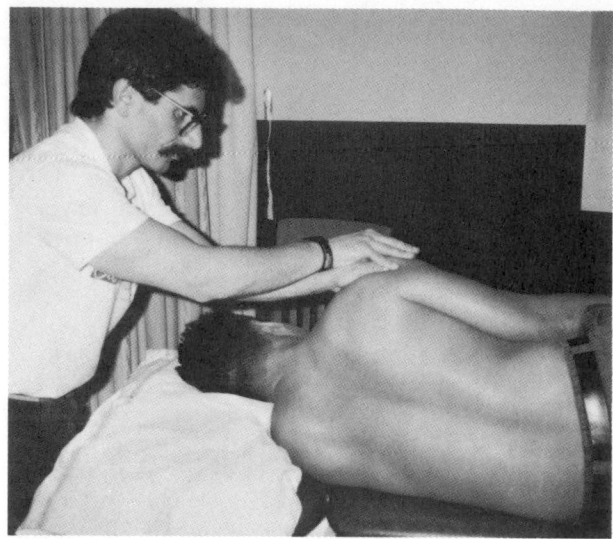

FIGURE 30–46   Start position for posterior elevation.

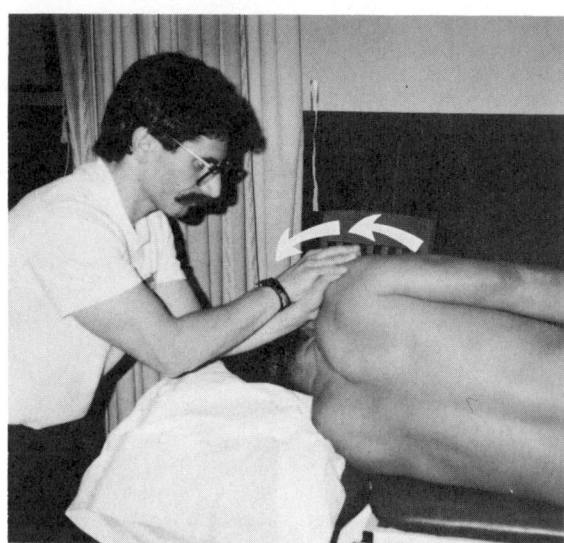

FIGURE 30–47   End position for posterior elevation.

V. Treatment

Using the Maitland concept, as described earlier in the chapter, involves following a methodical approach to treatment. The therapist initiates treatment from the subjective and objective portions of the examination. The subjective information provides the information necessary to determine how much treatment should be given initially as well as in follow-up visits. The following factors (SINS) are used in determining the type of treatment, the duration of each set, and how many sets of a technique will be performed:

- **S**everity (*eg*, the therapist may be attempting to change only the constancy of the symptoms).
- **I**rritability.
- **N**ature.
- **S**tability.
- **S**tage.

The therapist decides whether the patient is more of a pain patient (limited primarily by pain) or a dysfunctional patient (a structural dysfunction is the cause of the symptoms). These two different types of patients require different treatment approaches.

STEPS TO TAKE BEFORE COMMENCING WITH TREATMENT

1. Formulate a working hypothesis.
2. Establish baseline symptoms.
3. Reassess asterisk signs and symptoms (see operational terms and definitions)
   - One or two active physiological movements.
   - One or two passive physiological movements.
   - One or two passive accessory movements.
   - One or two special tests or cervical tests.

Three to four asterisks are an acceptable number for reassessment.

A. Treatment for the pain patient

1. Short of pain (P1).
2. Large-amplitude movement short of pain (P1).
3. Speed is slow (*ie*, 1/s).
4. Rhythm is smooth.
5. Few repetitions/few sets.

B. Treatment for the dysfunctional patient

1. Performing into the stiffness.
2. Movement is to the limit of the range (R2).
3. Speed is faster (*ie*, 2 to 3/s).
4. Rhythm is smooth to staccato.
5. Many repetitions/many sets.

C. Treatment options

Treatment selection can be based on the therapist's objective examination. A variety of techniques are available for use, but it is important that one procedure is performed and evaluated before adding any other technique. The value of a technique can be evaluated only by reassessment once that one technique has been performed. The following are treatment options dependent on SINS:

1. **Modalities.**
   a. Ice.
   b. Electrical stimulation.
   c. Ultrasound.

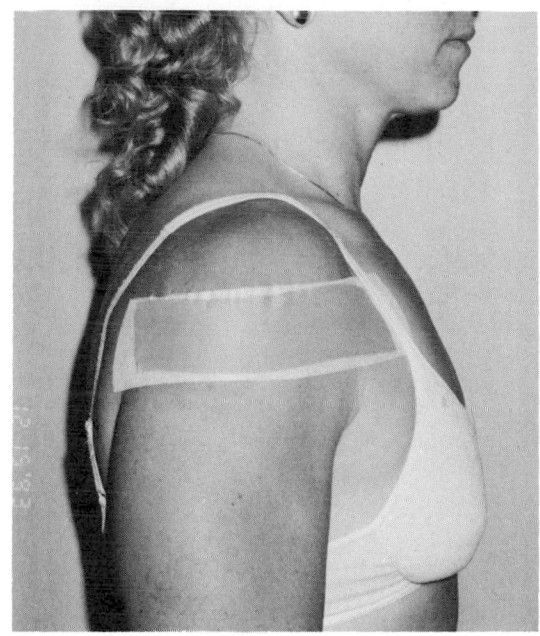

FIGURE 30–48   Taping for shoulder dislocations.

2. **Supports**
   a. Taping:
      (1). Glenohumeral taping for dislocations (see Figure 30–48).
      (2). Scapular taping for re-education (see Figure 30–49).
   b. Slings or supports to decrease traction on painful structures.

3. **Mobilization**
   a. Passive:
      (1). Passive physiological movements.
      (2). Passive accessory movements.
      (3). Passive accessory movements in physiological positions.
   b. Active:
      (1). Proprioceptive neuromuscular facilitation patterns.
      (2). Range of motion exercises.

4. **Friction massage**
   a. Positive palpation findings over tendon.
   b. Follow Cyriax's protocol for friction massage.[1]
   c. Teach patient how to perform at home.

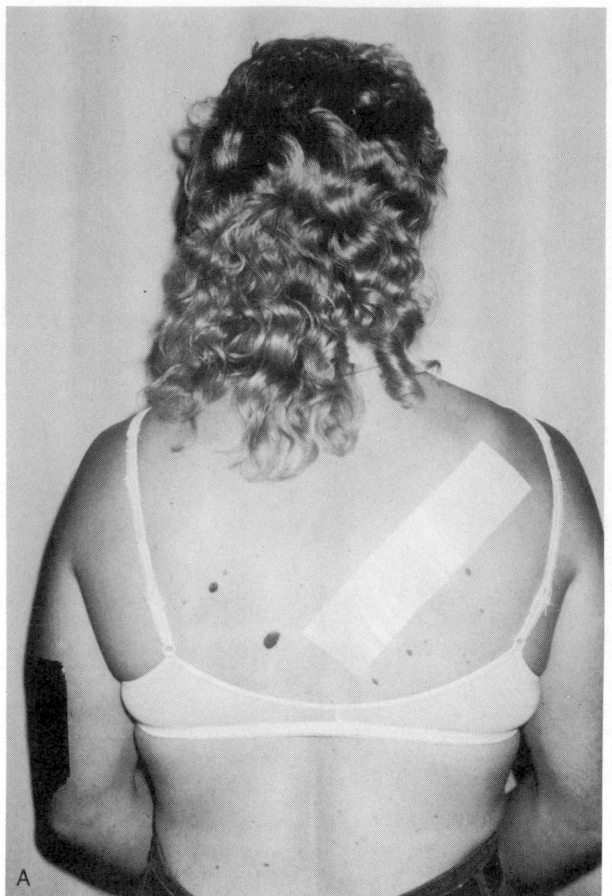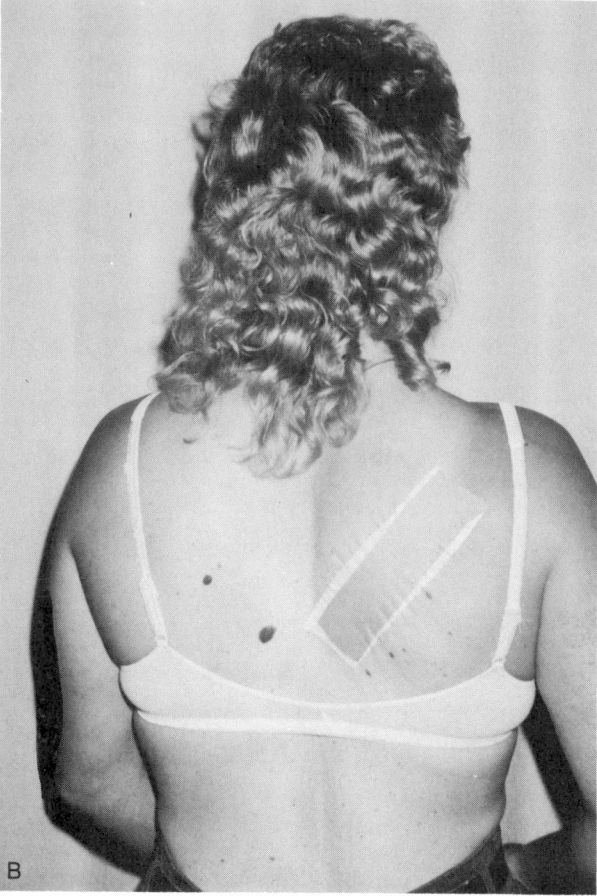

FIGURE 30–49   Taping for scapular re-education.

5. **Exercise programs** (see the section on rehabilitation exercises for the shoulder complex)
   a. Posture.

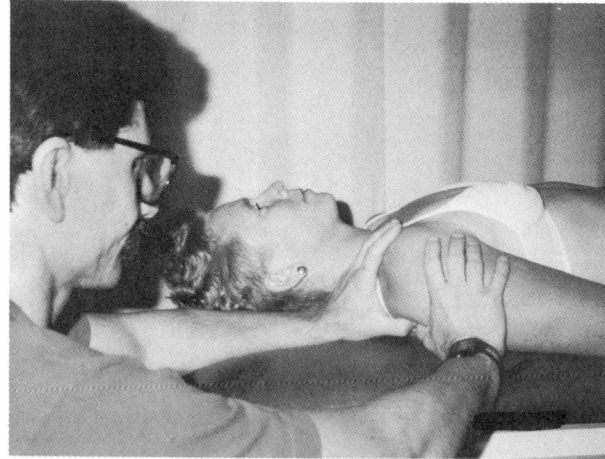

FIGURE 30–50   Posteroanterior pressure of the glenohumeral joint in a pain-easing position.

b. Flexibility exercises.
c. Strengthening exercises.

D. Examples of treatment options

The following are examples of possible treatment options. These are but a few options, as there is no one correct way to treat a patient.

1. **Irritable patient**
   a. Positioning (information from subjective examination on easing factors).
   b. Technique:
      (1). Modalities.
      (2). Manual techniques (*eg*, a passive accessory movement of the glenohumeral joint performed in the pain-free range. Use the parameters for the painful patient [see Figure 30–50]).

 PLEASE NOTE: Constantly reassess baseline symptoms for changes!

2. **Moderately irritable patient**
   a. Positioning:
      (1). Easing or neutral position for the shoulder.
   b. Technique:
      (1). Modalities.
      (2). Manual techniques (*eg*, a passive accessory movement of the glenohumeral joint performed in the pain-free range. Use the parameters for the painful patient; however, may be able to progress the positioning of the glenohumeral joint into a more functional range).
   c. Exercises (see the section on rehabilitation exercises for the shoulder complex).

3. **Mildly irritable to nonirritable**
   a. Positioning:
      (1). Easing or neutral position for the shoulder.
   b. Positioning (information from subjective examination on aggravating factors).
   c. Technique:
      (1). Modalities (*eg*, ultrasound for increasing tissue elasticity).
      (2). Manual techniques (*eg*, a passive accessory movement of the glenohumeral joint performed in the dysfunctional range. Use the parameters for the dysfunctional patient, increasing the vigor of the treatment [see Figure 30–51]).
   d. Exercises (see the section on rehabilitation exercises for the shoulder complex).

> PLEASE NOTE: All treatment, including exercise, should be appropriate for the patient's stage. Assessment is the key to success of any treat-

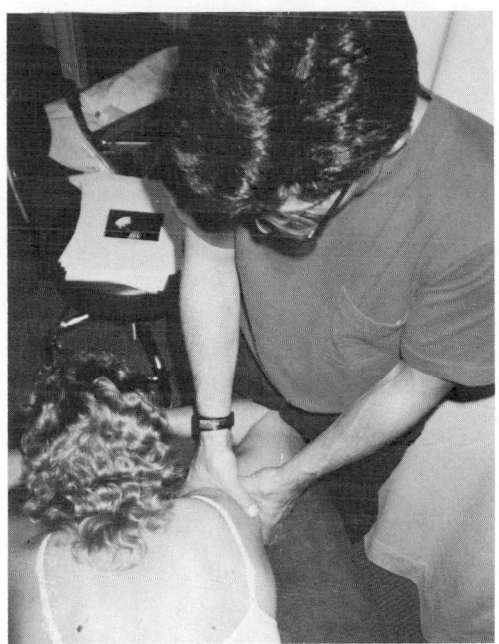

FIGURE 30–51   Anteroposterior pressure of the glenohumeral joint in the dysfunctional range.

ment program. If the patient is better subjectively and objectively, the treatment can be repeated. If significantly better, advance by repositioning the joint or increasing vigor. If the patient is worse, perform the same technique but in more of an easing position or decrease one of the treatment parameters. If the patient remains the same, perform the same technique more aggressively. If still unchanged, the therapist is perhaps performing the wrong treatment or treating the wrong area. The reader is encouraged to read the chapters on assessment in Maitland[5,19] for much more depth in treatment progression.

VI. Rehabilitation Exercises for the Shoulder Complex

The exercises provided in this section* follow the same format as that of the objective composite examination of the shoulder complex. The principles of the Maitland concept are applied. The subjective examination assists in deciding when to use exercises, which exercises, how much exercise, and when to add certain exercises and progress those exercises. The SINS are important factors to be

considered in the exercise program. For example, both irritable and nonirritable patients need to start exercise immediately. Principles of exercise can be used in evaluating, assessing, and initiating the program.

- Loading versus unloading the glenohumeral joint (intra-articular vs periarticular problems).
- Closed versus open kinetic chain exercises (scapula stability).
- Developmental sequence for treatment progression.[90,99,101,104]

---

*This exercise program is based on principles taught at the Kaiser Vallejo Proprioceptive Neuromuscular Facilitation residency program.[90]

A. Exercise goals

These goals are addressed in the rehabilitation exercise program that follows. All exercises should be performed in a pain-free range.

1. Decrease pain and symptoms.
2. Restore functional range of motion.
3. Increase functional strength through stability statically and dynamically.
4. Increase muscular endurance.
5. Improve sport/skill–specific activities as they relate to return to function.

B. Range of motion exercises

1. **Severe irritability**
   a. Pulley exercises in sitting position, spine in neutral position. Avoid scapula elevation. Pulley in following directions:
      (1). Flexion.
      (2). Abduction.
      (3). Hand behind back.
   b. Swiss ball exercises in sitting position, spine in neutral position. Perform easy horizontal movements in small, pain-free ranges.
   c. Codman's pendulum exercises.

2. **Mild irritability.** These exercises are added to the above exercises.
   a. *Swiss ball exercises*
      (1). *Sitting.* Spine in neutral position. Both hands on ball, rolling forward/backward.
      (2). *Prone.* Lying across ball, spine in neutral position. Both hands on floor, rolling forward/backward.
      (3). *Standing.* Spine in neutral position without arching. Both hands on ball, rolling up and down.
      (4). *Supine.* Spine in neutral position. Rolling ball up and down thoracic spine.

3. **Nonirritable.** Add the following:
   a. Trial of specific activity without resistance, *eg,* throwing motion without a ball or weighted object.
   b. Stretching capsular structures found restricted on examination:
      (1). Anterior capsule.
      (2). Posterior capsule.

◼ PLEASE NOTE: All exercises should be performed in the available range, respecting pain and the dysfunctional component. In other words, the patient should feel "a good stretch."

Ice should be applied after exercise in the irritable stage.

In the mild and nonirritable stages, heat can be used before exercise.

C. Shoulder re-education and strengthening program

1. **Goal.** To increase strength and stability in functional range with assumption of an acceptable posture.
   a. *Stage I: functional mobility*
      (1). This stage has been presented in the previous section on range of motion exercises.
      (2). Cervical/thoracic postural exercises.

2. **Goal.** To increase strength and stability of scapulae on thoracic cage for good function of rotator cuff.
   a. *Stage II: preparation for weight bearing*
      (1). *Stability*
         (a). Prone on Swiss ball (see Figure 30–52):
            (i). Increase lever of body by placing ball distal to arms.
         (b). Standing wall push-up in pain-free range:
            (i). "Push-up plus." [55]
         (c). Supine:
            (i). Bilateral horizontal extension and external rotation with tubing resistance for scapulae posterior depression.

3. **Goal.** To increase strength and stability of scapulae on thoracic cage while dynamically moving the extremity with good coordinated control.
   a. *Stage III: weight bearing*
      (1). *Mobility on stability*
         (a). Prone:
            (i). On elbows with head/neck in functional position:

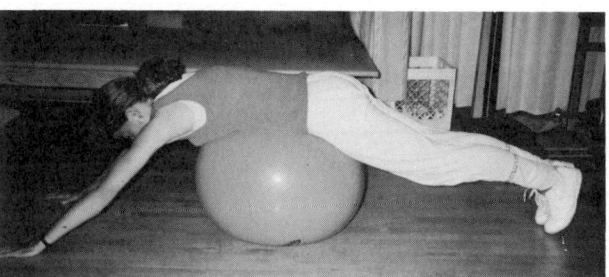

FIGURE 30–52   Patient is prone on the Swiss ball performing "push-up plus."

- Static positioning.
- Weight shift side to side.

(ii). Lying on table:
- Rowing motion with tubing for resistance.

(b). Sitting:
(i). Elbows slightly adducted/flexed resting on a supported surface:
- Resisted external rotation of shoulders with use of tubing.

(ii). Elbows on foam roller (see Figure 30–53):
- Static positioning.
- Weight shift side to side.
- Rolling foam roller forward and backward while maintaining functional position of cervical spine.

(iii). Elbow on Swiss ball:
- Scapula depression while rolling ball forward and backward in horizontal plane.
- Simultaneously, add external/internal rotation of arm.
- Do the above with tubing at wrist for resistance.

(iv). Treadmill walking on hands:
- Forward.
- Karioka.

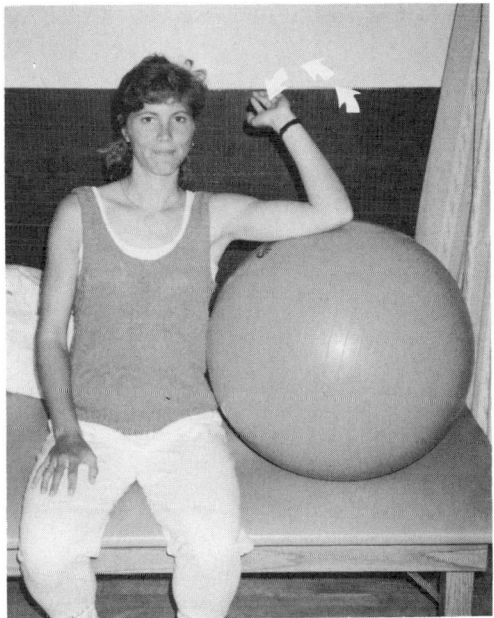

FIGURE 30–54 Throwing motion of external rotation to internal rotation at 90 degrees of abduction. Performing scapular depression simultaneously for stability.

4. **Goal.** Once mobility on stability achieved, to promote functional tasks in functional range.
   a. *Stage IV: skill*
   (1). *Prone*
      (a). On elbows with head/neck in functional position:
         (i). Lift extremity off supported surface.
         (ii). Lift objects and cross midline.
      (b). With elbows on foam roller/Swiss ball:
         (i). Lift extremity off supported surface.
         (ii). Lift objects and cross midline.
   (2). *Supine*
      (a). Lift extremity off supported surface.
      (b). Lift objects and cross midline using proprioceptive neuromuscular facilitation diagonals and tubing.
   (3). *Erect*
      (a). Unilateral extremity patterns
         (i). Tubing unilateral arm exercises crossing midline using proprioceptive neuromuscular facilitation diagonals.

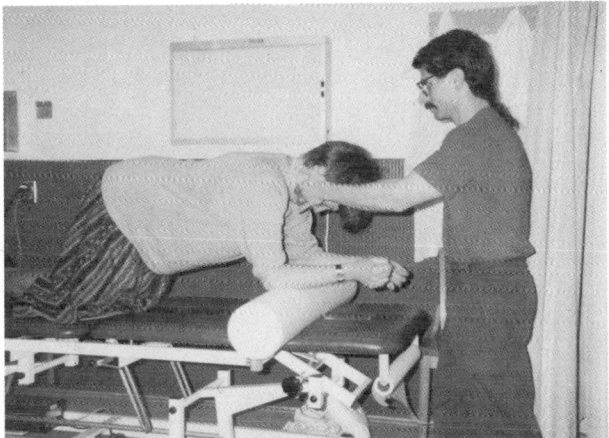

FIGURE 30–53 Quadruped on elbows supported by foam roller with cervical spine in good functional position.

(4). Incorporate specific sport activity into rehabilitation (see Figure 30–54).

5. **Goal.** To increase aerobic capacity while maintaining good functional stability.

D. Endurance

1. **Muscular**
   a. The *time* spent performing all of the exercises described above should increase; do not be concerned with the number of repetitions. Time = function!

2. **Aerobic**
   a. All exercises can be incorporated into a patient's specific sport or cardiovascular program.

 PLEASE NOTE: The SINS factors should be the guiding force in adding or deleting resistance or time as appropriate. Exercise progression will be determined by reassessment of the subjective and objective changes in the patient's condition on subsequent visits. Most important, the therapist needs to evaluate the performance of the exercise on follow-up visits and correct or modify appropriately.

VII. Conclusion

The primary emphasis in shoulder evaluation and treatment is on assessment. The concept of making a physical therapy diagnosis from the signs and symptoms found on examination is critical to reaching the root of the problem. Clinical decision making is a process that requires several steps until reaching and then proving a hypothesis. As a clinician acquires knowledge, whether through research of the literature or the examination of many, many patients, his/her database continues to grow. This is the stage at which the clinician develops expertise in finding patterns to problems and reaching correct conclusions quickly. This is achieved not by taking shortcuts in examination but by prioritizing what needs to be examined. The expert reassesses continually, searching for the best answer. Anatomy and biomechanics form a basic foundation for developing a plausible hypothesis, but it is the methodical examination that makes the features fit. The critical mind will accept only that which can be proven through repeated testing and measurement. Once this occurs, the therapist will be able to relate signs and symptoms to a hypothesis of what might be the cause of the problem.

Clinical Decision-Making Cases

The case studies presented here represent three different types of shoulder dysfunction. Each case study is accompanied by a body chart representing the area of symptoms as well as areas that are asymptomatic. An area that is cleared, subjectively asked of the patient, is marked with a check sign (✓✓) on the body chart or in the special questions section. The special questions comprise the patient's subjective complaints and the therapist's thoughts during the subjective examination of what possible structures are involved and what tests may be necessary to confirm the hypothesis. Before the objective portion of the examination, the SINS or behavior of the patient's complaints is determined. As explained in the discussion of the Maitland concept, clinical decision making plays an integral role in planning the examination. How the therapist interprets the subjective data in regard to SINS will determine the aggressiveness and extent of the objective examination. Also, the therapist's thoughts during the objective examination will be taken into account. This will eventually lead to a treatment approach based on the subjective examination, objective examination, and, finally, interpretation of findings.

The following are symbols commonly used in the objective portion of the examination:

Abd: abduction.
ER: external rotation.
F: flexion.
HBB: hand behind back.
HF: horizontal flexion.
IR: internal rotation.
Rot: rotation.

Case #1: Rotator Cuff Tear

SUBJECTIVE EXAMINATION

Patient Profile

The patient is a 50-year-old male carpenter; he is presently working although avoiding sustained overhead activities. He had done some light weight lifting prior to complaint three times a week but does not at present because of shoulder pain. He is right hand dominant.

His chief complaint is an intermittent, deep dull ache in the right shoulder. He has difficulty raising his right arm, "feels weak," and experiences a sharp pain when bringing arm to 90 degrees elevation. There are also complaints of an intermittent deep ache at the base of the right side of the neck (see Figure 30–55).

Aggravating Factors

1. Reaching forward or to the side produces a sharp pain, and he cannot lift right arm higher than mid-chest level because of weakness. (Test movements could include the functional movement, flexion, abduction, and horizontal flexion.)
2. Reaching for wallet out of back pocket causes anterior shoulder pain; once out of that position, symptoms subside. (Possible test movements to assess are hand behind back, internal rotation, and the lock position, taking into consideration the patient's severity and irritability.)
3. Neck soreness occurs if he tries to hold a bag of groceries for 2 to 3 minutes. The soreness remains

for about 5 minutes, but is not severe. (Test movement of cervical quadrant, palpation.)

Easing Factors

1. Avoiding overhead activities.
2. Providing some support to the shoulder. Also, not using or moving the arm.
3. Ice helps the shoulder when aching. Hot showers seem to free up the neck for range of motion.

24-Hour Day

1. Night: Sleeping or rolling over on to the right arm will awaken him. This occurs three to four times a night. He can return to sleep immediately.
2. Morning: The shoulder feels stiff, but he has no pain unless he moves it.
3. Day: The pain in the shoulder is more dependent on activity and use. The neck is more achy at the end of the day.

Present History

Two weeks previously, the patient slipped and fell down on his right elbow and experienced immediate sharp pain in the right shoulder. He noticed difficulty raising the right shoulder because of pain, but he also felt weakness. A few days later he noticed some achiness in the neck, but he feels that his primary problem is his shoulder. Presently, he still experiences the same sharp pain if attempting to elevate the shoulder. Additionally, he feels a deep ache in the shoulder if it hangs unsupported for 10-minute periods. The neck complaints have not changed from the initial onset of those symptoms. Present treatment includes medication and ice, which decreases some of the sharp pain; however, the feeling of weakness is unchanged.

Past History

The patient describes that he has had intermittent sharp pains in the right shoulder on and off for the past 20 years. He has had an episode approximately once each 2- to 3-year period for a duration of about 1 week to 1 month. These complaints have always resolved with medication, ice, and rest. He has never had strength problems in raising his arm. Also, on further questioning, he offers information of intermittent stiffness in the neck, which presents at times other than the shoulder episodes. He has never had any treatment in the past for his shoulder and/or neck. He denies other trauma to shoulder or neck.

Special Questions

General health: ✔✔
Weight loss/gain: ✔✔
Medications: ibuprofen, 800 mg three times a day
Steroids/Anticoagulants: ✔✔
Radiography/special tests: plain films of right shoulder normal

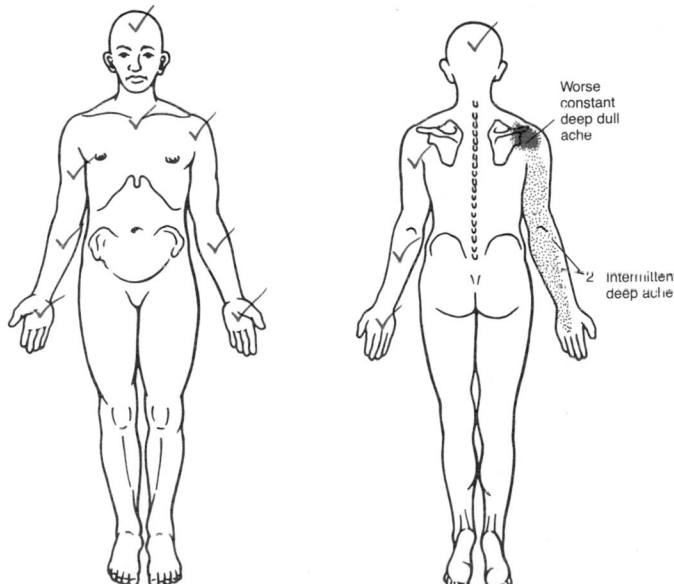

FIGURE 30–55   Body chart of painful shoulder case study.

Vertebral artery: ✔✔
Cord signs: ✔✔

SINS

Initial impressions from the subjective examination that will guide the objective examination for determining the vigor in testing are:

Severity: Mild. Pain is intermittent, and weakness seems to be more of a concern to the patient. He can still work.

Irritability: Mild. He can do a movement that brings on the sharp pain, but it is only present in that position.

Nature: Trauma to the shoulder with weakness. Possible sources of pain and weakness needing investigation are the glenohumeral structures, including capsule, ligaments, labrum, and rotator cuff muscles.

Stability: Worsening. He has had multiple episodes of shoulder pain with resolution, but never weakness.

Stage: Acute. Onset approximately 2 weeks previously; symptoms unchanged.

Examination instructions for patient: instruct patient to perform movements to available range.

OBJECTIVE EXAMINATION

Observation

Slightly overweight, round shouldered male. He experiences some difficulty removing right arm from sleeve of shirt.

Active Physiological Movements (Shoulder)

F: 80 degrees in right shoulder before sharp local pain and cannot maintain position because of pain and weakness.

Abd: 45 degrees produces sharp pain with some scapula elevation.

ER: 30 degrees, some anterior shoulder pain.

HBB: right hand to midbuttock region with sharp pain, settling to dull ache for 1 minute.

HF: immediate pain when attempted.

Resisted Cuff Tests

Abd: slight resistance given to patient caused increased local symptoms, and he immediately gave way because of pain.

ER: pain and weak 2−/5.

IR: strong and painless.

Elbow flexion: strong with slight pain in anterior shoulder.

Cervical Spine Clearing

Active physiological movements:

Right rot: full range, stiff with local pain in the right posterior region of C7 with overpressure to this movement.

Left rot: ✔✔

Lower cervical quadrant, left and right: local C7 region of posterior neck on the same pain.

Neurological

Reflexes: biceps and triceps jerk 2/2 brisk.

Motor: C5 deltoid on the right 4+/5 because of pain, C6 to T1 5/5.

Sensation: light touch intact.

Passive Physiological Movements (Shoulder)

F: onset of symptoms (P1) at 90 degrees.

Abd: onset of symptoms (P1) at 65 degrees.

ER: onset of symptoms (P1) at 30 degrees.

Shoulder quadrant: top of hill onset of symptoms at one half range.

Palpation (Shoulder)

1. Soft tissue: anterior and posterior portions of capsule tender and warm, supraspinatus and infraspinatus tendons at insertion painful.
2. Passive accessory movements, right glenohumeral joint:
   • Posteroanterior pressure: tight at end of range, slight pain.
   • Caudal glide: slight local stretch at end of range.

Palpation (Cervical Spine)

1. Soft tissue: thickening noted over the posterior articular pillars bilaterally C4–C5, C5–C6, and C6–C7.
2. Passive accessory movements:
   • Anteroposterior pressure: Unilateral left-right stiffness over C4 to T1 without any reproduction of any type of symptoms to area of pain.

Special Tests

Instability tests for shoulder: anterior drawer, posterior drawer, and inferior glide ✔✔. Isometric resisted abduction at 30 degrees of abduction performed with and without slight distraction of right arm produced same pain response. (This test is indicative of rotator cuff, specifically supraspinatus tendinitis. See the section on special tests.)

Reassessment After Objective Examination

No change in symptoms subjectively. Objectively, shoulder active movements and resistive tests are the same.

PHYSICAL THERAPY DIAGNOSIS

Right painful shoulder from traumatic injury leading to strain/tear of rotator cuff tendons. Although stability testing was negative, more specific diagnostic testing may be needed to rule out instability of capsule, labrum, and ligaments.

Prognosis

Although symptoms have not worsened, there has not been a change in the patient's pain or, more importantly, strength.

Expected Outcome

1. Pain control and improvement in range of motion in 3 to 4 weeks.
2. Return to 80% functional use of arm for activities of daily living, which will be dependent on integrity of the structures, particularly the rotator cuff. If partial tear, 4 to 6 weeks. If full tear without surgical intervention, 3 to 6 months.
3. A 95% full recovery will take 6 months to 1 year; again, this will be dependent on rotator cuff and its related structures.

TREATMENT

Day 1

Technique: physiological passive movement of shoulder flexion and/or external rotation.

Position patient: supine.

Therapist: perform technique to pain for 30 seconds to 1 minute, assessing for changes in symptoms. If tolerated, repeat same technique two to three times since irritability is mild.

Reassess:

Subjectively: patient's resting symptoms.

Objectively: one active movement and one passive accessory movement (eg, shoulder flexion and postero-anterior pressure on the glenohumeral joint). Assess one resisted test but do not expect any major changes, especially if the rotator cuff is torn.

Instructions and warning to the patient:

1. Ask patient to note symptoms over the next 2- and 24-hour time periods.
2. Warn patient of possible treatment soreness, which should be different from symptoms.
3. Instruct patient in icing, proper use of medication(s), and positions of ease.
4. Initiate exercise program with pulleys and light weight-bearing exercises.

Day 2

Reassess subjectively and objectively at 2- and 24-hour periods. If improved for short duration and symptoms returned, the treatment worked but not for a long enough period. Perform the same treatment. If worse, what is worse, when did it get worse, and how is it worse? If the patient is the same, perform the same technique and reassess. If unchanged, the therapist may be able to increase the technique by changing the position in which the technique is performed (eg, posteroanterior pressure on the glenohumeral joint with the shoulder in some flexion) or increase the vigor of the technique.

Follow-up visits should include the following:

1. Clearing of all shoulder physiological and accessory movements with overpressure. This includes the acromioclavicular joint and the thoracic spine.
2. Clearing of the rotator cuff muscles.
3. Completion of the neurological examination for the upper quarter.

The home program should address rotator cuff, scapular stabilizers, and postural exercises for improvement of thoracic spine extension.

Clinical decision making for the above physical therapy diagnosis is based on:

1. Age of patient (middle to older age); occupation and/or sport involving many overhead activities; and/or trauma of falling on shoulder.
2. Sudden onset of localized sharp pain with inability to raise arm.
3. Inability to raise arm and painful and weak to resistive testing.
4. Tendons can be thickened and painful on palpation; however, if complete rupture, this will not necessarily be the case.
5. Shoulder quadrant test can be positive, as rotator cuff tendons form part of capsule. If the cuff is affected, the other periarticular structures need to be examined.

Case #2: Painful Shoulder

SUBJECTIVE EXAMINATION

Patient Profile

The patient is a 60-year-old female, retired housewife, who is restricted in doing her normal household chores secondary to pain. Dressing and bathing are significantly limited because of pain and some restriction. She had walked 3 miles a day for aerobic activity but has decreased it to 1 mile a day because the swinging motion of the arm increases her symptoms. She is right hand dominant.

Her chief complaint is a constant, severe, deep dull ache in the right shoulder joint, which intermittently radiates down the entire arm and into the hand. The fingers do not have any symptoms (see Figure 30-56).

Aggravating Factors

1. Lifting arm overhead immediately increases symptoms; however, once the arm is back down by her side, symptoms return to resting pain level. (Test movements to assess are those involving elevation.)

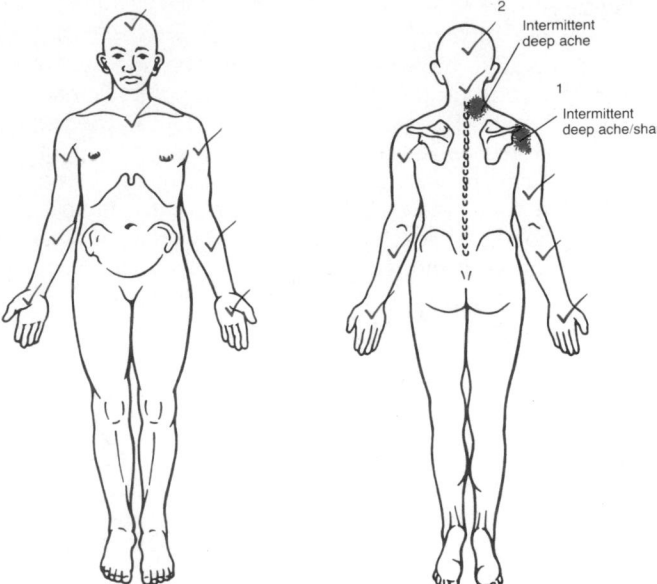

FIGURE 30–56   Body chart of rotator cuff tear case study.

2. Putting arm through sleeve of blouse, *ie*, hand behind back motion, produces severe increase in shoulder and arm symptoms. Once out of that position, it takes approximately 2 to 3 minutes to settle back to resting level. (Test movements to assess are hand behind back, internal rotation, and lock position, noting severity and irritability.)
3. Turning the steering wheel to the left; once out of position, symptoms return to resting pain levels. (Test horizontal flexion.)

Easing Factors
Rest (supporting arm by her side).

24-Hour Day
1. Night: Difficulty falling asleep. Cannot sleep on the right side; if rolls over on to right, will awaken. The pain awakens her two times a night. It takes 15 minutes to return to sleep.
2. Morning: The shoulder feels better because of less severe pain but feels stiff.
3. Day: The pain is more dependent on activity and use. However, generally feels better in the morning; by evening feels tired and more easily aggravated with movement.

Present History
One month previously, the patient slipped and fell but grabbed a railing with her right hand from behind, breaking the fall. Initially, she did not experience severe pain but did notice some soreness in the shoulder. A few days later, she could not lift her right arm without the same severe pain in shoulder that is present today. A few days after the initial shoulder pain, she started experiencing radiating pain down the arm and into the hand. The intensity of the symptoms has become progressively worse and is constant, whereas it had been only intermittent 1 week previously. She has not received any treatment other than medication and the use of a heating pad, which she feels provides temporary comfort only.

Past History
The patient reports that she had right local shoulder pain approximately 12 years previously. The details of this episode are vague, but she does remember that a cortisone injection provided total relief in 1 day. She denies any other incidents related to the shoulder or neck region.

Special Questions
General health: diabetes
Weight loss/gain: ✔✔
Medications: ibuprofen as needed for pain; glyburide for diabetes
Steroids/anticoagulants: ✔✔
Radiography/special tests: plain films of right shoulder normal; the cervical spine demonstrated multiple-level spurring and degenerative changes bilaterally from C4–C7.
Vertebral artery: ✔✔
Cord signs: ✔✔

SINS
Initial impressions from the subjective examination that will guide the objective examination for determining the vigor in testing are:

Severity: Severe. Constancy and the fear that any movement will increase the pain. She is limited in her normal daily activities.
Irritability: Moderately. She can do a movement that brings on the severe symptoms radiating down the arm, but they return to their resting level in a relatively short period of time.
Nature: Trauma to the shoulder with gradual increase in symptom intensity and peripheralization to the arm. Possible sources of pain needing investigation are the glenohumeral extra-articular and intra-articular structures.
Stability: Stable. Although the shoulder symptoms have progressed into the arm, this would be expected from the stage of the disorder. The patient has had only one other bout years ago with quick resolution of symptoms.
Stage: Acute. Onset approximately 1 month previously, but symptoms are intensifying and progressing.

Examination instructions for patient: instruct patient to perform movements to short of her increasing resting symptoms.

OBJECTIVE EXAMINATION

Observation

Slightly kyphotic female. She experiences difficulty undressing, with much guarding and avoidance in movement of the right arm.

Active Physiological Movements (Shoulder)

F: 70 degrees in right shoulder before increase in local symptoms.

Abd: 45 degrees, with majority of movement from scapula elevation; slight increase in local shoulder pain but settles immediately.

HBB: right hand to greater trochanter increases symptoms all the way into the hand; settles in 1 minute.

HF: not tested.

ER: not tested.

Resisted Cuff Tests

Abd: slight resistance given to patient caused increased local symptoms. (Pain may be causing inhibitory weakness such that an accurate assessment cannot be made.)

Cervical Spine Clearing[20]

Active physiological movements:

Right rot: three fourths range, stiff local pain in the right posterior region of C7 with overpressure to this movement.

Left rot: ✔✔

Lower cervical quadrant, left and right: local same-side soreness.

Neurological

Reflexes: biceps and triceps jerk 2/2 brisk.

Motor: not tested because of severity of symptoms.

Sensation: light touch intact.

Passive Physiological Movements (Shoulder)

F: onset of increase in resting symptoms (P1) at 70 degrees with muscle spasm.

Abd: onset of increase in resting symptoms (P1) at 45 degrees.

ER: onset of symptoms (P1) at 0 degrees when tested with arm at 0 degrees abduction.

Palpation (Shoulder)

1. Soft tissue: anterior and posterior portions of capsule tender and warm.
2. Passive Accessory Movements, right glenohumeral joint (position of ease, right arm at side with pillow under humerus for support):
   - Posteroanterior pressure: increase in resting symptoms at one half range.
   - Caudal glide: increase in resting symptoms at one fourth of available range.

Palpation (Cervical Spine)

One small pillow is used under head because of kyphotic posture.

- Anteroposterior pressure: bilateral stiffness over C4 to T1 without any reproduction of any type of symptoms to area.

Reassessment After Objective Examination

Patient has slight increase in resting symptoms from examination. Irritability is placed slightly higher in the moderate range, and examination and treatment will need to be more cautious. No objective tests will be performed, as subjectively the patient is worse and pain is the primary factor with this patient.

PHYSICAL THERAPY DIAGNOSIS

Right painful shoulder from traumatic injury leading to strain of periarticular and related structures of the glenohumeral joint.

Prognosis

The symptoms have spread distally and with greater intensity. Although symptoms are of gradual onset, trauma is the precipitating factor leading to the patient's problem.

Expected Outcome

1. Pain control and centralization of symptoms to shoulder region to be fairly quick, 1 to 2 weeks.
2. Return to 80% functional ability for activities of daily living, 6 to 8 weeks.
3. A 95% full recovery will take 6 months with a well-tailored home exercise program.

TREATMENT

Day 1

Technique: glenohumeral posteroanterior pressures short of pain.

Position patient: supine, one pillow under head and one under right humerus for support and easing of symptoms.

Therapist: perform technique to short of pain for 30 seconds, continually assessing resting symptoms for change in constant pain. If no change or improvement, perform one more repetition of 30 seconds.

Reassess:

Subjectively: patient's resting symptoms.

Objectively: one active movement short of onset of resting symptoms and one passive accessory movement (eg, shoulder flexion and posteroanterior pressure on the glenohumeral joint).

Instructions and warning to the patient:

1. Ask patient to note symptoms over the next 2- and 24-hour time periods.
2. Warn patient of possible treatment soreness, which should be different from symptoms.
3. Instruct patient in icing, proper use of medication(s), and positions of ease.

Day 2

Reassess subjectively and objectively at 2- and 24-hour periods. If improved for short duration and symptoms returned, the treatment worked but not for a long enough period. Keep the same treatment. If worse, may need to do less with present technique, even though condition had already been getting worse. If the patient is the same, perform the same technique and reassess. If still unchanged, the vigor with which the technique is performed.

Follow-up visits should include the following:

1. Clearing of all shoulder physiological and accessory movements with overpressure.
2. Clearing of the rotator cuff muscles.
3. Completion of the neurological examination for the upper quarter.

The home program should address rotator cuff, scapular stabilizers, and postural exercises for improvement of thoracic spine extension.

Clinical decision making for the above physical therapy diagnosis is based on:

1. Age of patient and female gender.
2. History of diabetes.
3. Trauma leading to gradual onset, possibly secondary to painful use.
4. Sleep significantly affected, patient not able to lie on shoulder.
5. Capsular pattern restrictions: lateral rotation most limited, followed by abduction.
6. Passive accessory movements of the capsule and its related structures significantly decreased.

Case #3: Instability Versus Impingement

SUBJECTIVE EXAMINATION

Patient Profile

The patient is a 25-year-old male, self-employed gardener, who is presently working. He plays softball twice a week but is currently unable to play because of shoulder pain. He is right hand dominant.

His chief complaint is an intermittent, deep sharp pain in the anterior portion of the right shoulder. He also complains of an intermittent deep ache after use of the right shoulder (see Figure 30–57).

Aggravating Factors

1. Reaching overhead when throwing a softball produces a catch type of sharp pain that goes away immediately once out of this position. (Possible test movements include the functional movement of throwing, the shoulder quadrant, and the rotator cuff.)
2. Turning a steering wheel to the left produces the sharp catch pain; symptoms resolve once out of this position. (Possible testing includes the impingement tests.)
3. Lifting gardening tools and placing them in the truck is associated with immediate onset of sharp pain. Sharp pain immediately goes away, but a dull ache remains for about 1 to 3 minutes depending on the weight of the object. (Test rotator cuff muscles at different ranges and speeds.)
4. Deep ache often comes on when putting weight through the arm. Ache can last up to 5 minutes once out of position. (Test for structures that might compress the subacromial space and the intra-articular structures of the glenohumeral joint. A quick test would be to have the patient perform a push-up.)

Easing Factors

1. Not using right shoulder.
2. If aggravated, a hot shower seems to help temporarily.

24-Hour Day

1. Night: Sleeping or rolling over onto the right arm will awaken him; he will also awaken if sleeping on the left side with his right arm hanging down. He

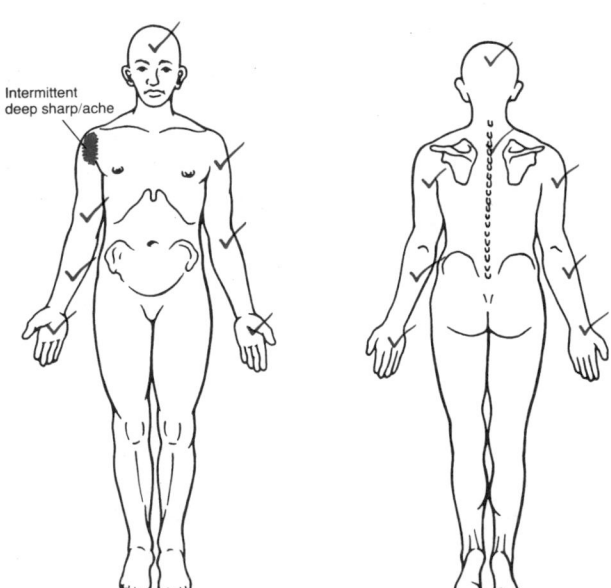

Intermittent deep sharp/ache

FIGURE 30–57 Body chart of impingement versus instability case study.

wakes up three to four times a night. He can return to sleep immediately.

2. Morning: The shoulder feels stiff but has no pain unless he moves it.
3. Day: The pain in the shoulder is more dependent on activity and use.

Present History

Approximately 1 month previously, while playing softball, the patient threw a ball from right field to home plate. He felt something "move in the joint" but denies an actual dislocation. He says it felt more like something was "loose." He did not experience any pain with this incident and continued to play the game. He had some soreness in the arm that evening, but the next morning the shoulder felt fine. He continued to play as usual that week. Two weeks ago, while walking on a wet lawn, he slipped and fell on his right elbow and experienced immediate sharp pain in the right shoulder. He noticed difficulty raising the right shoulder because of pain, but he also felt weakness. Presently, he still experiences the same sharp pain if attempting to elevate the shoulder. Additionally, he feels a deep ache in the shoulder if it hangs unsupported for greater than 30-minute periods. He denies any neck symptoms at this time.

Past History

The patient denies any past trauma to shoulder or neck.

Special Questions

General health: ✔✔
Weight loss/gain: ✔✔
Medications: tried ibuprofen, 800 mg three times a day, without change; stopped because no changes were noticed.
Steroids/anticoagulants: ✔✔
Radiography/special tests: plain films of right shoulder normal.
Vertebral artery: ✔✔
Cord signs: ✔✔

SINS

Initial impressions from the subjective examination that will guide the objective examination for determining the vigor in testing are:

Severity: Nonsevere. Pain is of an intermittent quality; the patient is able to continue with daily activities, eg, work a normal shift. Mild severity could be considered if looking at how it affects his sleep.
Irritability: Nonirritable. He can do a movement that brings on the sharp pain, but it is only present when in that position. The ache is also of short enough duration to be of a nonirritable character.

Nature: The disorder has the type of pain quality such that certain stabilizing structures of the joint, eg, capsule, labrum, and/or ligaments, would be indicated. The cuff could also be implicated.
Stability: Stable. He has not had any other episodes or trauma. However, the therapist must take into consideration his predisposition of joint laxity.
Stage: Acute. Recent onset with no other episodes.

Examination instructions for patient: instruct patient to perform movements to available range.

OBJECTIVE EXAMINATION

Observation

Questionable slight winging of the scapula, but this is not obvious.

Active Physiological Movements (Shoulder)

F: to 85 degrees before experiencing a catch pain in the right anterior shoulder and continuing the movement, finishing at 180. There is slight hiking of the scapula on the right just prior to the catch pain. When overpressure is applied at the end of range, the same local pain is elicited. On return from full flexion, the catch pain is more severe at 110 degrees, and he loses control of the arm, bringing it back to neutral quickly.
Abd: similar catch pain as flexion but at 75 degrees with some scapula hiking. Follows similar pattern as flexion movement.
ER: full 100 degrees discomfort with overpressure.
HBB: right equals left for range. When overpressure is applied, he experiences some right anterior shoulder pain different from complaint. Important note is that he does not feel that pain on the left with overpressure. The dull ache pain from this maneuver takes 1 minute to settle.
HF: on full range of motion, he experiences anterior sharp shoulder pain at end of range.

Resisted Cuff Tests

Abd: gradual buildup of resistance, slight pain at approximately 5 seconds holding in the right shoulder.
ER: same as abduction, but earlier onset of shoulder pain.
IR: strong and painless.
Elbow flexion: strong with slight pain in the anterior shoulder.

Cervical Spine Clearing

Active physiological movements:

Right rot: ✔✔
Left rot: ✔✔
Lower cervical quadrant, left and right: ✔✔

Neurological

Reflexes: biceps and triceps jerk 2/2 brisk.

Motor: C5 deltoid on the right 5−/5 because of pain; C6 to T1 5/5.

Sensation: light touch intact.

Passive Physiological Movements (Shoulder)

F: onset of anterior shoulder pain (P1) at 160 degrees.

Abd: onset of anterior and superior shoulder pain at 120 degrees.

ER: onset of anterior shoulder pain (P1) at 90 degrees.

IR: onset of anterior shoulder pain (P1) at 60 degrees.

HF: pain with overpressure in the anterior and posterior portions of the right shoulder.

Lock test: superior acromiohumeral area, pain with overpressure. Not the same pain, but no pain on the left side.

Quadrant: top of hill onset of anterior shoulder pain at end of range. (This maneuver was the most reproductive of the patient's complaint of pain.)

Palpation (Shoulder)

1. Soft tissue: anterior and posterior portions of capsule slightly tender; supraspinatus and infraspinatus tendons at insertion slightly thickened and painful. This was also similar to the sharp pain the patient experienced with certain movements.
2. Muscle testing:
   - Serratus anterior on the right 5/5, but when tested in a retracted position had difficulty stabilizing.
   - In sidelying, tested quality of muscle recruitment by performing scapula proprioceptive neuromuscular facilitation patterns. Weakness in performance of posterior depression and anterior elevation at end of scapula's available range.
3. Passive accessory movements:
   - Right glenohumeral joint: ✔✔
   - Anteroposterior pressure: ✔✔
   - Posteroanterior pressure: ✔✔
   - Caudal glide: slight local stretch at end of range. In shoulder quadrant position, anteroposterior pressure reproduced the pain.

Palpation (Cervical Spine)

1. Soft tissue: no obvious abnormalities or thickened swollen areas.
2. Passive accessory movements:
   - Anteroposterior pressure: on the right at C5–C6, slight hypomobility but no reproduction of symptoms.

Special Tests

1. Instability tests for shoulder:
   - Anterior drawer: at 120 degrees of abduction, some play was noted and tenderness in the anterior shoulder region as compared to the left.
   - Posterior drawer and inferior glide: ✔✔

2. Impingement test: with the arm in 90 degrees of flexion and internal rotation with overpressure, reproduced pain in anteromedial portion of the right shoulder.
3. Isometric resisted abduction at 30 degrees of abduction performed with and without slight distraction of right arm produced a slight pain response.
4. Testing for intra-articular compression of the glenohumeral joint: ✔✔
5. Testing for the acromiohumeral space was uncomfortable but did not reproduce symptoms.

Reassessment After Objective Examination

1. No change in symptoms subjectively.
2. Objectively, shoulder flexion had same arc of pain in both directions, but movement of the scapulohumeral rhythm was smoother.
3. Resistive test still positive for pain of the rotator cuff tendons.
4. Shoulder quadrant still painful, but onset is noted later in the range.

PHYSICAL THERAPY DIAGNOSIS

Instability appears to be the primary problem with static constraints; possibly the capsule and glenohumeral ligaments are affected. Also, normal timing of the scapulohumeral joint is off because of muscle imbalances and weakness of the scapula stabilizers. Impingement is secondary to the primary instability.

Prognosis

If the static stabilizers are still intact with some scarring of the capsule, good outcome can be expected. The patient has not had prior trauma, but aberrant movement patterns are possibly long-standing and need to be changed.

Expected Outcome

1. Painful arc to decrease 50% in 1 to 2 weeks.
2. Return to 80% function of use of arm for overhead activities, which will be dependent on integrity of the noncontractile structures, particularly the capsule and glenohumeral ligaments. Also, if partial tear or tendinitis of rotator cuff, 4 to 6 weeks. If full tear of cuff or lesion to capsule or ligaments without surgical intervention, 3 to 6 months.
3. A 95% full recovery will take 3 months to 1 year, depending on the rotator cuff and the dynamic stabilizers of the scapula and its related noncontractile structures.

TREATMENT

Day 1

Technique: right shoulder quadrant just into pain where symptom reproduction is most significant.

Position patient: supine.

Therapist: perform technique to pain for 30 seconds to 1 minute, assessing symptoms for changes in symptoms. If tolerated, repeat same technique two to three times since irritability is mild.

Reassess:

Subjectively: patient's resting symptoms.
Objectively: one active movement and one passive accessory movement (eg, shoulder abduction and posteroanterior pressure on the glenohumeral joint in the shoulder quadrant position). Reassess scapula movement with proprioceptive neuromuscular facilitation patterns.

Instructions and warning to the patient:

1. Ask patient to note symptoms over the next 2- and 24-hour time periods.
2. Warn patient of possible treatment soreness, which should be different from symptoms.
3. Instruct patient in icing and positions of ease.
4. Initiate exercise program with weight-bearing exercises for scapula stabilization, eg, push-up plus.
5. Optional: if the dependent position is bothersome, tape the humerus from anterior to posterior trunk to provide support and proprioception for shoulder stabilization.

Day 2

Reassess subjectively and objectively at 2- and 24-hour periods. If painful arc improved for short duration and symptoms returned, the treatment worked but not for a long enough period. Perform the same treatment for longer. If worse, what is worse, when did it get worse, and how is it worse? If the patient is the same, perform the same technique and reassess. If unchanged, the therapist may be able to increase the technique by changing the position in which the technique is performed (eg, posteroanterior pressure on the glenohumeral joint with the shoulder in the quadrant position) or increase the vigor with which the technique is performed.

Follow-up visits should include the following:

1. Clearing of all shoulder physiological and accessory movements with overpressure This includes the acromioclavicular joint, sternoclavicular joint, and special tests.
2. Strengthening of the rotator cuff and scapula muscles with eccentric and concentric control (closed and open kinetic chain exercises).

Strengthening needs to be performed in the position of instability, ie, 90 degrees abduction/flexion, for true functional strength.

Clinical decision making for the above physical therapy diagnosis is based on:

1. Pain deep in anterior shoulder, deep in joint.
2. Pain worse with overhead activities.
3. Horizontal flexion can compress anterior labrum and capsule.
4. Pain in an arc of movement, or of catch quality.
5. Pain reproduced with the shoulder quadrant test and worse when a posteroanterior pressure is applied in this position.
6. History of trauma.
7. Excessive joint laxity throughout.
8. Stability testing significant when compared to the affected side.
9. Positive impingement tests implicating subacromial structures.
10. Weakness of the scapula stabilizers when tested in the shortened position.

References

1. Cyriax J, Cyriax PJ: Illustrated Manual of Orthopaedic Medicine 2nd ed. London, Baillière Tindall, 1993.
2. Maitland GD: Passive movement techniques for intra-articular and periarticular disorders. Physiotherapy 1985, 31:3–8.
3. Farrell JP, Jensen GM: Manual therapy: a critical assessment of role in the profession of physical therapy. Phys Ther 1992, 72:843–852.
4. Jones MA: Clinical reasoning in manual therapy. Phys Ther 1992, 72:875–883.
5. Maitland GD: Peripheral Manipulation 3rd ed. London, Butterworth Publishers, 1991.
6. Myers RS, Rose SJ: Introduction: clinical decision making in physical therapy practice, education, and research. Phys Ther 1989, 69:523.
7. Higgs J: Developing clinical reasoning competences. Physiotherapy 1992, 78:575–581.
8. Higgs J: Fostering the acquisition of clinical reasoning skills. N Z J Physiotherapy 1990, 18:13–17.
9. Jette AM: Measuring subjective clinical outcomes. Phys Ther 1989, 69:580–584.
10. Rothstein JM: Manual therapy: a special issue and a special topic. Phys Ther 1992, 72:837–839.
11. Rothstein JM: On defining subjective and objective measurements. Phys Ther 1989, 69:577–579.
12. Delitto A, Shuylman AD, Rose SJ: On developing expert-based decision-support systems in physical therapy: the NIOSH low back atlas. Phys Ther 1989, 69:554–558.
13. Jensen GM, Shepard KF, Gwyer J, et al.: Attribute dimensions that distinguish master and novice physical therapy clinicians in orthopedic settings. Phys Ther 1992, 72:711–722.
14. Jensen GM, Shepard KF, Hack LM: The novice versus the experienced clinician: insights into the work of the physical therapist. Phys Ther 1990, 70:314–323.
15. Dekker J, Van Baar ME, Curfs EM, et al.: Diagnosis and treatment in physical therapy: an investigation of their relationship. Phys Ther 1993, 73:568–580.
16. Rose SJ: Physical therapy diagnosis: role and function. Phys Ther 1989, 69:535–537.
17. Sahrmann SA: Diagnosis by the physical therapist—a prerequisite for treatment: a special communication. Phys Ther 1988, 68:1703–1706.

18. Higgs J: Developing knowledge: a process of construction, mapping, and review. *N Z J Physiotherapy* 1992, 20:23–30.

19. Maitland GD: *Vertebral Manipulation* 5th ed. London, Butterworth Publishers, 1986.

20. Rothstein JM: The case for case reports. *Phys Ther* 1993, 73:492–493.

21. Gonnella C: Single-subject experimental paradigm as a clinical decision tool. *Phys Ther* 1989, 69:601–609.

22. Potter NA, Rothstein JM: Intertester reliability for selected clinical tests of the sacroiliac joint. *Phys Ther* 1985, 58:74–78.

23. Jones MA: Clinical reasoning. In Butler D (ed): *Mobilisation of the Nervous System*. New York, Churchill Livingstone, 1991, pp 91–106.

24. Watts NT: Clinical decision analysis. *Phys Ther* 1989, 69:569–576.

25. Echternach JL, Rothstein JM: Hypothesis-oriented algorithms. *Phys Ther* 1989, 69:559–564.

26. Maitland GD: The Maitland concept: assessment, examination, and treatment by passive movement. In Twomey LT, Taylor J (eds): *Physical Therapy of the Low Back*. New York, Churchill Livingstone, 1987, 135–155.

27. Silliman JF, Hawkins RJ: Current concepts and recent advances in the athlete's shoulder. *Clin Sports Med* 1991, 10:693–706.

28. Workman TL, Burkhard TK, Resnick D, *et al.:* Hill-Sachs lesion: comparison of detection with MR imaging, radiography, and arthroscopy. *Radiology* 1992, 185:847–852.

29. Ho CP: Applied MRI anatomy of the shoulder. *J Orthop Sports Phys Ther* 1993, 18:351–359.

30. Iannotti JP, Zlatkin MB, Esterhai JL, *et al.:* Magnetic resonance imaging of the shoulder. *J Bone Joint Surg* [Am], 1991, 73:17–29.

31. Recht MP, Resnick D: Magnetic resonance imaging studies of the shoulder. *J Bone Joint Surg* [Am], 1993, 75:1244–1253.

32. Stiles RG, Otte MT: Imaging of the shoulder. *Radiology* 1993, 188:603–613.

33. Harryman DT, Sidles JA, Clark JM, *et al.:* Translation of the humeral head on the glenoid with passive glenohumeral motion. *J Bone Joint Surg* [Am] 1990, 72:1334–1343.

34. Rockwood CA, Lyons FR: Shoulder impingement syndrome: diagnosis, radiographic evaluation, and treatment with a modified Neer acromioplasty. *J Bone Joint Surg* [Am], 1993, 75:409–423.

35. Fu FH, Harner CD, Klein AH: Shoulder impingement syndrome: a critical review. *Clin Orthop* 1991, 269:162–173.

36. Hawkins R, Abrams J: Impingement syndrome in the absence of rotator cuff tear. Stages 1 and 2. *Orthop Clin North Am* 1987, 18:373–382.

37. Neer CS: Impingement lesions. *Clin Orthop* 1983, 173:70–77.

38. Jobe FW, Pink M: Classification and treatment of shoulder dysfunction in the overhead athlete. *J Orthop Sports Phys Ther* 1993, 8:427–432.

39. Jobe FW, Bradley JP: The diagnosis and nonoperative treatment of shoulder injuries in athletes. *Clin Sports Med* 1989, 8:419–438.

40. Jobe FW, Kuitne RS, Giangarra CE: Shoulder pain in the overhand throwing athlete: the relationship of anterior instability and rotator cuff impingement. *Orthop Rev* 1989, 18:963–975.

41. Kamkar A, Irrgang JJ, Whitney SL: Nonoperative management of secondary shoulder impingement syndrome. *J Orthop Sports Phys Ther* 1993, 17:212–224.

42. Harryman DT, Sidles JA, Harris SL, *et al.:* The role of the rotator interval capsule in passive motion and stability of the shoulder. *J Bone Joint Surg* [Am] 1992, 74:53–66.

43. Matsen FA, Harryman DT, Sidles JA: Mechanics of glenohumeral instability. *Clin Sports Med* 1991, 10:783–788.

44. Bradley JP, Tibone JE: Electromyographic analysis of muscle action about the shoulder. *Clin Sports Med* 1991, 10:789–805.

45. Browne AO, Hoffmeyer P, Tanaka S, *et al.:* Glenohumeral elevation studied in three dimensions. *J Bone Joint Surg* [Am] 1990, 72:843–845.

46. Culham E, Peat M: Functional anatomy of the shoulder complex. *J Orthop Sports Phys Ther* 1993, 18:342–350.

47. Freedman L, Munro R: Abduction of the arm in the scapular plane: scapular and glenohumeral movements. *J Bone Joint Surg* [Am] 1966, 48:1503–1510.

48. Norkin CC, Levangie PK: *Joint Structure and Function: A Comprehensive Analysis* 2nd ed. Philadelphia, F. A. Davis Company, 1992.

49. Moseley JB, Jobe FW, Pink M, *et al.:* EMG analysis of the scapular muscles during a shoulder rehabilitation program. *Am J Sports Med* 1992, 20:128–135.

50. Kibler WB: Role of the scapula in the overhead throwing motion. *Contemp Orthop* 1991, 22:525–532.

51. Payne RM, Voight M: The role of the scapula. *J Orthop Sports Phys Ther* 1993, 18:386–391.

52. Poppen NK, Walker PS: Normal and abnormal motion of the shoulder. *J Bone Joint Surg* [Am] 1976, 58:195–201.

53. Poppen NK, Walker PS: Forces at the glenohumeral joint in abduction. *Clin Orthop* 1978, 135:165–170.

54. Saha AK: Mechanism of shoulder movements and a plea for the recognition of "Zero Position" of glenohumeral joint. *Clin Orthop* 1983, 173:3–10.

55. Townsend H, Jobe FW, Pink M, *et al.:* Electromyographic analysis of the glenohumeral muscles during a baseball rehabilitation program. *Am J Sports Med* 1991, 19:264–271.

56. Zuckerman JD, Masten FA III: Biomechanics of the shoulder. In Nordin M, Frankel VH (eds): *Basic Biomechanics of the Musculoskeletal System* 2nd ed. Philadelphia, Lea & Febiger, 1989, pp 235–247.

57. Andrews JR, Kupferman SP, Dillman CJ: Labral tears in throwing and racquet sports. *Clin Sports Med* 1991, 10:901–911.

58. Rames RD, Karzel RP: Injuries to the glenoid labrum, including SLAP lesions. *Orthop Clin* 1993, 29:45–53.

59. Kapandji IA: *The Physiology of Joints. Upper Limb* 5th ed. vol 1. New York, Churchill Livingstone, 1982.

60. Perry J: Anatomy and biomechanics of the shoulder in throwing, swimming, gymnastics and tennis. *Clin Sports Med* 1983, 2:247–270.

61. Kent BE: Functional anatomy of the shoulder complex. A review. *Phys Ther* 1971, 51:867–888.

62. Peat M: Functional anatomy of the shoulder complex. *Phys Ther* 1986, 66:1855–1865.

63. Elvey R: Functional anatomy of the shoulder joint. In *Proceedings of the Fourth Biennial Conference, Manipulative Therapists Association of Australia*. Brisbane, Australia, 1985.

64. Andrews JR, Gidamal RH: Shoulder arthroscopy in the throwing athlete: perspectives and prognosis. *Arthroscopy* 1987, 6:565.

65. Bigliani LU, Ticker JB, Flatow EL, *et al.:* The relationship of acromial architecture to rotator cuff disease. *Clin Sports Med* 1991, 10:823–838.

66. Epstein RE, Schweitzer ME, Frieman BG, *et al.:* Hooked acromion: prevalence on MR images of painful shoulders. *Radiology* 1993, 187:497.

67. Schneider G: Restricted shoulder movement: capsular contracture or cervical referral—a clinical study. *Aust J Physiotherapy* 1989, 35:97–100.

68. Shaffer B, Tibone JE, Kerlan RK: Frozen shoulder. *J Bone Joint Surg* [Am] 1992, 74:738–746.

69. Lundberg BJ: Glycosaminoglycans of the normal and frozen shoulder-joint capsule. *Clin Orthop* 1970, 69:279–284.

70. Lundberg BJ: The frozen shoulder. *Acta Orthop Scand* 1969, 119(suppl):1–59.

71. Hulstyn MJ, Weiss APC: Adhesive capsulitis of the shoulder. *Orthop Rev* 1993, 22:425–433.

72. Friedman NA, LaBan MM: Periarthrosis of the shoulder associated with diabetes mellitus. *Am J Phys Med Rehabil* 1989, 68:12–14.

73. Hawkins RJ: Cervical spine and the shoulder. *Instr Lect Notes* 1985, 34:191–195.

74. Macnab I: Cervical spondylosis. *Clin Orthop* 1975, 109:74.

75. Wells P: Cervical dysfunction and shoulder problems. *Physiotherapy* 1982, 68:71.

76. Moseley HF, Overgaard B: The anterior capsular mechanism in recurrent anterior dislocation of the shoulder. Morphological and clinical studies with special reference to the glenoid labrum and glenohumeral ligaments. *J Bone Joint Surg* [Br] 1962, 44:913–927.

77. Cooper DE, Arnoczky SP, O'Brien SJ, et al.: Anatomy, histology, and vascularity of the glenoid labrum: an anatomical study. *J Bone Joint Surg* [Am] 1992, 74:46–52.

78. Williams PL, Warwick R (eds): *Gray's Anatomy* 36th ed. London, Churchill Livingstone, 1980.

79. O'Connell PW, Nuber GW, Mileski RA, et al.: The contribution of the glenohumeral ligaments to anterior stability of the shoulder joint. *Am J Sports Med* 1990, 18:579–584.

80. Turkel SJ, Panio MW, Marshall JL, et al.: Stabilizing mechanisms preventing anterior dislocation of the glenohumeral joint. *J Bone Joint Surg* [Am] 1981, 63:1208–1217.

81. Cain P, Mutschler T, Fu F, et al.: Anterior stability of the glenohumeral joint. *Am J Sports Med* 1987, 15:144–148.

82. Ferrari DA: Capsular ligaments of the shoulder. *Am J Sports Med* 1990, 18:20–24.

83. Norwood LA, Barrack R, Jacobson K: Clinical presentation of complete tears of the rotator cuff. *J Bone Joint Surg* [Am] 1989, 71:499–505.

84. Brookes CH, Revell WJ, Heatley FW: A quantitative histological study of the vascularity of the rotator cuff tendon. *J Bone Joint Surg* [Am] 1992, 74:151–153.

85. Ozaki J, Fujimoto S, Nakagawa Y, et al.: Tears of the rotator cuff of the shoulder associated with pathological changes in the acromion. *J Bone Joint Surg* [Am] 1988, 70:1224–1230.

86. Warner JJP, Krushell RJ, Masquelet A, et al.: Anatomy and relationships of the suprascapular nerve: anatomical constraints to mobilization of the supraspinatus and infraspinatus muscles in the management of massive rotator-cuff tears. *J Bone Joint Surg* [Am] 1992, 74:36–45.

87. Mullen F: Locking and quadrant of the shoulder: relationships of the humerus and scapula during locking and quadrant. In *Proceedings of the Sixth Biennial Conference, Manipulative Therapist Association of Australia*. Adelaide, Australia, 1989. pp 130–137.

88. Slade S: The glenohumeral joint capsule: its role in the quadrant test. In *Proceedings of the Manipulative Therapist Association of Australia*. Adelaide, Australia, 1989, pp 130–137.

89. Inman VT, Saunders JB, Abbot L: Observations on the function of the shoulder joint. *J Bone Joint Surg* [Am] 1944, 26:1–30.

90. Proprioceptive neuromuscular facilitation lecture notes. Kaiser Residency Program. Vallejo, CA, 1987.

91. Goodman CC, Snyder TEK: *Differential Diagnosis in Physical Therapy. Musculoskeletal and Systemic Conditions*. Philadelphia, W. B. Saunders Company, 1990.

92. Graduate program in manipulative therapy course notes. Curtin University of Technology, Perth, Australia 1988.

93. Trott PH: Differential mechanical diagnosis of shoulder pain. In *Proceedings of the Fourth Biennial Conference, Manipulative Therapists Association of Australia*. Brisbane, Australia, 1985, pp 284–299.

94. Trott PH, Grant R: Shoulder in focus. Course notes. Kaiser Residency Program. Hayward, CA, 1990.

95. Cloward R: Cervical discography: a contribution to the etiology and mechanism of neck, shoulder, and arm pain. *Ann Surg* 1959, 150:1052.

96. Elvey RL: Brachial plexus tension tests and the pathoanatomical origin of arm pain. In Glasgow E, Twomey LT (ed): *Aspects of Manipulative Therapy*, 2nd ed. New York, Churchill Livingstone, 1985, pp 105–110.

97. Vargo MM, Flood KM: Pancoast tumor presenting as cervical radiculopathy. *Arch Phys Med Rehabil* 1990, 71:606–609.

98. Kendall FP, McCleary EK: *Muscles, Testing and Function*, 3rd ed. Baltimore, Williams & Wilkins, 1983.

99. Sullivan PE, Markos PD, Minor MA: *An Integrated Approach to Therapeutic Exercise. Theory and Clinical Application*. Reston, VA, Reston Publishing, 1982.

100. Voss DE, Ionta MK, Myers BJ: *Proprioceptive Neuromuscular Facilitation. Patterns and Techniques*, 3rd ed. Philadelphia, Harper & Row, 1985.

101. Dempsey D: Personal communication, 1989.

102. Watson M: Rotator cuff function in the impingement syndrome. *J Bone Joint Surg* [Br] 1989, 71:361–366.

103. Gerber C, Ganz R: Clinical assessment of instability of the shoulder with special reference to anterior and posterior drawer tests. *J Bone Joint Surg* [Br] 1984, 66:551–556.

104. Stockmeyer SA: An interpretation of the approach of Rood to the treatment of neuromuscular dysfunction. *Am J Phys Med* 1967, 46:900–949.

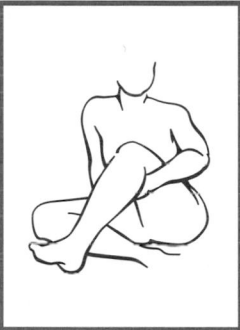

CHAPTER 31

Elbow, Forearm, Wrist, and Hand

Carolyn T. Wadsworth

To make precise clinical decisions regarding the management of disorders of the elbow, forearm, wrist, and hand, a clinician relies on knowledge and understanding of the clinical anatomy, kinesiology, pathomechanics, differential diagnoses, and treatments of choice of these highly specialized areas of the body. A competent therapist must also possess astute clinical observation skills and the technical ability to apply intricate manual testing and treatment maneuvers.

Throughout examination and treatment, a therapist must appreciate the complexity of upper extremity function and the delicate balance and interplay of the numerous parts that allow the hand to perform movements that require power or precision. Rarely is the position of one joint independent of those of the other joints; active and passive restraints, intrinsic and extrinsic motors, and sensory feedback loops all interact to produce the remarkable dexterity that characterizes this unit. This chapter addresses normal function and dysfunction of the elbow, forearm, wrist, and hand and discusses the current protocols for their evaluation and treatment.

I. Anatomy

A. Osteology

1. Humerus
  a. The distal end of the humerus widens and has epicondyles that project medially and laterally. Its lateral articular surface bears the dome-shaped capitulum, which articulates with the radius. Its medial articular surface is the pulley-shaped troch-

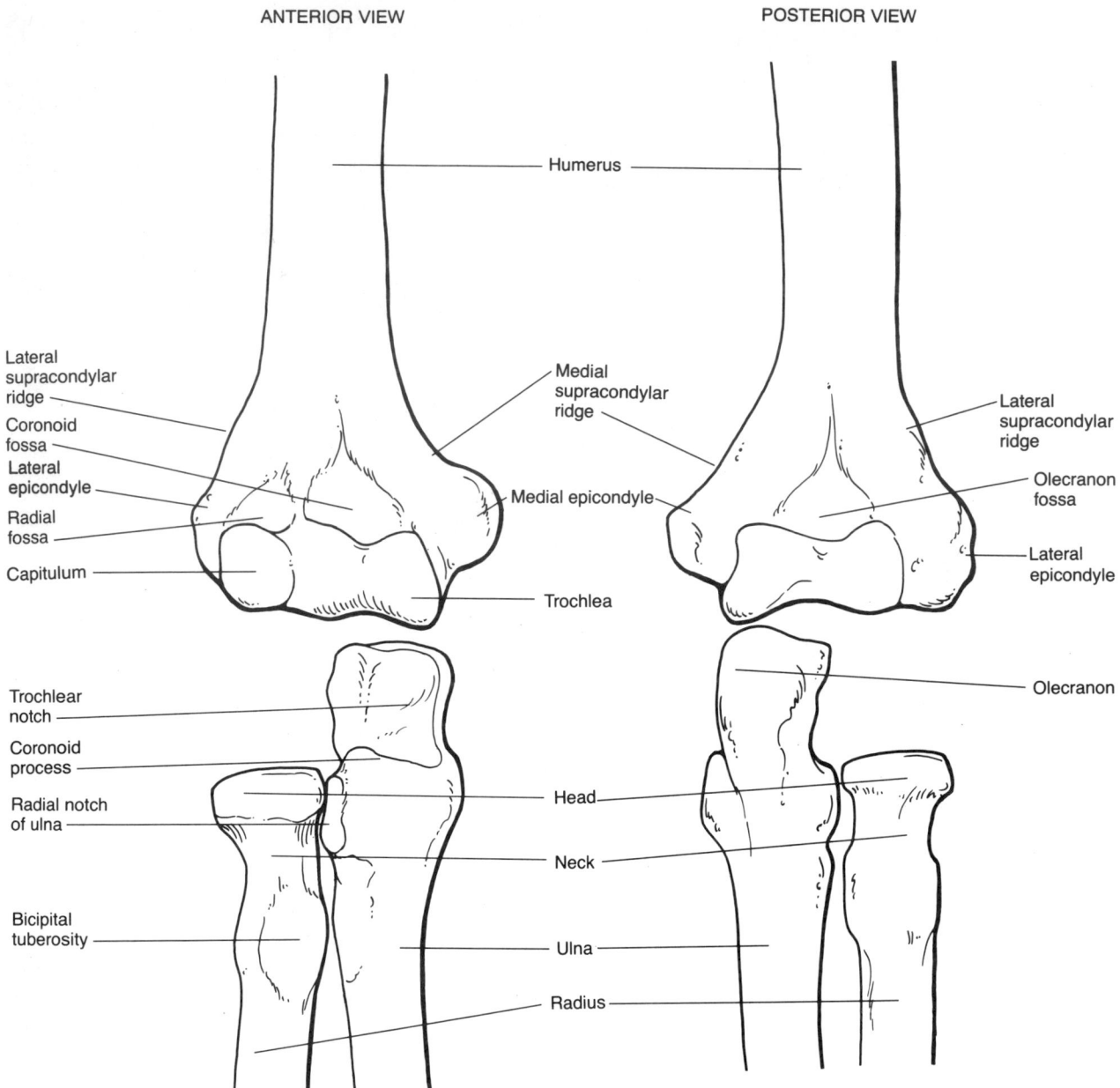

ANTERIOR VIEW

POSTERIOR VIEW

Humerus

Lateral
supracondylar
ridge

Coronoid
fossa

Lateral
epicondyle

Radial
fossa

Capitulum

Medial
supracondylar
ridge

Medial epicondyle

Trochlea

Lateral
supracondylar
ridge

Olecranon
fossa

Lateral
epicondyle

Trochlear
notch

Coronoid
process

Radial notch
of ulna

Bicipital
tuberosity

Olecranon

Head

Neck

Ulna

Radius

FIGURE 31–1   Bones of the right elbow, anterior and posterior views.

lea, which joins with the ulna (see Figure
31–1).

b. Three nonarticulating fossae increase
elbow range of motion (ROM) by delay-
ing bone impact.

  (1). The olecranon fossa is located on
  the posterior aspect of the humerus;
  it contains the tip of the olecranon
  during full extension.

(2). The coronoid fossa is found on the
anteromedial aspect of the humerus;
it receives the coronoid process of
the ulna during full flexion.

(3). The radial fossa is located on the
anterolateral aspect of the humerus;
it accommodates the radial head
during full flexion.

c. The transverse axis of the trochlea assumes a proximolateral to distomedial tilt, which produces a slight valgus angulation (5 degrees to 15 degrees) or "carrying angle" at the elbow. Angulation of greater than 15 degrees (cubitus valgus) may stretch the ulnar nerve excessively.[1]

2. Ulna
   a. The proximal end of the ulna assumes a hooklike shape; its large anteriorly concave surface is the trochlear notch; this notch is deepened by an anterior projection, the coronoid process, and a posterior projection, the olecranon process. A radial notch indents the lateral surface of the ulna, where the ulna contacts the radial head (see Figure 31–1).
   b. The two humeral epicondyles and the olecranon process of the ulna serve as landmarks that should lie in a straight line during elbow extension and form an isosceles triangle during elbow flexion.
   c. The distal end of the ulna is occupied by a small, rounded head that forms the convex articulation in the distal radioulnar joint; a distal projection on the medial aspect of the ulna is the ulnar styloid process (see Figure 31–2).

3. Radius
   a. The proximal end of the radius bears the disc-shaped head, which provides a shallow, concave surface for articulation with the capitulum; the circumference of the head is the convex articular surface in the proximal radioulnar joint. The radial neck is a constricted area just distal to the head. Slightly further distal is an anterior protrusion, the bicipital tuberosity, which offers insertion for the biceps tendon (see Figure 31–1).
   b. Laterally, the lateral humeral epicondyle, olecranon process, and radial head form a triangle. Deep within the center of the triangle lies the posterolateral aspect of the elbow joint capsule, where joint effusion from trauma or disease may be palpated or aspirated.
   c. Distally, the radius widens into a broad, concave articular surface, with indentations where it contacts the scaphoid and lunate bones; a medial indentation also provides the concave surface for articulation with the ulnar head in the distal radioulnar joint (see Figure 31–2). The radial styloid process projects distally from the lateral edge of the radius and lies one half inch more distally than the ulnar styloid process.

4. Carpus
   a. The scaphoid bears a prominent volar tubercle, to which the transverse carpal ligament attaches. The scaphoid is commonly fractured through its midsection, with the proximal fragment being susceptible to avascular necrosis.
   b. The lunate has a semilunar shape. It is the most frequently dislocated carpal bone.
   c. The triquetrum is three cornered and has an oval facet for articulation with the pisiform.
   d. The pisiform is the smallest carpal bone; it provides an attachment surface for several ligaments and tendons.
   e. The trapezium contains a prominent volar tubercle and groove in which lies the flexor carpi radialis (FCR) tendon. Its saddle-shaped articular surface joins the first metacarpal bone.
   f. The trapezoid is small with an irregular shape and four articular surfaces.
   g. The capitate is the largest carpal bone; it is centrally located in the wrist.
   h. The hamate contains a hooklike hamulus, which protects the ulnar artery and nerve.

5. Metacarpus. The metacarpus contains five bones that resemble long bones, with their shafts and expanded ends. The base of the first metacarpal bone is saddle-shaped for articulation in the sellar carpometacarpal joint. The other bases are flattened, articulating in plane joints with one another and the distal row of carpal bones. The head of the first metacarpal bone is pulley shaped for articulation in the hinged first metacarpophalangeal (MP) joint; other heads are biconvex and articulate in the biaxial MP joints (see Figure 31–2).

6. Phalanges. The phalanges include 14 bones that are also similar to long bones. The bases of proximal phalanges two through five are biconcave; the bases of the first proximal phalanx and all of the middle and distal phalanges contain two shallow depressions for articulation in the hinged first MP and all interphalangeal (IP) joints. The heads of proximal and middle phalanges possess two condyles, producing a pulley-shaped articular surface. The heads of the

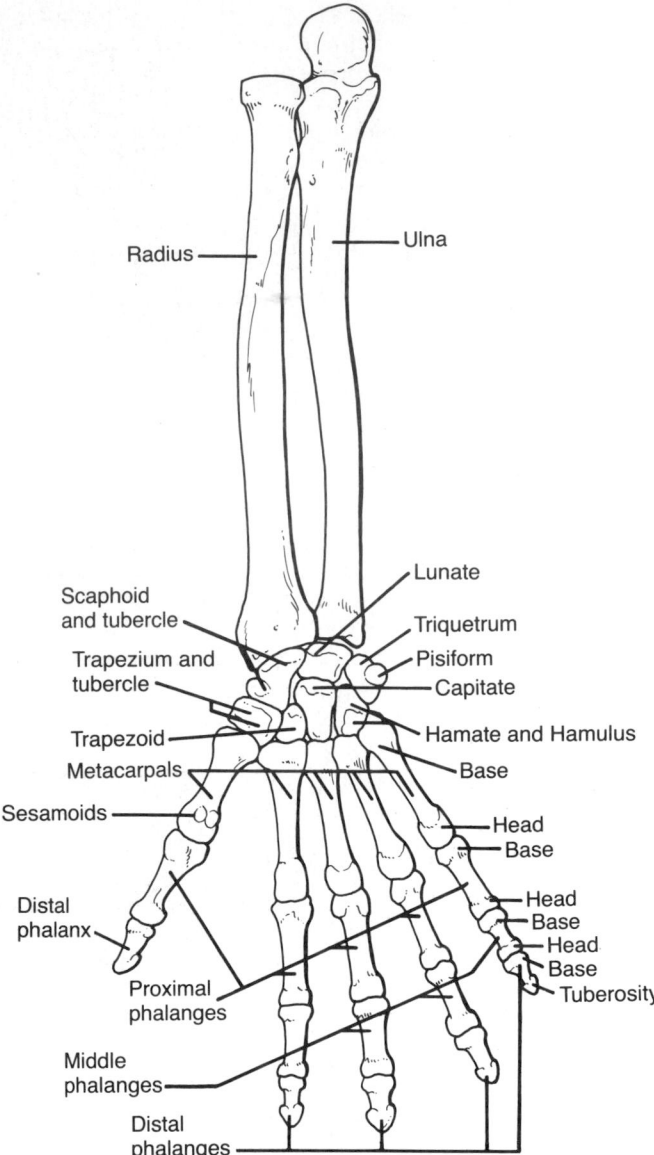

Radius — — Ulna

Scaphoid and tubercle
Trapezium and tubercle
Trapezoid
Metacarpals
Sesamoids

Distal phalanx

Proximal phalanges

Middle phalanges

Distal phalanges

Lunate
Triquetrum
Pisiform
Capitate
Hamate and Hamulus
Base

Head
Base

Head
Base
Head
Base
Tuberosity

FIGURE 31–2   Bones of the forearm, wrist, and hand, anterior view.

distal phalanges taper into points (see Figure 31–2).

7. **Arches.** Arches contribute to the hand's performance of prehensile activities (see Figure 31–3).[1]

a. The longitudinal arch spans the hand longitudinally; it is concave anteriorly.

b. The proximal transverse arch is created within the palmar concavity of the carpal bones. Volar projections of the scaphoid and trapezium bones laterally and of the pisiform and hamate bones medially create this fixed arch of bone. The transverse carpal ligament spans this arch and transforms it into the carpal tunnel.

c. The distal transverse arch is formed by the palmar concavity across the metacarpal heads; it is a relatively mobile arch that may be diminished (flattened) by nerve injuries and improper immobilization of the hand.

8. **Distal ulnar tunnel.** The distal ulnar tunnel is located in the space between the pisiform and hamate bones; its roof consists of the palmar carpal ligament, the palmaris brevis muscle, and the palmar aponeurosis; its floor is formed by the flexor retinaculum and the pisohamate and pisometacarpal ligaments (see Figure 31–3).[2]

B. Arthrology

1. Cubital complex

a. A single joint cavity encloses three joints: the humeroulnar and humeroradial joints, which operate about a common axis to produce elbow flexion and extension ($0°$–$150°$) in a hinged articulation; and the proximal radioulnar joint, which moves about an axis passing between the radial and ulnar heads to produce forearm rotation ($170°$) in a trochoid articulation (see Fig. 31–4).

b. The elbow's articular capsule is thinnest and weakest anteriorly and posteriorly but is reinforced by strong collateral ligaments medially and laterally (see Figure 31–4).

c. Ligaments

(1). The ulnar collateral ligament is the elbow's primary stabilizer, resisting valgus forces encountered in overhead throwing and other forceful motions; an anterior band runs between the medial humeral epicondyle and the coronoid process, and a posterior band runs to the olecranon process. An oblique band joins the others at the base of this triangle-shaped ligament (see Figure 31–4).

(2). The radial collateral ligament passes between the lateral epicondyle and the annular ligament, with some fibers also joining the ulna.

(3). The annular ligament encircles the radial head, maintaining it in contact with the ulna.

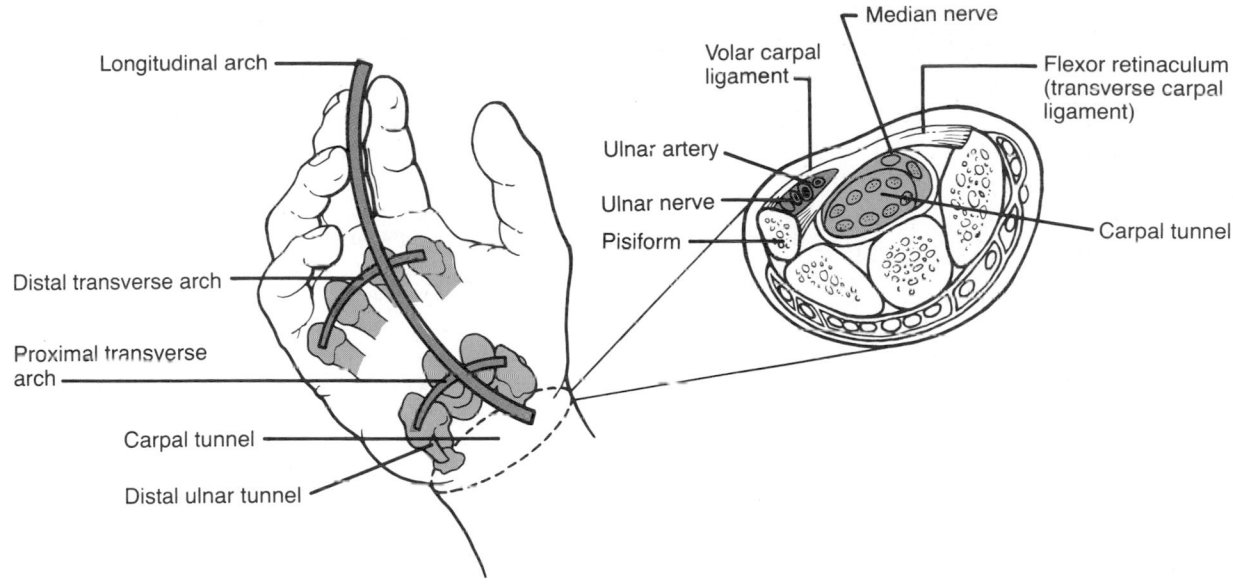

FIGURE 31–3   Arches of the hand and the carpal and distal ulnar tunnels.

(4). The quadrate ligament connects the radial notch (of the ulna) and the radius, reinforcing the inferior joint capsule and checking extreme ranges of pronation and supination.[3]

(5). The oblique cord runs obliquely,

proximomedial from the ulnar tuberosity to distolateral just beyond the radial tuberosity (perpendicular to the interosseous membrane).

(6). The interosseous membrane connects the adjacent radial and ulnar

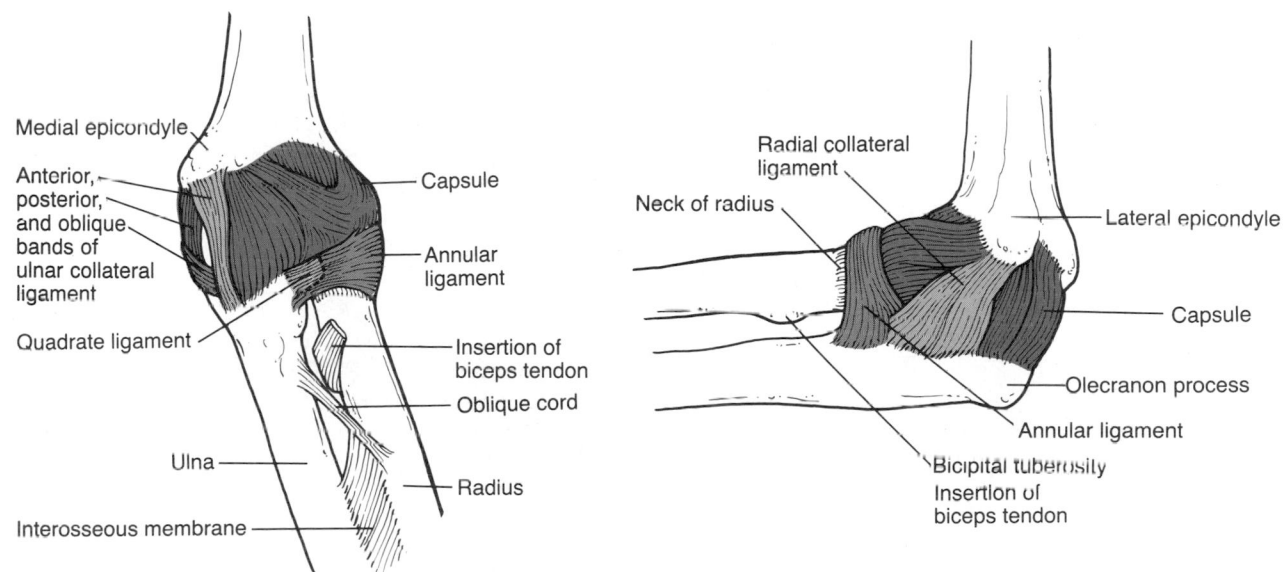

ANTEROMEDIAL VIEW   LATERAL VIEW

FIGURE 31–4   Elbow joint capsule and ligaments, anteromedial and lateral views.

borders; its fibers are oriented in a proximolateral to distomedial direction (see Figure 31–4).

2. Distal radioulnar joint
   a. This is a uniaxial pivot joint, in which the radius sweeps around the convex ulnar head, and the triangular fibrocartilage disc also pivots on the ulnar head; in full pronation (0°–85°) the distal radius crosses the ulna to lie in an anteromedial position, whereas the ulna moves slightly in a posterolateral direction. In full supination (0°–85°) the radius lies parallel and lateral to the ulna.
   b. The distal radioulnar joint's articular capsule attaches to margins of the radius, ulna, and disc, and projects proximally between the bones in a pouch named the recessus sacciformis (see Figure 31–5);

the capsule is lax in a neutral position and is tightened anteriorly during supination and posteriorly during pronation.
   c. The dorsal and volar radioulnar ligaments reinforce the capsule. The triangular fibrocartilage disc also binds the distal radius and ulna; the disc's apex attaches to the ulnar styloid process and its base to the radius. It separates the ulna from contact with the carpal bones (see Figure 31–5). The triangular fibrocartilage complex includes the dorsal and volar ligaments, the ulnar collateral ligament, the disc, and the sheath of the extensor carpi ulnaris (ECU) muscle.[4]

3. Carpal joints. The wrist "links" the forearm and hand through several superimposed segments whose composite movement surpasses that of the individual parts; the draw-

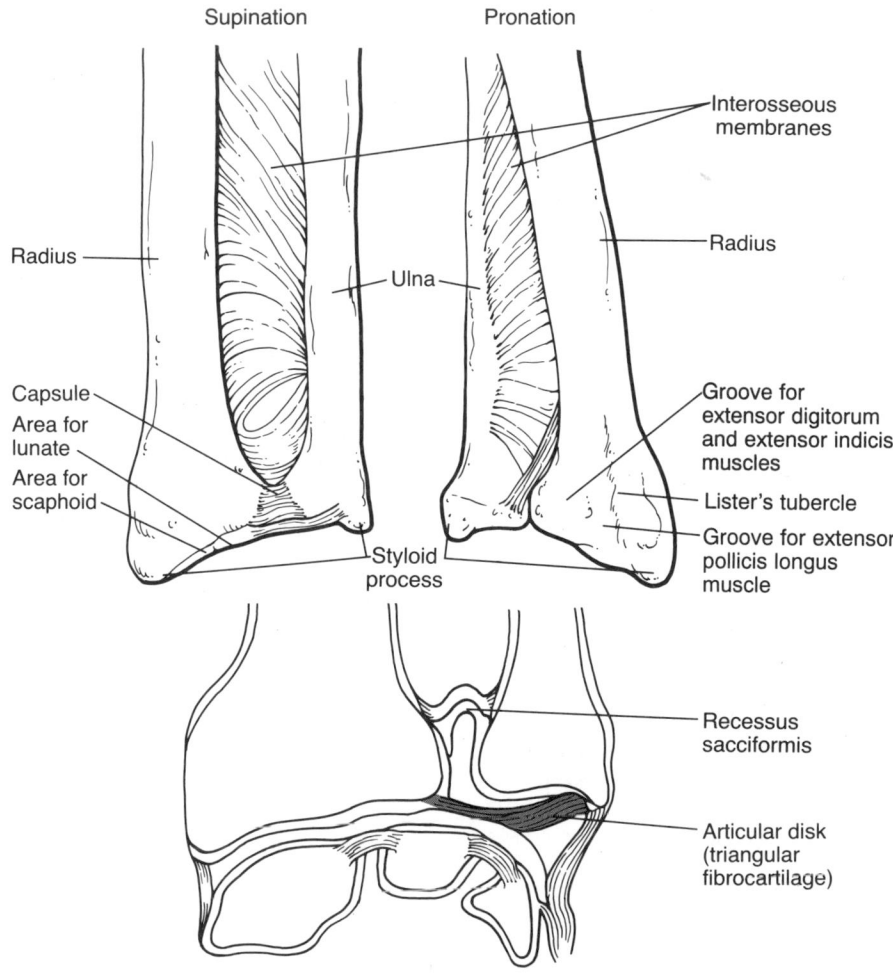

FIGURE 31–5   Distal radioulnar joint.

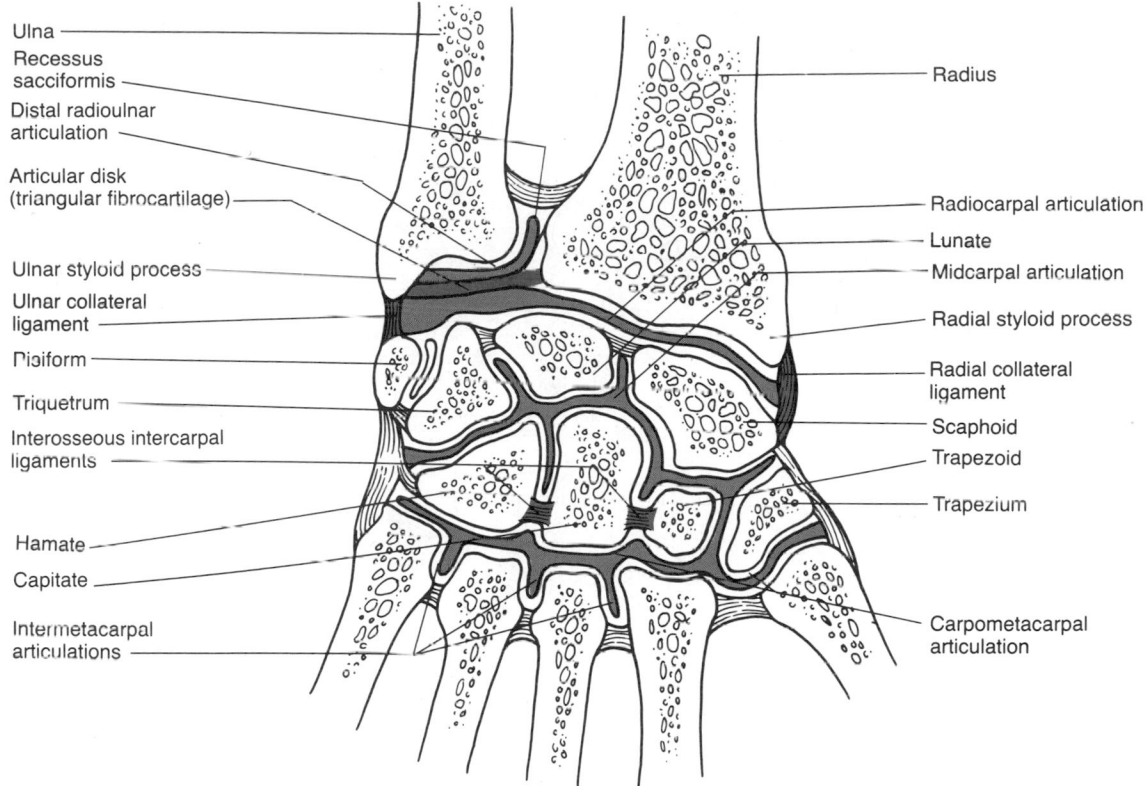

Ulna
Recessus sacciformis
Distal radioulnar articulation
Articular disk (triangular fibrocartilage)
Ulnar styloid process
Ulnar collateral ligament
Pisiform
Triquetrum
Interosseous intercarpal ligaments
Hamate
Capitate
Intermetacarpal articulations

Radius
Radiocarpal articulation
Lunate
Midcarpal articulation
Radial styloid process
Radial collateral ligament
Scaphoid
Trapezoid
Trapezium
Carpometacarpal articulation

FIGURE 31–6   Cross-section of the carpal joints.

back of this arrangement is the increased potential for instability. Numerous intercarpal ligaments, some of which are not named, bind the carpal bones together dorsally and volarly. One large synovial cavity encloses the wrist but is divided by interosseous ligaments into the following separate compartments (see Figure 31–6):

a. The radiocarpal joint is the articulation between the concave radius and the convex row of proximal carpal bones.

b. The midcarpal joint is the articulation between the proximal and distal rows of carpal bones; the proximal row is convex laterally and concave medially, with the distal row reciprocally shaped. Coupled with the radiocarpal joint, the midcarpal produces the biaxial wrist movements of 80 degrees of extension, 85 degrees of flexion, 20 degrees of radial deviation, and 35 degrees of ulnar deviation.

c. The common carpometacarpal joint is the plane articulation between the distal carpal bones and the bases of metacarpals two through five. It produces a slight

gliding that increases from the second to the fifth metacarpals, allowing cupping of the palm and enhancing the distal transverse arch.

d. The trapeziometacarpal joint is the sellar articulation between the trapezium and the first metacarpal; it permits thenar extension to 60 degrees, abduction to 50 degrees, and axial rotation to 17 degrees.

e. The pisiform-triquetral joint is a small plane joint that allows the pisiform to glide on the triquetrum.

4. MP joints

a. The MP joint of the thumb is a hinge joint that resembles the bone configuration of the interphalangeal joints with their inherent stability. The joint permits 0 degrees to 50 degrees of flexion. The articular capsule is reinforced by the volar and collateral ligaments (see Figure 31–7).

b. The MP joints of the fingers are biaxial joints that permit 20 degrees of abduction, 90 degrees of flexion, and 25 degrees of extension. The joint capsules are reinforced by the dorsal hood and volar

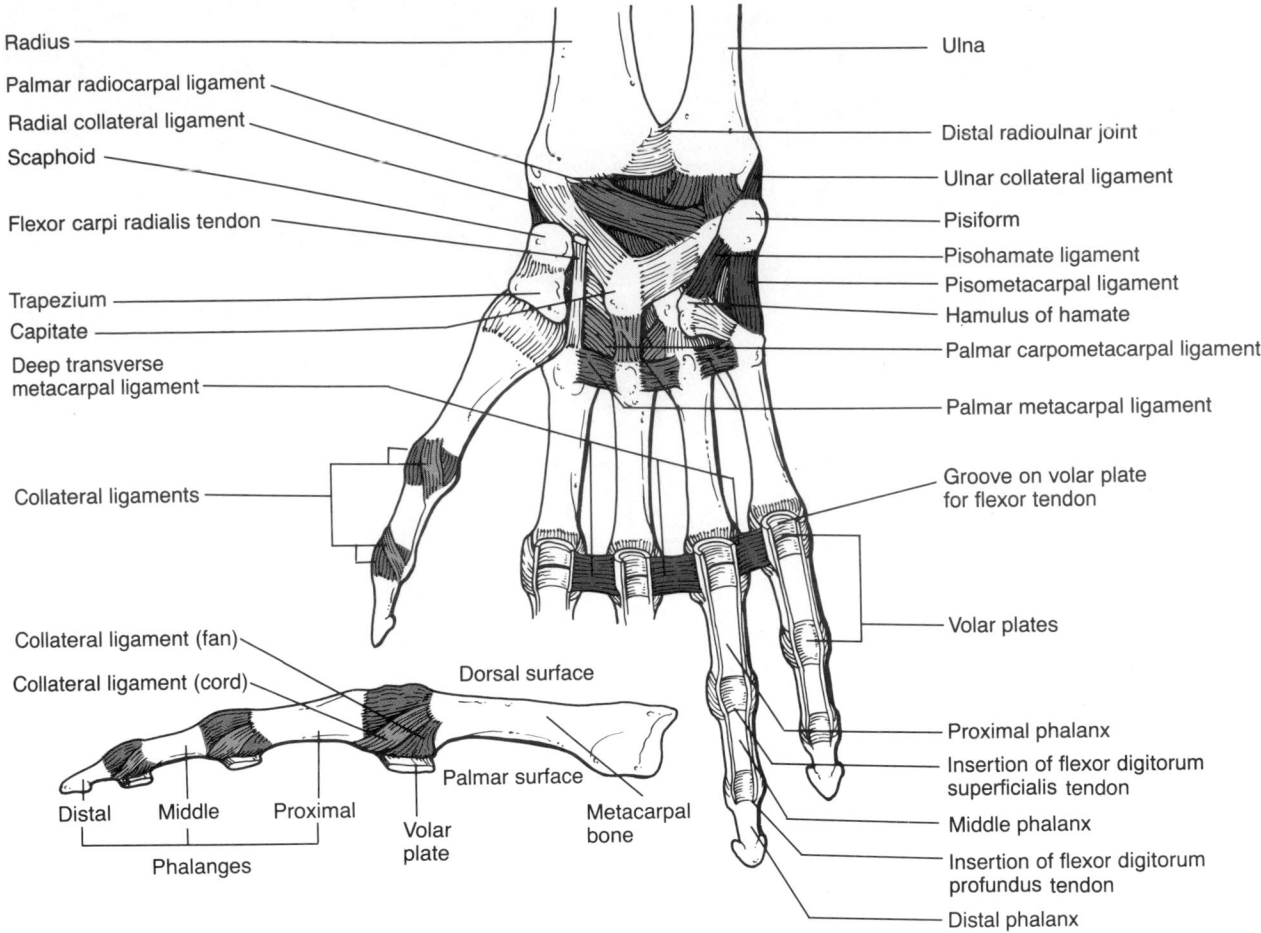

Radius

Palmar radiocarpal ligament

Radial collateral ligament

Scaphoid

Flexor carpi radialis tendon

Trapezium
Capitate
Deep transverse
metacarpal ligament

Collateral ligaments

Collateral ligament (fan)
Collateral ligament (cord)

Dorsal surface

Palmar surface

Distal   Middle   Proximal   Volar
plate
Phalanges

Metacarpal
bone

Ulna

Distal radioulnar joint
Ulnar collateral ligament
Pisiform
Pisohamate ligament
Pisometacarpal ligament
Hamulus of hamate
Palmar carpometacarpal ligament

Palmar metacarpal ligament

Groove on volar plate
for flexor tendon

Volar plates

Proximal phalanx
Insertion of flexor digitorum
superficialis tendon
Middle phalanx
Insertion of flexor digitorum
profundus tendon
Distal phalanx

FIGURE 31–7   Ligaments of the wrist and hand.

plates. The fibrocartilaginous volar plates attach firmly to the phalangeal bases but loosely to the metacarpal heads; this allows them to "pleat" during flexion. Strong collateral ligaments run obliquely from the dorsal aspect of the metacarpal head to the volar aspect of the phalangeal base; the ligaments are taut in flexion, the position in which they should be splinted to prevent contracture.

5. Interphalangeal (IP) joints. The IP joints are hinge joints that unite adjacent phalanges. Range of motion is 0 degrees to 110 degrees flexion at the proximal IP (PIP) joints, 90 degrees of flexion and 30 degrees of extension at the distal IP (DIP) joints, and 90 degrees of flexion and 50 degrees of extension at the thumb IP joint. Articular capsules enclose the joints and are reinforced by volar plates at the PIP joints (see Figure

31–7). Collateral ligaments, which offer some medial and lateral stability, are taut at 20 to 25 degrees of flexion. The recommended splint position to prevent contractures is near full extension.

C. Mechanics

1. Elbow and forearm
   a. The skin and subcutaneous tissue are loose and freely moving in the elbow and forearm; conversely, deeper fascia surrounds and firmly contains the flexor and extensor muscle compartments (see Figure 31–8). Following trauma, this inelastic deep fascia may entrap extravasated blood sufficiently to compromise circulation to the forearm (Volkman's ischemia).
   b. The muscles that power the elbow in-

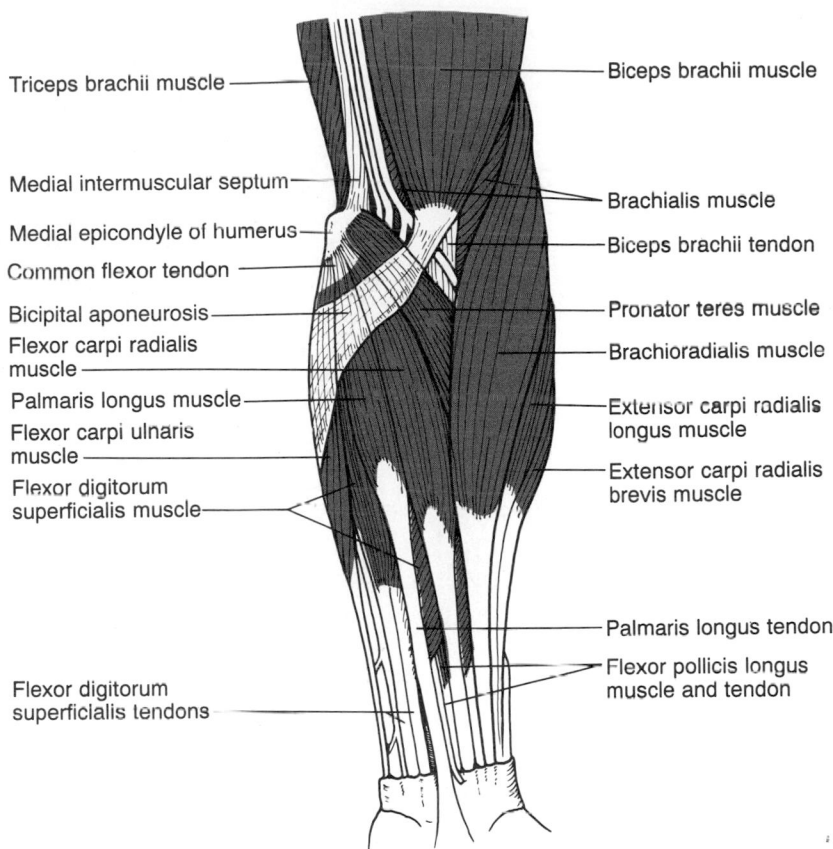

FIGURE 31–8 Superficial muscles of the anterior elbow and forearm.

clude the biceps brachii, brachialis, and brachioradialis muscles, which serve as flexors and the triceps brachii and anconeus muscles, which serve as extensors. The brachialis muscle is associated with a high incidence of myositis ossificans because of its large area of contact with bone.

c. Normal restraints to motion of the elbow are as follow: active flexion is checked by flexor muscle bulk, bone contact, and the posterior elbow joint capsule in this order; passive flexion is limited by bone contact, the posterior elbow joint capsule, passive triceps muscle tension, and flexor muscle bulk in this order; and active and passive extension are restrained by bone contact, the anterior elbow joint capsule, and passive flexor muscle tension in this order.[5,6]

2. Wrist and hand (tissues described from superficial to deep)
a. The skin and subcutaneous tissue of the wrist and hand are loosely attached and elastic over the dorsum (this facilitates a full fist position), but connected tightly to the palmar aponeurosis by strong fasciculi (this facilitates the firm gripping of objects in the palm).

b. The palmar aponeurosis is a dense fibrous structure, continuous with the palmaris longus (PL) tendon and the thenar and hypothenar fascia proximally. It attaches to the transverse metacarpal ligaments and the flexor tendon sheaths distally (see Figure 31–9). This aponeurosis offers some protection for the ulnar and digital arteries and nerves; it also is the site of nodule formation or contracture (Dupuytren's contracture).

c. The flexor retinaculum (transverse carpal ligament) spans the volar carpal area and forms the roof of the carpal tunnel. It offers a point of attachment for the thenar and hypothenar muscles, prevents bowstringing of the extrinsic flexor tendons, and protects the median nerve (see Figure 31–9).

d. The flexor tendon sheaths and the cru-

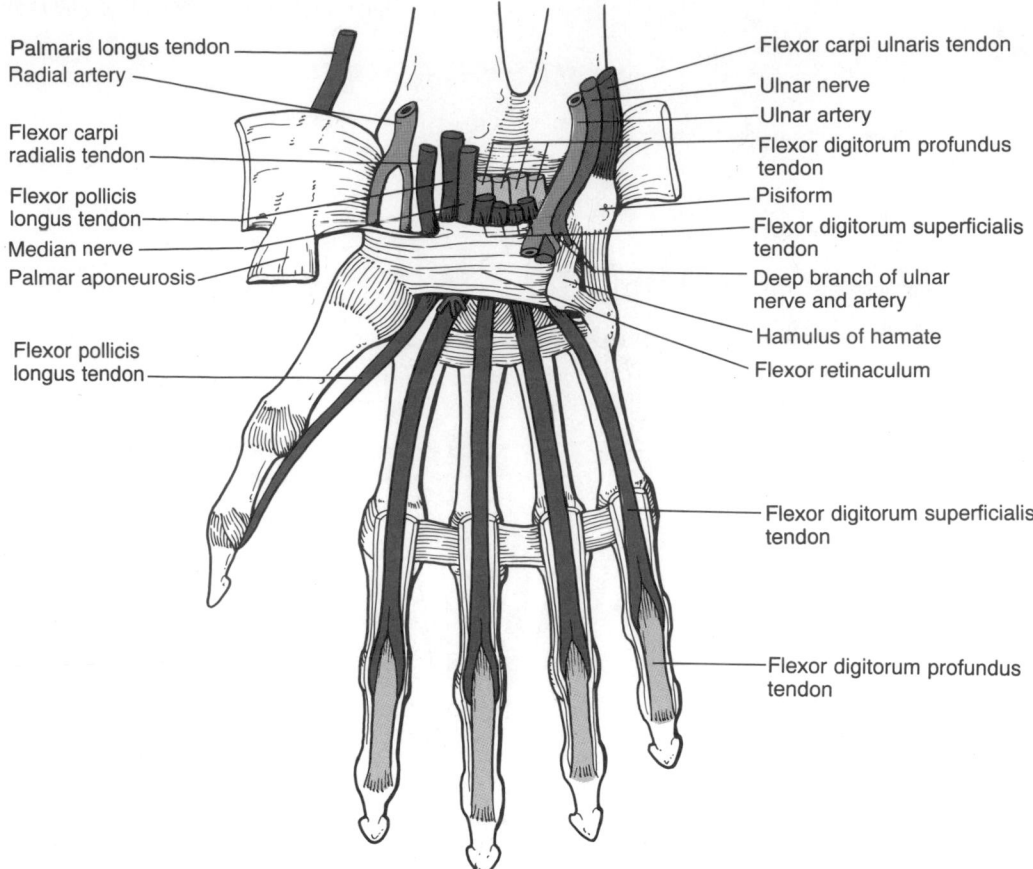

FIGURE 31-9 Soft tissues of the palm.

Palmaris longus tendon

Radial artery

Flexor carpi
radialis tendon

Flexor pollicis
longus tendon

Median nerve

Palmar aponeurosis

Flexor pollicis
longus tendon

Flexor carpi ulnaris tendon

Ulnar nerve

Ulnar artery

Flexor digitorum profundus
tendon

Pisiform

Flexor digitorum superficialis
tendon

Deep branch of ulnar
nerve and artery

Hamulus of hamate

Flexor retinaculum

Flexor digitorum superficialis
tendon

Flexor digitorum profundus
tendon

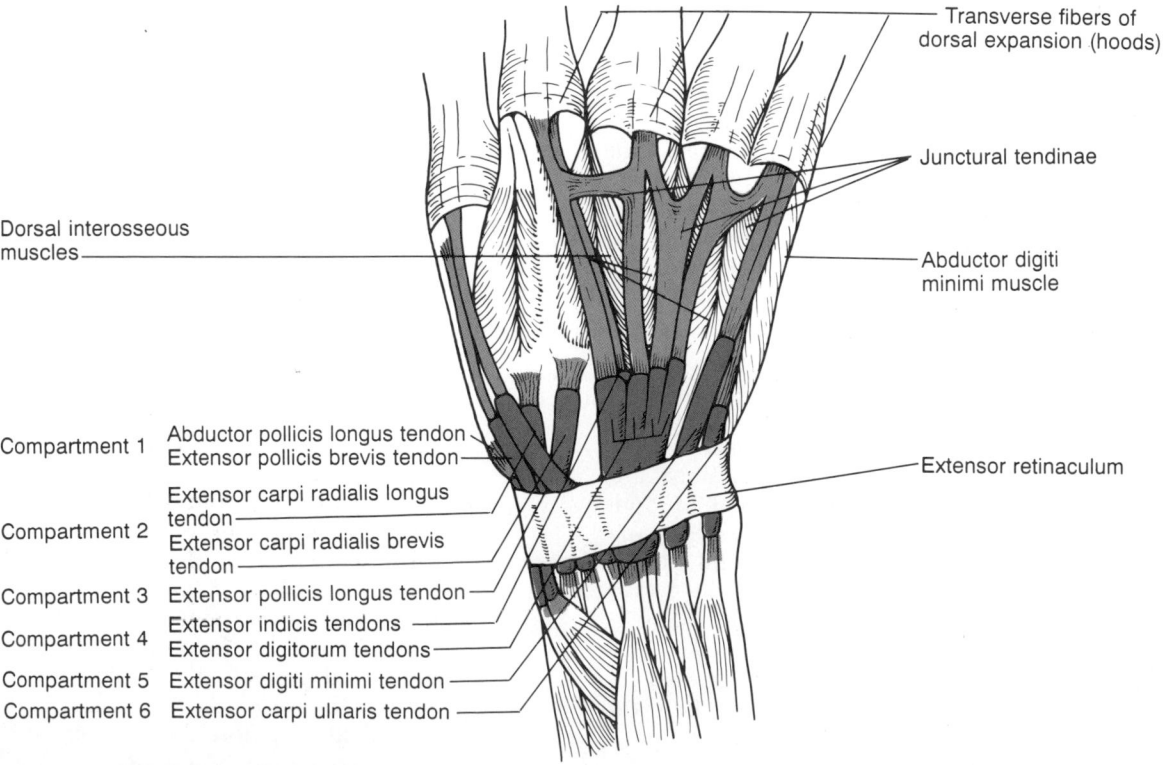

Transverse fibers of
dorsal expansion (hoods)

Junctural tendinae

Abductor digiti
minimi muscle

Extensor retinaculum

Dorsal interosseous
muscles

Compartment 1 Abductor pollicis longus tendon
Extensor pollicis brevis tendon

Compartment 2 Extensor carpi radialis longus
tendon
Extensor carpi radialis brevis
tendon

Compartment 3 Extensor pollicis longus tendon

Compartment 4 Extensor indicis tendons
Extensor digitorum tendons

Compartment 5 Extensor digiti minimi tendon

Compartment 6 Extensor carpi ulnaris tendon

FIGURE 31-10 Extensor tendons of the wrist and hand.

ciate and annular ligaments encase and anchor the extrinsic flexor tendons to the distal metacarpal bones and the phalanges.

e. The extensor retinaculum spans the dorsal carpal area; it is divided by fasciculi that separate the extrinsic extensor tendons into six compartments (see Figure 31–10).

(1). The first compartment contains the abductor policis longus (APL) and extensor policis brevis (EPB).

(2). The second compartment contains the extensor carpi radialis longus and brevis muscles.

(3). The third compartment contains the extensor policis longus (EPL) muscle.

(4). The fourth compartment contains the extensor indicis (EI) and extensor digitorum (ED).

(5). The fifth compartment contains the extensor digiti minimi.

(6). The sixth compartment contains the extensor carpi ulnaris.

f. The juncturae tendinae connect the extrinsic extensor tendons in the region of metacarpal heads, limiting their independent motion (see Figure 31–10).

g. The sagittal bands indirectly connect the

LATERAL VIEW

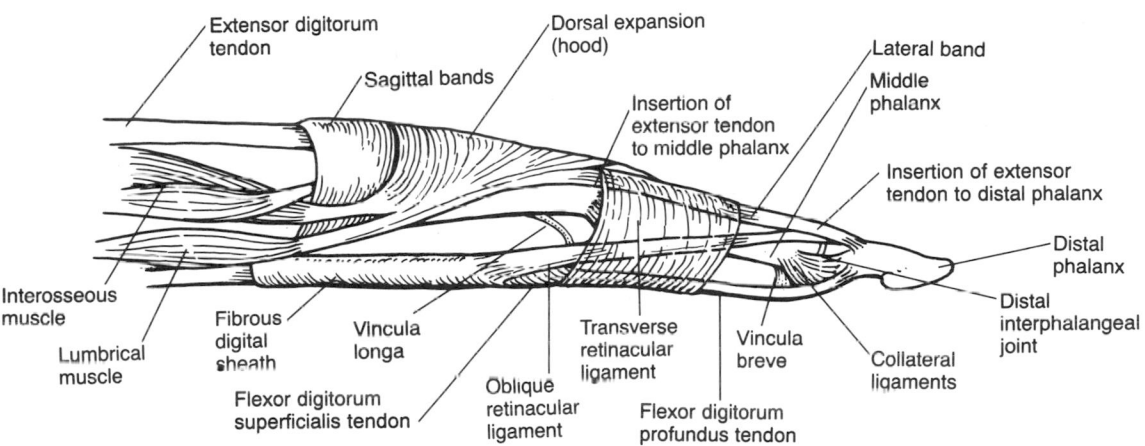

DORSAL VIEW

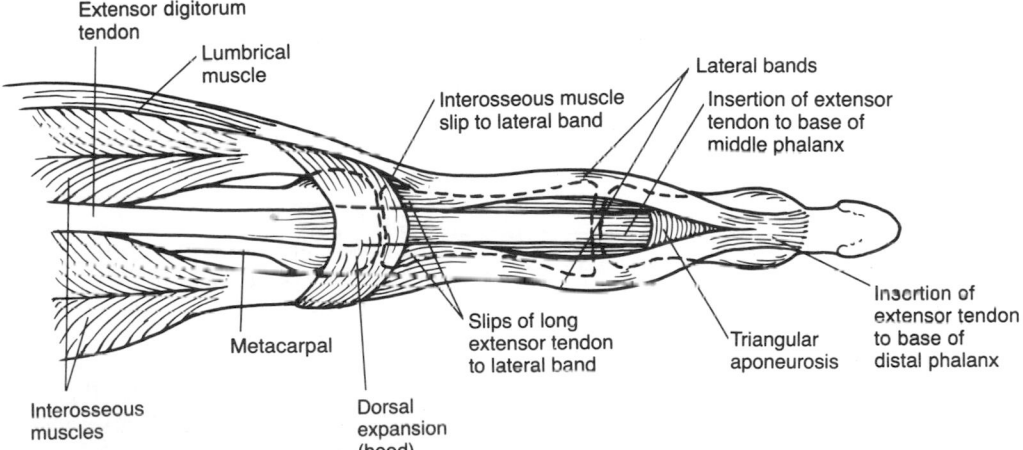

FIGURE 31–11   Extrinsic flexor and extensor tendons and intrinsic muscles.

extrinsic extensor tendons to the proximal phalanges by a sling mechanism that attaches to the volar plates. They prevent dorsal bowstringing of the extensor tendons (see Figure 31–11).

h. The dorsal hood, located between the MP and PIP joints, is the fibrous expansion from the union of the extensor digitorum tendon and the intrinsic musculature; the hood covers the dorsal proximal phalanx. The divisions of the dorsal hood include the central slip, which inserts into the base of the middle phalanx (its rupture results in a boutonnière deformity), and the lateral bands, which rejoin over the DIP joint into a terminal tendon that inserts into the distal phalanx (its rupture results in a mallet finger deformity).

i. The transverse retinacular ligaments link the lateral bands to the PIP joint volar plates and prevent their dorsal bowstringing (laxity of the transverse retinacular ligaments may contribute to the swan-neck deformity) (see Figure 31–11).

j. The oblique retinacular ligaments (Landsmeer's ligaments) run obliquely between the PIP joint volar plate and the terminal extensor tendon at the DIP joint; they exert passive extensor force to extend the DIP joint when the PIP joint is actively extended (see Figure 31–11).

k. The extrinsic and intrinsic muscles are listed in Table 31–1.

D. Neurology

1. The radial nerve (C5-8, T-1) spirals around the posterior humerus, where just proximal to the elbow it divides into superficial (sensory) and motor (posterior interosseous) branches that cross the elbow anteriolaterally. The posterior interosseous nerve supplies (in descending order) the brachioradialis muscle, the extensor carpi radialis longus (ECRL) and brevis (ECRB), the supinator, the ED, the ECU, the extensor digiti minimi (EDM), the APL, the EPL, the EPB, and the EI muscles. The sensory branch supplies the dorsolateral skin of the hand and the dorsal skin of the lateral three and one half digits to the level of the DIP joints (see Figure 31–12).

2. The median nerve (C5-8, T-1) travels anteromedial to the humerus and crosses anterior to the elbow under the lacertus fibrosis. In the forearm, it supplies (in descending order) the round pronator teres (PT), the FCR, the PL, and the flexor digitorum superficialis (FDS) muscles; the anterior interosseous nerve branches approximately 10 cm distal to the elbow and supplies the flexor digitorum profundus muscle (FDP) to the index and middle fingers, the flexor pollicis longus muscle (FPL), and the pronator quadratus (PQ) muscle and sends articular twigs to the wrist. A palmar branch arises 4 cm proximal to the wrist and descends to supply the skin over the lateral palm and thenar eminence. In the palm, the terminal motor branch of the median nerve innervates the abductor pollicis brevis (APB), the opponens pollicis (OP), the superficial head of the flexor pollicis brevis (FPB), and the first and second lumbrical muscles. Sensory branches innervate the skin over the palmar aspects and dorsal tips of the lateral three and one half digits (see Figure 31–13).

3. The ulnar nerve (C7-8, T-1) travels medial to the humerus and passes posterior to the medial epicondyle, providing an articular

Table 31–1. THE HAND'S EXTRINSIC AND INTRINSIC MUSCLES

Extrinsic Muscles

Flexor carpi radialis
Palmaris longus
Flexor carpi ulnaris
Flexor digitorum superficialis
Flexor pollicis longus
Flexor digitorum profundus
Extensor carpi radialis longus and brevis
Extensor carpi ulnaris
Extensor digitorum
Extensor digiti minimi
Extensor indicis
Extensor pollicis longus and brevis
Abductor pollicis longus

Intrinsic Muscles

Abductor pollicis brevis
Opponens pollicis
Flexor pollicis brevis
Adductor pollicis
Abductor digiti minimi
Opponens digiti minimi
Flexor digiti minimi
Palmaris brevis
Lumbricals
Dorsal and palmar interossei

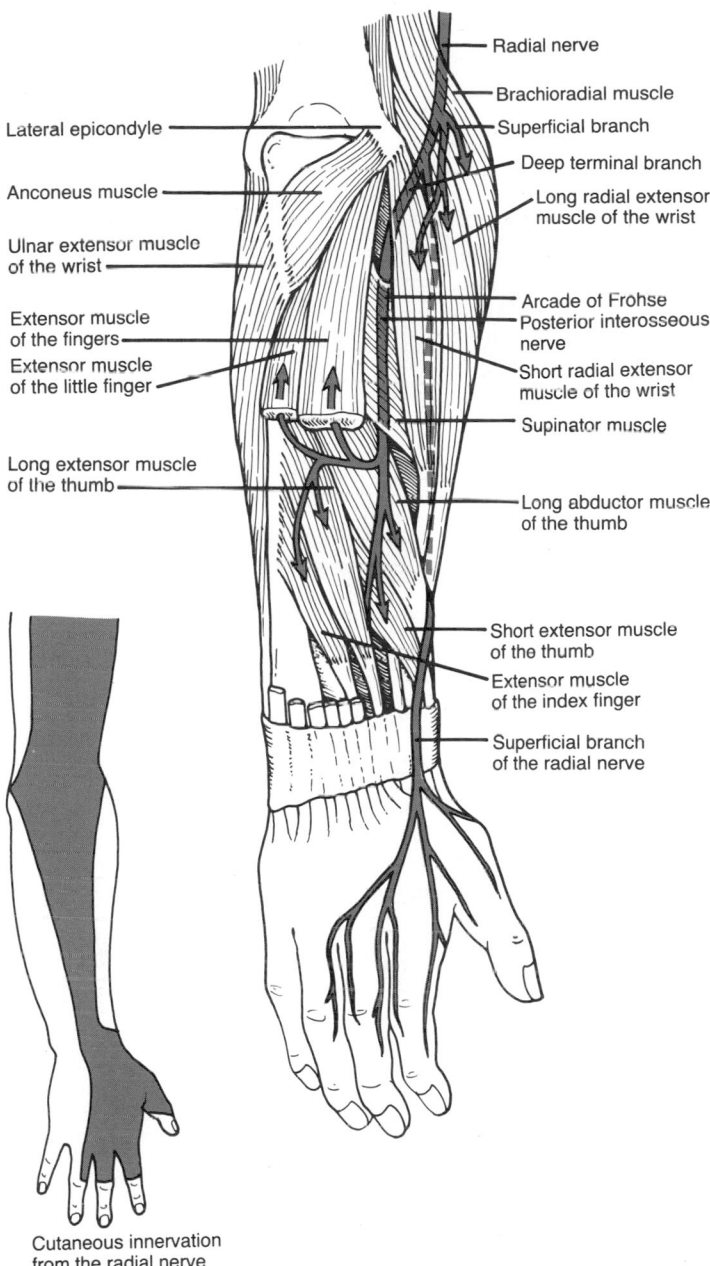

Radial nerve

Brachioradial muscle

Superficial branch

Deep terminal branch

Long radial extensor
muscle of the wrist

Arcade of Frohse
Posterior interosseous
nerve

Short radial extensor
muscle of tho wrist

Supinator muscle

Long abductor muscle
of the thumb

Short extensor muscle
of the thumb

Extensor muscle
of the index finger

Superficial branch
of the radial nerve

Lateral epicondyle

Anconeus muscle

Ulnar extensor muscle
of the wrist

Extensor muscle
of the fingers

Extensor muscle
of the little finger

Long extensor muscle
of the thumb

Cutaneous innervation
from the radial nerve

FIGURE 31–12 Radial nerve.

branch to the elbow. It then provides branches to the flexor carpi ulnaris (FCU) muscle of the wrist and to the FDP to the ring and little fingers; 5 to 10 cm proximal to the wrist, the dorsal and palmar sensory branches arise and supply the skin over the medial side of the back of the hand and medial one and one half fingers and the hypothenar area. After crossing the wrist, the ulnar nerve divides into the superficial and deep terminal branches. The superficial branch supplies the PB muscle and the skin over the medial palm and divides into three palmar digital nerves that supply the skin over the palmar surface of the little finger and the medial half of the ring finger. The deep branch of the ulnar nerve supplies the hypothenar muscles (the abductor, flexor, and opponens digiti minimi [ODM] muscle), the third and fourth lumbrical muscles,

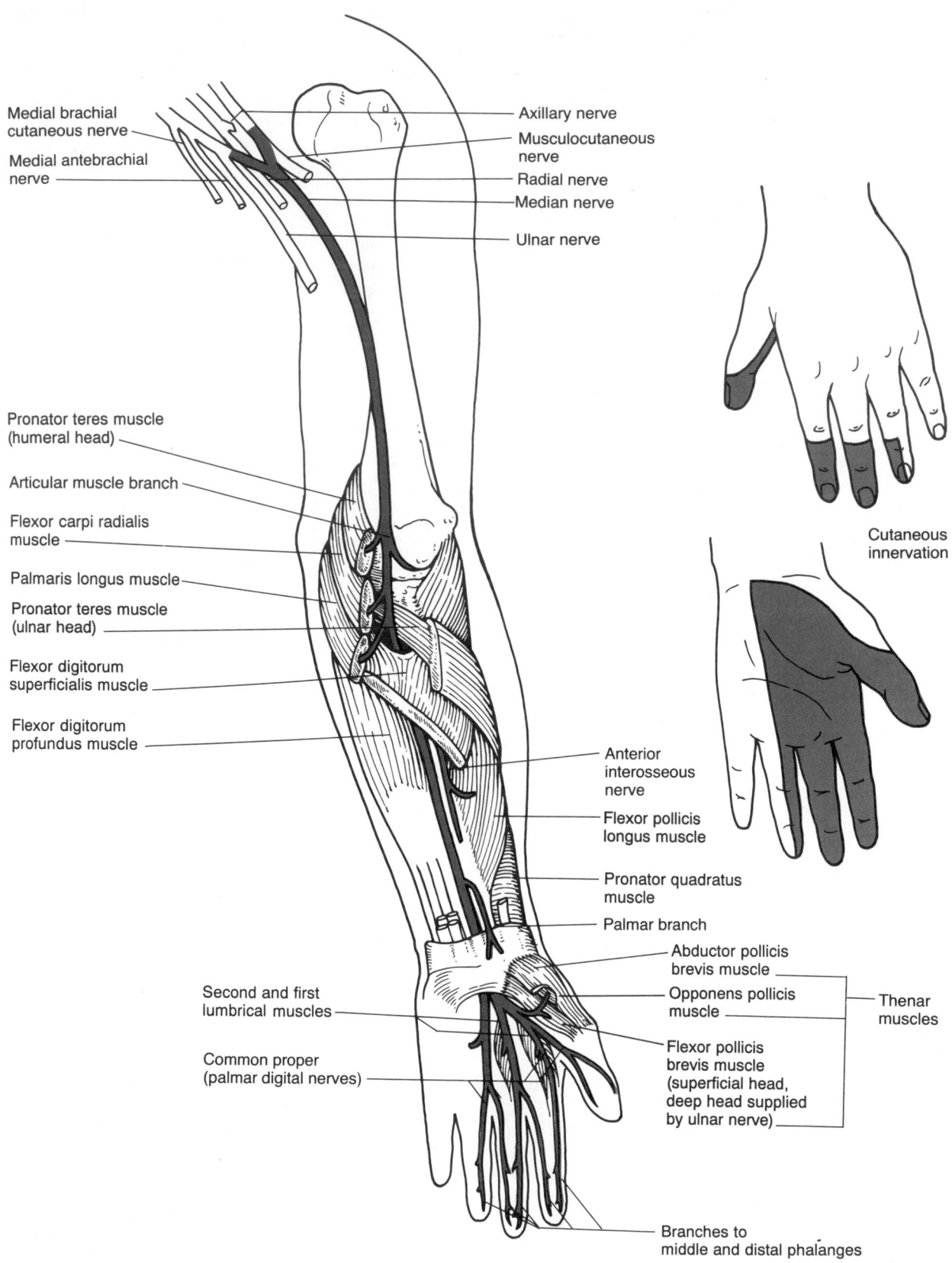

Medial brachial cutaneous nerve

Medial antebrachial nerve

Axillary nerve

Musculocutaneous nerve

Radial nerve

Median nerve

Ulnar nerve

Pronator teres muscle (humeral head)

Articular muscle branch

Flexor carpi radialis muscle

Palmaris longus muscle

Pronator teres muscle (ulnar head)

Flexor digitorum superficialis muscle

Flexor digitorum profundus muscle

Anterior interosseous nerve

Flexor pollicis longus muscle

Pronator quadratus muscle

Palmar branch

Abductor pollicis brevis muscle

Opponens pollicis muscle

Thenar muscles

Flexor pollicis brevis muscle (superficial head, deep head supplied by ulnar nerve)

Second and first lumbrical muscles

Common proper (palmar digital nerves)

Branches to middle and distal phalanges

Cutaneous innervation

FIGURE 31–13 Median nerve.

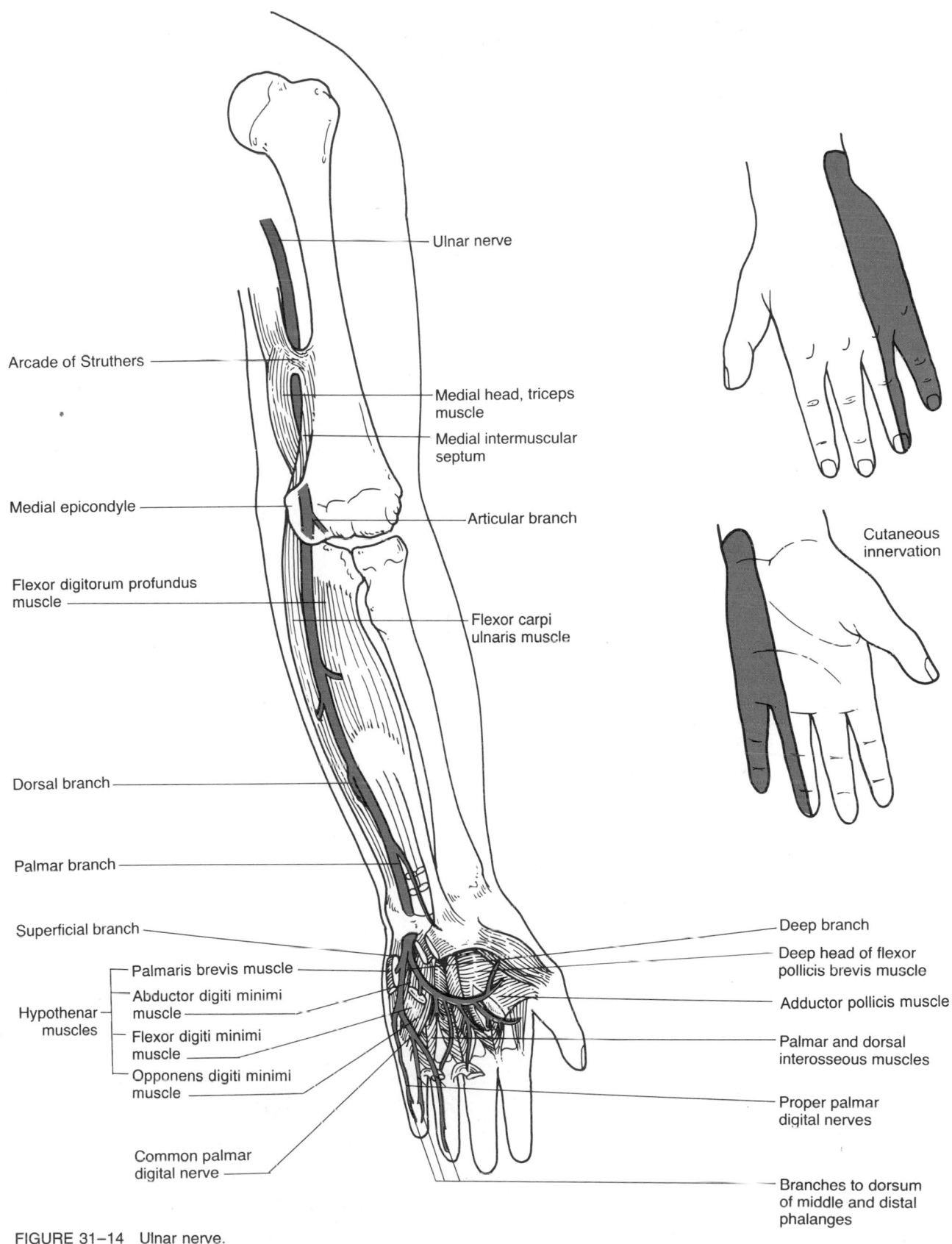

Ulnar nerve

Arcade of Struthers

Medial head, triceps muscle

Medial intermuscular septum

Medial epicondyle

Articular branch

Flexor digitorum profundus muscle

Flexor carpi ulnaris muscle

Dorsal branch

Palmar branch

Cutaneous innervation

Superficial branch

Deep branch

Deep head of flexor pollicis brevis muscle

Palmaris brevis muscle

Hypothenar muscles

Abductor digiti minimi muscle

Flexor digiti minimi muscle

Opponens digiti minimi muscle

Adductor pollicis muscle

Palmar and dorsal interosseous muscles

Proper palmar digital nerves

Common palmar digital nerve

Branches to dorsum of middle and distal phalanges

FIGURE 31–14 Ulnar nerve.

all of the interossei muscles, the adductor pollicis (AP) muscle, and the deep head of FPB muscle(see Figure 31–14).

E. Angiology

1. The brachial artery travels distally medial to the humerus and gives off three branches: the deep brachial artery and the superior and inferior ulnar collateral arteries. It then crosses the anterior elbow just medial to the biceps tendon and deep to the bicipital aponeurosis. At the level of the radial neck, the brachial artery divides into terminal branches, the radial and ulnar arteries (see Figure 31–15).

2. The radial artery courses along the lateral forearm to the wrist, where its pulse is palpable lateral to the FCR tendon. It then gives off a superficial palmar branch proximal to the scaphoid that anastomoses with the corresponding superficial ulnar branch from the ulnar artery; its deep branch winds posteriorly between the first and second metacarpals and joins the deep ulnar branch from the ulnar artery (see Figure 31–15).

3. The ulnar artery passes anterior to the ulna in the forearm and crosses the wrist anteromedially where its pulse is palpable just lateral to the FCU tendon. Just distal to the pisiform bone, it divides into a superficial branch that crosses the palm as the superficial palmar arch and a deep branch that completes the deep palmar arch (see Figure 31–15).

4. The palmar metacarpal arteries arise from the deep palmar arch.

5. The common palmar digital arteries arise from the superficial palmar arch.

6. The proper digital arteries are formed by the junction of the palmar metacarpal and common palmar digital arteries; they then branch into the medial and lateral digital arteries.

7. The superficial veins originate from the dorsal plexus in the hand; blood drains into the cephalic vein laterally and the basilic vein medially. Just distal to the elbow, the cephalic vein gives off the median cubital vein that connects with the deep venous system and also joins the basilic vein; this median cubital vein is commonly used for venipuncture (see Figure 31–16).

8. Pairs of deep veins (vena comicontes) are located in the hand; they accompany the local arteries as they ascend from the digits to the palmar plexi and forearm vessels.

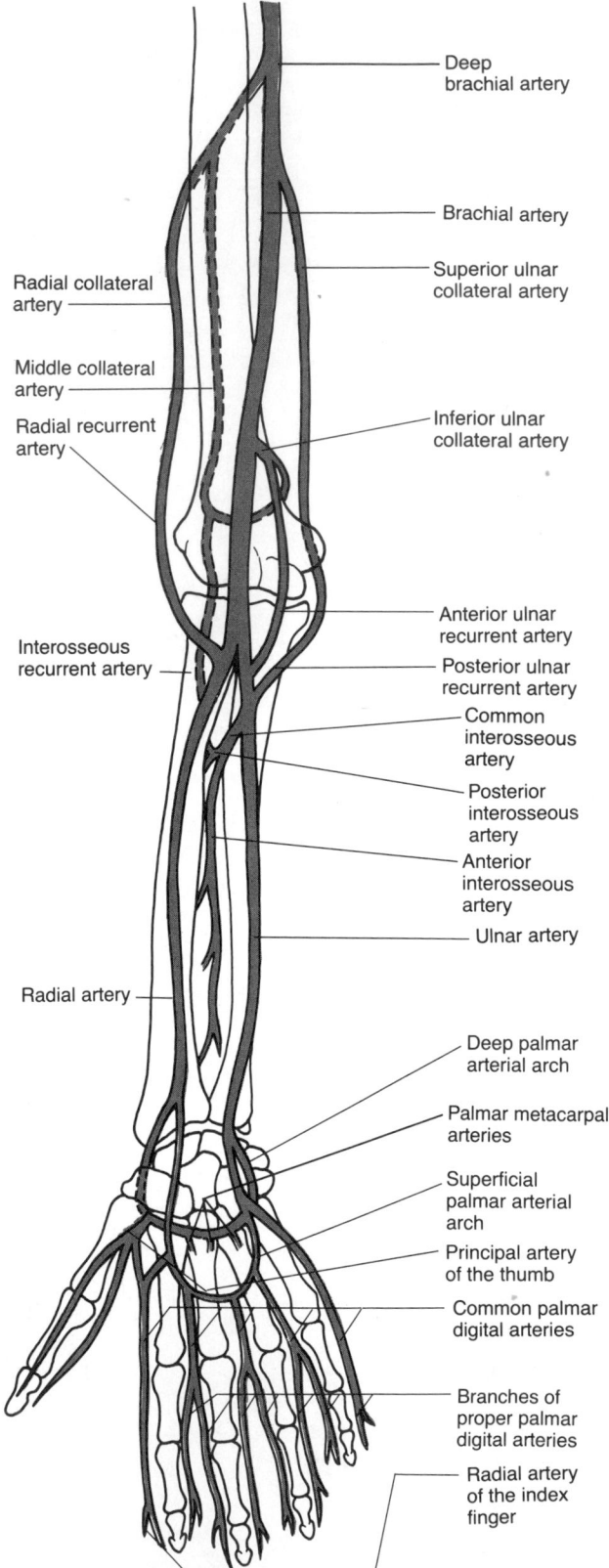

FIGURE 31–15 Arteries of the forearm and hand.

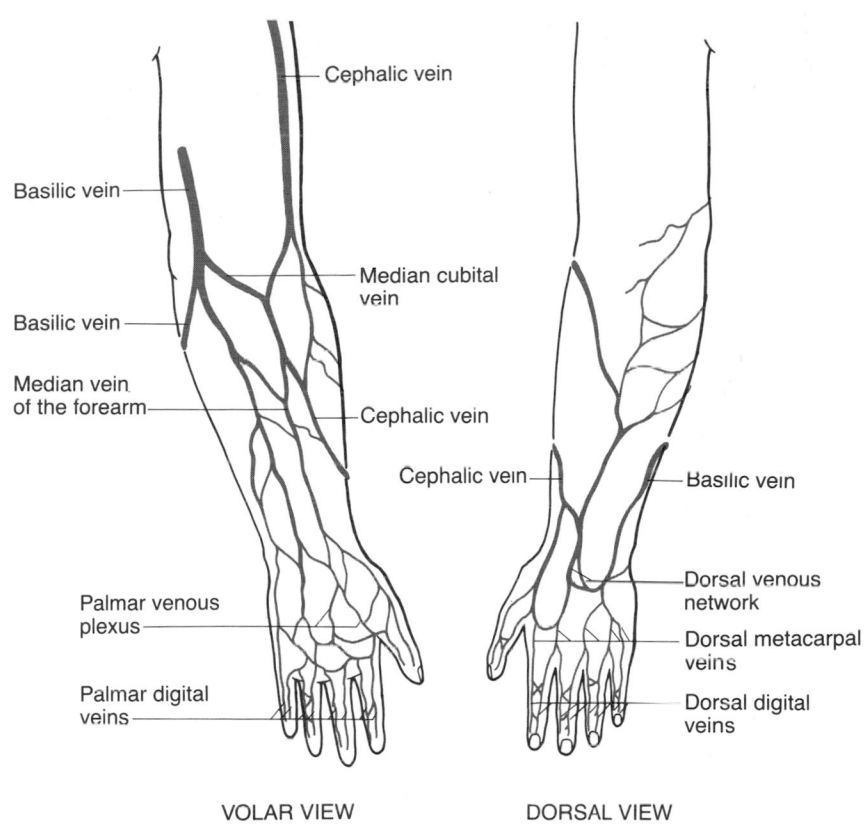

VOLAR VIEW   DORSAL VIEW

FIGURE 31–16   Veins of the forearm and hand.

II. Examination

A. General concepts

1. The primary objective of the examination is to determine a patient's functional capability.
2. Information from the examination is ultimately used to determine the means for restoring maximal use of the elbow, forearm, wrist, and hand.
3. A therapist must use thorough, accurate, reliable, and standardized procedures for testing a patient.
4. Photographs are often useful for documenting a patient's baseline status and progress.

B. History

1. Personal information. Record the patient's age, gender, hand dominance, and occupation.
2. Diagnosis. Note the patient's provisional diagnosis and any precautions (if the patient was referred).
3. Chief complaint. Record the patient's brief description of his/her condition and why he/she is seeking assistance; identify the "primary problem."

4. Present illness. Describe the *symptoms* associated with the primary problem (see Figure 31–17), including the following:
   a. Location—a body chart may be used
   b. Severity and impairment—analog scales may be used
   c. Nature, *eg*, aching, burning, and tingling
   d. Persistence, *ie*, constant versus intermittent; what worsens versus relieves symptoms (many musculoskeletal lesions are aggravated by activity and relieved by rest); whether irritated by mild versus vigorous activity
5. Onset of primary problem
   a. Acute versus insidious
   b. Mechanism of injury, if the problem is traumatic
   c. Sequence and progression of the symptoms
   d. Date of the initial onset and status of the problem up to the current visit
   e. Previous health care treatments (for this problem) and their results
   f. Condition worsening or improving?
   g. Associated deformity or disability?
   h. Prior condition of the involved body part

857

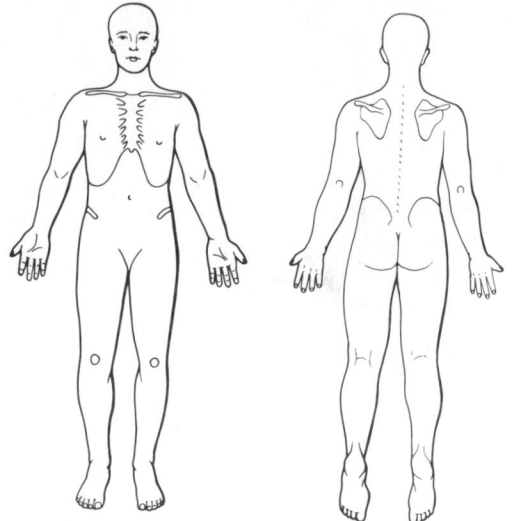

A. Indicate present symptoms on body chart.

B. Indicate severity of symptoms: 0 = none; 10 = worst

|---|
| 0   10 cm |

C. Indicate impairment related to condition: 0 = annoying;
   10 = completely disabling

|---|
| 0   10 cm |

D. Define nature of symptoms:

_____ aching _____ tingling _____ burning _____ throbbing

_____ cramping _____ other _____

E. Describe behavior of symptoms:

_____ constant _____ intermittent   aggravated by _____

relieved by _____ 24-hr pattern _____

FIGURE 31–17   Form used for describing symptoms.

6. Past history
   a. Previous episodes of the same problem; the dates when they occurred and their response to treatment
   b. Other affected body parts
   c. Familial, congenital, or developmental disorders
   d. Systemic diseases or other pathology (pre-existing pain or injuries may affect a patient's response to treatment)
   e. General health status
   f. Medications
   g. Radiographs
7. Lifestyle
   a. Profession or occupation
   b. Availability of assistance from family or friends
   c. Caregiving and occupational demands (dependent children or a dependent spouse or parent and job expectations may increase stress on the patient and affect goal setting)
   d. Activities of daily life, hobbies, sports
   e. Patient's concept of the impact of functional or cosmetic deficits, as well as economic factors (these factors may affect goals and management decisions such as reconstruction versus amputation)

C. **Physical examination**

1. Inspection
   a. On screening the therapist should:
      (1). Make a general observation of the involved part and its relation to the rest of the body; the patient may be overly protective or ignore it.
      (2). Observe the patient's resting posture, which may portray muscle imbalance, joint subluxation, structural deformities, or other problems (see Figure 31–18).
      (3). Note compensatory movement (hypomobility vs instability—both may alter movement patterns).
      (4). Note the patient's willingness and ability to use the involved limb for functional activities.
   b. Observe the shape of the affected body part—variations in shape often characterize specific hand disorders:
      (1). Thenar atrophy may signify median nerve dysfunction.
      (2). Intrinsic and hypothenar muscle atrophy is a sign of ulnar nerve dysfunction.
      (3). Wrist drop may indicate radial nerve dysfunction.
      (4). A flat hand, or loss of arches, may signify improper immobilization or neuromuscular dysfunction.
      (5). Drooping of the distal phalanx is a sign of mallet finger with distal extensor tendon rupture.
      (6). Drooping of the middle phalanx may indicate extensor lag, central slip rupture, or boutonnière deformity.
      (7). Nodules over the dorsal or volar forearm or wrist and the dorsal hand may be ganglion cysts.

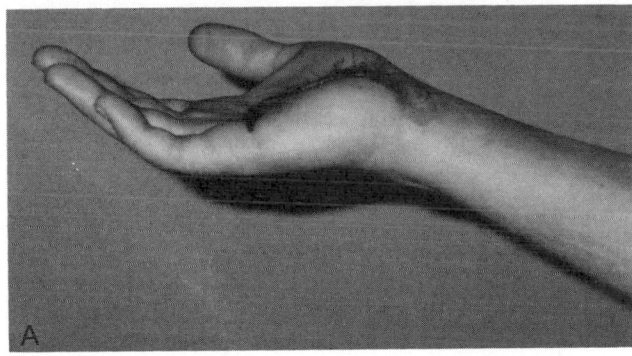

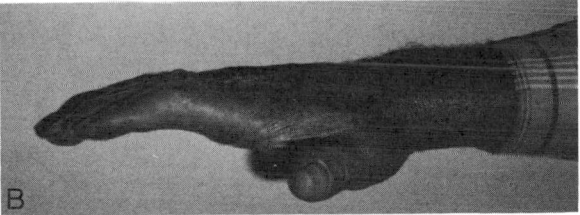

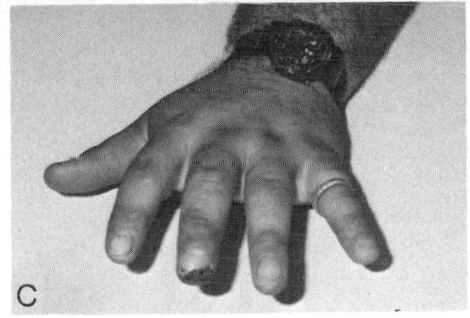

FIGURE 31–18 Inspection of resting posture. **A,** Three days after release of the carpal tunnel and the ring and little trigger fingers. **B,** Six months following crush injury. **C,** Two weeks after surgical repair of fingertip laceration.

(8). Mobile nodules in the palm near the MP joints may signify the presence of tenosynovitis or trigger finger.

(9). Dorsal nodules or enlargements over the PIP joints may be Bouchard's nodes secondary to rheumatoid arthritis.

(10). Dorsal nodules or enlargements over the DIP joints may be Heberden's nodes secondary to degenerative joint disease.

(11). Nodules over the proximal ulnar shaft may be rheumatoid nodules.

(12). "Boggy" swelling around the wrist area may mean that rheumatoid synovitis and pannus formation are present.

(13). Localized swelling over the olecranon is a sign of bursitis.

(14). A loss of continuity of any long bone may indicate a displaced fracture (acute) or malunion (chronic).

(15). Joint angulation or deformity is a sign of dislocation, subluxation, or contracture.

(16). Disruption of the bone landmarks at the elbow is indicative of elbow (humeroulnar) dislocation or fracture of the olecranon, humeral epicondyles, or humeral or ulnar joint surfaces (see Figure 31–19).

FIGURE 31–19 Bone landmarks at the elbow; in extension, the olecranon is bisected by a straight line connecting the medial and lateral epicondyles. In flexion, an isosceles triangle is formed by lines connecting the medial and lateral condyles with the olecranon.

PLEASE NOTE: At this point in the examination, it is recommended that the examiner stop and assess the findings at hand. Information from the history and initial inspection should be used to plan an appropriate, detailed examination so that valuable time and attention can be focused on specific problem areas. Depending on indications, some parts of the following format may be abbreviated or deleted.

c. Document combinations of joint deformities, generalized atrophy, or edema; describe the type and location of deviations in shape and other problems; for increased objectivity, use the following:

(1). Diagrams or photographs. Visualization aids in documenting the patient's initial condition and his/her progressive changes, especially in cases in which multiple joint involvement is difficult or too time consuming to describe.

(2). Circumferential measurements. Standardized norms are not available for hand circumference and volume, therefore, measurements are considered to be relative to the uninvolved limb or to subsequent measurements. Designated anatomical sites include the arm (7 cm proximal to the elbow flexion crease), the forearm (11 cm proximal to the distal wrist flexion crease), the wrist (the distal wrist flexion crease), and the hand (the distal palmar flexion crease) (see Figure 31–20).

(3). Volumetric measurements. The hand should be submerged in a volumeter filled with water to the level of the spout; with the middle and ring fingers "straddling" the dowel, the amount of displaced water is measured in a graduated

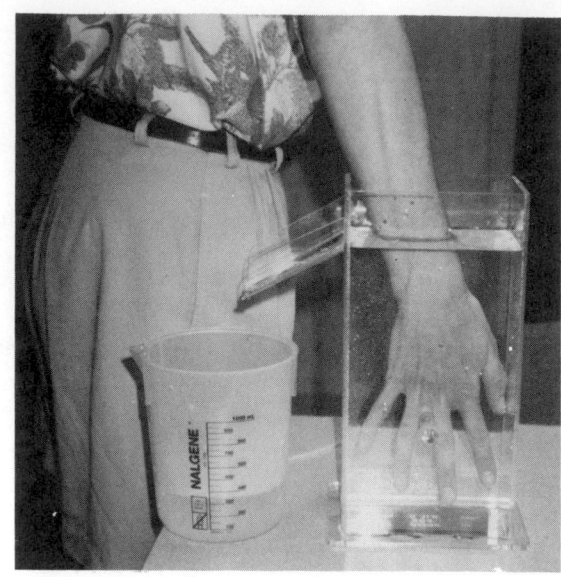

FIGURE 31–21 Volumetric measurement. With the hand submerged until the middle and ring fingers "straddle" dowel, the amount of displaced water is measured.

cylinder (for details, see manufacturer's instructions)[7] (see Figure 31–21).

d. Abnormalities of the skin may be recorded on a hand diagram or chart (see Figure 31–22).

(1). Superficial lesions. These include cuts, wounds, incisions (note the presence of sutures), blisters, scars, ulcerations, and grafts.

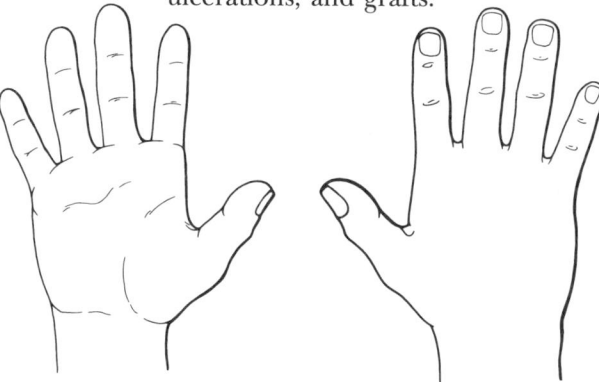

May indicate changes, ie

L = lesion
N = nail deformity
T = texture changed
H = abnormal hair pattern
R = reddened
C = cyanotic
W = whitened
S = scar

FIGURE 31–22 Chart for indicating superficial abnormalities of the hand.

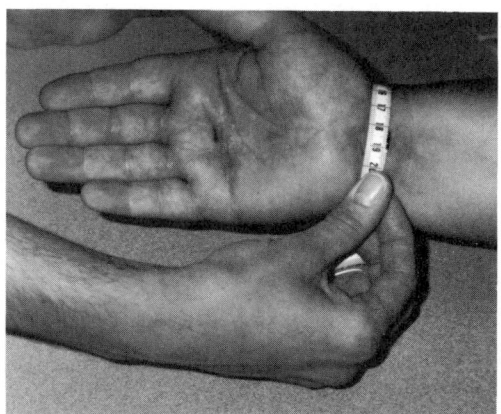

FIGURE 31–20 Circumferential measurement. Typical sites include 7 cm proximal to the elbow crease, 11 cm proximal to the distal wrist flexion crease, at the distal wrist flexion crease, and at the distal palmar flexion crease.

(2). Trophic changes. Trophic changes are indicated by thin, shiny skin, hair loss, and loss of papillary ridges (associated with vascular changes or denervation).

(3). Nail abnormalities. These include clubbing (a sign of a pulmonary disorder), psoriatic involvement, necrosis, an unusual growth pattern, or complete loss (associated with nail bed injury).

(4). Unusual color. Abnormalities may be indicated by a cyanotic color (from inadequate perfusion), redness (a sign of inflammation), or increased or decreased pigmentation (following grafting or caused by a chronic or sympathetic disorder).

(5). Use versus nonuse. Signs of use include callouses, abrasions, or a grimy hand, whereas an unused hand may appear soft and clean.

e. Any splints and adaptive devices should be noted.

(1). Describe the intended purpose of the splint or device.

(2). Ascertain its proper fit and application.

(3). Observe function with use of the splint or device.

(4). Note whether the splint or device is static or dynamic.

2. Palpation. Because of the superficial nature of most tissues of the elbow, forearm, wrist, and hand, structural and physiologic changes are relatively easy to detect; pro-gressively palpate from superficial to deeper layers, noting both the location and nature of any abnormality (see Fig 31–22).

a. Skin and subcutaneous tissues. Note any tenderness, edema, temperature alterations, decreased mobility (from scar adhesions or contracting graft), or dryness (caused by loss of sympathetic innervation) versus hyperhidrosis (from nerve regeneration or increased sympathetic flow).

b. Muscles and tendons. Look for tenderness, loss of continuity, adhesions, or changes in resting length, tone, or bulk.

c. Tendon sheaths and bursae. Note any tenderness, enlargement, or crepitation (tenosynovitis).

d. Bones and joints. Observe any tenderness, swelling, mechanical deformity, hypomobility, or hypermobility.

e. Arteries. Check for the presence of normal pulses. Perform Allen's test—check for patency of the radial and ulnar arteries at the wrist by compressing (occluding) both arteries after the patient has exsanguinated his/her hand by rapidly alternating opening and clenching his/her fist. Release one side to check the speed of filling, which is evidenced by a warm, pinkish flush; repeat, and release the pressure on the opposite side (see Figure 31–23). Repeat for the fingers if checking the digital arteries.[8]

f. Nerves. Check for neuromas or unusual sensitivity to pressure. Check for Tinel's sign, which identifies the level of regen-

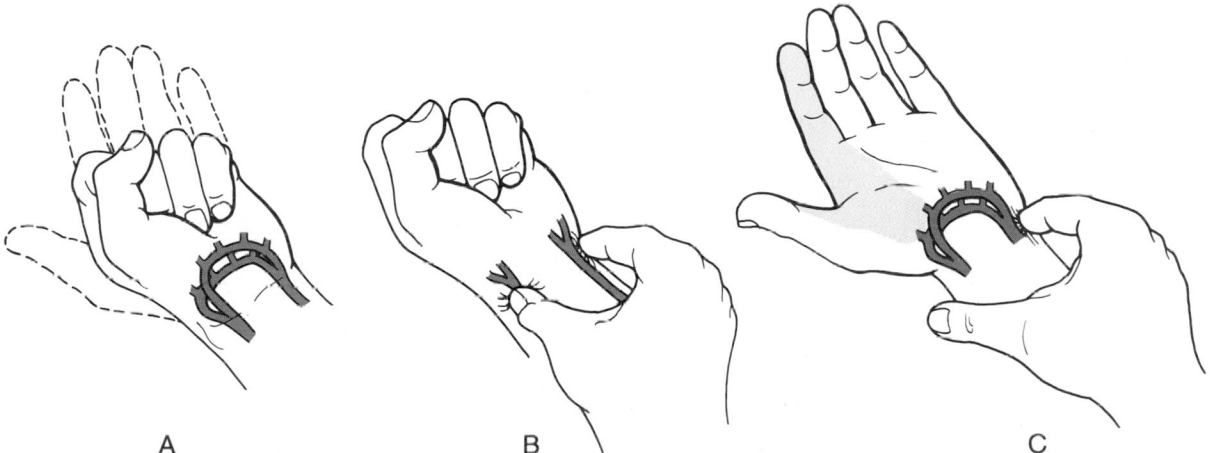

FIGURE 31–23 Allen's test. **A,** Patient exsanguinates blood by opening and closing the hand. **B,** Examiner occludes the radial and ulnar arteries. **C,** Examiner releases pressure from the radial artery and observes flush or filling.

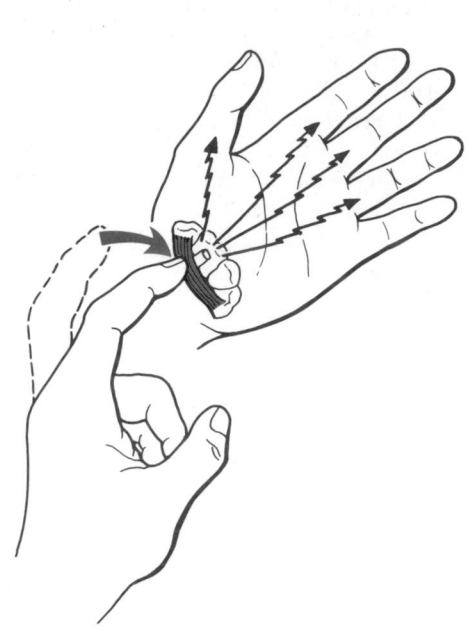

A   Carpal tunnel

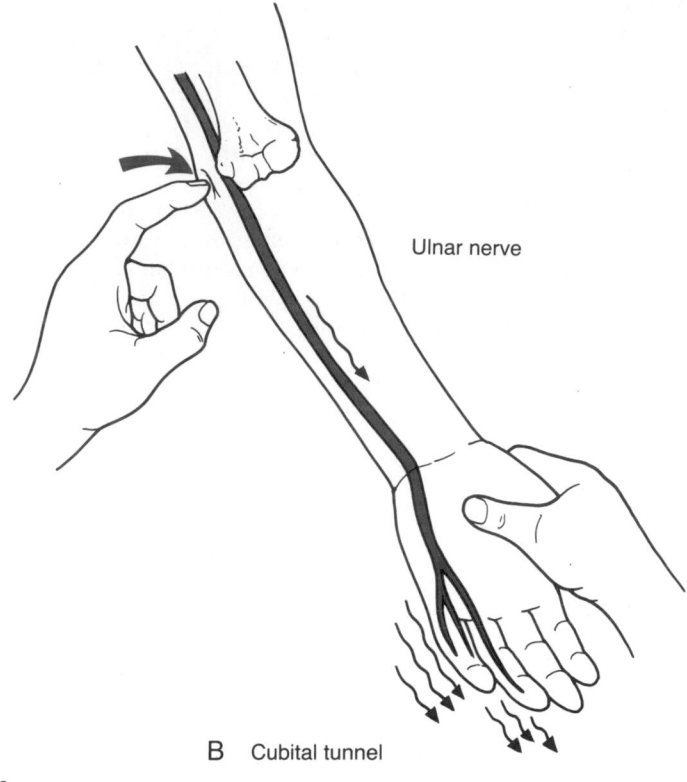

Ulnar nerve

B   Cubital tunnel

FIGURE 31–24   Tinel's sign, the carpal and cubital tunnels.

eration that has occurred following the repair of a nerve laceration. The test involves tapping along the nerve from distal to proximal toward the site of the injury; elicitation of paresthesia indicates the location to which regeneration has occurred. Paresthesia also may occur at the site of compression in peripheral nerve entrapment neuropathies; common sites include the following (see Figure 31–24):

   (1). Cubital tunnel. Tap posterior to the medial humeral epicondyle.

   (2). Carpal tunnel. Tap over the flexor retinaculum.

   (3). Distal superficial radial nerve. Tap dorsal to the radial styloid process.

   (4). Distal ulnar tunnel. Tap between the pisiform and the hook of the hamate.

3. Movement assessment

  a. Functional movement is the ability to perform basic types of grip and pinch activities. A therapist can assess a patient's functional movement by having him/her handle common objects, perform standardized hand function tests, or use a work simulator[9] (see Figure 31–25).

   (1). Examples of grip and pinch functional movements are as follow:

  (a). Power grip. This grip is associated with strongly gripping a handle. It requires finger flexion and rotation, particularly in the ulnar aspect of the hand. This grip requires integrity of the ulnar nerve.

  (b). Precision grip. Precision grip is associated with handling small objects, usually with prehension of the thumb, index finger and middle finger; it requires integrity of the median nerve.

  (c). Hook grip. This is associated with holding onto an object with contact at the PIP joints, which are flexed; it requires integrity of the median nerve.

  (d). Lateral pinch. Lateral pinch is associated with pinching or holding an object such as a key between the thumb pulp and the lateral aspect of the index finger; it requires integrity of the ulnar nerve.

  (e). Cylinder grasp. This grasp is associated with holding a rod with the fingers and thumb

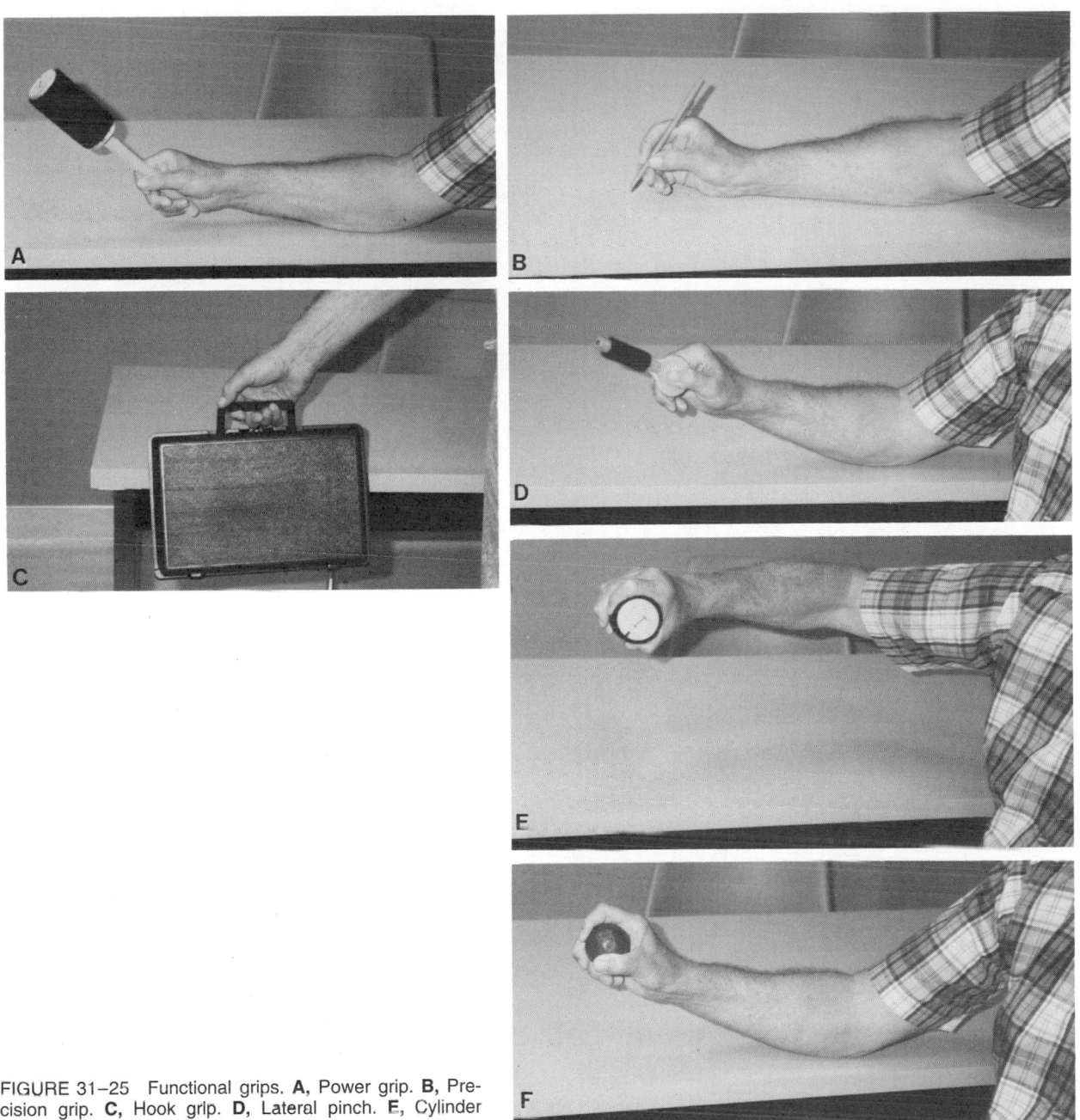

FIGURE 31–25 Functional grips. **A,** Power grip. **B,** Precision grip. **C,** Hook grip. **D,** Lateral pinch. **E,** Cylinder grasp. **F,** Spherical grasp.

flexed; it requires integrity of the median and ulnar nerves.

(f). Spherical grasp. This is associated with holding a ball with the fingers and thumb partially flexed and the thumb opposed; it requries integrity of the median and ulnar nerves.

(2). Gross strength is assessed with a Jamar dynamometer (Asimow Engineering, Los Angeles) and B & L pinch gauge (B & L Engineering, Sante Fe Springs, CA), for which norms have been established and published by Mathiowetz.[10]

(a). Grip strength is tested by placing the patient in a seated position with the arm at his/her side, the elbow flexed 90 degrees, the forearm in neutral rotation, and the wrist extended between 0 and 30 degrees and ulnarly deviated 15 degrees. The patient alternately grips a dynamometer with his/her right and left hands, performing three trials in each of the five handle positions.[11] Stokes[12] and Janda et al.[13] stated that graphed values should fall into a bell-shaped curve, peaking at the second or third handle position. Bechtol[14] reported that the coefficient of variance should not exceed 10% for adults (see Table 31–2 for normal values; see Figure 31–26).

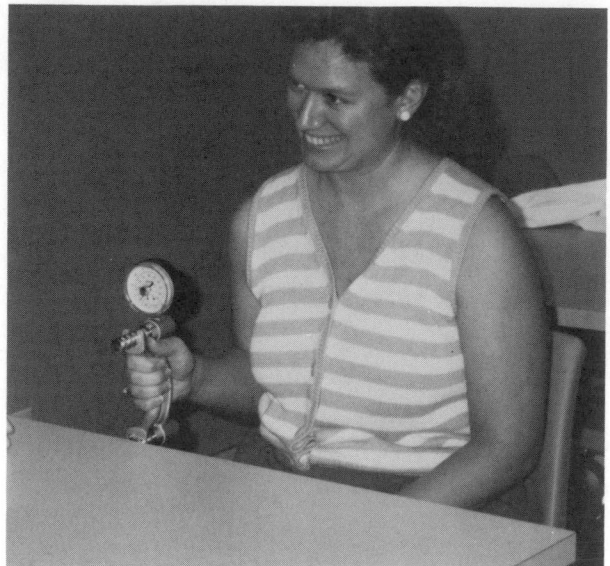

FIGURE 31–26   Testing grip strength.

(b). Pinch strength is tested by placing the patient in the same position as that used for testing grip strength. The examiner hands a pinch gauge to him/her in a comfortable position for pinching with the thumb, index finger, and middle finger (a three-point, or three-jaw, chuck). The patient alternates between his/her right and left hands for three trials; the tests are repeated for the key pinch (the thumb against the lateral index finger) and the tip pinch (the thumb tip against the index fingertip) (see Table 31–3 for normal values; see Figure 31–27).

(3). Composite ROM is assessed with a ruler or tape measure. The distance the patient *lacks* from reaching the following landmarks is recorded:

(a). Finger flexion to the proximal palmar crease. The distance from the fingertips to the proximal palmar crease when they are in flexion is indicative of combined MP, PIP, and DIP joint flexion (see Figure 31–28).

(b). Finger flexion to the MP crease. The distance from the fingertips to the MP crease when they are in flexion is indicative of combined PIP and DIP joint flexion.

(c). Finger extension to the dorsal plane. The distance from the

Table 31–2.   GRIP STRENGTH NORMS (IN POUNDS)

Sex	Hand	Age, y						
		16–19	*20–29*	*30–39*	*40–49*	*50–59*	*60–69*	*70+*
Male	Right	101	121	121	113	107	90	71
	Left	86	108	112	107	93	77	60
Female	Right	70	72	76	66	62	52	46
	Left	59	62	67	59	52	43	41

(Adapted from Mathiowetz V: Grip and pinch strength measurements. In Amundsen LR (ed): *Muscle Strength Testing*. New York, Churchill Livingstone, 1990.)

Table 31–3. PINCH STRENGTH NORMS (IN POUNDS)

Sex	Hand	Test	16–19	20–29	30–39	40–49	50–59	60–69
					Age, y			
Male	Right	Three-point	23	26	26	24	24	22
		Lateral	23	21	26	26	25	23
		Tip	16	18	18	18	17	16
	Left	Three-point	22	26	26	24	23	21
		Lateral	22	25	26	25	25	22
		Tip	15	17	18	18	16	15
Female	Right	Three-point	19	18	18	18	17	15
		Lateral	18	18	18	17	16	15
		Tip	13	12	12	12	12	10
	Left	Three-point	18	17	18	17	16	14
		Lateral	17	16	17	16	15	14
		Tip	12	11	12	12	11	10

(Adapted from Mathiowetz V: Grip and pinch strength measurements. In Amundsen LR (ed): *Muscle Strength Testing*. New York, Churchill Livingstone, 1990.)

fingertips to an extension of the plane of the dorsal hand when the fingers are in extension is indicative of combined MP, PIP, and DIP joint extension (see Figure 31–28).

b. Physiologic movement. In addition to testing for gross measures of function, strength, and motion, an examiner usually desires to know specific values for individual joints. To obtain such values, goniometric measurements and manual muscle testing are performed on isolated joints as indicated. It is often necessary to make a distinction between the *active* and *passive* ROM (AROM and PROM, respec-

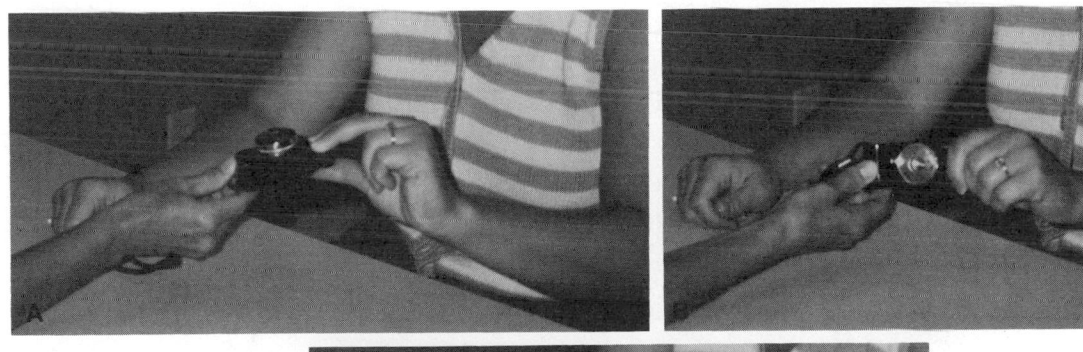

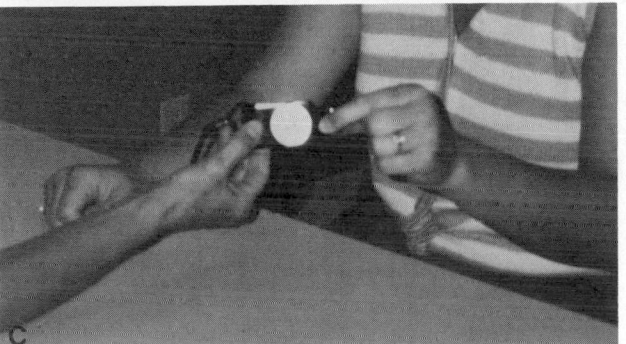

FIGURE 31–27   Testing pinch strength. **A,** Palmar (three-point pinch). **B,** Key pinch. **C,** Tip pinch.

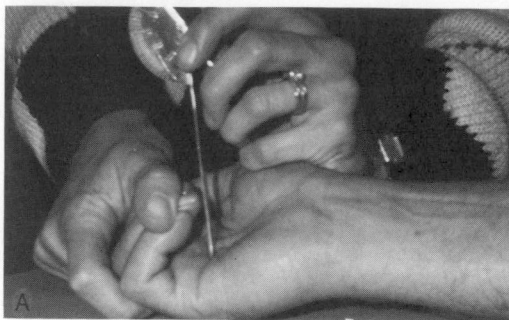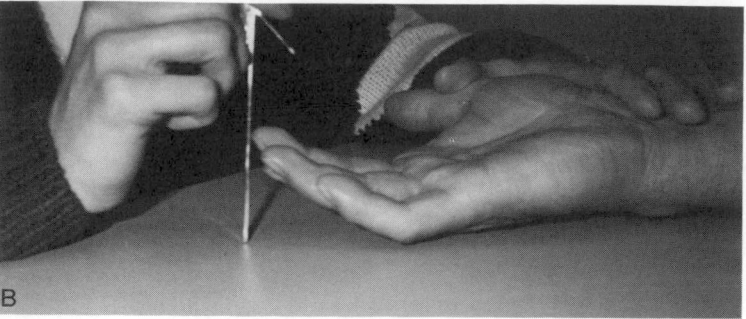

FIGURE 31–28   Measuring composite ROM. **A,** Flexion to proximal palmar crease. **B,** Extension to dorsal plane.

tively) available at a joint, as well as to identify the type of symptoms elicited by the various types of movement testing.

(1). AROM indicates the amount of movement that a patient can produce. This measurement demonstrates a combination of the patient's willingness to comply, joint mobility, tendon integrity and gliding, and neuromuscular integration. The examiner chooses an ap-

propriate goniometer, depending on the size of the joint to be tested, the examiner's preference for dorsal or lateral models, and the presence of edema, lesions, or other problems. Examples of common measurement techniques are illustrated in Figures 31–29 to 31–34 (see Table 31–4 for average ROM values). Because the finger tendons cross several joints, to measure ROM of any one particular joint, it is necessary to position the adjacent joints in positions that decrease the tension in the tendons. To measure composite mo-

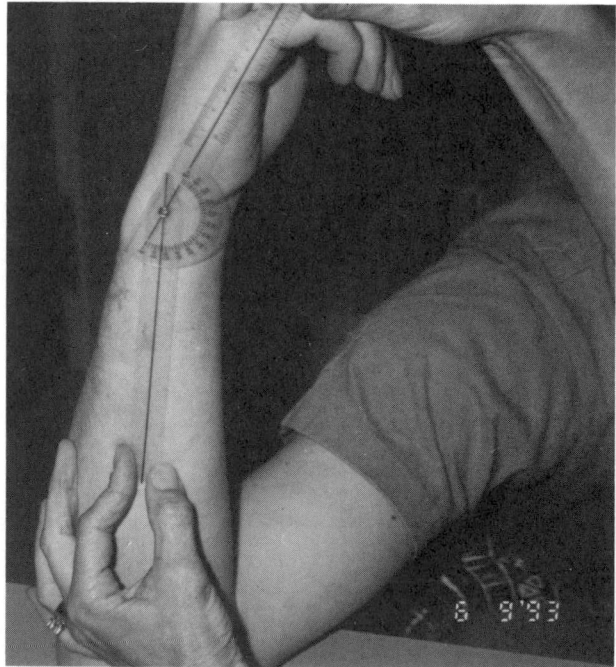

FIGURE 31–29 Measuring wrist flexion ROM—the axis of goniometer over the ulnar styloid process with the arms bisecting the ulna and fifth metacarpal bone.

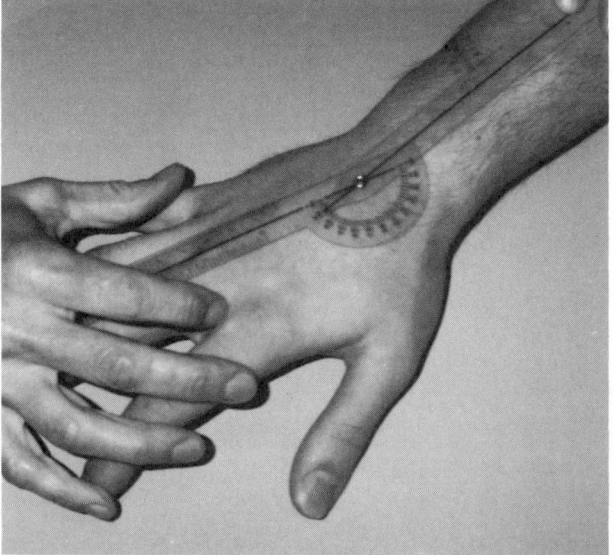

FIGURE 31–30 Measuring wrist ulnar deviation ROM—the axis of goniometer over the capitate with the arms bisecting the forearm and third metacarpal bone.

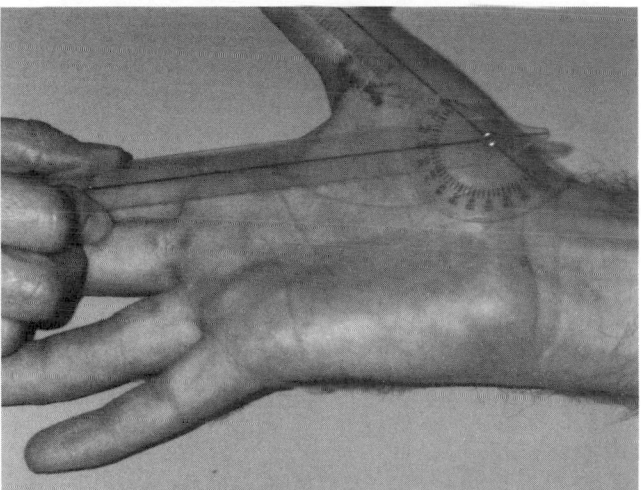

FIGURE 31–31   Measuring thumb extension ROM—the axis of goniometer over the volar CMC joint with the arms bisecting the first and second metacarpal bones.

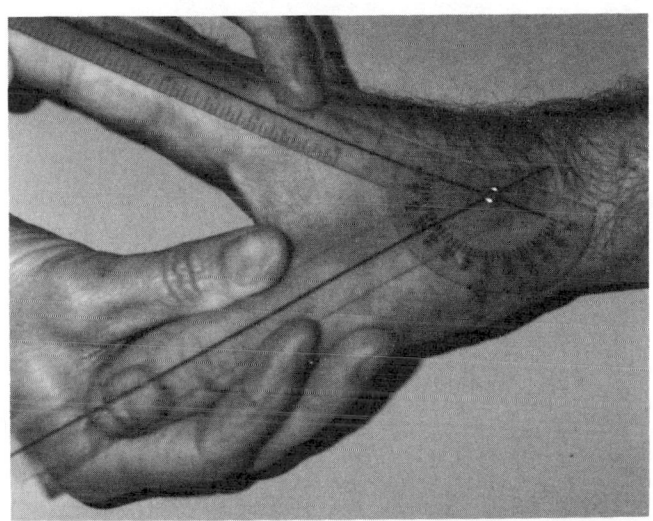

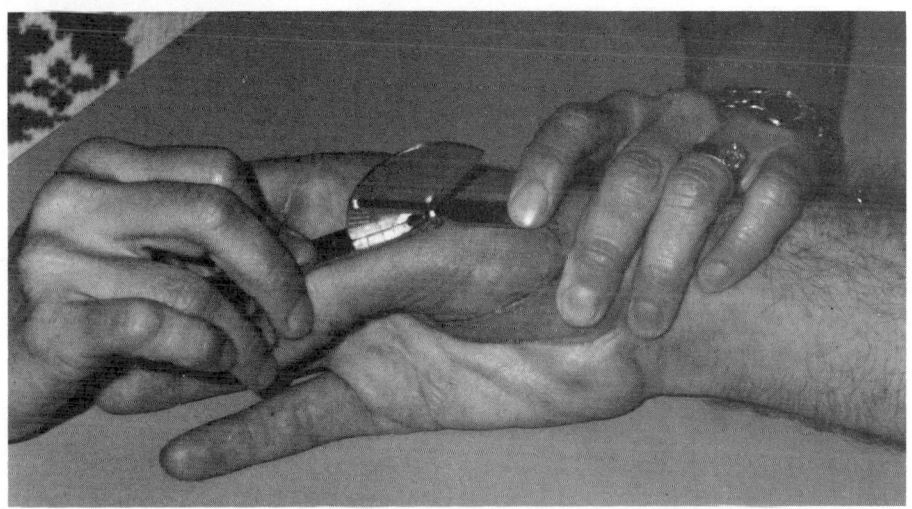

FIGURE 31–32   Measuring thumb abduction ROM—the axis of goniometer over the dorsal CMC joint with the arms bisecting the first and second metacarpal bones.

FIGURE 31–33   Measuring thumb MP joint ROM—the axis of goniometer over the dorsal MP joint with the arms resting on the first metacarpal bone and proximal phalanx.

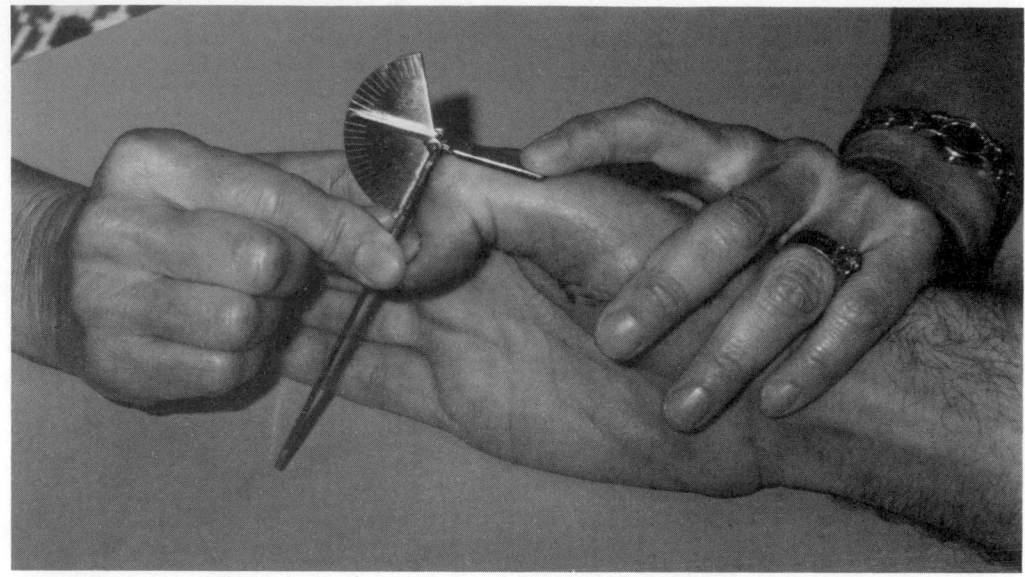

FIGURE 31–34 Measuring thumb IP joint ROM—the axis of goniometer over the dorsal IP joint with the arms resting on the proximal and distal phalanges.

tion, all joints are positioned to place maximum tension on the tendons.

(2). PROM indicates the amount of movement that can be produced in a joint by an outside force. This measurement primarily reflects the status of inert structures surrounding the joint, *ie*, the joint capsule

Table 31–4.   ROM

Joint	Motion	Range, Degrees
Elbow	Flexion	150
	Extension	0
Forearm	Supination	85
	Pronation	85
Wrist	Flexion	85
	Extension	80
	Ulnar deviation	35
	Radial deviation	20
Thumb CMC	Abduction	50
	Extension	60
Thumb MP	Flexion	50
	Extension	0
Thumb IP	Flexion	80
	Extension	50
Finger MP	Abduction	20
	Flexion	90
	Extension	25
Finger PIP	Flexion	110
	Extension	0
Finger DIP	Flexion	90
	Extension	30

and ligaments. Normally, PROM *slightly* exceeds AROM; differences of *greater* than 10 degrees signify a problem in AROM, *ie*, decreased tendon gliding or weakness. The principles for measuring passive individual joint movement and passive composite joint movement are the same as for AROM, except that movement is produced by an outside force.

(3). Active insufficiency denotes the failure of a musculotendinous unit that crosses two or more joints to shorten sufficiently to move all of the joints it crosses through their full excursion simultaneously (*eg,* the FDP muscle loses some mechanical efficiency when actively flexing the wrist and all finger joints simultaneously; consequently, grip strength is weaker when the wrist is flexed than when the wrist is extended).

(4). Passive insufficiency denotes the failure of a musculotendinous unit that crosses two or more joints to stretch sufficiently to passively allow all of the joints it crosses to reach their full excursion simultaneously (*eg,* the ED muscle is stretched maximally by passive wrist and finger flexion simultaneously; consequently, passive finger joint flexion is less when the wrist is flexed than when the wrist is extended).

(5). End feel imparts to the examiner the sensation of structures reaching the end of their ROM; this may help the examiner to identify the nature of the limitation.[15]

    (a). Bone: abrupt halt secondary to contact with hard surfaces, *eg*, during elbow extension.

    (b). Capsular: tight stretch as soft tissues are fully lengthened, *eg*, during MP joint extension.

    (c). Springy block: rebound or joint locking within ROM, *eg*, a loose body or meniscus tear.

    (d). Tissue approximation: involves a gradual "soft" limit as body surfaces engage, *eg*, during the performance of active elbow flexion.

    (e). Empty: no resistance to movement, *eg*, when a patient requests that the movement be stopped secondary to pain, or when a loss of restraints occurs in a hypermobile joint.

    (f). Spasm: muscle contraction limits ROM, *eg*, a spasm of the FCR muscle limits wrist extension.

(6). Resisted motion indicates the strength of specific muscles acting on designated joints, as well as symptoms elicited by their contraction. Standardized techniques for strength testing and documentation are presented in other sources and are not elaborated here.

An examiner usually isolates specific muscles during manual muscle testing; in the hand, specific maneuvers are needed to separate the FDS and FDP muscles (which both flex the PIP joint) and to separate the ED muscle and intrinsic muscles (which both extend the PIP joint). When testing the FDS muscle, the examiner holds all fingers not being tested in extension to anchor the FDP muscle distally. The patient then attempts to flex the PIP joint; this movement will now reflect solely the strength of the FDS muscle (see Figure 31–35). When the intrinsic muscles are being tested, the patient first actively extends all MP joints to anchor the ED muscle; he/she then attempts to extend the PIP joint; this movement will now reflect solely the strength of the intrinsic muscles (see Figure 31–36).

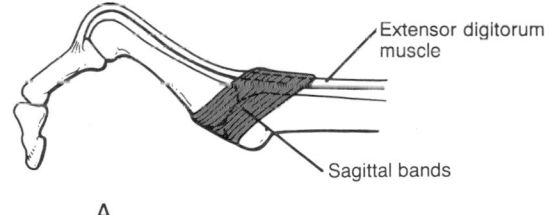

Extensor digitorum muscle

Sagittal bands

A

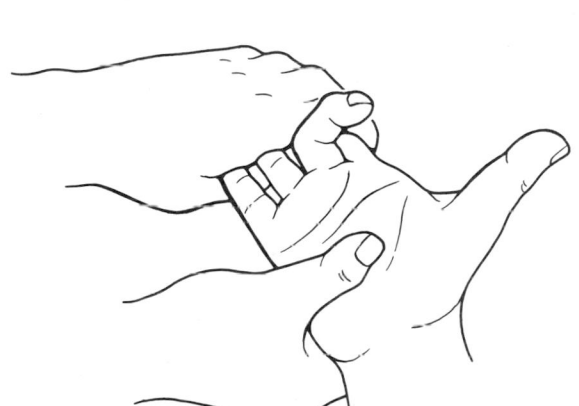

FIGURE 31–35 Isolated strength testing of FDS; the examiner holds the fingers not being tested in extension to anchor flexor digitorum profundus distally. Then the patient attempts to flex the PIP joint of the finger being tested, which is indicative of FDS strength.

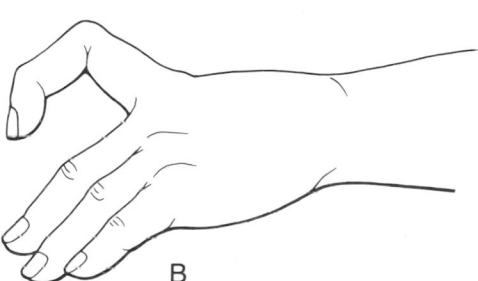

B

FIGURE 31–36 Isolated strength testing of intrinsic muscles. **A,** During active hyperextension of the MP joint, the sagittal bands anchor extensor digitorum at the MP joint, rendering it lax distally and incapable of extending the PIP joint. **B,** The patient attempts active extension of the PIP joint (while also holding the MP joint in hyperextension); in this position, only the intrinsic muscles can extend the PIP joint.

(7). Selective tissue tension testing is used to identify the lesioned tissue by reproduction of symptoms; pain arising from inert tissues usually occurs with active and passive movement in the *same* direction (*eg,* an anterior elbow capsular tear is painful with either *active* or *passive* extension, which both place tension on the anterior capsule). Pain from a contractile tissue usually occurs with active and passive movement in the *opposite* direction (*eg,* a biceps muscle tear is painful with *active elbow flexion* or *passive elbow extension,* which both increase tension in the muscle).[15]

(8). Accessory (arthrokinematic) movement assesses the passive capability of joint surfaces to move relative to one another. Traction and compression, gliding, and rotation are components necessary for normal, pain-free ROM, but they cannot be produced in isolation actively; an examiner assesses each joint's accessory movement on a scale from 0 to 6 (see Table 31–5) and notes any symptoms that are associated with the movement.

4. Neurologic evaluation reveals abnormalities in nerve conduction that may be the cause of a patient's problem, *eg,* weakness, sensory disturbance, pain, aberrant reflexes, or coordination difficulties. An examiner attempts to localize the source of involvement to a nerve root, peripheral nerve, or central nervous system lesion, keeping in mind that there may be overlaps and anomalies in innervation patterns. Compiling results from several tests facilitates the making of a differential diagnosis.

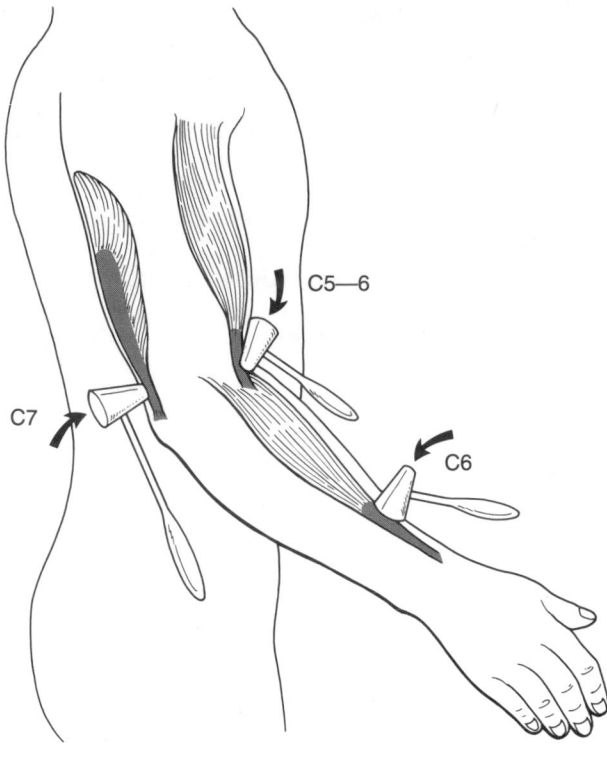

FIGURE 31–37 Testing deep tendon reflexes for the C5–C6, C6 and C7 root levels.

a. For general screening purposes, an examiner tests "key muscles," "key reflexes" (see Figure 31–37), and sensory changes to identify involvement of a particular nerve root level (see Table 31–6). "Sensory distributions" also help the examiner to distinguish between nerve root and peripheral nerve involvement (see Figure 31–38). An examiner hypothesizes about the source of a lesion and then completes the examination of the muscles and cutaneous area supplied by the nerve root or peripheral nerve to confirm the hypothesis. He/she must be aware that certain symptoms such as paresthesias, referred pain, and alterations of deep tendon reflexes may be produced by irritation of other tissues and do not always indicate nerve root or peripheral nerve involvement.

b. In the case of motor control disorders, which are manifested by spasticity, rigidity, flaccidity, and so forth, a thorough

Table 31–5. ACCESSORY JOINT MOVEMENTS

Grade	Movement
0	No movement; joint ankylosed
1	Considerable joint hypomobility
2	Slight joint hypomobility
3	Normal joint mobility
4	Slight joint hypermobility
5	Considerable joint hypermobility
6	Very unstable joint

Table 31–6.   MUSCLES, REFLEXES, AND SENSATION REPRESENTATIVE OF
NERVE ROOT LEVELS

Root Level	"Key Muscle"	Reflex	Sensory Distribution (Dermatome)
C5	Deltoid, biceps	Biceps (C5-6)	Lateral arm to wrist
C6	Biceps, brachioradialis	Brachioradialis	Lateral arm and thumb
C7	Triceps	Triceps	Middle of arm and index, middle, and ring fingers
C8	Flexor digitorum profundus	None	Medial arm and little finger
T1	Interossei	None	Medial arm to wrist

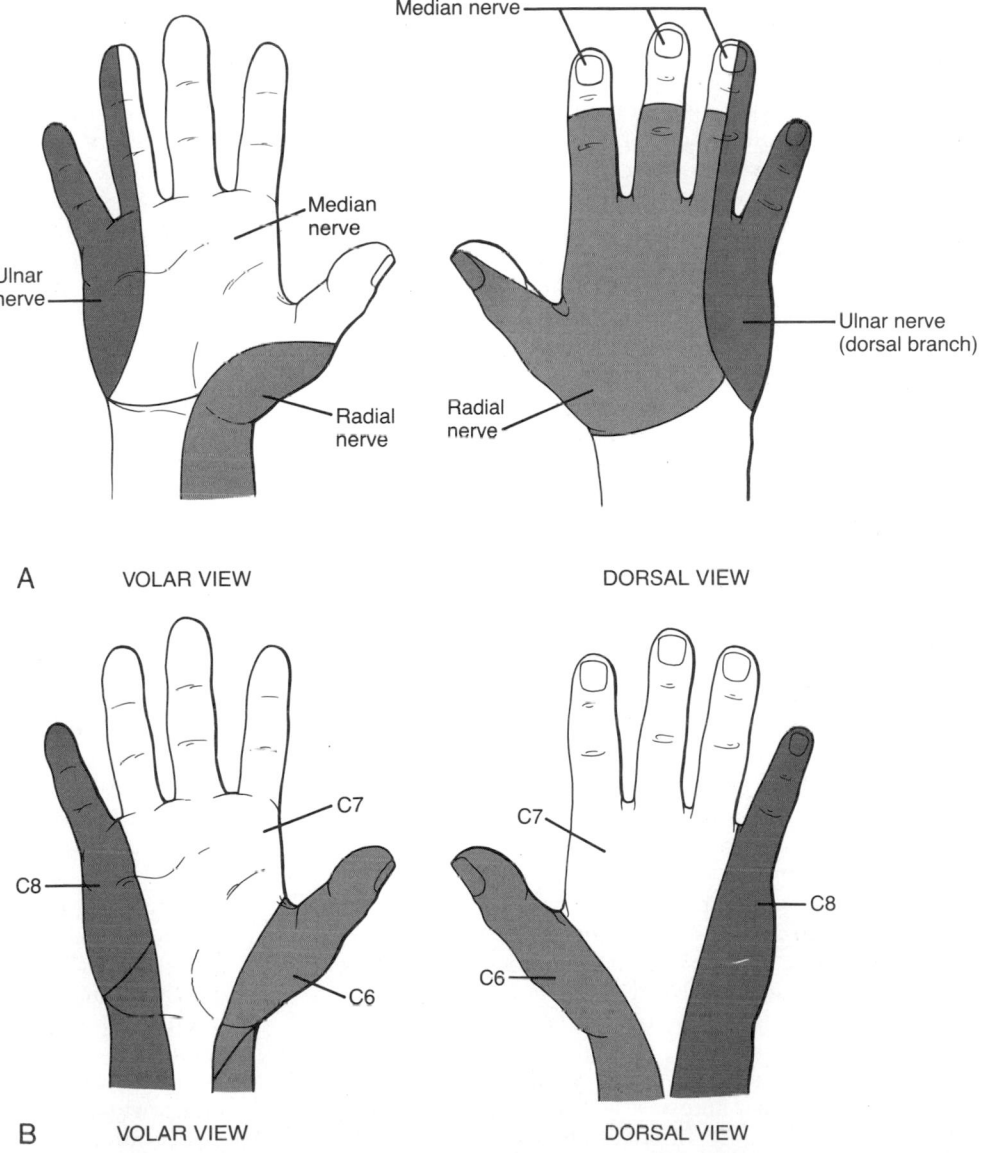

FIGURE 31–38   Comparison of sensory distributions supplied by the peripheral nerves **(A)** and cervical nerve roots **(B)**.

neurologic evaluation for upper motor neuron and spinal tract dysfunction is indicated.

c. Sensibility testing usually proceeds from a subjective description of any loss of or changes in nerve function to more objective tests and measurements. The results are used to identify the area of the lesion and the associated functional disability as well as the level of return in nerve regeneration. Return of sensibility with nerve regeneration usually occurs in the following order: pain, 30 cycles per second (cps), vibration moving touch and two-point discrimination, constant touch and two-point discrimination, and 256 cps vibration (see page 911 for reinnervation hypothesis).

(1). Modality tests include detection of light touch and discrimination between sharp versus dull and hot versus cold sensations; these tests initially help to determine the pattern of nerve involvement, *eg,* nerve root dermatome versus peripheral nerve cutaneous pattern.

(2). Tinel's sign monitors the progression of nerve regeneration (and may also signal the presence of compression neuropathy); an examiner percusses along a nerve distal to proximal until he/she reaches a point at which paresthesias are elicited. This is the level to which regeneration has progressed.

(3). Objective tests eliminate the subjectivity of a patient's response but the results may not correlate directly with functional return.[11]

(a). Sudomotor (sweat) test. Sympathetic nerve function corresponds to sensory nerve function only initially after a lesion or in cases of complete loss of nerve function. Ninhydrin applied to the palm reacts with certain amino acids in sweat, if present, to produce a colored print; areas devoid of color can be assumed to be denervated.[16]

(b). Wrinkle test. A hand is immersed in water at 104°F for 5 minutes; only innervated skin will wrinkle.[17]

(c). Nerve conduction velocity test. This test assesses the type, site, and degree of sensory nerve involvement by identifying loss or slowing of the conduction velocity or alteration in potential amplitudes; an electrical current stimulus is applied at the distal electrodes, and the action potential is recorded at the proximal electrodes.

(4). Subjective sensation is evaluated by several different types of tests.

(a). Vibratory testing evaluates the threshold of stimulus needed to elicit vibration perception; this test is useful for monitoring nerve compression.[18,19] The noninvasive nature of the test enhances patient receptivity. The test results are considered to correlate with the patient's functional ability. Vibrations are monitored with 30-cps or 256-cps tuning forks or vibrometers. Meissner receptors perceive 30 cps vibration, and Pacinian receptors perceive 256 cps. An examiner applies the vibratory instrument to one of the patient's fingertips and asks him/her to discern the differences between quality of vibration in involved and noninvolved areas. When a vibrometer is used, a patient reports when he/she detects vibration as the amplitude is gradually increased[20] (see Figure 31–39).

(b). Two-point discrimination tests a patient's ability to feel one versus two blunt points placed simultaneously on the skin. This test assesses innervation density and is useful in charting nerve regeneration. A caliper or discrimination device marked in millimeter increments should be used; it should be applied to the palmar surface of the supported hand while the patient's vision is occluded.[19,21]

(i). Static two-point discrimi-

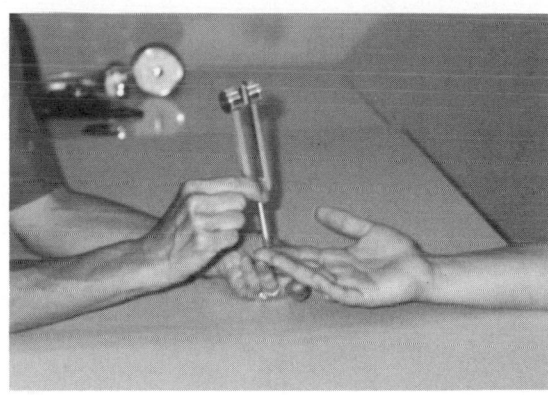

FIGURE 31–39 Testing vibratory sensation with a 256-cps tuning fork.

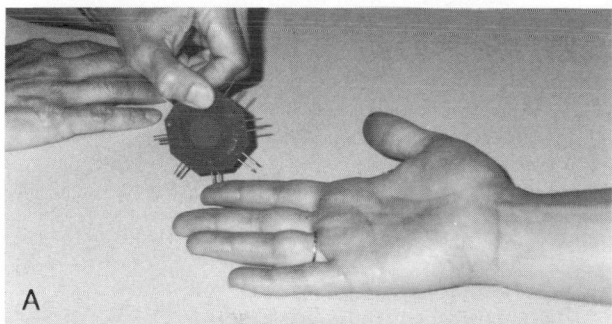

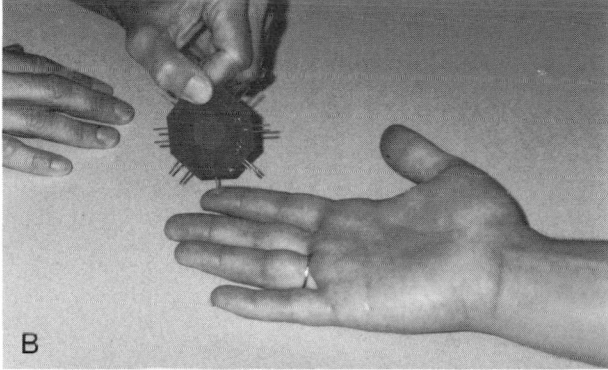

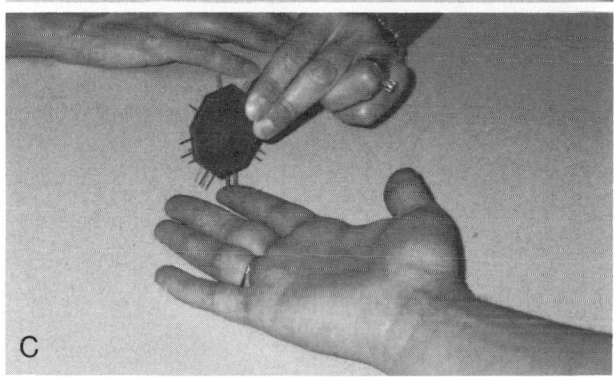

FIGURE 31–40 Testing two-point discrimination. **A,** Static two-point (points are applied parallel to long axis of finger). **B,** Application of one-point is randomly alternated with the application of two-points. **C,** Moving two-point (points are applied perpendicular to long axis of finger and moved from proximal to distal).

nation assesses a slowly adapting fiber receptor system. The examiner applies the points parallel to the long axis of the finger, randomly alternating between one and two points (see Figures 31–40A and 31–40B). The examiner narrows the interprong distance until the patient perceives only one point; the patient must provide 7 of 10 correct responses for the examiner to be able to document a discrimination distance (see Table 31–6 for standard values).

(ii). Moving two-point discrimination assesses the quickly adapting fiber receptor system; this test correlates best with tactile gnosis and function.[19] This test is applied in a similar manner to that of static tests, except that the instrument is moved in a stroking fashion from proximal to distal with the points aligned transverse to the long axis of the finger and moved parallel to the finger (see Figure 31–40C).

(c). The Semmes-Weinstein monofilament test is a threshold test that measures stimulus intensity. It is useful in assessing loss of sensory function associated with nerve compression. Calibrated sets of monofilaments are commercially available. An examiner touches the thinnest monofilament to the patient's fingertip until it bends; while the patient's vi-

Table 31–7. SENSORY NORMS

Monofilament Number	Two-Point Distance
Normal light touch: 1.65–2.83	Normal: <6 mm
Diminished light touch: 3.22–3.61	Fair: 6–10 mm
Diminished protective sensation: 3.84–4.31	Poor: 11–15 mm
Loss of protective sensation: 4.56–6.65	Protective: One point perceived
Deep pressure sensation: >6.65	Anesthetic: Nothing perceived

sion is occluded, he/she is asked to identify his/her perception of the stimulus. If it is not perceived after three applications, the next-thickest monofilament is applied; this progression is repeated until the stimulus is felt (see Table 31–7; see Figure 31–41).

(5). Functional tests range from manipulating common objects to sophisticated, standardized tests.

(a). A ridge sensiometer can be used to measure depth-sense limen.

(b). The Seddon coin test requires both motor and sensory integrity; the patient must manipulate the coin and recognize the smooth versus the milled edge.

(c). The Moberg pick-up test requires both motor and sensory integrity; it is a timed comparison of the ability of the involved and uninvolved hands to pick up objects and place them in a box.

(d). The Dellon modification of the Moberg test is the same as the Moberg test already discussed with the exception that it includes standardized items, and that the uninvolved fingers are taped to the palm to force the patient to use only the involved fingers.[19]

(e). Standardized tests, including the Perdue pegboard test, the Minnesota manual dexterity test, and the O'Connor finger dexterity test, are commercially available with instructions for application and documentation (see Figure 31–42).

5. Special tests may aid the examiner in clarifying a disorder or in isolating a lesion.

a. Elbow collateral ligamentous stress test. The examiner applies perpendicular force at the elbow joint; valgus force stresses the medial collateral ligament,

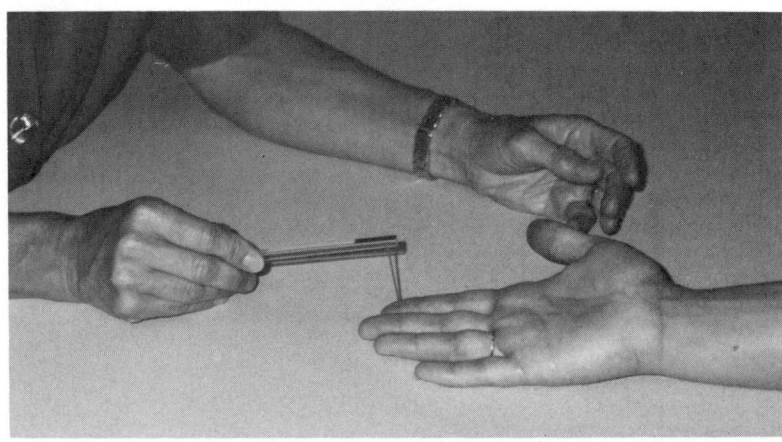

FIGURE 31–41 Testing threshold sensation with monofilaments.

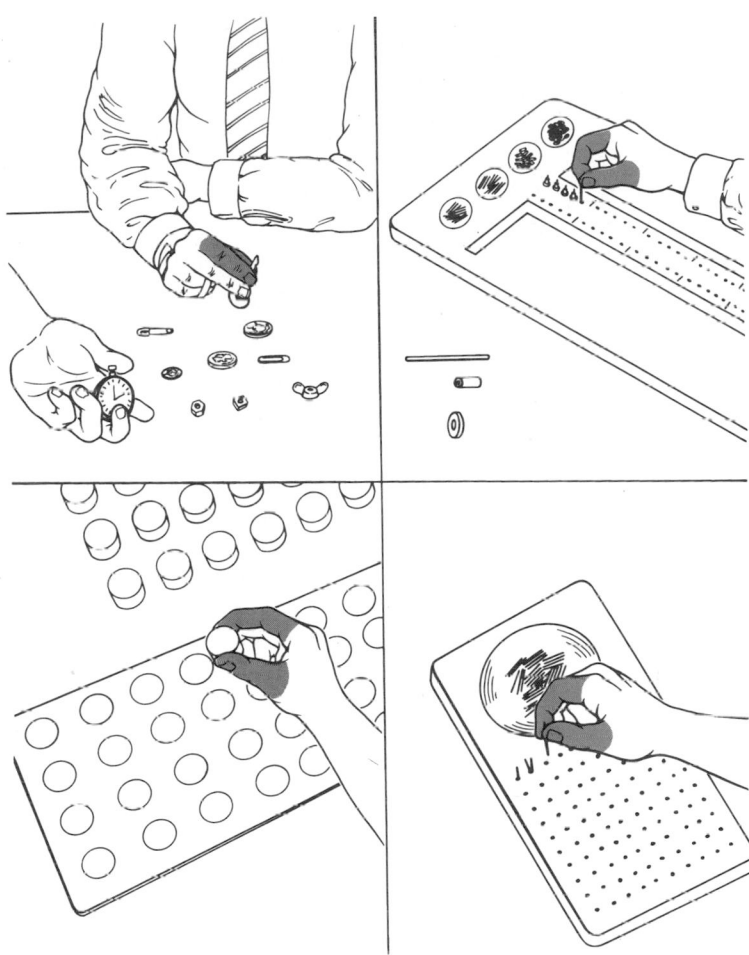

FIGURE 31–42 Functional tests of sensibility.
A, Modified Moberg pickup test. **B,** Purdue peg-
board test. **C,** Minnesota manual dexterity test.
D, O'Connor finger dexterity test.

reproducing symptoms of pain or laxity
following a sprain (see Figure 31–43).
The varus stress produces symptoms associated with a lesion of the lateral collateral ligament.

b. Lateral epicondylitis test. The examiner
resists wrist extension with the patient's
elbow extended and the forearm pronated (see Figure 31–44*A*); he/she then
passively flexes the wrist with the arm in
the same position (see Figure 31–44*B*).
Both maneuvers stress the ECRB muscle,
and, a positive test result occurs when the
patient reports pain over the lateral humeral epicondyle.

c. Medial epicondylitis test. The examiner
resists wrist flexion with the patient's
elbow extended and the forearm supinated; he/she then passively extends the

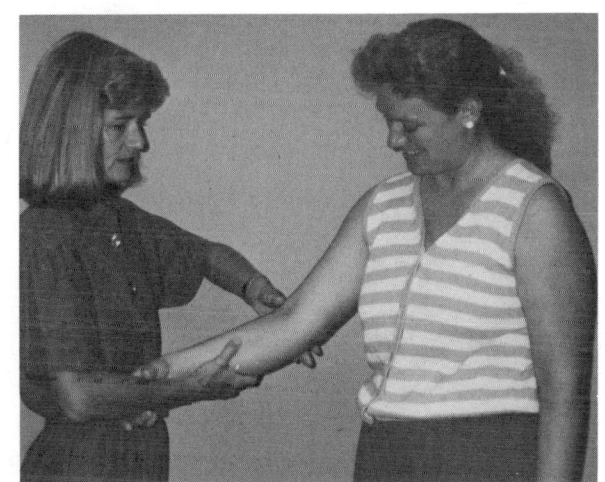

FIGURE 31–43 Stress testing of the medial collateral ligament of the elbow with valgus force on forearm.

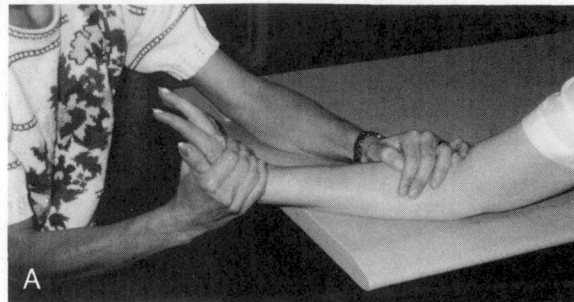

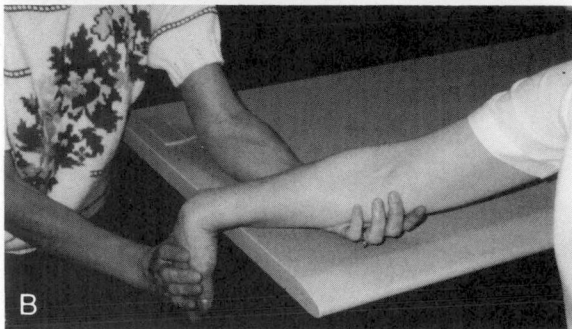

FIGURE 31–44   Lateral epicondylitis test. **A,** The examiner resists wrist extension while the elbow is extended and the forearm pronated. **B,** The examiner passively flexes the wrist while the elbow is extended and the forearm pronated. Pain over the lateral humeral epicondyle indicates a positive test.

wrist with the arm in the same position. Both maneuvers stress the FCR muscle and PT muscle. A positive test result occurs when the patient reports pain over the medial humeral epicondyle.

d. Finklestein test. The examiner resists thumb extension and abduction and then passively flexes the thumb and deviates the wrist in an ulnar direction. Both maneuvers stress the APL and EPB tendons.

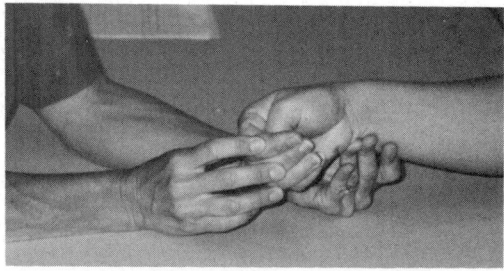

FIGURE 31–45   Finklestein test. The patient flexes the thumb and then ulnarly deviates the wrist. Pain over the radial styloid process indicates a positive test.

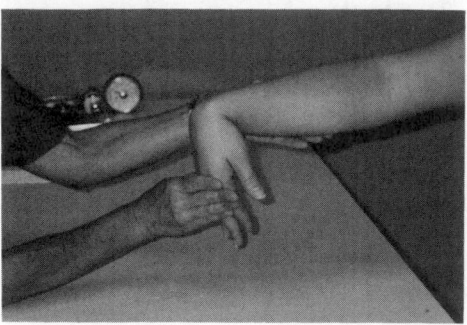

FIGURE 31–46   Phalen's test. Full wrist flexion with the elbow extended is maintained for 60 seconds. Pain or paresthesia in the median nerve distribution in the hand indicates a positive test.

A positive test occurs when the patient reports localized pain near the radial styloid process, which indicates DeQuervain's syndrome (see Figure 31–45).

e. Phalen's test. The examiner passively maintains full wrist flexion with the elbow extended for 60 seconds; reproduction of pain or sensory changes in the median nerve distribution in the hand is indicative of carpal tunnel syndrome (see Figure 31–46).

f. Bunnell-Littler test. The examiner attempts to passively flex the PIP joint, first with the MP joint passively extended and then with the MP joint passively flexed. If more PIP joint flexion is obtained when the MP joint is flexed, tightness exists in the intrinsic muscles (see Figure 31–47).

g. Oblique retinacular ligament test. The examiner attempts to passively flex the DIP joint, first with the PIP joint passively extended and then with the PIP joint passively flexed. If more DIP joint flexion is obtained when the PIP joint is flexed, tightness exists in the oblique retinacular ligament (see Figure 31–48).

h. Froment's sign. The patient performs a key pinch on an object such as a sheet of paper (see Figure 31–49). If the thumb "collapses" into flexion at the IP joint, then the FPL muscle has overpowered the thumb extensor mechanism; this usually indicates ulnar nerve involvement, with weakness in the AP muscle and the deep head of the FPB muscle. These muscles contribute to the dorsal hood of the thumb and assist in extension. Occasionally, Froment's sign may signify radial

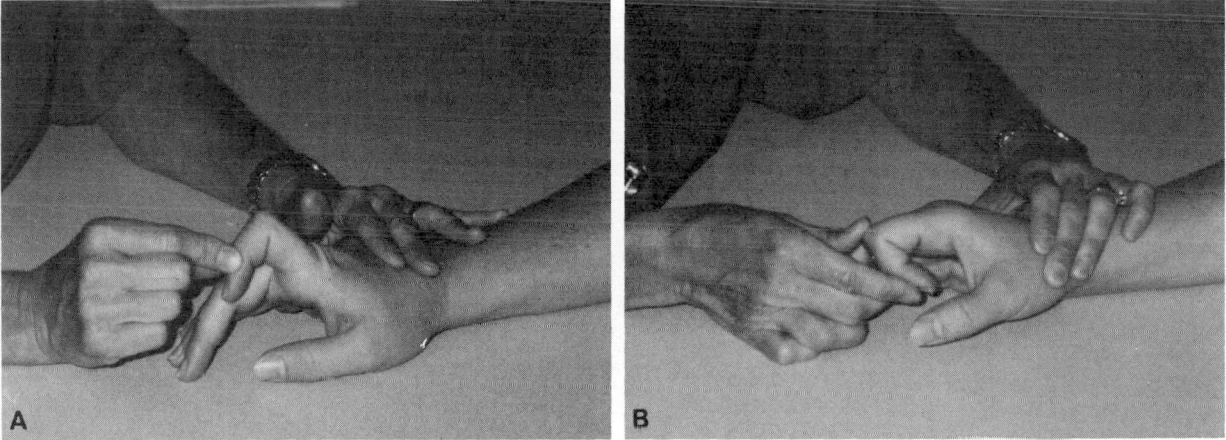

FIGURE 31–47   Bunnell-Littler test. **A,** The examiner passively flexes the PIP joint while the MP joint is extended. **B,** The examiner then passively flexes the PIP joint while the MP joint is flexed; if more PIP joint flexion occurs with the MP joint flexed, the test is positive for intrinsic muscle tightness.

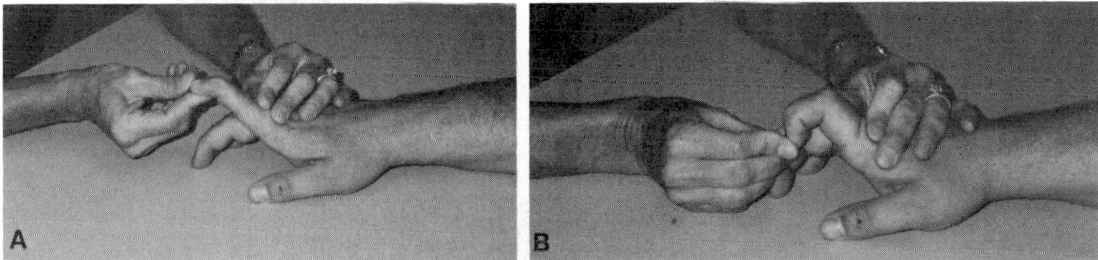

FIGURE 31–48   Oblique retinacular ligament test. **A,** The examiner passively flexes the DIP joint while the PIP joint is extended. **B,** The examiner then passively flexes the DIP joint while the PIP joint is flexed; if more DIP joint flexion occurs with the PIP joint flexed, the test is positive for oblique retinacular ligament tightness.

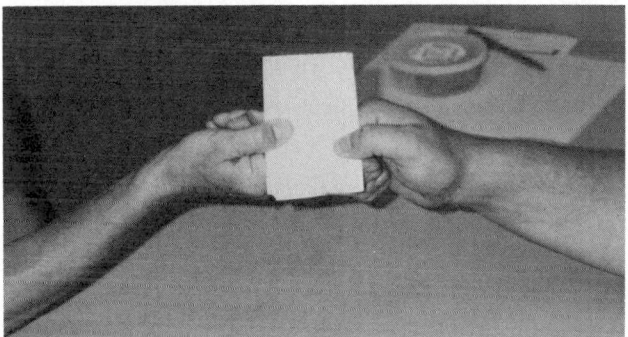

FIGURE 31–49   Froment's sign. The patient attempts to hold an object in a key pinch; if the thumb IP joint collapses into flexion (as on right side), there may be ulnar nerve involvement. Radial or median nerve involvement also may weaken IP joint extension.

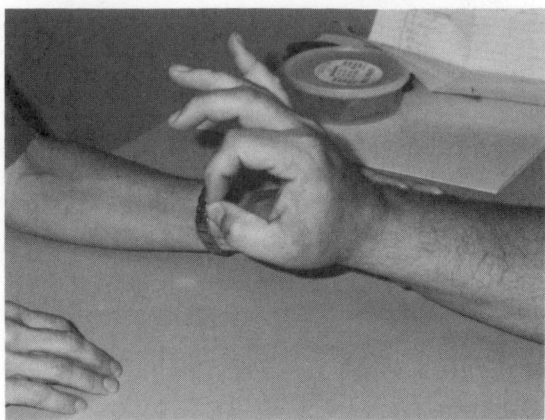

FIGURE 31–50   Circle formation. Opposition of the thumb tip to the index finger tip is a measure of median nerve function.

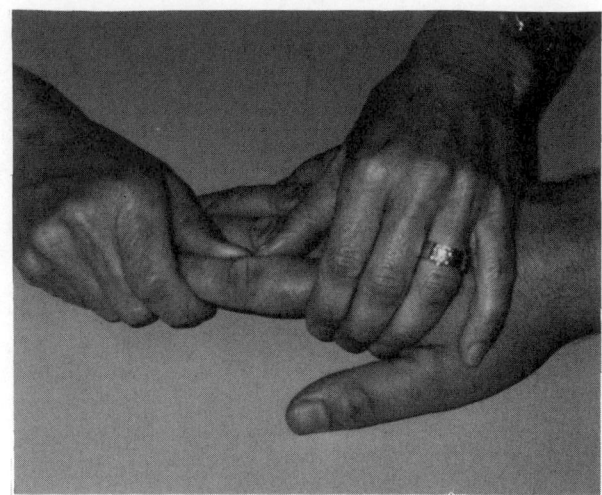

FIGURE 31–51   Stress testing the collateral ligament of the digit.

nerve involvement with weakness in the EPL muscle. Froment's sign may also occur with median nerve involvement, causing weakness in the superficial head of the FPB and APB muscles, which also contribute to the thumb's dorsal hood and assist in extension of the IP joint.[22]

i. Circle formation with tip opposition between thumb and index finger test. The patient attempts to form a circle by opposing the tips of his/her thumb and index finger (see Figure 31–50); a "flattened" circle with more pulp opposition is indicative of anterior interosseous involvement with weakness in the FDP and FPL muscles.

j. Digit collateral ligamentous stress test. Passive force is applied in an attempt to "gap" the MP or IP joints medially or laterally. Stress is placed on the respective ligaments; localized pain or laxity at the joint line may indicate the presence of a collateral ligament problem or a capsular injury (see Figure 31–51).

PLEASE NOTE: After completing the history and physical examination, an examiner must correlate and interpret the findings. Frequently, this requires the compilation of the results of numerous questions, tests, and measurements to make a definitive diagnosis or a prediction of the patient's functional capability. Occasionally, the examiner is not able to make a conclusive decision without obtaining further information. Parts of the examination may have to be repeated, or the patient may have to be referred to other specialists for consultation. Data from additional studies such as radiographic, electrodiagnostic, and laboratory may be required. On conclusion of all testing, the therapist proceeds to identification of the patient's specific problems and to implementation of the appropriate rehabilitation program.

III. Treatment of Common Disorders of the Elbow and Forearm

A. Introduction to elbow pathology

1. The elbow's role in upper extremity functions
   a. The elbow serves as a "link" in a mechanical chain of levers and ultimately determines the limits of hand positioning and accessibility to other body areas as well as to the environment.
   b. The elbow is an effective accelerator.
2. General disorders
   a. Degenerative. Syndromes caused by overuse and resulting in degeneration are common at the elbow.

b. Traumatic. The elbow is the most commonly injured joint in children and the second most frequently dislocated joint in adults.

c. Pattern of referred pain. The elbow may refer pain into the C-6 and C-7 dermatomes.

B. Peripheral nerve entrapment neuropathies

Isolated nerve injury may occur secondary to internal or external compression. The subsequent axon damage and conduction loss result from a combination of ischemia and mechanical distortion.[23,24]

1. Ulnar nerve

a. The history of the problem should be noted. Common sites of compression in and about the elbow and forearm (see Figure 31–52) are:

(1). Arcade of Struthers. This arcade is located between the medial head of the triceps muscle and the intermuscular septum 8 cm proximal to the medial humeral epicondyle.[25]

(2). Cubital tunnel. The cubital tunnel is posterior to the medial humeral epicondyle under the arcuate ligament that stretches between the olecranon and the epicondyle; flexion increases tautness in this ligament.

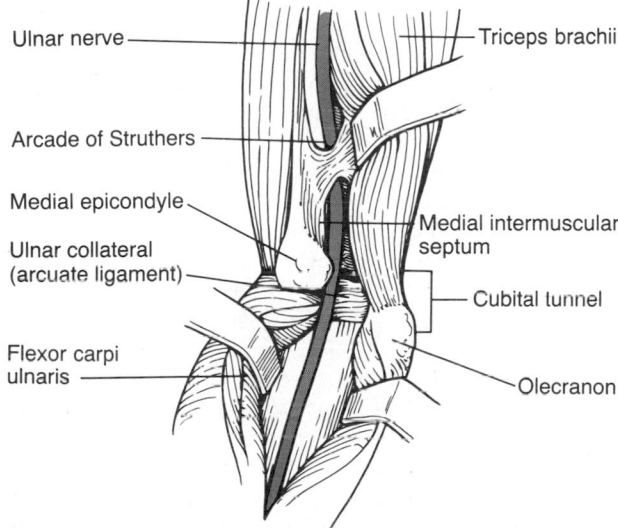

FIGURE 31–52 Ulnar nerve compression sites: the arcade of Struthers and the cubital tunnel.

b. Clinical presentation. The patient may experience vague pain over the medial elbow that may radiate proximally or distally; compression produces sensory changes over the ulnar side of the hand and the medial one and one half digits. Weakness may occur in the FCU muscle and the FDP muscle to the ring and little fingers and in the intrinsic muscles of the hand (except for the first and second lumbrical muscles and the APB, FPB, and OP muscles). Symptoms may be increased by the "elbow flexion test," *ie*, sustained maximum flexion for 1 to 5 minutes. Patients with chronic cases may demonstrate a clawing deformity, intrinsic muscle atrophy, and Froment's sign (see page 877 under subsection "Froment's sign").

c. Management

(1). Identify the patient's problems, which may include
   • pain
   • sensory changes
   • motor loss

(2). Conservative treatment. Have the patient avoid aggravating activity and repetitive motion.[26] Fabricate a Lister splint (the elbow close to full extension with the forearm and wrist in neutral positions) for wear during rest. A physician may prescribe nonsteroidal anti-inflammatory drugs (NSAIDs)[27]

(3). Surgical treatment and rehabilitation. Ulnar nerve transposition involves repositioning the nerve anterior to the medial humeral epicondyle. Rehabilitation includes splinting for 2 to 3 weeks at 90 degrees of elbow flexion, 30 degrees of pronation, and 30 degrees of wrist flexion. After the splint is discontinued, ROM exercises are initiated (possibly in conjunction with whirlpool treatment), along with measures for edema control and light scar massage. At week 6, the patient should begin stretching and strengthening exercises and work hardening; at week 12, the patient may return to heavy labor or sports[28,29] (see Figure 31–53).

2. Median nerve

a. The history of the problem should be

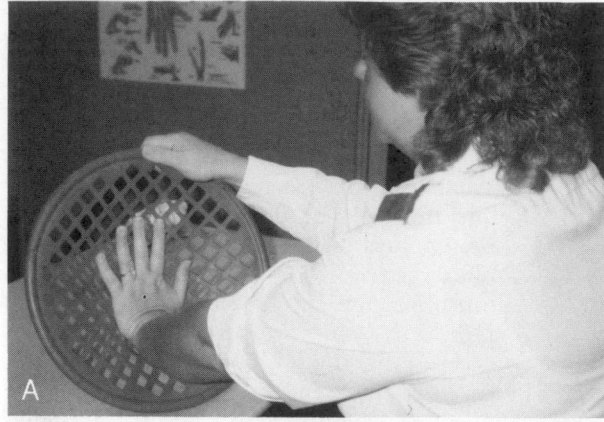

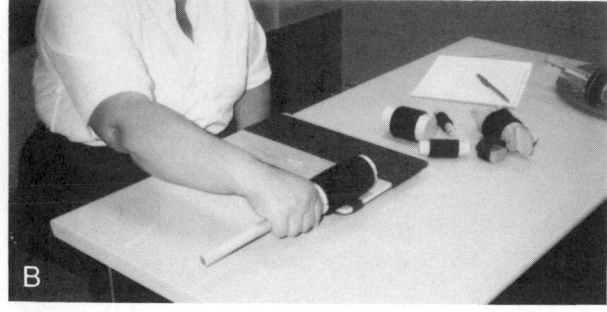

FIGURE 31–53 Exercising after cubital tunnel release. **A,** Stretching with the web. **B,** Strengthening with the Velcro board.

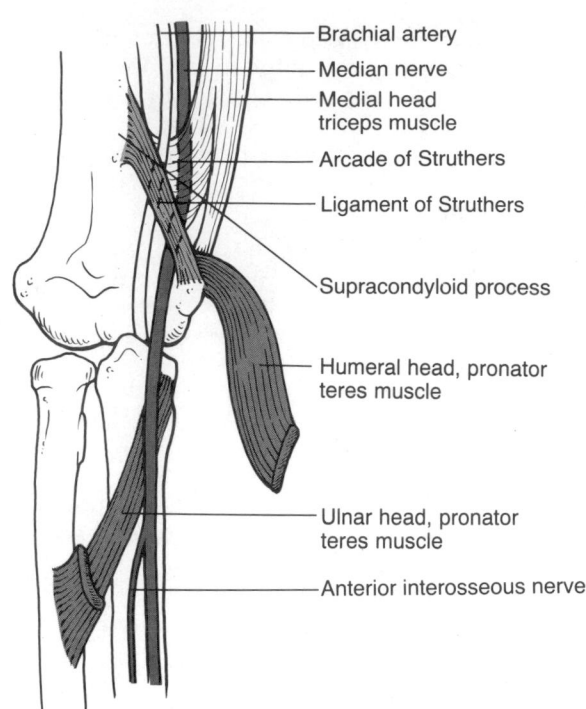

FIGURE 31–54 Median nerve compression sites: the ligament of Struthers and the PT muscle.

noted. Common sites of compression in and about the elbow and forearm (see Figure 31–54) are:

  (1). Ligament of Struthers. This is a vestigial ligament (found in 1% of the population) that stretches between a humeral bone spur 3 to 5 cm proximal to the medial humeral epicondyle and the medial humeral epicondyle.

  (2). Pronator teres muscle. Compression occurs under the lacertus fibrosus or between the two heads of the pronator muscle, or rarely, deep to both heads or to a solitary head of the PT muscle.

  (3). Anterior interosseous branch. This branch may be compressed by fibrous bands, a tendinous origin of the PT muscle, or the FDS muscle to the middle finger.

b. Clinical presentation of symptoms is as follows:

  (1). If the median nerve is compressed under the ligament of Struthers, vague pain may be present over the anterior surface of the elbow and forearm; sensory changes occur over the lateral area of the palm and lateral three and one half digits. Weakness occurs in the PT, the FCR, PL, FDS, FDP, to the index and middle fingers, FPL, PQ, the first and second lumbrical muscles, and the APB, FPB, and OP muscles. Symptoms may be reproduced by resisted elbow flexion at 120 to 135 degrees.

  (2). Pronator teres syndrome. The patient experiences pain over the anterior surface of the forearm that is elicited by repetitive elbow and forearm movement. Sensory and motor changes are the same as for compression under the ligament of Struthers, except that the PT, FCR, and PL muscles are not involved. Symptoms may be reproduced by resisted pronation and wrist flexion with the elbow extended, the forearm pronated, and the wrist flexed.

  (3). Anterior interosseous syndrome.

This disorder may produce vague pain over the anterior forearm, but it often is painless. Because the anterior interosseous branch of the median nerve is primarily a motor branch (with the exception of a few sensory fibers to the wrist joint capsule), compression is associated only with motor changes, *ie*, weakness in the PQ, FPL, and FDP muscles to the index and middle fingers. This compression causes a unique pathognomonic pinch pattern, with hyperextension of the thumb IP joint and the index finger DIP joint.

c. Management
  (1). Identify the patient's problems, which may include
     • pain
     • sensory changes
     • motor loss
  (2). Conservative treatment. Have the patient avoid aggravating activity and repetitive motion. Advise resting the limb or apply protective splints with the elbow flexed to 90 degrees, the forearm in a neutral position, and the wrist in 25 degrees of extension. A physician may prescribe NSAIDs.[18]
  (3). Surgical treatment. Surgical exploration of the involved nerves or branches and release of fibrous restrictions may be necessary.

3. Radial nerve
  a. The history of the problem should be noted. Common sites of compression in and about the elbow and forearm (see Figure 31–55) are:
  (1). Middle to distal humerus. The radial nerve spirals around the posterolateral humerus in the radial groove; it is susceptible to injury secondary to humeral shaft fractures, supracondylar humeral fractures, and elbow dislocations. The nerve also may be compressed during sustained pressure against the posterior humerus, *ie*, Saturday night palsy, in which a stuporous victim slumps in a chair with his/her arm stretched over the chair back.
  (2). Radial tunnel. The posterior interosseous branch of the radial nerve

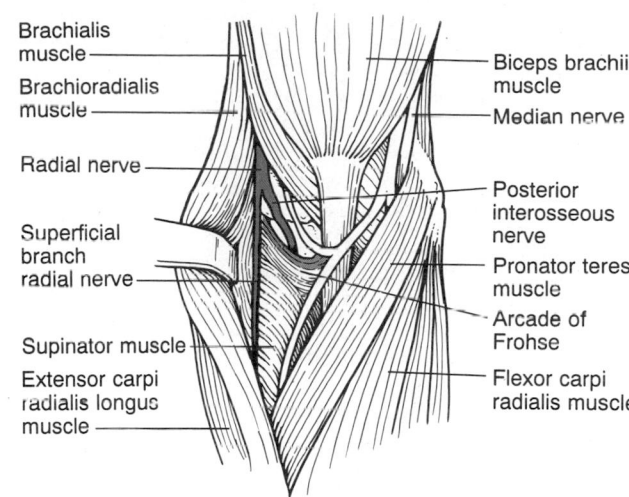

FIGURE 31–55 Radial nerve compression at the arcade of Frohse.

may be compressed by fibrous bands anterior to the radial head, a vascular arcade, the tendinous margin of the ECRB muscle, beneath the arcade of Frohse, or between the two heads of the supinator muscle.[30]
  (3). Distal radius. The terminal sensory branch of the nerve travels superficially over the dorsal lateral radius and across the wrist, where it may be subjected to external compression (*eg*, from a tight wrist watch or handcuffs).[27,31]

b. Clinical presentation
  (1). If the radial nerve is compressed in the area of humeral contact, pain radiating proximal or distal to the elbow may result. The patient may also experience sensory changes in the posterior regions of the arm and forearm, the dorsal area of the wrist, and the dorsal aspect of the lateral three and one half digits to the level of the DIP joints. Weakness occurs in the brachioradialis, ECRL, ECRB, supinator, ED, ECU, EDM, APL, EPB, EPL, and EI muscles.
  (2). Radial tunnel (posterior interosseous) syndrome. The patient experiences pain over the lateral elbow or the dorsal area of the forearm; symptoms are reproduced by resisted supination. The patient may have weakness in ED, ECU,

EPL, EPB, APL, EI, and EDM muscles.

    (3). Cheiralgia paresthetica (Wartenberg's syndrome). The patient experiences pain, burning, and sensory changes over the dorsal lateral area of the wrist and the dorsal aspect of the lateral three and one half digits to the level of the DIP joints.

  c. Management

    (1). Identify the patient's problems, which may include
- pain
- sensory changes
- motor loss

    (2). Conservative treatment. Apply a splint with the elbow in 90 degrees of flexion. A physician may prescribe NSAIDs. In patients with cheiralgia paresthetica, remove the constricting object, *eg*, wristwatch, cast.

    (3). Surgical treatment and rehabilitation. Decompress the nerve by removing hard- or soft-tissue constrictions or by dividing the arcade of Frohse. Immobilize the limb for 3 weeks at 90 degrees of elbow flexion with the forearm in a neutral position; begin ROM exercises.

C. Lateral epicondylitis (tennis elbow)

This condition is *tendinitis,* resulting from overuse or fatique stress to the tissue.

1. Etiology. The typical case involves repetitive trauma (*ie,* wrist extension) that produces microtears originating in the ECRB. These microtears heal with excessive granulation tissue and fibrosis; increased scar tissue and free nerve endings contribute to pain, decreased function, and susceptibility to reinjury.

2. Incidence. Tennis elbow is common in patients in their 20s and 30s; it is more frequent in males than in females, in the dominant arm than in the nondominant arm, in nonathletes than in athletes, and in whites than in blacks.

3. Clinical presentation. The patient may present with the insidious onset of dull or sharp lateral elbow pain and localized tenderness that is increased by resisted wrist and finger extension or passive flexion. The patient may have decreased wrist extension and grip strength (related to involve-

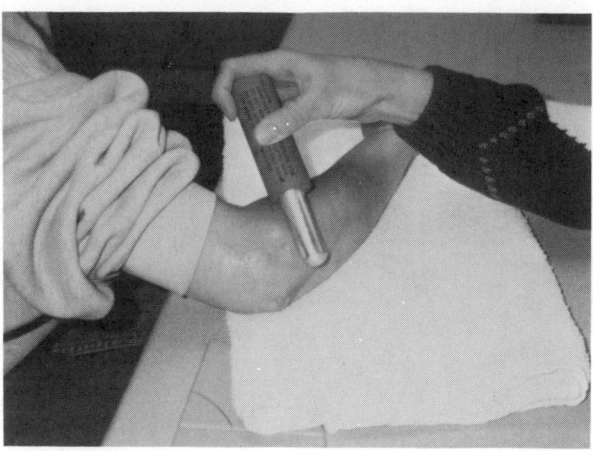

FIGURE 31–56 Cold application using the cryoprobe for tennis elbow.

ment of the synergistic wrist extensors) and localized swelling over the lateral humeral epicondyle.

4. Management

  a. Assess the patient's problems, which may include
- pain and inflammation
- decreased strength in wrist extension and, secondarily, in grip strength

  b. Acute treatment. A physician may prescribe NSAIDs. Apply cold pack or ice massage locally (see Figure 31–56). Prevent stress in wrist extension and during grasping with a wrist stabilizer splint in 25 degrees of wrist extension.[33]

  c. Subacute treatment. Apply ultrasound or phonophoresis over the area of the lateral epicondyle (see Figure 31–57). Fit the patient with a counterforce armband, which provides nonelastic restriction just distal to the elbow joint and assists in diffusing forces and in decreasing the amount of tension generated in wrist extension musculature,[34] (see Figure 31–58). Perform passive stretching (wrist flexion with elbow extended) and transverse friction massage.[15] Apply high-voltage galvanic stimulation (HVGS) (to promote healing and analgesia; apply for 20 minutes with negative polarity, 60–80 pulses).[35]

  d. Chronic treatment. Have the patient modify his/her activity (*eg,* increase the flexibility of tools and rackets, use a two-handed backhand stroke in tennis, adjust the handle size of tools and rackets)[36]

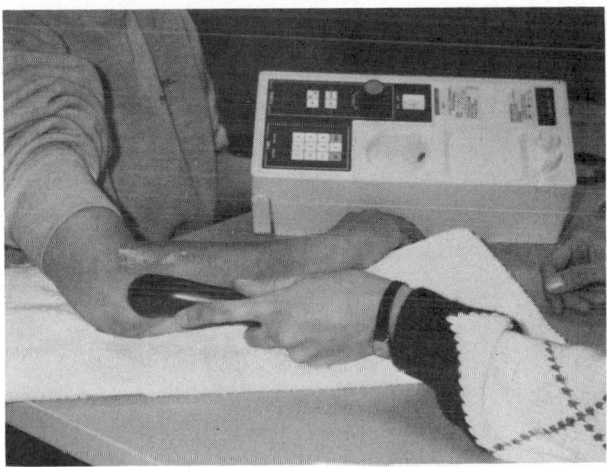

FIGURE 31–57   Ultrasound application for tennis elbow.

(see Figure 31–59). Recommend exercise for increasing flexibility, strength, and endurance.[37,38] A physician may administer a corticosteriod injection.[15]

e. Surgical treatment and rehabilitation. Excise nonhealing fibroblastic tissue and separate the extensor tendon origin from the epicondyle; rehabilitation following surgery involves gentle active movement for 3 weeks and then an increase in ROM and strengthening exercises[6] (see Figure 31–60).

D. Medial epicondylitis (baseball pitcher's or golfer's elbow)

This disorder is an overuse syndrome involving the tissues that lie over the medial aspect of the elbow.

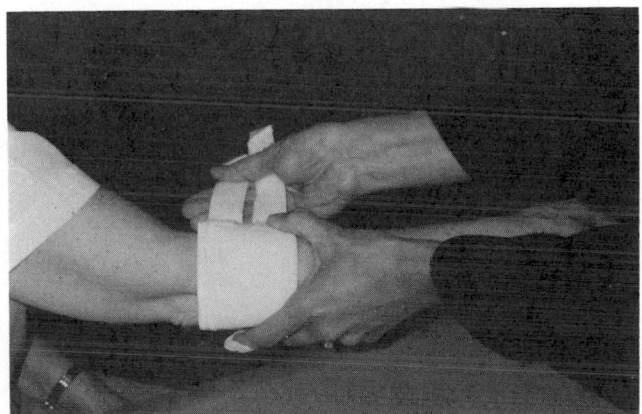

FIGURF 31–58   Counterforce armband application for tennis elbow.

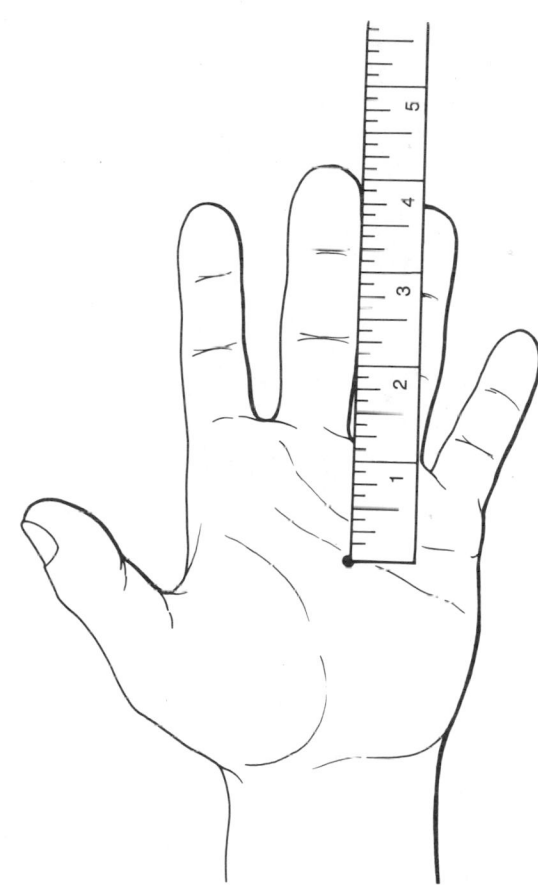

FIGURE 31–59   Measurement for proper handle circumference: distance between the proximal palmar crease and the tip of the ring finger.

1. Etiology. Repetitive trauma (ie, wrist flexion), often associated with baseball pitching, golfing, serving in tennis (in upper-level players) is the cause of medial epicondylitis. Trauma can result in avulsion of the medial epicondylar epiphysis, osteochrondosis, or tendinitis of the PT and FCR muscles.

2. Clinical presentation. The patient may describe an insidious onset of medial elbow pain that is increased by resisted wrist flexion or passive wrist extension.

3. Management
   a. Note the patient's problems, which may include
      • pain and inflammation
      • decreased wrist flexion strength
   b. Treatment is similar to that for lateral epicondylitis, except that it is applied over the medial humeral epicondyle and the origins of the FCR and PT muscles.[35]

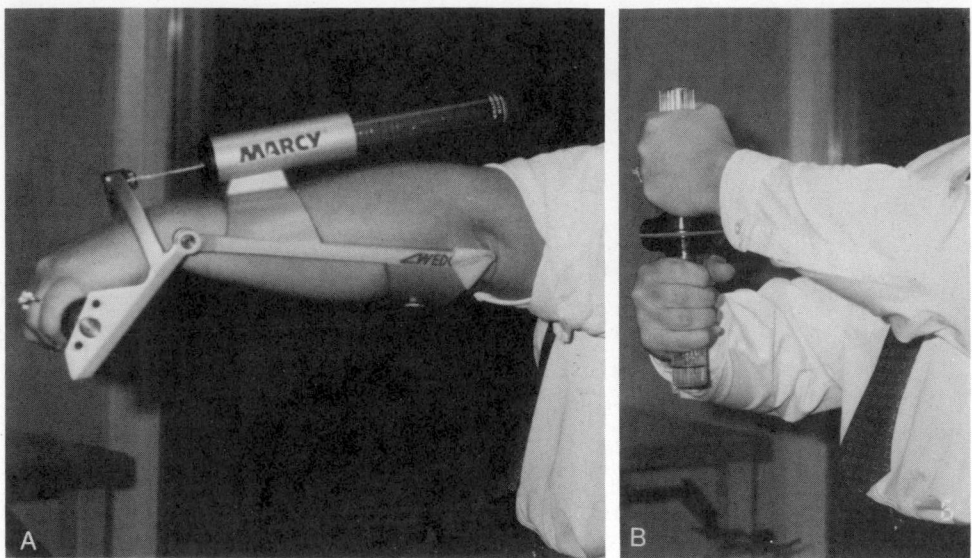

FIGURE 31–60   Strengthening exercises following surgical release of ECRB muscle. **A,** Resisted wrist flexion. **B,** Resisted wrist flexion and extension.

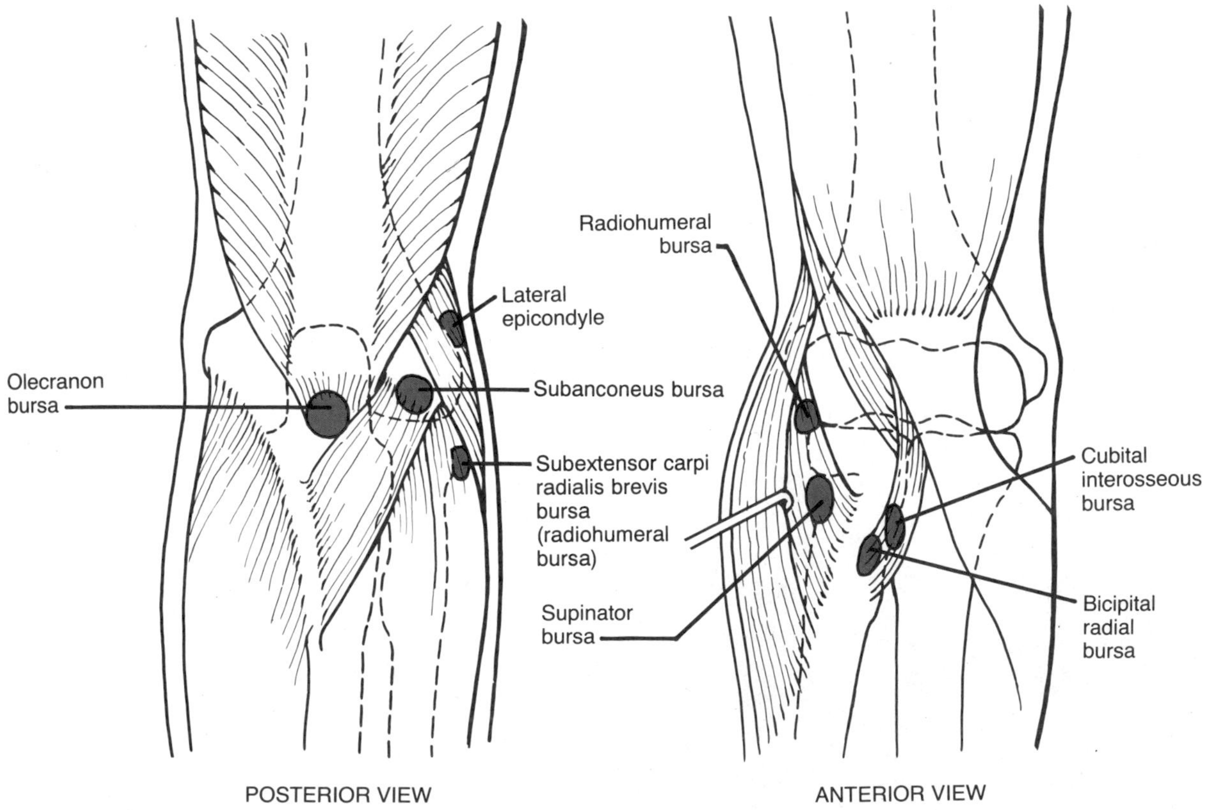

POSTERIOR VIEW

ANTERIOR VIEW

Olecranon bursa

Lateral epicondyle

Subanconeus bursa

Subextensor carpi radialis brevis bursa (radiohumeral bursa)

Supinator bursa

Radiohumeral bursa

Cubital interosseous bursa

Bicipital radial bursa

FIGURE 31–61   Bursae of the elbow region.

E. Bursitis

1. Bicipitoradial (see Figure 31–61)
   a. Etiology. Bicipitoradial bursitis is caused by repetitive elbow flexion or supination.
   b. Clinical presentation. The patient presents with pain in the anterior forearm and over the biceps muscle that increases with resisted flexion and supination and is tender to deep palpation.
   c. Management
      (1). Evaluate the patient's problems, which may include
         • pain, inflammation, and localized swelling
         • decreased function secondary to pain
      (2). Treatment should include immobilization of the limb, the application of ice, and a physician's prescription for anti-inflammatory medication.
2. Olecranon (see Figure 31–61)
   a. Etiology. Olecranon bursitis is caused by repetitive elbow extension or blunt trauma or compression over the olecranon.
   b. Clinical presentation. The patient has a painless, cystic swelling over the olecranon.
   c. Management
      (1). Assess the patient's problems, which may include
         • pain, inflammation, and localized swelling
         • decreased function secondary to pain
      (2). Treatment should include aspiration of the bursa and corticosteroid injection by a physician, followed by the application of a compressive wrap. The patient should be advised to protect the olecranon from repetitive trauma or contact pressure.

F. Nursemaid's elbow

1. Etiology. Sudden traction on a child's forearm can cause this condition. The radial head is displaced distally into the annular ligament. The ligament may partially rupture in older children.
2. Clinical presentation. The patient is protective of his/her arm and may hold it slightly pronated. Radiographic diagnosis may be difficult when the radial head is not ossified.

3. Management
   a. Note the patient's problems, which may include
      • pain
      • decreased function secondary to pain and mechanical block
   b. Treatment should include manual reduction by supinating the forearm and then flexing the elbow, or by flexing the elbow and then supinating the forearm. Immobilization is not necessary, and the patient is encouraged to resume normal function immediately.

G. Supracondylar fracture

This is the most frequent fracture in the elbow region; it presents a danger of complications and disability secondary to gross displacement (distal fragment posterior) or neurovascular compromise (see Figure 31–62).
1. Etiology. Supracondylar fracture is caused by a fall onto an outstretched hand.
2. Clinical presentation. Displacement may be

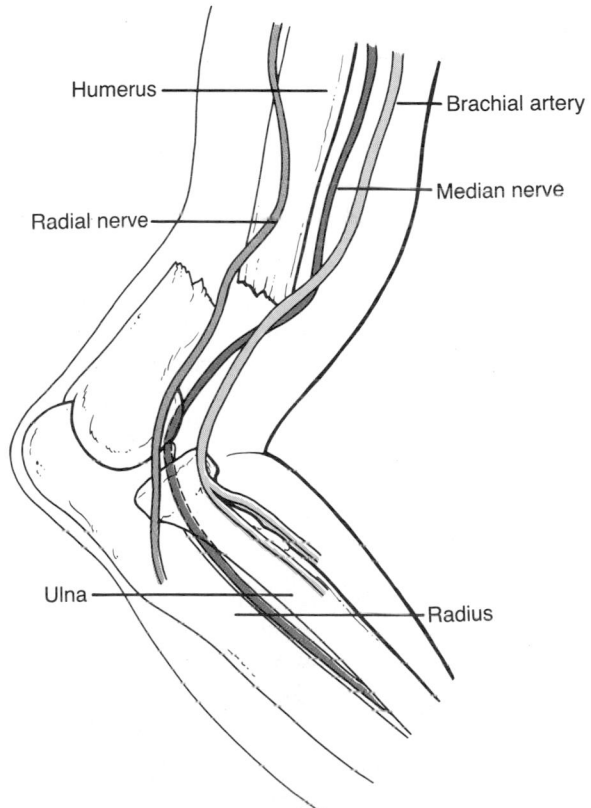

FIGURE 31–62 Supracondylar humeral fracture.

obvious; however, when it is not, diagnosis without radiographs is difficult (the condition may mimic dislocation). The fat pad sign is positive in patients with supracondylar fracture, and severe pain and loss of function are present.

3. Management
   a. Assess the patient's problems, which may include
      • pain and loss of function
      • displaced fragments
      • neurovascular compromise
      • potential deformity (cubitus varus is common)
   b. Surgical treatment. Neurovascular status is the first priority; reduction with traction, or closed manual reduction is followed with splinting at 120 degrees of flexion for 6 weeks. For displaced, unstable fractures immobilization is maintained with a Kirschner wire. For open fractures and fractures that have significant neurovascular compromise, open reduction and internal fixation is advocated.[39]
   c. Rehabilitation. Prescribe active and passive ROM exercises; progress to resistive strengthening exercise. Splint the limb if necessary to counteract a flexion contracture.

H. Dislocation

The elbow is the most frequently dislocated joint in children and the second most frequently dislocated joint in adults (second to the shoulder). This high incidence of injury may be attributed to general laxity, its large cartilaginous component, minimal osseous stability, and numerous ossification centers in children.

1. Etiology. A fall onto an outstretched hand or severe hyperextension is the main cause of elbow dislocation. A total of 10% of dislocations are complicated by radial head fractures.
2. Clinical presentation. The patient has severe pain and loss of function and may hold his/her elbow in a protected position, usually in semiflexion. If the dislocation is posterior, the olecranon is displaced and palpable posteriorly. Elbow dislocation is accompanied by extensive soft-tissue injury (medial collateral ligament rupture, avulsion of the musculature or brachial artery, or median or ulnar nerve severance) and instability. It may reduce spontaneously.

3. Management
   a. Note the patient's problems, which may include
      • pain and loss of function
      • displacement or instability
      • soft-tissue injury
      • loss of extension after healing[40]
   b. Treatment and rehabilitation
      (1). Initially, determine whether neurovascular injury or fracture is present and treat accordingly.
      (2). In teenagers and adults, reduce dislocation with traction from a weight dangling from the patient's hand in a prone position, with the arm hanging over a table edge. Apply a posterior splint in 90 degrees of elbow flexion and start active flexion within the confines of the splint after 1 week. Modify the splint to 60 degrees of flexion after 2 weeks. Remove the splint and start active flexion and extension exercise after 3 weeks.[40]
      (3). In children, use general anesthesia and anterior traction to reduce dislocation, aspirate the joint, and follow the splinting and exercise protocol described for teens and adults.

I. Volkman's ischemic contracture

This is a compartment syndrome secondary to pressure that produces muscle ischemia.

1. Etiology. The onset of this condition is often related to a major fracture or prolonged external pressure (eg, from a tight cast, or in the comatose patient or drug addict). The exact pathophysiology is under debate—it may involve arterial, venous, or neurologic factors, any of which may compromise circulation. Collateral circulation is sufficient to maintain hand vascularity, but the forearm musculature undergoes necrosis, fibrosis, and contracture.
2. Clinical presentation. The patient experiences pain within 2 hours of the onset of the condition, which is intensified by passive stretching of the wrist and finger flexor musculature. Pallor, pulselessness, paralysis, and eventual contractures are also pathognomonic.
3. Management
   a. Assess the patient's problems, which may include
      • pain and loss of function

- contracture with clawhand deformity
b. Prophylactic treatment. Relieve pressure that may obstruct circulation.[41]
c. Surgical treatment. A fasciotomy should be performed if indicated; reconstructive surgery (following necrosis and contracture) may include tendon transfers and releases.
d. Rehabilitation. Elevate the arm to reduce edema and apply a splint to counteract deformity. Prescribe functional exercise according to the symptomatic indications, *eg*, muscle re-education, stretching, and strengthening.

J. Traumatic myositis ossificans

1. Etiology. This disorder is caused by muscle trauma that is direct or secondary to a fracture or dislocation that produces hemorrhage within the muscle tissue. The proposed causes involve invasion of the hematoma by osteoblasts from the damaged periosteum or by fibroblasts; metaplasia of tissue; and calcification (may be resorbed) or ossification (irreversible) within the muscle.[42]
2. Clinical presentation. The patient has a rapidly enlarging painful mass that restricts motion. Occasionally, after 4 to 6 months of bone formation spontaneous regression occurs.
3. Management
   a. Assess the patient's problems, which may include
      - pain and loss of function
      - elbow flexion contracture
   b. Conservative treatment. The patient continues functional activities but avoids passive stretching.
   c. Surgical treatment. Excision may be performed only after maximal regression has occurred.

K. Reflex sympathetic dystrophy (post-traumatic dystrophy, Sudeck's atrophy, or shoulder-hand syndrome)

This condition is a neurovascular syndrome characterized by pain that is out of proportion to an inciting injury or disease and is accompanied by sudomotor and vasomotor changes, trophic changes of the skin and bone, stiffness, and decreased function.
1. Etiology. Although the etiology is not clearly understood, the proposed pathophysiology involves a "short circuit" between sympathetic efferent C fibers and sensory afferent C fibers; a vicious cycle develops because a patient experiencing pain has an increased sympathetic outflow through the efferents that is then transmitted through the sensory afferents; this enhances the pain sensation and stimulates additional sympathetic activity. Predisposing conditions include trauma, neurologic lesions and neuropathy, surgery, and other diseases involving the extremities. The onset of symptoms is rapid and not relative to the severity of the initiating event. Reflex sympathetic dystrophy is most common in patients who are 35 to 60 years of age. Women are afflicted three times more often than men.
2. Clinical presentation. The initial symptom is intense burning pain that later may be described as aching or crushing. Swelling, stiffness, and discoloration progress with time; the following stages are observed:
   a. At 0 to 3 months, the patient experiences burning pain and soft edema that may encompass the hand, wrist, and forearm; early vasomotor reflex spasm (sympathetic response) occurs with vasoconstriction and cool, pale, clammy skin followed by vasodilation (loss of sympathetic function) with warm, reddened, dry skin and increased hair and nail growth.
   b. At 3 to 9 months, the patient has pain associated with motion, brawny edema, and osteoporosis. The redness disappears, sweating and hair and nail growth decrease, trophic skin changes occur, and progressive stiffness develops.
   c. At 9 months and onward, the pain decreases, and fibrosis and atrophy of the skin with dry, cool extremities, joint stiffness or ankylosis, severe osteoporosis, and some irreversible functional loss may be present.
3. Management
   a. Evaluate the patient's problems, which may include
      - pain and loss of function
      - edema
      - stiffness and contractures
      - trophic changes
   b. Conservative treatment. Early diagnosis and treatment are essential to break the cycle; approach the patient with a positive, firm attitude and provide support

while encouraging independence. Provide a structured home program and supervised therapy sessions as needed to include edema control, pain management, early motion, activities of daily living, and total body conditioning.[43] A stress-loading program incorporating compression and traction is implemented by instructing the patient to bear weight on the affected extremity in a quadruped position initially 3 to 5 minutes three times a day. He/she is then to carry a weighted briefcase for at least 10 minutes three times a day. Compression and traction forces are increased as tolerated[44–46] (see Figure 31–63).

c. Drug therapy. A physician may prescribe analgesic medications, NSAIDs, corticosteroids, α- and β-blockers, and calcium channel blockers. Administer local anesthetics intravenously, or stellate ganglion block.

d. Surgical treatment. Regional sympathetic blocks or surgical stellate sympathectomy may be indicated for patients with resistant dysfunction.

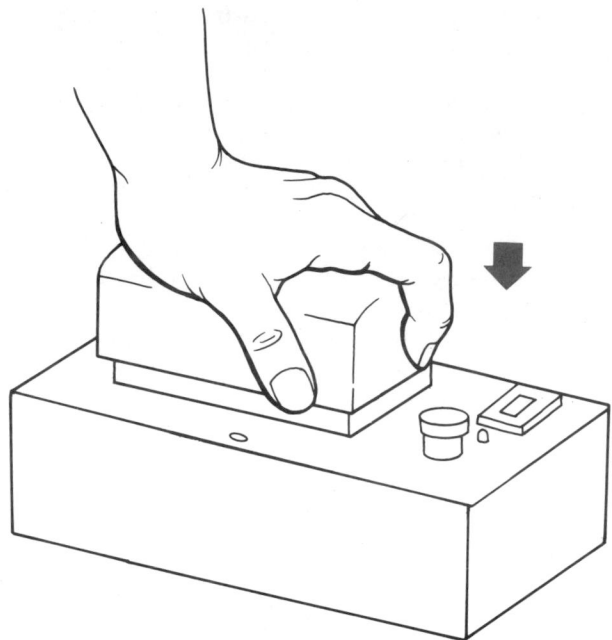

FIGURE 31–63   Stress-loading program with a dystrophile.

IV. Treatment of Common Disorders of the Wrist and Hand

A. The rheumatoid hand

1. Etiology and pathology
   a. Rheumatoid arthritis is a chronic, systemic, inflammatory disease that typically involves the synovial joints and other connective tissue. Although its etiology remains obscure, investigators hypothesize that an infectious agent may stimulate an immunologic response, and that genetic factors influence the expression of the disease.[47]
   b. Pathogenesis involves an inflammatory reaction that produces microvascular injury, edema, and eventual proliferation of synovial tissues. Rheumatoid pannus, a vascular granulation tissue, produces collagenase, which is activated by plasmin and is destructive to cartilage, ligaments, tendons, and bone.[42]
   c. Joint symptoms usually develop insidiously, although 20% of patients have an abrupt onset of polyarthritis. Any synovial joint may be affected, but those most commonly affected initially include the knees and the small joints of the hands, wrists, and feet.
   d. The general mechanisms producing deformity are external forces acting upon a system of links (wrist and fingers) that is simultaneously undergoing internal destruction.
      (1). The inert tissues are attacked by lysosomal enzymes from inflamed synovium that erode articular cartilage and destroy ligaments and joint capsules. Joint laxity and mechanical imbalance form a "vicious cycle," and collapse deformities become self-perpetuating.
      (2). The contractile structures also may be affected by lysosomal enzymes, which weaken tendons that may eventually rupture; painful inhibition also produces disuse atrophy and contractures in muscles. Con-

sider the functional length of finger motors, which may lose their mechanical advantage when joint contractures (*eg*, swan-neck and boutonnière deformities) develop.

2. Clinical presentation and typical deformities
   a. Distal radioulnar joint. In this joint, dorsal subluxation of the ulnar head and palmar displacement of the ECU tendon occur.
   b. Radiocarpal joint. Typical deformity in the radiocarpal joint involves flexion and radial deviation, and palmar subluxation of the carpals. Occasionally, spontaneous fusion of the wrist occurs. Ultimately, this disorder affects hand placement and stability and the functional length of the extrinsic finger tendons (*eg*, loss of wrist extension decreases grip strength).
   c. Finger metacarpophalangeal joints. Ulnar deviation and palmar subluxation of the proximal phalanges are due to (see Figure 31–64):
      (1). Anatomical predisposition. Because of the relative instability of the MP joints and the ulnar inclination of the metacarpal heads, ulnar deviation and palmar subluxation of the proximal phalanges may develop.
      (2). Extrinsic tendon forces. Functional gripping and pinching produce ulnar and palmar force. Furthermore, a loss of the flexor tendon pulleys contributes to bowstringing of the flexor tendons across the palm and increases their flexion force on the MP joints; extensor tendons lose stabilization over the dorsum of joints and slip into the sulci between the metacarpal heads, decreasing their effectiveness as MP joint extensors.
      (3). Role of intrinsic muscles. Contracture or spasm of the intrinsic muscles produces MP joint flexion ("intrinsic plus" deformity).
      (4). Collapse deformity. When the intercalated segments zigzag (*ie*, when the wrist radially deviates, and the MP joints ulnarly deviate), collapse deformity occurs.
   d. Finger interphalangeal joints. When intercalated bones zigzag within an unstable system, the following deformities may result:
      (1). Swan-neck deformity results from PIP joint extension with MP joint and DIP joint flexion (see Figure 31–65).
      (2). Boutonnière deformity results from PIP joint flexion with DIP joint extension (see Figure 31–65).
   e. Thumb carpometacarpal, MP, and PIP

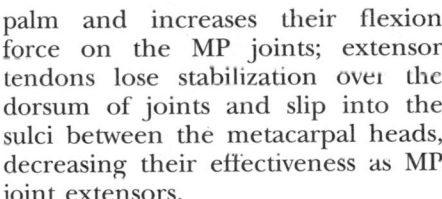

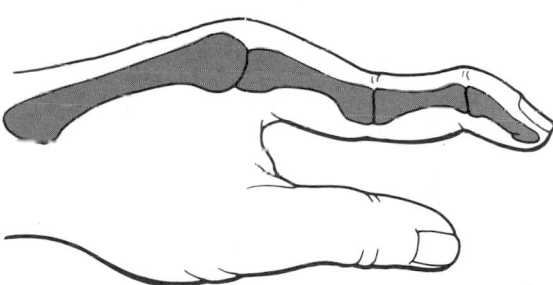

Swan-neck deformity

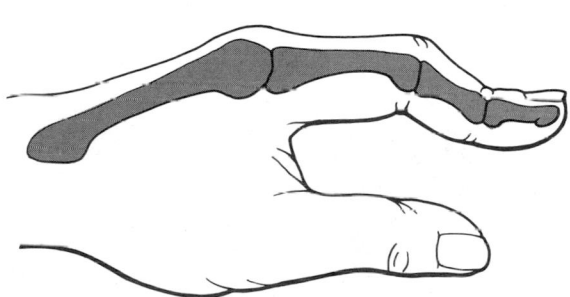

Boutonnière deformity

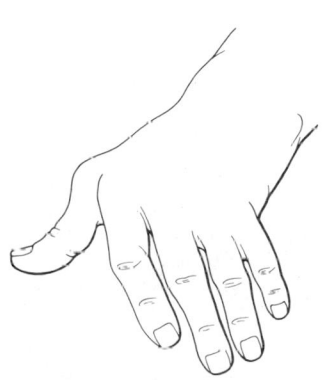

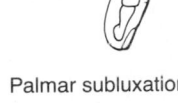

Ulnar drift   Palmar subluxation

FIGURE 31–64 Metacarpophalangeal joint ulnar drift and palmar subluxation.

FIGURE 31–65 Swan-neck and boutonnière deformities of the fingers.

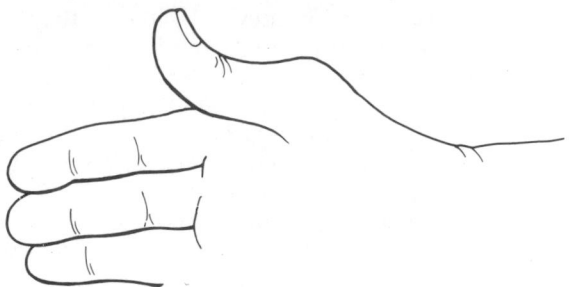

Thumb boutonnière deformity

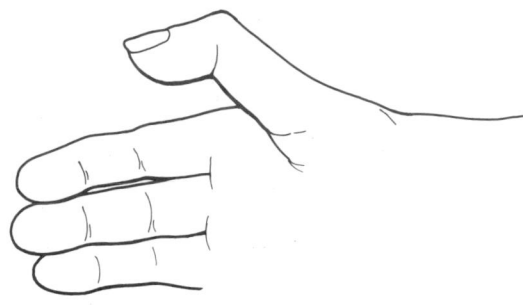

Thumb swan-neck deformity

FIGURE 31–66 Swan-neck and boutonnière deformities of the thumb.

joints. The following deformities can occur in the thumb joints.

(1). Boutonnière deformity results from MP joint flexion and IP joint extension (see Figure 31–66).

(2). Swan-neck deformity results from MP joint extension and IP joint flexion (see Figure 31–66).

3. Management

a. Assess the patient's problems, which can include
   - pain and inflammation
   - hyper- and hypomobility with deformity
   - weakness
   - loss of function
   - systemic disease with continual progression

b. During the acute phase (including exacerbations), management is as follows:

(1). Control pain and edema with medications and modalities.

(2). Apply splints to provide the joints with rest and protection until the patient is relatively free of pain; examples of resting splints include the cock-up, hand shell, ulnar deviation, and tri-point finger splints[48] (see Figure 31–67).

(3). Have the patient perform isometric exercises.

(4). Use gentle ROM exercises.

c. During the subacute phase, use the following methods of management:

(1). Continue pain management as needed.

(2). Have the patient avoid fatigue.

(3). Use functional and dynamic splinting.

(4). Initiate active assistive exercise and then progress to isotonic exercise, emphasizing MP joint extension.

(5). Initiate functional activities (may require adaptive devices); educate the patient on activities of daily living skills and on joint preservation principles.

d. During the chronic phase, management is as follows:

(1). Use splints to minimize contractures, *eg*, knuckle-benders, joint rings, reverse knuckle benders, spring wires, or spring coil splints.

(2). Use light isotonic resistive exercise.

(3). Surgery, including synovectomy, intrinsic release, tendon grafts and transfers, and joint reconstruction (arthrodesis, arthroplasty, or pros-

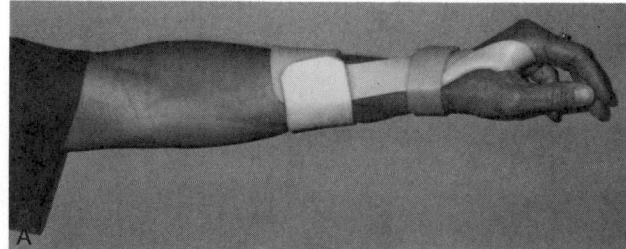
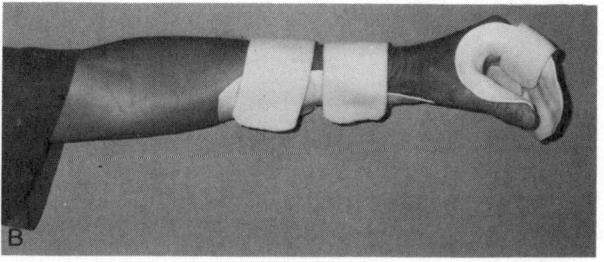

FIGURE 31–67 **A** and **B**, Resting splints.

thetic replacement), may be necessary.

e. The rehabilitation protocol following silicone joint arthroplasty includes controlled motion during encapsulation; for the MP joints, the patient should wear a dynamic splint from 3 to 5 days after surgery for 6 to 8 weeks; then continue to use it at night up to the 14th week; for the PIP joints, the patient should wear a splint for 1 week and then perform passive and active exercise.

B. Soft tissue pathology

1. Carpal tunnel syndrome. This is the most common peripheral nerve entrapment syndrome in the body; it is produced by any condition that decreases the area of the carpal tunnel or increases the volume of its contents. The symptoms of the syndrome are related to ischemia and mechanical compression of the median nerve.

   a. Etiology. The patient experiences the gradual onset of numbness and paresthesias in a median nerve distribution *distal* to the wrist; pain may radiate proximal or distal to the wrist; symptoms are aggravated by repetitive use of the hand, sustained or repetitive postures of wrist flexion and ulnar deviation, and vibration.

   b. Clinical presentation. In order of prevalence, the patient clinically presents with median nerve sensory disturbance, including numbness, paresthesias, and pain; a positive Phalen's test (60-second wrist flexion); the presence of Tinel's sign over the flexor retinaculum; thenar atrophy; decreased nerve conduction velocity; and volar swelling.[49]

   c. Management

   (1). Note the patient's problems, which may include
      • pain and sensory changes
      • weakness and clumsiness

   (2). Conservative treatment should proceed as follows:
      (a). Advise the patient to eliminate the activity that causes the problem (*eg*, sustained or repetitive wrist flexion or ulnar deviation).
      (b). Fit patient with a resting splint that positions the wrist in 20 degrees of extension (avoid

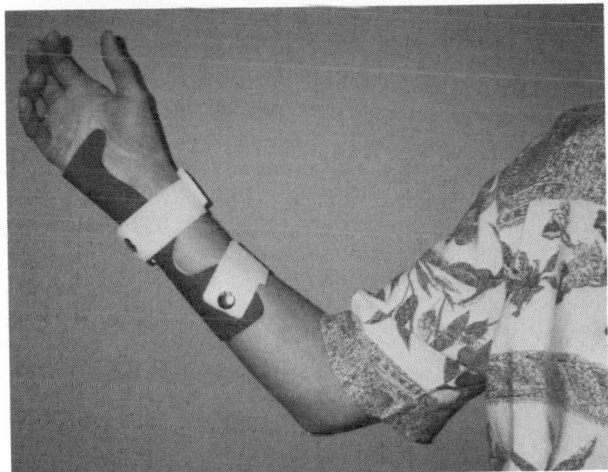

FIGURE 31-68   Carpal tunnel stop splint.

splint contact over the median nerve at the wrist)[50] (see Figure 31–68).
      (c). A physician may prescribe NSAIDs or administer a corticosteroid injection.

   (3). Surgical treatment and rehabilitation. Open release or endoscopic release of the transverse carpal ligament (flexor retinaculum) may be needed[51] (see Figure 31–69). The postoperative protocol is as follows:
      (a). Elevate the limb in postsurgical dressings for 3 to 4 days; initi-

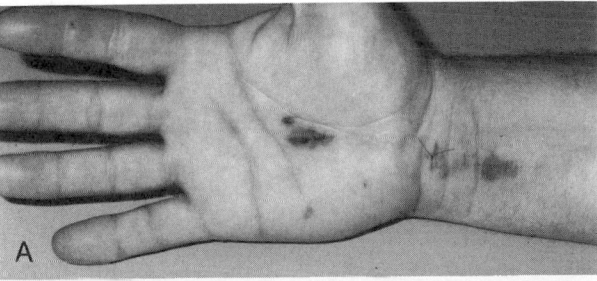

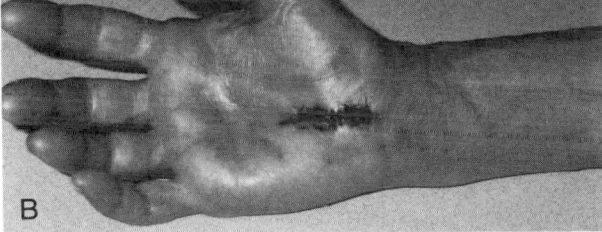

FIGURE 31–69   Surgical carpal tunnel release. **A,** Endoscopic. **B,** Conventional.

ate active finger exercises for up to 2 weeks. These exercises should include (1) making a full fist, which enhances maximal FDP gliding; (2) making a flat fist (MP and PIP flexion with DIP extension), which enhances maximal FDS gliding; (3) making a hook fist (MP extension with PIP and DIP flexion), which produces maximal excursion between the FDS and FDP; and (4) stretching the thumb into extension, which promotes median nerve gliding.[52]

(b). After 2 to 4 weeks, initiate light resistive exercise with exercise putty; the patient can return to full function in 4 weeks (after endoscopic release) or in 6 weeks (after open release) (see Figure 31–70).

2. Distal ulnar tunnel (Guyon's canal). Prob-

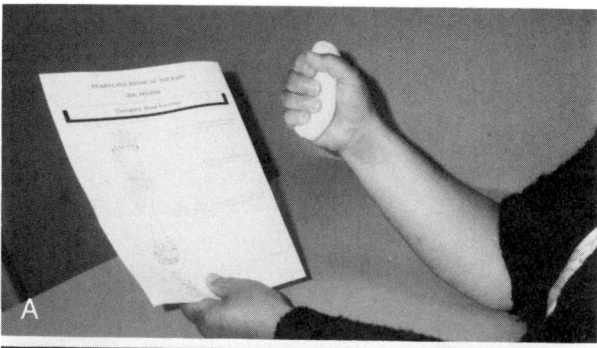
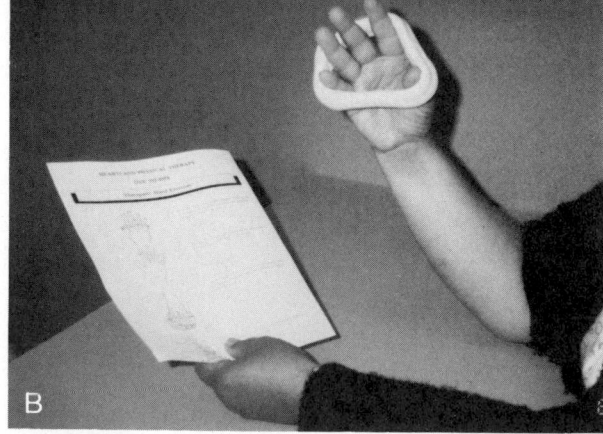

FIGURE 31–70 Light resistive exercise with exercise putty after carpal tunnel release. **A,** Flexion. **B,** Extension.

lems in this area are associated with numerous factors that may decrease the space within the tunnel, including thrombosis or aneurysm of the ulnar artery, a deep carpal ganglion, and fractures of the hamate or triquetrum, as well as occupational compression or blunt trauma.

a. Etiology. The patient experiences the insidious development of pain, paresthesia, or anesthesia over the ulnar side of the palm and the medial one and one half digits.

b. Clinical presentation. The patient presents with weakness in the third and fourth lumbrical muscles, the AP muscle, the interosseous muscles, and sometimes, the hypothenar muscles (unless compression occurs distal to the branch that supplies the hypothenar muscles); sensory changes, such as those described in the "Etiology" subsection, may be present.

c. Management

(1). Note the patient's problems, which may include
- pain and sensory changes
- weakness and clumsiness

(2). Conservative treatment

(a). Have the patient avoid trauma to the base of the palm.

(b). Advise the patient to eliminate repetitive motion; apply a wrist cock-up splint if necessary.

(c). A physician may prescribe NSAIDs.

(3). Surgical treatment and rehabilitation. Following release of the ulnar tunnel, the patient remains in postsurgical dressings for 3 to 4 days, then initiates gradual ROM and strengthening exercises similar to those used to manage carpal tunnel syndrome[53] (see Figure 31–71).

3. De Quervain's syndrome involves inflammation of the APL and EPB tendons' synovial sheaths in the first extensor compartment (see Figure 31–72).

a. Etiology. Trauma or overuse with repetitive thumb and wrist motion may cause this syndrome.

b. Clinical presentation. The patient has swelling and tenderness in the area of the radial styloid process and a positive Finkelstein's test (the thumb is held in flexion while the hand is ulnarly deviated, reproducing symptoms). Resisted

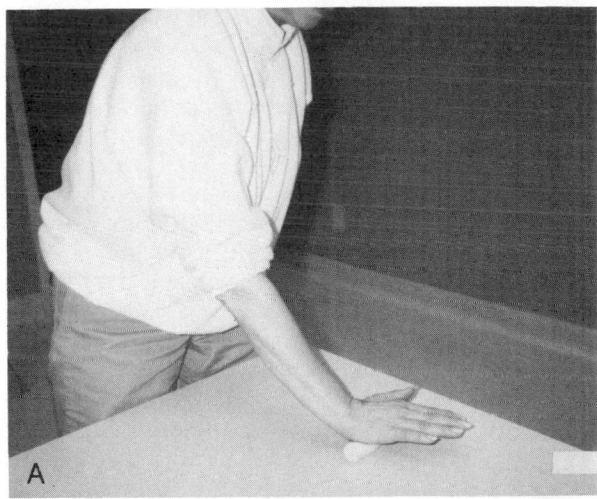

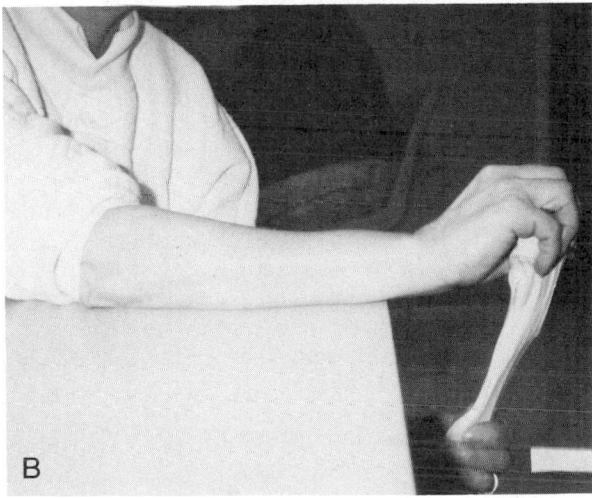

FIGURE 31–71 Exercise putty exercises after distal ulnar tunnel release. **A,** Rolling. **B,** Wrist extension.

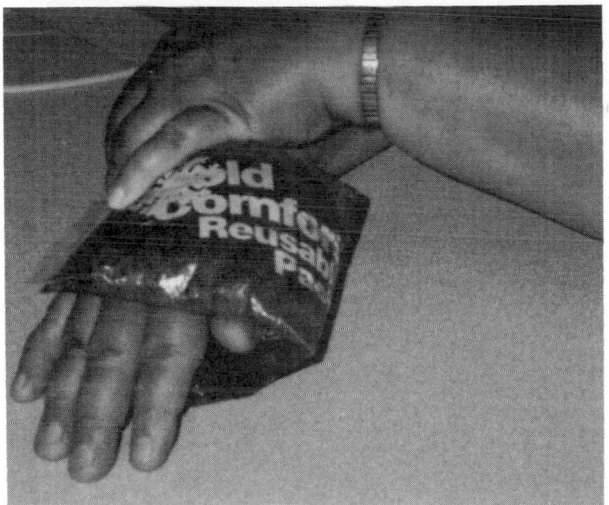

FIGURE 31–73 Cold pack application for deQuervain's disease.

- pain and inflammation
- decreased function secondary to pain

(2). Acute or conservative treatment

    (a). Apply ice and rest the wrist and hand with a thumb immobilizer forearm splint. A physician may prescribe NSAIDs, corticosteroids, or inject the sheath[36] (see Figures 31–73 and 31–74).

thumb abduction and extension also reproduce symptoms.

  c. Management

    (1). Assess the patient's problems, which may include

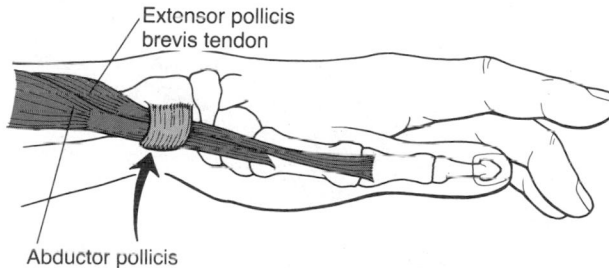

FIGURE 31–72 DeQuervain's disease, which involves EPB and EPL tendons in the first dorsal compartment.

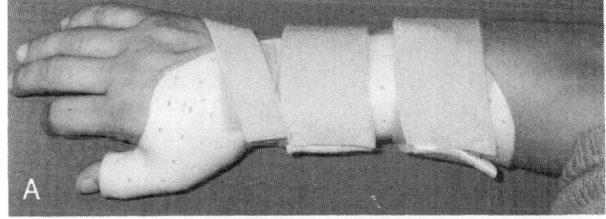

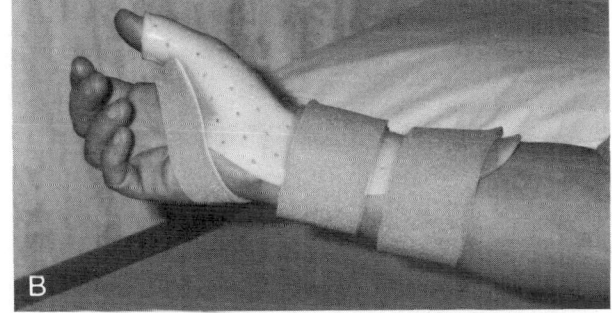

FIGURE 31–74 Resting splint for deQuervain's disease. **A,** Dorsal view. **B,** Volar view.

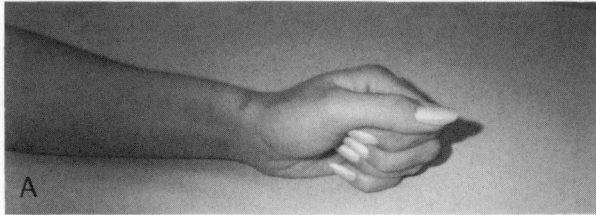

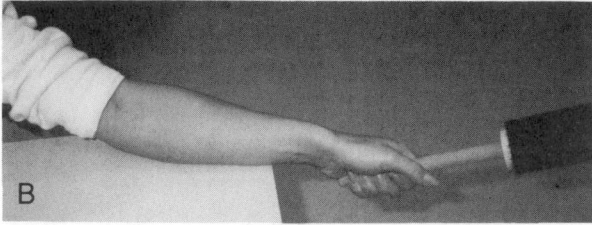

FIGURE 31–75 Surgical release of the first dorsal compartment for deQuervain's disease. **A,** Location of incision. **B,** Active exercises for stretching and strengthening.

       (b). In 1 to 2 weeks, begin applying heat, initiate phonophoresis and active exercise, and advise the patient to modify his/her activity to prevent recurrence.[54]
    (3). Surgical treatment and rehabilitation. Incision of the retinaculum and the first extensor compartment may be needed; initiate active exercise when the dressing is removed in 2 to 3 days[55] (see Figure 31–75).
  4. Dupuytren's disease involves progressive fibrosis of the palmar aponeurosis; it manifests as the formation of either a cellular, nodular lesion in the adipose tissue or collagenous bands in the palmar aponeurosis.
    a. Etiology. The patient experiences the insidious onset of a nodule or bands that may produce progressive contracture; there is a hereditary predisposition for this disease—it is more common in those of European descent.
    b. Clinical presentation. The patient presents with flexion contractures, typically involving the MP and PIP joints of the ring or little finger; the disease is commonly bilateral. A palpable lump or thickened palmar fascia may be present (see Figure 31–76).
    c. Management
      (1). The main problem associated with this disease is finger contractures.
      (2). Surgical treatment and rehabilitation includes fasciectomy; following the removal of the dressing in 3 days, apply a dorsal splint to enhance extension (see Figure 31–77). Active exercise and passive stretching should be initiated as indicated from day 3 to day 21 after surgery (see Figure 31–78).
  5. A ganglion is a cystic mass that protrudes from the tendon sheath or joint capsule.
    a. Etiology. The patient experiences the insidious development of a lump near the synovial structures of the forearm, wrist, or hand. Ganglia may be associated with repetitive trauma.
    b. Clinical presentation. A ganglion may be asymptomatic, or occasionally painful. A ganglion is firm and somewhat mobile. Typically, 50% disappear spontaneously.
    c. Management

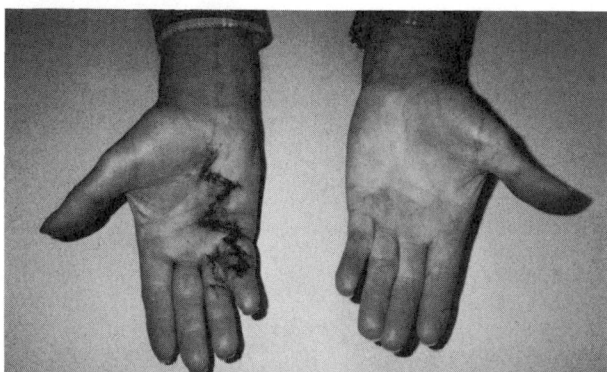

FIGURE 31–76 Patient with Dupuytren's contracture, shown after surgical release on the right hand; note mild contracture in the left hand.

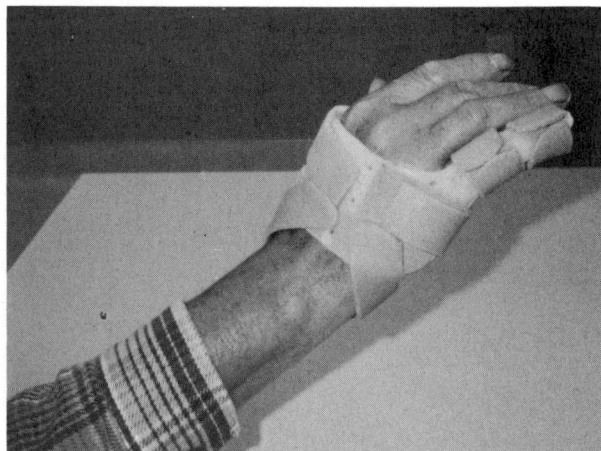

FIGURE 31–77 Dorsal splint to maintain extension after surgical release of Dupuytren's contracture.

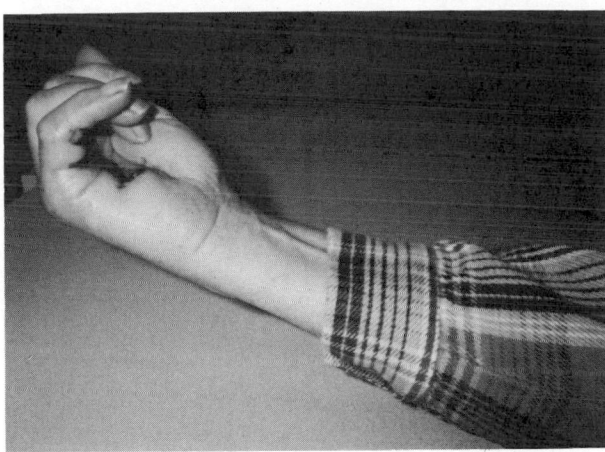

FIGURE 31–78 Exercise to increase ROM after surgical release of Dupuytren's contracture.

(1). The problems that a ganglion presents are as follow:
   • It may pose a cosmetic concern.
   • The patient may experience pain.
   • A ganglion may interfere with movement.
(2). Conservative treatment involves the application of pressure with conforming wrap, splinting, aspiration, and the administration of NSAIDs.[36]
(3). Surgical treatment and rehabilitation involves excision (resection) of the ganglion, then splinting for temporary immobilization for 2 to 3 weeks following surgery; the patient then begins ROM of the involved area.

6. Trigger finger is a thickening of the fibrous flexor tendon sheath in the area of a pulley (typically A1) (see Figure 31–79).
   a. Etiology. The patient's symptoms are insidious or secondary to repetitive trauma (eg, gripping tools with sharp edges or constant grasping).
   b. Clinical presentation. The patient presents with pain, stiffness, and swelling in the finger (or thumb) and palm; localized tenderness over the involved aspect of the flexor sheath; locking or snapping ("triggering") with attempted finger (or thumb) movement; and a mobile nodular enlargement proximal to the pulley.
   c. Management
   (1). Assess the patient's problems, which may include
      • pain with finger or thumb movement

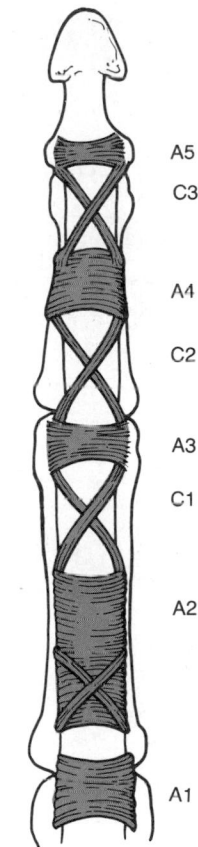

FIGURE 31–79 Annular (A) and cruciate (C) pulleys.

   • locking of the finger or thumb
(2). Conservative treatment involves local rest with a hand splint that holds the MP joint at 0 to 15 degrees and ends proximal to and allows full movement of the PIP joint, for 3 wks. A physician may also administer a hydrocortisone injection during this period.[56]
(3). Surgical treatment and rehabilitation involves release of the pulley. Rehabilitation involves active finger exercise from day 3 to day 14 and then the initiation of light resistive exercise, eg, with exercise putty. The patient can return to full function in 8 weeks (see Figure 31–80).

7. Crush injury
   a. Etiology. The finger or hand sustains a crushing blow or entrapment, resulting in relatively severe trauma (see Figure 31–81).
   b. Clinical presentation. The patient may

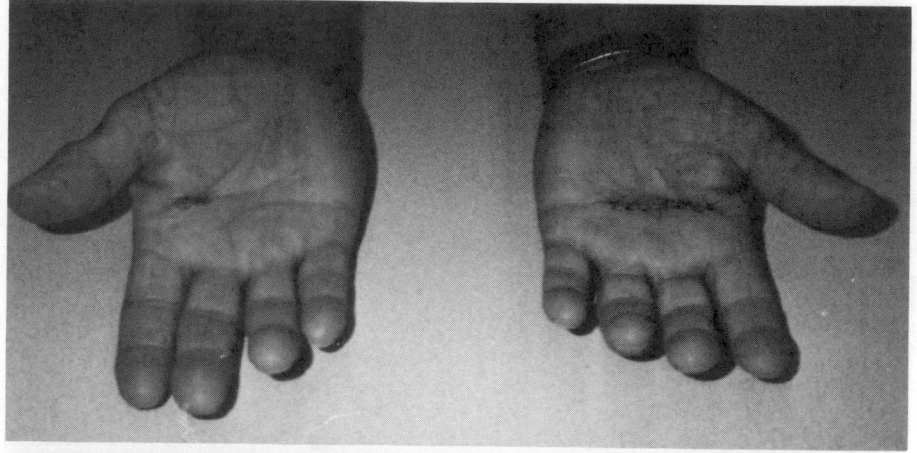

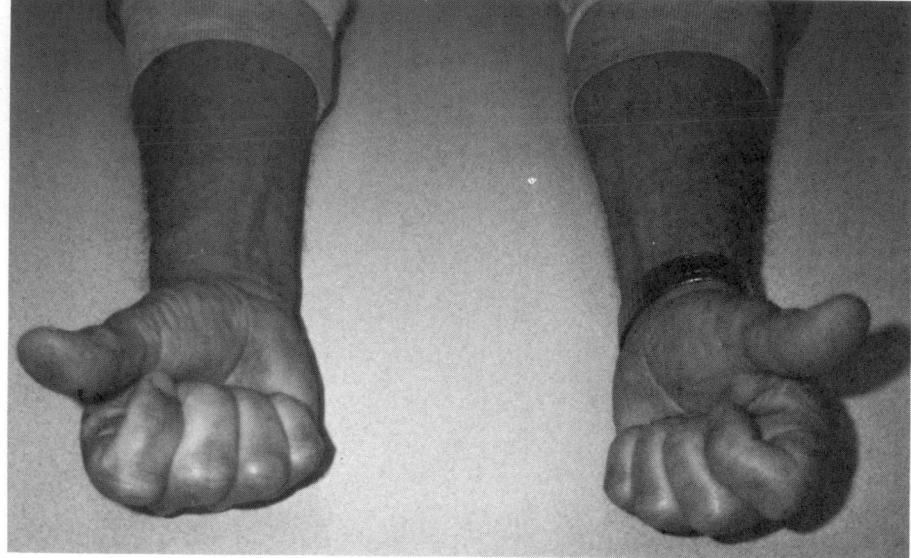

FIGURE 31–80   Surgical release of A1 pulleys. **A,** The right and left index fingers, left middle finger and ring finger. **B,** Initiating exercises.

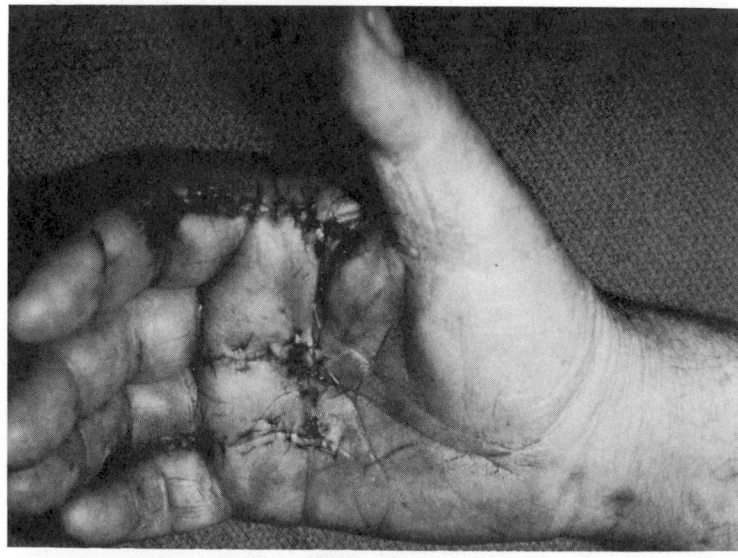

FIGURE 31–81   Acute crush injury.

have soft-tissue injury; widespread vascular damage and ischemia, fracture, or fingernail avulsion. Post-traumatic swelling is often a complication, and the "one wound–one scar" concept applies—after a hand injury, all damaged tissues respond with an inflammatory reaction and a marked tendency toward adhesion formation.

c. Management

(1). Note the patient's problems, which may include
- pain, inflammation, and edema
- possibly healing tendon, nerve, or vascular repairs, skin grafts, or fractures
- loss of passive motion
- loss of active motion

(2). Surgical treatment and rehabilitation[57]

(a). Thorough cleansing and débridement and surgical repair of damaged structures as necessary.

(b). Elevate the hand in a resting splint. Initiate continuous passive motion for as many digits as is appropriate. Progress to ROM exercises with *selective* movement of individual joints to enhance tendon gliding as early as possible.

(c). Institute measures for edema control such as retrograde mas-

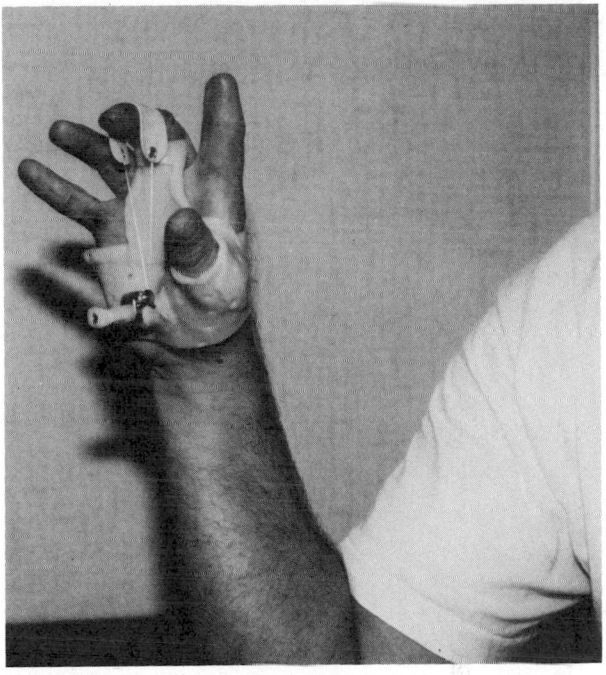

FIGURE 31–83 Splint with static progressive component to increase middle finger PIP joint flexion.

sage and the use of compression garments[58,59] (see Figure 31–82).

(d). Initiate functional activities as soon as healing status allows; a therapist should protect more involved fingers while promoting the use of the less involved; initiate passive stretching and dynamic splinting to minimize contractures (see Figure 31–83), and gradually progress to strengthening and endurance exercises (see Figure 31–84).

C. Dislocations and sprains

1. Lunate and perilunate dislocations

a. Etiology. A fall onto an outstretched hand with the wrist extended can cause an anterior dislocation of the lunate. More commonly, a perilunate dislocation occurs, which is a dorsal dislocation of the rest of the carpus relative to the lunate. Kienbock's disease (avascular necrosis of the lunate) may follow lunate trauma; it is characterized by decreased

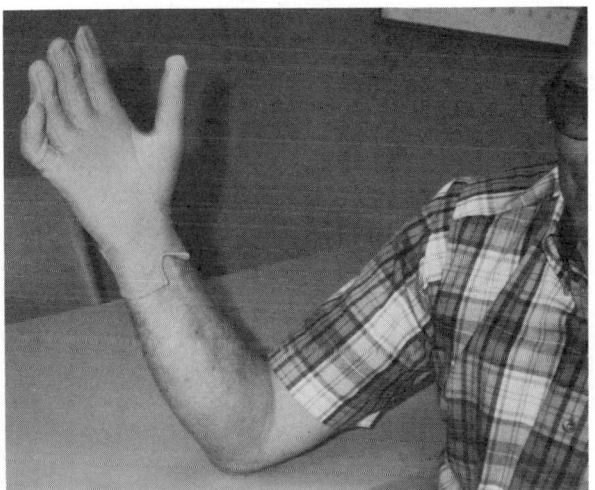

FIGURE 31–82 Compression glove for edema control following crush injury.

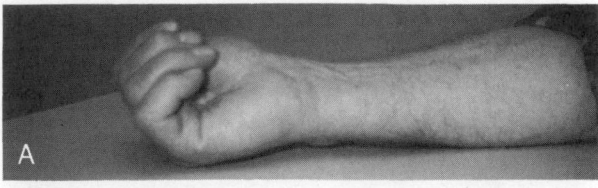

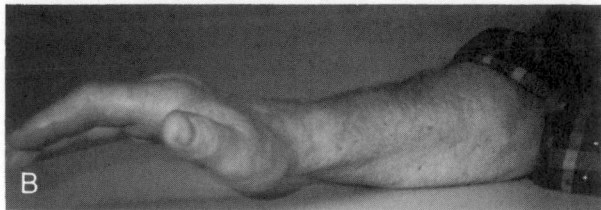

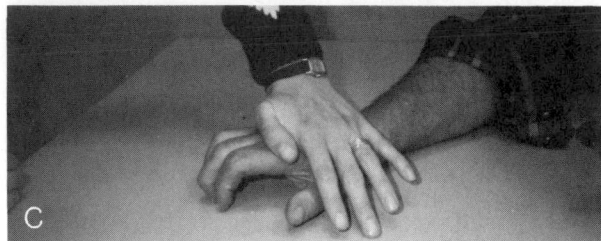

FIGURE 31–84   Exercises following crush injury. **A,** Attempted active flexion. **B,** Attempted active extension. **C,** Intrinsic stretching.

lunate vascularity, wrist pain, and lunate collapse.[31,42]

b. Clinical presentation. The dislocation may spontaneously reduce, leaving relatively little clinical evidence other than pain and instability from ligamentous damage. In some cases, palpable or visible lunate displacement and associated median nerve compression are present.

c. Management

(1). Assess the patient's problems, which may include

• wrist and palm pain, localized tenderness, and potential instability

• sensory and motor changes in the median nerve distribution distal to the wrist

(2). Treatment and rehabilitation

(a). Perform closed or open reduction with cast immobilization in slight wrist flexion for 4 to 6 weeks, during which time, finger, elbow, and shoulder function are maintained.[36]

(b). After removal of the cast, active thumb and wrist exercises are added to the program; attempts to restore motion lost secondary to immobilization must not stress the ligaments damaged by the initial injury. If complications such as median nerve palsy and flexor tendon restrictions occur, they must be treated accordingly.

2. First MP joint (Gamekeeper's thumb)

a. Etiology. Forceful hyperextension or abduction of the thumb ruptures the volar plate insertion or ulnar collateral ligament; this injury commonly occurs during skiing from a fall on an abducted thumb (see Figure 31–85).

b. Clinical presentation. Request a radiographic examination to rule out the possibility of fracture. Test the ulnar collateral ligament; if radial deviation is greater than 35 degrees (with the patient under local anesthesia) when the thumb is tested in 15 degrees of MP joint flexion, then complete rupture of the ligament is present. Partial ruptures may produce local tenderness but not instability.

c. Management

(1). Assess the patient's problems, which may include

• pain and inflammation

• instability and loss of function

(2). Treatment of partial rupture involves protected ROM and strengthening

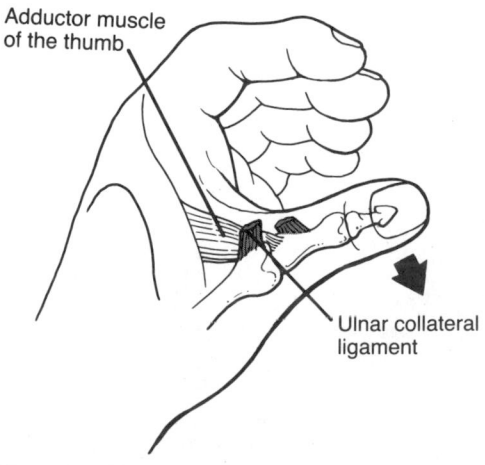

Adductor muscle of the thumb

Ulnar collateral ligament

FIGURE 31–85   Ulnar collateral ligament injury.

exercises of the thumb, with stability taking precedence over mobility.

(3). Treatment of complete rupture involves manual reduction followed by 2 to 6 weeks of immobilization; then follow the protocol for partial rupture. Open reduction is required if the adductor aponeurosis is trapped between the ligament and the proximal phalanx (Stenner lesion). Follow open reduction with 2 to 6 weeks of immobilization; then follow the protocol for partial rupture.

3. Second to fifth MP joints
  a. Etiology. Finger hyperextension, forcing the metacarpal head volarly, or twisting with lateral stress, may damage the capsule, collateral ligaments, or volar plates.
  b. Clinical presentation. The patient presents with volar projection of the metacarpal head and pain and instability in MP joint extension.
  c. Management
    (1). Note the patient's problems, which may include
      • pain and inflammation
      • instability and loss of function
    (2). Surgical treatment and rehabilitation involve open reduction with repair of the volar plate if indicated. Use a dorsal block splint to maintain 60 degrees of MP joint flexion; initiate and continue active flexion from this position for up to 5 weeks.[36]

4. PIP joints
  a. Etiology. Hyperextension or lateral angulation of the middle phalanx is the mechanism producing this injury. Dorsal dislocation is most common and may be associated with a fracture.
  b. Clinical presentation. The patient has localized tenderness over the collateral ligament or volar plate, instability, and edema.
  c. Management
    (1). Assess the patient's problems, which may include
      • pain, inflammation, and edema
      • instability and loss of function
    (2). Treatment of a stable sprain involves the use of protective splinting or buddy taping (to an adjacent finger) for 1 week.
    (3). An unstable sprain should be treated with closed reduction and splinting

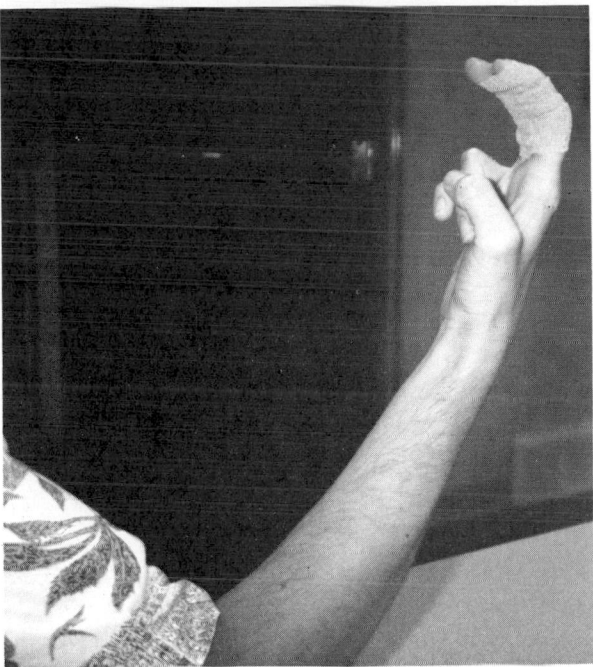

FIGURE 31–86 Buddy taping of the injured middle finger to the uninjured index finger; this allows mobility while providing protection.

(use a dorsal splint to block the last 25 degrees of extension, but permit active flexion from this position, for 3 weeks).[60] Active exercises are initiated 3 weeks postinjury, with buddy taping to protect the joint and to assist in the exercises for an additional 3 weeks (see Figure 31–86). Use coban wrap for edema control. Start intrinsic stretching and progressive resistive exercise at 6 weeks. Use a dynamic splint if a contracture develops. Restoration of full, pain-free motion may take as long as 6 to 9 months.[36]

    (4). A fracture and dislocation (coach's finger) requires surgical treatment and rehabilitation. Treatment involves Kirschner wire fixation for 7 to 10 days; then apply a dorsal splint to allow active flexion through the range of 70 to 110 degrees for 6 weeks. Attempt to regain full ROM after the dorsal splinting.

5. DIP joints
  a. Etiology. Hyperextension or lateral angulation of the distal phalanx is the mechanism of this injury.

b. Clinical presentation. The patient has pain, instability, and edema.
c. Management
  (1). Note the patient's problems, which may include
    • pain, inflammation, and edema
    • instability and loss of function
  (2). If closed injury, perform manual reduction followed by immobilization in a dorsal splint at 0 degrees for 1 to 3 weeks; follow this with active exercise and progressive resistive exercise.
  (3). If open injury, perform surgical reduction and Kirschner wire fixation for 3 weeks. Follow this with passive and active ROM and then progressive resistive exercise.

D. Avulsion injuries

1. Etiology.   Musculotendinous   contraction against sudden resistance may cause an avulsion of a tendon from the area it attaches to bone.
2. Clinical presentation. The patient has point tenderness and swelling over the area of the avulsion and functional loss directly related to the involved structure.
3. Management
  a. If avulsion of the central (slip) extensor tendon insertion onto the middle phalanx has occurred, proceed as follows:
    (1). Assess the patient's problems, which may include
      • loss of active PIP joint extension
      • development of boutonnière deformity and loss of DIP flexion (a major functional handicap)
    (2). Conservative   treatment   includes splinting the PIP joint in extension

for 4 weeks (the DIP is not splinted, and active movement of the DIP is encouraged).[61]
    (3). Surgical treatment involves reattaching the tendon, with Kirschner wire stabilization for 5 to 6 weeks. Then restore motion and prevent PIP joint extension lag by emphasizing active extension.
  b. If avulsion of the distal extensor tendon insertion onto the distal phalanx (see Figure 31–87) has occurred, proceed as follows:
    (1). Note the patient's problems, which may include
      • loss of active DIP joint extension
      • development of mallet finger (if the injury occurs with the DIP joint flexed more than 45 degrees, damage to both the ED muscle and the oblique retinacular ligament may occur. If the injury occurs with the DIP joint flexed less than 45 degrees, damage to only the ED muscle.
    (2). Conservative   treatment   involves splinting the DIP joint in extension for 6 weeks (while allowing the PIP joint to move). Have the patient start active motion and wear the splint at night and during athletic activity for 4 more weeks.[36]
    (3). Surgical treatment involves reattaching the tendon, then splinting the DIP joint in extension for 6 weeks. Have the patient start active motion and wear the splint at night for 4 more weeks.
  c. If avulsion of the FDP tendon inserted onto the distal phalanx has occurred, proceed as follows:
    (1). Assess the patient's problems, which may include loss of active DIP joint flexion.
    (2). Surgical treatment includes reattaching the tendon and placing the hand in a dorsal block splint with the MP joint at 70 degrees of flexion and the IP joints extended for 4 weeks (see tendon repair protocol). Initiate AROM in 4 to 6 weeks and progressive resistive exercise in 6 to 10 weeks. If a fracture is present, then wire the fragment into place and immobilize it for 1 week. There-

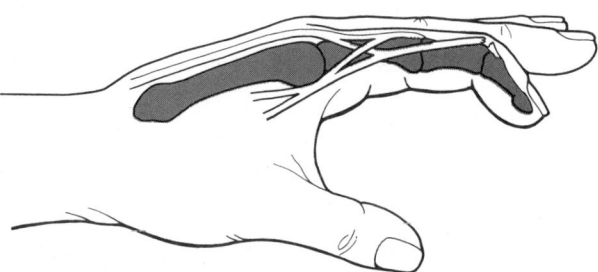

FIGURE 31–87   Mallet finger with rupture of the terminal extensor tendon.

after, follow the previously described protocol.

E. Tendon lacerations

1. Etiology. Tendon lacerations from a sharp cut may damage other soft tissues as well as the tendon. Tendon disruption may also result from attrition with delayed rupture, closed blunt trauma, and burns.
2. Clinical presentation. The patient has localized pain and immediate functional loss (with complete laceration).
3. Management. The principles of repair and management vary, according to the zone of injury (see Figure 31–88).
   a. Flexor tendons[62]
      (1). The zones of injury for the flexor tendons are as follow:

Zone	Location
I	Distal to the insertion of the FDS.
II	Between the A-1 pulley and the insertion of the FDS ("no man's land")
III	Area between the distal border of the carpal tunnel and the A-1 pulley
IV	Within the carpal tunnel; nine tendons are confined in a small space
V	Proximal to the carpal tunnel; may involve multiple tendons, arteries, and nerves. Injury in this zone commonly occurs when a hand breaks through a glass window
Thumb I	From the thumb IP joint distally
Thumb II	Between the thumb A-1 pulley and the IP joint
Thumb III	Area of the first metacarpal bone

(2). Assess the patient's problems, which may include
   • loss of flexion in a digit specific to the level of injury
   • decreased function secondary to adhesions, scarring, and loss of strength

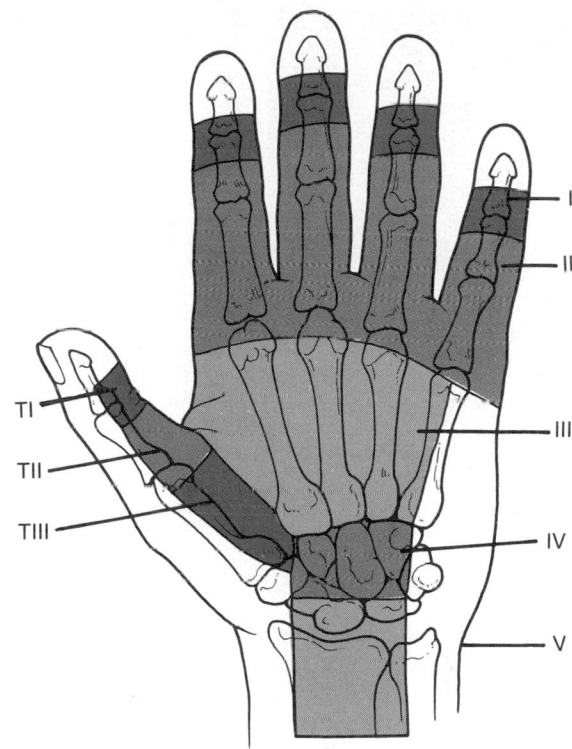

FIGURE 31–88 Flexor tendon zones.

(3). Surgical repair and rehabilitation involve direct primary repair or two-stage tendon reconstruction (see Figure 31–89). The patient's hand is placed in a dorsal blocking splint, with the wrist at approximately 30 degrees of flexion (this angle is lessened for injuries in zone V), the MP joints at 70 to 90 degrees of flexion, and the IP joints extended (see Figure 31–90). The fingers are *passively*

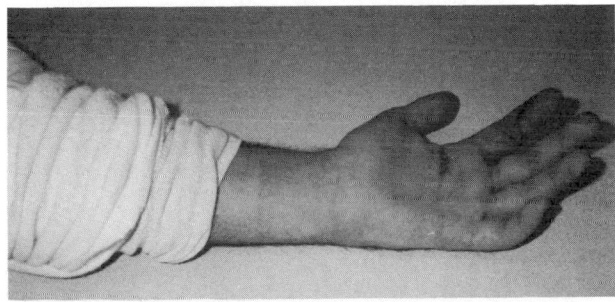

FIGURE 31–89 Surgical repair of laceration of the left index FDS and FDP.

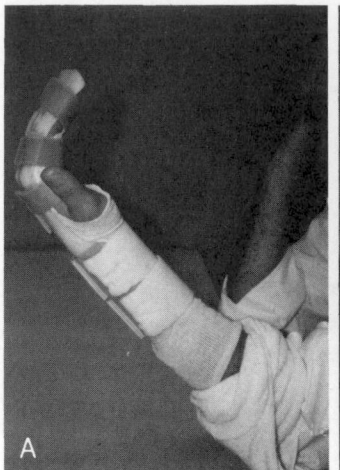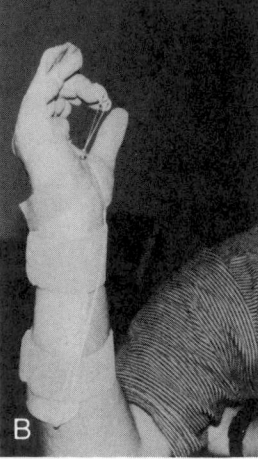

FIGURE 31–90 Dorsal blocking splint following flexor tendon repair. **A,** Static. **B,** Dynamic.

flexed within the splint, either manually (Duran protocol—"controlled passive motion") (see Figure 31–91) or by dynamic traction (Kleinert protocol) (see Figure 31–90*B*). A pully bar in the palm, used in conjunction with dynamic traction, assures flexion in all finger joints. The patient also *actively extends* his/her fingers within the confines of the splint.

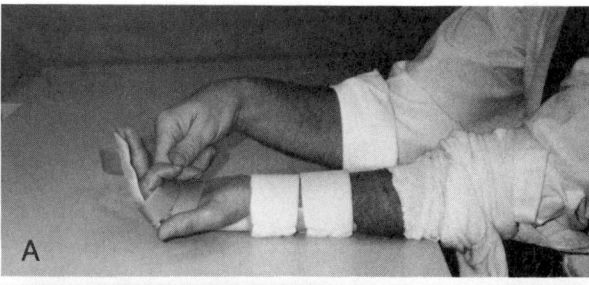
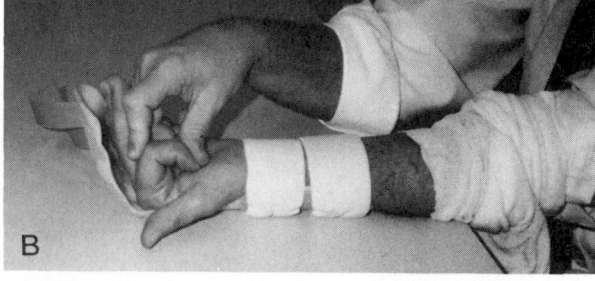

FIGURE 31–91 Duran protocol of controlled passive motion. **A,** PIP flexion. **B,** Composite flexion.

(4). The general protocol for progression is as follows:[63–66]

Time	Treatment
Day 0 through day 3 after surgery	Elevation in postsurgical dressing
Day 4 through week 3.5	Continuous wearing of a dorsal protective splint; protected passive flexion and active extension with both composite and isolated joint movement (eight repetitions every 2 hours); edema-control measures as indicated
Week 3.5 through week 5	Replace the splint with a wrist cuff, incorporating dynamic traction, or remold the splint with 45 degrees of wrist extension to minimize passive tension in the extensor tendons, thus decreasing the amount of active tension required to flex the fingers[67]; start *gentle* active finger flexion, active wrist extension with finger flexion, active finger extension with wrist flexion and composite wrist and finger extension *only* to a neutral position (10 repetitions per hour)
Week 6 through week 8	Discontinue use of the splint or wrist cuff; continue active wrist flexion and extension, and start digital blocking exercise to isolate flexion of the DIP, PIP, and MP joints and differential tendon gliding (12 repetitions per hour); do not forcefully stress the healing tendon, which is only 50%

Time	Treatment
	of its full strength; initiate scar management and contracture control measures as indicated (see Figure 31–92); passive wrist and digit extension or extension splinting for contractures may be initiated at week 7
Week 9 through week 12	Gradually increase resistive exercise and work therapy

b. Extensor tendons (see Figure 31–93)
   (1). The zones of injury for the extensor tendons are as follow:

Zone	Location
I	DIP joint and distal phalanx
II	Middle phalanx

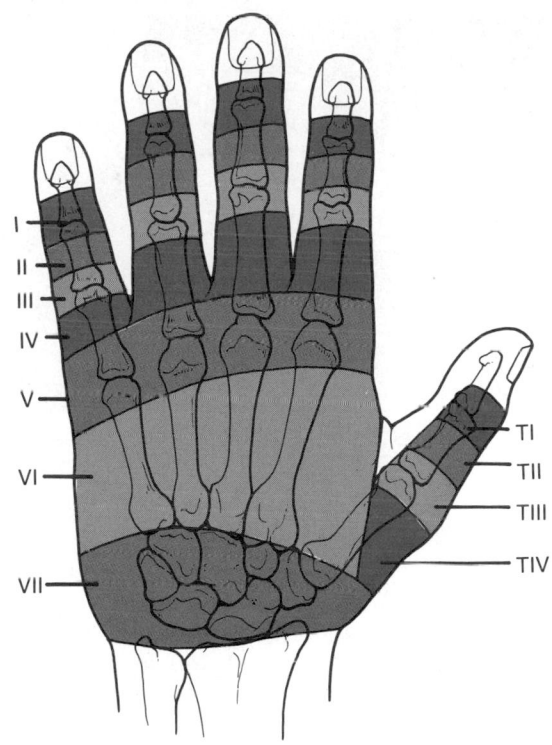

FIGURE 31–93   Extensor tendon zones.

Zone	Location
III	PIP joint
IV	Proximal phalanx
V	MP joint
VI	Metacarpal bone
VII	Wrist
Thumb I	IP joint and distal phalanx of the thumb
Thumb II	Proximal phalanx of the thumb
Thumb III	MP joint of the thumb
Thumb IV	Metacarpal bone of the thumb
Thumb V	Wrist

(2). Assess the patient's problems, which may include
   • loss of extension in the digit specific to the level of injury
   • decreased function secondary to adhesions, scarring, and loss of strength
(3). Surgical repair and rehabilitation involve approximating and suturing

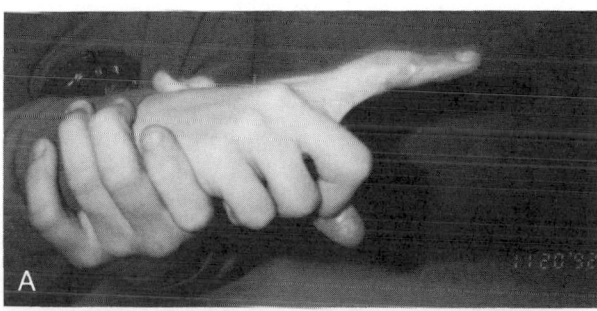

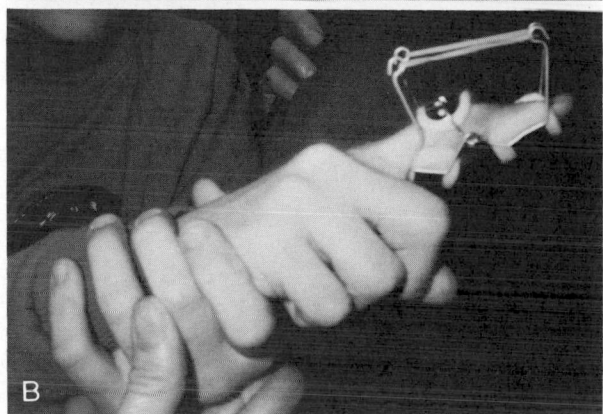

FIGURE 31–92   Healing flexor tendon repair. **A,** PIP flexion contracture. **B,** Dynamic splint to increase extension.

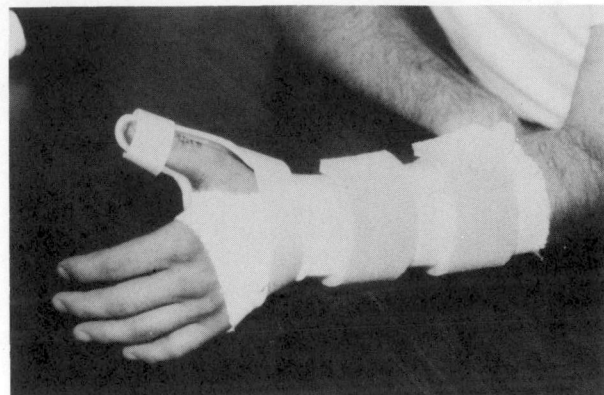

FIGURE 31–94 Splint for immobilization after surgical repair of the extensor pollicis longus muscle.

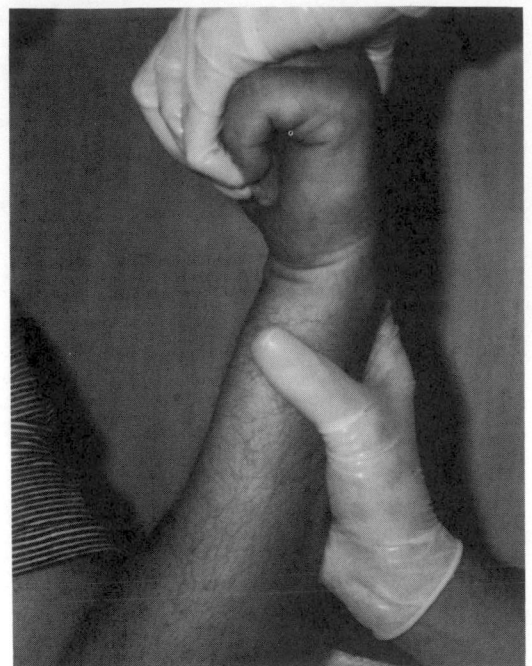

FIGURE 31–96 Composite flexion exercise to stretch the extensor tendons.

the lacerated ends of the tendons. The patient's finger or hand is placed in a volar blocking splint; (except a short dorsal splint may be used in zones I and II, and a cylinder may be used in zones III and IV.)

(4). The general protocol for progression is as follows[68–70] (see Figures 31–94 to 31–96).

Zone	Treatment
I, II	Day 0 through day 3, elevate the hand in postsurgical dressing; day 4 through week 7, splint the DIP joint in 0 to 10 degrees of hyperextension; week 8 through week 9, gradually wean the patient from the splint, but have him/her continue to wear it for heavy activity, and start

Zone	Treatment
	gentle active DIP flexion from 20 to 40 degrees; week 10 through week 11, the patient should progress to full ROM and function
III, IV	Day 0 through day 3, elevate the hand in postsurgical dressing; day 4 through week 6, splint the PIP joint at 0 degrees; if the patient has only a central slip injury, start DIP joint active exten-

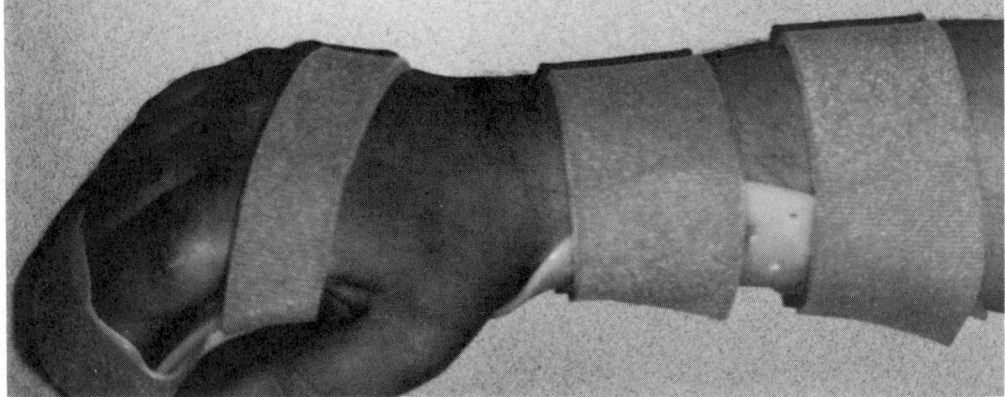

FIGURE 31–95 Splint for immobilization after surgical repair of the extensor digitorum muscle.

Zone	Treatment
	sion at 10 days; week 7 through week 8, gradually wean the patient from the splint, but have him/her continue to wear it for heavy activity, and start gentle active PIP joint flexion and extension with the MP joint in extension; week 9 through week 10, isolate the PIP joint active extension and increase resistance
V, VI	Day 0 through day 3, elevate the hand in postsurgical dressing; day 4 through week 4, apply a volar forearm-hand splint with 40 degrees of wrist extension, 40 degrees MP joint flexion, and IP joint extension; week 4, initiate active MP joint exercise and "clawing" exercise with wrist extension; week 5, modify the splint to neutral position of wrist and have the patient wear it for heavy activity through week 6; also initiate wrist ROM with fingers extended, and intrinsic muscle and clawing exercise; week 7 through week 9, initiate light resistive exercise; week 10 through week 11, initiate progressive resistive exercise
VII	Day 0 through day 3, elevate the hand in postsurgical dressing; day 4 through week 4, apply a volar forearm-hand splint with 40 degrees wrist extension; also splint the fingers 40 degrees of MP joint flexion and IP joint extension if the finger tendons are injured, in addition to the wrist extensor tendons; week 4, initiate wrist flexion exercise (with the fingers extended) and finger flexion (with the wrist extended); week 5 through week 6, have the patient wear the splint for heavy activity and initiate composite flexion and extension of the wrist and fingers; week 7 through week 9, initiate light resistive exercise; week 10 through week 11, initiate progressive resistive exercise

Zone	Treatment
Thumb I, II	Day 0 through day 3, elevate the hand in postsurgical dressing; day 4 through week 6, apply a splint with the IP joint at 0 degrees; week 7 through week 9, gradually wean the patient from the splint but have him/her continue to wear it for heavy activity; week 7 through week 8, start gentle active exercise; week 9 through week 11, the patient should progress to full ROM and function
Thumb III, IV	Day 0 through day 3, elevate the hand in postsurgical dressing; day 4 through week 4, splint the MP joint at 0 degrees and the wrist at 30 degrees of extension; week 5 through week 6, start AROM; week 7 through week 8, the patient should progress to full ROM and function
Thumb V	Day 0 through day 3, elevate the hand in postsurgical dressing; day 4 through week 4, splint the wrist at 40 degrees extension and the thumb extended and maintain the web; week 5 through week 6, start AROM; week 7 through week 8, the patient should progress to full ROM and function

F. Fractures

1. Monteggia's fracture
   a. Etiology. The mechanism of this injury is a direct blow to the proximal ulna or axial loading of the forearm in pronation.
   b. Clinical presentation. The patient presents with an angulated fracture of the upper third of the ulna and anterior dislocation of the proximal radioulnar and radiohumeral joints.
   c. Management
      (1). Assess the patient's problems, which may include
         • pain and instability
         • healing status of the fracture
      (2). In children, use closed reduction. Provide above-elbow plaster immo-

bilization; the plaster should not extend distal to the proximal palmar crease (PPC) in order to allow finger movement.

(3). In adults, use open reduction and internal fixation; provide fixation with a dynamic compression plate. Immobilize the limb in 70 to 90 degrees of elbow flexion for 2 to 3 weeks; brace at 45 degrees of flexion for up to 6 weeks.

(4). Exercise the uninvolved joints and treat the patient's symptoms when the cast is removed to allow him/her to regain full ROM and strength.

2. Galeazzi's fracture
   a. Etiology. A fall onto an outstretched hand may cause this fracture, which is common in young adults.
   b. Clinical presentation. The patient has a dorsally angulated fracture of the distal radius and dislocation of the distal radioulnar joint; it is best diagnosed with lateral radiography or computed tomography.
   c. Management
      (1). Note the patient's problems, which may include
         • pain and instability
         • healing status of the fracture
      (2). Provide open reduction and internal fixation with an intramedullary nail or plate.[42]
      (3). Exercise forearm and hand, progressing to functional activities as soon as the healing status will allow.

3. Colles' fracture
   a. Etiology. Colles' fracture is the most common of all fractures; it typically involves the elderly. It is caused by a fall onto an outstretched hand with the wrist extended.
   b. Clinical presentation. The patient presents with a dorsally-angulated fracture of the distal 2 in of the radius, with or without accompanying ulnar fracture; the fracture is often comminuted or impacted.
   c. Management
      (1). Assess the patient's problems, which may include
         • pain, instability, and edema
         • healing status of the fracture
         • complications may include malunion, subluxation of the distal radioulnar joint, joint stiffness

anywhere in the upper extremity, rupture of the EPL tendon, and reflex sympathetic dystrophy

(2). Use closed reduction (or open reduction if extensive displacement or malalignment is present); provide 3 to 4 weeks of immobilization in an above-elbow plaster cast. A below-elbow plaster cast should follow in healthy, active individuals for 2 to 4 more weeks.[71] (Immobilization is discontinued at 4 weeks in the elderly, and AROM is initiated.) Comminuted and unstable fractures are immobilized with an external fixator; elevation and coban wrapping of the fingers and accessible parts of the hand are useful for edema control. Initiate exercise of the uninvolved joints, and emphasize forearm, wrist, and thumb movements when the immobilization is removed. Passive stretching of the intrinsic musculature is accomplished in a position of MP joint extension and IP joint flexion; the extrinsic flexor tendons are stretched by composite extension of the fingers and wrist, and the extrinsic extensor tendons, by composite flexion. Joint mobilization is useful in lengthening inert tissues that limit the accessory motion of the joints[72] (see Figure 31–97). Use other modalities such as transcutaneous electrical nerve stimulation and functional electrical stimulation, as indicated, to decrease pain and enhance mobility.

4. Smith's fracture
   a. Etiology. The mechanism of this injury is a fall onto an outstretched hand with the wrist flexed and the forearm pronated.
   b. Clinical presentation. The patient presents with a volarly angulated radial fracture ("reverse Colles'").
   c. Management
      (1). Note the patient's problems, which may include
         • pain and instability
         • healing status of the fracture
      (2). Use closed reduction; the limb should be casted in supination with the wrist in a neutral position for 4 weeks. The limb should be rehabilitated as for Colles' fracture.[71]

5. Barton's fracture

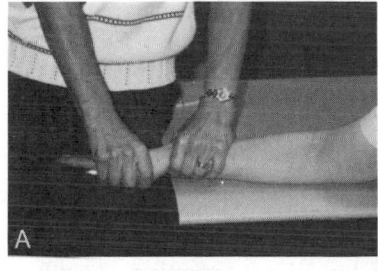
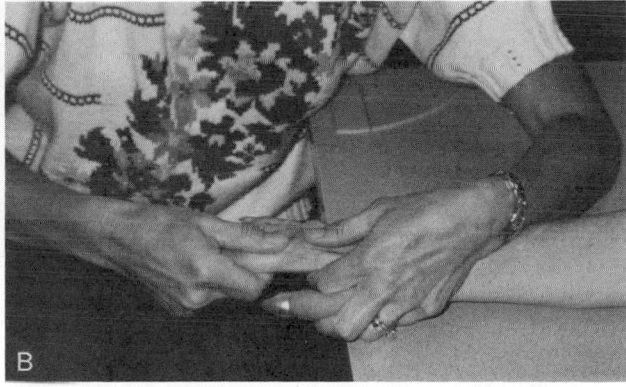

FIGURE 31-97   Joint mobilization. **A,** Volar glide radiocarpal joint. **B,** MP joint traction.

a. Etiology. The mechanism of this injury is a fall onto an outstretched hand with the wrist flexed.

b. Clinical presentation. The patient has an oblique fracture through the radial articular surface with dorsal or volar displacement of the fragment.

c. Management
   (1). Assess the patient's problems, which may include
      • pain
      • healing status of the fracture
   (2). One option is closed reduction and immobilization of the wrist toward the fracture to enhance stability, with slight extension for a dorsal fracture and slight flexion for a volar fracture.[71]
   (3). Another option is open reduction and internal fixation with a T-plate, percutaneous pins, or bone screws; initiate early active wrist motion.

6. Scaphoid fracture
   a. Etiology. The mechanism of this injury is a fall onto an outstretched hand with the wrist extended; it is more common in younger patients.
   b. Clinical presentation. The patient presents with a transverse fracture through the waist (most common), tuberosity, or proximal pole. He/she has localized tenderness in the snuffbox area. Taking an oblique-view radiograph is the best method of diagnosis; it may need to be repeated in 2 weeks if the results are negative initially.
   c. Management
      (1). Note the patient's problems, which may include

• pain
• healing status of the fracture
• complications may include delayed union, nonunion (which may necessitate a bone graft or prosthetic implant), avascular necrosis of the proximal pole, and osteoarthritis

   (2). Treat the problem as a fracture based on the history and clinical features, even if the radiographic diagnosis is initially uncertain; apply a long- or short-arm thumb spica cast in radial deviation with 10 degrees of wrist flexion and the thumb in full palmar abduction with the IP joint free for 8 to 12 weeks. Work to restore motion, strength, and endurance.[31,42]

7. Bennett's fracture dislocation
   a. Etiology. The mechanism of this injury is hyperabduction or hyperflexion of the thumb.
   b. Clinical presentation. The patient has an oblique articular fracture of the base of the first metacarpal, from which the large distal fragment is displaced by APL in a proximal, radial direction.
   c. Management
      (1). Note the patient's problems, which include
         • pain
         • healing status of the fracture
         • complications such as carpometacarpal joint arthritis
      (2). Use closed reduction and plaster immobilization for 5 to 8 weeks in a forearm cast, incorporating both joints of the thumb. Kirschner wire fixation is used if anatomical align-

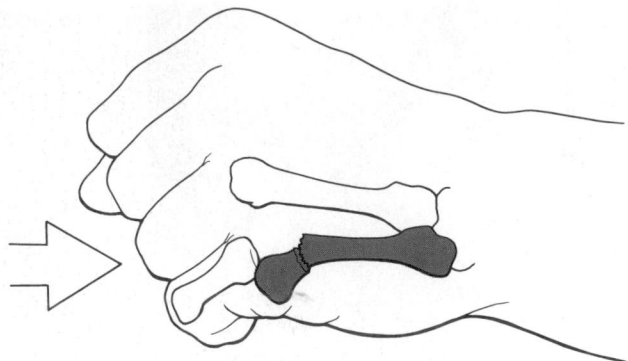

FIGURE 31–98   Boxer's fracture.

ment cannot be maintained, and a thumb spica cast is applied for 4 to 5 weeks, after which time, the cast is removed, and gentle active motion is started; the wires are removed 2 weeks later, at which time PROM can begin. At 7 to 8 weeks, start more aggressive stretching and joint mobilization.

8. Metacarpal fractures
   a. Etiology. A crushing blow, entrapment, or twisting of the hand may produce a metacarpal fracture; a boxer's fracture, which is a volarly angulated fracture of the metacarpal head, is caused by a compressive blow with the fist.
   b. Clinical presentation. A shaft fracture may be undisplaced, although they occasionally are rotated or angulated. Metacarpal neck fractures, such as boxer's fractures, typically display volar displacement of the metacarpal head and neck (see Figure 31–98).
   c. Management
      (1). Problems
         • pain
         • healing status of the fracture
         • edema
      (2). Apply a splint if the bones are in good alignment, or use open reduction and internal fixation if poor alignment is present. Immobilize the forearm and hand for 2 to 4 weeks with the wrist extended 35 degrees, the MP joints flexed 75 degrees, and the PIP joints free. Provide edema management throughout the course of treatment. Start exercise as soon

as the patient is stable, usually in 14 days. Use only active ROM exercise for the MP joints and wrist initially; initiate active and passive ROM for the IP joints and uninvolved parts.

9. Phalangeal fractures
   a. Etiology. A direct blow, twisting force, or a crushing injury (most common) may cause a phalangeal fracture.
   b. Clinical presentation. The bone is unstable, and displacement is common.
   c. Management
      (1). Assess the patient's problems, which may include
         • pain
         • healing status of the fracture
         • edema
         • complications may include tendon, skin, or other soft-tissue injuries
      (2). Use closed reduction with buddy taping (for spiral fractures); use a percutaneous pin or open reduction and internal fixation with Kirschner wire if the fracture is unstable (as in transverse fractures) and a cast or Alumafoam finger splint[72] (see Figure 31–99). Use coban wrapping of the finger for edema. Start AROM at 2 to 3 weeks; use joint mobilization and dynamic splinting to reduce contractures in 6 to 8 weeks. Diaphyseal fractures of the middle phalanx require 6 weeks of immobilization before initiating ROM, then 3 to 4 months of protection.

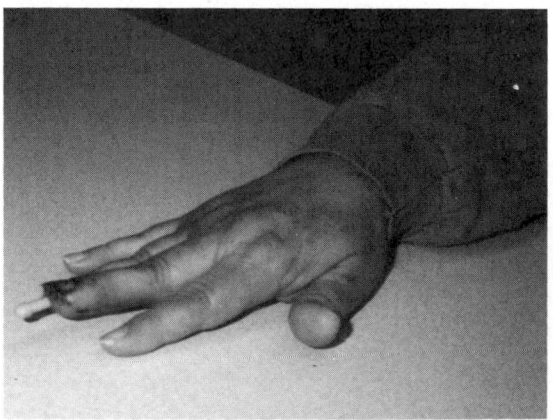

FIGURE 31–99   Distal phalangeal fracture with internal fixation and nail bed repair.

G. The burned hand

1. Etiology. Burn injuries often involve the hands because they are used to fight the fire, handle hot objects, protect the face, and so forth. Scarring is a major cause of disability after burns, and although it cannot be prevented, the object of treatment is to "control" scarring with exercise, pressure, contact, and splinting.

2. Clinical presentation. Burns are classified by the depth of injury.[58]
   a. Superficial partial-thickness burns are characterized by edema, blistering, pain, and erythema. They heal spontaneously with normal function and appearance.
   b. Deep partial-thickness burns result in damage to the dermis and epidermis.
   c. Full-thickness burns involve a complete loss of skin.

3. Management. The goal is to prevent deformity, enhance function, and improve cosmesis.
   a. Assess the patient's problems, which may include
      • potential for infection
      • pain
      • edema
      • healing status of burn wounds or skin grafts
      • hypertrophic scarring or keloids
      • contractures or deformity
   b. Treatment[58,74]
      (1). Emergent phase (up to 72 hours) Control edema by positioning the hand above the level of the heart and the shoulder at 100 degrees of abduction. After edema "peaks," apply a static splint in an antideformity position (the wrist at 20 to 30 degrees of extension, the MP joints at 70 to 90 degrees of flexion, the IP joints extended, and the thumb abducted). The splint initially is secured with nonrestrictive gauze wraps that should be reapplied frequently. Active motion should be performed during dressing changes with a forceful pumping motion (however, use precaution to protect against extensor tendon rupture with a dorsal burn over the proximal phalanges).
      (2). Acute phase (up to wound closure). Active exercise should be performed during hydrotherapy, emphasizing

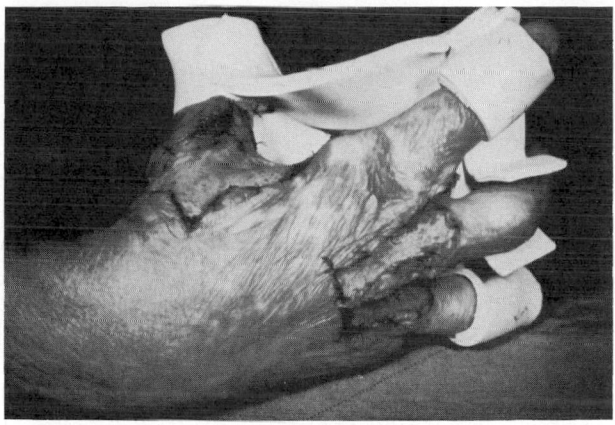

FIGURE 31–100 Splint to maintain web space after burn grafting.

the maintenance of muscle tone and ROM rather than strength. If limitations in PROM exist, perform gentle stretching and active assisted exercise (collagen in healing wounds possesses 20% of normal tensile strength after 3 weeks and 70% after 2 months). Protect exposed tendons and joints with moist dressings and immobilization. Encourage functional use of the hands throughout the day. Utilize custom splinting during rest periods and at night to counteract contractures. In general, the position of splinting is one in which burned surfaces are stretched, although other factors must be considered, eg, muscles spanning more than one joint; preservation of hand arches, web spaces, and prehension; the presence of fracture or nerve injury; and so forth.

(3). Skin graft phase. The hand should be immobilized for 5 to 7 days after surgery.[58] A splint may be applied in the operating room. The patient may continue hydrotherapy with soaking only. Initiate isometric exercise of grafted areas and continue full ROM exercise of nongrafted areas (see Figure 31–100).

(4). Rehabilitation phase (from wound closure until scar maturation [up to 2 years]).[75] Maintain scar pliability with massage, using oil-based mois-

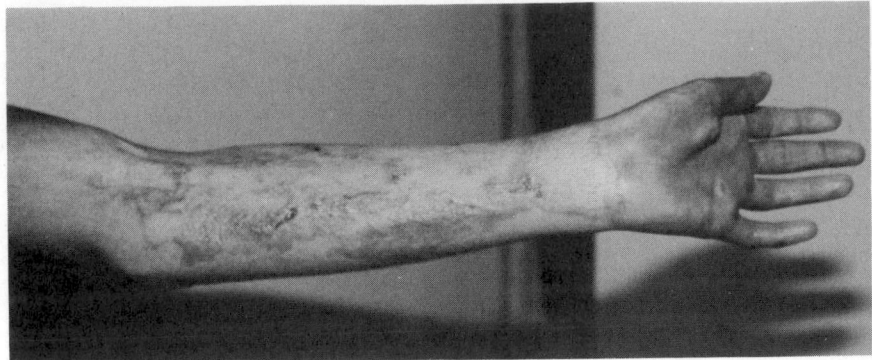
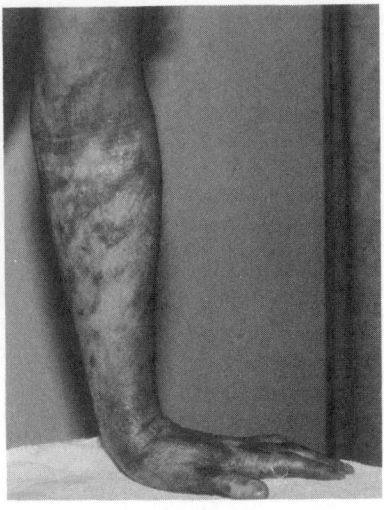

FIGURE 31–101   Burn wound. **A,** Hot tar burn on the arm and hand. **B,** The patient exercises to increase composite extension.

turizing lotion. For hypertrophic scarring apply pressure with custom-fit garments, or elastic wraps[76]; recent studies have found that contact of a Silastic or silicone gel sheet with scar tissue is effective in reducing hypertrophy.[77] Initiate an individualized exercise program with emphasis on both isolated and composite joint motion, increasing strength and endurance, and work hardening or job simulation, if indicated (see Figure 31–101).

H. Peripheral nerve injury

1. Review of fiber and receptor morphology
   a. The afferent (sensory) nerve fibers are as follow:

Fiber	Characteristics
Group I,a (A-alpha)	12 to 20 μm; myelinated; 70 to 120 m/s; annulo-spinal ending in muscle
Group I,b (A-alpha)	12 to 20 μm; myelinated; 70 to 120 m/s; Golgi tendon organ in muscle
Group II (A-beta, A-gamma)	6 to 12 μm; myelinated; 35 to 75 m/s; touch, pressure, movement, and position sense in skin and muscle
Group III (A-delta)	1 to 5 μm; myelinated; 5 to 30 m/s; pricking pain, temperature, and deep pressure in skin and muscle
B fibers	1 to 3 μm; finely myelinated; 30 to 60 m/s; pain, temperature, and proprioceptive in free nerve endings
C fibers	0.2 to 1.5 μm; unmyelinated; 0.5 to 2 m/s; aching and burning pain (50% are nociceptors); and total qualitative sensory receptors

b. The sensory receptors (end-organs) in glabrous (nonhairy) skin (see Figure 31–102)[19] are as follow:

Receptor and characteristics		Axon-to-receptor ratio
Merkel cell–neurite complex	Slowly adapting, constant touch, pressure, 2PD	$\frac{1}{>1} = <1$
Meissner's corpuscle	Quickly adapting, moving touch flutter, 30 cps, M2PD	$\frac{>1}{1} = >1$
Pacinian corpuscle	Quickly adapting, moving touch, vibration, 256 cps	$\frac{1}{1} = 1$

Cutaneous receptors in glabrous (nonhairy) skin:

axon
corpuscle ratio

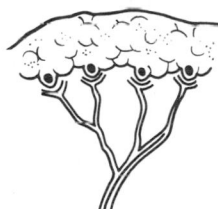

Merkel's cell–neurite complex:
slowly adapting; constant touch;
pressure, 2 PD

$$\frac{1}{>1} = <1$$

Meissner's corpuscle:
quickly adapting; moving touch;
flutter, 30 cps

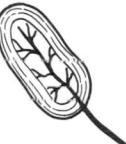

$$\frac{>1}{1} = >1$$

Pacinian corpuscle:
quickly adapting; moving touch;
vibration, 256 cps

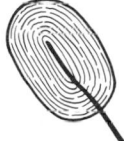

$$\frac{1}{1} = 1$$

FIGURE 31–102   Cutaneous receptors.

2. Etiology and pathology. Peripheral nerve injury occurs secondary to compression, crush, traction, or severance. The nerve injury classification (by Seddon)[18] is as follows:

  a. **Neuropraxia.** Caused by a crushing injury. It results in transient paralysis and sensory loss.

  b. **Axontomesis.** Axonal disruption due to stretch or compression. The Schwann sheath remains intact, but Wallerian degeneration occurs distal to the level of injury. The prognosis is good, but recovery depends on the distance between the injury and the receptors or muscle.

  c. **Neurotomesis.** A laceration produces division of the axons and epineurium and complete disruption of conduction. Surgical repair is indicated, and prognosis is guarded.

3. Clinical presentation

  a. Reinnervation hypothesis. The relative ease with which nerve *fibers* regenerate is related to their size. Nerve cell bodies in the dorsal ganglia produce axoplasm to fill regenerating nerves; therefore, the smallest (C) fibers regenerate fastest because they don't require as much exo-

plasm. The other factor determining whether reinnervation occurs is reconnection of the nerve fibers to the receptors. The greater the number of axons (fibers) supplying a *receptor*, the greater the chance of reinnervation; therefore, Meissner's corpuscles, whose axon:receptor ratio is >1, make contact first. They are followed by the Merkel cell–neurite complex (ratio, <1), then the Pacinian corpuscle, which theoretically should be ahead of the Merkel cell–neurite complex but is slowed by a mechanical barrier. Because of this feature, moving touch returns 2 to 6 months ahead of static touch following nerve repair. The nerve cell bodies in the dorsal ganglia will die in 9 to 12 months if the axon is not regenerated.[19]

  b. Typical hand postures associated with peripheral nerve loss (see Figure 31–103) are as follow:

    (1). Median nerve injury causes ape-hand deformity or "benediction attitude," with the thumb in the plane of the palm and an inability to flex the PIP and DIP joints of the index and middle fingers.

    (2). Damage of the ulnar nerve results in clawing of the ring and little fingers, with an inability to extend the PIP and DIP joints unless the MP joints are passively flexed.

    (3). Radial nerve injury results in wrist drop and loss of thumb and MP joint extension.

4. Evaluation following nerve injury or repair

  a. The goal is to identify loss from neuropathy or nerve injury, or the extent of return and functional ability following repair. The therapist should also determine the patient's readiness for sensory re-education.

  b. Modality tests are used to assess the presence or absence of specific modalities, but the results do not necessarily correlate with function. These tests are useful for identifying protective sensation and light touch, *eg*, a pinprick, discrimination between sharp and dull or hot and cold.

  c. Objective tests are those that the patient cannot control, but they may not correlate with function. Objective tests include sudomotor, wrinkle, and electrophysiologic tests.

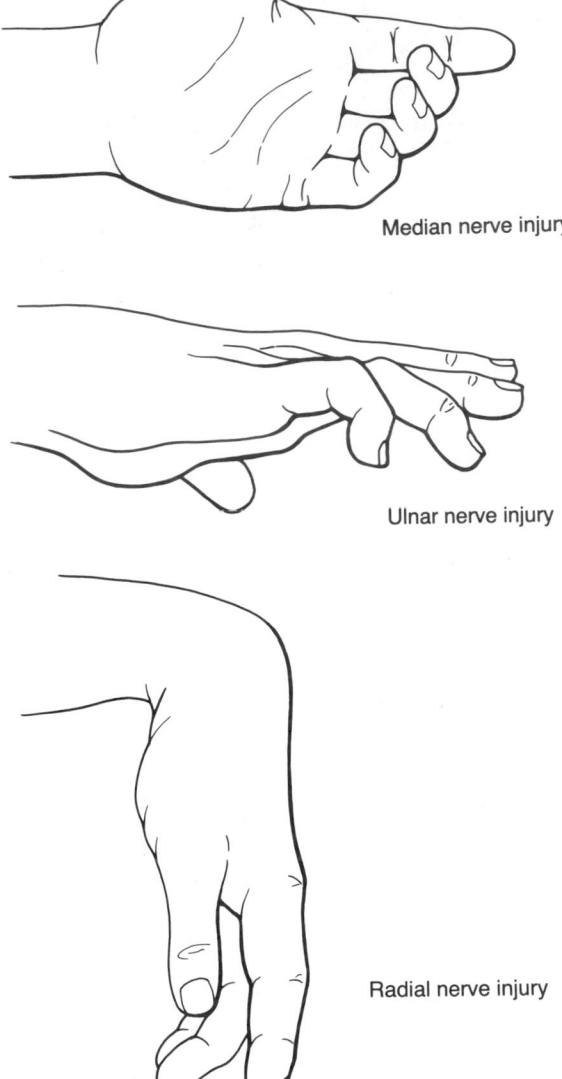

FIGURE 31–103   Hand postures after peripheral nerve injury.

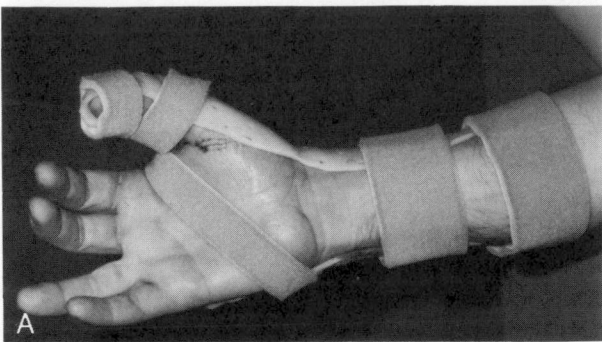

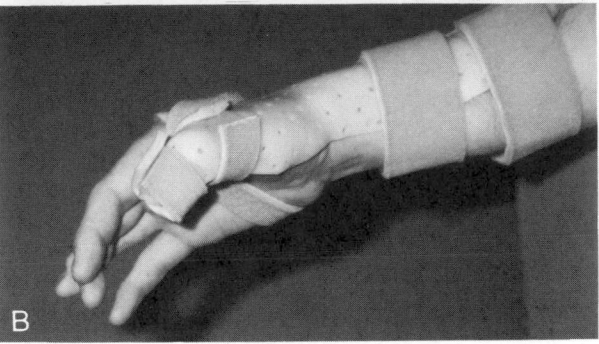

FIGURE 31–104   Surgical repair of the medial digital artery and nerve. **A,** Splint mobilization in moderate flexion, volar view. **B,** Dorsal view.

d. Functional tests assess quality and discriminatory ability and require a patient's cooperation and subjective responses. Examples include two-point discrimination, the Seddon coin test, and the Moberg pickup test.

e. Strength tests include manual muscle and dynametric tests and are administered according to standardized protocols.

5. Management

a. Assess the patient's problems, which may include
   • sensory changes
   • motor loss

b. Principles of rehabilitation
   (1). Splinting
      (a). Initially immobilize the limb for 3 to 4 weeks to minimize tension on the repair site and to protect the nerve from disruption. With compromised sensation, watch for skin breakdown under the splint (see Figure 31–104).
      (b). While awaiting complete reinnervation, proceed with the following:
         (i). Generally use a static splint to immobilize or stabilize joints, to protect and rest the limb, to prevent undesired motion, to resolve fixed joint contractures (*eg*, serial cylinder casting), and to substitute for lost muscle function.

(ii). Generally use a dynamic splint to mobilize the joints, to resolve tendon tightness and joint contractures, and to increase the AROM of given joints.

(c). Splints for specific nerve lesions are as follows:[11]

    (i). For radial lesions, use a wrist cock-up splint with or without an outrigger to assist with finger and thumb extension.

    (ii). For median lesions, use a thumb opponens splint to facilitate thumb and finger prehension and to preserve the thumb web space.

    (iii). For ulnar lesions, use a dorsal-based splint to block MP joint extension of the ring and little fingers to prevent clawing.

(2). Strengthening. Initiate exercise to combat deformities and functional deficiencies with a specific nerve loss; use graded exercise for increasing strength and endurance. Motor retraining, if indicated, can be used

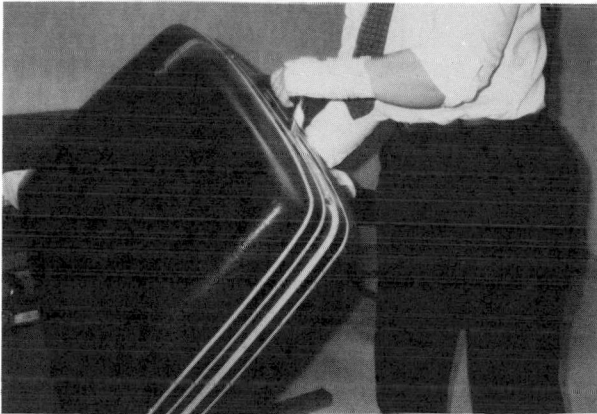

FIGURE 31–105   Work-hardening exercise: lifting a suitcase.

following tendon transfers. Patient education on compensatory movements may be required (see Figure 31–105).

(3). Sensory re-education or desensitization. Education enhances cortical correlation of sensory impulses with known stimuli; however, the patient must have some sensation to begin. Start with M2PD and progress to S2PD; the goal is to increase tactile gnosis.

Clinical Decision-Making Cases

Case #1

HISTORY

Patient #1 is a 33-year-old man who is a painter by trade. He sustained lacerations of his right (dominant) hand when he struck and broke a window pane. The lacerations occurred over the volar surface and on either side of the little finger. The patient underwent immediate surgical exploration and repair of severed FDP and FDS tendons in Zone II, the ulnar and radial digital nerves, and the radial digital artery. He was referred to physical therapy 2 days postoperatively.

Physical Examination

On removal of the dressings, inspection revealed incisions with sutures intact and some oozing blood. A dorsal forearm-hand splint was fabricated to immobilize the ring and little fingers with the IP joints flexed 20 degrees and the MP joints flexed 75 degrees, and the wrist extended 10 degrees. The fingers were secured in the splint with Velcro straps, and the patient was to wear the splint at all times, except for during brief periods of skin inspection and care. He was to return for daily physical therapy treatment.

Problems

1. The healing repairs of little finger FDP and FDS, the radial and ulnar digital nerves, and the radial digital artery required splint immobilization for proper positioning.

2. The patient required education in donning and doffing the splint and in skin care.

3. The patient lacked independence in his exercise program.

Treatment Goals

The goals of treatment were to initially provide immobilization during tendon, artery, and nerve healing, while maintaining tendon gliding with passive ROM; then to increase the ROM, strength, and function in the right hand's fifth digit; and to allow the patient to regain function in order to return to work.

Treatment

Several treatment options were available. Static and dynamic splints are both used following flexor tendon repair. In this case, a static splint was selected because the injury was complicated by nerve and artery repairs, which could not be stressed initially. Also, the IP joints might have been fully extended in the splint but instead were flexed 20 degrees to avoid stretching the nerve and artery repairs. The physical therapist's decision to passively flex and extend the fingers only once daily rather than to have the patient exercise on a more frequent basis was also made to protect the nerve and artery repairs, possibly at the expense of decreased tendon gliding. Plans were made to initiate the Duran protocol for controlled passive motion at 9 days postoperatively.

During postoperative days 2 through 9, the patient was followed daily for dressing changes and passive finger flexion by a physical therapist. Composite flexion with the fingertip to touch the PPC was achieved. Moderate edema persisted, and some wound drainage continued. The patient was admonished to maintain hand elevation and to wear his splint continually.

On the 9th postoperative day, the patient was instructed in a home program according to the Duran protocol for flexor tendon repairs. The frequency of supervised therapy sessions was decreased to once a week.

On the 14th postoperative day, the sutures were removed by the physician, who reported excellent Doppler results and finger coloration. The patient was instructed in light retrograde massage to decrease edema. His splint was modified to allow full IP joint extension. Passive ROM was as follows: 0 to 85 degrees for the MP joint; 15 to 72 degrees for the PIP joint; and 0 to 77 degrees for the DIP joint. The patient was to continue his program of passive flexion and active extension exercises.

At 3.5 weeks postoperatively, a callus over the incision was débrided by the physician. Splint use was limited to the night hours only. The patient was instructed in active finger flexion exercises according to the Duran protocol. He was to emphasize full active PIP extension while maintaining MP flexion to avoid excessive stress on the healing repairs.

At 4.5 weeks postoperatively, the incisions appeared well healed, with only a small scab remaining. The patient perceived dull sensation and paresthesias throughout his little finger. ROM was as follows: 0 to 95 degrees of active flexion for the MP joint and 0 to 100 degrees of passive flexion; 10 degrees of both active and passive extension for the MP joint; 20 to 75 degrees of active motion and 10 to 100 degrees of passive motion for the PIP joint; and 0 to 25 degrees of active motion and 0 to 70 degrees of passive motion for the DIP joint. The patient was instructed to initiate passive PIP joint extension exercise and to continue all other exercises, according to his home program. His splint use was discontinued.

At 6.5 weeks postoperatively, the incisions were completely healed, and edema was resolved. The patient continued to experience paresthesias in his finger. ROM was as follows: the MP joint was within normal limits; the PIP joint had 10 to 95 degrees of active motion and 10 to 100 degrees of passive motion; and the DIP joint had 0 to 40 degrees of active motion and 0 to 80 degrees of passive motion. The patient was fitted with a neoprene extension tube splint to be worn at night to decrease his 10-degree PIP joint flexion contracture. He was encouraged to continue active exercise, particularly blocking the middle phalanx to enhance pull through of the FDP of the finger.

At 8 weeks postoperatively, the patient was instructed in a home program of light resistive exercises using exercise putty and a foam gripper. He was also to begin desensitization of the finger, progressing from smooth to coarser surfaces. ROM was as follows: 5 to 105 degrees of active and passive motion for the PIP joint and 0 to 50 degrees of active motion and 0 to 80 degrees of passive motion for the DIP joint. The patient was allowed to return to work at 9 weeks but was cautioned to avoid forceful gripping.

Outcome

At 12 weeks postoperatively, sensation and ROM were within normal limits, with the exception of DIP joint flexion, which was only 60 degrees actively. The patient was pleased with these results and was discharged.

Case #2

HISTORY

Patient #2 is a 44-year-old male deputy sheriff who sustained a twisting injury to his left (nondominant) hand while arresting a suspected thief. He did not seek medical consultation until 1 week later, at which time radiographs revealed oblique and longitudinal fractures of the shaft of the fifth metacarpal. The patient underwent open reduction and internal fixation by means of a bone plate secured with four screws. The fracture was in good anatomical alignment following the surgical procedure. The patient was instructed by his physician to keep his hand clean, dry, and elevated and was referred to physical therapy 6 days postoperatively. He reported moderate pain and tenderness in his hand on attempts to flex and extend the fingers. He also experienced sensations of numbness and paresthesias over the dorsal medial aspect of his hand.

Physical Examination

On removal of the dressings, inspection revealed a healing incision over the dorsal medial aspect of the left hand, with sutures intact. Moderate edema was present over the dorsal area. Active ROM of the little finger was as follows: 0 to 44 degrees for the MP joint; 0 to 90 degrees for the PIP joint; 0 to 83 degrees for the DIP joint. An ulnar gutter splint was fabricated with the patient's wrist immobilized in a neutral position and the fingers left free to move; it was to be worn during any periods of moderate to heavy activity. The patient was to remove the splint every hour for skin inspection, and if any areas of pressure or irritation developed, he was to contact his therapist immediately. The patient was instructed in AROM exercises for individual finger joint and composite motions, according to a home program to be performed for 10 repetitions five times daily. He was scheduled to return in 4 days.

Problems

1. Healing of the fifth metacarpal fracture required splint protection.
2. The patient lacked full little finger motion and hand function.

Treatment Goals

The goals of treatment were to increase the patient's ROM, strength, and function in the left hand (specifically in the fifth digit); to help him to regain function; and to allow him to return to work.

Treatment

Several treatment options were available. Following open reduction and internal fixation with good alignment of the fracture fragments, a patient may be allowed to start active exercise. Stressful forces on the healing fracture should be minimized. Because this patient was anticipated to be overzealous, a splint was issued. Because the dorsal sensory branch of his ulnar nerve had to be temporarily displaced during surgery, the patient experienced some neuropraxia and had to be instructed in specific skin inspection and care. Also, the proximity of his extrinsic extensor tendons to the incision increased the possibility of adhesion formation; therefore, early repetitive exercise was recommended.

On the 10th postoperative day, the sutures were removed. The patient was instructed in retrograde massage with the hand elevated to reduce edema. He also started a regular physical therapy program 3 times weekly to gradually increase motion, strength, and function in his hand in preparation for returning to work. He performed active exercise of the individual finger joints as well as composite motion of the little finger.

Beginning on the 2nd postoperative week, gentle joint mobilization was performed on the finger joints for approximately 10 minutes per session. The patient was also instructed in light resistive exercises in which he used a variety of exercise devices for approximately 30 minutes per session. He was issued exercise putty for home use. Active ROM of the MP joint was 0 to 52 degrees; the other joints demonstrated normal ROM.

By the 3rd postoperative week, the patient had increased his active ROM in the MP joint to 0 to 80 degrees. Edema had resolved. He continued exercises, increasing resistance as tolerated. With heavy force, he would experience twinges of pain in the dorsum of his hand, which he recognized as a signal to decrease the resistance. He continued to wear his splint for heavy activities such as yard work.

Outcome

By the 4th postoperative week, the patient was experiencing only minimal pain with heavy resistance. He no longer felt numbness or paresthesias over the dorsum of his hand. Active ROM in the MP joint was 0 to 84 degrees. He returned to work with instructions to continue wearing the splint for protection for 2 more weeks.

References

1. Hoppenfeld S: *Physical Examination of the Spine and Extremities.* New York, Appleton-Century-Crofts, 1976.
2. Gross MS, Gelberman RH: The anatomy of the distal ulnar tunnel. *Clin Orthop* 1985, 196:238–247.
3. Stroyan M, Wilk KE: The functional anatomy of the elbow complex. *J Orthop Sports Phys Ther* 1993, 17:279–288.
4. Palmer AK, Werner FW: Biomechanics of the distal radioulnar joint. *Clin Orthop* 1984, 187:26–35.
5. Kapandji IA: *The Physiology of the Joints,* vol 1. Edinburgh, Churchill Livingstone, 1974.
6. Reid DC, Kushner S: The elbow region. In Donatelli R, Wooden MJ (eds): *Orthopaedic Physical Therapy.* New York, Churchill Livingstone, 1989.
7. Waylett-Rendall J, Seibly D: A study of the accuracy of a commercially available volumeter. *J Hand Ther* 1991, 1:10–13.
8. Hirai M, Kawai S: False positive and negative results in Allen test. *J Cardiovasc Surg* 1980, 21:353–360.

9. Magee DJ: *Orthopedic Physical Assessment,* 2nd ed. Philadelphia, W. B. Saunders Company, 1992.

10. Mathiowetz V: Grip and pinch strength measurements. In Amundsen LR (ed): *Muscle Strength Testing.* New York, Churchill Livingstone, 1990.

11. Fess EE: Rehabilitation of the patient with peripheral nerve injury. *Hand Clin* 1986, 2:207–214.

12. Stokes HM: The seriously uninjured hand: weakness of grip. *J Occup Med* 1983, 25:683–684.

13. Janda DH, Geiringer SR, Hankin FM, Barry DT: Objective evaluation of grip strength. *J Occup Med* 1987, 28:569–571.

14. Bechtol CO: Grip test: the use of a dynamometer with adjustable handle spacings. *J Bone Joint Surg* 1954, 36A:820–824.

15. Cyriax JH, Cyriax PJ: *Illustrated Manual of Orthopaedic Medicine.* London, O. M. Publications, 1983.

16. Jones LA: The assessment of hand functions: a critical review of techniques. *J Hand Surg* 1989, 14A:221–228.

17. Omer GE: Acute management of peripheral nerve injuries. *Hand Clin* 1986, 2:193–206.

18. Gerstner DL, Omer GE: Peripheral entrapment neuropathies in the upper extremity: part 1. Key differential findings, median nerve syndromes. *J Musculoskeletal Med* 1988, 5:14–29.

19. Dellon AL: *Evaluation of Sensibility and Re-Education of Sensation in the Hand.* Baltimore, Williams & Wilkins, 1981.

20. Tan AM: Sensibility testing. In Stanley BG, Tribuzi SM (eds): *Concepts in Hand Rehabilitation.* Philadelphia, F. A. Davis Company, 1992, pp 92–112.

21. Lovett WL, McCalla MA: Nerve injuries: management and rehabilitation. *Orthop Clin North Am* 1983, 14:767–778.

22. Lister G: *The Hand, Diagnosis and Indications,* 2nd ed. New York, Churchill Livingstone, 1984.

23. Jewell MJ: Peripheral nerve injuries: mechanisms and locations. *Top Acute Care Trauma Rehabil* 1988, 3:1–9.

24. Howard FM: Controversies in nerve entrapment syndromes in the forearm and wrist. *Orthop Clin North Am* 1986, 17:375–381.

25. Spinner M, Kaplan EB: The relationship of the ulnar nerve to the medial intermuscular septum in the arm and its clinical significance. *Hand* 1976, 8:239–242.

26. McPherson S, Meals R: Cubital tunnel syndrome. *Orthop Clin North Am* 1992, 23:111–123.

27. Gerstner DL, Omer GE: Peripheral entrapment neuropathies in the upper extremity: part 2. Recognizing and treating ulnar and radial nerve syndromes. *J Musculoskeletal Med* 1988, 5:37–49.

28. Spinner M, Linschild RL: Nerve entrapment syndromes. In Morrey BF (ed): *The Elbow and Its Disorders.* Philadelphia, W. B. Saunders Company, 1985, pp 691–712.

29. King P, Aulicino P: The postoperative rehabilitation of the Learmonth submuscular transposition of the ulnar nerve at the elbow. *J Hand Ther* 1990, 3:149–156.

30. Andrews JR, Whiteside JA: Common elbow problems in the athlete. *J Orthop Sports Phys Ther* 17:289–295.

31. Lichtman DM: *The Wrist and its Disorders.* Philadelphia, W. B. Saunders Company, 1988.

32. Nirschl R: Soft-tissue injuries about the elbow. *Clin Sports Med* 1986, 5:637–651.

33. Kamien M: A rational management of tennis elbow. *Sports Med* 1990, 9:173–191.

34. Wadsworth CT, Nielsen DH, Burns LT, et al.: Effect of the counterforce armband on wrist extension and grip strength and pain in subject with tennis elbow. *J Orthop Sports Phys Ther* 1989, 11:192–197.

35. Leach RE, Miller JK: Lateral and medial epicondylitis of the elbow. *Clin Sports Med* 1987, 6:259–272.

36. McCue FC III: The elbow, wrist, and hand. In Kulund DN (ed): *The Injured Athlete,* 2nd ed. Philadelphia, J. B. Lippincott Company, 1988.

37. Gellman H: Tennis elbow (lateral epicondylitis). *Orthop Clin North Am* 1992, 23:75–82.

38. Powell S, Burke A: Surgical and therapeutic management of tennis elbow: an update. *J Hand Ther* 1991, 4:64–68.

39. Kurer M, Regan M: Completely displaced supracondylar fracture of the humerus in children: a review of 1708 comparable cases. *Clin Orthop* 1990, 256:205–214.

40. Josefsson O, Johnell O, Wendeberg B: Ligamentous injuries in dislocation of the elbow joint. *Clin Orthop* 1987, 221:221–225.

41. Clement D, Phil D: Assessment of a treatment plan for managing acute vascular complications with supracondylar fractures of the humerus in children. *J Pediatr Orthop* 1990, 10:97–100.

42. Salter RB: *Textbook of Disorders and Injuries of the Musculoskeletal System,* 2nd ed. Baltimore, Williams & Wilkins, 1983.

43. Rothschild B: Reflex sympathetic dystrophy. *Arthritis Care Res* 1990, 3:144–153.

44. Carlson LK, Watson HK: Treatment of reflex sympathetic dystrophy using the stress-loading program. *J Hand Ther* 1988, 1:149–154.

45. Schutzer SF, Glossliny HR: The treatment of reflex sympathetic dystrophy. *J Bone Joint Surg* 1984, 66A:625.

46. Lankford LL, Thompson JE: Reflex sympathetic dystrophy, upper and lower extremity; diagnosis and management. Instructional course lectures. *Am Acad Orthop Surg* 1977, 26:163–178.

47. Rodnan GP, Schumacher HR (eds): *Primer on the Rheumatic Diseases,* 8th ed. Atlanta, Arthritis Foundation, 1983.

48. Phillips C: Management of the patient with rheumatoid arthritis: the role of the hand therapist. *Hand Clin* 1989, 5:291–309.

49. Phalen GS: The carpal-tunnel syndrome. *Clin Orthop* 1972, 83:29–40.

50. Bear-Lehman J, Bielawski T: The carpal tunnel syndrome: back to the source. *Rehabil Res* 1988, Oct:13–20.

51. Resnick C, Miller B: Endoscopic carpal tunnel release using the subligamentous two-portal technique. *Contemp Orthop* 1991, 22:269–277.

52. Baxter-Petralia PL: Therapist's management of carpal tunnel syndrome. In Hunter JM, Schneider L, Mackin E, et al. (eds): *Rehabilitation of the Hand: Surgery and Therapy,* 3rd ed. St. Louis, Mosby Year Book, 1989, pp 640–646.

53. Moneim MS: Ulnar nerve compression at the wrist: ulnar tunnel syndrome. *Hand Clin* 1992, 8:337–343.

54. Poole BC: Cumulative trauma disorder of the upper extremity from occupational stress. *J Hand Ther* 1988, 1:172–180.

55. Totten PA: Therapist's management of deQuervain's disease. In Hunter JM, Schneider L, Mackin E, et al. (eds): *Rehabilitation of the Hand: Surgery and Therapy,* 3rd ed. St. Louis, Mosby Year Book, 1989, pp 308–317.

56. Patel MR, Bassini L: Trigger fingers and thumb: when to splint, inject, or operate. *J Hand Surg* 1992, 17A:110–113.

57. Carter PR: Crush injury of the upper limb: early and late management. *Orthop Clin North Am* 1984, 14:719–747.

58. Miles WK, Grigsby L: Remodeling of scar tissue in the burned hand. In Hunter JM, Schneider L, Mackin E, et al. (eds): *Rehabilitation of the Hand: Surgery and Therapy,* 3rd ed. St. Louis, Mosby Year Book, 1989, pp 841–857.

59. Miles W: Soft tissue trauma. *Hand Clin* 1986, 2:33–43.

60. Wilson RL, Carter MS: Joint injuries in the hand: preservation of proximal interphalangeal function. In Hunter JM, Schneider L, Mackin E, et al. (eds): *Rehabilitation of the*

Hand: Surgery and Therapy, 3rd ed. St. Louis, Mosby Year Book, 1989, pp 295–309.

61. O'Brien ET: The sprained finger that isn't. *Am Fam Physician* 1981, 23:129–137.

62. Slattery PG: The modified Kleinert splint in zone II flexor tendon injuries. *J Hand Surg* 1988, 13B:273–276.

63. Edinburg MB, Widgrow AD, Biddulph SL: Early postoperative mobilization of flexor tendon injuries using a modification of the Kleinert technique. *J Hand Surg* 1987, 12A:34–38.

64. Chow JA, Thomes LJ, Dowelle SW, et al.: A combined regimen of controlled motion following flexor tendon repair in "no man's land." *Plast Reconstr Surg* 1987, 79:447–453.

65. Cannon NM, Strickland JW: Therapy following flexor tendon surgery. *Hand Clin* 1985, 1:147–155.

66. Gelberman RH, Manske PR: Factors influencing flexor tendon adhesions. *Hand Clin* 1985, 1:35–42.

67. Savage R: The influence of wrist position on the minimum force required for active movement of the interphalangeal joints. *J Hand Surg* 1988, 13B:262–268.

68. Calabro JJ, Hoidal CR, Susini LM: Extensor tendon repair in the emergency department. *J Emerg Med* 1986, 4:217–225.

69. Evans RB: Therapeutic management of extensor tendon injuries. *Hand Clin* 1986, 2:157.

70. Stewart KM: Tendon injuries. In Stanley BG, Tribuzi SM (eds): *Concepts in Hand Rehabilitation*. Philadelphia, F. A. Davis Company, 1992, pp 353–394.

71. Frykman GK, Flvert FN: Fractures and traumatic conditions of the wrist. In Hunter JM, Schneider L, Mackin E, et al. (eds): *Rehabilitation of the Hand: Surgery and Therapy*, 3rd ed. St. Louis, Mosby Year Book, 1989.

72. Mannarino SL: Skeletal injuries. In Stanley BG, Tribuzi SM (eds): *Concepts in Hand Rehabilitation*. Philadelphia, F. A. Davis Company, 1992, pp 274–321.

73. Widgerow A, Edinburgh M, Biddulph SL: An analysis of proximal phalangeal fractures. *J Hand Surg [Am]* 1987, 12A:134–139.

74. Puddicombe B, Nardone M: Rehabilitation of the burned hand. *Hand Clin* 1990, 6:281–292.

75. Fleegler EJ, Yetman RJ: Rehabilitation after upper extremity burns. *Orthop Clin North Am* 1983, 14:699–717.

76. "Management of the Burned Hand." Form 206. JOBST Institute, Toledo, Ohio.

77. Katz BE: Silastic gel sheeting is found to be effective in scar therapy. *Cosmetic Dermatol* 1992, 5:32–34.

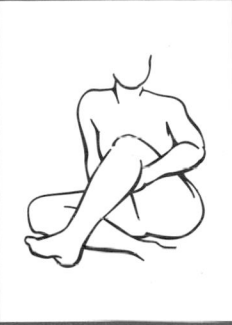

CHAPTER 32

Trunk

Peter I. Edgelow, Anna Conaway Lescak,
and Martha Jewell

I. Clinical Anatomy

A. Osteology

1. **Thoracic vertebrae.** The twelve thoracic vertebrae (T1–T12) increase in size from superior to inferior (see Figures 32–1 and 32–2). The body of a typical thoracic vertebra is approximately equal in its anteroposterior and transverse dimensions, but it is taller posteriorly than anteriorly. This height difference produces the thoracic curve.[1] There are four costal demifacets, two on the superior and two on the inferior edges of the body, for articulation with the heads of the ribs. The superior facets are just anterior to the vertebral notches. Two pedicles are attached to the upper half of the body posterolaterally. The pedicles become thicker from T1–T12. Laminae are short and thick and overlap the lamina below. The neural arch, which is composed of the two laminae and two pedicles, forms a relatively small, circular spinal canal.

The transverse processes are club-shaped projections that extend laterally from the junction of the pedicle and lamina. They decrease in length from T1–T12. Each of the 1st through 6th transverse processes has a concave facet that faces anteriorly and slightly laterally. The facets on the 7th through 10th transverse processes are flat and face somewhat superiorly, laterally, and slightly anteriorly.

At the junction of the two laminae, the spinous process is inclined posteriorly and inferiorly. The T7 spinous process has the greatest inclination. The T1–T3 and T12 spinous processes are on the same horizon-

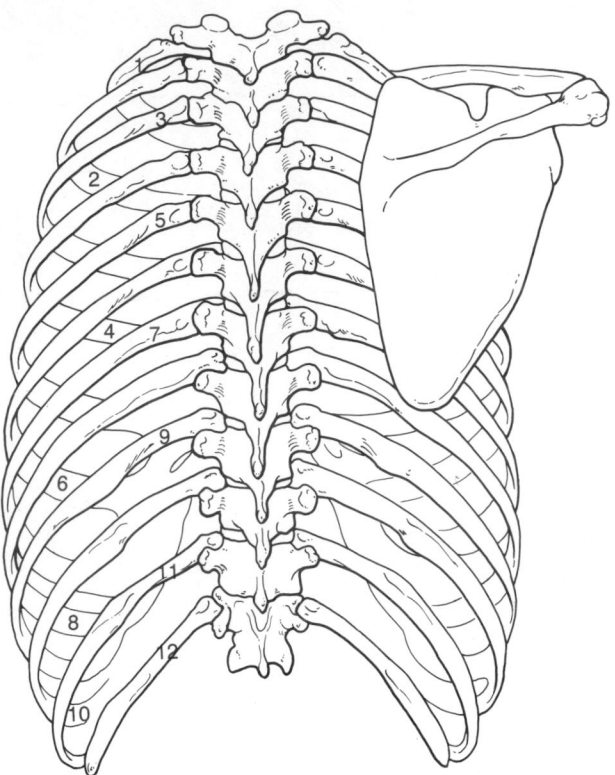

FIGURE 32–1   The thorax. (From Richardson JK, Iglarsh ZA: *Clinical Orthopaedic Physical Therapy.* Philadelphia, W. B. Saunders Company, 1994.)

tal plane as the transverse processes of the same vertebra. The T4–T6 and T11 spinous processes are on a horizontal plane halfway between the transverse processes at that

level and the ones below. The T7–T10 spinous processes are on a plane with the transverse processes of the vertebra below.

The articular processes are at the junction of the pedicle and lamina. The superior articular process is almost flat, faces posteriorly, slightly superiorly, and laterally. The inferior articular process faces anteriorly, slightly medially, and inferiorly. The plane of the thoracic zygapophyseal joints is 60 degrees to the horizontal plane and 20 degrees to the frontal plane.[2]

2. **Ribs.** There are twelve pairs of ribs, each of which includes a costal cartilage at its distal end. The first seven ribs are attached directly to the sternum via their costal cartilages. Costal cartilages 8 to 10 attach to the costal cartilage of the rib above. Ribs 11 and 12 end in the body wall. Rib length increases from the 1st to 7th ribs and then decreases in length to the 12th rib. The 9th rib has the most oblique angulation.

A typical rib includes a head with two facets separated by a crest, a neck, a tubercle, and a shaft or body. The facets on the head articulate with the demifacets of the vertebra of the same number and the vertebra above (see Figure 32–3). The crest of the head is attached to the intervertebral disk. The neck lies anterior to the transverse process of the vertebra of the same number. The tubercle is on the posterior surface of the rib at the junction of the neck and shaft. The tubercle includes a medial articular facet for articulation with the transverse pro-

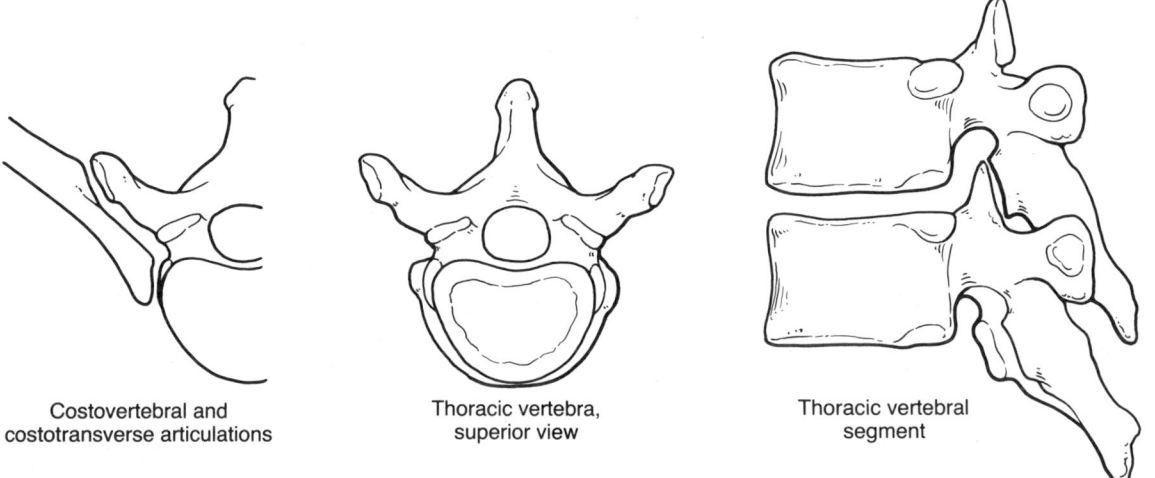

Costovertebral and costotransverse articulations

Thoracic vertebra, superior view

Thoracic vertebral segment

FIGURE 32–2   Distinguishing features of the thoracic spine. (From Richardson JK, Iglarsh ZA: *Clinical Orthopaedic Physical Therapy.* Philadelphia, W. B. Saunders Company, 1994.)

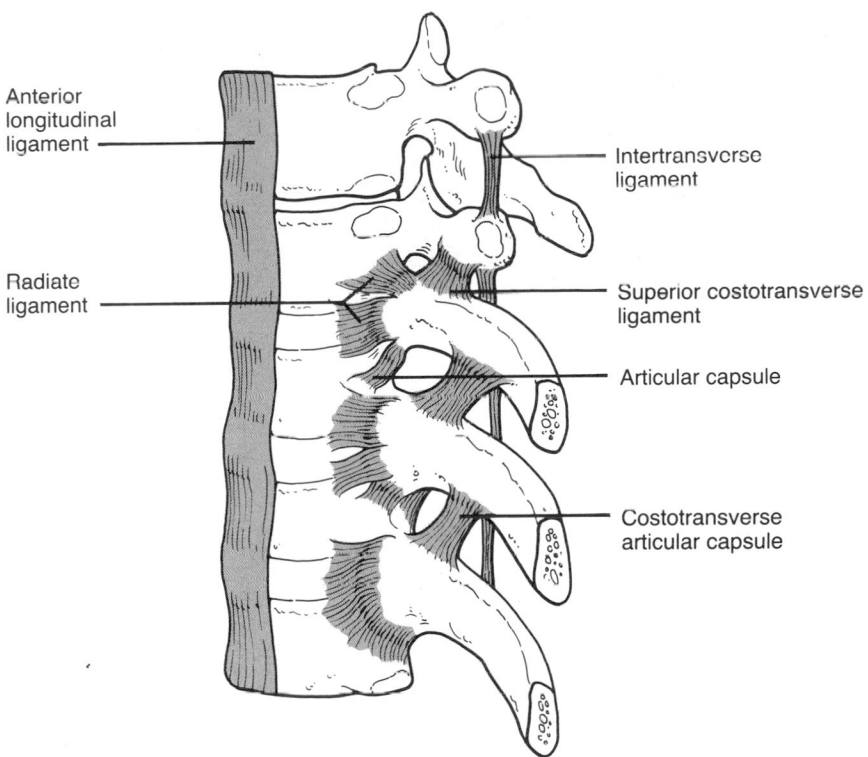

Anterior longitudinal ligament

Radiate ligament

Intertransverse ligament

Superior costotransverse ligament

Articular capsule

Costotransverse articular capsule

FIGURE 32-3 Costovertebral articulation and its ligamentous attachments. (From Richardson JK, Iglarsh ZA: *Clinical Orthopaedic Physical Therapy.* Philadelphia, W. B. Saunders Company, 1994.)

cess of the vertebra of the same number and a nonarticular area for attachment of the lateral costotransverse ligament. The shaft of a typical rib is flat and thin and is not only curved but twisted at the angle.

3. **Sternum.** The sternum is slightly convex anteriorly, broadest at the level of the 1st costal cartilage, and narrowest at the level of the 2nd costal cartilage. The sternum consists of three parts: manubrium, body, and xiphoid. The superior border of the manubrium is marked by the suprasternal or jugular notch in the midline and a clavicular notch on each corner. The clavicular notch faces superiorly, laterally, and slightly posteriorly. The lateral border of the manubrium has articular facets for the costal cartilages of the 1st and 2nd ribs. The junction of the manubrium and the body forms the sternal angle, which is a landmark for locating the costal cartilage of the 2nd rib. This manubriosternal junction is a symphysis joint that becomes ossified in the aged.

The body of the sternum is longer, narrower, and thinner than the manubrium and tapers to meet the xiphoid. The lateral border of the body has demifacets for artic-

ulation with the 2nd and 7th costal cartilages and facets for articulation with the 3rd to 6th costal cartilages.

The xiphoid varies in shape from triangular to bifid and includes a facet for the 7th costal cartilage.

4. **Lumbar vertebrae.** The five lumbar vertebrae (L1–L5) increase in size from superior to inferior. The bodies are massive and wider in transverse than anteroposterior diameters. The pedicles are short and attach to the upper part of the body. The laminae are broad, short, and strong. The transverse processes are flat, rectangular, and longer than the thoracic transverse processes. The spinous process is flat, somewhat quadrangular, and projects almost horizontally from the junction of the two laminae. An accessory process is at the root of each transverse process. The superior articular process extends upward from the junction of the lamina and pedicle. The mamillary process is a small, smooth process on the posterior edge of the superior articular process. The inferior articular process extends inferiorly from the lateral portion of the inferior border of the lamina. The spinal canal is oval to trian-

gular in shape and larger than the thoracic or cervical spinal canals.

5. **Sacrum and ilium.** The sacrum is composed of the five fused sacral vertebrae (S1–S5). It is somewhat triangular in shape, with the base or S1 segment forming the upper surface. The pelvic surface is concave both superior to inferior and side to side, with the anterior or pelvic surface of the S1 segment projecting anteriorly as the sacral promontory. The posterior surface is convex and marked by a median sacral crest with four spinous tubercles. Below the 4th tubercle is an inverted U-shaped gap, the sacral hiatus, that is present because the laminae of S5 do not fuse in the midline. Lateral to the median sacral crest are the dorsal sacral foramina for exit of the sacral dorsal primary rami. The lateral sacral crest is a low ridge lateral to the dorsal sacral foramina. The lateral surface of the sacrum is broader above and rapidly tapers. Part of the lateral surface is articular. The articular facet looks somewhat like an upside down L. The apex of the sacrum has a facet for articulation with the 1st coccygeal vertebra.

B. Arthrology

1. **Costovertebral and costotransverse articulations.** The costovertebral joints are synovial and fibrous (see Figure 32–3). The head of a typical rib (2nd to 10th ribs) articulates with the demifacet on the vertebra of the same number and the vertebra above. The crest of the head articulates with the intervening disc. The joint capsules are reinforced by radiate ligaments. The crest of the head of the rib is attached to the disc by an intra-articular ligament.

The costotransverse joints are synovial between the articular facet on the tubercle of the rib and the facet on the transverse process of the vertebra of the same number. The joint is reinforced by the superior costotransverse ligament from the crest of the neck of the rib to the transverse process of the vertebra above, the lateral costotransverse ligament from the apex of the transverse process to the nonarticular part of the tubercle of the rib, and the costotransverse ligament from the dorsum of the neck of the rib to the anterior surface of the trans-

verse process of the vertebra of the same number.

2. **Sternocostal, interchondral, and costochondral joints.** The joints between the first seven costal cartilages and the sternum are synovial, whose thin capsules are reinforced by sternocostal ligaments. The joints between the costal cartilages of the 7th to 10th ribs also have a synovial-lined capsule. These joints are strengthened by interchondral ligaments. The costochondral junctions are not true joints in that the costal cartilages are the unosssified anterior extremities of the ribs.

3. **Intervertebral joint**
   a. *Interbody joint.* The interbody joint is fibrocartilaginous. The intervertebral discs are thicker (higher) anteriorly at lumbar levels and of relatively equal height anterior to posterior at thoracic levels. The disc consists of three parts: the nucleus pulposus, annulus fibrosus, and end plate. The nucleus is a semifluid gel with a few cartilage cells and collagen fibers arranged irregularly in the ground substance.

   The annulus consists of 10 to 20 layers[3,4] of parallel collagen fibers oriented 65 to 70 degrees from vertical.[5,6] The collagen fibers of each lamella are oriented in the opposite direction of the adjacent lamella. Lumbar lamellae are thicker anteriorly and laterally and more finely packed posteriorly.[3,7,8] The outermost lamellae insert into the ring apophysis of the vertebral body. The rest of the annular fibers are continuous with the end plate.

   The end plate is a layer of hyalin cartilage covering the superior and inferior surfaces of the vertebral body, excluding the ring apophysis.
   b. *Zygapophyseal joints.* These are synovial joints between the articular portions of the superior and inferior articular processes of adjacent vertebrae. The somewhat loose joint capsule is attached to the articular processes beyond the margin of the articular cartilage. The thoracic joints are oriented 60 degrees to the horizontal plane and 20 degrees to the frontal plane.[2] The lumbar facets vary in their orientation. The L1, L2 joint is more like a thoracic zygapophyseal joint. The L2, L5 facet surfaces are somewhat L or J

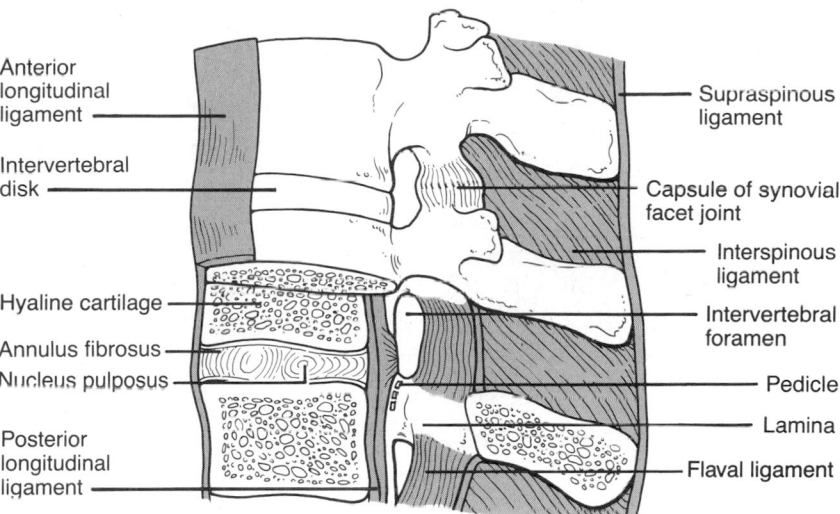

Anterior longitudinal ligament

Intervertebral disk

Hyaline cartilage

Annulus fibrosus

Nucleus pulposus

Posterior longitudinal ligament

Supraspinous ligament

Capsule of synovial facet joint

Interspinous ligament

Intervertebral foramen

Pedicle

Lamina

Flaval ligament

FIGURE 32–4 Ligaments of the spinal column. (From Richardson JK, Iglarsh ZA: *Clinical Orthopaedic Physical Therapy.* Philadelphia, W. B. Saunders Company, 1994.)

shaped, with the long part in the sagittal plane and the short piece in the frontal plane. The L5 to S1 facets are mostly flat and oriented somewhat obliquely, similar to thoracic zygapophyseal orientation. On average, the lumbar zygapophyseal joints are oriented 90 degrees to the horizontal plane and 45 degrees to the frontal plane.[2]

The joint capsules are reinforced anteriorly by the ligamentum flavum and posteriorly by the multifidus muscles, especially at lumbar levels. The L5 to S1 joint, and occasionally the L4–L5 joint, is also stabilized by the iliolumbar ligament, which runs from the 5th, and occasionally the 4th, transverse process to the anteromedial surface, inner lip, and crest of the ilium. Lumbar joint capsules are loose superiorly and inferiorly.

c. The intervertebral joints are further stabilized by the posterior and anterior longitudinal ligaments, the ligamentum flavum, and the supraspinous, interspinous, and intertransverse ligaments (see Figure 32–4). The anterior longitudinal ligament consists of both superficial fibers, which span multiple segments, and deep fibers, which span single segments. The fibers attach to the vertebral bodies and are only loosely attached to the discs. The anterior longitudinal ligament is thicker and narrower at thoracic levels.

The posterior longitudinal ligament consists of a relatively narrow band of collagen fibers over the posterior surface of the vertebral bodies. The collagen fibers expand over the posterior surface of the discs. The posterior longitudinal ligament is broader in thoracic levels and narrowest in lumbar regions.

The ligamentum flavum extends from the inferior border of one lamina to the superior border of the lamina below and is thickest at lumbar levels.

The supraspinous ligament connects the tips of the spinous processes, ends at L4 73% of the time,[9,10] and is actually more like tendinous fibers from the spinal muscles than a true ligament.[11]

The interspinous ligament consists of a pair of ligaments connecting adjacent spinous processes and separated by a small amount of fat. The intertransverse ligament connects transverse processes of adjacent vertebrae and is most developed at lumbar levels.

4. **Sacroiliac joint.** The sacroiliac joint is part synovial and part fibrocartilaginous. Both joint surfaces are covered with hyalin cartilage. The articular surface of the ilium includes some fibrocartilage.[12,13] The sacroiliac joint capsule is reinforced by the anterior capsular ligament, which is relatively thin; the interosseous sacroiliac ligament posteriorly and laterally; and the dorsal sacroiliac ligaments posteriorly. The interosseous sacroiliac ligament fills the irregular space posterior to the joint space and is covered by the

dorsal sacroiliac ligament. The dorsal sacroiliac ligament is attached from the intermediate and lateral sacral crests to the posterosuperior iliac spine and inner lip of the posterior part of the iliac crest. Accessory ligaments include the sacrotuberous and sacrospinous ligaments.

C. Myology

A detailed listing of muscle attachments can be found in depth in a comprehensive anatomy text. The purpose here is to list, not describe, the muscles to be evaluated (see Figures 32–5 to 32–8).

1. The superficial back muscles to be considered in thoracic and lumbar dysfunction include the trapezius, rhomboid major and minor, and the latissimus dorsi.
2. The intermediate back muscles are the serratus posterior superior and the serratus posterior inferior, which are actually accessory muscles of respiration.
3. The deep back muscles include the erector

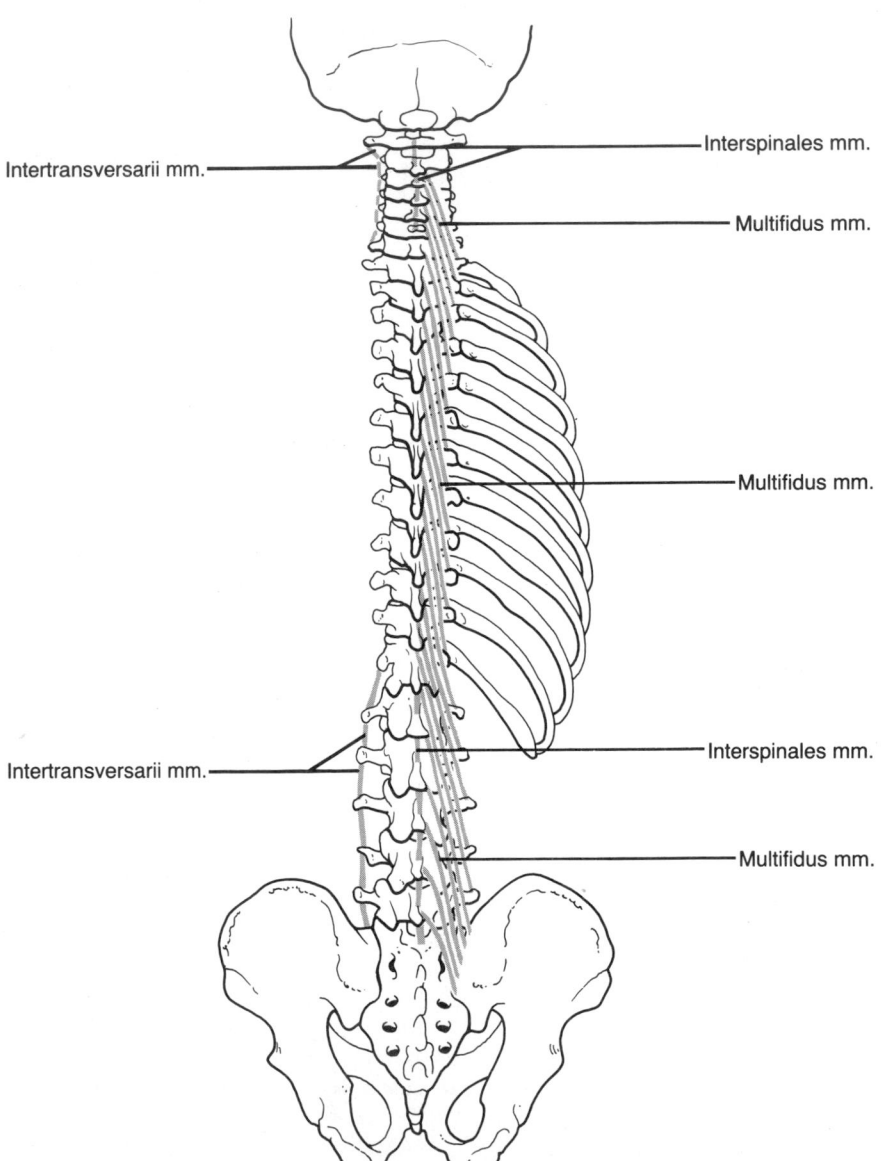

Intertransversarii mm.

Interspinales mm.

Multifidus mm.

Multifidus mm.

Intertransversarii mm.

Interspinales mm.

Multifidus mm.

FIGURE 32–5 Muscles of the spinal column: the multifidi, interspinales, and intertransversarii. (From Richardson JK, Iglarsh ZA: *Clinical Orthopaedic Physical Therapy.* Philadelphia, W. B. Saunders Company, 1994.)

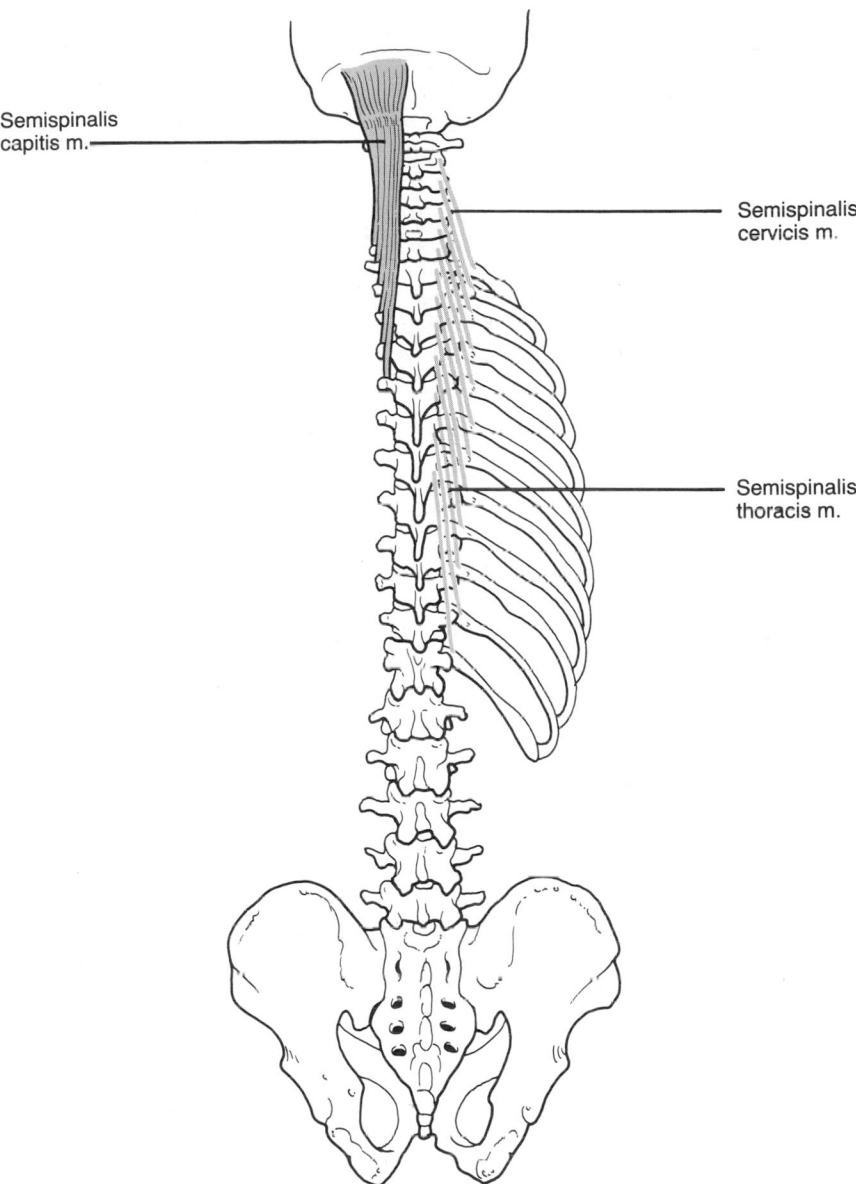

Semispinalis capitis m.

Semispinalis cervicis m.

Semispinalis thoracis m.

FIGURE 32–6 Muscles of the spinal column: the semispinales. (From Richardson JK, Iglarsh ZA: *Clinical Orthopaedic Physical Therapy*. Philadelphia, W. B. Saunders Company, 1994.)

spinae, the transversospinal group, and the interspinal and intertransverse muscles. The erector spinae consist of the iliocostalis, longissimus, and spinalis. The transversospinal group consists of the semispinalis, multifidus, and rotatores muscles.

4. The muscles of respiration to be considered are the diaphragm; external, internal, and innermost intercostals; transversus thoracis; subcostals; and levatores costarum.

5. The anterior abdominal wall musculature to be examined includes the external and in-

ternal oblique abdominals, the transversus abdominis, and the rectus abdominis.

6. The posterior abdominal wall muscles to be examined include the psoas, iliacus, and quadratus lumborum.

7. When evaluating patients with lumbar or sacral symptoms, the therapist should also consider muscles that cross the hip joint to attach to the os coxae because these muscles can affect the lumbar spine and sacroiliac joint. Muscles to consider include the gluteus maximus and medius, the hamstrings,

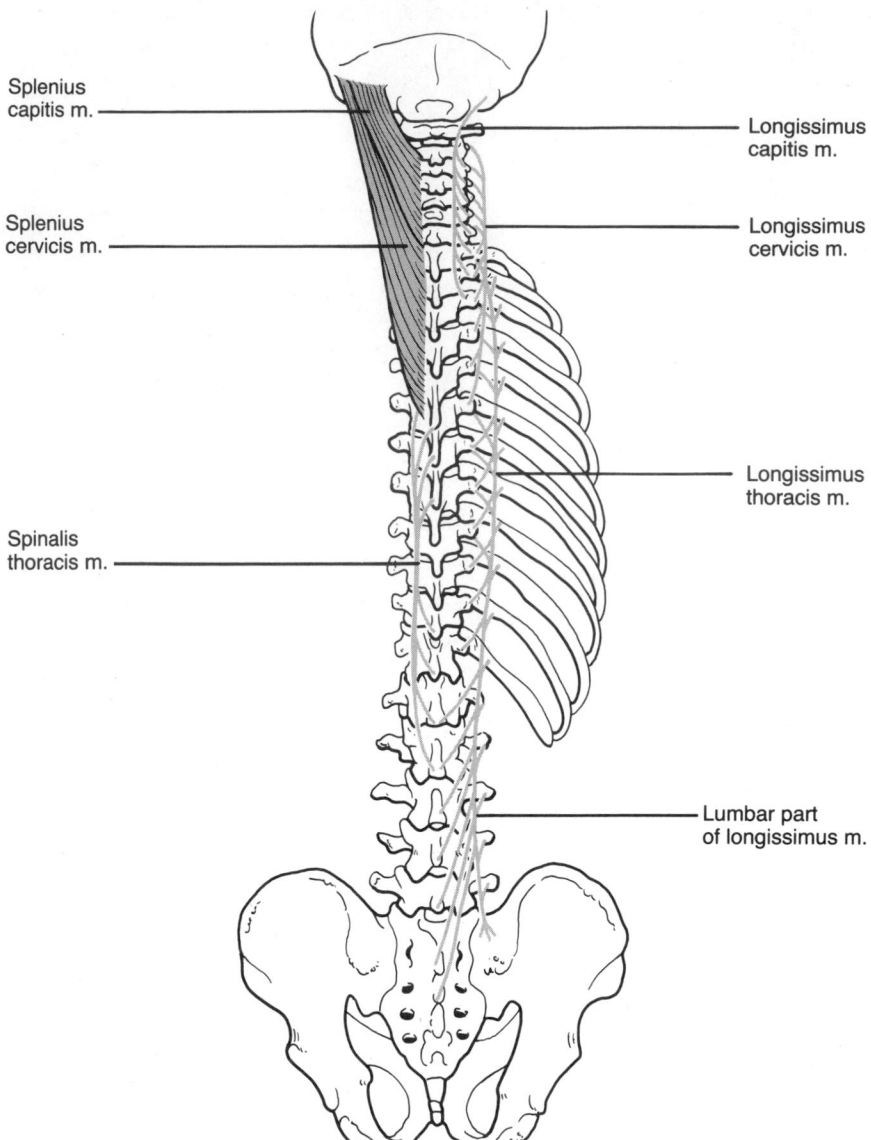

Splenius
capitis m.

Splenius
cervicis m.

Spinalis
thoracis m.

Longissimus
capitis m.

Longissimus
cervicis m.

Longissimus
thoracis m.

Lumbar part
of longissimus m.

FIGURE 32–7 Muscles of the spinal column: the spinalis, splenius, and longissimus. (From Richardson JK, Iglarsh ZA: *Clinical Orthopaedic Physical Therapy.* Philadelphia, W. B. Saunders Company, 1994.)

the rectus femoris, the tensor fascia lata, and the adductors, especially the adductor magnus.

D. Neurology

1. Thoracic nerve roots exit intervertebral foramina bounded anteriorly by the inferior half of the vertebral body of the same number, inferiorly by the pedicle of the vertebra below, posteriorly by the superior articular process of the vertebra below and the ligamentum flavum and superiorly by the pedicle of the vertebra of the same number. Lumbar nerve roots exit an intervertebral foramen bordered by pedicles superiorly and inferiorly, the ligamentum flavum posteriorly, and the bodies and intervening disc of the two vertebrae anteriorly. The lumbar nerve root normally exits high in the foramen and thus is not anatomically related to the disc at that level.

Both thoracic and lumbar roots (actually spinal nerves) divide immediately on exiting into dorsal and ventral primary rami. The dorsal primary ramus passes posteriorly to innervate deep and intermediate back muscles, posterior spinal structures (*eg,* ligamentum flavum, zygapophyseal joint, interspinous ligaments), and the skin over the deep back muscles. The ventral primary rami of T2–T11 continue as intercostal nerves. The ventral primary rami of T12 to S3 form the lumbosacral plexus in the substance of the psoas and anterior to the sacroiliac joint.

2. The sinuvertebral nerve is a recurrent branch of the ventral primary ramus, which receives a contribution from the sympathetic chain, re-enters the spinal canal by passing through the intervertebral foramen anterior to the spinal nerve, and divides into branches that ascend one to two segments on the posterior surface of the disc and posterior longitudinal ligament. The sinuverte-

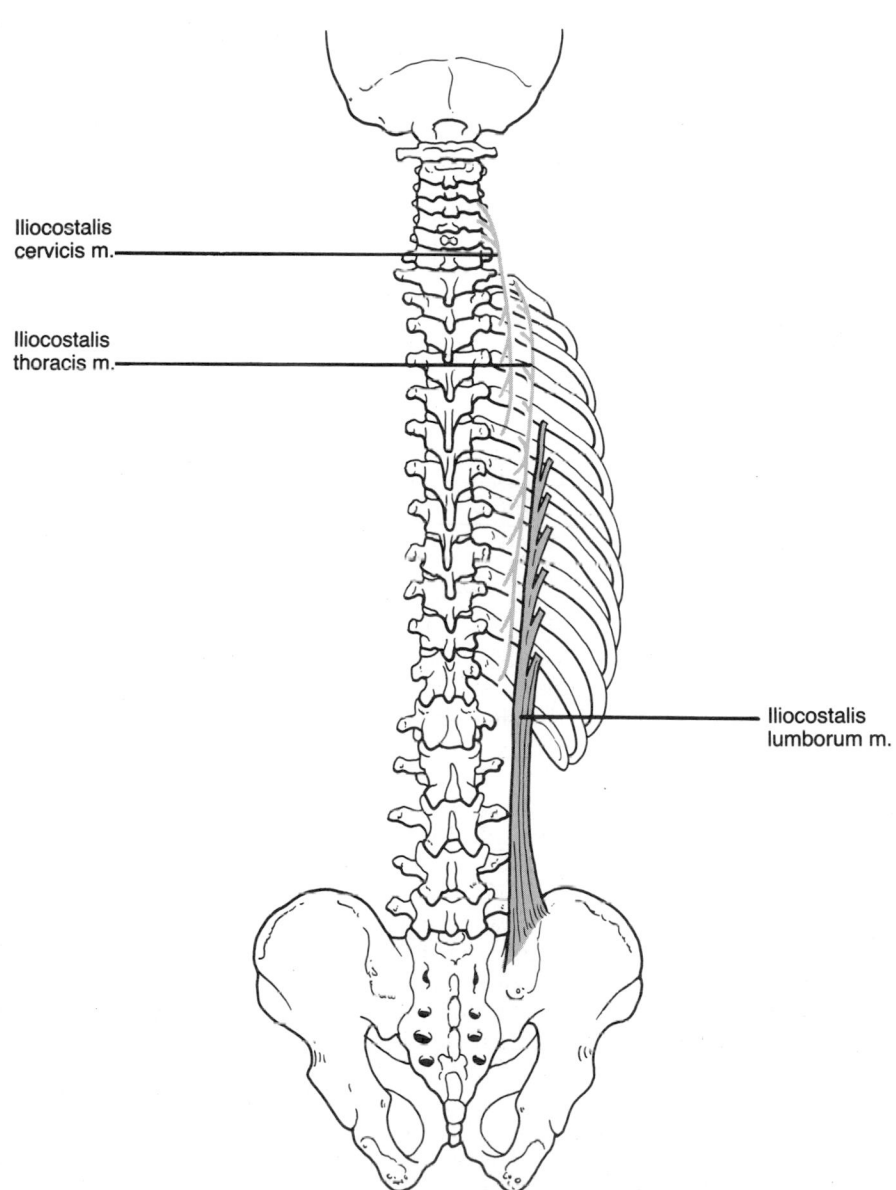

Iliocostalis cervicis m.

Iliocostalis thoracis m.

Iliocostalis lumborum m.

FIGURE 32–8 Muscles of the spinal column: the iliocostales. (From Richardson JK, Iglarsh ZA: *Clinical Orthopaedic Physical Therapy.* Philadelphia, W. B. Saunders Company, 1994.)

bral nerve carries sympathetic efferents and afferents from both encapsulated and unencapsulated receptors. From this, it can be inferred that the sinuvertebral nerve carries both proprioceptive and nociceptive information from the structures it innervates, which include the posterior longitudinal ligament, outer disc, anterior dura, epidural fat, and venous plexus.

E. Angiology

1. The arterial supply to spinal structures is mainly via radicular arteries, which are branches of segmental arteries (posterior intercostal and lumbar arteries). The lower cervical, lower thoracic, and upper lumbar radicular arteries are larger than the others. In other words, the upper thoracic and mid-thoracic roots and the spinal cord in those levels receive less segmental augmentation of the anterior and posterior spinal arteries. The anterior and posterior spinal arteries begin as branches of the vertebral artery and continue inferiorly to the conus medullaris.

2. An internal vertebral venous plexus is within the vertebral canal external to the dura, and an external vertebral venous plexus outside the vertebral canal. These plexuses have no valves and anastomose freely with each other. The venous return from the bone empties into the plexuses. The plexuses then empty into the iliac, azygos, and hemiazygos veins and the inferior vena cava. Because these plexuses are without valves, increased intra-abdominal pressure can back venous blood into the lumbar epidural venous plexus. Thus pelvic tumors (*eg*, prostatic), which tend to metastasize via the circulatory system, can spread to the epidural space and vertebrae.

II. Clinical Decision Making

1. **Overview**

Clinical decision making is a process based on theoretical knowledge and clinical data obtained through subjective and objective examinations. The therapist evaluates not only the patient's physical body but also his/her total environment. The whole person needs to be addressed. This involves recognizing the inter-relationship between all aspects of the patient: physical, intellectual, and emotional. Evaluation, treatment, and problem resolution create a cycle of processes, beginning with the patient's awareness of the problem and presentation for treatment. The physical therapist then has the job of identifying the problem through data collection and analysis. On the basis of this analysis, a treatment technique is selected and instituted. The effect of this treatment is assessed by re-examining one or more of the appropriate abnormal findings to see if they have changed. On the basis of this assessment, a decision is made as to whether to continue treatment at that time, to refer the patient to another health care practitioner, or to institute a home program. This cycle of examination, technique, assessment, and re-examination continues until the patient is normal or maximum progress has been attained.

The goal of the subjective examination is to quantify the patient's subjective complaints and establish functional tolerances to use in assessment. A judgment is made based on the subjective data regarding the severity, irritability, nature, and stage of the condition. Severity is related to the intensity of the symptoms and the relative degree of limitation of functional activities. Irritability refers to the duration/repetition/vigor of an activity or position required to provoke symptoms and the subsequent time for pain to ease. An irritable condition is provoked by minimal activity and requires a significant amount of time to ease. The nature of the condition is determined by the pathology or the structures at fault. The stage of the condition relates both to its chronicity or acuteness as well as to its stability.[14]

The goal of the objective examination is to determine the mechanical nature of the problem and to identify the structures at fault. The therapist seeks a comparable sign — the reproduction of the patient's symptoms via objective testing—or the establishment of a significant finding as a likely source of symptoms. Having determined the mechanical nature of the problem, the therapist must also identify the environmental and psychosocial factors that may influence treatment. If the condition does not appear amenable to physical therapy intervention, the decision must be made to refer to another health care professional.

III. Subjective Examination

A. Patient profile

A patient profile is established that includes age, occupation, physical requirements of occupation, recreational activities, forms of regular exercise, current activity level, and social status.

B. Record of patient's complaints

The patient's complaints are recorded on a body chart (see Figure 32–9). Complaints include pain, numbness/tingling, weakness, stiffness, and paresthesia. The therapist should

1. Mark in the area of symptoms, being specific as to the area and extent of symptoms.
2. Record the quality of the symptoms: burning, aching, throbbing, stabbing pain, etc.
3. Note whether each symptom is constant varying/nonvarying versus intermittent varying/non-varying. A constant nonvarying symptom may indicate a nonmechanical problem, such as cancer or other systemic medical disorder.
4. Record the depth of each symptom: deep versus superficial (gives information regarding the structure likely to be involved).
   a. If pain is described as superficial, it may involve muscle or ligament.
   b. If pain is described as deep, it may involve nerve roots or joints.
5. Identify each area of symptoms from most to least severe. Many mechanical dysfunctions have typical patterns of severity of symptoms; *ie*, acute nerve roots often present with distal pain that is more severe than proximal complaints.
6. Identify and record the relationship between

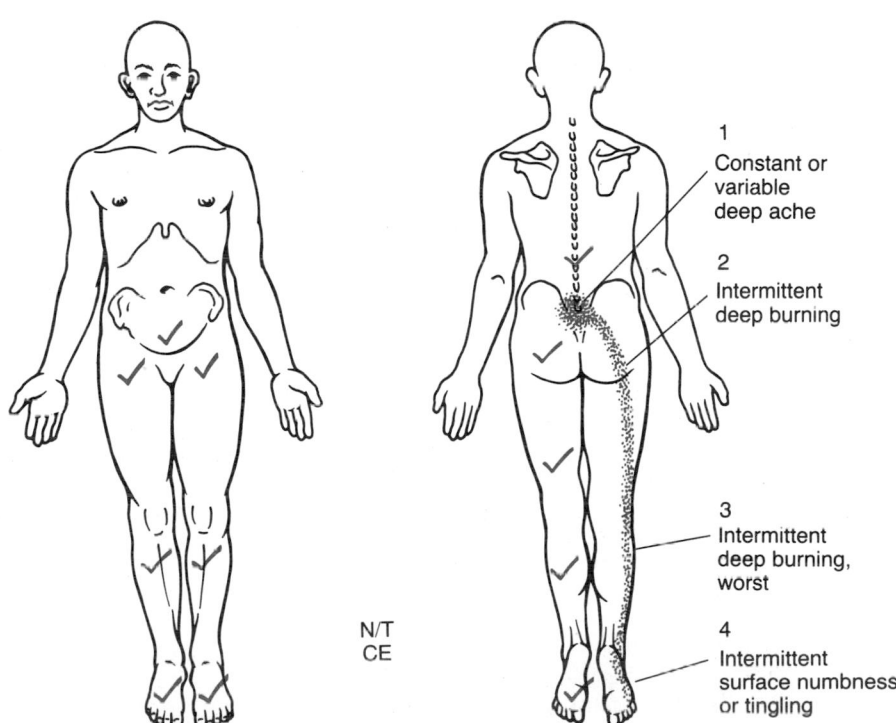

FIGURE 32–9 A body chart for recording a patient's complaints.

1
Constant or variable deep ache

2
Intermittent deep burning

3
Intermittent deep burning, worst

4
Intermittent surface numbness or tingling

N/T
CE

symptoms. This can aid in identifying syndromes and provide information pertaining to the behavior of symptoms.

7. Check off areas without symptoms. The therapist should ask the patient about structures above and below the area of complaint as well as areas of potential referral. Knowing where symptoms are not is as important as knowing where symptoms are.

C. Behavior of symptoms

1. **Aggravating/easing factors.** The therapist should ask the patient to describe activities or positions that consistently increase and decrease symptoms. These establish functional limitations, provide information regarding mechanical influences on pathology, and assist in classification into syndromes. Many mechanical dysfunctions present with classic patterns of aggravating/easing factors.

2. **Quantification of each factor.** The therapist determines how much activity produces how much increase in symptoms and how long it takes to ease so that information is gathered regarding the irritability of the symptoms. Establishing these factors allows the therapist to quantify the subjective complaint in order to evaluate progress over time.

3. **Behavior over 24 hours**
   a. The therapist determines how the pathology varies in a 24-hour period: patterns of increase/decrease in symptoms may be related to mechanical and inflammatory factors.
      (1). Position sensitive: consistent positions are associated with aggravation/ease of symptoms.
      (2). Weight-bearing sensitive: sensitive to the effects of loading/gravity.
      (3). Constrained-posture sensitive: intolerance of any one posture/position.
      (4). Static muscle-effort sensitive: intolerance of sustained contraction without consistent positions of aggravation/ease (may be seen in generally hypermobile people).
      (5). Pressure sensitive: sensitive to direct contact.[15]
   b. Behavior of symptoms over 24 hours describes the limitations of the patient within a 24-hour period.
   c. Description of the behavior of symptoms

over the 24-hour period may also be related to the psychological behavior of the individual and may provide insight into how he/she views the problem.
   d. Certain syndromes exhibit classic patterns of behavior over 24 hours.
      (1). Osteoarthritis patients tend to wake with stiffness, ease with movement during the course of the day, then worsen with overuse.[16]
      (2). If there is an inflammatory component, patients tend to have more pain/stiffness on arising.[17]

D. Special questions

The therapist determines contraindications and precautions to examination and treatment. The therapist should ask the patient

1. **About his/her general health.** This assists the therapist in gaining information about potential complicating factors, such as diabetes mellitus, high blood pressure (with respect to exercise consideration), and past history of cancer.

2. **About recent unexplained weight loss.** This may indicate cancer/systemic pathology.

3. **Cord questions.** Numbness/tingling in bilateral hands and/or feet and loss of balance during gait may indicate spinal cord compression/involvement.[16]

4. **Cauda equina questions.** Complaints of saddle paresthesia, retention of urine, or incontinence may indicate cauda equina involvement.[16]

5. **About use of steroids/blood thinners.** Prolonged use of steroids may lead to osteoporosis; use of anticoagulants may cause a patient to bleed easily and would preclude vigorous treatment.[16]

6. **What tests have been performed.** This is asked to rule out fracture or identify pathology: radiographs, computed tomographic scan, magnetic resonance imaging, nerve-conduction studies. The therapist also gains insight into what the patient understands about his/her problem.[16]

7. **About medications.** Dosage and frequency and the effect on symptom level should be noted. Is this patient taking medications as prescribed?

E. History

The history provides information about the nature of the pathology, the stage of pathology, the stability of the lesion, the direction and rate of change, the prognosis, and the anticipated rate and level of recovery.

1. The patient is asked to describe in detail the current episode. The therapist should
   a. Note whether the onset was sudden and related to a specific incident; the mechanism of injury in detail; the initial symptoms and whether there was immediate swelling/discoloration.
   b. Describe the area of initial symptoms and progression of symptoms.
   c. Note any predisposing factors: virus, overtired, new activity, stress, drafty environment.
   d. Note present status: getting better/worse/unchanging.
   e. Note any treatment to date and its effect.

2. **Previous history.** The patient is asked for information about past episodes. The therapist should
   a. Note episodes relative to current area of symptoms.
   b. Note relevant peripheral and vertebral joint involvement.
   c. Note other symptoms.
   d. Ask about frequency of episodes.
   e. Ask about the manner of onset and relative severity of other episodes.
   f. Note the time of recovery from prior episodes.
   g. Establish the level of recovery; note resting symptoms between episodes.
   h. Note treatment administered for other episodes and its effect.
   i. Note history of other musculoskeletal dysfunction, including childhood episodes and familial incidence.

F. Clinical decision making

1. On the basis of the data from the subjective examination, the therapist considers the structures that must be examined as possible sources of the symptoms.[14]
   a. Joints under the area of symptoms.
   b. Joints referring into the area of symptoms.
   c. Muscles underlying the area of symptoms.
   d. Other structures: neural tissue and vascular structures.
   e. Special tests: stability, vertebral artery.

2. A hypothesis is made based on the information from the subjective examination, and it is decided what structures are the most likely source of symptoms. The therapist should determine
   a. Whether a neurological examination is indicated (central vs peripheral vs segmental). With symptoms below the gluteal fold or if symptoms are secondary to trauma, a neurological examination should be performed. If there is a past history of symptoms below the gluteal fold, a neurological examination should be performed to establish a baseline.
   b. The severity, irritability, nature, and stage of each symptom.
      (1). The therapist determines whether the nature of the condition indicates caution or requires specific testing.
      (2). The therapist determines whether any part of the examination should be performed with caution and whether there are any contraindications to examination.
   c. The vigor of the examination. The therapist determines whether he/she will need to be gentle or vigorous in the examination in order to reproduce a comparable sign.

IV. Objective Examination

A. Purpose

The therapist

1. Establishes an interpretation of the patient's functional impairment in terms of the implicated structure(s).
2. Provides a baseline for assessment, reassessment, and treatment.
3. Confirms whether the subjective examination fits the objective findings.[14]

B. Components

1. **Observation.** The therapist observes and notes the patient's willingness to move and his/her ease of movement; the patient's pos-

ture from the front, back, and side; the symmetry of spinal curves, shoulder girdle, and pelvic girdle heights; muscle atrophy and hypertrophy; deviations/shifts.

2. **Quick tests.** The therapist has the patient perform a functional movement and/or assume a position that reproduces the patient's complaint. The quick test should be meaningful to the patient and used to make a reassessment following treatment throughout the course of treatment.

3. **Examination of active movements.** The therapist has the patient perform active movements, assessing the range of movement and the quality of movement; noting the point of increase/onset of symptoms through range and the deviation and effect of correction of deviations on symptoms and range. A relevant shift will alter symptoms/range with correction, whereas a structural deviation will have no effect. As applicable, the therapist corrects deformities, localizes to level, adds overpressure. Ask the patient to sustain, repeat, perform at speed or under load.

4. **Neurological examination.** A neurological examination is performed if there are current symptoms below the gluteal fold, a history of symptoms below the gluteal fold, or complaints of paresthesia/anesthesia. Neurological testing should include sensation, reflexes, and resisted static muscle contractions. Include Babinski and clonus tests if symptoms suggest possible upper motor neuron involvement. To establish a baseline, a neurological examination is performed in cases involving trauma.

5. **Examination of passive movements.** The therapist performs passive movements of peripheral joints above and below the areas of symptoms; and passive physiological interver-

tebral movements (flexion/extension/lateral flexion/rotation). The therapist notes the resistance to movement and symptom reproduction at the beginning/through/and end of range and the quality and quantity of movement.

6. **Palpation.** Use the back of the hand to feel for temperature and sweating. Increased temperature is found with inflammation, and increased sweating is found with sympathetic response. The therapist should feel for contours and symmetry and should palpate soft tissue (from superficial to deep and general to specific) and should assess bony alignment. Passive accessory intervertebral movements are performed.

7. **Clearing tests.** Clear the joints above and below the area of symptoms that refer into the area of symptoms using passive physiological and combined physiological movements as well as resisted static muscle contraction testing. To clear the hip in a situation in which the area of symptoms indicates that the hip as well as the sacroiliac joint and lumbar spine may be involved, the therapist would examine passive physiological hip flexion, then internal and external rotation with overpressure. If neither of these movements produced the complaint, the therapist would combine the physiological movement of hip flexion/adduction/internal rotation and compression. If this progression of stress testing does not elicit symptoms, the hip is considered to be noncontributing to the symptom complex, *ie*, it is clear.

8. **Special tests.** Tests of stability, vertebral artery, and neural element mobility should be performed as indicated. Testing should be performed with consideration of the irritability, severity, and stability of the lesion.

V. Examination by Anatomical Area

A. Thoracic spine

1. **Subjective examination**
   a. *Description of complaint*
      (1). Area of symptoms specific for the thoracic spine:
         (a). Central pain felt through the

chest or deep anterior chest/abdominal pain may implicate the thoracic intervertebral disc (see Figure 32–10).

      (b). Unilateral horizontal pain around the chest wall impli-

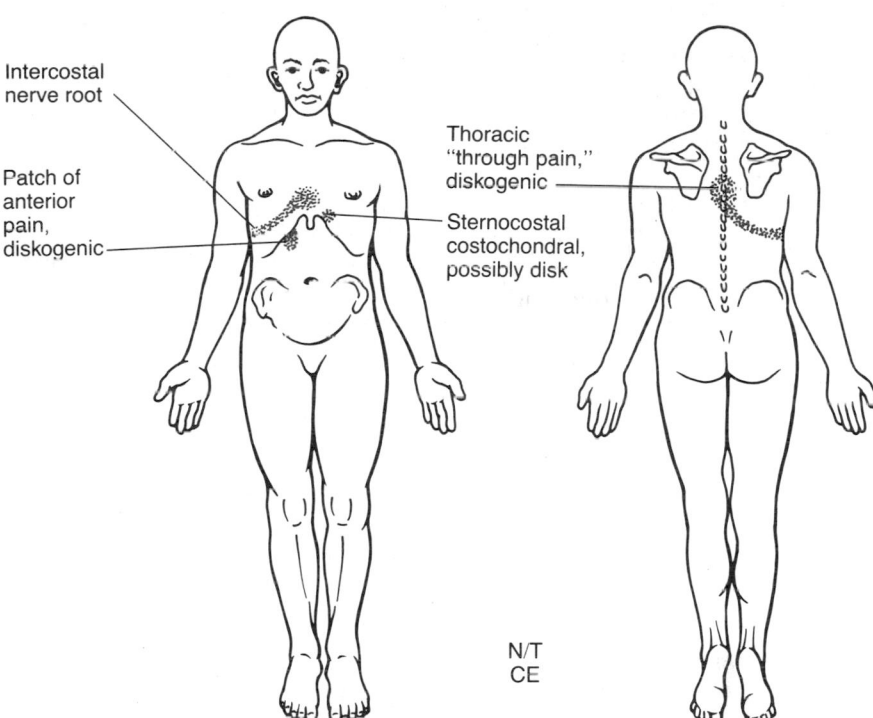

Intercostal
nerve root

Patch of
anterior
pain,
diskogenic

Thoracic
"through pain,"
diskogenic

Sternocostal
costochondral,
possibly disk

N/T
CE

FIGURE 32-10 Area of symptoms specific for the thoracic spine.

cates the costovertebral, costotransverse, or facet joints[14] (see Figure 32–10).

(2). Symptoms should be differentiated from cardiac chest pain that is often related to exertion: felt as pressure/crushing feeling; may have pain into the arm or jaw; frequently relieved by nitroglycerine; symptoms may include sweating, nausea.[17]

b. *Behavior of symptoms*
(1). For the thoracic spine, the patient should be asked about the following:
(a). Deep breathing: pain with inspiration implies rib involvement, especially 1st rib.
(b). Unsupported sitting: often aggravates symptoms.
(c). Twisting/reaching: frequently increases symptoms.
(d). Coughing/sneezing: if symptoms increase, possible involvement of thoracic disc or nerve root.
(e). Getting in and out of car: if an aggravating factor, may indicate adverse neural tension if aggravating component is neck flexion.[18]

c. *History*
(1). A history of thoracic surgery, sudden twisting movements under load, direct trauma, and sudden compression loading, especially in postmenopausal females, are typical in thoracic dysfunction patients.
(2). Predisposing factors include postural stress, sports, flu, vomiting/coughing spells, and lying in bed in an unusual or restricted position.

2. **Objective examination**
a. *Observation*
(1). The patient's posture is examined in sitting and standing, noting exaggeration of curves, shoulder girdle relationship, atrophy/hypertrophy, scoliosis, rib symmetry, and breathing pattern.
b. *Quick tests.* These include cough/deep breath, injuring movement, functional activity.
c. *Examination of active movements.* These are performed in sitting and/or standing, noting quality and pain.
(1). Flexion: with hands clasped behind the neck, the patient flexes forward, bringing elbows toward the groin.

(2). Extension: with hands behind the neck, the patient hollows out the upper back and extends.

(3). Lateral flexion: with hands behind the neck, the patient laterally flexes right and left.

(4). Rotation, in neutral, flexion, and extension as applicable: in sitting with arms crossed over the chest, and with the patient's knees stabilized between the therapist's knees, the patient rotates right and left.

(5). As applicable, the therapist
  (a). Corrects deformity.
  (b). Localizes to level.
  (c). Adds overpressure.
  (d). Sustains.
  (e). Repeats.
  (f). Performs movement at speed/loaded.
  (g). Combines movement tests.
  (h). Adds compression/distraction.

d. *Neurological examination*
  (1). Pinprick is performed over area of complaint of sensory changes.
  (2). Clonus and Babinski tests are performed with complaints of bilateral lower extremity symptoms, gait disturbance.
  (3). Muscle power tests are performed and reflexes checked with any complaints of extremity symptoms.

e. *Examination of passive movements*
  (1). Passive physiological intervertebral movements (PPIVM):
    (a). Flexion.
    (b). Extension.
    (c). Lateral flexion.
    (d). Rotation.

f. *Palpation*
  (1). Bony alignment: feel for rotation, scoliosis, deviations.
  (2). Passive accessory intervertebral movements (PAIVM): posteroanterior pressures are performed centrally over spinous processes and unilaterally over facet and costovertebral joints. Transverse pressures are applied to spinous processes.

g. *Clearing tests*
  (1). Cervical spine clearing.
    (a). Extension with overpressure.
    (b). Rotation bilaterally sustained 20 seconds.
    (c). Cervical quadrant bilaterally

sustained 20 seconds (a combined movement of extension and superimposed rotation and lateral flexion to the same side).

(2). Sacroiliac joint: compression and distraction.

(3). Glenohumeral joint: active flexion and with overpressure abduction, and hand behind back with overpressure; resisted static contractions of abduction, internal rotation, external rotation; shoulder quadrant.[14]

(4). Lumbar spine: flexion with overpressure, extension with overpressure, quadrant sustained 20 seconds bilaterally.

h. *Special tests.* Neural element mobility and other special tests are performed as applicable.
  (1). Upper limb tension tests (ULTT) to assess resistance and symptoms[18]: comparison made side to side.
    (a). ULTT 1: Median nerve dominant: blocked shoulder elevation, abduction to 90 degrees, supination, wrist and finger extension, external rotation, elbow extension, cervical lateral flexion away and toward.
    (b). ULTT 2a: Radial nerve bias: shoulder depression, elbow extension, internal rotation, pronation, wrist and finger flexion, shoulder abduction, cervical lateral flexion toward and away.
    (c). ULTT 2b: Median nerve bias: shoulder depression, elbow extension, external rotation, supination, wrist and finger extension, shoulder abduction, cervical lateral flexion away and toward.
    (d). ULTT 3: Ulnar nerve bias: shoulder depression blocked, wrist and finger extension, supination or pronation, elbow flexion, abduction to 90 degrees, cervical lateral flexion toward and away.

(2). Straight leg raise (SLR): comparison made side to side for resistance and symptom reproduction.

(3). Passive neck flexion: with one hand under the patient's head, the therapist passively flexes the neck on trunk while stabilizing at the sternum with the other hand; range and symptom reproduction are noted.

(4). Slump test: slump sitting with neck flexion; knee extension; ankle dorsiflexion. Symptoms and range are assessed and compared side to side; this test assesses mobility of structures within the spinal canal.

(5). Cervicothoracic differentiation: cervical spine rotation superimposed on thoracic rotation. Symptoms are assessed after each movement.
  (a). Thoracic rotation with overpressure is performed.
  (b). Cervical rotation with overpressure is performed.
  (c). Thoracic rotation with overpressure is performed with cervical rotation with overpressure superimposed.
  (d). Thoracic derotation is performed with cervical rotation maintained.
  (e). Findings are confirmed with thoracic rotation maintained while the cervical spine is derotated.[14]

(6). Tap test: performed over spinous processes when movement testing is negative; used to assess possibility of cancer or fracture.

B. Ribs

1. **Subjective examination**
  a. *Description of complaint*
    (1). Area of symptoms specific for the ribs (see Figure 32–10):
      (a). Often local.
      (b). Pain along the line of the rib implies intercostal nerve root compression.[14]
      (c). Pain at the anterior chest may be secondary to sternocostal or costochondral joint involvement.
      (d). First rib involvement may result in a pectoral ache or thoracic outlet symptoms, such as heaviness and clumsiness of the upper extremities.[16]
  b. *Behavior of symptoms*

    (1). For the ribs, the patient should be questioned about the following:
      (a). Effect of push/pull of arms: because of the attachment of the upper extremity muscles to the thorax and ribs.
      (b). Inspiration, especially deep breath: frequently provokes symptoms when ribs are involved.
      (c). Coughing: frequently painful because of the increase in intrathoracic pressure or the sudden movements involved.[14]

2. **Objective examination**
  a. *Observation*
    (1). Anterior/posterior/lateral views: the therapist looks for prominent ribs, accentuated curves, flattened interscapular region, scoliosis with rotation of rib cage.
  b. *Examination of active movement*
    (1). Quick test:
      (a). Deep breath.
      (b). Cough.
      (c). Injuring or aggravating movement.
    (2). In sitting:
      (a). Active spinal movements are performed as for thoracic (including cervical if upper four ribs are implicated; lumbar if lower four ribs).
        (i). Flexion.
        (ii). Extension.
        (iii). Lateral flexion, right and left.
        (iv). Rotation, right and left.
    (3). In standing: tests (glenohumeral joint for first rib); flexion; abduction hand behind back; with overpressure; resisted static contractions of abduction, internal rotation, external rotation.
  c. *Neurological examination.* If indicated, pinprick is performed for areas of sensation alterations.
  d. *Examination of passive movements*
    (1). Glenohumeral quadrant.
    (2). PPIVM: flexion, extension, lateral flexion, rotation.
  e. *Palpation*
    (1). Bony alignment:
      (a). First rib.

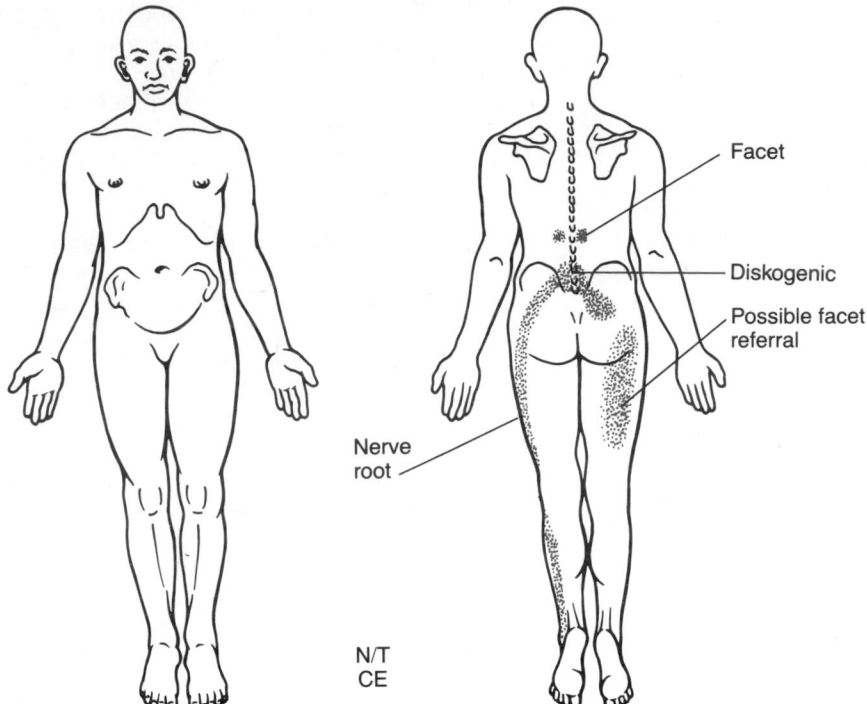

Facet

Diskogenic

Possible facet
referral

Nerve
root

N/T
CE

FIGURE 32–11 Area of symptoms
specific for the lumbar spine.

(b). Sternocostal joints.
(c). Costochondral joints.
(d). Costotransverse joints.
(e). Rib prominence, alignment, angle of ribs.
(f). Intercostal space.
(2). Passive accessory movements: posteroanterior, caudal, and rostral pressures over ribs lateral to costovertebral joint. Posteroanterior pressures over costovertebral joints.

f. **Clearing tests**
(1). Tap test to rule out potentially serious pathology, *eg*, bony metastasis or fracture.
(2). Glenohumeral joint (see 2.b.(3). and 2.d.(1).—glenohumeral quadrant above).

g. **Special tests.** Passive neck flexion, SLR, slump, ULTT.

C. Lumbar spine

1. **Subjective examination**
   a. *Description of complaint*
      (1). Area of symptoms specific for the lumbar spine (see Figure 32–11):

(a). A local unilateral symptom indicates a possible apophyseal problem.
(b). Central mid/lower lumbar pain may be discogenic, especially if it spreads into the buttocks.
(c). Bilateral mid/lower lumbar pain without central pain may be a bilateral apophyseal problem.
(d). Unilateral lumbar and lower limb symptoms indicate nerve root or possible facet involvement.

b. *Behavior of symptoms*
   (1). For the lumbar spine, the patient should be asked about the following:
      (a). Sitting: time until onset or increase in symptoms; frequently limited in discogenic problems/weight-bearing sensitive.
      (b). Standing: time until onset or increase in symptoms; may be aggravating in stenotic conditions and nerve root conditions.

(c). Walking: time until onset or increase in symptoms; often easing in discogenic problems, aggravating in stenotic conditions.

(d). Sitting to standing: pain may indicate possible discogenic involvement, as the fluid nature of the disc is unable to respond quickly to the transitional movement. May also indicate apophyseal involvement.

(e). Bending: frequently an aggravating factor in discogenic problems; if easing factor, may indicate a stenotic component; arcs of pain may indicate instabilities.

(f). Coughing/sneezing: may increase symptoms in discogenic and nerve root problems secondary to the increase in intra-abdominal pressure; may also be related to sudden flexion movements during coughing/sneezing.

(g). Half bending: frequently aggravating in discogenic problems.

(h). Twisting: may be low thoracic problem.

(i). The patient should be asked about the following to differentiate between lumbar spine and hip[14]:
  (i). Crossing legs: frequently increases symptoms in hip dysfunction.
  (ii). Squatting: frequently painful in those with hip dysfunction regardless of lumbar spine position.

2. **Objective examination**
  a. *Observation*
    (1). In standing: posture viewed from anterior, posterior, lateral; pelvic symmetry and leg length are noted.
    (2). In sitting: pelvic obliquity compared with standing in order to eliminate leg-length discrepancy as reason for spinal deviation.
  b. *Quick tests.* These include squat and functional movements.

c. *Examination of active movements*
  (1). In standing:
    (a). Lumbar movements: relevance of lateral deviation is assessed; side glides are performed as indicated. A deviation is relevant if correcting the deviation alters the symptoms.
      (i). Flexion and with neck flexion: patient bends forward and runs his/her hands down front of legs; neck flexion is superimposed.
      (ii). Extension: with knees straight, patient leans back from waist.
      (iii). Lateral flexion left and right: patient runs his/her hand down side of leg, keeping a pure lateral flexion movement.
    (b). As indicated:
      (i). Lumbar quadrant: combined movement of spinal extension, rotation to same side, side bend to same side, with compression.
      (ii). Repeated movements.
      (iii). Spinal compression/distraction.
      (iv). Neurological strength test of gastrocnemius/soleus (S1).
      (v). Hip/lumbar differentiation: trunk rotation in standing; symptoms assessed. Pelvis stabilized in rotation, and trunk derotated to neutral; symptoms assessed.[14]
  (2). In sitting:
    (a). Rotation: plus overpressure/sustained, etc., as indicated.
  (3). In supine:
    (a). Repeated flexion in lying.
  (4). In prone:
    (a). Repeated extension in lying.
    (b). Bilateral glutcus maximus contraction to assess for symmetry.
d. *Neurological examination*
  (1). Static muscle contractions:
    (a). L2: iliopsoas.

(b). L3: quadriceps.

(c). L4: tibialis anterior.

(d). L5: extensor hallucis longus; extensor digitorum longus.

(e). L5, S1: peroneals.

(f). S1: hamstrings, gastrocnemius/soleus.

(g). S2: toe flexors.

(2). Sensation: dermatomes L1–S2.

(3). Reflexes: knee jerk (L3–L4); ankle jerk (S1–S2)

(4). Upper motor neuron tests: Babinski reflex and clonus, as indicated.

e. *Examination of passive movements*

(1). PPIVM:

(a). Flexion.

(b). Extension.

(c). Lateral flexion.

(d). Rotation.

f. *Palpation*

(1). Alignment.

(2). Pelvic palpation for symmetry.

(3). Posteroanterior pressure on sacrum.

(4). Passive accessory intervertebral movement: posteroanterior pressure centrally over the spinous processes and unilaterally over the facet joints; transverse pressures to spinous processes.

g. *Clearing tests* (when indicated)

(1). Sacroiliac joint: compression/distraction.[14]

(2). Hip: flexion with overpressure, internal rotation with overpressure, flexion/adduction/internal rotation and compression with overpressure.[14]

(3). Knee: flexion with overpressure, extension with overpressure, extension/abduction and extension/adduction with overpressure.[14]

(4). Ankle: plantar flexion and dorsiflexion with overpressure.[14]

h. *Special tests*

(1). Passive neck flexion.

(2). SLR: with dorsiflexion and neck flexion as indicated.

(3). Prone knee bend.

(4). Instability test.

(5). Slump test.[14]

(6). Pulses: pedal pulses.

(7). Differentiation for peripheral neuropathy.

(8). Thomas' test.

(9). Length of the iliopsoas and the rectus femoris: hip extension (prone) with knee extended compared with knee flexed.

(10). Tensor fascia lata/iliotibial band length.

D. Sacroiliac joint

1. **Subjective examination**

a. *Description of complaint*

(1). Area of symptoms specific to the sacroiliac joint (see Figure 32–12):

(a). Typically unilateral, frequently in the absence of low back pain.

(b). Commonly in buttock, lower abdomen, groin (in the presence of buttock pain), and anteromedial or posterior thigh (symptoms may refer below the knee but rarely extend into the foot).

(c). Symptoms may include nondermatomal paresthesia, vague heaviness in the buttock or leg, and subjective numbness/tingling.[19]

(d). Symptoms may be in a sciatic distribution (proximity to sacral plexus should be noted).

(e). Pubic symphysis pain may occur in a severe sacroiliac joint problem.[14]

(f). Patients with sacroiliac problems may report sharp catches, clicking, or deep clunking and may state that the hip or back feels "out of place." [19]

b. *Behavior of symptoms*

(1). For the sacroiliac joint, the patient should be asked about the following:

(a). Single-legged stance: especially on affected side.

(b). Heel strike: stepping up/down stairs with affected leg.

(c). Transitional movements such as turning over in bed, getting out of bed, rising to standing (positive response could also implicate lumbar spine involvement).

(d). Crossing legs: patients with sacroiliac dysfunction complain of

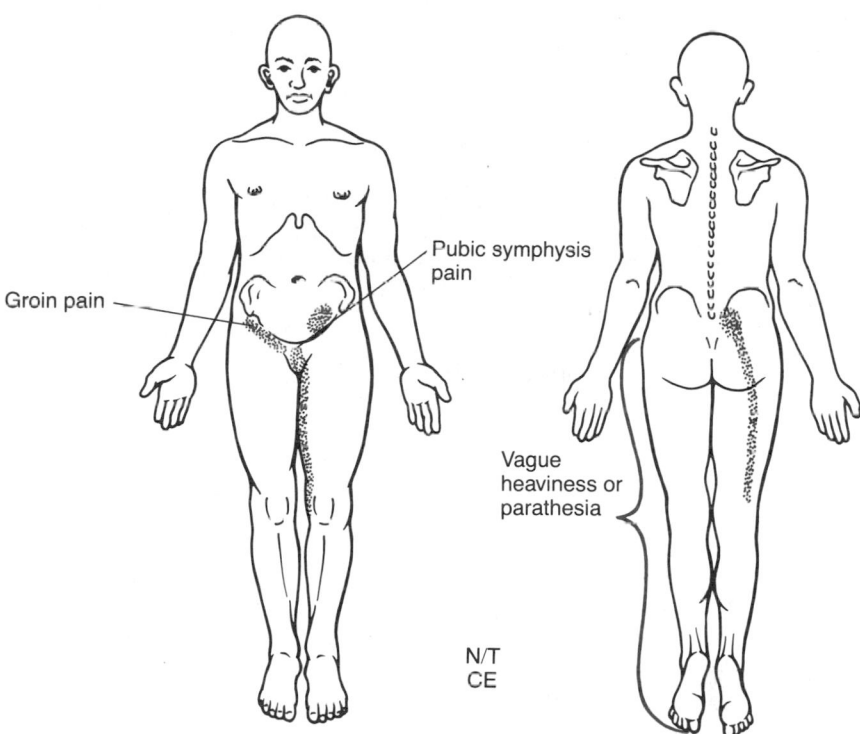

Groin pain

Pubic symphysis pain

Vague heaviness or parathesia

N/T
CE

FIGURE 32–12 Area of symptoms specific for the sacroiliac joint.

lateral pain more than groin pain compared with those with hip dysfunction.

(e). Pain with sexual intercourse (could also be lumbar spine involvement).

(f). Night pain or prolonged morning stiffness, especially in 30- to 40-year-old men: common in ankylosing spondylitis.

(g). Coughing/sneezing: usually negative.[14]

(2). Easing factors in sacroiliac problems:

(a). Sitting may ease symptoms and can help to differentiate from a lumbar spine problem, as sitting is frequently aggravating in lumbar spine conditions.[14]

(b). Lying supine with hips and knees flexed (could also be true in lumbar conditions).

c. *History*

(1). Habitual sloppy posture.

(2). Pregnant or up to 12 weeks post partum, or longer in women who are nursing.

(3). Specific job or sports activities (*eg,* stepping down out of a truck onto one leg, jumping hurdles in track) or work stance (*eg,* one-legged stance, sitting twisted).[14]

(4). Fall onto buttocks (can displace pubic symphysis)

(5). A motor vehicle accident in which the foot was on the brakes or the knee hit the dashboard.

(6). Long-standing lumbar spine or hip problems, especially stiffness.[19]

(7). Leg-length discrepancy (especially if acquired; *eg,* sacroiliac problems may develop if a walking cast is worn for a period of time because of gait and leg-length changes).

(8). Gynecological surgery.

2. **Objective examination**

a. *Observation*

(1). Standing posture

(a). Spinal contour and symmetry.

(b). Pelvic rotation.

(c). Buttock contour, level of gluteal folds, symmetry of cleft.

(d). Level of iliac crests; should be level and on the same plane.

(e). Swollen appearance of one or both joints.

(f). Posterosuperior iliac spine (PSIS).

(g). Anterosuperior iliac spine (ASIS).

(h). Lateral pelvic tilt (real or apparent leg-length shortening).

(2). Sitting: observation of posture repeated.

(3). Supine:

    (a). Leg lengths:

        (i). Hips and knees extended.

        (ii). Hips and knees flexed.

    (b). ASIS.

    (c). Pubic symphysis.

    (d). How hips fall into rotation.

(4). Prone:

    (a). Skyline views of gluteal mass.

    (b). Hip rotation.

b. *Quick tests*

(1). Squat.

(2). Functional movement.

c. *Examination of active movements*

(1). Standing:

    (a). Patient bends forward.

        (i). Skyline view of gluteal mass from front.

        (ii). Piedallu's sign: palpation is performed for symmetrical movement of PSIS during standing trunk flexion.[19]

    (b). Hip flexion: to 90 degrees while palpating the sacrum and the PSIS or ischial tuberosity: thumb on PSIS should move caudally with hip flexion and cephalically when foot returns to the ground; the ischial tuberosity should move laterally with hip flexion.[19]

    (c). Lumbar spine movement: with particular attention to

        (i). Deviation on flexion.

        (ii). Extension. Overpressure should be localized. Can be assessed with anterior pelvis tilt superimposed.

        (iii). Lateral flexion: toward the side of symptoms commonly reproduces or increases symptoms in pa-

tients with sacroiliac joint dysfunction.

(2). Sitting:

    (a). Palpation for Piedallu's sign should be repeated as signs of apparent leg-length discrepancies are eliminated.

(3). Supine:

    (a). Static contraction of abductors and adductors.

d. *Neurological examination.* Performed when indicated, as above.

e. *Examination of passive movement*

(1). Muscle length:

    (a). Abductors, iliotibial band.

    (b). Adductors.

    (c). Iliopsoas.

(2). Hip joint motion:

    (a). Extension/flexion.

    (b). Internal rotation/external rotation.

(3). Prone knee bend: femoral nerve tension sign should be differentiated from tight rectus femoris via side-lying passive knee flexion with hip extension and trunk slump.[18]

f. *Palpation*

(1). Supine:

    (a). Iliacus spasm (Baer's point): lateral one third of distance on a line from umbilicus to ASIS.[19]

    (b). Tenderness at adductor insertion.

    (c). Anterior acetabular region.

    (d). Pubic symphysis for symmetry and tenderness.

(2). Prone:

    (a). Attention to lumbosacral junction.

    (b). Unilateral posteroanterior pressures S1–S5, unilateral and transverse at PSIS, sacral apex pressure test, anteroposterior iliac gliding, longitudinal stress, torsional stress.

    (c). Palpation of sacroiliac joint:

        (i). Relative depth of sulci.

        (ii). Undue tenderness over PSIS.

        (iii). Symmetry and tenderness of sacrotuberous and sacrospinous ligaments (through gluteal mass, which may be tender).

(d). Examination of sacroiliac joint accessory movements:
  (i). Movement during hip rotation palpated.
  (ii). Sacral rocking at apex: movement on opposite side palpated.
  (iii). Sacrum stressed cephalad, ilium caudad; and the reverse.
  (iv). Compression/distraction.
  (v). Movement at sacroiliac sulcus palpated, with hip flexion, flexion/adduction repeated.
(3). Sidelying:
  (a). Approximation.
  (b). Torsion tests.
  (c). Torsion tests with hip flexion/extension.

g. *Clearing tests for hip*
(1). Flexion with overpressure.
(2). Internal rotation with overpressure.
(3). Flexion/adduction/internal rotation and with pressure along the line of the femur.

h. *Special tests*
(1). SLR: unilaterally or bilaterally. Not an exclusive sacroiliac joint test; it disturbs the lumbar joints as well as applying stress to the sacroiliac joints.
(2). Differentiation method: if SLR is restricted on the left to 70 degrees by pain and the other leg can be raised to 90 degrees, and bilateral SLR can be raised to a painless 90 degrees, this indicates that reduced range on the left side is due to unilateral torsional stress on the ipsilateral sacroiliac joint. This test does not preclude a coexisting lumbar problem.[19]

E. Clinical decision making

1. The physical therapist develops a provisional hypothesis from the subjective and objective data.
   a. The following are identified:
      (1). Severity: analogue pain scale and degree of disability are used to determine whether severity is mild, moderate, or severe.
      (2). Irritability: how much activity increases the symptoms, how much above resting level, and how long to settle to resting level.
      (3). Nature: the underlying mechanism or cause of the movement dysfunction is determined.
      (4). Stage: progression of the process (*eg,* acute, subacute, or chronic) and the overall progression of the pathology are determined.

2. The decision to treat or not to treat is based on indications and precautions suggested by the nature of the problem.
   a. Various nonmechanical/medical conditions may have contraindications or at least precautions for physical therapy intervention, which require consultation with a physician. As a general rule, conditions that present with severe, constant, unvarying pain that is not influenced by position or activity can be considered to be nonmechanical and outside the scope of physical therapy practice.
      (1). Angina: crushing pressure more than pain in the chest; pain may be in medial side of left arm, occasionally supraclavicular or temporomandibular. Aggravated by exertion, anxiety; may be accompanied by nausea, shortness of breath, lightheadedness, belching.
      (2). Dissecting aneurysm: low back pain that is constant; may be aggravated by increased activities and eased by rest. Dissection (expansion) may produce sudden, severe low back pain.
      (3). Pleurisy: sharp, stabbing pain with deep breath, usually well localized. Recent medical history is key.
      (4). Pancoast tumor: tumor in apex of lung, potentially puts pressure on lower trunk of brachial plexus. Cervical motions may be asymptomatic; scapular elevation may be painful. Mimics thoracic outlet syndrome with C8–T1 involvement but is less mechanical. History of gradual increase, possibly smoking, recent weight loss, or cancer (breast cancer with possibility of metastasis to lung).
      (5). Esophageal/hiatal hernia: more of

a burning pain in epigastric region, may refer to midthoracic levels, especially left. Should be aggravated by activities related to meal sequences, not to thoracic movement or postures.

(6). Gallbladder: may refer to right shoulder, inferior angle of right scapula; may be associated with fatty food intake; not clearly aggravated by thoracic or shoulder girdle position or movement.

(7). Herpes zoster: burning pain, tends to follow a single dermatome; may be accompanied by skin eruptions; patient often has history of recent upper respiratory infection, stress, or immune suppression.

(8). Metastasis to axial skeleton: involves lumbar and thoracic vertebral bodies, especially T4 and T11, secondary to breast, prostate, lung, kidney, or thyroid cancer. Pain is severe, constant, nagging, and deep; may be worse at night and unaffected by change in posture, position, or activity. Keys are quality and behavior of pain and any history of cancer or unexplained weight loss.

(9). Ankylosing spondylitis: pain and stiffness are much worse in the morning and decrease with activity; gradual onset, no specific incident in client who is under 40.

(10). Osteochondrosis (Scheuermann's disease): most common cause of back pain in adolescents; affects two times as many boys as girls.[16]

(11). Osteoporosis: may present as chronic back pain, especially thoracic, often in a kyphotic, postmenopausal female.

(12). Polymyalgia rheumatica: pain in the proximal joints and muscles in a client who is over 60. Client may know the date of onset because this pain is markedly different in quality from osteoarthritic symptoms. There is marked elevation of the erythrocyte sedimentation rate with mild malaise; these patients respond quickly to systemic corticosteroids.[16]

(13). Tietze's disease: local inflammation at sternocostal junction of 2nd and 3rd ribs; usually treated with hydrocortisone injection.[16]

(14). Rib-tip syndrome: pain localized to unilateral anterior costal margins of ribs 8 to 10; can be confused with pleurisy, coronary thrombosis, and gallbladder disease; usually a history of direct trauma to the costal margins.[16]

(15). Rheumatoid arthritis: may produce erosion of ribs and may affect costovertebral joint. Can lead to instability, nerve root compression, and vertebral collapse.[16]

b. Areas of referral from thoracic spine:

(1). T6–T7: epigastric, inferior ribs.

(2). T7–T8: right side, mimics gallbladder.

(3). T9: area over kidneys.

(4). T10–T11: urethra, bladder.

(5). T11 to L1: groin, lower abdomen—must be differentiated from bladder, urethra, testicular, hip pain, L2 nerve root.

(6). T9 to L2: low back pain, buttock pain, iliac crest.[16]

VI. Treatment

A. General treatment principles

1. Patient as therapist: the patient must be instructed to become his/her own therapist.

a. To accomplish this goal, it is necessary that the patient understand what is wrong and how the home program will promote, repair, and restore function.

(1). Stages of injury-repair:

(a). Inflammation.

(b). Consolidation.

(c). Scar formation.

(d). Remodeling (scar maturation).

(2). Circulation: good healing demands adequate circulation to all structures

Table 32–1. FLUID TRANSPORT SYSTEMS

System	Pump	Method
1. Arteries/veins	Heart	Walking
2. Lymph	Movement	Breathing with spinal motion
3. Synovial fluid	Movement	Walking
4. Cerebrospinal fluid	Movement	Breathing with spinal motion
5. Disc	Movement	Walking
6. Intraneuronal transport system	Movement	Ankle, knee, hip movement

(From Edgelow PI: *A Patient's Guide to Treatment of Thoracic Outlet Syndrome,* self-published.)

within the injured segment. Six fluid transport systems need maximum stimulus to promote circulation to structures within the mobile segment (see Table 32–1).[20]

(3). Dysfunctions of the musculoskeletal system that occur as a result of the injury repair process require specific treatments in a particular order to ensure maximum recovery. For example:

(a). Circulation—ice/heat, Grade II physiological movements, breathing with spinal motion.

(b). Flexibility—specific stretching using the 3-inch Ethafoam roll.

(c). Coordination—use of the 6-inch Ethafoam roll, walking.

(d). Endurance—use of the 6-inch Ethafoam roll, walking.

(e). Strength.

b. Patient understanding can be accomplished by the use of simple analogies (*eg,* a hinge that squeaks needs oil, a hinge that has loose screws needs stability, a hinge that is stiff needs stretching, and a swamp that needs draining has a problem of congestion/circulation).[21]

c. It is important to understand that pathological labels often do more to limit understanding from the patient's point of view. Also, the use of analogies saves one from the problem of defining a diagnostic label in a way that may not be consistent with the physician's mode of thinking or the patient's understanding.[21]

2. No pain/no gain:

a. The therapist should convey to the patient that remodeling necessitates small prolonged stresses spread out over a long time to promote maximum healing. An analogy to remodeling of bone is braces on the teeth. Too much remodeling causes damage; too little will not result in change, just irritation. Treatment focuses on pain when the pain response is dominant. Treatment focuses on flexibility, coordination, endurance, and strength when the movement characteristics are dominant.

b. In chronic conditions the adverse effects of immobilization and the pain withdrawal response and the vasomotor constriction response are made worse by ignoring pain and trying to work through it. Therefore, patients need to be taught to move in ways that promote circulation but do not cause a pain withdrawal response increasing their symptoms.

3. Common sense: patients often look for a quick fix and for the therapist to itemize exactly what they have to do in their home program. This assumes that the rate of progression of exercise in the home program can always be accurately predicted by the therapist. Instead, the patient must learn to evaluate his/her own progress and use his/her body's response to movement.

4. Ten-percent rule: with difficult problems, a good rule for progression of activity is to increase no more than 10% of what was done the day before. The percentage is not as important as is the concept of not overdoing the progression of activity as symptoms begin to ease.

5. Flares: patients can be taught to treat their symptoms in the acute stage. When a patient has a flare, he/she should revert to the acute treatment until the flare has subsided. Then the patient can resume his/her activities at 50% less than what he/she was doing before the flare and then progress as tolerated. Ultimately, effective treatment is that which guides the patient into becoming his/her own therapist.

6. The movements used by the therapist in treatment may be used by the patient in

his/her home program. These movements are not precisely the same but are effective.

7. Patients can be encouraged to take a positive view of treatment and to be in control of the treatment.

B. Treatment specifics: treating pain versus resistance

1. Treatment of pain: use Grade I, progress to Grade II, short duration of application.
   a. Accessory movement: loose-pack, pain-free position.
   b. Physiological movement: handling technique is critical so pain is not evoked.
   c. Exception: do not use through range techniques (Grade II) on a patient with an acute nerve root.
2. Treatment of resistance: use Grades III and IV as pain will allow. Use Grade IV if resistance is near the end of range. Use Grade III if resistance is early in the range.
3. Treatment of resistance respecting pain: use accessory movement if active range is less than 50%. Use physiological movement if active range is greater than 50%. The therapist may choose to provoke up to 20% of the pain.

C. Prognosis/discharge planning

1. Prior incidents: a past history of trauma/prior incidents may indicate that recovery may be limited; these should be related to persistent limitations and the overall stage of the pathology.
2. Level of recovery: if a patient has not fully recovered from prior incidents, recovery is not likely to exceed prior levels.
3. General health that might affect prognosis: diabetes mellitus can cause slower healing; cardiovascular conditions may limit a patient's ability to exercise; arthritis and systemic disease will have an impact on recovery.
4. Severity: more severe cases usually take longer to heal. Severity of injuring incident: the more severe the incident, the more involved the tissues.[14]
5. Age: the younger patients tend to heal more

quickly than the older patients; a young person who does not heal quickly is likely to have a more complex problem.
6. Psychosocial factors: stress, psychological components have an impact on a person's ability to heal.

D. Exercise/home program

The purpose of this section is to give an example of some home exercises to illustrate

---

Table 32–2.   BREATHING EXERCISES

1. Backlying on the floor without a pillow; knees bent. *Note:* If you have to use a pillow because of neck pain then do so, but understand that over time the goal is to slowly reduce the thickness of the pillow until you can perform the exercise without a pillow.

2. Place one hand on the abdomen and the other hand on the sternum (chest).

3. Breathe in through your nose and fill your lower lungs with air, which causes your abdomen to rise as if blowing up a balloon.

4. Breathe out through pursed lips as if you were playing the flute. This should be done by tightening your stomach muscles, which has the effect of lowering your rib cage.

5. Continue this rhythm of breathing in through the nose and out through the mouth, making sure that the only motion that occurs is in the stomach. This is breathing with your diaphragm.

6. Continue breathing with the diaphragm; add the movements of the spine noted in Step 7.

7. Slowly arch your low back as you breathe in and flatten the low back as you breathe out. These movements of the spine should feel like a wave motion up and down the spine. The movements should be gentle and relaxed.
   a. Relax neck.
   b. Breathing, the spine will shorten, causing the chin to nod down.
   c. Breathing out, the spine will lengthen, causing the chin to nod back up. *Note:* This should occur naturally. There should be no active movement of the neck.

8. Increase the range of motion of your spine until you are moving the spine through its maximum range of motion without pain.

9. Squeeze out the air from your stomach by using both your abdominal muscles and pelvic floor muscles (as if you were squeezing or tightening bladder and bowel).

10. Do this exercise protocol for breathing in sitting, on hands and knees, or standing.

(From Edgelow PI: *A Patient's Guide to Treatment of Thoracic Outlet Syndrome,* self-published.)

the principles described. It is not our purpose to cover all of the possible methods of conducting a home program. The reader can find good information in references 22 to 24.

1. Home exercises to treat dysfunctions of the thoracic and lumbar spines and sacroiliac joints:
   a. *Breathing.* Breathing exercises (see Table 32–2) can be the most important component of an exercise program for initial treatment of severe problems of the thoracic and lumbar spines and sacroiliac joints. Breathing promotes relaxation, can be trained in a gravity-eliminated position, and can include movements that stimulate circulation and coordination of the whole spine.
   b. *Walking.* One of the most effective methods for treating injuries to the lumbar spine is walking. A moderate walking program of 15 to 20 minutes, three to four times a day, is most effective at enhancing recovery. Visualization can assist in the effectiveness of walking. One method is to have the patient place his/her hands on his/her back and feel the contraction and relaxation of the muscles during walking so that the patient can visualize the pumping action of the muscles assisting in "lubricating" the injured area. The impact of walking is much broader than its effect on the mobile segment and the muscles and nerves of the spinal column (see Table 32–3).
   c. *Spinal mobilization*
      (1). Thoracic spine mobilization is achieved using a ball on a stick.
         (a). The patient assumes the back-lying position with bent hips and knees; the head and neck are supported with one hand placed behind the head; the ball is held on the stick in the other hand.
         (b). The patient rotates the trunk to one side; places the ball on the stick on the paraspinal area of the thoracic spine; rolls back over the ball.
         (c). The patient places the ball farther out to the side and applies

pressure to the ribs as he/she rolls over on the ball.[20]
      (2). Thoracic and lumbar spine mobilization is achieved using a 3-inch Ethafoam roll.[25]
      (3). Sacroiliac joint mobilization is achieved using a 3-inch Ethafoam roll.[25]
   d. Thoracic and lumbar spine exercises for coordination and endurance are performed using a 6-inch Ethafoam roll.[26]
   e. Spinal exercises are used for strengthening.
   f. Home modalities for pain relief:
      (1). Ice packs.
      (2). Hot packs.
   g. Posture: the physical therapist should emphasize the effect of breathing on posture, *ie*, sitting with lumbar spine in flexion facilitates scalene breathing. Sitting with lumbar spine in extension facilitates diaphragmatic breathing.

Table 32–3. BENEFICIAL EFFECTS OF WALKING

1. Stimulates circulation of the blood, the cerebrospinal fluids, and the lymphatics.
2. Benefits cardiovascular and cardiopulmonary fitness and stimulates the endocrine system.
3. Reduces the viscosity of the nucleus of the disk, allowing for a better fluid exchange within the nucleus itself.
4. Assists the exchange of fluid between the vertebrae and the nucleus mechanically by increasing and decreasing the pressure on portions of the disk.
5. Stimulates the mechanoreceptors, facilitating the normal neurophysiological status of the whole mobile segment.
6. Improves coordination and strength of the muscles necessary to control the movement of the mobile segment. This is accomplished through the reciprocal contraction and relaxation of the muscles engaged in walking.
7. Has a positive impact on the patient psychologically, maximizing the placebo effect.
8. Allows patients to get away from the environment of the home, where they are frequently confronted with stressful emotional and mental conditions.
9. Moves patient from role of passive victim to role of active healer—a crucially important psychological shift in the promotion of wellness.

(From Edgelow PI: *A Patient's Guide to Treatment of Thoracic Outlet Syndrome,* self-published.)

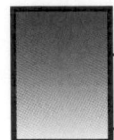

Clinical Decision-Making Cases

Case #1: Thoracic Spine/ Ribs

SUBJECTIVE EXAMINATION

Date

10/13.

Area of Symptoms

See Figure 32–13.

Patient Profile

The patient is a 36-year-old female; no recreational activities.

Occupation

Route sales/delivers bread from truck; off work since 8/19.

Aggravating Factors

Standing 1 hour increases all pains, eased by lying supine 15 minutes with one pillow under head.

Sitting 20 minutes increases all pains, eased by standing 5 minutes.

Stirring a pot with right hand 5 to 10 minutes increases all pains, gets shooting pain anterior chest, eased by 10 minutes lying supine.

Deep breath, cervical questions, shoulder questions, all negative.

Easing Factors

Stretching arms overhead, rubbing ointment onto back.

24 Hours

Morning: best time of day, pain 3/10 (3 on a scale of 10, where 10 is worst).

Course of day: after 3 hours of being up, pain in back increases to 8/10.

End of day: worst, regardless of activity.

Sleep: 30 minutes of difficulty getting comfortable, okay once asleep; sleeps on back with one pillow.

Special Questions

General health, weight loss, cord questions, vertebral artery questions: all negative.

Medication questions: prednisone, tapered dosage, as of yesterday.

Tests: radiographs within normal limits.

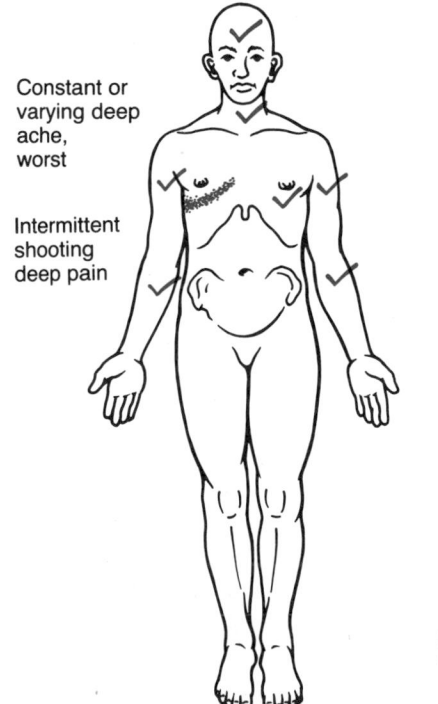

Constant or varying deep ache, worst

Intermittent shooting deep pain

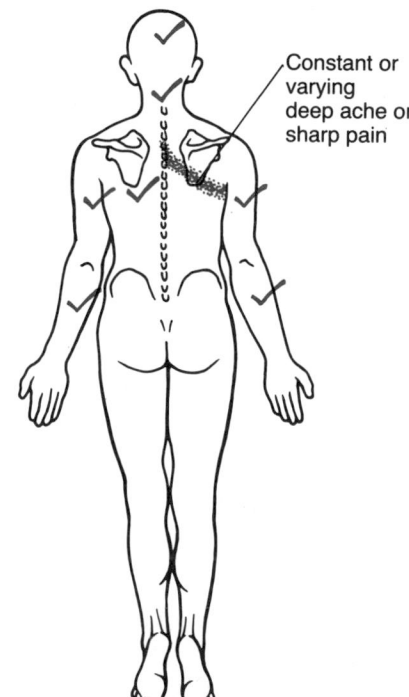

Constant or varying deep ache or sharp pain

N/T
CE

FIGURE 32–13 Case study 1: area of symptoms.

History

On 8/15, the patient was loading a 15-lb bread tray onto a rack while bent over at the waist. As she moved the tray from left to right, she felt a burning pain in the central midback. She continued to work the rest of the day and felt worse by the end of the day, with increased pain. By the next morning, the pain radiated around and down the ribs. She worked that day and the next, but only drove the truck. By the end of the 2nd day following the incident, the pain had radiated to the front of the chest. On 8/19, the patient went to see her physician and was taken off work. The patient had physical therapy three times a week until last week. Treatment consisted of heat, ice, ultrasound, phonophoresis, electrical stimulation, and light exercise during the last 2 weeks of treatment. At present, she states that she feels 30% better in that the bilateral upper thoracic pain (above the present area of pain) has been gone for 3 weeks. The rib and anterior and lateral thoracic pain is unchanged.

Past History

None for cervical, thoracic, or lumbar spine or shoulder.

Provisional Assessment

Severity: moderate.
Irritability: minimal.
Nature: midthoracic neurocentral joint dysfunction involving ribs, thoracic nerve root irritation.
Stage: chronic—unchanged over 3 weeks.

OBJECTIVE EXAMINATION

1. Observation: rounded shoulders, mild forward head, midthoracic flattened, kyphotic cervicothoracic junction.
2. Lumbar clearing tests (resting pain 7/10): flexion, extension, quadrant bilaterally sustained 20 seconds, all negative.
3. Cervical clearing tests: flexion, extension, quadrant bilaterally sustained 20 seconds, all negative.
4. Shoulder clearing tests:
   • Flexion: negative.
   • Abduction: left, negative; right, 170 degrees, pull chest wall.
   • Hand behind back: left wrist to T8, no symptoms; right wrist to T11, pain right lateral thoracic area.
5. Resisted static contractions: internal rotation, external rotation, abduction 5/5 bilaterally.
6. Thoracic active range of motion (resting pain 7/10):
   • Flexion: 80%, clear with overpressure.
   • Extension: 30 degrees, clear with overpressure, stiff midthoracic.
   • Left rotation: 30 degrees, clear with overpressure.
   • Right rotation, 20 degrees, pain right thoracic and lateral rib area.

7. Shoulder quadrant: left, clear; right, slight pull right anterior chest.
8. SLR: 90 degrees bilaterally, hamstrings stretch.
9. Palpation:
   • Central posteroanterior (PA) T5–T6: local pain with Grade IV .
   • Unilateral PA T5,6 > T6,7 > T7,8: local pain with Grade IV⁻.
   • Unilateral PA rib 5 > 6: pain spreads laterally with Grade IV⁻.

Treatment	Reassessment
1. Unilateral PA rib 5, Grade IV⁻	Resting pain: 6/10 Right rotation: 20 degrees, pain right thoracic only Glenohumeral abduction: right full, no pull Hand behind back: clear
2. Unilateral PA rib 5, Grade IV⁻, two more times	Resting pain: 4/10 Right rotation: 25 degrees, pain right thoracic less

Patient Instructions

Ice 10 to 15 minutes three times a day; sleeping, sitting, and standing posture. Patient to monitor symptoms over next 24-hour period and report at next visit. Patient to begin a walking program of 10 to 15 minutes, three times a day, if within tolerance; to stop short of increasing pain.

TREATMENT 2

Subjective

After the last treatment, the patient felt some decreased thoracic pain with sitting 20 minutes and was able to fall asleep in 20 minutes versus in 30 minutes previously. The next morning, the pain was the usual 3/10, but the pain has been 7/10 at its worst versus 8/10 previously. Stirring a pot: status quo. Standing 1 hour: status quo. Resting pain: 6/10 now.

Objective

1. Glenohumeral abduction: full bilaterally without symptoms.
2. Hand behind back: clear bilaterally.
3. Shoulder quadrant: clear bilaterally.
4. ULTT 1: clear bilaterally.
5. Left thoracic rotation: 30 degrees.
6. Right thoracic rotation: 25 degrees, pain right thoracic and lateral thoracic area.

Treatment	Reassessment
1. Transverse pressure T5,6, Grade IV⁻, first time	Resting pain 5/10 Right thoracic rotation: 25 degrees, pain right thoracic area

Treatment	Reassessment
2. Transverse pressure T5,6, Grade IV⁻, second time	Resting pain: 4/10 Right thoracic rotation: 30 degrees, pain right thoracic area
3. Unilateral PA rib 5, Grade IV⁻, first time	Resting pain: 3/10 Right thoracic rotation: 30 degrees, slight pain only
4. Unilateral PA rib 5, Grade IV⁻, second time	Resting pain: 2/10 Right thoracic rotation: 30 degrees, no increase in pain

Patient Instruction

Use of tennis balls for self-mobilization. TheraBand exercise for scapular retraction strengthening, stretches.

TREATMENT 3

Subjective

After the second treatment, the patient's pain was decreased for the rest of the day. She was able to sleep without difficulty. Stirring a pot: no symptoms.

Case #2: Lumbar Spine

SUBJECTIVE EXAMINATION

Date
10/15.

Area of Symptoms
See Figure 32–14.

Patient Profile
The patient is a 37-year-old male; recreational activities: jogging 4 miles/day but not able to jog now. He has been spending time lying on stomach all day, walking around apartment three times a day.

Occupation
Construction worker, cement and rock formation; off work since 10/13 owing to injury.

Aggravating Factors
Sit to stand: increases abdominal, leg, and lumbar pain; difficulty straightening.
Rolling over in bed: increases lumbar and abdominal pain, eased by 5 minutes prone.
Standing: has to lean against something, cannot stand straight.
Walking: 10 minutes increases lumbar and leg pain, eased by 20 minutes lying prone.
Sitting: 5 minutes increases lumbar and leg pain, eased by 10 minutes lying prone.

Sitting 1 hour: anterior chest pain. Standing: not limited. Pain no longer constant. Overall, she feels 80% improved. Will resume light duty next week.

Objective
1. Resting pain: 0.
2. Flexion: 85%, no pain.
3. Extension: 35 degrees, no pain.
4. Left thoracic rotation: 30 degrees, no pain.
5. Right thoracic rotation: 30 degrees, slight pain right lateral thoracic area with overpressure.

Treatment	Reassessment
1. Unilateral PA ribs 5 to 7, Grade IV, three times	Right thoracic rotation: 30 degrees, slight pain right lateral thoracic area
2. Unilateral PA T4,5–T7,8 Grade IV, three times	Right thoracic rotation: 30 degrees, no pain

Patient Instruction

Review home exercise program of self-mobilization, strengthening, and stretching. Follow-up at 1 week: the patient reports that she is able to perform all duties at work without symptoms. She states that she feels 100% improved and is continuing with home program.

Easing Factors
Ice to lumbar spine, lying prone, medications (hydrocodone bitartrate plus acetaminophen [Vicodin] three times a day; ibuprofen [Motrin], 600 mg, three times a day).

24 Hours
Morning: stiff in back for 5 minutes, eases with movement.
Course of day: same—lying around.
End of day: same—lying around.

Special Questions
General health, medications, weight loss, cord questions, cauda equina: negative.
Tests: none currently; magnetic resonance imaging of lumbar spine 7 years ago—"2 ruptured discs."

History
On 10/13, the patient was sitting at work and was spraying cement through a hose. He twisted right and felt a sharp pain in the right low back. He stopped working for 15 minutes, and the pain eased. Then the patient continued to work with the hose and had increased lumbar pain. He got up and tried to walk and had stomach pain. He sat in a chair for 2 hours because he could not walk, and a friend drove him to his physician while he lay in the back seat of the car. He was given medications and was taken off work. He has been at home and is doing better with bed rest and

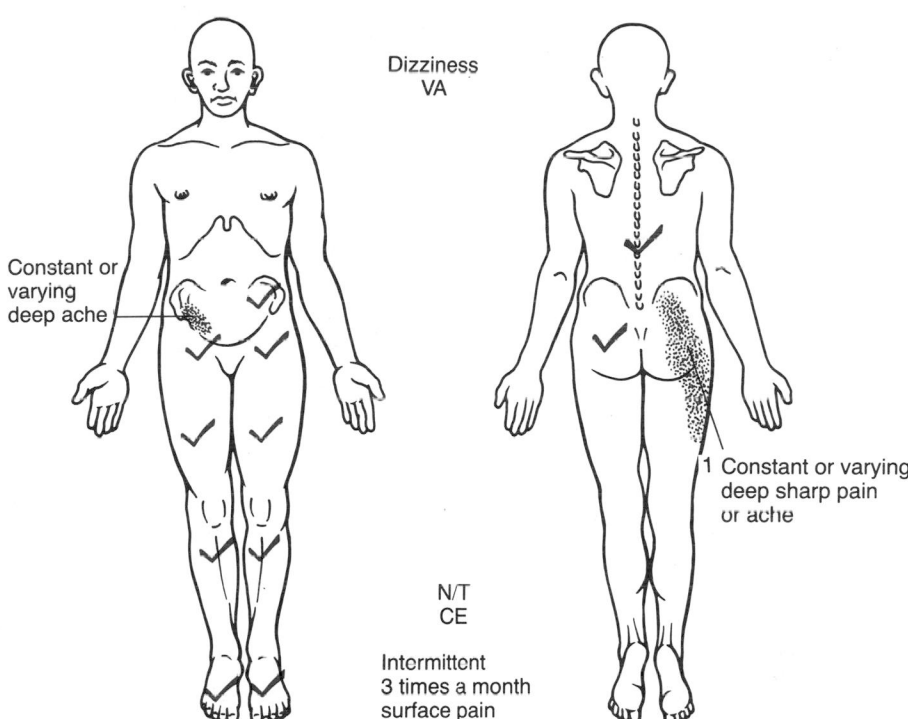

Dizziness
VA

Constant or
varying
deep ache

1 Constant or varying
deep sharp pain
or ache

N/T
CE

Intermittent
3 times a month
surface pain

FIGURE 32–14 Case study 2:
area of symptoms.

medications. Normally, he has low back pain by the end of a hard work day, but symptoms ease with a heating pad. Approximately three times a month he has numbness and tingling in the left leg.

Past History

Seven years ago, the patient was wheeling a wheelbarrow of cement and twisted to the right and hurt his low back—he does not remember which side. He had low back pain and leg numbness. He was on bed rest for 3 months and got better. He did not have any physical therapy. He has not had chiropractic or osteopathic treatment in the past.

Provisional Assessment

Severity: severe.
Irritability: moderate—difficult to determine secondary to patient's lack of activity.
Nature: discogenic with nerve root irritation.
Stage: acute.

Objective Examination

1. Observation: no weight bearing on the right leg, deviated left.
2. Resting pain: 8/10 abdominal, lumbar spine, and right leg.
3. Right side glide: 15%, increases right lumbar and abdominal pain; left side glide: 80%, increases lumbar pain.
4. SLR, left: 65 degrees, pain lumbar area.

5. SLR, right: 55 degrees, pain lumbar area.
6. Resisted static contractions:
   • L2: deferred.
   • L3: 5/5 bilaterally.
   • L4: 5/5 bilaterally.
   • L5: Extensor hallucis longus (right) 4+/5, (left) 5/5
   • S1: 5/5 bilaterally.
   • S2: 5/5 bilaterally.
7. Reflexes: knee jerk, clear; ankle jerk, decreased right.
8. Passive neck flexion: 90%, pain right lumbar area.
9. Prone knee bend: 120 degrees bilaterally, pressure lumbar spine.
10. Palpation: not shifted in prone or supine.
    • Central PA L3–L5: swollen, hot; L4 > L5: local pain and abdominal pain with Grade IV⁻.
    • Unilateral PA L4,5 > L5,S1: local pain with Grade IV⁻; slight leg pain with Grade IV.

Treatment	Reassessment
1. Ultrasound, ice, and interferential current to lumbar spine	Increased weight bearing right leg: patient estimates 20% Right side glide: 40%, increased pain right lumbar area and abdominal pain

Treatment	Reassessment
2. General rotation low lumbar, Grade IV⁻	Increased weight bearing right leg: patient estimates 50% Right side glide: 60%, increased pain right lumbar area
3. General rotation low lumbar, Grades IV⁻ to IV, two times	SLR, left: 70 degrees, increased pain right lumbar area SLR, right: 65 degrees, pain right lumbar area

Patient Instruction

Advised to ice every 1 to 2 hours at home for 10 to 15 minutes; instructed on sit to stand, log rolling, positioning, self-correction of shift if no peripheralization of symptoms, body mechanics for bending and putting on shoes.

TREATMENT 2

Subjective

The patient felt some decreased pain in the evening following treatment. He has intermittent abdominal and leg pain now. Walking: 10 minutes with increased lumbar pain, 15 minutes abdominal pain. Sit to stand: difficult straightening but easier. Standing: less crooked. Sitting: 5 to 10 minutes with increased lumbar and leg pain.

Objective

1. Resting pain: 6/10, right lumbar area only.
2. Observation: weight bearing right leg increased but not equal; shifted left but improved. Weight bearing: patient estimates 75%.
3. Left side glide: full, no increase in symptoms.
4. Right side glide: 75%, increased pain right lumbar area and slight abdominal pain.
5. Lumbar active movement:
   - Flexion: fingertips to midfemur, increased lumbar pain, deviation left; with correction of deviation, fingertips to midfemur with increased lumbar and abdominal pain.
   - Extension: 5 degrees, pain right lumbar area and leg.
   - Left lateral flexion: fingertips to 4 inches above joint line, pain right lumbar area.
   - Right lateral flexion: fingertips to 7 inches above joint line, pain right lumbar area and leg.
   - SLR, left: 70 degrees, pain right lumbar area.
   - SLR, right: 65 degrees, pain right lumbar area.
6. Resisted static contractions: L5, 4+/5 (right), 5/5 (left); L2, 5/5 bilaterally.
7. Ankle jerk: decreased right.
8. Palpation:
   - Central PA L4 > L5: local pain with Grade IV⁻, abdominal pain with Grade IV.
   - Unilateral PA L4–5: local pain with Grade IV⁻, slight buttock pain with Grade IV.

Treatment	Reassessment
1. Central PA L4–5, Grade IV⁻	Resting pain: 5/10 lumbar area only Weight bearing: 80% estimated, decreased shift left Right side glide: 80%, pain lumbar area Flexion: fingertips to 3 inches above knee, pain lumbar area, decreased deviation; with correction of deviation, fingertips to 4 inches above knee Extension: 10 degrees, pain right lumbar area Left lateral flexion: fingertips to 3 inches above joint line Right lateral flexion: fingertips to 5 inches above joint line L5: status quo Ankle jerk: slight increase
2. Central PA L4–5, Grades IV⁻ to IV	Resting pain: 4/10 lumbar area only Weight bearing: estimated 85%, decreased shift left Right side glide: 85%, pain right lumbar area Flexion: fingertips to knee, slight deviation left; with correction, fingertips to 2 inches above knee Extension: 10 degrees, pain right lumbar area Left lateral flexion: fingertips to 2 inches above joint line, pain lumbar area Right lateral flexion: fingertips to 4 inches above joint line, pain lumbar area L5: status quo Ankle jerk: slight increase SLR, left: 75 degrees, hamstrings stretch

Treatment	Reassessment
	SLR, right: 65 degrees, pain right lumbar area
3. Right rotation low lumbar, Grades IV⁻ to IV	Resting pain: 3/10 lumbar area only
	Weight bearing: estimated 90%, no shift
	Right side glide: 90%, pain right lumbar area
	Flexion: fingertips to inferior knee, pain right lumbar area, deviation left; with correction, fingertips to knee, pain right lumbar area
	Extension: 15 degrees, pain right lumbar area
	Lateral flexion: status quo
	L5: status quo
	Ankle jerk: status quo
	SLR, left: 75 degrees, hamstrings stretch
	SLR, right: 70 degrees, pain right lumbar area

Patient Instruction

The patient was instructed in repeated extension in lying, to be performed 10 times every 1 to 2 hours; the patient was warned about peripheralization of symptoms. Patient to begin walking 5 minutes three times a day short of increased pain/shifting.

TREATMENT 3

Subjective

The patient has been feeling much better. He no longer has any abdominal pain or leg pain. Sitting: 20 minutes, lumbar pain. Walking: 30 minutes, lumbar pain. Sit to stand: clear. Rolling over in bed: clear. Standing: 20 minutes, shifting weight deviations: occasional mornings if has been on feet a lot the day before. Overall, he feels 70% improved.

Objective

1. Observation: no shift.
2. Weight bearing: equal.
3. Side glide: equal bilaterally.
4. Flexion: fingertips to 4 inches below knee, pain right lumbar area.
5. Extension: 25 degrees, pain right lumbar area.
6. Left lateral flexion: fingertips to 2 inches above joint line, pull right lumbar area.
7. Right lateral flexion: fingertips to 3 inches above joint line, pain right lumbar area.
8. Passive neck flexion: clear.
9. SLR: 75 degrees bilaterally, hamstrings stretch.
10. Extensor hallucis longus: left, 5/5; right, 4+/5.
11. Ankle jerk: slightly decreased right.

12. Prone knee bend: 130 degrees bilaterally.
13. Palpation:
    - Central PA L4–5: local pain with Grade IV, abdominal pain with Grade IV⁺.
    - Unilateral PA L4,5 > L5,S1: local pain with Grade IV⁺.
    - Central PA L1–3: stiff with Grade IV⁺.

Treatment	Reassessment
1. Central PA L4–5, Grades IV⁻ to IV⁺	Flexion: fingertips to 5 inches below knees, no pain
	Extension: 25 degrees, painless
	Left lateral flexion: fingertips to 2 inches above joint line, painless
	Right lateral flexion: fingertips to 2 inches above joint line, pain right lumbar area
	Ankle jerk: status quo
	Extensor hallucis longus: status quo
2. Right rotation low lumbar, Grades IV⁻ to IV⁺	Flexion: fingertips to inferior half of tibia, painless
	Extension: 30 degrees, painless
	Lateral flexion: fingertips to 2 inches above joint line bilaterally, painless
	Ankle jerk: equal bilaterally
	Extensor hallucis longus: status quo

Patient Instruction

Home program of stretching, mobility, and stabilization exercises was reviewed.

TREATMENT 4

Subjective

The patient feels 90% of normal; he has lumbar pain only at the end of the day. He feels stiff in the mornings for 5 minutes. Sitting: 30 to 45 minutes. Walking: unlimited. Standing: unlimited. Shifting: none. The patient has been exercising daily. He will return to work on light duty (supervising and walking around job site) next week.

Objective

1. Flexion: fingertips to inferior one fourth of tibia, clear with gentle overpressure.
2. Extension: 30 degrees, no pain.
3. Lateral flexion: fingertips to 2 inches above joint line bilaterally, clear with overpressure.

4. Left quadrant: 80%, no pain.
5. Right quadrant: 75%, slight pain right lumbar area.
6. SLR: 80 degrees bilaterally, hamstrings stretch, with neck flexion no change.
7. Extensor hallucis longus: left, 5/5; right, 4+/5.
8. Ankle jerk: equal bilaterally.
9. Palpation:
   • Central PA L4–5: local pain only with Grade IV+.
   • Unilateral PA L4,5 L5,S1: local pain with Grade IV++.

Treatment	Reassessment
In right side bend: Central PA L4–5, Grade IV+	Flexion: status quo Extension: status quo Right quadrant: 80%, painless Extensor hallucis longus: status quo

Patient Instruction

Home program and body mechanics were reviewed.

Case #3: Sacroiliac Joint

SUBJECTIVE EXAMINATION

Date

10/15.

Area of Symptoms

See Figure 32–15.

Patient Profile

The patient is a 32-year-old female, 2 months post partum.

Recreational Activities

Walking 20 min/day, still doing so now.

Aggravating Factors

Climbing up curb: increases PSIS pain at left heel strike; eases within 2 minutes.

Walking on flat ground; rolling over in bed: feels left clunk and sharp pain; eases within 1 to 2 minutes of rest on back with knees bent.

Crossing leg with left over right for 15 minutes: gets heaviness/numbness in leg; eases within 3 minutes walking around.

Easing Factors

Heating pad, rubbing area, walking around helps leg symptoms.

24 Hours

Morning: stiff PSIS area for 15 minutes, eases with movement.

Course of day: burning in PSIS area.

End of day: burning in PSIS area.

Special Questions

General health medications, anticoagulants/steroids, weight loss, cord questions, cauda equina: within normal limits.

Tests: none.

History

The patient has had left PSIS pain for about 1 month, with the left leg heaviness/numbness and clunking for 2 weeks. Gradual onset of symptoms with no particular incident. Had some low back pain during pregnancy, but none prior or since. Did not have these symptoms during pregnancy. She feels as if the problem is getting worse because the pain is sharper and she has the leg symptoms and clunking now.

Past History

None for lumbar spine, leg, or hip.

Provisional Assessment

Severity: minimal.

Irritability: minimal.

Nature: sacroiliac joint hypermobility.

Stage: subacute, worsening overall.

OBJECTIVE EXAMINATION

1. Observation: right iliac crest slightly higher than left.
2. Palpation: right PSIS slightly higher than left; right ASIS slightly lower.
3. Quick tests: stepping onto a stool with left leg—pain left PSIS.
4. Piedallu's sign in standing: decreased movement left PSIS.
5. Piedallu's sign in sitting: results status quo.
6. Lumbar clearing tests:
   • Flexion: within normal limits.
   • Extension: within normal limits.
   • Quadrant: within normal limits bilaterally.
7. Neurological tests: within normal limits.
   • SLR, left: 80 degrees.
   • SLR, right: 90 degrees.
   • Passive neck flexion: within normal limits.
   • Prone knee bend: within normal limits.
8. Hip clearing tests:
   • Left flexion/adduction/internal rotation/compression: reproduces pain left PSIS.
   • Right: within normal limits.
9. Palpation:
   • Central PA L5: local pain with Grade IV+.
   • Central PA S2–S3: tender with Grade IV.
   • Unilateral PA left PSIS: tender with Grade IV.
   • Transverse PA left sacroiliac joint: thick, painful with Grade IV−.
   • PA sacrum: reproduces left PSIS pain with Grade IV.

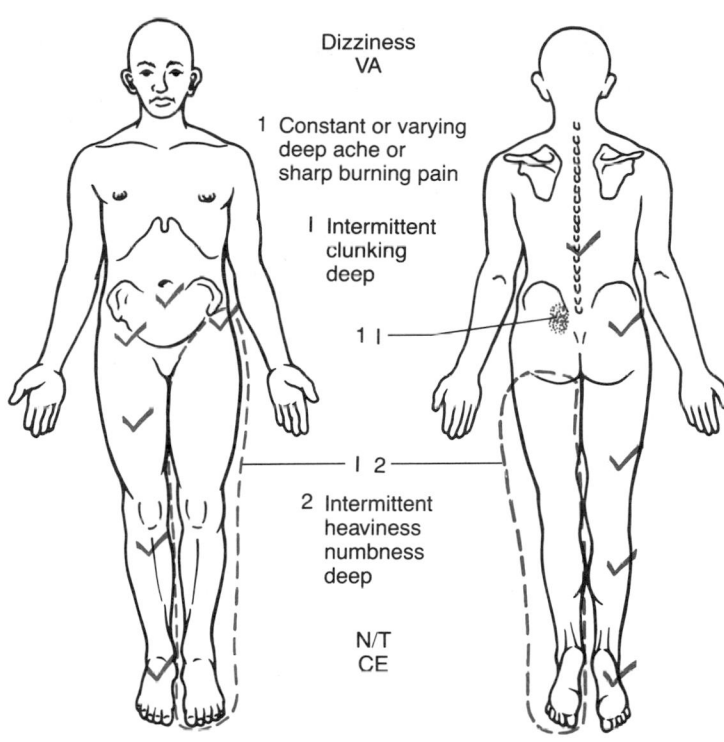

FIGURE 32–15 Case study 3: area of symptoms.

Treatment	Reassessment
1. PA L5, Grade IV⁺	Quick test: status quo
	Piedallu's sign: status quo
	Flexion/adduction/internal rotation/compression: status quo
	SLR: status quo
2. Same, three times	Status quo

Patient Instruction

The patient was instructed in proper body mechanics for bending and lifting.

TREATMENT 2

Subjective

The patient did not feel any differently that evening or the next morning after treatment. All subjective asterisks are status quo.

Objective

1. Quick tests: step stool with left PSIS pain.
2. Flexion/adduction/internal rotation/compression: left PSIS pain.
3. Palpation:
   • PA L5: painless with Grade IV⁺⁺.
   • PA S2–S3: tender with Grade IV.
   • Unilateral PA left PSIS: tender with Grade IV.
   • Unilateral PA left sacroiliac joint: thick and tender with Grade IV.

• Transverse pressure left sacroiliac joint: reproduces left PSIS pain with Grade IV.

Treatment	Reassessment
1. PA sacrum, Grade IV	Hip flexion/adduction/internal rotation/compression: within normal limits
	Quick test: decreased pain
	SLR, left: 85 degrees
	Piedallu's sign: status quo
2. PA sacrum, Grade IV, two times	Status quo

TREATMENT 3

Subjective

Following the last treatment, the patient felt decreased leg symptoms with crossing legs. She walked 20 minutes with less sharp pain when stepping onto curb. Clunking was the same; turning over in bed was the same.

Objective

1. Piedallu's sign: decreased mobility left.
2. SLR, left: 90 degrees.
3. SLR, right: 85 degrees.
4. Quick test: slight pain right PSIS.

5. Palpation:
- PA sacrum: painless with Grade IV^{++}.
- PA S2–3: local tender with Grade IV^{++}.
- Unilateral PA left sacroiliac joint: local pain with Grade IV^{+}.
- Unilateral PA left PSIS: local pain with Grade IV^{+}.
- Transverse pressure left sacroiliac joint: with Grade IV reproduces left PSIS pain.

Treatment	Reassessment
1. Transverse pressure left sacroiliac joint, Grades IV$^-$ to IV	Piedallu's sign: increased mobility left
	Quick test: slight pain only
	SLR: status quo
2. Same, two times	Piedallu's sign: 80% equal mobility
	Quick test: painless
	SLR, right: 90 degrees

TREATMENT 4

Subjective

After last session, the patient felt much better. She had no heaviness in the leg. She had only slight pain stepping onto curb. She had clunking only three times. Overall, she feels 80% improved.

Objective

1. Piedallu's sign: 80% equal mobility.
2. Quick test: painless.
3. Hop on left foot: pain left PSIS.
4. SLR: 90 degrees bilaterally.
5. Palpation:
- PA sacrum: painless with Grade IV^{++}.
- PA S2–3: painless with Grade IV^{++}.
- Transverse pressure left sacroiliac joint: reproduces left PSIS pain with Grade IV.
- PA left PSIS: slight pain with Grade IV^{++}.
- Unilateral PA left sacroiliac joint: decreased thickness and tenderness with Grade IV^{+}.

Treatment	Reassessment
1. Transverse left sacroiliac joint, Grade IV, three times	Piedallu's sign: 90% equal mobility
	Hop on left foot: decreased pain
2. Same, two times	Piedallu's sign: equal mobility
	Hop on left foot: painless

Patient Instruction

Body mechanics and stabilization and stretching exercises were reviewed.

References

1. Panjabi MM, Takata K, Goel V, et al.: Thoracic human vertebrae. Quantitative three-dimensional anatomy. *Spine* 1991, 16:888–901.
2. White AA, Panjabi MM: *Clinical Biomechanics of the Spine.* Philadelphia, J. B. Lippincott Company, 1990, p 31.
3. Armstrong JR: *Lumbar Disc Lesions.* Edinburgh, Churchill Livingstone, 1965, p 13.
4. Taylor JR: The development and adult structure of lumbar intervertebral discs. *J Man Med* 1990, 5:43–47.
5. Hickey DS, Hukins SWL: X-ray diffraction studies of the arrangement of collagen fibres in human fetal intervertebral disc. *J Anat* 1980, 131:81–90.
6. Hickey DS, Hukins DWL: Relation between the structure of the annulus fibrosus and the function and failure of the intervertebral disc. *Spine* 1980, 5:100–116.
7. Jayson MIV, Barks JS: Structural changes in the intervertebral disc. *Ann Rheum Dis* 1973, 32:10–15.
8. Peacock A: Observations on the prenatal development of the intervertebral disc in man. *J Anat* 1951, 85:260–274.
9. Heylings DJA: Supraspinous and interspinous ligaments of the human spine. *J Anat* 1978, 125:127–131.
10. Rissanen PM: The surgical anatomy and pathology of the supraspinous and interspinous ligaments of the lumbar spine with special reference to ligament ruptures. *Acta Orthop Scand Suppl* 1960, 46:1–100.
11. Bogduk N, Twomey LT: *Clinical Anatomy of the Lumbar Spine.* New York, Churchill Livingstone, 1991, p 40.
12. Walker JM: The sacroiliac joint: a critical review. *Phys Ther* 1992, 72:903–916.
13. Warwick R, Williams PI: *Gray's Anatomy.* London, Churchill Livingstone, 1980, p 473.
14. Maitland GD: *Vertebral Manipulation,* 5th ed. London, Butterworth Publishers, 1986.
15. Vollowitz E, personal communication.
16. Grieve GP: Common patterns of clinical presentation. In *Common Vertebral Joint Problems.* New York, Churchill Livingstone, 1988, pp 355–457.
17. Boissonnault WG: *Examination in Physical Therapy Practice: Screening for Medical Disease.* New York, Churchill Livingstone, 1991.
18. Butler DS: *Mobilization of the Nervous System.* Melbourne, Churchill Livingstone, 1991.
19. Wells P: The examination of the pelvic joints. In Grieve GP (ed): *Modern Manual Therapy of the Vertebral Column.* New York, Churchill Livingstone, 1986.
20. Edgelow PI: *A Patient's Guide to Treatment of Thoracic Outlet Syndrome,* Available from Peter Edgelow.
21. Donnattelli R, Wooden MJ: *Orthopedic Physical Therapy.* New York, Churchill Livingstone, 1989.
22. Home Exercises, Available from Peter Edgelow.
23. Home Exercises, Available from Peter Edgelow.
24. Home Exercises, Available from Peter Edgelow.
25. Video Tape 1, Available from Peter Edgelow.
26. Video Tape 2, Available from Peter Edgelow.

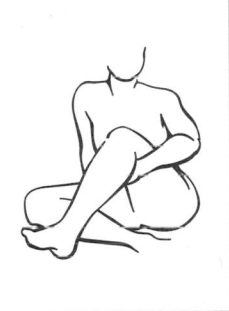

CHAPTER 33

Lower Extremity: Hip

Suzanne P. Hicklin and Miriam C. DePretis

The purpose of this chapter is to assist the clinician in the ability to make clinical decisions regarding the management of a patient with hip pain based on anatomy, biomechanics, critical observation skills, differential diagnosis, and treatments of choice.

Throughout the evaluation and treatment phases, the therapist must appreciate the interrelationship between the hip, sacroiliac joint, and lumbar spine. The hip joint plays an integral role in the facilitation of the body's movement through space in a controlled and efficient pattern. Therefore, if hip joint pathology exists, it is often seen with gait deviations or difficulty with household tasks and/or activities of daily living.

I. Anatomy

A. Structure

The hip is a ball-and-socket triaxial joint with spherical articulating surfaces.

1. **Bones** The ilium, ischium, and pubis form the acetabulum or socket of the joint. The head of the femur is considered the ball or sphere (see Figure 33–1).

   a. *Angle of torsion.* This is an approximately 15-degree angle formed by the neck of the femur and the transverse axis of the femoral condyles. An increased torsion angle causes excessive anteversion of the hip; a decreased angle is called retroversion (see Figure 33–2).

   b. *Angle of inclination.* This angle is formed

955

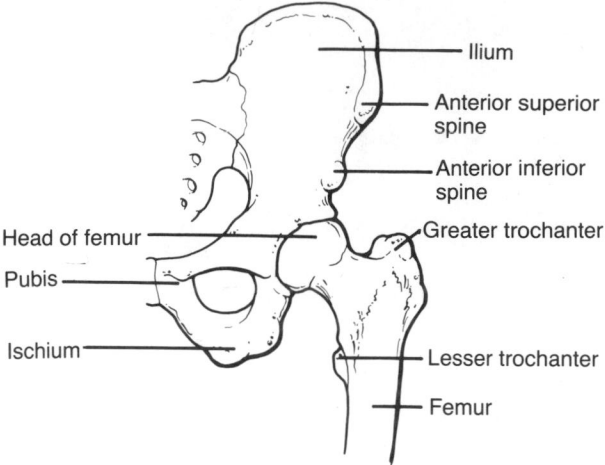

FIGURE 33–1   Structural components of the hip joint.

by the neck and shaft of the femur in the frontal plane. In children, the angle is approximately 150 degrees; it decreases to 125 degrees in adults. An increased degree of inclination in the hip is referred to as coxa valga; a decreased angle is called coxa vara. (These disorders are discussed later.)

c. ***Trabecular bone structure.*** The trabecular pattern of the hip joint is designed to withstand the normal forces of tension and compression. Three systems constitute the upper portion of the femur:

(1). The arcuate bundle runs from the lateral cortex and curves upward around the inferior border of the neck of the femur.

(2). The medial system runs relatively

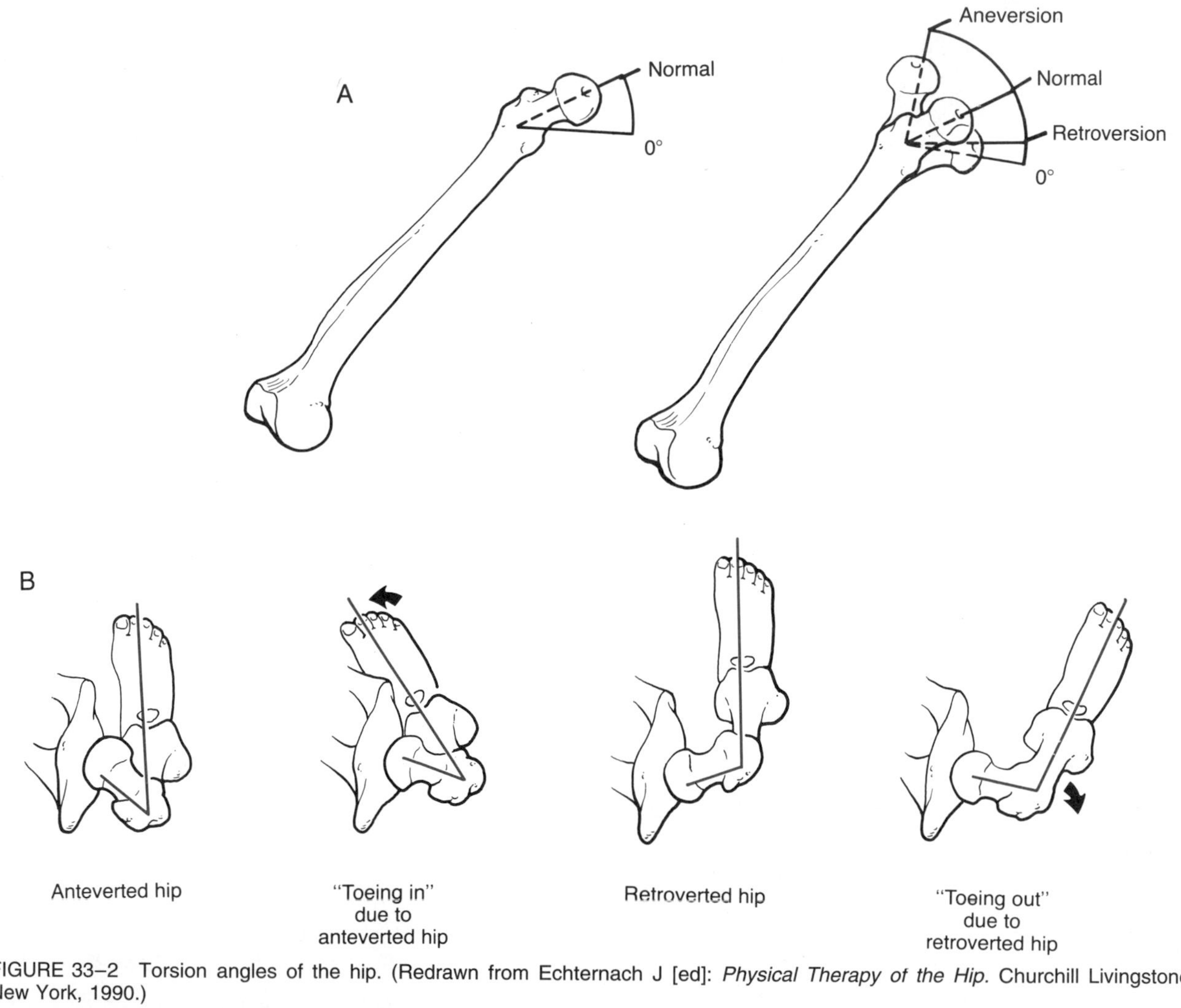

FIGURE 33–2   Torsion angles of the hip. (Redrawn from Echternach J [ed]: *Physical Therapy of the Hip.* Churchill Livingstone, New York, 1990.)

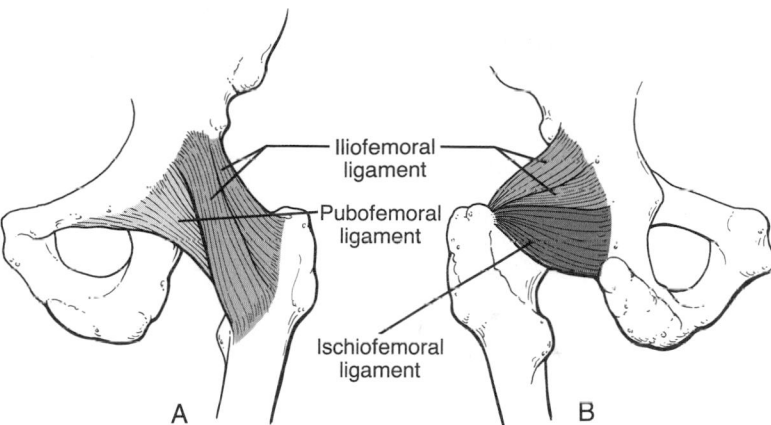

FIGURE 33–3 Ligamentous support of the hip joint. **A,** Anterior view. **B,** Posterior view.

straight from the medial cortex of the neck of the femur to the superior region of the head of the femur.

(3). The lateral system is weakest and runs between the lesser and the greater trochanters.

2. **Noncontractile tissues**
   a. *Capsule.* The hip joint has a strong articulating capsule that is reinforced by powerful ligaments anteriorly and posteriorly. The capsule encompasses the acetabulum and labrum and stretches to just proximal to the introchanteric crest. Thus, the neck of the femur is intracapsular.
   b. *Major ligaments* (see Figure 33–3)
      (1). Anteriorly, the iliofemoral ligament, one of the strongest ligaments in the body, checks internal rotation and extension. The ligament runs from the lower portion of the anteroinferior iliac spine (AIIS), with a slip to a portion of the ilium, to the superior and posterosuperior rim of the acetabulum.
      (2). The pubofemoral ligament tightens during abduction and helps check internal rotation. It attaches to the pubis, near the acetabulum, and runs to the lesser trochanter.
      (3). Posteriorly, the ischiofemoral ligament also checks internal rotation and extension. The ligament runs from an area of ischium posteroinferior to the rim of the acetabulum upward to the posterosuperior neck of the femur.

PLEASE NOTE: The ligaments lie in a clockwise position. Therefore, extension of the hip winds the ligaments around the neck of the femur and flexion unwinds them.

   c. *Bursae.* One or more trochanteric bursae lie over the greater trochanter. Bursae reduce friction between the gluteus medius muscle and the trochanter and are most extensive posterolateral to the trochanter.
      (1). Iliopectineal bursa overlies the anterior aspect of the hip joint just below the iliopsoas muscle.
      (2). Ischial bursa is found between the ischial tuberosity and the gluteus maximus.

3. **Contracticle tissues and muscles.** The muscles surrounding the hip capsule and their origin, insertion, and innervation are summarized in Tables 33–1 to 33–3. See Figure 33–4 for illustrations of the musculature.

4. **Major nerves.** Three nerves are of particular importance secondary to their involvement in hip pathology:
   a. *Sciatic nerve.* Irritation of this nerve may cause hip pain or sensory changes along the lateral and posterior portion of the leg and the dorsal and plantar surfaces of the foot. Prolonged irritation and entrapment may also cause progressive weakness in the hamstring muscles, a portion of the adductor magnus, and muscles of the leg and foot.
   b. *Obturator nerve.* Irritation of this nerve may cause referred pain and sensory changes along the medial thigh or knee.

Table 33–1. MUSCLES OF FLEXION AND EXTENSION AND THEIR INNERVATION, ORIGINS, AND INSERTIONS

	Innervation	Origin	Insertion
Muscles of flexion			
Psoas	Lumbar plexus L1,L2,L3,L4	Transverse processes and bodies T12–L4	Lesser trochanter
Iliacus	Femoral L2,L3	Iliac crest and fossa	Lesser trochanter
Sartorius	Femoral L2,L3	ASIS	Proximal medial tibia
Rectus femoris	Femoral L2,L3,L4	AIIS	Patella and patellar tendon into tibial tubercle
Gracilis	Obturator L2,L3,L4	Body and inferior portion of pubic ramus	Medial surface—proximal tibia
Adductor longus	Obturator L2,L3,L4	Anterior body of pubis below pubic tubercle	Linea aspera
Adductor brevis	Obturator L2,L3,L4	Body and inferior ramus of pubis	Proximal linea aspera
Pectineus	Femoral L2,L3	Pectineal of pubis	Pectineal line—posterior femur
Muscles of extension			
Gluteus maximus	Inferior gluteal L5,S1,S2	Posterior ilium and posterior gluteal line	Gluteal tuberosity and iliotibial tract
Semimembranosus	Sciatic L5,S1,S2	Posterolateral ischial tuberosity	Medial aspect—tibial body
Semitendinosus	Sciatic L5,S1,S2	Ischial tuberosity	Medial aspect—tibial body
Biceps femoris	Sciatic L5,S1,S2	Ischial tuberosity	Fibular head and lateral tibial condyle

c. *Femoral nerve.* Injury to this nerve is relatively uncommon; however, irritation may cause decreased sensation along the anterior and medial aspect of the thigh.

5. **Blood supply.** Primary vascularization to the head of the femur is derived from medial and lateral circumflex arteries (see Figure 33–5). Branches of these arteries form a ring surrounding the base of the femoral neck. The capsule receives its blood supply from branches of the arterial ring that enter through the capsule at its distal attachment to the femur and continue to run intracapsularly along the neck of the femur. Branches of the extracapsular ring supply the greater and lesser trochanter.

B. Biomechanics

1. **Functional stability.** The unique anatomy of the hip provides intrinsic stability. It includes the deep acetabulum and form-fitting

Table 33–2. MUSCLES OF ABDUCTION AND ADDUCTION AND THEIR INNERVATION, ORIGINS, AND INSERTIONS

	Innervation	Origin	Insertion
Muscles of abduction			
Gluteus medius	Superior gluteal L4,L5,S1	Ilium, posterior and anterior gluteal lines	Greater trochanter
Gluteus minimus	Superior gluteal L4,L5,S1	Ilium, anterior and inferior gluteal lines	Great trochanter
Tensor fasciae latae	Superior gluteal L4,L5,S1	ASIS and anterior iliac crest	Iliotibial tract
Sartorius	Femoral L2,L3	ASIS	Proximal medial tibia
Muscles of adduction			
Adductor longus	Obturator L2,L3,L4	Anterior body of pubis below pubic tubercle	Linea aspera
Adductor magnus	Obturator L2,L3,L4	Inferior pubic ramus, ischial ramus and tuberosity	Linea aspera and adductor tubercle
Adductor brevis	Obturator L2,L3,L4	Body and inferior ramus of pubis	Proximal linea aspera
Gracilis	Obturator L2,L3,L4	Body and inferior portion of pubic ramus	Medial surface—proximal tibia
Pectineus	Femoral L2,L3	Pectineal of pubis	Pectineal line—posterior femur
Gluteus maximus	Inferior gluteal L5,S1,S2	Posterior ilium and posterior gluteal line	Gluteal tuberosity and iliotibial tract

Table 33–3. MUSCLES OF EXTERNAL AND INTERNAL ROTATION AND THEIR INNERVATION, ORIGINS, AND INSERTIONS

	Innervation	Origin	Insertion
Muscles of external rotation			
Piriformis	Sacral plexus L5,S1,S2	Anterior surface of sacrum bodies of S2–S4	Greater trochanter
Obturator internus	Sacral plexus L5,S1,S2	Obturator membrane—internal surface	Trochanteric fossa
Obturator externus	Obturator L2,L3,L4	Obturator membrane and bones of obturator foramen	Trochanteric fossa
Gemellus superior	Sacral plexus L5,S1,S2	Ischial spine	Trochanteric fossa
Gemellus inferior	Sacral plexus L5,S1,S2	Superior aspect of ischial tuberosity	Greater trochanter
Quadrate femoris	Sacral plexus L5,S1,S2	Lateral aspect of ischial tuberosity	Quadrate tubercle
Sartorius	Femoral L2,L3	ASIS	Proximal medial tibia
Gluteus maximus	Inferior gluteal L5,S1,S2	Posterior ilium and posterior gluteal line	Gluteal tuberosity and iliotibial tract
Muscles of internal rotation			
Adductor magnus	Obturator L2,L3,L4	Inferior pubic ramus, ischial ramus and tuberosity	Linea aspera and adductor tubercle
Pectineus	Femoral L2,L3	Pectineal of pubis	Pectineal line—posterior femur
Gluteus minimus	Superior gluteal L4,L5,S1	Ilium, anterior and inferior gluteal lines	Greater trochanter
Gracilis	Obturator L2,L3,L4	Body and inferior portion of pubic ramus	Medial surface—proximal tibia

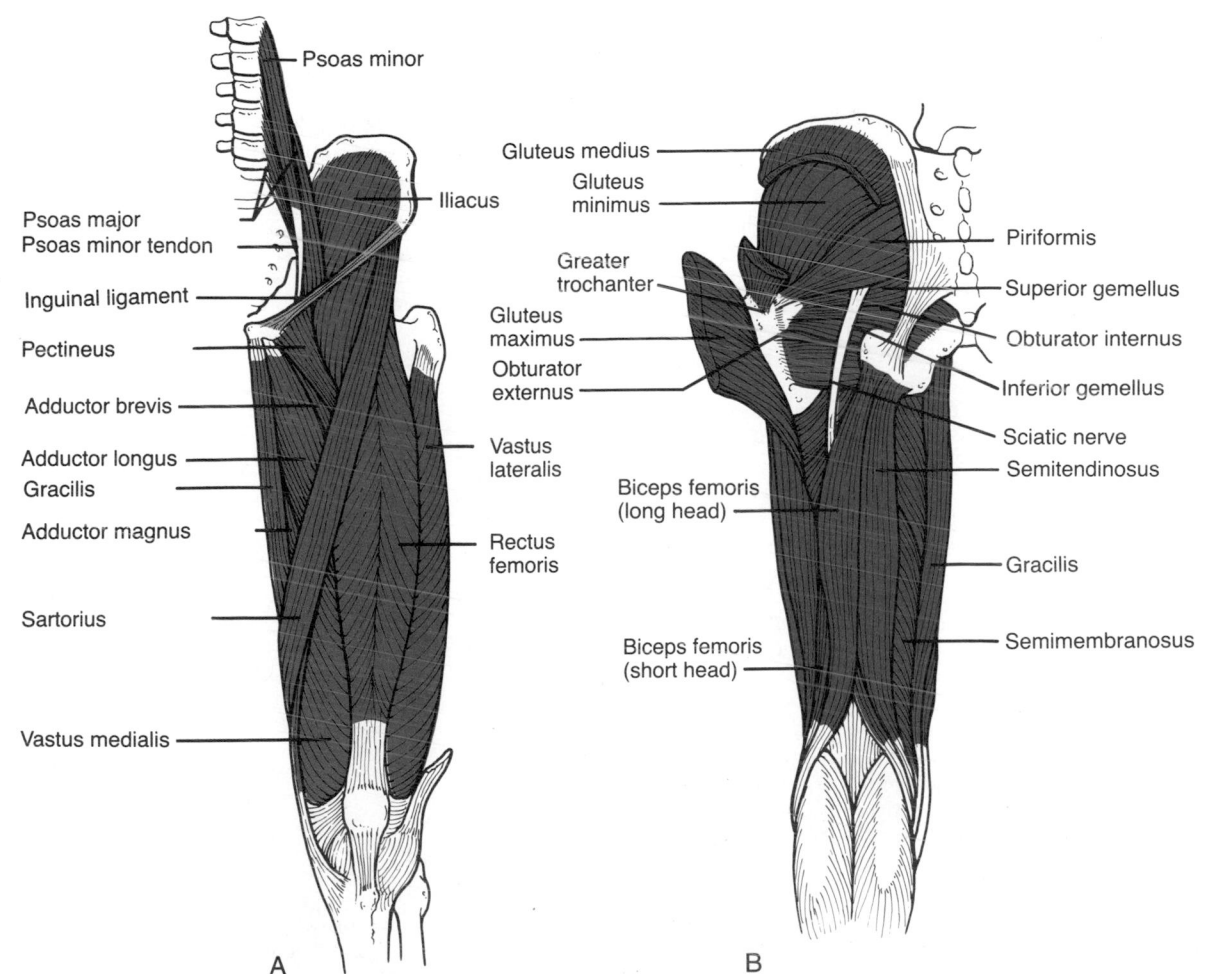

FIGURE 33–4 **A,** Anterior view of hip and thigh musculature. **B,** Posterior view of hip musculature.

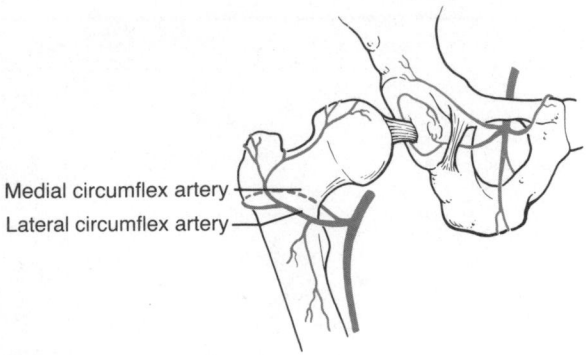

FIGURE 33–5 Blood supply to the head of the femur and surrounding capsule.

Medial circumflex artery
Lateral circumflex artery

Table 33–4. LIMITING STRUCTURES

Flexion	Anterior soft tissues
	Posterior capsule
Extension	Iliofemoral ligament
	Pubofemoral ligament
	Ischiofemoral ligament
Abduction	Adductor muscles
	Pubofemoral ligament
	Ischiofemoral ligament
Adduction	Abductor muscles
	Iliofemoral ligament
External rotation	Iliofemoral ligament
	Pubofemoral ligament
Internal rotation	Ischiofemoral ligament
	External rotator muscles

femoral head, a thick articulating capsule, a vacuum effect caused by coaptation of joint surfaces, ligamentous support, and muscular balance. Dynamic stability is provided by muscular balance seen in gait and is therefore an important consideration for the physical therapist.

BIOMECHANICS OF SINGLE-LEG STANCE

One example of the functional stability of the hip is seen in single-leg stance. "First, single-limb support occurs twice with every stride and therefore happens thousands of times a day in the normal individual. Second, analysis of forces sustained by a subject in a single-limb stance allows the reader to appreciate the significant loads the hip endures during a relatively sedate activity. Further analysis can provide a perspective of the enormous loads that the hip must sustain in such vigorous activities as running or jumping."[1]

The biomechanics of single-leg stance can be understood by visualizing the hip abductor muscles of the weight-bearing side, which must counter the large force created by the increased length of the moment arm. Counterforce occurs at the greater trochanter, which is closer to the femoral head (fulcrum) than the center of gravity line, which represents the force produced by the body weight (see Figure 33–6). Because the lever arm distance for the abductor's force is about one half of the ordinary distance, the abductors's pull must be at least two times body weight to prevent the pelvis from dropping. The force acting at the hip during single-limb stance is equal to the sum of the force of the abductor pull plus the force of the body weight, up to three times the body weight.[2] Under normal circumstances, the femoral head can withstand forces up to 12 to 15 times body weight without episode of fracture.[3]

2. **Functional mobility.** Although stability is an important function of the hip, the hip's unique structure allows for mobility without sacrificing stability.
   a. *Hip joint motion.* Ligaments around the joint limit excessive motion; the muscles in each plane may limit motion secondary to abnormal tightness (see Table 33–4).
   b. *Requirements for activity.* To establish realistic goals, the therapist must know the

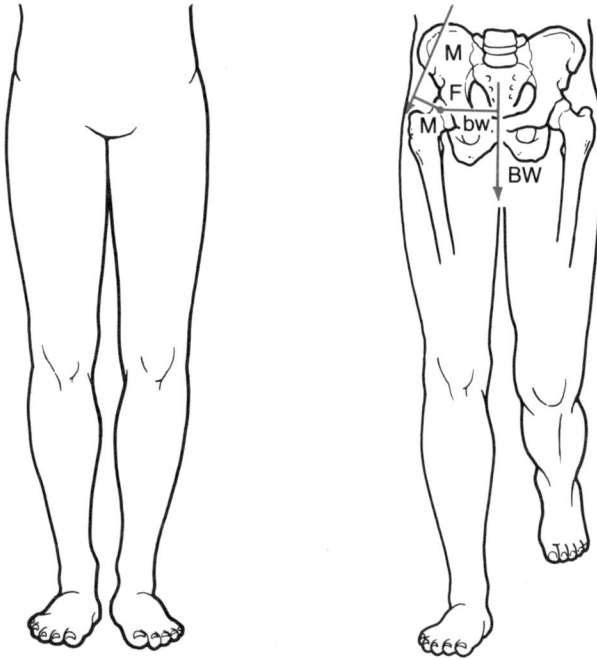

FIGURE 33–6 Hip abductor muscle force associated with single-leg stance. *Abbreviations:* BW = body weight; bw = lever arm for bodyweight force; f = center of femoral head (fulcrum); M = hip abductor force; m = lever arm for muscle force.

ranges of motion needed at the hip for certain tasks. The following mean degrees of motion have been documented in normal men:

(1). Walking:[4]
    (a). Extension: 15 degrees.
    (b). Flexion: 37 degrees.
    (c). Abduction: 7 degrees.
    (d). Adduction: 5 degrees.
    (e). Internal rotation: 4 degrees.
    (f). External rotation: 9 degrees.

(2). Tying shoe:
    (a). Flexion: 129 degrees.
    (b). Abduction: 18 degrees.
    (c). External rotation: 13 degrees.

(3). Stooping:
    (a). Flexion: 125 degrees.
    (b). Abduction: 21 degrees.
    (c). External rotation: 15 degrees.

(4). Ascending stairs:[5]
    (a). Flexion: 67 degrees.

(5). Descending stairs:[5]
    (a). Flexion: 36 degrees.

3. **Associated pelvic motions.**[6] Two hip joints are linked together through the pelvis and lumbosacral joint. The motion of the hip joint will cause other associated movement (see Figure 33–7).

a. *Anterior pelvic tilt.* This results in hip flexion and increased lumbar spine extension. The muscles involved are primarily the iliopsoas and the back extensors.

b. *Posterior pelvic tilt.* This results in hip extension and lumbar spine flexion. The muscles involved are the hip extensors and the rectus abdominis.

c. *Lateral pelvic tilt.* This results in hip adduction (hip hiking) on the elevated side and hip abduction (hip drop) on the opposite hip. The muscles involved are the quadratus lumborum on the side of the elevated pelvis and the gluteus medius

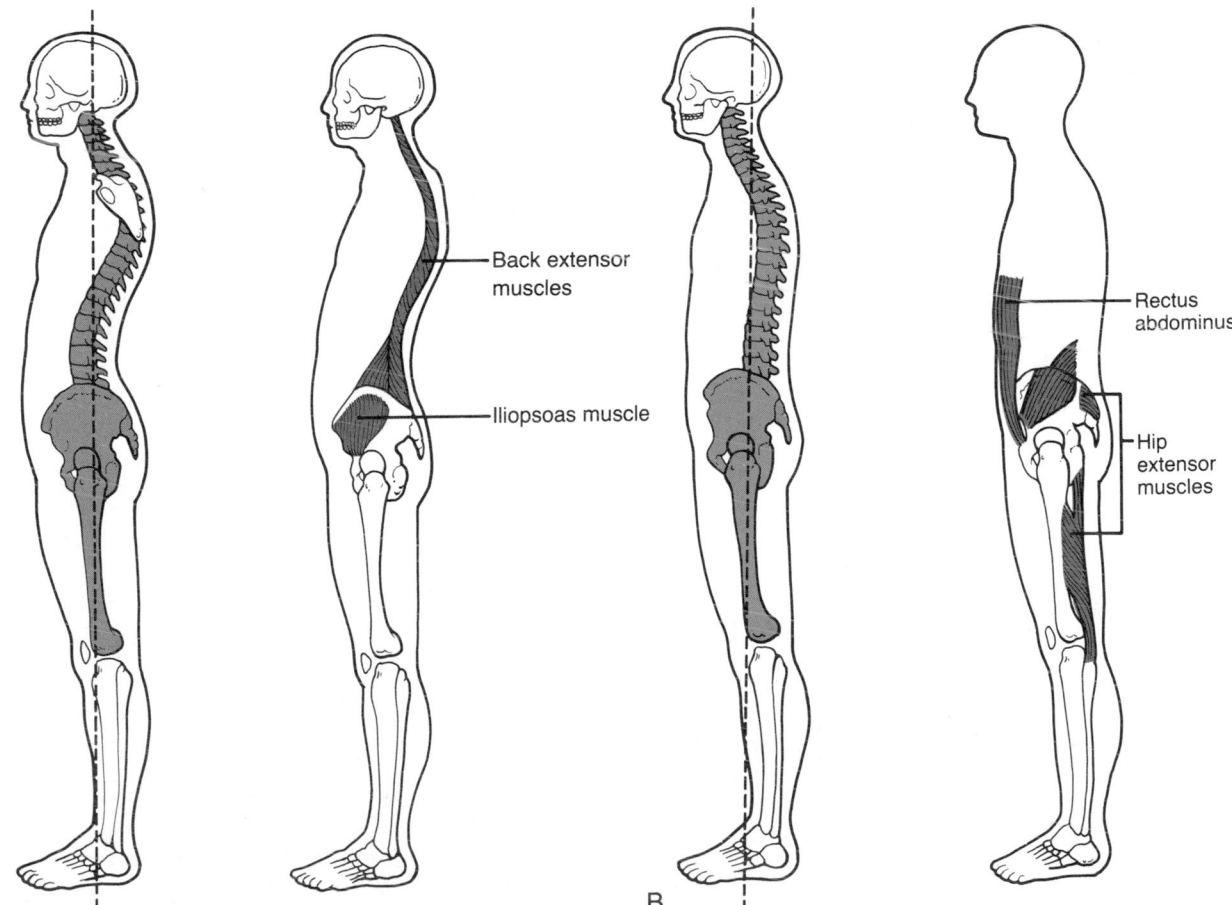

FIGURE 33–7   Associated pelvic motions. **A,** Anterior pelvic tilt. **B,** Posterior pelvic tilt.

acting with a reverse pull on the side of the lowered pelvis.

d. *Pelvic rotation.* This results in movement of the pelvis and unsupported extremity in the same direction. Forward movement of the unsupported leg results in forward rotation of the pelvis. Simultaneously, the femur on the stance leg rotates internally and the trunk rotates in the opposite direction.

II. Examination

A. History

The importance of the subjective portion of the evaluation should not be minimized. A thorough patient interview frequently provides enough information to establish a tentative diagnosis before clinical examination. The following information should be included during this portion of the examination:

1. Onset of symptoms.

2. Nature and location of symptoms.

3. Description of symptoms.

4. Change in symptoms since onset.

5. Previous history of similar symptoms (if yes, then previous treatment if any).

6. Thorough past medical and surgical history.

7. List of diagnostic tests that may have been performed and location of results.

8. Previous functional or activity level.

9. Effect, if any, symptoms have on present functional level.

10. Patient's occupation and age.

11. Present medications.

B. Physical examination

1. **Observation.** The examiner should begin to critically observe the patient from the point of initial introduction. Gross assessment of transfer status and gait can be achieved even before formal evaluation begins.
   a. *Gait.* The patient should be observed as he/she walks to the examination room. Special notice should be taken of weight bearing, step length, presence of a limp, use of assistive devices, etc. (A thorough review of gait dysfunction associated with hip pathology is presented later.)
   b. *Posture.* Gross postural asymmetries should be noted first, including pelvic levels and any obvious leg-length difference.

2. **Inspection.** The examiner looks for symmetry with the following bony and soft-tissue landmarks: anterosuperioriliac spine (ASIS), posterosuperior iliac spine (PSIS), iliac crests, greater trochanters, ischial tuberosities, gluteal folds, and popliteal creases. The examiner should also note the presence or absence of excessive hip rotation, genu varum or valgum, tibial torsion, and foot pronation or supination. Finally, any observable muscle atrophy, unusual swelling, or skin discoloration must be noted.

3. **Movement assessment**
   a. *Active.* Active range of motion (AROM) should be measured bilaterally. This should be compared with the uninvolved side and normal values. The examiner should also make note of the patient's willingness to move.
      (1). Normal range of motion (ROM) for the hip joint is as follows:
         (a). Flexion: 0 to 125 degrees, supine.
         (b). Extension: 0 to 10 degrees, prone.
         (c). Abduction: 0 to 45 degrees, supine.
         (d). Adduction: 0 to 15 degrees, supine.
         (e). External rotation: 0 to 45 degrees, prone or sitting.
         (f). Internal rotation: 0 to 40 degrees, prone or sitting.
   b. *Passive*
      (1). *Physiological.* Passive movement tests provide the examiner with information about full available motion and the end-feel. Normal end-feel for all hip motions is capsular or soft-tissue

approximation. Crepitus, snapping, and any other abnormal joint sounds will be appreciated during this portion of the evaluation.

    (2). *Joint play.* Three accessory motions are available at the hip joint: compression, distraction, and lateral distraction. Because of tight ligamentous support and large soft-tissue bulk, these motions can be quite difficult to assess. Joint play movements should be assessed and compared bilaterally.

  c. ***Resistive.*** Following active and passive movement tests, all movements should be tested against resistance to determine strength and to assess any symptoms that may be elicited with resistive movement. Careful attention should be given to proper positioning and stabilization to produce accurate results.

4. **Palpation.** Palpation of bony landmarks is accomplished during the inspection portion of the evaluation. The examiner should now palpate the soft tissues. Careful palpation will identify presence of muscle spasm, swelling, masses, or any unusually tender areas. It is important for the patient to remain relaxed during this portion of the examination.

5. **Special tests.** A number of special tests may reveal additional information about associated pathology. It is not necessary to perform all tests, only those that are appropri-

ate on the basis of the suspected pathology and clinical findings.

  a. ***Thomas test***
    (1). Purpose: To identify tightness of the iliopsoas muscle.
    (2). Test position: The patient is seated, with the thighs midway over the edge of the table. He/she is instructed to grasp one leg and pull it toward the chest while lying back on the table. The examiner assists by placing one hand on the back and the other hand under the patient's thigh (see Figure 33–8*A*). The position of the pelvis must be closely monitored to achieve full reduction of lumbar lordosis without creating a posterior pelvic tilt. The patient is asked to maintain this position[7] (see Figure 33–8*B*).
    (3). Positive result: If the opposite leg will not lie flat without overpressure, the angle between the thigh and the table should be measured. This represents the degree of hip flexor muscle tightness. If the addition of hip abduction allows the leg to lie flat, the tightness of the tensor fascia latae may be the cause. Ober's test should be performed.

  b. ***Two-joint hip flexor tightness test***
    (1). Purpose: To identify tightness of the two-joint hip flexor muscles.
    (2). Test position: Same as for Thomas test.

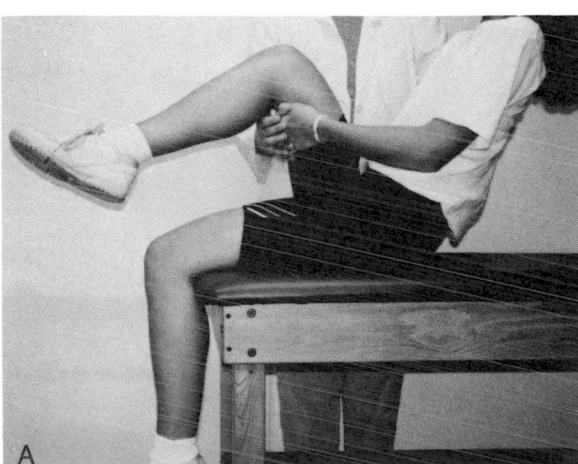 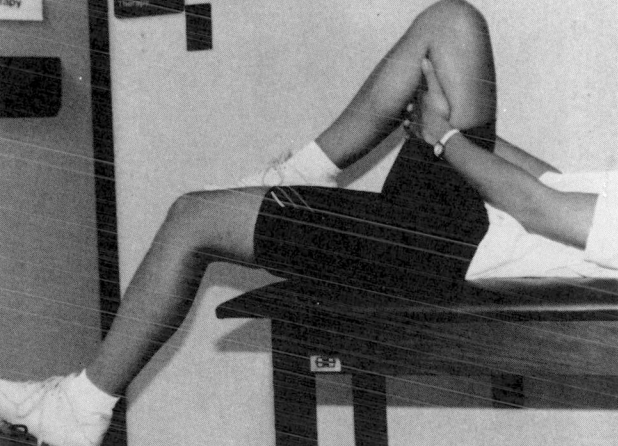

FIGURE 33–8 **A,** Thomas test starting position. **B,** End position demonstrating hip flexor muscle tightness.

(3). Positive result: At the conclusion of the Thomas test, the examiner should allow the patient's knee to flex. If the hip flexes passively while the knee is being flexed, this indicates a tightness of hip flexor muscles, which cross both hip and knee joints. Normal muscle length should allow for 80 degrees of knee flexion in this position.

c. **Quadrant or scouring test**
  (1). Purpose: To identify specific areas of the joint that may be causing symptoms.
  (2). Test position: The patient is placed supine. The examiner takes the hip into full flexion with the knee flexed. While the examiner places a compressive force through the long axis of the femur, the hip is slowly taken through full range of abduction and adduction while maintaining the flexion.
  (3). Positive result: Reproducible pain at a specific point in motion. This may indicate joint surface irregularities.

d. **Ober's test**
  (1). Purpose: To identify tightness in the iliotibial band.
  (2). Test position: The patient is placed sidelying with pelvis and shoulders perpendicular to the table. (The trunk should lie flat against the table or be supported with a towel roll to maintain a neutral position of the pelvis.) The examiner grasps the patient's upper leg, with the knee supported in 90 degrees of flexion. The upper leg is lifted into full abduction followed by hyperextension (see Figure 33–9). Care must be taken to maintain neutral hip rotation. The leg is lowered toward the table without allowing flexion or rotation.[7]
  (3). Positive result: The leg cannot be lowered to the table. Gentle rotation of the limb will usually produce a visible or palpable snapping as the taut iliotibial band is forced over the greater trochanter.

e. **Sacroiliac gap and compression test**
  (1). Purpose: To screen the sacroiliac joint.
  (2). Test position: The patient is placed supine. The examiner provides compression in an inward direction over both halves of the pelvis, putting pressure over the lateral anterosuperior portion of the iliac crests. This is followed by placing pressure in an outward direction from the medial anterosuperior iliac crests.
  (3). Positive result: The patient reports discomfort in the sacroiliac joint while force is being applied in either direction. This indicates that there is a need to further evaluate the sacroiliac joint. This test is important in a hip evaluation because the sacroiliac joint may refer pain to the hip region.

f. **Fabere or Patrick's test**
  (1). Purpose: To identify possible sacroiliac joint involvement or hip flexor and internal rotator tightness.
  (2). Test position: The patient is placed supine. The leg to be tested is placed in a position of hip flexion, with the foot placed on the opposite knee. The knee is lowered laterally so that the hip assumes a position of flexion, abduction, and external rotation.
  (3). Positive result: The knee does not passively fall to the level of the other leg. This may indicate tightness of the hip flexors or internal rotators. It is more indicative of sacroiliac joint dysfunction if gentle overpressure produces pain in the sacroiliac joint region.

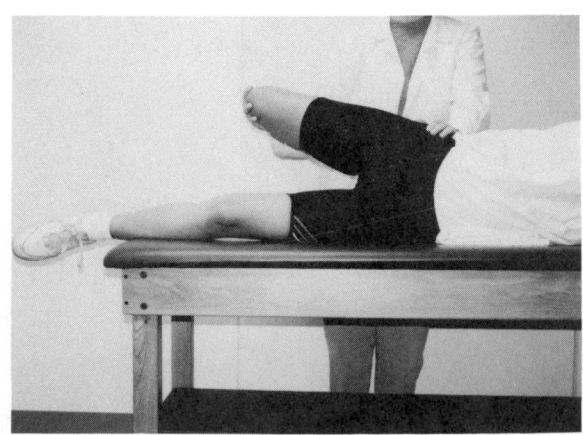

FIGURE 33–9   Ober's test position.

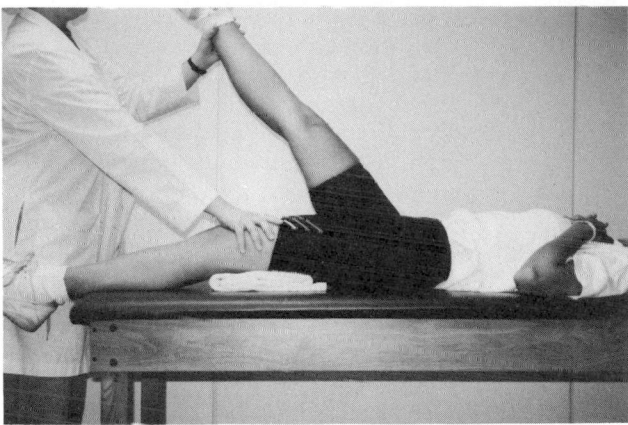

FIGURE 33–10 Straight-leg raise test position.

g. *Straight-leg raise*
   (1). Purpose: In addition to determining nerve root irritation, this test can be used to determine hamstring length.
   (2). Test position: The patient is placed supine. The pelvis should be in a neutral position. If the patient is unable to achieve this because of hip flexor tightness, a towel roll should be placed under the opposite thigh to allow flattening of the low back. The examiner lifts the patient's leg while the knee is maintained in full extension. (The patient may assist.) The other leg should be held down to stabilize the pelvis (see Figure 33–10). The end point is reached when the patient reports discomfort.[7]
   (3). Positive result: The leg is held in this position by the examiner and a goniometric measurement is taken of the hip angle. Normal hamstring length should allow 80 degrees of hip flexion.

h. *Tripod sign*
   (1). Purpose: To assess hamstring length.
   (2). Test position: The patient sits upright, with the pelvis level and the legs over the side of the plinth. The examiner passively extends one knee while observing the pelvis.
   (3). Positive result: The test is positive for tightness of hamstrings if the

pelvis is pulled into posterior tilt as the knee is extended.

i. *Femoral nerve stretch*
   (1). Purpose: To assess femoral nerve irritation secondary to tightness in surrounding structures.
   (2). Test position: The patient is placed prone, with one knee in 90 degrees of flexion. The examiner passively lifts the thigh while maintaining knee flexion.
   (3). Positive result: The patient experiences symptoms in the anterior thigh.

j. *Leg-length measurement*
   (1). Purpose: To determine an actual leg-length discrepancy.
   (2). Test position: The patient is placed supine, with the pelvis in a level position. The pelvis must be level before measurements are taken if results are to be accurate. The legs must be placed in an equivalent position in relation to the pelvis. If contracture is present in one leg, the other leg must be placed in identical relative position. Measurements are taken with a tape measure from the ASIS to the lateral malleolus. (The medial malleolus may also be used; however, if a significant amount of muscle atrophy is present, measurements to the lateral malleolus will yield more accurate results.) If a discrepancy is found, segmental measurements can be used to determine where the difference lies. Measurements should be taken from the crest of the ilium to the grater trochanter; from the greater trochanter to the lateral knee joint line; and from the lateral joint line to the lateral malleolus.
   (3). Positive result: Leg-length difference. Many people have a leg-length difference that is not symptomatic; however, even a slight difference may be symptomatic for other individuals.

k. *Piriformis test*
   (1). Purpose: To identify spasm or tightness of the piriformis muscle.
   (2). Test position: The patient is placed supine. The involved leg is posi-

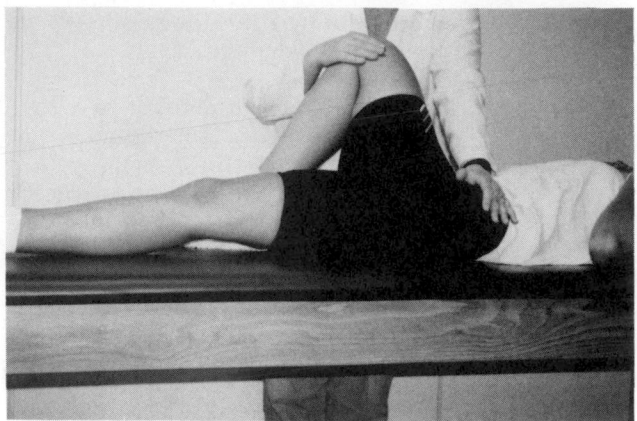

FIGURE 33–11   Piriformis test position.

tioned with the hip and knee flexed, and the involved foot is placed on the table lateral to the opposite knee. The examiner passively moves the involved hip and knee into adduction while blocking the ipsilateral pelvis to prevent trunk rotation (see Figure 33–11).

(3). Positive result: The patient reports discomfort across the buttocks; he/she may also experience onset of radicular symptoms if the piriformis is placing pressure on the sciatic nerve.

l. *Trendelenburg's test*

(1). Purpose: To assess the strength or functional ability of the hip abductors (especially the gluteus medius) to maintain stability of the pelvis.

(2). Test position: The patient is asked to stand on one leg while the examiner observes the position of the trunk and the opposite pelvis.

(3). Positive result: The pelvis drops on the opposite side or there is excessive lateral trunk flexion toward the same side. Normally, the pelvis should remain level or rise slightly on the opposite side. A positive test with patient standing on the right leg indicates weakness of the hip abductors on the right side.

m. *Femoral anteversion test*

(1). Purpose: To estimate amount of femoral anteversion.

(2). Test position: The patient is placed prone, with one knee flexed to 90 degrees. The examiner slowly rotates the leg while palpating the greater trochanter.

(3). Positive result: When the greater trochanter is positioned parallel to the table, the examiner measures the angle between the vertical and the lower leg. This provides an estimation of the degree of femoral anteversion.

6. **Pediatric tests**

a. *Telescoping sign*

(1). Purpose: To reveal a hip that can easily be dislocated.

(2). Test position: The child is placed supine. The examiner flexes the hip and knee to 90 degrees and applies alternate compression and distraction forces along the long axis of the femur. Both sides are compared (see Figure 33–12).

(3). Positive result: Greater amount of motion on one side compared with the other.

b. *Ortolani's test*

(1). Purpose: To reveal congenital hip dislocation.

(2). Test position: The infant is placed supine, with hips and knees flexed to 90 degrees. The examiner grasps both legs around the thighs, with one or two fingers lying over the greater trochanters. The hips are gently abducted and externally rotated, with light pressure over the greater trochanters (see Figure 33–13).

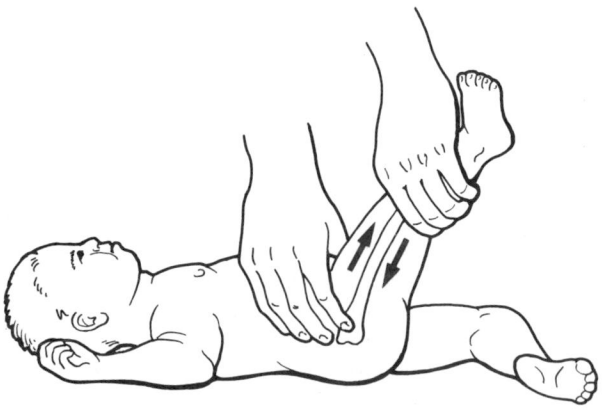

FIGURE 33–12   Telescoping test position.

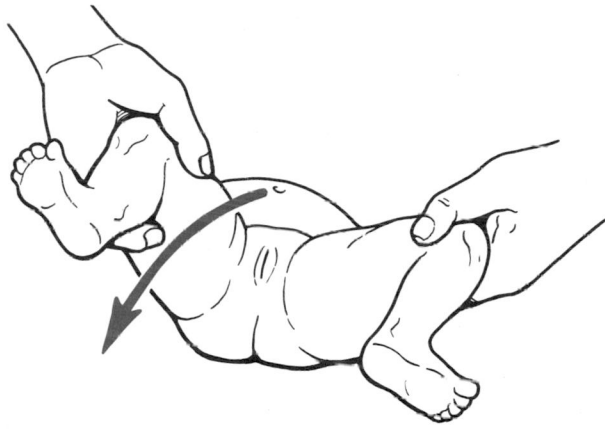

FIGURE 33-13 Ortolani's test position.

(3). Positive result: Resistance to external rotation and abduction. With gentle pressure beyond this point, the examiner may feel a "click" as the dislocated femoral head is reduced into the acetabulum. The test should not be repeated excessively as damage could occur to articular cartilage of the femoral head.

c. *Barlow's test*
(1). Purpose: To identify a hip that can be dislocated.
(2). Test position: Same as for Ortolani's test. The first part of the test is identical to Ortolani's test (see Figure 33–13).

   After Ortolani's test is completed, the examiner grasps one thigh, with the thumb over the proximal femur in the groin. The other hand is used to stabilize the pelvis. Pressure is applied in a posterior and lateral direction with mild adduction.
(3). Positive result: The hip can be dislocated with posterior pressure. Gentle anterior pressure should reduce the dislocation. The test should not be repeated beyond what is necessary as permanent dislocation or increased instability could result.

d. *Galeazzi sign*
(1). Purpose: To reveal congenital hip dislocation.
(2). Test position: The child is placed supine, with hips and knees equally

flexed and heels positioned evenly (see Figure 33–14).
(3). Positive result: The height of the knees is uneven. The test may appear negative in the case of bilateral dislocation. The examiner should also check for other possible causes of leg-length discrepancy before diagnosing congenital hip dislocation.

7. **Muscle imbalance and flexibility testing.**[8] The balance of force couples acting about a joint is determined by the length and pattern of recruitment of the musculature. "How the movement is accomplished is the most important factor, not just the end result."[8]
   a. *Common faults*
   (1). **Inadequate stability of trunk and pelvic girdle.** In nonexercising individuals, it is not uncommon to find that the abdominals and pelvic girdle musculature are unable to provide the stability necessary to maintain ideal alignment statically or dynamically when the musculature attached to these segments is con-

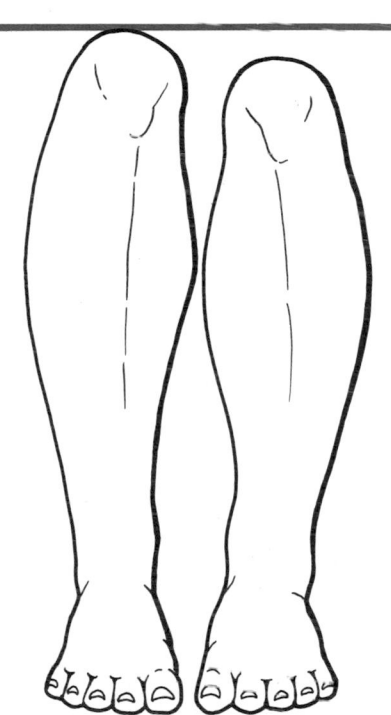

FIGURE 33–14 Galeazzi sign.

tracting; *eg*, in gait, lower extremity motions may be accompanied by excessive trunk and/or pelvic rotation.

(2). **Reduced flexibility of proximal joints.** The hip and glenohumeral joints become less flexible than some areas on the vertebral column with normal aging. The end result is that the vertebral joints become a site of excessive movement, often leading to pain. This is often found in individuals who are involved in activities that require exaggerated use of the lower extremities, *eg*, cycling or running. As the person develops excessive strength and tightness in the hip and thigh musculature, he/she may also develop decreased strength and mobility of the hip girdle.

b. *Hip joint imbalance*

Overworked Muscle	Underworked Muscle
Two-joint hip flexor	One-joint hip flexor
Tensor fasciae latae	Post gluteus medius
Hamstrings	Gluteus maximus
Pelvic rotators	Hip extensors

PLEASE NOTE: Faulty recruitment patterns can lead to overuse syndromes. In summary, each individual can develop different strategies to achieve the same task. However, these strategies may be faulty and predispose the person to an overuse injury. The key is to look at alignment and precision of movement.

c. *Evaluation for muscle imbalance*
  (1). *Standing hip drop test*
     (a). Purpose: To identify asymmetry of motion.
     (b). Test: The standing patient is asked to lift one leg and allow the stance leg to adduct. The examiner observes the quality of motion.
     (c). Positive result: The leg does not purely adduct but is accompanied by hip rotation (will fall in the path of least resistance, meaning the motion that offers the most flexibility).
  (2). *Forward bending with straight back test*

     (a). Purpose: To assess the patient's ability to dissociate hip movement from lumbar spine.
     (b). Test: The standing patient is asked to forward flex while keeping the spine straight.
     (c). Positive result: If the lumbar spine flexes before 50 degrees of hip flexion is achieved, the lumbar spine has greater flexibility than the hip joint.
  (3). *Two-joint hip flexor tightness test.* See description on page 963.
  (4). *Ober's test.* See description on page 964.
  (5). *Prone knee flexion test*
     (a). Purpose: To assess the flexibility of the rectus femoris and the balance of the hamstrings.
     (b). Test: The prone patient is asked to actively flex the knee through the full available range.
     (c). Positive result: Anterior pelvic tilt, limitation in knee flexion, or asymmetrical pull of medial or lateral hamstrings.
  (6). *Prone hip rotation test*
     (a). Purpose: To assess faulty associated movements and flexibility of hip rotation.
     (b). Test: The prone patient flexes one knee to 90 degrees. He/she is asked to perform medial and lateral hip rotation through full range.
     (c). Positive result: Pelvic rotation and excessive or limited motion in internal and external hip rotation.

8. **Neuromuscular tests**
   a. Sensation.
   b. Tendon reflexes.
   c. Muscle tone.
   d. Balance.
   e. Proprioception.

C. Differential diagnosis

Referred pain from disorders affecting the low back, abdominal, or retroperitoneal region, nerve roots, or other overlying structures may present as "hip pain." It is important to attempt to reproduce the patient's symptoms during evaluation to be sure the pain is of musculoskeletal origin and not because of

Hip Pain Decision-Making Flowchart

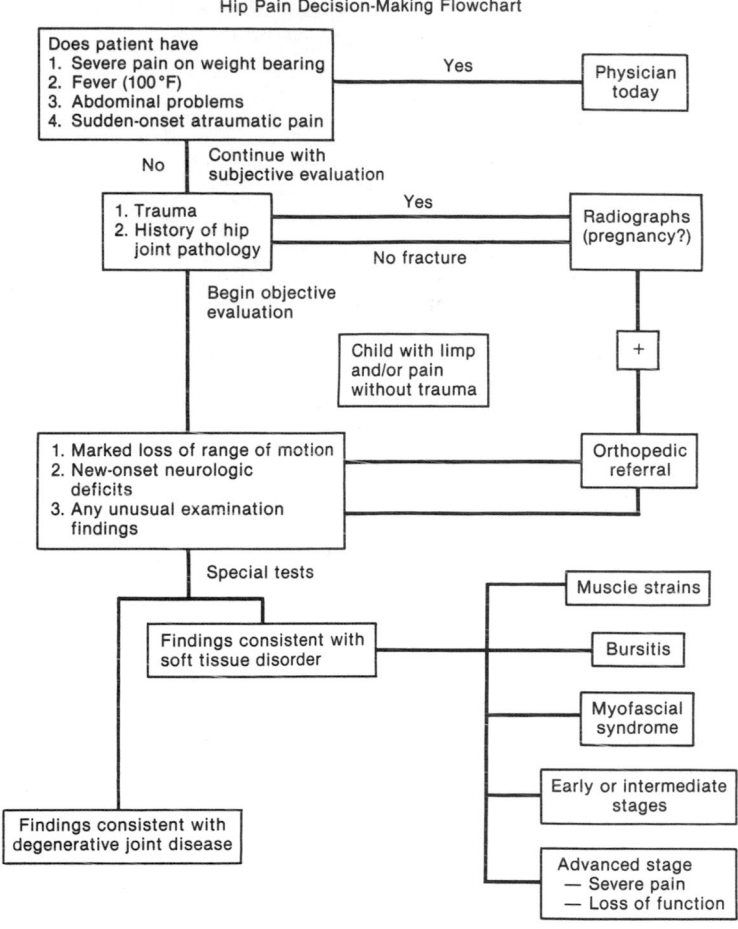

FIGURE 33–15 Hip pain decision-making flow-chart. (Adapted with permission from Echternach J [ed]: *Physical Therapy of the Hip*. Churchill Livingstone, New York, 1990.)

some systemic cause(s). (Figure 33–15 is a flow chart to aid the clinician in the evaluation and management of the patient presenting with hip pain.) The following are some systemic problems that may cause referred hip pain:[11]

1. Spinal metastases.

2. Iliopsoas abscess.

3. Tuberculosis.

4. Crohn's disease.

5. Ureteral colic.

6. Appendicitis.

7. Bone tumors.

8. Reiter's syndrome.

9. Sickle cell anemia.

10. Ankylosing spondylitis.

11. Pelvic inflammatory disease.

12. Hemophilia.

III. Radiology

As direct access to physical therapy/services becomes available in more states, it is increasingly important for therapists to have a basic knowledge of radiological principles. When choosing a form of diagnostic imaging, it remains important to take a thorough history and perform a careful evaluation. Imaging should be performed to confirm a suspected diagnosis or rule out specific pathology.

The appropriate test should provide the necessary information in the most timely and cost-effective manner.

IMAGING TECHNIQUES

Once considered the primary imaging tool for orthopedic disorders, conventional radiography is being replaced in many cases by more sophisticated techniques of imaging. These more advanced techniques include scintigraphy, computed tomography, magnetic resonance imaging, and diagnostic ultrasound. It is important for the therapist to have a basic knowledge of each technique as well as the information that each provides. A discussion of imaging techniques follows, including the advantages and special information provided by each. Summary tables are provided to assist the clinician in decision making (see Tables 33–5 and 33–6).

A. Conventional radiography

1. **Technique.** Conventional radiographs are produced when an x-ray beam is passed through the body. Various tissue types absorb differing amounts of x-rays; bony tissue has the highest absorption, air the lowest. Unabsorbed x-rays that pass through the body produce an image on film.

2. **Standard views.** Standard radiographical views of the hip are anteroposterior, posteroanterior, and axial, also called the frog-leg view. Anteroposterior and posteroanterior views are taken with the patient supine, with hips extended and legs placed parallel to each other. The x-ray beam is introduced from the anterior or posterior side, as indicated. The axial view is taken with the patient supine, with hips positioned in flexion, abduction, and external rotation.

PLEASE NOTE: Because radiographs generate a two-dimensional image of a three-dimensional object, all interposed tissue layers appear superimposed on film. This may be a drawback depending on the degree of differentiation needed. One way to improve three-dimensional viewing is to take another image of the same structure from a different angle (frequently 90 degrees).

3. **Advantages**
   a. Low cost.
   b. Easily obtained.

c. Excellent as a screening tool.

4. **Disadvantages**
   a. Exposure to radiation.
   b. Difficult to distinguish soft-tissue changes.
   c. Hard to evaluate joint surfaces.
   d. Cannot detect subtle changes in bone structure—50% of the bone must be destroyed before a lesion can be visualized radiographically.[9]

5. **General evaluation**
   a. Obvious fractures or dislocations.
   b. General bone density.
   c. Changes in bone density at specific locations.
   d. Contour of articular surfaces.
   e. Contour and integrity of joint space.
   f. General quality of cortex and cancellous bone.
   g. Irregularity of soft tissues.
   h. Integrity of growth plates, if appropriate.

6. **Specifics for hip radiographs**
   a. Fracture or dislocation.
   b. Shape of femoral head and articular surfaces (see Figure 33–16).
   c. Joint space.
   d. Angulation of femoral neck.
   e. Trabecular bone pattern.
   f. Presence of degenerative changes or bony overgrowths.
   g. Integrity of pelvis.
   h. Bilateral comparison, if possible.
   i. Teardrop sign: femoral head migration indicative of degenerative changes.

B. Scintigraphy (bone scan)

1. **Technique.** Small amounts of radioactive material, usually technetium, are injected into the bloodstream. After 3 to 4 hours, the radioactive material has circulated throughout the body and has concentrated in the skeletal system. A full-body radiograph is then taken.

2. **Evaluation.** Areas of bone with increased metabolic activity will have a higher concentration of radioactive substance and will appear bright on the film. These ''hot spots'' within the bone may represent an osteoblastic lesion, a recent fracture, degenerative changes, or an area of inflammation.

3. **Advantages**
   a. High sensitivity. Because nuclear imaging

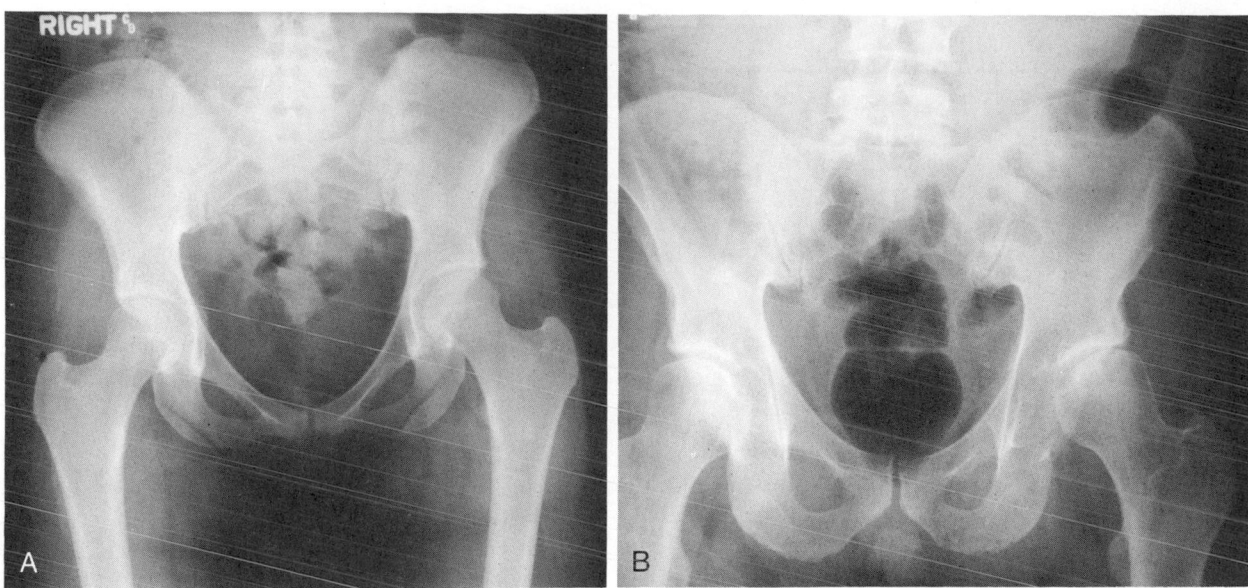

FIGURE 33–16   **A,** Radiograph of a normal hip. **B,** Radiograph of a hip with degenerative joint disease.

is a representation of metabolic activity, it is highly sensitive. Stress fractures that do not appear on conventional radiographs are visible on bone scans. In addition, osteoblastic lesions are detectable on bone scans long before they are visible on plain radiographs. Scintigraphy is the procedure of choice when screening for metastatic bone lesions.

b. Easily obtained.

4. **Disadvantages**
   a. Exposure to radiation.
   b. Slightly invasive.

C. Computed tomography (CT scan)

1. **Technique.** Computerized enhancement of x-ray images. X-rays are generated in a circular tube that rotates around the involved body part. The x-rays that pass through the body are recorded by a detector that is connected to a computer. The computer uses differential absorption data to recreate layers of the body, producing sequential cross-sectional "slices" of the body.

2. **Evaluation.** CT scans are detailed images of soft-tissue structures as well as joint surfaces. Sequential images allow the reader to recreate three-dimensional characteristics of the body.

3. **Advantages**
   a. Produces images of soft tissue as well as bone.
   b. Excellent resolution, with a density differential of 1%.[9]
   c. Allows visualization of articular surfaces.

4. **Disadvantages**
   a. Exposure to radiation.

D. Magnetic resonance imaging (MRI scan)

1. **Technique.** The most advanced imaging technique currently available. It offers excellent resolution for soft-tissue structures. To generate MRI scans, the body is placed inside a large magnetic field. The proton (nucleus) of the hydrogen atom (very prevalent because of the body's high water content) responds to the magnetic field by aligning within it. A second magnetic field is introduced for a short burst, causing different alignment of the hydrogen protons. When the second field is turned off, the protons resume their initial positions. As they realign, they emit a radio frequency signal that is detected and analyzed by computer. The image produced is based on the relative strength of the radio frequency signal.

Two tissue-specific constants are used to

Table 33–5. COMPARISON OF IMAGING TECHNIQUES

	Radiography	CT	Scintigraphy	MRI
Cost	Low	Moderate	Low	High
Availability	High	High	High	Moderate
Exposure to radiation	Yes	Yes	Yes	No
Screening value	Yes	No	Yes	No
Specificity	Low	High	Low	High
Soft-tissue imaging	Poor	High	None	High
Dimensions	2	3	2	3

provide further differentiation of structures. These are T1 (rate of realignment) and T2 (rate of signal decay). Altering the generation and repetition of the second magnetic field can produce images that are referred to as "T1 weighted" and "T2 weighted." With T1 weighting, cortical bone, fibrous tissue, and normal body fluid appear darkest; muscle, tumor, and infection appear intermediate; and fat appears whitest. With T2 weighting, fat, tumor, infection and all fluid (including edema) appear white, whereas muscle, bone, and fibrous tissue show the same appearance as on T1 weighting[10] (see Figure 33–17).

2. **Evaluation.** Clear and concise cross-sectional images are produced. MRI scans are similar to CT scans: sequential images allow recreation of three-dimensional characteristics of the body.

3. **Advantages**
   a. Excellent visualization of ligaments, meniscus, and other soft-tissue structures.
   b. Very effective for detecting early necrosis of the femoral head.
   c. No exposure to radiation.

4. **Disadvantages**
   a. Very costly.
   b. Actual test time is quite lengthy.

■ PLEASE NOTE: The presence of a metal joint prosthesis is not a definite contraindication to MRI. Metal is not affected by the magnetic field; however, it will produce an artifact on the image.

E. Ultrasound

Diagnostic ultrasound allows image production by way of reflected sound waves. No radiation exposure is required. It is not widely used for orthopedic diagnosis because sound waves cannot penetrate bone. Ultrasound has limited applications for differentiation of soft-tissue and muscle lesions. (see Tables 33–5 and 33–6).

Table 33–6. SUGGESTED IMAGING TECHNIQUES FOR VARIOUS PATHOLOGIES

	Radiography	CT	Scintigraphy	MRI
Fracture	+		+ stress	
Osteoarthritis	+			
Necrosis	+		+	+
Suspected metastatic lesion			+	
Trauma	+			
Soft-tissue injury (bursa, tendon, meniscus, ligament)		+		+
Articular fractures		+		

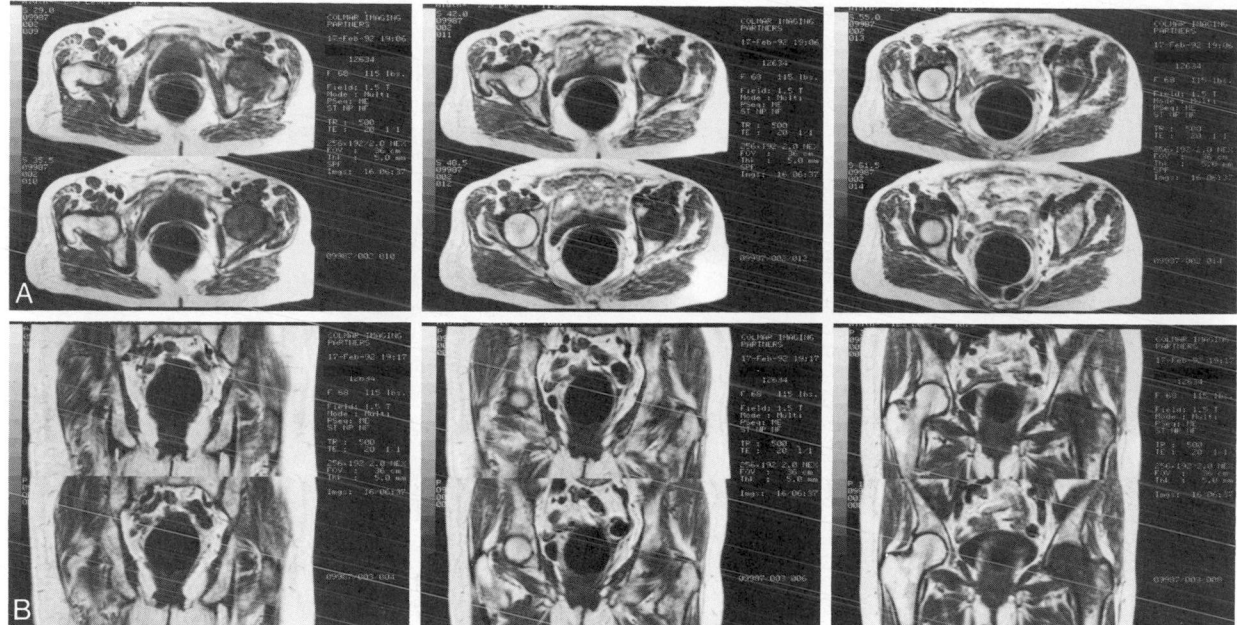

FIGURE 33–17 **A** and **B,** Magnetic resonance images displaying ischemic changes of the left femoral head.

IV. Treatment: Common Disorders of the Hip

In most cases of muscle strains and soft-tissue injuries, the clinician's treatment decision-making process should be based not only on the patient's functional needs, but also on the changes in soft-tissue properties (*ie,* tissue ischemia, fibrous reaction, altered arthrokinematics) and the cause of the dysfunction. Unlike specific treatment goals, generic goals for anticipated responses to treatment may be set, such as to increase circulation and nutrient flow, prevent abnormal joint mobility, improve normal length of contractile and noncontractile tissues, decrease pain. On the basis of these decisions, the clinician should choose a modality (if necessary) and an exercise plan that will most effectively coincide.

A. Muscle strains

1. **Hip adductors.** This is one of the most commonly strained muscle groups.
   a. *Etiology.* Vigorous twisting of the leg or trunk while the foot is planted on the ground. May also be caused by external forces or running with a pelvic imbalance.
   b. *Clinical presentation*[12]
      (1). Sharp pain in groin with acceleration.
      (2). Edema or ecchymosis.
      (3). A palpable defect and bony tenderness are possible in cases of severe rupture.
      (4). Muscle guarding.
      (5). Pain with resisted hip adduction.
   c. *Treatment and management.* Radiographs should be taken in severe cases to rule out avulsion fracture. Initial treatment should include rest, intermittent hip spica compression with ice, and elevation. In acute to subacute stages, modalities such as ultrasound and whirlpool may be included. The clinician should decide which modality will be most effective in assisting the patient to reach his/her physical therapy goal. For instance, if goals are to increase circulation and begin active ROM exercises, but the patient is anxious or exhibiting pain behavior, whirlpool may be more effective. The patient should be progressed from active ROM exercises to resistive exercise once pain-free motion has been achieved. Initial phases are critical because a "groin pull" can become chronic if mistreated.

2. **Hamstring strain.** This is also a commonly strained muscle group.

   a. *Etiology.* Many possible causes, both of insidious and/or traumatic origin. Insidious injury may be the result of poor posture, fatigue, or muscle imbalance. Traumatic injury may be a consequence of decreased flexibility, inappropriate quadricep to hamstring ratios, comparative limb-strength deficits, or forced hip flexion with the knee extended.

   b. *Clinical presentation*
     (1). Tenderness.
     (2). Increased stiffness.
     (3). Ecchymosis and hemorrhage in severe cases.
     (4). Muscle defect may be visible several days post injury.

   c. *Treatment and management.* Acutely, rest, ice, and compression are important in order to decrease effects of inelastic scar formation within the muscle belly. Cyriax and Cyriax,[13] encourage use of transverse friction massage for muscle or tendinous strains to maintain soft-tissue mobility and prevent random alignment of new collagen fibers. Also, gentle AROM, submaximal isometrics, and phonophoresis can be started in acute stages. When the patient can perform exercises with minimal pain, he/she can progress to stretching and a structured training program. Proper treatment is critical to avoid recurrent tears and the condition known as hamstring syndrome. Guidelines for possible rehabilitation time are 2 to 3 weeks for mild injuries and 2 to 6 months for severe cases. Most important, athletes should not return to full participation until full strength and flexibility have been achieved.[14]

     Prevention is key with this type of injury. Proper preseason evaluations and hamstring rehabilitation should place emphasis on quadricep to hamstring ratios, bilateral limb-strength equality, and hamstring stretching.[12]

3. **Gluteus medius strain**

   a. *Etiology.* Usually caused by overuse syndrome. Commonly seen in long-distance runners. Overload caused by weakness of surrounding muscles should also be considered.

   b. *Clinical presentation.* Pain over the region of the greater trochanter when resistance is applied. Trochanteric bursitis should be ruled out by pain-free active movement.

   c. *Treatment and management*
     (1). Heat modalities. Ultrasound may be chosen as the best modality secondary to depth of this tissue. This may be followed with moist heat for patient comfort and relaxation if the treatment goal is to begin gentle stretching.
     (2). Gentle stretching.
     (3). Progressive resistive exercises to strengthen hip extensors and external rotators. The program should include both open- and closed-chain activities as these muscles are active in both capacities during gait. Manual or mechanical resistance may be applied.

4. **Iliopsoas strain**

   a. *Etiology.* May be caused by forced extension of the lower extremity as the hip is actively being flexed. Common insidious onset occurs after repeated flexion as with an intense training session.

   b. *Clinical presentation*
     (1). The patient will usually hold the hip and thigh in a position of flexion, adduction, and external rotation.
     (2). Pain with resisted hip motions.
     (3). Increased stiffness.

   c. *Treatment and management*
   In adolescents, radiographs should be taken because of the risk of avulsion of the epiphyseal site.
     (1). Acutely, rest, ice, and compression are the treatments of choice.
     (2). Moist heat is added as the goal becomes mobilization and stretching to prevent hip flexion contracture.
     (3). Gentle progressive resistive exercise is begun when the patient has achieved pain-free active motion. Open- and closed-chain activities should be incorporated into the exercise program. Emphasis should be on hip extension exercises to prevent development of hip flexor tightness.

B. Bursitis

1. **Greater trochanteric bursitis.** This is the most common hip bursitis.

a. *Etiology.* Disorder is commonly seen in gymnasts, dancers, and runners who perform repetitive motions of flexion with external rotation. This may create imbalance of hip musculature, making the joint capsule and ligaments less stable. The result may be "snapping hip," which causes pain over the tensor fasciae latae and trochanteric bursa.[15]

Other causes include overstress secondary to function, occupation, or sports activity; iliotibial band tightness; muscle imbalance between hip abductors and adductors; poor posture; increased Q-angle; inadequate running shoes or surfaces; or leg-length discrepancy. The problem seems to occur more in the female population because of the wider pelvis, which may cause tensor fasciae latae to bow at a more acute angle.[16]

b. *Clinical presentation*

(1). Active and passive movements are within normal limits, except adduction may be limited by pain.

(2). Resisted hip abduction will increase symptoms.

(3). The differential test is palpable tenderness and increased temperature over the greater trochanter.

(4). An audible or palpable snap may occur with movement.

(5). The patient can usually point to the lateral hip as the source of pain and may even complain of pain down the lateral thigh if the iliotibial band is involved.

(6). Standing, walking, and sitting are usually all painful. Climbing stairs may aggravate symptoms.

(7). Positive Ober's test.

c. *Treatment and management.* Initial treatment should include rest, phonophoresis, and ice massage to reduce inflammation. Oral anti-inflammatory medication is often prescribed. Gentle stretching of tight musculature should soon follow. The patient should be educated about possible factors that may have caused irritation. The key to treatment is finding the cause that predisposed the patient to injury. Prognosis is usually excellent; however, some conditions become chronic and may require surgical excision of bursa and release of tensor fasciae latae.

2. **Psoas bursitis**

a. *Etiology.* Similar to trochanteric bursitis; causes include functional, occupational, and sports-related overstress.

b. *Clinical presentation*

(1). Report of pain in groin or anterior thigh.

(2). Occasional report of pain solely at area above patella.

(3). Active hip flexion with adduction reproduces pain.

(4). Passive hip flexion with adduction and passive external rotation are uncomfortable.

(5). Palpation may cause specific discomfort; however, area is very tender in most individuals.

(6). Muscle testing of psoas is without deficit, but tightness in muscle may be noted.

(7). Aggravated by activities requiring excessive hip flexion.

c. *Treatment and management.* Conservative treatment includes modalities such as ultrasound, phonophoresis, or interferential current. The initial goal is to decrease inflammation; therefore, the clinician's preference may be phonophoresis. If the patient does not respond favorably or show signs of progress, the therapist may choose to use another modality, such as interferential or electrical stimulation for pain control. As symptoms subside, it is important to begin stretching tight musculature. The patient should be educated on possible biomechanical factors that may have caused the irritation. Prognosis is excellent; however, if the condition becomes chronic, the physician may choose to inject the bursa. It is usually not advisable to inject a site more than three times during 6 months to 1 year.

3. **Iliopectineal bursitis**

a. *Etiology.* This disorder is relatively uncommon. Possible causes include osteoarthritis or iliopsoas muscle tightness.

b. *Clinical presentation*

(1). Resisted hip flexion is painful.

(2). Passive hip extension to end of range is painful.

(3). Report of pain in groin with occasional radiation into the L2 and L3 dermatomes.

c. *Treatment and management.* Symptomatic relief can usually be achieved with use of modalities such as ultrasound and ice. Ultrasound is usually the treatment of choice secondary to the depth of penetration required to reach the designated area. In combination with the above, the clinician may choose ice as a means of decreasing inflammation and providing an analgesic response. Another factor that must be considered when choosing a modality is favorable patient response. Stretching of tight musculature is indicated when the patient is less symptomatic. If osteoarthritis is thought to be the potential cause of the disorder, treatment of the original condition is important. (Treatment of osteoarthritis is discussed later.)

4. **Ischial bursitis**
   a. *Etiology.* This disorder is relatively uncommon, but bursa can become inflamed in individuals whose occupation requires prolonged sitting. It is commonly seen in males secondary to carrying a bulky wallet in the same back hip pocket.
   b. *Clinical presentation*
      (1). Palpable tenderness over ischial tuberosity.
      (2). Pain aggravated by stair climbing and walking.
      (3). Occasional radiating pain into hamstring muscles.
      (4). Person will sit on unaffected hip.
   c. *Treatment and management.* Treatment is similar to that for iliopectineal bursitis. Treatment goal: symptomatic relief using ice or heat. Appropriate positioning and pillow placement should be reviewed with the patient.

C. Piriformis syndrome

1. **Etiology.** Occurs almost six times as frequently in females as in males.[17] It is usually caused by a tight piriformis that compresses the sciatic nerve. It may also be caused by vigorous activity of the posterior hip muscles.

2. **Clinical presentation**
   a. Active and resisted hip external rotation is painful.
   b. Passive internal rotation is painful.
   c. Report of deep localized pain in posterior hip region.
   d. Occasional numbness and tingling into leg.
   e. Low back pain.

3. **Treatment and management.** Initial treatment should include rest, ice, and aspirin to decrease inflammation. Gentle stretching of the piriformis muscle in sitting or sidelying is added slowly.

D. Capsular tightness

1. **Etiology.** Possible causes are structural or muscle asymmetries of the hip, spine, or lower extremity, lack of exercise, and sedentary lifestyle.

2. **Clinical presentation**[18]
   a. Symptoms of stiffness and limitation of function.
   b. Pain with weight bearing on affected side.
   c. Active and passive hip motions are limited in flexion, abduction, and internal rotation.
   d. Passive accessory motions are limited in all directions, with greatest restriction being inferior glide and lateral distraction.
   e. Muscle tightness (tensor fasciae latae, rectus femoris, piriformis, and hip adductor muscles.)
   f. Positive quadrant or scouring test.

3. **Treatment and management.** Physical therapy intervention at this stage of joint pathology is critical. Capsular tightness has the potential to contribute to acceleration of hip degenerative changes.[19] This can be explained by the fact that the hip moves into a position of extension, internal rotation, and abduction with each step, which takes up

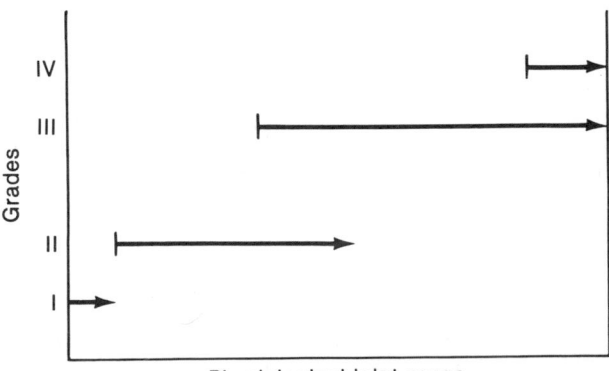

FIGURE 33–18 Grades of joint mobilization according to Maitland. Grade I mobilization is a small-amplitude oscillation performed at the beginning of the joint range. Grade II mobilization is a large-amplitude oscillation performed in the middle of the range but not reaching the end range. Grade III mobilization is a large-amplitude oscillation performed up to the limit of the joint. Grade IV mobilization is a small-amplitude oscillation performed at the end of the range.

the slack of the capsule. If the hip loses extensibility, the slack is taken up early and causes joint surfaces to approximate prematurely, which is known as "shock loading."[20]

a. *Treatment goals*[6]
(1). To decrease stiffness.
  (a). Active ROM of hip every day should be encouraged.
  (b). Gait training so that the patient learns to exercise hips with each step.
  (c). Joint mobilization (Grades I or II) in a pain-free position. Figure 33–18 provides a representation of grades of joint mobilizations as defined by Maitland.[21]

    Accessory joint glides should be initiated from the loose-pack position of the hip (30 degrees flexion, 30 degrees abduction, 15 degrees external rotation). Figure 33–19*A* to *D* illustrates specific hip joint mobilizations that may be used to assist in achieving the desired goal.
(2). To increase ROM.
  (a). Sustained Grade III mobilization.
  (b). Self-stretching techniques.
  (c). Self-mobilization.
(3). To decrease pain by decreasing mechanical stress.
  (a). Use of an assistive device. Most frequently a straight cane is appropriate at this stage to widen the base of support and to decrease the force of the hip abductors on the joint (see section on biomechanics).
  (b). If leg-length discrepancy creates asymmetry, gradually a shoe lift should be added.
  (c). Gentle strengthening, beginning with isometrics, for all supporting musculature.
(4). To decrease pain at rest.
  (a). Grade I or II oscillations.
  (b). Moist heat.

4. **Prognosis.** Fair to excellent depending on
a. The person's ability to change to a less sedentary lifestyle.
b. Collagen pathology.[18]

E. Degenerative joint disease or osteoarthritis

This is the most common painful condition of the hip joint.[17]

1. **Etiology.** Primary osteoarthritis is considered a result of the aging process. The term secondary osteoarthritis is used when an individual has a history of pre-existing joint disease (Legg-Calvé-Perthes disease, slipped capital epiphysis, or traumatic dislocations). Cartilaginous changes occur in "nonarticular" areas as part of the normal aging process. Another cause to consider is formation of osteophytes and capsular fibrosis in regions under the most stress.

2. **Clinical presentation.** A list of signs and symptoms in early and late stages of degenerative joint disease follows. The examiner should keep in mind that there are various intermediate stages, and, therefore, various presentations may be seen.
a. *Early stages*
  (1). Pain noticed with weight bearing at end of day or with fatigue.
  (2). Pain in groin or along L3 dermatome.
  (3). Mild limitation and pain at end of range of internal rotation, abduction, and extension.
  (4). Gait is usually asymptomatic.
b. *Advanced stages*
  (1). Constant aching, often awakened at night.
  (2). Morning stiffness.
  (3). Difficulty with functional activities such as climbing stairs, squatting, and dressing.
  (4). Gluteus medius muscle limp.
  (5). Use of assistive device.
  (6). Motion is limited in a capsular pattern.
  (7). Equilibrium and balance are impaired secondary to interruption of mechanoreceptor system as capsular tissue changes.[22]

3. **Treatment and management**
a. *Early stages.* The challenge for the physical therapist lies here. The majority of cases are not seen in the early stage, but in this stage the physical therapist has the most to offer the patient.[20]
  (1). Treatment of capsular tightness should be reviewed.
  (2). Heat modalities. The clinician must keep in mind the desired outcome of treatment. Ultrasound may be the preferred modality for its depth of penetration, whereas moist heat is widely used for its analgesic or com-

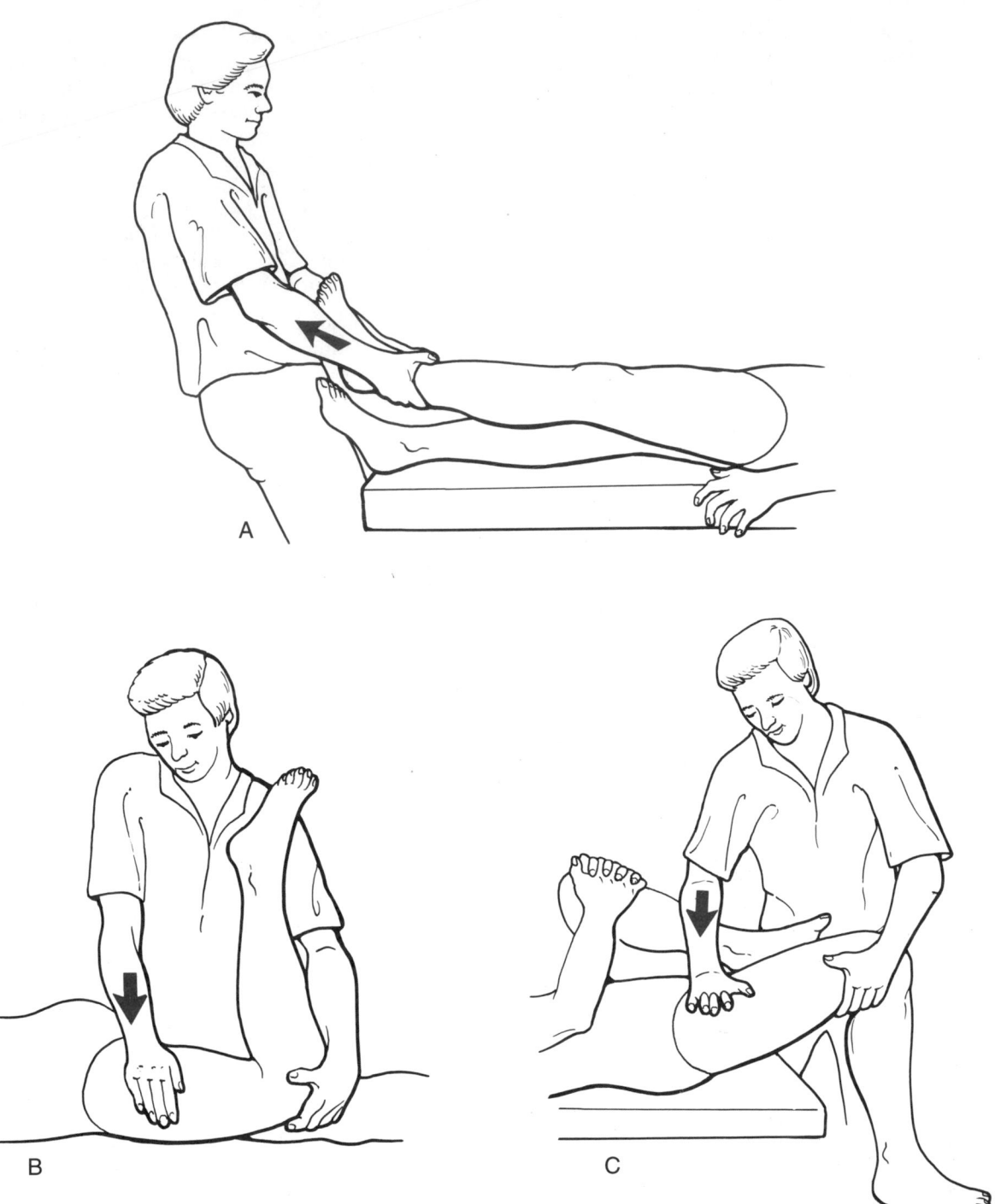

FIGURE 33–19 **A,** Hip joint distraction. Its uses are testing joint mobility and pain control. *Note:* force is exerted as therapist leans backward, using body weight. **B,** Anterior glide of the hip joint. Its use is to increase hip extension of external rotation. **C,** Posterior glide of the hip joint. Its uses are to increase flexion or internal rotation.

Continued

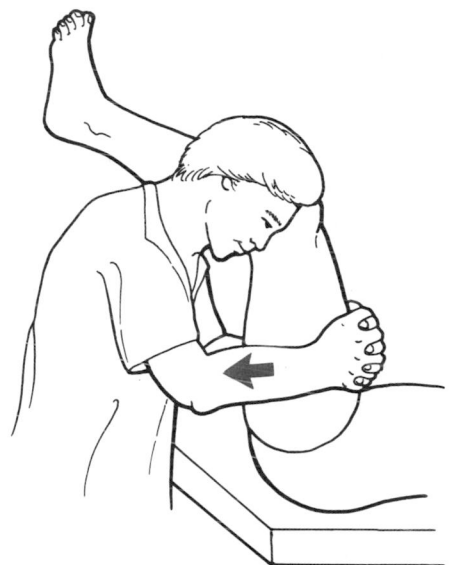

FIGURE 33–19 *(continued)* **D,** Inferior glide of the hip joint. Its uses are to increase hip flexion or abduction.

fort-inducing properties before exercise.

(3). Hip abductor strengthening should be emphasized.

(4). ROM exercises, to be done indefinitely, should be emphasized.

(5). The examiner continues to assess for biomechanical deficits that predispose the joint to abnormal stresses.

(6). A weight reduction program is enacted, if appropriate.

b. ***Advanced stages.*** Treatment must be comprehensive and vigorous. The goal is to restore the patient to optimal functional level and to regain (if possible) optimal joint mechanics.

(1). Treatment of capsular tightness should be reviewed. (Include Grade III joint mobilizations and muscle strengthening!)

(2). The patient should be instructed in the use of an assistive device if he/she has not begun using one. The clinician should choose an assistive device that best offers the patient the ability to decrease painful weight bearing and that provides for more erect posture.

(3). A raised toilet seat and other adaptive equipment should be considered.

4. **Surgical intervention.** This becomes an option after the patient has undergone adequate

conservative treatment without noticeable improvement in pain level, function, and quality of life. Good communication between the physical therapist and the physician is important. If the therapist has been working with a patient for a period of time, the decision to undergo surgery may be made more easily.

a. ***Total hip arthroplasty.*** This has been the procedure of choice for many years. Technology continues to improve, allowing surgeons to consider this option for the younger patient (< 60 years of age).

(1). *Prosthesis.* The femoral head is made of chrome-cobalt, and the stem of titanium alloy. The acetabular component is usually a combination of a metal shell with an ultra–high-molecular-weight polyethylene. Long-term fixation of components is achieved through bone ingrowth into the roughened porous surface on the implant or polymethyl methacrylate cement.

(2). *Indications.* Total hip arthroplasty is indicated in cases of severe osteoarthritis and rheumatoid arthritis in which conservative measures have been exhausted. It is also used in the management of chronic dislocations of the femoral head, avascular necrosis, and fractures of the femoral neck and acetabulum (especially in the elderly).

(3). *Contraindications*

(a). Active infection anywhere in the body.

(b). Progressive neurological disease.

(c). Skeletal immaturity.

(d). Precaution should be taken with individuals with multiple medical problems.

(4). *Complications.* Dislocation, infection, and component loosening.

(5). *Surgical approach.* The lateral (Watson-Jones) approach is the most widely used because it offers the easiest access for insertion of the prosthesis. It requires retraction of the greater trochanter, with a slight interruption of the attached muscles.

b. ***Treatment***

(1). *Preoperative.* Preoperative evaluation with instruction has proven beneficial for both the patient and the physical therapist. The therapist benefits because the patient's prior level of function, cognition, and attitude can be assessed before surgery, making goal setting and postoperative instruction easier. The patient benefits from a better understanding of the surgery and postoperative management. The patient can begin planning for any environmental changes that may ease the transition to home.

Preoperative examinations should include:

(a). Assessment of lower extremity ROM, strength, and functional level.

(b). Assessment of the patient's present living situation (stairs in the house, tub vs stall shower) and present occupation.

(c). Instruction in the use of an assistive device, possible weight-bearing precautions that may follow surgery, postoperative exercises, and estimated stages/goals that will be set for the patient. Total hip precautions (flexion < 90 degrees, adduction past midline, and internal rotation) should be emphasized.

(2). *Postoperative*

(a). The patient begins ankle pumps, quadricep and gluteal isometrics, and diaphragmatic breathing in the recovery room as a preventive measure against development of a pulmonary embolus.

(b). Transfer out of bed is made on postoperative day 1.

(c). Gait training varies depending on weight-bearing status and the patient's capabilities. Patients with uncemented hips should have partial or toe-touch weight bearing with crutches or a walker. They are progressed to a cane and should use it for at least 6 weeks to allow for bone growth and healing.

Patients with cemented hips are usually allowed to weight bear as tolerated. They begin ambulation with a walker or crutches and are then progressed to a straight cane. Stair climbing should be practiced several days prior to discharge to ensure safety and endurance.

(d). Transfer training should include transfers in and out of bed, on and off elevated chair and toilet, in and out of tub or shower. Car transfer should also be demonstrated and practiced prior to discharge.

(e). The patient is instructed in active ROM exercises for the involved extremity, such as heel slides, straight-leg raise, hip extension (standing), hip abduction, knee extension (sitting).

(f). Long term. At the end of 3 months, the patient is able to resume normal daily activities and may return to activities such as swimming, bicycling, and golf. The patient's main limitation is active involvement in high-impact sports.

F. Fractures

1. **Common types of hip fractures**

   a. *Subcapital femoral neck fracture (intracapsular).* This is the most common hip fracture seen in the elderly population (females more often than males). It is usually caused by a twisting motion during weight bearing.

   b. *Intertrochanteric fracture (extracapsular).* This is seen primarily in the elderly patient as a result of a fall. In addition to force directed through the femur from the fall, the iliopsoas and adductors add an indirect force on the lesser and greater trochanters.

   c. *Subtrochanteric fracture.* This is more often seen in the younger population. It is a direct result of traumatic mechanical stress to the femur, such as may occur in a motor vehicle accident.

   d. *Acetabular fracture.* This is often associated with a posterior dislocation of the hip.

2. **Surgical management.** Most hip fractures require a total hip replacement. Other hip fractures are most commonly treated with open-reduction internal fixation. A variety of procedures and various fixation devices exist. A fracture is considered stable postoperatively if the radiograph shows continuity of bone from the femoral head down the femoral neck into the subtrochanteric area. In

this case, partial weight bearing can be initiated on the 1st postoperative day. Most intertrochanteric fractures do not have a stable column. Therefore, the patient must maintain non–weight bearing in order to allow for fixation to heal. For the elderly patient, this causes significant functional limitations.

3. **Postoperative physical therapy treatment**
   a. The patient begins ankle pumps, gluteal and quadricep isometrics, and diaphragmatic breathing as early as possible as a preventive measure against thrombophlebitis.
   b. Transfers and gait training are initiated with a walker or crutches and appropriate weight-bearing precautions (as listed above) on postoperative day 1 unless otherwise specified by the surgeon.
   c. The patient is instructed on inactive ROM exercises of the involved extremity, such as heel slides, straight-leg raise, hip extension (standing), and knee extension (sitting). The patient should be progressed with gentle resistance as tolerated. Also, especially for those patients who must maintain non–weight bearing, upper body strengthening (scapular depressors and triceps) is very important.

PLEASE NOTE: Patients who have sustained a femoral neck fracture should avoid straight-leg raise and prone hip extension secondary to the force exerted at the hip.[23]

G. Athletic-related fractures

1. **Stress fracture**
   a. *Etiology*
      (1). Most often seen in runners.
      (2). Injury occurs near pubis symphysis of the femoral neck.
   b. *Clinical presentation*
      (1). Localized tenderness in inguinal area.
      (2). Pain at end of range of hip motion.
   c. *Treatment and management*
      (1). Diagnosis should be confirmed by radiograph or bone scan.[13]
      (2). Abstinence from athletic activity until there is no pain at rest.
      (3). The patient is progressed from partial weight bearing to full weight bearing with crutches.
      (4). Gentle progressive resistive exercises are initiated when the patient has achieved pain-free ambulation without an assistive device. Other suggested activities include swimming, walking, and bicycling, which should be done in quarter-mile increments.[24]

2. **Avulsion fracture**
   a. *Etiology*. Apophyseal avulsions of the pelvis and proximal femur occur in young male athletes (10 to 20 years old). Injury is the result of vigorous contractions of the sartorius or tensor fasciae latae that are not counterbalanced by a cocontraction.[24]
   b. *Clinical presentation*
      (1). Acute pain at onset.
      (2). Crepitus or hematoma.
      (3). Palpation over ASIS may show point tenderness, and a bony fragment may be detected.
      (4). Aggravated pain with active or passive hip flexion.
   c. *Treatment*
      (1). Ice and hip spica compression.
      (2). Bed rest, aspirin, and limited weight bearing with crutches.
      (3). Injury can possibly be prevented with thorough preseason screening for muscle imbalances.

H. Nerve entrapment syndrome—meralgia paresthetica

This syndrome involves entrapment of the lateral femoral cutaneous nerve. The compression site is usually around the ASIS, where the nerve passes through the inguinal ligament.

1. **Etiology**
   a. Sudden weight gain.
   b. Direct trauma.
   c. Overstress of abdominal musculature.
   d. Forced pelvic tilt.
   e. Abnormal tone of abdominal or hip musculature.
   f. Tight athletic undergarments.
   g. Leg-length discrepancy: short leg opposite side of symptoms.

2. **Clinical presentation**
   a. Pain, numbness, or burning sensation along anterior/lateral or posterior/lateral thigh.
   b. Full active and passive movement with pain at end of range of abduction.
   c. Decreased sensation to light touch and

pinprick along same areas where symptoms are felt.

d. Pain with palpation over above-mentioned areas.

3. **Treatment**
a. Modalities: ice for first 48 to 72 hours if secondary to an acute injury. Otherwise, the patient may get symptomatic relief from moist heat.
b. Heel lift for short leg (must be followed closely for patient needs).
c. Elimination of original cause (proper fitting of clothes).
d. The therapist may need to refer the patient to a physician for proper referral to a dietician.

I. Contusion—hip pointer

1. **Etiology.** Usually a result of athletic injury involving a direct blow to the iliac crest.

2. **Clinical presentation**
a. Bleeding and edema.
b. Pain on palpation, coughing, and active trunk flexion.

3. **Treatment**
a. Radiographs and other diagnostic studies should be performed to rule out avulsion fracture, intra-abdominal injury, or other serious injury.
b. Ice and anti-inflammatory medication during first 48 to 72 hours.
c. Gentle stretching may slowly be added.
d. Transcutaneous electrical nerve stimulation (TENS) may be used for pain control if sufficient rest from activity is not possible.
e. Prevention includes assessment of adequate padding.

J. Myofascial pain syndromes[25]

As defined by Travell and Simons,[25] myofascial syndrome is an automatic phenomenon, with pain and tenderness referred from hyperirritable spots in the skeletal muscle or fascia causing associated dysfunction. The hyperirritable foci are known as myofascial trigger points, which can be caused by acute or chronic overload of the muscle. These trigger points often refer pain in specific patterns. Almost all muscles in the body have the potential for developing trigger points; however, five muscles in par-

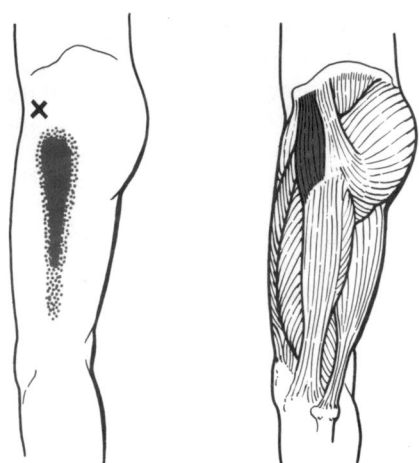

FIGURE 33–20 Tensor fasciae latae trigger points and referred pain patterns. (Redrawn from Travell J, Simons D: *Myofascial Pain and Dysfunction: The Trigger Point Manual. The Lower Extremities.* vol. 2. Baltimore, Williams & Wilkins, 1992, © 1992, the Williams & Wilkins Co., Baltimore.)

ticular should be kept in mind when evaluating a patient with hip pain.

PLEASE NOTE: The purpose of this section is to acknowledge that myofascial syndromes can exist, thereby making the reader aware of additional possibilities to consider.

1. **Tensor fasciae latae.**[25] The primary trigger point refers pain to the anterolateral thigh (see Figure 33–20). Referred pain is often misdiagnosed as trochanteric bursitis.
a. *Etiology*
(1). Acute trauma, such as falling from a significant height and landing on both feet.
(2). Overstress caused by running up-hill without appropriate footwear.
(3). Poor conditioning and warm-up time.
(4). Inappropriate muscle firing of gluteal musculature causing overuse of tensor fasciae latae for abduction.
b. *Clinical presentation*
(1). Pain worse with movement.
(2). Pain and tenderness in hip joint, especially over the greater trochanter.
(3). Pain aggravated by prolonged sitting if the hip is flexed more than 90 degrees.
(4). Inability to achieve comfortable side-lying secondary to pressure of the body over tender areas.

c. *Treatment and management*
   (1). The patient should be instructed in possible mechanical factors that may induce or aggravate trigger point(s) in this muscle (*eg*, walking/jogging uphill or on surfaces that slope side to side, prolonged flexion of hip beyond 90 degrees, and excessively worn shoes).
   (2). Ischemic compression. Digital pressure should be sustained over the trigger point until sensitivity of the trigger point decreases. Lengthening of the muscle should follow.
   (3). Ultrasound. This is particularly useful for deep trigger points that are difficult to work manually.
   (4). Moist heat. This should be used before and after treatment to provide vasodilation and relaxation to soft tissue.
   (5). Surface electromyogram (EMG) biofeedback. This is a relatively new treatment modality in the field of physical therapy. Further research and reliability testing are pending; however, the following procedure has been used with success at North Penn Hospital in Lansdale, Pennsylvania:
      (a). The patient is positioned in sitting with electrodes placed over the gluteal and tensor fasciae latae muscles. The patient is instructed to perform hip abduction using the gluteal muscles. At the same time, the patient is able to look at the screen, which will show asymmetries in muscle contractions. With this visual feedback, the patient is able to retrain inactive gluteal musculature.
   (6). Self-stretching. The patient is positioned in sidelying on the uninvolved side close to the edge of the table. The patient extends and laterally rotates the involved leg and then relaxes to allow for a gravity-assisted stretch (see Figure 33–21).

2. **Quadratus lumborum.**[25] Four trigger points may be responsible for referred pain into the sacroiliac area, buttocks, and hip region. The most proximal and superficial trigger point refers pain to the iliac crest. The sec-

ond superficial point refers pain to the greater trochanter or outer aspect of the thigh. The third deep and proximal point is responsible for referring pain to the sacroiliac joint, and the fourth point refers pain into the lower buttocks (see Figure 33–22).

a. *Etiology*
   (1). Awkward lifting of a heavy object.
   (2). Repetitive strain from activities such as gardening, walking, or jogging on a slanted surface or scrubbing the floor.
   (3). Motor vehicle accident.
   (4). Leg-length discrepancy.[26]
   (5). Soft hammocklike mattress.
   (6). Weak abdominal muscles.
   (7). Leaning over a low work area for a prolonged period.

b. *Clinical presentation*
   (1). Acute, debilitating low back pain forcing patient to crawl on hands and knees in the morning.
   (2). Persistent, deep, aching pain at rest,[27] which worsens in upright position.
   (3). Limited forward bending, side bending away from involved side, and rotation.

c. *Treatment and management*
   (1). The therapist should correct for biomechanical dysfunction, such as leg-length discrepancy.
   (2). Possible contributing factors that may aggravate trigger points should be explained to the patient. For example, the patient should be instructed to avoid sleeping on a soft mattress and activities that combine flexion with rotation. Also, if the patient sleeps supine, he/she should place a pillow under the knees. Most

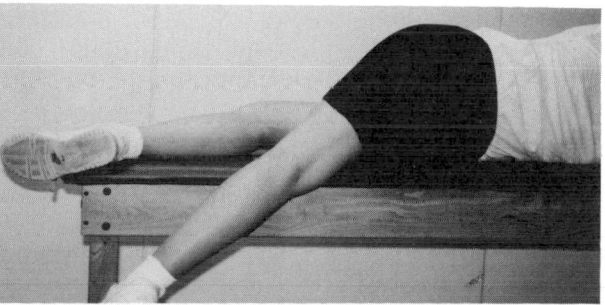

FIGURE 33–21 Tensor fasciae latae self-stretch position.

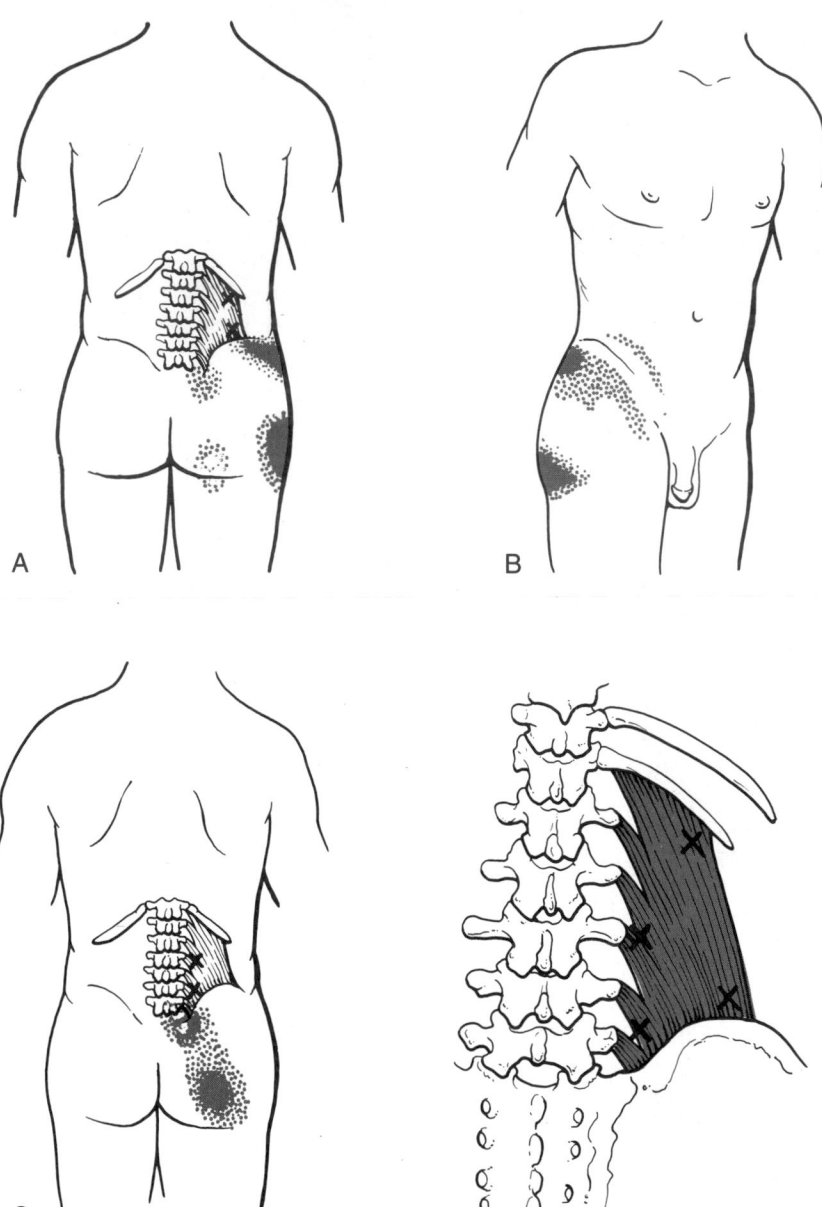

FIGURE 33–22 Quadratus lumborum trigger points and referred pain patterns. (Redrawn from Travell J, Simons D: *Myofascial Pain and Dysfunction: The Trigger Point Manual. The Lower Extremities.* vol. 2. Baltimore, Williams & Wilkins, 1992, © 1992, the Williams & Wilkins Co., Baltimore.)

important, the patient should be given a thorough explanation of the anatomy and function of the quadratus lumborum as a postural muscle. This may aid the patient in learning not to abuse the muscle.

(3). Moist heat before and after treatment.

(4). Self-stretching. The patient is positioned in hook lying. The uninvolved leg is crossed over the leg to be stretched. The involved leg is adducted as far as possible, then the patient performs a gentle isometric abduction contraction. Next, the patient allows both legs to relax on exhalation, which will allow the uninvolved leg to pull the involved leg downward and medial (see Figure 33–23).

(5). Hip-hike exercise. The patient is positioned in supine, with the hips and

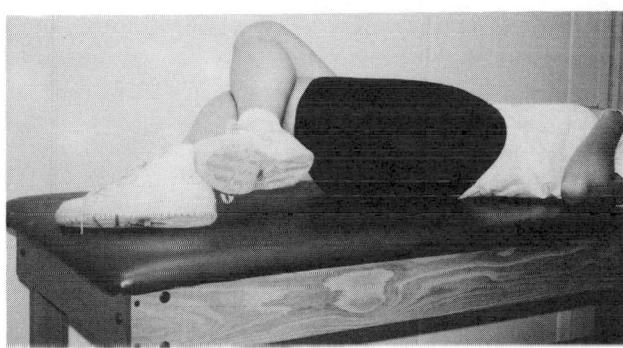

FIGURE 33–23 Quadratus lumborum self-stretch position.

knees straight. The exercise is initiated by first lowering one hip away from the shoulder while the other hip is pulled up in a "hiking" motion toward the opposite shoulder. This motion, in combination with slow, deep inhalations/exhalations, provides an adequate stretch to the quadratus lumborum.

(6). Trunk flexion exercises are included as another means of maintaining ROM. However, patients with weak abdominal muscles should begin with a lengthening contraction such as sit-backs and progress to abdominal curls as tolerated.

3. **Piriformis muscle.**[25] Two primary trigger points refer pain to the sacroiliac area, buttock, and posterior hip region. The piriformis myofascial syndrome commonly presents when the piriformis muscle syndrome, caused by entrapment of the sciatic nerve, is detected. Another component that may contribute is sacroiliac dysfunction (see Figure 33–24).

a. *Etiology*
   (1). Unusual overload of muscle, which may be caused by attempting to refrain from a fall.
   (2). Repetitive strain.
   (3). Direct trauma to the buttocks.
   (4). Sacroiliac dysfunction.

b. *Clinical presentation*
   (1). Pain aggravated by sitting with the legs crossed.
   (2). Pain increases with activity.[28]
   (3). Pain when rising from a sitting position.[29]

c. *Treatment and management*
   (1). The therapist corrects for biome-

chanical deficits, such as leg-length discrepancy.

(2). The patient is instructed in sleeping posture and other activities that may aggravate the muscle. The patient is instructed to sleep with a pillow between the legs, which provides support from the knees to the ankles. Long periods of immobilization should be avoided. Sports involving a quick braking motion with changes in direction may also perpetuate piriform trigger points.

(3). Intermittent cold spray with stretch. The patient is asked to perform active hip abduction and adduction, with the hip flexed at 90 degrees, and active rotation, with the hip straight. This is followed with application of moist heat to rewarm skin.

PLEASE NOTE: A good response to this procedure followed shortly thereafter by a reactivation of trigger points may be indicative of associated sacroiliac joint displacement.

(4). Ischemic compression. To avoid putting pressure over the sciatic nerve, the therapist should begin manual technique at the lateral end of the

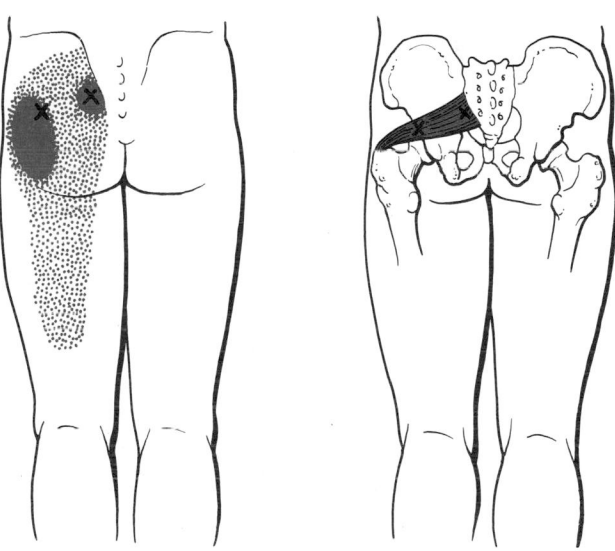

FIGURE 33–24 Piriformis trigger points and referred pain patterns. (Redrawn from Travell J, Simons D: *Myofascial Pain and Dysfunction: The Trigger Point Manual. The Lower Extremities.* vol. 2. Baltimore, Williams & Wilkins, 1992, © 1992, the Williams & Wilkins Co., Baltimore.)

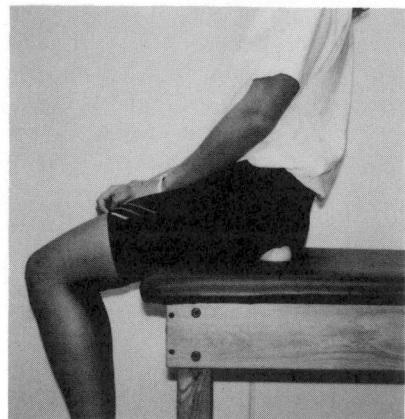

FIGURE 33–25   Use of a tennis ball for trigger-point pressure.

muscle. Travell and Simons[25] advocate use of a tennis ball for self-application of ischemic compression in sitting (see Figure 33–25).

(5). Ultrasound. Hallin[29] reports that 6 to 10 ultrasound treatments at 1.75 to 2 W/cm² for 5 to 6 minutes daily has relieved piriformis muscle syndrome.

(6). Surface EMG biofeedback. See explanation of EMG biofeedback under tensor fasciae latae. Inactive gluteal muscles may be related to an overactive piriformis on the ipsilateral side. In this case, electrodes are placed over the gluteal and piriformis muscles.

(7). Self-stretching. This is performed in sidelying on the uninvolved side. The uppermost thigh is adducted, with the hip at 90 degrees of flexion.

(8). Strengthening. The patient is positioned in sidelying on the uninvolved side, with the uppermost thigh flexed to 90 degrees. The involved leg is passively raised into abduction to allow the patient to perform a slow eccentric contraction. Gradually, the patient is progressed to a concentric contraction.

4. **Gluteus medius.**[25] Three primary trigger points can be found arranged in a fan shape at the anatomical attachment of muscle to iliac crest. The first trigger point refers pain to the posterior iliac crest and sacroiliac joint. The middle trigger point refers pain to the center of the iliac crest and downward to the midgluteal region. The third trigger point, rarely seen, refers pain to the lower lumbar area and sacrum (see Figure 33–26).

a. *Etiology*

(1). Running, sports injuries, prolonged tennis matches, and aerobics.

(2). Standing on one leg for a prolonged period.

(3). Injection of a medication into the muscle.

(4). Excessive pronation.

(5). Traumatic event such as a fall.

b. *Clinical presentation*

(1). Increased pain with walking.

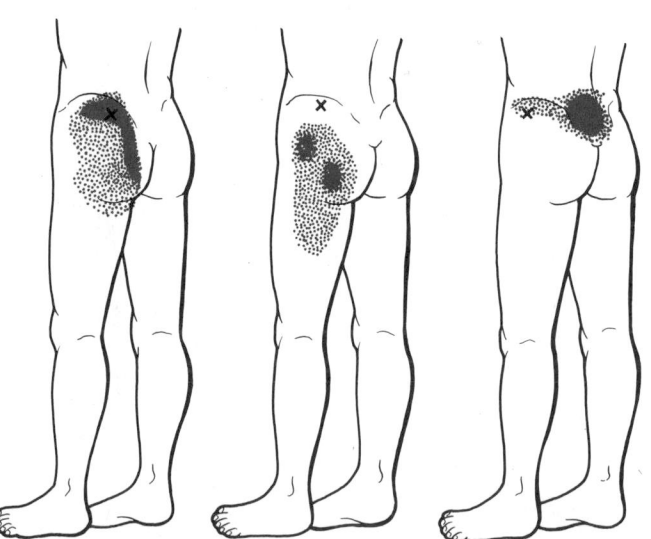
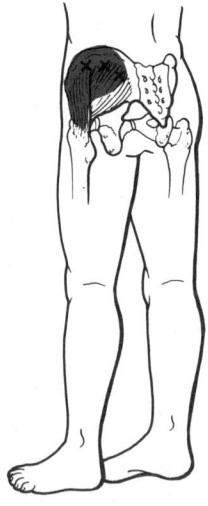

FIGURE 33–26 Gluteus medius trigger points and referred pain patterns. (Redrawn from Travell J, Simons D: *Myofascial Pain and Dysfunction: The Trigger Point Manual. The Lower Extremities.* vol. 2. Baltimore, Williams & Wilkins, 1992, © 1992, the Williams & Wilkins Co., Baltimore.)

(2). Difficulty sleeping secondary to being uncomfortable lying on affected side or supine.

c. *Treatment and management*

(1). The therapist corrects for biomechanical deficits that may perpetuate a trigger point (excessive pronation).

(2). The patient is instructed in postures to avoid, such as sitting with the legs crossed.

(3). Ultrasound.

(4). Ischemic compression. Travell and Simons[25] advocate lying supine on a tennis ball and rolling the ball forward across the tight muscle.

(5). Self-stretching. The patient is positioned in sidelying on the uninvolved side near the edge of the table. The involved leg is then placed in approximately 30 degrees of hip flexion, with the knee kept straight, which puts the hip in an adducted position. As the patient takes a slow breath in, the hip abductors gently contract. On exhalation, gravity aids in lengthening (see Figure 33–27).

(6). Strengthening. Progression to hip abductor strengthening is made when the patient does not show signs of active trigger points. Eccentric exercise is recommended as a starting point. For example, the patient lies on the uninvolved side and abducts the involved leg, with slight external

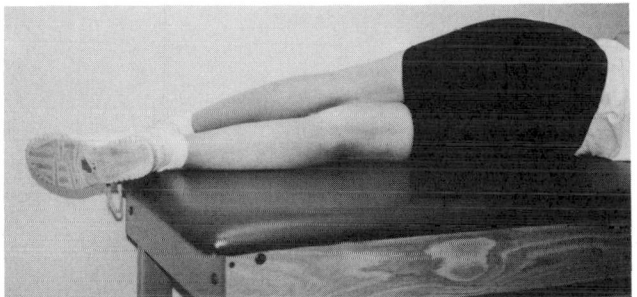

FIGURE 33–27 Gluteus medius self-stretch position.

rotation (false abduction). Then, the patient internally rotates the leg to neutral (true abduction) and proceeds to lower the extremity slowly.

5. **Gluteus minimus.**[25] Trigger points in the anterior fibers of the muscle refer pain into the lower lateral buttocks, the lateral thigh, and down into the perineal region. Posterior trigger points refer pain into the greater portion of the buttocks and into the posterior thigh and calf (see Figure 33–28).

a. *Etiology*

(1). Prolonged immobility caused by driving a car or standing.

(2). Sacroiliac dysfunction.

(3). Sitting with a full wallet in the back pocket.

(4). Acute overload secondary to a fall or walking or running too far without gradual conditioning.

(5). Intramuscular injection.

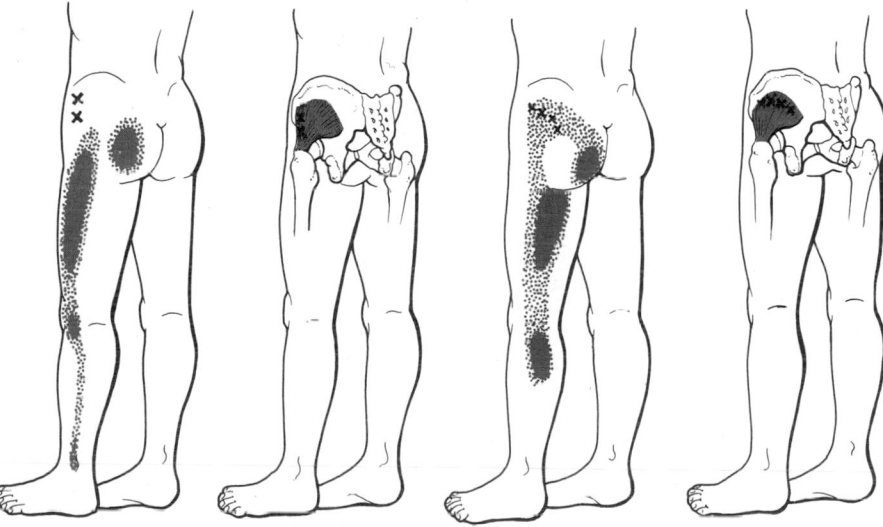

FIGURE 33–28 Gluteus minimus trigger points and referred pain patterns. (Redrawn from Travell J, Simons D: *Myofascial Pain and Dysfunction: The Trigger Point Manual. The Lower Extremities.* vol. 2. Baltimore, Williams & Wilkins, 1992, © 1992, the Williams & Wilkins Co., Baltimore.)

b. *Clinical presentation*

(1). Antalgic limp secondary to complaint of hip pain.

(2). Inability to tolerate sidelying on affected side.

(3). Difficulty rising from a sitting position and standing up straight secondary to pain.[30]

(4). Constant and excruciating pain.

c. *Treatment and management*

(1). Extrinsic factors that may aggravate trigger points should be corrected. For instance, an overweight patient may benefit from referral to a dietician.

(2). Unlike other trigger points discussed in this section, those in the gluteus minimus may be activated by direct icing of the muscle or cooling of the body as a whole. Therefore, the patient should be instructed to keep the body warm and may benefit from use of moist heat before and after exercise.

(3). The patient should be instructed in corrective postures. If trigger points are active, the patient should be instructed to sit whenever possible. The best sleeping posture is sidelying with a pillow between the knees and the legs.

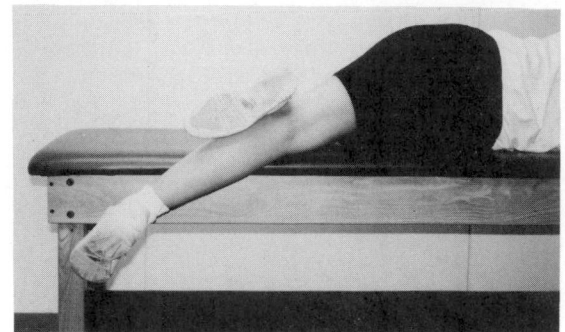

FIGURE 33–29   Gluteus minimus self-stretch position.

(4). Self-application of ischemic compression. A tennis ball should be placed under the tender area closest to the greater trochanter. The patient slowly slides the body downward. This rolling technique can also be done leaning against a wall.

(5). Self-stretching. The patient is positioned in sidelying on the uninvolved leg (back close to the edge of the mat). The bottom leg is flexed and crossed over the involved leg. The patient is instructed to perform a gentle isometric contraction. As the patient relaxes, the force of gravity assists the stretch into adduction (see Figure 33–29).

V. Treatment: Congenital and Developmental Disorders

A. Congenital hip dislocation (CDH)

1. **Etiology.** CDH may present as true congenital dislocation or as a femur that can easily be subluxed. Hips dislocated at birth may be classified as reducible or irreducible. The incidence of CDH in the United States is 1.55 in 1000 births and occurs six to eight times more frequently in girls than in boys.[31] Although the exact etiology is unknown, several potentially causative factors have been identified. Acetabular dysplasia or shallow malformation of the acetabular socket provides a mechanical mechanism for hip instability. Abnormal laxity of the hip capsule and ligaments also contributes to an unstable hip. Laxity may be the result of elevated levels of maternal estrogen that are present prior to delivery.[24] Additionally, the presence of CDH is more common after a breech delivery and therefore may be related to intrauterine positioning or trauma at birth.

2. **Clinical presentation.** Regardless of the exact etiology, early diagnosis and management of CDH are essential for positive outcome and prevention of further complication.

a. Positive results from the following special tests: Ortolani's test, Barlow's test, telescoping test, and Galeazzi sign. The ex-

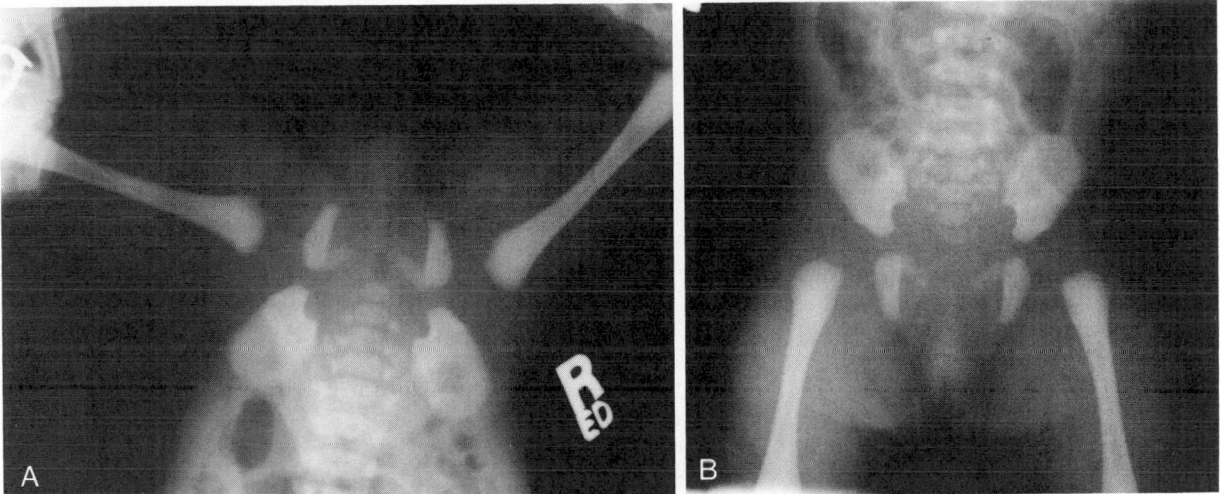

FIGURE 33–30   **A** and **B,** Radiograph demonstrating bilateral congenital hip dislocation.

aminer must remember that in cases of irreducible dislocation or bilateral dislocation there may be false-negative results.
b. Loss of abduction ROM.
c. Unequal folds in buttocks or medial thigh may be an indicator.
d. Radiographical analysis may or may not be helpful, depending on the degree of dislocation or subluxation (see Figure 33-30).

3. **Treatment.** Management for the infant with CDH involves splinting, with the hip placed in flexion and abduction. This position must be maintained to allow proper development of the acetabular socket. If the dislocation is not easily reducible, surgical intervention may be required. If diagnosis is not made at birth, and the child has begun to walk, he/she will demonstrate Trendelenburg's gait. Intervention at this point generally requires surgical reduction and an adductor tenotomy followed by application of a hip spica cast. Other surgical procedures that may be required include a derotational osteotomy if internal rotation deformity occurs, or innominate osteotomy as described by Salter to change acetabular position.[31]

B. Slipped capital femoral epiphysis

1. **Etiology.** This involves slippage of the femoral neck on the femoral head at or just dis-

tal to the epiphyseal plate. Displacement may be the result of a traumatic shearing force or, more commonly, chronic slippage of unknown origin. This condition is most common in adolescents aged 10 to 16, with a male to female incidence ratio of 2:1.[33] Slippage usually occurs in the posterior and inferior direction, with the growth plate ending up in a vertical and forward orientation.[32] The exact cause is unknown but may be related to unusual degeneration or weakening of developing bone. It has been suggested that an underlying endocrine imbalance, often seen in the very tall, slender child or obese child, may be a predisposing factor.[31]

2. **Clinical presentation**
a. Antalgic gait.
b. Pain in knee region.
c. Generally sudden onset, although there may not be traumatic history.
d. Limitation in internal rotation, abduction, and flexion. With passive flexion, femur will begin to abduct and externally rotate.[24]
e. Radiological evaluation will confirm diagnosis.

3. **Treatment.** Surgical fusion is needed to prevent further slippage. In advanced cases with complications, fusion of the hip joint itself may be necessary. Treatment following surgery is essentially identical to postfracture rehabilitation.

C. Legg-Calvé-Perthes disease

1. **Etiology.** Also known as coxa plana, this disease is a form of osteochondrosis of the femoral head. It is most frequently seen between the ages of 3 and 11 years and is four times more common in boys than in girls.[31] The etiology is unknown, but avascular necrosis of the femoral head is involved. Damage to the blood supply to the femoral head may be the result of chronic effusion with a traumatic or inflammatory condition.[31] It is a self-limited disease that ultimately resolves without intervention. Untreated, joint damage and functional limitation are likely outcomes.

   The disease process is divided into five stages: necrosis, fragmentation, revascularization (reossification), remodeling, and healed.

   a. Vascular damage occurs during the necrotic phase (see Figure 33–31A). Radiological signs that accompany this phase include small capital epiphysis, increased

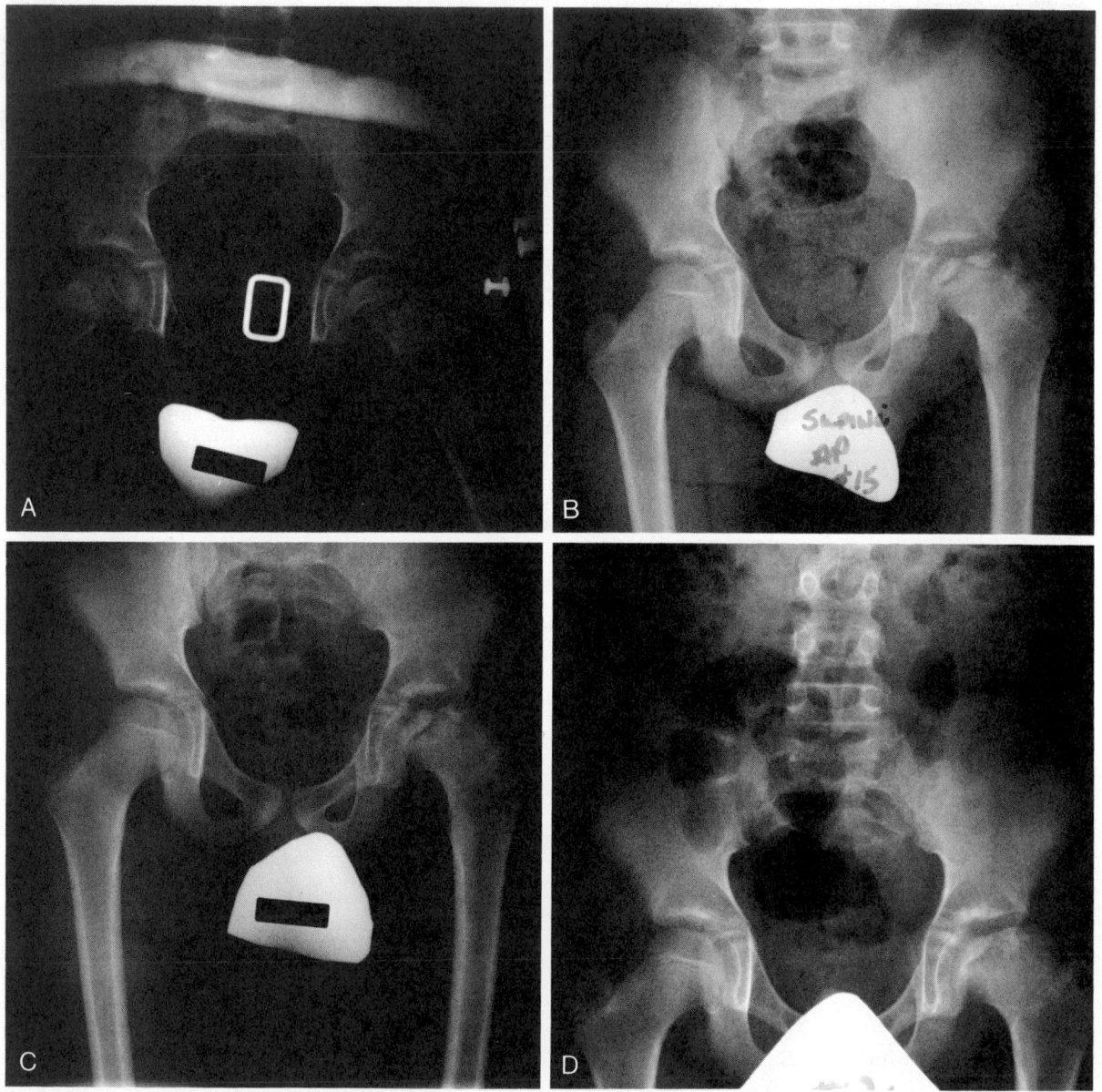

FIGURE 33–31   **A–E,** The radiographic stages of Legg-Calvé-Perthes disease.

Continued

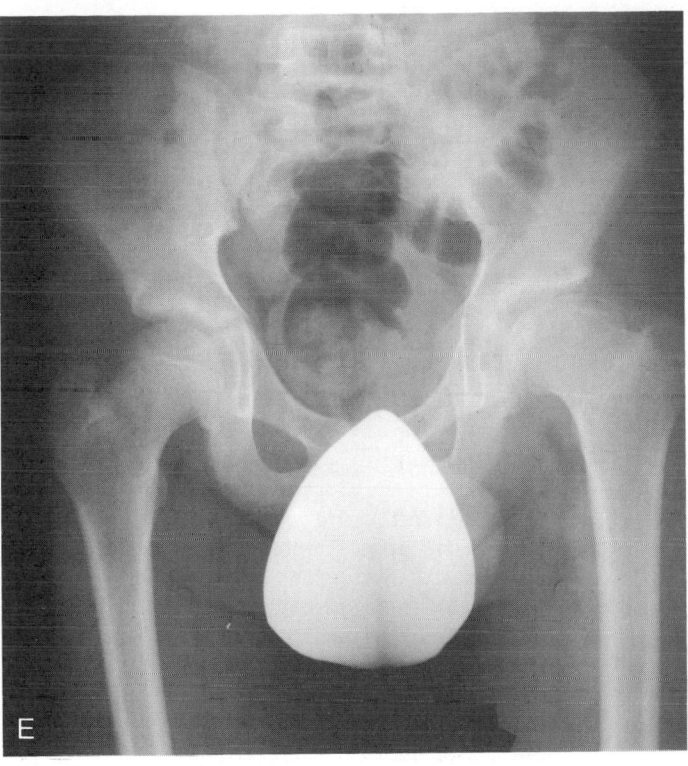

FIGURE 33–31 *(continued)*

radiodensity of the femoral head, and appearance of an osteopathic area in the medial aspect of the proximal femoral neck.

b. During the fragmentation stage, fibrous tissue invades the involved region and gradually resorbs the necrotic bone (see Figure 33–31*B*). Radiographic changes include enlargement of the femoral neck and severe deformity of the femoral head.

c. After all necrotic tissue has been resorbed, the revascularization or reossification stage begins (see Figure 33–31*C*). This gradual process is complete when the entire region has become reossified.

d. During the remodeling stage, some resultant deformity may resolve as the joint is subjected to weight bearing and normal joint forces[34] (see Figure 33–31*D*).

e. The healed stage represents the final outcome of the disease process. Bony tissue is once again viable, and further resolution of the deformity is minimal (see Figure 33–31*E*). Deformities that may result from Legg-Calvé-Perthes disease include enlarged femoral head, smaller than normal femoral head (secondary to an arrested growth plate), alteration in

femoral neck angle leading to leg-length discrepancy, or gross incongruency of articular surfaces.

2. **Clinical presentation.** Symptoms generally do not begin until the revascularization phase has begun.

a. The child may gradually develop a limp or complain of pain in the groin, medial thigh, or knee.

b. ROM limitations for internal rotation and abduction.

c. Definitive diagnosis only by radiograph, which will distinguish it from other disorders discussed in this section.

3. **Treatment.** The primary goal is to lessen the long-term damage and deformity of the femoral head. Incongruities of the joint surfaces will lead to pain and early degenerative changes. Past treatment consisted of strict bed rest with no weight bearing for several years if necessary. According to Salter,[31] carefully monitored weight bearing can be allowed as long as good joint position is maintained and treatment is initiated before significant damage has occurred. Braces or plaster casts may be applied to maintain the femoral head in the acetabulum, with the hip joint in a position of abduction and in-

ternal rotation. The prognosis is good for children who develop the disease at an early age (< 5 years) and are also diagnosed early. The outlook is better if less than half of the femoral head becomes involved. The prognosis is worse with increasing age and greater degree of involvement of the femoral head.

D. Rotational deformities

1. **Anteversion**
   a. *Etiology.* An orientation of the femoral neck and shaft whereby the neck lies in an anterior position. Because of intrauterine positioning, infants are born with an average of 30 degrees of femoral anteversion. With aging and normal development, the angle decreases to an average of 8 to 15 degrees by adulthood.[35] The developing femur is subject to torsional forces that affect its final orientation. Children who frequently sit in a W position are prone to developing excessive femoral anteversion.
   b. *Clinical presentation*
      (1). Toed-in gait.
      (2). Increased Q-angle.
      (3). Increased hip internal rotation and decreased external rotation.
      (4). Uncorrected, the condition may lead to the following:
         (a). Chondromalacia patellae.
         (b). Patellofemoral malalignment problems.
         (c). Excessive foot pronation.
         (d). Early degeneration of anterior aspect of femoral head because of concentrated weight bearing.
   c. *Treatment.* Treatment is aimed at preventing further deformity. The child will be instructed to use a "tailor" sit position instead of the W sit. If deformity is marked, night splints may be advised. As the child continues to grow, he/she may require foot orthotics to correct for overpronation and exercises to strengthen the vastus medialis oblique muscle to decrease likelihood of patellofemoral dysfunction.

2. **Retroversion**
   a. *Etiology.* This develops in a child who continually exposes the femurs to external torsional forces. Sleeping in a prone "frog" position with hips flexed, ab-

ducted, and externally rotated applies such a force.
   b. *Clinical presentation*
      (1). Toed-out gait.
      (2). Decreased Q-angle.
      (3). Increased hip external rotation and decreased internal rotation.
      (4). Uncorrected, may lead to increased internal tibial torsion and excessive foot supination.
   c. *Treatment.* As with anteversion, the treatment goal is to control abnormal forces. Changes in sitting and sleeping postures may be necessary. Bracing may be suggested only in extreme cases. Exercises to increase internal rotation may be prescribed. Corrective foot orthotics may be required as the child grows.

E. Coxa vara

1. **Etiology.** Change in femoral neck angle of inclination. At birth, this angle is 150 to 160 degrees. With normal development and weight bearing, it decreases to about 125 degrees by adulthood. Coxa vara refers to a developmental condition in which the angle of inclination continues to decrease and assumes a varus position. This bony defect may be congenital, a result of trauma, or secondary to slipped capital femoral epiphysis.

2. **Clinical presentation.** Generally not painful unless degenerative changes have begun.
   a. The patient will present with a limp associated with decreased leg length on the involved side. Segmental leg-length measurements should confirm the region of shortening.
   b. Trendelenburg's gait also will be noted as the abductors become less efficient.
   c. Decreased abduction and internal rotation.

3. **Treatment.** Treatment is conservative and involves protective weight bearing to prevent further deformity, strengthening of abductor muscles, and correction of leg-length difference if appropriate. The ultimate and most effective treatment is abduction subtrochanteric osteotomy.

F. Coxa valga

1. **Etiology.** The femoral neck angle of inclination is greater than the normal 125 degrees

in adulthood. This may be congenital, secondary to trauma or dislocation of the hip, a result of adductor spasticity, or related to lack of weight bearing in early childhood.[36] Bony changes often occur secondarily, including change in the weight-bearing surface of the femoral head, elongation of the acetabulum, and flattening of the upper acetabular rim secondary to increased forces placed there.[36]

2. **Clinical presentation**
   a. Gluteus medius limp caused by shortening of the abductor lever arm.
   b. Weakness of abductors on the involved side.
   c. Oblique position of the pelvis with leg-length difference (longer on the affected side).
   d. Radiographs needed to confirm diagnosis.

3. **Treatment.** The goal of nonsurgical management is to prevent secondary dysfunction by correcting leg-length difference. Uncorrected, dysfunction in the low back and sacroiliac joint may occur secondary to pelvic obliquity. Exercises to strengthen weak abductors and stretch tight adductors also may be indicated. In extreme cases, surgical correction by osteotomy may be necessary.

G. Infection

1. **Etiology.** Although uncommon in children, osteomyelitis can cause significant dysfunction and disability. The most usual route of entry for infective organisms is through the bloodstream. The most common organism after age 2 years is *Staphylococcus aureus*.[34]

2. **Clinical presentation.** The patient usually presents with a painful, swollen joint that may appear red and be warm to touch.

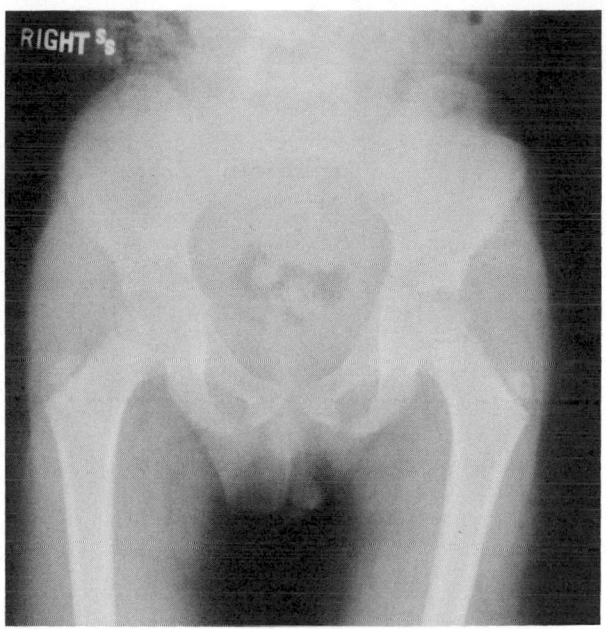

FIGURE 33–32 Radiograph demonstrating infection of the right hip joint. Note that distention of the joint capsule is consistent with the presence of excess fluid in the joint.

Range of motion is limited and painful. To confirm the suspected diagnosis, joint aspiration should be performed followed by culture of aspirated fluid. Radiographic changes may be visible (see Figure 33–32).

3. **Treatment.** Medical goals are to remove purulent fluid and to treat the patient with antibiotics. The patient may be placed in gentle traction to reduce joint pressure or be placed in a hip spica cast to immobilize the joint. Physical therapy goals are to restore joint ROM and to prevent disabling joint contracture. Strengthening exercises and gait training are also essential aspects of the program.

VI. Gait Disorders

Functional requirements (ROM) of the hip during gait were discussed earlier in this chapter, as well as the relationship between hip, pelvis, and lumbar spine. These are important concepts to keep in mind during the discussion of gait disorders.

A. Gluteus maximus lurch

1. **Cause.** Weakness of the hip extensors causes the trunk to lurch in a posterior direction at foot contact in order to shift the center of gravity posterior to the hip.

REVIEW OF NORMAL GAIT

Brief review of hip components during gait cycle: slight hip abduction and external rotation at heel strike, which rapidly moves toward adduction and internal rotation during loading. Adduction occurs secondary to drop of pelvis on the unsupported side and lateral trunk motion toward the supported side. At midstance, the pelvis is neutral, the hip is internally rotated, and the trunk begins to shift in order to load the opposite limb. The primary hip muscle groups responsible for a smooth normal gait cycle are the hip flexors, hip extensors, and hip abductors. The hip flexors contract to initiate swing and to control hip extension at the end of stance. The hip extensors provide a decelerating force after heel strike, then the greatest gluteal must initiate hip extension. During swing, the hip abductors (middle gluteal) are responsible for controlling excessive lateral pelvic tilt.

Most clinicians acknowledge that one faulty joint in the kinematic chain will cause changes throughout the lower extremity and body. This is especially true for the hip joint, which appears to be the driving force for the lower extremity. It is controlled by two-joint muscles that assist in energy conservation for the lower extremity.[29]

B. Trendelenburg's Gait

1. **Cause.** Weakness of the gluteus medius results in a lateral shift of the trunk to the weak side and a pelvis drop toward the uninvolved side. This usually occurs at the end of terminal stance as contralateral swing begins.

> PLEASE NOTE: Other possible causes of Trendelenburg's gait are painful hip, hip malalignment, or short leg.

C. Hip hiking

1. **Possible causes.** Hip flexor weakness, long leg on the involved side, or hip flexion contracture.

D. Abducted gait

1. **Possible causes.** Hip abduction contracture, pain, leg-length discrepancy.

E. Circumduction

1. **Possible causes.** Hip flexor weakness, long leg on the involved side.

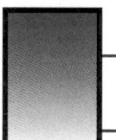

Clinical Decision-Making Cases

Case #1

EXAMINATION

Present History

CJ is a 30-year-old female who was referred to the physical therapist with a complaint of left hip and leg pain. She had undergone a dilation and curettage under general anesthesia 2 months before this evaluation. She reported sharp pain radiating from her left hip to left ankle, which began the day after the surgery. The intensity of the pain had decreased only slightly since onset, and the patient described it as severe. She also reported weakness in her left knee and calf associated with the pain. She reported an increase in symptoms with sitting and prolonged walking. Her stated position of comfort is supine, with hips and knees flexed.

Past Medical History

CJ has an unremarkable past medical history with no previous low back or lower extremity symptoms.

Social History

CJ is employed as a mail clerk/messenger at a large manufacturing company. Her job involves up to 6 hours of standing and walking daily. She is required to push up to 70 lb on the mail cart and must be able to lift up to 50 lb on an occasional basis.

Medical Evaluation

CJ initially reported to her surgeon, who ruled out any gynecological source of her symptoms. One week after onset, a radiographical evaluation revealed mild but unremarkable degenerative joint disease in the lumbar spine. An MRI scan also failed to reveal any significant lumbar spine pathology. CJ was referred to a neurologist for further work-up. Because her pain was now chronic, both conventional and surface EMG studies were performed to differentiate sciatic neuropathy from gluteal myofascial syndrome. Conventional EMG data were normal, with no signs of denervation or neuropathy. Baseline surface EMG data were collected, with electrodes placed bilaterally over the lumbar paraspinal and gluteus maximus muscles. For the test activities of lumbar flexion and gluteal isometrics, muscle activity was markedly asymmetrical, with decreased muscle activity on the involved left side.

Physical

1. Inspection.
   a. Moderately obese female with no remarkable postural deficits.
   b. Noted to stand frequently with her weight supported on her right leg.
2. Palpation.
   a. Exquisite point tenderness over the left piriformis and gluteus medius muscles.
   b. Deep pressure to trigger points in the piriformis reproduced the symptoms of left leg pain.
3. Active ROM.
   a. Marked to severe limitations in forward flexion and right lateral flexion, with severe left leg pain.
   b. Other trunk motions were moderately limited, with pain reported in the left gluteal region.
   c. Left hip internal rotation limited, with reproduction of symptoms as above.
   d. All other movements of both lower extremities within normal limits.
4. Strength.
   a. Both lower extremities 5/5.
   b. Significant discomfort with strength testing of left hip muscles.
5. Gait.
   a. Displayed an antalgic gait, favoring the involved extremity.
   b. Step length and cadence were both decreased.
6. Special tests.
   a. Lower extremity reflexes: normal and symmetrical.
   b. Straight-leg raise: positive on left at 70 degrees.
   c. Piriformis test: positive.
   d. Thomas, Ober's, scouring, and sacroiliac compression/distraction tests: negative.
7. Function.
   a. Independent mobility, but movements were slow and guarded during supine to sit and sit to stand transfers.
   b. Unable to drive secondary to exacerbation of symptoms.
   c. Reported difficulty sleeping secondary to pain.
   d. Out of work on medical leave since onset of symptoms.

ASSESSMENT/DIAGNOSIS

Correlation of surface EMG data (muscle asymmetry) with clinical evaluation (trigger points) confirmed the diagnosis of myofascial syndrome. The onset can be reasonably linked to the patient's surgery because of the prolonged positioning in hip flexion, abduction, and external rotation during the procedure; this places the piriformis in a shortened position. Palpation of trigger points in the piriformis reproduced the patient's symptoms of left buttock and lower extremity pain. Because piriformis trigger points may generate symptoms that mimic sciatic radiculopathy, use of conventional EMG testing as well as imaging is necessary to rule out lumbar spine/disc pathology. The decreased muscle activity on the involved side noted with the surface EMG test most likely represents inhibition caused by the painful trigger points.

Treatment Goals

Short-term goals for the patient included the following:

1. To achieve symmetry of the gluteal muscles (as evaluated by surface EMG).
2. To decrease sensitivity of the trigger points.
3. To decrease pain.
4. To improve function.

TREATMENT

CJ was initially seen three times a week because of the acute nature of her symptoms. The treatment plan included the use of surface EMG biofeedback, ischemic compression, massage, and thermal modalities. With the surface EMG biofeedback electrodes placed over the gluteal muscles, CJ performed isometric gluteal contractions bilaterally. (Because the piriformis muscle lies deep to the gluteal muscles, it is not possible using surface electrodes to record isolated activity of the piriformis.) The biofeedback provides visualization of the asymmetrical muscle contractions, allowing the patient to progress toward symmetry and therefore balanced contractions. Once able to perform symmetrical isometric contractions, CJ was instructed to perform functional activities such as partial squats and step-ups while being monitored by the biofeedback. As the patient achieved success, the visual feedback was used only as a tool for the therapist to monitor her progress (ie, CJ was not allowed to watch the screen while performing the tasks). This was the final assessment of her ability to produce symmetrical contractions.

Surface EMG biofeedback was used in this case as a modality to assist with neuromuscular re-education. The unique advantage it provides is the ability to identify and monitor asymmetrical muscle contractions that frequently accompany chronic pain. In clinics where this is not available, treatment using conventional modalities and stretching and strengthening exercises is also effective; however, underlying muscle imbalance may be overlooked.

Simultaneous treatment included ischemic compression and massage to the trigger points in the piriformis and gluteus medius muscles. CJ was also instructed to stretch these two muscles (see Figures 33–25 and 33–27). Moist heat was used before treatment sessions to increase local vasodilation and decrease muscle spasms associated with the trigger points. She was instructed to use heat and perform the stretches at home daily. Another option would be the use of ultrasound as a heating modality before treatment. Ultrasound was not used in this case because of a preference by the treating therapist to minimize passive therapy and encourage participation by CJ. Had the muscle spasm not responded to the selected treatment, ultrasound would have been added.

As CJ's pain resolved, her home program was advanced to include lumbar spine flexibility and strengthening exercises such as pelvic tilts, knee-to-chest stretching, bridging, and supine low back rotation exercises. She also began a light daily walking program, starting with 0.5 mile and progressing as tolerated. After 2 months, CJ had achieved her short-term goals. She now reported "minor twinges" of pain with overactivity or fatigue. Active ROM of the lumbar spine was now essentially normal. Straight-leg raise was also negative bilaterally. The piriformis muscle test continued to yield mildly positive results. Both lumbar paraspinals and gluteal muscles were now symmetrical based on surface EMG evaluation. CJ was advanced to the work-conditioning phase of her rehabilitation. Treatment frequency was increased to four times a week to maximize the strengthening and conditioning benefits. Her program included generalized conditioning activities using the treadmill, cross-country ski machine, and upper body ergometer. CJ was also instructed in proper body mechanics and lifting technique. Job-specific activities were designed, including mail sorting and stacking, push and pull activities with a weighted cart, and lifting drills.

OUTCOMES

After 4 weeks in this program, CJ was discharged to a home program that consisted of continuation of the low back flexibility and strengthening exercises and the walking program. She returned to work without restriction.

Case #2

EVALUATION

History

SM is a 9-year-old female who was admitted to the hospital with a fever and severe pain in her left hip. She underwent an arthrotomy of the hip for drainage of purulent fluid as well as a decompressive drilling of the femoral neck. SM was diagnosed with osteomyelitis and placed in mild traction, with the hip positioned in 25 degrees of abduction to maintain joint distraction. Physical therapy was initiated for ROM to the left hip and mobility training. She was discharged from the hospital with a continuous passive motion machine.

Two weeks later, SM underwent a second bone biopsy to rule out Ewing's sarcoma with subsequent fracture through the biopsy site. She underwent surgical repair and was placed in a spica cast for 6 weeks.

Following removal of the spica cast, she presented for initiation of outpatient therapy with a fibrotic hip joint.

Physical Examination

1. Dynamic posture characterized by retracted left hemipelvis and functional scoliosis.
2. Left hip maintained in external rotation.
3. Leg appears grossly equivalent.

	Passive ROM (Degrees)	Total Passive Motion (Degrees)
Left hip		
Flexion	0–42	
Extension	0–10	52
External rotation	30–55	
Internal rotation	(−)30	25
Abduction	0–35	
Adduction	0–5	40
Left knee	0–120	

	AROM (Degrees)	Total Active Motion (Degrees)
Left hip		
Flexion	0–25	
Extension	0	25
External rotation	45–50	
Internal rotation	(−)45	5
Abduction	0–25	
Adduction	0	25
Left knee	6–110	104

Strength	
Left hip	
Flexion	2−/5
Extension	2/5
External rotation	2+/5
Internal rotation	2−/5
Abduction	3−/5
Adduction	3/5
Left knee	
Extension	3−/5
Flexion	3/5

Mobility: independent with transfers and functional mobility.

Ambulation:

1. Ambulated with crutches, non–weight bearing on left lower extremity (although the patient is allowed to WBAT).
2. Left lower extremity maintained in external rotation.

ASSESSMENT/DIAGNOSIS

These results reveal substantial deficits in ROM and strength caused by fibrosis of the hip secondary to the joint infection followed by prolonged immobilization.

TREATMENT GOALS

1. Independent ambulation without assistive device.
2. Left hip flexion ROM 0 to 90 degrees.
3. Left hip internal rotation ROM 0 to 5 degrees.
4. Strength of left hip muscles 4+/5.

TREATMENT

1. Moist heat was applied to the anterior aspect of the hip, with SM in the supine position and the hip in full extension. Pelvic position was monitored closely to prevent anterior pelvic tilt (and associated hip flexion). Heat was chosen to provide vasodilation and increased extensibility of the fibrotic structures prior to stretching. Ultrasound was not used because of potential damage to the growth plate.
2. Joint mobilization.
   a. Distraction for pain relief and general capsular stretch.
   b. Posterior glide to increase hip flexion ROM.
3. Passive stretching was used for all limited motions.
4. A/AROM and AROM exercises. SM was placed in gravity-eliminated positions, using a powder board when necessary because of her strength deficits. As she improved, manual resistance was applied dur-

ing this activity, and she was progressed into positions requiring movement against gravity.
5. Weight-bearing activities.
   a. Weight bearing was initiated by means of weight shifts in a kneeling position. (Quadriped positioning was not effective because of the lack of hip flexion.) This was quickly advanced to standing weight shifts in the parallel bars.
   b. A limb-load monitor was used to provide auditory feedback for SM regarding her weight-bearing status in both kneeling and standing. The limb-load monitor was also used to increase the patient's weight bearing by gradually raising the threshold.
   c. Once SM was consistently partially weight bearing in standing, she was progressed to other activities to stimulate increased weight bearing. These included use of a balance/proprioception board, which allows gradual limb loading, and use of an isokinetic step machine with a load scale to provide visual weight-bearing feedback.
6. Functional activities. After 3 weeks, SM was beginning to ambulate short distances with only one crutch. She also reported gradual return to some normal play activities at home, including riding her bicycle and swinging her legs while using her playground swing. Her treatment was advanced to include locomotion sitting on a wheeled stool to encourage weight bearing, strengthening of knee muscles, as well as knee ROM. "Kick ball" was also added while the patient was seated on the stool.
7. An alternative treatment option would have been use of a therapeutic pool program. Water exercise would have provided the advantage of resistive exercise without the pain associated with weight bearing on the involved extremity. A therapeutic pool was not available in the clinic for use with SM.

At this point in treatment, follow-up radiographs ordered by the physician revealed the development of avascular necrosis of the femoral head. After consultation with the physician, physical therapy treatments continued with no restrictions.

Several weeks into her rehabilitation, SM was able to ambulate with a straight cane. Her gait was characterized by continued left hemipelvis retraction, with the left hip still held in abduction and external rotation (although markedly improved).

Treatment was progressed with more aggressive attempts to stabilize the pelvis during stretching and active ROM activities. This was accomplished by manual stabilization and use of stabilization straps on the treatment table. The goal was to increase dissociation of the hip and pelvis during gait, decreasing the pelvic retraction, and ultimately improving the quality of gait.

By 3 months, the patient presented with the following:

1. Passive ROM, left hip:
   a. Flexion: 0 to 65 degrees.
   b. Extension: 0 to 10 degrees.
   c. Abduction: 0 to 35 degrees.
   d. Adduction: 0 to 15 degrees.
   e. External rotation: 30 to 55 degrees.
   f. Internal rotation: (−)30 degrees.
2. Strength, left hip:
   a. Flexion, extension, abduction, adduction: 3+/5.
   b. External rotation, internal rotation: 3/5.

Treatment frequency was decreased to once per week in consultation with the physician to encourage increased activity at home and begin gradual weaning from formal therapy. Her program was advanced with an emphasis on stretching and strengthening. Special attention was placed on gait as the patient displayed Trendelenburg's gait when ambulating without the cane. Other new activities included weight-bearing exercises such as walking backwards and sideways and cross-over steps. The treadmill was introduced at this stage for additional gait training.

After 5 months, the patient was asymptomatic; however, she continued to have significant ROM and gait dysfunction. In consultation with the physician, it was agreed that she had reached a plateau and that further progress was unlikely. Re-evaluation revealed the following:

1. Passive ROM, left hip:
   a. Flexion: 0 to 80 degrees.
   b. Internal rotation: (−)15 degrees.
   c. Extension, abduction, adduction, external rotation: within normal limits.
2. Strength, left hip:
   a. All motions: 4−/5.
3. Gait:
   a. Independent without assistive device.
   b. Gluteus medius limp left with excessive left lower extremity external rotation.
   c. Stance phase shortened on left versus right.
   d. Able to perform light jog; however, gait dysfunction becomes more pronounced.

OUTCOMES

The patient was discharged to a water exercise program to include swimming and water walking twice a week. She was also encouraged to return to normal play activities as much as possible. She was to be seen by her surgeon in 2 months at which time the decision would be made about possible surgical intervention to address the external rotation contracture.

References

1. Oatis C: Biomechanics of the hip. In Echternach J (ed): *Physical Therapy of the Hip*. New York, Churchill Livingstone, 1990.
2. Lissner HR, Williams M: *Biomechanics of Human Motion*. Philadelphia, W. B. Saunders Company, 1962.
3. Rydell N: Biomechanics of the hip joint. *Clin Orthop* 1973, 92:6–15.
4. Johnston R: Mechanical considerations of the hip joint (1973). In Gould J, Davies G (eds): *Orthopedic and Sports Physical Therapy*. St. Louis, C. V. Mosby Company, 1985.
5. Johnston R: Hip motion measurements for selected activities of daily living. *Clin Orthop* 1970, 72:205–216.
6. Kisner C, Colby L: *Therapeutic Exercise: Foundations and Techniques*. Philadelphia, F. A. Davis Company, 1985.
7. Kendall F: Non-operative management of low back pain. Seminar notes. East Coast Continuing Education Center, Inc., Atlantic City, NJ, September 1991.
8. Sahrmann S: Diagnosis and treatment of muscle imbalances associated with musculoskeletal pain syndromes. Seminar notes. East Coast Continuing Education Center, Inc., Atlantic City, NJ, September 1991.
9. Karl R, Floberg J: Radiologic assessment of the musculoskeletal system. In Biossonnault WG (ed): *Examination in Physical Therapy Practice: Screening for Medical Disease*. New York, Churchill Livingstone, 1991.
10. Bassett L, Gold R, Seeger L: *MRI Atlas of the Musculoskeletal System*. London, Martin Dunitz Ltd., 1989 (distributed in the US by CRC press, Boca Raton, FL).
11. Goodman C, Snyder T: *Differential Diagnosis in Physical Therapy—Musculoskeletal and Systemic Conditions*. Philadelphia, W. B. Saunders Company, 1990.
12. Casperson PC, Kaverman D (eds): Groin and hamstring injuries (1982). In Echternach J (ed): *Physical Therapy of the Hip*. New York, Churchill Livingstone, 1990.
13. Cyriax J, Cyriax P: *Illustrated Manual of Orthopedic Medicine*. London, Butterworth Publishers, 1983.
14. American Academy of Orthopaedic Surgeons: *Athletic Training and Sports Medicine*, 2nd ed. Park Ridge, IL, American Academy of Orthopaedic Surgeons, 1991.
15. Klafs CE, Arnheim DD: Modern principles of athletic training (1989). In Echternach J (ed): *Physical Therapy of the Hip*. New York, Churchill Livingstone, 1990.
16. O'Donohue D: *Treatment of Injuries to Athletes*, 3rd ed. Philadelphia, W. B. Saunders Company, 1976.
17. Cailliet R: *Soft Tissue Pain and Disability*. Philadelphia, F. A. Davis Company, 1977.
18. Payton O (ed): Manual of Physical Therapy. New York, Churchill Livingstone, 1989.
19. Cameron HU, McNab I: Observations on osteoarthritis of the hip joint. *Clin Orthop* 1975, 108:31–40.
20. Hertling D, Kessler R: *Management of Common Musculoskeletal Disorders: Physical Therapy Principles and Procedures*, 2nd ed. Philadelphia. J. B. Lippincott Company, 1990.
21. Maitland GD: *Peripheral Manipulation*, 2nd ed. Boston, Butterworth Publishers, 1977.
22. Grieve G: Manual mobilizing techniques in degenerative arthrosis of the hip (1977). In Kisner C, Colby L: *Therapeutic Exercise: Foundations and Techniques*. Philadelphia, F. A. Davis Company, 1985.

23. Morris JM: Biomechanical aspects of the hip joint. *Orthop Clin North Am* 1971, 2:33–55.
24. Echternach J (ed): *Physical Therapy of the Hip.* New York, Churchill Livingstone, 1990.
25. Travell J, Simons D: *Myofascial Pain and Dysfunction: The Trigger Point Manual. The Lower Extremities.* vol 2. Baltimore, Williams & Wilkins, 1992.
26. Travell J: The quadratus lumborum muscle: an overlooked cause of low back pain. *Arch Phys Med Rehabil* 1976, 57:566.
27. Simons D, Travell J: Myofascial origins of low back pain. 2. Torso muscles. *Postgrad Med* 1983, 73:81–92.
28. Barton PM, Grainger WR, Nicholson RL, Bowler KL: Toward a rational management of piriformis syndrome. *Arch Phys Med Rehabil* 1988, 69:784.
29. Hallin RP: Sciatic pain and the piriformis muscle. *Postgrad Med* 1983, 74:69–72.
30. Travell J, Travell W: Therapy of low back pain by manipulation and of referred pain in the lower extremity by procaine infiltration. *Arch Phys Med* 1946, 27:537–547.
31. Salter R: *Textbook of Disorders and Injuries of the Musculoskeletal System,* 2nd ed. Baltimore, Williams & Wilkins, 1983.
32. Gruebel LD: *Disorders of the Hip.* Philadelphia. J. B. Lippincott Company, 1983.
33. Jacobs B: Diagnosis and history of slipped capital femoral epiphysis (1972). In Gould J, Davies G (eds): *Orthopedic and Sports Physical Therapy.* vol 2. St. Louis, C. V. Mosby Company, 1985.
34. Renshaw T: *Pediatric Orthopedics.* Philadelphia, W. B. Saunders Company, 1986.
35. Magee D: *Orthopedic Physical Assessment.* Philadelphia, W. B. Saunders Company, 1992.
36. Gould J, Davies G (eds): *Orthopedic and Sports Physical Therapy.* vol 2. St. Louis, C. V. Mosby Company, 1985.

Suggested Reading

American Academy of Orthopaedic Surgeons: *Athletic Training and Sports Medicine,* 2nd ed. Park Ridge, IL, American Academy of Orthopaedic Surgeons, 1991.

Boissonnault W: *Examination in Physical Therapy Practice: Screening for Medical Disease.* New York, Churchill Livingstone, 1991.

Debrunner H: *Orthopaedic Diagnosis,* 2nd ed. Stuttgart, Germany, Georg Thieme Verlag, 1982 (distributed in US by Year Book Medical Publishers, Chicago).

Gray H: *Anatomy, Descriptive and Surgical,* 15th ed. New York, Bounty Books, 1977.

Harris BA, Dyrek D: A model of orthopaedic dysfunction for clinical decision making in physical therapy practice. *Phys Ther* 1989, 69:548–553.

Hollinshead WH, Rosse C: *Textbook of Anatomy,* 4th ed. Philadelphia, Harper & Row, 1985.

Hoppenfeld S: *Physical Examination of the Spine and Extremities.* New York, Appleton-Century-Crofts, 1976.

Kapandji IA: *The Physiology of the Joints: Lower Limb.* vol 2. New York, Churchill Livingstone, 1982.

Kulund D: *The Injured Athlete.* Philadelphia, J. B. Lippincott Company, 1982.

Merritt C, Bluth E: Techniques for diagnostic imaging. *Postgrad Med* 1985, 77:56–71.

Renton P: *Orthopaedic Radiology—Pattern Recognition and Differential Diagnosis.* Chicago, Year Book Medical Publishers, 1990.

Richardson JK, Iglarsh ZA: *Clinical Orthopaedic Physical Therapy.* Philadelphia, WB Saunders Company, 1994.

Tachdjian M: *Pediatric Orthopedics.* vol 1. Philadelphia, W. B. Saunders Company, 1972.

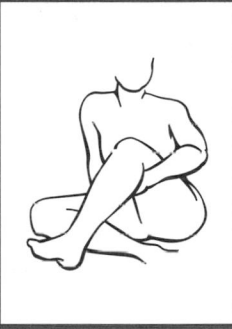

CHAPTER 34

Lower Extremity: Knee

Anthony Delitto

This chapter focuses on the assessment and treatment of common knee disorders. Conservative management is stressed. Screening procedures for injuries or severe pathologies are reviewed for the purpose of referring a patient to another health care professional, which in most cases will be an orthopedic surgeon.

Common diagnoses of the tibiofemoral as well as patellofemoral joints are reviewed. This chapter is designed to be a guide for the physical therapy treatment of the injured patient. After a brief review of anatomy, diagnosis and classification are stressed. Next, the major problems seen in knee injuries are delineated, including loss of motion, strength, endurance, and flexibility, and their significance is discussed. With each physical impairment, measurement and specific techniques to treat the resultant problems are elaborated. The pertinent literature is reviewed as needed. Finally, specific entities are discussed in case studies.

I. Epidemiology of Knee Injuries

Knee injuries rank second to low back pain as the reason people visit outpatient physical therapy clinics. The knee is the anatomical location of the most commonly seen injuries in such sports as ice hockey,[1] football,[2] wrestling,[3] cycling,[4] and soccer.[5,6] The incidence rate is equal in females and males[7,8] and certainly does not spare children and adolescents.[9,10] It is estimated that 100,000 acute knee injuries occur in the United States each year, costing millions of dollars in surgery and rehabilitation.

II. Anatomy

Thorough knowledge of the gross anatomy of the knee will aid the clinician during the diagnostic process. This section covers the gross anatomy pertinent to the musculoskeletal assessment of the knee. For more thorough coverage of anatomy, including circulation and integument, the reader is referred to other texts.[11]

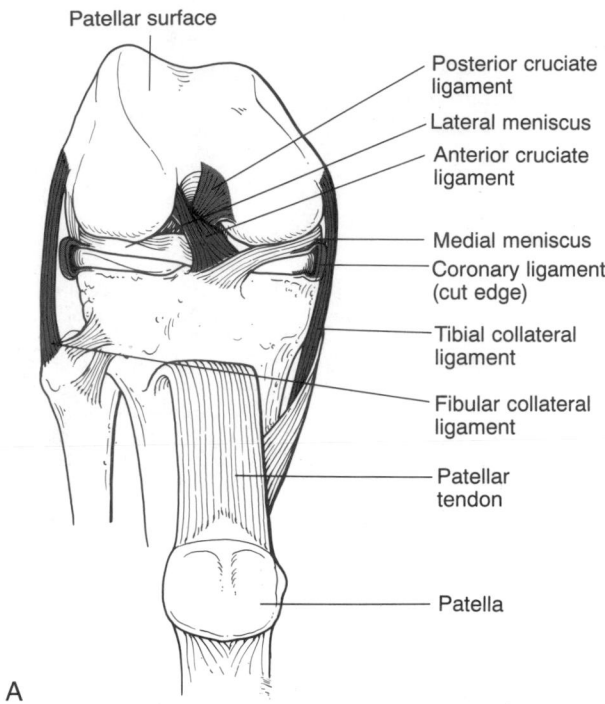

Patellar surface

Posterior cruciate
ligament

Lateral meniscus

Anterior cruciate
ligament

Medial meniscus

Coronary ligament
(cut edge)

Tibial collateral
ligament

Fibular collateral
ligament

Patellar
tendon

Patella

A

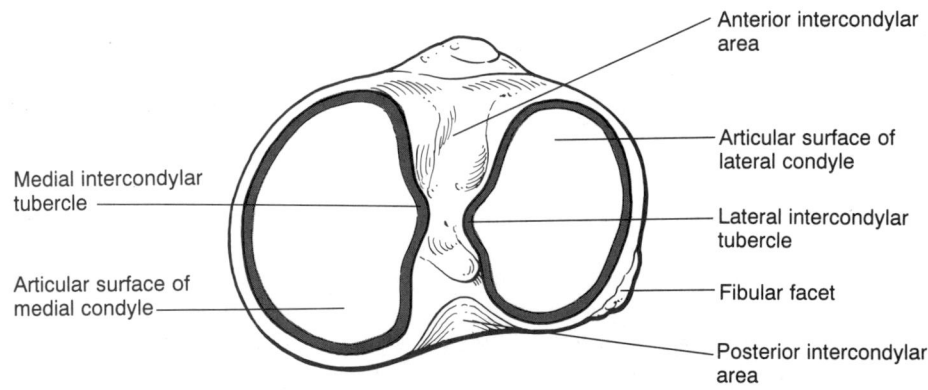

Anterior intercondylar
area

Articular surface of
lateral condyle

Lateral intercondylar
tubercle

Fibular facet

Posterior intercondylar
area

Medial intercondylar
tubercle

Articular surface of
medial condyle

B

FIGURE 34–1   **A**, Anterior view of the knee with the patellar tendon cut and drawn downward. Note the distal attachment for the anterior cruciate ligament, the proximal attachment of the posterior cruciate ligament, the coronary ligament attaching the menisci to the tibia, and the collateral ligaments.
   B, Superior view of the tibial condyles. Note the very small degree of concavity and the very small surface area of the tibial condyles.

A. Osteology

The knee joint is functionally two separate joints: the patellofemoral joint and the femorotibial articulation (referred to as the knee joint proper).

1. **Bony articulations**
   a. Distal femur.
   b. Proximal tibia.
   c. Patella, a sesamoid bone.

2. **Articulating surfaces**
   a. Distal femur: convex lateral and medial condyles and concave patellar articulating surface (see Figure 34–1A).
   b. Proximal tibia: minimally concave and relatively flat medial and lateral tibial condyles (see Figure 34–1B).

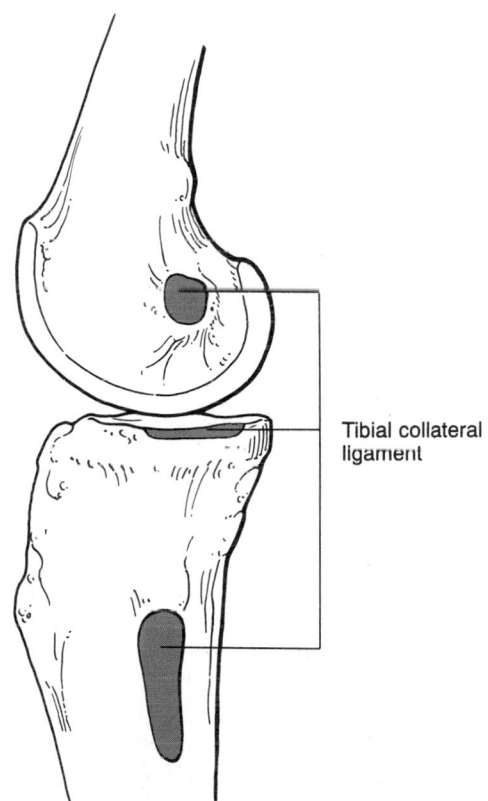

C

FIGURE 34–1 *(continued)* **C**, Sagittal view of the bones of the knee joint. Note the relative difference between joint surface area of the femoral and tibial condyles. Note two distinct distal attachments of the tibial (medial) collateral ligament.

c. *Patella:*
   (1). Undersurface, triangular shaped, fits well in the patellar articulating surface of the femur to provide a relatively stable joint.
   (2). Contributing to the static stability of the patellofemoral joint is a relatively high lateral portion of the patellar groove on the femur (see Figure 34–1A).

3. **Articulation weaknesses**
   a. Despite apparent static stability, patellar dislocations are seen with virtually all dislocations occurring laterally, with the patella overriding the lateral buttress of the patellar articulating surface of the femur.
   b. The femoral condylar surfaces of the knee joint proper are quite convex, articulating with relatively flat tibial condyles and not offering a great deal of static, bony stability to the knee. The femoral articulating surface area is much larger compared with the tibial surface area, and this has important ramifications in the arthrokinematics of the knee joint (see Figure 34–1C).
   c. The superior borders of the femoral articulating surfaces are not symmetrical when comparing medial to lateral condyles.
      (1). The medial border is higher (or more superior) than the lateral surface (see Figure 34–2A).
      (2). The higher medial border causes the medial tibial condyle to continue to move superiorly on the femoral condyle while the lateral condylar joint ceases movement, resulting in an apparent lateral rotation of the tibia on the femur at the terminal knee extension (the screw home mechanism; see Figure 34–2B).

B. Ligaments

1. The stability of the knee comes from ligamentous support.
2. Four major ligaments provide the bulk of support: the collaterals (medial and lateral) and the cruciates (anterior and posterior).
   a. *Medial collateral ligament.* This is a broad, fanlike structure that courses from the

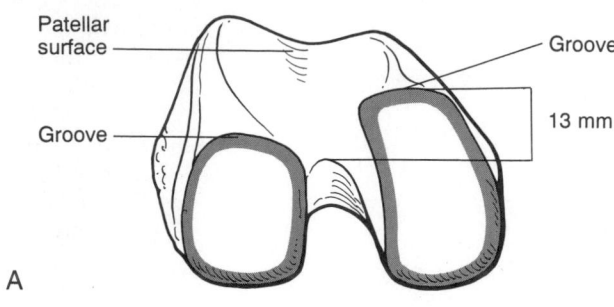

Patellar surface

Groove

Groove

13 mm

A

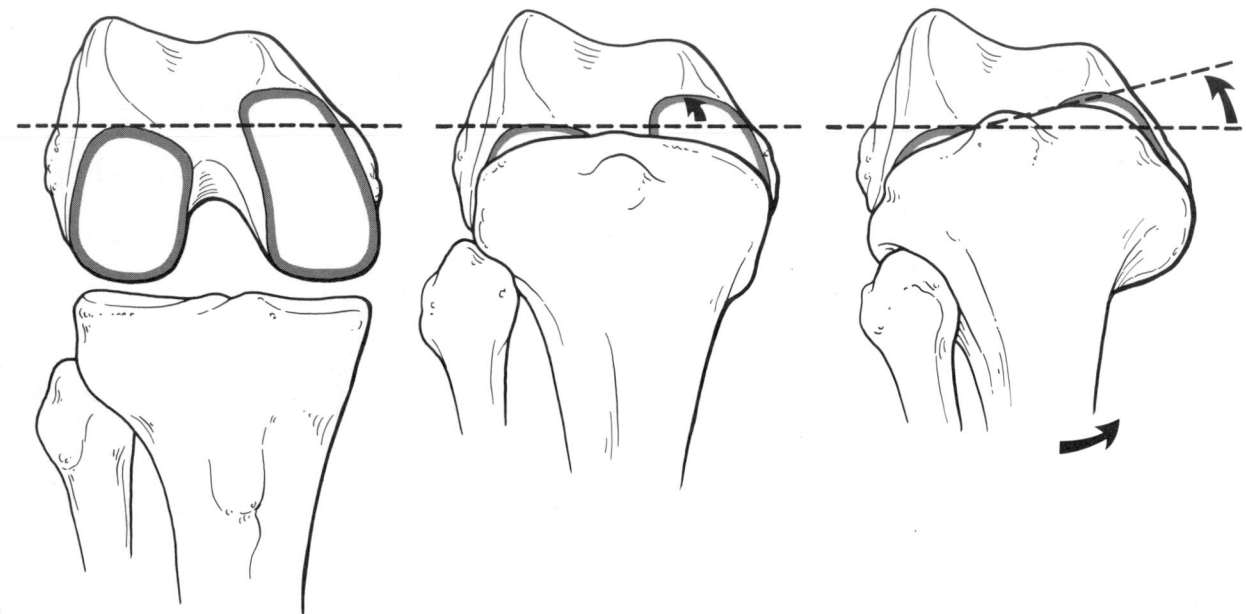

B

FIGURE 34–2 **A**, Joint surface of femoral condyles. Note the high lateral buttress of the lateral surface of the patellofemoral surface, which provides static medial stability to the patella, and the more superior border of the condylar surface on the medial side, which accommodates the medial tibial condyle and provides for external rotation of the tibia at terminal extension (the screw home mechanism).

B, The screw home mechanism of the knee joint at terminal extension.

medial femoral epicondyle to the medial tibial condyle (see Figure 34–3A). The superficial fibers attach distally on the pes anserinus, and the deeper fibers attach more proximally to the medial condyle as well as to the underlying joint structures, including the coronary ligament and the medial meniscus. The superficial fibers remain free of the proximal tibia (see Figure 34–1A), allowing lateral rotation of the tibia during terminal extension (screw home mechanism).

This ligament prevents the tibia from abducting (or prevents valgus stress).
  b. *Lateral collateral ligament.* This is a more cordlike structure than its medial counterpart; it courses from the lateral epicondyle to the head of the fibula (see Figure 34–3B). It does not articulate with the underlying knee joint structures. This ligament prevents the tibia from adducting (prevents varus stress).
  c. *Anterior cruciate ligament.* The proximal attachment is from the posterior portion

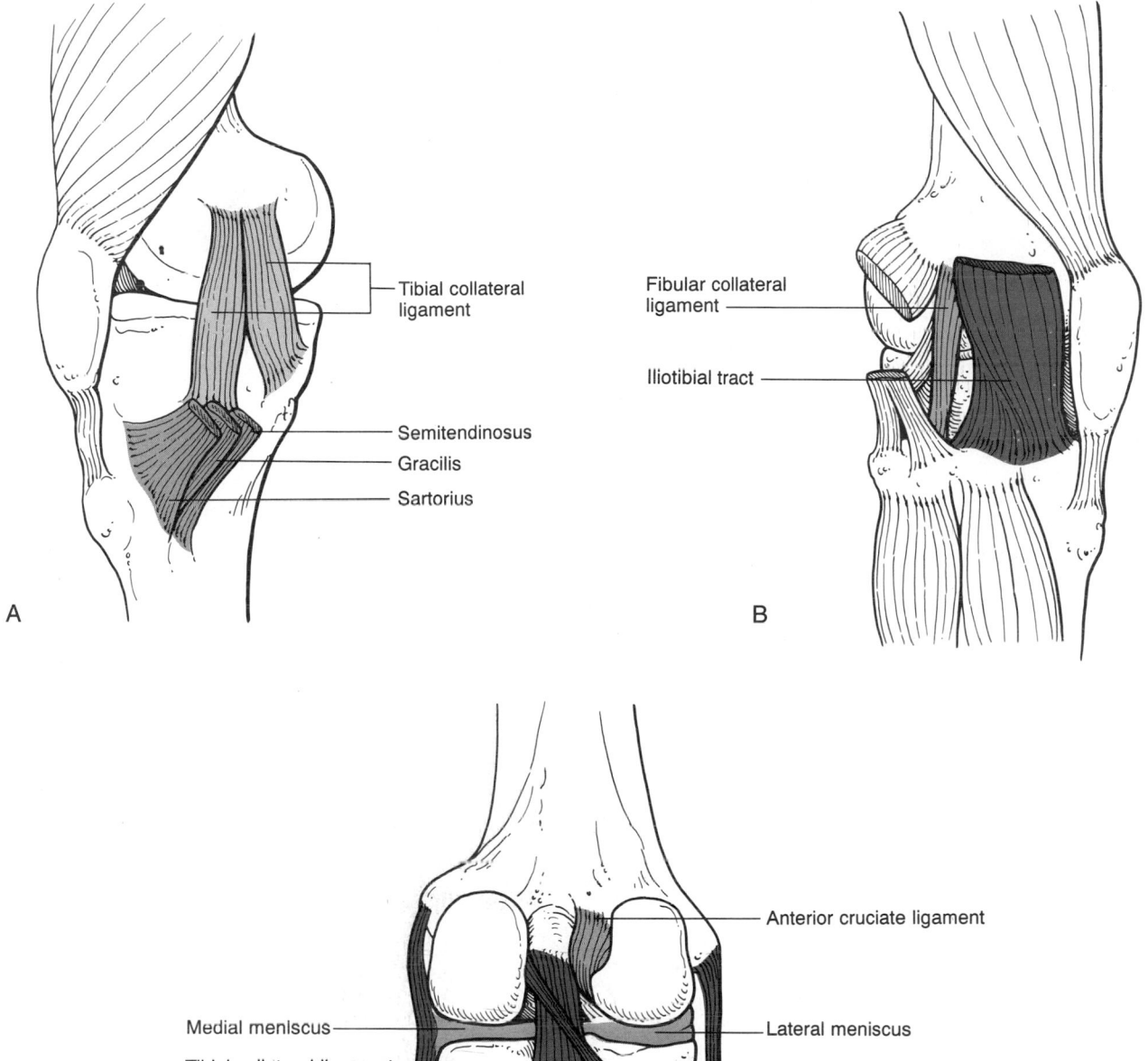

FIGURE 34–3 **A,** Medial view of the knee. Note the broad, fanlike tibial collateral ligament, whose superficial fibers have a distal attachment (along with the sartorius, semitendinosus, and gracilis muscles) on the pes anserinus whose deeper fibers have a distal attachment closer to the joint and joint structures.

B, Lateral view of the knee. Note the cordlike fibular (lateral) collateral ligament and its distal attachment on the fibular head. Also note the distal attachment of the iliotibial tract.

C, Posterior view of the knee. Note the distal attachment of the posterior cruciate ligament and the proximal attachment of the anterior cruciate ligament. Also, note the intimate arrangement between the tibial collateral ligament and the medial joint structures (*eg,* medial meniscus) and the absence of such an arrangement with the fibular collateral ligament.

of the medial surface of the lateral femoral condyle; it courses anteriorly and medially through the femoral intercondylar area to a distal attachment at the tibial intercondylar area just medial to the midline (see Figure 34–1A). It lies anterior to the posterior cruciate ligament.

   d. **Posterior cruciate ligament.** The proximal attachment is from the lateral surface of the medial femoral condyle; it courses posteriorly to a distal attachment at the posterior intercondylar area of the tibia (see Figure 34–3C).

3. The most commonly injured knee ligaments are the anterior cruciate and the medial collateral.

   a. Injury to the anterior cruciate ligament is the most common of all knee ligamentous injuries.

   b. It presents a particular challenge to health care professionals to return the patient to some degree of normal function.

C. Other joint structures: the menisci

A pair of fibrocartilaginous, semilunar menisci are located on the medial and lateral compartments. They are attached to the tibia via the coronary ligaments (see Figure 34–1A). The menisci are wedge shaped, thicker on the periphery, appearing to increase the concavity of the relatively flat tibial condylar surfaces. They are relatively avascular, making the viability of repair after injury (*eg*, tearing) questionable.

1. **Functional considerations: knee ligaments and menisci**

   a. The knee has two degrees of freedom, with the bulk of its motion being in the sagittal plane. Normally, it has no frontal plane motion because the collateral ligaments prevent abduction or adduction. Tear of either collateral ligament results in profound instability.

   b. The knee has minimal rotational motion, and only when in some degree of flexion. The bulk of its motion is sagittal, with the knee being able to extend fully and flex to greater than 130 degrees.

   c. The stable knee joint relies on the four major ligaments.

      (1). The role of collateral ligaments may be more obvious than that of the cruciate ligaments.

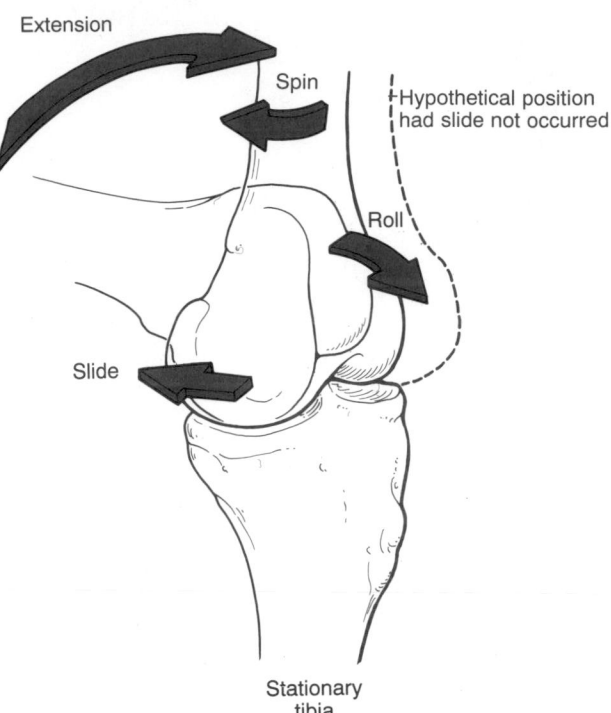

FIGURE 34–4 An analysis of the articular movements that are combined during extension at the knee joint.

      (2). The integrity of the cruciate ligaments is extremely important for normal knee function.

         (a). There is a greater area of femoral than tibial articulating surfaces.

         (b). The normal sagittal motion of the knee joint comprises a complex series of arthrokinematic movements, including rolling, spinning, and sliding (see Figure 34–4).

      (3). The critical role of both cruciate ligaments is to maintain normal arthrokinematics of the knee during flexion and extension, particularly during weight-bearing activities.

      (4). The major symptomatic complaint with anterior cruciate ligament insufficiency is the knee "giving way" during weight bearing with the knee near terminal extension.

   d. The major source of trouble involving the menisci is tearing and then impinging within the knee joint on the weight-bearing surfaces, resulting in knee "locking."

D. Musculature

Two basic muscle groups of major consequence around the knee are the hamstrings (semimembranosus, semitendinosus, and biceps femoris muscles) and quadriceps femoris (vastus medialis, vastus lateralis, vastus intermedius, and rectus femoris muscles). The oblique fibers of the vastus medialis serve to provide a medial pull to the patella, particularly during terminal extension. The quadriceps femoris muscle works through the extensor mechanism to extend the knee. The hamstring musculature is, for the most part, multijoint. The bulk of muscle crosses the hip joint. The quadriceps femoris muscle, with the exception of the rectus femoris muscle, crosses only the knee joint.

1. **Functional considerations of musculature**
   a. In a non–weight-bearing condition in which the distal segment is free to move, the quadriceps femoris muscle provides an extension moment to the knee while the hamstrings provide a flexion moment. Deficits in the function of the quadriceps femoris muscle are more prevalent in knee conditions, result in more deleterious effects on everyday function, and become the physical therapist's major target during rehabilitation.
   b. Disorders of the patellofemoral joint usually implicate lateral malalignment of the patella while in the patellofemoral groove of the femur. This results in vague anterior knee pain felt when any activity involving forceful knee extension (eg, climbing stairs) is attempted. Disorders contributing to this malady include
      (1). Femoral anteversion.
      (2). Patella alta.
      (3). Inherent weakness in the medial vastus muscle.
      (4). Chondromalacia.
   c. The patella (a sesamoid bone located within the quadriceps tendon) provides substantial mechanical advantage to the quadriceps extensor mechanism. Loss of all or part of the patella, a common occurrence with anterior blows resulting in fractures, will almost assuredly result in a physical limitation when forceful knee extension is required (eg, stooping, climbing stairs).

III. Diagnosis

Knee injuries appear inevitable and can be expected to occur with almost all sporting activities, especially those that involve contact. It is difficult to predict the outcome of any given injury; some are severe enough to disable a patient permanently, even with optimal intervention and rehabilitation. Incomplete or inadequate rehabilitation from injury will almost certainly result in compromised function. Therefore, an accurate diagnosis is of paramount importance. Two diagnostic perspectives follow: diagnosis by a referring physician and diagnosis by the physical therapist in direct access practice.

A. Diagnosis by physician

The patient is referred directly from an orthopedist after surgery or office visits. The clinician, the second contact, involved in rehabilitating the patient will already be aware of the diagnosis made by the orthopedist. Most severe diagnoses, such as complete tears of ligaments, will already be recognized, and primary management will be well under way. Problems of nonmusculoskeletal origin, such as malignancy of rheumatic diseases, should also have been screened for and ruled out. Clinicians should still be aware of signs or symptoms possibly inconsistent with the orthopedist's diagnosis. Any sign or symptom inconsistent with an initial diagnosis must be brought to the referring physician's attention, as alternative management strategies may be indicated. A list of signs and symptoms that should be considered and possibly brought to the attention of a primary care physician are included in Table 34–1.

B. Diagnosis by clinician

In selected other cases, the therapist involved in rehabilitating the patient may be the primary contact for the patient; therefore, the clinician must recognize signs and symptoms consistent with a severe knee injury.

Table 34–1. SIGNS AND SYMPTOMS INDICATING THAT THE KNEE PATIENT SHOULD BE RETURNED TO THE REFERRING PHYSICIAN

Locking of knee (true locking)
Progressive and unexplained swelling
Joint line tenderness, especially with extension and overpressure
Progressive loss of or failure to gain range of motion
Demonstrable instability
Pain that is severe and disproportionate to injury
Profound and sudden loss of sensory or motor function in the leg muscles

(From Delitto A, Lehman RC: Rehabilitation of the athlete with a knee injury. *Clin Sports Med* 1989, 8:805–840.)

1. Knee injuries can be divided into three categories of severity.
   a. *Injuries requiring emergency procedures.*
      (1). In cases involving trauma, dislocation of the knee with vascular compromise of the popliteal artery must be ascertained. Absence of pedal pulses and fullness in the popliteal space comprise the major signs. More subtle signs of vascular compromise include blanching, with increased time necessary for refilling of capillaries in the toes, and a coldness of the entire leg to the touch. Any question of vascular compromise after a knee injury constitutes an emergency situation. The patient must seek appropriate medical intervention immediately because the potential for limb loss exists.
      (2). Interruption of the common peroneal nerve is another injury problem seen with concomitant loss of function in the anterior compartment musculature.
      (3). Other severe injuries include subtle lateral tibial plateau fractures, which can be missed in the severely traumatized knee. Subtle depression of the lateral tibial plateau may not be evident, even with radiographs, and may require tomographical examination to define the bony pathology. Other clues to severe injury require invasive procedures, such as aspirating the joint. For example, fat globules must always be searched for in bloody knee aspirate. This is an important finding that suggests a possible fracture. Complete work-ups ruling out severe injuries require experienced medical care. To alleviate any doubt, the physical therapist must be sure that the patient had a thorough work-up before initiating treatment.
   b. *Injuries that should be seen by an orthopedist as soon as possible (within a day or so as opposed to immediately).*
      (1). Although the urgency is not as great as in the previously mentioned injuries involving vascular compromise, damage to ligamentous or meniscal structures should never be taken lightly. Referral to appropriate practitioners should be expedited. Signs and symptoms to look for are listed

DIAGNOSIS AND TREATMENT DECISION MAKING

A systematic approach to the history and physical examination of the patient with complaints of knee pain is important in making decisions concerning the diagnosis and subsequent treatment plan. For the physical therapist who sees a patient as a first contact, two major decisions have to be made: (1) to treat or to refer directly to an appropriate physician and (2) if the decision is treatment, to determine which is the best technique to use for the specific problem. In the three categories of knee injury described previously, the obvious decision in the first two categories is not to treat and instead to refer the patient. In the last category, the decision to treat or refer depends on what additional information is obtained from the history and physical examination.

The most conservative approach remains to refer the patient to an orthopedist or physician who is competent in knee care whenever there is a possibility of a severe knee injury.

Table 34–2. SIGNS AND SYMPTOMS IN THE ACUTE INJURY INDICATING THAT A SERIOUS INJURY HAS OCCURRED

Locked knee; inability to extend the knee fully without severe pain
Immediate swelling
Hearing a "pop" during the injury
Sensation of instability
Inability to do a straight-leg raise
History of rotational or valgus stress with foot planted
Pain with hyperflexion

(From Delitto A, Lehman RC: Rehabilitation of the athlete with a knee injury. *Clin Sports Med* 1989, 8:805–840.)

Table 34–3. MECHANISMS OF INJURY TO THE KNEE AND POSSIBLE STRUCTURES INJURED

Mechanism of Injury	Structure Possibly Injured
Varus or valgus contact without rotation	1. Collateral ligament 2. Epiphyseal fracture 3. Patellar dislocation or subluxation
Varus or valgus contact with rotation	1. Collateral and cruciate ligaments 2. Collateral ligaments and patellar dislocation or subluxation 3. Meniscus tear
Blow to patellofemoral joint, or fall on flexed knee, foot dorsi-flexed	1. Patellar articular injury or osteochondral fracture
Blow to tibial tubercle, or fall on flexed knee, foot plantar flexed	1. Posterior cruciate ligament
Anterior blow to tibia, resulting in knee hyperextension	1. Anterior cruciate ligament 2. Anterior and posterior cruciate ligament
Noncontact hyperextension	1. Anterior cruciate ligament 2. Posterior capsule
Noncontact deceleration	1. Anterior cruciate ligament
Noncontact deceleration, with tibial medial rotation or femoral lateral rotation on fixed tibia	1. Anterior cruciate ligament
Noncontact, quickly turning one way with tibia rotated in opposite direction	1. Patellar dislocation or subluxation
Noncontact, rotation with varus or valgus loading	1. Meniscus injury
Noncontact, compressive rotation	1. Meniscus injury 2. Osteochondral fracture
Hyperflexion	1. Meniscus (posterior horn) 2. Anterior cruciate ligament
Forced medial rotation	1. Meniscus injury (lateral meniscus)
Forced lateral rotation	1. Meniscus injury (medial meniscus) 2. Medial collateral ligament and possibly anterior cruciate ligament 3. Patellar dislocation
Flexion-varus-medial rotation	1. Anterolateral instability
Flexion-varus-lateral rotation	1. Anteromedial instability
Dashboard injury	1. Isolated posterior cruciate ligament 2. Posterior cruciate ligament and posterior capsule 3. Posterolateral instability 4. Posteromedial instability 5. Patellar fracture 6. Tibial fracture (proximal) 7. Tibial plateau fracture 8. Acetabular and pelvic fracture

(Adapted from Magee DJ: *Orthopedic Physical Assessment,* 2nd ed. Philadelphia, W. B. Saunders Company, 1992, p 375.)

in Table 34–2. An accurate history assists in the diagnosis. Various mechanisms of injury as related to possible structural pathology are given in Table 34–3.

c. ***Mild to moderate injuries of the joint and surrounding structures.***

  (1). These constitute the majority of knee cases requiring health care intervention.

IV. Examination

The examination consists of a history and physical examination, which ultimately lead to a classification that guides the physical therapist in treatment planning. The classification is merely a label placed on clusters of data obtained from the history and physical examination. Most often, the cluster contains obvious physical impairments that indicate obvious treatment. A list of common classifications, including the physical impairments, contributing factors, and differential classifications, is included in Appendix F.

A. History

1. **Mechanism of injury.** Patients can often reveal in great detail the mechanism of injury to the joint, including such invaluable information as whether the foot was planted, the occurrence of a valgus stress or direct blow, and so on. The patient should be interrogated closely to try to relate the mechanism of injury to possible structures that may be involved as a result of certain stresses to the joint. Table 34–3 lists mechanisms of injury to possible joint structures that may be involved.
   a. Patient heard a "pop." A distinct "pop" may denote serious injury, possibly involving the anterior cruciate ligament, especially if followed by immediate swelling.
   b. Patient remembers a misstep just before injury. Clicking, catching, or "true" locking point toward a possible meniscal injury. The complaint of locking must be specified.
      (1). True locking implicating the meniscus presents as an inability to extend with pain, as if something inside the joint has locked. Patients may further explain that when they internally or externally rotate the knee, motion is regained.
      (2). Clicking may indicate a meniscal injury but may also be associated with patellofemoral origin.
         (a). To differentiate the two, the therapist should ascertain where the click is and when it occurs. A medial or lateral joint line location implicates meniscal injury, whereas a parapatellar (usually lateral) location implicates a patellofemoral origin. Usually, clicking at end-range extension has a patellofemoral joint origin, whereas clicking with the knee in more flexion may be more indicative of a tibiofemoral joint problem.

PLEASE NOTE: True locking and clicking at the joint line with the knee in flexion, as described, strongly implicates either a meniscal injury or a loose body in the joint. These patients should be referred to an orthopedist if they have not already been sent there. Even if the patient was referred, it is important to review these findings with the physician. Before proceeding with rehabilitation, a meniscal injury or a loose body impinging in the joint should be ruled out.

2. **Swelling.** The most beneficial diagnostic marker for swelling will be the contents of the aspirate.
   a. The therapist should ascertain when the swelling occurred. Immediate swelling (within 6 hours of the injury) may indicate an acute, serious ligamentous injury.
   b. Delayed swelling (next day) may result from articular damage, meniscal injuries, loose bodies, overuse, or systemic disorders.

3. **Instability.** The patient should be asked to describe "giving way" in his/her own words. True instability of the rotatory type must be distinguished from the "giving way" that the patient feels owing to such signs as weakness in the quadriceps muscle or swelling in the knee. Most patients with true instability due to an anterior cruciate ligament deficiency can explain very well the pivot shift phenomenon, either verbally or with graphic displays using their hands.
   a. True instability due to an anterior cruciate deficiency usually occurs with a rotational motion with the knee close to end-range extension.
   b. Instability due to quadriceps muscle

weakness will manifest in activities such as stair descent (when the knee is flexed to a greater degree and greater quadriceps power is necessary).

4. **Overuse syndrome.** The clinician should ascertain whether the intensity of activity being performed was suddenly increased immediately before the patient sustained injury. This line of questioning is helpful in diagnosing any overuse syndromes that may be causing the patient's problem.

5. **Magnitude of dysfunction.** The patient should be questioned about the magnitude of dysfunction the injury causes. If the patient is able to continue playing, the injury is probably not as severe as if the injury forced him/her to stop playing. Valuable clinometric indices are available to quantify a patient's perceived disability, such as the Lysholm scale.[12] These scoring scales quantify what the patient feels is his/her disability, an often ignored component of the patient assessment.

V. Measuring Outcome

A few scales are used to assess the overall function of the patient with a predominant knee problem. General health status indices include the functional status questionnaire, the sickness impact profile, and the SF-36. The advantage of general health status indices is that these tools capture the overall function of the patient in a comprehensive manner and therefore are most beneficial with patients who have systemic problems (*eg*, rheumatoid arthritis).

Disease-specific measures of health status examine a patient's functional disabilities related to a specific diagnostic entity. An example of a disease-specific health status report is the Lysholm knee rating scale, which is designed to rate a patient with an anterior cruciate deficiency. The Lysholm knee rating scale is included in a modified form (so that it can be used as a self-report) in Table 34–4.

Table 34–4. MODIFIED LYSHOLM KNEE SCORE

Please check the statement that best describes the way you walk.
___ I never walk with a limp.
___ I rarely walk with a limp, or I walk with a slight limp.
___ I walk with a constant and severe limp.

Which of the following do you presently use as a support while you walk?
___ I can walk without crutches or a cane.
___ I can put some weight on my leg, but I need at least one crutch or a cane to walk.
___ I cannot put any weight on my leg when walking.

Do you experience LOCKING of your knee?
___ No, never.
___ My knee catches but does not lock.
___ Yes, my knee locks occasionally.
___ Yes, my knee locks frequently.
___ Yes, my knee is locked all the time.

Do you experience slipping or giving way of your knee?
___ No, never.
___ Yes, rarely during sporting activities or other severe exertion.
___ Yes, frequently during sporting activities or other severe exertion.
___ Yes, occasionally during daily activities.
___ Yes, frequently during daily activities.
___ Yes, on every step.

Which of the following best describes your level of pain?
___ I have no pain in my knee.
___ I have occasional pain, which is slight and present only after severe exertion.
___ I have marked pain during severe exertion.
___ I have marked pain after walking more than 2 mi.
___ I have marked pain after walking less than 2 mi.
___ I have constant pain.

Which of the following best describes swelling in your knee?
___ I have no swelling.
___ I have swelling only after severe exertion.
___ I have swelling after ordinary exertion.
___ I have constant swelling.

Which of the following best describes your ability to climb stairs?
___ I have no problems on stairs.
___ I am only slightly impaired on stairs.
___ I can negotiate stairs, but only one at a time.
___ I cannot go up or down stairs.

Can you get into a full squat position?
___ Yes, with no problems.
___ No, but I am only slightly impaired.
___ No, I cannot squat with my knee past 90 degrees.
___ No, I cannot squat at all.

VI. Treatment Problems

A. Swelling

Swelling should be treated as quickly as possible, certainly before any strengthening of the quadriceps muscle is attempted. DeAndrade *et al.* demonstrate convincingly the deleterious effects of knee effusions and the reflex inhibition to the quadriceps caused by swelling-induced joint distention.[13] Young *et al.* illustrate how this cycle can be circuitous, with continued attempts to use the quadriceps muscle of the thigh compounding the existing reflex inhibition.[14] Consider:

- The majority of functional activities require knee control at end-extension range.
- Therapists elicit quadriceps contractions routinely for this junction.

A swollen knee is a problem to the patient not only while attempting quadriceps exercises in rehabilitation but more so when performing everyday activities such as walking.

When the patient presents with a swollen knee and is seen for the first time, the knee must be assessed by a physician to determine the cause of the swelling. Because aspiration of the joint and its contents can yield invaluable diagnostic data, the patient should see a physician immediately. In many overuse injuries, the patient presents with a swollen knee and the physical therapist usually attributes the cause of the swelling to a sudden increase in activity compared with a baseline level. Even in the latter case, the patient who presents with swelling should be referred to a physician for determination of any intra-articular cause.

1. **Measurement: quantitative methods**
   a. *Tape measure.* Cheap and quick to administer. Accuracy is a problem. The clinician must be sure
      (1). To measure the same level each time.
      (2). To pull with the same tension consistently.
      (3). To take a cross-section while measuring.

PLEASE NOTE: Intra- and inter-rater reliability with circumferential measurement of the limbs has yet to be reported, so error associated with this measurement technique has not been determined.

   b. *Water displacement*
      (1). Convenient for more distal extremity assessment (*eg*, foot and ankle or wrist and hand).
      (2). Quite cumbersome for assessment of conditions such as knee effusion.

2. **Treatment**
   a. *Aspiration.* The most effective means of treatment is to aspirate the joint. This technique provides immediate relief for the patient and is diagnostic once the contents of the effusion are analyzed. Possible diagnoses associated with specific contents of knee joint aspirates after an injury to the knee are given in Table 34–5.

PLEASE NOTE: In addition to treating swelling, some techniques are used prophylactically. For example, a patient will first carry out exercise programs using various devices, and then modalities such as ice in combination with high-voltage pulsed currents will be used after workouts. The clinician should avoid the patient's having a swollen knee during physical therapy at all costs.

   b. *Cryotherapy.* Ice is usually applied for 20-minute intervals after exercise sessions, especially those designed to gain range of motion in the knee. Ice massage, ice packs, cold packs, or other cryotherapy machines are used. Ease of home use is the greatest advantage of cryotherapy.
   c. *Pressure bandaging.* This is often used to prevent swelling prophylactically.

PLEASE NOTE: Both cryotherapy and pressure bandaging have yet to be shown effective through well-designed clinical trials. Widespread

Table 34–5. DIAGNOSTIC MARKERS ASSOCIATED WITH ASPIRATE FROM AN ACUTELY INJURED KNEE

Aspirate	Diagnosis
Dark venous blood	Patellar dislocation
Light arterial blood	Anterior cruciate ligament
Synovial fluid, blood tinged	Peripheral meniscus
Pus	Infection
Clear synovial fluid	Nonspecific intra-articular damage

(From Delitto A, Lehman RC: Rehabilitation of the athlete with a knee injury. *Clin Sports Med* 1989, 8:805–840.)

use, logical mechanism of action, economy, and low potential harm to the patient make them acceptable additions to therapy. Few would argue against their use.

　　d. ***Transcutaneous electrical nerve stimulation/ stimulator (TENS).*** Many types of TENS are available for use by the clinician.
　　　　(1). *Monophasic current.* The most often used clinical modality is the so-called high-voltage pulsed current (HVPC) stimulator.
　　　　(2). *Biphasic current.* This type constitutes most other TENS used for both muscle training and pain control.

PLEASE NOTE: No reports are in the literature demonstrating the effectiveness of HVPC in decreasing knee swelling. HVPC is, however, a widely used modality for this purpose. HVPC has been shown by Kloth and Feeder in a controlled clinical trial to have positive effects on wound closure in humans.[15] Brown *et al.* have clearly demonstrated that electrical stimulation effects on wound healing are *polarity specific.*[16,17] Thus, the clinician should be aware that differential polarity effects have been substantiated with high-voltage galvanic current. If the swelling is of superficial origin concomitant with the surgical wound, HVPC may be an effective adjunct to therapy.

　　e. ***Compression pumps.*** These include Jobst extremity pumps.

B. Range of motion: extension

The knee should normally extend to neutral position, or 0 degrees. The importance of attaining full extension whenever possible in patients with knee disorders cannot be overemphasized. First, flexion contractures of the knee can have obvious detrimental effects on performance. Second, the position of full extension of the knee is the point of maximal joint congruity. Morrissey has shown that loading between the tibial and the femoral condyles approaches three times body weight at early and late phases of stance.[18] Inability to extend the knee fully during initial weight acceptance (*eg,* heel strike of gait) causes further increases in the force per unit area on the surfaces of the tibial and femoral condyles owing to the incongruence of the joint surfaces. Third, a flexion contracture functionally shortens the lower extremity, with resultant abnormal forces affect-

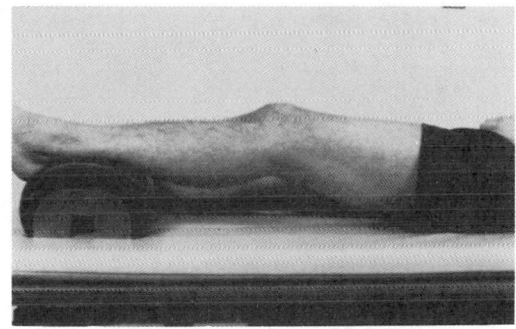

FIGURE 34–5 Positioning of the knee to assess passive extension. Any limitation seen in this position can be attributed to joint structures of the knee (as opposed to being attributed to muscle). (Reprinted from Delitto A, Lehman RC: Rehabilitation of the athlete with a knee injury. *Clin Sports Med* 1989, 8:805–840.)

ing the kinetic chain, especially at the pelvis and lumbar spine.[19]

　　1. **Measurement of knee extension**
　　　　a. *Patient supine:*
　　　　　　(1). The hamstring musculature is slackened; thus, assessment of the knee joint can be made.
　　　　　　(2). The examiner rests the patient's foot on his/her knee or a towel roll.
　　　　　　(3). The weight of the lower extremity segment is allowed to straighten the knee (see Figure 34–5).
　　　　　　(4). Goniometric measurement can be obtained easily with the patient in this position (see Figure 34–6).
　　　　b. Patient standing (if weight bearing is possible), with involved knee silhouetted in front of a normal, uninvolved knee:

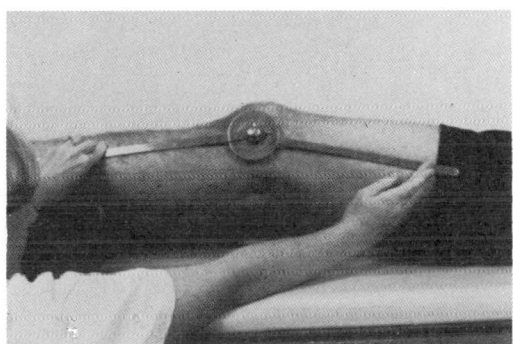

FIGURE 34–6 Measurement of passive extension of the knee with a standard goniometer. (Reprinted from Delitto A, Lehman RC: Rehabilitation of the athlete with a knee injury. *Clin Sports Med* 1989, 8:805–840.)

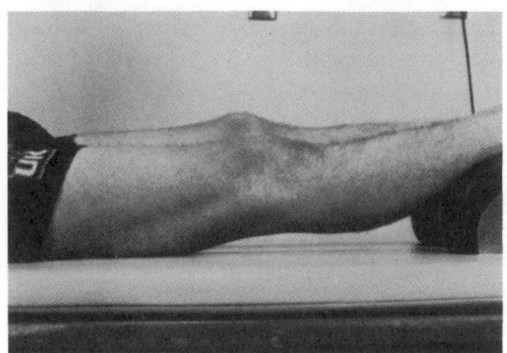

FIGURE 34–7 Qualitative assessment of lack of knee extension by superimposing uninvolved extremity. (Reprinted from Delitto A, Lehman RC: Rehabilitation of the athlete with a knee injury. *Clin Sports Med* 1989, 8:805–840.)

(1). Measurement using a goniometer becomes more difficult as the knee is assessed in the final 10 to 15 degrees of extension. This is due to the screw home mechanism of the knee in terminal extension, where motion is rotational as opposed to sagittal, especially in the last 5 degrees of movement.[20] For a better marker of how close the knee is getting to full extension, the position of the involved knee should be compared with that of the normal uninvolved knee (see Figure 34–7). The knees should be placed in the same position and their positions compared. That the knee does not screw home fully may be the best judgement rather than attempting to ascertain that the knee is 2 or 3 degrees from full extension as measured goniometrically. Because of the greater error associated with goniometric measurement of knee extension compared with other joint measurements, the knee comparison technique may be best.[21]

(2). Finally, even if the knee joint measures or looks to be fully extended, overpressure must be applied to the joint without reproduction of symptoms before a knee joint can be judged to have normal extension. This can be accomplished using the supine setup described above and applying overpressure to the joint in the direction of extension. This po-

sition is held briefly. At most, the patient should feel a stretch behind the knee similar to what is felt on the normal, uninvolved side. If pain is produced, it is usually indicative of either tightness in the capsule (where the pain can be decreased with application of techniques to increase knee extension) or an internal derangement (*eg*, loose body impinging inside the joint), in which the pain will worsen when implementing knee extension techniques.

2. **Knee flexion contractures**

PLEASE NOTE: For clarity, any joint limitation not involving a loose body impingement or meniscal injury is referred to as a flexion contracture.

a. *Prevention*
(1). It is best to allow motion of the knee as early as feasibly possible. Immobilization or partial immobilization times should be minimal. Immobilization should be supplemented with gentle passive range of motion of the knee, with the lower extremity out of any orthotic device. The potential for damage to intra-articular reconstruction or meniscal repair occurs when the patient or therapist is not *gentle*. With anterior cruciate ligament grafts that are isometric, a fixation loss is unlikely, even in the bone-tendon-bone anterior cruciate ligament reconstructions. Although the importance of early motion cannot be denied, surgeons can be reluctant to leave this treatment up to the discretion of the physical therapist or patient.
(2). Continuous passive motion (CPM) has been purported to be effective in the prevention of contractures as well as in decreasing pain and swelling after knee surgery.[22] The use of CPM may not be free of risks in certain cases, as illustrated in cadaver knees involving bone-to-bone fixation.[23] Excessive cost is another disadvantage. However, CPM can be a positive adjunct if used discriminately in gaining extension in postoperative cases.

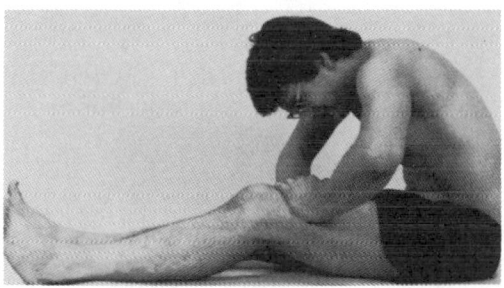

FIGURE 34-8 Patient whose hamstrings are so tight that they cannot effectively push the knee into passive extension. (Reprinted from Delitto A, Lehman RC: Rehabilitation of the athlete with a knee injury. *Clin Sports Med* 1989, 8:805–840.)

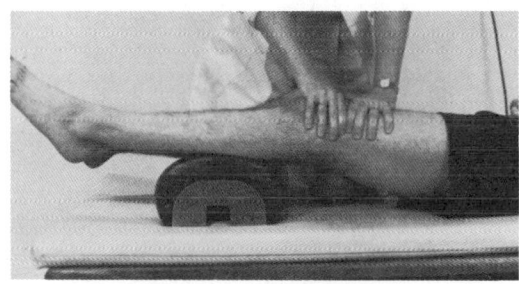

FIGURE 34-10 If higher forces are used to extend a flexion contracture, the counterforce should be moved up to the proximal tibia. This causes the patient to feel stretching behind the knee rather than deep inside the knee. (Reprinted from Delitto A, Lehman RC: Rehabilitation of the athlete with a knee injury. *Clin Sports Med* 1989, 8:805–840.)

PLEASE NOTE: The preceding techniques work well for acute knee injury when immediate intervention is possible; however, the clinician can always expect to see a large number of patients later, after contracture has occurred. Other techniques requiring more forceful pressure applied by the clinician must be used to regain extension.

    b. *Forceful passive extension.* This is reserved for times when the contraindications mentioned above (*eg,* graft fixation) are no longer a worry. The force can also be applied by the patient, although some patients may not be able to apply sufficient forces because of tight hamstrings (see Figure 34-8). Alternative exercise programs for such patients are accomplished with the hip in extension (see Figure 34-9). An extension force applied directly over the knee joint with the counterforce at the heel is often ineffective, usually resulting in little true knee

extension motion and a resultant pain "deep inside the knee." Applying a counterforce proximally on the tibia (see Figure 34-10) is helpful in inducing an anterior roll and slide on the tibia relative to the femur, an accessory motion necessary in normal knee extension. The patient should feel a stretching in the posterior area of the knee. Usually, lower-amplitude forces applied for long periods, as opposed to high-amplitude, short-duration bouts, are tolerated best by patients. Clinicians can use body weight or weight cuffs.

    c. *Posterior capsule stretch.* Muscular attachments are used (semimembranous and gastrocnemius).

       (1). *Contract relax method*

          (a). The patient is prone with the knee off the table (see Figure 34-11).

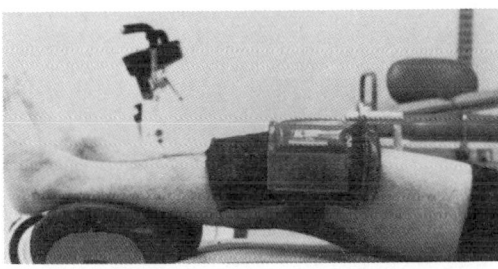

FIGURE 34-9 Alternative position, using the weight of an ice pack to apply extension force. This technique should use small forces for extended periods (*eg,* 5 lb for 25 minutes, at least three times a day). (Reprinted from Delitto A, Lehman RC: Rehabilitation of the athlete with a knee injury. *Clin Sports Med* 1989, 8:805–840.)

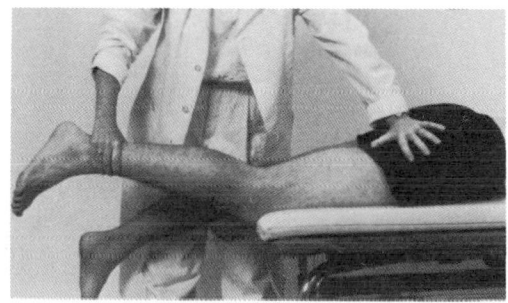

FIGURE 34-11 Positioning for the contract-relax technique to increase passive extension of the knee. The stretch should be felt in the posterior knee area. This should be repeated five times, for at least three sets. (Reprinted from Delitto A, Lehman RC: Rehabilitation of the athlete with a knee injury. *Clin Sports Med* 1989, 8:805–840.)

(b). The knee is placed in full extension with overpressure.

(c). The patient is instructed to bend the knee against resistance applied at the posterior shank.

(d). This is held for 8 to 10 seconds, then the patient relaxes.

(e). The therapist ascertains whether the patient truly relaxes by observing the hamstring musculature.

(f). When the hamstrings relax, slight pressure is exerted in the direction of knee extension.

(g). This process is repeated at least 8 to 10 times.

(h). Excessive pressure should not be exerted toward extension; the patient will resist with hamstring contraction.

(2). *"Wall lean" method*

(a). The patient stands in a "wall lean" position, with the knee in maximal extension.

(b). The foot is dorsiflexed maximally while maintaining full knee extension.

(c). The foot is then plantar flexed slightly for 8 to 10 seconds while maintaining knee extension.

(d). The patient relaxes.

(e). Then knee extension and ankle dorsiflexion are attempted.

(f). This process is repeated 8 to 10 times.

d. *Patient participation.* The patient must be an active participant in the process to gain full extension. This includes doing exercises as well as getting rid of habitual activities that reinforce the contracture. While sitting at home or work, the knee should be passively extended with slight overpressure at least 10 times per hour when awake. The patient must be encouraged to use increased range of motion as it is gained. Usually, this involves eliminating a postural habit resulting from the knee problem.

(1). Full extension at heel strike should be encouraged rather than walking almost flatfooted with the knee in 15 to 20 degrees of flexion at initial stance.

(2). The therapist should also encourage standing with body weight on the involved extremity, with the knee as straight as possible, rather than carrying most weight on the uninvolved side.

e. *Serial casting*

(1). Used if knee extension is not progressing as anticipated.

(2). A cylinder cast is applied.

(3). Gentle extension pressure is applied until the plaster hardens.

(4). Care should be exercised; the knee should not be pushed into extension or the patient will not tolerate the technique.

(5). Moderate discomfort may occur but there should not be severe pain, numbness, or any other signs of cast tightness.

(6). Every other day, the cast is removed and a new one applied.

(7). The goal is to stretch the knee slowly to full extension, within a week to 10 days.

(8). Major disadvantage: the patient will lose most of regained flexion.

3. **Contraindications to aggressive passive extension.** The clinician should consult with the referring physician concerning restrictions on full passive extension. Full extension may be contraindicated in some conditions, such as

a. Collateral ligament injuries (both surgically repaired and treated conservatively). The greatest potential for damage with passive full extension occurs during the first 6 weeks after injury or surgery.

b. Postsurgical anterior cruciate ligament grafts that have less stable fixation (*eg*, semitendinous).

C. Range of motion: flexion

Full knee flexion occurs when the calf touches the hamstrings with the heel pushed up against the buttock. The goal should be full flexion. Most ligamentous repairs or reconstructions, however, will not reach full flexion. With aging, flexion will probably decrease. Slight decreases in flexion do not have as drastic an effect on performance as decreases in extension do.

1. **Measurement of knee flexion**

a. *Patient supine:*

(1). The hip and knee are simultaneously

flexed to keep the rectus muscle of the thigh slack; this eliminates the rectus from causing a flexion deficit.

   (2). If measured in prone position, a tight rectus will always limit knee excursion.

   b. *Alternative technique:*

   (1). The patient steps onto a step stool.

   (2). The patient then leans forward, flexing hip and knee, applying gentle force with controlled body weight (see Figure 34–12).

   c. With either technique, a goniometer measurement can be precise, with little associated intra- or inter-rater error.

2. **Treatment: lack of knee flexion.** Physical therapy for a knee that does not bend fully should be avoided. A program of early gentle motion should be implemented. CPM can be used with the same precautions as mentioned earlier. More aggressive techniques are required for patients with flexion deficits.

   a. *Passive motion*

   (1). *Step-stool technique:*

      (a). As described previously, the patient steps onto a step stool and then leans forward, flexing the hip and knee simultaneously.

      (b). Simultaneously, the patient mobilizes the patellofemoral joint.

         (i). Pressure is applied after placing the pisiform muscle on the superior pole of the patella.

         (ii). The patella is pushed distally down the patellofemoral groove.

      (c). Patients should perform this exercise hourly.

      (d). A compliant patient may need only this technique to regain knee flexion.

   b. *Active motion*

   (1). *Stationary bicycle technique:*

      (a). This may be especially useful if available and can be used at home.

      (b). The seat height should be raised so that the patient can achieve just enough flexion to complete an excursion of the pedal.

      (c). As pedaling becomes easier, the seat height is lowered 0.5 in.

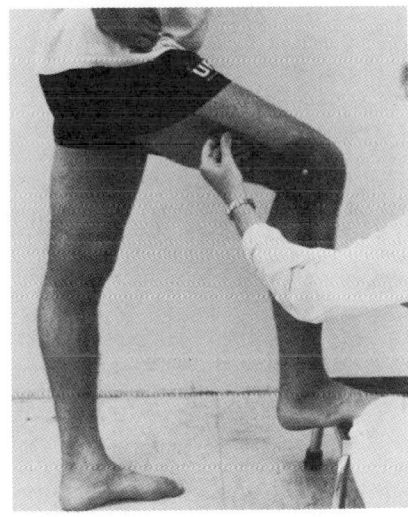

FIGURE 34–12 Alternative method for determining passive flexion of the knee. Controlled body weight adds to the external force. There always is more flexion with this technique than in the measurement described in Figure 34–11. (Reprinted from Delitto A, Lehman RC: Rehabilitation of the athlete with a knee injury. *Clin Sports Med* 1989, 8:805–840.)

      (d). The patient works to increase knee flexion by completing full excursion of the pedals.

      (e). The procedure is repeated until about 110 degrees of knee flexion is obtained.

      (f). This technique is not effective in regaining full flexion.

      (g). Substitutions such as hip hiking at the top of the excursion and plantiflexion while approaching the top of the excursion should be noted and discouraged.

   (2). *Prone knee flexion technique:*

      (a). A rope is attached to the ankle.

      (b). The rope is pulled over the shoulder to stretch the joint and rectus muscle of the thigh (see Figure 34–13).

      (c). The contract-relax technique is used.

   (3). *Squat technique:*

      (a). Squats are effective for regaining end range of flexion (110 to 135 degrees).

      (b). Weight bearing on the involved extremity must be encouraged.

   c. *Manipulation under general anesthesia*

   (1). Employed as a last resort if conservative techniques are unsuccessful.

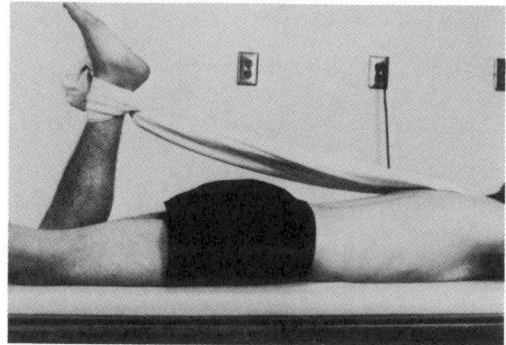

FIGURE 34–13 Rope over the shoulder. This method is not as effective as that described in Figure 34–12 for stretching the knee joint structures but provides an excellent tool to stretch the rectus muscle of the thigh. The contract-relax technique is an effective addition to this stretch. The therapist should watch for excessive anterior tilt to the pelvis. (Reprinted from Delitto A, Lehman RC: Rehabilitation of the athlete with a knee injury. *Clin Sports Med* 1989, 8:805–840.)

    (2). Following manipulation, as soon as feasible, the physical therapist aggressively intervenes.

    (3). The techniques described previously are used to maintain flexion of the knee.

D. Muscle performance

1. Of the major muscle groups around the knee, the quadriceps group is the most seriously affected by knee joint injuries and subsequent surgery. In addition to reflex inhibition induced by injury, the quadriceps group is selectively weakened after major knee ligament injury.[24–26] The disparity between quadriceps and hamstring loss of function probably arises from anatomical considerations; *ie,* the bulk of the hamstring muscles cross the hip joint, where they undergo lengthening and shortening during their action of hip extension. In contrast, of the quadriceps group, only the small strap muscle of the rectus muscle of the thigh crosses the hip. Thus, the quadriceps group is the primary target of deleterious and well-documented effects of immobilization and disuse.[27]

2. The task at hand for the physical therapist is twofold: the harmful effects of immobilization and disuse must be minimized and further injury to the knee joint must be prevented while it is immobilized or partially immobilized.

3. The task becomes quite a dilemma considering the following:

  a. *Functional overload* is the most widely respected and documented theory of strengthening muscle. The muscle must be stressed to a greater degree than it is used to being stressed for the muscle to respond by increasing its contractile force capability.[28] Usually, forces of near-maximal voluntary contractile efforts are used for short duration, or high-resistance and low-repetition exercises.

  b. Grafts not as strong as the original ligament are used in reconstructive surgeries, such as of the anterior cruciate ligament. Muscular force outputs, because of their elongation effect on the ligament grafts, are deleterious to the surgical repair. For example, heavy resistive exercises of the quadriceps muscle of the thigh should not be permitted in the range of 0 to 45 degrees in patients after anterior cruciate ligament injury repair.

  c. The most effective exercises are dynamic, with the muscle shortening or lengthening. Immobilization precludes using these types of contractions. Alternatively, isometric exercises can be used. Isometric exercise, however, purportedly only strengthens within the specific training range. This may not be optimal. For example, strength gain by training the quadriceps involves isometric exercise at greater than 45 degrees of flexion to protect an anterior cruciate ligament graft. Because most functional activities are performed with the knee at end-extension range, how effective can this technique be if it is specific to only this range of motion?

■ PLEASE NOTE: The best techniques to strengthen muscles (*eg,* heavy resistive, dynamic exercise) are contraindicated in treating the patient with knee disorders. All require high contractile forces that potentially can injure already compromised joint structures. Alternative techniques are described beginning on p 1020.

4. **Measurement of muscle performance deficits**

  a. Quantitative assessment of quadriceps strength is easily and reliably obtained using

    (1). Cable tensiometers.

(2). Strain gauge devices.

(3). Isokinetic dynamometers.[29]

PLEASE NOTE: Measurements are obtained either isometrically (peak force or peak torque) or isokinetically (work and power). Judgements concerning strength are best made by comparison with the uninvolved side. Caution should be used in making judgements based on ratios to body weight or another muscle group. It has been shown on numerous occasions that formation of such ratios is problematic and error prone.[30–32]

b. A ratio based on gravity corrected isokinetic work of the involved quadriceps to the uninvolved quadriceps is probably the most sensitive measurement of quadriceps strength.

(1). On the basis of a test-retest (3 days apart) model of more than 300 people with knee disorders, in our past work we found reliability coefficients to be greater than 0.90 (intraclass correlation coefficient) and standard error of measurement (SEM) to be 4% using a LIDO isokinetic dynamometer.

(2). The SEM is a useful indicator of error associated with measurement and is helpful in interpreting a single score.

(3). In a conservative estimate of error, the score obtained ± 2 SEM should be used.

(4). It is assumed that a meaningful change (greater than that associated with error in the measurement) occurred in quadriceps strength if the quadriceps ratio was greater or less than 8% of the initial score.

c. Our test protocol includes 60, 120, 180, and 240 degrees/s.

(1). Strength scores obtained at all speeds are highly correlated with one another (all Pearson correlation coefficients are >0.95).

(2). Because of the high correlations at all speeds, we question the need to assess strength isokinetically at multiple speeds.

(3). Some investigators have related velocity-specific isokinetic deficits in patients with rheumatic diseases[33] and fiber-type distribution in healthy subjects.[34]

(4). No studies with appropriate research designs document any velocity-specific deficits in patients with knee injuries.

d. In sum, a variety of quantitative methods exist to measure quadriceps muscle function of the knee.

(1). This myriad of instruments and techniques can be confusing.

(a). With computer technology, isokinetic assessments can yield pages of data detailing the torque production of the patient.

(b). The clinician should bear in mind that the major decision to be made from the data obtained is "is the quadriceps muscle of the thigh weak?"

(2). If the opposite extremity is truly uninvolved, it is the best "normal" measurement with which to compare the strength of the involved quadriceps.

(3). Judgements of deficits of 20%, 30%, 40%, and greater in quadriceps weakness are easy. The clinician has a good basis on which to diagnose quadriceps weakness.

(4). Judgements of deficits of ≤10% provide little basis to substantiate quadriceps weakness.

(5). The gray area is in the 10% to 20% range: does this constitute a deficit?

(a). Some say a deficit does exist in this range, and they will keep the patient out of participation in sports solely on the basis of the isokinetic assessment.

(b). Others will consider the actual numbers from the isokinetic assessment as well as the data based on the subject's performance of functional maneuvers, such as running figure eights, cutting 90 degrees at various speeds, and so on.

(c). The latter approach should be used. For example, elite athletes participate in practices and drills specific to their sport with up to 20% deficits; ie, they demonstrate that they have knee control in the assessment of functional activities.

5. **Treatment: quadriceps muscle performance deficits.** We will approach quadriceps weakness treatment by first dealing with the very weak muscle (*eg*, post surgery) and later with less involved quadriceps weakness.

a. *Electrical stimulation*

(1). Of all techniques, this is the most widely documented. Case reports, single-case experiments, and randomized clinical trials have addressed muscle stimulation in both patients and healthy subjects.

(2). Unfortunately, muscle stimulation is viewed generically despite clear and important differences in published studies.

(3). The term electrical stimulation alone inadequately explains this modality's effects.

(4). Differences in current generators and population generalizations can lead to misconceptions if not understood.

(a). Differences in current generators:

(i). Battery-operated units generally produce pulses of short duration (≤ 200 μs).

(ii). Console units (plug into the wall) can produce wider pulse widths with greater pulse charges.

(iii). Most battery-operated units cannot produce contractile forces in the muscles as high as those produced by the console units.

(iv). Differences in the use of current generators alone can explain some of the discrepancies found in the literature.

(v). Electrical stimulation treatment should be based on the same logic used in determining voluntary exercise protocols. Is electrical stimulation being used to increase strength or to increase endurance? If the answer is strength, sound biological principles should be applied in using electrical stimulation. For example, is the intent to over-

---

USE OF CURRENT GENERATORS ALONE

Morrissey *et al.* found modest increases in quadriceps strength with electrical stimulation compared with no treatment initially.[35] A battery-operated electrical stimulator adjusted to "highest tolerable output" was used. At maximal output, the unit used in this study produced 6 mA of true root mean square current when passed through a 2000-ohm resistance.

Delitto *et al.* used a unit that produces 200 MA true RMS current through a 2000-ohm resistance.[36] Stimulation was significantly better than exercise alone in producing strength gains after anterior cruciate ligament surgery. Measurement of quadriceps deficit was 21% in the electrical stimulation groups compared with 50% in the voluntary exercise group.

The disparate results between the two studies can possibly be explained by the different stimulators' effects. The battery-operated unit cannot cause as high a contractile force in the muscle as the console unit. In other words, it does not overload the muscle as effectively.

Additional controlled studies comparing the units in quadriceps muscle treatment must be done to ascertain whether this is indeed the reason for the disparate results.

---

load the muscle (high resistance, low repetition)? If so, will the current generator accomplish this? Or is the intent to increase endurance (low resistance, high repetition)? For functional overload, we have found that some console units are able to elicit sufficient contractile levels to overload the muscle for all patients. Some battery-operated units can also accomplish this in some patients, provided that the muscle area is small. The quadriceps area, however, is large. The battery-operated units produce, at best, contraction levels of only 30% to 40% of maximal voluntary contraction. On the other hand, for endurance protocols, battery-operated units are by far the most effective because low-level contractions are necessary for extended periods. Cost-effective treatment is accomplished by renting a current generator for the patient's home use.

(b). Population generalizations:

　(i). Making inappropriate inferences to patients by generalizing from studies done on healthy, mostly male college students leads to misconceptions. Studies on healthy individuals without muscle weakness show exercise and electrical stimulation to have equivalent strengthening effects.[37-41] Sweeping generalizations are often made that exercising and electrical stimulation are interchangeable as muscle strengthening techniques. This may be true in normal, young, male college students.

　(ii). Substantial literature exists comparing voluntary exercise with electrical stimulation in patients with demonstrated weakness that suggests that electrical stimulation is more effective in producing strength gains.[34,41-43] Perhaps the inconsistency between patients and normals is due to the more effective muscle overload with electrical stimulation. Patients may be unable or unwilling to exert enough effort to contract the muscle sufficiently to cause overload. Alternatively, Delitto and Snyder-Mackler have proposed that neurophysiological differences between electrically versus voluntarily elicited muscle contractions may be the answer.[44] Compared with voluntary exercise, electrical stimulation produces higher firing frequencies and has a greater propensity to elicit Type II motor units.[44]

(c). In summary, the clinician must be aware of the different experimental electrical stimulation protocols and the subjects used in the studies before generalizations can be made in support or not of electrical stimulation as a strength-improving technique. When faced with conflicting results, the clinician can treat effectively with electrical stimulation by using sound biological principles.

(5). *Electrical stimulation protocol for muscle strengthening.* Electrical stimulation can be beneficial in decreasing the debilitating effects of complete or partial immobilization immediately after surgery. Patients should be treated three to five times a week. A high-intensity (contractile force) electrical stimulation protocol should be employed.

DETERMINATION OF ELECTRICAL STIMULATION DOSAGE

Dosage should be determined by comparing electrically elicited torque measures with a maximal voluntary isometric torque measure. For example, if the subject can voluntary contract to 100 ft-lb, and the electrical stimulation causes a contraction level of 60 ft-lb, the dose of current given to the patient is 60% of maximal voluntary contraction. This is consistent with the voluntary muscle strengthening exercise literature (*eg*, the DeLorme protocol).[51,52]

A milliamperage reading on a current generator does not reflect contractile intensities in the quadriceps muscle. Gauge readings cannot predict the electrically elicited percentage of maximal voluntary contraction when assessed between subjects or between sessions with the same subjects. The reading serves little purpose in documenting an electrical stimulation dose. Additionally, visible muscle contractions produced with electrical stimulation can mislead the clinician into thinking the intensity of stimulation is sufficient. A visible contraction can be a weak contraction in muscle force and serves little purpose in strengthening the muscle.

Protocol:

(a). Flex the knee between 45 and 70 degrees.

(b). Place electrodes on the quadriceps muscle of the thigh using bipolar placement.

(c). Remove any orthotic device, if necessary, and observe any range of motion restrictions while the patient is out of the device.

(d). In anterior cruciate deficient knees, flex the knee to at least 60 degrees. This ensures that extension will not exceed 45 degrees.

(e). To ensure patellar stability, place one electrode over the medial oblique vastus muscle belly.

(f). The patient should be seated, preferably at an isokinetic device so that contractile intensity can be measured.

(g). Hip, thigh, and shank should be stabilized firmly.

(h). With the isokinetic device in an isometric mode, gradually increase the current intensity *to as high as tolerable.*

(i). Muscle contraction should be not only visible but measurable in torque production.

(j). With subsequent contractions, increase intensity to tolerable levels.

(k). Ten contractions per session are sufficient.

b. **Biofeedback (myofeedback).** During early postoperative periods, biofeedback has been shown to be an effective adjunct to exercise for strengthening the quadriceps. Krebs conducted a randomized clinical trial on patients post knee arthrotomy using myofeedback plus exercise or exercise alone.[45] The quadriceps function was significantly greater in the myofeedback plus electrical stimulation group. Draper recently replicated Krebs' result in anterior cruciate ligament patients. Myofeedback was an effective adjunct in exercise training. The quadriceps deficit in the myofeedback group was reduced to 20%.

(1). *Biofeedback protocol for muscle strengthening*

(a). Place the electromyographic electrodes over the quadriceps muscle of the thigh belly(s).

(b). An audio and/or visual signal is displayed that corresponds in intensity to the magnitude of the electrical muscle activity.

(c). Valuable and almost immediate feedback on how strong the quadriceps muscle is voluntarily contracting is given.

(d). The patient learns through feedback how to elicit vigorous muscle contractions.

(e). More efficient overload of the muscle can be elicited as effort and contractile force increase, thus producing greater strength gains.

(f). The patient should work in sets of 10 to 15, resting for short periods as needed.

(g). After each set, the patient should rest alone (in a quiet area if possible) for short periods, usually 20 to 30 minutes.

(h). Console as well as portable units are available. Portable units can be used by the patient at home.

(i). Myofeedback is labor intensive and requires patience in training the patient. This disadvantage partially explains why myofeedback is not often used, despite its documented effectiveness.

c. **Isokinetics.** The isokinetic dynamometer was originally developed as a treatment device in the late 1960s to more effectively overload the muscle throughout the entire range of motion.[46,47] In isokinetic treatment, the patient's shank is secured to a lever arm attached to the dynamometer. The angular velocity can be preset; any attempt to exceed preset velocity is resisted to maintain the lever arm at the preset velocity.

Resistance is variable, depending on the patient's effort to exceed the preset velocity. The term *accommodating resistance* was coined to describe resistance that changes as the joint moves through ranges in which the biomechanics, length tension, and so on are not optimal. Hislop and Perrine showed that accommodating resistance allows the muscle to be stressed maximally throughout the entire range of motion.[46] Implications for functional overload are obvious if the subject produces a maximal effort.

Some early studies claiming the superiority of isokinetic exercise to alternative exercise forms (*eg*, weights) have methodological problems. For example, Thistle *et al.* claimed that isokinetic exercise led to superior strength gains compared with a progressive resistive exercise program.[47] The authors, however, tested strength in all groups isokinetically and did not control for practice effects. The strength gain in the isokinetic group could easily be attributed to practice. Methodological flaws such as these should be noted in studies that attempt to document the "superiority" of one exercise paradigm over another.

(1). *Devices*. Isokinetic dynamometers are available in a variety of shapes and sizes. The most commonly used today include the Cybex II,* LIDO,† Kin-Com,‡ and BIODEX.§ All devices offer concentric, isokinetic exercise at velocities from 0 to 300 degrees/s; some exceed the upper end of this range. In addition, all but the Cybex offer eccentric training. That is, the units move the joint passively while the patient resists the movement, causing a resistive, *lengthening* contraction. The Kinetron, made by Cybex, provides excellent exercise to the quadriceps and the hip extensors.

(2). *Isokinetic exercise protocols*

    (a). Almost all isokinetic exercise protocols involve exercise with maximal or near maximal effort through an entire or restricted range of motion.

    (b). Each set includes 10 to 20 contractions and is usually begun at relatively high speeds.

    (c). More than one speed is typically included in a treatment session. For example, Davies described an exercise regimen with a ve-

locity spectrum that begins at 240 degrees/s and moves down to 90 degrees/s in increments of 30 degrees/s, then moves back up to 240 degrees/s in reciprocal fashion.[48]

    (d). Most dynamometers are equipped with range-limiting devices, controlled by computer hardware or software.

    (e). Higher isokinetic speeds are usually tolerated better than lower speeds, especially in the acute injury phase. Additionally, some evidence exists that training at higher speeds may be more beneficial than training at lower speeds. Moffroid and Whipple noted that subjects who trained at lower speeds improved their strength at lower speeds only, whereas those who trained at higher speeds improved strength measures at both higher and lower speeds.[49] Smith and Melton found carry-over effects from high-speed isokinetic exercise to gains in vertical leap and 40-yard dash.[50] Both studies involved healthy people (noninjured) with strength deficits. Similar results have yet to be demonstrated with muscular weakness. Further study is indeed needed.

d. *Weight training*. Progressive resistive exercise (PRE) programs using weights have been used to increase quadriceps strength for decades. DeLorme is credited with initiating PRE.[51,52] Unfortunately, many clinicians misuse the term PRE, calling any resistive exercise program employing weights a "progressive resistive exercise." A true PRE program requires

(1). Determining the 10 repetition maximum (or 10 RM).

(2). Exercising at high percentages of the 10 RM (as described by DeLorme, 50%, 75%, 100%).[51,52]

(3). Periodically redetermining the 10 RM and adjusting the weights accordingly. Using a 5-lb weight in 3 sets of 10 exercise repetitions is *not* a progressive resistive exercise in the true sense.

---

* Cybex, Division of Lumex, Ronkonkoma, NY.
† Loredan Biomedical Company, Davis, CA.
‡ Chattex, Division of Chattanooga Medical Company, Chattanooga, TN.
§ BIODEX Corporation, Shirley, NY.

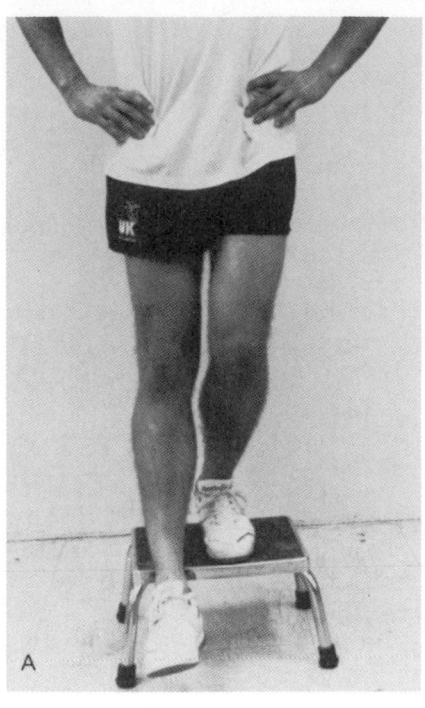 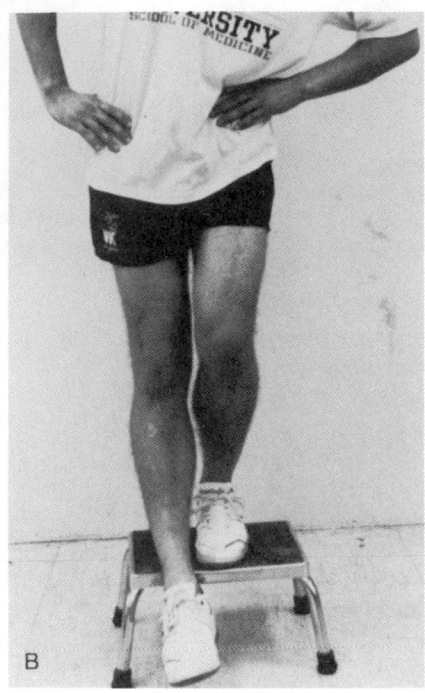

FIGURE 34–14 **A**, Step-down test to assess knee control. The patient is asked to step down *slowly* from a height of 18 in. The knee must remain over the great toe and not drift medially, and the patient should not feel as though the knee will give out. This test is recommended before any functional activities are considered.

B, Typical posturing of a patient who demonstrates lack of knee control during descent of a step. The pelvis tilts downward in the frontal plane in an attempt to lengthen the leg that is stepping down, so that the weight-bearing knee does not have to flex as much. (Reprinted from Delitto A, Lehman RC: Rehabilitation of the athlete with a knee injury. *Clin Sports Med* 1989, 8:805–840.)

(a). Knee extension exercises with weights:
  (i). Nautilus machines can be used for both knee extension and leg presses, working the quadriceps sufficiently to cause overload if a true PRE program is employed.
  (ii). Free weights can be used.
  (iii). Full squats with weights should be limited to individuals accustomed to this type of training.
e. ***Weight-bearing, multijoint training.*** It may be preferable to use weight-bearing, multijoint exercises, which are commonly misnamed "closed kinetic chain" exercises. The Stair-master (Stair-master 4000 Pt, Trilech, Inc, Tulsa, OK) is one of the more commonly used devices, but other options include running stairs and jumping rope. Although these exercises may not always supply an overload stimulus to the quadriceps muscle, they do assist in regaining neuromotor control of the knee. They do so by supplying stresses short of those experienced in full competition, yet greater than those experienced since the injury or surgery.

(1). Before performing weight-bearing, multijoint exercises, the patient must meet the following criteria. The patient should demonstrate
  (a). At least 10 to 120 degrees of motion.
  (b). Walking without a limp with good evidence of knee control throughout the gait cycle.
  (c). No hesitancy in bearing full weight on the involved extremity.
  (d). Ascending and descending stairs confidently, foot over foot, in a symmetrical pattern.
(2). Slowly descending a high (18 in) step with the involved leg high (see Figure 34–14) is a useful test to determine whether there is sufficient knee control to begin functional exercises. A patient without sufficient muscle strength for adequate knee control will almost certainly fail. If the patient passes this test, the following activities should be started:
  (a). Straight-line activities, such as jogging. While the patient jogs, the therapist
    (i). Views from the front, looking for equal weight distri-

bution on both legs during stance. Also, both knees should flex symmetrically and the patient should feel in control as the knee accepts weight.
   (ii). Views from the side, ensuring that the knee is fully extending at initial stance.
   (iii). Views from behind, ensuring that the knees are flexing symmetrically at push-off and early swing. This is especially important when running speed is increased.
   (b). Slow turning activities such as figure eights; speed is slowly increased around figure eights, and the distance between the turns is slowly decreased.
   (c). Ninety-degree cuts; first around known markers, then on the clinician's command.

6. **Hamstring muscle performance deficits**
   a. These are extremely rare. Many long-term studies that evaluated thigh muscle performance showed quadriceps muscle performance deficits but did not find similar deficits in the knee flexors.
   b. At one time, hamstring strength was thought to be extremely important in the rehabilitation of anterior cruciate ligament injuries. In fact, physical therapists were encouraged to target hamstring musculature until a 1:1 ratio existed between knee flexor and knee extensor peak torque measures. This notion, coined the "hamstring myth" by Minkoff and Sherrin,[54] is now in dispute. The major clinical problems the hamstrings present are tears and pulls, which can best be related to lack of flexibility not to muscle performance.
   c. **_Hamstring flexibility measurement_**
      (1). Straight-leg raise.
      (2). "90-90" test. The patient lies supine, with the hips at 90 degrees flexion and the knee extended maximally.

 PLEASE NOTE: No standard based on sound evidence exists for interpreting hamstring flexibility measures. Therefore, the therapist relies on normal values based on clinical experience. Generally, in the 90-90 position, women should be able to extend knees to at least 30 degrees and men to at least 50 degrees.

   d. **_Treating hamstring injuries._** Perhaps one of the most difficult patients to treat is the patient with chronic hamstring strains.
      (1). _First-degree strains._ No noticeable ecchymosis, no loss of strength, but pain with resistive testing.
      (2). _Second-degree strains._ Presents with loss of strength and may or may not have ecchymosis.
      (3). _Third-degree strains._ Profoundly weak (commonly unable to move the leg against gravity), ecchymosis almost always present, can be quite debilitating.

Clinical Decision-Making Cases

Case #1

HISTORY

Screening
Symptoms checked: none.

Demographics
A reputable orthopedist refers a patient with a diagnosis of a sprain of the left medial collateral ligament. The patient is a 19-year-old male who plays Division III college football, and he sustained the injury during a game 5 days previously. He is a senior and in his last year of eligibility and is most anxious to return to football as soon as possible. Approximately 2 months remain in the season. Other pertinent information: weight, 190 lb; height, 6 ft; right-foot dominant.

Present Symptoms
The patient's chief complaint is that he cannot play football. At present, he has no complaint of pain. In the morning, he has pain along the medial side of the knee. The pain decreases with time, and, by the time he is out of the shower, he is once more asymptomatic. There are no radicular symptoms.

Chronology/Timing

The pain has been present since the injury. It has been improving since the injury. The pain is worse in the morning and after he sees the orthopedist, who "manipulates the knee around." The pain does not affect his sleep pattern nor does it cause him to change his position.

Quality

When the pain is there, it is described as sharp.

Severity

The pain is described as 1 to 2 on a scale of 10. It is intermittent.

Grade

None of the choices are applicable.

Setting/Onset

The patient was injured during a game when he attempted to tackle someone and was hit on the side of his leg with his foot planted. He described a valgus stress to the knee. There was a great deal of pain, and he could not continue playing. In fact, he had to be helped from the field and could not bear weight on the left lower extremity. He saw the orthopedist immediately and was placed in a limited-mobility splint (30 to 90 degrees). He will be reassessed in 2 weeks and weekly afterward for ligamentous stability. Mechanism of Injury: valgus stress to knee.

There are no factors influencing the symptoms and no associated symptoms.

Relevant Test Results

Positive valgus stress test with minimal gapping, a solid end-feel, and pain. Negative Lachmann, anterior drawer, posterior sag tests. There was never an effusion.

Past Medical History

Noncontributory. No history of previous knee problems.

Social History

The patient wishes to return to competitive, high-level sports, including football and rugby.

Review of Patient's Concerns/Goals

To return to high level competitive football as soon as possible.

PHYSICAL EXAMINATION

Range of motion:	Passive range is 30 to 90 degrees.
Strength:	A 35% quadriceps muscle of the thigh deficit on isometric assessment, with knee in 60 degrees of flexion. No pain with knee extension testing. A 45% deficit when attempting to test the hamstrings, but there is medial joint line pain with attempts to actively flex the knee against resistance.
Gait:	Ambulates without assistive device with knee limited to 30 to 90 degrees excursion, so there is lack of knee extension in stance and lack of flexion during early swing.
Special tests:	Point tender along medial collateral ligament, especially from the medial joint line to the pes anserinus. There is no effusion.

STATUS IN THREE WEEKS

The patient has come to see the physical therapist 1 day after seeing the orthopedist. There is no pain. He is now wearing a smaller brace with lateral and medial uprights that allows full range of motion of the knee. He walks exactly as he did with the limited-motion brace, however.

Physical Examination

The patient's motion is unchanged. His quadriceps strength is now 115% of his other side when measured isometrically with the knee in 65 degrees flexion. His hamstring testing is still painful in the medial side of the knee at the distalmost insertion of the medial collateral ligament, and the flexion deficit is measured at 30%. His gait is unchanged. No atrophy or swelling is noted.

PHYSICAL THERAPY PROTOCOL

1. Diagnosis: Second-degree medial collateral ligament sprain.
   a. Decision to treat: Yes.
   b. Factors supporting diagnosis: Mechanism of injury, results of valgus stress test, location of symptoms.
   c. Diagnoses ruled out (and reasons): Anterior cruciate ligament (no swelling, negative Lachmann test); posterior cruciate ligament (no posterior sag).
2. Problem to be treated: Quadriceps strength deficit must be addressed. Must use restricted range, no straighter than 30 degrees.
   a. Isometric strengthening.
   b. Isokinetic training.
   c. Electrical stimulation.
   d. Nautilus.
   e. Anything else that is a convincing strength-training strategy.
3. Prognosis: Excellent.
   a. Time frame: 6 ± 2 weeks.
   b. Moderators: Diagnosis, degree of motivation, age, no previous history.
4. Goals

a. Long term: Return to football in 6 to 8 weeks; full range of motion (after restriction) in 4 to 6 weeks; pain-free active knee flexion.

b. Short term: Normal quadriceps strength in 2 to 4 weeks.

5. Plan: Frequency of two to three times a week. Treat with any strengthening protocol for quadriceps as above. Of minor consequence, ultrasound and deep friction massage may be applied to the proximal medial portion of the tibia over the distal portion of the medial collateral ligament.

6. Progression

a. Justification: Ligament is now healed sufficiently to allow full motion to the knee.

b. New plan: Work should be toward full extension of the knee. Mobilization techniques may be incorporated to gain extension. Also, deep friction massage may be applied to the distal medial collateral ligament. Physiological stretching also can be performed. Also, work should be done on gait: full extension at heel strike, and flexion at heel off.

Case #2

HISTORY

The referred patient in this study is a 56-year-old female who, 1 month previously, sustained a knee injury while "stepping off a curb." She noticed immediate swelling and could not bear full weight on the involved extremity. After seeing an orthopedist, she underwent arthroscopy. Subsequently, it was determined that she had torn her anterior cruciate ligament and also had sustained a tear of her medial meniscus. The latter was taken care of while undergoing the arthroscopy. The orthopedist decided that, "because of her age," reconstruction of the anterior cruciate ligament was not an option. The patient works as a technician in her husband's laboratory.

Presently, she is ambulating using crutches and partial weight bearing with a knee immobilizer. Her biggest complaint now is the inability to ambulate without the crutches, stating that her knee will just "buckle under unexpectantly." Although she continues to work, the necessity of using crutches in the laboratory has become a nuisance, taking its toll on her productivity. She also states that her knee swells after being on her feet for a while, and this causes her knee to "ache." She has become more irritable since the knee problem arose, and she feels that the knee pain is mostly responsible for this.

Physical Examination

On physical examination, the therapist notes obvious thigh atrophy (1.5-in deficit in thigh circumference 8 in above patella), positive anterior drawer sign, positive Lachmann test, positive pivot shift. There is also calf atrophy (1-in deficit 4 in below fibular head). Varus and valgus stresses are negative. Range of motion is 10 to 110 degrees. There is swelling in the knee (1.5-in increase in circumference taken around superior pole of patella with knee in full extension). An isokinetic test of the quadriceps and hamstring musculature show the following work measurements:

	Involved (degrees)	Uninvolved (degrees)
Quadriceps	125	250
Hamstrings	100	145

Problems

1. Instability of the knee that limits job performance and activities of daily living.
2. Pain in the knee that is bothersome and interferes with functional activities.

Contributing Factors

1. Positive Lachmann test.
2. Positive anterior drawer sign.
3. Positive pivot shift.
4. Limited strength.
5. Limited motion.
6. Swelling.

DIAGNOSIS

Anterior cruciate deficient knee, treated nonoperatively. The decision is to treat.

GOALS

Long-Term Goals (Within 4 to 6 Weeks)

1. To ambulate without assistive device and without incidence of instability.
2. To be pain free during normal activities of daily living.

Short-Term Goals (Within 2 to 3 Weeks) and Plans

1. Problem #1:
   a. To progress patient to ambulation with full weight bearing with a cane in 2 weeks (gait training, progressive ambulation, weight shifting, etc.).
   b. To improve quadriceps and hamstring strength to 70% and 90%, respectively (PRE, muscle stimulation, stationary bicycle).
2. Problem #2:
   a. To reduce incidence of knee pain concomitant

with swelling to zero incidence by decreasing and controlling swelling so that there is no circumferential difference with measures around the knee (positive pressure [*eg*, Jobst extremity pump, wrapping], modalities [HVPC], patient education [*eg*, ice, elevation]).

b. To improve range of motion of the knee to 0 to 125 degrees (mobilization, home program, stretching toward extension and flexion with techniques demonstrated in class).

PROGRESSION

The patient returns after 2 weeks, and the following are noted: She is now ambulating with a cane and is full weight bearing. Her swelling is under control, and she is compliant with the treatment regimen for this. Her quadriceps strength is now 70% and hamstring strength 100% of the other side (using work as a dependent measure). She states that her aching episodes are now diminished and are not a problem unless she is on her feet for an extended period. She also notes that she cannot ambulate for greater than 1 block before the knee feels as though it is "getting wobbly" again. The quadriceps "fatigue index" on an isokinetic assessment is 40% on the involved side and 75% on the uninvolved side.

Reasons for Progression

The patient has a complaint related to lack of endurance.

New Short-Term Goal

Within 2 to 3 weeks, to improve endurance of the knee extensors so that the fatigue index is 50% and the patient can ambulate with a cane for normal (for her) distances without complaints of fatigue.

New Program Plan

Resistive endurance exercises using interval training on any exercise device that uses the lower extremity muscles (*eg*, ergometer).

References

1. Lorentzon R, Wedren H, Pietila T: Incidence, nature and causes of ice hockey injuries. A three-year prospective study of a Swedish elite ice hockey team. *Am J Sports Med* 1988, 16:392–396.
2. Culpepper MI, Niemann KM: High school football injuries in Birmingham, Alabama. *South Med J* 1983, 76:873–875.
3. Wroble RR, Mysnyk MC, Foster DT, Albright JP: Patterns of knee injuries in wrestling: a six year study. *Am J Sports Med* 1986, 14:55–56.
4. Weiss BD: Nontraumatic injuries in amateur long distance bicyclists. *Am J Sports Med* 1985, 13:187–192.
5. Ekstrand J, Gillquist J: Soccer injuries and their mechanisms: a prospective study. *Med Sci Sports Exerc* 1983, 15:267–270.
6. Strauss RH, Lanese RR: Injuries among wrestlers in school and college tournaments. *JAMA* 1982, 248:2016–2019.
7. DeHaven KE, Lintner DM: Athletic injuries: comparison by age, sport, and gender. *Am J Sports Med* 1986, 14:218–224.
8. Kannus P, Niittymaki S, Jarvinen M: Sports injuries in women: a one year prospective follow-up study at an outpatient sports clinic. *Br J Sports Med* 1987, 21:37–39.
9. Pediatric and adolescent sports injuries: recent trends. *Exerc Sport Sci Rev* 1986, 14:359–374.
10. Pritchett JW: A claims-made study of knee injuries due to football in high school athletes. *J Pediatr Orthop* 1988, 8:551–553.
11. Moore KL: *Clinically Oriented Anatomy* 2nd ed. Baltimore, Williams & Wilkins, 1985.
12. Tegner Y, Lysholm J: Rating systems in the evaluation of knee ligament injuries. *Clin Orthop* 1984, 173:43–49.
13. DeAndrade JR, Grant C, Dixon SJ: Joint distension and reflex muscle inhibition in the knee. *J Bone Joint Surg* 1965, 47A:313–322.
14. Young A, Stokes M, Iles JF: Effects of joint pathology on muscle. *Clin Orthop* 1987, 219:21–27.
15. Kloth LC, Feeder JA: Acceleration of wound healing with high voltage monophasic pulsed current. *Phys Ther* 1988, 60:503–508.
16. Brown M, McDonnel MK, Menton DN: Electrical stimulation effects on cutaneous wound healing in rabbits. *Phys Ther* 1988, 6:955–960.
17. Brown M, McDonnell MK, Menton DN: Polarity effects on wound healing using electrical stimulation in rabbits. *Arch Phys Med Rehabil* 1989, 70:624–627.
18. Morrisson JB: Mechanics of the knee joint in relation to normal walking. *J Biomechanics* 1970, 3:51–61.
19. Vink P, Kamphuisen HAC: Leg length inequality, pelvic tilt and lumbar back muscle activity during standing. *Clin Biomechanics* 1989, 4:115–117.
20. Warwick R, Williams PL: Arthrology. In *Gray's Anatomy* 35th ed. Philadelphia, W. B. Saunders Company, 1973, pp 455–458.
21. Rothstein JM, Miller PJ, Roetgger RF: Goniometric reliability in a clinical setting: elbow and knee measurements. *Phys Ther* 1983, 1611–1615.
22. Frank C, Akeson WH: Physiology and therapeutic value of passive joint motion. *Clin Orthop* 1984, 185:113–125.
23. Burks C, Daniel D, Losse G: The effect of continuous passive motion on anterior cruciate ligament reconstruction and stability. *Am J Sports Med* 1984, 12:323–327.
24. Vegso JJ, Genuaro SE, Torg JS: Maintenance of hamstring strength following knee surgery. *Med Sci Sports Exerc* 1985, 17:376–379.
25. Gerber C, Hoppeler H, Claassen H, *et al.*: The lower extremity musculature in chronic symptomatic instability of the anterior cruciate ligament. *J Bone Joint Surg* 1985, 67A:1034–1043.
26. Dvir Z, Eger G, Halperin N, Shklar A: Thigh muscle activity and anterior cruciate ligament insufficiency. *Clin Biomechanics* 1989, 4:87–91.
27. Rose SJ, Rothstein JM: Muscle mutability. Part 1. General concepts and adaptations to altered patterns of use. *Phys Ther* 1982, 62:1773–1787.
28. Astrand P-O, Rodahl K: *Textbook of Work Physiology* 2nd ed. New York, McGraw-Hill, 1977, p 393.
29. Mayhew TP, Rothstein JM: Measurement of muscle performance with instruments. In Rothstein JM (ed): *Clinics in Physical Therapy: Measurement in Physical Therapy*. vol 7. New York, Churchill Livingstone, 1985, pp 57–102.
30. Winter DA, Wells RP, Orr GW: Errors in the use of isokinetic dynamometers. *Eur J Appl Physiol* 1981, 46:397–408.

31. Rothstein JM, Lamb RL, Mayhew TP: Clinical uses of isokinetic measurements: critical issues. *Phys Ther* 1987, 67:1840–1844.

32. Delitto A, Crandell CE, Rose SJ: Peak torque to body weight ratios in the trunk: a critical analysis. *Phys Ther* 1989, 69:138–143.

33. Rothstein JM, Delitto A, Sinacore DR, Rose SJ: Muscle function in rheumatic disease patients treated with corticosteroids. *Muscle Nerve* 1983, 6:123–131.

34. Thorstensen A, Grimby G, Karlsson J: Force velocity relations and fiber composition in human knee extensor muscles. *J Appl Physiol* 1976, 40:12–21.

35. Morrissey MC, Brewster CE, Shields CL, Brown M: The effects of electrical stimulation on the quadriceps during postoperative knee immobilization. *Am J Sports Med* 1985, 13:40–45.

36. Delitto A, Rose SJ, Lehman RC, *et al.:* Electrical stimulation versus voluntary exercise in strengthening the thigh musculature after anterior cruciate ligament surgery. *Phys Ther* 1988, 68:660–663.

37. Currier DP, Mann R: Muscle strength development by electrical stimulation in healthy individuals. *Phys Ther* 1983, 63:915–921.

38. Laughman RK, Youdas JW, Garrett TR: Strength changes in normal quadriceps femoris muscle as a result of electrical stimulation. *Phys Ther* 1983, 63:494–499.

39. Selkowitz DM: Improvement in isometric strength of the quadriceps femoris as a result of electrical stimulation. *Phys Ther* 1985, 65:186–196.

40. McMiken DF, Todd-Smith M, Thompson C: Strengthening of human quadriceps muscles by cutaneous electrical stimulation. *Scand J Rehabil Med* 1983 15:25–28.

41. Eriksson E, Haggmark T: Comparison of isometric muscle training and electrical stimulation supplementing isometric muscle training in the recovery after major knee ligament surgery. *Am J Sports Med* 1979, 7:169–171.

42. Godfrey CM, Jayawardena H, Quance TA, Welch P: Comparison of electrostimulation and isometric exercises in strengthening the quadriceps muscle. *Physiother Can* 1979, 31:265–267.

43. Grove-Lainey C, Walmsley RP, Andrew GM: Effectiveness of exercise alone versus exercise plus electrical stimulation in strengthening the quadriceps muscle. *Physiother Can* 1983, 35:5–11.

44. Delitto A, Snyder-Mackler L: Two theories explaining strength augmentation using electrical stimulation [In press].

45. Krebs DE: Clinical electromyographic feedback following meniscectomy. A multiple regression experimental analysis. *Phys Ther* 1981, 61:1017–1021.

46. Hislop HJ, Perrine JJ: The isokinetic concept of exercise. *Phys Ther* 1967, 47:114–119.

47. Thistle HG, Hislop HJ, Moffroid M, Lowman EW: Isokinetic contraction: a new concept of resistive exercise. *Arch Phys Med Rehabil* 1967, 48:279–284.

48. Davies GJ: *A Compendium of Isokinetics in Clinical Usage and Rehabilitation Techniques*, 3rd ed. La Crosse, WI, S & S Publishing Inc, 1987, pp 37–39.

49. Moffroid MT, Whipple RH: Specificity of speed of exercise. *Phys Ther* 1970, 50:1692–1700.

50. Smith MJ, Welton P: Isokinetic versus isotonic variable resistance training. *Am J Sports Med* 1981, 9:275–279.

51. DeLorme TL: Restoration of muscle power by heavy resistance exercise. *J Bone Joint Surg* 1945, 27:645–652.

52. DeLorme TL, Watkins AL: Technics of progressive resistive exercise. *Arch Phys Med Rehabil* 1948, 49:263–271.

53. Minkoff J, Sherman OH: Considerations pursuant to the rehabilitation of the anterior cruciate injured knee. *Exerc Sport Sci Rev* 1987, 15:297–349.

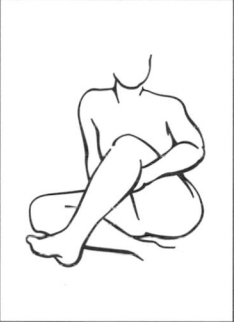

CHAPTER 35

Lower Extremity: Ankle

Lisa M. Giallonardo

The ankle functions as a hinge, allowing the tibia to move over the foot during gait. Dorsiflexion of this joint lowers the center of gravity and increases the shock absorption capability of the entire lower extremity.

I. Normal Anatomy and Biomechanics

A. Talocrural joint axis and motions (see Figure 35–1)

  1. The convex talus moves on the concave tibia and fibula (mortise); the mortise spreads during dorsiflexion to allow talar movement.[1]

  2. The ankle is a modified hinge joint; its axis is oblique, and it is 80 degrees from the vertical axis of the tibia.[2]

  3. The range of motion (ROM) is 20 degrees of dorsiflexion to 50 degrees of plantar flexion; the loose packed position is 10 degrees of plantar flexion.[1]

B. Muscles

  1. **Dorsiflexors**
    a. Tibialis anterior[3–6] (see Figure 35–2)

      (1). This muscle is a primary muscle in moving the ankle; it secondarily inverts the foot.

      (2). It joins the superior two thirds of the lateral tibia and the interosseous membrane to the base of the first metatarsal and medial cuneiform bones.

      (3). The deep peroneal nerve (L4 and L5) innervates the tibialis anterior, and the anterior tibial artery supplies it with blood.

    b. Extensor hallucis longus[3–6] (see Figure 35–3)

      (1). This is a secondary muscle in moving the ankle; it primarily extends first toe.

      (2). It joins the middle third of the me-

1031

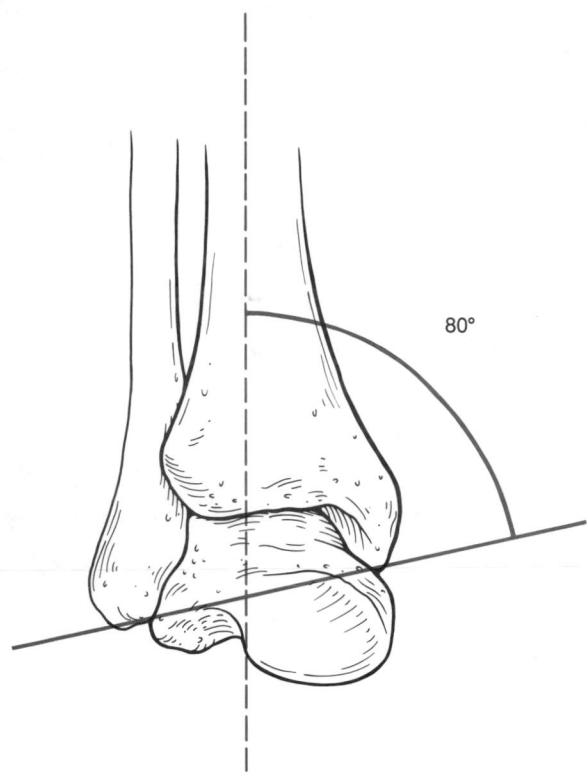

80°

FIGURE 35–1   Talocrural (ankle) joint and axis at approximately 80° from vertical.

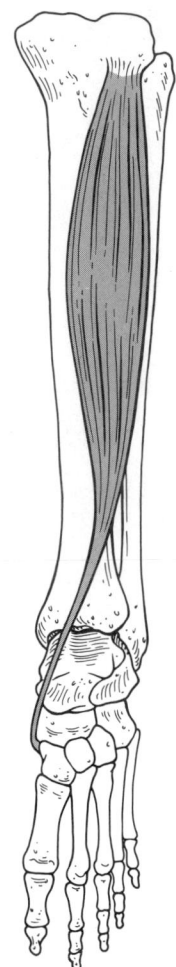

FIGURE 35–2   Tibialis anterior.

dial fibula to the base of the first toe distal phalanx.

(3). The deep peroneal nerve (L5 and S1) innervates the extensor hallucis longus, and the anterior tibial artery supplies it with blood.

c. Extensor digitorum longus[3–6] (see Figure 35–4)

(1). This is a secondary muscle in moving the ankle; it primarily extends toes two through five.

(2). It joins the superior two thirds of the medial fibula to a tendon on digits two through four for the middle and distal phalanges.

(3). The deep peroneal nerve (L5 and S1) innervates the extensor digi-

torum longus, and the deep peroneal branch of anterior tibial artery supplies it with blood.

d. Peroneus tertius[3–6] (see Figure 35–5)

(1). This is a secondary muscle in moving the ankle; it primarily everts the foot.

(2). It joins the inferior third of the medial fibula (the continuation of the

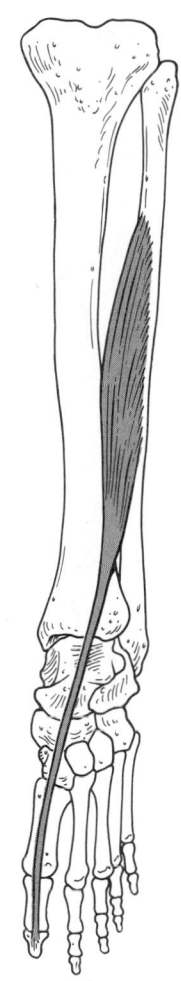

FIGURE 35-3   Extensor hallucis longus.

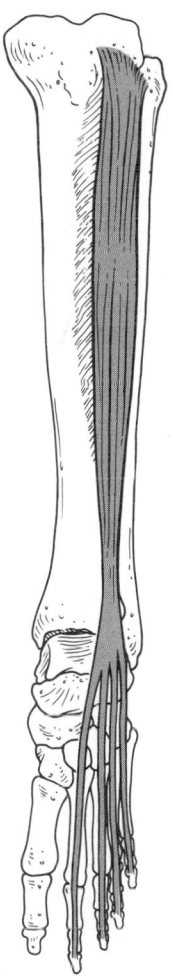

FIGURE 35-4   Extensor digitorum longus.

extensor digitorum longus) to the base of the fifth metatarsal bone.

   (3). The deep peroneal nerve (L5 and S1) innervates the peroneus tertius, and the deep peroneal branch of the anterior tibial artery supplies it with blood.

2. Plantar flexors

  a. Gastrocnemius[3-6] (see Figure 35-6)

   (1). This is a primary muscle in moving

the ankle; it secondarily flexes the knee.

   (2). Its medial head joins the posterosuperior medial femoral condyle to the Achilles tendon.

   (3). Its lateral head joins the lateral femoral condyle to the Achilles tendon.

   (4). The Achilles tendon inserts into the middle posterior calcaneus.

   (5). The tibial nerve (S1 and S2) inner-

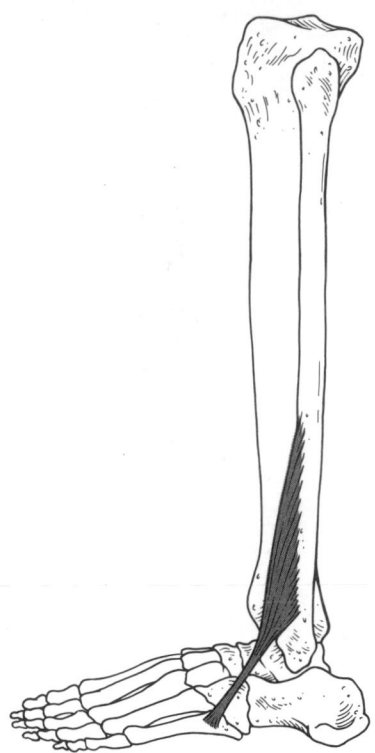

FIGURE 35–5   Peroneus tertius.

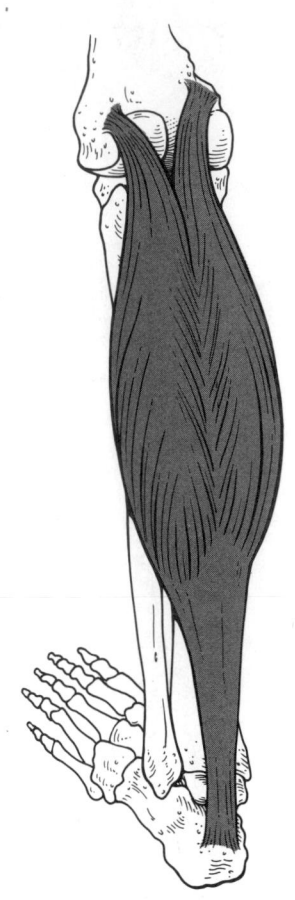

FIGURE 35–6   Gastrocnemius.

vates the gastrocnemius, and the sural branches of the popliteal artery supply it with blood.

b. Soleus[3–6] (see Figure 35–7)

(1). It is a primary muscle in moving the ankle.

(2). It joins the soleal line, medial border of the tibia, and posterior surface of the fibula to the Achilles

tendon (with the gastrocnemius muscle).

(3). The Achilles tendon inserts into the middle posterior calcaneus muscle.

(4). The tibial nerve (S1 and S2) innervates the soleus muscle, and the posterior tibial, peroneal, and sural branches of the popliteal arteries supply it with blood.

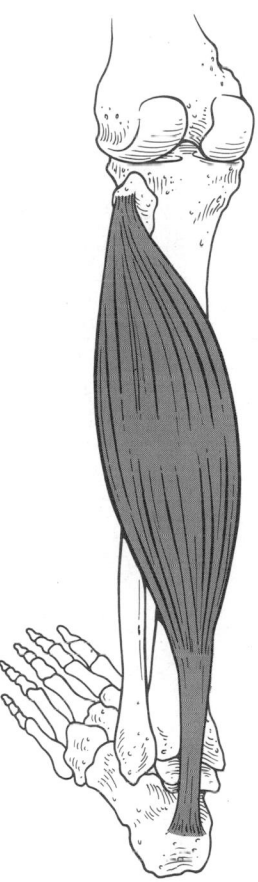

FIGURE 35–7   Soleus.

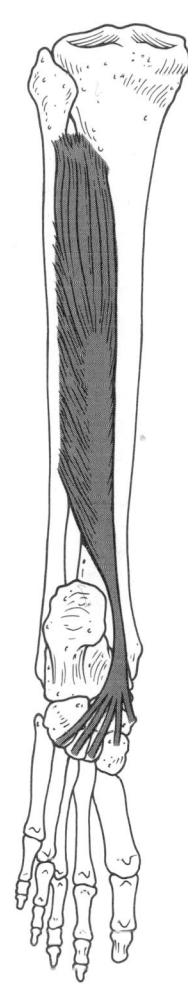

FIGURE 35–8   Tibialis posterior.

c. Tibialis posterior[3–6] (see Figure 35–8)
   (1). It is a secondary muscle in moving the ankle; it primarily inverts the foot.
   (2). It joins the posteromedial tibia, fibula, and interosseous membrane to the navicular tuberosity, and the cuboid bone, three cuneiform bones, and metatarsal bones two through four.

   (3). The tibial nerve (L4 and L5) innervates the tibialis posterior, and the peroneal artery supplies it with blood.
d. Flexor hallucis longus[3–6] (see Figure 35–9)
   (1). It is a secondary muscle in moving the ankle; it primarily flexes the first toe.
   (2). It joins the inferior two thirds of the

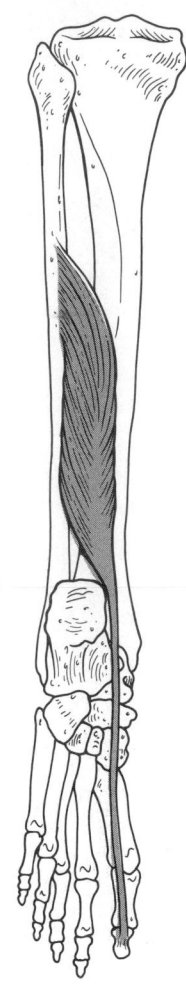

FIGURE 35–9   Flexor hallucis longus.

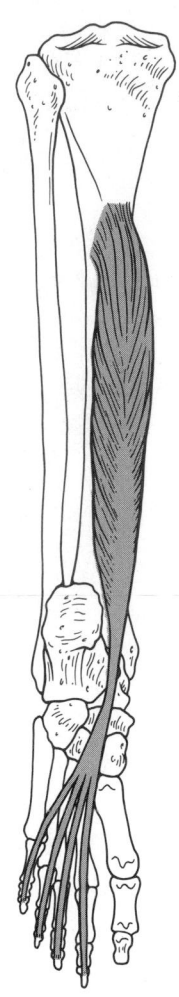

FIGURE 35–10   Flexor digitorum longus.

posterior fibula to the plantar surface of the base of the first distal phalanx.

(3). The tibial nerve (S2 and S3) innervates the flexor hallucis longus, and the peroneal artery supplies it with blood.

e. Flexor digitorum longus[3–6] (see Figure 35–10)

(1). It is a secondary muscle in moving the ankle; it primarily flexes toes two through five.

(2). It joins the medial posterior tibia to a tendon on phalanges two through five and the plantar surface to the base of the distal phalanx.

(3). The tibial nerve (S2 and S3) innervates the flexor digitorum longus, and the posterior tibial artery supplies it with blood.

f. Peroneus longus[3–6] (see Figure 35–11)

(1). It is a secondary muscle in moving the ankle; it primarily everts the foot.

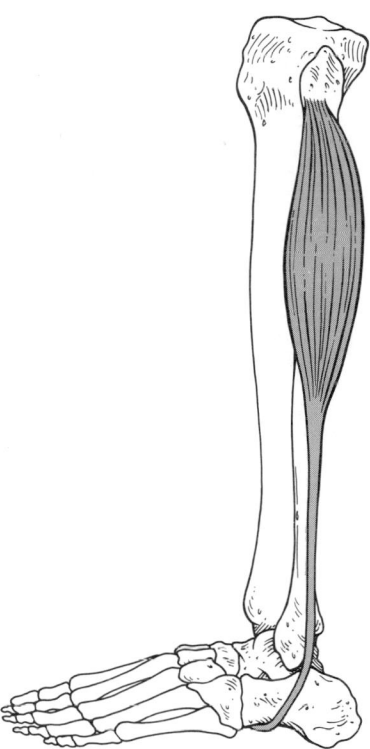

FIGURE 35–11   Peroneus longus.

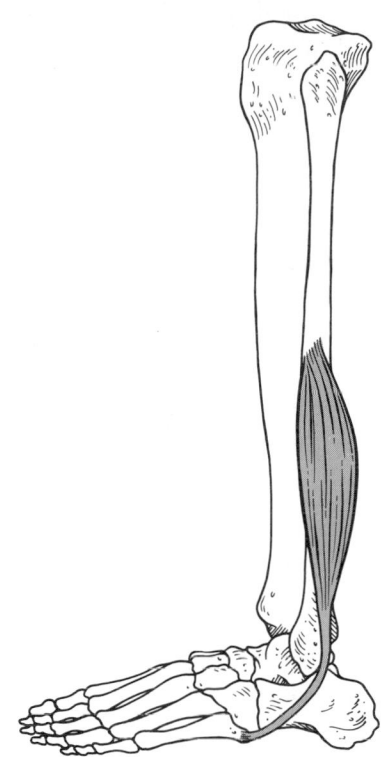

FIGURE 35–12   Peroneus brevis.

(2). It joins the superior two thirds of the lateral fibula to the first cuneiform bone and the base of the first metatarsal bone.

(3). The superficial peroneal nerve (L5, S1, and S2) innervates the peroneus longus, and the anterior tibial and peroneal arteries supply it with blood.

g. Peroneus brevis[3–6] (see Figure 35–12)

(1). It is a secondary muscle in moving the ankle; it primarily everts the foot.

(2). It joins the inferior two thirds of the lateral fibula to the tuberosity of the first metatarsal base.

(3). The superficial peroneal nerve (L5, S1, and S2) innervates the peroneus brevis, and the peroneal artery supplies it with blood.

h. Plantaris[3–6] (see Figure 35–13)

(1). It is a secondary muscle in moving the ankle; it primarily flexes the knee.

(2). It joins the lateral supracondylar line of the femur to the medial Achilles tendon.

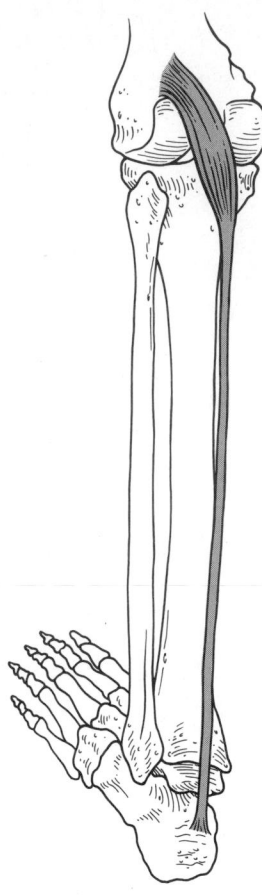

FIGURE 35–13   Plantaris.

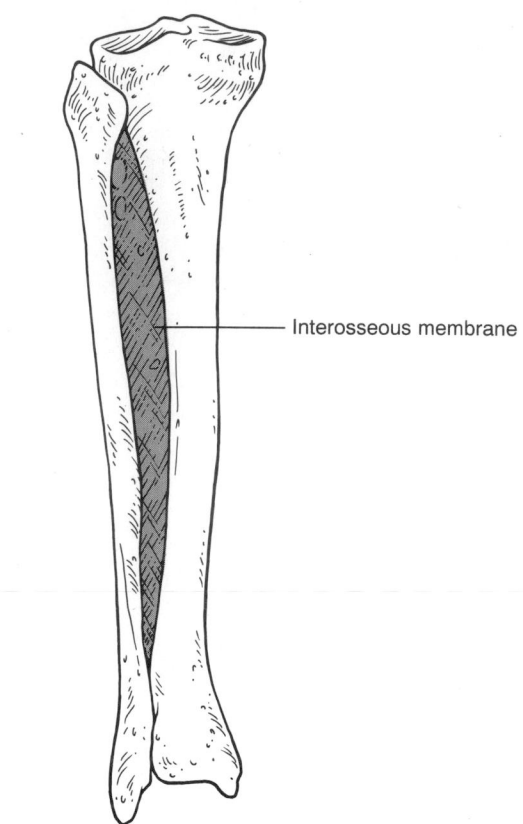

Interosseous membrane

FIGURE 35–14   Interosseous membrane.

(3). The tibial nerve (S1 and S2) innervates the plantaris, and the sural
branches of the popliteal artery supply it with blood.

C. Ligaments and fascial structures

1. Fascial structures

a. Interosseous membrane[3–6] (see Figure
35–14). This is an oblique membrane
that extends distal and lateral from the
interosseous crests of the tibia and fibula
to the inferior tibiofibular articulation.

b. Extensor retinaculum[3–6] (see Figure 35–
15)

(1). The superior retinaculum is attached laterally to the fibula and
medially to the tibia, and it encompasses the tendons of the tibialis anterior, the extensor hallucis and digitorum longus, the peroneus tertius,
the anterior tibial artery, and the
deep peroneal nerve.

(2). The inferior retinaculum is a y-
shaped band from the lateral surface
of the calcaneus to the superomedial
tibia and the inferomedial tibia. It
encompasses the tendons of the tibialis anterior, the peroneus tertius,
the extensor hallucis and digitorum

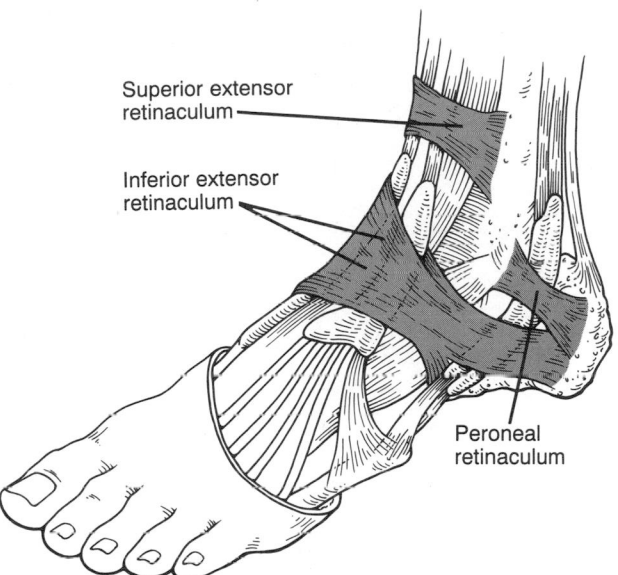

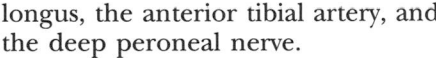

FIGURE 35–15 Superior and inferior extensor retinaculum covering the tibialis anterior, extensor digitorum longus, and extensor hallucis longus; peroneal retinaculum covering the peroneal tendons.

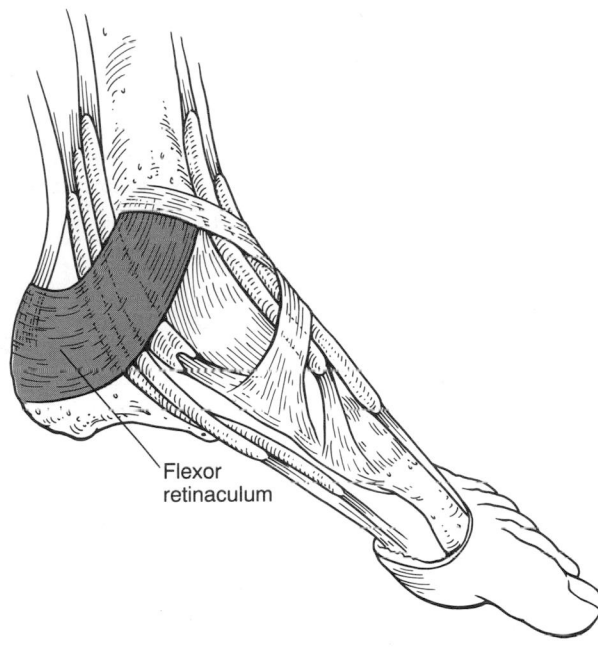

FIGURE 35–16 Flexor retinaculum covering the tendons of tibialis posterior, flexor digitorum longus, and flexor hallucis longus.

longus, the anterior tibial artery, and the deep peroneal nerve.

c. Peroneal retinaculum[3–6] (see Figure 35–15)

   (1). The superior retinaculum runs from the lateral malleolus bone to the lateral calcaneus and encompasses the tendons of the peroneus longus and brevis.

   (2). The inferior retinaculum is continuous with the inferior extensor retinaculum and then attaches to the posterolateral calcaneus. It also encompasses the tendons of the peroneus longus and brevis.

d. Flexor retinaculum[3–6] (see Figure 35–16). This is a strong band that extends from the medial malleolus to the distal calcaneus and encompasses the tendons of the tibialis posterior, the flexor hallucis and digitorum longus, the posterior tibial artery, and the tibial nerve.

2. **Medial ligamentous structures (collectively, the deltoid ligament)**

a. Anterior talotibial ligament[3–6] (see Figure 35–17). This ligament courses from the tip of the medial malleolus to the medial tibia.

b. Posterior talotibial ligament[3–6] (see Figure 35–17). This ligament courses from the medial malleolus to the inner side of the talus and to the tubercle on the posterior talus.

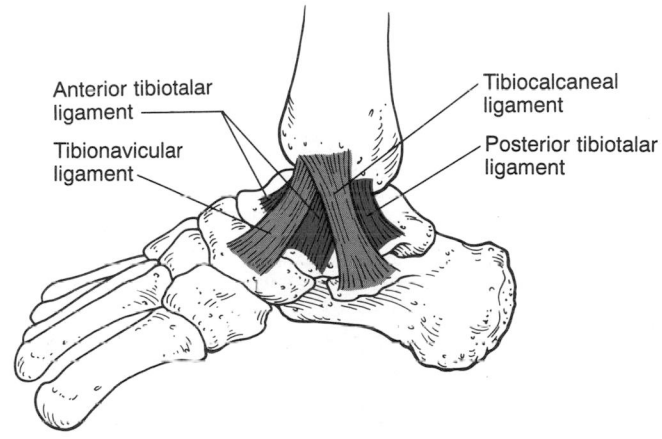

FIGURE 35–17 The four medial collateral (deltoid) ligaments.

c. Tibiocalcaneal ligament[3–6] (see Figure 35–17). This ligament courses from the medial malleolus to the sustentaculum tali.

d. Tibionavicular ligament[3–6] (see Figure 35–17). This ligament courses from the medial malleolus to the navicular tuberosity.

3. **Lateral ligamentous structures**

a. Anterior talofibular ligament[3–6] (see Figure 35–18). This ligament courses from the anterior margin of the lateral malleolus to the lateral facet on the anterior talus.

b. Posterior talofibular ligament[3–6] (see Figure 35–18). This ligament courses from the posterior margin of the lateral malleolus to the tubercle on the posterior talus.

c. Calcaneofibular ligament[3–6] (see Figure 35–18). This ligament courses from the lateral malleolus to the tubercle on the lateral calcaneus.

D. Functional significance

1. **Dorsiflexion** of the ankle (in combination with subtalar and midtarsal joint pronation) lowers the body's center of mass, thus facilitating shock absorption and decreasing energy expenditure.[1,2]

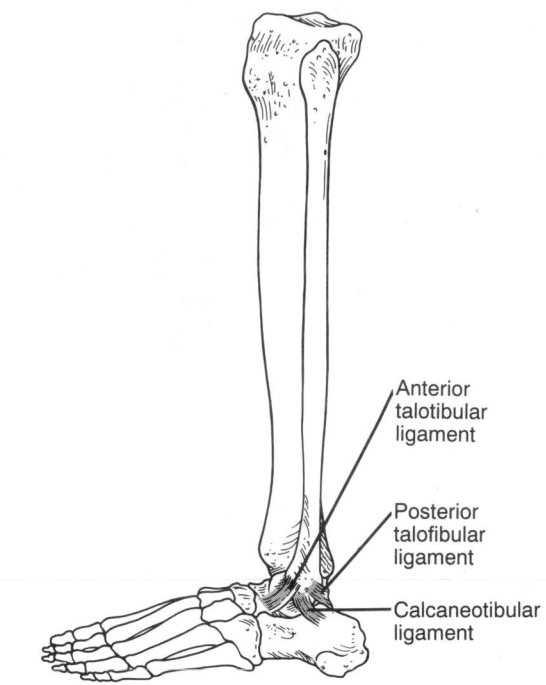

FIGURE 35–18   The three lateral collateral ligaments.

Anterior talotibular ligament

Posterior talofibular ligament

Calcaneotibular ligament

2. **Plantar flexion** of the ankle (in combination with subtalar and midtarsal joint supination) facilitates the rigid lever action of the ankle and foot during push off to help propel the body forward.[1,2]

II. Examination

A. Subjective

1. Ask patient about his/her perception of the problem(s) to better focus the objective evaluation.

a. Ask whether the patient thinks that the problem (or problems) is related to activity (leading the therapist to focus on contractile tissue).

b. Ask whether the patient thinks that the problem (or problems) is chronic (leading the therapist to attempt to reproduce the exact symptoms during evaluation).

2. Discuss the patient's goals so that they may be combined with the therapist's goals and incorporated into the treatment planning process.

a. Ask whether the patient wants to participate in a particular activity that requires certain muscle strength or joint ROM.

B. Objective

1. **History**

a. Elicit information concerning any trauma, including a complete description of the mechanism of injury.

b. Discuss symptom presentation[7] (see Table 35–1).

Table 35–1. SYMPTOM PRESENTATION IN PATIENTS WITH ANKLE PROBLEMS

How long ago did symptoms begin?
What makes the symptoms worse, and what makes them better?
How do the symptoms affect physical activity?
What is done to alleviate the symptoms?
Has a change in the symptoms occurred?
Has any previous treatment been rendered for this injury?
Have any previous injuries occurred to the back or lower extremities?
Have any surgical procedures been performed on the lower extremity?
Does any history of diabetes, circulatory disorders, heart disease, neurological disease, or arthritis exist?
Are any medications being taken? For what conditions?
Has any testing been done on the ankle (*eg*, radiography, magnetic resonance imaging, bone scanning)?
Has a change in body weight occurred over the last year?
Should any other information be noted?

2. **Inspection and palpation**
   a. **Posture** evaluation begins as the patient walks into the examining room.
      (1). Note varus or valgus deformities of the hip, knee, and tibia as well as pronation or supination of the foot in the frontal plane.
      (2). The sagittal plane is observed and any spinal curves, pelvic rotation, and hip, knee, and ankle flexion or hypertension is noted.
      (3). Note rotation abnormalities of the spine, femur, and tibia in the transverse plane.
      (4). Any noted abnormalities should be inspected further to detect their possible relationship to ankle dysfunction (see "Posture," Chapter 37).
   b. **The skin** of the lower leg and foot is examined for extensibility, swelling, discoloration, trophic changes, and temperature.
      (1). Note the nail bed condition and whether calluses, blisters, warts, and ulcerations are present.
      (2). Examine the dorsalis pedis (between extensor hallucis and digitorum tendons on the dorsum) and posterior tibial (posterior to the medial malleolus and anterior to the Achilles tendon)[3,4] **pulses** are assessed and graded as present, absent, or weak-

ened, compared with those on the other side.
   c. **Orthotic** use should be noted with a description of the purpose, characteristics, and effectiveness of the device.
   d. **Footwear** is evaluated for wear patterns and proper style and fit for the patient. Note heel counter, toe box, arch support, sole, heel, and material.

C. Measurement

1. Assess talocrural **joint play** including:[8–10]
   a. Fibula and tibia dorsal and ventral glides (see Figures 35–19 and 35–20), tibiofibular dorsal and ventral glides (see Figure 35–21), talocrural dorsal and ventral glides (see Figures 35–22 and 35–23), and talar distraction and rocking (see Figures 35–24 and 35–25).
   b. Note the **capsular pattern;** if the gastrocsoleus is tight, dorsiflexion is more restricted and exhibits a soft end feel; if not, plantar flexion is more restricted.[11]
2. Measure ankle **ROM** in plantar flexion and dorsiflexion.

   PLEASE NOTE: Keep the subtalar and midtarsal joints in a neutral position when measuring ankle dorsiflexion[12] (see Figure 35–26).

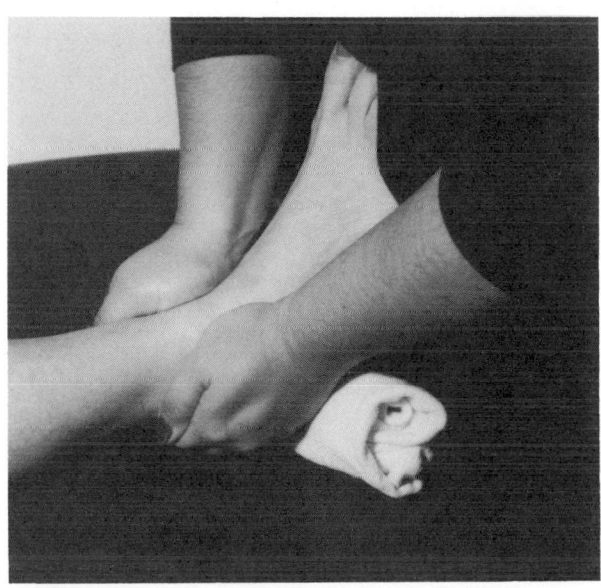

FIGURE 35–19 Fibula dorsal glide.

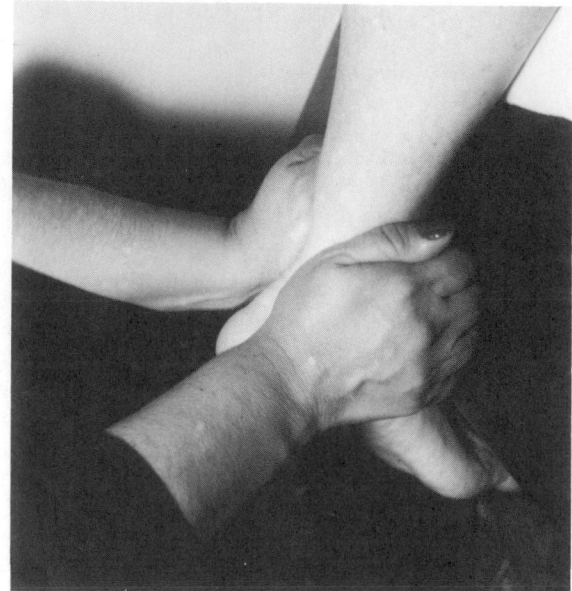

FIGURE 35–20 Tibia ventral glide.

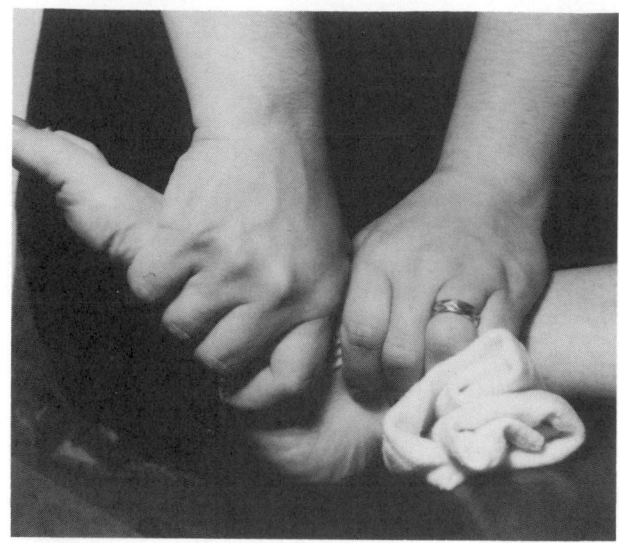

FIGURE 35–22 Talocrural dorsal glide.

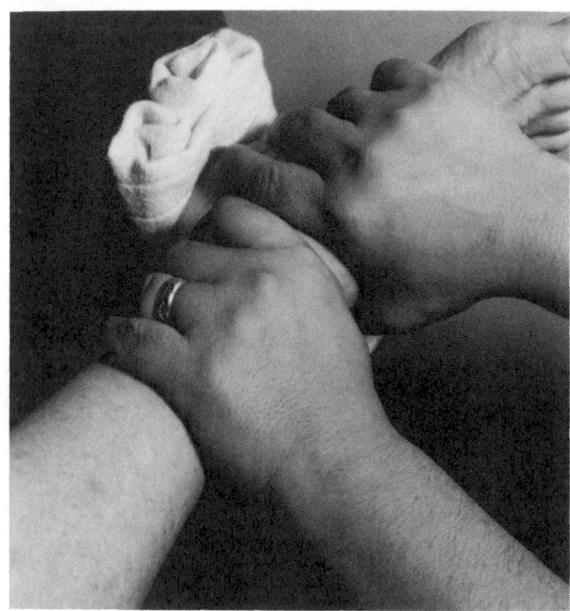

FIGURE 35–21 Tibiofibular dorsal glide.

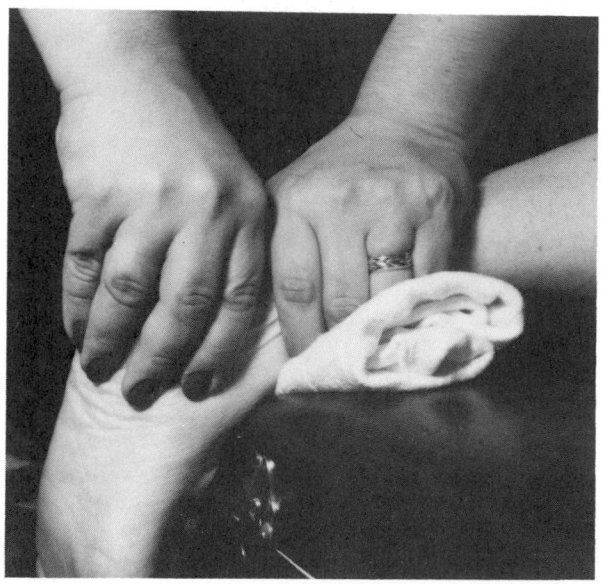

FIGURE 35–23 Talocrural ventral glide.

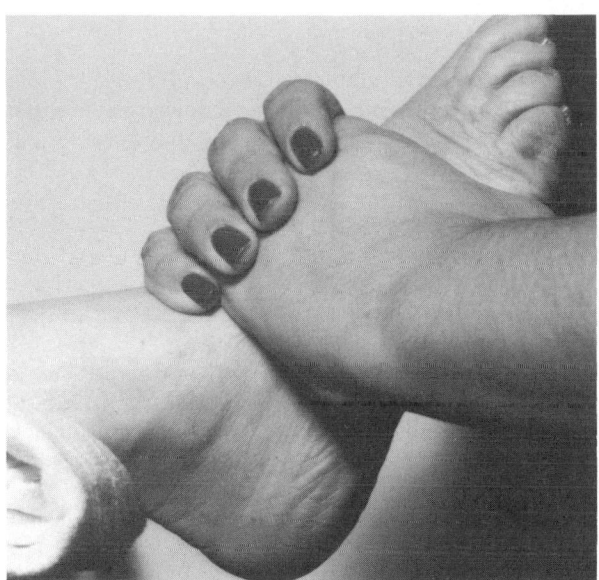

FIGURE 35–24   Talar distraction.

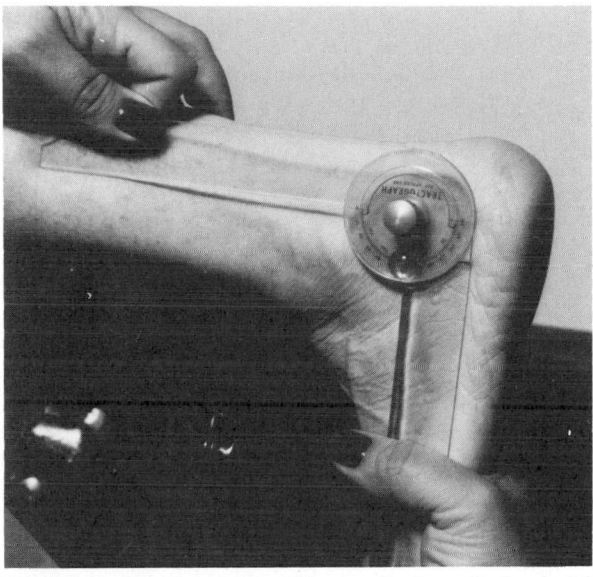

FIGURE 35–26   Measuring ankle dorsiflexion with the foot in slight supination.

3. **Muscle strength** is evaluated with function in mind. Along with **manual muscle test positions**[13,14] (tibialis anterior and posterior, and the gastrocnemius, soleus, and peroneals), assess the patient's **strength in weight bearing,** eg, rising up and down on the toes both quickly and slowly; walking on the toes and on the heels.

1. Test two point discrimination, light touch, and temperature of the lower leg and foot as a gross assessment of **sensation.**

5. **Stability** of the joint should be assessed.[7,15]
   a. Use the anterior drawer sign to test the anterior talofibular ligament (see Figure 35–27).
   b. Examine the medial and lateral glides of the talus in the mortise for general lateral collateral, and deltoid ligament laxity (also known as talar tilt).

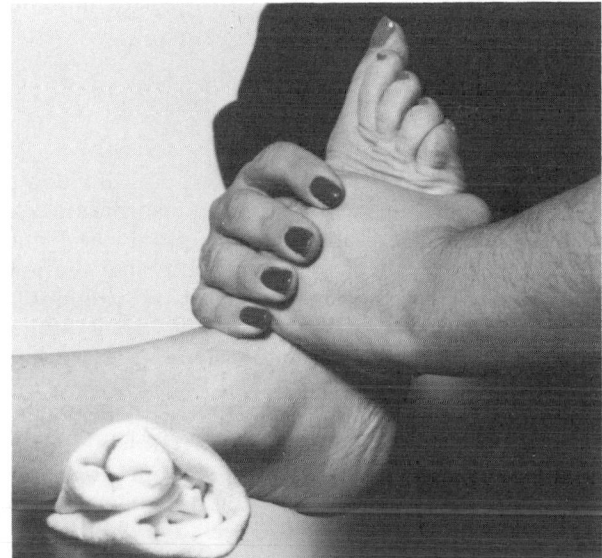

FIGURE 35–25   Talar rocking.

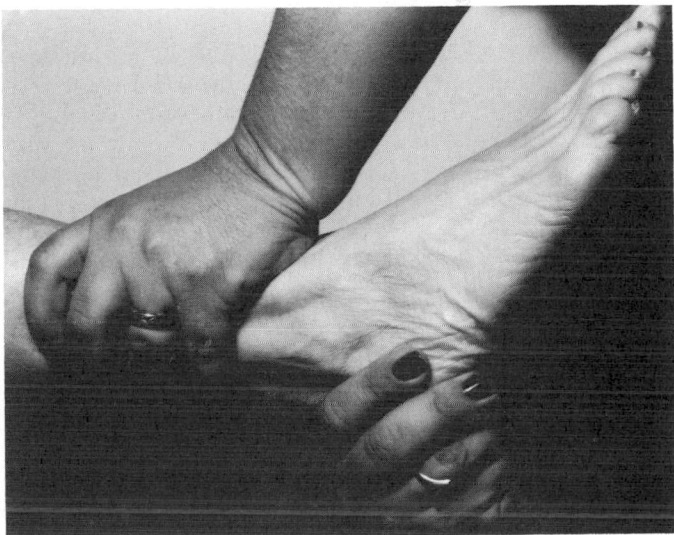

FIGURE 35–27   Anterior drawer sign with dorsal tibial pressure and ventral calcaneal pressure.

c. Note the degree and ease of movement as well as pain.

6. Test **double-limb and single-limb balance** on both mobile and stable surfaces.
   a. Move a balance board for a mobile surface.

b. Gently push the patient off balance on a stable surface.

c. Note the patient's reaction time and use of the head, upper and lower extremities, and trunk to assist in balance.

7. **Gait.** See "Gait," Chapter 38.

III. Assessment

Evaluate the objective findings, considering the following factors.

A. Mobility

The patient should have sufficient ROM for movement and assumption of correct posture.[16,17]

1. Assess whether the ankle has sufficient ROM and joint play.
2. If the ankle lacks ROM, determine whether restriction stems from the joint, soft tissue, or muscle tissue (use end-feel as a guide).
3. If the ankle lacks joint play, it must be restored again for gains in ROM to be achieved.

B. Stability

The muscles should be able to perform tonic holding and cocontraction.[16,17]

1. Determine whether any muscle weakness is present isometrically, concentrically, or eccentrically.
2. Assess whether a difference in torque production exists isokinetically (when appropriate) and in what positions the muscle is weak; if muscle force production is lacking, determine whether sufficient ROM exists in the joint for the muscle to contract efficiently.

C. Controlled mobility

The muscles should have the ability to move the proximal joints over the fixed distal end.[16,17]

1. Determine whether the patient can bear weight and move over his/her foot and ankle with and without assistance; the patient's inability to perform these functions may indicate a continued problem in stability.

2. Determine whether the patient can accept challenges to bear weight in a double-limb or single-limb stance; if the patient lacks weight-bearing ability, a need for increased joint movement may exist to allow him/her to detect motion changes in the foot and ankle.[17]

D. Skill

The muscles should be able to move and stabilize the proximal joints when the distal end is mobilized.[16,17]

1. Determine whether the patient can walk on level and uneven surfaces. Assess whether he/she can run and whether he/she can walk step over step up and down stairs.
   a. If the patient lacks the ability to walk on even surfaces, mobility and stability may be lacking.
   b. If he/she is unable to walk on uneven surfaces or to run, controlled mobility may be lacking.

E. Diagnosis and prognosis

Based on your initial judgement, including the relationship of all anomalous findings to each other and at what structural level the problem is occurring, make a **physical therapy diagnosis** and a **physical therapy prognosis.** This allows you to set reasonable goals and a treatment plan. **Musculoskeletal dysfunction** should be the focus of your diagnosis and the basis of your treatment plan. Examples of physical therapy diagnoses include Achilles tendinitis, shin splints (anterior or posterior tibial tendinitis), and talocural dysfunction. Goals must be **measurable** and **time related.** Formulate long-term goals from a functional perspective. Keep in mind the patient's goals.

IV. Treatment Plan

A. Management of mobility dysfunction

1. Soft-tissue management
   a. Release (or minimize) soft-tissue restrictions first. Move from superficial to deep, breaking up surface scar tissue first, and gradually move into deeper connective tissue, and, then into muscle. Use superficial and deep myofascial release techniques, traditional effleurage and petrissage methods, friction massage, or deep acupressure to alleviate the restrictions[18-20] (see Figure 35-28).
   b. Modalities are used to decrease swelling, pain, and calcification, as well as to increase blood flow and metabolism. Therapeutic heat is used as a precursor to massage, mobilization, and exercise, and it includes the use of hot packs, paraffin baths, hydrotherapy, ultrasound, short-wave and microwave diathermy, and fluidotherapy. Cryotherapy, with its local vasoconstriction effect, helps to alleviate swelling. It also decreases nerve conduction velocity, diminishing the pain response to therapy. Cold is beneficial in the treatment of acute lesions by aiding in the management of pain and swelling; cryotherapy can also be used as an ending to treatment to minimize trauma to tissues caused by mobilization and exercise. Electrical stimulation in its various forms is used to modulate pain, to reduce swelling and muscle spasm, and to re-educate muscles. These forms of electrical stimulation include transcutaneous electrical nerve stimulation; high-voltage, interferential, galvanic stimulation and iontophoresis; and functional (neuromuscular) electrical stimulation. All modalities are used as **adjuncts** to enhance or modulate the effects of treatment.

      The skin at the distal end of the tibia and fibula is thin. Consider this when working with soft-tissue tightness. Pressure must be commensurate with tissue integrity. Darkened skin color; hair loss; shiny, dry skin; or skin lucency may indicate fragile tissue. Extreme caution should be used when applying forces to fragile tissues.[21]
   c. Wound problems are not uncommon in the distal tibiofibular area because of thin tissue and diminished circulation in this region. Accurate description of the wound facilitates proper management. Wounds (or ulcers) may be superficial, partial thickness, or full thickness and can be traumatic, vascular (venous stasis), arteriosclerotic, or metabolic (diabetic) in origin. Relate sensation and surrounding skin changes to ulcerations; full-thickness wounds result in a complete loss of pain sensation, whereas partial-thickness wounds leave pain sensation intact. Note changes in the size, depth, color, and odor of the wound; purulent drainage and pungent odor are indicative of bacterial infection.[21-23]

      Treatment for ulcers and wounds includes hydrotherapy with an appropriate antiseptic solution for cleaning; eschar removal with sterile instruments or with high-pressure water and hydrophilic pellets (Debrisan); and the application of a clean and sterile dressing (gauze or Kling), with or without topical enzymatic ointments (collagenase or sutilains [Travase]). Treatment with hyperbaric oxygen and cold laser is also used for the management of decubiti.[21-23]

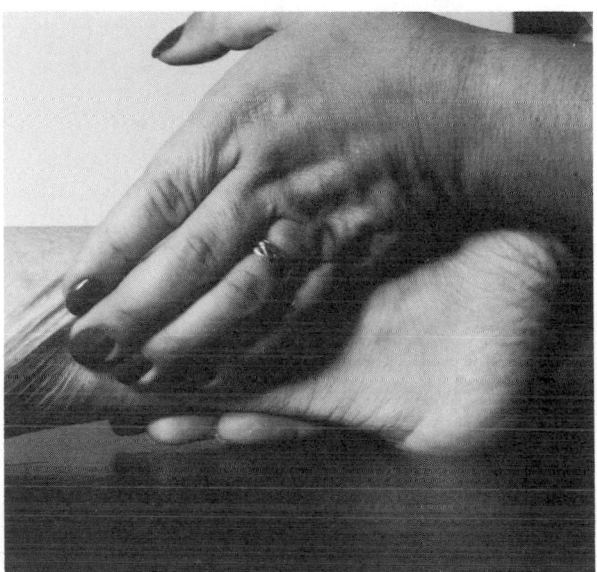

FIGURE 35-28 Soft tissue manipulation of the peroneal area.

2. **Joint management**
   a. Warm the joint before attempting mobilization (eg, with heat, massage, or passive or active ROM exercise). To determine the patient's tolerance to mobilization, use the Cyriax sequence of pain and limitation:[11]
      (1). Pain *before* tissue resistance indicates that an acute or extraarticular lesion may be present (the capsule and soft-tissue do not tolerate stretching).
      (2). Pain *with* tissue resistance indicates the presence of a subacute lesion (gentle stretching of the capsule and soft-tissue may begin).
      (3). Pain *after* tissue resistance indicates that a chronic lesion may be present (stretching can be performed to gain length in the capsule and soft tissue).
   b. Begin with grade 1 mobilization (small oscillations at the beginning of the capsular range) for pain modulation. In the subacute stage, progress into grade 2 mobilization (large oscillations at the middle of the capsular range) as the patient tolerates. As the problem becomes chronic, use grades 3 and 4 mobilizations (large oscillations toward the end of the capsular range and small oscillations at the end of the capsular range, respectively) to cause more permanent deformation of (and therefore to stretch) the joint capsule.[9,10]
   c. Joint mobilization techniques include fibula and tibia dorsal and ventral glides (see Figures 35–19 and 35–20), tibiofibular dorsal and ventral glides (see Figure 35–21), talocrural dorsal and ventral glides (see Figures 35–22 and 35–23), talar distraction and rocking (see Figures 35–24 and 35–25). Calcaneal distraction and rocking also should be done because of the attachment of the triceps surae to the calcaneus.[8–10]
   d. Acutely inflamed joints should be managed with the use of ice, compression, elevation, and rest. As the swelling diminishes, grade 1 mobilization can be attempted. If the patient complains of sharp pain or if swelling increases, the techniques should be discontinued. Gradually increase the intensity and grade of mobilization as the patient's tolerance and reactivity allow. Patients with long-standing joint hypomobility secondary to trauma (eg, from complex tibiofibular fractures, prolonged healing time of fractures, and elongated immobilization) require slow increases in both the intensity and duration of mobilization. Even in the chronic stage, patients with these problems tend to be more reactive to specific joint techniques, and their condition can easily become worse with protracted treatment sessions. These patients are also prone to the development of osteoarthritic changes in the joint, which is atypical for the general population. Educate the patient on the levels and types of activities to minimize stress and to maximize function of the arthritic ankle joint.

3. **Muscle length management**
   a. Muscle tightness plays a significant role in lack of mobility at the ankle. The most common form of tightness is that of the gastrocsoleus muscle. **Stretching** should be done with the subtalar joint positioned in neutral to slight supination (which prevents substitution of foot motion) and can be done when the patient is either weight bearing (see Figure 35–29) or non weight bearing (see Figure 35–30). If the patient's foot is not al-

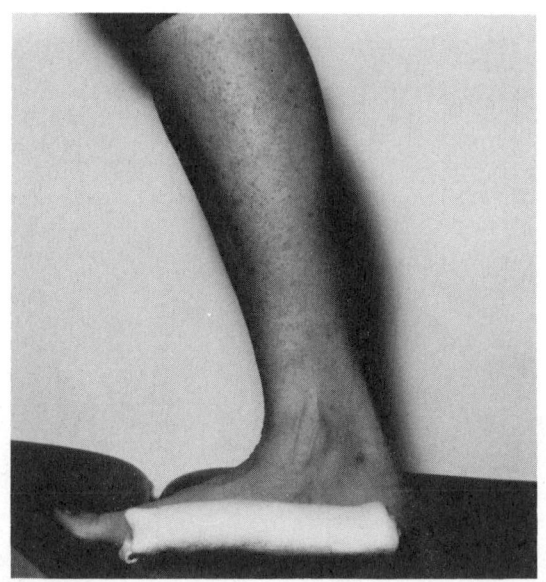

FIGURE 35–29 Gastrocnemius stretch in weight-bearing position with elevation of the medial arch (foot in neutral).

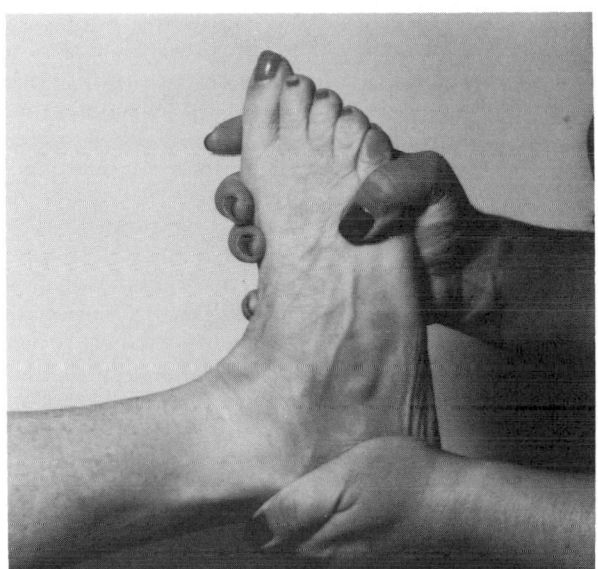

FIGURE 35–30 Non–weight-bearing gastrocnemius stretch with the foot in slight supination.

lowed to pronate, elongated stretching is effective in either position.[12]

b. Peroneal and tibialis anterior stretching should be done with a knowledge of the integrity of the lateral collateral ligaments, especially the anterior talofibular and calcaneofibular ligaments. Stretching is most easily accomplished in a non–weight-bearing posture.

4. **Progression of mobility management**

Some degree of soft-tissue mobility must be restored before treatment can proceed to include deeper joint and muscle structures. Shift back and forth between techniques for the tissues, muscles, and joints as the patient begins to loosen up. Instruct the patient in a home program to help him/her to maintain the mobility that is gained during physical therapy sessions. Most patients with primary mobility problems have secondary stability concerns that must be addressed before they can function at controlled mobility and skill levels.

B. Management of stability and controlled mobility dysfunction

1. **Overview of stability dysfunction**

Stability dysfunction is primarily caused by ligament laxity and muscle weakness. There are no techniques to tighten or strengthen ligaments other than immobilization. Muscle strengthening is fairly easy to accomplish because of constant functional demands on the joint. Begin treatment with the patient non weight bearing to eliminate the body mass's force of gravity on the muscles. Move on to weight-bearing exercises as soon as the patient and the injured structures can tolerate it.

2. **Muscle strength management**

Patients with a muscle strength grade that is fair (3/5) or worse should begin **strength training** in a non–weight-bearing posture. As strength increases, cardinal-plane and diagonal motions can be used while manual resistance is superimposed at the foot (see Figure 35–31), while rubber tubing or exercise bands are applied at the foot (see Figure 35–32), free weights are placed on the foot, or isokinetic exercises are performed. Keep the patient's functional needs (eg, prolonged standing, excessive walking, side-to-side running, or jumping) in mind when you design an exercise program; also focus on the specificity of training. Many repetitions of a movement with limited (low-level) resistance can be used to improve muscle endurance, whereas few repetitions with increased (high-level) resistance can be used to bring about greater force production by the muscle. Eccentric training of the tibialis

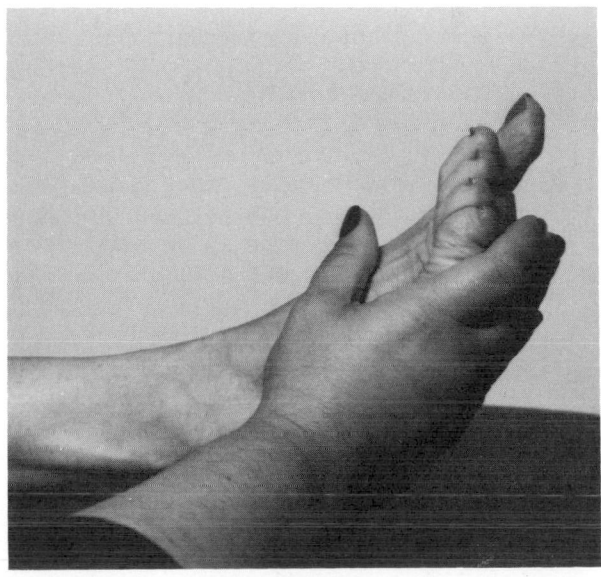

FIGURE 35–31 Manual resistance to peroneal muscle group.

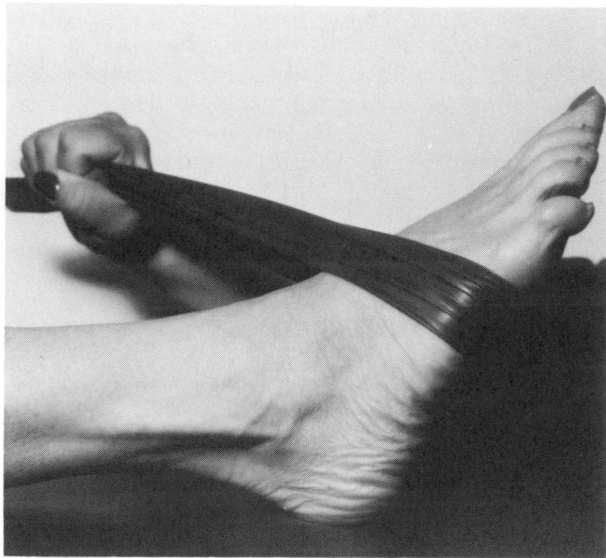

FIGURE 35–32 Resistance with rubber tubing to peroneal muscle group.

be accomplished through protected weight bearing with rhythmic stabilization at the pelvis; through weight shifting with and without rhythmic stabilization (see Figure 35–33); through unilateral weight bearing; and through balance board activities. Enhance the patient's somatosensory feedback by providing training with and without the patient being able to see. The Biomechanical Ankle Platform System (BAPS) Board (Camp International) is a relatively inexpensive balance board system that has balls of varying size to alter stress and motion on the ankle. The activities should progress from exercise with an orthotic device to exercise with a high-top sneaker and, finally, exercise with bare feet. For a patient who has chronic laxity, it may be prudent to have him/her run, jump, and perform other sporting activities with an orthotic to im-

anterior, extensor hallucis and digitorum longus, and gastrocsoleus is important for improving the patient's gait.

3. **Ligament laxity management**
   a. Ankle ligament laxity, specifically lateral collateral instability, is a frustrating and often recurrent problem. Once the diagnosis has been made, **management of acute symptoms** consists of the application of ice, orthotics or cast immobilization, and rest (non–weight-bearing ambulation). Once initial swelling has subsided, gradual protected weight bearing can occur. **Orthotics** can consist of rigid plastic bilateral uprights that surround the malleoli for a moderate to severe ankle sprain or an ankle sleeve, ace wrap, or tape for a minor sprain. The plastic splint (Aircast), is a commonly stocked item that allows air to be blown into a bladder lining of hard plastic uprights for the management of swelling as well as to provide stability. All such braces that provide total contact also contribute to proprioceptive input of the ankle joint. Adhesive taping can also be used to increase the proprioceptive input and to provide some protection for the lateral collateral ligaments during athletic activities.
   b. Management of ligament laxity also involves **proprioceptive training.** This can

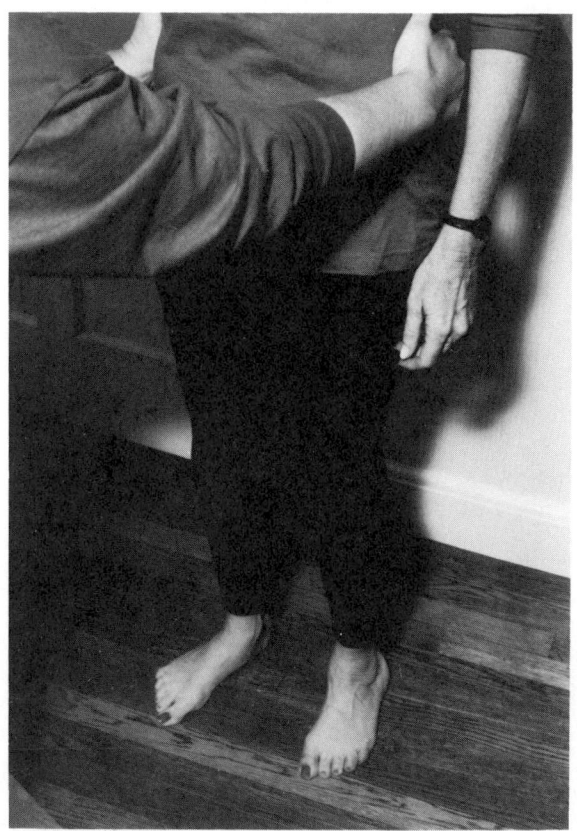

FIGURE 35–33 Rhythmic stabilization with manual contacts at the pelvis.

prove proprioceptive input to the joint and to protect it.

4. **Management of controlled mobility dysfunction**

Trauma, immobilization, and weakness lead to problems in weight bearing. Easing a patient into weight bearing involves **gradual protected weight bearing** with shoes and orthotic devices in a sitting position or on parallel bars. Have the patient sit in a chair (a rocker works well) and move the tibia over the foot. Having the patient move the tibia back and forth over the foot helps to improve ROM in a functional movement and prepares the patient for gait.

Have the patient stand with a wide base of support and shift his/her weight over the foot. Have him/her move side to side and front to back. Work slowly, gradually having the patient increase his/her speed and decrease the base of support. As the patient progresses, have him/her begin to perform a single-limb stance, increasing time and perturbation as his/her ability improves. Again, use a balance board or BAPS system to improve proprioceptive input to the joint. Add stable footwear or orthotics to enhance feedback and to supply external support to the joint.

C. Management of skill dysfunction

As the patient's weight-bearing ability on stable surfaces improves, transfer him/her on to uneven surfaces (use foam, a pillow, or ramps) and stairs. Have the patient step up and down on a stair or short stool, moving the tibia over the foot and increasing weight bearing onto the foot. As the patient is able to bear full weight, have him/her progress to walking step over step. Jogging with progression to running is a further option. Use an elastic bungee-type cord to apply more resistance. Keep in mind that the ground reaction forces for jogging and running are three to four times body weight force, and the talocrural joint should be mobile and stable before the patient undertakes this activity. Generalized lower extremity training tools such as the Fitter, Snowbounder, and Russian Leaper functionally train the lower extremities and provide activity-specific training. Plyometrics (fast and powerful movements that use the stretch reflex to facilitate muscle action)[24] also train the lower extremity in activities such as jumping, running, and squatting.

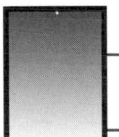

Clinical Decision-Making Cases

Case #1

HISTORY

At the time of presentation, SC was a 30-year-old engineer who had been involved in a motor vehicle accident 6 months earlier. She sustained open, comminuted distal tibia and fibula fractures of the right lower extremity. She was casted for 12 weeks, but her fractures did not heal. Skin grafting was performed at 14 weeks because the wound would not close. After the graft had healed 4 weeks later, a plate and screws were attached to the fracture site for stabilization. A week later, SC was discharged from the hospital on crutches with a toe-touch gait. She was referred to physical therapy for gait training and ROM exercise. When SC first started therapy, she was limping quite badly and was in a lot of pain. This was only the 3rd week she had been able to bear weight in 6 months, and she was supposed to increase the amount of weight bearing as much as she could tolerate. In addition, her left leg and back were sore, and she was very discouraged.

EXAMINATION

SC's soft tissue was thin and fragile along the distal shin; discoloration (reddish black) of the distal shin was also present, with mild swelling of the foot and ankle. On a scale of 0 (no pain) to 10 (unbearable pain), SC had scores of 8 in her ankle during walking, 3 in her ankle when she was not bearing weight, and 5 in the incision area all of the time. SC's ROM was as follows:

Motion	Range In Right Side, Degrees	Range In Left Side, Degrees
Plantar flexion	5	40
Dorsiflexion	−10	5
Knee flexion	100	125
Knee extension	−5	0

Joint play on the right was as follows: tibia and fibula glides were grade 1⁻; the talus on tibia and fibula glide was grade 1⁻; the calcaneal glides were grade 1; the intertarsal glides were grade 1; the metatarsal glides were grade 2; and all glides on the left were grade 3. The therapist was unable to test the patient's strength because of pain. SC was working full time (she sat during the day), and she used crutches safely on all surfaces.

ASSESSMENT AND DIAGNOSIS

SC had significant pain and dysfunction caused by a lack of joint play and by soft-tissue tightness, which in turn limited her ROM. She also had proprioceptive loss because of the extent of the injury and the length of time that she could not bear weight.

TREATMENT GOALS

Short-Term Goals

- To eliminate SC's ankle swelling in 3 weeks.
- To increase SC's ROM in plantar flexion by 15 degrees, in dorsiflexion by 5 degrees, in knee flexion by 25 degrees, and in knee extension by 5 degrees in 3 weeks.
- To increase SC's joint play in the tibiofibular and talocrural joints by 1 grade in 3 weeks.
- To allow SC to ambulate with a cane with a pain score of 3 out of 10 in 4 weeks.

Long-Term Goal

SC wants to be able to ambulate on all surfaces without an assistive device in 6 months.

TREATMENT OUTCOME

Initially, SC needed to regain mobility. Soft-tissue and joint mobilization (mobility) was initiated, with close attention paid to her reactivity to the treatment. Over the course of 3 to 4 weeks, her ankle motion improved enough to allow her to perform gentle isometric exercises (stability) of the plantar flexors and dorsiflexors in non–weight-bearing positions; gradually, SC progressed to weight-bearing activities (controlled mobility) after 4 to 6 weeks. Her pain continually decreased, and her function improved. An extensive home exer-

cise plan was initiated at the outset of treatment; she would demonstrate her program as a part of each treatment session. Joint mobilization intensity increased as the overall motion improved, which, in turn, allowed even more range and function. If the mobilization was too vigorous (with respect to either intensity or duration), SC would experience increasingly more pain, and as a result, less function. This was a dilemma with regard to treatment planning. She needed to increase her mobility, but her talocrural joint cartilage was so severely compromised that it was easily irritated by specific mobilizations. It was unrealistic to attempt to regain normal joint play; rather, treatment focused on optimizing function. After 3 months of intensive treatment, SC was making remarkable gains. Now 9 months after her injury, she was ambulating with a cane, bearing 90% of her weight, with pain occurring only at the end of the day.

THREE MONTH RE-EXAMINATION

The soft tissue on SC's distal shin was more pliable and stronger; the discoloration and swelling were no longer present in the foot, but a minimal amount remained around the ankle. SC's pain score was 1 out of 10 in the fracture area and in the ankle when she bore weight (she described it as a dull ache); she also occasionally had severe pain after treatment, but she stated that such pain "disappeared in a day or so." SC's ROM was as follows:

Motion	Range In Right Side, Degrees
Plantar flexion	25
Dorsiflexion	0
Knee flexion	120
Knee extension	0

Joint play on the right was as follows: the tibia and fibula glides were grades 1⁺ and 2⁻, respectively; the talus on the tibia and fibula was grade 2; the calcaneal glide was grade 2⁺; and the intertarsal and metatarsal glides were grade 3.

The results of strength testing in the right extremity were as follows (on a scale of 0 to 5, with 5 indicating the greatest level of strength):

1. Gastrocsoleus—3 (through available range).
2. Tibialis posterior—3 (through available range).
3. Tibialis anterior—3 (through available range).
4. Peroneals—3 (through available range).
5. Toe flexors—4.
6. Toe extensors—3⁺.

TREATMENT GOALS

Short-Term Goals

- To increase SC's ROM in plantar flexion by 15 degrees and in dorsiflexion by 5 degrees in 6 weeks.
- To increase SC's joint play to grade 3 in the tibiofibular and talocrural joints in 4 weeks.
- To increase SC's strength to normal in the ankle and foot musculature in 8 weeks.

Long-Term Goal

SC wants to be able to ambulate on all surfaces without an assistive device in 3 months.

TREATMENT OUTCOMES

Treatment focused on continued restoration of mobility and stability but concentrated on controlled mobility and skill. More weight-bearing activities were emphasized, including weight-shifting, balance-board, and, gradually, single-limb stance exercises.

After 2 more months of treatment, the patient was able to ambulate without an assistive device on all surfaces with minimal to no swelling or pain. She regained good to normal strength and balance. The tissue around the ankle remained discolored but swelled only if she spent many hours standing.

Case #2

HISTORY

On presentation, GL was a 31-year-old male who had stepped backward into a pothole while playing softball 3 weeks earlier and had laterally sprained his left ankle. He was given an Aircast and crutches in the emergency room at the local hospital, along with instructions to rest and elevate the ankle and to apply ice to it. He openly admits that he did not use the crutches or the Aircast brace, nor did he follow the acute-care instructions. He was referred to physical therapy because of continued pain and dysfunction. He was taking codeine for the pain and Ibuprofen for the swelling.

EXAMINATION

GL's soft tissue on the left foot and ankle was swollen and red; the skin appeared to be slightly dry. On a scale of 0 (no pain) to 10 (unbearable pain), GL had scores of 8 at rest and 10 when the foot was dependent. He also had pin-point pain over the anterior talofibular ligament. The ROM in GL's right ankle was within normal limits; his left ankle had *no* movement in dorsiflexion, plantar flexion, inversion, or eversion. The therapist was unable to test joint play and strength because of the presence of pain and swelling. GL is a telephone repairman but was out of work for 2.5 weeks after his injury. At the time of referral, he was using crutches and was not bearing weight on the left side because of pain.

ASSESSMENT AND DIAGNOSIS

GL had significant soft-tissue changes and pain that increased over time instead of decreasing with normal healing. The extremes of his symptoms (unbearable pain when the ankle was in a dependent position; redness, swelling, and dry skin; and pin-point pain) suggested that he either had a fracture that was not detected (no radiographs had been taken) or that he was beginning to develop reflex sympathetic dystrophy (RSD; a neurovascular disorder that results in excessive sympathetic nervous system activity). Before any physical therapy treatment was initiated, GL was sent back to his physician for further testing.

One week later, GL returned with a note from the physician stating that radiographs and bone scans had produced negative results. The physician was concerned about reflex sympathetic dystrophy and asked that GL be evaluated and treated by a physical therapist. A re-evaluation did not reveal that any changes had occurred since the previous evaluation. With a tentative diagnosis of reflex sympathetic dystrophy, the treatment was to be focused on decreasing the sympathetic response through desensitization, gradual increases in mobility and stability, and slow increases in weight bearing, as tolerated.

TREATMENT GOALS

Short-Term Goals

- To eliminate GL's redness and swelling in the left foot in 4 weeks.
- To decrease GL's pain score at rest to 4 out of 10 in 4 weeks.
- To increase GL's ROM in dorsiflexion and eversion by 5 degrees and in plantar flexion and inversion by 15 degrees in 4 weeks.
- To increase GL's weight bearing on the left side with crutches to 50 lb of force in 4 weeks.

Long-Term Goal

GL wanted to be able to ambulate without pain and without an assistive device in 3 months.

TREATMENT OUTCOME

Treatment included the use of a home transcutaneous electrical nerve stimulation unit (with electrodes on the L5, S1, and S2 spinal segments); gentle massage to the entire left lower extremity, beginning at the hip region and gradually moving distally, as tolerated; active ROM exercises, and active lower-extremity proprioceptive neuromuscular facilitation (PNF) patterns bilaterally. After 2 weeks, the redness and swelling were beginning to subside, and the pain score had decreased to 6 out of 10. Treatment then could begin to address the stability problem; the treatment consisted of gentle setting exercises, progressing to isometric exercises. These exercises were tolerated well, and GL improved rapidly over the next week, walking with a toe-touch gait and allowing the limb to rest more frequently in a dependent position.

After 2 more weeks, GL was working on partial weight bearing after having gained 30 degrees of plantar flexion and 5 degrees of dorsiflexion. He was performing isometric and resistive exercises using light rubber tubing. The redness and swelling were minimal, and his pain score in weight-bearing positions had decreased to 4 out of 10; the pain score was minimal in non–weight-bearing positions.

Two months after the injury, GL was able to return to work, but he needed to use a cane for ambulation. He was to continue a home physical therapy program that consisted of ankle and foot ROM exercises, PNF lower-extremity diagonal exercises with rubber tubing, weight-bearing exercises in a rocking chair, and the use of an ankle sleeve brace. Physical therapy in the clinic stressed weight-bearing exercises on the BAPS Board to improve function and proprioception and included more active stretching and strengthening exercises for the left lower extremity. GL was discharged from therapy 3 months after the injury; he was able to ambulate without an assistive device and was fully functional at work. He still had minor deficits in strength and ROM and was put on a maintenance home program to correct these concerns.

It was very clear to the patient that had he listened to the emergency room physician and followed the acute-care instructions to promote normal healing, the RSD probably would not have occurred. Nevertheless, he was able to achieve full function by a careful progression through mobility, stability, and controlled-mobility exercises that would allow the sympathetic nervous system to decrease its firing rate and the soft tissue, joints, and muscles to heal at their own pace.

References

1. Norkin CC, Levangie PK: *Joint Structure and Function,* 2nd ed. Philadelphia, F. A. Davis Company, 1992, pp 380–388.
2. Inman VT: *Joints of the Ankle.* Baltimore, Williams & Wilkins, 1976, pp 3–10.
3. Goss CM (ed): *Gray's Anatomy of the Human Body,* 29th ed. Philadelphia, Lea and Febiger, 1973, pp 356–358, 504–514.
4. Riegger CL: Anatomy of the ankle and foot. *Phys Ther* 1988, 68:2–14.
5. Warfel JH: *The Extremities: Muscles and Motor Points.* Philadelphia, Lea and Febiger, 1985, pp 88–100.
6. McMinn RMH, Hutchings RT, Logan BM: *Color Atlas of Foot and Ankle Anatomy.* Norwalk, CT, Appleton-Century-Crofts, 1982.
7. Giallonardo LM: Clinical evaluation of foot and ankle dysfunction. *Phys Ther* 1988, 68:50–56.
8. Kaltenborn FM: *Manual Mobilization of the Extremity Joints,* 4th ed. Oslo, Olaf Norlis Bokhandel, 1989, pp 152–159.
9. Maitland GD: *Peripheral Manipulation,* 4th ed. London, Butterworth Publishers, 1977.
10. Paris SV: Extremity mobilization and dysfunction [Course Notes], 1979.
11. Cyriax J: *Textbook of Orthopedic Medicine.* vol 1. *Diagnosis of Soft Tissue Lesions.* London, Baillière Tindall, 1975.
12. McPoil TG, Brocato RS: The foot and ankle: biomechanical evaluation and treatment. In Gould JA (ed): *Orthopedic and Sports Physical Therapy,* 2nd ed. St. Louis, C. V. Mosby Company, 1990, pp 293–321.
13. Kendall FP, McCreary EK: *Muscles: Testing and Function,* 4th ed. Baltimore, Williams & Wilkins, 1993.
14. Daniels L, Worthingham C: *Muscle Testing Techniques of Manual Examination.* Philadelphia, W. B. Saunders Company, 1972.
15. Magee DJ: *Orthopedic Physical Assessment,* 2nd ed. Philadelphia, W. B. Saunders Company, 1992, pp 438–513.
16. Stockmeyer SA: Personal communication, 1993.
17. Sullivan PE, Markos PD, Minor MA: *An Integrated Approach to Therapeutic Exercise: Theory and Application.* Reston, VA, Reston Publishing Company, 1982.
18. Tappan FM: *Healing Massage Techniques.* Reston, VA, Reston Publishing Company, 1978.
19. Manhiem CJ, Lavett DK: *The Myofascial Release Manual.* Thorofare, NJ, Slack, 1989.
20. Cantu RI, Grodin AJ: *Myofascial Manipulation.* Gaithersburg, MD, Aspen, 1992.
21. Birke JA, Sims DS: The insensitive foot. In Hunt GC (ed): *Physical Therapy of the Foot and Ankle.* New York, Churchill Livingstone, 1988, pp 133–168.
22. McGarvey CL: Skin and toenail problems. In Hunt GC (ed): *Physical Therapy of the Foot and Ankle.* New York, Churchill Livingstone, 1988, pp 169–198.
23. Sims DS, Cavanagh PR, Ulbrecht JS: Risk factors in the diabetic foot: recognition and management. *Phys Ther* 1988, 68:87–102.
24. Voight ML, Draovitch P: Plyometrics. In Alpert MA (ed): *Eccentric Muscle Training.* New York, Churchill Livingstone, 1991.

Suggested Reading

Bucholz R, Lippert F, Wenger D, *et al: Orthopedic Decision Making.* St. Louis, C. V. Mosby Company, 1984.

Cyriax J, Cyriax P: *Illustrated Manual of Orthopedic Medicine.* London, Butterworth Publishers, 1983.

Cyriax J: *Textbook of Orthopedic Medicine: Treatment by Manipulation, Massage, and Injection,* 8th ed. vol 2. London, Baillière Tindall, 1971.

Donatelli R: *The Biomechanics of the Foot and Ankle,* Philadelphia, F. A. Davis Company, 1990.

Edmond SL: *Manipulation and Mobilization.* St. Louis, C. V. Mosby Company, 1993.

Hoppenfeld S: *Physical Examination of the Spine and Extremities.* Norwalk, CT, Appleton-Century-Crofts, 1976.

Kapandji IA: *Physiology of the Joints.* vol 2. New York, Churchill Livingstone, 1970.

Hertling D, Kessler R: *Management of Common Musculoskeletal Disorders,* 2nd ed. Philadelphia, J. B. Lippincott Company, 1990.

Kissner C, Colby LA: *Therapeutic Exercise: Foundations and Principles,* 2nd ed. Philadelphia, F. A. Davis Company, 1990.

Mennel J: *Joint Pain: Diagnosis and Treatment Using Manipulative Techniques.* Boston, Little, Brown and Company, 1964.

Wadsworth CT: *Manual Examination and Treatment of the Spine and Extremities.* Baltimore, Williams & Wilkins, 1988.

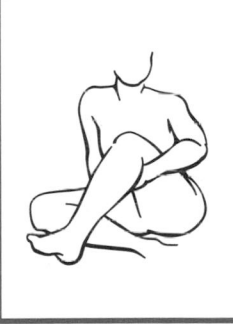

CHAPTER 36

Lower Extremity: Foot

Lisa M. Giallonardo

The foot, with its complex triplanar joints and multijoint muscles, makes initial contact with the ground during gait. It acts as a base of support for the body, as a shock absorber when it lowers into pronation, and as a stiff lever to propel the body forward in push off.

I. Normal Anatomy and Biomechanics

A. General osteology

1. The foot has 26 bones.
   a. The seven tarsal bones are the calcaneus, the talus, the navicular [scaphoid], the cuboid, the medial cuneiform, the intermediate cuneiform, and the lateral cuneiform.
   b. The foot also has five metatarsal bones and 14 phalanges[1] (see Figure 36–1).
2. The foot has three arches[2-4] (see Figure 36–2).
   a. The **medial** arch comprises the calcaneus, the talus, the navicular, the three cuneiforms and the first three metatarsal bones.
   b. The **lateral** arch comprises the calcaneus, the cuboid and fourth and fifth metatarsal bones.
   c. The **transverse** arch stretches across the metatarsal heads.
3. The plantar aponeurosis (plantar fascia), short and long plantar ligaments, and spring ligament (plantar calcaneonavicular) passively bind the bones together; they tighten during weight-bearing activities to prevent failure of the longitudinal arches.

B. Subtalar joint axis and motions (see Figure 36–3)

1. The subtalar joint is the biconvex calcaneus on the biconcave talus; individual differences between people result in two or three talar facets (the posterior, anterior, and, occasionally, middle facets).[5,6]
2. The joint axis is oblique, moving at 45 de-

1055

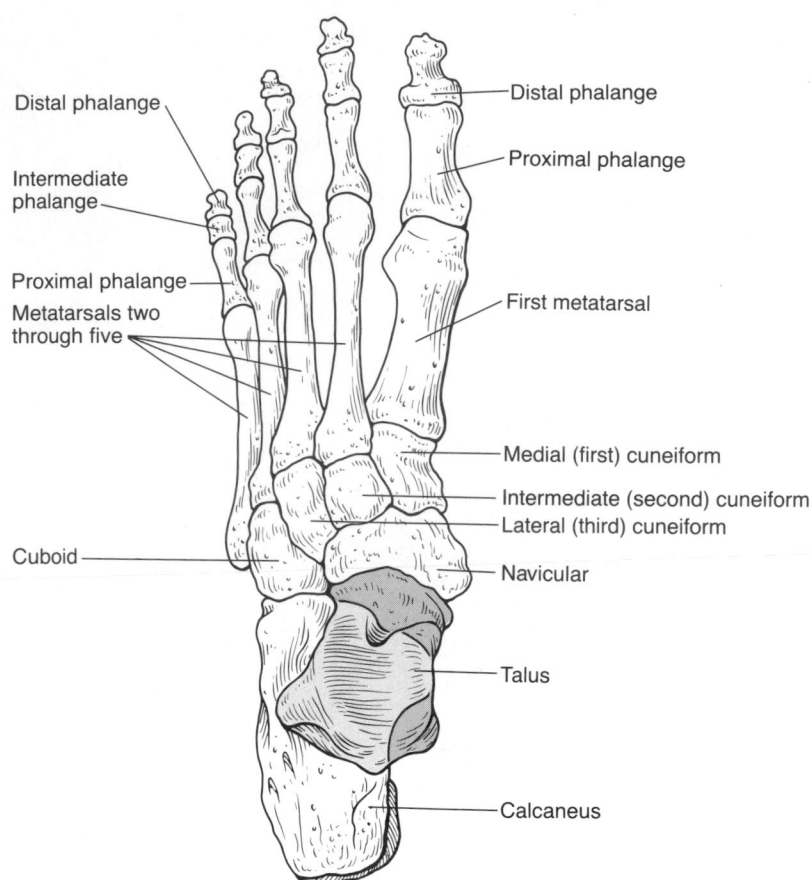

Distal phalange

Intermediate phalange

Proximal phalange

Metatarsals two through five

Cuboid

Distal phalange

Proximal phalange

First metatarsal

Medial (first) cuneiform

Intermediate (second) cuneiform

Lateral (third) cuneiform

Navicular

Talus

Calcaneus

FIGURE 36–1 General osteology of the foot.

grees (coursing downward, posterior, and lateral), resulting in triplanar motion.[5–8]
  a. **Supination** is subtalar adduction and inversion.
  b. **Pronation** is subtalar abduction, eversion, and dorsiflexion.
3. The calcaneus moves posterior, superior, and lateral during pronation, appearing as eversion of the calcaneus during gait.

C. Transverse tarsal (or midtarsal) joint axis and motions (see Figure 36–4).

1. The transverse tarsal axis is made up of two joints (it has an S-shaped appearance when observed from above).[4]
  a. One joint is the biconvex talus on the biconcave navicular bone.
  b. The other is the saddle-shaped calcaneus on a reciprocally shaped cuboid bone.
2. Two functional axes can be noted, with resulting triplanar motion.[6–8]
  a. Eversion/inversion and abduction/adduc-

tion occur to a greater degree around a longitudinal axis similar to the subtalar joint.
  b. Dorsiflexion and plantar flexion occur to a greater degree around an oblique axis similar to the talocrural joint.
  c. Therefore, overall movement is pronation and supination.

D. Tarsometatarsal joints (see Figure 36–5)

1. The articulation is between the first to fifth rays (metatarsal bones) and the medial, intermediate, and lateral cunieform bones (rays one through three) and the cuboid bone (rays four through five).[1,3,4]
2. The articulation is similar to the articulations between the tarsal bones, where gliding and joint separation occurs.[3,4]
3. The second ray has strong contact with all three cuneiform bones for load transmission during gait.[4]

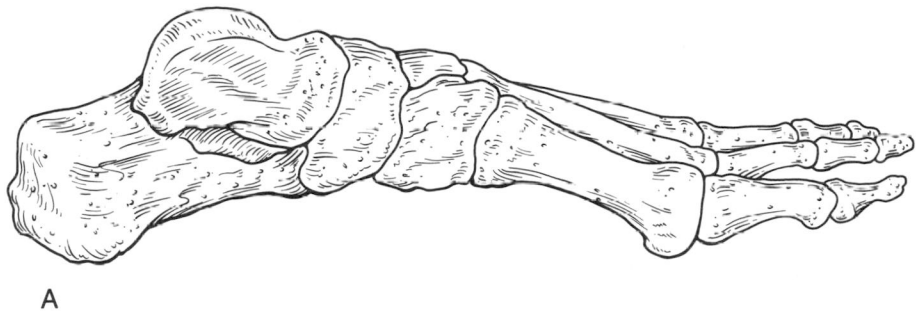

A

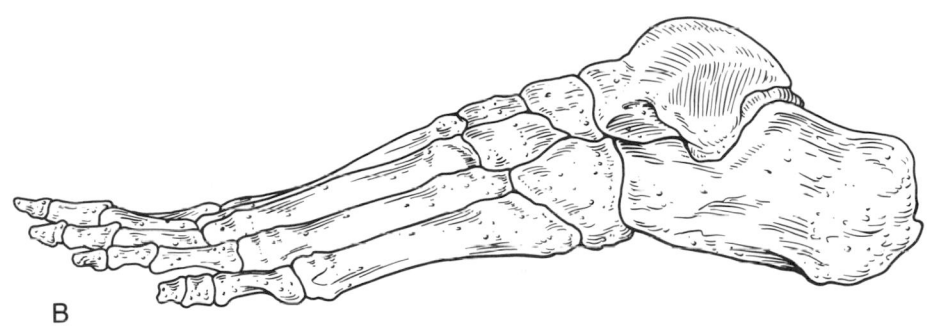

B

FIGURE 36-2 **A**, Medial longitudinal arch (calcaneus, talus, navicular, three cuneiforms, metatarsals one through three). **B**, Lateral longitudinal arch (calcaneus, cuboid, metatarsals four and five).

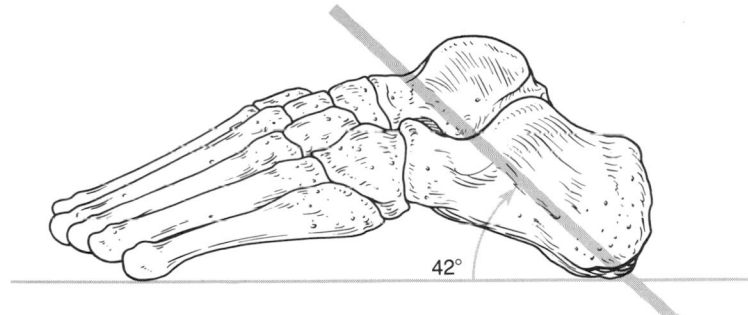

FIGURE 36-3   Subtalar joint (talus on calcaneus), with joint axis approximately 42° from horizontal.

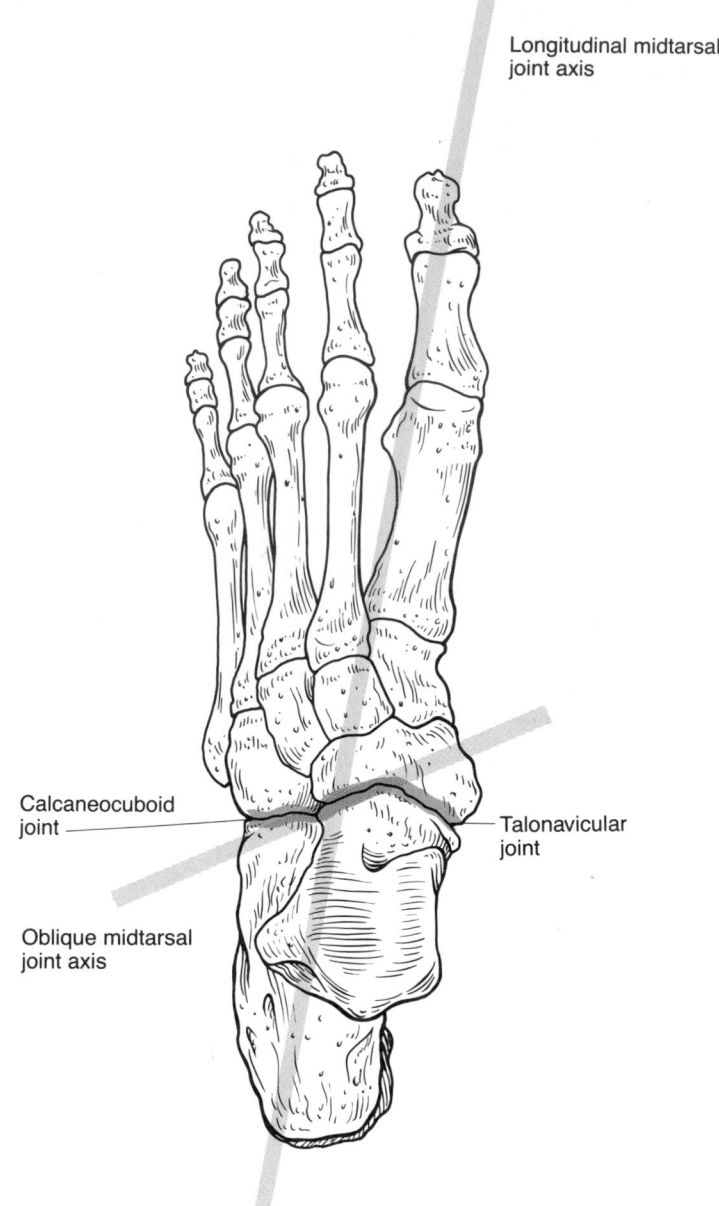

FIGURE 36-4   Midtarsal joints and the two joint axes.

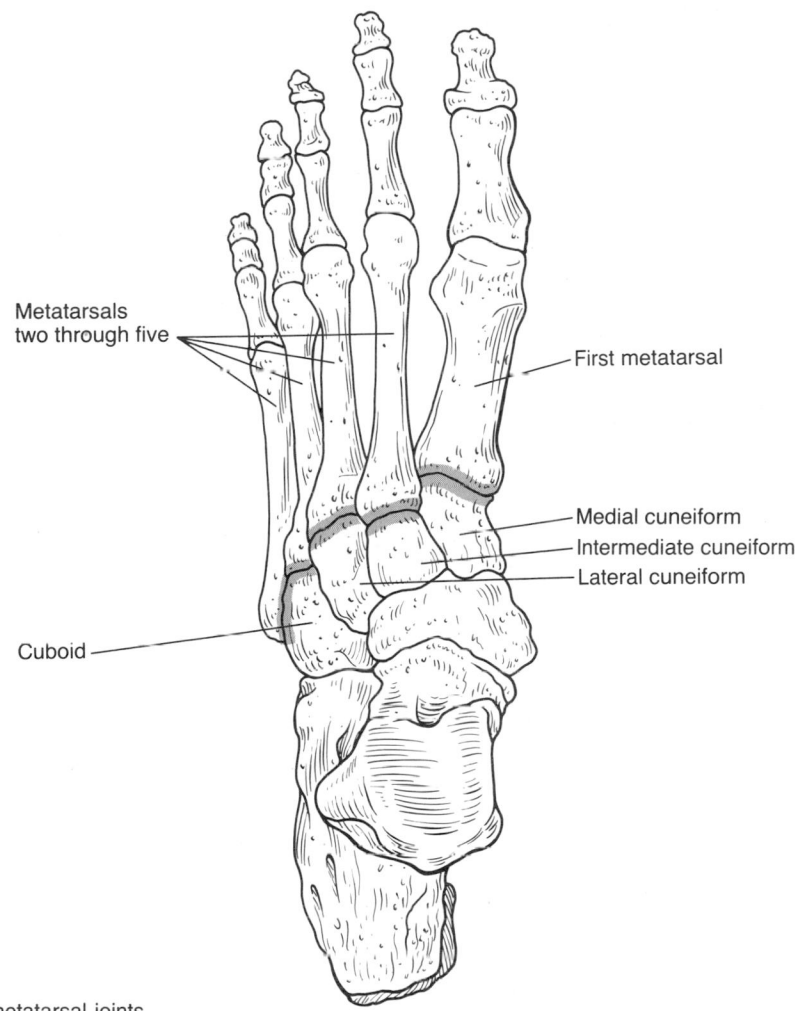

Metatarsals
two through five

First metatarsal

Medial cuneiform
Intermediate cuneiform
Lateral cuneiform

Cuboid

FIGURE 36–5   Tarsometatarsal joints.

E. Metatarsophalangeal joints (see Figure 36–6)

1. These joints are formed by the convex metatarsal bones on the concave proximal phalanges, allowing flexion/extension and abduction/adduction, as well as circumduction.[4]
2. The first metatarsophalangeal joint takes greater stress during gait, requiring full extension for push off.

F. Phalangeal joints (see Figure 36–7)

1. Digits two through five have proximal and distal interphalangeal joints.
2. The first digit has only one interphalangeal joint.
3. The proximal surfaces of the interphalangeal joints are convexoconcave with the distal surfaces reciprocally shaped, allowing the same motions as those allowed by the metatarsophalangeal joints.[3,4]

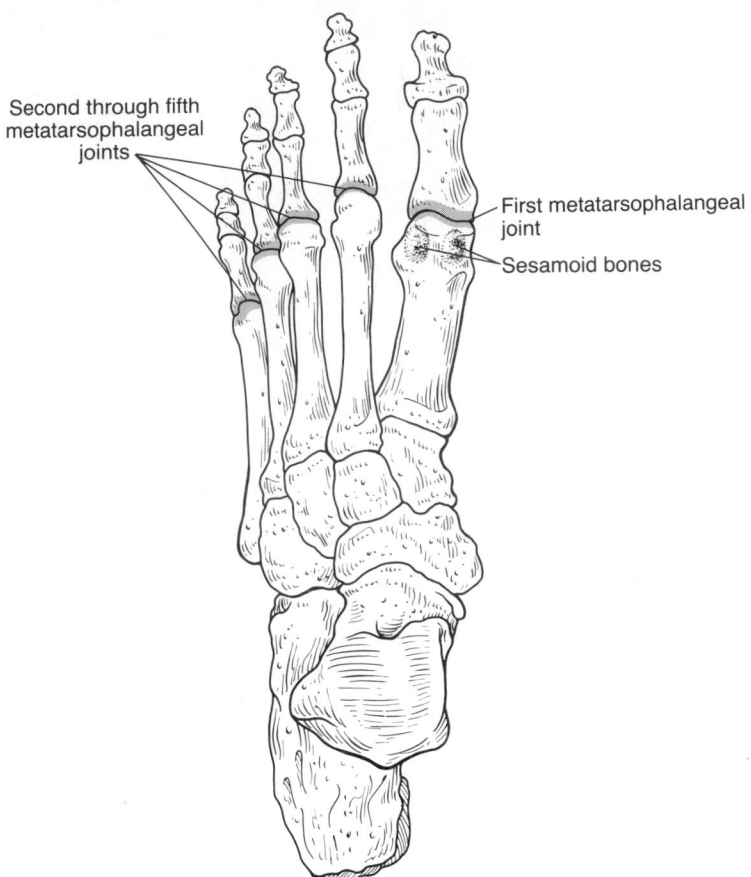

Second through fifth metatarsophalangeal joints

First metatarsophalangeal joint

Sesamoid bones

FIGURE 36–6   Metatarsophalangeal joints.

G. Muscles moving the foot

1. **Invertors**

a. Tibialis posterior[1,4,9,10] (see Figure 35–8)

(1). The tibialis posterior is the primary muscle for inversion of the foot; it secondarily adducts the foot and plantar flexes the ankle.

(2). It joins the posteromedial surface of the tibia, fibula, and interosseous membrane to the navicular tuberosity, cuboid bone, three cuneiform bones, and metatarsal bones two through four.

(3). The tibial nerve L4–L5 innervates this muscle, and the peroneal artery supplies it with blood.

2. **Evertors**

a. Peroneus longus[1,4,9,10] (see Figure 35–11)

(1). The peroneus longus is the primary muscle for eversion of the foot; it secondarily abducts the foot and plantar flexes the ankle.

(2). It joins the superior two thirds of the lateral surface of the fibula to the first cuneiform bone and to the base of the first metatarsal bone.

(3). The superficial peroneal nerve (L5, S1, S2) innervates this muscle, and the anterior tibial and peroneal arteries supply it with blood.

b. Peroneus brevis[1,4,9,10] (see Figure 35–12)

(1). The peroneus brevis is a primary muscle for eversion of the foot; it

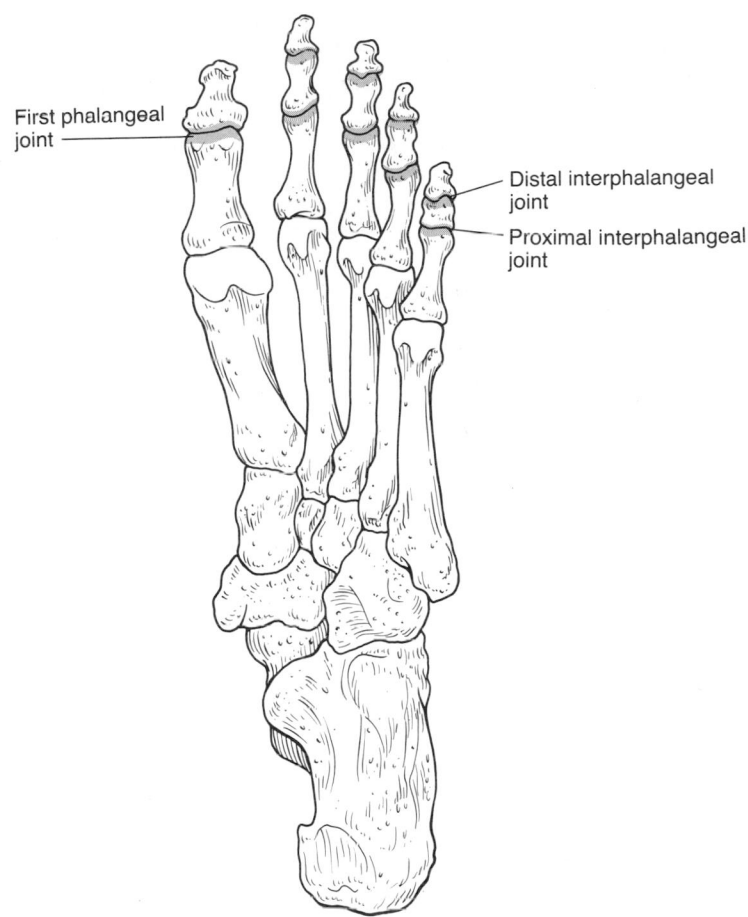

First phalangeal joint

Distal interphalangeal joint

Proximal interphalangeal joint

FIGURE 36-7 Phalangeal joints.

secondarily abducts the foot and plantar flexes the ankle.

(2). It joins the inferior two thirds of the lateral surface of the fibula to the tuberosity of the first metatarsal base.

(3). The superficial peroneal nerve (L5, S1, S2) innervates this muscle, and the peroneal artery supplies it with blood.

3. **Toe flexors**

a. Flexor hallucis longus[1,4,9,10] (see Figure 35–9)

(1). The flexor hallucis longus is the primary muscle for flexion of the interphalangeal joint of the first toe; it secondarily inverts and adducts the foot and plantar flexes the ankle.

(2). It joins the inferior two thirds of the posterior surface of the fibula to the plantar surface of the base of the first distal phalanx.

(3). The tibial nerve (S2, S3) innervates this muscle, and the peroneal artery supplies it with blood.

b. Flexor digitorum longus[1,4,9,10] (see Figure 35–10)

(1). The flexor digitorum longus is the primary muscle for flexion of the interphalangeal joints of toes two through five; it secondarily inverts and adducts foot and plantar flexes the ankle.

(2). It joins the medial posterior surface of the tibia to a tendon on phalanges two through five and the plantar surface to the base of the distal phalanx.

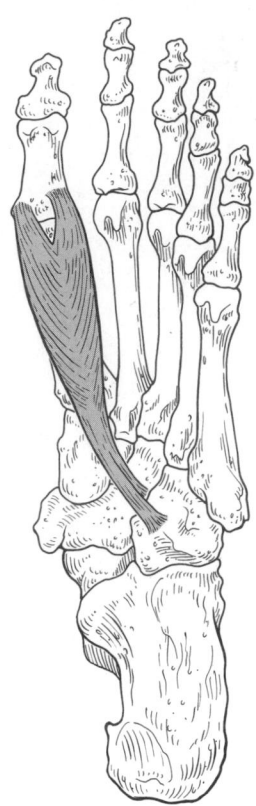

FIGURE 36–8   Flexor hallucis brevis.

(3). The tibial nerve (S2, S3) innervates this muscle, and the posterior tibial artery supplies it with blood.

c. Flexor hallucis brevis[1,4,9,10] (see Figure 36–8)

(1). The flexor hallucis brevis is the primary muscle for flexion of the metatarsophalangeal joint of the first toe.

(2). It joins the medial plantar cuboid bone, lateral cuneiform bone, and tibialis posterior tendon to the medial and lateral part of the first proximal phalanx base.

(3). The first plantar digital nerve (S2, S3) innervates this muscle, and the plantar metatarsal artery supplies it with blood.

d. Lumbricales[1,4,9,10] (see Figure 36–9)

(1). The lumbricales are primary muscles in flexion of the metatarsophalangeal joints of toes two through five.

(2). They join the two adjacent tendons

of the flexor digitorum longus to the base of the distal phalanx with the extensor digitorum longus.

(3). The medial and deep lateral plantar nerves (S2, S3) innervate these muscles, and the plantar metatarsal artery supplies them with blood.

e. Flexor digitorum brevis[1,4,9,10] (see Figure 36–10)

(1). The flexor digitorum brevis is the primary muscle in flexion of the metatarsophalangeal joints of toes two through five.

(2). It joins the medial tuberosity of the calcaneus and the plantar fascia to the middle phalanges of toes two through five.

(3). The medial plantar nerve (S2, S3) innervates this muscle, and the medial plantar artery supplies it with blood.

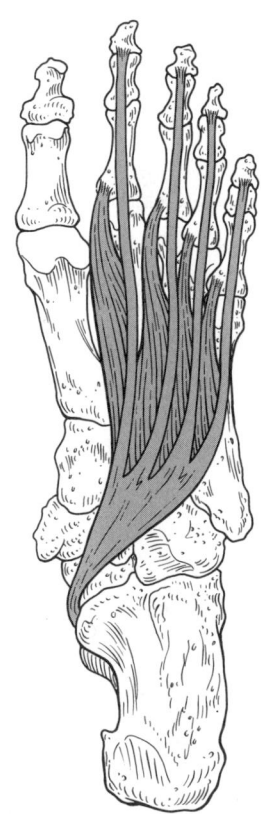

FIGURE 36–9   Lumbricales.

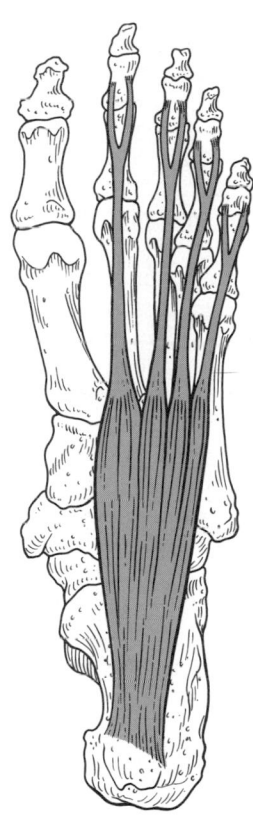

FIGURE 36–10   Flexor digitorum brevis.

4. **Toe extensors**
   a. Extensor hallucis longus[1,4,9,10] (see Figure 35–3)
      (1). The extensor hallucis longus is the primary muscle for extension of the metatarsophalangeal joint of the first toe.
      (2). It joins the middle third of the medial surface of the fibula to the base of the first toe distal phalanx.
      (3). The deep peroneal nerve (L-5, S-1) innervates this muscle, and the anterior tibial artery supplies it with blood.
   b. Extensor digitorum longus[1,4,9,10] (see Figure 35–4)
      (1). The extensor digitorum longus is the primary muscle in extension of the metatarsophalangeal joints of toes two through five.

(2). It joins the superior two thirds of the medial surface of the fibula to a tendon on digits two through four for the middle and distal phalanx.
(3). The deep peroneal nerve (L-5, S-1) innervates this muscle, and the deep peroneal branch of the anterior tibial artery supplies it with blood.
   c. Lumbricales[1,4,9,10] (see Figure 36–9)
      (1). The lumbricals are primary muscles in extension of the interphalangeal joints for toes two through five.
      (2). See the previous description of the lumbrical muscles for origins and insertions and for nerve and blood supply.
   d. Interossei[1,4,9,10] (see Figure 36–11)
      (1). The interossei muscles are primary muscles in extension of the in-

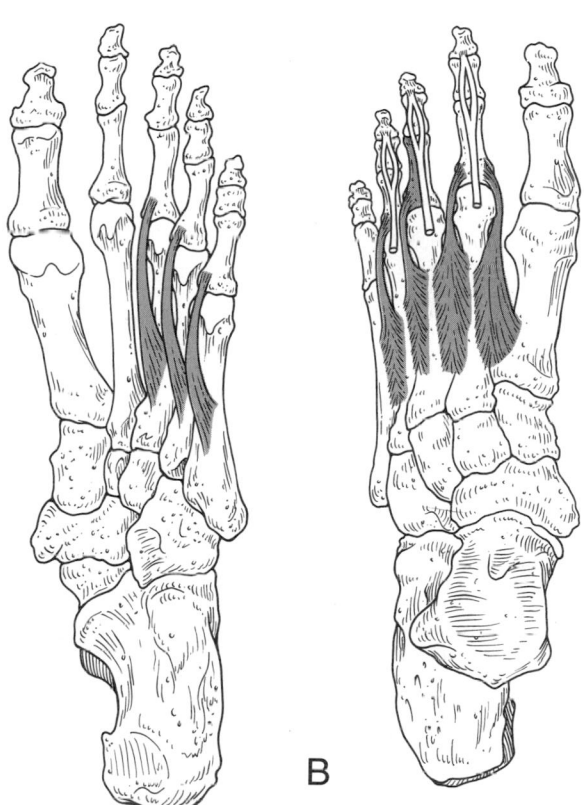

FIGURE 36–11   **A,** Plantar interossei. **B,** Dorsal interossei.

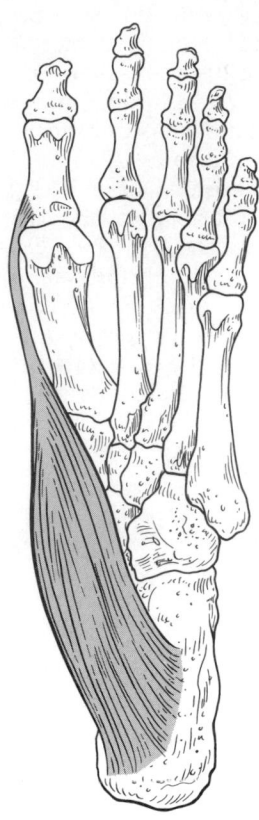

FIGURE 36–12   Abductor hallucis.

terphalangeal joints of toes two through five.

(2). The dorsal interossei join the two heads from the adjacent sides of the metatarsal bone to the medial and lateral sides of metatarsal bones two through four.

(3). The plantar interossei join the base and medial side of metatarsal bones three through five to the medial base of proximal phalanges three through five.

(4). The superficial and deep lateral plantar nerves (S-2, S-3), respectively, innervate these muscles, and the dorsal and plantar metatarsal arteries, respectively, supply them with blood.

5. **Toe abductors**
   a. Dorsal interossei[1,4,9,10] (see Figure 36–11 B)
      (1). The dorsal interossei muscles are the

primary muscles in abduction of the metatarsophalangeal joints for toes two through five.

(2). See the previous discussion of the interossei muscles for origins and insertions, and the nerve and blood supply.

b. Abductor hallucis[1,4,9,10] (see Figure 36–12)
   (1). The abductor hallucis is the primary muscle in abduction of the metatarsophalangeal joints of the first toe.
   (2). It joins the medial calcaneal tuberosity and plantar fascia to the medial base of the proximal phalanx of the first toe.
   (3). The medial plantar nerve (S-2, S-3) innervates this muscle, and the medial plantar artery supplies it with blood.

c. Abductor digiti minimi[1,4,9,10] (see Figure 36–13)
   (1). The abductor digiti minimi is the

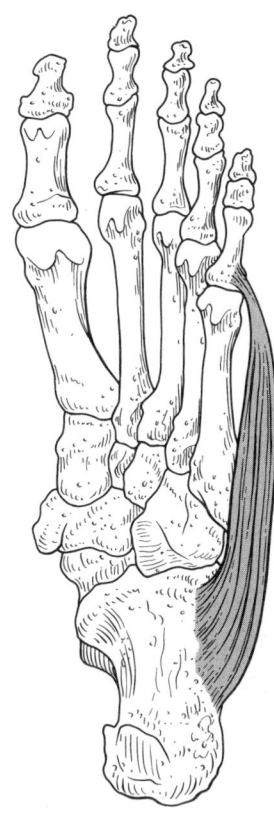

FIGURE 36–13   Abductor digiti minimi.

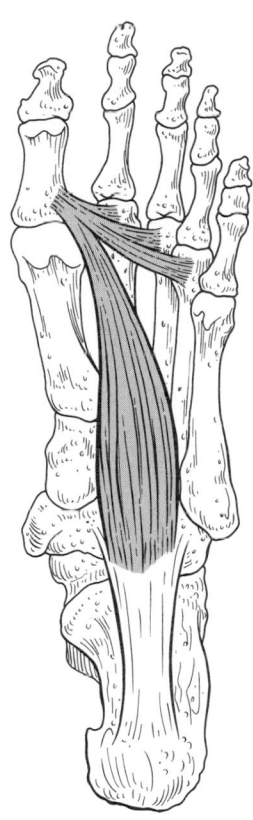

FIGURE 36-14   Adductor hallucis.

primary muscle in abduction of the metatarsophalangeal muscles of the fifth toe.

(2). It joins the medial and lateral calcaneal tuberosity to the lateral base of the fifth proximal phalanx.

(3). The lateral plantar nerve (S2, S3) innervates this muscle, and the lateral plantar artery supplies it with blood.

6. **Toe Adductors**

a. Plantares interossei[1,4,9,10] (see Figure 36-11)

(1). The plantares interossei are primary muscles in adduction of the metatarsophalangeal joints of toes two through five.

(2). See the previous discussion of the interossei muscles for origins and insertions and the nerve and blood supply.

b. Adductor hallucis[1,4,9,10] (see Figure 36-14)

(1). The adductor hallucis is the primary muscle in adduction of the metatarsophalangeal joints of the first toe.

(2). It joins the base of metatarsal bones two through four and the metatarsal ligaments to the lateral base of the first proximal phalanx.

(3). The lateral plantar nerve (S2, S3) innervates this muscle, and the first plantar metatarsal artery supplies it with blood.

H. Ligaments and fasciae of the foot

1. **Fascial structure**

a. Plantar aponeurosis (fascia)[1,2,4,10] (see Figure 36-15)

(1). The plantar aponeurosis has three portions: the central, the lateral, and the medial.

(2). It originates at the sustentaculum tali (medial tuberosity of calcaneus), splays over the sole, and inserts into the ligaments near the metatarsal heads.

(3). It supports the medial longitudinal arch and covers all soft-tissue structures.

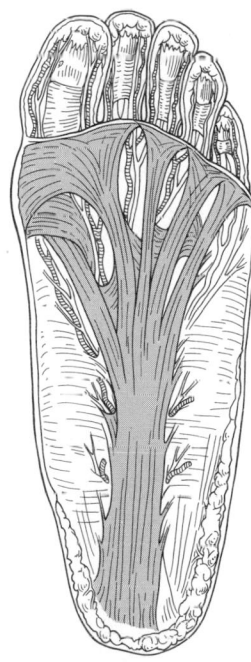

FIGURE 36-15   Plantar aponeurosis.

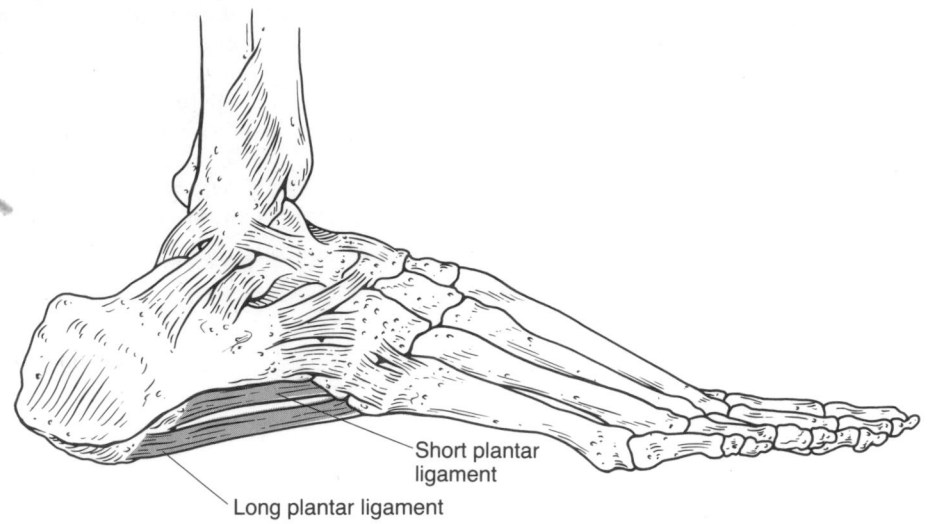

Short plantar
ligament

Long plantar ligament

FIGURE 36–16 Long and short plantar ligaments.

2. **Plantar ligaments**
   a. Long and short plantar ligaments[1,4,10] (see Figure 36–16)
      (1). The long plantar ligament joins the calcaneus (anterior to tuberosity) to the bases of digits three through five.
      (2). The short plantar ligament is a short, wide, strong band; it lies close to the bone and joins the distal surface of the calcaneus to the cuboid bone.

   (3). It supports the lateral arch.
   b. Plantar calcaneonavicular (or spring) ligament[1,4,10] (see Figure 36–17)
      (1). The plantar calcaneonavicular ligament connects the calcaneus at the sustentaculum tali to the navicular bone, thus supporting the head of the talus and maintaining the medial arch.
      (2). It has a high content of elastic fibers and gives "spring" to the arch during weight bearing.

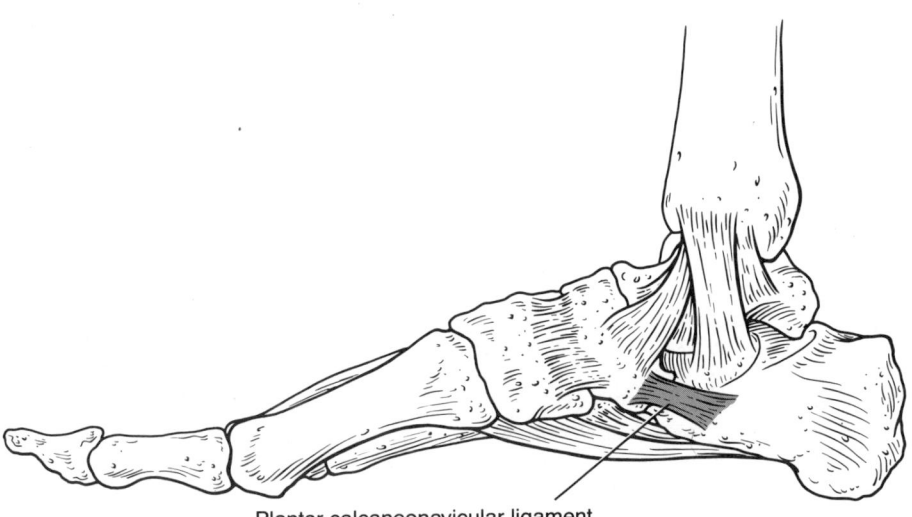

Plantar calcaneonavicular ligament

FIGURE 36–17 Plantar calcaneonavicular or spring ligament.

I. Functional significance of the foot

1. **Three basic requirements for smooth and efficient gait are as follows:**[11,12]
   a. The lower extremity must absorb ground reaction force.
      (1). This is accomplished through flexion of the hip, knee, and ankle at heel strike.
      (2). It is further assisted by pronation of the foot when it moves into the flat foot stage of gait.
   b. The joints of the lower extremity should be in a state of balance at midstance.
      (1). The distal third of the lower leg should be perpendicular to the floor.
      (2). The calcaneus should be perpendicular to the floor.
      (3). All five metatarsal heads should be in equal contact with the floor.
   c. The foot must be able to function as
      (1). A base of support (accomplished through foot flat to midstance).
      (2). A mobile adapter (accomplished through pronation during foot flat).
      (3). A rigid push-off lever (accomplished through supination at push off).

II. Examination

A. Subjective

1. Ask the patient about his/her perception of any problems to help narrow the focus of the examination.
   a. Determine whether the patient can relate the problem to an activity or a change in activity (leading the therapist to focus on contractile tissue rather than on noncontractile tissue).
   b. Determine whether the patient relates the problem as chronic (leading the therapist to specifically reproduce the symptoms because of uncertainty regarding the cause of the problem.)
2. Discuss the patient's goals; they should be incorporated into the therapist's statement of goals, and also into the treatment-planning process.
   a. Determine whether the patient has a need or desire to perform a particular activity that requires a certain amount of weight bearing, range of motion (ROM), or strength.

B. Objective

1. **History**
   a. Elicit information concerning any trauma, including the complete mechanism of injury.
   b. Discuss changes in activity level, footwear, and body weight, which could account for idiopathic foot pain.
   c. Discuss symptom presentation (see Table 35–1).
2. **Inspection and palpation**
   a. **Posture** evaluation should begin as the patient walks into the examining room.
      (1). Note varus or valgus deformities of the hip, knee, and tibia, as well as spinal curvatures.
      (2). Sagittal plane observation is done to learn whether hyperflexion or extension of the spine, hip, knee, or ankle is present.
      (3). Rotational components in the transverse plane include the pelvis, femur, tibia, and foot pronation or supination.
      (4). Note foot deformities such as pes planus (flatfoot), pes cavus (high-arched foot), claw toes, hammer toes, hallux valgus, talipes equinovarus (supinated foot), or talipes equinus (plantar flexed foot). (For more information, see ''Posture,'' Chapter 37.)
   b. Examine the **skin** of foot (and lower leg) for extensibility, swelling, trophic changes, and temperature.
      (1). Note the condition of nail bed and whether calluses, blisters, plantar warts, or ulcerations are present.
      (2). The pulses at the top of the foot (between the extensor hallucis longus and extensor digitorum longus on the dorsum) and poste-

rior tibialis (posterior to the medial malleolus and anterior to the Achilles tendon)[3,4] **pulses** are assessed and graded as present, absent, or weakened, compared with the pulses on the other side.

c. **Footwear** is evaluated for wear patterns and for proper style and fit for a patient.

    (1). Note the heel counter, toe box, arch support, sole, heel, and material of the shoe.

        (a). Determine whether the shoe supports and controls movement.

        (b). Determine whether shoe material accommodates or irritates the skin.

    (2). The use of an **orthotic** device should be noted, with a description of the purpose, characteristics, and effectiveness of the device.

        (a). Issues on which to focus when assessing orthoses include[13]

            (i). Purpose of the orthosis, *eg,* stabilization, total contact, softness, shock absorption, balance, and whether it fulfills its purpose.

            (ii). Whether the patient's symptoms are alleviated when the orthosis is worn at the appropriate time.

            (iii). Whether the orthosis fits

the patient properly (it should be sufficiently wide and long, and the heel cup should be sufficiently deep), especially in a weight-bearing position.

            (iv). Whether it is worn down and not functioning properly.

            (v). Whether footwear used with the orthosis is appropriate, *eg,* it should not be excessively worn, should have a low heel and sufficient eyelets to hold the foot snugly, should have a rigid or soft midfoot and heel counter, depending on the patient's foot type, and should be deep enough to accommodate the foot and the orthosis without pistoning.

            (vi). Whether posting (or wedging) exists on the orthosis.

            (vii). Whether the medial heel wedge is too high (the patient is unbalanced laterally).

            (viii). Whether the medial heel wedge is incapable of

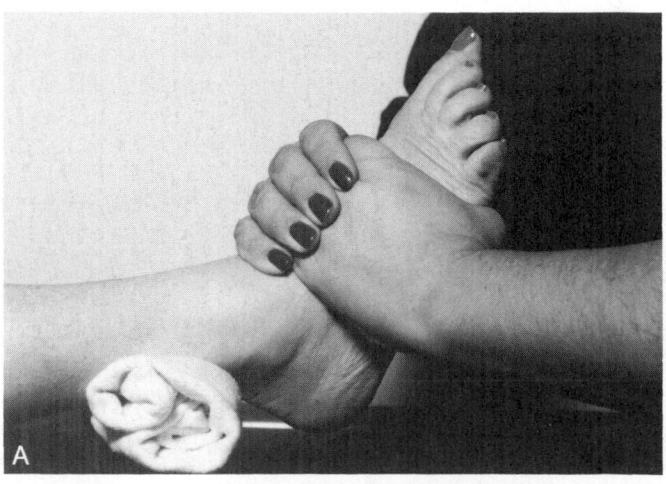 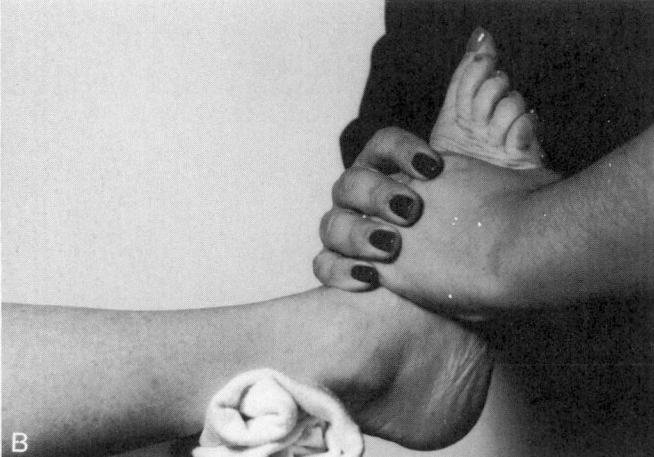

FIGURE 36–18   **A,** Talar distraction. **B,** Talar rocking.

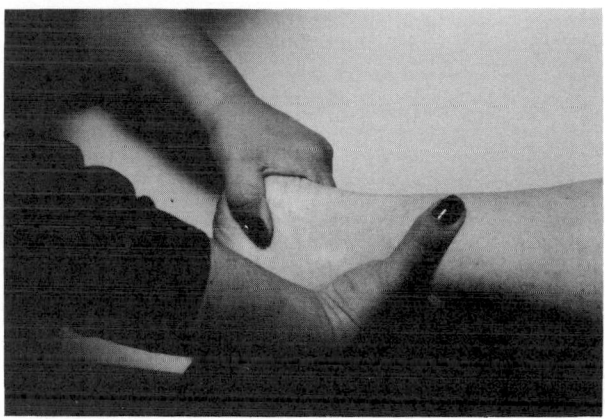

FIGURE 36–19 Calcaneal distraction and rocking.

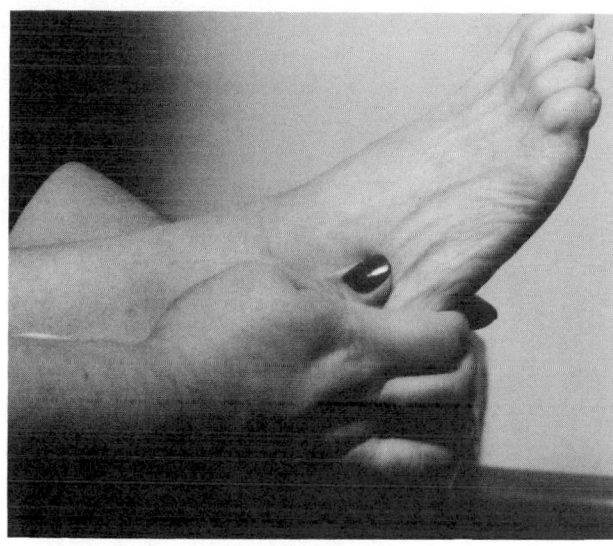

FIGURE 36–21 Calcaneocuboid glide.

controlling excessive pronation.

(ix). Whether the forefoot post is uncomfortable, *eg*, it is too far proximal or distal or not sufficiently beveled.

(x). Whether the heel lift is of the appropriate height (for balancing pelvic landmarks).

(xi). Whether the rocker bottom is positioned just proximal to the metatarsal heads.

3. **Measurement**
   a. Assess **joint play**[14–16]
      (1). At the subtalar joint: talar distraction and rocking (see Figure 36–18) and calcaneal distraction and rocking (see Figure 36–19).
      (2). At the transverse tarsal joints: talonavicular glide (see Figure 36–20) and calcaneocuboid glide (see Figure 36–21).
      (3). At the intertarsal joints: do the navicular, three cuneiform (see Figure 36–22), and cuboid bones (see Figure 36–21) glide on each other?
      (4). At the tarsometatarsal joints: glides

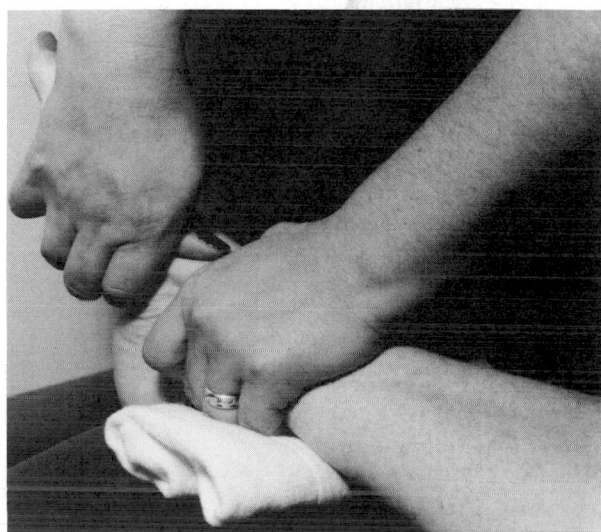

FIGURE 36–20 Talonavicular glide.

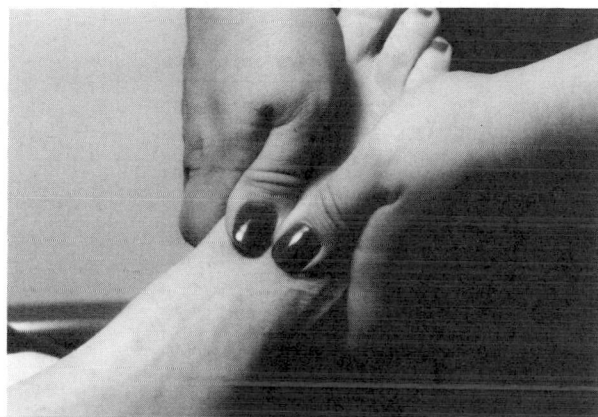

FIGURE 36–22 Cuneiform glide.

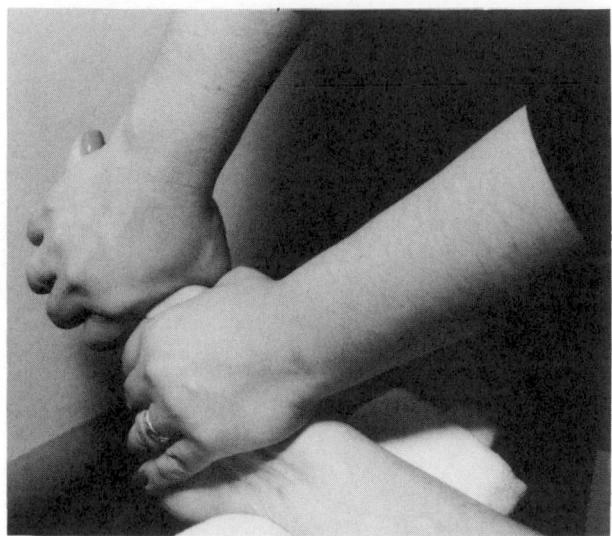

FIGURE 36–23   Tarsometatarsal glide.

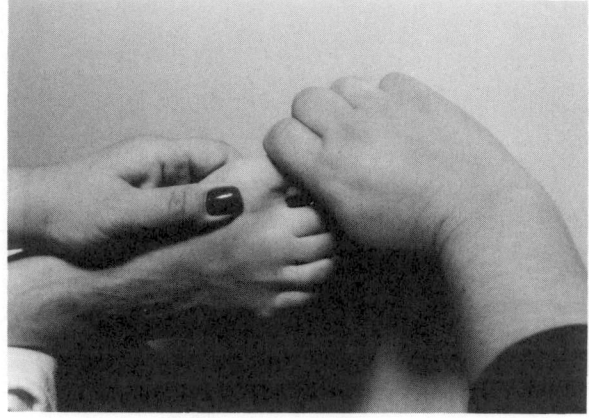

FIGURE 36–25   First metatarsophalangeal glide.

of each metatarsal bone on the cuboid and three cuneiform bones (see Figure 36–23).

(5). At the metatarsophalangeal joints: glides between each metatarsal bone (see Figure 36–24), and distraction and dorsal and ventral glides between the metatarsal and phalangeal bones (see Figure 36–25).

(6). At the phalangeal joints: distraction, dorsal and ventral glides, and tilts between the proximal and distal interphalangeal joints (see Figure 36–26).

PLEASE NOTE: Motions are graded from 0 to 6, with 0 indicating ankylosis, 3 indicating normal motion, and 6 indicating dislocation.[14,16]

b. Measure the ROM of the foot and of those joints that directly affect the foot.
   (1). **Tibial torsion** is the relationship of the transverse axis of the knee to the frontal plane axis of the ankle[12,13,17] (see Figure 36–27).
      (a). Measurement is done with the

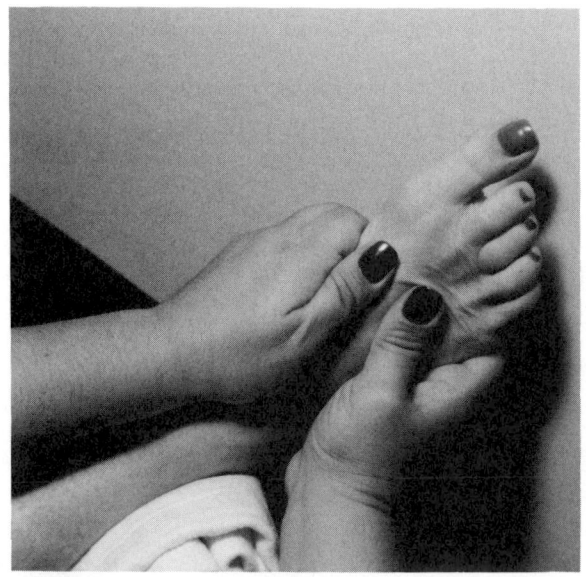

FIGURE 36–24   Metatarsal glide.

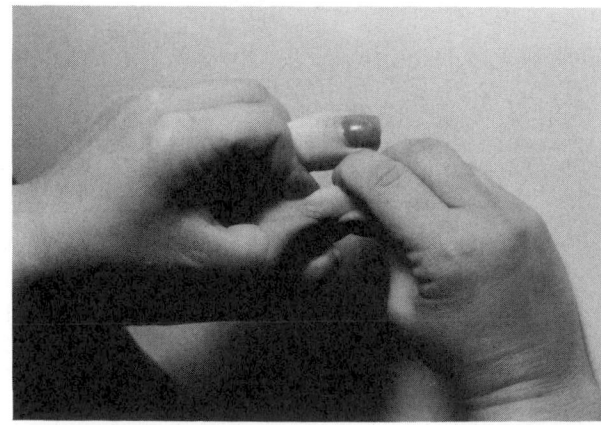

FIGURE 36–26   Interphalangeal glide.

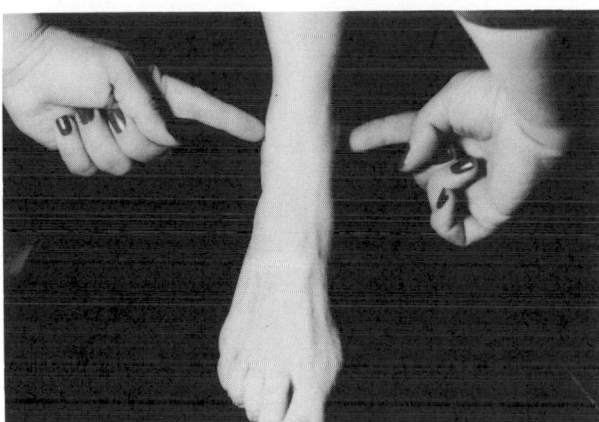

FIGURE 36–27   Evaluating tibial torsion.

patient sitting over the edge of a table.

(b). The patella is in the frontal plane; angulation of the malleoli is used as a landmark.

(c). Palpate the apex of the medial malleolus and the anterior border of the lateral malleolus.

(d). Internal or external torsion is noted by the direction of a line between the palpating fingers.

(e). The normal range is approximately 15 degrees of external tibial torsion.[11]

(2). **Tibial varum** is detected by measuring the frontal plane angle of the tibia in relation to the floor when the patient is standing[12,13,17] (see Figure 36–28).

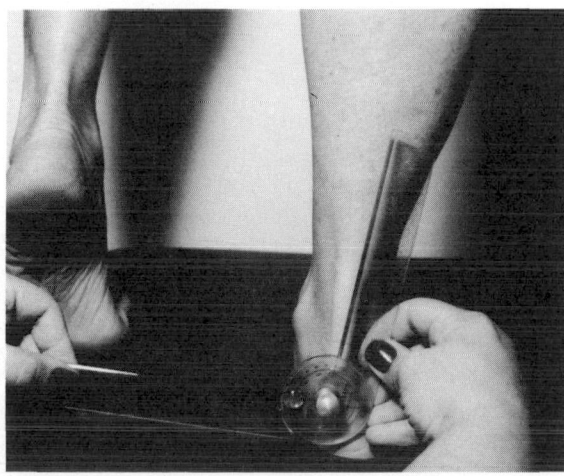

FIGURE 36–28   Measuring tibial varum.

(a). The degree of tibial varum is measured with the midline of the distal one third of the tibia and the floor as points of reference.

(b). When the patient is standing in the normal base position of gait, have him/her stand on one foot (on the side being measured), with the opposite side establishing balance with toe contact.

(c). The stance foot is placed in a neutral position by equal palpation of the talar heads while the patient rotates his/her trunk.

(3). **Neutral calcaneal stance** is the amount of movement needed from the subtalar joint during midstance.[12,13,17]

(a). The foot is placed in a neutral position (see the procedure for measuring tibial varum).

(b). A protractor is used to measure the angle between vertical (perpendicular to the support surface) and the angle of the calcaneal midline during stance.

(c). A straight edge is placed along the support surface with the center aligned with the calcaneal midline; the angle is the deviation of the midline from the center.

(4). **Calcaneal eversion and inversion.** The calcaneus is used as an extension of the subtalar joint for evaluating one component of pronation and supination.[12,13,17]

(a). A goniometer's stationary arm is placed on the midpoint of the distal third of the tibia and moved along the midpoint of the calcaneus.

(b). Full eversion is determined by passively moving the calcaneus laterally (see Figure 36–29).

(c). Calcaneal inversion is measured in the same position by passively moving the calcaneus medially (see Figure 36–30).

(5). **Great toe extension** is measured by noting the extension of the metatar-

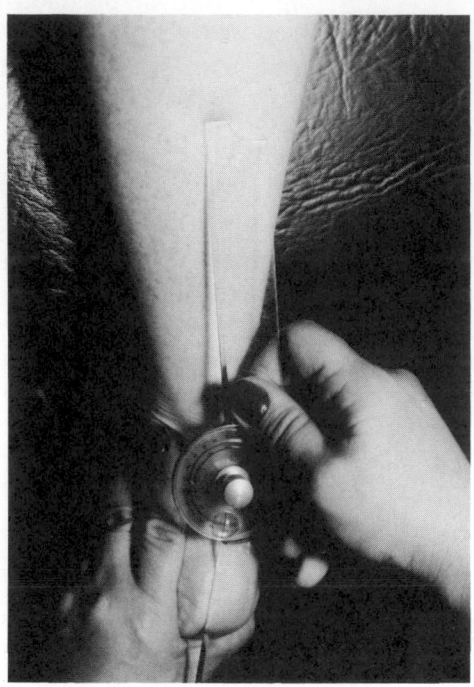

FIGURE 36–29   Measuring calcaneal eversion.

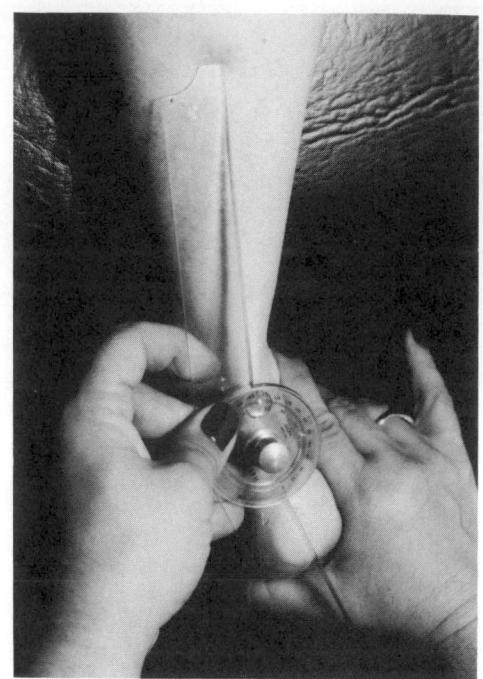

FIGURE 36–30   Measuring calcaneal inversion.

sophalangeal joint[12,13,17] (see Figure 36–31).

(a). It can be measured in both non–weight-bearing and weight-bearing positions.

(b). Align a goniometer's moveable arm with the lateral border of the first phalanx and the stationary arm with the first metatarsal bone.

c. **Muscle strength** screening should be done with the patient in more functional weight-bearing positions as well as in **manual muscle test positions**[18,19] (for testing the tibialis anterior and posterior, the peroneus longus and brevis, and the toe flexor muscles).

(1). Some examples of screening techniques are as follow:[13]

(a). Have the patient rise on his/her toes several times rapidly in succession.

(b). Instruct him/her to walk on the heels.

(c). Have him/her slowly lower the body from a toe-rise position several times in succession.

(d). Advise the patient to rise slowly

on his/her toes in an inverted position (see Figure 36–32).

(e). Have him/her resist dorsiflexion and plantar flexion of the tibia on the foot.

(f). Instruct the patient to gather a towel together with his/her toes and to perform towel scrunches (see Figure 36–33).

(g). Have him/her pick up objects

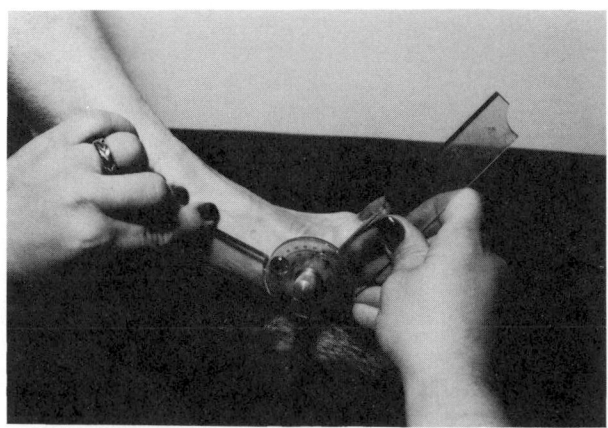

FIGURE 36–31   Measuring great toe extension.

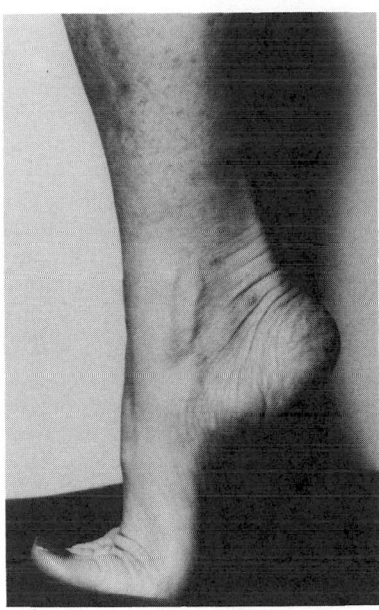

FIGURE 36–32   Rising on toes in with foot inverted.

of different sizes with his/her toes.

(2). Test the muscles' reactions to different types of contractions.[13]

(a). Have the patient hold an isometric contraction at various points in the range.

(b). Have him/her perform different patterns of facilitation in weight bearing (*eg*, rhythmic

stabilization or alternating isometric exercises); note the reaction and compare it with that on the other side (see Figure 36–34).

(c). In bridging, note the ability of the foot and ankle to stabilize with and without proximal resistance.

(d). Instruct the patient in the performance of isokinetic techniques for the invertor and evertor muscles.

(3). Stabilize the lower extremity to prevent substitution and overflow from the proximal musculature.

(4). Always compare values with those of the other lower extremity.

d. Other tests

(1). **Sensation** testing is important for all patients, especially those with neurologic or circulatory disorders. Two-point discrimination and temperature and light-touch testing should be performed.

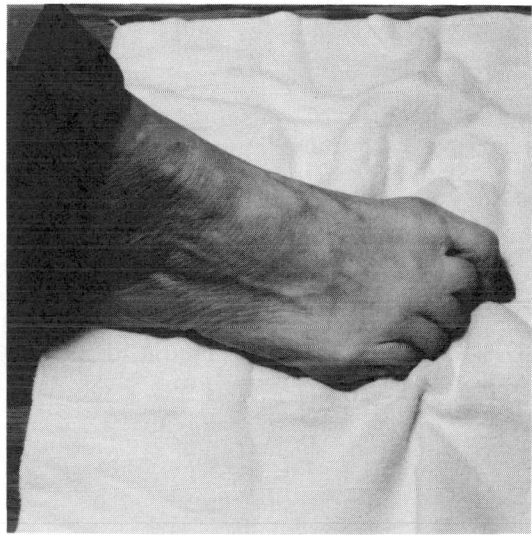

FIGURE 36–33   Towel scrunches.

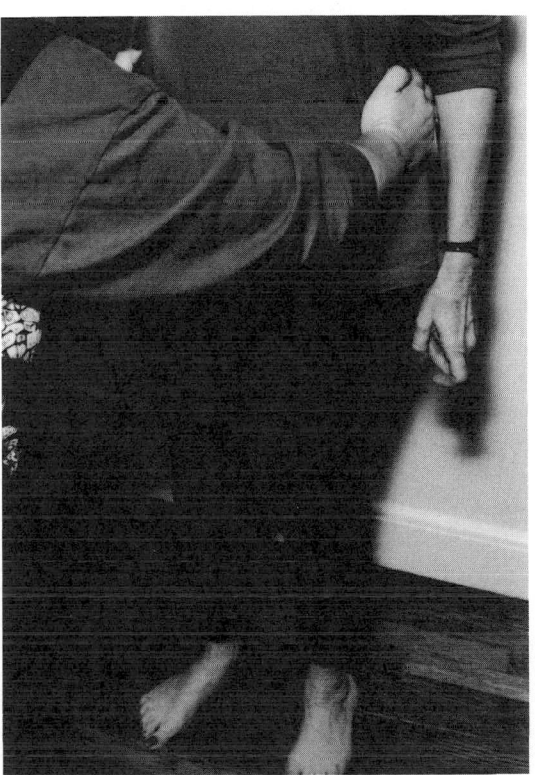

FIGURE 36–34   Rhythmic stabilization with manual contacts at the pelvis.

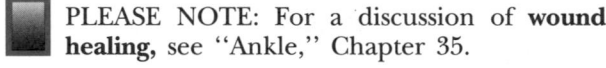

PLEASE NOTE: A commonly used tool to measure light touch is the nylon monofilament. Monofilaments are graded as follows: if a patient feels pressure induced by a #5.07 monofilament, protective sensation is present. A patient sensing pressure from a monofilament of #6.10 or greater indicates a loss of protective sensation.[20]

(2). **Proprioception** (position sense) can be tested by assessing the patient's response to movement or spatial relations.[21]

(a). Movement is evaluated by having the patient close his/her eyes and moving a toe up or down; the patient then describes the direction of toe movement.

(b). Spatial relationship is also evaluated with the patient's eyes closed; the therapist moves one of the patient's lower limbs into a certain position. The patient is then asked to imitate that position with the other limb.

PLEASE NOTE: For a discussion of **wound healing,** see "Ankle," Chapter 35.

e. Alignment
(1). Forefoot and rearfoot positions[11–13,17]

(a). Forefoot and rearfoot measurements are taken with the subtalar joint placed in a neutral position (see Figure 36–35).

(b). The neutral position is determined by equal palpation of the lateral and medial margins of the talar head (the lateral margin is felt anterior to the lateral malleolus toward the midline; the medial margin is slightly inferior and anterior to the medial malleolus).

(c). The talus is prominent medially during pronation (because it is adducting and plantar flexing); the opposite is true during supination.

(d). The patient should be in the prone position with the foot being examined hanging over the table edge; the opposite limb should be flexed, abducted, and externally rotated at the hip and flexed at the knee.

(e). Palpation of the talus is done with the thumb on the medial margin and the index finger on the lateral margin; the opposite hand grasps the forefoot to maintain a neutral position.

(f). The forefoot and rearfoot are evaluated with the metatarsal heads and the midline of the calcaneus acting as landmarks; in a neutral subtalar joint position, the *forefoot* (five metatarsals) should be perpendicular to the midline of the calcaneus (see Figure 36–36).

(g). An *inverted* position is considered a *varus* deformity; an *everted* position is a *valgus* deformity (see Figure 36–36).

(h). The *rearfoot* (midline of the calcaneus) should be a continuation of the distal third of the tibia (see Figure 36–37).

(i). The rearfoot is in a *varus* position when the midline of the calcaneus is angled *medially;* when the calcaneus is angled *laterally,* it is considered to be in a *valgus* position (see Figure 36–37).

(j). A relative position should be noted, or a goniometric measure can be taken with same alignment as that used for calcaneal inversion or eversion.

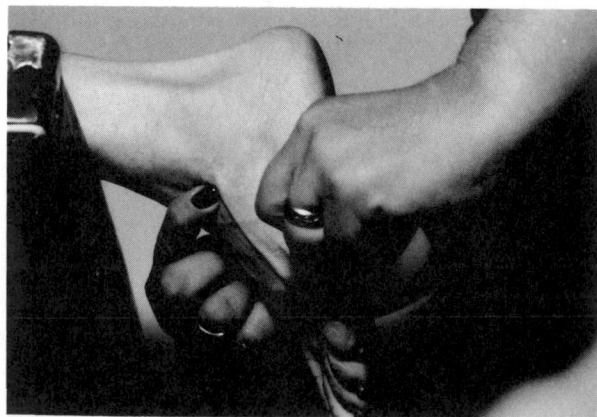

FIGURE 36–35 Assessing subtalar neutral position.

NEUTRAL   VALGUS   VARUS

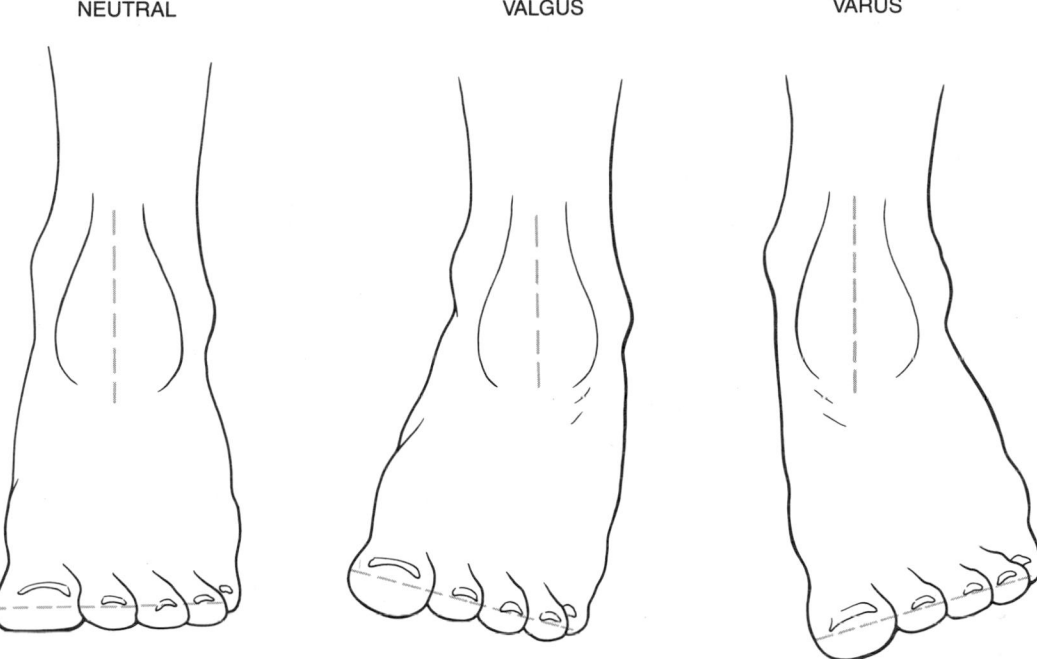

FIGURE 36–36   Left forefoot postures.

(2). Feiss' line[13,22] (see Figure 36–38)
   (a). Test to assess a flexible versus a true flatfoot (pes planus).
   (b). The navicular should be in line with the medial malleolus and the first metatarsal head.

   (c). If the navicular is depressed in *both* non–weight-bearing and weight-bearing positions, the patient has a *true pes planus*.
   (d). If the navicular is depressed *only* in weight bearing, a *flexible*

NEUTRAL   VALGUS   VARUS

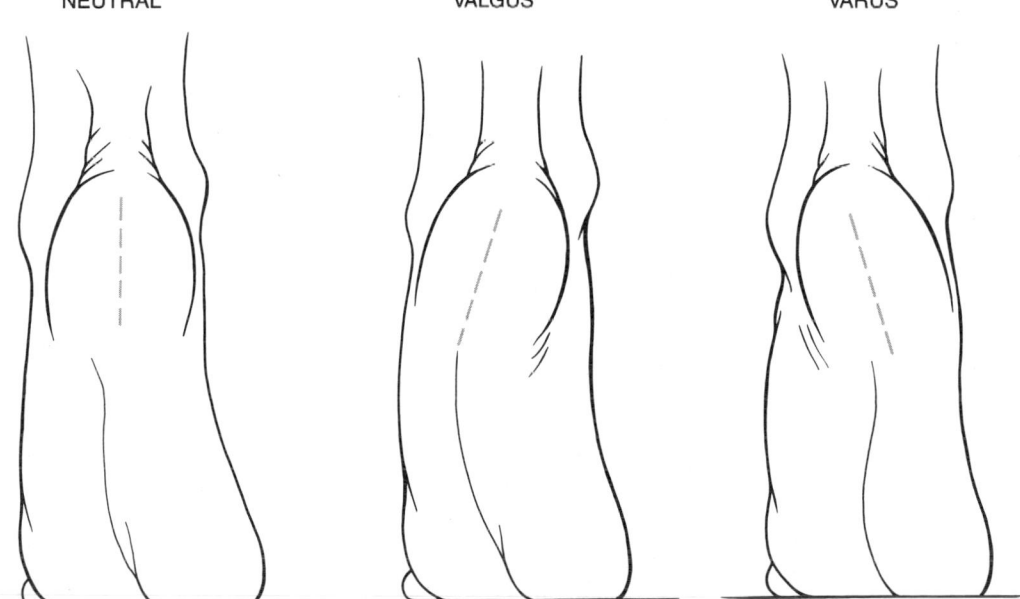

FIGURE 36–37   Left rearfoot postures.

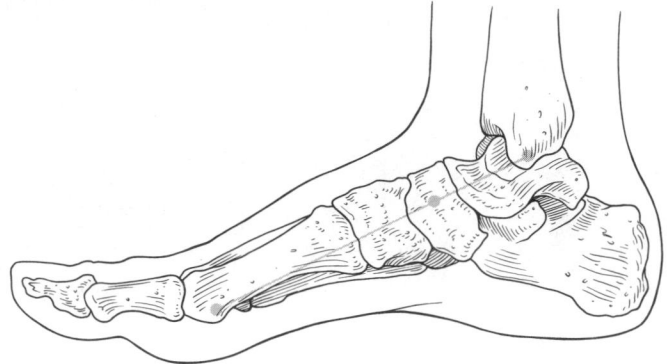

FIGURE 36–38   Feiss's line.

flatfoot exists (and possible causes should be investigated).

(3). Assessment of plantar pressure[11,13,17,20]

(a). A method to assess weight-bearing forces involves the use of pressure-sensitive devices and materials, *eg*, a podoscope, Harris footprint mat (Smith's Industries Medical Systems, Ontario, Canada), and slipper-socks (Slipper Sock Project, Carville, LA).[6]

(i). A podoscope uses lights and mirrors to show the pressure distribution of the plantar surface during unilateral or bilateral stance. Darker areas are associated with increased pressure (with foot insensitivity, high-pressure areas can be potential sites of skin breakdown).

(ii). The Harris footprint mat and microcapsular slipper-socks qualitatively measure weight-bearing forces. Darkened areas signify sites of increased pressure.

(b). Compare both sides of the body; normal or even distribution of force on the sole of the foot occurs from the postero-lateral rearfoot to the antero-medial forefoot.

f. For a discussion of balance, see "Ankle," Chapter 35.

g. For a discussion of gait, see "Gait," Chapter 38.

III. Assessment

Evaluate the objective findings, considering the following factors:

A. Mobility. Sufficient ROM for movement and the assumption of correct posture must exist.[23,24]

1. Evaluate whether the foot joints have ROM and joint play.
   a. If they lack ROM, determine whether the restriction originates in the joint, soft tissue, or muscle tissue (use end-feel as a guide).
   b. If they lack joint play, it must be restored for gains in ROM to be achieved.
2. Determine whether the foot pronates while it is flat.
   a. If not, determine whether the subtalar joint is moving or whether the patient has pes cavus.
   b. If the subtalar joint is not moving and pes cavus is not present, determine whether the patient's lower extremity is shorter on the affected side, causing the patient to supinate to lengthen the limb.

B. Stability. The ability of the muscle to perform tonic holding and cocontraction.[23,24]

1. Determine whether muscle weakness exists isometrically, concentrically, or eccentrically.
2. Determine whether a difference in torque production exists isokinetically (when it is appropriate to measure).
3. Determine in what positions the muscle is weak.
   a. If muscle force production is lacking, determine whether sufficient ROM is present in the joint for the muscle to contract efficiently.
4. Determine whether the patient has pes planus or excessive pronation.
   a. If he/she has pes planus, determine whether the patient has supportive footwear or orthoses to externally stabilize the foot.
   b. If the foot is excessively pronated, determine whether patient has an imbalance in:
      • hip rotation range or strength
      • tibial rotation range or strength
      • ankle dorsiflexion range (equinus foot)
      • an increased Q-angle or excessive tibial varum

C. Controlled mobility. The ability of the muscles to move the proximal joints over the fixed distal end.[23,24]

1. Determine whether the patient can bear weight and move over the foot (assisted and unassisted).
   a. An inability to bear weight and to move over the foot may indicate a continued stability problem.
   b. If pain persists at the distal surface of the tibia, excessive pronation (increased foot mobility) may be present.
   c. If pain persists at the medial surface of the knee or in the patellofemoral joint, excessive pronation (increased foot mobility) may be the problem.
   d. If the patient has metatarsalgia or heel pain, excessive pronation (increased foot

mobility) or excessive supination (decreased foot mobility) may be the problem.
2. Determine whether the patient can accept a challenge to weight bearing (in a double- or single-limb stance).
   a. If the patient lacks weight-bearing ability, a need for increased joint movement to detect motion changes in the foot may exist for him/her.

D. Skill. The ability of the muscles to move and stabilize the proximal joints with the distal end mobilized.[23,24]

1. Determine whether the patient can walk on level surfaces and on uneven surfaces and whether he/she can run. Determine whether he/she can walk in a step-over-step manner up and down stairs.
   a. If the patient lacks the ability to walk on even surfaces, mobility and stability may be lacking.
   b. If he/she is unable to walk on uneven surfaces or run, controlled mobility may be lacking.

E. Diagnosis and prognosis

Based on your initial judgement (including consideration of the relationship among all anomalous findings and at what level the cause of the problem is occurring), make a **physical therapy diagnosis** and a **physical therapy prognosis,** allowing you to set reasonable goals and to plan treatment.

Musculoskeletal dysfunction is at the root of your diagnosis and is the basis of your treatment plan. Examples of physical therapy diagnoses include shin splints (anterior or posterior tibial tendinitis), plantar fasciitis, metatarsalgia, forefoot or rearfoot deformity, and hallux rigidus. Goals must be *measurable* and *time related.* Formulate a long-term goal that includes a functional outcome. Keep in mind the patient's goals.

IV. Treatment Plan

A. Management of mobility dysfunction
1. Soft-tissue management
   a. Release (or minimize) soft-tissue restrictions first. Move from superficial to deep, breaking up surface scar tissue first and gradually moving into deeper connective

tissue and muscle. Use superficial and deep myofascial release, traditional effleurage and petrissage, friction massage, or deep acupressure points to alleviate the restriction.[25-27]

Plantar structures such as plantar fascia are prone to tightening from weight-bearing forces. Deep massage or modalities such as ultrasound can be used to soften tissue and to facilitate stretching. Extension of toes with cross-friction massage on the fascia also improves extensibility. Heel and arch pain should decrease as the length of plantar fascia increases.

b. Insensitivity in patients with peripheral nerve lesions, diabetes, vascular disease, and Hansen's disease can lead to skin breakdown and possible gangrenous lesions and to the need for amputation. Monitor the limbs for muscle weakness that commonly accompanies lack of sensation.

c. Proper skin care[20]

   (1). Scrupulous inspection of the plantar surface, toes (including between the toes), nails, and skin temperature (with the back of hand) is necessary. Note red areas, blisters, calluses, or wounds as well as maceration between the toes.

   (2). Toenails should not be thickened or ingrown.

   (3). The patient's socks and shoes should be inspected before he/she wears them to ensure that the socks are wrinkle free and that the socks and shoes are devoid of foreign objects and protrusions.

   (4). Shoes should be constructed of leather and with a wide and deep toe box to allow for expansion of the feet; this is especially important for patients with toe deformities such as hammer toes, claw toes, and hallux valgus that causes the toes to rub against the toe box unless sufficient room exists. Friction and repetitive stress result in the development of blisters and calluses, respectively, with the first and fifth metatarsals as common sites.

   (5). Skin care also includes daily soaks in warm water followed by the application of petroleum jelly or mineral oil to maintain moisture.

   (6). The patient should not walk barefoot, even in his/her home.

d. For **wound management,** see "Ankle," Chapter 35.

e. Various modalities are used to decrease swelling, pain, and calcification as well as to increase blood flow and metabolism.

   (1). Therapeutic heat is used as a precursor to massage, mobilization, and exercise; it can be applied through the use of hot packs, paraffin baths, hydrotherapy, ultrasound, shortwave and microwave diathermy, and fluidotherapy.

   (2). Cryotherapy, with its local vasoconstricting effect, helps to alleviate swelling. It also decreases nerve conduction velocity, diminishing the pain response to therapy. It is beneficial in patients with acute lesions for swelling and pain management and as an ending to treatment to minimize trauma to tissues from mobilization and exercise.

   (3). Electrical stimulation in its various forms is used for pain modulation, swelling and muscle spasm reduction, and muscle re-education. Various forms of electrical stimulation include transcutaneous electrical nerve stimulation; high-voltage, interferential, galvanic stimulation and iontophoresis; and functional (neuromuscular) electrical stimulation.

f. All modalities are used as *adjuncts* to enhance or modulate the effects of treatment.

2. **Joint management**

a. **Mobilize joints** to promote proper function of the foot. Warm the joints (with heat, massage, or passive or active ROM exercise) before attempting mobilization.

   (1). To determine the patient's tolerance to mobilization, use the Cyriax sequence of pain and limitation:[28]

      (a). Pain *before* tissue resistance indicates the presence of an acute or extra-articular lesion (the capsule and soft tissue do not tolerate stretching).

      (b). Pain *with* tissue resistance indicates the presence of a subacute lesion (gentle stretching to the capsule and soft tissue may begin).

(c). Pain *after* tissue resistance indicates the presence of a chronic lesion (stretching can be performed to gain length in the capsule and soft tissue).

(2). Begin with grade 1 mobilization (small oscillations at the beginning of the capsular range) for pain modulation.

(3). In the subacute stage, progress to grade 2 (large oscillations at the middle of the capsular range) as the patient tolerates.

(4). As the problem becomes chronic, use grades 3 and 4 (large oscillations toward the end of the capsular range and small oscillations at the end of the capsular range, respectively) to cause more permanent deformation of (and therefore to stretch) the joint capsule.[14,16] Because of functional demands, mobility of the intertarsal joints and first metatarsophalangeal joint is key.

(5). Joint mobilization techniques include
 (a). Talar distraction and rocking.
 (b). Calcaneal distraction and rocking.
 (c). Intertarsal glides.
 (d). Tarsometatarsal glides.
 (e). Metatarsophalangeal distraction and dorsal and ventral glides and tilt.
 (f). Phalangeal distraction and dorsal and ventral glides and tilt.[14-16]

(6). Talocrural joint mobility is also important in such cases and should be included in management, as necessary. Having the patient roll a tennis ball or a similar ball under the foot will help him/her to maintain gains in mobility of the intertarsal and metatarsal joints.

b. An **acutely inflamed joint** should be managed with the application of ice and with compression, elevation, and rest of the joint. As the swelling goes down, grade 1 mobilization can be attempted. If the patient complains of sharp pain, or if swelling increases, the techniques should be discontinued. Gradually increase the mobilization intensity and grade as the patient's tolerance and reactivity allow. Patients with **long-standing joint hypomo-**

bility secondary to trauma (such as complex subtalar fractures, fractures with a prolonged healing time, and prolonged immobilization) require slow increases in both the intensity and duration of mobilization techniques. Even in the chronic stage, such patients tend to be more reactive to specific joint techniques, and their condition can easily become worse with protracted treatment sessions. These patients are also prone to developing osteoarthritic changes in the joint, which is atypical for the general population. Educate the patient on the levels and types of activities that minimize stress and maximize function of an arthritic foot.

3. **Muscle length management.** Gastrocsoleus tightness affects foot mechanics by causing the subtalar and transverse tarsal joints to compensate by excessively pronating. Stretching of this muscle is done with the foot in a neutral position to slight supination. Toe flexor and extensor muscle tightness can result in dorsal and plantar pressure problems, leading to the development of callouses or skin breakdown. Stretch the toe muscles by stabilizing the metatarsal joints and then extending or flexing the toes.

4. **Progression of mobility management.** Some degree of soft-tissue mobility must be restored before therapy can proceed into the deeper joint and muscle structures. Shift back and forth between techniques for the tissue, muscles, and joints as the patient begins to loosen up. Instruct the patient to perform a home program, such as rocking over the foot in a rocking chair and rolling the foot over a ball, to maintain gained mobility. Most patients with primary mobility problems have secondary stability issues that must be addressed before they can function at adequate controlled mobility and skill levels.

B. **Management of stability and controlled mobility dysfunction**

1. **Overview of stability dysfunction**
 Stability dysfunction is primarily caused by ligament laxity and muscle weakness. No techniques to tighten or strengthen ligaments other than immobilization exist. Muscle strengthening is fairly easy to accomplish because of constant functional demands on

the joint. Begin treatment in a non–weight-bearing position to eliminate the body mass force of gravity on the muscles. Progress to exercises in a weight-bearing position as soon as the patient and the injured structures can tolerate it.

2. **Muscle strength management**
   a. Patients with muscles that have a fair strength grade (3 of 5) or a lower grade should begin **strength training** in a non–weight-bearing posture. As the muscle strength increases, cardinal plane and diagonal motions can be used while manual resistance is superimposed at the foot (see Figure 36–39); rubber tubing or exercise bands are applied at the foot (see Figure 36–40); free weights are used on the foot; or isokinetic exercises are performed. Keep in mind the patient's functional needs and the specificity of training (eg, prolonged standing, toe raises, excessive walking, side-to-side running, or jumping) when designing an exercise program. Many repetitions and low-level resistance can be used to improve muscle endurance, whereas few repetitions and high-level resistance can be used to encourage greater force production by the muscle. Towel scrunching with and without weight is good exercise for the plantar muscles (see Figure 36–41).
   b. Proprioceptive neuromuscular facilitation (PNF) diagonal exercises are used successfully to strengthen the foot and entire lower extremity.[29] Use timing for emphasis; slow reversal and slow reversal hold, repeated contractions, and rhythmic sta-

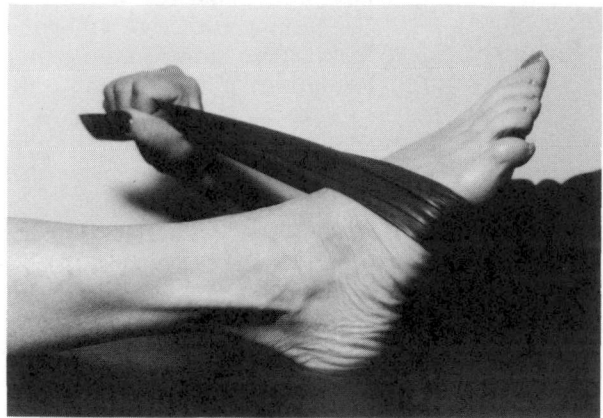

FIGURE 36–40   Rubber tubing resistance to everters.

bilization for the facilitation of weak muscle through isometric contraction; and quick stretch, cocontraction, and overflow from stronger muscles. Eccentric training must be done to improve gait activities. Special attention should be paid to the tibialis anterior and posterior, toe extensors, and gastrocsoleus muscle.

3. **Ligament laxity management**
   Ligament laxity is commonly manifested by the collapse of the longitudinal arches in weight-bearing (excessive pronation) and non–weight-bearing (pes planus) postures. Treatment includes adhesive taping and orthotic management.
   a. **Adhesive taping** is one technique that is inexpensive and is often used as a predictor for success with orthotics. Two techniques to control excessive pronation

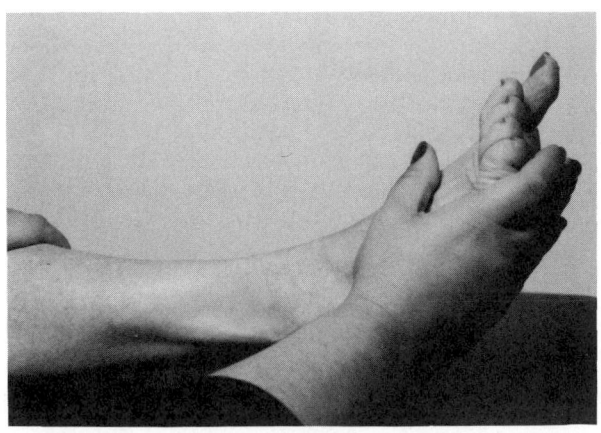

FIGURE 36–39   Manual resistance to everters.

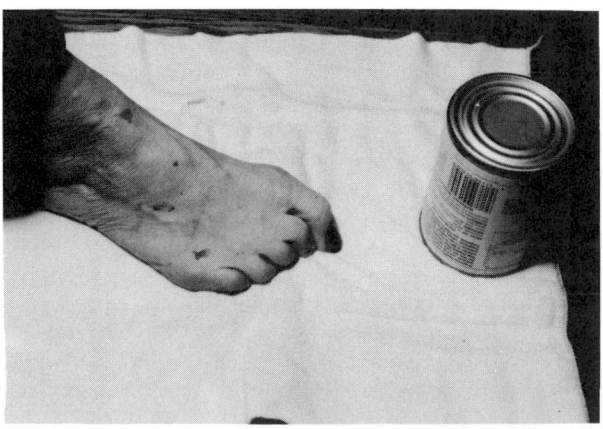

FIGURE 36–41   Towel scrunches with added resistance.

by stabilizing the subtalar and midtarsal joints in stance are the Low Dye and cross X techniques.[30]

b. **Orthotic management**[31] stabilizes a hypermobile foot, provides shock absorption, decreases friction, or maintains a neutral subtalar joint position in midstance. There are three types of orthoses: soft, semirigid, and rigid. Each has a unique purpose and function.

(1). *Soft orthoses*[12,31] are used for reducing shear forces and for relieving pressure-sensitive areas. They are constructed from cushioned materials that are not custom molded; effectiveness requires them to be 3 mm thick. They are highly compressible and have a limited duration of usability. Examples are the Spenco (Spenco Medical Corp.) and Sorbethane orthoses.

(2). *Semirigid orthoses*[12,31] are designed to provide softness and shock absorption, together with control. Patients who require them have some rigidity to their foot structure but need restraint from excessive pronation when moving from midstance to the heel-off position. These orthoses may be fabricated directly over the foot or over a plaster foot model. They provide total contact and may be posted or wedged to correct forefoot or rearfoot deformities. These orthoses are commonly used by athletes. Examples of materials used in construction are 10A Aliplast (Nimed), Plastazote, Thermacork, and Alimold (Alimed Corp.).

(3). *Rigid orthoses*[12,31] are made from hard thermoplastic material and are designed to provide total support for a foot without inherent control. Patients with pes planus have intrinsic shock absorption but need maximum control of intertarsal movement from external material. Care in choosing footwear with resilient soles is important.

c. Goals of orthotic management[12] include:

(1). Rearfoot control and medial wedging. The orthosis is used to slow down excessive pronation by allowing a near-neutral position; it also provides some shock absorption during heel strike.

(2). Rearfoot control and heel counter. The orthosis is used to enhance medial wedging by controlling the rearfoot from midstance to the heel-off position. A reinforced medial heel counter is more effective in impact activities like running and jumping. Lateral heel counters can be used to provide support for lax ankle lateral collateral ligaments.

(3). Forefoot control and medial or lateral wedging. The orthosis is used to correct forefoot varus and valgus deformities by bringing the floor up to the deformity. Wedges are placed just proximal to the metatarsal heads and must be angled and beveled so that they are not felt when in the shoe. Posting for varus deformity is done medially; posting for valgus deformity and a plantar flexed first ray is done laterally.

PLEASE NOTE: Orthoses should be used to correct foot deformities and should be comfortable when put into a shoe. Excessive pronation or supination may also be caused by tibial or femoral dysfunction. Orthoses used to correct foot *compensations* result in a need to compensate at some other joint. Excessive control at the foot can cause knee, hip, or back pain.

d. Management of ligament laxity also involves **proprioceptive training.** This can be accomplished through protected weight bearing with rhythmic stabilization at the pelvis; weight shifting with and without rhythmic stabilization; unilateral weight bearing; and balance board activities. Enhance somatosensory feedback by having the patient undergo training with and without vision. The Biomechanical Ankle Platform System (BAPS) Board (Camp International, Inc.) is a relatively inexpensive balance board system that has balls of varying size that alter stress and motion on the foot and ankle. Activities should progress from the patient exercising with an orthotic in place to exercising while wearing a high-top sneaker, and, finally, to exercising barefoot. For patients with chronic laxity, it may be prudent to advise them to run, jump, and perform other sporting activities with an orthotic in place to improve proprioceptive input to the joints and to offer some protection.

4. **Management of controlled mobility dysfunction**

Trauma, immobilization, and weakness lead to problems in weight bearing. Easing the patient into weight-bearing activities involves **gradual protected weight bearing** with shoes and orthoses and during sitting or on parallel bars. Have the patient sit in a chair (a rocker works well) and move the tibia over the foot. Moving back and forth over the foot helps to improve the ROM in a functional movement and is preparatory for gait.

Have the patient stand with a wide base of support and shift his/her weight over the foot. Instruct him/her to move side to side and front to back. Work slowly, gradually increasing the speed and decreasing the base of support. As the patient progresses, have him/her begin to perform single-limb stance; increase time and perturbation as the patient improves. Again, use a balance board or BAPS-type system to improve proprioceptive input to the joints. Add stable footwear or orthoses to enhance

feedback and to supply external support to the joints.

C. Management of skill dysfunction

As the patient's ability to bear weight on stable surfaces improves, move him/her onto uneven surfaces (use foam, a pillow, or ramps as an alternative) and stairs. The patient should step up and down on a stair or short stool, moving the tibia over the foot and increasing weight bearing onto the foot. As the patient is able to bear full weight, have him/her progress to a step-over-step movement. Jogging with a progression to running is a further option. Use an elastic, bungee-type cord to apply more resistance. Keep in mind that ground reaction forces for jogging and running are three to four times greater than body weight force, and that the foot and ankle joints should be mobile and stable before the patient undertakes this activity. General lower extremity training tools such as the Fitter, Snowbounder, and Russian Leaper functionally train the lower extremities and provide activity-specific training. Plyometrics (fast and powerful movements that use the stretch reflex to facilitate muscle action)[32] also train the lower extremity in activities such as jumping, running, and squatting.

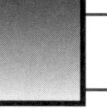

Clinical Decision-Making Cases

Case #1

HISTORY

NK is a 35-year-old pharmacist who has severe right medial knee pain. An arthroscopic examination yielded negative results. He is a recreational runner, averaging 25 to 35 miles a week on the side of a road. He recently started a training program for a marathon, increasing his mileage from 15 miles a week slowly and methodically to a high of 40 miles. His running shoes were fairly new, standard, and without any unusual features.

EXAMINATION

Manual muscle testing for strength showed no difference in the strength of NK's quadriceps and hamstring muscles. Isokinetic testing reported equal strength bilaterally, in both quadriceps and hamstring muscles,

with good time factors and a normal 3:2 muscle strength ratio, respectively. His quadriceps torque was 90% of his body weight (NK is 6 ft 3 in and 230 lbs).

ROM was as follows:

Motion	Range on right side	Range on left side
Hip internal rotation	45°	35°
Hip external rotation	30°	35°
Straight leg raising	65°	70°
Knee flexion	Within normal limits (pain at end of range medial joint line)	Within normal limits

Motion	Range on right side	Range on left side
Tibial external torsion	5°	7°
Tibial varum	10°	10°
Ankle dorsiflexion	3°	8°
Foot, calcaneal eversion	5°	5°
Foot deformity	Rearfoot and forefoot varus	Rearfoot varus

Examination of the soft tissue of the right foot demonstrated a thickened callous under the second and third metatarsal heads.

Gait showed excessive pronation bilaterally from midstance through toe-off; increased internal femoral moment was present from midstance through toe-off on the right.

ASSESSMENT AND DIAGNOSIS

NK excessively pronates during gait, causing increased varus force at the knee joint; this results in medial pain. He is pronating for several reasons:

- Increased right internal hip rotation is present.
- Decreased calcaneal eversion exists compared with tibial varum bilaterally.
- Decreased ankle dorsiflexion is present bilaterally.
- Rearfoot and forefoot varus exist on the right side, and rearfoot varus is present on the left.

The right side is worse than the left because of the hip internal rotation (from tight medial hamstrings). NK has a forefoot and rearfoot deformity on the right side that is the primary diagnosis with a secondary diagnosis of internal femoral rotation tightness. The secondary diagnosis must be treated aggressively. If the foot deformities are corrected and the hip continues to internally rotate too much, the torque originally dissipated through the excessive pronation at the foot will be felt more frequently at the knee.

TREATMENT GOALS

Short-Term Goals

- To increase NK's right hip external rotation to equal right hip internal rotation in 4 weeks.
- To increase NK's straight leg raising bilaterally by 10 degrees in 4 weeks.
- To increase NK's right ankle dorsiflexion by 5 degrees in 4 weeks.
- To increase NK's calcaneal rocking into eversion (joint play) from grade 2 to grade 3 in 4 weeks.

Long-Term Goal

- NK wants to demonstrate no gait deviations when he wears running shoes and orthoses in 6 weeks.

TREATMENT OUTCOME

NK was put on an aggressive stretching program for the medial hamstring muscle and gastrocsoleus muscles. The muscles were heated and then stretched by the use of a hold-relax technique. The patient performed a vigorous home stretching program twice a day as well. He refused to stop running during the time he participated in the treatment program but agreed to cut his mileage to 15 miles a week. A Sorbothane insole was added to his running shoes at first to assist in shock absorption. As the medial hamstring gained length and as the gap between internal and external rotation lessened (their ratio should be 1:1), a semi-rigid orthosis was used in both shoes. The left orthosis was posted with a medial heel wedge to correct for the rearfoot varus deformity. The right orthosis was also posted with a medial heel wedge but it had a medial forefoot wedge to correct for both the rearfoot and forefoot varus. The wedging was built up very slowly as NK continued to stretch the medial hamstring and gastrocsoleus muscles. The knee pain gradually disappeared because he wore the orthosis in his work shoes as well (he stood all day on concrete floors). He built up his running mileage over several months. The running shoes were changed to a model with a firmer heel counter to give added resistance to the excessive pronation. Because of his size, NK wore down the orthoses in 6 months' time and needed replacements to continue to run without experiencing pain.

Case #2

HISTORY

MB is a 45-year-old woman who has had a 2-year history of leg and foot pain, with the pain worse on the left side. She has no recollection of any specific trauma,

but the onset of pain did follow an extended period during which she took antidepressant medication, which resulted in a weight gain of 30 lbs (she is 5 ft 2 in, 140 lb). She has a very petite frame with small bones and mobile joints. The psychiatrist suggested that she begin walking to help lose the weight; the symptoms of pain came on after her exercise program had begun. She is a professional weaver, and the use of large looms has begun to increase her symptoms.

EXAMINATION

The pain began on the plantar surface of both heels only; on examination, MB also had pain in the posterior medial tibia (pain greater on the left side). An examination of the soft tissue revealed a thickened callus under the first and fifth metatarsal heads on the left side, with mild swelling along the posterior medial tibia and malleolus. On the right, a thickened callus was present under the second and third metatarsal heads and lateral aspect distal first toe. On examination of MB's strength it was discovered that she had pain on toe raising, non–weight-bearing dorsiflexion and plantar flexion, and inversion and eversion; strength grading was not valid at that point of the examination. ROM was as follows:

Motion	Range on left side	Range on right side
Tibial varum	15°	10°
Tibial external rotation	5°	5°
Ankle dorsiflexion	0°	5°
Foot eversion	12°	15°
Deformity	Rearfoot varus; forefoot varus	Rearfoot varus; forefoot valgus
Hip motions	Within normal limits	Within normal limits
Knee motions	Within normal limits	Within normal limits

Gait showed excessive pronation bilaterally; MB pushed off on the great toe only on the right side.

ASSESSMENT AND DIAGNOSIS

MB originally developed mild plantar fasciitis as a result of her weight gain and the increase in her activity level. She always excessively pronated (from decreased ankle dorsiflexion and rearfoot and forefoot deformities); however, the pronation was not problematic because her weight-bearing forces were not sufficient to elicit injurious forces on her soft tissue. Given that walking places a force equal to that of body weight through each foot with each step, MB's plantar fascia was unable to bear the load when her body weight increased. The shin splint pain was caused by the excessive force production by the posterior tibial muscle to eccentrically control her excessive pronation

during gait. Her physical therapy diagnosis was plantar fasciitis and posterior tibial tendinitis.

TREATMENT GOALS

Short-Term Goals

- To eliminate swelling in MB's posterior medial shin and malleolus in 2 weeks.
- To increase MB's left ankle dorsiflexion by 10 degrees and her right dorsiflexion by 5 degrees in 4 weeks.
- To increase MB's aerobic capacity sufficiently to lower her resting heart rate by 5 beats per minute in 8 weeks.

Long-Term Goal

MB wants to demonstrate pain-free and deviation-free gait with shoes and orthoses in 6 weeks.

TREATMENT OUTCOME

MB was put on an exercise program to stretch her Achilles tendon; she also was put on a non–weight-bearing aerobic program of swimming and referred to a podiatrist for orthotic fabrication. She has a rare blood disorder that causes her to have an allergic reaction to anti-inflammatory drugs and also causes her to bruise easily. This contraindicated ultrasound and massage as treatments for her acute inflammatory process. She was able to use ice, which she applied to the distal medial tibia and heel before and after weaving and walking for more than 5 or 10 minutes. Her symptoms began to abate.

Two months later MB informed the therapist that her heel pain was almost gone but that she had terrible pain in her fifth metatarsal head that radiated throughout the right foot. The shin splint pain had diminished slightly, but it was difficult to determine by what extent because she was still unable to stand and walk for any distance. Evaluation of her orthoses revealed that she used a standard semirigid orthosis with medial posting from the heel to just proximal to the metatarsal heads bilaterally. The wedging at the heel was approximately 5 degrees on the left and half that on the right. She wore Nike Air (Nike Inc.) running shoes (at the podiatrist's suggestion). She admitted to wearing her Reebok (Reebok USA Ltd., Inc.) walking shoes most of the time because the Nike shoes increased her pain.

REASSESSMENT

The medial forefoot wedging on the right orthosis was feeding into MB's forefoot valgus deformity, causing her midfoot to supinate (to decrease the pressure on the great toe) and her rearfoot to remain in a neutral position because of the medial forces of the orthosis.

The supination was putting excessive force on the fifth metatarsal head and thus caused her pain. The running shoes were too rigid in the forefoot and did not allow enough movement for her. The right orthosis was changed to accommodate the forefoot valgus deformity (it had a lateral wedge), and new shoes with a flexible forefoot were recommended. She had near complete resolution of her symptoms within a month.

References

1. Goss CM (ed): *Gray's Anatomy of the Human Body,* 29th ed. Philadelphia, Lea and Febiger, 1973.
2. Hoppenfeld S: *Physical Examination of the Spine and Extremities.* Norwalk, CT, Appleton-Century-Crofts, 1976.
3. Kapandji IA: *Physiology of the Joints,* vol. 2. New York, Churchill Livingstone, 1970.
4. Riegger CL: Anatomy of the ankle and foot. *Phys Ther* 1988, 68:2–14.
5. Inman VT: *Joints of the Ankle.* Baltimore, Williams & Wilkins, 1976, pp 3–10.
6. Root ML, Orien WP, Weed JH: *Clinical Biomechanics: Normal and Abnormal Function of the Foot,* vol. 2. Los Angeles, Clinical Biomechanics Corporation, 1977.
7. Manter JT: Movements of the subtalar and transverse tarsal joints. *Anat Rec* 1941, 80:397–409.
8. Oatis CA: Biomechanics of the foot and ankle under static conditions. *Phys Ther* 1988, 68:15–21.
9. Warfel JH: *The Extremities: Muscles and Motor Points.* Philadelphia, Lea and Febiger, 1985, pp 88–100.
10. McMinn RMH, Hutchings RT, Logan BM: *Color Atlas of Foot and Ankle Anatomy.* Norwalk, CT, Appleton-Century-Crofts, 1982.
11. Hunt GC: Examination of lower extremity dysfunction. In Gould JA (ed): *Orthopedic and Sports Physical Therapy.* 2nd ed. St. Louis, Mosby, 1990, pp 395–421.
12. McPoil TG, Brocato RS: The foot and ankle: biomechanical evaluation and treatment. In Gould JA (ed): *Orthopedic and Sports Physical Therapy,* 2nd ed. St. Louis, Mosby, 1990, pp 293–321.
13. Giallonardo LM: Clinical evaluation of foot and ankle dysfunction. *Phys Ther* 1988, 68:50–56.
14. Kaltenborn FM: *Manual Mobilization of the Extremity Joints,* 4th ed. Oslo, Olaf Norlis Bokhandel, 1989, pp 152–159.
15. Maitland GD: *Peripheral Manipulation,* 4th ed. London, Butterworth, 1977.
16. Paris SV: Extremity Mobilization and Dysfunction [Course Notes], 1979.
17. Fromherz, WA: Examination. In Hunt GC (ed): *Physical Therapy of the Foot and Ankle.* New York, Churchill Livingstone, 1988, pp 133–168.
18. Kendall FP, McCreary EK, Provance PG: *Muscles, Testing and Function,* 4th ed. Baltimore, Williams & Wilkins, 1993.
19. Daniels L, Worthingham C: *Muscle Testing Techniques of Manual Examination.* Philadelphia, W. B. Saunders Company, 1972.
20. Birke JA, Sims DS: The insensitive foot. In Hunt GC (ed): *Physical Therapy of the Foot and Ankle.* New York, Churchill Livingstone, 1988, pp 133–168.
21. Magee DJ: *Orthopedic Physical Assessment,* 2nd ed. Philadelphia, W. B. Saunders Company, 1992, pp 438–513.
22. Norkin CC, Levangie PK: *Joint Structure and Function,* 2nd ed. Philadelphia, F. A. Davis Company, 1992, pp 380–388.
23. Stockmeyer SA: Personal communication, 1993.
24. Sullivan PE, Markos PD, Minor MA: *An Integrated Approach to Therapeutic Exercise: Theory and Application.* Reston, VA, Reston Publishing, 1982.
25. Tappan FM: *Healing Massage Techniques.* Reston, VA Reston Publishing, 1978.
26. Manheim CJ, Lavett DK: *The Myofascial Release Manual.* Thorofare, NJ, Slack, 1989.
27. Cantu RI, Grodin AJ: *Myofascial Manipulation.* Gaithersburg, MD, Aspen, 1992.
28. Cyriax J: *Textbook of Orthopedic Medicine: Diagnosis of Soft Tissue Lesions,* vol. 1. London, Baillière Tindall, 1975.
29. Voss DE, Ionta MK, Myers BJ: *Proprioceptive Neuromuscular Facilitation,* 3rd ed. Philadelphia, Harper and Row, 1985.
30. McPoil TG, McGarvey TC: The foot in athletics. In Hunt GC (ed): *Physical Therapy of the Foot and Ankle.* New York, Churchill Livingstone, 1988.
31. Lockard MA: Foot orthoses. *Phys Ther* 1988, 68:50–56.
32. Voight ML, Draovitch P: Plyometrics. In Alpert MA (ed): *Eccentric Muscle Training.* New York, Churchill Livingstone, 1991.

Suggested Reading

Bateman J, Trott A: *The Foot and Ankle.* New York, Thieme-Stratton, 1980.

Bucholz R, Lippert F, Wenger D, *et al.: Orthopedic Decision Making,* St. Louis, Mosby, 1984.

Cailliet R: *Foot and Ankle Pain.* Philadelphia, F. A. Davis Company, 1968.

Cyriax J, Cyriax P: *Illustrated Manual of Orthopedic Medicine.* London, Butterworth, 1983.

Cyriax J: *Textbook of Orthopedic Medicine: Treatment by Manipulation, Massage, and Injection,* 8th ed. vol. 2. London, Baillière Tindall, 1971.

Donatelli R: *The Biomechanics of the Foot and Ankle.* Philadelphia, F. A. Davis Company, 1990.

Edmond SL: *Manipulation and Mobilization.* St. Louis, Mosby, 1993.

Hertling D, Kessler R: *Management of Common Musculoskeletal Disorders,* 2nd ed. Philadelphia, J. B. Lippincott Company, 1990.

Kissner C, Colby LA: *Therapeutic Exercise: Foundations and Principles,* 2nd ed. Philadelphia, F. A. Davis Company, 1990.

Mennel J: *Joint Pain: Diagnosis and Treatment Using Manipulative Techniques.* Boston, Little, Brown and Company, 1964.

Wadsworth CT: *Manual Examination and Treatment of the Spine and Extremities.* Baltimore, Williams & Wilkins, 1988.

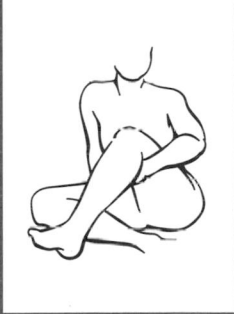

CHAPTER 37

Posture

Lisa M. Giallonardo

I. Introduction to Posture

A. General Information

1. Posture is "a position or attitude of the body, a relative arrangement of body parts for a specific activity, or a characteristic manner of bearing the body."[1] Posture also can be defined as a relative alignment of body segments in relation to each other and to the support surface.[1]

2. "**Good posture** is that state of muscular and skeletal balance which protects the supporting structure of the body against injury or progressive deformity irrespective of the attitude (erect, lying, squatting, stooping) in which these structures are working or resting."[2]

3. "**Poor posture** is a faulty relationship of the various parts of the body which produces increased strain on the supporting structures and in which there is less efficient balance of the body over its base of support."[2]

4. Good posture involves using energy in the most efficient manner, because each body movement begins and ends with a posture.[1]

5. When resting posture is not "normal," more energy is needed to perform or control movements, *eg*, forward head posture puts increased stress on the cervicothoracic spine and requires more work from the erector spinae muscles if an erect posture is to be maintained.[3]

6. Posture neutralizes the effects of gravity with internal, and sometimes external, forces, making it easier to maintain the recumbent position.[4]

7. Electromyography studies show that healthy people who do not tense their muscles constantly can sit comfortably and rest in a variety of positions. Nervous subjects cannot relax and cannot change position without significant energy expenditure.[4]

8. Very little muscle activity is required to maintain an upright position. The antigravity muscles of humans are not used as much to maintain normal standing or sitting positions as they are to produce powerful movements that are necessary when people change position, *eg*, from a sitting to a standing position.[4]

9. Basmajian and DeLuca[4] theorize that most fatigue associated with standing is related to venous and arterial problems or to pressure and tension on inert structures. Also, a Swedish study showed walking to be less fati-

guing than standing because the constant shifting of weight during walking acts as a relief mechanism to the muscles and inert structures.

B. Forces affecting posture

1. Gravitational forces[5]
   a. **Gravitational moment** is defined as torque that is produced by the force of gravity acting on the body.
      (1). When the line of gravity falls anterior to the joint axis, the resulting torque causes motion of the proximal segment in an anterior direction (see Figure 37–1).
      (2). When the line of gravity falls posterior to the joint axis, the resulting torque causes motion of the proximal segment in a posterior direction (see Figure 37–2).
      (3). **Flexion moment** occurs when gravitational torque produces flexion of an involved joint.
      (4). **Extension moment** occurs when gravitational torque produces extension of an involved joint.
      (5). Examples of gravitational effects
         (a). Extension moment at the hip allows the iliofemoral (Y) ligaments to support the body from falling backward.
         (b). Extension moment at the knee allows the joint to lock and

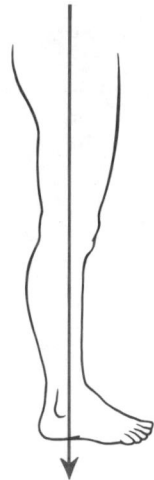

FIGURE 37–2 Line of gravity falling posterior to the knee joint, resulting in a flexion moment.

cease to require muscle action to maintain extension.
         (c). Extension moment at the ankle requires counteraction by the gastrocsoleus muscle.
   b. Gravitational forces act through the body's center of gravity or mass **(COG),** allowing the body's equilibrium to be maintained by the COG within the base of support.
2. Ground reaction forces (GRFs)[5]
   a. GRFs are the forces that react to the body's weight on the ground.
   b. One vertical and two horizontal forces exist; their resultant force is equal and opposite to the force of gravity.
   c. GRFs can be problematic if the **shock-absorbing** capability of the foot, ankle, tibia, knee, femur, hip, pelvis, or lumbosacral spine is not adequate.
3. Balance[5,6]
   a. Three patterns of muscle action for maintaining balance in an upright posture have been identified: **ankle, hip, and stepping patterns.**
   b. The muscles surrounding the ankle and hip react to changes in body position and readjust the body to place the COG within the body's base of support.
   c. When a movement exceeds the limit of a person's ankle and hip muscles to respond, he/she can maintain an upright position and thus re-establish balance by stepping forward or backward.

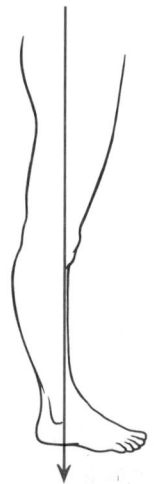

FIGURE 37–1 Line of gravity falling anterior to the knee joint, resulting in an extension moment.

C. Definitions

1. Spinal positions[3]

   a. **Lordosis.** Lordosis is an extension of the spine that is seen as an anterior curve; lordosis normally occurs in the cervical and lumbar spine. *Exaggerated* anterior curvature is *not* normal.

   b. **Kyphosis.** Kyphosis is flexion of the spine that is seen as a posterior curve; it normally occurs in the thoracic spine. *Exaggerated* posterior curvature is *not normal.*

   c. **Scoliosis.** Scoliosis involves curvature of the spine, seen as a lateral curve; it may be accompanied by a rotation component. Lateral curvature is *not* normal.

   d. **Forward head posture.** This posture involves flexion of the lower cervical spine in combination with extension of the upper cervical spine. It is often accompanied by protracted scapulae and increased thoracic kyphosis (see Figure 37–3).

   e. **Swayback posture.** A posterior shift of the upper trunk (flexion of the thoracic spine on the lumbar spine) and an anterior shift of the pelvis (extension of the hip) result in a swayback posture. Decreased lumbar lordosis (flattened spine), posterior *tilt* of the pelvis, and increased kyphosis of the thoracic spine also are present (see Figure 37–4).

   f. **Lordotic posture.** Lordotic posture combines an increase in the lumbosacral angle with an increase in lumbar lordosis, anterior pelvic tilt, and hip flexion (see Figure 37–5).

   g. **Flat back posture.** The absence of curvature in the lumbar spine (flexion) with posterior pelvic tilt results in a flat back posture. It is often accompanied by a flat upper back (caused by a decrease in thoracic and cervical curve) (see Figure 37–6).

2. Extremity positions[3]

   a. **Elbow-carrying angle.** This angle is the lateral deviation of the radius and ulna from the humerus at the elbow joint; 10 to 20 degrees is its normal measurement, especially in women.

   b. **Coxa vara.** Coxa vara is a deviation of the femur toward the midline (medially).

   c. **Coxa valga.** Coxa valga is a deviation of the femur away from the midline (laterally).

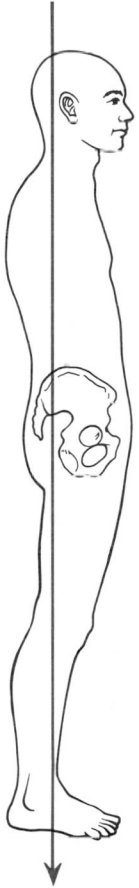

FIGURE 37–4   Swayback posture.

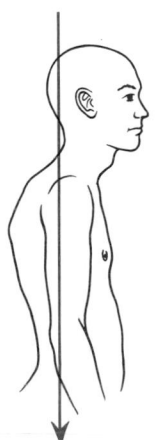

FIGURE 37–3   Forward head posture.

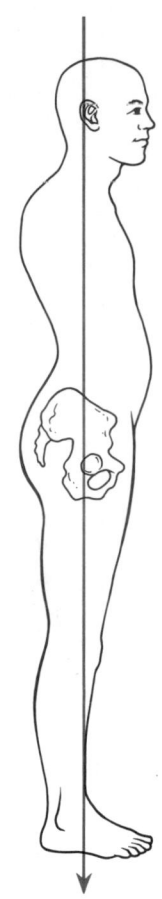

FIGURE 37–5   Lordotic posture.

i. **Pelvic posterior torsion (tilt).** Angulation of the pelvis dorsal; the plane of the ASIS is posterior to the plane of the pubic symphysis.

j. **Femoral anteversion.** Internal rotatory angulation of the femur due to anterior angulation of the femoral neck causes femoral anteversion.

k. **Femoral retroversion.** External rotatory angulation of the femur due to posterior angulation of the femoral neck causes femoral retroversion.

l. **Tibial internal (medial) torsion.** Internal rotatory angulation of the tibia.

m. **Tibial external (lateral) torsion.** External rotatory angulation of the tibia results in this position; up to 15° of external torsion is considered normal.

d. **Genu varum.** Genu varum is a deviation of the tibia toward the midline (medially) that results in bowleg deformity.

e. **Genu valgus.** Genu valgus is a deviation of the tibia away from the midline (laterally) that results in knock knee deformity.

f. **Tibial varum.** A frontal plane angulation of the distal third of the tibia in relation to the floor during standing results in tibial varum.

g. **Metatarsus adductus.** This deformity involves the angulation of the metatarsal bones toward the midline (medially).

h. **Pelvic anterior torsion (tilt).** Pelvic anterior torsion involves the angulation of the pelvis ventrally; the plane of the antero-superior iliac spine (ASIS) is anterior to the plane of the pubic symphysis.

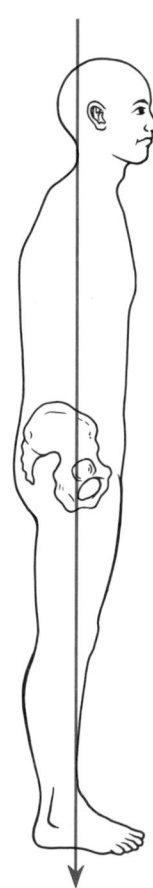

FIGURE 37–6   Flat back posture.

n. **Foot pronation.** Foot pronation is the result of triplanar motion of the subtalar and midtarsal joints. It involves dorsiflexion, abduction, and eversion.

o. **Foot supination.** Foot supination is the result of triplanar motion of the subtalar and midtarsal joints. It involves plantar flexion, adduction, and inversion.

II. Examination

A. Subjective

1. Ask the patient to relate his/her perception of the problem (or problems) to better focus your objective evaluation.
   a. Determine whether the patient thinks that the problem is related to activity (leading the therapist to focus on contractile tissue).
   b. Ask the patient whether he/she thinks that the problem is chronic (leading the therapist to attempt to reproduce the exact symptoms during the evaluation).
2. Discuss the patient's goals so that they may be incorporated into the therapist's goals and into the treatment-planning process.
   a. Determine whether the patient wants to participate in a particular activity that requires certain muscle strength or joint range of motion (ROM).

B. Objective

1. **History**
   a. Elicit information concerning any trauma that the patient might have experienced, including a complete description of the mechanism of injury.
   b. Discuss the symptom presentation (see Table 35–1).
2. **Inspection and palpation**
   a. *Measurement*
      (1). A **plumb line** is a string with a weight on the end that may be hung next to a standing patient. It allows the evaluation of his/her posture in relation to the line. For a frontal plane view, the patient stands with the line midway between the heels; for a sagittal plane view, the patient stands with the line anterior to the lateral malleolus.
      (2). A **grid** is a framework of evenly placed horizontal and vertical lines in front of which the patient stands. With a grid, the patient's posture can then be evaluated in relation to ideal posture.
   b. *Standing (anterior, posterior, or frontal view)*[1,4,5] (see Figure 37–7)
      (1). *Head and neck.* Measure the line of gravity (LOG) through the forehead, nose, and chin that divides the head into two equal parts; the cervical spine should be in a neutral position, with no lateral flexion or rotation.
      (2). *Trunk.* The LOG should divide the trunk into two equal parts; no scoliotic curves (lateral flexion or rotation) should be present in the cervical, thoracic, or lumbar spine nor in the lateral tilt of the pelvis.
      (3). *Upper quarter.* The scapulothoracic, glenohumeral, elbow, forearm, and wrist joints should all be in neutral positions.
      (4). *Lower quarter.* The hip should be in neutral rotation; the tibia may be in as much as 15 degrees of external rotation; the patellae and toes should be pointed forward.
   c. *Standing (lateral or sagittal view)*[1,4,5] (see Figure 37–8)
      (1). *Head and neck.* The LOG should pass through the ear, anterior to the atlanto-occipital joints, and posterior to the remainder of the cervical spine; if it does, the extension moment (and normal anterior curve) results.
      (2). *Trunk.* The LOG should pass posterior to the thoracic spine and anterior to the lumbar spine and pelvis; if it does, a flexion moment of the

Table 37-1. SUMMARY OF TYPES OF MUSCLE WEAKNESS AND TIGHTNESS (SHORTENING) WITH POSTURAL DEVIATIONS[3,5]

Postural Defect	Joints	Short Muscle	Weak Muscle
Forward head posture	Atlanto-occipital joint Cervical spine Temporomandibular joint Scapulothoracic joint Glenohumeral joint	Levator scapulae Sternocleidomastoid Scalenes Suboccipital muscles Upper trapezius Pectoralis major and minor	Hyoid muscles Lower cervical and thoracic erector spinae Middle and low trapezius Rhomboids
Swayback posture	Thoracolumbar spine Pelvic joints Hip joint	Upper abdominals Internal intercostals Hip extensors Lower lumbar extensors	Lower abdominal muscles Lower thoracic extensor muscles Hip flexor muscles
Lordotic posture	Thoracolumbar spine Pelvic joints Hip joint	Lumbar extensors Tight hip flexors	Abdominal muscles
Kyphotic posture	Thoracic spine	Intercostales Pectoralis major Serratus anterior Levator scapulae Upper trapezius	Thoracic erector spinae Rhomboids Middle and lower trapezius
Flat back posture	Lumbar spine Pelvic joints	Abdominals Hip extensors	Lumbar extensor muscles Hip flexor muscles
Flat upper back posture	Cervicothoracic spine Scapulothoracic joint	Thoracic erector spinae Scapula retractors	Scapula protractor muscles Anterior intercostal muscles
Scoliosis	Cervicothoracolumbar spine Pelvic joints Hip joint Foot joints	Muscles on the concave side Hip adductors Foot supinators on the short side	Muscles on the convex side Hip abductor muscles Foot pronation muscles on the long side

thoracic spine, extension moment of the lumbar spine, and a slight forward tilt (torsion) of the pelvis result.

(3). *Upper quarter.* The LOG should pass through the glenohumeral joint.

(4). *Lower quarter.* The LOG should fall posterior to the hip and anterior to the knee and ankle joints, resulting in an extension moment at the hip and knee and in a dorsiflexion moment at the ankle.

3. **Measurement**
   a. *Introduction.* When changes from the ideal posture are present, areas of tightness and weakness must be noted to allow changes in aberrant posture to be made. Use end-feel to guide the evaluation of structures (*ie*, bony, muscular, capsular, springy, or empty end-feel).
   b. *Joint Play.*[7-9] When capsular end-feel is detected, evaluate the joint play (for rolls, glides, and slides that allow a full,

normal, pain-free range but are beyond the patient's voluntary control). All synovial joints may be examined for capsular tightness.

▪ PLEASE NOTE: Motions are *graded* from 0 to 6, with 0 indicating ankylosis, 3 indicating normal status, and 6 indicating dislocation.

   c. *ROM.* Measure ROM to ensure that the patient has enough motion to make postural corrections. Evaluate range in the spine as well as in the extremities.
   d. *Muscle length*
      (1). A muscular end-feel may detect a tightness in the muscles that must be alleviated before postural correction can be achieved. Evaluate a muscle's length by elongating it over all of the joints that it crosses (increasing the distance between the origin and the insertion) and by noting changes in joint motion.

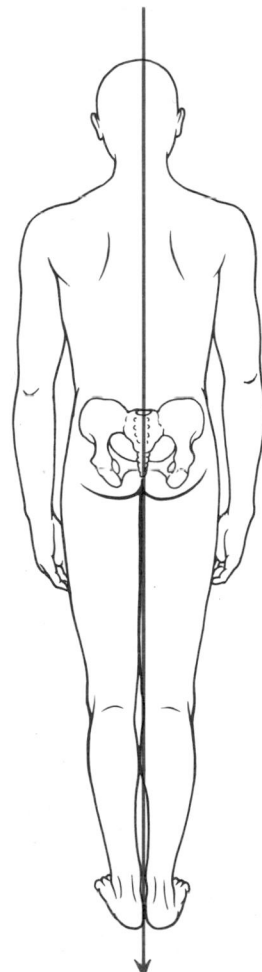

FIGURE 37–7   Center of gravity line in the frontal plane.

(2). A muscle may also be excessively long; evaluate it with the same technique as for a tight muscle.

(3). A shortened (tight) muscle requires stretching; a lengthened muscle requires strengthening.[3]

e. ***Muscle strength.*** To regain and maintain good postural alignment, normal muscle strength is required. Use manual muscle testing positions and grades to evaluate the muscles of the extremities, trunk, and face.[3,10]

f. ***Function.*** The patient should be observed as he/she performs daily activities, including work-related activities. This will allow the physical therapist to assess the ability of the muscles and joints to perform during specific activities. Analysis of the patient's physical needs helps the physical therapist to determine whether sufficient ROM and strength are present. Bad postures that lead to pain and overuse syndromes should also be noted.

g. ***Sensation.*** Balance, proprioception, and sensation should be evaluated if any deficits are suspected, because these functions affect the patient's ability to maintain and use proper posture.

(1). To test **sensation,** perform an evaluation of the patient's two-point discrimination and ability to sense temperature and light touch.

(2). Test **balance** on both mobile and stable surfaces; move a balance board to provide a mobile surface, and gently push the patient off balance on a stable surface. Note his/

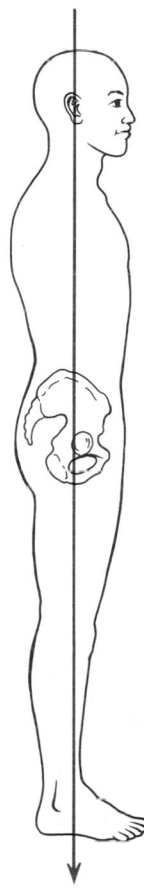

FIGURE 37–8   Center of gravity line in the sagittal plane.

her reaction time and use of the head, upper and lower extremities, and trunk to assist in achieving balance.

(3). **Proprioception** (position sense) can be tested by examining the patient's ability to detect movement and to perceive spatial relations.[11]

(a). Movement is evaluated by instructing the patient to close his/her eyes while the therapist moves one of the patient's toes up or down; the patient then describes the direction of the toe movement.

(b). Spatial relationship is also evaluated with the patient's eyes closed; the therapist moves the patient's lower limb into a certain position, and the patient is asked to imitate that position with the other limb.

III. Assessment

Evaluate the objective findings, considering the following factors:

A. Mobility (sufficient ROM for movement and assumption of posture)[12,13]

1. Determine whether the extremity and trunk joints have sufficient ROM and joint play.
   a. If the patient lacks ROM, determine whether the restriction stems from a joint, from soft tissue, or from muscle tissue (use end-feel as a guide).
   b. If the patient lacks joint play, it must be restored for gains in ROM to be achieved.
   c. If the patient lacks mobility, proper posture cannot be attained.

B. Stability (the ability of the muscle to perform tonic holding and cocontraction)[12,13]

1. Determine whether muscle weakness is present isometrically, concentrically, or eccentrically; whether a difference in torque production exists isokinetically (when appropriate); and in what positions the muscle is weak.
   a. If the patient lacks muscle force production, determine whether sufficient ROM exists in the joint to allow the muscle to contract efficiently.
   b. If the muscle cannot contract efficiently, proper posture cannot be maintained.

C. Controlled mobility (the ability of the muscles to move the proximal joints over the fixed distal end)[12,13]

1. Determine whether the patient can bear weight and move over the lower extremity (assisted and unassisted).
   a. An inability to perform these functions may indicate a continued problem in stability.
2. Determine whether the patient can maintain proper posture during weight bearing and whether he/she can accept challenges to weight bearing (in a double-limb stance or a single-limb stance).
   a. If the patient lacks weight-bearing ability, a need for increased joint movement may exist to allow the detection of motion changes in the lower extremity.
   b. If the patient is unable to maintain proper posture, stability may be lacking in the trunk.

D. Skill (the ability of the muscles to move and to stabilize the proximal joint or joints, with the distal end mobilized)[12,13]

1. Determine whether the patient can walk on level surfaces and on uneven surfaces and whether he/she can run. Assess whether the patient can walk in a step-over-step manner up and down stairs.
   a. If the patient lacks the ability to walk on even surfaces, mobility and stability may be lacking.
   b. If the patient is unable to walk on uneven surfaces or to run, controlled mobility may be lacking.
   c. If the patient is unable to maintain proper posture during walking, controlled mobility may be lacking.

E. Diagnosis and prognosis

Based on your initial judgement (including your assessment of the relationship among all anomalous findings and at what level the problem occurs) make a **physical therapy diagnosis** and a **physical therapy prognosis**. This will allow you to set reasonable goals and a treatment plan.

Musculoskeletal dysfunction is the focus of your diagnosis and the basis of your treatment plan. Examples of physical therapy diagnoses include forward head syndrome, scoliosis, and excessive lordosis or kyphosis.

PLEASE NOTE: Treatment goals must be *measurable* and *time related*. Formulate long-term goals with a functional outcome. Keep in mind the patient's goals.

IV. Treatment Plan

A. Management of mobility dysfunction

1. Soft-tissue management
    a. Release (or minimize) soft-tissue restrictions first. Move in a superficial to deep direction, breaking up surface scar tissue first. Gradually move toward deeper connective tissue and then muscle. Use superficial and deep myofascial release, traditional effleurage and petrissage, friction massage, or massage of deep acupressure points to alleviate the restrictions.[14–16]

    Correction of postural deviations in the neck requires management of soft-tissue dysfunction in the anterior as well as in the posterior sides of the neck and consideration of the temporomandibular muscles. Anterior neck muscles such as the sternocleidomastoid and scaleni become shortened and often spasm in patients with forward head syndrome and thus require some type of massage and stretching. Proper head and neck posture can not be maintained if these muscles are unable to function normally.

    b. Various **modalities** are used to decrease swelling, pain, and calcification as well as to increase blood flow and metabolic rate.
        (1). Examples of these modalities are as follows:
            (a). Therapeutic heat is used as a precursor to massage, mobilization, and exercise and includes the use of hot packs, paraffin baths, hydrotherapy, ultrasound, shortwave and microwave diathermy, and fluidotherapy.
            (b). Cryotherapy, with its local vasoconstricting effect, helps to alleviate swelling. It also decreases nerve conduction velocity, diminishing the pain response to therapy. It is beneficial in the treatment of acute lesions because it aids in the management of swelling and pain; it is also good as an ending to treatment to minimize trauma to tissues from mobilization and exercise.
            (c). Electrical stimulation, in its various forms, is used for pain modulation, swelling and muscle spasm reduction, and muscle re-education. The forms of electrical stimulation include transcutaneous electrical nerve stimulation; high-voltage, interferential, galvanic stimulation and iontophoresis; and functional (neuromuscular) electrical stimulation.
        (2). All modalities are used as *adjuncts* to enhance or modulate the effects of treatment. The postural muscles, many of which are small with phasic function, are prone to overuse, imbalance in length and strength, and spasm. This is especially true of the paraspinals in the thoracolumbar spine and the scapular stabilizers.

Before these muscles can be stretched, strengthened, and retrained, the surrounding soft tissue must be made healthy. Modalities can assist in this process.

2. **Joint management**
   a. Warm the joint (with heat, massage, or passive or active ROM exercises) before attempting **mobilization**. To determine the patient's pain tolerance, use the Cyriax sequence of pain and limitation.[17]
      (1). Pain *before* tissue resistance indicates the presence of an acute or extra-articular lesion (the capsule and soft tissue do not tolerate stretching).
      (2). Pain *with* tissue resistance indicates the presence of a subacute lesion (gentle stretching to capsule and soft tissue may begin).
      (3). Pain *after* tissue resistance indicates the presence of a chronic lesion (stretching can be performed to gain length in the capsule and soft tissue).
   b. Begin with Grade 1 mobilization (small oscillations at the beginning of the capsular range) for pain modulation. In the subacute stage, progress to Grade 2 mobilization (large oscillations at the middle of the capsular range) as the patient tolerates. As the problem becomes chronic, use Grades 3 and 4 mobilization (large oscillations toward the end of the capsular range and small oscillations at the end of the capsular range, respectively) to cause more permanent deformation of (and therefore to stretch) the joint capsule.[7,9]

      See "Craniomandibular Examination and Treatment," Chapter 28; "Cervical Spine," Chapter 29; "Upper Extremity: Shoulder," Chapter 30; and "Trunk," Chapter 32 for specific mobilization techniques.
   c. **Acutely inflamed joints** should be managed with the application of ice and with compression, elevation, and rest. As the swelling goes down, Grade 1 mobilization can be attempted. If the patient complains of sharp pain or if swelling increases, the techniques should be discontinued. Gradually increase the intensity and grade of mobilization as the patient's tolerance and reactivity allow.
   d. Patients with **long-standing joint hypomobility** secondary to trauma and elongated immobilization (severe sprains, muscle or ligament tears, or bracing) require slow increases in both the intensity and duration of mobilization techniques. Even when in the chronic stage such patients tend to be more reactive to specific joint techniques, and their condition can easily become worse with protracted treatment sessions. These patients are also prone to developing osteoarthritic changes in the joints, which is commonly seen in the cervical and lumbar spine regions and can result in chronic pain and dysfunction. Educate these patients on the levels and types of activities that are available to minimize stress and to maximize the function of arthritic joints, including the use of proper posture in standing, sitting, working, and sleeping.

3. **Muscle length management**
   Just as joint mobility must allow the patient to assume correct postures, so must muscle be sufficiently long to allow postural correction to be realized. Especially affected by postural malalignment are the pectoralis major and minor, the sternocleidomastoid and hyoid muscles, the hip flexor muscle group, and the hamstring muscles (see Table 37–1). A tight muscle is elongated to the point at which the patient feels a stretch and held there for a minimum of 15 to 30 seconds to gain length. Bouncing should be avoided.

   See "Craniomandibular Examination and Treatment," Chapter 28; "Cervical Spine," Chapter 29; "Upper Extremity: Shoulder," Chapter 30; "Trunk," Chapter 32; "Lower Extremity: Hip," Chapter 33; and "Lower Extremity: Ankle," "Lower Extremity: Knee," Chapter 34; Chapter 35 for specific stretches.

B. Progression of mobility management

1. Some degree of soft-tissue mobility must be restored before treatment can proceed into the deeper joint and muscle structures. Shift back and forth between techniques for tissue, muscles, and joints as the patient begins to loosen up. Instruct the patient to follow a home exercise program to maintain gained mobility. Encourage the patient to begin to

move into more neutral postures. Most patients with primary mobility problems have secondary stability dysfunction that must be addressed before they can function at high levels of controlled mobility and skill, including the ability to *maintain* proper posture. This phase should emphasize *shifting* from faulty positions toward more normal and less stressful postures.

2. Feldenkrais[18] developed a technique that stresses movement as a means of improving posture. His principles include the idea that all muscular activity is movement and that movement is the basis of awareness. The purpose of his exercises is to improve a patient's kinesthetic awareness and therefore to improve the patterns in which he/she moves. This is accomplished through the performance of small, isolated movements that are always comfortable and within the patient's ability. One example of these exercises is a pelvic rocking technique in which the patient slowly and gently moves the pelvis back and forth from an anterior to a posterior tilt. This *small* movement occurs at the lumbar spine, pelvis, and hips and is useful in both encouraging motion and finding neutral posture. It can be done in any position; this movement can be helpful in overcoming stiffness in a patient who has been sitting for long periods of time.

C. Management of stability and controlled mobility dysfunction

1. **Overview of stability dysfunction**

   Stability dysfunction is caused primarily by ligament laxity and muscle weakness. No techniques to tighten or strengthen ligaments exist other than immobilization. Muscle strengthening is fairly easy to accomplish because of the constant functional demands that are placed on the joints. Have the patient begin treatment in a proper (or near proper) non–weight-bearing posture to eliminate the body mass's force of gravity on muscles. Have the patient proceed to weight bearing in a proper posture as soon as the injured or irritated structures tolerate it. Increase the time that the posture is held, concentrating on isometric holds to reset the gamma bias and to improve the muscle's ability to maintain a neutral or normal posture.

2. **Muscle strength management**

   Patients with muscles with a strength grade of fair (3 of 5) and lower should begin **strength training** in a non–weight-bearing posture. Keep in mind that postural muscles that are abnormally long or short are not able to function properly. Isometric exercising of these muscles in a neutral position helps to reset the muscles' gamma bias and allows them to maintain the position. As their strength increases, cardinal plane and diagonal motions can be used while manual resistance is superimposed. Developmental sequence positions such as sidelying, pivot prone, prone on elbows, quadriped, and high kneeling are also good positions for alternating isometric exercises and rhythmic stabilization at the trunk.[19] Keep in mind the need for balance of agonist and antagonist muscle strength; functional needs when designing an exercise program; and the importance of specificity of training. Many repetitions and limited (low-level) resistance can be used to improve muscle endurance, whereas few repetitions and increased (high-level) resistance can be used to stimulate greater force production by the muscle. Consider that the majority of postural muscles are slow-twitch muscles with phasic function that function in relation to the body's aerobic capacity, which guides how weak muscles should be strengthened.

   See "Craniomandibular Examination and Treatment," Chapter 28; "Cervical Spine," Chapter 29; "Upper Extremity: Shoulder," Chapter 30; "Trunk," Chapter 32; "Lower Extremity: Hip," Chapter 33; "Lower Extremity: Knee," Chapter 34; "Lower Extremity: Ankle," Chapter 35; Chapter 35 for specific strengthening exercises.

3. **Ligament laxity management**

   Management of ligament laxity involves strength training and **proprioceptive training.** It can be accomplished through protected weight bearing with rhythmic stabilization at the shoulder or pelvis, weight shifting with and without rhythmic stabilization, unilateral weight bearing, and balance-board activities. Enhance somatosensory feedback by performing training exercises on the patient with and without his/her being able to see. As a progression, the Biomechanical Ankle Platform System (BAPS) board (Camp International, Inc.) is a relatively inexpensive balance-board system that has balls of varying size to alter stress and motion on the lower extremity and trunk. **Proper posture should be maintained to enhance the muscle response in proprioception.**

D. Management of controlled mobility dysfunction

Trauma, immobilization, and weakness lead to problems in weight bearing. Utilizing his/her enhanced mobility and stability, the patient should assume a neutral posture. Easing the patient into weight bearing involves **gradual protected weight bearing** during sitting and then with the use of parallel bars. While standing with a wide base of support, the patient should shift his/her weight over the foot. He/she should then move from side to side and from front to back. *The therapist should continue to stress the need for proper posture.* Isometric holds should be superimposed on the patient's shoulder or pelvis. Progress slowly, gradually increasing the patient's speed and decreasing the base of support. As the patient progresses, he/she should begin to perform a single-limb stance, increasing the time and perturbation as he/she improves. Again, use a balance board or BAPS-type system to improve proprioceptive input to the joints. Use of total-contact braces enhances the tactile input and proprioception.

E. Management of skill dysfunction

As the patient's ability to bear weight on stable surfaces improves, transfer him/her onto uneven surfaces (use foam, a pillow, or ramps as alternatives) and stairs. **Begin by having the patient assume a neutral posture.** He/she should step up and down on a stair or short stool, moving the tibia over the foot and increasing weight bearing by the foot. As the patient is able to bear full weight, he/she should progress to moving step over step. Jogging with progression to running is a further option. Use an elastic, bungee-type cord to apply more resistance. Keep in mind that ground reaction forces for jogging and running are three to four times greater than body weight force; therefore, the patient needs to be both mobile and stable in the lower extremities and spine. For more athletic rehabilitation, generalized lower extremity training tools such as the Fitter, Snowbounder, and Russian Leaper functionally train the lower extremities and trunk while enabling the patient to perform activity-specific training. Functional stabilization of the spine involves isometric, concentric, and eccentric training of the trunk with the patient in a relatively neutral spinal position. These exercises improve the ability of the trunk muscles to maintain stationary posture as well as to move the body safely through space.[20]

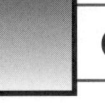

Clinical Decision-Making Cases

Case #1

HISTORY

At presentation, DM, a 64-year-old left-handed man, had pain in the left shoulder for many years. Eighteen months previously, the pain became worse, and he sought relief. Five months earlier he had undergone an acromioplasty on the left side to decrease the impingement. The pain decreased minimally after surgery but then returned to its presurgery level or worse. DM's medical history includes gallbladder surgery, previous right hip fracture, and stomach irritation from the use of nonsteroidal anti-inflammatory drugs. He is married with three grown children and lives in a ranch-style home. He is the vice president of sales for a major paintbrush company and travels 2 to 3 days a week, setting up displays.

EXAMINATION

Posture

See Figures 37–9 to 37–12 for DM's posture. DM's right shoulder was low (he stated that he had always had this problem). His shoulders are positioned forward bilaterally and he is in a forward head position. His scapulae are protracted and rotated upward bilaterally; they move too quickly, with glenohumeral elevation occurring on the left side. DM has V-shaped clavicles.

Soft Tissue

Maximal tissue tension was present in the anterior side of the chest and the posterolateral side of the neck. Tightness was also detected along the left distal biceps muscle region.

Trigger points were located throughout the scapula region, especially in the medial area (in the rhomboid muscles and the levator scapulae). The left side was worse than the right side.

Pain

DM had a pain score of 9 out of 10 (with 10 representing unbearable pain) in the left shoulder when he performed abduction activities (eg, reaching for a ticket at a toll booth). He had a pain score of 5 out of 10 in the upper trapezius region bilaterally, especially at the end of the day.

Joint Play	Joint Play on the Left Side	Joint Play on the Right Side
Glenohumeral inferior glide	1/3	2/3
Glenohumeral posterior glide	1/3	2/3
Glenohumeral anterior glide	2/3	2/3
Scapulothoracic retraction	1/3	2/3
Scapulothoracic down rotation	1/3	2/3
Scapulothoracic protraction	3/3	3/3
Sternoclavicular glides	1/3	2+/3
Acromioclavicular glides	2/3	2/3

ROM

Motion	Range on Left, Degrees	Range on Right, Degrees
Glenohumeral flexion	115	135
Glenohumeral abduction	85	115
Glenohumeral internal rotation	60	60
Glenohumeral external rotation	30	80
Elbow extension	−5	0

Strength

DM's strength scores on a scale of 0 to 5 (with 5 representing normal strength) were as follows:

Hypertrophied anterior and middle deltoid muscle strength bilaterally—5/5.
Atrophied left posterior deltoid—2/5.
Atrophied left middle trapezius—3/5.
Atrophied left rhomboids—1/5.
External rotators—2/5.

DM was unable to assume the test position for lower trapezius muscle testing, and his right upper extremity tested grossly within normal limits.

ASSESSMENT AND DIAGNOSIS

DM was diagnosed with severe adhesive capsulitis of the left glenohumeral joint with mild capsulitis on the right side secondary to chronic impingement syndrome. The impingement syndrome stemmed from the chronic postural changes and the activities at work that required him to move both of his upper extremities greater than 90 degrees in the sagittal and coronal planes. The physical therapist believed that DM would benefit from mobilization and scapula exercises to increase strength, ROM, and joint play. The prognosis was good that DM should be able to function with a tolerable level of pain.

TREATMENT GOALS

Short-Term Goals

DM would demonstrate balanced strength in his bilateral shoulder girdle in 5 months.
He would demonstrate equal ROM and joint play in his bilateral shoulder girdle in 5 months.
DM would demonstrate a decrease in the pain score associated with function to a level of 5 out of 10 in 2 months.

Long-Term Goal

The patient would demonstrate equal function in his right and left shoulder girdle in 6 months.

TREATMENT PLAN

Treatment consisted of connective-tissue massage to the anterior chest wall and shoulder joint; joint mobilization for the glenohumeral, sternoclavicular, acromioclavicular, and scapulothoracic joints; exercise of the scapula and shoulder musculature; and massage with ice. DM was also to perform a home program that focused on scapula stability and glenohumeral mobility.

RE-EVALUATION

DM made some significant gains in strength and ROM over a 3-month period.

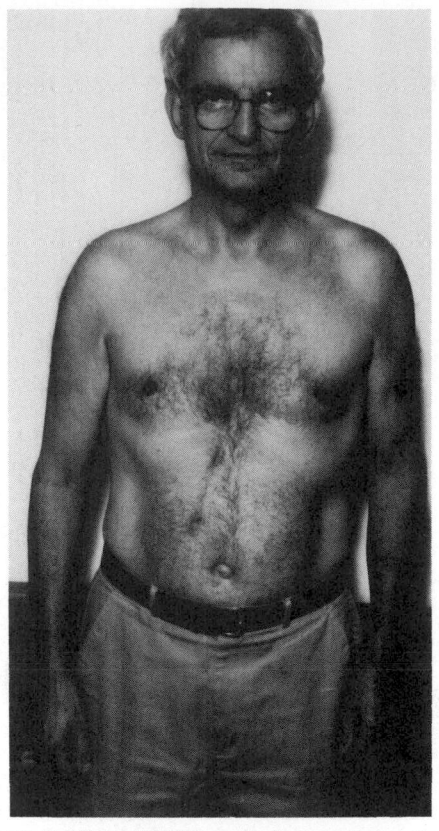

FIGURE 37–9   Patient DM: frontal plane, anterior view.

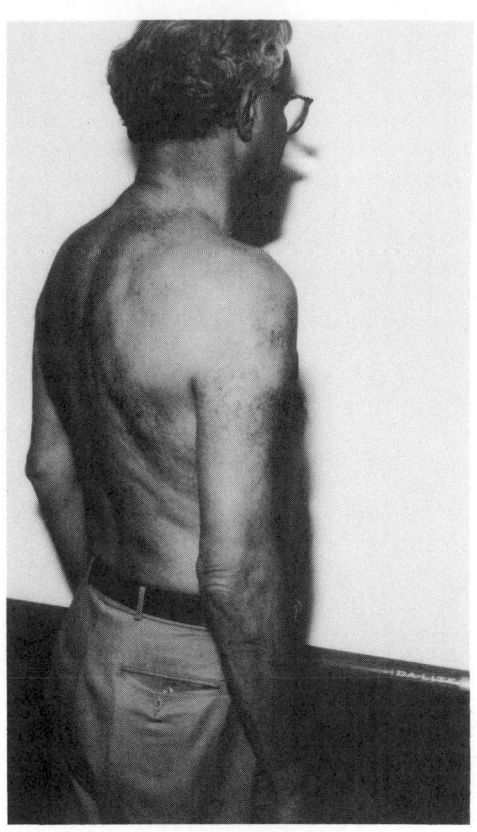

FIGURE 37–11   Patient DM: oblique view

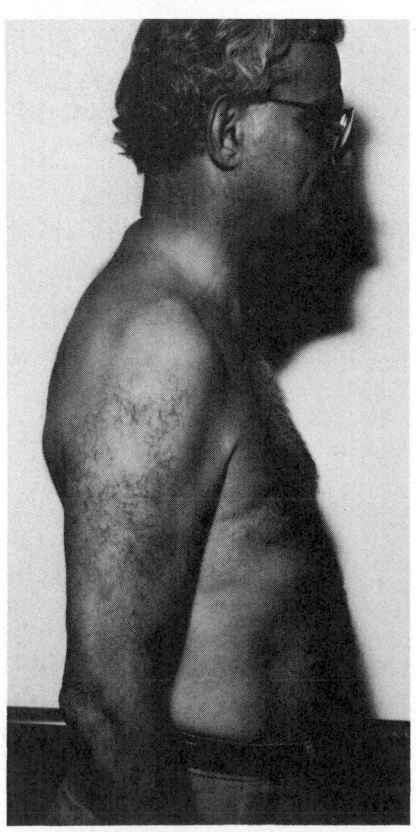

FIGURE 37–10   Patient DM: sagittal plane view.

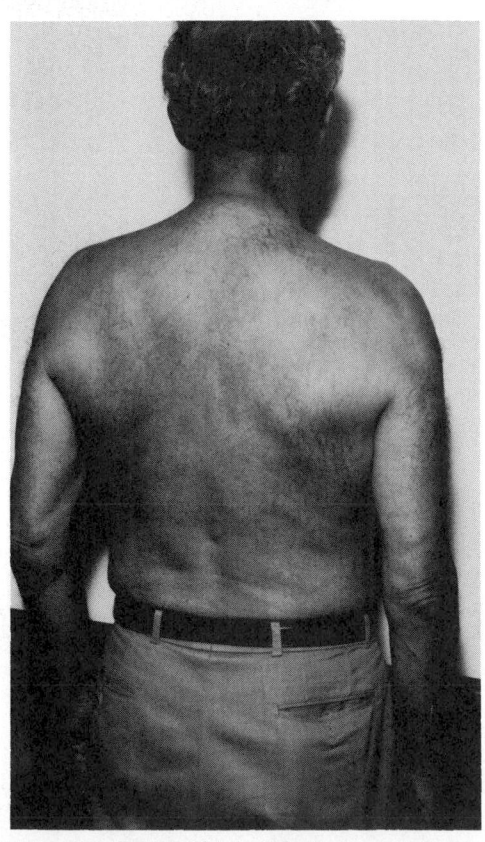

FIGURE 37–12   Patient DM: frontal plane, posterior view.

Joint Play

Joint Motion	Joint Play on the Left Side	Joint Play on the Right Side
Glenohumeral inferior glide	2/3	2/3
Glenohumeral posterior glide	2/3	2/3
Glenohumeral anterior glide	4/3	3/3
Sternoclavicular glides	3/3	2/3
Scapulothoracic medial glide	3/3	3/3

ROM

Motion	Range on Left Side, Degrees	Range on Right Side, Degrees
Glenohumeral flexion	135	140
Glenohumeral abduction	105	115
Glenohumeral external rotation	70	90

Strength

DM's strength scores were as follows:

The deltoid, biceps, triceps, and pectoralis major muscles—5/5 bilaterally.
The rotator cuff muscles on the left—3/5.
The rhomboid muscles had become equal bilaterally (5/5).
The lower trapezius—3/5 on the left and 4/5 on the right.

Pain

DM was sensitive to palpation along the posterolateral capsule. Infrequent impingement was present in the acromioclavicular area (only when the joint was at extremes of abduction and external rotation). DM felt achiness after treatment, but this sensation went away after several hours.

Assessment

The major problems continued to be decreased inferior capsule joint play and restricted abduction, tightness and hypertrophy of the anterior shoulder and chest muscles, decreased scapula stabilization, and significant weakness of the rotator cuff muscles. DM continued to experience impingement, although the intensity and duration of his pain had decreased, especially within 48 to 72 hours after the initiation of therapy.

At that point, the therapist wanted to improve the mobility of both glenohumeral joints to normal (3/3) and to see the strength of the lower trapezius muscle increase, because the left scapula was still too mobile too quickly during elevation. The therapist worked toward accomplishing these goals within 2 months. DM was very compliant with his exercise program, which made the therapist's work a lot simpler. Physical therapy sessions took place once or twice a week (depending on DM's availability) and included joint mobilization, stretching, strengthening, myofascial work, and the application of ice.

OUTCOME AND DISCHARGE SUMMARY

DM made significant gains and was able to stop seeing the physical therapist after 5 months of therapy; he was to continue with an aggressive home program.

Joint Play

Joint Motion	Joint Play on the Left Side	Joint Play on the Right Side
Glenohumeral inferior glide	3/3	3/3
Glenohumeral posterior glide	3/3	3/3
Glenohumeral anterior glide	4/3	3/3
Sternoclavicular glides	3/3	3/3
Scapulothoracic medial glide	3/3	3/3

ROM

Motion	Range on the Left Side, Degrees	Range on the Right Side, Degrees
Glenohumeral flexion	135	140
Glenohumeral abduction	115	115
Glenohumeral external rotation	80	90

Strength

DM's muscle strength scores were as follows:

The deltoid, biceps, triceps, and pectoralis major muscles—5/5 bilaterally.
The rotator cuff muscle—5/5 on the left side.
The rhomboid muscles were equal bilaterally (5/5). The lower trapezius muscle—5/5 on the left and 5/5 on the right.

Pain

Infrequent impingement was present in the acromioclavicular area, but only when the joint was at the extremes of abduction and external rotation.

Case #2

HISTORY

At presentation, GS was a 54-year-old chief executive for a major utility company. He had back and radiating right buttock and leg pain; he consulted a physical therapist to request "an exercise program." He was having trouble coping with the pain, given the demands of his work (he sits for long hours in meetings and also travels once or twice a month).

GS had pain for more than 15 years, with no specific trauma. He had spent several years in a concentration camp as a child, where he had been forced to perform heavy labor and had been beaten periodically. He had also suffered numerous injuries while fighting in the Hungarian Revolution during his late teens. He said that his back had never been totally pain free, but over the previous few years, it had definitely become worse. He liked to jog for stress release. Radiographs and magnetic resonance imaging demonstrated moderate lumbar and mild thoracic osteoarthritic changes and mild herniation at L5, S1 on the right side. GS had never had spinal surgery, and numerous physicians have suggested that he is not a candidate for such surgery.

EXAMINATION

Posture

GS had flat back posture with no scoliotic curves. He was of average size and build. His back musculature appeared tight, and his abdominal muscles appeared to have adequate tone.

Active Movements

GS's movements showed significantly decreased forward and backward flexion with lumbar pain. Lateral flexion was somewhat restricted bilaterally. The straight leg raising test demonstrated a range of 60 degrees bilaterally; a modified Thomas test showed abduction and external rotation of the limb on the right side and abduction of the limb on the left. Both sides showed hip flexor muscle tightness.

Soft Tissue

Tissue along the spine was extremely dense and very difficult to stretch. A temperature increase also was noted along the lumbar paraspinal and the spinous processes.

Passive Movements

GS's intervertebral joint movement score was 1/3 in the lumbar spine. Pain was noted on movement at L5, S1. The thoracic spine intervertebral movement score was 2/3.

Strength

Weakness was present in the trunk and hip muscles; the muscle strength scores were generally 3+/5, although it was difficult to determine whether GS was weak because he had pain or had pain because he was weak when doing trunk motions. His abdominal muscles appeared to be toned. (GS stated that he does 25 sit-ups a day when not in extreme pain.)

Neurological Factors

No numbness or tingling was noted, and no gross lower extremity weakness or dermatomal changes were present. Lower extremity reflexes were slow but equal bilaterally.

Pain

GS had a very high pain tolerance. Sitting was his worst position; lying flat on his back was his best. His mattress was very firm, allowing him to get comfortable at night.

ASSESSMENT AND DIAGNOSIS

GS was diagnosed as having long-standing spinal dysfunction that probably stemmed from injuries sustained in his youth. His flat back posture rendered his spine relatively noncompliant to stresses from prolonged sitting at work and jogging in the morning. The more GS sat and the more emotional stress he had, the worse his symptoms became. On diagnosis, GS was having an acute exacerbation of the chronic lumbar dysfunction. Therefore, he first required acute management, followed by a home maintenance program.

TREATMENT GOALS

Short-Term Goals

GS would demonstrate a decrease in his lumbar spine pain score from 8/10 to 4/10 in 1 month.

He would demonstrate no temperature or color changes in the lumbar tissue in 2 weeks.

He would demonstrate full hip ROM in 10 weeks.

The patient would demonstrate strength scores of 5/5 in his trunk extensor, abdominal (rectus and oblique) and gluteus maximus muscles in 10 weeks.

GS would demonstrate lumbar joint play with a score of 2/3 and minimal restriction in active trunk ROM in 10 weeks.

He would demonstrate knowledge of proper body mechanics, including how long he could comfortably sit and in what position, how long he could stand and in which postures, and which exercises would be most effective in 1 week.

Long-Term Goal

GS would return to functioning at work with a tolerable pain level in 3 months.

TREATMENT OUTCOMES

GS responded well to treatment. The acute symptoms resolved over 2 weeks with myofascial release, gentle trunk ROM exercises, and the application of ice. Once the inflammatory condition subsided, Grade 2 to 3 spinal joint mobilization and more vigorous strengthening of the hip extensor, back extensor, and abdominal oblique muscles was begun. He stretched his hip flexor and hamstring muscles on a daily basis. GS performed strengthening exercises in the developmental sequence, starting with the pivot prone position and moving to a position on the hands and knees, using functional stabilization techniques. As GS gained more lumbar mobility, he worked on achieving a neutral position and was able to gain slight lordosis. He then attempted to exercise in the neutral position. A pool was available in which GS could walk, swim, and exercise. This improved his aerobic capacity and caused his pain to diminish dramatically. After 2 months, GS had normal strength in the trunk, and his lumbar intervertebral motion score had improved to 2/3. He had lengthened his hamstring muscle by 20 degrees and his hip flexor length by 10 degrees. He was swimming 30 minutes three to four times a week, and his pain score had decreased to 2/10.

GS did not expect all of his pain to resolve. A significant part of the treatment process involved educating the patient on how to help himself. He was able to perform 15 to 20 minutes of strengthening and stretching exercises each day along with the swimming. He was educated on the proper sitting and standing postures, and he used a lumbar roll in his car and at work. It was suggested that he not perform high-impact activities such as jogging, but rather walk or swim on a regular basis. If he were able to maintain trunk strength and mobility and to keep his cardiovascular state healthy, he would be able to keep his pain at a tolerable level. These methods also gave him some degree of control over his symptoms, increasing his responsibility and reducing that of the therapist.

References

1. Lehmkuhl LD, Smith LK: *Brunnstrom's Clinical Kinesiology*, 4th ed. Philadelphia, F. A. Davis Company, 1984.
2. Posture and Its Relationship to Orthopedic Disabilities. A Report of the Posture Committee of the American Academy of Orthopedic Surgeons. vol. 1. 1947.
3. Kendall FP, McCreary EK: *Muscles Testing and Function*, 4th ed. Baltimore, Williams & Wilkins, 1993.
4. Basmajian JV, DeLuca CJ: *Muscles Alive*, 5th ed. Baltimore, Williams & Wilkins, 1993.
5. Norkin CC, Levangie PK: *Joint Structure and Function*, 2nd ed. Philadelphia, F. A. Davis Company, 1992.
6. Nashner LM: Concepts for understanding sensory and motor components of human balance. Presented at the Massachusetts Chapter of the American Physical Therapy Association Conference, Boston, MA, 1991.
7. Kaltenborn FM: *Manual Mobilization of the Extremity Joints*, 4th ed. Oslo, Olaf Norlis Bokhandel, 1989.
8. Maitland GD: *Peripheral Manipulation*, 4th ed. London, Butterworth, 1977.
9. Paris SV: Extremity mobilization and dysfunction [Course notes]. 1979.
10. Daniels L, Worthingham C: *Muscle Testing Techniques of Manual Examination*. Philadelphia, W. B. Saunders Company, 1972.
11. Magee DJ: *Orthopedic Physical Assessment*, 2nd ed. Philadelphia, W. B. Saunders Company, 1992, pp. 438–513.
12. Stockmeyer SA: Personal communication, 1993.
13. Sullivan PE, Markos PD, Minor MA: *An Integrated Approach to Therapeutic Exercise: Theory and Application*. Reston, VA, Reston Publishing Company, 1982.
14. Tappan FM: *Healing Massage Techniques*. Reston, VA, Reston Publishing Company, 1978.
15. Manheim CJ, Lavett DK: *The Myofascial Release Manual*. Thorofare, NJ, Slack, 1989.
16. Cantu RI, Grodin AJ: *Myofascial Manipulation*. Gaithersburg, MD, Aspen, 1992.
17. Cyriax J: *Textbook of Orthopedic Medicine: Diagnosis of Soft Tissue Lesions*. vol. 1. London, Baillière Tindall, 1975.
18. Feldenkrais M: *Awareness Through Movement*. San Francisco, Harper & Row, 1977.
19. Voss DE, Ionta MK, Myers BJ: *Proprioceptive Neuromuscular Facilitation*, 3rd ed. Philadelphia, Harper & Row, 1985.
20. Saal JA: Dynamic muscular stabilization in the nonoperative treatment of lumbar pain syndromes. *Orthop Rev* 1990, 19:691–700.

Suggested Reading

Bucholz W, Lippert FG: *Orthopedic Decision Making*. St. Louis, C. V. Mosby Company, 1984.

Cailliet R: *Low Back Pain Syndrome*, 2nd ed. Philadelphia, F. A. Davis Company, 1983.

Cailliet R: *Neck and Arm Pain*. Philadelphia, F. A. Davis Company, 1983.

Cyriax J, Cyriax P: *Illustrated Manual of Orthopedic Medicine*. London, Butterworth, 1983.

Cyriax J: *Textbook of Orthopedic Medicine: Treatment by Manipulation, Massage, and Injection*, 8th ed. vol. 2. London, Baillière Tindall, 1971.

Edmond SL: *Manipulation and Mobilization*. St. Louis, C. V. Mosby Company, 1993.

Hertling D, Kessler R: *Management of Common Musculoskeletal Disorders*, 2nd ed. Philadelphia, J. B. Lippincott Company, 1990.

Kissner C, Colby LA: *Therapeutic Exercise: Foundations and Principles*, 2nd ed. Philadelphia, F. A. Davis Company, 1990.

Mennel J: *Joint Pain: Diagnosis and Treatment Using Manipulative Techniques*. Boston, Little, Brown and Company, 1964.

Palmer ML, Epler M: *Clinical Assessment Procedures in Physical Therapy*. Philadelphia, J. B. Lippincott Company, 1990.

Wadsworth CT: *Manual Examination and Treatment of the Spine and Extremities*. Baltimore, Williams & Wilkins, 1988.

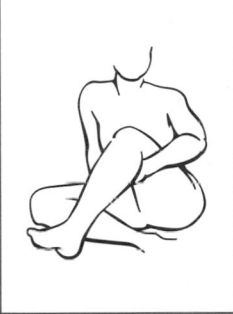

CHAPTER 38

Gait

Lisa M. Giallonardo

I. Introduction to Gait

A. General Information

1. Normal gait is a rhythmic movement of the body that propels it from one point to another with the most efficient use of energy.[1]

2. The center of gravity (COG) is the most important factor in gait; the body has a 2-in excursion horizontally and vertically to absorb ground reaction force and to shift weight from one foot to the other, respectively. Through each step, the COG remains inside the pelvis. The COG movement can be described as a smooth sinusoidal curve that should not deviate more than a few centimeters.[2]

3. The majority of muscle action during gait is eccentric, which means that it is used to slow down the effects of gravity and momentum.[1–3]

4. Nelson[4] suggested that there are three phases of gait that require certain fundamental skills for ambulation ability. Each phase has musculoskeletal and neuromuscular requirements, and without the successful execution of each phase, gait is not smooth and efficient.[4]

   a. First phase. The first phase of gait involves the "ability to provide a stable base of support for the body while standing on both limbs and also on each limb separately with and without hand support."[4] This phase occurs during heel strike to foot flat (initial contact and loading response in the phases of gait described by the Ranchos Los Amigos Gait Laboratory [RLA]).

   b. Second phase. During the second phase, "efficient transfer of weight from one limb to the other in a rhythmic and relatively rapid fashion" takes place.[4] This occurs during foot flat to midstance and during midstance to heel off (midstance and terminal stance in RLA).

   c. Third phase. The third phase consists of "alternating weight transfer during forward progression."[4] It occurs during toe off to acceleration; acceleration to midswing; and midswing to deceleration (preswing, initial swing, midswing, and terminal swing in RLA).

B. Definitions[1,2,5,6]

1. **Gait cycle.** The period between ipsilateral foot contacts (essentially, two steps).

2. **Temporal (time-related) variables**
   a. **Cycle time.** The time (in seconds) of one complete gait cycle.
   b. **Stance time.** The stance time is the time (in seconds) that one foot is in contact with the support surface.
   c. **Single-support time.** The time (in seconds) that one foot is the sole contact with the support surface during one gait cycle.
   d. **Double-support time.** The total time (in seconds) that both feet have contact with the support surface.
   e. **Step duration.** The time (in seconds) between contralateral foot contacts.
   f. **Stride duration.** The time (in seconds) between ipsilateral foot contacts.
   g. **Cadence.** The number of steps per unit time; normal cadence ranges from 70 to 130 steps per minute.

3. **Spatial (distance-related) variables**
   a. **Step length.** The distance (in centimeters) between heel strikes of contralateral feet; normal range is 37.5 to 50 cm.
   b. **Stride length.** The distance (in centimeters) between heel strikes of ipsilateral feet; the normal range is 75 to 100 cm.
   c. **Stride width.** The distance (in centimeters) between the midline of contralateral heel strikes; the normal range is 7.5 to 15 cm.
   d. **Toe out.** The angulation of the long axis of the foot (in degrees) to the line of walking progression; the normal range is up to 15 degrees.

4. **Walking velocity.** The number of centimeters per second walked or the rate of forward body motion.

5. **Phases of gait cycle (traditional)**
   a. **Heel strike.** The initial contact of the foot with the support surface.
   b. **Heel strike to foot flat.** The initial contact of the foot with the support surface to when the foot is in total contact with the support surface.
   c. **Foot flat to midstance.** The movement of body weight directly over the supporting limb.
   d. **Midstance to heel off.** The movement of body weight in front of the stance limb as a preparation for push off.

e. **Toe off.** The phase when the toe is in contact with the support surface.
f. **Toe off to acceleration.** When the foot leaves the ground and the limb moves toward alignment with the stance limb.
g. **Acceleration to midswing.** When the swing limb moves in line with the stance limb.
h. **Midswing to deceleration.** When the swing limb moves in front of the trunk and begins to slow down in preparation for heel strike.

6. **Phases of gait (RLA)**
   a. **Initial contact.** The point at which the foot strikes the support surface is the initial contact.
   b. **Loading response.** Shock absorption occurs as the foot becomes flat while the body moves forward; ends when the contralateral limb leaves the support surface.
   c. **Midstance.** Begins at single-limb support and progresses to when the body is over and in front of the stance limb.
   d. **Terminal stance.** The phase from the end of midstance to the point of heel off (just before the contralateral limb strikes the ground).
   e. **Preswing.** The phase from heel off to when the toe pushes off of the support surface.
   f. **Initial swing.** Begins at toe off and continues until maximal knee flexion occurs.
   g. **Midswing.** Extends from maximal knee flexion to when the tibia is vertical.
   h. **Terminal swing.** Involves the slowing of swing limb just prior to its contact with the support surface.

7. **Determinants of gait**
   a. Inman and colleagues[2] described six essential elements for smooth and efficient gait.
      (1). The first element is **pelvic rotation.**
         (a). Description. The pelvis rotates right and left around a vertical axis about 4 degrees in each direction; rotation increases markedly with an increase in the speed of gait.
         (b). Purpose. Rotation negates the need for excessive horizontal trunk motion and also decreases the impact of ground reaction forces.
         (c). Two problems related to pelvic rotation are as follows:

(i). When pelvic rotation is diminished or absent, the need for hip flexion increases to propel the body forward (increasing energy expense); diminished or absent rotation also would increase ground reaction force through the lower extremities and trunk.

(ii). When pelvic rotation is increased, too much energy is expended in rotating the pelvis while the body moves forward.

(2). The second element is **pelvic list.**

(a). Description. The pelvis drops down slightly on the side of the swing limb.

(b). Purpose. Lowers the COG and contributes to the effectiveness of the abductor mechanism by producing relative abduction of the swing limb.

(c). Problems. Weakness of the abductor mechanism causes Trendelenburg gait (excessive lowering of the pelvis on the swing side, which lengthens that limb and makes ground clearance difficult).

(3). The third element is **knee flexion in stance.**

(a). Description. Knee flexion occurs at heel strike and again at heel off.

(b). Purpose. Knee flexion smooths the transition between the swing and stance phases, flattens out COG shifts, and increases shock absorption of ground reaction force.

(c). Problems related to knee flexion include the following:

(i). If the quadriceps femoris is weak and the body does not compensate, then too much knee flexion may occur; this results in knee buckling. If the body does compensate, stiff-legged gait may result to prevent knee buckling. The latter disorder causes problems with shock absorption.

(ii). Weak hamstring muscles

may result in genu recurvatum (knee hyperextension). This disorder results in problems with shock absorption.

(4). The fourth element is **ankle dorsiflexion in stance.**

(a). Description. Ankle dorsiflexion is the movement of the tibia over the foot during the foot flat to midstance and midstance to heel off phases.

(b). Purpose. Ankle dorsiflexion lowers the COG and propels the body forward.

(c). Two problems related to ankle dorsiflexion are as follow:

(i). A weak tibialis anterior causes the foot to slap at the heel strike to foot flat phase and requires more energy to propel the body forward.

(ii). Decreased ankle dorsiflexion requires subtalar and midtarsal compensation through excessive pronation.

(5). The fifth element is **coordinated knee, ankle, and foot motion.**

(a). The movement can be described as follows:

(i). The knee flexes, the ankle plantar flexes, then dorsiflexes, and the foot pronates from heel strike to midstance.

(ii). The knee extends, the ankle plantar flexes, and the foot supinates from midstance to heel off.

(b). The purpose of this movement is as follows:

(i). The effective coordination of the movement of the knee, ankle, and foot lowers the COG and increases shock absorption of the entire lower extremity; it also prevents abrupt changes in the COG, keeping its motion in a smooth sinusoidal curve.

(ii). Extension of the limb slows depression of the COG by lengthening the limb during push off.

(c). Problems. Diminished motion at one joint requires overcompensation by the other (*eg*, weak hamstring muscles and the resultant genu recurvatum cause more ankle dorsiflexion or increased foot pronation if the COG is to be lowered sufficiently).

(6). The sixth element is **lateral trunk displacement.**

(a). Description. The stride width (width of the base of support) and the tibiofemoral angle (with slight genu valgum) permits the tibia to remain vertical and the feet relatively close together.

(b). Purpose. Lateral trunk displacement prevents the need for horizontal excursion.

(c). Two problems related to lateral trunk displacement are:

(i). A decreased tibiofemoral angle results in genu varum (bowed legs); this increases the body's side-to-side movement.

(ii). An increased tibiofemoral angle results in genu valgum (knock knees); this causes the base of support to be too wide and more energy to be used to shift from one limb to another.

8. For a summary of kinematic and kinetic forces of normal gait, see Tables 38–1 to 38–4.[7]

Table 38–1. SUMMARY OF JOINT MOTIONS AND FORCES DURING STANCE PHASE: FOOT AND ANKLE

	Kinematic Motion		Kinetic Motion	
Phase	**Foot**	**Ankle**	**External Forces**	**Internal Forces**
Heel strike	Supination: (rigid) at heel contact	Moving into plantar flexion	Reaction forces behind joint axis; plantar flexion moment at heel strike	Dorsiflexors (the tibialis anterior, extensor digitorum longus, and the extensor hallucis longus) contract eccentrically to slow down plantar flexion
Foot flat	Pronation: adapting to support surface	Plantar flexion to dorsiflexion over a fixed foot	Maximum plantar flexion moment is reached; reaction forces begin to shift anterior, producing a dorsiflexion moment	Dorsiflexion activity decreases; the tibialis posterior, the flexor hallucis longus, and the flexor digitorum longus are working eccentrically to control pronation
Midstance	Neutral	3° of dorsiflexion	Slight dorsiflexion moment	Plantar flexor muscles (gastrocsoleus and peroneal muscles) are activated to control dorsiflexion of the tibia and fibula over a fixed foot contracting eccentrically
Heel off	Supination as foot becomes rigid for push off	15° dorsiflexion toward plantar flexion	Maximal dorsiflexion moment	Plantar flexor muscles are beginning to contract concentrically to prepare for push off
Toe off	Supination	20° plantar flexion	Dorsiflexion moment	Plantar flexor muscles are at peak activity but become inactive as foot leaves the ground

Table 38–2. SUMMARY OF JOINT MOTIONS AND FORCES DURING STANCE PHASE: KNEE AND TIBIA

| Phase | Kinematic Motion | | Kinetic Motion | |
	Knee	Tibia	External Forces	Internal Forces
Heel strike	In full extension before heel contact; flexes as heel strikes floor	Slightly externally rotated	Rapid increase in reaction forces behind knee joint causing flexion moment	Quadriceps femoris contracts eccentrically to control rapid knee flexion and to prevent buckling
Foot flat	In 20° flexion moving toward extension	Internally rotating	Flexion moment	After foot flat, quadriceps femoris activity becomes concentric to bring femur over tibia
Midstance	In 15° flexion moving toward extension	Neutral	Maximum flexion moment	Decrease in quadriceps femoris activity, gastrocnemius working eccentrically to control excessive knee extension
Heel off	In 4° flexion moving toward extension	Externally rotated	Reaction force moves anterior to joint; extension moment	Gastrocnemius begins to work concentrically to start knee flexion
Toe off	Moves from near full extension to 40° flexion	Externally rotated	Reaction forces move posterior to joint as knee flexes; flexion moment	Quadriceps femoris contracting eccentrically

Table 38–3. SUMMARY OF JOINT MOTIONS AND FORCES DURING STANCE PHASE: HIP

| Phase | Kinematic Motion | Kinetic Motion | |
		External Forces	Internal Forces
Heel strike	20°–40° of hip flexion moving toward extension Slight adduction and external rotation	Reaction force in front of joint-flexion moment moving toward extension forward pelvic rotation	Gluteus maximus and hamstrings working eccentrically to resist flexion moment Erector spinae working eccentrically to resist forward bend
Foot flat	Hip moves into extension, adduction, internal rotation	Flexion moment	Gluteus maximus and hamstrings contracting concentrically to bring hip into extension Erector spinae resist trunk flexion
Midstance	Moving through neutral position Pelvis is rotating posterior	Reaction force is posterior to hip joint; extension moment	Iliopsoas works eccentrically to resist extension Gluteus medius contracting in reverse action to stabilize opposite pelvis
Heel off	10°–15° extension of hip abduction, external rotation	Extension moment decreases after double-limb support begins	Iliopsoas activity continues
Toe off	Moves toward 10° extension, abduction, external rotation	Decrease of extension moment	Adductor magnus works eccentrically to control or stabilize pelvis Iliopsoas activity continues

Table 38–4. SUMMARY OF JOINT MOTION AND FORCES DURING SWING PHASE: ACCELERATION TO MIDSWING AND MIDSWING TO DECELERATION

| Joint | Acceleration to Midswing | | Midswing to Deceleration | |
	Kinematic Motion	Kinetic Motion	Kinematic Motion	Kinetic Motion
Hip	Slight flexion (0°–15°) moving to 30° flexion and external rotation to neutral	Hip flexors work concentrically to bring limb through; contralateral gluteus medius concentrically contracts to maintain pelvis position	Continues to flex around 30°–40°	Gluteus maximus contracts eccentrically to slow hip flexion
Knee	30°–60° knee flexion and lateral rotation of tibia moving toward neutral	Hamstrings concentrically contract	Moving to near full extension and slight external tibial rotation	Quadriceps femoris contracts concentrically and hamstrings contract eccentrically
Ankle/foot	20° dorsiflexion and slight pronation	Dorsiflexors contract concentrically	Ankle in neutral; foot in slight supination	Dorsiflexors contract isometrically

II. Examination

A. Subjective

1. Ask the patient about his/her perception of the problem or problems to better focus the objective evaluation.
   a. Determine whether the patient thinks that the problem is related to a particular activity, such as walking certain distances, climbing stairs, or running (leading you to focus on contractile tissue).
   b. Determine whether the patient thinks that the problem is chronic (leading you to reproduce the exact symptoms during the evaluation).
2. Discuss the patient's goals so that they may be incorporated into your goals as well as into the treatment-planning process.
   a. Determine whether the patient wants to participate in a particular activity, such as running, that requires a certain level of muscle strength or joint range of motion (ROM).

B. Objective

1. **History**
   a. Elicit information concerning any trauma; this includes a complete description of the mechanism of injury.
   b. Discuss symptom presentation (see Table 35–1).

2. **Inspection.** Normal gait requires normal joint play and ROM as well as normal muscle length and strength. Lower extremity and trunk evaluation must be performed to pinpoint the causation of gait faults. See "Cervical Spine," Chapter 29; "Lower Extremity: Hip," Chapter 33; "Lower Extremity: Knee." Chapter 34; "Lower Extremity: Ankle," Chapter 35; and "Lower Extremity: Foot," Chapter 36 for techniques.
   a. *Observational gait analysis*
      (1). Note the patient's standing posture, including the base of support, and observe overall the way that the patient walks.
      (2). Information should then be gathered **systematically;** evaluate **one joint** at a time and **one view** (frontal or sagittal) at a time. Start at the foot and work upward.
      (3). Use of an analysis form is very helpful (see Figure 38–1); the RLA form is an alternative that includes a delineation of significant gait deviations at each joint.[5]
      (4). Have the patient walk without shoes, with shoes, and with shoes and orthoses, if applicable, making note of any differences, both positive and negative.
      (5). Other types of gait, including race

Gait Limb	Heel Strike, Foot Flat	Foot Flat, Midstance	Midstance, Heel Off	Heel Off, Toe Off	Acceleration, Midswing	Midswing, Deceleration
Trunk						
Hip						
Knee						
Tibia						
Ankle						
Foot						

FIGURE 38–1 Gait analysis form.

Table 38–5.   COMMON GAIT PATHOLOGIES

Deviation	Phase	Cause
Excessive foot pronation	Midstance through toe off	Compensated forefoot or rearfoot varus deformity; uncompensated forefoot valgus deformity; pes planus; decreased ankle dorsiflexion; increased tibial varum; long limb; uncompensated internal rotation of tibia or femur; weak tibialis posterior
Excessive foot supination	Heel strike through midstance	Compensated forefoot valgus deformity; pes cavus; short limb; uncompensated external rotation of tibia or femur
Bouncing or exaggerated plantar flexion	Midstance through toe off	Heel cord contracture; increased tone of gastrocsoleus muscle
Insufficient push off	Midstance through toe off	Gastrocsoleus weakness; Achilles tendon rupture; metatarsalgia; hallux rigidus
Foot slap	Heel strike to foot flat	Dorsiflexor weakness
Steppage gait (hip and knee flex to clear foot)	Acceleration through deceleration	Dorsiflexor weakness
Excessive knee flexion	Heel strike through toe off	Hamstring contracture; decreased ROM ankle dorsiflexion; plantar flexor muscle weakness; lengthened limb; hip flexion contracture
Genu recurvatum (knee hyperextension)	Heel strike through midstance	Quadriceps femoris weak or short; compensated hamstring weakness; Achilles tendon contracture; habit
Excessive medial or lateral femur rotation	Heel strike through toe off	Medial or lateral hamstrings tight, respectively; or opposite muscle group weakness; anteversion or retroversion, respectively
Increased base of support (BOS) (greater than 4 in)	Heel strike through toe off	Abductor muscle contracture; instability; genu valgum; leg length discrepancy
Decreased BOS (less than 2 in)	Heel strike through toe off	Adductor muscle contracture; genu varum
Circumduction	Acceleration through deceleration	Increased limb length; abductor muscle shortening or overuse
Hip hiking	Acceleration through deceleration	Increased limb length; hamstring weakness; quadratus lumborum shortening
Inadequate hip flexion	Acceleration through heel strike	Hip flexor muscle weakness; hip extensor muscle shortening; increased limb length
Inadequate hip extension	Midstance through toe off	Hip flexion contracture; hip extensor muscle weakness
Excessive trunk back-bending	Heel strike through midstance	Hip extensor or flexor muscle weakness; hip pain; decreased knee ROM
Excessive trunk forward bending	Deceleration through midstance	Quadriceps femoris and gluteus maximus weakness
Excessive trunk lateral flexion (compensated Trendelenburg gait)	Foot flat though heel off	Gluteus medius weakness
Pelvic drop	Foot flat through heel off	Contralateral gluteus medius weakness

walking, jogging, and running, can also be observed in a similar manner.

(6). Videotaped gait analysis is helpful because it allows the therapist to observe certain sections repeatedly or in slow motion; the use of a treadmill, although somewhat artificial and difficult for some patients, aids in observation with and without videotaping. Start the patient on the treadmill at a slow pace, and gradually increase the speed to approximate the patient's normal cadence. The patient's arms should hang down and should be allowed to swing naturally. The patient should be videotaped from anterior and posterior frontal plane views as well as from a sagittal view. Stabilizing the camera on a tripod is also useful.

b. *Gait analysis systems*

(1). Several techniques are available for more complex gait analysis. Choice depends on equipment availability, cost, patient diagnosis (pathology), and desired functional data. Perry[5] provides a detailed analysis of available techniques. All systems begin with observational gait analysis as the core technique.

(a). **Motion analysis** gives quantifiable and detailed data on the intricacies of joint motion in all three planes. Several tools are used to measure and record motion. Electrogoniometers (single-axle and multiaxial types that are attached to recorders) are used to gather specific ROM values. The addition of cameras or computers allows the therapist to record motion visually and to digitize values.[5,8]

(b). **Dynamic electromyography,** with surface or fine wire electrodes, is used to measure the timing and intensity of muscle function during gait activities. Occasionally, some approximation of muscle force may be made. Generally, electromyography is used as a method to determine which muscles should be the focus of the treatment of gait dysfunction. It can be used to determine when and how strenuously a muscle is working as well as how its function corresponds to that of other muscles and to that of the opposite limb.[3,5,9]

(c). **Ground reaction force and vector analysis** can aid in gait analysis. The ground reaction forces are the vertical, horizontal, and rotatory forces that are transmitted through the lower extremity during each step. These forces can be measured with a force plate and transducers on a walkway. The center of pressure and shear forces can also be determined. This information can be used in the management of patients with diminished sensation.[2,5,10] Orthotic fabrication, with wedging to offset increased pressure, is just one example of how treatment is influenced by this gait tool.

(d). **Stride analysis** can also be used to analyze gait. The temporal and spatial characteristics described (in the definitions section of this chapter) are a measure of the combined musculoskeletal and neuromuscular function. Tools such as a stopwatch, foot switch, or sensored walkway can measure stride and step width, length, and duration as well as cadence and velocity. Even simple tools like paper and a sole marking device can measure distance parameters.[1,5]

(e). **Energy expenditure** is another measurement that can aid in gait analysis. The function of the cardiopulmonary system can be evaluated during walking and running activities. Metabolic energy measures such as oxygen cost, heart and respiratory rate, and blood pressure are evaluated while the patient is ambulating on a treadmill.[5,11]

III. Assessment

Evaluate the objective findings, considering the following factors:

A. Mobility (sufficient ROM for movement and assumption of posture)[12,13]

1. Determine whether the foot, ankle, knee, hip, and trunk have adequate ROM and joint play (see Table 38–5).
   a. If the patient lacks ROM, determine whether restriction stems from the joint, soft tissue, or muscle tissue (use end-feel as a guide).
   b. If the patient lacks joint play, it must be restored for gains in ROM to be achieved.
   c. If he/she lacks mobility at one joint, compensation occurs at another joint (eg, decreased ankle dorsiflexion results in excessive foot pronation).

B. Stability (the ability of the muscle to perform tonic holding and cocontraction)[12,13]

1. Determine whether muscle weakness is present isometrically, concentrically, or eccentrically.
2. Determine whether a difference in torque production exists isokinetically (when appropriate).

3. Determine in what positions the muscle is weak.
   a. If the patient lacks muscle force production, determine whether sufficient ROM is present in the joint for the muscle to contract efficiently.
   b. If the muscle cannot contract efficiently, normal gait mechanics are not possible.
   c. If the muscle is not strong enough eccentrically, compensatory action by muscles and joints occurs.

C. Controlled mobility (the ability of the muscles to move the proximal joints over the fixed distal end)[12,13]

1. Determine whether the patient can bear weight and move over the lower extremity (assisted and unassisted).
   a. An inability to do so may indicate a continued problem in stability.
2. Determine whether the patient can maintain proper posture during weight bearing.
3. Determine whether the patient can accept challenges to weight bearing (in a double-limb stance and in a single-limb stance).
   a. If the patient lacks weight-bearing ability, increased joint movement may be needed to allow the detection of motion changes in the lower extremity.
   b. If the patient is unable to maintain proper posture, mobility or stability is lacking in the trunk.

D. Skill (the ability of the muscles to move and to stabilize the proximal joint or joints with the distal end mobilized)[12,13]

1. Determine whether the patient can walk on level surfaces and on uneven surfaces, whether he/she can run, and whether he/she can walk step over step up and down stairs.
   a. If he/she lacks the ability to walk on even surfaces, mobility and stability may be absent.
   b. If the patient is unable to walk on uneven surfaces or to run, controlled mobility may be lacking.
   c. If he/she is unable to maintain proper posture during walking, controlled mobility may be lacking.
   d. If stability is lacking in the trunk, the lower extremity joints have difficulty performing mobility activities (proximal stability is necessary for distal mobility), and walking on all surfaces is compromised.

E. Diagnosis and Prognosis

Based on your initial judgement (including your assessment of the relationship among all anomalous findings and of the level at which the problem is occurring), make a **physical therapy diagnosis** and a **physical therapy prognosis.** This allows you to set reasonable goals and plan. *Musculoskeletal dysfunction* is the focus of your diagnosis and the basis of your treatment plan. Examples of physical therapy diagnoses include Trendelenburg gait, excessive foot pronation, talipes equinus deformity, drop foot disorder, or a variety of muscle weaknesses.

Goals must be **measurable** and **time related.** Formulate a long-term goal with a functional outcome. Keep in mind the patient's goals.

IV. Treatment Plan

A. Management of mobility dysfunction

1. Given that sufficient ROM is necessary for normal gait activities, joint play as well as soft tissue problems and muscle length must be addressed first.
2. **Joint mobilization, soft-tissue mobilization, and passive and active stretching techniques** should be employed to loosen the restricted structures.
3. Great toe extension, subtalar and midtarsal pronation, ankle dorsiflexion, knee flexion, and hip flexion are vital motions for normal gait. See "Lower Extremity: Hip," Chapter 33; "Lower Extremity: Knee," Chapter 34; "Lower Extremity: Ankle," Chapter 35; and "Lower Extremity: Foot," Chapter 36 for specific techniques.

B. Progression of mobility management

1. Some degree of soft-tissue mobility must be restored before therapy can proceed to the deeper joint and muscle structures.

2. Shift back and forth between techniques for tissue, muscle, and joint as the patient begins to loosen up. Instruct the patient to perform a home program to maintain gained mobility. For example, have the patient sit in a rocking chair with a foot on the floor and gently rock over the foot to increase foot pronation, ankle dorsiflexion, and (to a lesser extent) knee flexion.

3. Most patients with primary mobility problems have secondary stability issues that must be addressed before they can function at adequate controlled mobility and skill levels.

C. Management of stability dysfunction

1. Stability dysfunction is caused primarily by ligament laxity and muscle weakness. No techniques to tighten and strengthen ligaments exist other than immobilization. Particular problem sites for normal gait function are the plantar ligaments, lateral collateral ankle ligaments, cruciate and collateral ligaments of the knee, and sacroiliac ligaments. Providing **bracing** in a near-neutral posture for these structures allows healing and, hopefully, scarring, resulting in a more shortened position. Bracing may be required during all activities that tend to stress the previously injured structure, such as contact sports or even running. See "Orthotic Management for Lower Extremity Disorders," Chapter 17 for more details.

2. **Muscle strengthening** is fairly easy to accomplish because of the constant functional demands on the joint. Begin treatment with the patient in a non–weight-bearing position to eliminate the body mass force of gravity on the muscles. Transfer him/her to a weight-bearing position as soon as he/she and the injured structures tolerate it. Major muscles involved in gait activities must perform **eccentrically** for normal ambulation. Included in this group are the tibialis anterior and tibialis posterior, the gastrocsoleus, the quadriceps femoris, the gluteus maximus, the hamstrings, and the iliopsoas. These muscles must be trained (strengthened) eccentrically if they are to be used with greatest efficiency during gait. See "Lower Extremity: Hip," Chapter 33; "Lower Extremity: Knee," Chapter 34; and "Lower Extremity: Ankle," Chapter 35 for techniques.

D. Management of controlled mobility dysfunction

Trauma, immobilization, and weakness lead to problems in weight bearing. Have the patient assume a neutral posture utilizing his/her enhanced mobility and stability. Easing the patient into weight bearing involves **gradual protected weight bearing** during sitting, and then on parallel bars. While the patient is standing with a wide base of support have him/her shift weight over the foot and move from side to side and from front to back. **Continue to stress the importance of proper posture.** Superimpose isometric holds on the shoulder or pelvis. Work slowly, gradually increasing the patient's speed and decreasing the base of support. As the patient progresses, have him/her begin to perform a single-limb stance, increasing the time and perturbation as he/she improves. **Rhythmic stabilization** and **alternating isometric exercises** improve the muscles' ability to hold during single-limb stance when manual contacts are present at the pelvis or shoulder.[14] As the patient tolerates isometric exercises, have him/her advance to manually resisted forward advancement of the limb. Have the patient work forward *and* backward. Braiding (side stepping with alternating forward and backward step-over-step motion), with resistance applied to the pelvis or femur of the advancing limb, provides further advancement and is a good method for strengthening the gluteus medius. Use a balance board or BAPS (Camp International, Inc.) type system to **improve proprioceptive input** to the joints. Total-contact braces enhance the tactile input and proprioception.

E. Management of skill dysfunction

As the patient's weight bearing on stable surfaces improves, transfer him/her onto uneven surfaces (use foam, a pillow, or ramps as alternatives) and stairs. Begin by having the patient assume a neutral posture. Instruct him/her to step up and down on a stair or short stool, while he/she moves the tibia over the foot and increases weight bearing onto the foot. As the patient is able to bear full weight, have him/her progress to a step-over-step movement. Jogging with progression to running is a further option. Use an elastic, bungee-type cord to apply more resistance. Keep in mind that the ground reaction forces for jogging and running are three to four times body weight force; this requires the patient to be both mobile and stable in the lower extremities and spine. For more athletic rehabilitation, generalized lower extremity training tools such as the Fitter, Snowbounder, and Russian Leaper functionally train the lower extremities and trunk while providing activity-specific training.

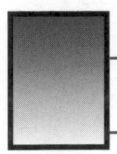

Clinical Decision-Making Cases

Case 1: Excessive Pronation and Peripheral Neuropathy

HISTORY

At presentation, BG was a 63-year-old man with a 2-month history of foot and knee pain during walking. He avoided standing and walking for more than 5 to 10 minutes because of the pain. He was working full time as a small-town police chief. He lived with his wife in a two-story home.

BG's medical history was significant in that he had adult onset diabetes mellitus for 15 years; he controlled it with daily insulin injections. He had coronary artery disease but no history of myocardial infarction. He had periodic ulcerations on the soles of both feet that healed slowly but completely.

EXAMINATION

Posture

The patient was overweight (he was 6 ft, 2 in; 255 lb) and had a forward head and flat back posture and slight genu varum bilaterally.

Soft Tissue

Both feet were pale, cold, and hairless. A thick callus was present under the second and third metatarsal heads bilaterally; some calluses also were noted under the lateral border of the right great toe.

ROM

BG had full active ROM in both lower extremities, with the exception of right dorsiflexion (the patient was unable to bring the foot past a neutral position). Passively, full right dorsiflexion was achieved.

Muscle Strength

The muscles of the lower extremities were found to have a good strength grade, except for the right tibialis anterior, which tested at a fair minus grade. The patient stated that he had been tripping going up stairs over the previous few months.

Special Tests

Knee ligament and cartilage test results were negative. The left foot had rearfoot varus and forefoot varus deformities, and the right foot had rearfoot varus and forefoot valgus deformities.

Gait

Bilateral excessive subtalar and midtarsal pronation were present at foot flat through toe off.

A slight foot slap on the right side at heel strike to foot flat that increased with increases in walking time was noted.

Slightly exaggerated right knee flexion was present on swing.

A slight trunk lean toward the left to clear the right foot on swing was seen after the patient had walked for 5 minutes on a treadmill.

All deviations increased with increases in the time spent on the treadmill and with increases in the incline of the treadmill.

ASSESSMENT AND DIAGNOSIS

BG had significant gait deviations that could be clearly linked to his foot and knee pain. The excessive pronation bilaterally was due to compensated rearfoot varus deformity plus compensated forefoot varus deformity on left and uncompensated forefoot valgus deformity on the right. He also demonstrated signs of diabetic neuropathy with tibialis anterior weakness and quick fatigue of the muscle during gait with increases in both time on and incline of the treadmill. His prognosis was good for continued function with improved foot position, orthoses, and exercise.

TREATMENT GOALS

Short-Term Goals

BG would demonstrate:

A working knowledge of proper foot care in 1 week.
An increase in the strength of the tibialis anterior by a half of a grade in 4 weeks.

An elimination of excessive pronation from midstance to toe off with the use of foot orthoses in 2 weeks.

An increase in the duration and incline of treadmill walking without symptoms from 10 minutes at 5 degrees of incline and an increase in heart rate of no more than 10 beats per minute from resting heart rate in 6 weeks.

Long-Term Goal

BG would stand and ambulate for 30 minutes without pain in 8 weeks.

TREATMENT PLAN

BG was fitted with bilateral full-length, semi-rigid foot orthoses with medial wedging. He was instructed in proper foot care, including daily monitoring of the skin (on the plantar and dorsal surfaces and between the toes) and was instructed to wear white cotton socks and well-fitting, leather footwear with a crepe sole. A home exercise program was prescribed to increase his lower extremity collateral circulation (with Buerger-Allen exercises). He was also performing active dorsiflexion

exercises against gravity but was unable to progress to exercising the muscle with increased resistance. BG was instructed to use the treadmill three times a week for 1 month; he was to incorporate increases in time and incline in an attempt to lower his heart rate. He was also walking around his neighborhood twice a week.

OUTCOMES

BG was discharged on an extensive home program after 2 months of treatment. His endurance had increased, and he was walking 20 minutes a day with no symptoms. He was also more comfortable when standing on the cement floors at work. Six months later, BG returned to the physical therapist complaining of continually tripping over his right foot, despite his daily performance of exercise. He demonstrated poor strength of the tibialis anterior at that time and was fitted for a total-contact ankle-foot orthosis to stabilize the ankle in a neutral position. His physician had little hope that BG would experience any return of muscle function because of his increasingly poor circulation.

Case 2: Scoliosis and Leg Length Discrepancy

HISTORY

At presentation, PG was a 20-year-old physical therapist student who had been diagnosed with right thoracic scoliosis at age 13. An exercise program was prescribed, and PG was monitored for 18 months. When she was re-evaluated, the curve had progressed to 25 degrees, and she was given a CTLSO (Boston Brace) to be worn 23 hours a day (it was not worn for the 1 hour that she performed pool exercises) for 2 years. The curve did not progress further, and the final radiograph showed the curve to be stable at 22 degrees. PG also had a compensatory left lumbar curve and a longer left limb. She was very active, doing aerobics four times a week, running three to four times a week, and performing Nautilus weight training (Nautilus Sports/Medical Industries) three times per week. She had a negative medical history and was taking birth control pills as prescribed and ibuprofen when necessary.

PG presented in physical therapy class one day with low back pain. She had central pain moving across the back that increased with activity and significantly diminished with non–weight bearing and rest. She was training for the Boston Marathon and had significantly increased her mileage over the previous month and was running more on the side of the road and less on a track. She was also trying out new running shoes,

which were more flexible and lighter than her old ones. There were no other changes in her activity level and no trauma was noted.

EXAMINATION

Posture

Right thoracic and left lumbar scoliosis were present, and a mild left cervical curve was necessary to orient the head to a neutral position. The left side of the pelvis (the anterior and posterior superior iliac spine, iliac crests, and pubic symphysis) was lower than the right, and the left lower extremity was functionally longer (by ~1 in).

The right foot was supinated, the left knee was slightly flexed, and the left foot was pronated.

Soft Tissue

Severe paraspinal spasm was noted throughout the lumbar spine, and tenderness was present along the iliac crest and deep into the quadratus lumborum and the lumbodorsal fasciae; the left side was more painful than the right.

Joint Play

Spinal joint play in all segments was within normal limits; some pain was present during posteroanterior glides in the lumbar spine.

The sacral, ilial, and hip joints were unremarkable.

ROM

ROM was limited in forward trunk flexion by half with pain; left lateral trunk flexion and right trunk rotation were significantly limited and painful.

Muscle Strength

Trunk strength was difficult to assess because of the presence of pain; the abdominal muscles appeared to be toned.

On screening, gross lower extremity strength was within normal limits.

Gait

Excessive pronation was noted on the left from midstance through toe off; excessive supination was seen on the right from heel strike through midstance.

Excessive knee flexion (~10 degrees greater than normal) was seen on the left throughout the gait cycle.

Slight trunk lateral flexion on the right was noted during the swing phase of the left lower extremity.

ASSESSMENT AND DIAGNOSIS

PG was diagnosed as having an acute muscle strain in the lumbar paraspinal muscles secondary to stress from running. She had successfully accommodated to her postural abnormalities, as evidenced by her joint play, muscle tone and strength, and activity level. Normally, the combination of her strength and mobility kept her symptom free. However, the change in running mileage and terrain as well as the use of more flexible and less supportive shoes was enough to increase the ground reaction force and to cause her spinal muscles to take up more slack. PG was pronating on the left to try to functionally shorten that limb and she was supinating on the right to try to functionally lengthen that limb. The excessive pronation resulted in PG's pushing off on a flexible foot, whereas the excessive supination resulted in a decrease in shock absorption. Given her previous level of activity, PG should be able to return to running, aerobics, and weight training without problems.

TREATMENT GOALS

Short-Term Goals

The patient would demonstrate:

A decrease in lumbar paraspinal muscle spasm from severe to minimal in 2 weeks.

An increase in trunk ROM to normal in 5 weeks.

Elimination of left foot pronation from midstance to toe off in 4 weeks.

Elimination of right foot supination from heel strike to midstance in 4 weeks.

An increase in running mileage from 10 miles per week to 30 miles per week in 4 weeks.

Long-Term Goal

The patient would return to marathon training without symptoms in 6 weeks.

TREATMENT PLANS

The initial focus of PG's therapy was the elimination of her acute symptoms. The decreased mobility of her soft tissue had been limiting her trunk ROM and causing pain; this was addressed first. Treatment consisted of myofascial release, gentle stretching, and positioning while PG was sitting and sleeping. She was using ice at home after activity.

The mobility concern with her left foot pronation that was a result of her longer limb also existed. The pronatory motion functionally shortened the limb. Correction of this problem required a change in PG's leg length discrepancy. However, the discrepancy was a result of the scoliosis, which, at that point, was not going to change (she had reached skeletal maturity). Therefore, correction of the leg length change would affect the spine, increasing the compressive forces on that side. Consequently, *full* correction was not appropriate; a heel lift was added on the right side, and its size was gradually increased to 0.5 in. Thermacork (Alimed) was used because it has shock-absorbing qualities. Because the leg length was more manageable, the need for supination by the right foot became unnecessary.

Before PG began her marathon training again, a change in her footwear was necessary. She required a running shoe that had heel counter-support and shock absorption. She also needed to choose her running surface carefully; the roadside in the city was very uneven, and the concrete was jarring to her body. She returned to running on the school track and was able to increase her mileage gradually. Her gait improved to the point where there was no need for increased knee flexion or lateral trunk flexion and the pronation and supination were minimal.

OUTCOMES

PG returned to running, aerobics, and weight training within 4 weeks. Her trunk range returned to normal, and her muscle spasm disappeared. The heel lifts, with 0.125 in of height added at a time, were well tolerated. The full 0.5 in lift was so comfortable that PG did not feel it in her shoe. She also put lifts in her other shoes. She felt that the lift improved her running time by making her muscles work more efficiently. She continued her active lifestyle and did not have recurrence of symptoms.

References

1. Norkin CC, Levangie PK: *Joint Structure and Function,* 2nd ed. Philadelphia, F. A. Davis Company, 1992.
2. Inman VT, Ralston HJ, Todd F: *Human Walking.* Baltimore, Williams & Wilkins, 1981.
3. Basmajian JV, DeLuca CJ: *Muscles Alive,* 5th ed. Baltimore, Williams & Wilkins, 1993.
4. Nelson AJ: Functional ambulation profile. *Phys Ther* 1974, 54:1059–1065.
5. Perry J: *Gait Analysis, Normal and Pathological Function.* Thorofare, NJ, Slack, 1992.
6. Smidt GL: Rudiments of gait. In Smidt GL (ed): *Gait in Rehabilitation.* New York, Churchill Livingstone, 1990, pp 1–20.
7. Giallonardo LM, Lake D: Clinical kinesiology [Course notes]. Boston, Northeastern University, 1985–1986.
8. Kadaba MP, Ramakaishnan HK, Wootten ME: Measurement of lower extremity kinematics during level walking. *J Orthop Res* 1990, 8:383–392.
9. Winter DA: Pathologic gait diagnosis with computer-averaged electromyographic profiles. *Arch Phys Med Rehabil* 1984, 65:393–398.
10. Brand PW, Ebner JD: Pressure sensitive devices for denervated hands and feet. *J Bone Joint Surg* 1969, 51A:109–116.
11. Åstrand PO, Rodahl K: *Textbook of Work Physiology,* 2nd ed. New York, McGraw-Hill, 1977.
12. Stockmeyer SA: Personal communication, 1993.
13. Sullivan PE, Markos PD, Minor MA: *An Integrated Approach to Therapeutic Exercise: Theory and Application.* Reston, VA, Reston Publishing Company, 1982.
14. Voss DE, Ionta MK, Myers BJ: *Proprioceptive Neuromuscular Facilitation,* 3rd ed. Philadelphia, Harper and Row, 1985.

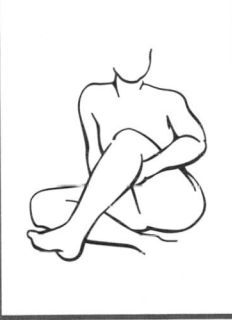

Prosthetics

David G. Patrick

Physical therapists involved in the rehabilitation of individuals following an amputation face a challenging yet rewarding task. Reduced length of rehabilitation intervention necessitates efficiency and accuracy in patient management. The rapidly evolving field of prosthetics requires clinicians to stay abreast of new technologies and innovations.

Based on existing literature and the author's ex-perience, this chapter will assist clinicians to problem solve a wide range of clinical situations related to the rehabilitation of the patient with amputation. An overview of current prosthetic componentry and biomechanical principles is provided as a basis for analyzing and resolving specific clinical issues.

I. Prosthetic Treatment Planning

A. Physical therapy evaluation[1-5]

1. **Age**
   a. A patient's chronological age is not as important in predicting outcomes and treatment planning as is overall wellness/

conditioning, functional abilities, and motivation.

2. **Diagnoses**
   a. Date of amputation.
   b. Cause of amputation.
   c. Level of amputation.

d. Medications.

3. **Secondary diagnoses**
   a. Other pertinent medical conditions/surgeries.
   b. Medications.

4. **Precautions**

5. **Social history**
   a. *Living arrangement prior to amputation*
      (1). A home assessment form should be completed by the patient and/or family within the 1st week of rehabilitation admission.
      (2). The therapist determines whether the prior home setting will be a realistic living setting after discharge.
      (3). Functional and activities of daily living (ADL) skills are prioritized based on the requirements needed to function in the home.
      (4). Equipment needs are identified.
   b. *Support system*
      (1). The therapist determines whether the patient must function independently or to what degree assistance will be available.
         (a). This should be considered when setting outcome requirements for discharge.
         (b). Education and training of individuals providing support should be included.
   c. *Work history*
      (1). Prior work history is determined.
      (2). If the patient was working before the amputation, the therapist determines the patient's vocational goals.
         (a). If expectations appear reasonable, the therapist should consider the related needs when making recommendations for prosthetic prescription and therapeutic program goals.
         (b). If expectations appear unrealistic, the patient should be referred for vocational counseling.

6. **Functional level**
   a. *Wheelchair*
      (1). Expected outcomes will vary depending on the amputee's overall wellness/conditioning, functional abilities, and motivation in general.
         (a). Unilateral lower extremity amputee:

(i). May use a wheelchair for long-distance transportation.
(ii). May use a wheelchair if not fitted with a prosthesis or if skin problems or prosthetic problems develop that prohibit the use of the prosthesis and if ambulation with an assistive device without a prosthesis is difficult for long distances.
   (b). Bilateral amputee, particularly at the above-knee or more proximal level will use a wheelchair as a primary means of mobility.
(2). Considerations:
   (a). An amputee frame or frame in which the rear axle can be adjusted posteriorly should be used when the extent of limb loss results in a tendency for the wheelchair to tip backward when the patient leans back, aggressively propels the wheels forward, or negotiates ramps or curbs.
   (b). Legrests/footrests should be included unless the amputee has an above-knee or more proximal amputation and is not a candidate for a prosthesis.
      (i). Elevated legrests are indicated for the amputee with a below-knee or more distal amputation to allow for proper positioning of the residual limb in an elevated position with the knee in extension when not wearing the prosthesis.
      (ii). Footrests are less bulky and are indicated for the amputee with an above-knee or more proximal amputation for use while wearing the prosthesis.
      (iii). Legrests/footrests should be the swing-away and removable type to facilitate transfers, to promote safety during sit to stand activities, and to allow for

easier management in and out of a vehicle.

(c). Armrests should be removable.

(d). The physical therapist determines whether the amputee's home environment will dictate wheelchair size and accessories.

(e). If the wheelchair is to be used primarily for long-distance mobility, it should be lightweight and easy to transfer in and out of a vehicle.

(f). An appropriate wheelchair cushion should be acquired and training in skin monitoring and pressure relief provided if the wheelchair is to be the primary means of mobility.

(g). The amputee's insurance coverage should be considered in the equipment planning process.

(h). The amputee should participate in the equipment planning process and, whenever possible, try the wheelchair/accessories before permanent acquisition.

B. Transfers

1. **Expected outcome.** In general, independence is an appropriate goal for level transfers for all lower extremity amputation levels.

2. **Methods**
   a. *Unilateral.* Stand-pivot transfer with or without prosthesis. Wearing a prosthesis for a below-knee or distal amputation will facilitate the transfer because weight can be borne through the flexed anatomical knee. The prosthesis does not actively assist in transfers for amputation levels above the knee because of the inability to bear weight through the prosthetic knee in a position of extreme flexion.
   b. *Bilateral*
   (1). *Below knee.* Stand-pivot transfer with prosthesis. Sliding transfer with or without a sliding board without prosthesis (side approach, front approach).
   (2). *Above knee or proximal.* Modified stand-pivot transfer (sitting push-up) with prosthesis. Sliding/sitting push-up transfer without prosthesis. Sliding board used if necessary.

3. **Considerations**
   a. The therapist should attempt to level transfer surfaces (*ie*, bed height should be lowered or raised to match wheelchair height).
   b. If needed, a drop-arm commode can facilitate side-sliding transfers to the toilet.
   c. The term sliding transfer is a misnomer. A sliding transfer should consist of a series of lifts (sitting push-ups), moving from one surface to another.

C. Bed mobility

1. **Expected outcome.** Independence for all lower extremity amputation levels for sit to supine, supine to sit, and rolling.

2. **Considerations**
   a. The greater the extent of lower extremity loss, the greater the tendency to fall backward during supine to sit and sit to supine activities. The amputee can compensate by lowering and raising the trunk to the side versus straight forward or backward.
   b. Rolling can be difficult to initiate. Training can be initiated from a three-quarter completed roll position and progressed back to full supine position as ability improves. Cuff weights can be applied to the wrists initially to assist in rolling and then eliminated as ability improves.

D. Ambulation

1. **Expected outcome.** In general, independence in ambulation on level and unlevel surfaces is an appropriate goal for unilateral amputees with or without a prosthesis. The bilateral amputee will generally be a limited ambulator, with the extent of limitation correlating with the extent of amputation loss.

2. Three-point gait training principles are followed for training the unilateral amputee without a prosthesis.

3. **Considerations.** When amputation is a result of vascular disease, the therapist should consider protecting the unaffected lower extremity by
   a. Using a more conservative assistive device.

b. Limiting ambulation distance without a prosthesis.

c. Closely monitoring the skin condition of the remaining lower extremity.

4. Outcome expectations and interventions for gait training with the prosthesis are discussed as they apply in the sections on below-knee, above-knee, and other prostheses.

5. Donning/doffing is discussed as it applies in the sections on below-knee, above-knee, and other prostheses.

E. Range of motion

1. **Expected outcome.** Range of motion within normal limits in all upper extremity and lower extremity joints.

2. Range of motion is assessed in all major upper and lower extremity joints. The therapist should screen specifically for

   a. Partial foot amputation: plantar flexor contractures of ankle.

   b. Below-knee amputation: knee flexion, hip flexion contracture.

   c. Above-knee amputation: hip abduction, hip external rotation, hip flexion contracture.

3. **Intervention for areas of limitation**

   a. *Positioning.* Positioning of the residual limb should be assessed when the prosthesis is removed (*eg,* in the wheelchair and bed).

(1). The patient, family, and support personnel, should be instructed in proper positioning.

(2). Low-temperature plastic shell or bivalve casting could be used for serial low-load prolonged stretching.

 PLEASE NOTE: Careful skin monitoring is essential to prevent skin breakdown.

b. *Range of motion program*

   (1). An appropriate therapeutic program to increase joint range of motion should be designed.

   (a). Deep heat modalities (*eg,* ultrasound) are used to increase tissue extensibility before therapeutic exercise.

   (b). Joint mobilization is used to restore joint assessory motions as indicated.

   (c). A passive, active assisted, active stretching (*eg,* contract-relax, contract-relax-contract) exercise program is used.

   (d). The patient should be instructed in a self–range of motion program. The patient's family and support personnel should be instructed to carry out the program if the patient is unable.

II. Residual Limb Assessment and Preparation

A. Volume containment

1. **Goals**

   a. To facilitate girth reduction of the residual limb until size stabilizes. Once stabilized, a definitive prosthesis can be fit.

   b. To assist in shaping the residual limb in preparation for prosthetic fitting.

   c. To reduce pain associated with edema formation in the residual limb.

   d. To facilitate healing by reducing edema in the residual limb.

2. **Methods**

   a. *Elastic bandages*

   (1). Advantages:

   (a). Pressure can be customized.

(i). Increased pressure can be applied distally with decreasing pressure applied proximally to facilitate edema reduction.

(ii). Pressure can be adjusted to patient tolerance (initially, less pressure may be tolerated).

(b). Dog ears or other residual limb-shape abnormalities can be specifically molded to improve shape.

(c). Easily acquired and inexpensive.

(2). Disadvantages:

(a). Difficult to apply correctly.

(b). Pressures exerted vary according to how applied.

(c). Fails to sustain constant pressures, loosening over time and requiring reapplication.

(d). Quickly loses compressibility after washing.

(3). Indication:

(a). Appropriate option for any lower extremity amputee; however, successful volume containment requires a patient or support system skilled in application technique and reliable in monitoring and reapplying bandage.

b. *Residual limb shrinkers*

(1). Advantages:

(a). Easily applied.

(b). More consistent pressure over a longer period of time.

(c). More consistency in the amount of compression applied.

(d). Significantly easier to apply and maintain position in the above-knee application.

(2). Disadvantages:

(a). Loses compressibility over time after washing.

(b). More expensive than elastic bandages.

(c). Acquisition of a new shrinker may be required to maintain adequate compression as shrinkage occurs (lack of adjustability).

(3). Indication:

(a). Appropriate option for any lower extremity amputee. Particularly indicated when ease of application is a priority or reliability to monitor the need for reapplication is questionable.

c. *Rigid dressings*

(1). Advantages:

(a). Protects the residual limb from trauma.

(b). Allows early weight bearing.

(c). Removable rigid dressing allows

(i). Observation of the residual limb.

(ii). Progressive shrinking by adding socks.

(2). Disadvantages:

(a). Not as readily available as shrinkers or elastic bandages.

(b). Requires skill in fabrication.

(c). Requires skill to don correctly.

(d). Heavier and bulkier than other methods.

(e). Requires monitoring and skill to maintain appropriate compression by adjusting the number of socks.

(3). Indication:

(a). Most appropriate for the below-knee amputee with the ability and "gadget tolerance" to learn to don correctly and adjust socks as required.

d. *General principles*

(1). Volume-containment devices should be worn whenever the prosthesis is removed.

(2). They can be discontinued when the residual limb volume has stabilized. The amputee should be instructed to leave the device off over night. If the prosthesis can be donned the next morning with the same number of sock plys as the previous day, the volume-containment device may be discontinued. If residual limb volume increases and a reduction of sock plys is necessary, use of the device should continue.

(3). A cylindrically shaped residual limb should be the goal.

B. Length measurements

1. **Method**

a. Starting reference point:

(1). Above knee: adductor longus tendon origin (as proximal as can be palpated) or greater trochanter.

(2). Below knee: medial tibial plateau (do not use patella because of its mobility).

b. Measure to the end of the residual limb and end of bone.

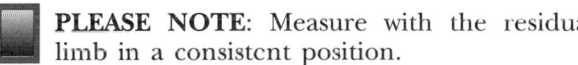 **PLEASE NOTE**: Measure with the residual limb in a consistent position.

2. **Clinical considerations**

a. *Below knee.* The shorter the residual limb

(1). The more difficult it is to accomplish mediolateral stability of the prosthesis during the stance phase.

Supracondylar, supracondylar-supra-patellar (SCSP), or, in extreme cases, joint and corset prosthetic design should be considered during prescription recommendation. Alignment should be adjusted to decrease the inset of the prosthetic foot.

(2). The less surface area there is to distribute weight-bearing forces, resulting in increased pressure and greater susceptibility to skin breakdown. Therefore, the skin should be monitored more closely during prosthetic training. SCSP or joint and corset prosthetic designs in extreme cases may be considered to assist in force distribution.

(3). The more difficult it is to effectively suspend the prosthesis.

b. *Above knee*

(1). Very long above-knee residual limbs can result in difficulty matching the prosthetic knee center to the anatomical knee center of the remaining residual limb. A polycentric knee should be considered with long residual limbs.

(2). The shorter the residual limb, the more difficult it is to accomplish mediolateral pelvic stability during the stance phase. The following should be considered:

(a). Ischial containment socket design.

(b). High lateral wall socket design with Silesian belt.

(c). In extreme cases, hip joint and pelvic band.

(3). Prosthetic alignment should be adjusted to decrease the inset of the foot.

(4). With above-knee prostheses, there is more difficulty maintaining suspension. Use of auxiliary suspension should be considered (*ie*, suction suspension primary with Silesian belt suspension secondary).

C. Girth measurements

1. **Method**
   a. Use a consistent position when measuring.
   b. Measure and document at least weekly.
   c. Place tape at a standardized starting point:

(1). Transtibial: medial tibial plateau.

(2). Transfemoral: long adductor tendon origin.

d. Mark with a skin pencil every 1 or 2 inches (depending on length of residual limb).

e. Measure circumference at these points in millimeters, exerting consistent tension on the tape measure. (Do not compress skin.)

PLEASE NOTE: Weekly girth measurements should indicate the effectiveness of the volume-containment program.

2. **Clinical considerations**
   a. Circumference reduced: program effective. Program should be continued.
   b. Circumference increasing: program ineffective. The therapist should determine whether

(1). There is a compliance problem; if so, it should be corrected.

(2). An alternative volume-containment approach would be more effective (*eg*, elastic bandage falls off after 2 hours and is not reapplied, whereas residual limb shrinkers would be worn more consistently).

(3). An underlying medical condition is causing volume fluctuations (*eg*, hemodialysis, congestive heart failure). Consider referral for a medical evaluation or management.

c. Circumference stable: residual limb size may have stabilized.

(1). Stable circumference over a 3- to 4-week period is usually indicative of girth stability. It is appropriate to pursue definitive prosthesis.

PLEASE NOTE: A practical clue that residual limb girth has stabilized is the use of the same number of sock plys for 3 to 4 weeks while using the temporary prosthesis.

d. Larger distal circumference than proximal circumference: indicative of a bulbous-shaped residual limb that is unsuitable for prosthetic fitting. An aggressive volume-containment program is indicated.

(1). Removable rigid dressing should be considered.

(2). Intermittent compression may be used (unless contraindicated).

D. Anteroposterior and mediolateral knee stability*

1. **Method**
   a. *Anteroposterior stability.* Perform anterior and posterior drawer sign test to determine integrity of anterior and posterior cruciate ligaments.
   b. *Mediolateral stability.* Perform knee varus and valgus stress test to determine the integrity of the medial and lateral collateral knee ligaments.

2. **Clinical considerations**
   a. In the presence of anteroposterior instability:
      (1). An SCSP, or, in extreme cases, joint and corset prosthetic design should be considered to facilitate anteroposterior knee stability at stance.
   b. In the presence of mediolateral instability:
      (1). Inset of the prosthetic foot should be reduced to decrease knee varus moment at stance.
      (2). Socket designs with higher mediolateral walls should be considered during the prescription process to facilitate mediolateral knee stability at stance:
         (a). Supracondylar.
         (b). SCSP.
         (c). In extreme cases, joint and corset.

E. Shape

1. Cylindrical: ideal shape for prosthetic fitting.
2. Bulbous: larger distal circumference than proximal circumference.
   a. Inappropriate for prosthetic prescription because there will be problems donning and doffing (large distal end unable to pass through smaller proximal end) of prosthetic socket.
   b. Resolution: see section on residual limb volume containment.
3. Conical: may be indicative of an absent or short fibula.
   a. Results in loss of an important lateral force-bearing area between the fibular head and the distal end of the fibula used to control knee varus at stance.

* Below-knee amputation only.

b. May be necessary to reduce the amount of foot inset to reduce the knee varus moment at stance.
c. Socket designs with higher medial and lateral walls should be considered to facilitate mediolateral knee control.

F. Incision

1. **Location.** Clinically, the location of the incision is indicative of the type of amputation surgery and may provide insight into the cause of amputation and the condition of the extremity preoperatively. The incision location has particular clinical significance if it is located over a pressure-bearing area or prominent bony area. Close monitoring is required to avoid breakdown over the incision line.
   a. Mediolateral anterior: indicative of a posterior flap (most common).
   b. Mediolateral midline: indicative of a "fish-mouth" amputation.
   c. Mediolateral posterior: indicative of an anterior flap.
   d. The incision may be oriented in a direction other than medial to lateral. This may be indicative of a traumatic amputation or a complicated closure.

2. **Condition**
   a. *Inflamed*
      (1). Reddened, warm, hypersensitive.
      (2). Response:
         (a). Determine whether there is active infection.
         (b). Whirlpool.
         (c). Prosthetic use may continue with careful monitoring to ensure that the incision condition does not worsen.
   b. *Open area*
      (1). Size, location, and drainage quality and amount are noted.
      (2). Response:
         (a). Whirlpool
         (b). Water Pik irrigation.
         (c). Débridement if necrotic tissue present.
         (d). High-volt pulsed current (HVPC).
         (e). Small open area does not necessarily prohibit use of prosthesis.
         (f). Ultrasound.
            (i). Eliminate cause of open

area if prosthetic in nature.

(ii). Protect area with a thin protective barrier (*eg*, Telfa pad or Steri-Strips [3M Corp.]).

(iii). Consider use of prosthetic sheath.

(iv). Monitor area closely.

c. *Scabbed area*

(1). Response:

(a). Note location and condition.

(b). Monitor area closely. If the scab falls off, the skin in this area is more fragile. Close monitoring and a cover such as a thin Telfa pad or adhesive bandage should initially be considered when gait training.

d. *Adhesion*

(1). Adhesions make the incision line more prone to breakdown and pain.

(2). Response: mobilize adhesions using gentle friction massage.

e. *Blister*

(1). Superficial water blisters often form during the initial prosthetic training period as a result of shear/friction forces.

(2). Response:

(a). Typically, prosthetic training can continue by covering superficial water blisters with an adhesive bandage or thin Telfa pad.

(b). Consider using a nylon sheath to reduce shear forces.

(c). Monitor blisters closely and discontinue prosthetic use if the underlying skin integrity is violated.

f. *Sutures*

(1). Prosthetic use is typically not initiated while sutures are in place.

(2). Measuring for the temporary prosthesis is appropriate while sutures are in place if the residual limb shape is not bulbous.

G. Skin

1. The classifications of residual limb skin are used to aid in anticipating resiliency to shear/friction and pressure forces within the prosthetic socket.

2. Method: observe.

a. *Delicate*

(1). Vascular insufficiency responses (tissue quality such as shiny skin, hair loss, or discoloration).

(2). Individuals with light complexions.

(3). Decreased tolerance to shear and pressure forces.

b. *Average*

(1). Majority of white individuals without vascular problems.

(2). Average tolerance to shear and pressure forces.

c. *Tough*

(1). Individuals with dark coloring.

(2). High tolerance to shear and pressure forces.

H. Bones

1. The therapist determines whether the cut end of bone is beveled.

a. If not beveled, there is increased susceptibility to pain and skin breakdown.

(1). The skin should be monitored more closely during prosthetic training.

(2). Increased relief is necessary in socket to avoid pain and skin problems.

2. In below-knee amputees, the therapist determines whether the fibula is present and fibula length in comparison to tibia.

a. If not present or significantly shortened in comparison to tibia, a conical-shaped residual limb can be expected and resultant decreased mediolateral socket control at stance.

3. The therapist determines whether there is heightened sensitivity to palpation.

a. This may be indicative of bone spurs.

(1). Increased relief is required in socket to avoid pain during prosthetic use.

I. Subcutaneous tissue

1. The classifications of residual limb subcutaneous tissue are used to aid in anticipating amount of shrinkage and potential sensitivity to pressure.

2. Method: grasp tissue between thumb and index fingers at lateral fibula.

a. *Heavy*

(1). Greater than 1.5 inches grasped.

(a). Expect greater shrinkage.

(b). Expect greater tolerance to pressure in prosthetic socket.

  b. *Average*
   (1). Approximately 1.0 inch grasped.
    (a). Expect average shrinkage.
    (b). Expect average tolerance to pressure in prosthetic socket.
  c. *Light*
   (1). Less than 0.5 inch grasped.
    (a). Expect little shrinkage.
    (b). Expect sensitivity to pressure in prosthetic socket.

J. Sensation

 1. Method: test light touch and sharp/dull.
  a. Results are used to predict the individual's ability to detect abnormal pressures and/or shear forces during prosthetic use.
  b. If sensation is impaired or absent, visually monitor the skin more closely during prosthetic training.
   (1). Rely on visual skin inspection regardless of the results of sensory testing, especially during the initial prosthetic training period.

K. Phantom pain/sensation

 1. **Phantom pain.** Debilitating pain that interferes with prosthetic rehabilitation and the general ability of the amputee to function.
  a. True phantom pain is rare.
  b. It should be differentiated from other causes of pain.
   (1). Neuromas.
   (2). Adherent scars.
   (3). Bursitis.
   (4). Vascular insufficiency.
   (5). Infection.
  c. Treatment:
   (1). Prosthetic wear.
   (2). Gentle massage.
   (3). Volume-containment device.
   (4). Mild heat or cold.
   (5). Ultrasound.
   (6). Trancutaneous electrical nerve stimulation (TENS).
 2. **Phantom sensation.** The sensation or awareness that the amputated body part still exists.
  a. Very common.
  b. Specific treatment is not necessary; however, it is important to discuss with the patient to alleviate concerns that the sensation is abnormal.

  c. More common in early postoperative period.
  d. Tendency to dissipate over time as residual limb becomes desensitized.

L. Description of prosthetic appliance

 1. The current prosthetic device should be described if applicable.
 2. Nomenclature strategy:
  a. An overall general description should be made followed by a description of componentry organized from proximal to distal.
   (1). General description by level (*ie*, above knee, below knee).
   (2). Definitive or temporary.
   (3). If definitive, exoskeleton or endoskeleton.
   (4). Type of socket with or without insert interface.
   (5). Type of suspension.
   (6). Type of hip joint (if indicated).
   (7). Type of knee joint (if indicated).
   (8). Type of foot.

   Example 1:
   Components: Above-knee prosthesis, SACH (solid ankle cushioned heel), foot, safety knee, ischial containment flexible socket, endoskeletal, suction suspension, definitive.
   Description: Above-knee definitive endoskeletal prosthesis with ischial containment flexible socket, suction suspension, safety knee, and SACH foot.

   Example 2:
   Components: Below-knee prosthesis, PTB (patellar tendon bearing) socket, SACH foot, pylite insert, temporary, supracondylar cuff suspension.
   Description: Below-knee temporary prosthesis with PTB socket, pylite insert, supracondylar cuff suspension, and SACH foot.

M. Condition of remaining lower extremity

 1. **Objective.** To examine and monitor the remaining lower extremity to prevent/correct problems that can result in further amputation.

2. **Method**
   a. Inspect for evidence of vascular insufficiency.
      (1). Determine whether pulse is palpable.
         (a). Femoral.
         (b). Popliteal.
         (c). Posterior tibial.
         (d). Dorsalis pedis.
      (2). Evaluate for integrity of sensation to anticipate the individual's ability to detect soft-tissue trauma.
         (a). Light touch.
         (b). Sharp/dull.
   b. Inspect skin integrity for current breakdown or signs of soft-tissue trauma.
      (1). Pursue aggressive treatment for open areas of skin.
         (a). Whirlpool.
         (b). Water Pik irrigation.
         (c). Débridement if necrotic tissue present.
         (d). Total contact casting.
         (e). HVPC.
         (f). Medical management.
         (g). Nutritional management.
      (2). Eliminate cause of problem.
         (a). Proper shoe wear.
         (b). Accommodative foot orthotics.
      (3). Monitor potential problem areas closely.
         (a). Discoloration.
         (b). Bony prominences.
         (c). Edema.

III. Below-Knee Prostheses

A. Biomechanics of below-knee prostheses[1-3]

An understanding of below-knee prosthetic biomechanical principles is required to gait train and problem solve gait deviations effectively. The biomechanics of below-knee prostheses can be summarized into three basic principles:

- Maximization of the weight-bearing capacity of the residual limb within the prosthetic socket.
- Maintenance of the mediolateral stability of the knee during weight bearing on the prosthesis while striving to mimic the biomechanical principles of normal gait and reducing energy expenditure.
- Maintenance of the anteroposterior stability of the knee throughout the stance phase of gait while striving to mimic biomechanical principles of normal gait.

1. Maximization of the weight-bearing capacity of the residual limb within the prosthetic socket.
   a. During weight-bearing activities, forces are generated at the residual limb–prosthetic socket interface.
   b. The prosthetist strives to design a socket whose shape promotes optimum comfort and residual limb tolerance to the forces generated during weight-bearing activities.
   c. The magnitude of the forces generated during weight-bearing activities are determined by the amputee's weight and the acceleration of the body's mass during activity.
   d. Pressure equals force per unit area. Therefore, the greater the available area to distribute forces, the greater the potential to reduce pressure in any one area.
   e. Different areas of the residual limb vary in their ability to tolerate pressure before discomfort and/or skin breakdown occurs.
   f. Three strategies are pursued to maximize the residual limb's ability to tolerate pressure:
      (1). The socket is designed to distribute greater forces over areas of the residual limb capable of greater force tolerance (pressure-tolerant areas) and less force over areas with less tolerance (pressure-sensitive areas). (See Section III.C.1., p 1133.)
      (2). The socket is tilted anteriorly (flexed) to increase the effectiveness of the surface area of the anterior residual limb to accept weight.
      (3). Sockets are designed to contact the residual limb completely to maximize the area over which to spread forces. Because pressure equals force per unit area, this results in a reduc-

tion of overall pressure on the residual limb tissues.

2. Maintenance of mediolateral stability of the knee during weight bearing on the prosthesis.

a. Prosthetic alignment is defined as the orientation of prosthetic components in relationship to each other.

b. Frequently, the goal of prosthetic alignment is to arrange the prosthetic components to mimic the biomechanics of normal gait.

c. Analysis of the biomechanics of normal gait in the frontal plane during the stance phase of gait reveals an anatomical alignment that is integral to an energy-efficient and cosmetic gait pattern.

(1). Relative medial positioning of the foot in relationship to the proximal leg and thigh results in a narrowing of the base of support during gait.

(2). A narrow base of support reduces the horizontal displacement of the body's center of gravity during gait, resulting in energy efficiency and improved gait appearance.

d. A similar strategy is pursued with below-knee prostheses to improve cosmesis and reduce energy consumption during gait.

(1). The midpoint of the prosthetic foot is inset approximately 0.5 inch in relation to the midpoint of the posterior socket as a starting point in prosthetic alignment.

(a). In normal biomechanics, the medial position of the foot results in the ground reaction forces passing medial to the knee axis when viewed in the frontal plane.

(b). This results in a knee varus moment, which is normally controlled by the lateral knee ligaments, tendons, and capsule.

(c). Medial placement of the foot in below-knee prosthetic alignment also results in a varus moment at the knee.

(d). A difference exists, however, in the control of the varus moment because the extremity is no longer directly attached to the floor; rather, a pseudo-arthrosis exists between the prosthetic socket and the residual limb.

(e). A varus moment results in a tendency for the knee to move into varus within the prosthetic socket.

(f). This tendency is controlled by the medial proximal socket above the knee axis and the lateral distal socket below the knee axis.

(2). The extent to which the foot may be inset in relationship to the midpoint of the posterior socket wall is dependent on two factors:

(a). A greater varus moment can be controlled in the presence of a longer residual limb and a prosthetic socket designed with higher medial socket support, because of the longer lever arm over which forces can be exerted.

(b). The magnitude of the varus moment can be determined by multiplying the right-angle distance of the floor reaction line from the axis of rotation (ie, amount of foot inset) by the force applied (ie, body weight/acceleration relationship).

(c). The prosthetic foot may be inset while maintaining control of the resultant knee moment more successfully in the presence of a longer residual limb, prosthetic socket designed with higher proximal trim lines, and a lighter-weight individual.

3. Maintenance of anteroposterior stability throughout the stance phase of gait.

a. Gait studies reveal that the knee is maintained in a position of varied flexion throughout the stance phase.[6]

b. Knee flexion serves a shock absorption function at initial stance from heel strike to foot flat.

c. Knee flexion assists in minimizing the vertical displacement of the center of gravity during gait, which assists in reducing energy expenditure.

d. Three strategies are followed to promote controlled knee flexion during the stance phase of gait:

(1). The socket is flexed, resulting in a flexion moment at the knee during stance.

(2). The socket is positioned ahead of

the ankle bolt of the prosthetic foot, resulting in a knee flexion moment during stance.

(3). A harder heel bumper is used in the foot to maintain floor reaction forces behind the knee longer, resulting in a knee flexion moment from heel strike to foot flat.

e. Flexion moment at the knee is controlled by quadriceps musculature to promote an appropriately controlled degree of knee flexion.

f. Extent of socket flexion, anterior socket placement, and heel bumper stiffness must be properly adjusted to accomplish a smooth, flowing gait pattern.

B. Prosthetic components

1. **Interim prosthesis**

   a. An interim prosthesis consists of all the componentry of a definitive prosthesis, except the shank is not cosmetically completed to look like an anatomical leg.

   b. Its purpose is

   (1). To allow early prosthetic fitting before the residual limb volume has stabilized. Wearing the prosthesis assists in residual limb shrinkage and shaping and allows early gait and functional training with the prosthesis.

   (2). To maintain availability of alignment adjustments to allow fine-tuning of the alignment as the amputee's gait progresses. Initially during gait training, the amputee may bear less weight on the prosthetic side because of discomfort and/or lack of confidence. As more symmetrical weight bearing occurs, alignment adjustments may be necessary to promote an optimal gait pattern.

2. **Definitive prosthesis**

   a. A definitive prosthesis is completed cosmetically and is intended to be worn for an extended period of time.

   b. A definitive prosthesis is prescribed when the residual limb volume is stable.

   c. Two major types of definitive prostheses are available:

   (1). *Endoskeletal.* An endoskeletal prosthesis gains its structural integrity from the inner endoskeleton. A soft foam

cover is used to complete the cosmetic finish (see Figure 39–1).

(a). Advantages of this design include the availability of the alignment adjustments and the ability to interchange components by removing the foam cover.

(b). The disadvantages of this design are the lack of durability of the foam cover and patient weight restrictions imposed by some systems.

(2). *Exoskeleton.* An exoskeleton prosthesis gains its structural integrity from the outer laminated shell (see Figure 39–2).

(a). Durability is its greatest advantage.

(b). Lack of alignment adjustability is its greatest disadvantage.

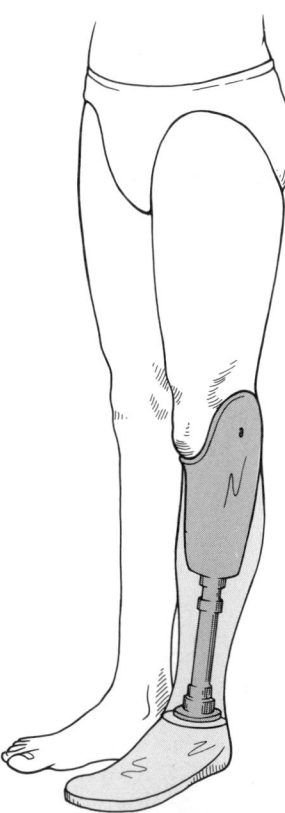

FIGURE 39–1 Below-knee endoskeletal prosthetic design. The strength is derived from the inner endoskeleton.

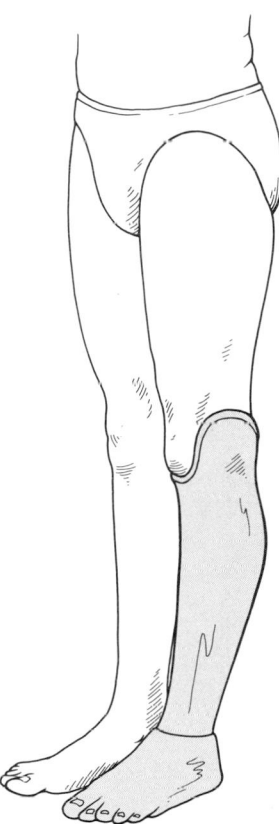

FIGURE 39–2 Below-knee exoskeletal prosthetic design. The strength is derived from the outer exoskeleton.

C. Socket designs

1. The PTB socket is the most common below-knee socket design. It incorporates a total contact fit of the residual limb, distributing greater pressure to pressure-tolerant areas and less pressure to pressure-sensitive areas.
   a. *Pressure-tolerant areas*[1,2]
      (1). Patellar tendon.
      (2). Pretibial muscle mass between the tibial crest and the fibula.
      (3). Lateral surface of the fibula.
      (4). Inferior surface of the medial tibial condyle.
      (5). Popliteal fossa.
   b. *Pressure-sensitive areas*[1,2]
      (1). Patella.
      (2). Tibial tubercle.
      (3). Crest of the tibia.
      (4). Anterior distal end of the tibia.
      (5). Distal end of the tibia.
      (6). Head of the fibula.
      (7). Hamstring tendons.

      (8). Lateral distal end of the fibula.
      (9). Common peroneal nerve.
   c. Proper function of the PTB socket is dependent on maintaining correct antero-posterior and mediolateral socket dimensions.
      (1). Correct anteroposterior socket dimension ensures proper patellar tendon weight bearing and is determined by anatomical distance between the patellar tendon and the popliteal fossa at the level of the medial tibial plateau.
      (2). Correct mediolateral socket dimension is required for proper mediolateral stability of knee at stance and is determined by anatomical width of the femoral condyles.
2. The total surface–bearing socket design is less frequently used.
   a. The concept of the total surface–bearing socket is to customize pressure distribution within the socket through a careful check of socket fitting procedures (transparent socket evaluation), ensuring that each area of the residual limb is accommodating as much pressure as it is able.
   b. The objective of this design is to improve comfort and skin tolerance to prosthetic use by efficiently distributing forces over all areas of the residual limb, as tolerated, thereby reducing pressure in any one particular area.
   c. Although in theory this approach would appear to have advantages over the traditional PTB fitting approach, results may not always justify the extensive fitting procedures required.
      (1). This may be because of the constantly changing skin-socket interface pressure distribution during active use of the prosthesis as well as the dynamic nature of the residual limb, which changes in size and shape with factors such as weight loss or gain, edema, and muscle function.

D. Suspension[3,4,6]

1. **Supracondylar cuff suspension** (see Figure 39–3)
   a. The supracondylar cuff grips over the proximal patella anteriorly and wraps circumferentially above the femoral condyles.

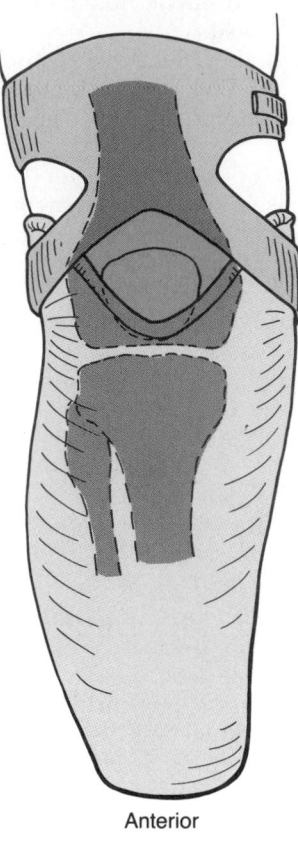

Anterior

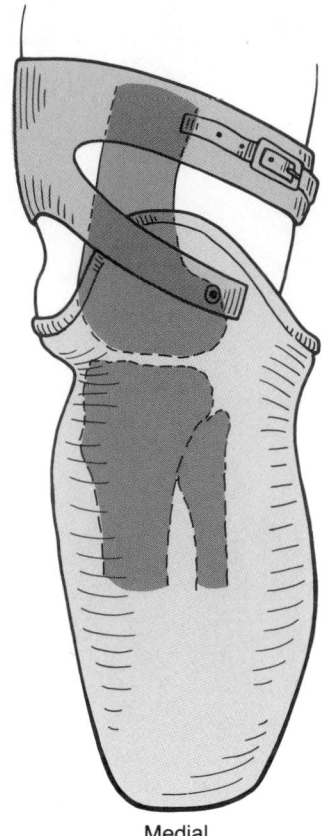

Medial

FIGURE 39–3 Below-knee prosthesis with supracondylar cuff suspension.

b. The cuff is connected to the socket via tabs.
   (1). The attachment points of tabs to socket are positioned so that the tabs are taut with the knee in a position of full extension to 60 degrees of flexion. This maintains the cuff's grip over the proximal patella, accomplishing effective suspension.
   (2). From 60 to 90 degrees of flexion, the tabs loosen, allowing comfortable sitting by relaxing the cuff.

c. Indications:
   (1). The patient requires simplicity in donning and doffing (Velcro can be utilized in place of buckles when required).
   (2). The ability to adjust the suspension is a priority.

d. Examples:
   (1). New amputees in whom residual limb shrinkage is anticipated.
   (2). Limited access to prosthetist.
   (3). Limited ambulators who spend the majority of time sitting. Cuff is comfortable for the amputee during sitting.

e. Contraindications:
   (1). Mediolateral knee instability or short residual limbs where problems with mediolateral knee control are anticipated. Lower socket trim lines are used with a supracondylar cuff suspension in comparison with other below-knee socket suspension designs.
   (2). A patient who is opposed to the appearance or use of straps on prosthesis.
   (3). Fleshy residual limbs with poor bony definition make gripping over the patella or femoral condyles for suspension difficult.

2. **Supracondylar cuff with fork strap and waist belt suspension** (see Figure 39–4)
   a. The fork strap is attached to the prosthesis distally and to the waist belt proximally.

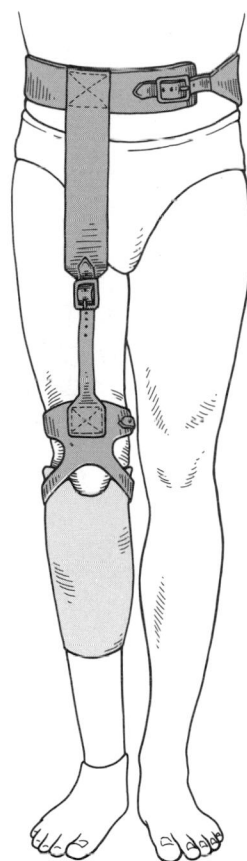

FIGURE 39–4 Below-knee prosthesis with a supracondylar cuff with waist belt suspension.

b. A portion of the fork strap is always elastic to allow for the knee to flex during ambulation while maintaining tension for suspension at all times.

c. Indications:
   (1). Serves well as auxiliary suspension to the supracondylar cuff in early prosthetic fittings, when effective suspension is essential to protect the skin from shear forces during gait.
   (2). Active amputees benefit from its use during vigorous activities, when additional suspension is required (*ie,* athletic activities).
   (3). Where the need for adjustability of the suspension is anticipated (*ie,* new amputees).

d. Contraindications:
   (1). When auxiliary suspension is not required.
   (2). When the patient is opposed to the use of belts, particularly around the waist.

3. **Supracondylar suspension (PTS)** (see Figure 39–5)
   a. Medial and lateral walls extend higher than the traditional PTB socket with cuff suspension, thereby providing greater mediolateral stability of the knee.
   b. Suspension is gained primarily over the medial femoral condyle by the medial socket wall, with the lateral socket wall acting as a counterforce.
   c. Patellar area is cut out.
   d. Indications:
      (1). Patients opposed to using straps or belts for prosthetic suspension.
      (2). Patients with mild to moderate mediolateral knee instability or short residual limb who would benefit from the higher medial proximal socket trim lines.
      (3). Patients with well-defined femoral condyles.
   e. Contraindications:
      (1). Patients who spend the majority of time sitting. Discomfort may result on the proximal femoral condyles as the knee tries to lift out of the socket during knee flexion and the suspension wedge is attempting to maintain the knee within the socket by gripping the femoral condyles (primarily medial femoral condyle).
      (2). Moderate to severe mediolateral knee instability that requires a joint and corset prosthetic design.
      (3). Knee hyperextension instability that requires a PTS (supracondylar), SCSP, or joint and corset prosthetic design for control.
      (4). Higher proximal socket trim lines are frequently noticeable through clothing and may be inappropriate for the individual who is particularly concerned about cosmetic appearance.
      (5). Although not a contraindication, new amputees in whom shrinkage is expected may require more frequent adjustments to the suspension wedge as the residual limb shrinks.
      (6). Suspension over the femoral condyles may be difficult to obtain in residual limbs with flabby muscula-

Anterior

Medial

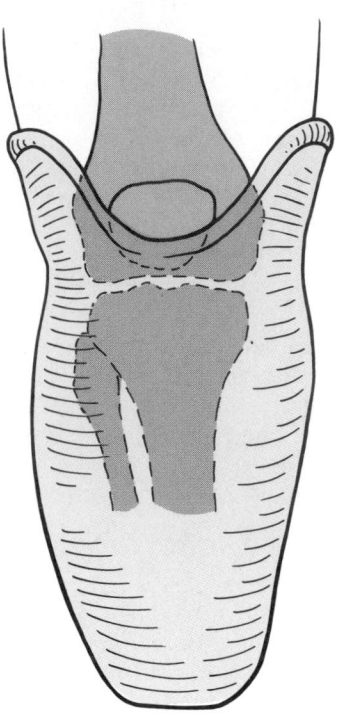
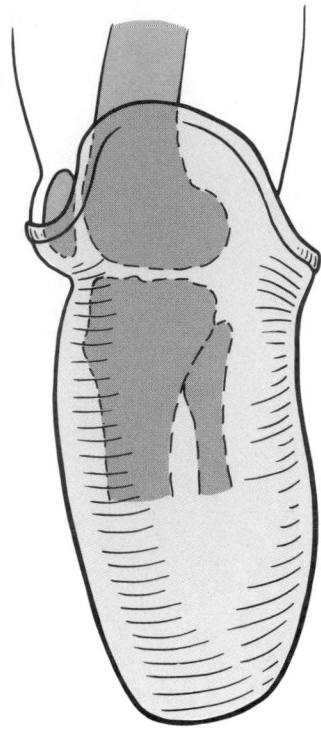

FIGURE 39–5 Below-knee   prosthesis with supracondylar suspension (PTS).

ture or very firm musculature around the femoral condyles.

4. **SCSP suspension** (see Figure 39–6)
   a. This design is similar to the supracondylar socket design except that the patella is enclosed and the proximal anterior socket forms a "quad bar" proximal to the patella.
   b. Patellar closure tends to add structural integrity to the mediolateral walls (stiffness), thereby increasing their effectiveness in providing mediolateral knee stability and suspension over the femoral condyles.
   c. The quad bar serves as a counterforce to the posterior popliteal area. This acts as a knee hyperextension stop, shunting weight from the remainder of the residual limb and providing additional suspension over the patella.
   d. Indications:
      (1). Short residual limbs that benefit from
         (a). Increased mediolateral control.
         (b). The weight-shunting feature of the quad bar to reduce forces

on the remainder of the residual limb.
         (c). Additional suspension gained over the patella.
         (d). More effective suspension and mediolateral knee control owing to additional stiffness of medial and lateral walls.
      (2). Amputees with mild to moderate knee hyperextension.
   e. Contraindications:
      (1). Patients whose lifestyle includes frequent kneeling, which can be inhibited by patellar enclosure.
      (2). Patients with longer residual limbs who do not require the benefits of this design may dislike the quad bar pressure generated during activities that require full knee extension (ascending/descending stairs and ramps, running).
      (3). Suspension over the femoral condyles may be difficult to obtain in residual limbs with flabby musculature or very firm musculature around femoral condyles.

Anterior   Medial

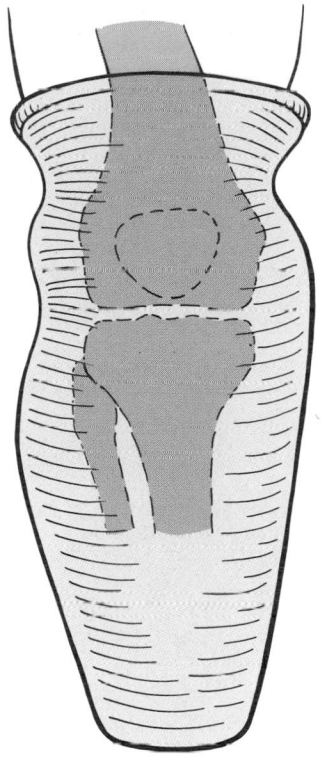
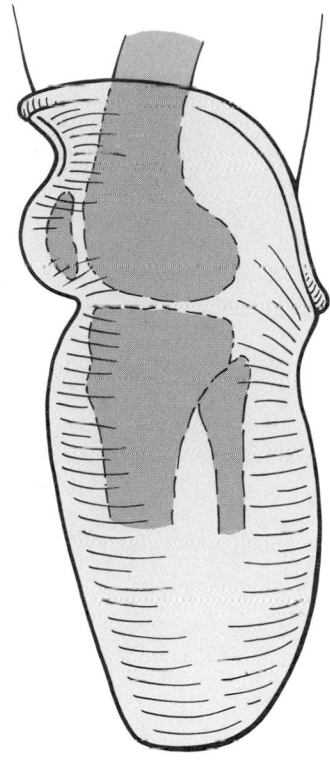

FIGURE 39–6 Below-knee prosthesis with supracondylar-suprapatellar suspension (SCSP).

5. **Sleeve suspension** (see Figure 39–7)
   a. A suspension sleeve may be made of latex, neoprene, or other elastic material.
   b. It may be used as the primary suspension of a prosthesis or in conjunction with another suspension (*ie*, supracondylar design).
   c. The distal end of the sleeve is rolled over the prosthetic socket, whereas the proximal sleeve is rolled up over the thigh (extending a few inches above the prosthetic sock).
   d. Suspension is accomplished through a combination of longitudinal tension in the sleeve and negative pressure during the swing phase, which results in a suction-type effect.
   e. Indications:
      (1). As an auxiliary suspension when added security is desired, control of positioning is essential, or high activity levels create higher suspension demands.
      (2). May be utilized as a primary suspension with standard PTB trim lines for same population that benefits from a supracondylar cuff.
   f. Contraindications:
      (1). Should not be used as a primary suspension with standard PTB trim lines when
         (a). Mediolateral knee stability is questionable.
         (b). Hyperextension control is required.
         (c). Residual limbs are short.
      (2). Patients who perspire excessively; they may experience additional sweating, which can result in skin irritation.
      (3). Patients who lack the hand dexterity or strength to manipulate a sleeve.

6. **Suction suspension** (see Figure 39–8)
   a. A silicone liner is worn directly against the skin and "plugged" into the prosthesis by means of a shuttlecock arrangement in the distal end.

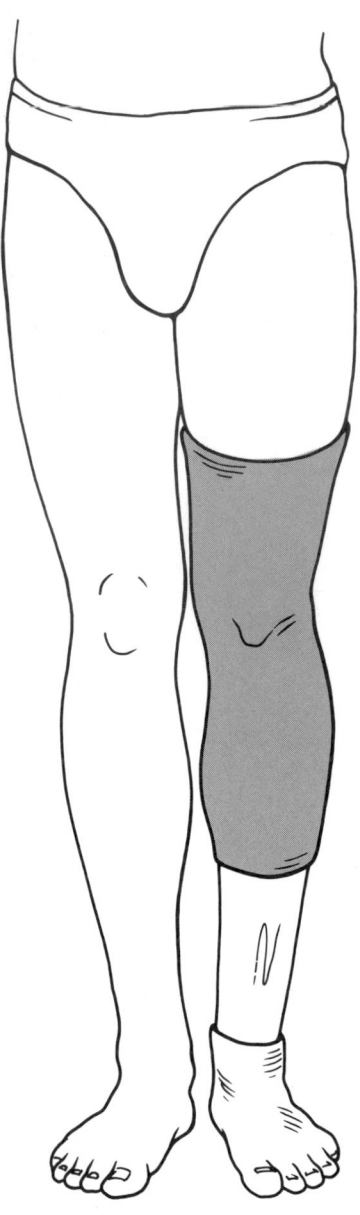

Anterior

Medial

FIGURE 39–7 Below-knee prosthesis with sleeve suspension.

b. Suspension is accomplished through
   (1). Longitudinal tension in the sleeve.
   (2). Tension between the sleeve and the residual limb.
   (3). Negative pressure, resulting in a suction effect between the residual limb and the liner.
c. The liner may be incorporated into a socket with a soft interface material (liner) or a hard socket.
d. Prosthetic socks are worn over the liner to accommodate changes in socket fit.

e. Standard PTB trim lines are commonly used, which allows for the combination of a secure suspension with relative freedom of knee movements.
f. Indications:
   (1). Applications where standard PTB trim lines are adequate for knee stability.
   (2). Short residual limbs for which suspension may be difficult to obtain and standard PTB trim lines are adequate for stability.

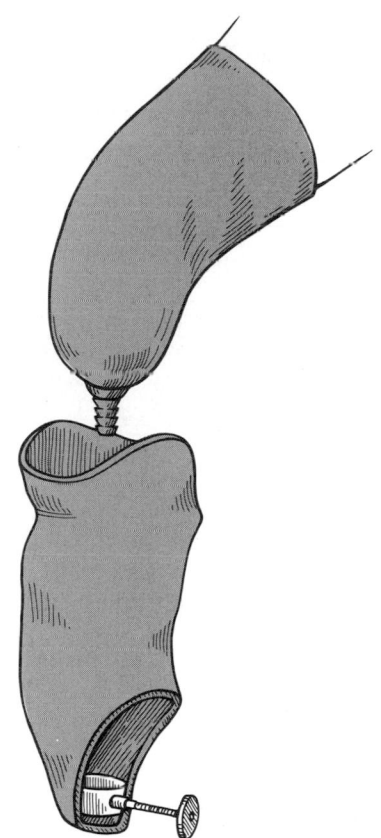

FIGURE 39–8 Below-knee prosthesis with suction suspension.

(3). Patients with high activity levels, and therefore greater suspension demands.

(4). Residual limbs when skin integrity is susceptible to shear forces and would benefit from a secure inherent suspension.

g. Contraindications:

(1). Patients with knee stability problems who would benefit from an alternative socket design with higher proximal socket walls.

(2). Patients who lack the hand dexterity or strength to manipulate the silicone liner.

(3). Patients with little "gadget tolerance" to care for the liner and manage the donning/doffing procedure.

7. **Joint and corset design** (see Figure 39–9)

a. A leather thigh corset is connected to the prosthesis via metal joints and side bars.

b. A thigh corset is a poor suspensory

mechanism for the prosthesis because of the conical shape of the thigh. Suspension is gained through the corset by its grip over the proximal patellar area. Typically, an auxiliary suspension such as a fork strap and waist belt is used.

c. Indications:

(1). To reduce weight bearing on the residual limb when comfort and/or skin integrity cannot be accomplished through a corsetless design. Forty to 60% of the body weight can be shunted from the residual limb to the thigh.

(2). To control moderate to severe mediolateral knee instability. Joint and corset design effectively extends the length of the medial and lateral

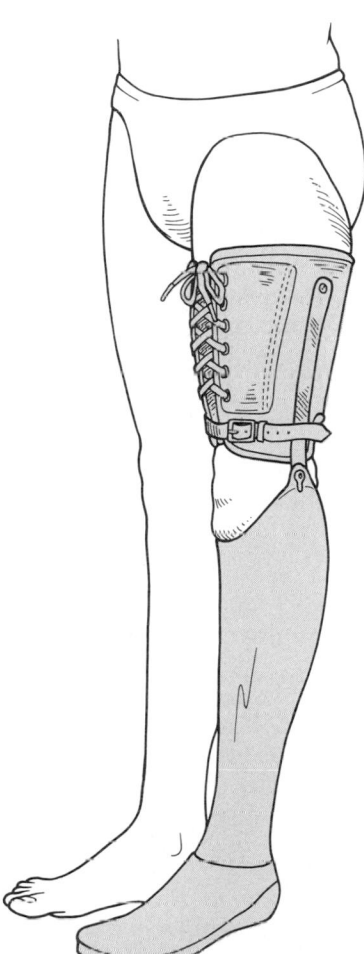

FIGURE 39–9 Below-knee prosthesis with joint and corset design.

socket walls, providing a significant mechanical advantage in controlling knee instability.

(3). To control moderate to severe knee recurvatum. Prosthetic joints limit knee extension. A check strap can be added to the posterior socket to prevent excessive prosthetic knee joint wear and to adjust the degree of knee hyperextension control.

(4). An experienced wearer who is satisfied with this design is probably better off continuing with its use.

E. Prosthetic feet[7-9]

Prosthetic feet can be categorized into one of five classes based on the function of the foot.

1. **SACH foot**
   a. The cushioned heel simulates ankle plantar flexion from heel strike to foot flat.
   b. The flexible toe and internal keel allow rollover at terminal stance.
   c. No ankle dorsiflexion, inversion, or eversion is allowed.
   d. Advantages:
      (1). Simple design makes it durable.
      (2). Cosmetically acceptable.
      (3). Inexpensive.
   e. Disadvantages:
      (1). Rigidity of foot makes it less desirable on uneven surfaces.
      (2). Energy consuming owing to rigid keel.
   f. Indications:
      (1). Level-surface ambulators.
      (2). Limited ambulators.
      (3). Financial constraints.

2. **Single-axis foot**
   a. Similar to a SACH foot with the exception of a single-axis ankle joint with an adjustable plantar flexion bumper, which allows the foot to plantar flex more easily from heel strike to foot flat.
   b. Advantages:
      (1). Increased stability in early stance as a result of getting the foot to the floor faster. This can be a significant advantage in above-knee amputees with an unlocked knee as it results in moving the floor reaction forces anterior to the knee more rapidly, thereby promoting knee extension stability.

c. Disadvantages:
   (1). Heavier.
   (2). More expensive than SACH foot.
   (3). Requires more maintenance. (Can be noisy.)
   (4). Energy consuming.
d. Indications:
   (1). Above-knee amputees with unlocked knee requiring assistance with knee stability.
   (2). Less aggressive above-knee amputees to promote stability and cosmesis of gait.

3. **Multiple-axis foot**
   a. Like SACH foot but includes a multiple-axis ankle joint, which allows plantar flexion, dorsiflexion, inversion, eversion, and transverse rotation.
   b. Advantages:
      (1). Accommodates uneven surfaces.
      (2). Multiple plane motion may reduce forces on the soft tissues of the residual limb.
   c. Disadvantages:
      (1). Heavier.
      (2). More expensive than SACH foot.
      (3). Requires more maintenance than SACH foot.
      (4). Dissipates energy, therefore more energy consuming.
   d. Indication:
      (1). Lifestyle in which ambulation on uneven surfaces is a high priority.

4. **Elastic keel**
   a. Like the SACH foot, but the keel is made of a flexible material that allows rollover at terminal stance and facilitates ambulation by providing limited push-off.
   b. Advantages:
      (1). Accommodates rollover.
      (2). Some designs accommodate inversion, eversion, and torsional damping.
      (3). Lighter weight.
      (4). Nonarticulated, therefore low maintenance.
   c. Disadvantages:
      (1). Unable to accommodate the demands of high activity.
      (2). More expensive.
   d. Indication:
      (1). Moderately active ambulators.

5. **Dynamic response**
   a. Characterized by a keel that is capable of

deflecting during rollover and providing active push-off at terminal stance at a variety of activity levels. Some designs accommodate inversion, eversion, and torsional damping.

  b. Advantages:
    (1). Provides active push-off.
    (2). Most energy efficient.
    (3). Promotes a natural gait at a variety of activity levels.
    (4). Facilitates high-impact activities (*eg*, running).
    (5). May be lighter weight.
  c. Disadvantage:
    (1). Most expensive.
  d. Indications:
    (1). Moderate to highly active individuals.
    (2). May improve the energy efficiency and appearance of gait in less active individuals but cost-benefit ratio is questionable.

F. Prosthetic evaluation[3,10]

Physical therapy prosthetic intervention begins with an evaluation of the fit and function of the prosthesis. This evaluation serves as a baseline to identify deviations from clinical standards. This alerts the clinician to potential problems that may warrant more intensive monitoring or intervention. It is important to realize that deviations from a clinical standard alone do not necessarily warrant prosthetic revision. The quality of prosthetic fit and function is a critical indicator of prosthetic success. When fit and function are affected and can be improved, prosthetic revision is warranted.

1. Evaluation with prosthesis off patient prior to donning.
  a. Is the prosthesis as prescribed?
    (1). The componentry of the prosthesis should be checked against the prescription.
    (2). If specific components have been ordered, substitution should not be made without an order from the prescribing physician.
    (3). The prosthetist should be contacted to determine the rationale for deviations from the prescription and to determine whether the prescribing physician approved the change.
    (4). If substitution has not been prescribed, the physician should be contacted to determine whether the

substitution is acceptable or if revisions are required to comply with the original prescription.

2. Evaluation with patient standing in parallel bars wearing prosthesis.
  a. Is the patient experiencing discomfort while standing with equal weight on each side with the feet 4 to 6 inches apart?
    (1). The patient is asked if any discomfort is being experienced.
    (2). If yes, the clinician differentiates between pain and pressure.
    (3). If pressure, it is explained to the amputee that a general feeling of pressure is expected because of the intimate fit of the socket required for prosthetic control. The therapist should rely on visual inspection to determine whether areas of abnormal concentrated pressure are present.
    (4). If pain, the therapist determines whether the complaint is concentrated in a small area or diffuse. Diffuse pain is of less concern. Concentrated pain should be explored immediately to ensure that skin integrity is not at risk (see section on management of skin problems).
    (5). If complaints of pain are localized to the lateral distal residual limb, the clinician determines whether the foot is excessively inset, creating an excessive varus moment and resulting in pressure at the lateral distal fibula.
      (a). Resolution: refer to prosthetist to reduce inset of foot.
    (6). The therapist determines whether relief of the lateral distal fibula is inadequate as evidenced by localized skin discoloration and/or prominent sock marks left on the skin over the distal fibula after weight bearing.
      (a). Resolution: refer to prosthetist to adjust socket.
    (7). If complaints of pain are on the distal residual limb, the therapist determines whether there is adequate total contact on the distal residual limb. Lack of total contact can cause discomfort.
      (a). Evaluation procedure. Wrap a small ball of clay in plastic (piece of trash bag). Place in the bottom of the insert or

1142 Part Seven • Musculoskeletal System

hard socket. The prosthesis is carefully donned to maintain clay in distal socket. The patient stands and weight shifts onto the prosthesis. Remove prosthesis. Flattened clay indicates contact at distal socket. Excessively flattened clay indicates excessive distal contact. Intact clay indicates lack of total contact.

(b). Resolutions:

(i). Lack of total contact. Following consultation with the prosthetist, wad up a small plastic trash bag and place in the distal insert or socket (hard socket) to determine whether distal contact reduces discomfort. If effective, refer to prosthetist to add a distal end pad to the socket or an insert to provide total contact.

(ii). Excessive total contact. Determine if the residual limb is sinking too far into the socket by evaluating the position of the patellar tendon weight-bearing mark on the skin after weight bearing. If the mark is too proximal, it indicates that the residual limb is too far into the socket. Add socks and/or refer to prosthetist to tighten the antero-posterior dimension of the socket. This increases patellar tendon weight bearing, which helps suspend the residual limb correctly in the socket, reducing excessive distal pressure.

(8). It is important to communicate to the patient that some discomfort is not unusual and does not necessarily indicate a problem with the prosthesis.

b. Is the length of the prosthesis correct?

(1). In unilateral below-knee prosthetic applications, the goal is to equalize length in both extremities.

(2). In bilateral below-knee prosthetic applications, the height is determined by choice. Typically, height is reduced to lower the patient's center of gravity, which makes walking easier and more stable. The goal of equal height is maintained.

(3). The therapist ensures that the patient is standing with the feet 6 inches apart, equal weight bearing, and hips and knees in full extension.

(4). The iliac crests are palpated to determine whether they are level.

(5). The magnitude of any discrepancy is determined by placing boards of various thicknesses under the shorter side until the iliac crests are level.

(6). A referral is made to the prosthetist to make required changes in length. A shoe lift may be used on the short side in the interim and to verify the amount of change in length required.

(7). New amputees frequently complain of feeling long on the prosthetic side. If no objective evidence is present, changes in length should be avoided. This subjective complaint typically resolves within the first few weeks.

c. Is the knee stable without the feeling that it is being pushed into excessive flexion or extension?

(1). The sole of the shoe should be flat when observed in the sagittal plane.

(2). The sensation of the knee being forced into flexion may be caused by

(a). Excessive socket flexion. The therapist should observe the amputee walking toward him/her. If the toe on the prosthetic side at heel strike is noticeably higher than the sound side, excessive socket flexion is suspected.

(i). Resolution: refer to prosthetist to adjust alignment.

(b). Excessive anterior placement of the socket. A plumb line is dropped from the midpoint of the lateral socket at the patellar tendon level. Typically, the socket should not exceed 1.5 inches anterior to the prosthetic ankle (ankle bolt).

(i). Resolution: refer to prosthetist to adjust alignment.

(c). A shoe with a higher heel height than appropriate for the prosthetic foot. This effectively tips the prosthesis forward, resulting in excessive socket flexion and excessive anterior socket placement.

    (i). Resolution: obtain a shoe with a lower heel or refer to prosthetist to exchange foot with one appropriate to accommodate shoe with a higher heel.

(3). The sensation of the knee being forced into extension may be caused by

(a). Inadequate socket flexion. The therapist observes the amputee walking toward him/her. If the toe on the prosthetic side at heel strike is noticeably lower than the sound side, insufficient socket flexion is suspected.

    (i). Resolution: refer to prosthetist to adjust alignment.

(b). Inadequate forward placement of the socket.

    (i). Resolution: refer to prosthetist to adjust alignment.

(c). A shoe heel that is too low or a prosthetic foot with an accommodation for a higher heel height.

    (i). Resolution: add a heel lift to level the prosthetic foot so that the top of the foot is parallel to the floor.

(d). Heel bumper on the prosthetic foot too soft, which excessively compresses with weight bearing.

    (i). Resolution: place paper toweling or newspaper into the toe of the shoe to tighten the fit around the heel bumper, effectively firming it. If inadequate, refer to prosthetist to exchange the foot for one with a firmer heel durometer.

(4). If the patient is unable to maintain the heel on the floor when observed in the sagittal plane, a knee flexion contracture may be present, which is not adequately accommodated for in the degree of socket flexion.

(a). Resolution: use heel lift to evaluate and correct temporarily or in cases in which gains in knee extension range of motion are anticipated. Consult with prosthetist regarding alignment adjustment.

d. Does the sole of the shoe evenly contact the floor when observed at midstance in the frontal plane (mediolateral alignment)?

(1). The prosthesis is aligned so that the foot is flat on the floor when 100% of the patient's weight is on the prosthesis at midstance. When standing in double support, weight may be shifted more onto the medial border of the shoe because only partial weight bearing is being exerted on the prosthesis.

(2). If the varus or valgus angulation of the socket does not match the natural angulation of the patient's knee, the sole of the shoe may be excessively on the medial or lateral border. Whether the sole of the shoe becomes flat on the floor at midstance during gait will ultimately determine whether a socket angulation problem exists. If weight bearing remains on the medial border of the foot throughout the stance phase, a socket angulation problem is suspected.

(a). Resolution: refer to prosthetist to evaluate the varus or valgus angulation of the socket.

(3). If weight bearing is shifted to the lateral border of the foot at midstance, an excessive knee varus moment is suspected. This may be the result of an excessive inset position of the prosthetic foot or a loose socket mediolateral dimension.

e. Is suspension adequate, minimizing pistoning of the residual limb in the socket when the prosthesis is raised off the floor?

(1). With the knee extended, the patient hikes up the hip on the prosthetic side, raising the prosthesis off the floor, while the therapist palpates at the anterior proximal socket brim to detect whether the residual limb raises out of the socket.

(2). Completely eliminating pistoning is nearly impossible. It should be remembered that pistoning is one of the primary causes of skin breakdown secondary to the resultant shear/friction forces.

(3). Resolutions:

(a). Supracondylar cuff: check to determine that the cuff around the leg is snug and the tab extensions are taut with the knee in extension.

(b). Supracondylar or SCSP suspension: determine whether the mediolateral dimension of the socket above the femoral condyles is adequately snug to maintain suspension. Following consultation with prosthetist, slide a piece of pylite or cork wedge between the insert and the medial socket wall. If suspension is improved, refer to prosthetist for a permanent adjustment. If not improved, determine whether additional socks are required or discuss the appropriateness of an auxiliary suspension with prosthetist.

(c). Sleeve suspension: determine whether a hole is present in the sleeve, resulting in a loss of suction, or whether the sleeve is worn, reducing its longitudinal resiliency. Have the sleeve replaced or determine whether additional socks or an auxiliary suspension is required.

(d). Silicone suction suspension: determine whether a hole is present in the sleeve, resulting in a loss of suction. If so, have the sleeve replaced. If not, determine whether additional socks over the silicone sleeve reduce pistoning.

(e). Joint and corset design: determine whether the inferior anterior aspect of the corset grips over the patella adequately. If not, refer to prosthetist to ad-

just corset position and/or recommend adding fork strap and waist belt if not present. If fork strap and waist belt are present, determine whether

(i). The fork strap is taut with the patient standing and the hip and knee extended. If not, tighten fork strap.

(ii). The waist belt is adequately tightened to prevent the fork strap from pulling the belt down with resultant loss of tightness of the fork strap. If not, tighten waist belt.

(iii). The elastic portion of the fork strap/waist belt is worn out, resulting in loss of suspension. If so, refer to prosthetist to replace.

(iv). The corset is too loose (ends of corset butt up against each other when attempting to snug the laces). If so, refer to prosthetist to add a liner to the inner corset, trim the corset to prevent the edges from meeting, or replace the corset.

3. Evaluation with patient wearing prosthesis.

a. Can the patient sit comfortably with the knee flexed to 90 degrees and the shoe flat on the floor?

(1). If discomfort is experienced in the popliteal area, the tissue in this area should be palpated with the knee flexed to determine whether the posterior wall is too high, resulting in compression of soft tissue. Patients with short residual limbs will experience more problems because of the need to keep the posterior wall higher for increased counterpressure for the patellar tendon bar anteriorly.

(a). Resolution: refer to prosthetist to lower or flare posterior wall.

(2). If discomfort is experienced in the hamstring tendon area only, the posterior wall is inspected for inadequate flaring of the corners, resulting in inadequate relief of the hamstring tendons.

  (a). Resolution: refer to prosthetist to increase flaring of corners to provide relief for hamstring tendons. (The posterior wall may be angled with the medial corner lower than the lateral corner to accommodate the lower position of the medial hamstring tendon with the knee flexed.)

(3). If discomfort exists over the medial femoral condyle when using a supracondylar or SCSP design socket, determine whether the suspension wedge is improperly positioned (too low) or the mediolateral dimension is too tight.

  (a). Resolution: refer to prosthetist to adjust position of suspension wedge or loosen socket mediolateral dimension, balancing its effect on suspension.

b. Is the anterior gap of the socket minimal?

(1). The larger the gap, the more noticeable the prosthesis through clothing. The therapist should determine whether the cosmetic result is acceptable to the patient. Some gapping will typically be present.

  (a). Resolution: refer to prosthetist to adjust if unacceptable to patient.

4. Evaluation with patient sitting and prosthesis removed.

a. Are the forces appropriately distributed over the residual limb?

(1). It is determined whether the patellar tendon bar of the PTB socket is contacting residual limb at the patellar tendon.

  (a). Resolutions: if the weight-bearing area is too high (toward the patella), reduce plys of prosthetic socks to lower the residual limb in the socket. If the weight-bearing mark is too low (toward the tibial tubercle), add plys of prosthetic socks to raise the residual limb in the socket.

    (i). If unable to don the soft insert completely after re-

ducing to 1 ply, an attempt may be made to don the insert wearing only a nylon sheath, or a hole may be placed in the bottom of the insert (after consulting with prosthetist) and a 1-ply stockinette used as a pull sock, reflecting the external portion back over the insert.

    (ii). If unable to don the insert using a pull sock, it may be necessary to don the prosthesis without an insert, adding required ply of socks to accomplish appropriate positioning of the residual limb within the socket. A suspension sleeve or fork strap and waist belt may be required if suspension was an integral portion of the insert (*ie*, supracondylar or SCSP design).

(2). It is determined whether excessive pressure is noted in pressure-sensitive areas. Significant discoloration or prominent sock marks are indicative of excessive pressure.

  (a). Resolution: refer to prosthetist to adjust socket or insert to relieve pressure.

PLEASE NOTE: Activities should be reduced or terminated until adjustment is made if skin integrity is questioned. Abrasions warrant an immediate termination of activity until an adjustment is made or the area is protected.

b. Is the prosthesis generally acceptable to the patient?

(1). Any concerns should be discussed with the prosthetist to determine whether modifications are possible to better meet the patient's expectations.

G. Prosthetic management[3,4]

1. **Donning/doffing procedure.** Patient sitting.

Remove volume-containment device and initiate donning sequence.

a. Sequence—supracondylar cuff:
  (1). Apply nylon sheath, if indicated, to reduce shear forces against skin.
  (2). Apply prosthetic socks individually, keeping the higher-ply socks closer to the skin to take advantage of their tighter, smoother weave. Do not allow multiple socks to be applied simultaneously because wrinkles may occur, causing skin pressure within the socket.
  (3). Apply insert, if present, aligning patella with patellar cutout.
  (4). Place soft insert and residual limb into prosthesis, aligning patellar cutout.
  (5). Tighten supracondylar cuff suspension.
  (6). Doffing: unfasten supracondylar cuff. Remove insert and residual limb as one unit and reverse steps 1 through 3 above.

b. Sequence—supracondylar or SCSP suspension:
  (1). Follow steps 1 through 4 as described for supracondylar cuff. Note that resistance will be encountered as the widest portion of the femoral condyles move past the narrow supracondylar portion of the proximal socket brim. The patient places foot on floor and pushes on top of knee into prosthesis. If unable to don
    (a). Ensure that there is a stockinette over the insert to facilitate sliding into the socket.
    (b). Apply baby powder to the outside of the insert.
    (c). Refer to prosthetist to widen the supracondylar portion of the socket, being careful to maintain enough tightness to accomplish socket suspension.
  (2). Doffing: grasp sock over insert with one hand and push away anterior brim of socket with the other hand. Reverse steps 1 through 3 as described for supracondylar cuff.

c. Sequence—sleeve suspension:
  (1). Roll sleeve down over proximal brim of prosthesis.
  (2). Follow steps 1 through 4 as described for supracondylar cuff.
  (3). Roll sleeve up over the thigh, ensuring that the sleeve extends over the prosthetic sock onto the skin a few inches to accomplish an air seal. If difficult to roll on sleeve, consult with prosthetist to determine if a different size sleeve is indicated.
  (4). Doffing: roll down sleeve over proximal brim of prosthesis. Reverse steps 1 through 4 as described for supracondylar cuff.

d. Sequence—silicone suction suspension:
  (1). Powder sleeve.
  (2). Roll sleeve flat.
  (3). Roll up sleeve directly over skin.
  (4). Place prosthetic socks, if indicated, over sleeve.
  (5). Apply insert, if using one, over sleeve.
  (6). Insert sleeve into socket as far as possible, clicking the shuttlecock fully into place.
  (7). Doffing: push shuttlecock release button and remove silicone liner and residual limb. Reverse steps 1 through 5.

e. Sequence—joint and corset design:
  (1). Follow steps 1 through 4 as described for supracondylar cuff.
  (2). If the objective is to reduce weight bearing, tighten laces while sitting with residual limb fully positioned in socket but in a non–weight-bearing position. This method shunts more weight from the residual limb to the thigh corset.
  (3). If the objective is to improve mediolateral control, have the patient stand and tighten laces, with the residual limb positioned in socket in a weight-bearing position. This method promotes weight bearing on the residual limb but should be avoided if the patient's balance is impaired and it is unsafe for the patient to stand while donning.

H. Gait training

1. **General principles**
  a. The majority of below-knee amputees will be able and eager to immediately stand and initiate ambulation activities with the prosthesis.
  b. The below-knee amputee is highly sus-

ceptible to skin breakdown because of the relative bony configuration of the residual limb and thin soft-tissue protection.

c. In addition to teaching the amputee how to ambulate with a natural gait pattern, controlling and methodically progressing gait training to prevent skin breakdown is a major responsibility of the therapist.

(1). Progression procedure:

(a). Increase wearing time (*ie*, progress prosthetic wearing tolerance from 15 minutes to 30 minutes, etc.).

(b). Increase ambulation distance (*ie*, progress from one length of the parallel bars to two lengths of the parallel bars, etc., before visually checking skin).

(c). Progress assistive devices (*ie*, visually check residual limb more frequently after progressing from a more supportive assistive device like the parallel bars to a less supportive assistive device like a walker, etc.).

d. Visual inspection of the residual limb should be relied on as opposed to subjective feedback to ensure that skin integrity is not being compromised during prosthetic wear and activity.

e. Advancements in socket and feet technology have made more advanced skills possible (*eg*, running) for the aggressive amputee.

2. **Gait training progression (new amputee in parallel bars)**

a. Patient standing. Feet equal distance from midline. Symmetrical weight bearing. Shifts weight alternately onto prosthetic and sound side.

(1). Problem: patient reluctant to accept weight onto prosthetic side.

(a). Resolutions:

(i). Patient maintains hips and knees in extension. Place hands on side of each hip and cue patient to alternately shift hips toward each hand in gradually increasing increments.

(ii). Use biofeedback limb-load monitors to encourage weight shifting.

(iii). Use bathroom scale to promote visual feedback regarding amount of weight bearing.

(iv). If discomfort continues to interfere, see section III.F.2.a., p 1141.

b. Patient steps forward and places swing foot into heel strike position. Alternates prosthetic and sound side.

(1). Problem: asymmetrical step lengths.

(a). Resolution: encourage heel-to-toe step length initially as a cue. Step lengths will naturally increase as gait velocity progresses.

c. Patient advances from heel strike to a foot flat position.

(1). Problem: patients often maintain hip and knee in extension and roll over the heel to a foot flat position.

(a). Resolution: manually cue patient to flex the hip and knee slightly to assist the foot to the foot flat position.

d. Patient progresses from foot flat to midstance position.

(1). Problem: hip and knee extension are not achieved at midstance.

(a). Resolution: cue the patient to extend the hip and knee (within the alignment constraints of the prosthesis) at midstance. Patient holds this position to reinforce its importance prior to initiating swing on the sound side.

e. Patient steps through on sound side.

(1). Problem: short step length on the sound side.

(a). Resolution: reinforce heel-to-toe step length.

f. Sequence is repeated as skin tolerance allows.

(1). Speed is increased as tolerated without losing quality of gait sequence.

(2). Methodical progression is made to less restrictive assistive devices.

(3). The focus should be on maintenance of skin integrity as assistive devices are advanced (walker, crutches, wide-based quadripod cane, narrow-based quadripod cane, straight cane, no device).

I. Gait analysis[3,10]

1. **Sagittal analysis**

   a. Deviation: abrupt knee flexion on heel strike to foot flat.

Potential Causes	Resolutions
(1) Excessive socket flexion.	(1) Refer to prosthetist to reduce socket flexion.
(2) Socket too far anterior.	(2) Refer to prosthetist to move socket posterior.
(3) Heel bumper too hard.	(3) Refer to prosthetist to reduce plantar flexion resistance of foot or to exchange foot with one with softer heel durometer.

   b. Deviation: knee extension or hyperextension on heel strike to foot flat.

Potential Causes	Resolutions
(1) Insufficient socket flexion.	(1) Refer to prosthetist to increase socket flexion.
(2) Insufficient anterior placement.	(2) Refer to prosthetist to move socket anterior in relation to the foot.
(3) Heel cushion too soft.	(3) Tighten heel in shoe by placing paper toweling or newspaper in toe. Refer to prosthetist to replace foot with one with harder heel durometer.
(4) Heel of shoe too low to accommodate prosthetic foot.	(4) Place wedge under heel to level top of foot parallel with floor. Acquire higher-heel shoes. Refer to prosthetist to exchange foot for one properly accommodating heel height of shoe.

   c. Deviation: jerky movement of knee into flexion and extension from foot flat to midstance.

Potential Causes	Resolutions
(1) Excessive socket flexion.	(1) Refer to prosthetist to reduce socket flexion.
(2) Weak knee extensors.	(2) Strengthen knee extensors.

   d. Deviation: early excessive knee flexion (drop off) from midstance to heel off.

Potential Causes	Resolutions
(1) Excessive socket flexion.	(1) Refer to prosthetist to reduce socket flexion.
(2) Socket too far anterior.	(2) Refer to prosthetist to move socket posteriorly.

   e. Deviation: prolonged knee extension moment (hill climbing).

Potential Causes	Resolutions
(1) Insufficient socket flexion.	(1) Refer to prosthetist to increase socket flexion.
(2) Socket too far posterior.	(2) Refer to prosthetist to move socket anterior.

   f. Deviation: knee remains extended throughout early stance phase.

Potential Cause	Resolution
(1) Typically a gait performance versus a prosthetic cause.	(1) Retrain gait, incorporating slight knee flexion from heel strike to foot flat.

g. Deviation: early heel rise.

Potential Causes	Resolutions
(1) Insufficient socket flexion in the presence of a knee flexion contracture.	(1) Refer to prosthetist to increase socket flexion to accommodate contracture. Intervention to reduce contracture.
(2) Amputee unweights prosthesis early.	(2) Gait training, concentrating on maintaining hip and knee extension longer from mid-stance to heel off while maintaining weight on prosthesis.

h. Deviation: unequal step length.

Potential Causes	Resolutions
(1) Typically a gait performance versus a prosthetic cause.	(1) Retrain symmetry of step length (verbal and visual cues).
(2) Discomfort during weight bearing on the prosthetic side, resulting in a shorter step on the sound side.	(2) See section III.F.2.a., p 1141
(3) Possible hip flexion contracture on opposite side of short step.	(3) Increase range of motion—affected hip.

2. **Frontal analysis**
   a. Deviation: toe out asymmetrical compared with sound side.

Potential Cause	Resolution
(1) Improper toe out alignment.	(1) Refer to prosthetist to correct toe out alignment.

b. Deviation: abducted gait on prosthetic side.

Potential Causes	Resolutions
(1) Patient habit; ambulating without prosthesis with sound side directly underneath trunk (three-point gait).	(1) Gait training with visual midline cues, stressing symmetry of gait width.
(2) Patient feels unstable and widens base of support for increased security.	(2) Use assistive device or more supportive assistive device for stability. Gait training, stressing skills to improve balance (braiding, side stepping, etc.).
(3) Prosthesis too long.	(3) Place lift on sound side to evaluate whether length is a problem. Refer to prosthetist to shorten prosthesis if lift successful.

c. Deviation: excessive varus moment at midstance on prosthetic side.

Potential Causes	Resolutions
(1) Foot excessively inset.	(1) Refer to prosthetist to outset foot.
(2) Mediolateral dimension of socket too loose at femoral condyle.	(2) Place pylite wedge between socket and insert at medial proximal socket to evaluate whether this reduces excessive varus moment. Refer to prosthetist to tighten mediolateral dimension of proximal socket if this is successful.

d. Deviation: valgus moment at knee at mid-stance.

Potential Cause	Resolution
(1) Foot outset too far. Valgus moment should be avoided as it results in pressure on wrong areas of residual limb.	(1) Refer to prosthetist to inset foot.

e. Deviation: foot on medial or lateral border throughout stance phase (as opposed to thrusting motion at midstance).

Potential Cause	Resolution
(1) Valgus or varus angulation of socket does not appropriately match patient's anatomical knee alignment.	(1) Refer to prosthetist to adjust socket angulation in frontal plane. Do not wedge shoe.

f. Deviation: vaulting on sound side.

Potential Causes	Resolutions
(1) Prosthesis too long.	(1) Place lift on sound side to evaluate.
(2) Inadequate suspension, resulting in a relative extremity-length increase during swing.	(2) Correct suspension (see section III.F.2.e., p 1143).
(3) Habit.	(3) Gait training with mirrors and cueing to keep heel down.

g. Deviation: external rotation of prosthesis on heel strike to foot flat.

Potential Causes	Resolutions
(1) Amputee not bearing full weight on prosthetic side.	(1) Gait training, reinforcing symmetrical weight transfer to prosthetic side. Use limb-load monitor.
(2) Heel cushion or plantar flexion mechanism too stiff.	(2) Refer to prosthetist to reduce stiffness of heel (plantar flexion mechanism) or to exchange foot.

h. Deviation: pelvis rises or lowers during midstance on prosthetic side.

Potential Cause	Resolution
(1) Prosthesis too short (pelvis lowers) or long (pelvis rises).	(1) Evaluate height (see section III.F.2.b., p 1142). Use shoe lift to evaluate effect of length change. Refer to prosthetist to adjust length if lift improves.

i. Deviation: unequal stance time.

Potential Causes	Resolutions
(1) Discomfort during stance on prosthetic side.	(1) See section III.F.2.a., p 1141.
(2) Lack of confidence during stance on prosthetic side.	(2) Gait training, stressing symmetry in weight shifting and prosthetic stance activities.

J. Management of skin problems[3]

1. **General principles**
   a. Below-knee amputees are highly susceptible to skin problems during prosthetic training (particularly early prosthetic training).
   b. Skin integrity should be monitored closely through visual inspection as activity is progressed.
   c. The therapist should identify abnormal discoloration, prominent sock marks over pressure-sensitive areas, abrasions, blisters.
   d. The underlying cause is determined and addressed. The therapist should consider
      (1). Alignment factors generating abnormal forces.
      (2). Inadequate relief of pressure-sensitive areas.
      (3). Inadequate suspension or socket fit resulting in pistoning and abnormal shear forces.
      (4). Incorrect number of socks resulting

in improper position of residual limb in socket.

(5). Wrinkles in prosthetic socks.

e. When abrasion or blister occurs, if underlying cause is determined and corrected, prosthetic training can often continue by protecting the affected area. Covering should be as thin as possible to avoid increasing pressure over the area within the socket. Options include adhesive bandages, Telfa pads under nylon sheath, and Op-Site dressing.

2. **Common skin problems**
   a. *Abrasion, anterior distal tibia*

Potential Causes	Resolutions
(1) Alignment: excessive socket flexion, excessive anterior placement of socket relative to prosthetic foot, heel cushion too hard, increased heel height of shoe. All result in an excessive flexion moment requiring the quadriceps to work more forcefully, resulting in increased pressure of the anterior distal tibia against the anterior socket wall.	(1) Refer to prosthetist to adjust alignment. Correct heel-height problem or refer to prosthetist to exchange foot for proper heel-height match.
(2) Improper relief within the socket.	(2) After consulting with prosthetist, evaluate by adding moleskin strips to socket wall or insert around the area of pressure (redistributes pressure to the surrounding pressure-tolerant areas). Prosthetist makes permanent adjustment if successful (see Figure 39–10).

Potential Causes	Resolutions
(3) Pistoning resulting in shear/friction forces.	(3) See section III.F.2.e, p 1143. Use nylon sheath.
(4) Incorrect number of socks resulting in improper position of residual limb in socket. Pressure-relief areas do not match pressure-sensitive areas of residual limb and loss of skin integrity can result.	(4) When applying insert, palpate patellar tendon bar of insert and determine whether it is properly located over patellar tendon. If too low, remove insert and reduce socks. If too high, remove insert and add socks. If no insert, have patient weight bear, then remove prosthesis and examine position of patellar tendon weight-bearing area. Proceed as above.
(5) Wrinkles in prosthetic socks.	(5) Remove prosthesis and reapply socks individually to remove wrinkles.

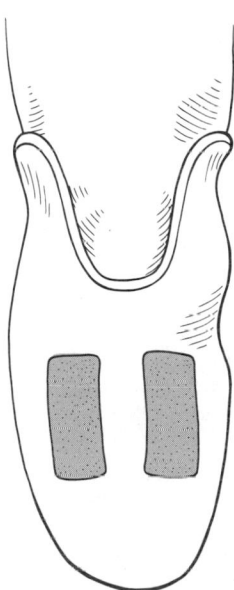

FIGURE 39–10 Moleskin strips added to socket insert of below-knee prosthetic to reduce pressure on anterior tibial crest.

b. *Breakdown, tibial tubercle*
(1). Potential causes/resolutions: see 2 through 5 above.
c. *Fibular head*
(1). Potential causes/resolutions: see 2 through 5 above.
d. *Inferior patella*
(1). Potential causes/resolution: see 4 above.
e. *Breakdown, soft-tissue area*
(1). Potential causes/resolution: see 3 and 5 above.
f. *Breakdown, hamstring areas*

Potential Causes	Resolutions
(1) See 4 above.	(1) See 4 above.
(2) Inadequate flaring of posterior wall corners.	(2) Refer to prosthetist to increase flaring of corners of posterior wall. Use nylon sheath.

g. *Breakdown, patellar tendon*

Potential Cause	Resolution
(1) Anteroposterior dimension of socket too tight, causing excessive patellar tendon weight bearing.	(1) Refer to prosthetist to remove material at patellar tendon bar or popliteal area.

h. *Breakdown, suture line*

Potential Cause	Resolution
(1) See 3 and 4 above.	(1) See 3 and 4 above. Use adhesive bandage or Steri-Strips to close area and reinforce tissues during activity (consult physician).

i. *Water blister on suture line*

Potential Cause	Resolution
(1) Typically due to shear forces. See 3 and 4 above.	(1) See 3 and 4 above. Cover area with adhesive bandage to eliminate shear/friction. Do not puncture blister. Blister typically resolves under bandage. Monitor closely. Discontinue use of prosthesis if skin integrity becomes worse. Consult prosthetist.

K. **ADL training**[3]

1. **Stairs**
a. *Method.* Initially repeat sequence of leading with sound side and bringing prosthetic side to the same step. Progress to step over step.
b. *Potential problems*
(1). Skin breakdown due to increased demand on residual limb tissues when raising or lowering body weight with prosthetic side.
(2). Lack of dorsiflexion on prosthetic ankle when descending.
c. *Resolutions*
(1). Monitor skin closely and discontinue step-over-step method if skin integrity is questioned. Use railing and/or assistive device whenever possible for balance and reduction of forces on residual limb.
(2). Place only prosthetic heel on step to allow prosthetic foot to roll forward, mimicking dorsiflexion.

2. **Inclines**
a. *Method.* Directly ascending and descending steps in a forward position is the most natural method.
(1). Start ascending, leading with sound step and stepping to level of the sound step with prosthetic side.
(2). Progress to step over step as able.
(3). Start descending, leading with the prosthetic side followed by the sound side.
(4). Progress to step over step as able.
b. *Potential problem.* Lack of prosthetic ankle

dorsiflexion interferes with forward approach.
  c. *Resolutions*
    (1). Shorten steps.
    (2). Ascend and descend on an angle across the ramp.
    (3). Side-stepping approach, leading with the sound step when ascending and leading with the prosthetic step when descending.

3. **Curbs.** Follow procedure for stairs.

4. **Uneven surfaces** (*eg,* grass, gravel, unlevel surfaces)
  a. *Method.* Shorten steps and decrease speed, progressing step length and speed as skill level improves.
  b. *Potential problem.* Can be difficult secondary to prosthetic foot that does not accommodate uneven surfaces and lack of proprioceptive cues through residual limb.
  c. *Resolutions*
    (1). May consider prosthetic foot with multiple-axis ankle function if amputee's lifestyle demands frequent management of uneven surfaces.
    (2). Use of assistive devices.
    (3). Repetitive practice to increase skill level.

5. **Kneeling**
  a. *Method.* Place sound foot forward and lower to prosthetic side knee, keeping weight on sound side. Assume same position and extend sound hip and knee to arise.
  b. *Potential problems*
    (1). Loss of balance.
    (2). Inadequate strength of sound hip and knee extensors.
  c. *Resolutions*
    (1). Kneel, holding onto object when possible. Therapeutic exercise to improve balance and technique.
    (2). Strengthening hip and knee extensors. Place hand on top of sound knee to assist if there is no assistive device or other object to grasp.

6. **Rising from floor**
  a. *Method.* Assume quadruped position. Progress to kneeling position with sound side forward and foot flat on floor. Extend sound hip and knee forcefully and push up with hands.

  b. *Potential problems*
    (1). Weakness of hip and knee extensors.
    (2). Balance difficulties.
  c. *Resolutions*
    (1). Strengthen hip and knee extensors.
    (2). Use an object (*eg,* chair) to assist.

7. **Stepping over objects**
  a. *Method.* Direct approach. Lead with the sound side over the obstacle and step through with the prosthetic side.
  b. *Potential problems*
    (1). Obstacle too large.
    (2). Balance difficulties.
  c. *Resolutions*
    (1). Use side-stepping approach, leading with sound side and following with prosthetic side.
    (2). Balance drills with prosthesis (side stepping, braiding, etc.).

8. **Car transfers**
  a. *Method.* Easiest to approach car so that sound side leads into car. Use reverse procedure to exit car.
  b. *Potential problem.* Unable to lead with sound side and difficulty flexing hip and knee sufficiently to lead into car.
  c. *Resolution.* Back into seat. Slide back onto seat until able to swing legs into car. Reverse procedure to exit car.

L. **Bilateral below-knee prosthetic considerations**[2]
  1. **Problems**
    a. Skin breakdown.
      (1). The bilateral below-knee amputee must bear all weight through the prostheses while in the upright position.
      (2). When performing elevations and ADL, one prosthetic extremity must accept the higher force normally borne on the sound side in a unilateral amputee. This places the bilateral below-knee amputee at more risk for skin integrity problems.
      (3). Resolutions:
        (a). Monitor skin more frequently during gait training and progress weight-bearing activities more conservatively.
        (b). Consider recommending a soft insert fabricated with more shock-absorptive, shear-resistive

materials (*eg*, gel, silicone) during the prescription process.

(c). Monitor skin closely during elevation activities. Determine whether one extremity should serve the role of the sound limb based on residual limb length, skin integrity, strength, etc.

b. Tendency to fall backward.

(1). The absence of ankle dorsiflexors on either extremity results in a susceptibility to falling backward if the amputee's center of gravity moves too far posteriorly.

(2). Resolutions:

(a). The prosthetic socket should be aligned in more flexion to promote a more anterior position of the center of gravity (a small wedge can be positioned inside the shoe under the heel of the foot to evaluate the effect of increasing socket flexion).

(b). Harder heel cushions should be used (paper toweling may be placed in toe of shoes to tighten the fit of the prosthetic foot in the shoes. This has the effect of stiffening the heel cushion and is helpful in determining whether the heel cushion is contributing to tendency to fall backward).

c. Loss of balance.

(1). The bilateral below-knee amputee is more susceptible to balance problems owing to lack of a sound residual limb to help recover from balance upsets and the lack of a sound ankle when managing uneven terrain.

(2). Resolutions:

(a). Feet should be less inset to increase width of amputee's base of support.

(b). If lifestyle results in frequent encounters with uneven terrain, multiple-axis feet should be considered during the prescription process.

(c). Height of center of gravity can be lowered by lowering the overall height of the prosthesis. Particularly for a person who is struggling during the training period with temporary prostheses, reducing prosthetic length can greatly assist in balance, gait training, and prosthetic control.

■ **PLEASE NOTE:** An average prosthesis height for an adult below-knee amputee is 18 inches from the floor to the knee center. This allows the feet to sit flat on the floor with the knees level in an average-height chair.

d. Difficulty with toe clearance at swing.

(1). The bilateral below-knee amputee is more susceptible to clearance problems at swing owing to a lack of a sound ankle gaining height for the prosthetic side to initiate swing.

(2). Resolution:

(a). Use of shorter feet can sometimes assist in clearance at swing.

IV. Above-Knee Prostheses[1-3]

A. Biomechanics of above-knee prostheses

1. Maximal weight-bearing capacity of the residual limb within the prosthetic socket.

a. The principle of total contact is used to take advantage of the entire residual limb to distribute forces.

b. Less emphasis is placed on differentiating pressure-tolerant and pressure-sensitive areas owing to the adequate soft-tissue covering and lack of bony prominences of the above-knee residual limb.

c. In the quadrilateral socket design, weight bearing is concentrated on the ischial tuberosity, which rests on top of the posterior socket wall.

d. In the ischial containment socket design, weight bearing is more generally shared over the ischial tuberosity located within the posteromedial corner of the socket and the remaining residual limb musculature, particularly the lateral aspect. This is accomplished by increasing the socket adduction angle and aggressively narrowing the mediolateral socket dimension.

2. Achievement of energy efficiency during gait by reducing the lateral displacement of the center of gravity.
   a. The prosthetic foot is inset to narrow the base of support during ambulation to
      (1). Improve gait appearance.
      (2). Promote energy efficiency by reducing the horizontal oscillation of the center of gravity during gait.
   b. Insetting the foot results in the floor reaction forces passing medial to the hip joint, resulting in a hip varus moment.
   c. Hip abductors are responsible for controlling the tendency of the pelvis to move laterally at stance. With above-knee prostheses, this stabilizing mechanism is complicated by the fact that
      (1). The residual limb is a shorter lever arm through which the hip abductors work.
      (2). The hip abductors' stabilizing mechanism is no longer directly attached to the floor. The effectiveness of the hip abductors to provide stability of the pelvis during stance is dependent on the prosthetic socket's ability to stabilize the femur within the prosthesis when the muscles are active.

3. Maintenance of the anteroposterior stability of the knee joint during the stance phase.
   a. Alignment stability consists of positioning the prosthetic knee joint in a position relative to the socket and foot, which results in maintaining the floor reaction forces anterior to the knee joint, promoting knee extension throughout the stance phase.
   b. The knee joint is positioned so that the axis is slightly posterior to a line connecting a point on the socket representing the trochanter and a point on the foot representing the ankle (trochanter/knee/ankle [TKA] line).
   c. Positioning the knee joint too far posteriorly results in difficulty initiating knee flexion.
   d. Locating the knee joint anterior to this line can result in the knee buckling during stance.

4. Control of the prosthetic knee during swing phase to promote symmetry of heel rise.
   a. Mechanical knees have a friction adjustment that is set to promote equal heel rise at the most popular walking speed (set for one speed).
   b. Increasing gait velocity increases the forces acting on the knee at swing. Because the mechanical knee cannot adjust to this change, the result is an asymmetrically high heel rise. Decreasing speed has the opposite effect, resulting in an asymmetrically low heel rise.
   c. Hydraulic and pneumatic knee joints accommodate changes in gait velocity, resulting in the maintenance of a symmetrical heel rise regardless of changes of velocity.

5. Socket alignment allowing symmetrical step length.
   a. Hip extension on the stance side is required to accomplish a normal-length step on the opposite side.
   b. Aligning the prosthetic socket in flexion allows a normal-length step on the sound side while requiring less extension range of motion of the anatomical hip on the amputated side.
   c. A hip flexion contracture must be accommodated in the initial socket flexion angle to accomplish a normal-length step on the opposite side.

B. Prosthetic components

- Interim/definitive: see sections III.B.1. and III.B.2., p 1132.
- Endoskeletal/exoskeletal: see section III.B.2.c., p 1132.

1. **Socket designs**[1,2,8] (see Figures 39–11 and 39–12)
   a. *Socket shape*
      (1). *Quadrilateral* (see Figure 39–13)
         (a). This design is based on providing proper contour for functioning muscles (quadrilateral shape).
         (b). "Quadrilateral variant" sockets are more commonly used. The same principles as for the traditional quadrilateral socket are followed, but quadrilateral variant sockets are "rounder" in shape and therefore tend to be more comfortable.
         (c). Adducting the lateral socket wall attempts to re-establish the

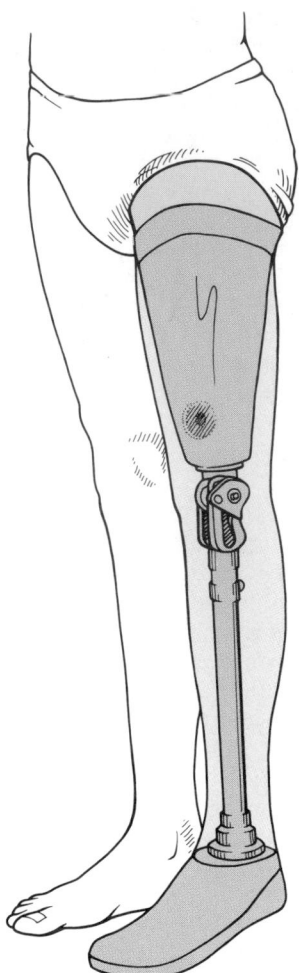

FIGURE 39-11   Above-knee endoskeletal prosthetic design.

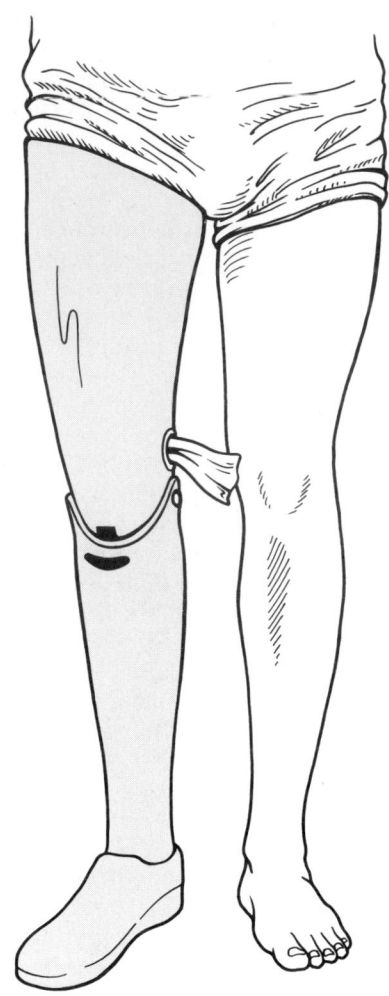

FIGURE 39-12   Above-knee exoskeletal prosthetic design.

''normal'' operating tension of the hip abductors necessary for mediolateral stability of the pelvis at stance.

(d). Primary weight bearing is on the ischial tuberosity, which is positioned on top of the posterior socket wall.

(e). Narrow anteroposterior dimension is based on a skeletal measurement (distance from the long adductor origin to the ischial tuberosity). This is relied on to maintain the ischial tuberosity properly positioned on the posterior wall (prevents ischial tuberosity from sliding forward off the posterior wall).

(f). Mediolateral socket dimension is larger than anteroposterior

socket dimension. It is based on a circumferential measurement of the residual limb (*ie,* the larger the volume of the residual limb, the larger the mediolateral dimension of the socket).

PLEASE NOTE: The quadrilateral socket design has been criticized for its questionable ability to stabilize the femur during forceful contraction of the hip abductors at stance. The common gait deviations of lateral trunk bending and abducted gait are cited as evidence of the quadrilateral socket's ineffectiveness in providing mediolateral stability of the hip/pelvis at stance. Criticism has centered on the large mediolateral dimension of the quadrilateral socket and the ischial tuberosity's position on top of the posterior wall.

The large mediolateral dimension is theorized to

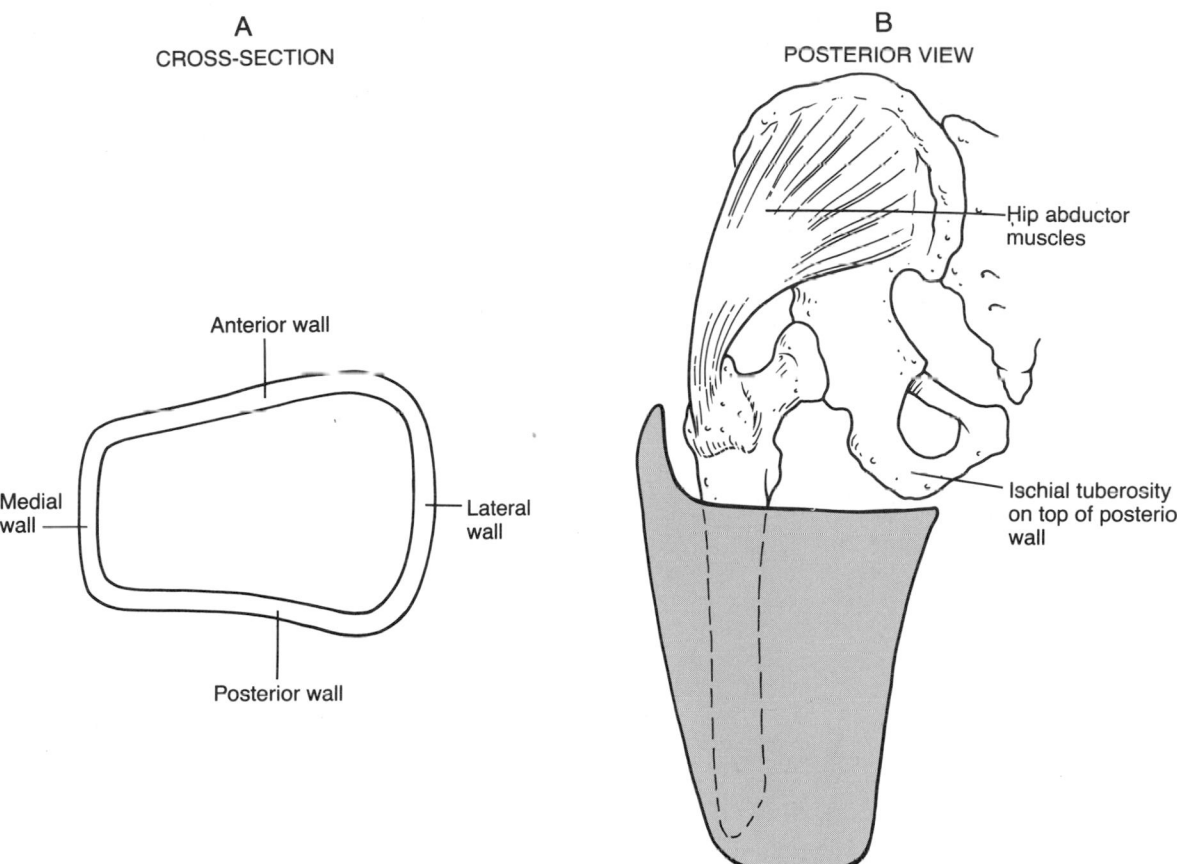

A
CROSS-SECTION

Anterior wall

Medial wall

Lateral wall

Posterior wall

B
POSTERIOR VIEW

Hip abductor muscles

Ischial tuberosity on top of posterior wall

FIGURE 39–13 **A** and **B**, Quadrilateral socket shape.

reduce the effectiveness of the lateral socket wall to maintain the femur in adduction. The normal operating tension of the hip abductor muscles is not maintained, resulting in their ineffectiveness in controlling the hip/pelvis during stance. Concern over the ischial tuberosity's position on top of the posterior wall centers around the principle of a system following the "path of least resistance." When the hip abductors contract, it is theorized that it is easier for the ischial tuberosity to slide medially than for the femur to stabilize the pelvis by maintaining forceful abduction against the lateral socket wall. Sliding of the ischial tuberosity allows the femur to move into abduction, reducing the effectiveness of the hip abductors to control the hip/pelvis during stance. Lateral trunk bending toward the prosthetic side and an abducted gait on the prosthetic side are strategies used by the amputee to reduce the demand on the hip abductors during the stance phase of gait by moving the floor reaction forces closer to the hip joint (reduces varus moment at the hip).

(2). *Ischial containment socket* (see Figure 39–14)
  (a). This design was inspired by the perceived inadequacies of the quadrilateral socket to provide mediolateral stability of the hip during the stance phase of gait.
  (b). Narrow mediolateral socket dimension provides more direct skeletal control of the femur by the lateral socket wall during forceful hip abductor muscle activity. This is designed to improve the effectiveness of the hip abductor mechanism to stabilize the pelvis during stance.
  (c). The ischial tuberosity is positioned inside the socket in the posteromedial corner, creating a "bony lock" that prevents sliding during forceful hip abductor muscle activity at stance.
  (d). Locking the position of the

A
CROSS-SECTION

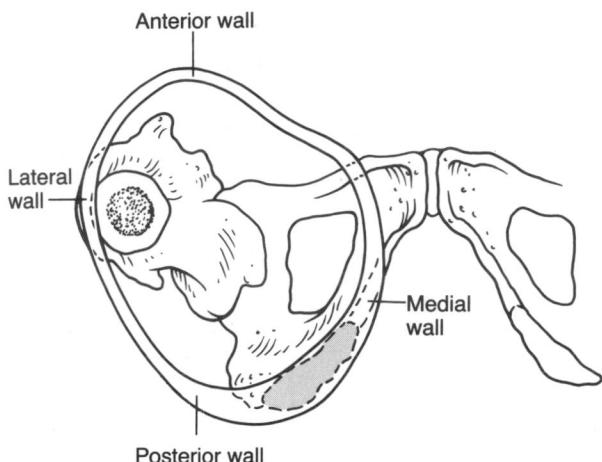

Anterior wall

Lateral
wall

Medial
wall

Posterior wall

B
POSTERIOR VIEW

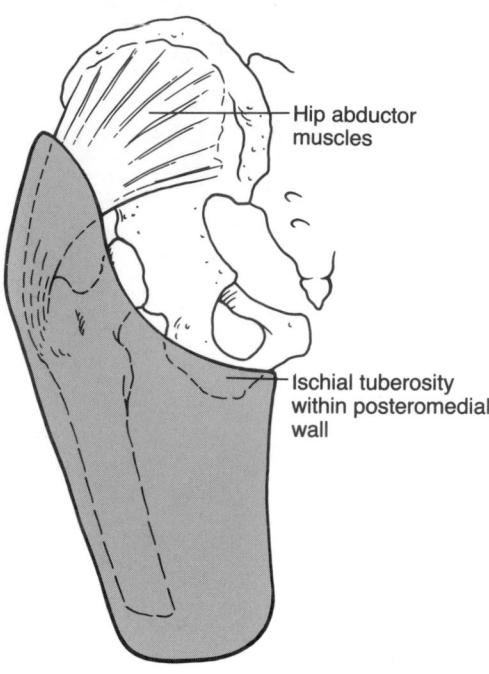

Hip abductor
muscles

Ischial tuberosity
within posteromedial
wall

FIGURE 39–14   **A** and **B**, Ischial containment socket shape.

pelvis and narrowing the medio-lateral dimension of the socket are theorized to result in an effective environment for the hip abductor musculature to stabilize the hip at stance. This in turn allows the foot to be more aggressively inset medially under the socket, improving gait cosmesis and energy efficiency.

b. *Materials.*[8] Both the quadrilateral and the ischial containment sockets can be fabricated as a rigid or a flexible socket.

  (1). Objectives of the flexible socket (see Figure 39–15):

    (a). Increased comfort.

      (i). Flexible aspect of socket accommodates to any changes in muscle size and shape during activity.

      (ii). When sitting, flexible socket accommodates to the sitting surface.

    (b). Improved suspension. Plastic clings to the skin and accommodates changes in shape, improving the suction suspension's effectiveness.

    (c). Improved heat dissipation.

  (2). Potential disadvantages:

    (a). Increased cost of fabrication.

    (b). Increased bulk of flexible socket within rigid frame design.

    (c). Decreased durability of flexible socket compared with rigid.

c. *Suspension* (see Figure 39–16)

  (1). *Suction suspension*

    (a). The prosthesis is maintained in place by an intimate fitting socket worn directly against the skin with an air-expulsion valve. During the swing phase, the socket is airtight, creating negative pressure that holds the prosthesis in place. Very positive suspension results in improved control of the prosthesis.

    (b). Suction suspension is most effective in medium to long residual limbs owing to the greater surface contact area but can be used in shorter limbs as a primary suspension or with an axillary suspension.

    (c). Donning requires greater skill and effort than with other sus-

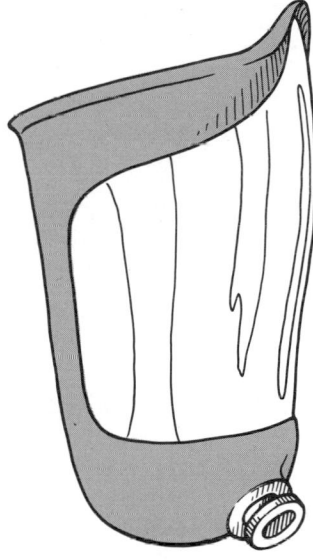

Anterior

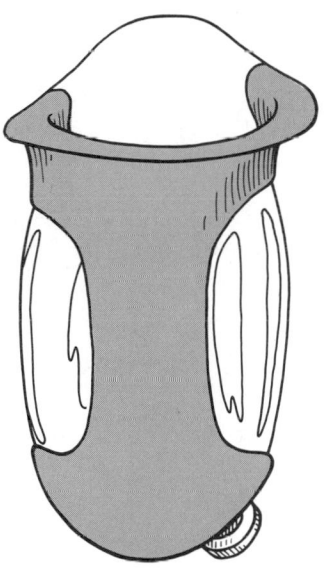

Medial

FIGURE 39–15   Above-knee prosthesis with flexible socket design.

pension options; therefore, it may be contraindicated in the presence of balance deficits, hand dexterity problems, weakness, and cardiac problems.

(d). Irregularities in residual limb tissue contour (*ie,* scarring) can cause loss of suction as a result of air loss through invaginated areas.

(e). Fluctuations in residual limb volume can result in the inability to don the prosthesis or loss of suction, contraindicating its use. Other above-knee suspension alternatives incorporate the use of socks, which allows for accommodations of fluctuations in volume.

(2). *Partial suction suspension*
  (a). Same principles as suction suspension apply, except that the socket is designed to be worn with a sock or nylon sheath. Air can move through the sock, reducing the suction effect, but suspension is improved through the partial negative pressure that is produced.
  (b). Used as an auxiliary suspension versus a primary suspension.

(3). *Silesian belt suspension* (see Figure 39–17)
  (a). Flexible belt attached to the lateral proximal socket. Wraps posteriorly around the waist, gripping primarily over the iliac crest. Attaches to the anterior proximal socket wall.
  (b). Used as a primary or secondary suspension.
  (c). Less restrictive than hip joint and pelvic band. More comfortable in sitting. Lightweight.
  (d). Provides reasonably good suspension. Reduced contribution to mediolateral stability of pelvis during stance unless attached to a high lateral wall. Provides rotational abduction and adduction control of prosthesis.
  (e). Some designs have confusing strap arrangements and can be more difficult to use.
  (f). Patients who engage in aggressive activities should consider the use of an auxiliary suspension to prevent loss of prosthetic suspension.

(4). *Neoprene belt suspension*
  (a). Consists of an elastic neo-

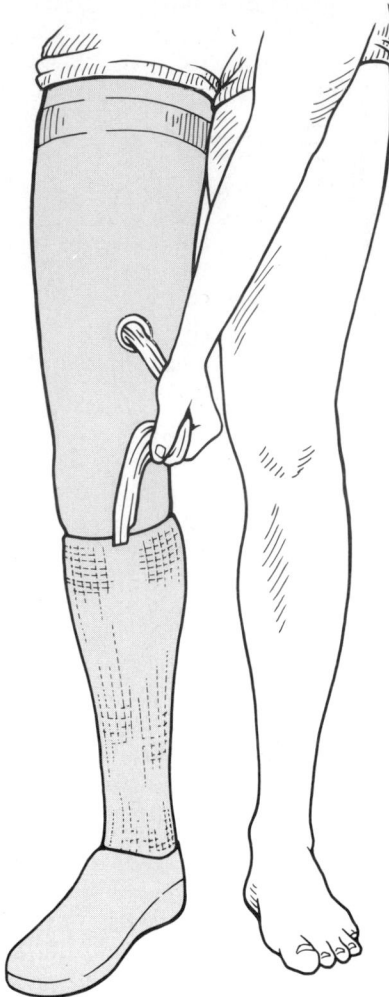

FIGURE 39–16   Above-knee prosthesis with suction suspension.

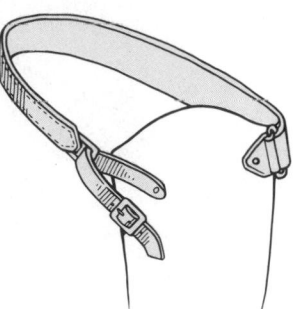

FIGURE 39–17   Above-knee prosthesis with Silesian belt suspension.

(b). More restrictive and less comfortable, especially in sitting. Adds weight and bulk to the prosthesis.

(c). Indicated in cases requiring aggressive mediolateral, rotational, abduction and adduction control of the prosthesis, including short residual limbs, flabby/obese residual limbs, weak hip abductors. Used frequently for geriatric patients. Indicated when simplicity of donning is a priority.

d. **Knee joints**[1–4,6,8,10,11]

(1). Prosthetic knee joints are designed to provide

(a). Stability at stance.

(b). Controlled flexion and exten-

prene sleeve that slides over the proximal socket. Elastic neoprene waist belt wraps around the waist and fastens with Velcro overlap (see Figure 39–18).

(b). Simple, comfortable, effective suspension.

(c). Elastic materials provide moderately effective suspension and rotational control.

(d). Durability is limited. May require periodic replacement.

(5). *Hip joint and pelvic band suspension* (see Figure 39–19)

(a). Provides suspension, mediolateral control of the hip and pelvis at stance, and rotational control of the prosthesis.

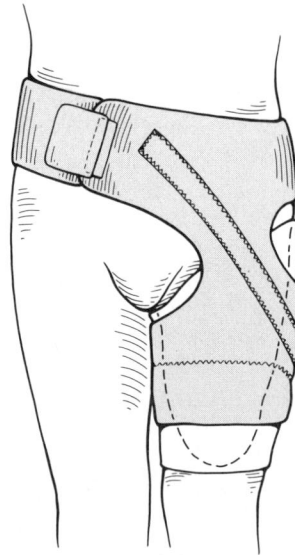

FIGURE 39–18   Above-knee prosthesis with elastic suspension belt.

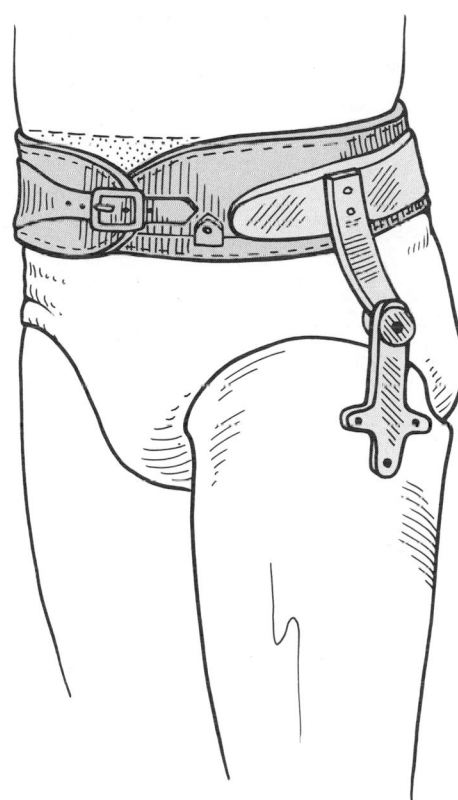

FIGURE 39–19 Above-knee prosthesis with hip joint and pelvic band suspension.

sion to provide as natural a swing phase as possible.

(c). Required knee flexion for functional activities (*eg,* sitting, kneeling).

(2). Major differences in prosthetic knees are the methods used to provide stance-phase stability and that allow smooth and natural knee flexion during the swing phase, especially as the patient changes gait velocity.

(3). Appropriateness of the knee depends on the patient's ability to control the knee, activity level, durability and maintenance requirements, and stability requirements to prevent buckling during use.

(4). Innovations in knee joint design have resulted in greater inherent mechanical contributions to knee stability.

(5). The weight of some knee units has been reduced by using carbon graphite and titanium materials.

(6). *Single-axis constant friction knee*

(a). Low cost. Simple, reliable design.

(b). Stance stability depends completely on alignment.

(c). Should be used cautiously in the presence of

(i). Hip extensor weakness.

(ii). Balance problems.

(iii). Significant hip flexion contracture causing alignment problem.

(iv). Patients who are susceptible to serious consequences should they fall.

(d). Swing phase adjusted to one velocity of walking. This can be adjusted by friction screw (applies friction to the knee bolt); however, heel rise will be symmetrical only when walking at the velocity for which the knee is adjusted.

(e). Indications:

(i). Children, owing to durability and cost advantages.

(ii). Low-activity ambulators who maintain a relatively consistent gait velocity and do not require an inherent mechanical contribution from the knee joint to maintain knee stability at stance.

(7). *Stance-control knee*

(a). Provides improved knee stability at stance through a weight-activated friction brake that engages as weight is applied to the prosthesis at stance. Friction brake sensitivity is adjustable.

(b). At swing phase functions as a single-axis constant friction knee.

(c). Indications:

(i). Short residual limb.

(ii). Hip musculature weakness.

(iii). Geriatric applications.

(iv). Balance deficits.

(d). Disadvantages: Must reduce or remove weight from the prosthesis to flex knee (can interfere with functional activities, *eg*, sitting).

(8). *Polycentric knee*

(a). Offers a knee axis with an instantaneous center of rotation that shifts position to provide greater stability at stance and facilitates the initiation of knee flexion at swing.

(b). Some designs improve the cosmetic result for individuals with long above-knee residual limbs or knee disarticulation by allowing the shank to fold under the thigh section when sitting, assisting to match the length of the thigh and leg sections with those of the sound leg.

(c). Shank section shortens during knee flexion, which facilitates foot clearance at swing.

(d). Same indications as stance-control knee plus long above-knee residual limbs and knee disarticulation.

(e). Disadvantages:

(i). Increased cost.

(ii). Weight.

(iii). Maintenance requirements.

(9). *Manual-lock knee*

(a). Provides maximum knee stability when locked. May offer the option to walk with knee unlocked.

(b). Must unlock to sit and relock when standing.

(c). Remains locked during ambulation activities, resulting in a less natural and more energy-consuming gait pattern (exchange cosmetic result for stability).

(d). Manual lock may be used for specific applications, such as uneven terrain, hunting, and climbing.

(10). *Hydraulic/pneumatic knee*

(a). Accommodates changes in gait velocity, maintaining a symmetrical heel rise at swing by creating more resistance to flexion and extension at fast velocities and less resistance at slower velocities.

(b). Dampens and smooths the swing component of gait, providing the most natural-appearing gait of all knee units.

(c). Most units control knee flexion and extension at swing phase only. Some knees can be combined with any of the aforementioned stance-phase control options (*ie*, hydraulic swing-phase control combined with a polycentric stance-control unit).

(d). Most expensive, heaviest, highest maintenance requirements.

(e). Indicated for active amputees who change gait velocity routinely or participate in activities in which the benefits of this knee unit outweigh the disadvantages (considerations include vocational and avocational activities and athletics).

e. ***Prosthetic feet.***[3,10] See section on prosthetic feet, p 1140.

C. Prosthetic evaluation

1. Evaluation with prosthesis off patient before donning.

a. Is the prosthesis as prescribed?

(1). See section III.F.1.a., p 1141.

2. Evaluation with patient standing in parallel bars wearing prosthesis.

a. Is the patient experiencing discomfort while standing with equal weight on each side with the feet 4 to 6 inches apart?

(1). See section III.F.2.a., p 1141.

(2). The patient may complain of discomfort in the perineum area from pressure during weight bearing. The medial brim should not contact the ischial or pubic rami.

(3). Resolutions:

(a). Add socks if it is suspected that the residual limb is sinking into the socket too far. Refer to prosthetist to add a liner to the socket if 15 ply of socks is insufficient to raise the residual limb to the proper position in the socket.

(b). Refer to prosthetist to flare the medial wall to improve comfort. As a last resort, consult with prosthetist about lowering the medial wall. This can result in loss of containment of the adductor tissues as well as a reduction in the length of the proximal medial lever arm for stabilizing the pelvis during stance.

(c). If discomfort is localized to the anteromedial corner (long adductor groove), there may be insufficient relief for the long adductor. Ensure that long adductor tendon is properly located in the groove. Refer to prosthetist to increase relief for long adductor tendon if required.

b. Is the length of the prosthesis correct?

(1). The goal in unilateral applications with a free knee unit at swing is to equalize length in both extremities.

(2). When using a manual-lock knee, the prosthetic side is typically shortened up to 0.5 inch to assist in swing-phase clearance by reducing the necessary extent of hip hiking.

(3). The goal for bilateral above-knee prostheses is equal height, adjusting as required if difficulty is experienced in clearing one side versus the other.

(4). The goal for above-knee–below-knee combination prostheses is to shorten the above-knee prosthesis up to 0.5 inch to assist in swing-phase clearance.

(5). To determine whether the prosthetic length is correct, see section III.F.2.b., p 1142.

c. Is the ischial tuberosity properly located?

(1). *Quadrilateral socket.* While the patient bends forward, the therapist palpates the ischial tuberosity. While the patient stands erect, the therapist maintains his/her finger on the ischial tuberosity. The finger should be compressed between the ischial tuberosity and shelf of the posterior wall, indicating that it is bearing weight.

(a). Problem: ischial tuberosity position too high.

(i). Resolution: reduce number of sock plies until properly located. Use only a nylon sheath if necessary, or pull the residual limb into the socket using

an extended length of stockinette. If still unable to don properly, recheck circumference of residual limb against initial evaluation. If greater circumference, attempt to reduce edema by elevating the residual limb, intermittent compression (unless contraindicated), and/or volume-containment techniques. If circumference measurements are not greater, consult with prosthetist concerning socket fit.

(b). Problem: ischial tuberosity too low inside socket.

(i). Resolution: add sock plys until properly positioned. If approximately 15 plys not adequate, refer to prosthetist to add liner to socket to reduce socket volume and/or tighten anteroposterior socket dimension.

(2). *Ischial containment socket.* The same procedure is used to palpate ischial tuberosity. The ischial tuberosity should be located *within* the socket in the posterior medial corner.

(a). Problem: ischial tuberosity is too high. Proceed as above.

(b). Problem: ischial tuberosity is too low. Proceed as above.

d. Is the adductor longus channel properly located in the socket?

(1). While the patient stands with equal weight bearing on both legs, the therapist palpates the adductor longus (patient should be asked to isometrically contract hip adductors if difficulty locating). The tendon should be located in the channel, indicating that the socket is in its proper rotational orientation.

(a). Problem #1: tendon too far anterior.

(i). Resolution: indicates prosthesis is excessively internally rotated. Loosen suspension while standing and externally rotate prosthesis. Have patient put weight on prosthesis as suspension is retightened to prevent rotating internally as suspension is tightened.

(b). Problem #2 (less common): tendon too far posterior.

(i). Resolution: indicates prosthesis excessively externally rotated. Loosen suspension while standing and internally rotate prosthesis until tendon in groove. Reapply suspension.

e. Is the knee stable on weight bearing?

(1). The patient stands with equal weight distributed on each leg. The therapist *carefully* taps the posterior thigh. (For safety reasons, it is recommended to have an additional person guard the patient during this test.) The knee should remain stable and not demonstrate a tendency to buckle.

(a). Problem: knee demonstrates a tendency to buckle.

(i). Resolution:

• Safety knee: consult with prosthetist to evaluate alignment stability and adjust the stance control adjustment to increase sensitivity.

• Manual-lock knee: malfunctioning locking mechanism (evaluate cable from the release to the knee unit to determine whether too taut, creating inadvertent unlocking).

• Hydraulic knee with stance control: consult with prosthetist to evaluate alignment stability and adjust stance control.

• Single-axis / polycentric knee: consult with prosthetist to evaluate alignment stability before proceeding with gait training.

f. Has total contact been achieved in the socket fit?

(1). *Suction socket.* This is crucial to successful prosthetic use. Lack of total contact can result in a pocket of ex-

cessive negative pressure, resulting in edema formation or skin breakdown. The valve of the socket should be removed. Tissue should protrude into the valve hole area. If it does not, the therapist should palpate into the valve hole area to determine the extent of the void.

(2). *Semisuction or nonsuction socket.* Total contact is preferable to prevent edema formation and to more effectively distribute forces in the socket (improve comfort/skin integrity). Air moving within the socket reduces the degree of negative pressure created and the incidence of skin problems resulting from lack of total contact.

(a). Problem: lack of total contact.

(i). Resolution: determine whether the residual limb is correctly located within the socket by checking the position of the ischial tuberosity and long adductor tendon. Correct any problems with position (see section III.C.2.c.,d., p 1133). If positioned correctly:

• Suction socket: refer to prosthetist to correct void.

• Nonsuction socket: evidence of secondary problems associated with lack of contact? If so, refer to prosthetist to correct problem. If not, monitor skin socket comfort and request correction if development of a secondary problem occurs.

g. Is suspension adequate to minimize pistoning of the residual limb when the prosthesis is raised off the floor?

(1). To detect whether the residual limb rises out of the socket, the patient should hike the hip on the prosthetic side, raising the prosthesis off the floor, while the therapist palpates at the brim of the posterior wall.

(2). Pistoning is expected to be absent in a suction suspension. Minimal pistoning is expected when other suspensions are used.

PLEASE NOTE: The acceptability of pistoning is based on whether it is contributing to skin problems, discomfort, or creating functional problems such as clearance during the swing phase.

(a). Problem: excessive pistoning.
  (i). Resolution (suction suspension):
  • Ensure that prosthesis has been donned correctly.
  • Ensure that valve is properly tightened and functioning. To evaluate, place clay over valve area if it is suspected that air is leaking into socket through valve hole.
  • Loss of suction indicates a loss of intimacy of fit of socket. Refer to prosthetist to evaluate socket fit and to modify socket to re-establish suction seal in socket if indicated.
  (ii). Resolution (Silesian belt suspension):
  • Determine whether belt is properly tightened and lying between iliac crest and greater trochanter on sound side.
  • Determine whether socks need to be added by checking position of ischial tuberosity (if inside socket on quadrilateral or positioned too low in ischial containment socket, add socks). Often it is necessary to work in reverse. After adding socks, determine whether ischial tuberosity has been improperly raised out of position. If not, it is appropriate to use additional socks to tighten fit of socket.
  (iii). Resolution (neoprene belt suspension):

  • Determine whether belt is adequately tightened.
  • Determine whether belt has lost its elasticity. If so, pursue replacement.
  • See discussion on socks under Silesian belt suspension above.
  • Determine whether Velcro is properly overlapping and is adequately functioning.
  (iv). Resolution (hip joint and pelvic band suspension):
  • Determine whether belt is adequately tightened.
  • Determine whether pelvic band lies flat between iliac crest and greater trochanter of amputated side. If not, refer to prosthetist to correct contour.
  • See discussion on socks under Silesian belt suspension above.
3. Evaluation with patient sitting.
  a. Does the socket maintain its position on the residual limb?
  (1). Problem: prosthesis is pushed off when sitting.
  (a). Resolutions:
  (i). Anterior wall may be too high, pushing against the abdomen or pelvis, especially when leaning forward. Refer to prosthetist to evaluate and to lower or flare anterior wall if indicated.
  (ii). With hip joint and pelvic band suspension, if the hip joint is improperly located (proper location is approximately 0.5 inch anterior and 1 inch proximal to the greater trochanter) such that the anatomical and mechanical joint congruencies do not coincide, the socket will be either pushed off or pulled on too tightly when sitting. Refer to prosthetist to evaluate and correct.

b. Do the lengths of the prosthetic leg and thigh sections approximate those of the sound side?

   (1). Problem: thigh too long and leg section short (foot may be off floor).

      (a). Resolutions:

         (i). Once the prosthesis is fabricated, this is a difficult problem to resolve.

         (ii). Discuss the reason for this inequality with the prosthetist.

         (iii). May be unavoidable in long residual limbs and knee disarticulation, although the use of appropriate componentry should minimize the problem.

c. Does the shin section remain perpendicular to the floor when seated (vertical)?

   (1). Problem: shin is turned in or turned out.

      (a). Resolution: indicative of socket rotation on the residual limb. Instruct amputee to manually correct the socket rotation so that shin assumes a vertical position.

d. Does the knee remain flexed during sitting?

   (1). Problem: knee tends to extend.

      (a). Resolutions:

         (i). The foam cover of an endoskeletal prosthesis can act as an extension aid. Instruct patient to store the prosthesis with knee flexed at night in order to stretch cover at knee, reducing the extension bias.

         (ii). If knee has an extension aid, it may be too strong. Refer to the prosthetist to decrease strength of extension aid.

e. Does the patient experience pressure on posterior thigh corresponding to top of posterior socket wall?

   (1). Problem: discomfort.

      (a). Resolution: posterior shelf may be too wide, concentrating pressure in this area during sitting. Refer to prosthetist to evaluate and narrow wall as necessary.

4. Evaluation with patient sitting and prosthesis removed.

a. Are the forces appropriately distributed over the residual limb? The therapist should evaluate for abrasions and discoloration.

   (1). Problem #1: discoloration of distal residual limb.

      (a). Resolution: most likely caused by a lack of total contact. See section III.F.2.a.(7), p 1141.

   (2). Problem #2: discoloration of anterior distal residual limb over end of femur.

      (a). Resolution: most likely inadequate relief in the socket for the anterior distal femur. In consultation with the prosthetist, evaluate the need for socket relief in this area by padding the anterior socket wall proximal to end of femur using moleskin or removable adhesive foam. Refer to prosthetist for definitive resolution if this is effective in reducing discomfort.

   (3). Problem #3: discoloration of lateral distal femur.

      (a). Resolution: most likely inadequate relief in socket for lateral distal femur. Proceed as described above for anterior distal femur problem.

   (4). Problem #4: skin breakdown on ischial tuberosity.

      (a). Resolutions:

         (i). Increase sock plys to relieve pressure from ischial tuberosity.

         (ii). Determine whether posterior wall is angled up on medial side during standing (not parallel to floor), increasing pressure on ischial tuberosity. If so, refer to prosthetist to determine whether socket alignment can be adjusted to relieve ischial tuberosity pressure without adversely affecting gait.

         (iii). Posterior wall can be padded either around the ischial tuberosity or the entire posterior wall to relieve pressure. Evaluate with removable padding. Refer to prosthetist for definitive solution.

D. Gait training[1-4,12]

1. **General principles**
   a. Learning to ambulate with an above-knee prosthesis is more difficult and requires more training than with a below-knee prosthesis.
   b. The above-knee amputee is less susceptible to skin problems than the below-knee patient.
   c. Properly donning the above-knee prosthesis can be difficult and can limit long-term successful use of the prosthesis.
   d. Less emphasis is placed on controlling the progression of gait training to protect the skin integrity of the residual limb. Ambulation progression is encouraged and prosthetic donning skills are emphasized in the early rehabilitation stages.
   e. Advancements in technology of knee, feet, and socket componentry make possible more advanced skills (*eg*, running) for the more aggressive amputee.

2. **Gait training progression (new amputee in parallel bars)**
   a. Weight shifting: see section III.H.2.a., p 1147.
   b. Patient steps forward and places swing foot into heel strike position (see section III.H.2.b., p 1147).
   c. Patient advances from heel strike to foot flat position.
      (1). Problem: knee buckles from heel strike to foot flat.
         (a). Resolution: emphasize hip extension from heel strike to foot flat to move floor reaction forces anterior to knee joint as rapidly as possible and to assist in holding knee joint in extension.
   d. Patient progresses from foot flat to midstance.
      (1). Problem: knee buckles from foot flat to midstance.
         (a). Resolution: cue patient to maintain hip extension and erect trunk.
   e. Patient steps through on sound side.

   (1). Problem: patient relaxes hip extension, leans forward with trunk, short stance time on prosthetic side.
      (a). Resolution: emphasize a continuation of hip extension, progressing the pelvis forward as a step is taken on the sound side.
   f. Sequence is repeated as skin tolerance allows.
      (1). Speed is progressively increased as tolerated without losing quality of gait sequence.
      (2). Methodical progression is made to less supportive assistive devices.
      (3). The focus should be on gait quality to avoid regression as assistive devices are advanced.

E. Gait analysis

1. **Sagittal analysis**
   a. Deviation: knee unit buckles or appears unstable at stance.

Potential Cause	Resolution
(1) Foot delays moving from heel strike to foot flat.	(1) Emphasize hip extension from heel strike through stance phase. Foot mechanism responsible for controlling plantar flexion from heel strike to foot flat may be too rigid. Refer to prosthetist to evaluate. Knee unit may be aligned too close or ahead of TKA line. Refer to prosthetist to evaluate. Hip extension may be weak. Initiate strengthening exercises. Hip flexion contracture may be present. Increase range of motion of affected hip.

b. Deviation: uneven step lengths.

Potential Causes	Resolutions
(1) Pain during weight bearing on prosthetic side.	(1) Determine whether socket fits appropriately by assessing position of ischial tuberosity and adductor longus tendon (see sections IV.C.2.c. and IV.C.2.d., p 1163).
(2) Insecurity during weight bearing.	(2) Gait training drills, emphasizing stance on the prosthetic side (static weight shifting, side stepping, braiding, etc.).
(3) Hip flexion contracture or insufficient socket flexion resulting in a shorter step on the sound side.	(3) Concentrate on increasing range of motion of affected hip. Consult with prosthetist to determine need to increase socket flexion to accommodate contracture.

c. Deviation: rapid plantar flexion from heel strike to foot flat resulting in foot slap.

Potential Causes	Resolution
(1) Foot mechanism responsible for controlling plantar flexion from heel strike to foot flat is too soft.	(1) If foot has cushioned heel, stuff paper towel into toe of shoe, tightening fit, which will limit heel expansion and effectively stiffen heel. If ineffective, consult with prosthetist to evaluate need to change foot.

Potential Causes	Resolutions
	(2) Consult with prosthetist to determine whether plantar flexion resistance can be adjusted.

d. Deviation: vaulting (rising up on the toe of sound foot during swing phase of prosthetic side).

Potential Causes	Resolutions
(1) Prosthesis too long.	(1) Determine whether posthesis too long following procedures in sections III.F.2.b., p 1141, and IV.C.2.b., p 1163.
(2) Inadequate suspension resulting in the prosthesis being relatively too long at swing.	(2) Determine whether suspension problem following procedure in section IV.C.2.g., p 1164.
(3) Inadequate knee flexion at swing due to excessive friction on knee unit; improperly adjusted hydraulic or pneumatic knee swing-phase control; extension aid too strong.	(3) Consult with prosthetist.
(4) Residual limb not properly seated in socket (ischial tuberosity too high).	(4) Determine whether ischial tuberosity properly positioned (see section IV.C.2.c., p 1163).

e. Deviation: unequal height of heel rise during swing.

Potential Causes	Resolutions
(1) Inadequate friction on prosthetic knee during swing; improperly adjusted swing-phase control of hydraulic or pneumatic knee; knee extension aid too strong or too weak.	(1) Consult with prosthetist.
(2) Amputee is changing gait velocity using a prosthesis with a mechanical knee joint (not hydraulic or pneumatic).	(2) Uneven heel rise is to be expected because the knee bolt friction on a mechanical knee can be set only for one velocity. Teach amputee to hop/skip run with a mechanical knee.

f. Deviation: Excessive force of impact of knee at terminal swing.

Potential Causes	Resolutions
(1) Inadequate friction on prosthetic knee during swing; improperly adjusted swing-phase control of hydraulic or pneumatic knee; extension aid too strong.	(1) Consult with prosthetist.
(2) Amputee may be forcefully extending knee to obtain secure feeling that knee is in full extension before stance.	(2) Ensure that knee is stable with weight bearing (see section IV.C.2.e., p 1164). Gait training with cueing to reduce forceful extension of knee.

2. **Frontal analysis**

a. Deviation: prosthesis maintained in abduction throughout gait cycle.

Potential Causes	Resolutions
(1) Discomfort, proximal medial socket (perineal area).	(1) Determine whether medial socket wall is too high. Attempt to place finger on top of medial wall between top of wall and pubic ramus while patient is standing. If ramus is contacting medial wall brim, ensure that residual limb is not too deep in socket (assess location of ischial tuberosity as described in section IV.C.2.c., p 1163).
(2) Prosthesis too long.	(2) Evaluate and address as described in sections III.F.2.b. and IV.C.2.b., pp 1142 and 1163.
(3) Hip abductor mechanism unable to adequately maintain hip and pelvic mediolateral stability at stance. May be due to inadequate support of the femur by the lateral wall during active hip abduction and or sliding of the ischial tuberosity medially in a quadrilateral socket at stance. Abducting the prosthesis effectively reduces the demand on the hip abductors by moving the floor reaction forces closer to axis of rotation (hip joint) and reducing the moment causing mediolateral instability.	(3) Strengthen hip abductors. Short, fleshy, residual limbs may benefit from an ischial containment socket design (see section IV.B.1.b., p 1158).

Potential Causes	Resolutions
(4) Amputee habitually maintains an abducted position during gait.	(4) Determine whether amputee can volitionally correct the abducted position during gait without increasing discomfort or creating mediolateral hip instability at stance. If yes, correct through gait training. If no, pursue either discomfort or mediolateral instability problem to determine cause.
(5) Pelvic band may be improperly contoured to the body and not lying flat on the hip between the iliac crest and greater tronchanter.	(5) Determine whether a gap exists between the pelvic band and the pelvis when the prosthesis is correctly positioned during standing and the waist belt loosened. If gap exists, tightening waist belt results in abducting prosthesis by pulling proximal socket toward body. Refer to prosthetist to recontour waist band to pelvis with prosthesis in correct position.

b. Deviation: lateral bending of trunk.

Potential Causes	Resolutions
(1) Prosthesis too short.	(1) Assess and address as described in sections III.F.2.b. and IV.C.2.b., pp 1142 and 1163.

Potential Causes	Resolutions
(2) Discomfort, proximal medial socket (perineal area).	(2) See a.(1) above.
(3) Hip abductor mechanism unable to adequately maintain hip/pelvic mediolateral stability at stance.	(3) Consider mediolateral dimension of socket; position of ischial tuberosity; adduction angle of socket. Consult with prosthetist.

c. Deviation: amputee circumducts prosthesis during swing phase.

Potential Causes	Resolutions
(1) Prosthesis too long. Excessive friction on knee bolt; improperly adjusted hydraulic or pneumatic knee swing-phase control; knee extension aide too strong.	(1) See a.(2) above. Consult with prosthetist to determine whether adjustment is indicated.
(2) Inadequate socket suspension.	(2) Determine whether suspension is adequate, following procedures in section IV.C.2.g., p 1164.
(3) Residual limb not properly seated in socket (ischial tuberosity too high).	(3) Determine whether ischial tuberosity is properly positioned in socket. (see section IV.C.2.c., p 1163).

d. Deviation: external rotation of prosthetic foot from heel strike to foot flat.

Potential Causes	Resolutions
(1) Patient not bearing adequate weight at initial stance for the foot plantar flexion mechanism to operate properly.	(1) Cue patient to increase weight bearing at initial stance. Use limb-load monitor to encourage weight bearing at initial stance.

Potential Causes	Resolutions
(2) Foot mechanism responsible for controlling plantar flexion from heel strike to foot flat is too rigid.	(2) Refer to prosthetist to adjust or change to foot with less plantar flexion resistance.
(3) Socket may be loose fitting or residual limb musculature may be weak and flabby, allowing for rotation between residual limb and socket.	(3) Suction socket: refer to prosthetist to evaluate by adding temporary pads to tighten socket fit. Nonsuction socket: determine whether more sock plys are required (see section IV.C.2.c., p 1163, to evaluate proper number of socks). Ensure that suspension is effective (see section IV.C.2.g., p 1164).

e. Deviation: improper tracking of heel during swing phase (whips).

Potential Causes	Resolutions
(1) Improper position of knee bolt. Normally when standing, knee bolt is slightly externally rotated in relation to line of progression of walking. During swing phase, hip internally rotates, bringing knee bolt perpendicular to line of progression, resulting in heel tracking straight in line of progression at swing. If knee bolt is too externally rotated, it does not reach a perpendic-	(1) Ensure that socket is donned properly (assess rotational orientation; see section IV.C.2.d., p 1163). (2) Consult with prosthetist if knee bolt improperly oriented to line of progression.

Potential Causes	Resolutions
ular position to line of progression at swing, and heel whips medially at initial swing. If knee bolt is not adequately externally rotated, it assumes position of internal rotation at swing, and heel whips laterally at initial swing.	
(2) Socket may be loose fitting or residual limb musculature may be weak and flabby.	(2) See d.(3) above.

F. ADL training

1. **Stairs**
   a. *Method.* Ascending, lead up with sound side and bring prosthetic side to the same step. Descending, lead down with prosthetic side and bring sound side to the same step. If the prosthetic knee unit incorporates a hydraulic stance control, a step-over-step method of descending is possible. The aggressive amputee may descend in a step-over-step fashion with a mechanical knee by placing the heel only of the prosthetic foot on the lower step and "jackknifing" (volitionally buckling) the knee once the sound side is in place to assume the next lower step.
   b. *Potential problems*
      (1). Loss of balance.
      (2). Knee instability.
   c. *Resolutions*
      (1). Use rails whenever possible.
      (2). Emphasize hip extension on the prosthetic side during stance to promote knee stability.

2. **Inclines**
   a. *Method.* Directly ascend or descend in a forward position.
      (1). Ascend: lead with the sound side followed by stepping to the level of the sound step with the prosthetic side.

(2). Descend by leading with the prosthetic side followed by stepping to the level of the prosthetic side with the sound step. The prosthetic step is shortened to reduce the chance of the floor reaction forces moving posterior to the knee axis, promoting knee instability. If the knee incorporates a hydraulic stance control, a step-over-step method of ascending and descending is possible. Jackknifing may also be used by the aggressive amputee to descend ramps.

b. *Potential problem.* Prosthetic knee instability.

c. *Resolutions.* Shorten the length of the prosthetic step. Emphasize hip extension on the prosthetic side during stance. Ascend and descend on an angle across the ramp. Side-stepping approach, leading with the sound step when ascending and leading with the prosthetic step when descending.

3. **Curbs.** Follow procedure for stairs.

4. **Uneven surfaces.** See section III.K.4., p 1153. Additionally, uneven surfaces increase the potential for knee buckling.

   a. *Resolutions*

   (1). Shorten steps.

   (2). Emphasize hip extension at stance.

   (3). If the patient's lifestyle includes frequent walking on uneven surfaces, a knee unit with inherent stance stability or stance control should be considered.

5. **Kneeling.** See section III.K.5., p 1153.

6. **Rising from floor.** See section III.K.6., p 1153.

7. **Stepping over objects.** See section III.K.7., p 1153.

8. **Car transfers.** See section III.K.8., p 1153.

G. Bilateral above-knee prosthetic considerations

1. **Problem.**

   a. Knee stability, particularly when managing elevations and ADL.

   (1). The absence of a sound extremity with active knee extension places

the bilateral above-knee amputee at a great disadvantage.

(2). Resolutions:

   (a). Recommend at least one manual-lock knee.

   (b). Recommend hydraulic knees with stance-phase control for the more active amputee.

   (c). An unlocked knee should be aligned to promote more stance-phase stability.

PLEASE NOTE: An endoskeletal unit provides the option of interchanging knee units if the amputee is unsuccessful with prosthetic knee control.

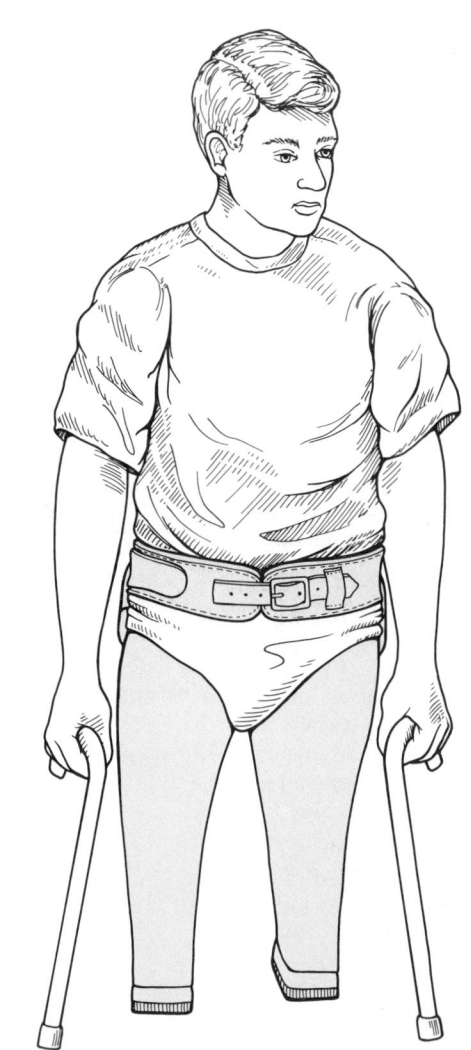

FIGURE 39–20 Above-knee "stubbies."

b. Loss of balance.
  (1). See section III.L.1.c., p 1154. In addition, the above-knee amputee faces the potential of an unlocked knee buckling when balance is upset.
  (2). Resolutions:
    (a). See section III.L.1.c., p 1154.

> ▮ **PLEASE NOTE:** Lowering prosthetic height has a significant effect on improving balance, gait, and prosthetic control (lowers the center of gravity). Height can be progressively lengthened as tolerated if using an endoskeletal system.

    (b). A foot with a stiffer plantar flexion mechanism is used to reduce the chance of falling backward.
  c. Use of bilateral above-knee prostheses unsuccessful or determined to be inappropriate, but patient desires or needs to be able to get out of wheelchair and ambulate short distances.
    (1). Resolutions: "stubbies" may be indicated to allow short-distance ambulation or ambulation trial. Stubbies consist of an above-knee socket with rocker bottom, which eliminates the knee joint and lowers the amputee's center of gravity. Balance, gait, and prosthetic control are improved, and energy costs are reduced. Full-length prosthesis may be used for cosmetic reasons or special occasions (see Figure 39–20).
  d. Lack of space in the perineum area, creating impingement.
    (1). This is a frequent problem with quadrilateral socket wearers because of the large mediolateral dimension of the socket in comparison to an ischial containment socket.
    (2). Resolutions:
      (a). When appropriate, recommend ischial containment sockets. Consider a flexible socket brim design.
      (b). Males may benefit from use of an athletic supporter.

V. Other Prostheses

A. Partial foot prosthesis[1,2,4,6]

1. Biomechanical purposes of partial foot prosthesis:
   a. Reproduces lever arm of normal foot for push-off at terminal stance phase.
   b. Distributes force on residual limb so that soft tissue is capable of withstanding the direct and shear pressures that occur during activity.
   c. Provides mediolateral stability of the shortened midfoot.
   d. Prevents anterior migration of the foot in the shoe.
   e. Provides resistance to creasing of the shoe vamp.
   f. Provides shoe-size symmetry.
2. Choice of prosthetic design depends on
   a. Amputation level.
   b. Condition of remaining soft tissue.
   c. Activity level requirements.
   d. Ankle joint condition.
3. Three basic design criteria:
   a. Comfort.
     (1). Shock-absorbing materials used when shock-absorbing mechanisms of foot and ankle are compromised.
     (2). Total contact distribution over residual limb to reduce pressures.
   b. Cosmesis.
     (1). Typically advantageous to use the least amount of prosthetic intervention required.
   c. Function (three primary losses).
     (1). Push-off at terminal stance: lose at higher speeds after great toe lost. Decreased push-off as residual limb length shortens.
     (2). Weight bearing: two primary arches of foot—longitudinal and transverse. Lost arches result in a splayed foot, creating problems in fitting the residual limb in the shoe and resulting in alterations in weight bearing. There is also a tendency toward muscle imbalance as the residual limb shortens. Plantar flexors tend

to overpower the dorsiflexors, resulting in equinus, which can result in pressure concentrations on the anterior residual limb. Muscle transfer is sometimes used to correct this problem.

(3). Suspension: as the residual limb shortens, it becomes more difficult to suspend a shoe on it.

4. Toe amputation:
   a. Minimal functional loss unless great toe involved, reducing the ability to push off.
   b. Effect is primarily cosmetic.
   c. Prosthetic management: toe filler sometimes used to prevent shoe from deforming and/or migration of other toes toward voided area.

5. Longitudinal ray amputation:
   a. Loss of surface area over which to distribute forces.
   b. Loss of push-off if first ray involved.
   c. Mediolateral foot instability may result if 1st or 5th ray involved.
   d. Prosthetic management:
      (1). Total-contact shoe insert promotes distribution of forces. Semirigid forefoot promotes push-off if 1st ray involved.
      (2). Simple toe filler may be all that is required.

6. Transmetatarsal amputation:
   a. Results in bony knuckle–like anterior foot.
   b. Arches disrupted, forefoot tends to flatten over time, resulting in weight-bearing problems.
   c. Loss of push-off at terminal stance.
   d. The shorter the residual limb, the greater the tendency for motion between the prosthesis and the residual limb during terminal stance.
   e. Prosthetic management:
      (1). Total-contact shoe insert and arch support with toe filler.
      (2). Semirigid forefoot or steel shank in shoe to simulate push-off and prevent shoe from bending and pressing on distal residual limb.
      (3). Rocker-bottom sole could be used to promote rollover at proper area of shoe and protect distal residual limb from pressure.

7. Tarsometatarsal amputation:
   a. Further loss of balance and weight bearing. Increased tendency toward equinus contractures at ankle.
   b. Increased problem with suspension of shoe resulting from loss of anterior surface area of foot.
   c. Prosthetic management:
      (1). Typically, most proximal level that a shoe filler can be successfully used. If ankle retains dorsiflexion and plantar flexion range of motion, this should not be limited.
      (2). Posterior leaf-spring ankle-foot orthosis or laminated prosthetic design with toe filler that extends above ankle, creating a counterforce to resist anterior migration of the residual limb during rollover at terminal stance.
      (3). Slipper-type prosthesis that encompasses the residual limb but does not extend significantly above the ankle joint.

8. Transtarsal amputation:
   a. Foot has strong tendency toward equinus.
   b. Prosthetic management:
      (1). A PTB-level prosthesis to protect anterior tibial crest from excessive pressure during rollover at terminal stance.
      (2). If ankle motion available, may be able to fit with an above-the-ankle boot-height prosthesis (ie, Chicago boot-type: ankle motion prevents concentration of pressure anteriorly).
      (3). Extra-depth shoes help correct leg-length discrepancy by removing inlay (removable insert) on prosthetic side and maintaining inlay on sound side.

9. Biomechanical purposes of semirigid forefoot or extended sole stiffener:
   a. Directs where the sole of the shoe bends during rollover at terminal stance so that forces are not concentrated at distal amputation site.
   b. Serves as a lever arm to control the torque produced by body weight at rollover of terminal stance.

B. Syme-level prosthesis

1. Advantage of Syme-level amputation:
   a. Direct end-bearing capabilities result in greater comfort and prosthetic control with fewer skin problems.

b. Long residual limb (lever arm) results in greater prosthetic control and power.

c. Ambulation is possible without a prosthesis.

d. Suspension is inherently provided by the bulbous end of the residual limb.

2. Disadvantages of Syme-level amputation:

a. Cosmetic result is often inferior to a below-knee amputation because of the bulbous end of the residual limb.

3. Syme prosthetic designs:

a. Removable window design: (see Figure 39–21).

(1). Window typically placed distal medially.

(2). Indicated for residual limbs with a larger bulbous end to aid in donning.

b. Closed double wall with expandable inner sleeve design (see Figure 39–22).

(1). Stronger structurally because no cut-out required.

(2). Indicated for a residual limb with a smaller bulbous end or cosmesis of finished prosthesis sacrificed to provide large enough circumference to allow donning.

c. Solid single wall with expandable, slit, soft insert design (see Figure 39–23).

(1). Insert is designed to maintain an adequate inner socket circumference to allow for donning.

(2). Insert is applied to residual limb and then placed into socket.

(3). Intimate fit of insert in socket is typically adequate suspension.

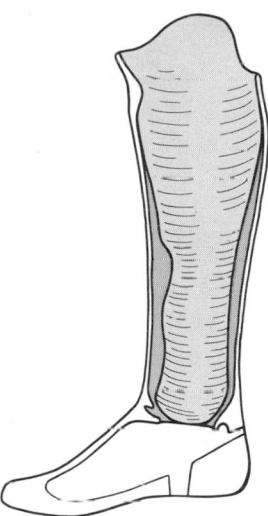

FIGURE 39–22 Syme prosthesis with expandable inner sleeve design.

(4). Structurally sound design but, like the expandable inner sleeve design, it can create a "stovepipe" appearance if the bulbous end is too large.

4. Objectives of Syme prosthetic fitting:

a. Suspension of the prosthesis on the residual limb. Suspension is typically accomplished by the intimate fit above the bulbous end. A supracondylar cuff or suspension sleeve may be added if required.

b. Equalization of limb-length discrepancy. A specialized foot is used that accommodates the long residual limb without creating leg-length discrepancy.

c. Replacement of lost foot function.

d. Maintenance of proper position of heel pad for end bearing. Heel pad may have a tendency to drift medially and posteriorly during weight bearing.

5. Problem: difficulty donning and/or doffing.

a. Resolutions:

(1). Medial opening door design: determine whether door size is adequate to allow the bulbous end to pass through the narrow portion of the prosthetic socket. The door is typically located from the widest circumference point of the bulbous end to an area 0.5 inch above the same circumference proximally. The width of the door is typically one quarter of the bulbous end's circumference.

(2). Insert design:

(a). Adjust number of sock plys

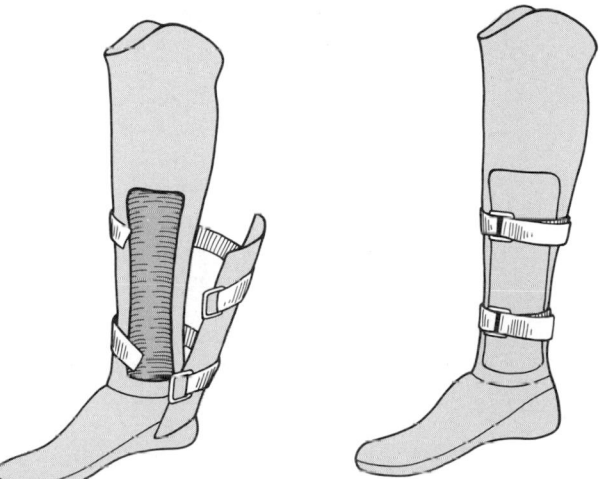

FIGURE 39–21 Syme prosthesis with removable window design.

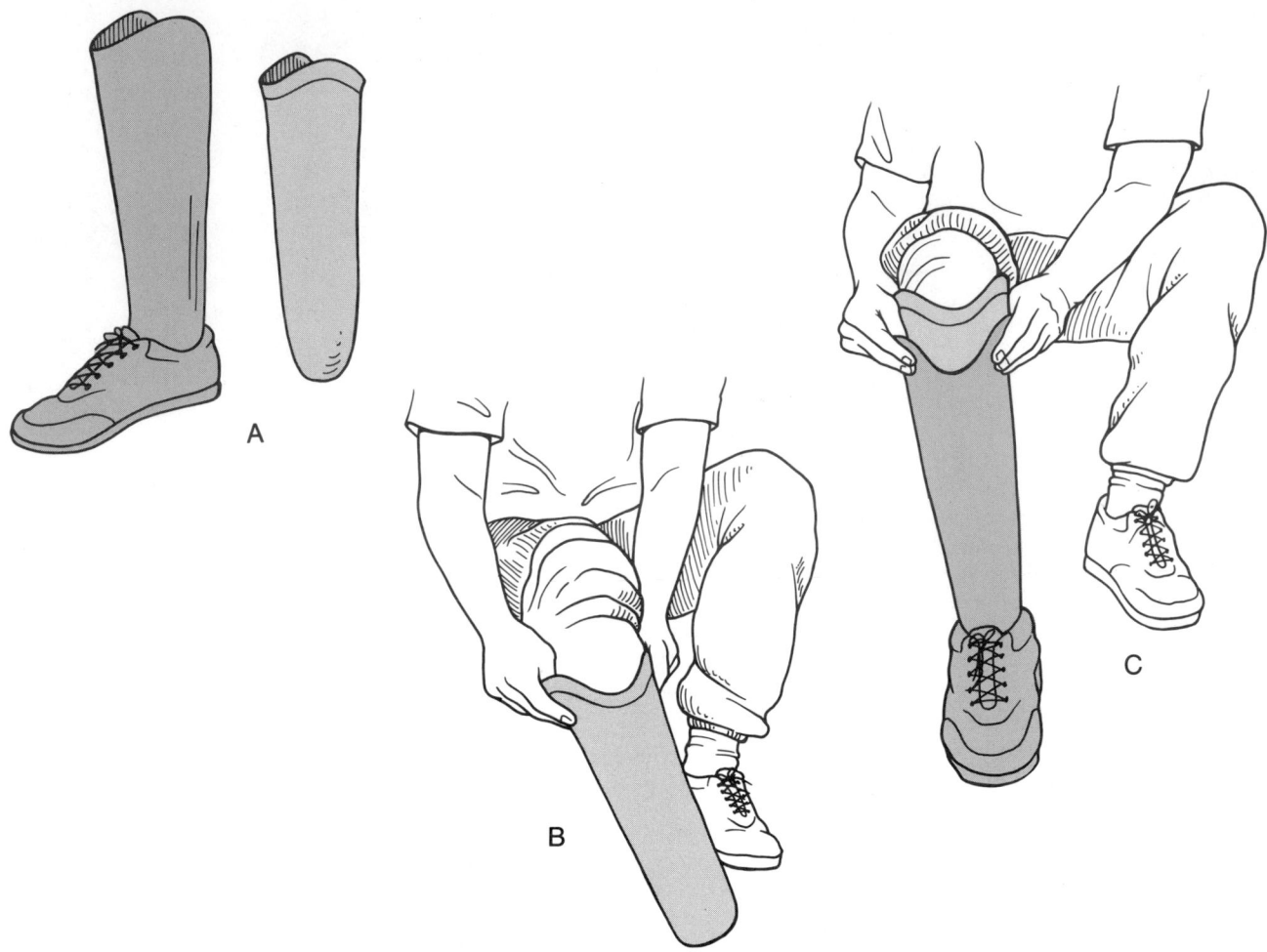

FIGURE 39–23 **A–C**, Syme prosthesis with expandable soft insert design.

until insert is positioned correctly on residual limb (patellar tendon bar should be appropriately located over the patellar tendon, and the distal end should be in contact with the distal insert).

    (b). Apply powder to outside of insert to facilitate donning.

    (c). Apply stocking to outside of insert to facilitate donning.

6. Problem: excessive varus moment during gait.

  a. Resolutions:

    (1). This is a common prosthetic challenge because the long residual limb limits space to outset the foot. Consult with prosthetist.

    (2). Determine whether mediolateral dimension of socket is loose (see section III.I.2.c.(2), p 1149).

7. Problem: difficulty rolling over anterior lever arm of foot from midstance to push-off.

  a. Resolution:

    (1). Assess prosthetic alignment to determine whether

      (a). Foot has been moved as posterior as possible.

      (b). Foot has been toed out as much as is cosmetically acceptable (a little more than on the sound side). This shortens the anterior lever arm.

      (c). Socket is set in adequate flexion (~ 7 degrees).

      (d). Foot has a flexible or rigid keel. A flexible keel will facilitate the rollover process.

8. Problem: rotation of foot at heel strike.

  a. Resolution: This may be due to rotational instability of the socket on the residual limb. The socket should be triangular in shape anteriorly and flattened posteriorly. Discuss problem with prosthetist to determine whether socket modifications can be made to eliminate the rotational problem.

9. Problem: leg-length discrepancy.
   a. Resolution: Assess using procedure described in section III.F.2.b., p 1142. Correction will require referral to prosthetist.

10. Problem: inadequate suspension of residual limb in socket when the prosthesis is raised off floor.
    a. Resolutions:
       (1). Assess using procedures described in section III.F.2.b., p 1142.
       (2). Medial door design: after consultation with prosthetist, assess by temporarily adding foam or layers of moleskin to the inside of the removable door. If improved suspension, refer to prosthetist to make permanent correction.

11. Problem: pressure experienced on proximal aspect of bulbous end when sitting.
    a. Resolution: assess whether posterior wall is too high, forcing the residual limb proximally in the socket when sitting. Consult with prosthetist.

12. Problem: foot not flat on floor at midstance.
    a. Resolution: most likely secondary to a prosthetic alignment problem. Consult with prosthetist.

13. Problem: skin integrity problem or complaint of anterior tibial discomfort during gait.
    a. Resolutions:
       (1). Ensure that anterior distal socket extends to patellar tendon to protect anterior tibial crest, particularly from heel off to toe off, when forces are concentrated anterior proximal and posterior distal.
       (2). Use procedure in section III.F.2.a., p 1141.

C. Hip disarticulation/hemipelvectomy prosthesis[2,3,6,13] (see Figure 39–24)

Early hip disarticulation/hemipelvectomy designs incorporated a locked hip joint. The Canadian design was later introduced and allowed for the use of unlocked hip and knee joints that were stabilized at stance through alignment stability.

1. **Components**
   a. Socket:
      (1). Incorporates the ischial tuberosity for weight bearing.
      (2). Provides suspension at swing by gripping the iliac crest.
      (3). Provides mediolateral stability by extending around the pelvis on the sound side.
   b. Hip joint:
      (1). Standard single-axis joint located anteriorly on socket forward of weight-bearing line. Results in stability at stance phase and facilitates flexion during swing phase.
   c. Knee joints:
      (1). Single-axis constant friction knee.
         (a). Commonly used because of its durability, affordability, and relatively light weight.
         (b). Knee bolt friction can be minimized to facilitate knee extension as rapidly as possible to prepare for heel strike at stance.
      (2). Weight-activated stance-control knee.
         (a). Also commonly used: inherent stability, retains most of the advantages of the single-axis constant friction knee.
         (b). Requires the ability to remove weight from the prosthesis in order to flex the knee to sit. (Can be somewhat more difficult with a hip disarticulation/hemipelvectomy design.)
      (3). Polycentric knee.
         (a). Excellent stance-phase stability.
         (b). Facilitates toe clearance at initial swing because shank section shortens when knee flexes.
         (c). Somewhat heavier and less durable.
      (4). Manual-lock knee.
         (a). Must unlock to sit.
         (b). Use only when necessary.
      (5). Hydraulic (fluid-controlled) knee.
         (a). Proposed to allow greater hip flexion during gait and faster velocity.

2. **Feet**[14]
   a. SACH: moderate weight, low cost, excellent durability.
   b. Single axis: used where greater knee stability is required.
   c. Multiple axis: see section III.E.3., p 1140.

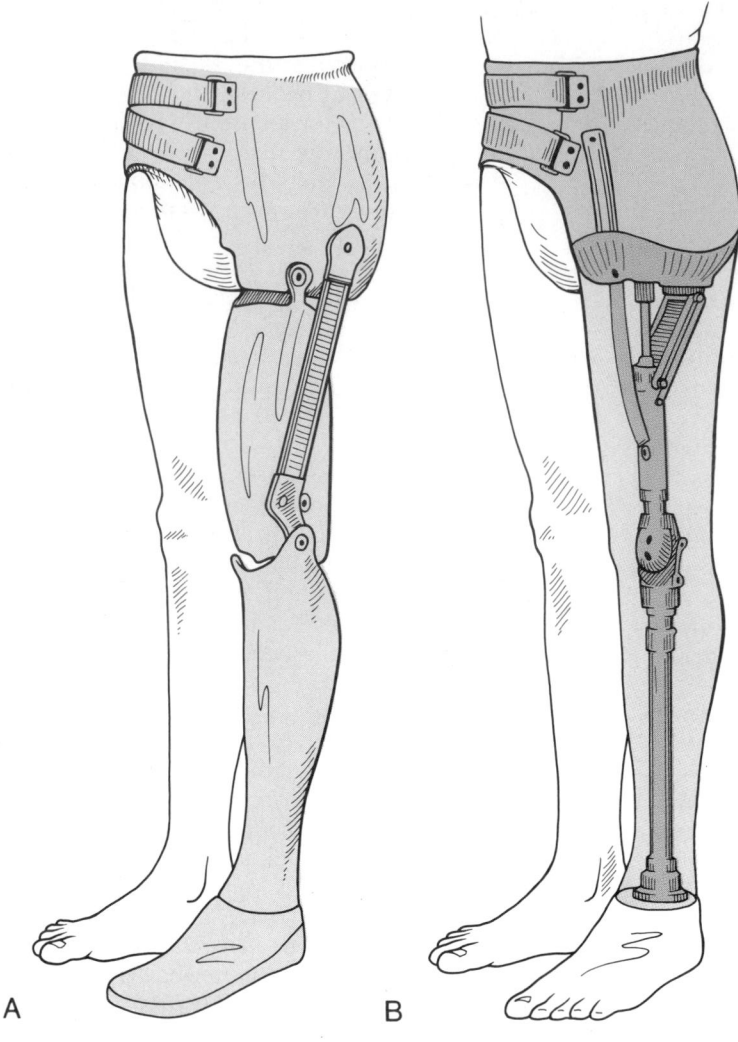

A   B

FIGURE 39–24   Exoskeletal (**A**) and endoskeletal (**B**) hip disarticulation prostheses.

d. Elastic keel: see section III.E.4., p 1140.
e. Dynamic response:
   (1). May facilitate faster gait velocity with hip disarticulation.
   (2). Recommended in combination with a fluid-controlled knee or knee with strong friction adjustment to take best advantage of gait momentum.

3. **Stride length control strap**
   a. Attaches posterior to hip joint proximally and anterior to knee joint distally.
      (1). Controls stride length.
      (2). Controls heel rise at swing.
      (3). Flexes knee when sitting.
      (4). Prevents excessive hip and knee flexion.

4. **Torque absorbers**
   a. Frequently recommended to reduce shear forces on patient and components.
   b. Major objective is to assist the patient to compensate for the normal rotation of ambulation.

5. **Biomechanics of hip disarticulation/hemi-pelvectomy prosthesis**
   a. Heel strike: period of double support.
      (1). Hip joint: reduced moment at hip owing to period of double support. Tendency toward extension because center of gravity posterior to floor reaction line owing to double support.
      (2). Knee: extension moment stabilizes knee.
      (3). Ankle: plantar flexion moment.

b. Foot flat: advantageous for fast transition from heel strike to foot flat to further stabilize the knee by moving the ground reaction line anterior.
   (1). Hip joint: tendency toward extension continues as described above.
   (2). Knee joint: increased extension moment at knee as ground reaction force moves further anteriorly.
   (3). Ankle: decreased plantar flexion moment as ground reaction line moves anteriorly.
c. Midstance:
   (1). Hip: floor reaction line posterior to hip increases hip extension stability.
   (2). Knee: strong extension moment.
   (3). Ankle: dorsiflexion moment at ankle must be controlled to prevent the knee from moving anteriorly, resulting in instability.
d. Heel off:
   (1). Hip: extension moment maintained as long as amputee maintains an erect trunk.
   (2). Knee: extension moment maintained but reduced as floor reaction line moves closer to the knee axis.
   (3). Ankle: dorsiflexion moment increased and continues to require control to prevent knee instability.
e. Toe off:
   (1). Hip: strong extension moment.
   (2). Knee: floor reaction force close to knee axis. Amputee sits in socket and performs posterior pelvic tilt to flex knee. Trunk is maintained in an erect position and hip/pelvis is stabilized while gravity pulls leg forward.
f. Initial swing phase:
   (1). Hip: in the presence of a stride length control strap, the hip is unable to flex until the knee reaches full extension. The stride length control strap can flex the hip after the knee reaches full extension as part of swing phase. For this reason, the length of the prosthesis must be shortened to allow toe clearance at initial swing.
   (2). Knee: stride length control strap limits heel rise initially and then initiates knee extension.
g. Terminal swing phase:
   (1). Hip: stride length control strap can now flex hip.

(2). Knee: stride length control strap and gravity have accomplished full knee extension.

PLEASE NOTE: Stride length control strap controls length of stride to prepare for heel strike.

h. Frontal view at midstance:
   (1). Floor reaction line is medial to primary point of support in the socket (ischial tuberosity), resulting in a tendency for the pelvis to move laterally.
   (2). Forces generated at area where the socket encompasses the contralateral (sound) hip, counteracting the tendency for the pelvis to move laterally (toward the prosthetic side) (maintains mediolateral pelvic stability).
   (3). The foot can be outset approximately 1 inch, which moves the ground reaction line closer to the ischial tuberosity, reducing the magnitude of the moment tending to rotate the hip laterally. This reduces the amount of force between the socket and the contralateral (sound) hip area required to provide mediolateral stability. (Results in a less cosmetic and more energy-consuming gait).

6. **Evaluation of hip disarticulation/hemipelvectomy prosthesis**
   a. *Patient standing*
      (1). The lateral stability of the prosthesis is assessed.
         (a). Method: support the prosthesis against a chair and instruct the patient to raise the sound leg without lateral trunk bending (leaning) over the prosthesis.
         (b). Problem: lateral instability.
         (c). Resolutions:
            (i). Drop a plumb line from the socket where the ischial tuberosity rests and determine whether the foot is outset approximately 1 inch. Discuss alignment adjustment with prosthetist if foot is more inset.

(ii). Ensure that socket fits snugly around the contralateral hip. Discuss adjustment with prosthetist if loose.

(2). The anteroposterior alignment stability of the prosthesis is assessed.

(a). Method: drop a plumb line through the hip axis and prosthetic knee center. The line should fall 1.5 inches behind the prosthetic heel.

(b). Problem #1: line falls less than 1.5 inches behind heel.

(c). Resolution: potential knee instability problem. Discuss with prosthetist if instability evident at knee.

(d). Problem #2: line falls greater than 1.5 inches behind heel.

(e). Resolution: potential difficulty initiating knee flexion at swing. Discuss with prosthetist if difficulty evident.

(3). The therapist ensures that the extension stride length control strap, if present, is anterior to the prosthetic knee center.

(a). Method: observe.

(b). Problem: posterior to knee center.

(c). Resolution: strap will flex knee rather than extend knee. Discontinue training and refer patient to prosthetist.

(4). The therapist ensures that no friction is present in the knee joint.

(a). Method: manually flex and extend knee joint to determine whether friction present.

(b). Problem: friction present.

(c). Resolution: friction may delay knee from extending rapidly enough at terminal swing. The foot and knee are not in position soon enough for heel strike. Discuss adjustment of friction with prosthetist if this problem is evident.

(5). The therapist ensures that the hip bumper and stop are in contact.

(a). Method: observe with patient standing with erect trunk.

(b). Problem: hip bumper and stop are not in contact.

(c). Resolution: this may allow hyperextension at the hip, which can result in knee instability as the ground reaction forces move posterior, following the center of gravity. Consult with prosthetist if knee instability evident.

(6). The patient's posture while in the prosthesis is assessed.

(a). Method: observe during standing.

(b). Problem: patient forced into lordosis or feels proximal back pressure.

(c). Resolution: the hip bumper may be contacting the stop too soon. Consult with prosthetist.

b. *Patient sitting*

(1). The therapist ensures that there is adequate clearance between the socket and the thigh section anteriorly.

(a). Method: observe.

(b). Problem: inadequate clearance.

(c). Resolution: may result in the patient's being unable to sit with the hip flexed to 90 degrees. Consult with prosthetist.

(2). Assess the patient's sitting posture.

(a). Method: observe.

(b). Problem: lean to the amputated side.

(c). Resolution: place temporary shims under the exterior gluteal socket area. If effective in balancing sitting posture, refer to prosthetist to add material to this area.

(3). The therapist inspects for pressure between the proximal end of the socket and the rib cage.

(a). Method: palpate perimeter of proximal socket edge and inspect for reddened pressure areas.

(b). Problem: increased pressure area.

(c). Response: foam or padding may be temporarily added around the pressure area. Refer to prosthetist to relieve pressure by heating and remolding or padding the socket.

(4). The therapist ensures that the shank of the prosthesis is vertical.
   (a). Method: observe in sitting on firm surface.
   (b). Problem: shank internally or externally rotated.
   (c). Resolution: ensure that socket is not rotating. Request alignment adjustment.
(5). It is determined whether the prosthetic knee protrudes excessively.
   (a). Method: compare thigh length with sound side for symmetry.
   (b). Problem: knee protrudes excessively.
   (c). Resolutions:
     (i). Ensure that the pelvis is not rotated forward on the prosthetic side.
     (ii). The hip joint may be located too far anterior. Consult with prosthetist.
(6). It is determined whether the amount of toe out of the prosthetic foot is correct.
   (a). Method: compare prosthetic toe out with sound side for symmetry.
   (b). Problem: asymmetry.
   (c). Response: refer to prosthetist to correct toe out.

7. **Donning/doffing of hip disarticulation/hemipelvectomy prosthesis**
a. Patient applies body sock or underwear.
   (1). Wrinkles or seams over bony prominences should be avoided.
b. Application of prosthesis (three methods):
   (1). Lean prosthesis in standing position against an object. Stand and push into socket. Tighten suspension straps.
   (2). Place prosthesis in a sitting position in a chair, wheelchair, or edge of bed. Transfer into the prosthesis. Snug suspension. If possible, stand and, while pushing into socket, complete tightening of suspension straps.
   (3). Lay prosthesis down on bed. Transfer into prosthesis and tighten suspension straps. Sit and, if possible, stand and tighten suspension.
   (4). Velcro closures should be snugly fastened.

(5). Socket adjustments may be required if the amputee is unable to snug the socket securely around the trunk.

8. **Gait training**
a. The patient is instructed to initiate swing phase with a posterior pelvic tilt. The patient practices pelvic tilts while lying supine on a mat.
b. Gait training in parallel bars is initiated.
c. The patient weight shifts from prosthetic to sound side and back. Weight bearing on prosthetic side should be emphasized by instructing the patient to "sit" in socket. It should be explained to the patient that hip and knee stability are accomplished through proper alignment when weight is borne on the prosthesis.
d. The patient practices stepping with the prosthetic side. Swing is initiated by means of a posterior pelvic tilt. The patient is instructed that the length of the prosthetic step is controlled by the stride length control strap, if present.
e. After advancing the prosthesis forward and attaining heel strike, the patient is instructed to shift weight forward over the prosthesis and sit in socket.
f. The patient progresses to holding a midstance position, emphasizing an erect trunk.
g. The patient steps forward with the sound side.
h. The gait sequence is repeated.
i. The patient progresses to increase speed and fluency of gait.
j. Gait deviation: vaulting.
   (1). Description: the patient raises up on the toe of the sound side. May be an effort to ensure clearance of the prosthetic foot at initial swing or a strategy to "bide time" while waiting for the prosthesis to advance forward for the next step.
   (2). Resolutions:
     (a). Increase the patient's awareness of the deviation using videotape or mirrors.
     (b). Practice advancing the prosthetic side without vaulting.
     (c). If toe clearance problems exist, determine whether the prosthesis is appropriately shortened (~ 0.5 inch). A temporary lift on the sound side may be used

to assess whether prosthetic length is contributing to vaulting. If the prosthesis appears appropriately shortened, determine whether a relative leg-length discrepancy is occurring owing to inadequate suspension.

References

1. Staff, Northwestern University Prosthetic-Orthotic Center: Lower and upper limb prosthetics for physicians, surgeons, and therapists. Continuing education course. Chicago, IL, Northwestern University Medical School, 1982.
2. Course notes: Northwestern University Prosthetic Certificate Program. Northwestern University Prosthetic-Orthotic Center. Chicago, IL, Northwestern University Medical School, 1986.
3. Karacoloff LA: *Lower Extremity Amputation: A Guide To Functional Outcomes in Physical Therapy Management.* Rockville, MD, Aspen Publishers Inc, 1985.
4. Sanders GT: *Lower Limb Amputations: A Guide To Rehabilitation.* Philadelphia, F. A. Davis Company, 1986.
5. Schmidt M: Prosthetics-orthotics I. Course manual. Hahneman University Graduate School Program in Physical Therapy. Philadelphia, Hahneman University, 1988.
6. Bowker JH, Michael JW: *Atlas of Limb Prosthetics: Surgical, Prosthetic, and Rehabilitation Principles,* 2nd ed. St. Louis, C. V. Mosby Company, 1992.
7. Michael JW: Energy storing feet: a clinical comparison. *Clin Prosthet Orthot* 1987, 11:154–168.
8. Michael JW: State of the art prosthetic components and socket designs: a comprehensive review. Continuing education course: Striding into the 21st century: the art and science of amputee running, sports, and advanced rehabilitation. [Course notes.] JFK Johnson Rehabilitation Institute, Iselin, NJ, May 1993.
9. Michael JW: Lower limb prosthetics. *Top Geriatr Rehabil* 1992, 8:30–38.
10. Staff, Faculty Prosthetics and Orthotics, New York University School of Medicine and Post-Graduate Medical School: *Lower-Limb Prosthetics.* New York, New York University, 1980.
11. Michael JW: Overview of prosthetic knee mechanisms [Submitted for publication].
12. Gailey RS, McKenzie A: Prosthetic gait training program for lower extremity amputees. [Course notes.] Department of Orthopaedics and Rehabilitation Division of Physical Therapy. Miami, University of Miami School Of Medicine, 1989.
13. Michael JW: Component selection criteria: lower limb disarticulations. *Clin Prosthet Orthot* 1988, 12:99–108.
14. Michael JW: Overview of prosthetic feet. In Greene WB (ed): *Instructional Course Lectures.* vol. 39. Chicago, American Academy Of Orthopaedic Surgeons, 1990, pp 367–372.
15. Kreuter P: Aggressive physical therapy for lower extremity amputees: beyond basic training. Continuing education course: Striding into the 21st century: the art and science of amputee running, sports, and advanced rehabilitation.
16. Balsley D: Exercise techniques and use of exercise equipment for lower extremity amputees. Continuing education course: Striding into the 21st century: the art and science of amputee running, sports, and advanced rehabilitation. [Course notes.] JFK Johnson Rehabilitation Institute, Iselin, NJ, May 1993.

Suggested Reading

Beekman CE, Axtell LA: Prosthetic use in elderly patients with dysvascular above-knee and through-knee amputations. *Phys Ther* 1987, 67:1510–1516.
Krebs DE, Edelstein JE, Thornby MA: Prosthetic management of children with limb deficiencies. *Phys Ther* 1991, 71:920–934.
Lehneis HR: Beyond the quadrilateral. *Clin Prosthet Orthot* 1985, 9:6–8.
Long IA: Normal shape–normal alignment (NSNA) above-knee prosthesis. *Clin Prosthet Orthot* 1985, 9:9–14.
Manella KJ: Comparing the effectiveness of elastic bandages and shrinker socks for lower extremity amputees. *Phys Ther* 1981, 61:334–337.
Michael JW: New developments in prosthetic feet for sports and recreation. *Palaestra* 1989, Winter:21–35.
Michael J: Pediatric prosthetics and orthotics. *Phys Occup Ther Pediatr* 1990, 10:123–146.
Mitchell CA, Versluis TL: Management of an above-knee amputee with complex medical problems using the CAT-CAM prosthesis. *Phys Ther* 1990, 70:389–393.
Mueller MJ: Comparison of removable rigid dressings and elastic bandages in preprosthetic management of patients with below-knee amputations. *Phys Ther* 1982, 62:1438–1441.
Mueller MJ, Delitto A: Selective criteria for successful long-term prosthetic use. *Phys Ther* 1985, 65:1037–1040.
Sabolich J: Contoured adducted trochanteric-controlled alignment method. *Clin Prosthet Orthot* 1985, 9:15–26.
Staros A, Rubin G: Prescription considerations in modern above-knee prosthetics. *Clin North Am Phys Med Rehabil* 1991, 2.
Waters RL, Perry J, Antonelli D, Hislop H: Energy cost of walking of amputees: the influence of level of amputation. *J Bone Joint Surg* 1976, 58-A:42.
Wu Y, Krick H: Removable rigid dressing for below-knee amputees. *Clin Prosthet Orthot* 1987, 11:33–44.

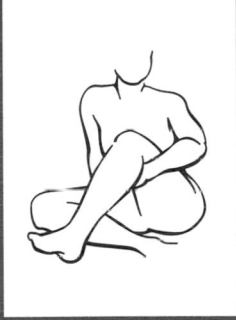

CHAPTER 40

Orthoses

Joan E. Edelstein

Physical therapists who practice in rehabilitation centers, long-term care facilities, schools, and in patients' homes often use orthoses as part of a treatment plan. An orthosis is a device worn on the body for therapeutic purposes, particularly to reduce or assist motion or to alter the alignment of a body segment. Most often, an orthosis is a shoe insert, an ankle-foot orthosis (AFO), or a corset. Occasionally, an upper-limb orthosis is prescribed for a patient who has paralysis or pain. Orthoses are sometimes termed "braces" or "supports"; contemporary terminology, however, incorporates the word "orthosis" (*eg,* lumbosacral orthosis). "Splint" connotes a temporary orthosis. Although widely used as a noun, particularly with regard to the foot, "orthotic" is an adjective (*eg,* orthotic device).

Unlike other modes of treatment, orthotic management usually requires that the physical therapist cooperate with an orthotist, who constructs and fits the orthosis. Foot orthoses may also be provided by a pedorthist. The physical therapist and the orthotist or pedorthist examine the patient and formulate an orthotic prescription, often in association with a physician. When the orthosis is delivered, the physical therapist should evaluate its fit, function, and construction before permitting the patient to wear it.

Therapists should be able to use new technological advances when they formulate goals based on a comprehensive assessment of a patient to provide the most effective care. With the increasing use of plastics, it is not uncommon for therapists to participate in orthotic design. By understanding the general principles that pertain to virtually all orthoses, a therapist can create practical designs. This chapter emphasizes the assessment, planning, and evaluation of the most widely used contemporary lower-limb, trunk, and upper-limb orthoses. Many patients can benefit from various orthotic options; however, only the most efficacious orthoses are featured here.

I. General Principles of Orthoses

The following principles apply to most orthoses, regardless of the body segment on which the orthosis is worn.[1-4]

A. Forces

Orthoses apply forces to limit or to assist in motion.

1. Rigid material spanning a joint prevents motion.

    Example: A solid AFO prevents foot and ankle motion in all planes.

2. A leaf spring or a coil spring is stressed by one motion and then recoils to assist in the opposite, desired motion.

    Examples: (1) A plastic posterior leaf spring is tensed in early stance and in midstance and recoils as the wearer unloads the braced leg and proceeds into the swing phase. (2) A coiled metal dorsiflexion-assist spring is compressed in early stance and in midstance and recoils as the wearer unloads the braced leg and proceeds into the swing phase.[5]

B. Pain

Pain may be reduced by limiting motion.

Examples: (1) Metatarsalgia may be lessened by a metatarsal bar, which prevents hyperextension at the metatarsophalangeal joints. (2) Arthritic wrist pain is often reduced when a patient wears a rigid wrist-hand orthosis.

C. Flexible deformity

Flexible deformity may be corrected by an orthosis.

1. Corrective force must be balanced by proximal and distal counterforces. An orthosis applies one or more three-point force systems.

    Examples: (1) An orthosis for left thoracic scoliosis applies a right-directed force at the apex of the curve, counterbalanced with left-directed forces above and below the apex. (2) An elbow orthosis for a flexion contracture applies an anteriorly directed force in the vicinity of the elbow and posteriorly directed forces to the arm and forearm.

2. The greater the distance between the force and the counterforces, the less counterforce is required.

    Example: Genu valgum (knock-knee deformity) may be controlled with a knee orthosis that applies a laterally directed force at the knee and medially directed forces at the thigh and leg; however, a knee-ankle-foot orthosis (KAFO) can apply the medially directed forces at a greater distance from the knee, thus reducing the force at the ends of the orthosis.

D. Fixed deformity

Fixed deformity must be accommodated by an orthosis; an orthosis may prevent the progression of the deformity.

Example: A patient with pes cavus is more comfortable with a shoe insert that fills the space between the plantar surface of the foot and the insole of the shoe; the insert, however, does not change the alignment of the foot.

E. Pressure reduction

1. **Increased area of skin contact**

    Examples: (1) A resilient shoe insert cushions the entire foot throughout the stance phase, unlike a rigid insert. (2) A broad band on a wrist-hand orthosis applies lower unit pressure to the forearm than would a narrow strap.

2. **Decreased force achieved by increasing the distance between force and counterforce**

    Example: A wrist-hand orthosis that has its proximal forearm band relatively close to the elbow is more comfortable than one that has its proximal forearm band relatively closer to the wrist.

F. Heat

Greater skin contact retains more heat.

Example: A plastic thoracolumbar jacket may be uncomfortable during the summer. The broad shells cover much more of the trunk than do narrow plastic or upholstered metal uprights and bands.

G. Adjustability

Orthotic adjustability is indicated for children to accommodate growth and for patients with progressive or resolving disorders.
1. Plastic may be heated and reshaped or ground away.
2. Metal is reformed by bending or grinding.
3. Some orthotic joints can be adjusted, but these types of joints tend to be relatively bulky or fragile.

   Example: A dorsiflexion spring-assist ankle joint has a metal coil spring that the therapist can remove. If the spring channel is left empty, then the ankle joint moves freely. If the therapist puts a rod in the spring channel, then no motion occurs at the ankle joint.

H. Weight

Orthoses should be as lightweight as possible but should have reasonable durability.[6]

I. Appearance

Orthotic appearance is important, particularly if the orthosis is to be worn on the job or at school.

J. Maintenance

Ease of orthotic maintenance is essential.[7] Breakage and malfunction deprive the client of the functional benefits of the orthosis and exact the costs of repair and travel to the orthotist. These problems also result in time lost from work, school, or preferred activities by the client and often a family member. Durability depends on:
1. Suitable materials and construction.
2. No or few moving parts.

K. Cleaning

The orthosis should be readily cleaned, preferably by the client.

1. **Hygiene**

   Example: An incontinent client may develop dermatitis from urine-soaked leather upholstery; semirigid plastic shells do not retain fluids.

2. **Aesthetics.** Most individuals regard a clean orthosis as being more attractive than a soiled one.

L. Application

The client should be able to apply the orthosis correctly and rapidly. Difficulty in donning is a major reason why some patients discard an orthoses.[6,7]

II. Lower-Limb Orthoses

In contemporary practice, lower-limb orthoses are classified by the joint or body segment that they cover. Formerly, an AFO was known as a "short leg brace" or a "below-knee orthosis." A KAFO was called a "long leg brace" or an "above-knee orthosis."

A. Principles

In addition to the general principles listed previously, lower-limb orthoses should satisfy the following requirements:
1. The client must be able to sit comfortably while wearing the orthosis.

   Example: KAFO should not impinge on the popliteal fossa when the knee is flexed 90 degrees.

2. A form-fitting orthosis may not be appropriate in the presence of edema.

   Example: A client with peripheral vascular disease or gastrocnemius muscle paralysis who develops dependent edema requires either an AFO with metal uprights that do not contact the leg or a plastic AFO that the client can adjust during the day. Otherwise, the orthosis may impose excessive pressure.

3. An orthosis should improve gait.

   a. During the stance phase, orthoses can aid in loading or in load transition.

      Example: Rocker-soled shoes reduce the distance that the wearer must travel over the stance foot, thereby lessening demand on the triceps muscle of the calf; this benefits the patient with multiple sclerosis or with peripheral vascular disease.[8,9]

   b. During the swing phase, orthoses can aid in clearance.

      Example: An AFO with a posterior stop prevents the foot from dragging during the swing phase, thus obviating fatiguing compensations such as exaggerated hip flexion.

B. Physical assessment

Because every client has distinctive physical and psychosocial attributes, a thorough assessment is imperative before the prescription of an orthosis. The conscientious physical therapist thus avoids recommending a so-called "hemiplegic orthosis" or a "poliomyelitis brace." The orthosis that suits one patient with hemiplegia may be inappropriate for someone else with the same diagnosis. The first individual may need only a slight dorsiflexion assist, whereas the second patient may have substantial foot and ankle instability, requiring a solid-ankle AFO. Similarly, poliomyelitis affects patients with many different patterns of weakness and deformity; additionally, many clients have a long orthotic history, which profoundly influences their preferences.

  1. **Limb alignment**

    a. *Toe*

      (1). Hallux valgus may be present.

      (2). Hammer, claw, or mallet toes may be present.

      (3). The patient may have metatarsal head prominence on the plantar surface of the toes.

    b. *Foot.* The patient may have pes valgus, varus, cavus, equinus, or calcaneus.

    c. *Knee*

      (1). Genu valgum, varum, or recurvatum may be present.

      (2). The patient may have flexion contracture.

    d. *Hip*

      (1). The patient may have flexion contracture.

      (2). Abduction or adduction contracture may be present.

      (3). Malrotation may occur.

    e. *Pelvis*

      (1). Frontal plane obliquity may be present.

      (2). The patient may have anterior or posterior tilt.

  2. **Joint range**

Particular emphasis should be placed on the ranges of the following joints:

- Ankle.
- Knee.
- Hip.

  3. **Muscle power**

Particular emphasis should be placed on the power of the following muscles:

- Tibialis anterior.
- Triceps surae.
- Quadriceps.
- Iliopsoas.
- Gluteus medius.

  4. **Coordination and spasticity**

Observe the following in the patient:

- Unipedal stance.
- Extensor synergy.
- Flexor synergy.

  5. **Sensory status**

Test the patient's status:

- Tactile sensation.
- Proprioceptive sensation.

  6. **Skin condition**

Observe the skin for the presence of:

- Ulcerations.
- Abrasions.
- Dermatitis.
- Other lesions.

  7. **Posture**

Evaluate the patient's posture during:

- Standing.
- Walking.

  8. **Gait**

Observe the patient's gait, keeping the following factors in mind:

- Need for assistive devices.
- Duration of gait.
- Deviations in gait.
- Ability to rise from various types of chairs.
- Ability to climb stairs and ramps.

  9. **Manual dexterity**

Observe the patient's ability to manage hose, shoes, laces, buckles, and other fasteners.

10. **Vision**

The patient's visual ability should be sufficient to allow performance of the following tasks:
- Walking safely indoors and outdoors.
- Dressing independently.
- Reading typewritten instructions.

C. Subjective assessment

1. **Comprehension**
   a. The client should indicate an understanding of oral instructions.
   b. The client should indicate an understanding of written instructions.
   c. The patient's language preference should be noted.

2. **Complaints**
   a. *Pain*
      (1). Determine where pain occurs.
      (2). Evaluate when the pain occurs (*ie*, whether it is constant or occasional).
      (3). Record the character of the pain (*eg*, throbbing, burning, dull, or sharp).
      (4). Note the date of the onset.
      (5). Record any aggravating factors.
      (6). Note any diminishing factors.
   b. *Performance*
      (1). The patient may have difficulty maneuvering at home.
      (2). He/she may have difficulty maneuvering outdoors and at work or at school.
      (3). Fatigue should be evaluated in relation to the duration of activity.
      (4). The patient may limp (*ie*, may experience undesirable motions during walking).
      (5). Evaluate falling.
         (a). Determine when the fall occurs.
         (b). Evaluate why the fall occurs (*eg*, limb failure or balance failure).
   c. *Appearance*
      (1). Evaluate the contour of the limb with and without an orthosis while the patient is standing and sitting.
      (2). Note the skin condition.

(3). Determine whether the orthosis causes clothing abrasion or style limitation unacceptable to the patient.

3. **Previous orthotic experience**
   a. *Preferred orthosis.* The patient may have a preference with regard to:
      - Material.
      - Weight.
      - Fit.
      - Design.
      - Durability and maintenance.
   b. *Disliked orthosis.* The patient may have disliked certain features of previous orthoses, including:
      - Material.
      - Weight.
      - Fit.
      - Design.
      - Durability and maintenance.

4. **Goals.** The patient's goals may include:
   - Reduced pain.
   - Improved stability.
   - Improved gait.
   - Improved appearance.

5. **Economic considerations**
   a. Consider the funding source of the treatment.

   Examples: (1) A client who depends on Federal medical insurance can only be provided with orthotic components that are approved by the government. In addition, a therapist must consider the patient's funding for transportation to the orthotist for measurement, fitting, and repairs, as well as for transportation to the training site. Orthotic replacement needs to be scheduled to allow time for financial authorization and for other administrative requirements. (2) An elderly client who lives alone on a limited pension may attempt to conserve funds by ignoring incipient signs of irritation from the misfit or erosion of a shoe or of an orthosis.

   b. Be aware of the patient's social environment.
      (1). Home, work, and school accessibility should be factors in treatment decisions.
      (2). The role of the patient's peers, family, work, school, and social activities in motivating compliance must be considered.

1. **Foot orthoses**
   a. *Shoes and hose.*
      (1). The most versatile shoe for adults with foot disorders has an extra-depth, Blucher upper with a laced or pressure tape closure and a low heel.[10-20] Such shoes, manufactured in men's and women's styles and sizes, are especially spacious, because they contain a top insole that can be removed to accommodate foot orthoses, edema, or dressings. The Blucher shoe, in which the distal portion of the opening consists of two separate flaps, permits greatest opening into the shoe and maximum adjustment of closure. Canvas athletic shoes often are suitable. The term "orthopedic shoe" should be avoided: rather, the therapist should select shoes with the features that suit the specific client. Shoes should accommodate fixed deformities.
      (2). Hose should fit each foot without binding the toes or wrinkling. Holes tend to concentrate pressure at the fabric periphery, whereas mended holes are apt to be abrasive; consequently, hose that develop holes should be discarded.
      (3). Foot orthoses may be placed inside the shoe (*eg,* removable inserts and stationary internal modifications) or outside the shoe (*eg,* stationary external modifications).
   b. *Rearfoot disorders*
      (1). *Heel spur*
         (a). The goal: reduce pressure on the tender site.
         (b). Option: prescribe a viscoelastic plastic heel wedge with a central depression under the tender site.
         (c). The rationale for this option:
            (i). The material absorbs shock at heel contact.
            (ii). The depression reduces stress at the tender site.
            (iii). The wedge shifts the load to the forefoot.
      (2). *Achilles tendinitis*
         (a). The goal: reduce, then gradually increase tensile stress on the tendon.
         (b). Option: prescribe an AFO with limited-motion ankle joints worn with a shoe with a heel lift.
         (c). The rationale for this option is as follows:
            (i). The heel lift reduces tension on the Achilles tendon; as healing progresses, heel lift is diminished.
            (ii). The AFO limits mediolateral foot motion, thus preventing instability caused by painful tendinitis and the plantar flexed posture of the foot.
      (3). *Flexible pes valgus*
         (a). The goals:
            (i). Realign the foot, restoring neutral position of the subtalar joint.
            (ii). Reduce hypermobility during midstance.
         (b). Option one: prescribe the University of California Biomechanics Laboratory insert[21] (see Figure 40-1).
         (c). The rationale for this option is that the custom-molded semi-rigid orthosis maintains the calcaneus and talus in corrected alignment, applying upward and laterally directed force at the medial border of the midfoot and hindfoot and medially directed force at the lateral border of the heel.

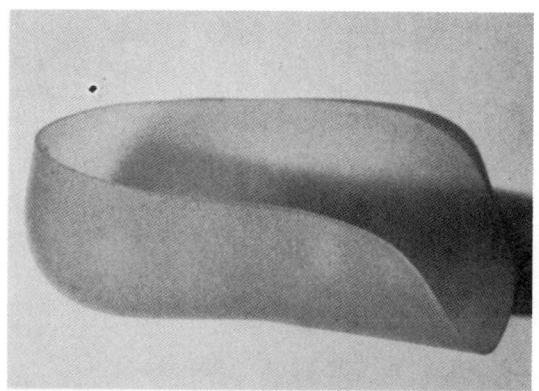

FIGURE 40–1   UCBL insert. (From Palmer, Toms: *Manual for Functional Training,* 3rd ed. F. A. Davis Company, p 771.)

(d). Option two: prescribe a semi-rigid scaphoid pad affixed to a shoe or incorporated into an insert.

(e). The rationale for this option is that this is a less expensive orthosis that applies upward force at the medial border of the midfoot and hindfoot.

(f). Option three: prescribe a medial heel wedge, with or without a medial forefoot wedge, either as an insert or in a shoe sole.

(g). The rationale for this option is that it redirects weight bearing laterally.

(h). Option four: prescribe a valgus correction strap on an AFO that has a lateral metal upright.

(i). The rationale for this option is that the strap applies laterally directed force at the medial malleolus; however, the strap is conspicuous and adds to donning time.

(4). *Fixed pes valgus*

(a). The goal: reduce excessive loading on the medial border of the foot.

(b). Option: prescribe a lateral heel wedge, with or without a lateral forefoot wedge, either as an insert or in a shoe sole.

(c). The rationale for this option is that it increases the plantar-bearing area.

(5). *Flexible pes varus*

(a). The goal: realign the foot, restoring the neutral position of the subtalar joint.

(b). Option one: prescribe a lateral heel wedge, with or without a lateral forefoot wedge, either as an insert or in a shoe sole.

(c). The rationale for this option is that it redirects weight bearing medially.

(d). Option two: prescribe a varus correction strap on an AFO that has a medial metal upright.

(e). The rationale for this method is that the strap applies medially

directed force at the lateral malleolus.

(6). *Fixed pes varus*

(a). The goal: reduce excessive loading on the lateral border of the foot.

(b). Option: prescribe a medial heel wedge, with or without a medial forefoot wedge, either as an insert or in a shoe sole.

(c). The rationale for this option is that it increases the plantar-bearing area.

(7). *Flexible pes equinus*

(a). The goal: realign the foot to achieve a neutral ankle position.

(b). Option one: prescribe an AFO with dorsiflexion assist—either a plastic posterior leaf spring or a metal coiled spring.

(c). The rationale for this option is that it assists in dorsiflexion and also permits slight plantar flexion during early stance.

(d). Option two: prescribe an AFO with a posterior stop.

(e). The rationale for this option is that it prevents plantar flexion.

(8). *Fixed pes equinus*

(a). The goals:

(i). Reduce excessive loading on the forefoot.

(ii). Cover the foot with a shoe.

(b). Option: prescribe a heel lift; high-top shoe may be required.

(c). The rationale for this option is that a lift increases plantar-bearing area.

c. **Midfoot disorder: plantar fasciitis**

(1). The goal: reduce pain.

(2). Option: prescribe an insert with heel elevation, a scaphoid pad, and a resilient top cover.[15–18]

(3). The rationale for this option is as follows:

(a). This orthosis reduces tension on the plantar fascia.

(b). It also absorbs shock.

d. **Forefoot disorder**

(1). *Metatarsalgia*

(a). The goal: reduce pain.

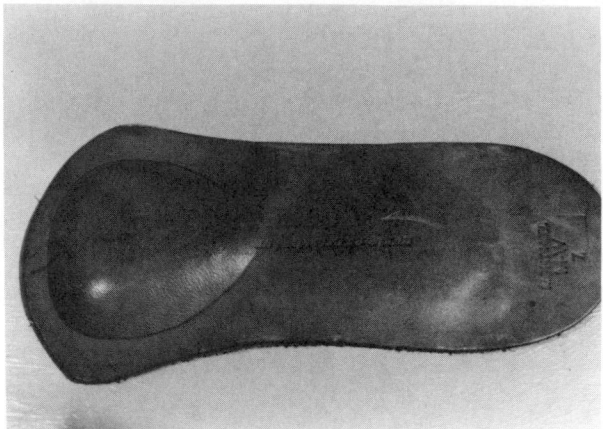

FIGURE 40–2   Metatarsal pad.

(b). Option one: prescribe a metatarsal pad in a shoe insert (see Figure 40–2).

(c). The rationale for this option is that it transfers the load from the metatarsophalangeal joints to the metatarsal shafts.

(d). Option two: prescribe a metatarsal bar on a shoe sole (see Figure 40–3).

(e). The rationale for this option is that it transfers the load from the metatarsophalangeal joints to the metatarsal shafts and reduces forefoot motion.

(2). *Hallux valgus with a bunion*

(a). The goal: to reduce pain.

(b). Option one: recommend an accommodative shoe with adequate width and a pliable leather balloon patch to be worn at the bunion site.

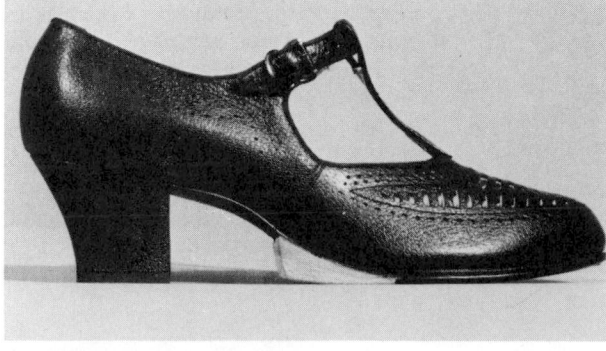

FIGURE 40–3   Metatarsal bar.

(c). The rationale for this option is that it prevents abrasion and compression of the medial forefoot.

(d). Option two: prescribe a resilient bunion shield to be worn over the first toe at the bunion site.[22]

(e). The rationale for this option is that it broadens the area for load application over the bunion site.

(3). *Hammer toe, claw toe, and mallet toe*

(a). The goal: reduce pain.

(b). Option: prescribe an accommodative shoe with a spacious toe box; a heat-moldable shoe also may be required.[23]

(c). The rationale for this option is that it prevents abrasion and compression of the dorsal toe surfaces.

e. ***Diabetic peripheral vascular disease***

(1). The goal: prevent ulceration.

(2). Option: prescribe an accommodative shoe with a resilient insert and a rocker sole.[9,24–37]

(3). The rationale for this option is as follows:

(a). The shoe insert absorbs shock and reduces repetitive shear.

(b). The rocker sole rigidity reduces stress on the metatarsal heads and aids in late stance.

f. ***Length discrepancy***

(1). Foot length discrepancy can disturb gait.

(a). The goal: reduce gait deviation, particularly asymmetrical timing.

(b). Option: prescribe a rigid insert with a toe filler and a scaphoid pad.

(c). The rationale for this option is as follows:

(i). The insert permits the client to wear a pair of shoes sized for his/her larger foot; otherwise, he/she would have to wear split-sized shoes or buy two pairs of shoes and discarding the extra shoes.

(ii). The scaphoid pad supports the medial longitudinal arch, which is compromised with the loss of distal attachment of the plantar aponeurosis to the proximal phalanges.

(2). Leg length discrepancy disturbs gait.

(a). The goal: reduce gait deviation, particularly lateral trunk bending.

(b). Option: prescribe a lift equal in size to the size of the discrepancy minus 1 cm. The lift can be lodged partially inside of a low shoe (approximately 1 cm), and the remainder can be placed externally at the heel and sole. The sole should have a rocker convexity with the apex posterior to the metatarsophalangeal joints.

(c). The rationale for this option is as follows:

(i). The 1-cm discrepancy aids in the swing phase transition.

(ii). The rocker sole aids in the late stance phase.

2. **AFOs**

An AFO consists of a foundation, an ankle control, a foot control, and a superstructure. The foundation consists of the shoe and either an insert foot plate or a steel stirrup, which is riveted to the shoe. The ankle-control components limit or assist in dorsiflexion and plantar flexion. The foot-control components restrict mediolateral motion.[5,38-41] The superstructure includes the plastic shell or metal uprights and the proximal band. In view of the many permutations of the AFO, the term "conventional" is not useful. Similarly, the terms "floor reaction" and "inhibitory bracing" are not specific; various designs have been described by those terms. All lower-limb orthoses are influenced by the floor reaction during stance phase. Patients with spasticity caused by cerebral palsy, head injury, or cerebrovascular accident may benefit from an orthosis that inhibits the extensor or flexor synergy and prevents contracture.

a. *Dorsiflexor muscle paralysis*

(1). The goals:

(a). Reduce gait deviation; in par-

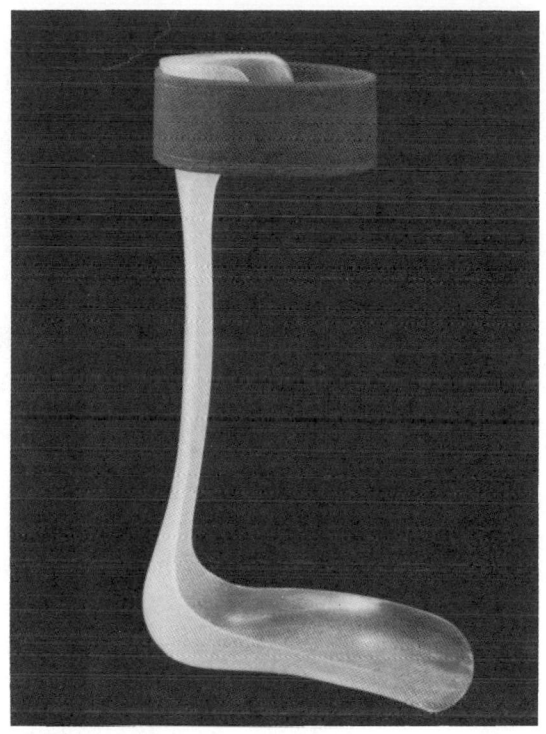

FIGURE 40–4 Posterior leaf-spring AFO. (Courtesy of AliMed, Inc, Dedham, MA.)

ticular, provide aid for swing-phase clearance.

(b). Prevent contracture of the Achilles tendon.

(2). Option one: prescribe a dorsiflexion assist—either a plastic posterior leaf spring (see Figure 40–4) or a metal coiled spring. The plastic posterior leaf-spring AFO includes an insert that facilitates the donning of the orthosis and enables the client to wear different shoes (assuming that all of the shoes have the same heel height). If the shoe's heel is too high, the client's knee tends to flex excessively; if it is too low, the client has difficulty flexing the knee during the stance phase.[42] The posterior leaf-spring AFO is relatively rigid in both plantar flexion and dorsiflexion.[43] With a dorsiflexion spring assist, it is important to ensure that the client wears appropriate shoes with the orthosis; otherwise, spring response can be adjusted, or the spring can be replaced with a dowel to limit motion.

(3). The rationale for this option is as follows:
  (a). The spring prevents the foot from dragging during swing.
  (b). The spring also permits slight plantar flexion during early stance, thereby enabling the client to achieve a foot flat position without undue knee flexion.
  (c). Tension on the Achilles tendon counteracts any tendency to form contracture.
(4). Option two: prescribe a metal and leather AFO with a posterior ankle stop.
(5). The rationale for this option is as follows:
  (a). The AFO limits plantar flexion, both during the swing phase and also during early stance, thus jeopardizing knee stability.
  (b). The posterior ankle stop is simpler than the dorsiflexion spring assist. The orthosis prohibits ankle plantar flexion, thus preventing Achilles contracture.

b. **Plantar flexor paralysis**
(1). The goal: to reduce gait deviation; in particular, to aid in late stance transition.
(2). Option one: prescribe an AFO with limited-motion ankle joints and a shoe with a rocker sole (see Figure 40–5).
(3). The rationale for this option is that the rigid sole enables the wearer to pivot over the rocker, which has its apex slightly posterior to the metatarsophalangeal joints.
(4). Option two: prescribe a metal and leather AFO with an anterior stop that is set in slight plantar flexion.
(5). The rationale for this option is that the stop prevents dorsiflexion, thus aiding in advancement during late stance. The patient's body weight pivots over the metatarsal heads; slight plantar flexion prevents inadvertent knee flexion during early stance.

c. **Ankle and foot paralysis**
(1). The goals:

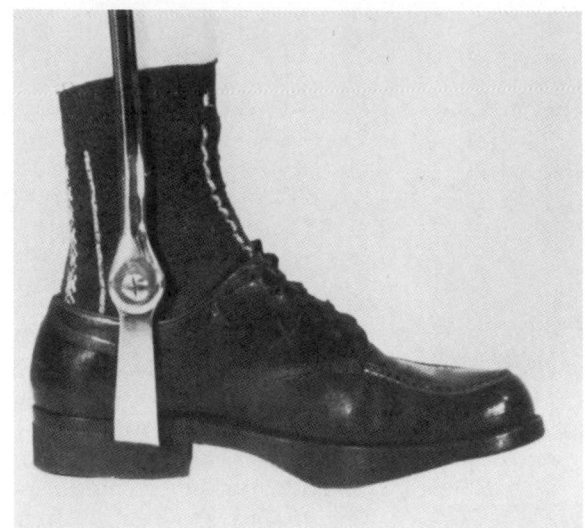

FIGURE 40–5 AFO with limited-motion ankle joints and rocker bar. (From American Academy of Orthopaedic Surgeons: *Atlas of Orthotics,* 2nd ed. C. V. Mosby Company, p 209.)

  (a). Provide stability in all planes.
  (b). Reduce gait deviations during the swing and stance phases.
(2). Option one: prescribe a plastic solid-ankle AFO to be worn with a shoe with a resilient heel or a beveled heel.
(3). The rationale for this option is as follows:
  (a). The rigidity of the plastic prevents the foot from dragging during swing; the brace rigidity also prevents ankle dorsiflexion during midstance and late stance, thus assisting in the transition of weight over the braced limb.
  (b). A resilient or beveled heel enables the foot to approach the floor more readily, thus reducing the risk of inadvertent excessive knee flexion during early stance.[44]
(4). Option two: prescribe a plastic hinged AFO (see Figure 40–6). Adjustable hinges enable the clinician to alter the range of ankle excursion.
(5). The rationale for this option is as follows:
  (a). The AFO provides mediolateral stability.

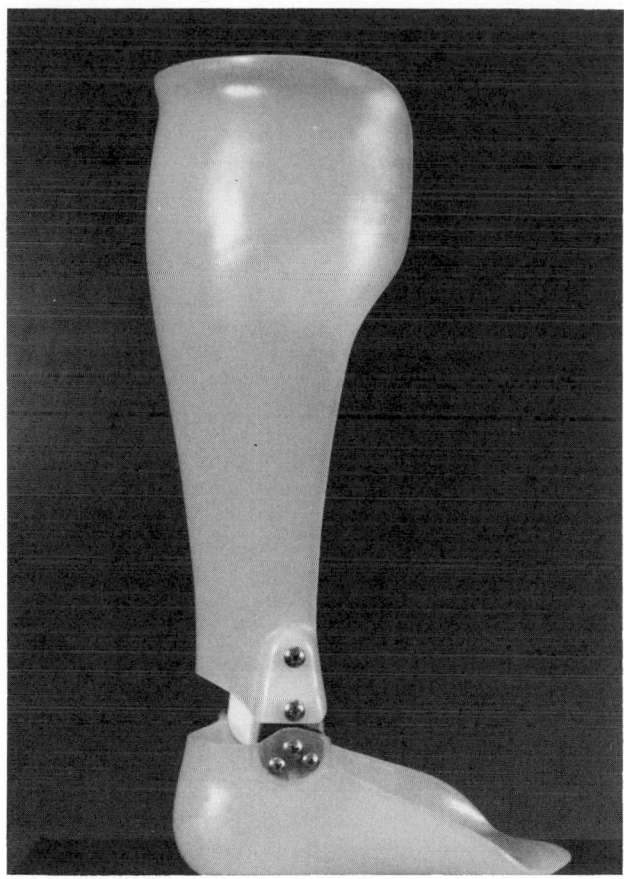

FIGURE 40–6   Hinged AFO. (Courtesy of Becker Orthopedic Co, Inc, Troy, MI.)

(b). It prevents toe drag during the swing phase.

(c). It assists during late stance somewhat, depending on the extent of dorsiflexion limitation.

(d). The motion at the ankle assists in the gait of some children with cerebral palsy.[45]

(6). Option three: prescribe a metal and leather AFO with plantar flexion- and dorsiflexion-adjustable ankle joints; a valgus (varus) correction strap may be added.

(7). The rationale for this option is as follows:

(a). The AFO provides some mediolateral stability.

(b). It prevents toe drag during the swing phase and assists in late stance.

(c). The adjustable joints may be converted to rigid dorsiflexion

or plantar flexion stops. When adjusted to permit slight plantar flexion, the orthosis increases knee extension torque; the orthosis set in dorsiflexion causes the knee to flex during early stance.

d. *Hypertonicity*

(1). The goals:

(a). Reduce gait deviation, particularly during the swing phase.

(b). Stabilize the foot during early stance.

(2). Option one: prescribe a plastic solid-ankle AFO; the proximal trim line may be lowered.

(3). The rationale for this option is as follows:

(a). The orthosis prevents plantar flexion, thus stopping toe drag during the swing phase.

(b). The side walls of the orthosis control pes varus during early stance.

(4). Option two: prescribe a plastic tone-inhibiting AFO. This orthosis has a foot plate that maintains the toes slightly hyperextended; it also has a small pad on each side of the Achilles tendon.[46–50]

(5). The rationale for this option is as follows:

(a). The rigid orthotic ankle prevents toe drag during the swing phase.

(b). The pads at the toes and at the Achilles tendon tend to cause fatigue of spastic muscles during grasping and during extensor synergy.

e. *Limited weight bearing*

(1). The goal: reduce loading on the leg and foot.

(2). Option: prescribe an AFO with a weight-relieving brim and limited-motion ankle joints (see Figure 40–7).

f. *Knee extensor muscle paralysis*

(1). The goals:

(a). Provide stability during standing.

(b). Reduce gait deviation at early stance.

(2). Option: prescribe a metal and leather AFO with plantar flexion- and dorsiflexion-adjustable ankle

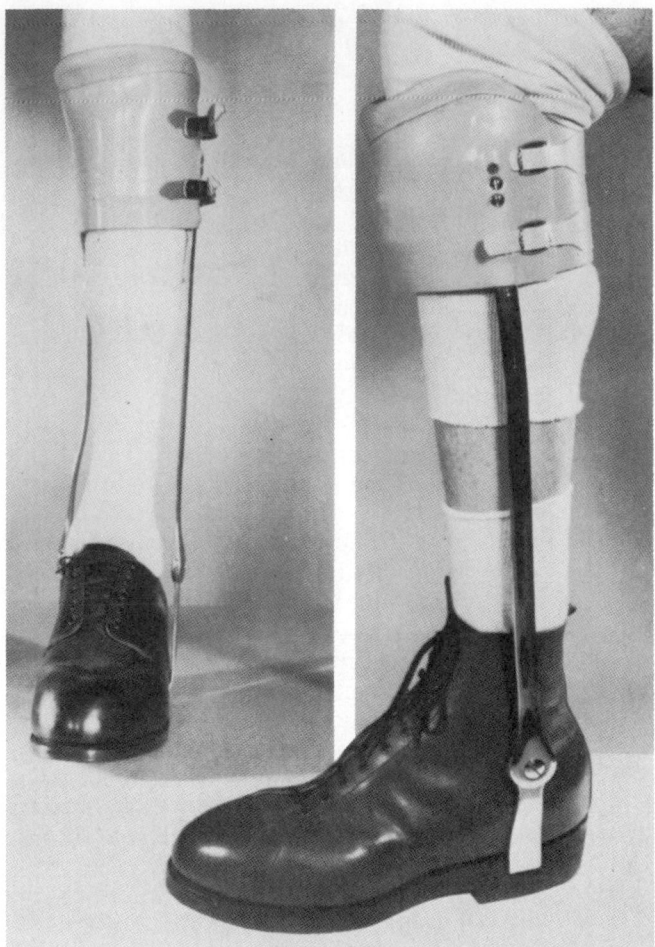

FIGURE 40–7   AFO with weight-relieving brim. (From American Academy of Orthopaedic Surgeons: *Atlas of Orthotics*, 2nd ed. C. V. Mosby Company, p 208.)

joints and an anterior band[51] (see Figure 40–8). The limited-motion ankle joint may be solid plastic, or it may have adjustable plantar flexion and dorsiflexion stops.

(3). The rationale for this option is that:

(a). The anterior band provides posteriorly directed force near the knee, thus preventing flexion, which is especially important during early stance.

(b). The ankle joints prevent foot drag during swing phase and aid transition during stance by preventing dorsiflexion.

g. *Knee hyperextension control*

(1). The goal: reduce knee pain caused by hyperextension.

(2). Option: prescribe an AFO with a limited-motion ankle and posterior (calf) band. The limited-motion joint may be solid plastic, or it may have adjustable plantar flexion and dorsiflexion stops.

(3). The rationale for this option is as follows:

(a). The posterior band provides anteriorly directed force near the knee, which is especially important during early stance.

(b). The orthotic ankle prevents the plantar flexion associated with genu recurvatum.

3. **KAFOs**

a. *Knee extensor muscle paralysis*

(1). The goals:

(a). Provide stability during standing.

(b). Reduce gait deviation at early stance.

(2). Option: prescribe a plastic and metal KAFO with a knee lock (either a drop ring or a pawl with bail release and an anterior leg band)[52–54] (see Figure 40–9).

(3). The rationale for this option is as follows:

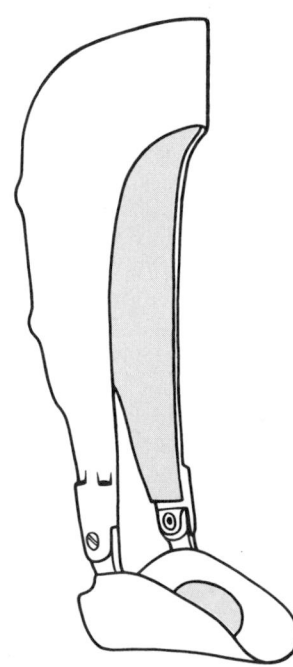

FIGURE 40–8   AFO with plantar flexion and dorsiflexion adjustable ankle joints and anterior band. (Courtesy of Eastern Orthotics & Prosthetics, Spring Valley, NY.)

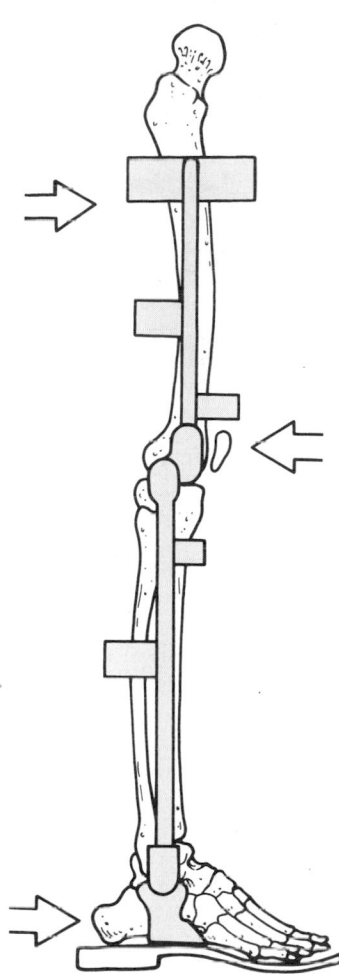

FIGURE 40–9 KAFO three-point force system. (From Lehmann JF, Warren CG: Restraining forces in various designs of knee ankle orthoses: their placement and effect on the anatomical knee joint. *Arch Phys Med Rehabil* 1976, 57:430–437.)

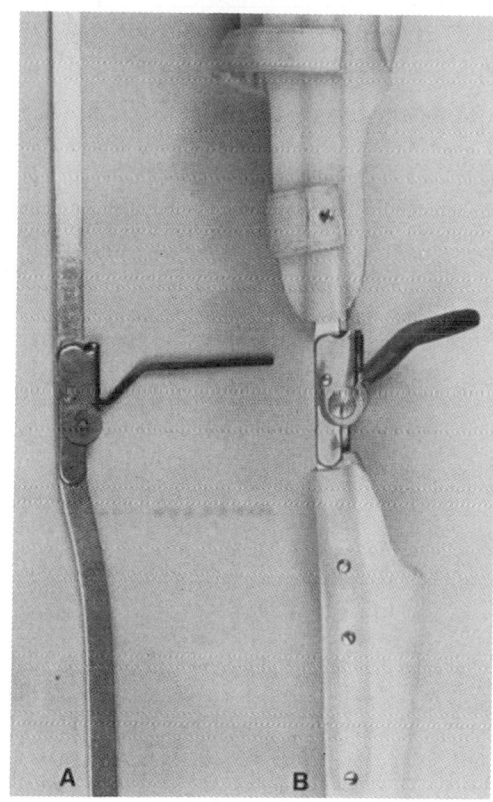

FIGURE 40–10 Pawl lock with bail release. (From O'Sullivan SB, Schmitz TJ: *Physical Rehabilitation: Assessment and Treatment,* 3rd ed. F. A. Davis Company, p 665.)

(a). An AFO with an anterior band usually suffices on level surfaces, but it may not be adequate when the client walks on ramps.

(b). Knee locks, when engaged, prohibit all knee motion, regardless of the walking surface. They must be disengaged when the client wishes to sit. A drop-ring lock is simple and inexpensive but somewhat difficult to manage when it is used on the medial and lateral uprights.

(c). A pawl lock with a bail release (see Figure 40–10) provides automatic locking of both uprights; however, the bail adds bulk to the orthosis.

(d). A plastic and metal KAFO with an insert footplate is lighter in weight and easier to don than the leather and metal version that has a stirrup riveted to the shoe.[55]

(e). The anterior leg band resists knee flexion effectively and is faster to don than a buckled leather knee pad.

(f). The plastic and metal orthosis may incorporate carbon fiber to reduce its weight.[56,57]

b. *Genu valgum and genu varum*

(1). The goal: reduce mediolateral instability and pain.

(2). Option: prescribe a KAFO with a plastic calf shell extended proximally on the medial side (for valgum control or on the lateral side (for varum control).

(3). The rationale for this option is that proximal extension provides counterforce opposing the deformity; valgum control requires laterally directed force at the knee.

c. *Limited weight bearing*
   (1). The goal: eliminate loading on the thigh, leg, and foot.
   (2). Option: is to prescribe a KAFO with a quadrilateral or ischial containment brim,[58] a locked knee, limited-motion ankle joints, and a patten bottom. The opposite shoe requires a lift to equalize leg length.
   (3). The rationale for this option is that the brim transmits loading to the brace uprights and ultimately to the patten. Because the shoe does not touch the floor, no weight is borne through the lower limb.

4. **Hip-knee-ankle-foot orthoses (HKAFOs)**
   a. *Hip rotation control*
      (1). The goal: reduce gait deviation—particularly toeing in—that is attributable to faulty hip control.
      (2). Option: prescribe KAFOs with Dacron (duPont) webbing hip rotation control straps.[59]
         (a). To limit internal rotation, the client wears a webbing waist belt; secured to the posterior midline of the belt are two straps, each having its distal attachment on the proximolateral upright of the KAFO (see Figure 40–11).
         (b). To limit external rotation, a strap doubled on itself passes anteriorly between the left and right lateral uprights (see Figure 40–12).
      (3). The rationale for this option is that the straps resist the tendency of the hips to rotate by applying transverse plane force to each braced leg.
   b. *Hip abduction, adduction, and rotation control*
      (1). The goal: reduce gait deviation that is attributable to faulty hip control.
      (2). Option: prescribe an HKAFO.
      (3). The rationale for this option is that the bilateral hip joints control frontal and transverse plane motion.
   c. *Hip abduction, adduction, rotation, and flexion control*
      (1). The goal: reduce gait deviation that

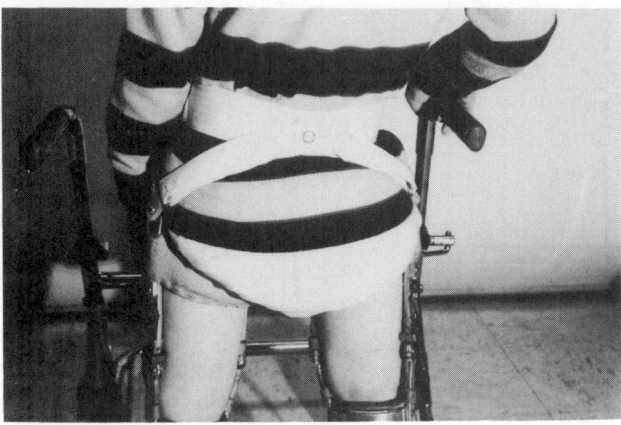

FIGURE 40–11   Internal rotation control strap. (From Hoffman E: Hip-rotation control straps. *Inter-Clin Info Bull* 1983, 18:1–4.)

is attributable to faulty hip control — particularly crouch gait.
   (2). Option: prescribe an HKAFO that has drop ring locks at the hip joints.
   (3). The rationale for this therapy is as follows:
      (a). Locked hip joints prevent all hip motion.
      (b). Ambulation is restricted to trunk rotation or swing-to or swing-through crouch gait.

5. **Trunk-hip-knee-ankle-foot orthoses (THKAFOs)**
   Several orthotic alternatives are available to provide clients with the physiological and psychological benefits of standing, which include the following:
   • Skeletal stress promotes growth in children and reduces osteoporosis in adults.
   • Urinary and bowel function is aided.
   • The risk of decubitus ulceration is lessened.
   • The risk of forming contractures is lessened.
   • The risk of obesity is lessened.
   • The cardiovascular benefits of moderate aerobic activity are gained.
   • Self-esteem is enhanced (*eg*, the patient can meet peers at eye level).
   • The patient's work area is expanded vertically.
   Traditional THKAFOs are so difficult for the client to don that they are rarely used following the patient's discharge from the rehabilitation center. Rather than orthoses, some clients prefer a wheelchair that has a mechanism that enables the user to stand.
   a. *Juvenile paraplegia*
      (1). The goals:

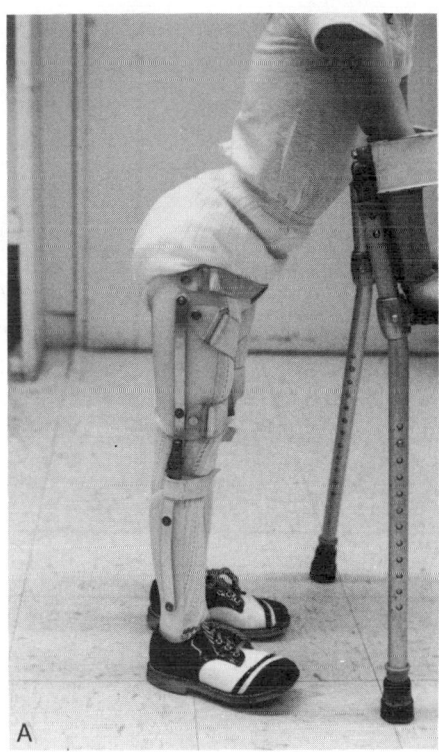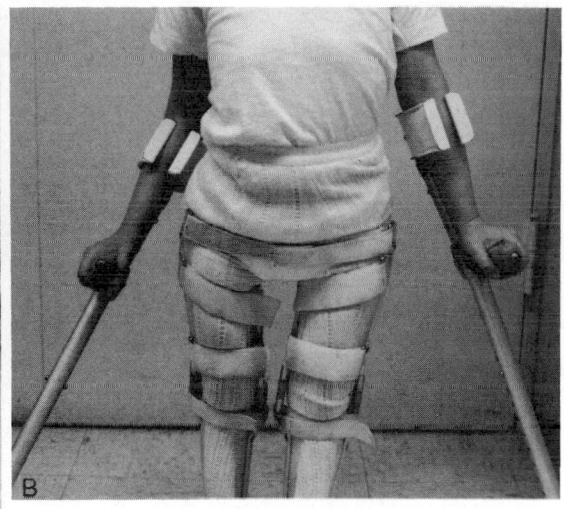

FIGURE 40–12   External rotation control strap. **A**, Lateral view. **B**, Anterior view. (From Hoffman E: Hip-rotation control straps. *Inter-Clin Info Bull* 1983, 18:1–4.)

(a). Foster development of upright posture and balance.

(b). Facilitate walking.

(2). Option one: prescribe a standing-frame THKAFO. This mass-produced frame consists of a base to which is attached a pair of posterior uprights that terminate in the upper thorax. Attached to the frame are a dorsolumbar band, a chest band, and a band that secures both knees. The child wears any low-heeled shoes, which are strapped to the base.

(3). The rationale of this option is as follows:

(a). During standing, the child is supported by the rigidity of the frame and the three-point stabilizing systems, which consist of a broad posterior dorsolumbar band counteracted by chest and knee bands.

(b). During gait, many children discover that by shifting weight to one corner of the base of the frame, they can pivot and thereby maneuver indoors.

(4). Option two: prescribe a parapodium THKAFO[60] (see Figure 40–13). This mass-produced orthosis has a frame similar to a standing frame; the child wears shoes that are held to the base by spring-loaded clips. Handles on the frame enable the wearer to lock and unlock the joints for sitting, bending at the hips, and standing.

(5). The rationale for this option is as follows:

(a). During standing, the same support system is used as in a standing frame. The parapodium also permits sitting.

(b). During gait, a pivot gait is possible, as with a standing frame. For longer distances, the child uses crutches for a swing-to or swing-through gait.

(6). Because the parapodium must be worn on the outside of slacks, school-aged children become dissatisfied with its appearance. Op-

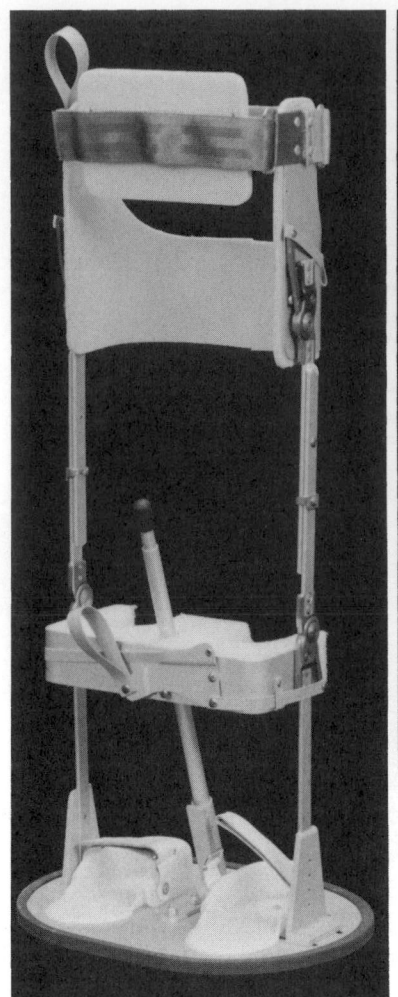
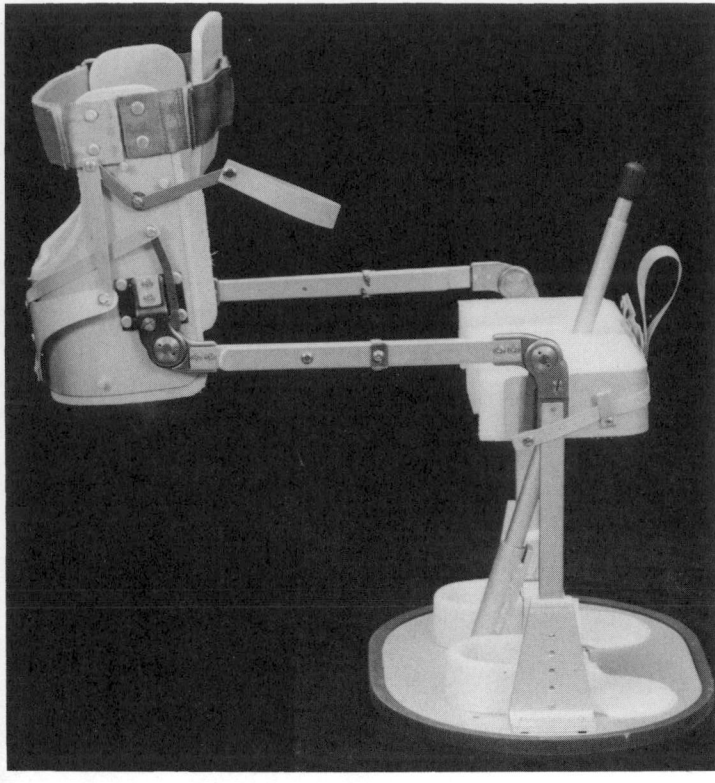

FIGURE 40–13 Parapodium.

tions for children and adults are as follows:

(a). A swivel walker can be used.

(b). A reciprocating-gait orthosis may be helpful.

(c). A ParaWalker can be prescribed.

b. **Adult paraplegia.** Adults with paraplegia have many orthotic options, none of which restores the individual to the premorbid level of function.

(1). The goals: to allow standing and walking.

(2). Orthotic fitting is predicated on:

(a). High motivation of the patient to persist with an intensive training program.

(b). The patient's physical condition.

(i). The patient must be relatively slender.

(ii). No, or minimal, contractures can be present.

(iii). No marked spasticity can be present.

(iv). No ligamentous laxity can be present.

(v). The patient must be able to tolerate the upright posture.

(vi). Individuals with incomplete lesions or with relatively low levels of lesions fare better.

(3). *Limitations.* Long-term use of orthoses is unlikely because most orthotic systems limit clients in one or more ways.[61]

(a). Independence. The client should be able to don the orthosis independently and rapidly, rise from a chair, and traverse obstacles commonly found at home and at the workplace, such as door sills and carpets.

(b). Energy cost. The client should not be so fatigued after walking that other activities, such as those required on the job, cannot be readily performed. Walking must not take so much time as to interfere with other activities.

(c). Appearance. The client may be embarrassed by the awkward appearance of his/her gait and by the bulges caused by orthoses worn under slacks. Orthoses may tear or stain clothing.

(d). Durability. The active wearer imposes high torsional forces on the orthoses, leading to breakage and malfunction.

(e). Cost. Public or private insurance may not reimburse the client for the full cost of the orthoses and their maintenance.

(4). Option one: prescribe a swivel walker THKAFO[62] (see Figure 40–14). Available in child and adult sizes, this nonarticulated orthosis has two swiveling plates on the base. The client wears any low-heeled shoes, which are strapped to the base of the walker.

(5). The rationale for this option is as follows:

(a). During standing, the same support system is used as in the juvenile standing frame. A posterior chute-like design facilitates donning. Sitting is impossible with the swivel walker.

(b). During gait, a pivot gait is possible, as with standing frame or parapodium. Swiveling plates increase the wearer's security because the plates always contact the floor. For walking longer distances, the wearer uses crutches for a swing-to or swing-through gait. The swivel walker must be worn on the outside of slacks.

(6). Option two: prescribe a Vannini-Rizzoli stabilizing boot AFO[63,64] (see Figure 40–15). Each boot has

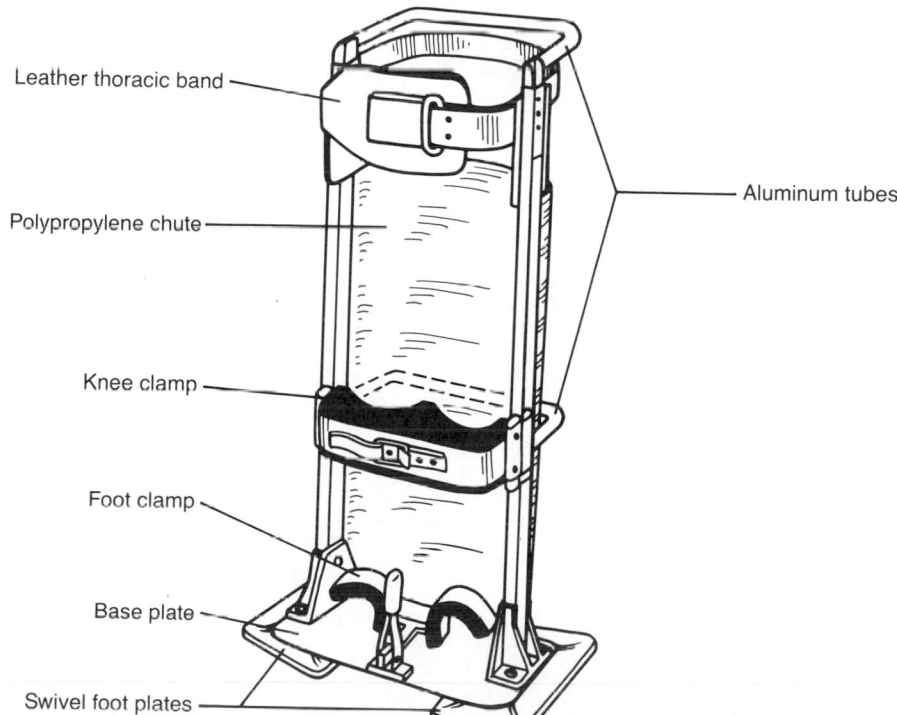

Leather thoracic band

Aluminum tubes

Polypropylene chute

Knee clamp

Foot clamp

Base plate

Swivel foot plates

FIGURE 40–14 Swivel walker. (From Seymour RJ, Knapp CF, Anderson TR, Kearney JT: Paraplegic use of the ORLAW swivel walker: case report. *Arch Phys Med Rehabil* 1982, 63:490–494.)

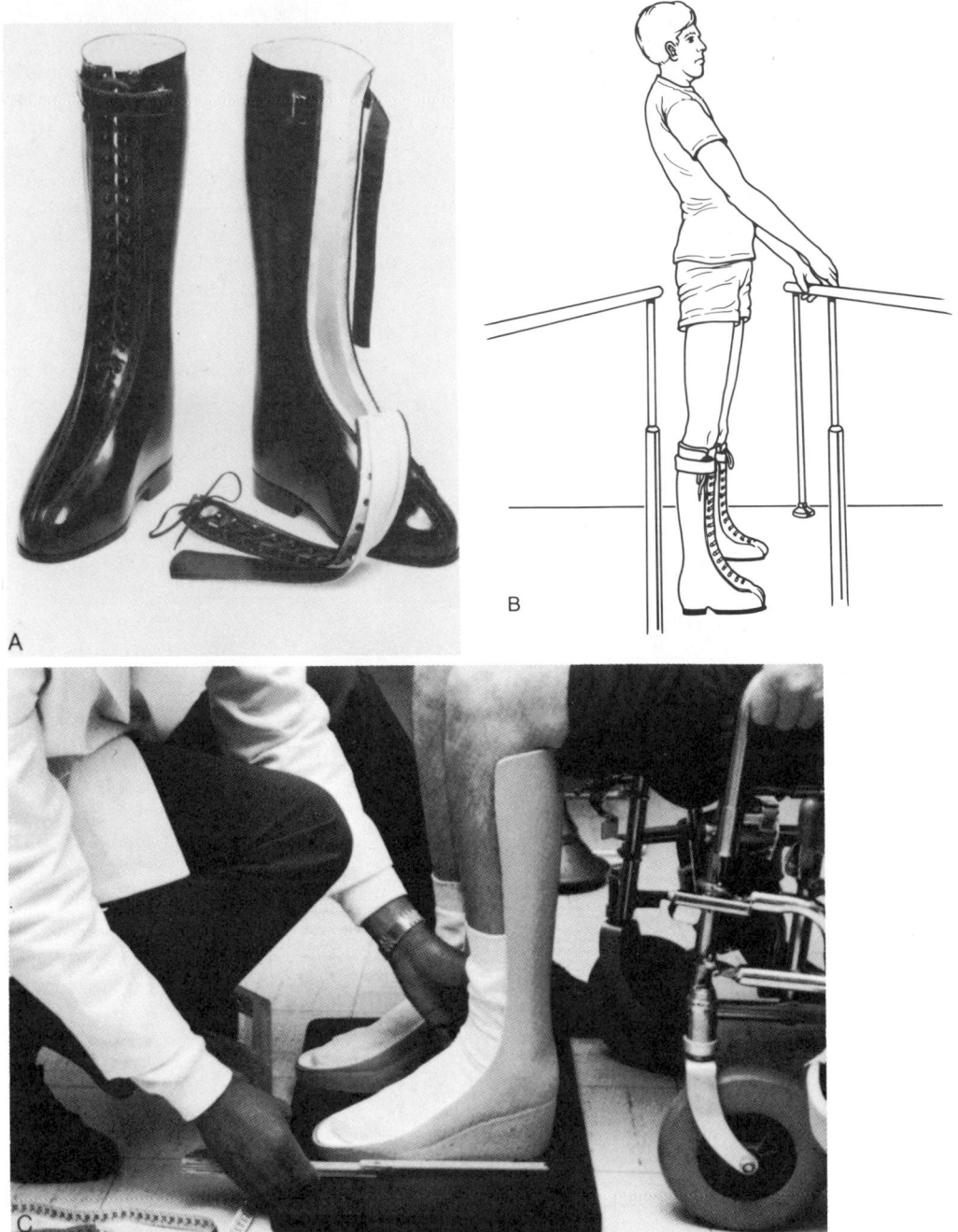

FIGURE 40–15   **A**, Vannini-Rizzoli stabilizing boots. (From Lyles M, Munday J: Report on the evaluation of the Vannini-Rizzoli stabilizing limb orthosis. *J Rehabil Res Dev* 1992, 29:77–104.) **B**, Client's posture. (From Kent HO: Vannini-Rizzoli stabilizing orthosis (boot): preliminary report on a new ambulatory aid for spinal cord injury. *Arch Phys Med Rehabil* 1992, 73:302–307.) **C**, Fitting the wedge. (Courtesy of St. Joseph Hospital, Memphis, TN.)

an inner rigid posterior calf shell continuous with a footplate angled at approximately 15 degrees. The most frequently used model has a leather exterior, which closes with two longitudinal zippers in the front.

(7). The rationale for this option is as follows:

   (a). During standing, the feet are maintained in plantar flexion on flat-based boots. The client's center of gravity is shifted anterior to the ankles and knees. Rigidity of the posterior shell of the boots, together with the anterior leather, prevents dorsiflexion. Posterior knee ligaments resist genu recurvatum, and the iliofemoral ligaments resist hip hyperextension. Standing posture requires that the shoulders be retracted and that the thoracic spine be extended.

(b). During gait, the client walks with a walker, canes, or crutches in a four-point gait pattern by shifting the upper trunk to the right or by contracting the left quadratus lumborum to allow the left leg to swing forward; the wearer then shifts the trunk to the left or uses the right quadratus lumborum to advance the right leg. Trunk fusion limits the client's ability to rotate the trunk, the maneuver needed to advance the legs.

(8). Option three: prescribe Craig Scott KAFOs[65] (see Figure 40–16). Each orthosis consists of a reinforced shoe with a solid stirrup that terminates in a pair of metal plantar flexion and dorsiflexion stops, an anterior leg band, knee locks, and a single posterior thigh band. Alternatively, a plastic solid ankle may be substituted for the stirrups and the plantar flexion and dorsiflexion stops.[66]

(9). The rationale for this option is as follows:

(a). During standing, the knees and feet are kept rigid by the orthosis. The hips are stabilized by thoracic extension; hip hyperextension is limited by the iliofemoral ligaments.

(b). Gait is similar to that achieved with Vannini-Rizzoli stabilizing boots. Although the shoe sole must be rigid, either by means of longitudinal and transverse plates or by means of a rigid insert foot plate, the shoes should have resilient soling to absorb impact shock, particularly during the swing-to or swing-through gait.[67] A temporary version of the Craig Scott orthoses is manufactured to

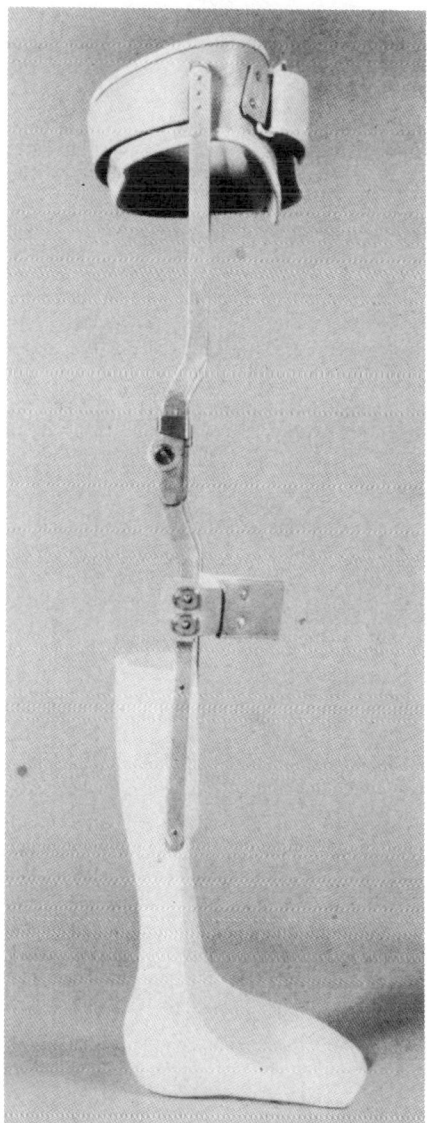

FIGURE 40–16 Craig-Scott KAFO. (Reprinted from Lobley S, Rogerson J, Cullen J, Freed M: Orthotic design from the New England Regional Spinal Cord Injury Center. *Phys Ther* 1985, 65:492–493 with the permission of the American Physical Therapy Association.)

enable the patient to try ambulation with the orthoses.

(10). Option four: prescribe a reciprocating gait orthosis,[68,69] a type of THKAFO (see Figure 40–17). The KAFO section consists of a reinforced plastic solid-ankle foot plate, an anterior leg band, a knee lock, and an optional thigh band. The thoracic-hip unit has right and left hinged hip joints that can be set by

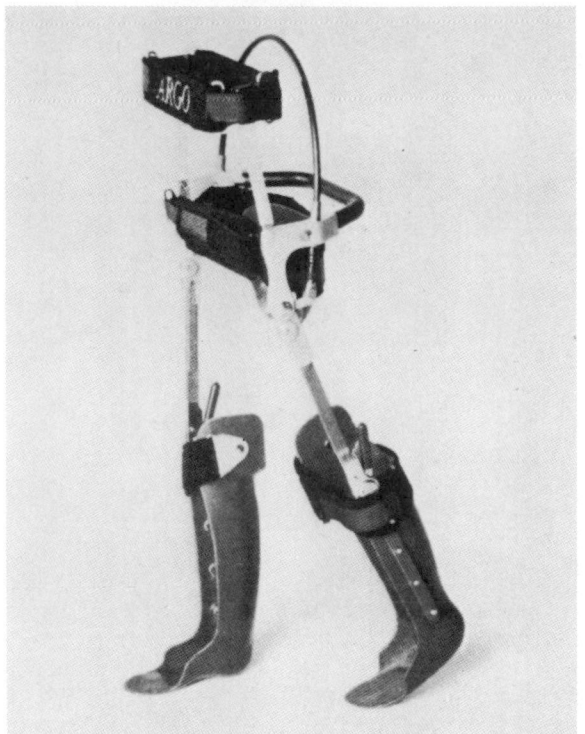

FIGURE 40–17   Reciprocating gait orthosis. (Courtesy of Liberty Mutual Research Center, Hopkinton, MA.)

the wearer to unlock for sitting; for walking, the hip joints are either locked at 180 degrees or set to flex approximately 25 degrees. The hip joints are connected posteriorly by one or two steel cables. Hip extension on one side causes hip flexion on the opposite side. Trunk uprights from the hip joints support a posterior pelvic girdle with an anterior strap and a circumferential chest strap.

An improved version of the orthosis includes a spring mechanism that enables the wearer to sit and to stand more easily; the mechanism causes the orthotic knee joints to unlock and to lock automatically.

(11). The rationale for this option is as follows:
(a). During standing, the knees and feet are kept rigid by the orthosis. Hip excursion is limited by the hinged hip joints and by the iliofemoral ligaments. Additional stabilization is provided by crutches.

(b). Gait is a four-point, reciprocal gait, similar to that achieved with Vannini-Rizzoli stabilizing boots or with a Craig Scott AFO. The gait sequence is as follows:
  (i). Shift: diagonal weight shift to the right leg is achieved by trunk rotation to the right.
  (ii). Tuck: the trunk and hip extend to gain clearance for the left leg.
  (iii). Push: vigorous elbow extension enables the client to push on the walker or on the crutches.
  (iv). Kick: swift trunk rotation to the right permits the left leg to advance like a pendulum.
  (v). The sequence is then repeated, with the client shifting weight to the left leg.

(12). Option five: prescribe a Para-Walker, originally called a hip-guidance orthosis,[70–72] a type of THKAFO (see Figure 40–18). The KAFO section consists of a foot plate with a rocker sole to which the shoe is strapped, an anterior leg band, a knee lock, and a thigh band. The thoracic-hip unit has very large right and left hinged hip joints that can be set by the wearer to unlock for sitting; for walking, the hip joints are set to flex and to hyperextend through a total arc of approximately 25 degrees. Trunk uprights from the hip joints support a posterior pelvic girdle and a circumferential chest strap.

(13). The rationale for this option is as follows:
(a). During standing, the knees and feet are kept rigid by the orthosis. Hip excursion is limited by the orthotic hip joints and by the iliofemoral ligaments. Additional stabilization is provided by crutches.

(b). Gait is a four-point, reciprocal gait, similar to that achieved with Vannini-Rizzoli stabilizing boots or with a reciprocating gait orthosis.

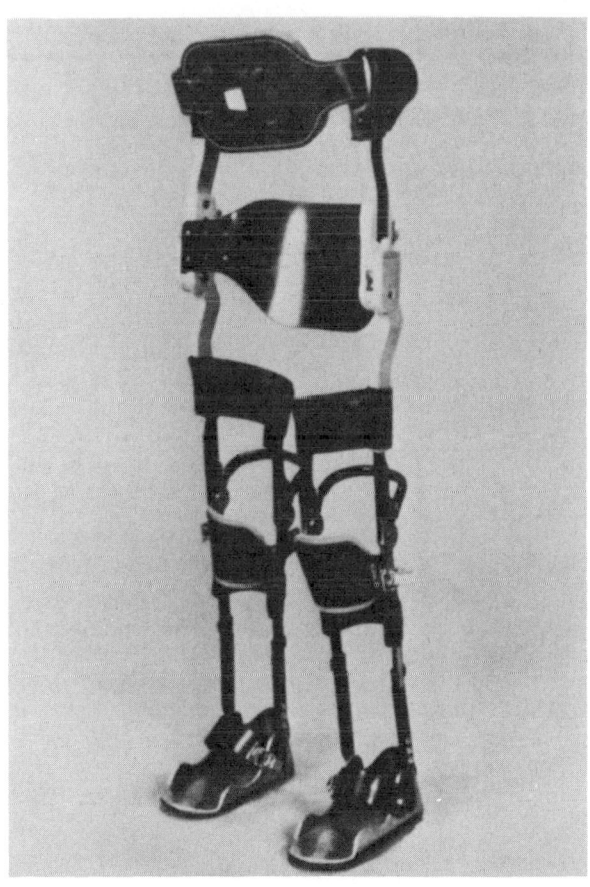

FIGURE 40–18   ParaWalker. (Courtesy of ORLAU Publishing, with permission.)

(14). Option six: prescribe an orthosis plus functional electrical stimulation.[76-81] Various hybrids are used, including the reciprocating gait orthosis and the ParaWalker. Surface electrical stimulation may be applied to both the gluteal musculature and to the quadriceps or to either muscle group. A commercial system applies stimulation to the quadriceps, peroneal nerves, and gluteus maximus without orthoses, enabling the user to stand, walk slowly with a special walker, and sit.

(15). The rationale for this option is as follows:

  (a). To aid with standing, stimulation with the orthosis enables the clients to rise from a chair more easily. The rigidity of the orthosis and the use of a hand support appear to be the major factors in helping the patient to maintain standing balance.

  (b). With stimulation, gait is somewhat faster with less cardiopulmonary demand.

  (c). The patient walks with less deviation.

  (d). Deformity is controlled or reduced.

  (c). As compared with the reciprocating gait orthosis, the ParaWalker is heavier and less flexible, and wearers experience more difficulty maneuvering over curbs and slopes. Walking velocity is slow with either orthosis, and energy requirements with both are similarly high.[73-75]

E. Static evaluation

Table 40–1 describes the key elements in the assessment of the fit, function, and construction of lower-limb orthoses.

F. Dynamic evaluation

Table 40–2 indicates the most common gait deviations and their orthotic and anatomic causes.

Table 40–1. LOWER-LIMB ORTHOTIC EVALUATION

1. Is the orthosis as prescribed?
2. Can the client don the orthosis easily?

Standing

3. Is the shoe satisfactory and does it fit properly?
4. Are the sole and heel of the shoe flat on the floor?
5. If a shoe insert is used, does minimal rocking exist between insert and shoe?

Ankle

 6. Do the mechanical ankle joints coincide with the anatomic ankle?

7. Does adequate clearance exist between the anatomic ankle and the mechanical ankle joints?
8. Does the valgus or varus correction strap control the foot position?

Knee

 9. Do the mechanical knee joints coincide with the anatomic knee?
10. Does adequate clearance exist between the anatomic knee and the mechanical knee joint?
11. Is the knee lock secure and easy to operate?

Table 40–1. LOWER-LIMB ORTHOTIC EVALUATION *(Continued)*

Shells, Bands, Cuffs, and Uprights

12. Do the shells, bands, cuffs, and uprights conform to the contours of the leg and thigh?
13. Does adequate clearance exist between the top of the calf shell or band and the head of the fibula?
14. Does adequate clearance exist between the orthosis and the perineum?
15. Is the orthosis below the greater trochanter but at least 2.5 cm higher than the medial shell or upright?
16. Are the uprights at the midline of the leg and thigh?
17. Do the shells, bands, and cuffs conform to the contours of the leg and thigh?
18. Is any flesh roll above the shell or band minimal?
19. Are the bottom of the thigh shell or distal thigh band and the top of the calf shell or band equidistant from the knee?
20. In a child's orthosis, does adequate provision exist for lengthening the orthosis?

Weight-Relieving Components

21. In a patellar-tendon–bearing brim, does adequate relief exist for the head of the fibula?
22. With a quadrilateral brim, is the client free from excessive pressure in the anteromedial and medial aspect of the brim?
23. With a quadrilateral brim, does the ischial tuberosity rest on the ischial seat?
24. With a patellar-tendon–bearing or proximal thigh brim, does adequate reduction exist in weight-bearing through the orthosis?

Hip

25. Is the center of the pelvic joint slightly above and ahead the greater trochanter?
26. Is the hip lock secure and easy to operate?
27. Does the pelvic band fit the torso accurately?

Stability

28. Does the orthosis provide adequate stability to the client

Sitting

29. Can the client sit comfortably with the hips and kne flexed 90 degrees?
30. Can the client lean forward to touch the shoes?

Walking

31. Is the client's performance in level walking satisfactory?
32. Is the client's performance on stairs and ramps satisfacto
33. Is the orthosis sufficiently rigid?
34. Does the varus or valgus correction strap provide ad quate support?
35. Does the orthosis operate quickly?
36. Does the client consider the orthosis to be satisfactory regard to comfort, function, and appearance?

Orthosis Off the Client

37. Is the skin free of abrasions or other discolorations att utable to the orthosis?
38. Is the construction satisfactory?
39. Do all components function satisfactorily?

Table 40–2. ORTHOTIC GAIT ANALYSIS

Phase	Deviation	Orthotic Causes	Anatomical Causes
Early stance	Foot slap (forefoot slaps the ground)	Inadequate dorsiflexion assist Inadequate plantar flexion stop	Weak dorsiflexors
	Toes first (tiptoe posture may or may not be maintained throughout stance)	Inadequate heel lift Inadequate dorsiflexion assist Inadequate plantar flexion stop Inadequate relief of heel pain	Short leg Pes equinus Extensor spasticity Heel pain
	Flat foot contact (entire foot contacts ground initially)	Inadequate traction from sole Requires walking aid, *eg,* cane Inadequate dorsiflexion stop	Poor balance Pes calcaneus
	Excessive medial (lateral) foot contact (medial [lateral] border contacts floor)	Transverse plane malalignment	Weak invertors (evertors) Pes valgus (varus) Genu valgum (varum)
	Excessive knee flexion (knee collapses when foot contacts ground)	Inadequate knee lock Inadequate dorsiflexion stop Plantar flexion stop Inadequate contralateral shoe lift	Weak quadriceps Short contralateral leg Knee pain Knee or hip flexion contracture Flexor synergy Pes calcaneus
	Hyperextended knee (knee hyperextends as weight is transferred to leg)	Genu recurvatum inadequately controlled by plantar flexion stop Excessively concave calf band Pes equinus uncompensated by contralateral shoe lift Inadequate knee lock	Weak quadriceps Lax knee ligaments Extensor synergy Pes equinus Short contralateral leg Contralateral knee or hip flexion contracture

Table 40–2.   ORTHOTIC GAIT ANALYSIS *(Continued)*

Phase	Deviation	Orthotic Causes	Anatomical Causes
	Anterior trunk bending (patient leans forward as weight is transferred to leg)	Inadequate knee lock	Weak quadriceps Hip flexion contracture Knee flexion contracture
	Posterior trunk bending (patient leans backward as weight is transferred to leg)	Inadequate hip lock Knee lock	Weak gluteus maximus Knee ankylosis
	Lateral trunk bending (patient leans toward stance leg as weight is transferred to leg)	Excessive height of medial upright of KAFO Excessive abduction of hip joint of HKAFO Insufficient shoe lift Requires walking aid, *eg,* cane	Weak gluteus medius Abduction contracture Dislocated hip Hip pain Poor balance Short leg
	Wide walking base (heel centers more than 10 cm [4 in] apart)	Excessive height of medial upright of KAFO Excessive abduction of hip joint of HKAFO Insufficient lift on contralateral shoe Knee lock Requires walking aid, *eg,* cane	Abduction contracture Poor balance Short contralateral leg
	Internal (external) rotation (limb internally [externally] rotated)	Uprights incorrectly aligned in transverse plane Requires orthotic control, *eg,* rotation control straps, pelvic band	Internal (external) hip rotators spastic External (internal) hip rotators weak Anteversion (retroversion) Weak quadriceps (external rotation)
Late stance	Inadequate transition (delayed or absent transfer of weight over the forefoot)	Plantar flexion stop Inadequate dorsiflexion stop	Weak plantar flexors Achilles tendon sprain or rupture Pes calcaneus Forefoot pain
Swing	Toe drag (toes maintain contact with ground)	Inadequate dorsiflexion assist Inadequate plantar flexion stop	Weak dorsiflexors Plantar flexor spasticity Pes equinus Weak hip flexors
	Circumduction (leg swings outward in a semicircular arc)	Knee lock Inadequate dorsiflexion assist Inadequate plantar flexion stop	Weak hip flexors Extensor synergy Knee or ankle ankylosis Weak dorsiflexors Pes equinus
	Hip hiking (leg elevated at pelvis to enable the limb to swing forward)	Knee lock Inadequate dorsiflexion assist Inadequate plantar flexion stop	Short contralateral leg Contralateral knee or hip flexion contracture Weak hip flexors Extensor synergy Knee or ankle ankylosis Weak dorsiflexor muscles Pes equinus
	Vaulting (exaggerated plantar flexion of contralateral leg to enable the limb to swing forward)	Knee lock Inadequate dorsiflexion assist Inadequate plantar flexion stop	Weak hip flexors Extensor spasticity Pes equinus Short contralateral leg Contralateral knee or hip flexion contracture Knee or ankle ankylosis Weak dorsiflexors

III. Trunk Orthoses

The term "spinal orthosis" is widely used; nevertheless, it is misleading because orthoses are applied on the outside of the body. Although an orthosis may be prescribed to stabilize the spine (*eg*, the vertebral column), the orthosis exerts its force through the skin, soft tissue, and ribs. Contemporary nomenclature emphasizes the region covered by the orthosis (*eg*, lumbosacral) and the motions controlled by the orthosis (*eg*, flexion). Thus, trunk orthoses include cervical orthoses, lumbosacral orthoses (LSO), thoracolumbosacral orthoses (TLSO), and cervicothoracolumbosacral orthoses.[82,83] In some instances, particularly with regard to scoliosis orthoses, the generic name does not indicate design distinctions; consequently, eponyms are used.

A. Principles

In addition to the general principles applicable to nearly all orthoses, trunk orthoses should satisfy the following requirements:

1. The client must be able to sit comfortably while wearing the orthosis.

   Example: A lumbosacral orthosis must be designed to allow a slight clearance between the chair and the inferior edge of the orthosis. When the wearer sits, the pelvis tilts, thus altering the alignment and position of the orthosis. Consequently, the orthosis must be evaluated in both sitting and standing positions.

2. A form-fitting orthosis must not restrict breathing, digestion, or chewing.

   Example: Although the purpose of the orthosis may be to immobilize the site of vertebral fusion, provisions must be made for thoracic and abdominal motion during respiration and digestion; for example, an anterior opening may be placed over the thorax and abdomen. Similarly, a cervical orthosis that has a mandibular plate should be fitted to allow the client to move the jaw.

3. Although the short-term use of lumbosacral orthoses promotes reduction of muscle spasm, prolonged orthotic wear fosters:
   a. Atrophy.
   b. Weakness.
   c. Lessened flexibility.
   d. Psychological dependence.

Examples: (1) The patient with a lower-back disorder may appreciate the immediate pain relief provided by a corset or rigid orthosis; however, the patient should be re-examined regularly to determine when to discontinue use of the orthosis and to institute therapeutic exercise. (2) The adolescent with idiopathic scoliosis should participate in an exercise program to complement brace wear to help maintain motor power and flexibility.

B. Physical assessment

1. **Trunk alignment and posture**
   a. Sitting.
   b. *Standing*. The following postural disorders may be present:
      (1). Kyphosis.
      (2). Lordosis.
      (3). Scoliosis.
      (4). Shoulder and pelvic asymmetry.
      (5). Head not over the buttocks.
   c. Walking.
2. Flexibility.
3. Muscle power.
4. **Sensory status**
   a. *Tactile sensation*. The patient should be able to determine whether the orthosis is impinging on bone prominences.
5. **Skin condition.** Examine the patient for the presence of:
   a. Abrasions.
   b. Ulcerations.
   c. Dermatitis.
   d. Other lesions.
6. **Manual dexterity.** The patient should possess the ability to manage the fastening of laces, buckles, and other fasteners.
7. **Vision**
   a. The patient should have the ability to dress independently.
   b. The patient should possess the ability to read typewritten instructions.

C. Subjective assessment

1. **Comprehension:** the client should
   a. Indicate an understanding of oral instructions.
   b. Indicate an understanding of written instructions.
   c. Express a language preference.

2. **Complaints**
   a. *Pain*
      (1). Assess where pain occurs.
      (2). Determine when it occurs (*eg*, whether it is constant or occasional).
      (3). Assess the character of the pain (*eg*, whether it is throbbing, burning, dull, or sharp).
      (4). Record the date of onset of pain.
      (5). Note any aggravating factors.
      (6). Note any diminishing factors.
   b. *Performance*
      (1). The patient may have difficulty maneuvering at home, at work, at school, or during recreation.
      (2). Evaluate the patient's fatigue in relation to the duration of activity.
   c. *Appearance*
      (1). Examine the trunk contour with and without the orthosis, both when the patient is standing and when sitting.
      (2). Note the patient's skin condition.
      (3). Determine whether the orthosis causes any clothing abrasion or style limitation unacceptable to the patient.
3. **History of disorder**
   A chronic painful disorder may be less amenable to orthotic management than an acute disorder.
4. **Previous orthotic experience**
   a. *Preferred orthosis.* The patient may have a preference for certain features of an orthosis, including:
      (1). Material.
      (2). Weight.
      (3). Fit.
      (4). Design.
      (5). Durability and maintenance.
   b. *Disliked orthosis.* The patient may have disliked certain features of a previous orthosis, including:
      (1). Material.
      (2). Weight.
      (3). Fit.
      (4). Design.
      (5). Durability and maintenance.
5. Other therapeutic options include:
   a. Medications.
   b. Surgery (previous and contemplated).
   c. Therapeutic exercise, including relaxation techniques.
   d. Electrotherapy.
   e. Other physical modalities.
6. The goals include:
   a. Reduced pain.

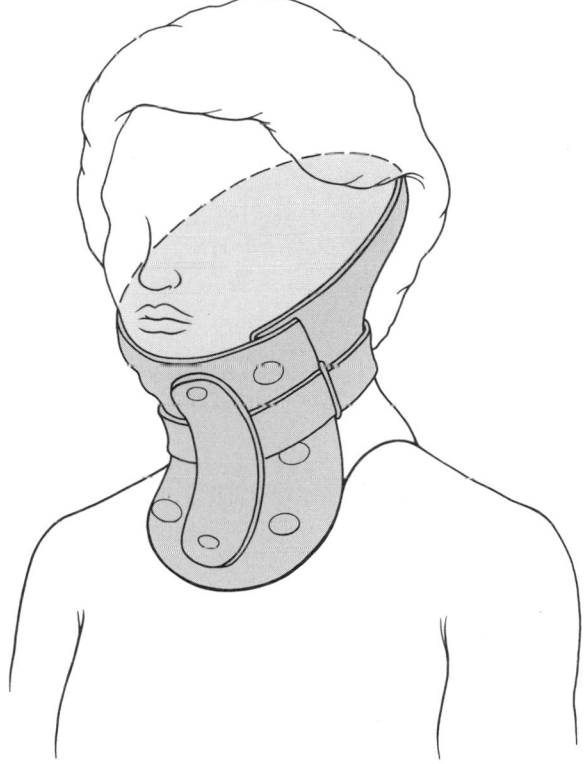

FIGURE 40–19 Philadelphia collar. (From Fisher SV: Cervical orthoses. *Phys Med Rehabil Clin N Am* 1992, 1:29–44.)

   b. Improved appearance.
   c. Improved respiration.
7. **Economic considerations.** Particularly in patients with lower-back disorders and neck trauma, evaluate secondary financial or emotional benefits realized through the continuation of symptoms.

D. **Planning and implementation**

   1. **Cervical orthoses**
      a. *Sprain, strain, or arthritis*
         (1). The goal: reduce pain.
         (2). Option one: prescribe a collar made of soft fabric, foam plastic, or rigid plastic.[84-86] For example, the Philadelphia collar (see Figure 40–19) is made of foam plastic, encompasses the lower jaw and occiput, and has rigid anterior and posterior struts.
         (3). The rationale for this option is as follows:
            (a). The least motion limitation is achieved with a soft collar; a rigid collar and the Philadelphia collar restrict motion—es-

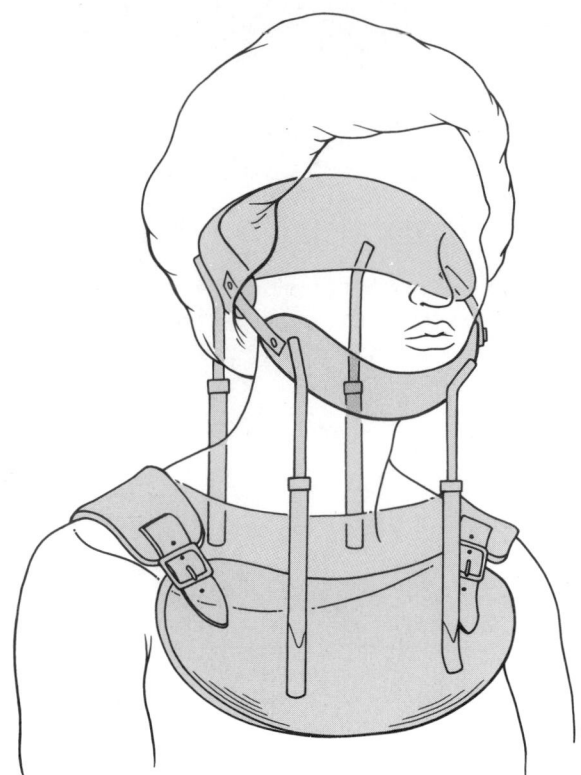

FIGURE 40–20   Four-post orthosis. (From Fisher SV: Cervical orthoses. *Phys Med Rehabil Clin N Am* 1992, 1:29–44.)

pecially neck flexion—slightly more.

(b). A collar reminds the wearer not to move abruptly, thus reducing stress on the damaged tissues.

(c). A collar retains body heat, which enhances circulation to the injured structures.

(4). Option two: prescribe a post orthosis (see Figure 40–20). This mass-produced orthosis has mandibular and occipital plates connected to sternal and thoracic plates by two, three, or four posts.

(5). The rationale for this option is as follows:

(a). This orthosis provides greater motion limitation—especially the four-post orthosis, which limits motion in all planes.

(b). The clinician can adjust the length of the posts, thereby selecting the optimal alignment of the head on the neck.

(c). Post orthoses are cooler than collars but are generally bulkier.

b. *Paralysis with or without fracture*

(1). The goals:

(a). Support the head to allow the patient to see, speak, and eat more easily.

(b). In the presence of vertebral fracture, foster spontaneous healing or healing of surgical arthrodesis.

(2). Option one: prescribe a Philadelphia collar or a four-post orthosis.

(3). The rationale for this option is that these orthoses:

(a). Produce the least obtrusive motion limitation.

(b). May be adequate in the later stages of healing.

(4). Option two: prescribe a Minerva orthosis.[87] This mass-produced or custom-made orthosis includes a rigid posterior shell that extends from the midthorax to the upper portion of the head. Anteriorly, the orthosis has a forehead strap that secures the upper posterior shell and a rigid mandibular plate that extends to a chest plate that is strapped to the posterior plate. A tracheostomy opening is usually made in the anterior plate.

(5). The rationale for this option is as follows:

(a). This orthosis provides excellent motion limitation.

(b). Unlike a cast, the orthosis can be removed for skin care.

(6). Option three: prescribe a halo-vest orthosis[88,89] (see Figure 40–21). This mass-produced orthosis is applied surgically. A rigid halo is secured to the skull with four pins. The halo supports four posts that terminate in hardware attached to the front and back of the vest.

(7). The rationale for this orthosis is as follows:

(a). It provides maximal motion limitation, particularly for high fractures.

(b). This orthosis is usually cooler and lighter in weight than a Minerva orthosis.

(c). The risk of pin-site infection, pin loosening, and pressure sores is present.

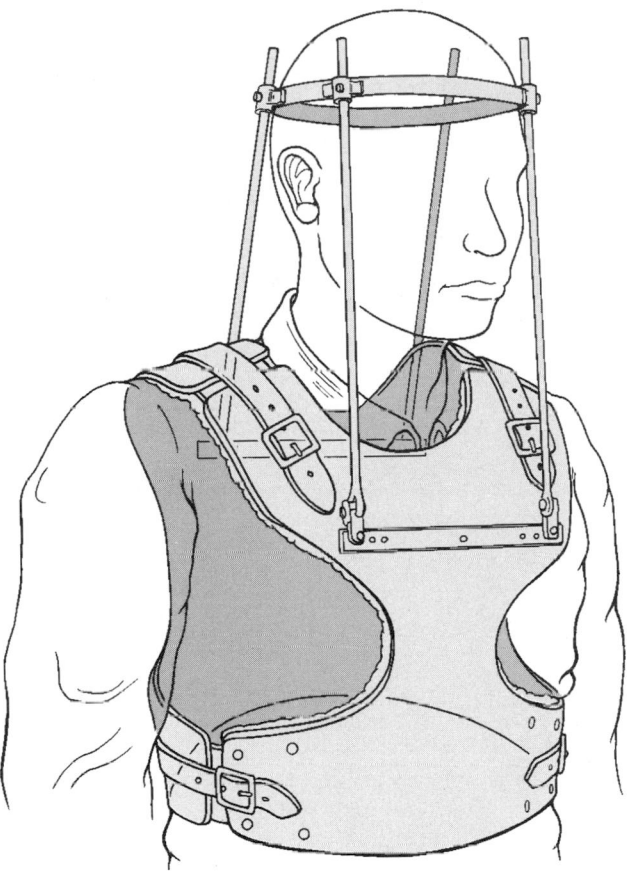

FIGURE 40–21 Halo vest orthosis. (From Fisher SV: Cervical orthoses. *Phys Med Rehabil Clin N Am* 1992, 1:29–44.)

      (d). The orthosis may interfere with rehabilitation activities such as rolling.
2. **LSOs and TLSOs.** Increasingly, manufacturers construct the rigid components of LSOs and TLSOs of rigid or semirigid plastic, lined with resilient foam plastic. This construction enables the orthosis to be lighter in weight and easier to keep clean than the more traditional leather-upholstered aluminum or steel orthosis. In addition, the thermoplastic material can be adjusted by the application of heat, which makes reshaping relatively easy. Orthoses that are custom made by orthotists, however, may be constructed of either plastic or leather-upholstered aluminum.[90–92]
  a. *Lower-back pain, spondylolisthesis, intervertebral disc disease, nonoperative and postoperative management*
    (1). The goal: reduce pain.
    (2). Option one: prescribe a lumbosacral corset.[93–96] A corset may have vertical

reinforcements or a rigid posterior plate, but it has no rigid horizontal bands.
(3). The rationale for this option is as follows:
    (a). The corset reminds the wearer to avoid abrupt motion.
    (b). It increases intra-abdominal compression, thereby reducing contraction of the erector spinae and consequently reducing compression of the intervertebral discs.
    (c). This is the best tolerated, least expensive option.
    (d). Intermittent use of a corset may reduce incidence of work-related injuries.[97]
(4). Option two: prescribe resilient shoe soles with or without resilient shoe inserts.[98]
(5). The rationale for this option is that the soles absorb impact shock that occurs during walking.
(6). Option three: prescribe an LSO.[99][101] Although the term "orthosis" refers to any external appliance worn for therapeutic purposes and would therefore include corsets, the term is usually reserved for trunk orthoses that have rigid horizontal bands.
    (a). Lumbosacral flexion and extension are controlled by one type of LSO (*ie*, a chair-back brace), which has pelvic and thoracic bands, two posterior uprights, and a fabric abdominal front.
    (b). Lumbosacral flexion, extension, and lateral motion are controlled by another LSO (*ie*, a Knight brace) (see Figure 40–22) which has pelvic and thoracic bands, two posterior uprights, two lateral uprights, and a fabric abdominal front.
    (c). Lumbosacral flexion and lateral motion are controlled by a third type of LSO (*ie*, a Williams brace), which has pelvic and thoracic bands, two lateral uprights, and a fabric abdominal front.
    (d). The lumbosacral jacket (*ie*, Boston Overlap Brace) (see

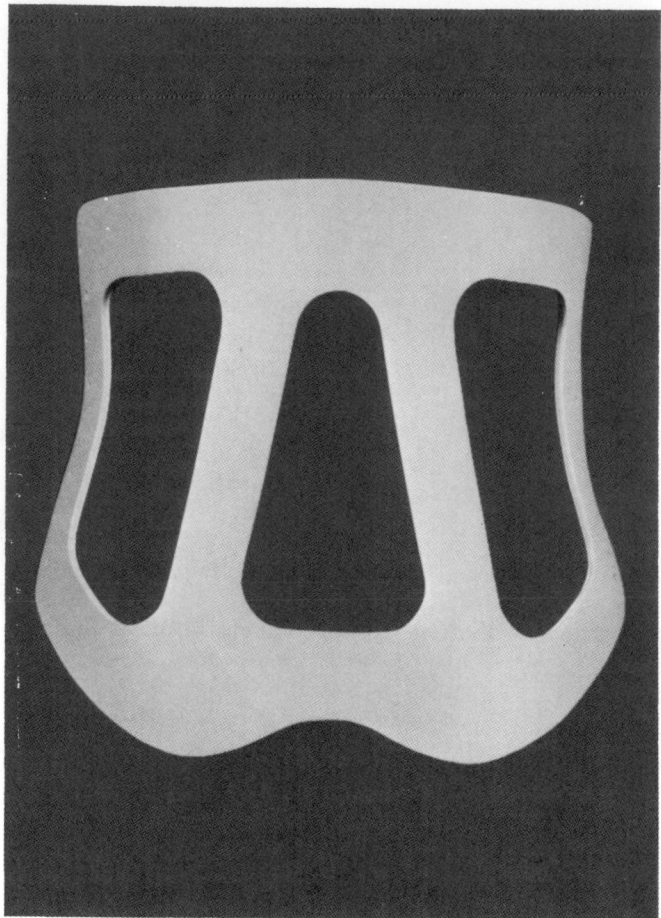

FIGURE 40–22 Lumbosacral flexion-extension-lateral control orthosis. (Courtesy of Orthomedics, Inc, Brea, CA.)

Figure 40–23) is made of semi-rigid plastic and encases the lower trunk. It controls all lumbosacral motion.

(7). The rationale for this option is as follows:

(a). The orthosis reminds the wearer to avoid abrupt motion.

(b). Motion control is achieved by means of various three-point force systems.

(i). Flexion control is achieved through the posterior uprights, which provide anteriorly directed force, and through the top and bottom of the abdominal front, which provide posteriorly directed force.

(ii). Extension control is achieved through the abdominal front, which provides posteriorly directed force, and through the pelvic and thoracic bands, which provide anteriorly directed force.

(iii). Lateral control (the restriction of left lateral flexion) is achieved through the top and bottom of the left lateral upright, which provides right-directed force, and through the midportion of the right lateral, which provides left-directed force.

(c). The orthosis increases intra-abdominal compression.

(d). It reduces trunk muscle activity.

(e). Except for the lumbosacral jacket, LSOs may be cooler than corsets.

b. *Trunk paralysis and instability*

(1). The goal: stabilize the trunk.

(2). Option one: prescribe a TLSO.

(a). A thoracolumbosacral corset is rarely adequate.

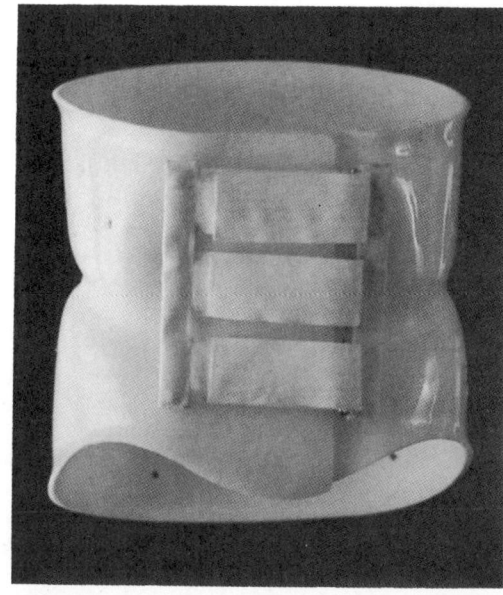

FIGURE 40–23 Lumbosacral jacket (Boston Overlap Brace). (Courtesy of Boston Brace International, Inc, Avon, MA.)

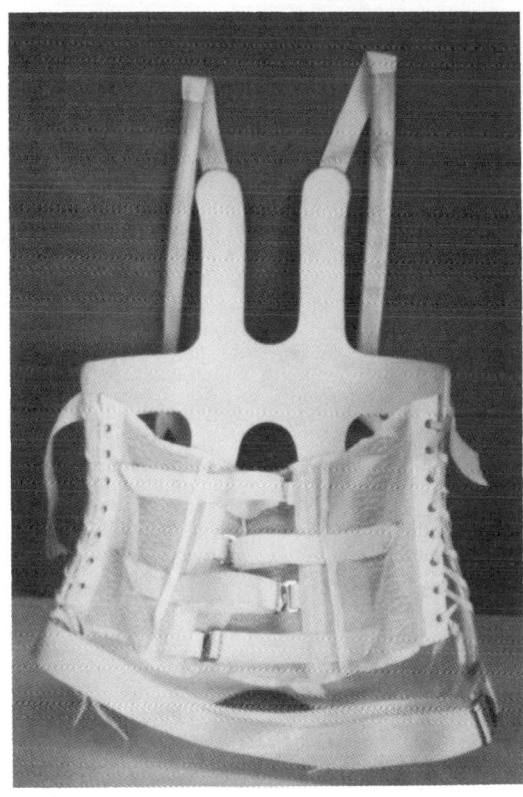

FIGURE 40–24 Thoracolumbosacral flexion/extension/lateral control orthosis. (Courtesy of Orthomedics, Inc, Brea, CA.)

(b). Thoracolumbosacral flexion and extension are controlled by one type of TLSO (*ie*, a Taylor brace), which has a pelvic band and two posterior uprights that extend to the midscapular level and are secured to the trunk with axillary straps. The orthosis also has an interscapular bar and an abdominal front.

(c). Thoracolumbosacral flexion, extension, and lateral control are achieved with another type of TLSO (*ie*, a Knight-Taylor orthosis) (see Figure 40–24), which has a pelvic band, a thoracic band, two lateral uprights two posterior uprights extending to the midscapular level that are secured with axillary straps, and an abdominal front.

(d). Thoracolumbosacral flexion is controlled by another TLSO (*eg*, a Becker/Jewett TLSO [see Figure 40–25] and the cruci-

form anterior spinal hyperextension orthosis).

(i). The Becker/Jewett TLSO has a sternal plate, a suprapubic plate, a dorsolumbar plate, and lateral uprights.

(ii). The cruciform anterior spinal hyperextension TLSO has an anterior upright that joins the sternal and suprapubic plates and a dorsolumbar plate that is strapped to the horizontal band at the midpoint of the anterior upright.

(e). A thoracolumbosacral jacket[102,103] (see Figure 40–26) may be made of relatively thick rigid polyethylene or polypropylene; alternatively, a thinner layer of rigid polyethylene can be sandwiched between two layers of polyethylene foam, creating a semirigid orthosis.

(3). The rationale for this option is as follows:

(a). Motion control is achieved by means of various three-point force systems.

(i). Flexion control is achieved through the posterior uprights or the dorsolumbar plate, which provide anteriorly directed force, and through the axillary straps and the bottom of the abdominal front, or through the sternal and suprapubic plates, which provide posteriorly directed force.

(ii). Extension control is achieved through the abdominal front, which provides posteriorly directed force, and through the pelvic and thoracic or interscapular bands, which provide anteriorly directed force.

(iii). Lateral control (the restriction of left lateral flexion) is achieved through the top and bottom of the

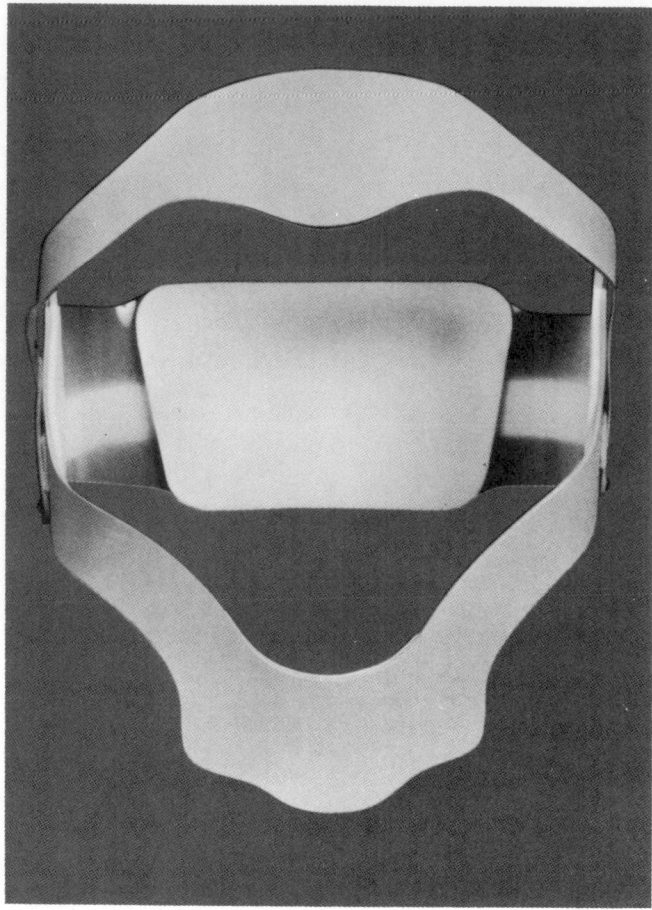

FIGURE 40–25   Thoracolumbosacral flexion-control orthosis. (Courtesy of Orthomedics, Inc, Brea, CA.)

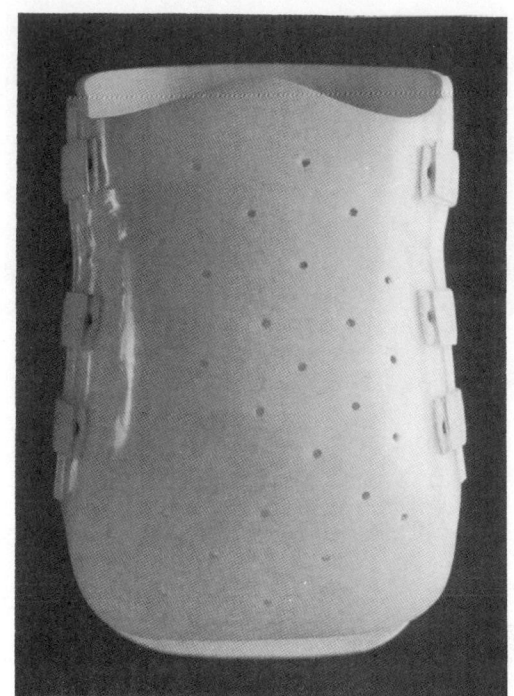

FIGURE 40–26   Thoracolumbosacral jacket. (Courtesy of Boston Brace International, Inc., 20 Ledin Drive, Avon, MA.)

left lateral upright, which provide right-directed force, and through the midportion of the right lateral upright, which provides left-directed force.

(b). TLSOs increase intra-abdominal compression (except for the flexion-control TLSO).

(4). Another goal of physical therapy is to improve respiration.

(5). Option two: prescribe a lumbosacral corset.[104]

(6). The rationale for this option is that vital capacity is increased by increased resistance provided to the diaphragmatic component of respiration.

c. *Scoliosis*

(1). The goal: to prevent the progression of moderate deformity (approximately 20 to 45 degrees of curva-

ture) until the patient reaches skeletal maturity.[105–108]

(2). Option one: prescribe a Boston orthosis TLSO[109–111] (see Figure 40–27). This symmetrical rigid plastic jacket is fitted with interior pads to apply corrective forces. A superstructure may be added to control higher curves.

(3). The rationale for this option is as follows:

(a). Left thoracic scoliosis is controlled by the following factors:

(i). A thoracic pad is placed over the rib just below the apex.

(ii). A right lumbar pad is also included.

(iii). The right superior margin of the orthosis also helps to control this deformity.

(b). Vertebral rotation is reduced by the following:

(i). Lumbar flexion (*ie*, reduction of lumbar lordosis).

(ii). Pressure on the abdomen.

(c). The symmetrical contour of the jacket encourages symmetrical posture.

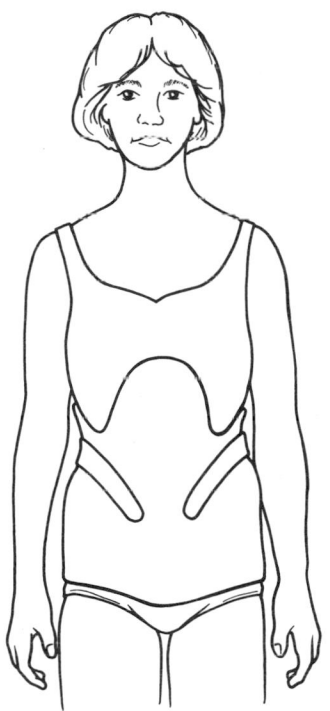
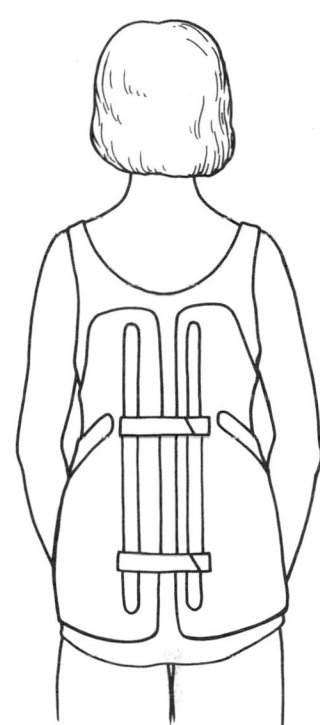

FIGURE 40–27   Boston orthosis. (From King HA: Orthotic management of idiopathic scoliosis. *Phys Med Rehabil Clin N Am* 1992, 1:45–56.)

(d). Part-time wear (*eg*, 16 hours per day appears to yield results comparable to those from full-time use (*eg*, 23 hours per day).

(e). Exercise is useful to counteract disuse weakness and loss of flexibility.

(4). Option two: prescribe a Milwaukee cervicothoracolumbosacral orthosis[112,113] (see Figure 40–28). This rigid

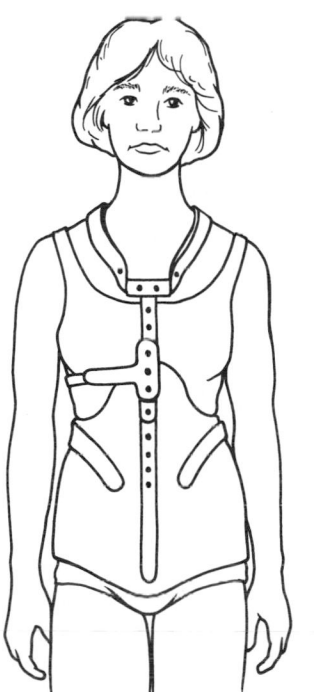
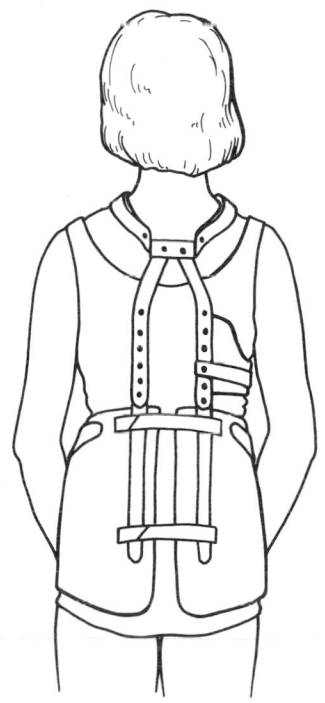

FIGURE 40–28   Milwaukee orthosis. (From King HA: Orthotic management of idiopathic scoliosis. *Phys Med Rehabil Clin N Am* 1992, 1:45–56.)

Table 40–3. TRUNK ORTHOTIC EVALUATION

Standard to Be Checked	Possible Deficiencies
Dons orthosis easily	1. Orthosis too tight 2. Thoracic band too long 3. Technique improper
Stands comfortably	1. Pelvic or thoracic band too narrow or not conforming to torso 2. Pelvic band at or above posterior superior iliac spines 3. Pelvic band terminates posterior to lateral midline of torso 4. Thoracic band above inferior angles of scapulae 5. Thoracic band not horizontal 6. Posterior uprights press on vertebrae 7. Interscapular band too short, too long, or too high 8. Subclavicular extensions of the thoracic band, if present, too high or too low 9. Abdominal support too small 10. Suprapubic pad, if present, impinges on pelvis 11. Sternal plate, if present, too high 12. Occipital plate, if present, too low
Appearance is satisfactory	Orthosis design or construction excessively bulky or shoddy
Sits comfortably	1. Pelvic band below greater trochanters or contacting chair 2. Thoracic band too high 3. Interscapular band too low 4. Abdominal support too large, or inferior border too low or too high 5. Posterior uprights press on vertebrae 6. Pads impinge on clavicles
With orthosis removed, construction is satisfactory	1. Edges rough 2. Metal nicked 3. Stitching inadequate 4. Rivets not flush with surface 5. Plastic molding not uniform
Skin unblemished by orthosis 10 minutes after removal	1. Orthosis too tight 2. Pelvic or thoracic band improperly contoured
Wearer satisfied	1. Any deficiency noted above 2. Discomfort within the trunk or neck 3. Psychosocial dysfunction

Table 40–4. SCOLIOSIS ORTHOTIC EVALUATION

Standard to Be Checked	Possible Deficiencies
Dons orthosis easily	1. Orthosis too tight 2. Technique improper 3. Pelvic girdle straps too short 4. Pelvic girdle opening insufficient
Stands comfortably	1. Pads too snug or too small 2. Pelvic girdle too tight 3. Pelvic girdle anteroinferior border contacts pubis 4. Pelvic girdle anterosuperior border too low or too high 5. Pelvic girdle superolateral border contacts ribs 6. Pelvic girdle does not accommodate iliac spines 7. Thoracic pad strap not centered on pad 8. Thoracic pad spans fewer than three ribs 9. Lumbar pad impinges on pelvis or vertebrae 10. Shoulder ring or sling improperly contoured 11. Sternal pad too high 12. Pads or frame interfere with deep breathing or arm motion
Appearance satisfactory	1. Pelvic girdle superolateral border gaps 2. Uprights not contoured to the torso 3. Shoulder ring or sling improperly contoured
Sits comfortably	1. Pelvic girdle anteroinferior border too low, contacting chair 2. Pelvic girdle anteroinferior border too low, impinging on thighs 3. Pelvic girdle lateral border impinges on greater trochanters
With orthosis removed, construction satisfactory	1. Uprights not covered with plastic or leather 2. Edges rough 3. Metal nicked 4. Stitching inadequate 5. Rivets not flush with surface 6. Plastic molding not uniform
Skin unblemished by orthosis 10 minutes after removal (Painless reddening is satisfactory just above the ilium and beneath pads)	1. Pads impinge on bony prominences 2. Pelvic girdle too tight or too loose
Wearer satisfied	1. Any deficiency noted above 2. Discomfort within the trunk or neck 3. Psychosocial dysfunction

plastic pelvic girdle is connected to a neck ring over the upper thorax by one anterior and two posterior uprights. Pads are strapped to the uprights to apply corrective forces.

(5). The rationale for this option is that it provides the same force systems as the Boston orthosis. The Milwaukee orthosis is prescribed for curves that are slightly higher and for thoracolumbar and lumbar scolioses.

E. Expected outcomes

1. The patient should achieve pain relief.

2. The patient should function with less fatigue.

3. The deformity should be controlled or reduced.

F. Evaluation

Table 40–3 is an orthotic assessment form that indicates the key points related to the fit and construction of trunk orthoses. Table 40–4 illustrates a checklist intended to aid in the evaluation of scoliosis orthoses.

IV. Upper-Limb Orthoses

A. Principles

In addition to the general principles, upper-limb orthoses should satisfy the following requirements:[114-121]

1. The orthosis may assist with residual motor power or substitute for absent motor power.

   Examples: (1) The patient with radial neuropathy can use ulnar- and median-innervated muscles more effectively if an orthosis supports the wrist in a neutral or slightly dorsiflexed position. (2) The patient with C5 quadriplegia may benefit from an orthosis that provides prehension.

2. Prehension force should be adequate to enable the client to perform daily activities but not so forceful as to jeopardize anesthetic fingers.

3. Orthoses that substitute motor power provide only one grasp pattern, either three-jaw chuck grasp or lateral, key pinch grasp.

4. With an electrically powered orthosis, the client must be able to operate the control actuator reliably. The control site, often on the shoulder, should have normal sensation and good motor power.

5. Hand orthoses obscure tactile sensation over the areas that they cover.

   Example: The patient with C7 quadriplegia may not wear a wrist-hand orthosis even though the orthosis improves prehension, because its bands deprive the individual of some of the residual sensation.

6. The orthosis may protect the body segment against pain or deformity.

   Examples: (1) The patient who is experiencing exacerbation of rheumatoid arthritic pain in the wrist is likely to achieve some comfort from an orthosis that prevents motion of the hand and wrist. (2) The patient with elbow burns requires an orthosis to prevent formation of flexion contracture.

7. A patient may benefit from several orthoses rather than from one complex orthosis.

   Example: A patient with quadriplegia may need a utensil holder to hold a pencil. The same person may also need an opponens orthosis to maintain the normal bone architecture of the hand.

8. The orthosis may correct deformity.

   Example: Claw hand deformity (ie, hyperextension contractures of the metacarpophalangeal joints) may be reduced with the consistent wearing of an orthosis that applies force dorsalward to the metacarpophalangeal joints and palmarward to the dorsal hand and dorsal proximal phalanges.

B. Physical assessment

1. **Limb alignment.** Evaluate the entire upper limb.

2. **Joint range**

   Example: The patient with quadriplegia who has hand contractures may not be able to operate a prehension orthosis even though the orthotic joints have unimpeded excursion.

3. **Muscle power**
   a. Evaluate the patient's prehension ability.
   b. Evaluate the patient's ability to position the hand throughout the work space.
4. **Coordination and spasticity**
5. **Sensory status**
   a. Assess the patient's pain discrimination to determine whether the orthosis or any object in contact with the limb is exerting excessive pressure.
   b. Adequate pressure discrimination is necessary for the patient to prevent the use of excessive force when holding objects to prevent them from slipping.
   c. Temperature discrimination protects the individual from burns and from cold injury.
   d. Proprioception is used to position joints easily.
6. **Skin.** Examine the patient for the presence of:
   a. Trophic changes.
   b. Abrasions.
   c. Dermatitis.
   d. Atrophy.
   e. Scars, including keloids.
7. **Manual dexterity**
   a. *Dominance*
      (1). A patient who has sustained an injury to the dominant hand may be compliant because the injury interferes with daily and vocational activities. However, the patient may not tolerate excessive orthotic bulk or complexity.
      (2). A patient who has sustained an injury to or has a disability of both hands usually is more motivated to use the dominant hand. Rather than fitting a pair of complex orthoses, the therapist should fit the patient's dominant hand and allow the individual time to gain proficiency with the single orthosis. Then, the patient and therapist should consider the advisability of trying a second orthosis.
   b. *Ability to manage buckles, straps, and other fasteners*

8. **Vision**
   a. The patient should have sufficiently good vision to be able to dress independently.
   b. The patient also should possess the ability to read typewritten instructions.
9. **Other disabilities.** Upper-limb orthotic acceptance is influenced by any other disabilities that the patient may have.

   Example: The ambulatory patient with arm paralysis is unlikely to accept a heavy orthosis. In contrast, the individual who uses a wheelchair may accept the same orthosis because the wheelchair can support its bulk and weight.

C. **Subjective assessment**

1. **Comprehension:** the patient should
   a. Indicate an understanding of oral instructions.
   b. Indicate an understanding of written instructions.
   c. State a language preference.
2. **Complaints**
   a. *Pain*
      (1). Determine where pain exists.
      (2). Assess when it occurs (*eg,* constant or occasional).
      (3). Note the character of the pain (*eg,* throbbing, burning, dull, or sharp).
      (4). Determine the date of onset.
      (5). Note any aggravating factors.
      (6). Note any diminishing factors.
   b. *Performance:* the patient may
      (1). Have difficulty performing daily activities.
      (2). Have difficulty performing vocational and avocational activities.
      (3). Experience fatigue related to the duration of activity.
   c. *Appearance*
      (1). Note the skin condition.
      (2). Determine whether the orthosis causes clothing abrasion or style limitation unacceptable to the patient.
3. **Previous orthotic experience**
   a. *Preferred orthosis.* The patient may have preferences regarding certain features, including:
      (1). Material.
      (2). Weight.
      (3). Fit.
      (4). Design.
      (5). Durability and maintenance.

b. ***Disliked orthosis.*** The patient may dislike certain features of a previous orthosis, including:

    (1). Material.

    (2). Weight.

    (3). Fit.

    (4). Design.

    (5). Durability and maintenance.

4. **Gadget tolerance.** The willingness of the patient to accept an orthosis is influenced by many psychological factors. As a rule, an individual who has a relatively minor disability is less likely to accept an orthosis as compared with a more severely disabled person.

5. The goals:

    a. Reduced pain.

    b. Improved prehension.

    c. Improved appearance.

6. **Economic considerations.** Funds are needed for the purchase of the orthosis and for associated care. In general, the more complex the orthosis, the more training is required. In addition, resources must be available for the repair of the orthosis, particularly if it has moving parts.

D. Planning and implementation

1. **Wrist-hand orthoses**

    a. *Paralysis: median neuropathy*

        (1). The goals:

            (a). Reduce pain.

            (b). Maintain the thumb web space.

            (c). Maintain the thumb in abduction and opposition, preventing deformity in which the thumb lies in the plane of the other fingers.

            (d). Maintain the transverse palmar arch.

            (e). Assist in prehension.

        (2). Option one: prescribe a basic opponens wrist-hand orthosis (see Figure 40–29).

        (3). The rationale for this option is as follows:

            (a). The orthosis reminds the wearer to reduce motion while healing occurs; if additional motion restriction is required, a forearm bar and bands may be added to the orthosis.

            (b). The abduction bar maintains the web space by preventing thumb adduction.

            (c). The opposition bar applies an ulnar force against the first metacarpal bone.

            (d). Palmar and dorsal bars support the transverse arch.

            (e). Maintaining the thumb in opposition enables the client to use residual motor power more effectively.

        (4). Option two: prescribe an opponens wrist-hand orthosis with wrist control.

        (5). The rationale for this option is that the forearm bar prevents wrist motion that may otherwise aggravate hand disability.

    b. *Paralysis: ulnar or combined median and ulnar neuropathy*

        (1). The goals:

            (a). Stabilize the first metacarpophalangeal joint.

            (b). Prevent clawing (*ie*, hyperextension of the metacarpopha-

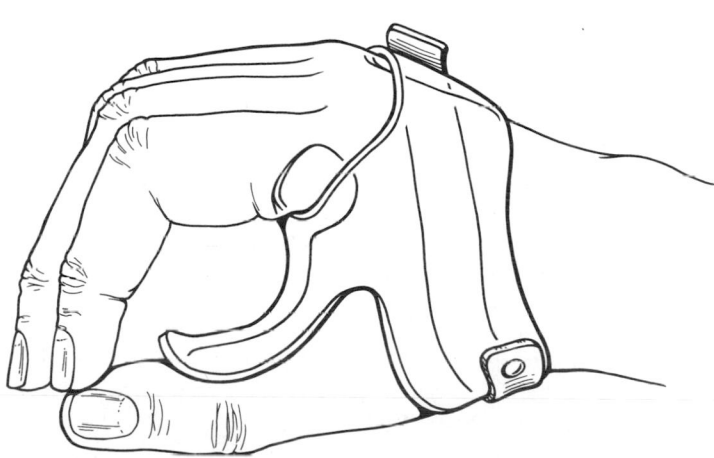

FIGURE 40–29 Basic opponens orthosis. (Courtesy of Rusk Institute of Rehabilitation Medicine, New York, NY.)

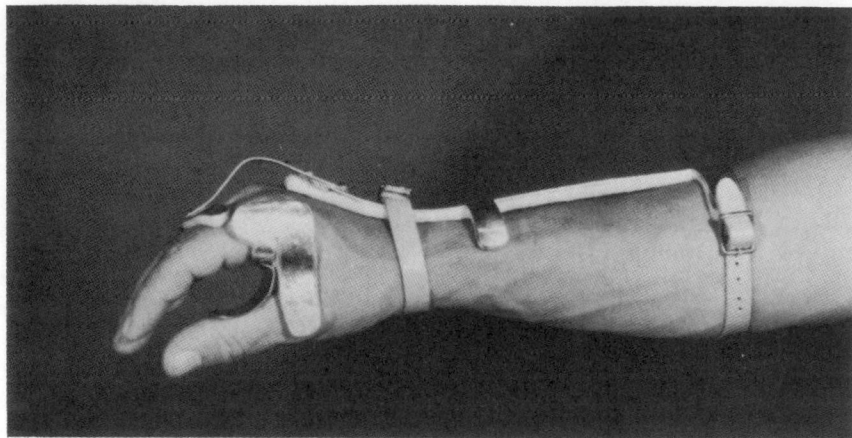

FIGURE 40–30   Opponens wrist-hand orthosis with metacarpophalangeal extension stop. (From American Academy of Orthopaedic Surgeons: *Atlas of Orthotics,* 2nd ed. C. V. Mosby Company, p 166.)

langeal joints and flexion of the proximal interphalangeal joints); ulnar neuropathy can result in claw deformity of the fourth and fifth fingers. Combined median and ulnar neuropathy may cause deformity in the second, third, fourth, and fifth fingers.

(c). Maintain the transverse palmar arch.

(d). Assist in prehension.

(2). Option: prescribe an opponens orthosis with a metacarpophalangeal extension stop (see Figure 40–30). The orthosis may include a forearm bar and bands.

(3). The rationale for this option is as follows:

(a). The metacarpophalangeal extension stop applies a palmarward force on the proximal phalanges, preventing hyperextension.

(b). The opponens and abduction bars maintain the thumb in a functional position.

(c). The palmar and dorsal bars maintain the transverse palmar arch and apply dorsalward force to prevent metacarpophalangeal hyperextension.

c. *Paralysis: radial neuropathy*

(1). The goals:

(a). Prevent wrist flexion muscle contracture.

(b). Prevent finger extension muscle contractures.

(c). Assist prehension.

(2). Option: prescribe a wrist-flexion–control orthosis (cock-up wrist splint) (see Figure 40–31).

(3). The rationale for this option is as follows:

(a). The orthosis prevents the wrist from flexing, thereby preventing contracture at the wrist and fingers.

(b). Prehension is assisted by maintaining adequate tension on the finger flexor muscles.

d. *Complete paralysis: C6 quadriplegia*

(1). The goals:

(a). Provide prehension.[123–125]

(b). Maintain flexibility of the hand, wrist, and elbow.

(2). Option: prescribe a wrist-driven prehension orthosis (see Figure 40–32). This orthosis stabilizes the interphalangeal joints of the thumb, index, and middle fingers. Hinge joints are located at the second metacarpophalangeal joint and wrist, with a spring-loaded button near the wrist.

(3). The rationale for this option is as follows:

(a). Prehension. Linkage between the fingers and the wrist enables the wearer to achieve grasp by active wrist extension; release occurs by passive wrist

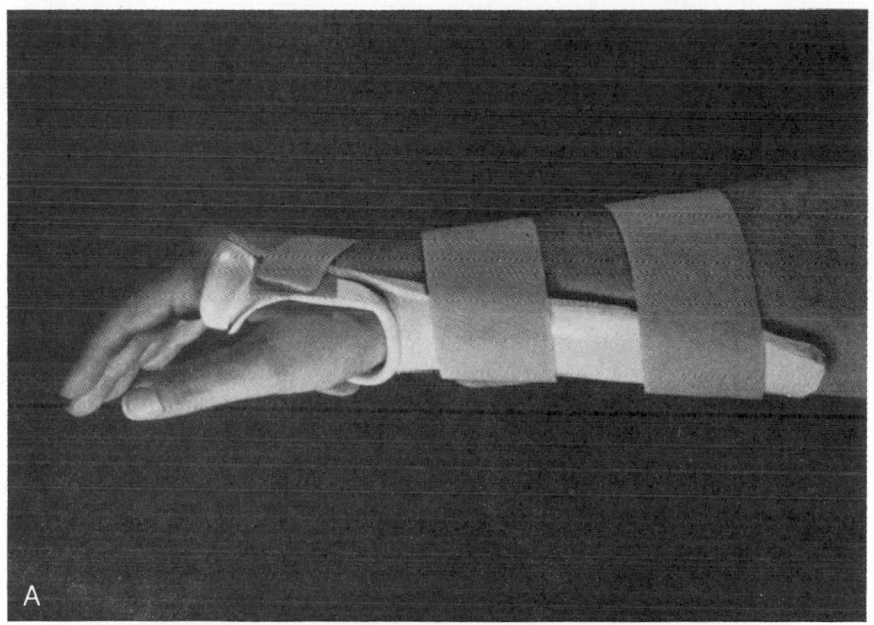

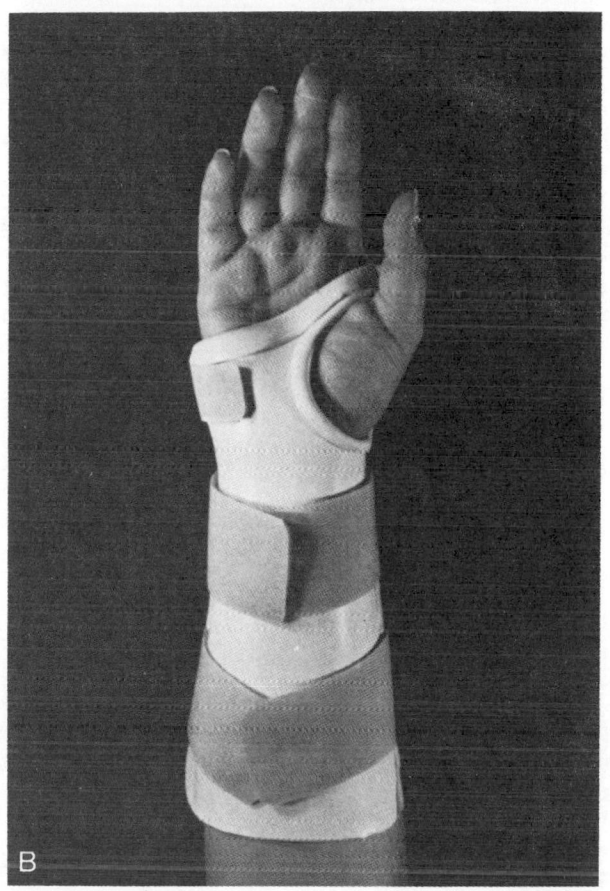

FIGURE 40–31 Volar wrist flexion–control orthosis. **A**, Radial view. **B**, Palmar view. (From *Atlas of Hand Splinting.* Tenney CG, Lisak JM. Published by Little, Brown and Company, p. 32.)

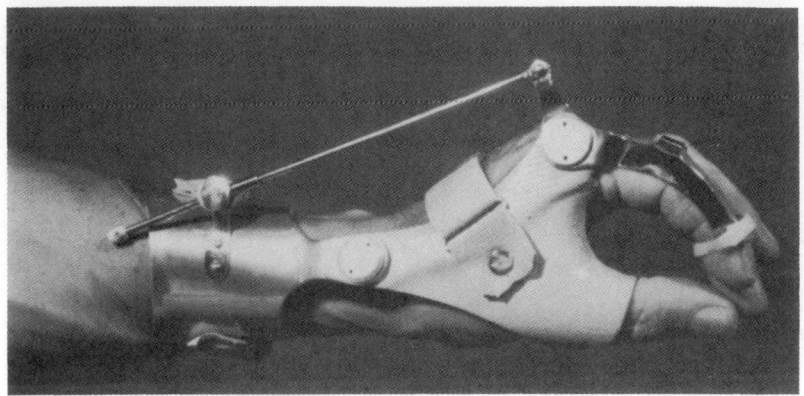

FIGURE 40–32 Wrist-driven prehension orthosis. (From American Academy of Orthopaedic Surgeons: *Atlas of Orthotics,* 2nd ed. C. V. Mosby Company, p 171.)

flexion by means of tenodesis action. The patient must have full mobility of the wrist and fingers, as well as a minimum of fair plus power in the wrist extensor muscles. Prehension is in the three-jaw chuck pattern, in which the thumb tip opposes the palmar tips of the index and middle fingers. This pattern is suitable for handling most eating, writing, and grooming tools.

By pressing the spring-loaded button, the wearer adjusts the prehension range to the size of the object being handled.

Example: To handle a sheet of paper, the individual would either have to extend the wrist fully or to press the button to reduce the prehension range.

PLEASE NOTE: Although patients with C7 and C8 quadriplegia have reduced hand function, they rarely accept orthoses, preferring to use residual motor power and utensils with enlarged handles. In addition, the wrist-driven prehension orthosis and similar devices interfere with manual wheelchair propulsion.

    (b). Flexibility: the palmar bar and hand activity counteract joint stiffness.

e. *Complete paralysis: C5 quadriplegia*
    (1). The goals:
        (a). Provide prehension.
        (b). Maintain flexibility of the hand, wrist, and elbow.

(2). Option one: prescribe an electrically-driven prehension orthosis. This orthosis stabilizes the interphalangeal joints of the thumb and of the index and middle fingers. The hinge joint is located at the second metacarpophalangeal joint. A steel cable pulls the fingers toward the thumb; a spring allows the fingers to extend when cable tension is released. The wearer causes the cable to move by pressing a control lever, usually located near the shoulder. Shoulder elevation against the lever turns on the motor to which the cable is attached. The motor is battery operated; hence, the battery should be recharged daily.

(3). The rationale for this option is that the orthosis allows the wearer to actively control grasping and releasing. Because the system depends on a motor-and-cable system, maintenance is an ongoing problem.

(4). Option two: prescribe a utensil holder (see Figure 40–33). This orthosis may be mass produced or custom made. It consists of a handcuff that has a palmar pocket. Wrist bands are optional; they balance the weight of the hand and the object being held. Objects of suitable width may be placed directly in the pocket. Alternatively, objects such as a spoon or a fork may be fitted with an adaptor that is put in the pocket.

(5). The rationale for this option is that the orthosis allows the patient to grasp suitably sized utensils, including most of those used for eating,

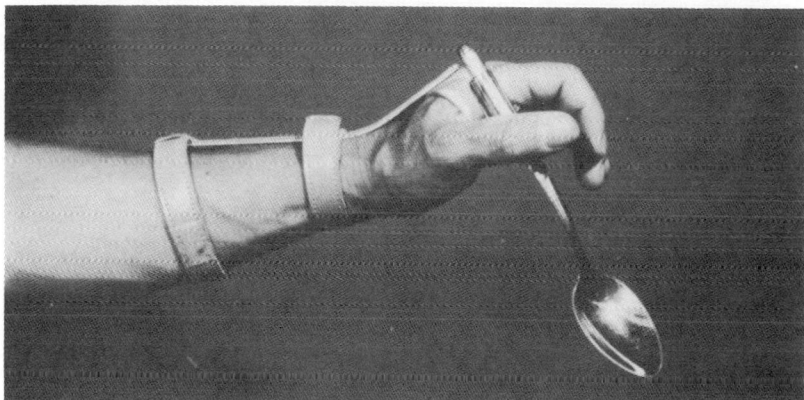

FIGURE 40–33 Utensil holder. (From American Academy of Orthopaedic Surgeons: *Atlas of Orthotics,* 2nd ed. C. V. Mosby Company, p 175.)

writing, and grooming. The wearer may need assistance with inserting and removing the utensil; often, clients use their teeth for this purpose. The orthosis is much less expensive than the electrical alternative; furthermore, because it has no moving parts, the utensil holder is very durable.

f. *Spasticity*
  (1). The goals:
    (a). Prevent thumb adduction and wrist flexion contractures.
    (b). Reduce spasticity.[126–129]
  (2). Option one: prescribe a volar wrist–hand–stabilizing orthosis (a resting hand splint) (see Figure 40–34).
  (3). The rationale for this option is that the orthosis maintains the thumb in abduction and the wrist in neutral alignment. Orthotic management of spasticity, whether caused by cerebrovascular accident or cerebral palsy, is controversial. Spasticity appears to diminish after the application of an orthosis, perhaps because it causes the spastic musculature to be less sensitive to stretch. It is unclear whether the rigid portion of the orthosis should be on the dorsal or on the volar surface of the hand and forearm. Stimulation of the dorsally located extensor muscles would appear to be beneficial; however, both types of orthoses are secured to the opposite surface by straps that also provide sensory stimulation. The volar orthosis accommodates any edema and is generally easier to

fit because of the thicker palmar subcutaneous tissue.
  (4). Option two: prescribe an inflatable pressure splint.[130] The mass-produced transparent plastic splint is slipped over the hand and then inflated to a maximum pressure of 40 mm Hg. It is worn for approximately 30 minutes several times a day.
  (5). The rationale for this option is that inflatable splints reduce spasticity by passive positioning and the slow continuous stretch of muscles in a reflex-inhibiting posture as well as through the warmth of the encased hand.

g. *Pain from arthritis or repetitive stress*
  (1). The goal: to reduce pain.
  (2). Option one: prescribe a volar wrist–hand–stabilizing orthosis.
  (3). The rationale for this option is that the orthosis prevents wrist and finger motion, thereby allowing synovitis to resolve. This orthosis also counteracts the tendency toward wrist and finger deformity.
  (4). Option two: prescribe an inflatable pressure splint.[131]
  (5). The rationale for this option is that this orthosis reduces edema by accelerating the absorption of tissue fluid by the capillaries and lymphatic vessels.

2. Elbow and shoulder orthoses

The major function of the forearm and upper arm is to transport the hand within the work space. When the entire upper limb is disabled, orthotic

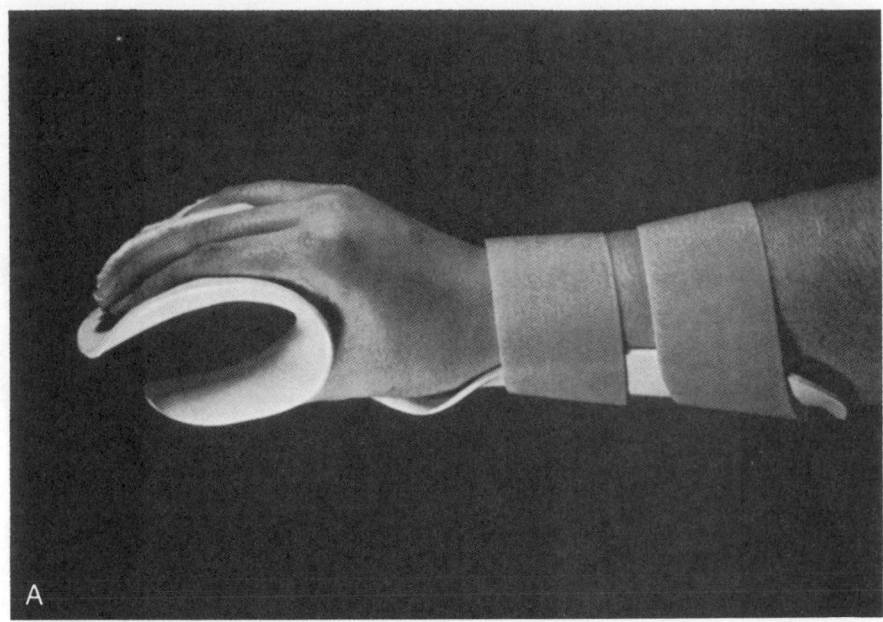

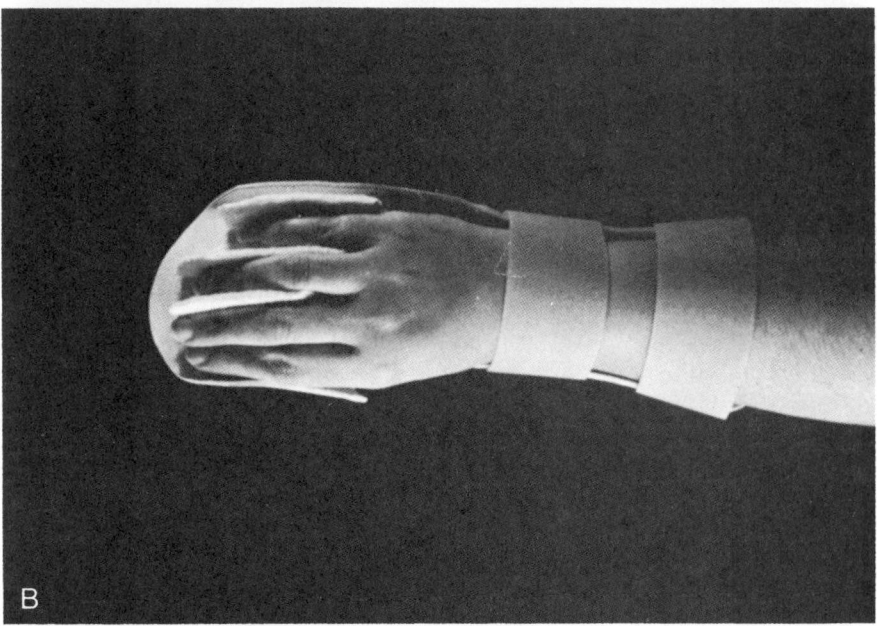

FIGURE 40–34   Volar wrist-hand–stabilizing orthosis. **A**, Radial view. **B**, Dorsal view. (From *Atlas of Hand Splinting.* Tenney CG, Lisak JM. Published by Little, Brown and Company, p 56.)

restoration of hand function takes priority over that of the elbow or shoulder.

   a. ***Forearm, elbow, and shoulder paralysis***

      (1). The goal: transport the hand in the work space.

      (2). Option one: prescribe a balanced forearm orthosis[132] (see Figure 40–35). This mass-produced orthosis consists of a forearm trough and a pivoting bar screwed to the trough and attached to the distal link. The link joins the proximal link with a ball-bearing joint. The proximal link is connected to a wheelchair bracket by another ball-bearing joint.

      (3). The rationale for this option is that

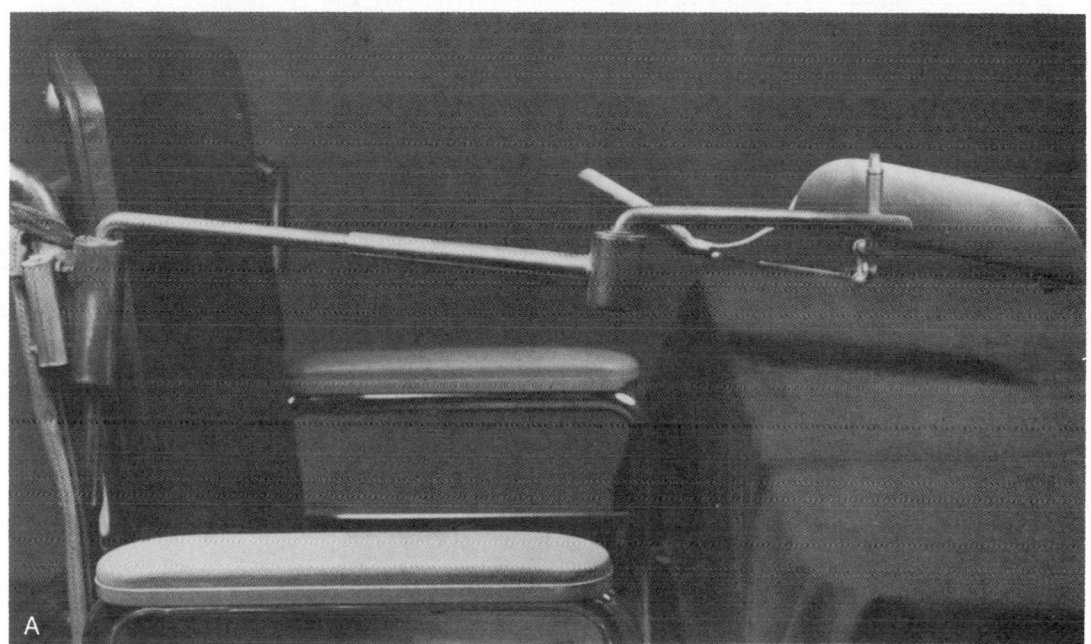

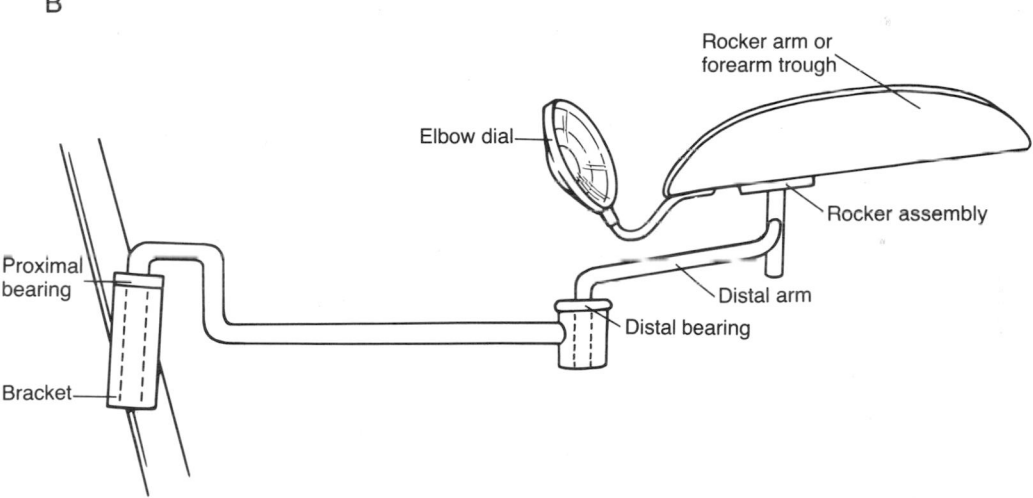

FIGURE 40–35 Balanced forearm orthosis. (**A**, from American Academy of Orthopaedic Surgeons: *Atlas of Orthotics,* 2nd ed. C. V. Mosby Company, p 194.)

for the nonambulatory client, the balanced forearm orthosis is an inexpensive, practical orthosis. Slight head or trunk motion causes the linkage system to move the limb horizontally. The trough rests on a first-class lever that the therapist adjusts to favor elbow flexion or extension, depending on the patient's muscle power; the patient causes vertical motion by head or trunk motion.

b. *Shoulder pain or subluxation*

(1). The goal: to reduce pain or subluxation.

(2). Option one: prescribe a sling.[133,134]

(3). The rationale for this option is that most slings are mass produced, and they vary according to the number of straps and the number and type of cuff that they have, which affects the ease of donning. When properly fitted, the sling resists gravitational force that tends to cause painful subluxation.

Table 40–5. UPPER LIMB ORTHOTIC EVALUATION

Standard to Be Checked	Possible Deficiencies	Standard to Be Checked	Possible Deficiencies
Dons orthosis easily	1. Orthosis too tight 2. Orthosis too complex 3. Technique improper 4. Fastenings unsuitable		provide desired grasp (either three-jaw chuck or lateral grasp) 9. Forearm bar too long or too short 10. Forearm bar does not maintain wrist in desired position 11. Electric microswitch actuator unsatisfactory 12. Battery inadequately charged 13. Utensil holder too large or too small
Wearing orthosis, moves fingers comfortably	1. Mechanical joints not congruent with anatomic joints 2. Components press on bone prominences 3. Wrist strap does not lie between metacarpal bases and wrist crease		
Orthosis promotes maximum function (except for orthosis intended to promote rest)	1. Palmar surface of fingertips obstructed 2. Opponens bar does not provide adequate ulnar-directed force on thumb metacarpal bone 3. Opponens bar does not extend to palmar edge of thumb metacarpal bone 4. Thumb abduction bar does not maintain adequate abduction 5. Thumb abduction bar restricts thumb interphalangeal or index metacarpophalangeal joint motion 6. Palmar or dorsal bars do not conform to contour of distal transverse arch 7. Metacarpophalangeal extension stop ineffective 8. Thumb and index and middle fingers not aligned to	Appearance satisfactory	Orthosis excessively bulky, complex, or shoddy construction
		With orthosis removed, construction satisfactory	1. Edges rough 2. Plastic molding not uniform 3. Rivets not flush with surface 4. Mechanical joints bind when moved
		Skin unblemished by orthosis 10 minutes after removal	1. Orthosis too tight 2. Orthosis too loose, permitting slippage during function 3. Edges rough
		Wearer satisfied	1. Any deficiency noted above 2. Discomfort within the upper limb 3. Psychosocial dysfunction 4. At final evaluation, insufficient training

E. Expected outcomes

1. The patient should achieve pain relief.
2. Therapy should improve the patient's dexterity.
3. Limb transport ability should improve.
4. Deformity should be controlled or reduced.

F. Evaluation

Table 40–5 is a guide to the assessment of upper-limb orthoses. It includes a description of possible deficiencies.

References

1. Good DC, Supan T: Basic principles of orthotics in neurological disorders. In Aisen ML (ed): *Orthotics in Neurologic Rehabilitation.* New York, Demos, 1992, pp 1–24.
2. Redford JB: Principles of orthotic devices. In Redford JB (ed): *Orthotics Etcetera,* 3rd ed. Baltimore, Williams & Wilkins, 1986, pp 1–20.
3. Rose GK: *Orthotics: Principles and Practice.* London, Heinemann, 1986.
4. Smith EM, Juvinall RC: Mechanics of orthotics. In Redford JB (ed): *Orthotics Etcetera,* 3rd ed. Baltimore, Williams & Wilkins, 1986, pp 21–51.
5. McHugh B, Campbell J: Below-knee orthoses. *Physiotherapy* 1987, 73:380–385.
6. Kohn JG, Mortola P, Le Banc M: Clinical trials and quality control: checkpoints in the provision of assistive technology. *Assist Technol* 1991, 3:67–74.
7. Phillips B, Zhao H: Predictors of assistive technology abandonment. *Assist Technol* 1993, 5:35–45.
8. Perry J, Gronley JK, Lunsford T: Rocker shoe as walking aid in multiple sclerosis. *Arch Phys Med Rehabil* 1981, 62:59–65.
9. Richardson JK: Rocker-soled shoes and walking distance in patients with calf claudication. *Arch Phys Med Rehabil* 1991, 72:554–558.
10. Bordelon RL: *Surgical and Conservative Foot Care.* Thorofare, NJ, Slack, 1988.
11. Edelstein JE: Physical therapy for elderly patients with foot disorders. *Top Geriatr Rehabil* 1992, 7:24–35.
12. Finlay OE: Footwear management in the elderly care programme. *Physiotherapy* 1986, 72:172–178.
13. Lockard MA: Foot orthoses. *Phys Ther* 1988, 68:1866–1873.
14. Newell SG: Functional neutral orthoses and shoe modifications. *Phys Med Rehabil Clin N Am* 1992, 3:193–222.
15. Pfeffinger LL: Foot orthoses. In American Academy of Or-

thopaedic Surgeons: *Atlas of Orthotics,* 2nd ed. St. Louis, C. V. Mosby Company, 1985, pp 346–357.

16. Ragnarsson KT: Orthotics and shoes. In DeLisa JA (ed): *Rehabilitation Medicine: Principles and Practice.* Philadelphia, J. B. Lippincott Company, 1988, pp 307–329.

17. Reed JK, Theriot S: Orthotic devices, shoes and modifications. In Hunt G (ed): *Physical Therapy of the Foot and Ankle.* New York, Churchill Livingstone, 1988, pp 285–313.

18. Riegler HF: Orthotic devices for the foot. *Orthop Rev* 1987, 16:293–303.

19. Wu KK: *Foot Orthoses: Principles and Clinical Application.* Baltimore, Williams & Wilkins, 1990.

20. Zamosky I, Redford JB: Shoes and their modifications. In Redford JB (ed): *Orthotics Etcetera,* 3rd ed. Baltimore, Williams & Wilkins, 1986, pp 388–452.

21. Mereday C, Dolan CM, Lusskin R: Evaluation of the University of California Biomechanics Laboratory shoe insert in flexible pes planus. *Clin Orthop* 1972, 82:45–48.

22. Bottomley JM, Herman H: Making simple, inexpensive changes for the management of foot problems in the aged. *Top Geriatr Rehabil* 1992, 7:62–77.

23. Moncur C, Ward JR: Heat-moldable shoes for management of forefoot problems in rheumatoid arthritis. *Arthritis Care Res* 1990, 3:222–226.

24. Brand PW: Repetitive stress in the development of diabetic foot ulcers. In Levin ME, O'Neal LW (eds): *The Diabetic Foot.* St Louis, C. V. Mosby Company, 1988, pp 83–90.

25. Brodsky JW, Kourosh S, Stills M, Mooney V: Objective evaluation of insert material for diabetic and athletic footwear. *Foot Ankle* 1988, 9:111–116.

26. Chantelau E, Kushner T, Spraul M: How effective is cushioned therapeutic footwear in protecting diabetic foot? A clinical study. *Diabet Med* 1990, 7:355–359.

27. Edelstein JE: Foot care for the aging. *Phys Ther* 1988, 68:1882–1886.

28. Helfand AE: Health promotion and podogeriatrics: a conceptual design for preventive services. *J Am Podiatr Med Assoc* 1990, 80:100–103.

29. Hogan-Budris J: Choosing foot materials for the elderly. *Top Geriatr Rehabil* 1992, 7:49–61.

30. Holewski JJ, Moss KM, Stess RM, et al.: Prevalence of foot pathology and lower extremity complications in a diabetic outpatient clinic. *J Rehabil Res Dev* 1989, 26:35–44.

31. Johnson GR: The effectiveness of shock-absorbing insoles during normal walking. *Prosthet Orthot Int* 1988, 12:91–95.

32. Michael JW, Isbell MA, Harrelson JM: Orthotic management of diabetic neuropathic arthropathy. *J Prosthet Orthot* 1992, 4:45–55.

33. Mueller MJ, Minor SD, Diamond JE, Blair VP 3rd: Relationship of foot deformity to ulcer location in patients with diabetes mellitus. *Phys Ther* 1990, 70:356–362.

34. Nawoczenski DA, Birke JA: Management of the neuropathic foot in the elderly. *Top Geriatr Rehabil* 1992, 7:36–48.

35. Nemchik R: From research to practice: saving the diabetic foot. *Diabet Spectrum* 1990, 153–155.

36. Pratt DJ: Long term comparison of some shock attenuating insoles. *Prosthet Orthot Int* 1990, 14:59–62.

37. Schaff PS, Cavanagh PR: Shoes for the insensitive: the effect of a "rocker-bottom" shoe modification on plantar pressure distribution. *Foot Ankle* 1990, 11:129–140.

38. Fishman S, Berger N, Edelstein JE: Lower-limb orthotics. In American Academy of Orthopaedic Surgeons: *Atlas of Orthotics,* 2nd ed. St Louis, C. V. Mosby Company, 1985, pp 199–236.

39. Halar E, Cardenas DD: Ankle-foot orthoses: clinical implications. *Phys Med Rehabil: State Art Rev* 1987, 1:45–66.

40. Lehmann J, de Lateur BJ, Price R: Ankle-foot orthoses for

41. Perkins KE: Lower extremity orthotics in geriatric rehabilitation. In Guccione AA (ed): *Geriatric Physical Therapy.* St Louis, C. V. Mosby Company, 1993, pp 269–282.

42. Cook TM, Cozzens B: The effects of heel height and ankle-foot-orthosis configuration on weight line location: a demonstration of principles. *Orthot Prosthet* 1976, 30:43–46.

43. Yamamoto S, Ebinu M, Iwasaki M: Comparative study of mechanical characteristics of plastic AFOs. *J Prosthet Orthot* 1993, 5:59–64.

44. Wiest DR, Waters RL, Bontrager EL: The influence of heel design on a rigid ankle-foot orthosis. *Orthot Prosthet* 1979, 33:3–10.

45. Middleton EA, Hurley GR, McIlwain JS: The role of rigid and hinged polypropylene ankle-foot-orthoses in the management of cerebral palsy: a case study. *Prosthet Orthot Int* 1988, 12:129–135.

46. Bronkhorst AJ, Lamb GA: An orthosis to aid in reduction of lower limb spasticity. *Orthot Prosthet* 1987, 41:23–28.

47. Diamond MF, Ottenbacher KJ: Effect of a tone inhibiting dynamic ankle-foot orthosis on stride characteristics of an adult with hemiparesis. *Phys Ther* 1990, 70:423–430.

48. Embrey DG, Yates L, Mott DH: Effects of neuro-developmental treatment and orthoses on knee flexion during gait: a single-subject design. *Phys Ther* 1990, 70:626–637.

49. Harris SR, Riffle K: Effects of inhibitive ankle-foot orthoses on standing balance in a child with cerebral palsy: a single-subject design. *Phys Ther* 1986, 66:663–667.

50. Lohman M, Goldstein H: Alternative strategies in tone-reducing AFO design. *J Prosthet Orthot* 1993, 5:1–4.

51. Yang GW, Chu DS, Ahn JH: Floor reaction orthosis: clinical experience. *Orthot Prosthet* 1986, 40:33–37.

52. Condie DN: Long leg braces. *Physiotherapy* 1987, 73:276–279.

53. Lehmann J, de Lateur BJ, Price R: Knee-ankle-foot orthoses for paresis and paralysis. *Phys Med Rehabil Clin N Am* 1992, 3:161–185.

54. Merritt JL: Knee-ankle-foot orthoses, long leg braces and their practical applications. *Phys Med Rehabil: State Art Rev* 1987, 1:67–82.

55. Krebs DE, Edelstein JE, Fishman S: Comparison of plastic/metal and leather/metal knee-ankle-foot orthoses. *Am J Phys Med Rehabil* 1988, 67:175.

56. Granata C, DeLollis A, Campo G, et al.: Analysis, design and development of a carbon fibre reinforced plastic knee-ankle-foot orthosis prototype for myopathic patients. *Proc Inst Mech Eng [H]* 1990, 204:91–96.

57. Heckmatt JZ, Dubowitz V, Hyde SA, et al.: Prolongation of walking in Duchenne muscular dystrophy with lightweight orthoses: a review of 57 cases. *Dev Med Child Neurol* 1985, 27:149–154.

58. Hoehne JA: Weight-bearing KAFO utilizing modern prosthetic above-knee socket design. *J Prosthet Orthot* 1989, 2:82–93.

59. Hoffman E: Hip-rotation control straps. *Inter-Clinic Information Bull* 1983, 18:1–4.

60. Gram M: *Using the Parapodium: A Manual of Training Techniques.* New York, Eterna Press, 1984.

61. Stallard J, Major RE, Patrick JH: A review of the fundamental design problems of providing ambulation for paraplegic patients. *Paraplegia* 1989, 27:70–75.

62. Stallard J: The ORLAU VCG (variable centre of gravity) swivel walker for muscular dystrophy patients. *Prosthet Orthot Int* 1992, 16:46–48.

63. Kent HO: Vannini-Rizzoli stabilizing orthosis (boot): preliminary report on a new ambulatory aid for spinal cord injury. *Arch Phys Med Rehabil* 1992, 73:302–307.

64. Lyles M, Munday J: Report on the evaluation of the Vannini-Rizzoli stabilizing limb orthosis. *J Rehabil Res Dev* 1992, 29:77–104.

65. Scott BA: Engineering principles and fabrication techniques for the Scott-Craig long leg brace for paraplegics. *Orthot Prosthet* 1971, 28:14–19.

66. Lobley S, Rogerson J, Cullen J, Freed M: Orthotic design from the New England Regional Spinal Cord Injury Center. *Phys Ther* 1985, 65:492–493.

67. Bierling-Sørensen F, *et al.*: Shock absorbing material on the shoes of long leg braces for paraplegic walking. *Prosthet Orthot Int* 1990, 14:17–32.

68. Beckman J: The Louisiana State University reciprocating gait orthosis. *Physiotherapy* 1987, 73:386–392.

69. McCall RE, Schmidt WT: Clinical experience with the reciprocal gait orthosis in myelodysplasia. *J Pediatr Orthoped* 1986, 6:157–161.

70. Butler PB, Major R: The ParaWalker: a rational approach to the provision of reciprocal ambulation for paraplegic patients. *Physiotherapy* 1987, 73:383–387.

71. Nene AV, Major RE: Dynamics of reciprocal gait of adult paraplegics using the ParaWalker (hip guidance orthosis). *Prosthet Orthot Int* 1987, 11:124–127.

72. Summers BN, McClelland MR, el Masri WS: A clinical review of the adult hip guidance orthosis (ParaWalker) in traumatic paraplegics. *Paraplegia* 1988, 26:19–26.

73. Heinemann AW, Magiera-Planey R, Schiro-Geist CN, Gimines G: Mobility of persons with spinal cord injury: an evaluation of two systems. *Arch Phys Med Rehabil* 1987, 68:90–93.

74. Jefferson RJ, Whittle MW: Performance of three walking orthoses for the paralysed: a case study using gait analysis. *Prosthet Orthot Int* 1990, 4:103–110.

75. Whittle MW, Cochrane GM, Chase AP, *et al.*: A comparative trial of two walking systems for paralysed people. *Paraplegia* 1991, 29:97–102.

76. Campbell JM, Meadows PM: Therapeutic FES: from rehabilitation to neural prosthetics. *Assist Technol* 1992, 4:4–18.

77. Jaeger RJ: Lower extremity applications of functional neuromuscular stimulation. *Assist Technol* 1992, 4:19–30.

78. Kralj A, Bajd T, Turk R: Enhancement of gait restoration in spinal injured patients by functional electrical stimulation. *Clin Orthop* 1988, 233:34–43.

79. McClelland M, Andrews BJ, Patrick JH, *et al.*: Augmentation of the Oswestry ParaWalker orthosis by means of surface electrical stimulation: gait analysis of three patients. *Paraplegia* 1987, 25:32–38.

80. Petrofsky JS, Smith J: Physiological costs of computer-controlled walking in persons with paraplegia using a reciprocating gait orthosis. *Arch Phys Med Rehabil* 1992, 72:890–896.

81. Phillips CA, Hendershot DM: Functional electrical stimulation and reciprocating gait orthosis for ambulation exercise in a tetraplegic patient: a case study. *Paraplegia* 1991, 29:268–276.

82. Fishman S, Berger N, Edelstein JE, *et al.*: Spinal orthotics. In American Academy of Orthopaedic Surgeons: *Atlas of Orthotics*, 2nd ed. St Louis, C. V. Mosby Company, 1985, pp 238–256.

83. Sypert GW: External spinal orthotics. *Neurosurgery* 1987, 20:642.

84. Beavis A: Cervical orthoses. *Prosthet Orthot Int* 1989, 13:6–13.

85. Fisher SV: Cervical orthoses. *Phys Med Rehabil Clin N Am* 1992, 3:29–44.

86. Harris JD: Cervical orthoses. In Redford JB (ed): *Orthotics Etcetera*, 3rd ed. Baltimore, Williams & Wilkins, 1986, pp 100–121.

87. Millington PJ, Ellingsen JM, Hauswirth BE, Fabian PJ: Thermoplastic Minerva body jacket—a practical alternative to

current methods of cervical spine stabilization. *Phys Ther* 1987, 67:223–225.

88. Krag MH, Beynnon BD: A new halo-vest: rationale, design and biomechanical comparison to standard halo-vest designs. *Spine* 1988, 13:228–235.

89. Pringle RG: Halo versus Minerva—which orthosis? *Paraplegia* 1990, 28:281–284.

90. Hart DL: Spinal immobility: braces and corsets. In Gould JA (ed): *Orthopaedic and Sports Physical Therapy*, 2nd ed. St Louis, C. V. Mosby Company, 1990, pp 265–289.

91. Kumar VN: Corsets and soft supports. In Redford JB (ed): *Orthotics Etcetera*, 3rd ed, Baltimore, Williams & Wilkins, 1986, pp 80–99.

92. Stillo JV, Stein AB, Ragnarsson KT: Low-back orthoses. *Phys Med Rehabil Clin N Am* 1992, 3:57–94.

93. Alaranta H, Hurri H: Compliance and subjective relief by corset treatment in chronic low back pain. *Scand J Rehabil Med* 1988, 20:133–136.

94. Borenstein DG, Wiesel SW: *Low Back Pain: Medical Diagnosis and Comprehensive Management*. Philadelphia, W. B. Saunders Company, 1989.

95. Million R, Nilsen KH, Jayson MI, Baker RD: Evaluation of low back pain and assessment of lumbar corsets with and without back supports. *Ann Rheum Dis* 1981, 40:449–454.

96. Lucas DB, Jacobs RR, Trautman P: Spinal orthotics for pain and instability. In Redford JB (ed): *Orthotics Etcetera*, 3rd ed. Baltimore, Williams & Wilkins, 1986, pp 122–152.

97. Walsh NE, Schwartz RK: The influence of prophylactic orthoses on abdominal strength and low back injury in the workplace. *Am J Phys Med Rehabil* 1990, 69:245–250.

98. Wosk J, Voloshin AS: Low back pain: conservative treatment with artificial shock absorbers. *Arch Phys Med Rehabil* 1985, 66:145–148.

99. Gavin TM, Boscardin JB, Patwardhan AG: Preliminary results of orthotic treatment for chronic low back pain. *J Prosthet Orthot* 1993, 5:5–9.

100. Lantz SA, Schultz AB: Lumbar spine orthosis wearing: I. Restriction of gross body motions. *Spine* 1986, 11:834–837.

101. Willner SW: Test instrument for predicting the effect of rigid braces in cases with low back pain. *Prosthet Orthot Int* 1990, 14:22–26.

102. MacMillan M, Stauffer ES, Barth G: Orthotic management of the surgically stabilized spine in quadriplegic and paraplegic patients. *Clin Prosthet Orthot* 1987, 11:210–214.

103. Turner MS, Carus DA, Troup IM: Custom moulded plastic spinal orthoses. *Prosthet Orthot Int* 1986, 10:83–86.

104. Maloney FP: Pulmonary function in quadriplegia: effects of a corset. *Arch Phys Med Rehabil* 1979, 60:261–265.

105. Asher MA, Whitney WH: Orthotics for spinal deformity. In Redford JB (ed): *Orthotics Etcetera*, 3rd ed. Baltimore, Williams & Wilkins, 1986, 153–197.

106. Bunch WH, Patwardhan AG: *Scoliosis: Making Clinical Decisions*. St Louis, C. V. Mosby Company, 1989.

107. Cassella MC, Hall JE: Current treatment approaches in the nonoperative and operative management of adolescent idiopathic scoliosis. *Phys Ther* 1991, 71:897–909.

108. King HA: Orthotic management of idiopathic scoliosis. *Phys Med Rehabil Clin N Am* 1992, 3:45–56.

109. Emans JB, Kaelin A, Bancel P: The Boston bracing system for idiopathic scoliosis: follow-up results in 295 patients. *Spine* 1986, 11:792–801.

110. Letts M, Rathbone D, Yamashita T: Soft Boston orthosis in management of neuromuscular scoliosis: a preliminary report. *J Pediatr Orthop* 1992, 12:470–474.

111. Micheli LJ: The use of the modified Boston brace system (B.O.B.) for back pain: clinical indications. *Orthot Prosthet* 1985, 39:41–46.

112. Cochran T, Nachemson A: Long-term anatomic and func-

tional changes in patients with adolescent idiopathic scoliosis treated with the Milwaukee brace. *Spine* 1985,
10:127–132.

113. Wallace S, Madigan R, Wasserman J: Low profile contoured ring. *Orthot Prosthet* 1986, 39:13–15.

114. Duncan RM: Basic principles of splinting the hand. *Phys
Ther* 1989, 69:1103–1116.

115. Fess EE, Phillips CA: *Hand Splinting: Principles and Methods,*
2nd ed. St. Louis, C. V. Mosby Company, 1987.

116. Fishman S, Berger N, Edelstein JE: Upper-limb orthoses.
In American Academy of Orthopaedic Surgeons: *Atlas of
Orthotics,* 2nd ed. St. Louis, C. V. Mosby Company, 1985,
pp 163–198.

117. Gribben MG: Splinting principles for hand injuries. In
Moran CA (ed): *Hand Rehabilitation.* New York, Churchill
Livingstone, 1986, pp 159–189.

118. Hunter JM, Schneider LH, Macklin EJ (eds): *Rehabilitation
of the Hand: Surgery and Therapy,* 3rd ed. St. Louis, C. V.
Mosby Company, 1990.

119. Irani KD: Wrist and hand orthoses. *Phys Med Rehabil: State
Art Rev* 1987, 1:137–160.

120. Schutt AH: Upper extremity and hand orthotics. *Phys Med
Rehabil Clin N Am* 1992, 3:223–242.

121. Tenney CG, Lisak JM: *Atlas of Hand Splinting.* Boston, Little, Brown, and Company, 1986.

122. Basford JR, Allen EM: Adaptive equipment for C6 quadriplegia: an approach to effective, simple, and inexpensive
devices. *Arch Phys Med Rehabil* 1985, 66:829–831.

123. Garber SA, Gregoria L: Upper extremity assistive devices:
assessment of use by spinal cord-injured patients with
quadriplegia. *Am J Occup Ther* 1990, 44:126–131.

124. Makaran JE, Dittmer DK, Buchal RD: The SMART wrist-

125. Rosen WR, McColey JJ, Bowker JH: The team approach to
orthotic management in quadriplegia. *Clin Prosthet Orthot*
1987, 11:201–209.

126. Langlois S, Mac Kinnon JR, Pederson L: Hand splints and
cerebral spasticity: a review of the literature. *Can J Occup
Ther* 1989, 56:113–119.

127. McPherson JJ, Kreimeyer D, Aalderks M, Gallagher T: A
comparison of dorsal and volar resting hand splints in the
reduction of hypertonus. *Am J Occup Ther* 1982, 36:664–
670.

128. Mills V: Electromyographic results of inhibitory splinting.
Phys Ther 1984, 64:190–193.

129. Neuhaus BE, Ascher ER, Coullon BA, *et al.*: A survey of
rationales for and against hand splinting in hemiplegia.
Am J Occup Ther 1981, 35:83–90.

130. Poole JL, Whitney SL: Inflatable pressure splints (Air-
splints) as adjunct treatment for individuals with strokes.
Phys Occup Ther Geriatr 1992, 11:17–27.

131. McKnight PT, Shomburg FL: Air pressure splint effects on
hand symptoms of patients with rheumatoid arthritis. *Arch
Phys Med Rehabil* 1982, 63:560–564.

132. Yasuda YL, Bowman K, Hsu JD: Mobile arm supports:
criteria for successful use in muscle disease patients. *Arch
Phys Med Rehabil* 1986, 67:253–256.

133. Prevost R: Bobath axillary support for adults with hemiplegia: a biomechanical analysis. *Phys Ther* 1988, 68:228–232.

134. Williams R, Taffs L, Minuk T: Evaluation of two support
methods for the subluxated shoulder of hemiplegic patients. *Phys Ther* 1988, 68:1209–1214.

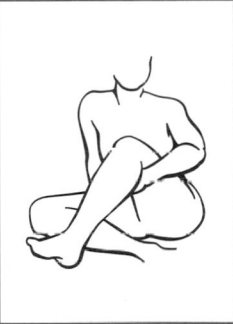

CHAPTER 41

Age-Related Considerations: Pediatric

Susan K. Brenneman, Meg Stanger, and Dolores B. Bertoti

Children need to be viewed in a different light from adults: not only in the cognitive, social, and psychological realms but also in the physiological realm. The musculoskeletal impairments of children are unique because of the changes that occur during growth and development. The authors hope to convey the importance of being aware of those changes and the impact on the types of musculoskeletal impairments found in children.

The information is organized according to common pediatric diagnoses because that is how children present to physical therapists. A child is seldom seen with an isolated musculoskeletal problem. The authors have attempted to focus on the musculoskeletal aspects of those diagnoses; when other information is presented, its purpose is to give the clinician enough information to make appropriate referrals for further evaluation if a diagnosis has not been made.

I. Anatomical and Physiological Considerations: Growth and Development

A. Introduction

1. An understanding of the processes of the growth and development of the musculoskeletal system will assist the clinician in providing sound interventions.
2. *Development* can be defined as maturational change from a lower to a higher stage of complexity.[1]
3. *Growth* connotes a normal process of increase in size and volume of an organism.[1]
4. An interplay of several factors affects growth and development:
   a. Genetic—prenatal
   b. Mechanical—latter third trimester and postnatal
   c. Nutrition
   d. Hormones
   e. Drugs

B. Terminology describing morphological abnormalities[2]

1. Malformations
   a. The defects occurring when normal organogenesis is interrupted, which are generally genetic in origin, thus arising at the moment of conception.
   b. Examples: cleft lip and palate and polydactyly.
2. Disruptions
   a. Defects that are the result of the breakdown of normal developmental processes; development is disrupted at the cellular level by an external factor.
   b. Examples: amniotic bands, thalidomide embryopathy.
3. Deformations
   a. Abnormalities in form, shape, or position of body parts caused by unusual mechanical forces; these forces may be intrinsic, such as fetal hypomobility, or extrinsic, such as uterine constraint.
   b. Mechanical forces are important in the morphogenesis of muscles, cartilage, and bone.[1–4]
   c. Modifications are more readily achieved when tissues are easily pliable and in periods of rapid growth.
   d. Examples: Clubfoot and tibial torsion.
4. Dysplasias
   a. Problems stemming from abnormal organization of cells into tissues leading to abnormal tissue differentiation; these are not necessarily recognizable at birth.
   b. Example: the connective tissue defect that produces osteogenesis imperfecta.

C. Embryology

1. Most of the tissues of the musculoskeletal system develop from the mesenchymal cells: the skeleton, tendons, joints, and muscles.[5]
2. Mesoderm—somite
   a. Myotome—muscle
   b. Dermatome—skin and nerve endings
   c. Sclerotome—bone

D. Limb development

1. Critical periods.[5]
   a. Lower limb—28 days
   b. Upper limb—26 days
2. Mechanism
   a. Mesenchymal cells accumulate and form a bulge over which the ectoderm becomes a specialized and thickened rim called the *apical epidermal ridge* (AER) along the anteroposterior axis of the future limb.
   b. By 33 days, mesenchymal cells differentiate into cartilage in the proximal upper extremity.
3. Pattern formation
   a. Structures are laid down in a proximal to distal sequence.
   b. The AER is essential for limb outgrowth and development of the pattern along the proximodistal axis.
      (1). Removal of the AER results in truncated limbs.[5]
      (2). It is thought that an interaction between the underlying mesenchyme and the AER is necessary for continued growth.[5]
   c. A group of mesenchymal cells called the *polarizing region* is the reference to anteroposterior pattern formation.
   d. Little is known about pattern formation across the dorsoventral axis.

E. Skeletal development

1. The skeletal matrix is formed during the first fetal month.
2. In the second month, bone formation begins.
3. Mechanisms of ossification[4,6]
   a. Endochrondral bone formation
      (1). Cartilage is laid down to form the template, the basic outline of which resembles adult bone.
      (2). The diaphysis is the primary center of ossification.
         (a). Ossification begins in the middle of the cartilage in long bones.
         (b). Continues until the epiphyseal region is reached.
      (3). The proliferation and hypertrophy of the epiphyseal cartilage provide for the longitudinal growth of the long bones.
   b. Membranous bone formation
      (1). Develops directly from mesenchymal cells through deposition of bone mineral: endosteal or periosteal ossification.
      (2). Skull, clavicle, scapula, and mandible.
   c. Appositional growth
      (1). Refers to the increase in diameter and density of bone.
4. Factors that influence skeletal growth
   a. Mineral content plays an important role in prenatal, perinatal, and postnatal development.[6]
   b. Hormones and vitamins appear to play a larger role in development postnatally.[6]
5. Mechanical forces
   a. Applied forces, or loading, affect both the amount and the direction of tissue growth.[3]
      (1). Appropriate magnitude, direction, and duration are necessary.
         (a). A minimum effective stimulus is required
         (b). Unknown how much or what kind
      (2). A biological range exists for each tissue type.[7]
   b. Endochrondral growth
      (1). Compression—tension
         (a). Essential for conversion of cartilaginous tissue into bone.

         (b). An excess of compression–tension inhibits growth.
         (c). Unequal loading may lead to angulation of the epiphyseal plate and change the direction of growth.[8,9]
         (d). Duration[10]
            (i). Intermittent—growth
            (ii). Constant of great magnitude leads to bone atrophy
            (iii). Persistent, gentle loads (creep)—deformity or correction of deformity.
         (e). When perpendicular to the direction of growth, displacement of the epiphyseal plate and deflection of growth along the line of the deforming force may occur.
      (2). Torsional force
         (a). Bone is least resistant to torsion.
         (b). Causes rotational deflection of the growth columns.[11]
   c. Appositional growth
      (1). *Flexure-drift principle*[12]
         (a). Compression with bending creates positive and/or negative potentials on either side of the bone, which results in modeling
            (i). Affects size and alignment
         (b). Compression and tension stimulate appositional growth
            (i). Increase—an increase in the thickness and density tibial shaft is observed[9,13]
            (ii). Decrease—results in bone atrophy[9]
   d. Trabecular growth
      (1). Internal structure of bone developed to resist the loads they bear.
      (2). Compression stimulates the development of trabeculae.[10,14]
      (3). Related to the forces of both weight bearing and muscle pull.
   e. Cartilage
      (1). Intermittent compression of appropriate magnitude results in growth
      (2). Constant or excessive compression results in the degeneration of cartilage
      (3). Lack of compression results in atrophy

(4). Congenital deformities that result in abnormal forces may lead to early degenerative joint disease[3,13]

f. Fibrous tissue

(1). Tissue properties are affected by changes in tension[15]

(2). *Stretch-creep rule*[16]

(a). Elongation over time with the application of a load

(b). Implications for the development and treatment of deformities

g. The effect of dynamic stimulus has implications for stationary standing versus mobility for skeletal growth

h. The application of abnormal loads during periods of rapid growth results in permanent deformity.

(1). Positioning

(2). Muscle pull

6. Rate of growth

a. Growth is rapid in the early fetal period

b. A deceleration of growth is seen in the last prenatal trimester

7. Postnatal bone and chondral modeling

a. During the first 2 years of life, it is thought that all primary bone has been remodeled.[6]

b. Remodeling persists until adulthood at the rate of 5% per annum.[6]

c. Correction of deformity is possible because of this growth process.

(1). Appropriate management of forces

(2). Knowledge of biomechanical and growth principles[3]

F. Joint formation

1. Embryonic stage

a. Region of cells forms between two areas that are differentiating into cartilage[17]

(1). Genetically driven

(2). Initial form not dependent on mechanical pressure

b. Differentiation of structures from synovial mesenchyme

(1). Synovial membrane

(2). Fibrous capsule

(3). Intra-articular structures

c. Cavitation[18]

(1). Formation of the joint cavity

(2). Differentiation occurs over a relatively short period of time

(a). Week 4½ to 7

(b). Individual differences in timing do occur

(i). Sacroiliac joint—10th week to 7th month[4]

(ii). Hands and feet—early fetal period[18]

d. Development is susceptible to teratogens during this time period[4]

2. Fetal period

a. Increase in size and maturation of structures

(1). The amount of collagen

(2). Differentiation of ligaments

(3). Extension of the joint cavity

(4). Development of bursae

b. Innervation occurs

3. Movement is an important factor in maintaining the molding of the articular form once established.[6]

G. Muscular development

1. Stages

a. Mesenchyme

b. Myoblast cell

c. Primary myotubules—5 weeks

d. Early muscle fibers—11 weeks

e. Striated myofibrils—20 weeks

(1). Muscle fibers packed with myofibrils

(2). Have peripheral nuclei and are similar to those of adult muscle[19]

2. Myogenesis

a. Nerve independent less than 9 weeks

(1). Genetic differentiation

(2). Noninnervated

(3). Primary myotubes show a greater number of slow-twitch fibers as opposed to fast-twitch fibers

(a). Type I

(b). Clear distinction cannot be made between the two[4]

b. Nerve dependent after 9 weeks

(1). Neural elements

(a). Tenth week: primitive nerve branches ramify among muscle fibers

(b). Eleventh week: myoneural junction with early motor end-plate formation

(c). Twelfth week: golgi tendon organ (GTO) commences innervation

(d). Fourteenth week: muscle spindle shows all components

(e). Sixteenth week: GTO is encapsulated and myelination of its fibers begins

(2). Enhances muscle development and differentiation

(3). Secondary and tertiary myotubes have more fast-twitch than slow-twitch fibers

(4). At term there is an equal number of fast-twitch and slow-twitch fibers

c. Full-term infant

(1). Skeletal muscle contains less than 20% of adult number of cells.

(2). Accounts for about 25% of the weight of the infant.[19]

d. Postnatal growth

(1). Subsequent growth occurs through hypertrophy of existing fibers.

(2). Steady increase in number of fibers up to the middle of the fifth decade.

H. Lower limb alignment

1. Both movement and positioning are important contributors to initial limb alignment and to changes in alignment.

2. Acetabulum

a. Pre- and postnatal shape is related to the size and shape of the femoral head.[1]

(1). Initially, the head is spherical and deeply set.

(2). Slowly becomes hemispherical and less deeply positioned.

(3). After week 12, the acetabulum grows more slowly than the femoral head.

(4). At birth, the joint is shallow, with 65% coverage of femoral head.

(5). Postnatally, the depth increases, creating a mature ball-and-socket joint, with coverage by 3 years of age.[20,21]

b. At birth, acetabular roof faces downward and forward at an angle of 7 degrees with the vertical plane.[1]

(1). Makes it more at risk for the femur to dislocate up and back.

(2). Increases to 17 degrees by 3 years.[22]

c. Displays a variable anterior/posterior orientation[23]

(1). Posterior orientation results in increased risk of dislocation

3. Hip

a. Prenatal position contributes to range of motion limitations

b. There are 50 degrees of physiological hip flexion contracture at birth; by 9 months there are virtually none[24]

c. Abduction and external rotation tightness[24]

4. Femur

a. Angle of inclination: coxa valga[24,25]

(1). In utero 175 degrees

(2). Birth: 135 to 145 degrees

(3). Adult: 125 degrees

b. Angle of declination: the angle the femoral neck makes with the femoral condyles[25]

(1). Changes from retro to ante in utero

(2). Birth: 20 to 30 degrees antetorsion

(3). Maturity: 8 to 16 degrees

c. These changes occur through

(1). The differential growth of the three epiphyseal zones in the proximal femur[14]

(2). Normal compression and tension of weight bearing and muscles[26]

5. Knee

a. Femorotibial axis undergoes changes from relative varus at birth to extreme valgus (160 degrees) at 3 years of age to normal valgus 171 degrees) by 7 years[3,27,28]

b. Physiological flexion contracture at birth of 20 to 30 degrees[29]

6. Tibial shaft torsion changes from 0 degree to 23 to 25 degrees of lateral torsion by maturity.[30]

7. Ankle

a. Term infants have as much as 45 degrees of physiological ankle dorsiflexion contracture[1]

b. The complex positional and rotational changes of the ankle–foot complex have been well documented and reviewed in the literature; those readers who desire more in-depth treatment are referred to Cusick[31]; Bernhardt[1]; and LeVeau and Bernhardt.[3]

8. Foot[1,3]

a. Weight-bearing calcaneal valgus of 5 to 10 degrees until age 5 to 7 years

b. No apparent arch in weight bearing until age 2 to 3 years

c. Forefoot varus at birth changes to neutral by age 1 to 2 years

d. Metatarsus adductus of 5 to 10 degrees up to age 1 to 2 years

II. Age-Related Considerations in Musculoskeletal Assessment

Pediatric musculoskeletal assessment requires an integration of physical therapy assessment procedures and an appreciation of normal growth and development.
- Knowledge of what skeletal appearances are normal or abnormal at given ages
- Understanding of the possible causative factors in the development of impairments
- Determination of the primary deficiencies and secondary compensations.

A. Goniometry

1. Age-related considerations
   a. Changes in joint mobility are age related and parallel changes in locomotor abilities.
   b. Table 41–1 highlights the differences in range of motion
      (1). Full-term neonate shows physiological limitations[4,29,32–34]
         (a). Hip and knee extension
         (b). Ankle plantar flexion
      (2). Premature infants may show no limitations with hypermobility of most joints.[4]
2. Joint-specific considerations
   a. Evaluation of the spine
      (1). Assessment of active and passive spinal mobility.
      (2). Techniques using distance measurements have been described in the literature.[35–38]
   b. Evaluation of the hip
      (1). Extension
         (a). Physiological flexion contracture is common[33,39]
            (i). Newborn: 28 degrees
            (ii). Six weeks of age: 19 degrees
            (iii). Three to 6 months of age: 7 degrees
         (b). Measurement[35,40,41]
            (i). Thomas test
            (ii). Staheli prone extension test. (Fig. 41–1)
      (2). Medial and lateral rotation. (Fig. 41–2)

   a. Medial rotation[42]
      (i). Greatest in infants younger than 1 year
      (ii). Gradually decreases to a mean of 50 degrees in males and 40 degrees in females.
   (b). Lateral rotation[42]
      (i). Mean value in infants of 70 degrees
      (ii). Gradually decreases to a mean of 45 degrees
   c. Hamstring range of motion
      (1). Child lies supine with hip at 90 degrees, slowly extend knee, measure popliteal angle.
      (2). Normal is less than 20 degrees[35]

B. Muscle strength

1. Some differences exist in methods used to evaluate muscle strength in the pediatric population.
2. Factors that affect the results of strength assessment[43]
   a. Growth with developmental muscle tissue changes
   b. Neuromuscular status
   c. Maturation and cognition
3. Because of the effect of changing lever lengths during growth, the report of strength by torque values is more meaningful.
   a. Comparative value reports of strength is limited without documentation of weight and length of the lever arm.[43]
4. In children younger than 2 years[43–45]
   a. Observations of function and spontaneous movement
   b. Palpation
   c. Description of muscle bulk and contour
5. Options for quantitative strength testing in the child older than 2 years
   a. Manual muscle test
      (1). Results of one study question the ability to quantify strength deficits or increases objectively[43]
      (2). Acceptable reliability has been demonstrated in the grading range of *trace* through *fair*[46–48]

Table 41–1. DEVELOPMENTAL FEATURES OF THE LOWER EXTREMITY*†

	Newborn	Child	Adult
Femur and hip	Antetorsion[1,2,3,4,7,16] ... 35°–40°	Antetorsion[1,3,4,5,8,24]	Antetorsion[4,8,13,14] ... 5°–16°
	Anteversion[3,7,14] ... 40°–60°	Age 1 ... 31°–37°	Anteversion ... 5°–16°
	Total Range of Rotation[7,11,21] ... 120°–150°	Age 2 ... 28°–32°	Femoral Neck/Shaft Angle[1,7,8,16] ... 125°
	Lateral Rotation[21,23] ... 60°–92°	Age 5 ... 23°–28°	Total Hip Rotation Range[8] ... 90°–100°
	Medial Rotation[21,23] ... 40°–76.9°	Ages 8–12 ... 15°–26°	(lat.≥med.)
	Flexion Contracture[5,6,8,21] ... 30°–50°	Age 15 ... 5°–16°	Transcondylar Axis[7] ... 0°–10°
	Coxa Valga[1,2,7,16] ... 145°–150°	Femoral Neck/Shaft Angle	(relative to frontal plane)
	Transcondylar Axis[7] ... 20°–30°	(Age 6)[1] ... 135°	
	(lateral to the frontal plane)	Range of Hip Rotations	
	Anterior (and Lateral) bowing	Age 2[10] ... 52° medial, 47° lateral	
	Abduction in 90° flexion[21] ... 79.3°(63–86)	Age 7[23] ... 50° medial, 45° lateral	
	Abduction "extended" to 30°[21] ... 38.9°(26–58)	... (25–65)	
	Adduction "extended"[21] ... 17.3°(11–30)	Hip Flexion Contracture[10]	
		Age 1 ... 10°–20°	
		Age 2 ... 3°	
		Age 5 ... 0°	
Knee	Axial Tip-fib Rotation (total M/L) (in knee flexion)[3] ... 90°–155°	Axial Tip-Fib Rotation Frontal Plane Deviation (tibiofemoral angle)[5,9]	Axial Tib-Fib Rotation (medial<lateral rotation by 1:2 ratio)
	[Medial Rotation often exceeds lateral through age 24 months]	Ages 6–36 months ... 0°–12° valgum	Knee extended[13] ... 0°–5°
		Ages 3–6 ... 12°–5° valgum	Knee flexed[28] ... 40°
	Flexion Contracture[5,8] ... 20°–30°	Ages 6 and up ... 5°–7° valgum	Frontal Plane Deviation (tibiofemoral angle)[9] ... 5°–7° valgum
	[Resolves within 6 months]	Popliteal Angle (in Israel)[9]	(lower leg on sagittal plane)
	Frontal Plane Deviation (Varum) (tibiofemoral angle)[5,8] ... ≤17°	Ages 1–3 ... −6°(0°–15°)	
		Age 4 ... F: −17°(−5° to −45°)	
		M: −27°(−10° to −45°)	
		Ages 5–10 ... −26°(0° to −50°)	

Table continued on following page

Table 41–1. DEVELOPMENTAL FEATURES OF THE LOWER EXTREMITY*† *(Continued)*

	Newborn	Child	Adult

Tibia	Tibiofibular Torsion (AJA)[7,20] .... 0°–20°
	Proximal Tibial Plateau[2] .... 27° retroversion
	Tibial Plafond[27] .... everted
		Apparent (ideal) Leg Varum[7] Age 5 (major resolution by age 2) 0°–2°
		
		Tibiofibular torsion:
		Valmassy (1989)[29] [N=281 children]
		              Mean Values
		18 mos (N=3) .... 5.5°
		2–2.5 yrs (N=6) .... 6.3°
		2–5.3 yrs (N=7) .... 5.7°
		3–3.5 yrs (N=38) ...... 7.7°
		3.5–4 yrs (N=25) ...... 8.1°
		4–4.5 yrs (N=81) ...... 8.5°
		4.5–5 yrs (N=55) ...... 9.3°
		5–5.5 yrs (N=53) ...... 9.7°
		5.5–6 yrs (N=13) ...... 11.2°
		[All SD between 1.2°–2.7°]
		
		Sutherland, et al (1988)[30] [N=435 children]
		              Median
		1 yr (N=44) .... 4°
		18 mos (N=41) ...... 6°
		2 yrs (N=48) .... 8°
		2.5 yrs (N=58) ...... 7°
		3 yrs (N=52) .... 7°
		3.5 yrs (N=41) ...... 6°
		4 yrs (N=41) .... 9°
		5 yrs (N=39) .... 9°
		6 yrs (N=46) .... 10°
		7 yrs (N=45) .... 10°
			Apparent (ideal) Leg Varum[7] .... 0°–2°
			
			Tibiofibular Torsion (AJA) (lateral to frontal plane)
			         12°–18°[12]
			         20°–30°[0.0]
			     average 22°[4]

Ankle	Dorsiflexion[22] .... 58.9° (36.7°–71.7°) (Reduces to 45°–50° within 3 months) past neutral Plantarflexion[22] .... 25.7° (10°–41.7°) (calcaneo-fibular angle)	Dorsiflexion (in STN)[7,8,15,30] (maximum passive range) Age 1 .... 25°–45° Age 4 .... 15°–26° Age 5 .... 10°–20° Age 7 .... 15° Plantarflexion (calcaneofibular angle)[7] Age 1 .... 45°+ Age 5 .... 45°+	Dorsiflexion (with STN)[6,12] .... 8°–15° Minimum normal passive end range: Knee extended .... 5°–10° Knee flexed .... 5°–10°

Foot		
Average Neutral STJ[28]	22.4° varus	
(Drops to 10° by age 1 yr)[7,14]		
Total STJ Range of Motion[7]	45°	
(1:1 inversion:eversion)		
Forefoot Varus[7,14]	12°–15°	
Metatarsus Primus Adductus[7] ...	8°–15°	

Ideal STN[12]	0°	
(calcaneus to distal lower leg)		
Actual Average STN[17,28]	2°–3.5° varus	
Total STJ Range of Motion[12]	5°–10°	
(2:1 inversion:eversion around STN)		
Age 4	3°–8°	
Age 5	1°–6°	
Age 6	0°–5°	
Age 7 and up	±2°	

Relaxed Calcaneal Stance (eversion relative to saggital plane)

Ages 15–36 mos[12]	25°–30°
Age 7 or more years	25°–30°
Geriatric	18°
Minimum range needed (on level surface)	8°–12°
Forefoot Varus[12] (ideal)	0°–2°

Subtract: the child's age from 7[18]

* This chart was used with the written permission of Beverly D. Cusick, MS, PT. The chart was compiled by Ms. Cusick for use as a handout for two courses which she has developed and offers internationally: 1) Casts and Splints: New Concepts in the Management of Lower Extremity Deformity in Individuals with CNS Dysfunction; and 2) Developmental Biomechanics: A Study of Growing Lower Extremity Structures and Related Assessment Procedures. Contact Telluride Wordcraft, P.O. Box 62, Placerville, CO 81430 (303/728/3304) for information about the availability of these courses.

† Sources:
1. Beals (1969)
2. Bernhardt (1988)
3. Engel and Stahell (1974)
4. Fabry, McEwen, and Shands (1973)
5. Hensinger and Jones (1982)
6. Hoffer (1980)
7. Jordan, Cusack, and Resseque (1983)
8. McCrea (1985)
9. McDade (1977)
10. Phelps, Smith, and Hallum (1985)
11. Pitkow (1975)
12. Root, Orien, Weed, and Hughes (1971)
13. Schafer (1987)
14. Sgariato (1971)
15. Tardieu and Tardieu (1987)
16. Tax (1985)
17. Tiberio (1988)
18. Valmassy (1984)
19. Wilkins (1986)
20. Badelon et al. (1989)
21. Forero et al. (1989)
22. Waugh et al. (1983)
23. Stahell et al. (1985)
24. Shands et al. (1958)
25. Kate et al. (1992)
26. Soderburg (1986)
27. Tachdjian (1985)
28. Strauss (1927)
29. Valmassy (1989)
30. Sutherland (1988)

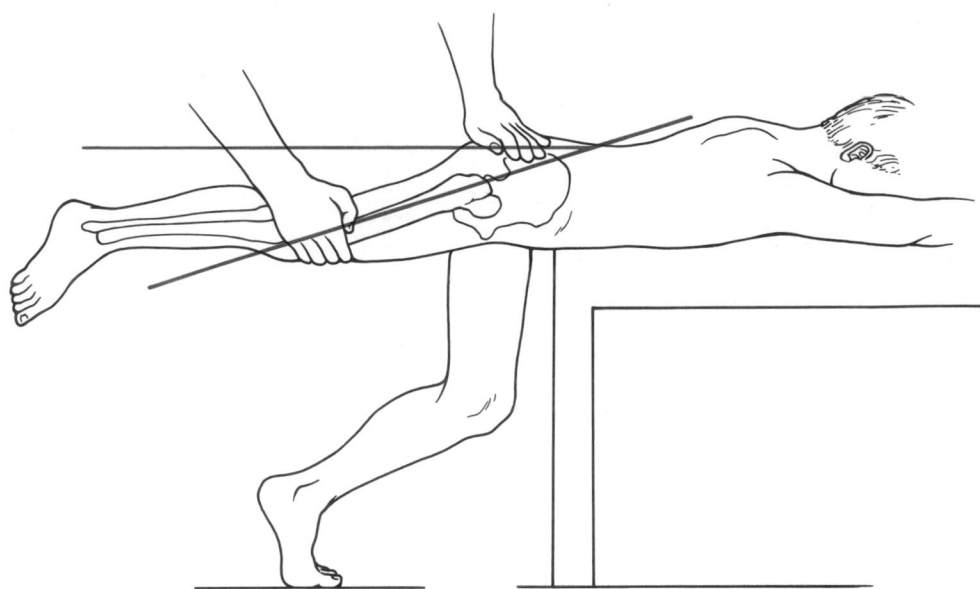

FIGURE 41–1   Prone hip flexion contracture test. (From Bleck EE: *Orthopaedic Management in Cerebral Palsy.* London, MacKeith Press, 1987.)

(3). Criteria for grades *good* and *normal* are ambiguous.

(4). Grades *good* through *normal* sometimes exceed resistance offered by the examiner.

b. Hand-held dynamometer or myometer
   (1). Isometric strength
   (2). Appears to be reliable in pediatrics[46]
   (3). Inexpensive, easy to use
   (4). Most models limited to 27.2 kg recording capacity, which may not be sufficient for children with mild strength losses[46]

c. Force gauge system
   (1). Isometric strength
   (2). Reliability as adapted for the pediatric population has been demonstrated[49]

d. Isokinetic dynamometer systems
   (1). Demonstrated to be reliable and useful in the pediatric population.[50-53]
   (2). Reliability of results is dependent on positioning, clarity of instructions, and testing precision.[54]

6. The efficacy of muscle strength testing in patients with neurological impairment is controversial.[55,56]

a. A gauge of strength and function is an important aspect of recording change in all patients.

b. Factors such as motor control and basic physiological changes associated with central nervous system (CNS) lesions as they influence strength and performance continue to be under study.

C. Skeletal assessment

1. Skeletal maturity
   a. Corresponds to the real age of the majority of individuals of the same sex who have reached the same degree of skeletal maturation[6]
   b. Determined radiographically
   c. Used in determining timing for surgical intervention

2. Leg length
   a. Position of test
      (1). Level pelvis
      (2). Hips in extension, neutral abduction/adduction, and neutral rotation
      (3). Knees fully extended
   b. Measure from anterosuperior iliac spine (ASIS) to top of medial malleolus.

3. Hip instability
   a. Asymmetrical gluteal folds
   b. Leg-length discrepancy: dislocated or subluxed hip may be shorter.
   c. Galeazzi's sign[57] (see Fig. 32–14)
      (1). Supine with hips and knees flexed and feet flat on table; positive test

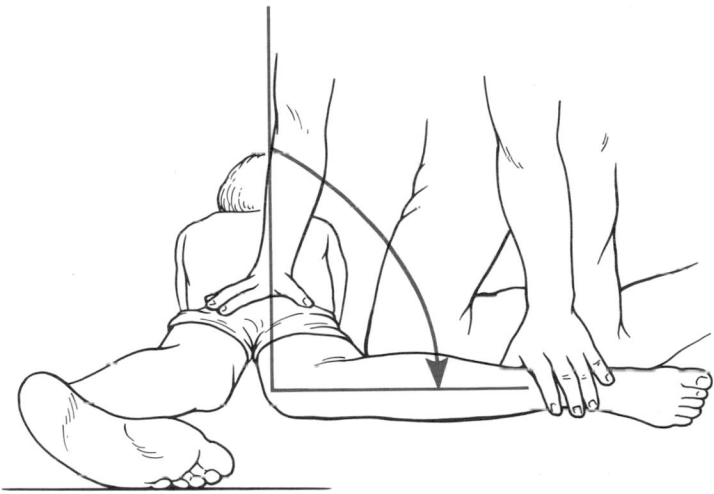

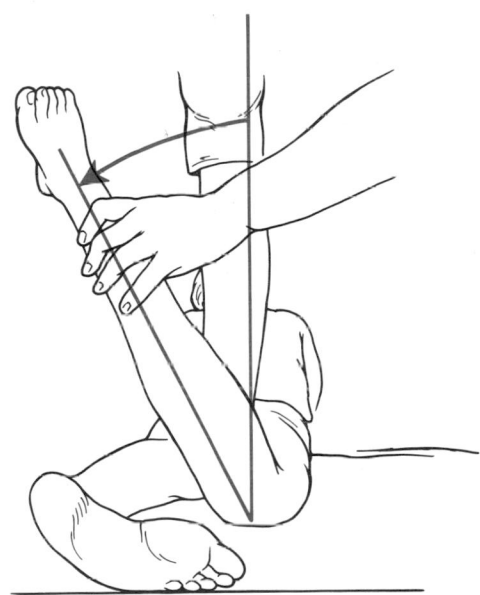

FIGURE 41–2 **Top panel,** Measurement of internal rotation of the hip in extension with the patient in a prone position. One hand should always be firmly placed on the pelvis to stabilize it and to minimize pelvic rotation. **Bottom panel,** Measurement of external rotation of the hip. (From Bleck EE: *Orthopaedic Management in Cerebral Palsy.* London, MacKeith Press, 1987.)

indicated by one knee higher than the other.
   (2). Use with children 3 to 18 months of age.
   (3). Assessment of unilateral dislocation only.
  d. Ortolani's sign[57] (Fig. 41–3)
   (1). Supine position, examiner flexes hips and knees and abducts the hips; positive test indicated by a palpable click.
   (2). Valid only for first few weeks after birth.
  e. Telescoping sign[57] (see Fig. 32–12)

   (1). Supine with hips and knees flexed to 90 degrees, push down on femur toward table, and lift up.
   (2). Positive test indicated by excessive movement.

D. Alignment

1. Femoral anteversion[35]
   a. Torsion or internal rotation of the femoral shaft on the femoral neck
   b. Clinically assessed by internal rotation far exceeding (greater than 7 degrees) external rotation (less than 20 degrees)

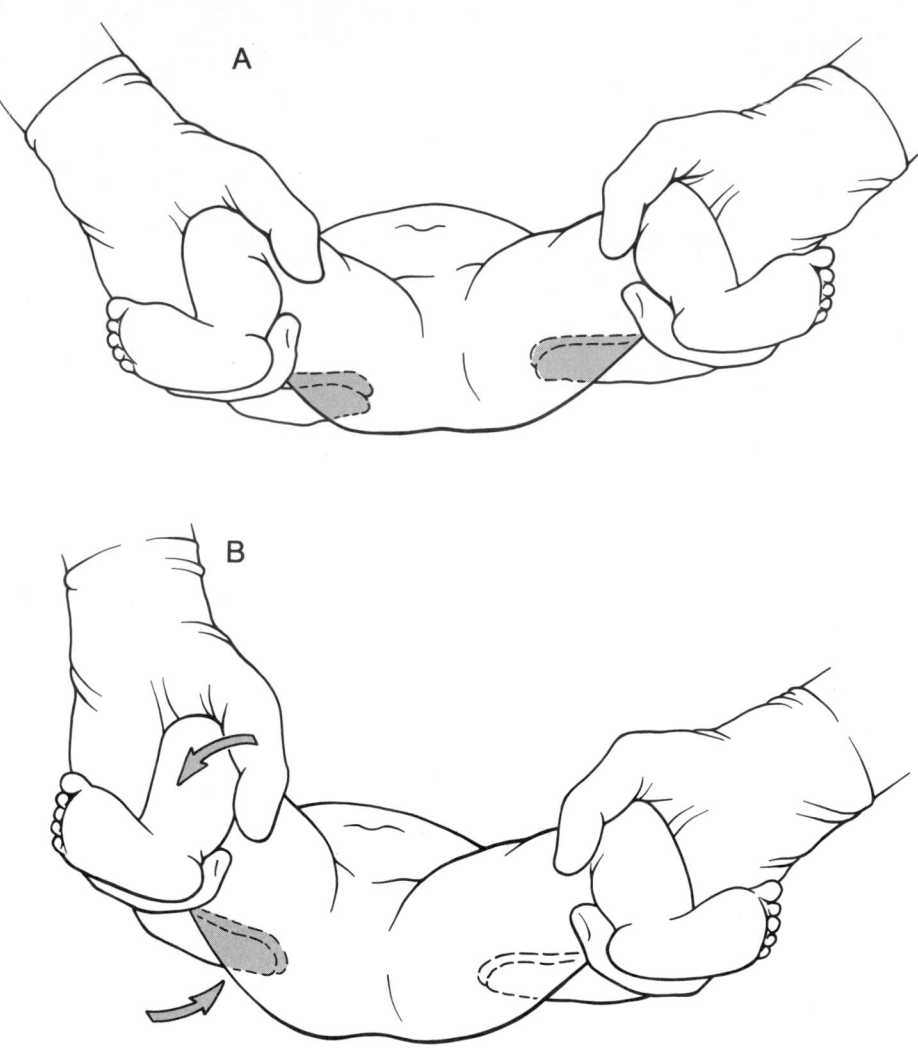

FIGURE 41–3 Testing for Ortolani's sign. In the newborn, the two hips can be equally flexed, abducted, and externally rotated without producing a "click." **A,** Normal. **B,** Ortolani's sign.

2. Tibial torsion
   a. The normal mean angles are:[35]
      (1). Zero to 12 months: 7 degrees (± 4.1 degrees)
      (2). Three to 24 months: 10 degrees (± 2 degrees)
      (3). Twenty-five months to 13 years: 13 degrees (± 3 degrees)
      (4). Thirteen years to adults: 22 degrees
   b. Photographic measurement of the transmalleolar axis used by Staheli *et al.* produced the following values:[42]
      (1). Younger than 1 year: 0 degrees (± 20 degrees)
      (2). Eight years of age: 20 degrees (0–35 degrees)
      (3). Skeletally mature: 20 degrees (0–45 degrees)
3. Foot progression angle
   a. Variability is normal for all ages.
   b. Greater variability in those younger than 2 years.
   c. Toeing in resolves by 4 years of age.
      (1). Greater than 15 degrees is considered severe.
   d. Toeing out of greater than 15 degrees creates stress on the medial structures.

E. Gait

1. Methods of assessment[58]
   a. Observation

(1). Qualitative descriptions of gait parameters, fluidity of movement, and postural control.

(2). Include ambulation on uneven terrain, elevations, and in natural environments.

b. Video analysis
   (1). Supplement to observational analysis
   (2). Allows clinician more time to observe gait.

c. Cinematography

d. Electromyograph (EMG)
   (1). Provides information about the timing and intensity of a muscle contraction.
   (2). Useful in evaluating causes of abnormal movements and determining surgical intervention.

e. Kinematics provides measures of joint motions.

2. Age-related changes in gait[59,60]

a. One year
   (1). Arms in high, on-guard position
   (2). Lack of reciprocal arm swing
   (3). Excessive anterior pelvic tilt
   (4). Elevation of the pelvis during swing
   (5). Wide base of support
   (6). Hip external rotation during swing
   (7). Lack of full hip extension in terminal stance
   (8). Knee flexion throughout stance
   (9). Lack of heel strike
   (10). Rapid walking cadence with short step length

b. Two years
   (1). Arms in medium, on-guard position
   (2). Reciprocal arm swing near fully developed
   (3). Decrease in anterior pelvic tilt
   (4). Narrowing base of support
   (5). Decreased external hip rotation during swing
   (6). Full hip extension present in terminal stance
   (7). Knee extension during but less than seen in mature gait pattern
   (8). Heel strike beginning
   (9). Cadence decreased

c. Three years
   (1). Reciprocal arm swing movements with arms at side
   (2). Base of support normal
   (3). Heel strike present
   (4). Step length remains limited

d. Seven years
   (1). Adult gait components
   (2). Increased step length secondary to increased limb length

3. Mature components are requirements for an efficient gait
   a. Minimize the translation of the body's center of gravity.
   b. Impairments that prevent the development of gait into its mature components will result in an inefficient, ineffective gait pattern.

III. Pediatric Neuromuscular Disorders

A. Cerebral palsy

1. A chronic, nonprogressive movement disorder with early onset.[61,62]

2. Abnormalities in muscle tone and muscle imbalance with the secondary effects of immobility and positioning problems contribute to significant musculoskeletal impairments.[35]
   a. Children with cerebral palsy frequently present with deformity and contractures in many combinations.
   b. Prevalance and distribution of musculoskeletal impairments closely correlate with the type of cerebral palsy and the distribution of muscle tone.[35,63-65]

3. Associated problems secondary to musculoskeletal impairments.
   a. Oculomotor problems[62,66,67]
      (1). Strabismus
         (a). Incidence of 20 to 60% of children with cerebral palsy
         (b). Highest incidence in those with diplegia and quadriplegia.
      (2). Esotropia, deviation of eyes toward midline, is more prevalent than exotropia.
   b. Oral motor control difficulties[62]
      (1). Secondary to abnormal tone and poor control of the muscles of the face, mouth, and respiratory system.

(2). Problems with feeding and communication.

c. Growth disturbances[26,62,68,69]

(1). Growth disturbances in both longitudinal and cross-sectional directions are seen in the involved limbs of children with hemiplegia.

(2). Disturbances in longitudinal growth were greatest in the radius, followed by the humerus and tibia.

(3). Cross-section area of the involved limb segments was decreased by 16 to 19%.

(4). Limb muscle atrophy increases with age; the causes may include neurotrophic and vascular changes.

d. Respiratory complications/inefficiency.

(1). Lung expansion is often compromised in children with cerebral palsy.

(a). Results from abnormal muscle tone and lack of antigravity control/strength of the muscles of the trunk.

(2). Limited antigravity control and delayed maturation of upright mobility results in the following:

(a). Lack of full development of the normally downward slant of the ribs.

(b). Therefore, the intercostals and/or the diaphragm do not have their full mechanical advantage.

(3). Weakness of the abdominals and lack of balance between the trunk flexors and extensors further limit thoracic strength and expansion.

(4). It is important to assess thoracic movement and muscle strength in functional positions.

(5). Interventions are directed at increasing antigravity control and increasing the tone and strength of the thoracic muscles.

(6). Goal: improve respiratory efficiency.

4. Musculoskeletal assessment

a. Frequent and sequential in the lifelong management of the child with cerebral palsy.

b. Knowledge of the sequences of problems seen in abnormal motor development, and the patterns and types of cerebral palsy, alerts the clinician to those joints and muscles that are significantly at risk for contracture and bony deformity.[70]

c. Mechanisms of deformity

(1). Persistent shortening of a muscle or group of muscles from spasticity without adequate activation of antagonists

(2). Abnormal reflex activity

(3). Weakness

(4). Static positioning

d. Differentiating between primary deforming factors and secondary compensations is vital.

(1). Presurgically

(2). Preventive, ongoing management

(3). Table 41–2 offers a problem-solving process for assessing and managing the musculoskeletal problems

e. Goniometric assessment

(1). Positioning of the child is important.

(a). Minimize the effect of extensor or flexor tone.

(b). Negate the influence of reflexes.

(c). Isolate true passive joint movement.

(2). Move the limb slowly to avoid eliciting a stretch reflex, thereby increasing spasticity.

(3). Document clonus, sustained or unsustained.

(4). Common range of motion deficits, assessment strategies, and management options are depicted in Table 41–2.

f. Gait

(1). An understanding of the determinants of both immature and mature gait gives a basic framework for understanding and evaluating gait dysfunction in children with cerebral palsy.[71]

(2). A review of the current literature highlights the following key points:

(a). EMG studies of gait show:

(i). Less activity in the muscles of children with cerebral palsy; not more, as is sometimes suspected.[72]

(ii). Abnormalities in timing and phasing of muscle contraction, not just a lack of or excess of muscle activity.[73]

(b). There are mechanical changes in spastic muscle fibers.[72]

(i). The increase in tension noted in the plantar flex-

Text continued on page 1251

Table 41-2. MUSCULOSKELETAL MANAGEMENT OF CEREBRAL PALSY

Shoulder: Common Problems and Management Options

Adduction and internal rotation contractures of the shoulder in cerebral palsy can present significant problems in positioning of the extremity in space.[177] Most common surgical correction is a lengthening of pectoralis major tendon and subscapularis lengthening or myotomy.[35,177] Fixed contractures not frequently addressed with soft-tissue release because weakening of capsular structures can result in shoulder instability or dislocation.

Elbow: Common Problems and Management Options

Significant elbow flexion contractures can prevent adequate hand function. Surgical release may be necessary when contractures are > 60°, are exaggerated during activity and interfere with function.[177] Most frequent need is in spastic hemiplegia.[35] Combinations of lengthenings of the biceps tendon, brachialis, and wrist flexor pronator origin can be used.[177] Release of capsule only necessary in severe, long-standing contractures.[177]

Forearm: Common Problems and Management Options

Pronation spasticity and early contracture are common.[177] Posterior subluxation of the radial head often accounts for the fixed deformity, which also limits elbow extension.[35] Pronator teres tenotomy is often the procedure of choice.[35,177] Mild contractures do not require surgical intervention. Indications for both elbow and forearm surgery should be based primarily on hand position and function rather than on elbow position.[35,177-179]

Wrist/Hand: Common Problems and Management Options

Excessive wrist flexion preventing adequate hand grasps and release is the most common reason for surgical intervention at the wrist.[177] According to Bleck,[35] it is quite impossible to offer a complete picture of the options and decisions, and he offered that Zancolli, Goldner, and Swanson[180] did give some guidelines depending on the three most common hand patterns seen in cerebral palsy:

Pattern 1: Mild flexion spasticity, especially of the flexor carpi ulnaris and the finger flexors. Option: Tenotomy of flexor carpi ulnaris and musculoaponeurotic release of the flexor origins.

Pattern 2: If wrist extensors are weak or absent option is to transfer the flexion flexor carpi ulnaris to the extensor carpi radialis brevis.
If finger extension is possible with < 50° of wrist flexion, option is to do a musculoaponeurotic release of flexor origins.
If finger extension is possible only with > 50° wrist flexion option is to do a more extensive release of flexor origins with a pronator teres release.

Pattern 3: Severe flexion of the fingers and inability to extend with full flexion of the wrist option is to do multiple tendon lengthenings.
Improved function is the main criteria for surgical intervention. Physical therapy management is covered in another section of this text.

Common Problems	Possible Causes	Assessment	Physical Therapy Management	Surgical Candidate	Surgical Options
Spine					
1. Exaggerated curvatures: Lordosis Kyphosis 2. Scoliosis	Postural defects, usually flexible; secondary to muscle imbalance, weakness, poor antigravity control, compensation for balance deficits Can become structural; also seen in combination with limitations in range at shoulders, hips	1. Spinal mobility (clinical assessment) A. Passive: Assess with child sitting by passively rotating upper trunk and with child supine or prone by rotating lower trunk while maintaining upper trunk in stable posture[62]	1. Exercise Exercise alone will not prevent progression nor will it correct scoliosis or exaggerated curves;[183] physical therapy management is combination of positioning, orthotic management, patient education, and exercise; exercises	In curves > 40° and certainly > 50°, orthosis not likely to be effective;[35] however, if risk or potential surgical benefit are substantial, surgery is an option in CP; generally, the following reasons in addition to significant curvature (> 40-50°) are indications for corrective	Possible surgical choices in CP include but are not limited to Harrington rod instrumentation (requires postoperative body cast)[35] Other posterior element arthrodeses[35] Anterior spinal fusion and instrumentation

Table continued on following page

1243

Table 41-2. MUSCULOSKELETAL MANAGEMENT OF CEREBRAL PALSY (Continued)

Common Problems	Possible Causes	Assessment	Physical Therapy Management	Surgical Candidate	Surgical Options
		B. Active: Use distance measurements taken by tape measure of changes in bony landmark relationships. Assess anterior and lateral flexion, right and left[35-38,181,182] C. Clinical assessment: Thoracic kyphosis and lumbar lordosis can be estimated by placing a ruler against the midthoracic spine and the sacrum; when significant thoracic kyphosis is suspected, the ruler deviates posteriorly from the perpendicular;[35] the distance between the edge of the ruler and the midlumbar spine is a clinical measure of lordosis (norm no more than 4 cm)[35] 2. Scoliosis screening and clinical assessment A. Posterior view: Drop plumb line from 1st thoracic vertebra or assess visually; note inequality of height of shoulders or pelvis; also note prominence of scapula, rib B. To differentiate structural from flexible scoliosis, child is to flex forward, hips at 90°, upper extremities downward and forward with palms together; asymmetry of thorax is assessed visually; a rib hump	have value in that they can improve posture, general muscle tones, and flexibility,[183] antigravity exercises as needed are indicated for kyphosis and scoliosis; attention to tilt of pelvis and hip flexor tightness is important in management of lordosis 2. Positioning: to prevent progression of curvature 3. Electrotherapy: Use is controversial and of questionable success;[184,185] electrotherapy with surface stimulators to stimulate activation of weak muscles may be of value[185] 4. Orthotics A. TLSO;[35,186-188] in cerebral palsy, orthotics usually used to delay definitive treatment (delay fusion as long as possible because spinal fusion stops growth) but probably do not prevent progression of curvature	surgery for scoliosis in CP: Pain Compromises with sitting or makes sitting painful/uncomfortable 2° to pelvic obliquity Compromise of respiratory function/cardiac function but not where respiratory function is so compromised that surgery is too much of a risk Where function would be improved through surgery[35]	(eg, Dwyer)[189] Spinal fixation with interlaminar wires at each segment attached to 2 semirigid rods laterally (Luque procedure)[190] For further details and surgical options, see chapter on scoliosis

		denotes rotation of thoracic vertebrae to convex side of structural scoliosis.[35] C. Scoliometer:[132] Specially designed inclinometer, which objectively measures angle of trunk rotation; minimum significant rotation justifying referral for orthopedic evaluation is a 5° level of rotation at any level of the spine D. Radiographics: See chapter on scoliosis		

Hip

| Hip subluxation and dislocation | Muscle imbalance and the effect of muscle action on the shape of the femur causing increased coxa valga[191,192]
 Persistent femoral[191–193] anteversion
 Spastic iliopsoas[192]
 Spastic adductors
 Combined spasticity adductors and iliopsoas[91]
 Incidence also directly related to ambulation ability: In child with quadriplegic CP (nonambulatory), lateral subluxation without acetabular dysplasia is often followed by dislocation; children who are weight bearing or household ambulators usually retain the subluxation and acetabular dysplasia and do not progress to dislocation[191] | Spasticity and contracture, especially into hip flexion and adduction
 Femoral anteversion (judged clinically by increased internal rotation as compared with external rotation; judged roentgenographically by a decreased neck shaft angle)[192]
 Often complicated by spastic medial hamstrings
 Clinical signs
 Shortening of one lower extremity in Thomas position
 Shortening accompanied by posture into flexion or flexion with adduction or internal rotation
 Asymmetrical gluteal folds
 Unstable hips often are accompanied by pelvic obliquity[191] | Prevention
 Range of motion
 Positioning to decrease or prevent contracture, especially to preserve hip abduction, external rotation
 Adaptive equipment including seating adaptations
 Weight-bearing program
 Orthotics/splints
 Treatment to decrease overactivity of spastic hip flexors, adductors, internal rotators, and medial hamstrings with simultaneous activation and strengthening of antagonists
 Postoperative PT management:
 Soft-tissue surgery only usually requires no cast; abduction splinting or orthotic may be appropri- | Subluxation
 1. Release or lengthening of unbalanced muscle pull in an effort to prevent dislocation: adductor or iliopsoas myotomy or tenotomy
 2. Often no surgery is indicated: conservative management (PT) used to prevent progression to dislocation
 Dislocation
 Hip subluxation may require soft-tissue release, especially in ambulatory child and to prevent progression to dislocation
 Indications for surgery
 Pain (more often associated with subluxation than dislocation)[192]
 Impaired sitting balance
 To improve perineal care
 To prevent progression of hip deformity (coxa valga)
 To reduce or prevent incidence of fractures of femoral shaft or neck (severe nonambulatory CP)
 To improve functional activity status[192]
 Soft-tissue surgery may be done
 Adductor myotomy, tenotomy, or transfer
 Iliopsoas tenotomy or recession
 Obturator neurectomy (usually anterior branch)
 Soft-tissue surgery only after 5 years age considered to be less successful; bone surgery |

Table continued on following page

Table 41–2. MUSCULOSKELETAL MANAGEMENT OF CEREBRAL PALSY *(Continued)*

Common Problems	Possible Causes	Assessment	Physical Therapy Management	Surgical Candidate	Surgical Options
	Retention of neonatal reflexes[192]	Hip on high side is prone to dislocate[194] Audible click Painful sitting, especially in nonambulatory child Radiographic evidence	ate to maintain position; depending on surgeon and type of surgery, hip spica cast may be used PT postoperative management consists of Positioning to maintain surgical correction Adaptive equipment to maintain surgical correction Weight bearing as ordered		often indicated, which may include the following: Varus derotation subtrochanteric osteotomy to correct excessive femoral anteversion Salter innominate osteotomy, perhaps in combination with femoral osteotomy Iliac osteotomy (*ie*, Pemberton, Chiari) Acetabular augmentation "shelf procedure"
Adduction deformity	Spastic adductors with contracture Medial hamstring spasticity with contracture	Assess hip abduction with extension in supine Phelps-Baker test to try to isolate the medial hamstrings as the possible deforming force[195]	Positioning into abduction Adaptive equipment Abduction orthotics/splints with long-term night use (6–12 months) Treatment to decrease overactivation hip adductors and simultaneously to activate abductors	In the ambulatory child, <20° abduction bilaterally[191] usually clinically accompanied by scissoring In the nonambulatory child, significant contracture accompanied by hygiene concerns or threatening hip stability	Adductor longus tenotomy Adductor origin transfer to ilium Gracilis myotomy often with adductor longus tenotomy Anterior branch obturator neurectomy or intrapelvic obturator neurectomy
Hip flexion deformity	Spastic hip flexors, usually iliopsoas Spastic rectus femoris, usually in combination with spasticity entire quadriceps group[191,196] Combination of flexion/adduction deformity	Thomas test[197] Often unreliable, especially in presence of hamstring spasticity[35] Often unreliable in spastic diplegia[196] Prone hip extension test[40,197] More reliable Rectus femoris stretch test (Ely test)[35] Hip flexion deformity often is accompanied by biomechanical adaptation to the deformity such as Posterior inclination of pelvis Anterior inclination of pelvis Dependent on position of knee[35]	Positioning especially prone Adaptive equipment Orthotics/splints Treatment to decrease overactivation of hip flexors and simultaneously activate/strengthen hip extensors Postoperative management In soft-tissue release alone, usually no cast is used; position to maintain surgical correction with emphasis on prone positioning; weight bearing in upright alignment; activities to activate hip extension	In ambulatory patients, contractures >40° which interfere with posture of hip and knee[40] In nonambulatory patients, significant contractures which threaten hip integrity Some texts continue to say that flexion contracture of 15–20° (Thomas test) is an indication for surgery[191] Clinicians are reminded of unreliability of Thomas test in spasticity;[195–198] Prone hip extension test more accurate in this population[135]	(nonambulatory patients) Iliopsoas tenotomy (nonambulatory patients)[35] Iliopsoas lengthening (ambulatory patients) Iliopsoas recession (ambulatory patients with concomitant hip subluxation) Rectus femoris transfer

Deformity	Mechanism/Etiology	Clinical/Diagnostic Findings	Characteristics	Treatment/Prevention	Surgical
Internal rotation deformity (femoral anteversion)	Main mechanism is thought to be excessive femoral anteversion for age of child possibly biomechanically caused in CP by lack of normal hip extension, which then decreases the torque strains on femur so that age-related derotation cannot occur[35] Contributory influence is from several possibilities: Dysphasic and prolonged activity medial hamstrings[35,199] Spasticity medial hamstring[200] Hamstring contracture	Clinically, increased hip internal rotation as compared with external rotation;[192] where clinically internal rotation is in 70–90° range with external rotation less than 20°[35] Roentgenographically, decreased neck shaft angle[192] CT scan and MRI most effective diagnostic tool[35]	Internal rotation of 70–90° with external rotation <20° Significant scissoring during internal rotation gait	Prevention: Physical therapy to increase active hip extension with hip abduction in attempt to normalize biomechanical forces on femur and thereby facilitate age-related derotation[2 35] Positioning to emphasize hip abduction, extension, and external rotation Decreased spasticity and movement postures into hip flexion, adduction, internal rotation Range of motion; splinting Postoperative management: Use of plaster immobilization dependent on surgeon and type of surgery Generally: Weight bearing as ordered Strengthening especially of hip extension, abduction, and external rotation Gait training and weight shift activities onto externally rotated, abducted LES Avoid excessive rotation or torsion on femur; no passive rotation	Medial hamstring lengthening: tenotomy of semitendinosus and gracilis with lengthening of semimembranosus[194] In older child (7–8 years age), derotation osteotomy either subtrochanteric or supracondylar[35,194,199]

Table continued on following page

Table 41–2. MUSCULOSKELETAL MANAGEMENT OF CEREBRAL PALSY *(Continued)*

Knee

Common Problems	Possible Causes	Assessment	Physical Therapy Management	Surgical Candidate	Surgical Options
Flexion deformity: most common knee deformity in cerebral palsy	Fixed flexion deformity Inability to achieve full knee extension passively with hips/knees extended (supine) Cause is contracture of posterior joint capsule usually secondary to long-standing hamstring contractures[201] Contracted hamstrings with or without fixed knee flexion contracture[201] Contracture of hip flexors, which pulls proximal end femur into flexion Triceps surae: contracture or weakness Coactivation of spastic quadriceps and hamstrings[194] Frequent sitting, especially sitting in posterior pelvic tilt	Hamstring range of motion: Measure popliteal angle with hip at 90° (normal is <20°)[2] Check posterior capsule with hip/knee extended When assessing the dynamic causes of knee flexion or crouch gait, assess the hip flexors, triceps surae, rectus femoris, and hamstrings as a group[201] Dynamic EMG	Prevention: Range of motion Positioning especially with hip flexed, knee extended with pelvis in neutral Serial casting[202] Night splints or use of long leg immobilizers as night splints and for long sit positioning Therapy to balance strength and activity of hamstrings and quadriceps Attention to effect of hip and ankle position on knee position; weakened triceps surae will increase crouch in stance; hip flexion with inadequate hip extension/pelvic control will increase crouch in stance In absence of fixed knee contracture floor reaction, AFOs can be effective to increase the extensor moment at knee Postoperative PT management After surgery, child often placed in long leg casts or below-knee casts or immobilizers with AFO, depending on surgeon's preference	Depending on surgeon and text: Fixed flexion deformity >15° with hip in extension[35] Knee flexion deformity >15° during stance[35] Popliteal angle >30°[194]	Fractional lengthening of hamstrings is most common current surgical option[35,204] For fixed deformity, hamstring lengthening with posterior capsulotomy[35]

Foot/Ankle

Equinus: most common static and dynamic deformity in children with cerebral palsy;[194] seen alone or in combination with varus or valgus; hemiplegia typically produces equinus or equinovarus; diplegia and quadriplegia more commonly produce equinus or equinovalgus[154,204]

Probably from premature or prolonged activity of either gastrocnemius or soleus[194,205]

Fixed deformity is usually due to position and gravity with limited voluntary movement control[206]

Dynamic deformity results from contraction of muscle in response to abnormal neural control; caused by spasticity and varies with posture[206]

Silverskiold test for gastrocnemus versus soleus contracture[35]

Often unreliable because flexing the knee also relaxes the soleus as well as the gastrocnemius[154]

Differentiated from idiopathic toe walking:

Children with CP usually present with dynamic equinus, heel cord contractures, and hamstring

Main Treatment Goals

Maintain full length hamstrings especially with hip flexed, pelvis in neutral; avoid posterior pelvic tilt

Standing activities to activate knee and hip extension

Strengthening activities for hip and knee extension

Gait training and weight-shifting activities with neutral pelvis, hip extension and abduction, knee in extension; gait training with graded knee flexion

Attempt to balance activity of quadriceps and hamstrings during movement[203]

Preventive:

Manual stretching, ROM

Serial casting

Inhibitive casting[208,209]

AFO (most preferred for dynamic equinus)

Casting also helpful to negate dynamic equinus so therapist can assess effect of hip and knee as the deforming force

Treatment to activate and strengthen dorsi-

General indications for surgery:

Increasing deformity and lack of functional improvement in spite of adequate therapy[206]

Contracture of triceps surae that will not allow foot to be passively dorsiflexed to neutral while being held in supination with knee extended[194]

Interference with functional weight bearing

Fractional hamstring lengthening may resolve dynamic equinas[35]

Achilles tendon lengthening (cast should be only to neutral to avoid over-correction, which could predispose to a calcaneus deformity)[194,207–210]

Table continued on following page

Table 41-2. MUSCULOSKELETAL MANAGEMENT OF CEREBRAL PALSY *(Continued)*

Common Problems	Possible Causes	Assessment	Physical Therapy Management	Surgical Candidate	Surgical Options
	Children with CP often present with mixed deformity: combination fixed and dynamic[206]	tightness with sustained knee flexion at terminal stance; children with idiopathic toe walking may present with dynamic equinus, heel cord contractures, but usually minimal or no hamstring tightness, and, more often than not, knee extension is present in stance[207]	flexion during functional activity and during balance activities Post-Operative Therapy Weight bearing may be limited while in casts—sometimes short leg walking casts (surgeon preference) Maintain new range of motion into dorsiflexion Treatment to activate and strengthen dorsiflexion with appropriate activation of triceps surae during stance, weight shift and ambulation with special attention to alternating dorsiflexion or plantarflexion appropriately during gait cycle Electrotherapy to activate dorsiflexion if excessively weak		
Foot Spastic pes valgus Equinus and eversion; inclination of calcaneus and abduction of midfoot, which results in a prominence of head of talus medially[35] Most common in spastic diplegia[35]	Major deforming force probably is spastic peroneal[35] Hyperactive peroneal muscles with strong posterior tibialis[211] Hyperactive peroneals with weak posterior tibialis[211] Hyperactive extensor digitorum longus[212] Persistent fetal medial deviation of talus[35] Variations in ligamentous laxity among children may account for early development of pes valgus[35] Contributing factor may be gastrocnemius–soleus contracture[35]	Often flexible even until adolescence: Until time of fixed changes, foot can be passively corrected by stabilizing subtalar joint and plantar flexing the ankle with inversion of foot[35] Lateral radiographs in stance will show greater than normal plantar flexion of talus and varying degrees of loss of dorsiflexion of calcaneus[35] Antero/posterior radiograph in weight bearing[35]	Preventive: Orthotic/splint management: AFO Supramalleolar ankle/foot splint Obvious and severe pes valgus can only be corrected surgically	Fixed deformity documented by radiographs	Peroneal tendon transfer or lengthening Subtalar arthrodesis Calcaneal osteotomy Triple arthrodesis Peroneal and posterior tibialis transfers or lengthenings Try to delay surgery until 7 years when there is some skeletal maturity but not to delay to where deformity is rigid[35]

Abbreviations: AFO = ankle-foot orthosis; CP = cerebral palsy; CT = computed tomography; EMG = electromyography; MRI = magnetic resonance imaging; PT = physical therapy; ROM = range of motion.

ors after initial contact is due to passive mechanical stretching of the triceps surae.

(ii). It is not because of an increased activity level in the muscle itself.

(c). Olney[74] contended that defect of the plantar flexors is one of the most important mechanical deficiencies in gait of the child with cerebral palsy.

(i). Many of the other characteristic features of gait disturbances result from biomechanical and musculoskeletal compensations for this primary defect.

(ii). An inadequate force moment is generated by weak plantar flexors, decreasing the amount of work that can be done through the gait cycle.

(iii). Intervention: exercises to strengthen the plantar flexors without stimulating adverse muscle activity in other parts of the body.

(d). Movement, including gait, is characterized by coactivation or reciprocal excitation instead of smooth reciprocal inhibition.

(i). There is evidence of reflex irradiation and reciprocal excitation in the impaired ambulation in children with cerebral palsy.[73]

g. Presurgical assessment

(1). The planning and timing of surgical procedures must be appropriate for the overall management of the child.

(2). Factors to be considered include the following:

(a). Growth and development stages.

(b). Psychosocial concerns.

(c). Educational timing.

(d). The primary musculoskeletal impairment.

(3). Presurgical planning includes the following:

(a). Family education.

(b). School consultation.

(c). Postsurgical equipment and orthotic needs.

(4). Table 41–2 can be used as a general guideline for assessing the common impairments seen in cerebral palsy.

(a). Careful analysis of one joint at a time and one motion at a time.

(b). Analysis of movement patterns, gait, and transitional movement.

(c). Determination of the primary deforming force.

(i). Occasionally, it may be difficult to elucidate which force is most deforming or out of phase.

(ii). Therefore, EMG gait analysis can be valuable to help define the pathomechanics of the gait disturbance and objectively delineate the best surgical choice.[71]

5. Orthotic management

a. Determinaton of the appropriate orthotic.[75]

(1). Assessment of range of motion, joint stability and alignment, and function.

(2). The anticipated effects of an orthotic on both mobility and stability.

b. The use of low-temperature plastic splints.[75]

(1). The exact orthotic needed has not been determined.

(2). The child is very young.

(3). Assessment of the effect of an orthosis on the gait and function of a child.

(4). Can be fabricated by a therapist and thus less expensive.

(5). Easily modified according to the evolving needs of the child.

c. Orthotics commonly used in children with cerebral palsy.

(1). Molded ankle foot orthosis (MAFO) is most common.

(a). For control of the following:

(i). Flexible, functional equinus.

(ii). Genu recurvatum that occurs during stance secondary to a flexible equinus.

(iii). Flexible pes valgus, thereby stabilizing foot position.

(b). Modifications within the MAFO
  (i). Extension of the footplate to the end of the toes to inhibit toe flexion or clawing.
  (ii). Footplate raised slightly to decrease hypertonus.
  (iii). Footplate ends behind the metatarsal heads to permit a smooth toe off during gait.
(2). Articulating ankle–foot orthosis.
  (a). Indicated when a child requires a plantar flexion stop with some degree of movement desired.
  (b). Limitation of plantar flexion to decrease gastrocnemius and soleus hypertonus.
  (c). Remaining ankle musculature can still be activated and strengthened.
(3). Anterior shell ankle–foot orthosis: floor reaction ankle–foot orthosis.
  (a). Use is indicated when active knee extension cannot be maintained in stance.
  (b). Contraindicated when full passive knee extension is not available in stance with the foot and ankle in neutral alignment.
(4). Supramalleolar ankle–foot orthosis
  (a). This orthosis provides less support than a MAFO.
  (b). Malleoli and hindfoot support.
(5). Shoe orthotics
  (a). Indicated to maintain the calcaneus, subtatar, and metatarsal joints in alignment.[62]
  (b). Contraindicated when isolated control of the knee and ankle is not present.

B. Congenital hypotonia

1. Definition: clinical presentation of the "floppy baby," characterized by poverty of movement, reduction in muscle tone, and an assumption of abnormal postures.[76]
  a. Three main subgroups
  b. Characteristics of each group are outlined in Table 41–3 in order for the clinician to make appropriate referrals for

Table 41–3. CHARACTERISTICS OF CONGENITAL HYPOTONIA

Suprasegmental Factors	Benign	Prader-Willi Syndrome
Also termed "cerebral hypotonia"	Classically "floppy baby"	"Floppy" at birth
Brain abnormalities	Onset infantile period	Low birth weight
Associated with history of perinatal hypoxia	Hypermobility of joints	Significant neonatal feeding difficulties
DTRs: sometimes absent but often brisk	Uniform delay of motor milestones	Striking weight gain at age 3 years
Mental function delay as well as motor delay	DTRs depressed or absent	Small hands and feet
Muscle biopsy shows selective atrophy of Type 2 fibers	Muscle biopsy normal	Characteristic facial features almond shaped eyes frequent strabismus
	Abnormal muscle tone only finding	
	Good prognosis for independence	Hypogonadism; often undescended testicles
		Mental retardation
		Short stature, bone age retarded
		Hypothalamic dysfunction or abnormality in growth hormone

Abbreviation: DTR = deep tendon reflex.

further testing and to develop the physical therapy program.
2. Musculoskeletal impairments
  a. Contracture formation secondary to immobility, low muscle tone, weakness, habitual positioning.
  b. Associated problems include hip dislocation, kyphosis, scoliosis, foot deformities.
  c. Limited mobility: may see delays with motor skills.
3. Physical therapy management[77]
  a. Improve muscle tone and strength, especially antigravity.
  b. Facilitate attainment of developmental skills.
  c. Prevent contracture and deformity through use of appropriate splinting and positioning aids.

C. Down's syndrome

1. Definition: a common chromosomal disorder with 47 chromosomes instead of 46,

resulting in neuropathology, hypotonia, musculoskeletal differences, and, at times, sensory and/or cardiopulmonary anomalies.[78]

2. Musculoskeletal impairments
   a. Linear growth deficits
      (1). Velocity of growth in stature shows the greatest deficiency between 6 and 24 months of age.[79-81]
      (2). Major deficiency in stature is due to leg-length reduction.[82]
      (3). Metacarpal bones and phalanges are 10 to 30% shorter.
   b. Ligamentous laxity
      (1). Probably caused by a collagen deficit.
      (2). Results in pes planus, patellar instability, scoliosis.[79,83]
   c. Atlantoaxial instability caused by increased laxity of transverse ligaments between the atlas and odontoid process.
      (1). Diagnostic indicator by radiograph is a distance of 5 mm or more between the posteoinferior aspect of the anterior arch of the atlas and the adjacent anterior surface of the odontoid process.[79]
      (2). Incidence is 12 to 20% in persons with Down's syndrome.[84]
      (3). Symptomatic when joint interval is 6 to 10 mm.
         (a). Pyramidal tract signs
         (b). Hyper-reflexias
            (i). Positive Babinski sign
            (ii). Ankle clonus
         (c). Muscle weakness
         (d). Abnormal gait
         (e). Limitation of cervical range of motion with torticollis
         (f). Pain
      (4). Follow with radiographs at 2 years of age, middle childhood, adolescence, and adulthood.
      (5). Treatment of instability by surgical fusion.
      (6). Contact sports, gymnastics, diving, and any activity that can lead to cervical spine injury are contraindicated.[85,86]
   d. Muscle variations that may be present are:[87]
      (1). Absent palmarus longus.
      (2). Extra supernumerary forearm flexors
      (3). Lack of differentiation of distinct muscle bellies for zygomaticus major and minor and levator labii superior.

   e. Weakness of neck and trunk antigravity musculature.
   f. Acetabular dysplasia[83]
      (1). Widening or flaring of iliac wings
      (2). Flattening of roof of acetabulum
      (3). Long, tapered ischia, resulting in decreased acetabular and iliac angles
3. Physical therapy management
   a. Improve strength, especially antigravity.
   b. Facilitate attainment of developmental skills
   c. Appropriate splinting or orthotic intervention
   d. Refer for orthopedic assessment as needed.

D. Muscular dystrophies

1. Definition: generally defined as a familial disease characterized by progressive atrophy and wasting of muscles.[88]
   a. There may be differing ages of onset and different courses of progression.
   b. Some of the congenital dystrophies are not considered progressive.
2. Knowledge of the differences and patterns of weakness among the muscular dystrophies that affect children and understanding of the course of the specific disorder will help to direct the physical therapy management (Table 41–4)
3. Musculoskeletal impairments[76]
   a. Muscle weakness
      (1). Atrophy
      (2). Asymmetrical muscle development
      (3). Primary involvement of neck and proximal musculature
      (4). Contributes to feeding difficulties and dysphagia
   b. Contractures
      (1). Joints involved are dependent on the pattern of muscle weakness.
      (2). At risk in the child with Duchenne's muscular dystrophy are the following:
         (a). Hip flexors
         (b). Iliotibial band
         (c). Knee flexors
         (d). Ankle plantar flexors
      (3). Shoulder and scapular limitations are found in the child with fascioscapulohumeral dystrophy.
   c. Spinal deformities
      (1). Scoliosis
      (2). Lordosis

Table 41–4. PROGRESSIVE MUSCULAR DYSTROPHIES AND THEIR CHARACTERISTIC PATTERNS OF WEAKNESS

Duchenne's	Becker's	Fascioscapulohumeral	Limb Girdle	Congenital
Proximal to distal Hypertrophy	Proximal to distal Hypertrophy	Proximal to distal Initially face and shoulder girdle	Proximal to distal Generalized	Varied according to type Significant weakness of neck and trunk musculature
Gastrocnemius, deltoid, infraspinous Rapid progression	Gastrocnemius Slow progression	Eventually pelvis Early onset (infantile) = rapid progression	Early onset = rapid progression	Severe hypotonia Spinal deformities

4. Physical therapy management[89,90]
   a. Assessment
      (1). Serial strength assessment to monitor the following:[91]
         (a). Progression of disease
         (b). Influence of strength on functional ability
         (c). Effectiveness of medical treatment and physical therapy
      (2). Serial goniometric assessments to enhance prevention of contractures.[89,92]
   b. Goals of physical therapy treatment
      (1). Prevention of deformity and contracture.
         (a). Anticipate progression pattern and rate.
      (b). Appropriate range of motion and strengthening activities.
      (c). Additional use of positioning, splinting, orthotics, and adaptive equipment.
      (2). Energy conservation techniques as appropriate.
      (3). Maintain functional abilities with support of orthotics and equipment.
      (4). Family education.
5. Medical treatment may include steroids (prednisone)
   a. Positive effect on muscle strength.
   b. Awareness of the effect of steroids on bone density.[93]

IV. Juvenile Rheumatoid Arthritis (JRA) and Other Systemic Disease Processes

A. Cause, incidence, and classification[94,95]

1. JRA is the most common type of chronic arthritis in children.
2. There are three main subtypes, which are outlined in Table 41–5.
   a. The importance of subdividing these groups relates to their differing complications and prognosis.[95]
   b. The common feature is that they produce a destructive disease and deformity in a growing skeleton.

B. Musculoskeletal impairments[95–98]

1. Joints
   a. Inflammation with loss of motion.
      (1). Increased amounts of synovial fluid and thickening of synovial tissues.[96]
      (2). Joint is edematous and warm to the touch.
   b. Morning stiffness
      (1). Joints tend to "gel" during periods of inactivity.
   c. Direct damage to joint structures
      (1). Loss of articular cartilage.
      (2). Bone destruction and collapse.
      (3). Adhesions, osteophytes, bone spurs.
      (4). Avascular necrosis is sometimes present.[95]
   d. Most commonly affected joints[97]
      (1). Knee and ankle more than hip.
      (2). Wrist and fingers more than elbow and shoulder.

Table 41-5. TYPES OF ONSET OF JUVENILE RHEUMATOID ARTHRITIS*

	Polyarthritis	Oligoarthritis	Systemic Disease
Relative frequency	40%	50%	10%
Number of joints involved	≥5	≤4	Variable
Sex ratio (F:M)	2:1	6:1	1:1
Extra-articular involvement	Moderate	Not prominent	Prominent
Chronic uveitis	5%	20%	Rare
Seropositivity			
Rheumatoid factors	10%	Rare	Rare
Antinuclear antibodies	40%	75%†	10%
Clinical course	Systemic disease generally mild; articular involvement often unremitting	Systemic disease absent; major cause of morbidity is uveitis	Systemic disease often self-limited; arthritis chronic and destructive in 50%
Prognosis	Moderately good	Excellent	Moderate

* From Cassidy JT. Juvenile rheumatoid arthritis. In Kelley WN *et al.* (eds): *Textbook of Rheumatology.* 3rd ed. Philadelphia, W. B. Saunders Company, 1989, p 1291. Used with permission.

† In girls with uveitis.

(3). Cervical spine: limitation of extension, rotation, and lateral flexion may be seen.

2. Muscles
   a. Disuse atrophy of muscles that surround the affected joint leaves joints less protected from external forces.
   b. Muscle tightness contributes to joint contractures.
      (1). Tensor fascia lata
      (2). Hamstrings
      (3). Gastrocnemius
3. Skeleton
   a. Immature skeletal system is susceptible to the abnormal forces; its development may be permanently altered.
   b. Postural deformities from muscle imbalance and abnormal weight bearing.
      (1). Scoliosis, kyphosis, torticollis, cervical lordosis
      (2). Genu valgum
      (3). Valgus and varus ankle deformities
   c. Growth disturbances
      (1). Epiphyseal plates are open in children.
      (2). Overgrowth of femur or tibia caused by increased blood flow near the knee joint results in leg-length discrepancy.[95]
      (3). Limb shortening when joint destruction causes closure of an adjacent epiphysis.[95]

C. Functional limitations

1. Gait deviations[99]

   a. Decreased velocity, cadence, and stride length.
   b. Anterior pelvic decreased throughout the gait cycle.
   c. Lack of hip extension and ankle plantar flexion at toe off.
   d. May be due to one or a combination of impairments such as contractures, weakness, and pain.
2. Activities of daily living (ADLs)
3. Functional mobility

D. Assessment: unique factors to be considered for juvenile rheumatoid arthritis

1. Cervical spine range of motion: use active motion only, with manual stabilization of shoulders.
2. Muscle examination
   a. Modify to allow for inflammation and pain.
   b. Resistance only when pain allows.
   c. Break test with isometrics.
   d. Girth measurements of thigh and calf.
   e. Observation of muscle atrophy.
3. Standardized tests to assess ADL skills
   a. Modified version of the adult Arthritis Impact Measurement Scales (AIMS)[100]
   b. Juvenile Arthritis Functional Assessment Scale[101]

E. Management

1. Medical management focuses on the use of anti-inflammatory agents to suppress joint inflammation.[94-96]

2. Physical therapy
  a. Goals
    (1). Maintain or increase range of motion
    (2). Maintain or increase strength
    (3). Prevention of deformity
    (4). Independence in ADL and mobility
    (5). Control of pain
  b. The need for daily therapeutic management makes the implementation of a home program essential.
    (1). Simple, realistic, and accommodating to family's schedule.
    (2). Therapist monitors and revises as needed.
  c. Progression
    (1). Individualized for each child because of the nature of the phases of the disease.
    (2). Acute phase
      (a). Resting in therapeutic positions
      (b). Encourage ADLs
      (c). Application of heat for relief of swelling/pain
    (3). Subacute phase (under medical control)
      (a). Moderate exercise
      (b). Positioning
      (c). Heat for morning stiffness
      (d). Avoid fatigue and exacerbation of symptoms
    (4). Chronic phase
      (a). Progressive resistive exercise
      (b). Increase in activity level
      (c). General conditioning and recreational activities
  d. Range of motion
    (1). All joints should be moved through their available range at least once a day.
    (2). Stretching can be done during the subacute/chronic phases.
    (3). Prevention of flexion contractures in lower extremities (LEs)
      (a). Daily positioning program of prone for 20 minutes.[97,98]
    (4). May allow joints to fuse in functional positions.
    (5). Vary positions frequently throughout the day.
    (6). Sleep without a pillow to prevent cervical flexion.
  e. Strength
    (1). Focus on antigravity muscles, particularly the LE stabilizers, which function during gait.
    (2). Isometrics recommended
      (a). Minimized pain
      (b). Protect damaged joints
    (3). Play activities
      (a). Bike riding
      (b). Aquatics
  f. Use of modalities to ease joint symptoms.
    (1). Moist heat in form of tub, whirlpool, hot packs, swimming.
    (2). Retention of body heat with appropriate clothing.
    (3). Cold during the acute phase.
    (4). Deep heat (ultrasound or diathermy) is contraindicated.
      (a). Potential increase of inflammation.
      (b). Unknown effect on the epiphyseal plate.
  g. Gait training
    (1). Seek to minimize or eliminate observed deviations.[102]
    (2). Postural training, weight-bearing activities.
    (3). Use of assistive devices.
  h. ADLs
    (1). Modification of environment through the use of assistive devices, such as dressing stick and adaptive utensils.
    (2). Principles of joint protection.
      (a). Reduce physical and mechanical stress on inflamed joints.
      (b). Use large joints rather than small joints.
  i. The use of splints and orthotics is dependent on the therapeutic goal and the phase of the disease.[97,98]
    (1). Resting splint
      (a). Used in the acute phase to rest inflamed joint.
      (b). Maintained in a functional position.
      (c). Usually worn during sleep.
    (2). Corrective splint
      (a). Serial and/or dynamic splinting.
      (b). Used to improve range of motion
      (c). Able to apply a prolonged stretch in a position of proper alignment.
    (3). Functional splints or orthoses.
      (a). Support and protect a joint during ADL.

(b). MAFOs or shoe inserts.
(c). Wrist splint.
3. Surgical interventions[95,102]
  a. Soft-tissue releases
    (1). Performed if joint integrity is present.
    (2). Adductor and psoas muscle tenotomics.
      (a). Increase in range of motion and relief of pain.
    (3). Hamstring muscle releases.
      (a). Perform early to prevent contractures and subluxation of knee joint.
  b. Arthroplasty
    (1). Hip
      (a). Marked functional impairment or severe disabling pain.
      (b). Component wear not a significant problem because of small stature of children with JRA.
    (2). Knee
      (a). Older children
      (b). Preservation of ambulation
      (c). Effective in reducing pain and increasing functional mobility
  c. Postoperative rehabilitation is extensive.

(1). Functional range of motion.
(2). Positioning after hip arthroplasty.
(3). Strengthening
  (a). Disuse atrophy is present.
  (b). Osteoporosis.
(4). Gait training.

F. Other systemic disorders

There are a number of other systemic rheumatic disorders in children.

1. Examples: ankylosing spondylitis, dermatomyositis, scleroderma.
  a. Each has unique characteristics.
  b. Overall joint, muscle, and skeletal impairments are present.
2. The joint complications of hemophilia also result in musculoskeletal impairments similar to those described for JRA.
3. The treatment principles described for the child with JRA are applicable to these diseases.
  a. However, it is crucial to be aware of the characteristic problems manifested in each individual.
  b. Intervention is modified according to assessment findings.

V. Congenital Anomalies

Classification of congenital anomalies by their pathology and time of occurrence provides the clinician with a model for understanding and, therefore, assists in evaluation and management. Congenital anomalies can be subdivided into a classification system as follows: (1) malformations, (2) disruptions, (3) dysplasias, and (4) deformations.[2]

A. Malformations

A defect of tissue, organ, or larger region of the body occurring when normal morphogenesis is interrupted; malformations are often genetic in origin and are present from the time of organogenesis.[2]

1. Myelodysplasia
  a. Definition: a complex congenital anomaly that primarily affects the nervous system and secondarily affects the musculoskeletal and urologic systems.[103]

  b. A general term encompassing a variety of neural tube defects.[104]
    (1). Spina bifida occulta: vertebral defect resulting from failure of the two halves of the vertebral arch to fuse.
    (2). Spina bifida cystica: protrusion of the spinal cord and/or meninges through the defect in the vertebral arch.
      (a). Meningocele
        (i). Protrusion of the meninges and cerebrospinal fluid (CSF)
        (ii). Spinal cord and spinal roots remain in normal position in the vertebral canal.
        (iii). May be spinal cord anomalies.
      (b). Myelomeningocele
        (i). Protrusion of the spinal

cord, nerve roots, meninges, and CSF.

(ii). Marked neurological damage at the level and caudal to the lesion.

c. Musculoskeletal impairments

(1). Spinal deformities present in 90% of children with myelomeningocele.[105]

(a). May be caused by structural defects of the vertebral bodies, muscle imbalance, and asymmetrical postures.[105,106]

(b). Kyphosis

(i). By early adolescence, just over one third of patients have kyphotic curves greater than 65 degrees.[107]

(ii). Can severely limit sitting and ambulation abilities, lead to skin ulcerations, and impair respiratory function.

(c). Scoliosis

(i). One percent of children with thoracic-level lesion have a scoliosis of greater than 30 degrees at birth and eventually exhibit the greatest increase in severity of scoliosis.[107]

(ii). May interfere with sitting balance and ambulation potential, lead to skin ulcerations, and affect respiratory function.

(d). Lordosis develops as a secondary impairment to hip flexion contractures or weak hip extensors.[108]

(2). Hip deformities may occur as the result of muscle imbalances and/or dysplasia of the acetabulum, femoral head, or femoral neck.

(a). Adduction contracture

(i). Occurs with spasticity of the hip adductor musculature.

(ii). Higher level lumbar lesions

(a). Result in flaccid or weak hip abductor and hip extensor musculature.

(b). Unopposed hip adductor muscle action.

(iii). Unilateral adduction contracture produces pelvic obliquity with resultant hip subluxation or dislocation and possible scoliosis.

(b). Flexion contracture

(i). High lumbar/thoracic-level lesions

(a). Unopposed action of the hip flexors.

(b). Positioning in sitting or supine with legs flexed for extended periods of time.

(ii). Can interfere with bracing and ambulation.

(iii). May cause increased pelvic tilt with excessive lumbar lordosis.[109]

(iv). May be associated with knee flexion contractures.[105]

(c). Subluxation and dislocation may be the result of several factors.[105]

(i). Congenital, teratological, resulting from a dysplastic acetabulum and/or femoral head.

(ii). Paralytic, resulting from muscle imbalance.

(3). Knee deformities are most often seen in children with high lumbar and thoracic lesions.[109]

(a). May occur as result of muscle imbalances and static postures.

(b). Flexion contracture

(i). Supine lying with legs in frog-legged posture.

(ii). Sitting in wheelchair for extended periods of time.

(iii). Crouched stance posture as result of weak ankle plantar flexors.

(iv). Hamstring spasticity accompanying tethered cord syndrome.

(c). Extension contracture

(i). Children born with breech presentation, often associated with knee recurvatum.[110]

(ii). Fibrosis of quadriceps mechanism.

(iii). Muscle imbalance with quadriceps overpowering hamstring musculature.

(d). Genu valgus
   (i). High lumbar lesion
   (ii). Contracture of iliotibial band
   (iii). May interfere with fitting of orthotics if severe

(4). Foot and ankle deformities
   (a). May be congenital as a result of intrauterine positioning and paralysis.
   (b). May be acquired, resulting from muscle imbalances, spasticity, and the influence of positioning, gravity, and growth.
   (c). Common deformities include clubfoot, equinus, equinovarus, calcaneovalgus, and a vertical talus.

(5). Pathological fractures
   (a). Occur in 20% of children with thoracic and high lumbar lesions.[108,111]
   (b). Diminished properties of bone are seen, which could explain the cause of pathological fractures.[112]
      (i). Decreases in square area, cortical thickness, and circumference of bones, which indicate bone thinning and atrophy.
      (ii). Decreased numbers of haversian systems and bone remodeling cavities indicate an increased amount of osteoid tissue.
   (c). Prolonged immobilization after casting increases incidence of fractures.[113]
   (d). Ambulatory children have higher bone densities than nonambulators.[114]

d. Management of musculoskeletal impairments
(1). Spinal deformities
   (a). Goal of treatment is to slow or limit progression of the deformity, prevent skin breakdown, and improve functional posture for sitting or standing activities.
   (b). Orthotics
      (i). Management of kyphosis

through use of orthotics is not feasible secondary to skin breakdown and lack of control of the progression of the deformity.[103,105,108,115]
      (ii). Two conflicting viewpoints regarding the use of orthotics with scoliosis: orthotics may be beneficial in limiting or slowing the progression of a scoliosis and are indicated if curve is greater than 20 degrees;[105,108,109] orthotics to limit scoliosis may be incorporated into the child's bracing system for ambulation or standing and for positioning when seated; others state that an orthotic has little role in scoliosis secondary to the inability to halt progression of a curve and the difficulty of maintaining pressure over insensitive skin.[103]
   (c). Surgical
      (i). Kyphectomy and anterior and/or posterior fusion with internal fixation;[108,109,115,116] when performed on a subject younger than 3 years, will preserve spinal length.[108,115]
      (ii). Sufficient stabilization to control or correct scoliosis is best achieved with anterior and posterior spinal fusion.[117]

(2). Hip subluxation/dislocation
   (a). Goal of treatment is a level pelvis and free motion of the hips.[118]
   (b). Infants with hip subluxations or dislocations are generally not treated with abduction splints such as a Pavlik harness or Frejka pillow; hip flexor and iliotibial band tightness may develop.[109,110]
   (c). Complications of hip-reduction surgery include infection, pathological fractures, skin ulceration, loss of range of motion,

decrease in function, and failure to maintain relocation of the hip.[109,117,118]

(3). Joint contractures
  (a). Range of motion exercises
  (b). Positioning
    (i). Alternatives to supine or prone lying with lower extremities in frog-legged posture and periods of prolonged sitting.
    (ii). Prone or supine lying with towel rolls to limit hip abduction and external rotation.
    (iii). If hip flexion contractures of greater than 20 degrees or greater are present, prone lying may accentuate a lordosis.
    (iv). Standing with the use of orthotics to maintain lower extremity joint mobility.[119]
  (c). Serial casting
    (i). Not recommended for children with impaired sensation secondary to possibility of skin breakdown.
    (ii). Neuropathic fractures may occur after immobilization with casts.[113]
    (iii). Indicated for initial treatment of a clubfoot deformity.
  (d). Splinting
    (i). Fabrication of splints from low-temperature materials for prevention or limitation of joint contractures.
    (ii). Knee immobilizers used at night for children who tend to sleep in excessive hip and knee flexion.
  (e). Surgical correction of contractures that are limiting function or causing postural deformities.
    (i). Hip flexion contractures of 25 to 30 degrees or greater as a result of interference with orthotic fit and ambulation.[109]
    (ii). Hip adduction contractures causing hip subluxation, pelvic obliquity, and asymmetrical trunk posture.[105]
    (iii). Knee flexion contractures greater than 25 degrees;[109] ambulation with knee flexion weakens the strength of the quadriceps.[120]
    (iv). Foot deformities that either are present at birth or develop over time;[109,110] it is important to maintain foot position after surgery through the use of orthotics.

(4). Pathological fractures
  (a). Surgical reduction kept to minimum.
  (b). Immobilization should be well padded
  (c). Initiate weight bearing as soon as fracture is stable.

e. Functional limitations
  (1). Mobility is impaired secondary to paralysis at and below the level of the lesion.
    (a). Related to the level of the lesion and muscle strength and function.[121]
    (b). Infants and toddlers may use rolling, crawling on their belly, or scooting on their bottom as means of mobility.
    (c). Assistive devices are available as alternate means of mobility.
      (i). Prone carts
      (ii). Scooter boards
      (iii). Hand-propelled carts
      (iv). Toddler-size wheelchairs
    (d). Use of varied mobility methods increases position changes and possible prevention of joint contractures.

  (2). Ambulation
    (a). Ambulation and standing may be achieved with a variety of orthotic devices ranging from foot orthosis, thoracic–hip–knee–ankle–foot orthosis to parapodiums and standing frames (Fig. 41–4).
    (b). School-aged children with low lumbar and sacral lesions are usually community ambulators.[122]
    (c). Most school-aged children with

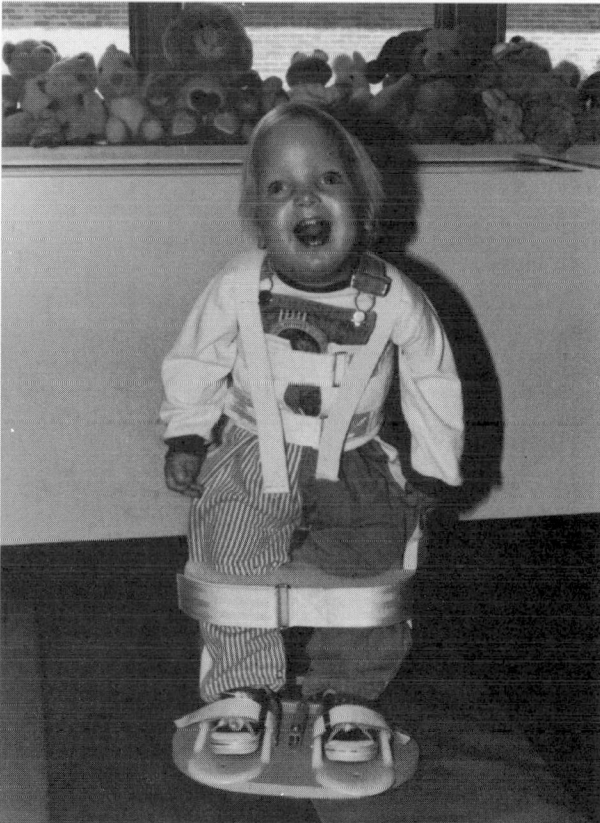

FIGURE 41–4   Standing with a parapodium.

thoracic and high lumbar lesions are not ambulatory.[121,122]

(d). High-energy expenditure and musculoskeletal impairments contribute to limited ambulation as children age.[118,121,123–125]

(e). Physical therapy provides gait training, transfer training, and parent and school instruction for ambulation and standing activities.

2. Longitudinal limb deficiencies

a. A reduction or absence of an element or elements within the long axis of the limb.

(1). Normal skeletal elements may be present distal to the affected bones.

(2). Described by naming the bones affected in a proximal to distal sequence and stating whether each affected bone is totally or partially absent[126] (Fig. 41–5).

b. Musculoskeletal impairments

(1). Occurs as a partial or total deficiency of a long bone.

(2). Abnormal or dysplastic structure of nearby joints.

(3). Associated deficiencies of soft tissue.

c. Common presentations

(1). Proximal femoral focal deficiency (PFFD)[127,128]

(a). Includes absence or hypoplasia of the proximal femur with varying degrees of involvement of the acetabulum, femoral head, patella tibia, and fibula.

(b). Shortened thigh, which is held in flexion, abduction, and external rotation.

(c). Hip and knee flexion contracture.

(d). Severe leg-length discrepancy, with the foot often at the level of the opposite knee.

(e). Instability of knee joint secondary to absent or deficient cruciate ligaments.

(f). Total longitudinal deficiency of the fibula is frequently associated.

(2). Total longitudinal deficiency of the fibula[129]

(a). Absence of the fibula, tibia may be bowed, and the distal epiphysis of the tibia may be abnormal.

(b). Other possible sequelae

(i). Shortening of femur

(ii). Absence of lateral rays, metatarsals, and tarsals.

(iii). Deficiency of soft tissue.

(c). With unilateral involvement, progressive limb-length discrepancy develops because of abnormal distal epiphysis of tibia.

(3). Longitudinal deficiency of the radius.[130]

(a). Partial or complete absence of radius.

(b). Hand often positioned in severe radial deviation.

(c). Absent or dysplastic thumb.

(d). Radial digits are often stiff with limited active flexion.

d. Management of musculoskeletal impairments

(1). Goal: to improve the child's functional ability

(2). Upper extremity

(a). Splinting

(i). To decrease elbow flexion

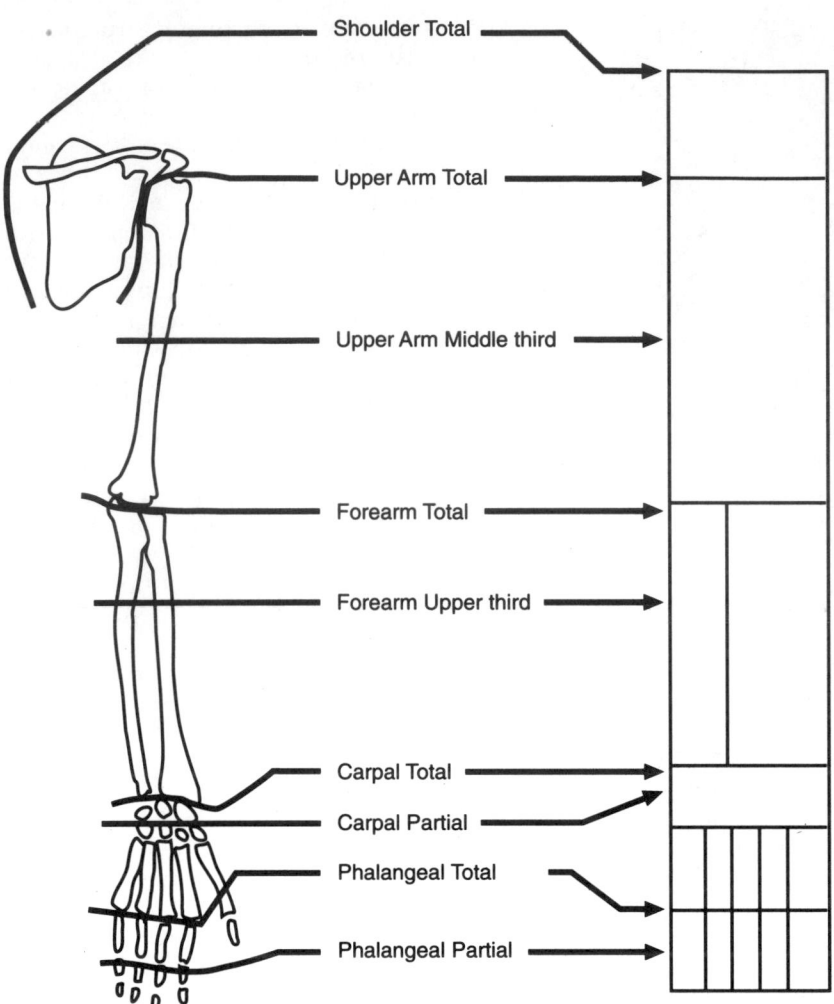

Shoulder Total

Upper Arm Total

Upper Arm Middle third

Forearm Total

Forearm Upper third

Carpal Total

Carpal Partial

Phalangeal Total

Phalangeal Partial

FIGURE 41–5 Examples of transverse deficiencies at various levels are shown in a realistic (left) and a stylized (right) representation. (From Day HJB: The ISO/ISPO classification of congenital limb deficiency. In Bowker JH, Michael JW (eds): *Atlas of Limb Prosthetics: Surgical, Prosthetic and Rehabilitation Principles,* 2nd ed. Philadelphia, Mosby Year Book, 1992.)

contracture, splinting must be performed before surgical procedures to the hand and before significant growth of the ulna.[131]
  (ii). Splinting or serial casting to position hand in center of forearm.
(b). Surgical
  (i). Hand surgically centered on the forearm
    (a). Full elbow flexion required.
    (b). Lack of full elbow flexion limits hand to face activities.
  (ii). Reconstruction of thumb.
(3). Lower extremity

(a). Surgical alternatives
  (i). Amputation of the foot recommended if significant leg-length discrepency exists: A child with a fibular deficiency can then be fitted with a prosthesis; a child with a PFFD may benefit from a fusion of the knee joint to increase lever arm of residual limb.
  (ii). Limb-lengthening techniques are alternatives to amputations: Adequate limb length is necessary; for viable correction of PFFD, 60% of predicted

femoral length must be present.[132]

(iii). Rotation plasty or a turn-about procedure may be an option for PFFD.[133,134] Involves excision of the distal femur and proximal tibia, 180-degree rotation of the residual limb, including the distal tibia, ankle joint, foot, and neurovascular supply, and reattachment to the proximal femur; ankle then functions as a knee joint (plantar flexors extend the knee; ankle dorsiflexion flexes the knee).

(4). Physical therapy
  (a). Range of motion exercises
    (i). Positioning and stretching program to decrease contractures and promote later prosthetic fit.
    (ii). Increase in ankle range of motion is crucial after a rotation plasty: Ankle dorsiflexion of 0 to 20 degrees for ambulation and sitting; optimally 45 to 50 degrees of ankle plantar flexion to achieve greater extension of knee.
  (b). Prosthetic fitting and training at developmentally appropriate age—8 to 12 months for lower extremity prosthesis.
    (i). Children younger than 2 years fitted with prosthesis without a knee with a goal to begin weight-bearing and ambulation activities.
    (ii). Progress to control of prosthetic knee closer to 3 years of age.

B. Disruptions

Morphological defect of an organ or body part resulting from the breakdown of a previously normal process or tissue. Normal development is disrupted at the cellular level by an external factor such as an infection, teratogen, or traumatic event.[2]

1. Transverse limb deficiencies
  a. The limb has developed normally to a particular level beyond which no skeletal elements exist; digital buds may be present.
  b. Described by naming the segment where the limb terminates and then describing the level within the segment beyond which no skeletal elements exist (Fig. 41–6).
  c. Common presentations
    (1). Most are unilateral
    (2). Transverse deficiency of the forearm upper third.[131]
    (3). Transverse deficiency of the leg; middle third (transtibial) may be associated with constriction band syndrome.[129]

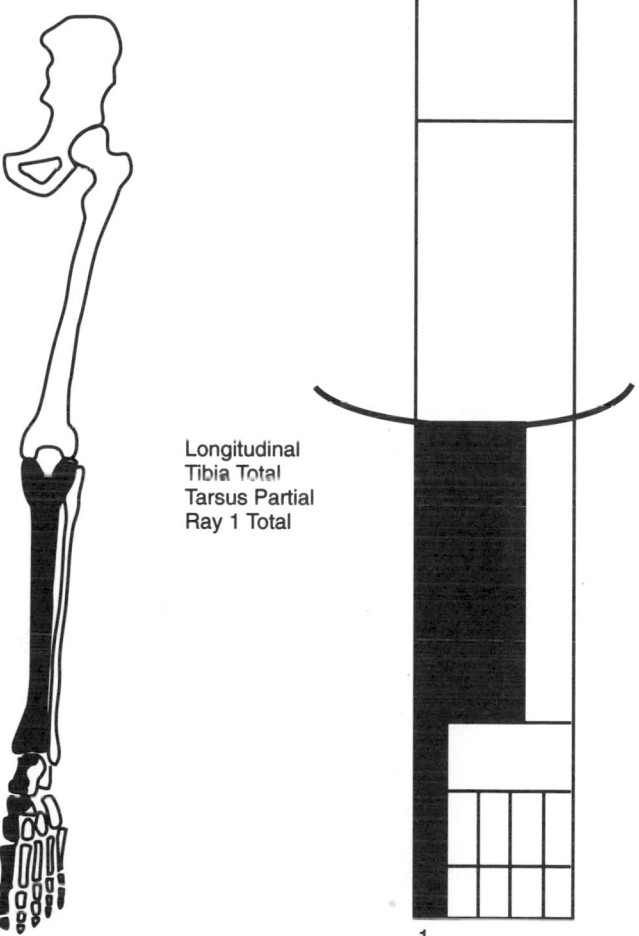

Longitudinal
Tibia Total
Tarsus Partial
Ray 1 Total

FIGURE 41–6 An example of longitudinal deficiency is shown in a realistic (left) and a stylized (right) representation; the stylized version shows not only the original deficiency but also the treatment by knee disarticulation. (From Day HJB: The ISO/ISPO classification of congenital limb deficiency. In Bowker JH, Michael JW (eds): *Atlas of Limb Prosthetics: Surgical, Prosthetic and Rehabilitation Principles,* 2nd ed. Philadelphia, Mosby Year Book, 1992.)

d. Management
 (1). Range of motion of joints immediately proximal to the deficiency should be monitored.
 (2). Knee flexion contracture may be present at birth with transverse deficiencies of the leg, requiring surgery before prosthetic fitting.
 (3). Prosthetic fitting and training should occur at a developmentally appropriate age.
  (a). Upper extremity
   (i). Fit with prosthesis to assist with weight-bearing skills in prone position or with early playing skills while sitting.
   (ii). Between 6 and 8 months of age or when child begins to sit independently.[135,136]
   (iii). Terminal device initially may be a passive hand or mitt.
   (iv). Progress to terminal device for grasping when child begins to engage in bimanual play.
   (v). Training to operate terminal device begins by about 18 months of age.
  (b). Lower extremity
   (i). Fit with prosthesis when weight bearing is appropriate and child begins to pull to stand: 8 to 10 months of age.
   (ii). Physical therapy emphasizes controlled weight shifting and balance activities to promote symmetrical posture and movement with developmental activities.

C. Dysplasias

Disorders that originate from the abnormal organization of cells into tissues leading to abnormal tissue differentiation.[2]

1. Osteogenesis imperfecta[137,138]
 a. Disorder of collagen synthesis affecting all connective tissue.

b. Failure to produce organized collagen results in brittleness of bones.
c. Classified according to clinical, radiologic, and genetic findings into four types (Table 41–6).[138]
d. Musculoskeletal impairments.[139]
 (1). Fractures
  (a). Bone trabeculae are thin and lack organized pattern.
  (b). Cortex of long bones is very thin with disproportionately large epiphyseal ends.
 (2). Bowing of long bones
  (a). Muscles pull across bone
  (b). Fractures of long bones
 (3). Compression and deformities of spine due to the following:
  (a). Compression fractures
  (b). Wedging of vertebral bodies
 (4). Short stature
  (a). Trauma and compression of epiphyses
  (b). Growth retardation when cartilaginous skeleton is being replaced by bone
e. Management
 (1). Goals
  (a). Prevent or limit skeletal deformities
  (b). Prevent cardiorespiratory compromise
  (c). Maximize a child's functional ability
 (2). The observation that immobilization after fracture or as prevention causes additional osteoporosis and muscle wasting, resulting in more fractures, has an impact on the nature of physical therapy intervention.[137]
 (3). Physical therapy
  (a). Parental instruction for handling and positioning the child.
  (b). Positioning emphasizes symmetry of head and spine and alignment of extremities (Fig. 41–7).
   (i). For infants, towel rolls may be used: Encourage symmetrical postures; avoid positions of malalignment that may promote deformities.
   (ii). As child grows, supported

Table 41–6. SILLENCE CLASSIFICATION OF OSTEOGENESIS IMPERFECTA (OI) SYNDROMES*

Type	Genetics	Description
I	Autosomal dominant	Mildest form of OI Mild-to-moderate bone fragility without deformity Associated with blue sclerae, early hearing loss, easy bruising May have mild to moderate short stature Type IA: Dentinogenesis Imperfecta Absent Type IB: Dentinogenesis Imperfecta Present
II	Autosomal dominant or recessive	Perinatal lethal Extreme fragility of connective tissue, multiple *in utero* fractures, usually interuterine growth retardation Soft, large cranium Micromelia, long bones crumped and bowed, ribs beaded
III	Autosomal recessive	Progressive deforming phenotype Severe fragility of bones, usually have *in utero* fractures Severe osteoporosis Relative macrocephaly with triangular facies Fractures heal with deformity and bowing Associated with white sclerae and extreme short stature, scoliosis
IV	Autosomal dominant	Skeletal fragility and osteoporosis more severe than type I Associated with bowing of long bones; light sclerae, ± moderate short stature, ± moderate joint hyperextensibility Type IVA: Dentinogenesis Imperfecta Absent Type IVB: Dentinogenesis Imperfecta Present

* From Marin JC. *Osteogenesis Imperfecta: Comprehensive Management. Advances in Pediatrics.* Chicago, Year Book Medical, 1988, p. 393. Used with permission.

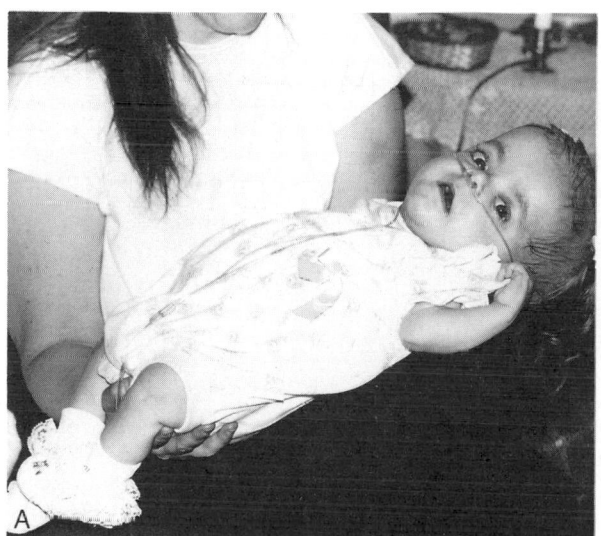
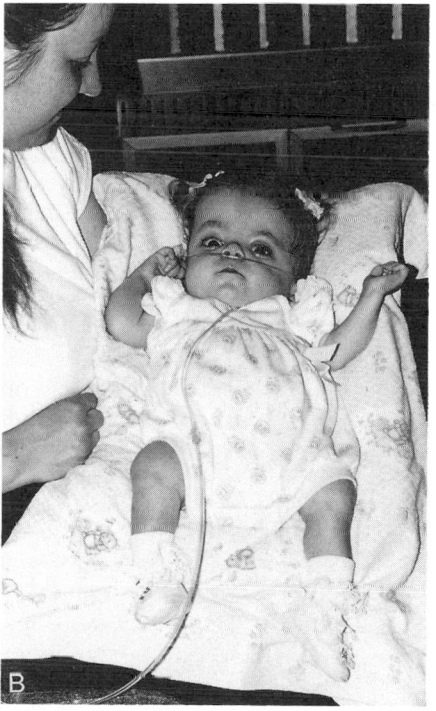

FIGURE 41–7 Handling an infant with osteogenesis imperfecta. **A,** Handling a young child with osteogenesis imperfecta with hands supporting the neck and shoulders and the pelvis; do not lift the child from under the arms. **B,** Placing the child on a pillow may make lifting and holding easier.

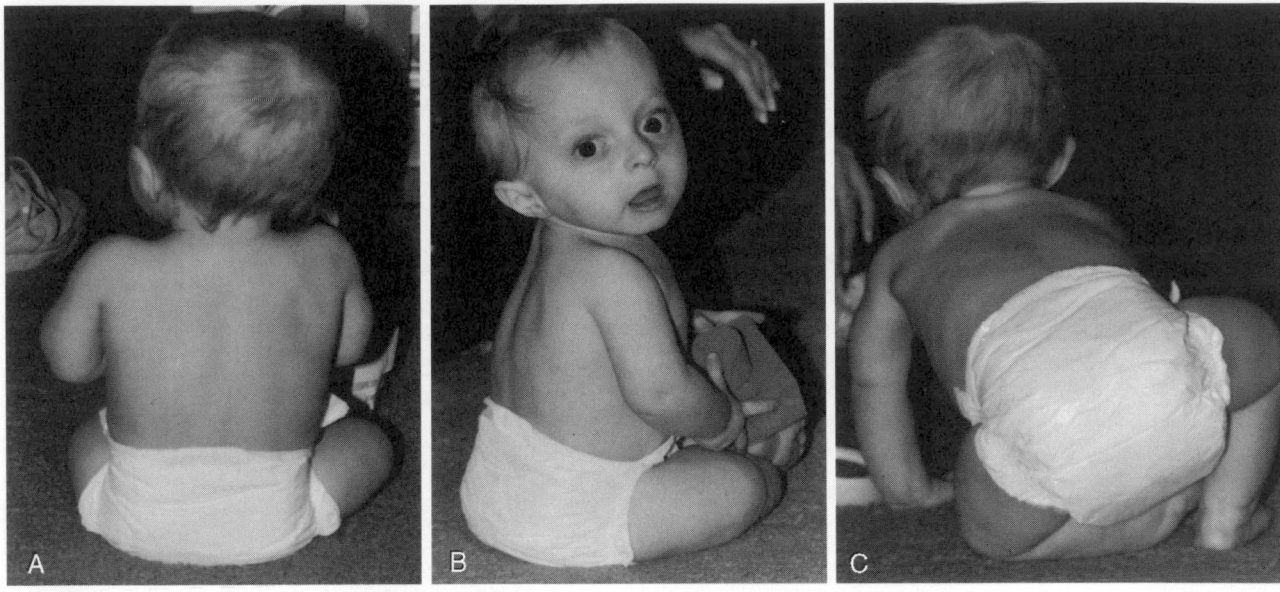

FIGURE 41–8 Developmental activities for a child with osteogenesis imperfecta. **A,** Emphasis on sitting with erect trunk. **B,** All rotations should be active, not passive. **C,** Weight bearing as tolerated on arms and legs.

seating in strollers and wheelchairs is important to promote head and trunk alignment.

(c). Developmental activities (Fig. 41–8)

  (i). Infants placed in a variety of positions including prone and side lying.

  (ii). Prone positioning promotes development of neck and upper trunk musculature, leading to head control.

  (iii). Reaching is encouraged from supine and side lying to develop upper extremity strength.

  (iv). Rolling must be done with care to avoid trapping an arm under the child's trunk.

  (v). Trunk extension and symmetry are important when sitting.

(d). Strengthening is achieved through active movement.

  (i). Resistive weights can be initiated with preschool-aged children: Increase weight in small increments; place weights near large joints to avoid a long lever arm and potential fractures.[137]

  (ii). Water is an excellent medium to incorporate active movement.

(e). Ambulation

  (i). Unsupported ambulation discouraged for children with Type III osteogenesis imperfecta.[137]

  (ii). Fitting for braces to be used for standing and ambulation is usually between 2 and 3 years of age.[138]

  (iii). Braces should be lightweight, clamshell type with quadrilateral cuffs to support the long bones fully.

  (iv). Pneumatic trouser splints have been used but may not be tolerated as well by children with osteogenesis imperfecta because of their tendency to sweat profusely.[140]

(v). Eventual progression to ambulation with an assistive device.

(f). Mobility often requires the use of a manual or power wheelchair for independence and function.

(4). Orthopedic surgery

(a). Fracture management

(i). Immobilization in plaster or soft casts to maintain bony alignment.

(ii). Less immobilization is favorable to prevent cycle of osteoporosis and increased fractures.[139]

(b). Bowing deformities of the lower extremities, which can impair standing and ambulation abilities.

(i). Osteotomies and insertion of intramedullary rods to correct bowing and prevent fractures:[139] Rods may be solid or extensible; complications include fracture and migration of rods, extensive osteoporosis, nonunion, and fractures adjacent to rod ends.

(ii). Osteotomies and insertion of plate and screws to provide support to the femur, which may decrease cortex shrinkage and osteoporosis.[138]

(c). Scoliosis is present in 80 to 90% of individuals with osteogenesis imperfecta.

(i). Orthotics are ineffective in controlling scoliosis.[141]

(ii). Spinal fusion:[142] may be indicated for rapidly progressing curves and those that affect respiratory function; complications often accompany spinal surgery (eg, respiratory compromise and internal fixation of osteoporotic bone).

2. Arthrogryposis (multiple congenital contractures)

a. Congenital complex characterized by joint contractures secondary to

(1). Weakness and/or fibrosis of muscles.

(2). Thickening and shortening of periarticular cartilage and ligamentous tissues.

(3). Immobility of joints during fetal development leading to contractures and abnormal development of joint surfaces.[143,144]

b. Musculoskeletal impairments vary among individuals, but five common clinical features exist.[144]

(1). Featureless extremities: cylindrical or spindle-shaped extremities with absent skin creases and thin, subcutaneous tissue.

(2). Joint rigidity

(a). Any combination of flexion and extension contractures may be seen.

(i). Equinovarus deformities of the feet

(ii). Fixed flexion or extension contractures of the knees

(iii). Flexion contracture of the hips

(iv). Medial rotation of the shoulders

(v). Extension or flexion contractures of the elbows

(vi). Forearm pronation

(vii). Wrist flexion contracture

(viii). Contracture of proximal interphalangeal joints

(ix). Adducted thumbs

(x). Scoliosis

(b). Involvement is usually symmetrical with distal greater than proximal.

(3). Joint dislocation of the hip is most common.

(4). Muscle atrophy or absence of muscles

(a). Normal embryological development

(b). During fetal period, muscle tissue is replaced by fibrous and fatty tissue.[145]

(5). Intact sensation, although deep tendon reflexes may be diminished.

c. Management

(1). Goal is to maximize the child's functional abilities.

(2). Treatment is variable because the disorder is complex and its manifestations are variable.

(3). Serial splinting and casting
    (a). Deformities are initially managed with serial casts or splints.
    (b). To improve the function of the joint
        (i). Casting an equinovarus deformity to achieve a plantigrade foot for weight bearing and shoe fit.
        (ii). Serial splinting or casting of elbow and knee flexion to improve self-help skills and mobility, respectively.
    (c). Vigorous stretching is contraindicated because damage to articular cartilage and soft tissues can occur.
(4). Surgical correction is often necessary to improve function.[146,147]
    (a). Tendon transfers to improve muscle imbalances
    (b). Lengthening of soft tissues, including capsulotomy and capsulectomy
    (c). Joint arthrodesis
    (d). Osteotomy.
(5). Deformities frequently recur after casting or surgery and should be managed by prolonged postoperative splinting to prevent or limit recurrence.[148]
(6). Functional mobility is determined by the extent of the musculoskeletal involvement.
    (a). Floor mobility is often bottom scooting
    (b). Ambulation training with orthotics is appropriate for some children.
    (c). Powered wheelchair mobility may be necessary for children with severe lower extremity involvement.

D. Deformations

Abnormalities in form, shape, or position of body parts caused by mechanical forces and molding; deformations may resolve spontaneously or with simple therapeutic interventions.[2]

1. Causes
  a. Extrinsic
    (1). Uterine constraint secondary to large or multiple fetuses, small pelvis, increased uterine tone, and oligohydramnios.
    (2). Fetal positioning (*ie,* breech) in late stages of pregnancy.
    (3). Muscle imbalances and positioning during postnatal and childhood growth.
  b. Intrinsic
    (1). Malformations such as myelomeningocele predispose the infant to deformations secondary to muscle imbalances and limited active kicking movements.
    (2). CNS or muscle diseases with hypotonia increase the fetus's susceptibility to extrinsic forces.
2. Patterns of deformations
  a. Common deformations as a result of uterine constraint include torticollis, compressed face, thoracic compression, hip dislocation, metatarsus, equinovarus, and small-for-gestational-age infants[149]
  b. Breech presentation is associated with increased incidence of dislocated hips, excessive hip flexion and hyperextended knees, equinovarus deformity, metatarsus adductus, and torticollis.[2]
3. Management
  a. Passive exercises to counteract abnormal postures.
  b. Serial casting or splinting to counteract the abnormal posture and maintain the joint in alignment.
  c. Surgical correction may be necessary to correct deformity secondary to significant muscle imbalances or prolonged abnormal positioning.
  d. Postoperatively, passive and active exercises and splinting are recommended to maintain the correction of the deformity.

VI. Bony Abnormalities

Several pediatric disorders are caused by the results of rapid growth, alterations, or stresses to the physes or disturbances of chondrosis or osteogenesis.

A. Osteochondroses

A group of self-limiting disorders in which both chondrosis and osteogenesis are deranged.[150]

1. Legg-Calvé-Perthes disease
   a. Self-limiting disease of the hip produced by ischemia and varying degrees of necrosis of the femoral head.
   b. Subchondral stress fracture of the necrotic bone initiates the clinical onset of the disease and the process of resorption of dead bone; natural progression of the disease is through four stages:
      (1). Initial phase of vascular compromise and fragmentation of the femoral head with possible deformation.
      (2). Healing or reossification, which can last up to 2 years.
      (3). Remodeling of the femoral head and acetabulum.
      (4). The definitive period in which the femoral head is revascularized but permanent deformity may exist.[150,151]
   c. Clinical picture
      (1). Limping
      (2). Complaint of mild pain often referred to the groin, anteromedial thigh, and knee, which is aggravated by activity and relieved by rest.
      (3). Decreases range of motion of the hip, especially hip abduction and internal rotation, with hip flexion contracture.
   d. Management
      (1). Goal is to produce a normal congruent hip joint with full range of motion and prevention of secondary degenerative arthritis.
      (2). Milder forms with less than 25% involvement of the femoral head may only require close monitoring.
      (3). Treatment is aimed at restoration of range of motion, containment of the femoral head in the acetabulum, and resumption of weight bearing.[150]
         (a). Restoration of full hip motion through traction.
         (b). Maintenance of hip range of motion through active motion of the hip while wearing a containment orthosis.
      (4). Containment orthosis
         (a). Aim is to reduce forces acting on the femoral head and contain the femoral head in the acetabulum.
         (b). Examples: Scottish-Rite, Newington abduction, Robert's and trilateral hip abduction orthosis.
         (c). Use of orthotics gradually discontinued after healing process is established (12–18 months)
      (5). Surgery
         (a). Containment can be achieved through femoral and/or innominate osteotomy.
         (b). Surgery is an option that allows faster return to normal activities (~3 months).
2. Osgood-Schlatter disease
   a. Caused by prolonged overuse and chronic avulsion of fragments of the patellar tendon at the insertion on the tibial tubercle.[151]
      (1). During a rapid growth spurt when the tibial tubercle is susceptible to stress.
      (2). Self-limiting and ceases when the tibial tubercle ossifies to the diaphysis of the tibia.[151]
   b. Clinical picture
      (1). Complaint of localization at the knee.
      (2). Pain aggravated by physical activity or direct pressure over the tibial tubercle.
      (3). Tightness of gastrosoleus complex, hamstring, and quadriceps musculature often present but without contractures.
   c. Management
      (1). Rest and decreased activity level resolve acute symptoms
      (2). Stretching of tight musculature, especially quadriceps mechanism, to decrease the pull over the tibial tubercle.
      (3). Immobilization in long leg cast if symptoms persist.
      (4). Surgery is rarely indicated but may

include excision of the tubercle or excision of loose ossicles.[150,151]

B. Slipped capital femoral epiphysis

1. Displacement of the femoral head from normal position on the femoral neck as the result of weakening and shear stresses on the proximal femoral physis.[150,151]
2. Clinical picture
   a. Dull pain radiating to the groin, anteromedial aspect of the thigh, and the knee.
   b. Limited motion of hip internal rotation and hip flexion.
   c. Antalgic gait
3. Management
   a. Goal of treatment is prevention of further slippage of the femoral head and secondary deformities caused by avascular necrosis.[150,151]
   b. Weight bearing should be immediately stopped.
   c. Immobilization through traction, orthotics, and casting is usually ineffective.
   d. Surgical options include pinning, epiphysiodesis, osteotomy, and reconstruction.

C. Leg-length discrepancy

1. Marked leg-length discrepancy is usually the result of congenital or developmental abnormalities or the arrest of growth from trauma or infection at the physis.[152]
2. Functional limitations[133]
   a. Back pain
   b. Awkward gait with increased energy expenditure
   c. Assistive device for ambulation if shortened leg does not reach the floor.
3. Management
   a. Shoe lift[133]
      (1). Difference of 1 to 2 cm: lift placed inside shoe
      (2). Difference of 2 to 4 cm: lift placed on outside of shoe
      (3). Shoe lift of greater than 5 cm can be fabricated but is unstable and cosmetically unappealing.
   b. Surgical treatment[133]
      (1). Arrest of growth of the longer leg
         (a). Epiphysiodesis of one or more physis
         (b). Indicated for discrepancies of 2 to 5 cm
         (c). Must be timed accurately
      (2). Shortening of the longer leg
         (a). Tibial or femoral shortening achieved through excision of portion of the bone.
         (b). Not recommended for skeletally immature children.
      (3). Limb lengthening[133,152]
         (a). Recommended for discrepancies greater than 5 cm
         (b). Requires patient and family compliance for frequent follow-up, care of external fixator, and participation in physical therapy program.
         (c). Requisites include the following:
            (i). Stable joints above and below the lengthened bone.
            (ii). Normal neuromuscular function and vascular circulation.
            (iii). Normal bone density.
         (d). Techniques
            (i). Osteotomy with slow distraction of bone fragments
               (a). Requires additional surgery to plate the distraction gap.
               (b). Correction in one plane only.
            (ii). Corticotomy with distraction
               (a). Ilizarov is the most widely used technique.
               (b). Correction of rotational deformities possible.
4. Postoperative management of limb lengthening
   a. Child and family perform daily self-distraction of the device.
   b. Daily care of pin sites by child and family.
   c. Physical therapy
      (1). Gait training with assistive device
         (a). Osteotomy technique: non-weight bearing
         (b). Corticotomy technique: weight bearing to tolerance.
      (2). Passive and active exercise to maintain and increase range of motion and to increase strength.[153]
         (a). Flexion contractures proximal to fixator

(b). Extension contractures distal to fixator.

(3). Splinting

(a). Resting splint to maintain ankle dorsiflexion range if the ankle is not incorporated into the external device.

(b). Knee extension splint to limit knee flexion contracture with tibial lengthening procedure.

VII. Musculoskeletal Aspects of Pediatric Oncology

A. Musculoskeletal tumors

1. Bone
   a. Osteosarcoma
      (1). Primary malignant bone tumor derived from bone forming mesenchyme in which the malignant cell produces osteoid tissue or immature bone.[154,155]
      (2). Peak incidence coincides with pubertal growth spurt.
      (3). Most common sites are the distal femur, proximal tibia, and proximal humerus.
   b. Ewing's sarcoma
      (1). Undifferentiated round cell tumor, which infiltrates bone marrow and adjacent soft tissue.[156]
      (2). Primary sites are weight-bearing bones of the lower extremity or pelvis.

2. Soft-tissue sarcomas
   a. Tumor derived from skeletal muscle (*rhabdomyosarcoma*) or connective tissue.
   b. Nonrhabdomyosarcoma soft-tissue sarcomas of young children exhibit benign behavior and may be managed with surgery alone.

3. Initial complaint and diagnosis
   a. Initial complaint is usually pain at the site of the tumor with or without a palpable mass; may be present for several months.
   b. Systemic symptoms rare unless widespread metastatic disease is present.
   c. Fever present in 25% of children with Ewing's sarcoma at time of diagnosis; may be mistaken for chronic osteomyelitis.[154,155]
   d. Children presenting to a physical therapist with complaint of pain, often chronic, negative history of trauma, and no evidence of musculoskeletal abnormalities should be referred for further medical workup.

   e. Diagnosis by radiologic evaluation.
   f. Definitive diagnosis is through biopsy and histological examination.

4. Management
   a. Medical
      (1). Radiotherapy
         (a). Energy from radiation disrupts the structure of atoms and damages essential molecules, especially the chromosomes; reproductive capacity is compromised, and cellular metabolism is disrupted, leading to cell death.[157]
         (b). Osteosarcoma unresponsive to radiotherapy.[155]
         (c). Ewing's sarcoma very responsive to radiotherapy.[156]
      (2). Chemotherapy
         (a). Used to control size of the primary tumor and to control micrometastatic disease.
         (b). Chemotherapy agents circulate in the bloodstream and therefore are delivered to all tissues; they enter the cells and disrupt metabolic processes, especially cell division.[157]
   b. Surgical
      (1). Amputation
         (a). Surgical margin usually 6 to 7 cm above the most proximal medullary extent of the tumor.[154]
         (b). Last resort for tumors of the upper extremity secondary to severe loss of function that results from loss of a hand.
         (c). Considerations in children:
            (i). Skeletal immaturity: physes should be preserved when possible to ensure growth of the limb.
            (ii). Terminal overgrowth: painful spikelike prominence of new bone that develops

from osteogenic activity of the periosteum of the transected bone.[158]

(2). Limb-sparing procedures

(a). Procedures that involve resection of the tumor and reconstruction of the limb to preserve function without amputation of the limb.

(i). Use of cadaver allografts.

(ii). Autologous grafts.

(iii). Excision of tumor without replacement.

(iv). Excision of bone with implantation of endoprosthetic devices.

(v). Rotation plasty procedure

(b). Contraindications[159]

(i). Tumor has invaded surrounding soft tissue to a large extent.

(ii). Involvement of the neurovascular supply.

(iii). A wide surgical margin cannot be achieved.

(iv). The very young skeletally immature child.

B. Musculoskeletal implications of oncology treatment

1. Radiotherapy

   a. Acute side effects[154]

   (1). Seen in rapidly dividing tissues such as the skin, bone marrow, and gut.

   (2). Irradiation of the extremities produces few acute side effects.

   b. Late side effects[160]

   (1). Fibrosis of soft tissues.

   (2). Osteoporosis and possible fractures.

   (3). Damage to the physis, which may lead to bowing of the metaphysis and growth disturbances.

2. Chemotherapy (see Table 41–7)

3. Surgical

   a. Amputation

   (1). Wide surgical margins may result in very short residual limb.

   (2). Terminal overgrowth

   (a). May interfere with weight bearing and wearing of prosthesis.

   (b). Usually requires surgical revision or bone capping to alleviate the overgrowth.

b. Limb-sparing procedures

(1). Physes removed

(a). Severe leg-length discrepancy

(b). Nonfunctional lower extremity, if young skeletally immature child.

(2). Endoprosthetic devices

(a). Problems include loosening of the device, fracture, infection, and failure of the implant.

(b). Most devices do not allow for growth of the young child.

C. Physical therapy management

1. Goals

   a. Maintain or increase range of motion postsurgically.

   b. Prevent secondary deformities resulting from chemotherapy regimen.

   c. Maintain or increase strength and activity level.

   d. Independence with mobility and ADL.

2. Progression of treatment program.

   a. Individualized for each child because of the complexity of medical status and needs.

   b. Physical therapy may range from very intensive to only consultative.

3. Range of motion

   a. Children may be more lethargic secondary to effects of radiotherapy and chemotherapy and therefore may spend more time resting in bed.

   b. Emphasis on maintaining hip and knee extension and hip adductor range of motion of the residual limb.

   c. Resting knee extension splints for child with below-knee amputation.

   d. Important after limb-sparing procedures.

4. Management of secondary deformities related to chemotherapy agents.

   a. Knowledge of chemotherapy regimen and possible side effects.

   b. Monitoring of skin very closely if wearing prosthesis.

   c. Preventive splinting of wrist or ankles if initial symptoms of peripheral neuropathy develop.

5. Strength

   a. May begin with isometrics and progress to resistive exercises as appropriate.

   b. Emphasis on hip extensors and abductors for children with above-knee amputation.

Table 41–7.   CHEMOTHERAPY AGENTS*

Agent	Side Effects/Adverse Reactions	Therapy Concerns
Adriamycin (doxorubicin)	Alopecia (hair loss), myelosuppression, oro-GI reactions (oral reddening, ulcers, nausea, vomiting; more serious include diarrhea, dysphagia, GI bleeding), myocardial toxicity (can lead to cardiac failure)	Extravasation can occur with IV administration; reactions include stinging and burning sensation, possible cellulitis, blistering, tissue necrosis Life-threatening arrhythmias during or within few hours of administration Cardiac failure not often favorably affected by medical or physical therapy support; cardiac failure must be detected early for successful treatment.
Blenoxane (bleomycin)	Toxic to skin and lung tissues; skin reactions include erythema, tenderness, hyperpigmentation; pulmonary toxicities occur in 10% of patients; pneumonitis may progress to pulmonary fibrosis and death	Dyspnea is earliest symptom of pulmonary toxicity; fine rales on auscultation; pulmonary function test changes include decrease in total lung volume, decrease in vital capacity, but not predictive of development of pulmonary fibrosis; pulmonary toxicity monitored through x-ray changes
Cosmegen (dactinomycin, actinomycin D)	Oro-GI reactions, alopecia, myelosuppression, liver toxicity	Can impair wound healing Corrosive to soft tissue; if extravasation occurs, severe damage to soft tissues will occur and can lead to contractures Severe skin reactions occur where there has been previous irradiation
Cytoxan (cyclophosphamide)	Alopecia, nausea and vomiting, myelosuppression, hemorrhagic cystitis	Can impair wound healing Must force liquids to control cystitis
DTIC (dacarbazine)	Myelosuppression, anorexia, nausea and vomiting, myalgias, malaise, alopecia	Extravasation after IV administration produces severe local pain and stinging; can result in tissue damage
Methotrexate	Potential for serious toxicity; toxicity is function of dose and duration of treatment; oro-GI reactions, myelosuppression, hepatic and/or renal damage with prolonged use; leukoencephalopathy reported in patients with osteosarcoma; neurological effects include behavioral changes, abnormal reflexes, focal sensorimotor signs; pulmonary symptoms include dry, nonproductive cough; fever; dyspnea; hypoxemia; chest x-ray infiltrate	After discontinuation of methotrexate, complete recovery not always seen with leukoencephalopathy; blurred vision, headaches, aphasia, and hemiparesis are other neurological adverse reactions seen with methotrexate Seizures have led to coma in children; may be administered anticonvulsants if on large dose
Oncovin (vincristine)	Alopecia, constipation, nausea and vomiting, hypertension and hypotension, neuromuscular side effects, cranial nerve manifestations, seizures	Monitor cardiovascular status Neuromuscular side effects include pain distally, loss of deep tendon reflexes, footdrop, with progression to contractures, gait abnormalities, ataxia; splinting may be helpful to avoid contractures Extravasation during administration can lead to cellulitis Paralysis of cranial nerves may be seen; most commonly affected muscles are extraocular and laryngeal
Platinol (cisplatin)	Nausea and vomiting, myelosuppression, cumulative renal toxicity, ototoxicity, peripheral neuropathies; ototoxic effects can be more severe in children than adults	Ototoxicity may include tinnitus and/or hearing loss in high-frequency range, occasionally may affect ability to hear normal conversation Peripheral neuropathies may be irreversible and can include loss of motor function.

* From Campbell SK, Van der Linden D, Palisano R (eds.): *Physical Therapy for Children.* Philadelphia, W.B. Saunders, 1994; data obtained from *Physician's Desk Reference.* Oradell, NJ, Medical Economics Company, 1993.
Abbreviation: GI = gastrointestinal.

c. Extremity strengthening after limb-sparing procedure.

d. Increase overall strength and activity level secondary to effects of bed rest and general malaise.

6. Gait training
a. Minimize gait deviations, especially compensations of the trunk.
b. Emphasis on symmetrical posture.
c. Progression with assistive devices as needed.

VIII. Mechanisms and Examples of Sports Injuries

A. Classification of injuries secondary to recurrent microtrauma

1. Can be thought of as overuse injuries
2. Becoming increasingly common in pediatrics.[161]
3. Although many sports injuries in children are similar to those found in adults, two major differences have been identified.[162,163]
   a. Trauma to a joint may cause fracture of epiphyseal growth site plate instead of a ligamentous injury.
   b. Stress injuries related to differential growth or strength of musculoskeletal structures.[161,163]
      (1). Length changes in the musculotendinous system and the skeletal system do not occur concurrently.
      (2). Imbalance of muscle strength around individual joints.
      (3). Decrease in flexibility as growth occurs.

B. Risk factors[161–163]

1. Training errors/maltraining
2. Musculotendinous imbalance
   a. Second most important risk factor
   b. Increase in strength may not be uniform across all joints or on either side of a given joint.
3. Anatomical malalignment including leg-length discrepancy, abnormal hip rotation, coxa valga or varus, abnormal foot pronation, and flat feet.[162–166]
4. Footwear and playing surface.
5. Associated musculoskeletal disease states such as Legg-Calvé-Perthes, osteogenesis sarcoma, slipped capital epiphysis.
6. Immature structures
   a. Clinical and biomechanical evidence that growth cartilage is less resistant to repetitive trauma than is adult cartilage.[167]
   b. Child's articular cartilage is more susceptible to shear forces, especially at the elbow, knee, and ankle.[161]
   c. Tight musculotendinous units at the traction apophysis.[168]
7. Growth process
   a. The effect of growth process on the tissues themselves.
   b. Periods of rapid growth, "growth spurts," appear to be correlated with injury occurrence.[161]

C. Types of injuries

1. Stress fracture
   a. Not known in children before advent of organized sports training in the early 1950s.[161,169,170]
   b. Associated with maltraining, anatomical malalignment, tight musculotendinous junction.
   c. Most often seen in long bones of lower extremity and the metatarsals: can occur in any weight-bearing bone of lower extremity and spine.[164]
   d. Signs.
      (1). Severe pain and skin irritation over injury site.
      (2). Relief of pain with rest from activity.
   e. Roentgenograms often negative for 2 to 3 weeks after onset of pain.[171]
   f. General rule is that a stress failure requires as long to heal as it did to occur (*ie,* complaint of pain for 5 months; 5 months to heal).[163]
2. Tendinitis and bursitis
3. Joint disorders: subluxation or dislocation as result of overuse.[161]

D. Common sites of overuse injuries

1. Spine
   a. During growth spurts, there is a tendency to develop lordosis accompanied by relative hip flexion contracture and tight hamstrings.
      (1). Enhanced growth anterior in the vertebral bodies.
      (2). Secondary tethering of the spine posteriorly by heavy lumbodorsal fascia.[161]
   b. Characteristic injuries
      (1). Compression fractures of vertebral bodies.
      (2). Juvenile round back.
      (3). Pain at thoracolumbar junction.
2. Shoulder

a. "Little League shoulder" refers to micro-fracture of proximal humeral growth plate from repetitive training.[172]

b. Impingement of rotator cuff musculature.

c. Repetitive stress of the articular cartilage of proximal humerus.

   (1). Hypertrophy of the humeral head.

   (2). Secondary decreased capacity for excursion of the rotator cuff tendons.[161,173]

3. Elbow

a. "Little League elbow" is the general label applied to overuse injury.

b. Caused by repetitive valgus strain, with compression medially and laterally, applied to the elbow during throwing.[161,174]

4. Hip and pelvis

a. Stress during childhood may predispose individual to adult osteoarthritis.[161,175]

   (1). Small, undetected slipping of the capital femoral epiphysis at the growth plate results in deformation of the femoral head.

   (2). Leads to abnormal stress on the articular cartilage.

b. Apophyseal pain at the site of major muscle insertions.

5. Knee

a. The most frequent site of overuse injury.[161]

   (1). Usually involves the extensor mechanism.

   (2). With growth, muscles crossing the knee joint must adjust to the most rapidly growing bones in the body.

b. Patellofemoral stress syndrome

   (1). Presence of heavy fascia lata laterally and relatively lighter tissues medially results in a lateral longitudinal traction on the patella.[161,176]

   (2). Soft-tissue imbalances may actually deform and alter shape of patella itself, predisposing child to femoral stress syndrome symptoms.

   (3). Abnormal anatomical factors most often identical include femoral anteversion, genu valgum, tibia vara, increased Q angle, and compensatory foot pronation.[166]

c. Osgood-Schlatter disease

   (1). Excessive traction on tibial tubercle in skeletally immature bone, resulting in an epiphysitis.[163,177]

6. Ankle and foot

a. Heel pain with tenderness over os calcis apophysis at insertion of Achilles tendon.[161]

   (1). Frequently bilateral

   (2). Associated with growth spurts

b. Growth plate fracture of distal tibia[178]

   (1). Most common injury at ankle in skeletally immature athlete.

   (2). Of all the joints in body, injuries to the ankle joint differ the most between the child and the adult.

     (a). Distal tibial and fibular growth plates create a plane of weakness.

     (b). Children's ligaments are usually stronger than bone.

     (c). Results in injury to the growth plate rather than injury to ligaments or soft tissue.

Clinical Decision-Making Cases

Congenital Right Proximal Femoral Focal Deficiency (PFFD)

EXAMINATION

History

RJ is a 3½-year-old boy with a congenital right PFFD, Aitken type B. Aitken type B involvement signifies presence of a femoral head and acetabulum; the acetabulum may be dysplastic, the femoral neck contains defective cartilage that fails to ossify at maturity, and the shaft of the femur is short. Previous radiological assessments have revealed an absent right distal femoral epiphysis and absent right proximal tibial and fibular epiphyses. A Boyd amputation of the right foot was performed at 8 months of age to promote the fitting of RJ's first prosthesis and beginning weight bearing in standing. By 2 years of age RJ ambulated independently wearing a prosthesis without a knee joint; no assistive device was used. An arthrodesis of the right knee was performed at 3 years of age to increase the length of the lever arm needed for an efficient gait. A metaphyseal epiphyseal synostosis with bone grafting was also performed at that time to improve the stability of the proximal femur. RJ was then fitted with a new prosthesis with a knee joint.

DIAGNOSIS AND ASSESSMENT

Diagnosis

RJ is diagnosed with a congenital right PFFD, status-post arthrodesis of his right knee and a metaphyseal epiphyseal synostosis of his right femur.

Assessment

Significant range of motion measurements include a 10-degree right hip flexion contracture and right hip abduction limited to 35 degrees. All joint motions of the right foot and left leg are within normal limits.

The strength of the right hip is measured as follows: iliopsoas 5/5, gluteus maximus 3/5, and gluteus medius 3/5. The left leg musculature exhibits normal strength. Functionally, RJ is able to advance his prosthesis using his hip flexors; a Trendelenberg is present during assisted ambulation.

RJ is independent with all transfers and floor mobility. He stands independently with his prosthesis, but weight bearing is minimal through his prosthetic leg. RJ ambulates with a walker and his prosthesis.

TREATMENT AND GOALS

Treatment goals included (1) elimination of the right hip flexion contracture, (2) increased strength of right hip musculature, and (3) independent ambulation without an assistive device. A home program of passive stretching exercises was implemented. Increases in prosthetic wearing time and ambulation activities were also encouraged. Strengthening activities included active and resistive exercises to appropriate muscle groups. Functional strengthening activities included standing with hips extended and no forward trunk bending. Lateral weight shifting skills were added to the standing activities to develop a weight shift without lateral trunk flexion. Gait training activities also included lateral weight shifting skills as well as control of the prosthetic knee during stance and weight shift forward over the extended knee. RJ progressed from ambulation with a walker to forearm crutches to independent ambulation without an assistive device. Gait training also included running skills and stair climbing.

OUTCOME: 6 MONTHS AFTER ONSET OF PHYSICAL THERAPY

Full hip extension range of motion was achieved. Strength of right hip musculature is as follows: iliopsoas 5/5, gluteus maximus 5/5, and gluteus medius 4/5.

Functionally, RJ ambulates independently without an assistive device but uses forearm crutches or a stroller for long distance ambulation or when in crowds. Gait is characterized by a mild Trendelenberg, good prosthetic knee control in stance, knee flexion during swing, and no falling secondary to prosthetic knee instability. RJ ascends and descends stairs nonreciprocally using a rail. He is not yet running.

Spastic Diplegic Cerebral Palsy

EXAMINATION

History

CB is a 7½-year-old girl with spastic diplegic cerebral palsy. She was born at 33 weeks gestation; pregnancy and delivery were complicated by placenta previa with subsequent neonatal distress. She has been involved in preschool programming with therapy intervention. CB currently attends a special needs classroom in her local school district and is partially mainstreamed.

Physical

The patient's general health is good. CB wears corrective lenses. Her hearing is normal. CB has a mild cognitive impairment. She wears molded ankle foot orthotics.

ASSESSMENT

The following chart presents the assessment data for goniometry.

Variable	Right (Degrees)	Left (Degrees)
1. Hip		
Extension	Full	Full
Flexion	0–150	0–150
Internal rotation	70	80
External rotation	10	10
Abduction	40	40
2. Knee		
Popliteal angle	40	50
Extension in supine (hip extended)	Full	Full
3. Ankle		
Dorsiflexion knee extended	15	15
Dorsiflexion knee flexed	25	25

Left forefoot adduction is noted with inversion and slight supination. The upper extremity range of motion is within normal limits. Spinal alignment is normal. Leg lengths are equal, and hips are clinically stable.

Regarding strength, CB is able to isolate voluntary antigravity knee extension within range limitations. Active hip extension against gravity is present. Poor hip and knee extension is evident in stance.

The neurological assessment provided several findings. Mild to moderate spasticity is present in both lower extremities. Hyper-reactive DTRs are noted at the knee and ankle (3+). There is no clonus, and a low tone is noted in the trunk. Upper extremity tone and strength are within normal limits.

Regarding posture/movement, retracted scapulae, extended shoulders, and limited reciprocal arm swing are noted in the patient's gait. The trunk is in slight hyperextension, with increased lumbar lordosis, protruding abdomen, and anterior pelvic tilt. There is hip and knee flexion with significant internal rotation; the left is greater than the right. Crouched posture throughout the gait cycle is evident, with the lower extremities in internal rotation and frequent scissoring. The foot is stable on the right, but the left foot is inverted and adducted. Gait cycle is brief, with significant difficulty with weight shift. The base of support is narrow, and stride length is short.

Floor and transitional movement is characterized by poor trunk cocontraction, weak abdominals, and limited disassociation between shoulders and trunk and trunk and pelvis. Weight shift is poor in quadruped while kneeling and in stance. The patient uses plantigrade to transition floor to stand. A limited ability to shift weight, decreased range of motion of lower extremities, and poor disassociation contribute to difficulty with transitional movements.

Regarding function, the patient ambulates independently without assistive devices, although she falls frequently. CB uses stairs nonreciprocally with close supervision and support of two railings.

The diagnosis is as follows: spastic diplegic cerebral palsy with bilateral femoral anteversion, bilateral hamstring contractures, and left forefoot adductus. CB is referred for orthopedic assessment and subsequent surgical intervention, including bilateral femoral derotation osteotomies, bilateral fractional hamstring lengthenings, and left split posterior tibialis tendon transfer.

TREATMENT GOALS AND TREATMENT

Surgery was performed as just discussed. CB was discharged to home 3 days postoperatively with long leg immobilizers (no plaster casts). CB underwent physical therapy daily for 2 weeks postoperatively. Therapy was decreased to three times weekly for 2 months and then one to two times weekly to complete the 6-month postoperative period. A home program, which was to be done daily, included positioning, range of motion, and strengthening activities. This was updated frequently.

Positioning

The patient was placed in a prone position, with hips and knees extended and hips abducted and externally rotated. The use of abduction splint and knee immobilizers was optional. The patient was then placed in a long sitting position, with neutral pelvis, hips at 90 degrees flexion and abducted, and knees extended. Initially knee immobilizers were used and removed as able.

Weight bearing was allowed per physician's orders on prone or supine stander with appropriate foot orthotics. Seating equipment was adapted as needed: Knees were extended, pelvis was in a neutral position (to prevent posterior pelvic tilt), and hip flexion was at 90 degrees.

Range of Motion

For the hamstrings, full knee extension with hips at 90 degrees was achieved with an erect trunk over a neutral pelvis. Passive range of motion exercises were performed in the first few weeks postoperatively. Knee immobilizers were used to maintain a new range. Regarding the ankle/foot, full passive range of motion was maintained or increased. Split posterior tibialis was activated to re-educate motion to dorsiflexion and eversion. Rotation/torsion at hips is contraindicated after a derotation osteotomy. Full hip abduction, extension, and flexion were maintained according to the surgeon's recommendations.

Strength

The patient underwent selective strengthening of hip and knee extension, hip abduction, and re-education of tibialis posterior:

1. Quadriceps sets progressing to progressive resistive exercises
2. Gluteal sets progressing to progressive resistive exercises
3. Hip abduction against gravity
4. Posterior tibialis—functional electrical stimulation and active exercise
5. Functional activities for selective strengthening (bridging, bridging with unilateral knee extension, quadruped with and without unilateral hip/knee extension, weight shift activities, and gait training).

Functional Movement Patterns

Maintain neutral pelvis with erect trunk and weight shift over extended hip and knee: kneeling, half-kneel, squat to stand; grading of muscle strength during transitional movement.

Gait Training

The goal of gait training is safe and independent ambulation with or without an assistive device.

OUTCOMES

The outcome data for range of motion after 6 months of postoperative therapy are as follows:

Variable	Right (Degrees)	Left (Degrees)
1. Hip		
Extension	Full	Full
Flexion	0–150	0–150
Internal rotation	40	40
External rotation	55	55
Abduction	50	50
2. Knee		
Popliteal angle	10	10
Extension in supine	Full	Full
3. Ankle		
Dorsiflexion knee extended	15	15
Dorsiflexion knee flexed	25	25

The left foot is in neutral alignment with the hindfoot and forefoot. Orthotics are no longer required.

Regarding the 6-month outcome data for function, the patient is ambulating independently without assistive devices: She ascends and descends stairs reciprocally with support of one railing. CB is now able to ride an adapted four-wheel bicycle.

Regarding gait pattern, there is slight trunk extension and slight anterior pelvic tilt. CB swings through with hip external rotation and abduction. Knee extension is present throughout appropriate portions of the gait cycle. Heel strike is evident on initial contact, with progression over aligned foot/ankle. Speed, timing, and smoothness of gait continue to be difficult for CB.

References

1. Bernhardt DB: Prenatal and postnatal growth and development of the foot and ankle. *Phys Ther* 1988; 68:1831–1839.
2. Dunne KB, Clarren SK: The origin of prenatal and postnatal deformities. *Pediatr Clin North Am* 1986; 33:1277–1297.
3. LeVeau BF, Bernhardt DB: Effect of forces on the growth, development, and maintenance of the human body. *Phys Ther* 1984, 64:1874–1881.
4. Walker JM: Musculoskeletal development: a review. *Phys Ther* 1991; 71:878–889.
5. Tickle C, Wolpert L: Limb development. In Davis JA, Dobbing J (eds): *Scientific Foundations of Paediatrics.* 2nd ed. Baltimore, MD. University Park Press, 1981. pp 544–564.
6. Royer P: Growth and development of bony tissues. In Davis JA, Dobbing J (eds): *Scientific Foundations of Paediatrics.* Baltimore, MD. University Park Press, 1981. pp 565–589.
7. Albright J, Brand R (eds): *Scientific Basis of Orthopedics.* New York, Appleton-Century-Crofts, 1979.
8. Davenport C: Postnatal development of the human extremities. *Proc Am Philosophical Soc* 1944, 88:375–455.
9. Arkin A, Katz J: The effects of pressure on epiphyseal growth. *J Bone Joint Surg* [Am] 1956, 38:1056–1076.

10. Scott JH: The mechanical basis of bone formation. *J Bone Joint Surg* [Br] 1957, 39:134–144.

11. Ogden JA: *Skeletal Injury in the Child*. Philadelphia, Lea & Febiger, 1982, pp 16–40.

12. Frost HM: A chondral modeling theory. *Calcif Tissue Int* 1979, 28:181–200.

13. Storey E: Growth and remodeling of bone and bones. *Dent Clin North Am* 1975, 19:443–454.

14. Siffert RS: Patterns of deformity of the developing hip. *Clin Orthop* 1981, 160:14–29.

15. Lanyon LE: Adaptive mechanics: the skeleton's response to mechanical stress. In Stokes IA (ed): *Mechanical Factors and the Skeleton*. London, John Libbey, 1981, pp 72–82.

16. Frost HM: The physiology of cartilaginous, fibrous, and bony tissue. In *Orthopaedic Lectures*. vol. 2. Springfield, IL, Charles C Thomas, 1972.

17. Holder N: An experimental investigation into the early development of chick elbow. *J Embryol Exp Morph* 1977, 39:115–127.

18. O'Rahilly R, Gardener E: The embryology of moveable joints. In Skoloff L (ed): *The Joints and Synovial Fluid*. vol. 1. New York, Academic Press, 1978, pp 29–103.

19. Mastaglia FL: Growth and development of skeletal muscle. In Davis JA, Dobbing J (eds): *Scientific Foundations of Paediatrics*. 2nd ed. Baltimore, MD, University Park Press, 1981, pp 590–620.

20. Ralis Z, McKibbin B: Changes in shape of the human hip joint during its development and their relation to its stability. *J Bone Joint Surg* [Br] 1973, 55:780–785.

21. Harris NH: Acetabular growth potential in congenital dislocation of the hip and some factors upon which it may depend. *Clin Orthop* 1976, 119:99–106.

22. Hensinger R, Jones E: Developmental orthopaedics: 1. The lower limb. *Dev Med Child Neurol* 1982, 24:95–116.

23. Stuberg W: Musculoskeletal development and flexibility: assessment and intervention. Paper presented at the Annual Conference of the American Physical Therapy Association, Cincinnati, OH, June 14, 1993.

24. Phelps E, Smith LJ, Hallum A: Normal ranges of hip motion of infants between nine and 24 months of age. *Dev Med Child Neurol* 1985; 27:785–792.

25. Gibson D: Torsional variations in the lower limbs of children. *Appl Ther* 1966, 8:326–330.

26. Stahili L, Duncan W, Schaefer E: Growth alteration in the hemiplegic child. *Clin Orthop* 1968, 60:205–212.

27. McDade W: Bowlegs and knock knees. *Pediatr Clin North Am* 1977, 24:825–839.

28. Cozen L: Knock-knee deformity in children. *Clin Orthop Rel Res* 1990, 258:191–203.

29. Hoffer MM: Joint motion limitations in newborns. *Clin Orthop Rel Res* 1980, 148:94–96.

30. Bleck E: Developmental orthopedics: 3. toddlers. *Dev Med Child Neurol* 1982, 24:533–555.

31. Cusick BD: *Progressive Casting and Splinting for Lower Extremity Deformities in Children with Neuromotor Dysfunction*. Tuscon, AZ, Therapy Skill Builders, 1990.

32. Waugh KG, Mendel JL, Parker R, Coon VA: Measurement of selected hip, knee, and ankle joint motions in newborns. *Phys Ther* 1983, 63:1616–1621.

33. Haas SL, Epps CH, Adams JP: Normal ranges of hip motion in the newborn. *Clin Orthop Rel Res* 1973, 91:114–118.

34. Forero N, Okamura LA, Larson MA: Normal ranges of hip motion in neonates. *J Pediatr Orthop* 1989, 9:391–395.

35. Bleck EE: *Orthopaedic Management in Cerebral Palsy*. Philadelphia, J. B. Lippincott Company, 1987.

36. Haley SM, Tada WL, Carmichael EM: Spinal mobility in young children: a normative study. *Phys Ther* 1986, 66:1697–1703.

37. Moll JMH, Liyange SP, Wright V: An objective clinical method to measure lateral spinal flexion. *Rheumatol Phys Med*, 1972, 11:225–239.

38. Macrae IF, Wright V: Measurement of back movement. *Ann Rheum Dis* 1969, 28:584–589.

39. Coon V, Donato G, Hauser C, Bleck EE: Normal ranges of motion of the hip in infants, six weeks, three months and six months of age. *Clin Orthop Rel Res* 1975, 110:256–260.

40. Staheli LT: Prone hip extension test: method of measuring hip flexion deformity. *Clin Orthop Rel Res* 1977, 123:12–15.

41. Barttet MD, Wolf LS, Shurtleff DB, Staheli LT: Hip flexion contractures: a comparison of measurement methods. *Arch Phys Med Rehabil* 1985, 66:620–625.

42. Staheli LT, Corbett BS, Wyss C, King H: Lower extremity rotational problems in children. *J Bone Joint Surg [Am]* 1985, 67:39–47.

43. Hinderer K, Hinderer S: Strength: assessment and intervention approaches. Paper presented at the Annual Conference of the American Physical Therapy Association, Cincinatti, OH, June 14, 1993.

44. Kendall F, McCreary E: *Muscle Testing and Function*. 3rd ed. Baltimore, MD, Williams & Wilkins, 1983.

45. Daniels L, Worthingham C: *Muscle Testing: Technique of Manual Examination*. 5th ed. Philadelphia: W. B. Saunders Company, 1986.

46. Stuberg WA, Metcalf WK: Reliability of quantitative muscle testing in healthy children and in children with Duchenne muscular dystrophy using a hand-held dynamometer. *Phys Ther* 1988, 68:977–982.

47. Iddings DM, Smith LK, Spencer WA: Muscle testing: part 2. Reliability in clinical use. *Phys Ther Rev* 1961, 41:249–256.

48. Lilienfeld AM, Jacobs M, Willis M: A study of the reproducibility of muscle testing and certain other aspects of muscle scoring. *Phys Ther Rev* 1954, 34:279–289.

49. Brussock CM, Haley SM, Munsat TL, Bernhardt DS: Measurement of isometric force in children with and without Duchenne's muscular dystrophy. *Phys Ther* 1992, 72:105–114.

50. Alexander J, Molnar GE: Muscular strength in children: preliminary report on objective standards. *Arch Phys Med Rehabil* 1973, 54:424–427.

51. Molnar GE, Alexander J: Objective quantitative muscle testing in children: a pilot study. *Arch Phys Med Rehabil* 1973, 54:224–225.

52. Molnar GE, Alexander J, Gutfeld N: Reliability of quantitative strength measurements in children. *Arch Phys Med Rehabil* 1979, 60:218–221.

53. Gilliam TB, Villanacce JF, Freedson PS, et al: Isokinetic torque in boys and girls ages 7–13: effect of age, height and weight. *Res Q* 1979, 50:599–609.

54. Burnett CN, Betts EF, King WM: Reliability of isokinetic measurements of hip muscle torque in young boys. *Phys Ther* 1990, 70:244–249.

55. Bohannon RW: Is the measurement of muscle strength appropriate in patients with brain lesions? A special communication. *Phys Ther* 1989, 69:225–230.

56. Rothstein JM, Riddle DL, Finucone SD: Commentary to #57. *Phys Ther* 1989, 69:230–235.

57. Magee DJ: *Orthopedic Physical Assessment*. Philadelphia, W. B. Saunders Company, 1992, pp 347–349.

58. Rose SA, Ounpuu S, DeLuca PA: Strategies for the assessment of pediatric gait in the clinical setting. *Phys Ther* 1991, 71:961–980.

59. Sutherland DH: *Gait Disorders in Children and Adolescents*.

Baltimore, MD, Williams & Wilkins Company, 1984, pp 14–27.

60. Sutherland DH, Olshen R, Cooper L, Woo SL: The development of mature gait. *J Bone Joint Surg* [Am] 1980, 62:336.

61. Nelson K: What proportion of cerebral is related to birth asphyxias? *J Pediatr* 1988, 113:572–574.

62. Styer-Acevedo J: Physical therapy for the child with cerebral palsy. In Tecklin JS (ed): *Pediatric Physical Therapy.* 2nd ed. Philadelphia, J. B. Lippincott Company, 1993, pp 89–134.

63. Sharrard WJW: The mechanism of deformity in cerebral palsy. *Proc R Soc Med* 54:1016.

64. Fulford GE, Brown JK: Position as a cause of deformity in children with cerebral palsy. *Devel Med Child Neurol* 1976, 18:305–314.

65. Bobath B, Bobath K: *Motor Development in the Different Types of Cerebral Palsy.* London, Heinemann Medical Books, 1975.

66. Molnar GE (ed): *Pediatric Rehabilitation.* Baltimore, MD, Williams & Wilkins, 1972.

67. Brett EM (ed): *Pediatric Neurology.* New York, Churchill Livingstone, 1983.

68. Holt KS: Growth disturbances: Hemiplegic cerebral palsy in children and adults. In Clinical Developmental Medicine. No 4. London, Heinemann Medical Books, 1961.

69. Stanley FS, English DR: Prevalence and risk factors for cerebral palsy in a total population cohort of low birth weight infants. *Dev Med Child Neurol* 1986, 28:559–568.

70. Bly L: Abnormal motor development. In Slaton DS (ed): *Proceedings: Development of Movement in Infancy.* Chapel Hill, NC, University of North Carolina at Chapel Hill, Division of Physical Therapy, 1980.

71. Sutherland DH: Gait analysis in cerebral palsy. *Dev Med Child Neurol* 1978; 20:807–813.

72. Berger W, Quintern J, Dietz V: Pathophysiology of gait in children with cerebral palsy. *Electroencephalogr Clin Neurophysiol* 1982, 53:538–548.

73. Mykebust BM: A review of myotatic reflexes and the development of motor control and gait in infants and children: a special communication. *Phys Ther* 1990, 70:188–203.

74. Olney SJ: New developments in the biomechanics of gait in children with cerebral palsy: lesson I. In *Touch Topics in Pediatrics:* Lesson 1: Department of Education, APT A, Alexandria, VA, American Physical Therapy Association, 1989.

75. Cusick B: Casts and splints: their changing role in the management of foot deformity. Continuing education packet (Unpublished data). 1988.

76. Brook MH: 2nd ed. Baltimore, MD, Williams & Wilkins, 1986.

77. Boehme R: *The Hypotonic Child: Treatment for Postural Control, Endurance and Sensory Organization.* Milwaukee, WI, Boehme Workshops, 1987.

78. Harris SR: Down syndrome. In Campbell SK (ed): *Pediatric Neurologic Physical Therapy.* 2nd ed. New York, Churchill Livingstone, 1991, pp 131–168.

79. Shea AM: Growth and developments in Down syndrome in infancy and early childhood: implications for the physical therapist. In *In Touch Topics in Pediatrics;* Lesson 5. Department of Education, A PTA, Alexandria, VA, American Physical Therapy Association, 1990.

80. Cronk CE: Growth of children with Down's syndrome: birth to age 3 years. *Pediatrics* 1981, 61:564–568.

81. Cronk CE, Crocker AC, Pueschel SM, et al: Growth charts for children with Down syndrome: 1 month to 18 years of age. *Pediatrics* 1988, 81:102–110.

82. Rarick GG, Seefeldt V: Observations from longitudinal data on growth in stature and sitting height of children with Down syndrome. *J Ment Defic Res* 1974, 18:63–78.

83. Dummer GM: Strength and flexibility in Down's syndrome. In American Association for Health, Physical Education and Recreation (ed): *Research Consortium Papers: Movement Studies.* vol. 1. book 3. Washington, DC, American Association for Health, Physical Education and Recreation, 1978.

84. Whaley WJ, Gray WD: Atlantoaxial dislocation and Down's syndrome. *Can Med Assoc J* 1980, 123:35.

85. American Academy of Pediatrics, Committee on Sports Medicine: Atlantoaxial instability in Down syndrome. *Pediatrics* 1984, 74:152–153.

86. Giblin PE, Michele LJ: The management of atlanto-axial subluxation with neurologic involvement in Down's syndrome: a report of two cases and review of the literature. *Clin Orthop* 1979, 140:66.

87. Bersu ET: Anatomical analysis of the developmental effects of aneuploidy in man: the Down syndrome. *Am J Med Genet* 1980, 5:399.

88. Thomas CL: *Taber's cyclopedic medical dictionary.* 17th ed. Philadelphia: F. A. Davis Company, 1993.

89. Allsop K, Tecklin JS: Physical therapy for the child with myopathy and related disorders. In Tecklin JS (ed): *Pediatric Physical Therapy.* Philadelphia, J. B. Lippincott Company, 1989, pp 303–317.

90. Eng GD: Rehabilitation of children with neuromuscular diseases. In Molnar GE (ed): *Pediatric Rehabilitation.* 2nd ed. Baltimore, MD, Williams & Wilkins, 1992, pp 363–380.

91. Hosking GP, Bhat US, Dubowitz V, Edwards RHT: Measurements of muscle strength and performance in children with normal and diseased muscle. *Arch Dis Child* 1976, 51:957–963.

92. Johnson ER, Fowler WM, Lieberman JS: Contractures in neuromuscular disease. *Arch Phys Med Rehabil* 1992, 73:807–810.

93. Griffin MG, Avioli LV, Florence J, Pestronk A: *The Long-Term Effect of Prednisone Treatment for Duchenne's Muscular Dystrophy on Bone Density* [Abstract]. St. Louis, MO, The Jewish Hospital of St. Louis and the Irene Johnson Institute of Rehabilitation at Washington University Medical Center, 1991.

94. Cassidy JT: Juvenile rheumatoid arthritis. In Kelley WN, Harris ED, Ruddy S, Sledge CB (eds): *Textbook of Rheumatology.* 3rd ed. Philadelphia, W. B. Saunders Company, 1989, pp 1289–1311.

95. Swann M: Juvenile chronic arthritis. *Clin Orthop Rel Res* 1987, 219:38–49.

96. Schaller JG: Arthritis in children. *Pediatr Clin North Am* 1986, 33:1565–1580.

97. Scull SA, Dow MB: Physical and occupational therapy for children with rheumatic diseases. *Pediatr Clin North Am* 1986, 33:1053–1077.

98. Scull SA: Juvenile rheumatoid arthritis. In Tecklin JS (ed): *Pediatric Physical Therapy.* Philadelphia, J. B. Lippincott Company, 1989, pp 216–236.

99. Lechner DE, McCarthy CF, Holden MK: Gait deviations in patients with juvenile rheumatoid arthritis. *Phys Ther* 1987, 67:1335–1341.

100. Coulton CJ, Zborowsky E, Lipton J, Newnan J: Assessment of the reliability and validity of the arthritis impact measurement scales for children with juvenile arthritis. *Arthritis Rheum* 1987, 30:819–824.

101. Lovell DJ, Howe S, Shear E, Hartner S, *et al.*: Development of a disability measurement tool for juvenile rheumatoid arthritis: the juvenile arthritis functional assessment scale. *Arthritis Rheum* 1989, 32:1390–1395.

102. Rhodes VJ: Physical therapy management of patients with juvenile rheumatoid arthritis. *Phys Ther* 1991, 71:910–919.

103. Ryan KO, Ploski C, Emans JB: Myelodysplasia: the musculoskeletal problem. Habilitation from infancy to adulthood. *Phys Ther* 1991, 71:935–946.

104. Moore KL: *The Developing Human.* 3rd ed. Philadelphia, W. B. Saunders Company, 1982, pp 375–412.

105. Dias LS: Myelomeningocele. In Canale ST, Beaty JH (eds): *Operative Pediatric Orthopedics.* Philadelphia, C. V. Mosby Company–Year Book, 1991, pp 683–715.

106. Piggott H: The natural history of scoliosis in myelodysplasis. *J Bone Joint Surg [Br]* 1980, 62B:54.

107. Shurtleff DB, Goiney R, Gordon LH, Livermore N: Myelodysplasia: the natural history of kyphosis & scoliosis. A preliminary report. *Dev Med Child Neurol* 1976, 18(Suppl):126.

108. Menelaus MB: *The Orthopedic Management of Spina Bifida Cystica.* 2nd ed. New York, Churchill Livingstone, 1980, pp 125–187.

109. Tachdjian MO: Myelomeningocele. In Tachdjian MO (ed): *Pediatric Orthopedics.* 2nd ed. Philadelphia, W. B. Saunders Company, 1990, pp 1773–1871.

110. Carroll NC: Assessment and management of the lower extremity in myelodysplasia. *Orthop Clin North Am* 1987, 18:709–724.

111. Lock TR, Aronson DD: Fractures in patients who have myelomeningocele. J Bone Joint Surg [Am] 1989; 71: 1153–1157.

112. Ralis ZA, Ralis HM, Randall M, Watkins G, Blake PD: Changes in shape, ossification and quality of bones in children with spina bifida. *Dev Med Child Neurol* 1976, 18(Suppl):29–41.

113. Drummond DS, Moreau M, Cruess RL: Post-operative neuropathic fractures in patients with myelomeningocele. *Dev Med Child Neurol* 1981, 23:147–150.

114. Rosenstein BD, Greene WB, Herrington RT, Blum AS: Bone density in myelomeningocele: the effects of ambulatory status and other factors. *Dev Med Child Neurol* 1987, 29:486–494.

115. Hall JE, Poitras B: The management of kyphosis in patients with myelomeningocele. *Clin Orthop Rel Res* 1977, 128:33–40.

116. Heydemann JS, Gillespie R: Management of myelomeningocele kyphosis in the older child by kyphectomy and segmental spinal instrumentation. *Spine* 1987, 12:37–41.

117. Drummond DS, Moreau M, Cruess RL: The results and complications of surgery for the paralytic hip and spine in myelomeningocele. *J Bone Joint Surg [Br]* 1980, 62:49–53.

118. Feiwell E, Sakai D, Blatt T: The effect of hip reduction on function in patients with myelomeningocele. *J Bone Joint Surg [Am]* 1978, 60:169–173.

119. Garber JB: Myelodysplasia. In Campbell SK (ed): *Pediatric Neurologic Physical Therapy.* 2nd ed. New York, Churchill Livingstone, 1991, pp 169–212.

120. Perry J, Antonelli D, Ford W: Analysis of knee joint forces during flexed knee stance. *J Bone Joint Surg [Am]* 1975, 57:961–967.

121. Asher M, Olson J: Factors affecting the ambulatory status of patients with spina bifida cystica: *J Bone Joint Surg* 1983, 65:350–356.

122. DeSouza LJ, Carroll NC: Ambulation of the braced myelomeningocele patient. *J Bone Joint Surg* 1976, 58:1112–1118.

123. Mazur JM, Shurtleff D, Menelaus M, Colliver J: Orthopedic management of high-level spina bifida: Early walking compared with early use of a wheelchair. *J Bone Joint Surg [Am]* 1989, 71:56–61.

124. Lough LK, Nielsen DH: Ambulation of children with myelomeningocele: parapodium versus parapodium with orlav swivel modification. *Dev Med Child Neurol* 1986, 28:489–497.

125. Dudgeon BJ, Jaffe KM, Shurtleff DB: Variations in midlumbar myelomeningocele: implications for ambulation. *Pediatr Phys Ther* 1991, 3:57–62.

126. Day HJB: The ISO/ISPO classification of congenital limb deficiency. In Bowker JH, Michael JW (eds): *Atlas of Limb Prosthetics: Surgical, Prosthetic and Rehabilitation Principles.* 2nd ed. Philadelphia, C. V. Mosby Company–Year Book, 1992, pp 743–748.

127. Aitken GT: Proximal femoral focal deficiency: definition, classification and management. In Aitken GT (ed): *Proximal Femoral Focal Deficiency: A Congenital Anomaly.* Washington, DC, Natural Academy of Sciences, 1969, pp 1–22.

128. Epps CH: Current concepts review proximal femoral focal deficiency. *J Bone Joint Surg [Am]* 1983, 65:867–870.

129. Kruger LM: Lower limb deficiencies: surgical management. In Bowker JH, Michael JW (eds): *Atlas of Limb Prosthesics: Surgical, Prosthetic and Rehabilitation Principles.* 2nd ed. Philadelphia, C. V. Mosby Company–Year Book, 1992, pp 795–834.

130. Light TR: Upper-limb deficiencics: surgical management. In Bowker JH, Michael JW (eds): *Atlas of Limb Prosthetics: Surgical, Prosthetic and Rehabilitation Principles.* 2nd ed. Philadelphia, C. V. Mosby Company–Year Book, 1992, pp 749–760.

131. Wright PE, Jobe MT: Congenital anomalies of the hand. In Canale ST, Beaty JH (eds): *Operative Pediatric Orthopedics.* Philadelphia, C. V. Mosby Company–Year Book, 1991, pp 253–330.

132. Gillespie R: Principles of amputation surgery in children with longitudinal deficiencies of the femur. *Clin Orthop Rel Res* 1990, 256:29.

133. Herzenberg JE: Congenital limb deficiency and limb length discrepancy. In Canale ST, Beaty JH (eds): *Operative Pediatric Orthopedics.* Philadelphia, C. V. Mosby Company–Year Book, 1991, pp 187–251.

134. Kotz R, Salzer M: Rotation-plasty for childhood osteosarcoma of the distal femur. *J Bone Joint Surg [Am]* 1982, 64:959–969.

135. Krebs DE, Edelstein JE, Thornby MA: Prosthetic management of children with limb deficiencies. *Phys Ther* 1991, 71:920–934.

136. Setoguchi Y, Rosenfelder R (eds): *The Limb Deficient Child.* Springfield, IL, Charles C Thomas, 1982.

137. Binder H, Hawks L, Graybill G, Gerber NL, Weintrob JC: Osteogenesis imperfecta: rehabilitation approach with infants and young children. *Arch Phys Med Rehabil* 1984; 65:537.

138. Marin JC: Osteogenesis imperfecta: comprehensive management. *Adv Pediatr* 1988, 35:391.

139. Tachdjian MO: Osteogenesis imperfecta. In Tachdjian MO (ed): *Pediatric Orthopedics.* 2nd ed. Philadelphia, W. B. Saunders Company, 1990, pp 758–786.

140. Morel G, Houghton GR: Pneumatic trouser splints in the treatment of severe osteogenesis imperfecta. *Acta Orthop Scand* 1982, 53:547–552.

141. Benson DR, Newman DC: The spine and surgical treatment in osteogenesis imperfecta. *Clin Orthop* 1981, 159:147–153.

142. Cristofaro RL, Hock KJ, Bonnet CA, Brown JC: Operative treatment of spine deformity in osteogenesis imperfecta. *Clin Orthop* 1979, 139:40–48.

143. Swinyard CA, Bleck EE: The etiology of arthrogryposis (multiple congenital contracture). *Clin Orthop Rel Res* 1985, 194:15–29.

144. Thompson GH, Bilenker RM: Comprehensive management of arthrogryposis multiplex congenita. *Clin Orthop Rel Res* 1985, 194:6–14.

145. Hall JG: Genetic aspects of arthrogryposis. *Clin Orthop Rel Res* 1985, 194:44–53.

146. Beaty JH: Neuromuscular disorders. In Canale ST, Beaty

JH (eds): *Operative Pediatric Orthopedics.* Philadelphia, C. V. Mosby Company–Year Book, 1991, pp 731–733.

147. Tachdjian MO: Arthrogryposis. In Tachdjian MO (ed): *Pediatric Orthopedics.* 2nd ed. Philadelphia, W. B. Saunders Company, 1990, pp 2086–2119.

148. Drummond DS, Siller TN, Cruess RL: The management of arthrogryposis multiplex congenita. In American Academy of Orthopedic Surgeons (ed): *Instructional Course Lectures.* vol. 23. St. Louis, MO, C. V. Mosby Company, 1974, pp 79–95.

149. Dunn PM: Congenital postural deformities. *Br Med Bull* 1976, 32:71–76.

150. Tachdjian MO: Osteochondrosis and related disorders. In Tachdjian MO (ed): *Pediatric Orthopedics.* 2nd ed. Philadelphia, W. B. Saunders Company, 1990, pp 932–1081.

151. Canale ST: Osteochondrosis. In Canale ST, Beaty JH (eds): *Operative Pediatric Orthopedics.* Philadelphia, C. V. Mosby Company–Year Book, 1991, pp 743–776.

152. Tachdjian MO: Limb length discrepancy. In Tachdjian MO (ed): *Pediatric Orthopedics.* 2nd ed. Philadelphia, W. B. Saunders Company, 1990, pp 2850–3012.

153. Burdick P: Personal communication, March, 1993.

154. Link MP, Grier HE, Donaldson SS: Sarcomas of bone. In Fernbach DJ, Vietti TJ (eds): *Clinical Pediatric Oncology.* 4th ed. St. Louis, MO, C. V. Mosby Company–Year Book, 1991, pp 545–575.

155. Meyers PA: Malignant bone tumors in children: osteosarcoma. *Hematol Oncol Clin North Am* 1987, 1:655–666.

156. Meyers PA: Malignant bone tumors in children: Ewing's sarcoma. *Hematol Oncol Clin North Am* 1987, 1:667–673.

157. Link MP: Cancer in childhood. In *Physically Handicapped Children.* New York, Grune & Stratton, 1982, pp 43–58.

158. Gillespie R: Principles of amputation surgery in children with longitudinal deficiencies of the femur. *Clin Orthop Rel Res* 1990, 256:29–38.

159. Finn HA, Simon MA: Limb-salvage surgery in the treatment of osteosarcoma in skeletally immature individuals. *Clin Orthop Rel Res* 1991, 262:108–118.

160. Goldwein JW: Effects of radiation therapy on skeletal growth in childhood. *Clin Orthop Rel Res* 1991, 262:101–107.

161. Micheli LG: Overuse injuries in children's sports: the growth factor. *Orthop Clin North Am* 1983, 14:337–360.

162. Micheli LG, Smith AD: Sports injuries in children. *Curr Probl Pediatr* 1982, 12:4–54.

163. McPoil TG: Considerations in the management of pediatric and adolescent sports injuries. In *In Touch Topics in Pediatrics;* Lesson 3, Department of Education, A PTA, Alexandria, VA. American Physical Therapy Association, 1990.

164. O'Neill DB, Micheli LG: Overuse injuries in the young athlete. *Clin Sports Med* 1988, 7:591–610.

165. Subotnick SS: Podiatric aspects of children in sports. *J Am Podiatr Assoc* 1979, 69:443–454.

166. James SL: Chondromalacia of the patella in the adolescent. In Kennedy JC (ed): *The Injured Adolescent Knee.* Baltimore, MD, Williams & Wilkins, 1979, pp 205–251.

167. Bright RW, Burstein AH, Elmore SM: Epiphyseal plate cartilage: A biomechanical and histological analysis of failure modes. *J Bone Joint Surg* [Am] 1974, 56:668–703.

168. Ogden JA, Southwick WD: Osgood-Schlatter's disease and tibial tubercle development. *Clin Orthop* 1976, 116:180–189.

169. Devas MB: Stress fractures in children. *J Bones Joint Surg* [Br] 1963, 45:528.

170. Walters NE, Wolf MD: Stress fractures in young athletes. *Am J Sports Med* 1977, 5:165–170.

171. McPoil TG Jr, McGarvey TC: The foot in athletics. In Hunt GC (ed): *Physical Therapy of the Foot and Ankle.* vol. 15. New York, Churchill Livingstone, 1988, pp 199–230.

172. Cahill BR, Tullos HS, Fair RH: Little league shoulder. *J Sports Med* 1974, 2:150–153.

173. Jobe F: Personal communication to Micheli LG: Relates to reference 161.

174. Bennett G: Elbow and shoulder lesions of baseball players. *Am J Surg* 1959, 98:484–488.

175. Murray RO, Duncan C: Athletic activity in adolescence as an etiological factor in degenerative hip disease. *J Bone Joint Surg* [Br] 1971, 53:406–419.

176. Ficat RP, Hungerford DS: *Disorders of the Patello-Femoral Joint.* Baltimore, MD, Williams & Wilkins, 1977.

177. Irrgang J: Associated pathologies. In Mangine RD (ed): *Physical Therapy of the Knee.* vol. 19. New York, Churchill Livingstone, 1988, pp 57–74.

178. McMonoma GB, Jr: Ankle injuries in the young athlete. *Clin Sports Med* 1988, 7:547–562.

179. Koman LA, Gelberman RH, Toby EB, Poehling GG: Cerebral palsy: management of the upper extremity. *Clin Orthop Rel Res* 1990, 253:62–74.

180. Colton CL, Ransford AO, Lloyd-Roberts GC: Transposition of the tendon of the pronator teres in cerebral palsy. *J Bone Joint Surg* [Br] 1976, 58:220.

181. Gelberman RH: The upper extremity in cerebral palsy. In Bora W (ed): *Pediatric Upper Extremity Surgery.* Philadelphia, W. B. Saunders Company, 1986, p 323.

182. Zancolli EA, Goldner JL, Swanson AB: Surgery of the spastic hand in cerebral palsy: report of the Committe on Spastic Hand Evaluation. *J Hand Surg* 1983, 8: 766–772.

183. Lonstein JE: Natural history and school screening for scoliosis. *Orthop Clin North Am* 1988, 19:2, 227–237.

184. Bunnell WP: An objective criterion for scoliosis screening. *J Bone Joint Surg* [Am] 1984, 66:1381–1387.

185. Calliet R: *Scoliosis: Diagnosis and Management.* Philadelphia, F. A. Davis Company, 1975.

186. Bobechko WP, Herbert MA; Totally implantable stimulators for treatment of scoliosis in children with CP. *Orthop Trans* 1986, 10:156.

187. Nelson RM, Currier DP: *Clinical Electrotherapy.* Norwalk, CT, Appleton and Lange, 1991.

188. Bunnel WP, MacEwen GD: Non-operative treatment of scoliosis in cerebral palsy: preliminary report on the case of a plastic jacket. *Dev Med Child Neurol* 1977, 19:45–49.

189. Moe JH, Winter RB, Bradford DS, Lonstein JE: *Scoliosis and Other Spinal Deformities.* Philadelphia, W. B. Saunders Company, 1978.

190. Zimbler S, Craig C, Harris J, *et al.*: Orthotic management of severe scoliosis in spastic neuromuscular disease—results of treatment. *Orthop Trans* 1985, 9:78.

191. Dwyer AF, Newton C, Sherwood AA: On anterior approach in scoliosis: a preliminary report. *Clin Orthop Rel Res* 1969, 62:192–202.

192. Cardoso A: Paralytic scoliosis. In Luque ER (ed): *Segmental Spinal Instrumentation.* NJ, Slack, 1984, pp 119–146.

193. Brookes M, Wardle EN: Muscle action and the shape of the femur. *J Bone Joint Surg* [Br] 1962, 44:398–411.

194. Samilson RL, Tsou P, Aamoth G, Green WM: Dislocation and subluxation of the hip in cerebral palsy. *J Bone Joint Surg* [Am] 1972, 54:863–873.

195. Beals RK: Developmental changes in the femur and acetabulum in spastic paraplegia and diplegia. *Dev Med Child Neurol* 1969, 11:303–313.

196. Jones ET, Knapp DR: Assessment and management of the lower extremity in cerebral palsy. *Orthop Clin North Am* 1987, 18:725–738.

197. Thomas HO: *Diseases of Hip, Knee and Ankle Joints with their*

Deformities, Treated by New and Efficient Method. 2nd ed. Liverpool, Dobb, 1986, p 17.

198. Csongradi J, Bleck EE, Ford WF: Gait electromyography in normal and spastic children with special reference to the quadriceps, femoris and hamstring muscles. *Dev Med Child Neurol* 1979, 21:738–748.

199. Bartlett MD, Wolf LS, Shartle DB, Stahell LT: Hip flexion contractures: a comparison of measurement methods. *Arch Phys Med Rehab* 1985, 66:620–625.

200. Hoffer MM, Knoebel RT, Roberts R: Contractures in cerebra palsy. *Clin Orthop Rel Res* 1986, 219:70–77.

201. Hoffer MM, Prietto C, Koffman M: Supracondylar derotational osteotomy of the femur for internal rotation of the thigh in the cerebral palsied child. *J Bone Joint Surg* [Am] 1981, 63:389.

202. Bleck EE, Ford F, Stevik AC, et al.: EMG telemetry studies of spastic gait patterns in cerebral palsy children. *Dev Med Child Neurol* 1975, 17:307.

203. Gage JR: Surgical treatment of knee disfunction in cerebral palsy. *Clin Orthop Rel Res* 1990, 253:45–54.

204. Phillips WE, Audet M: Use of serial casting in the management of knee joint contractures in an adolescent with cerebral palsy. *Phys Ther* 1990, 70:521–523.

205. Harryman SE: Lower extremity surgery for children with cerebral palsy: physical therapy management. *Phys Ther* 1992, 72:16–24.

206. Girolomi GL, Hertz K: Early mobilization and postsurgical management after hamstring or gracilis muscle release in children with cerebral palsy. In *In Touch Topics in Pediatrics, Lesson 8*. Alexandria, VA, American Physical Therapy Association, 1990.

207. Bennett GC, Rang M, Jon D: Varus and valgus deformities of the foot in cerebral palsy. *Dev Med Child Neurol* 1982, 24:499.

208. Hoffer MM, Perry J: Pathodynamics of gait alterations in cerebral palsy and the significance of kinetic electromygraphy in evaluating foot and ankle problems. *Foot Ankle* 1983, 4:128.

209. Banks HH: Equinus and cerebral palsy. *Foot Ankle* 1983, 4:149.

210. Duncan WR, Mott DH: Foot reflexes and the use of the "inhibitive cast." *Foot Ankle* 1983, 4:145.

211. Bertoti DB: Effect of short leg casting on ambulation in children with cerebral palsy. *Phys Ther* 1986, 66:1522–1529.

212. Fulford GE: Surgical management of ankle and foot deformities in cerebral palsy. *Clin Orthop Rel Res* 1990, 253:55–61.

213. Hicks R, Durinick N, Gage FR: Differentiation of idiopathic the walking and cerebral palsy. *J Pediatr Orthop* 1988, 8:160–163.

214. Skinner SR, Lester DK: Dynamic EMG findings in valgus hindfoot deformity in spastic cerebral palsy. *Orthop Trans* 1985, 9:91.

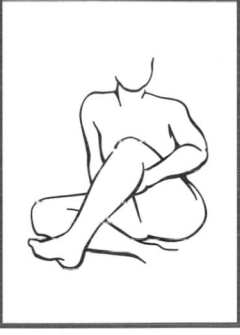
Age-Related Considerations: Geriatric

Mary Ann Wharton, Terry R. Holley, and Kathryn P. Medlin

Chronic and acute musculoskeletal disorders associated with aging are a challenge to the physical therapist. An understanding of the pathophysiology of normal and pathological aging is imperative for making effective clinical decisions. The foundation for understanding the aging musculoskeletal system is in understanding the sequence of normal musculoskeletal development, which begins prenatally. In this chapter, the foundation of normal musculoskeletal development is used to inspect closely development and aging of the musculoskeletal system. From the perspective of physical therapy, prevention and rehabilitation strategies are discussed.

I. Skeletal Considerations

A. Ossification process
1. **Osteogenesis**
   a. Describes the process of bone formation, which begins prenatally, approximately 3 months after fertilization of the ovum.
      (1). Hyaline cartilage precursor forms the skeleton.
      (2). Fibrous membrane precursor makes up the prebone structures of the skull, including the mandible.
   b. These hyaline cartilage and membranous precursors set the stage for the calcium deposition process known as ossification.
2. **Endochondral ossification**
   a. Begins with the cartilagenous skeletal precursor.
      (1). Derived from mesoderm.
      (2). Avascular and aneural.
   b. Periosteum, called perichondrium at this early stage, is present.

(1). Cells on the inner surface of the perichondrium differentiate into osteoblasts.

(2). These osteoblasts begin forming a ring of bone in the diaphysis called the subperiosteal collar.

c. Blood vessels begin entering the avascular cartilage, enhancing the ossification process.

d. Diaphyseal ossification spreads toward each epiphysis.

e. Chondroclastic (cartilage destroying) activity soon begins formation of the medullary cavity.

f. Secondary ossification centers begin in the epiphysis, growing toward the diaphysis.

g. An area of cartilage remains between the epiphysis and diaphysis known as the epiphyseal cartilage or growth plate.

(1). Facilitates growth in bone length until approximately 18 to 25 years of age.

(2). Disappears at the end of longitudinal long-bone growth, allowing the diaphysis to co-ossify with the epiphysis.

(3). *Intramembranous ossification*

(a). Primary ossification sites occur within a fibrous membrane.

(b). Ossification sites represent each bone in the skull.

(c). Ossification sites enlarge and grow through a process known as appositional growth.

(i). Because of lack of a growth plate, intramembranous ossification occurs with the addition of osseous tissue to the outer surface.

(ii). Intramembranous ossification sites either co-ossify or form highly congruent joints.

B. Microscopic structure of bone

1. **Compact bone**

a. Found in the cortical region of all bones.

b. Is responsible for diaphyseal strength of long bones.

c. Microscopic structure consists of highly vascular, metabolically active cells that play an important role during osteogenesis and bone remodeling throughout life.

d. *Haversian system (osteone)*

(1). Thousands of haversian systems make up compact bone within each long bone's diaphysis, giving rise to the structural integrity of the bone.

(2). Each osteone is arranged along lines of mechanical stress, producing a bone precisely shaped for maximum structural integrity able to withstand forces transmitted through it.[1]

(3). *Composition*

(a). Lamellae

(i). Concentric, cylindrical layers of calcified matrix primarily containing collagen, calcium, and phosphorus.

(ii). Help make up the structural integrity and strength of each osteone.

(b). Lacunae

(i). Small spaces arranged within the concentric lamellae.

(ii). Contain tissue fluid in which bone cells such as osteocytes lay imprisoned.

(c). Canaliculi

(i). Ultra-small canals radiating out in many directions.

(ii). Connect each lacuna to a multitude of other lacunae, which communicate with the larger haversian canal.

(iii). Enable nutrients and gases to travel from the circulatory system through the bone to the various bone cells.

(iv). Serves as an intrabone circulation system that allows the metabolically active bone cells to receive nutrients and dispose of metabolic byproducts.

(d). Haversian canal

(i). Channel containing blood and lymphatic vessels.

(ii). Forms the pathway in which blood cells enter bone. A blood cell travels through the haversian canal, enters a canaliculi before arriving at its destination, a bone cell housed within the lacuna.

2. **Cancellous bone**
   a. Found primarily in the ends of long bones, vertebral bodies, and flat bones such as the skull and pelvis.
   b. Consists primarily of trabeculae with a covering of compact bone (Fig. 42–1).
      (1). Trabeculae make up approximately 20% of the skeleton.[2]
      (2). Creates a lighter skeleton with high structural integrity.[2]
         (a). Trabeculae are arranged in vertical and horizontal patterns, which maximizes strength.[3]
         (b). Trabecular strands are highly metabolic and depend on available calcium coupled with load bearing to develop and maintain tensile strength.[4]

3. **Osteocytes (bone cells)**
   a. Make up less than 20% of bone.[1]
   b. Play a very important roll in osteogenesis and maintenance of structural integrity throughout life.
   c. *Composition*
      (1). *Osteoblasts*
         (a). Bone-forming cells are under hormonal influence.
         (b). Appear to respond to load-bearing forces.[3,4]
         (c). Found throughout bone, housed inside lacunae and the inner layer of periosteum.
         (d). Remove calcium and phosphate from blood and form crystals of apatite called hydroxyapatite.
         (e). Form and secrete collagen into the extracellular space, forming the haversian system.
         (f). Are very active during osteogenesis, and remain active during life through bone remodeling.[2]
      (2). *Osteoclasts*
         (a). Bone removing cells.
            (i). Break down hydroxyapatite.
            (ii). Return calcium and phosphate to the blood.
            (iii). Process reverses osteoblastic development of haversian systems.
         (b). Have potential of becoming very active with age.[5]
            (i). Hormonal and dietary changes, coupled with decreased physical activity, may result in decreased available calcium.
            (ii). With decreased available calcium, osteoclasts will shift calcium from bone to the blood, ensuring that blood-borne calcium is available for other important cellular processes.[3]
            (iii). The resultant unbalancing can be detrimental to the aging skeletal system.[6]

4. **Bone matrix**
   a. *Collagen—organic matrix*
      (1). *Composition*
         (a). Collagenous fibers
         (b). Ground substance—mixture of protein and polysaccharides

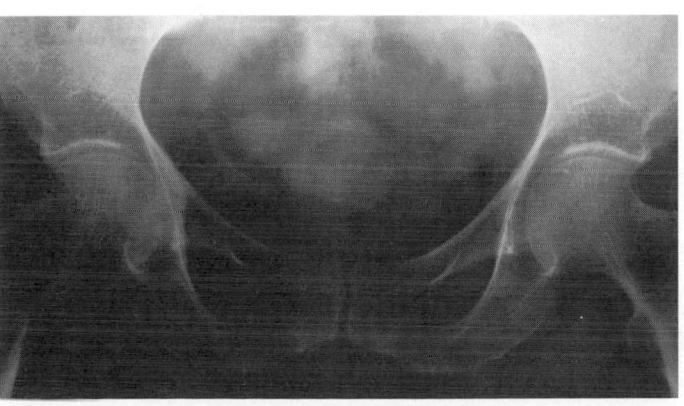

FIGURE 42–1 A radiograph of a woman older than 80 years with degenerative joint disease. Note the pattern of proximal femur trabeculae system. Also note the decreased joint space in the right hip.

(2). Role—combines with inorganic matrix to aid in maintaining the structural integrity and strength of bones.[1]

b. *Apatite—inorganic matrix*

(1). *Composition*

(a). Calcium

(b). Apatite (phosphate)

(i). Chemical crystals that adhere to sides of collagen fibers.

(ii). Forms hardness and structural rigidity of bones.[1]

C. Function of bones

1. **Supportive framework**

a. Tensile strength is nearly equal to cast iron but less than one third of iron's weight.[1]

b. Tensile strength is the result of relationship of the microscopic structure of bone.

2. **Protection**

a. Provides protective covering for brain and visceral organs of thoracic, abdominal, and pelvic cavity.

b. Loss in structural integrity can subject organs to decreased function and/or injury.

3. **Movement**

a. In combination with the neuromuscular system, plays an important role in allowing the organism to move within its environment.

b. Movement can be highly compromised with fractures or other skeletal anomalies associated with bone decalcification.

4. **Mineral reservoir**

a. Serves as a major storage depot for calcium and phosphorus.

b. Assists in maintaining homeostasis of blood calcium concentrations.[2,3,7]

5. **Hemopoiesis**

a. Blood cell formation at red marrow sites.

b. In the adult, red marrow sites of hemopoiesis are located primarily in the proximal humerus, proximal femur, vertebral bodies, and flat bones of the skull, pelvis, and rib cage.

D. Structural integrity

1. **Factors influencing the development and maintenance of a healthy skeletal system**

a. *Genetics*[8]

b. *Diet*

(1). *Calcium*

(a). Dietary intake is important in maintaining calcium homeostasis.[9,10]

(i). Extracellular ionized calcium represents less than 1% of the body's calcium stores.[10]

(ii). Extracellular ionized calcium is instrumental in enzymatic reactions such as mitochondrial function, cell membrane maintenance, intercellular communication, interneuronal transmission, neuromuscular transmission, muscular contraction, and blood clotting.

(iii). Because calcium is instrumental in all of these physiological processes, the bones will give up calcium if adequate intake is not sufficient to meet these demands.

(iv). This serum ionized calcium concentration is maintained within a very narrow physiological range.

(b). National Research Council of the National Academy of Sciences recommended dietary allowances for calcium of all age groups (average amount of calcium needed to maintain a neutral calcium balance and prevent the body from drawing on the mineral stores in bone).[11]

(i). Young adults: 750 to 1000 m per day.

(ii). Healthy premenopausal women older than 30 years: 1000 m per day.

(iii). Pregnant women and/or postmenopausal women: 1500 m per day.[12]

(2). *Vitamin D*

(a). Vitamin D is converted to active vitamin D (1,25-dihydroxyvitamin D).

(i). Active hormone that helps maintain normal serum calcium and phosphate levels.

(ii). Works by increasing calcium absorption from the

intestine and resorption from the bone and kidney.

(b). Source

(i). Approximately one half comes from dietary sources;[13] RDA is 400 IU;[14] RDA increases to 800 IU in the elderly;[13] most milk in the United States is fortified with 400 IU of vitamin D.

(ii). Approximately one half comes from an endogenous reaction in skin stimulated by ultraviolet radiation.[13]

c. *Hormones*

(1). Play important roles in maintaining adequate extracellular ionized calcium concentrations.

(2). Many are primarily concerned with resorption of calcium from the bone to maintain proper serum calcium levels.

(3). Their demands have priority over the potential for structurally deleterious effects on the skeletal system.

(a). Parathyroid hormone (PTH)

(i). PTH is secreted by the four parathyroid glands.

(ii). Chief function is to help maintain homeostasis of blood calcium concentration by promoting calcium absorption into the blood, preventing hypocalcemia.

(iii). PTH acts on the intestine, bones, kidneys, and kidney tubules to accelerate calcium absorption into the blood.

(iv). Output by the parathyroid glands is normally regulated by the concentration of calcium in the blood.[10]

(v). It causes increased blood concentration of calcium.

(vi). Osteoclasts seem to be very sensitive and responsive to PTH.[2]

(b). Active vitamin D

(i). Is very important for ab-

sorption of calcium from the intestines into the circulatory system.

(ii). Is derived from ingested vitamin D or sunlight.

(c). Estrogen

(i). Important in bone growth; researchers have recently discovered estrogen receptor sites on bone cells;[14] although mode of action awaits further study, it seems to reduce osteoclastic activity.[6]

(ii). At menopause and after menopause, there is a dramatic loss of calcium of both the cortical and trabecular bone, alluding to the important roll of estrogen in bone and calcium concentration.[2,5,13–15]

(d). Calcitonin

(i). Secreted by the thyroid gland.

(ii). Primary role is to prevent hypercalcemia; acts quickly to decrease the blood calcium concentration by either inhibiting resorption of calcium from the bone or promoting calcium deposition into the bone.

(iii). Although action is opposite that of PTH, it works synergistically to maintain blood calcium homeostasis.[10]

d. *Physical activity and bone growth*

(1). Physical activity has been shown to be a direct stimulant for bone development and growth.[16,17]

(2). Mechanical stress activates bone cell remodeling to help ensure structural competence.

(a). The consensus of many physical activity studies seems unanimous: Increased skeletal loading through exercise and activity is associated with increased bone mass; decreased functional loading through decreased exercise and activity is associated with decreased bone mass.

(b). Skeletal weight bearing or load bearing, in the presence of sufficient calcium, is associated with cortical thickness and the number and thickness of trabeculae.[3,16,17]

(i). Wolff's law[18] states that changes in bone mass accompany a change in the load through the process of skeletal remodeling. Current research documenting the negative effects of weightlessness, inactivity, and/or immobilization on bone[19–21] serves as validation of Wolff's law.

(ii). Modeling: Skeletal growth, which is considered to be a general change in the size and shape of the bone by formation and resorption of bone;[2,3,13,22] primarily hormonally and mechanically produced coupled with sufficient minerals

(iii). Remodeling: occurs throughout life. Maintenance of skeletal integrity and mineral homeostasis occurs throughout life through a continuous process of bone resorption by osteoclasts and formation by osteoblasts.[14] Ideally maintains a general balance between osteoblastic and osteoclastic activity.[2,3,5,8]

(iv). Peak bone mass: describes the amount of calcium in the skeletal system around the ages of 28 to 35 years;[23] bone bank develops throughout life and is affected by such factors as diet, hormones, activity, and genetics; individuals can no longer increase their bone bank account after they achieve peak bone mass around the ages of 28 to 35 years; automatic age-related bone loss seems to begin in the third decade of life; on the average, women lose 35 to 40% of their cortical bone and 55 to 60% of their trabecular bone throughout life.[14]

(v). Fracture threshold:[14,23,24] the concept of a fracture threshold has been identified by various authors; at levels greater than this threshold, osteoporotic-related fractures seldom occur; at levels lower than this threshold, there is a progressive probability that an osteoporotic-related fracture will occur; the higher the peak bone mass, the later in life the individual will drop below the fracture threshold.

2. **Demineralization contributing factors**
   a. *Calcium availability*
      (1). *Ingestion*
         (a). As discussed earlier, the average American female ingests less than 500 mg of calcium daily.[10]
         (b). RDA for calcium, also noted previously, is 1000 m per day for healthy premenopausal women older than 30 years and 1500 m per day for postmenopausal women.[11]
      (2). *Absorption*
         (a). Calcium is absorbed partially by diffusion and partially by active transport from active vitamin D.[8,25]
         (b). Absorption seems to decrease with age.
         (c). Calcium malabsorption results in hypocalcemia.
            (i). This triggers the parathyroid glands to secrete PTH, discussed earlier.
            (ii). This leads to secondary hyperparathyroidism manifested by increased bone resorption by osteoclasts.
      (3). *Caffeine effects*
         (a). Generally, it appears that caf-

feine does not detrimentally affect calcium.

> (b). Increased caffeine does increase urinary output of calcium, which is important for people who are borderline regarding calcium intake and serum levels.[26]

(4). *Alcohol effects*

> (a). Alcohol causes undesirable urinary loss of calcium.
>
> (b). Chronic alcoholics present with markedly increased decalcification, which seems most pronounced in the proximal femur.[27,28]

b. *Cigarette smoking*

(1). Studies have shown that female smokers have lower cortical bone mass than nonsmokers.

(2). As a result, female smokers have a greater risk of osteoporosis-related fractures than women who do not smoke.[29-33]

c. *Genetics*

(1). In the United States, blacks have bones of greater density with markedly less osteoporosis than people of other ethnic origins.[8]

(2). Age-specific fracture rates for white women are more than twice those for black women at any given age.[29]

d. *Gender*

(1). Data from most available studies support the conclusion that women older than 50 years are more than twice as likely to experience osteoporosis-related fractures from bone demineralization than men at any given age as a result of the role of estrogen and menopause.[34,35]

(2). Men in the eighth or ninth decade of life also experience osteoporotic fractures resulting from bone demineralization.

e. *Advanced age*

(1). Incidence rates for hip fracture resulting from bone demineralization increase rapidly after age 50 for white women.

(2). In the early 60s, the incidence rate is approximately 2 per 1000 per year, whereas at age 85 and older, the incidence rate is greater than 3% per year.[36]

f. *Physical inactivity*

(1). Decreased bone mass occurring in response to decreased mechanical stress may result in disuse osteoporosis.

> (a). Focal loss may occur after immobilization, such as casting secondary to a fracture of a limb.
>
> (b). General loss may result from decreased activity.

(2). Bone density decreases rapidly with as much as 30 to 40% of the initial total bone mass lost after 6 months of complete immobilization.[20]

(3). Movement alone does not protect against osteoporosis and must be coupled with weight-bearing activity and the use of the antigravity muscles.[17]

3. **Postmenopausal demineralization prevention strategies**

a. *Estrogen replacement therapy (ERT)*

(1). Research reports that ERT may be the most effective single means of preventing and treating osteoporosis.[6,13]

(2). *Associated problems*

> (a). Resumption of menses: may be eliminated by the physician prescribing estrogen and progestin continuously.[37]
>
> (b). Increase in endometrial carcinoma: can be largely alleviated by coadministration of progestin.[10,37]
>
> (c). Prompt acceleration of loss of bone mineral density when ERT is discontinued.

(3). *Optimal management*

> (a). Initiation of ERT shortly after menopause.[38]
>
> > (i). Many studies showed that once the decalcification process has occurred, it is very difficult to regain bone calcium.
> >
> > (ii). ERT is known to be very effective in arresting progressive loss of bone mineral density.[37,38]
> >
> > (iii). Consensus is that ERT prevents both cortical and trabecular bone loss.
> >
> > (iv). Appears to work primarily

by reducing osteoclastic bone resorption.

(b). It appears that ERT is safe and well tolerated until approximately age 75 years; because of the prompt acceleration of loss of bone mineral density when ERT is discontinued, many physicians elect to continue prescribing after age 75 if it is well tolerated.[6,37]

(c). The optimal daily dose is 0.625 mg.[6,37]

(d). Some studies have shown ERT to be most effective with calcium carbonate.[38]

(4). ERT also appears to decrease cholesterol low-density lipoproteins and increase high-density lipoproteins, thereby preventing or diminishing cardiovascular disease.[6]

b. *Calcitonin*

(1). Calcitonin can be used when ERT is contraindicated.[8,34]

(2). Drawback: it must be injected.

(3). It is thought to work by inhibiting osteoclastic bone resorption.[34]

(4). Side effects: Nausea and vomiting occur in approximately 10% of the patients when treatment is first initiated.[7]

4. **Problems associated with low bone density**

a. *Osteoporosis* (Fig. 42–2)

(1). *Type 1: postmenopausal*

(a). A 1 to 2% cortical bone loss and 3 to 10% trabecular bone loss per year is superimposed over type 2 (age-related) bone loss.[34,39]

(b). More bone is lost in the first 5 years postmenopausally than in the subsequent 15 years.[35,37]

(c). With women living 25 years after menopause, one third of these postmenopausal women will experience osteoporosis-related fractures, which will typically occur 15 to 20 years after menopause.[35,37]

(d). As discussed previously, this postmenopausal pronounced demineralization can be largely eliminated with administration of ERT.

(2). *Type 2: age related*

(a). Slow yet consistent loss of .3 to .5% of both cortical and trabecular bone throughout life.[35]

(b). Occurs in both men and women beginning in the third decade of life.[35]

(3). *Exercise and osteoporosis*

(a). The consensus of the plethora of research is that a decrease in weight bearing coupled with decreased stress on the bones, often occurring with age, results in calcium resorption with subsequent loss of bone.[2,3,4,34]

(b). To help prevent this disuse osteoporosis, individuals need to maintain weight-bearing and/or stress exercises.

(i). Because this strain-related remodeling is essentially a local response, each bone must literally experience some form of a high strain.

(ii). Research has shown that, to attain and maintain bone mass, this high-intensity, short-duration strain should occur daily

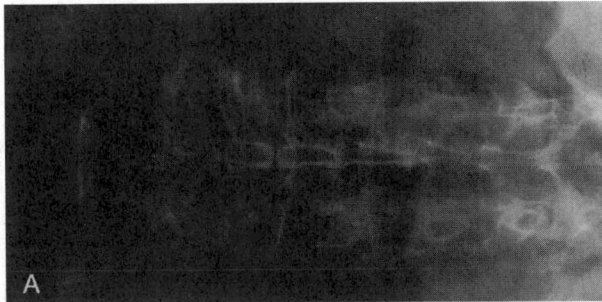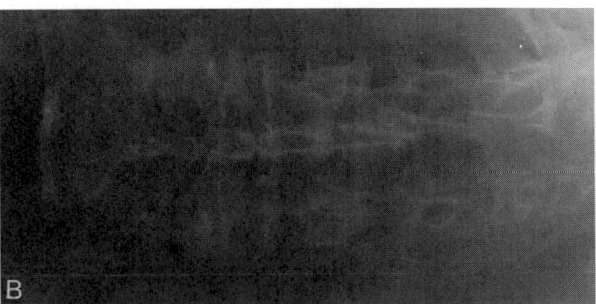

FIGURE 42–2 **A,** A radiograph of a woman older than 80 years with progression of osteoporosis. This anteroposterior view of the lumbar spine shows diffuse demineralization with narrowing in multiple intervertebral disc spaces. **B,** A radiograph taken 1 year later shows progression of the osteoporosis with multiple compression fractures.

to help offset bone demineralization caused by the calcium-regulating hormones.[3,4,34]

(c). There is sufficient evidence for individuals to engage in a load-bearing, safe exercise program premenopausally, preosteoporotically, or even after an osteoporosis-related fracture.

(i). It is important that load-bearing exercises affect the entire skeletal system.[3]

(ii). Research has shown that even postmenopausal, post-fracture women can gain bone mass with appropriate exercise. In one study, 35 postmenopausal women took part in a dynamic bone-loading exercise program of walking, jogging, and stair climbing at 70 to 90% of maximal oxygen uptake for 50 to 60 minutes three times per week; bone mineral content increased 5.2% above baseline levels after short-term training with no change in the control group; after 22 months of exercise, bone mineral content was 6.1%; after 13 months of decreased activity, bone mass was 1.1% above baseline levels in the detraining group.[40]

b. *Fractures*
(1). *Incidence*
(a). Approximately 1.2 to 1.5 million osteoporosis-related fractures occur in the United States each year.[35]
(b). Approximately 44% affect the vertebrae, 19% affect the hip, 14% result in a radial fracture, and the remaining 23% affect other limb sites.[35]
(c). In general, areas of osteoporosis-related fractures affect the areas of high trabecular bone remodeling.[21,34,35]

(2). *Location*
(a). Distal radius (Colles) (Fig. 42–3)
(i). Bone composition: 30% cortical bone; 70% trabecular bone.
(ii). Incidence: approximately 172,000 per year in the United States.[34]
(iii). Cause: primarily the result of a low-impact fall to an outstretched arm or palm.
(iv). Management: correction through either closed or open reduction.
(b). Vertebral (Fig. 42–4)
(i). Bone composition: 35% cortical bone; 65% trabecular bone.
(ii). Incidence: approximately 538,000 per year in the United States;[34] one third of women older than 65 years will experience a vertebral compression fracture.[8]
(iii). Cause: can be associated

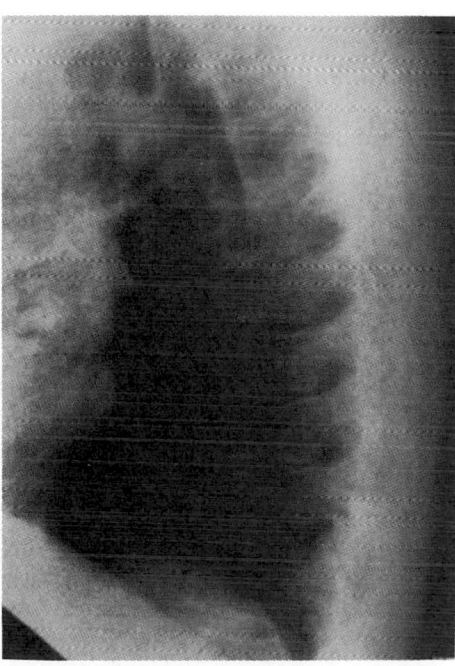

FIGURE 42–3 A radiograph of a distal radius fracture. (From Barth RW, Lane JM: Osteoporosis. *Orthop Clin N Am,* 1988, 19:845–858.)

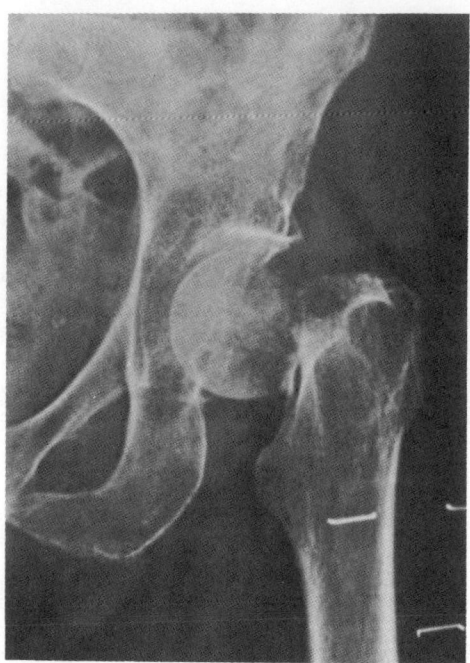

FIGURE 42–4 A radiograph showing a vertebral fracture. (From Barth RW, Lane JM: Osteoporosis. *Orthop Clin N Am,* 1988, 19:845–858.)

with a fall, stepping off of a step, or any other routine daily activity.

(iv). Clinical presentation: these fractures usually manifest themselves with an episode of acute pain in the middle to low thoracic area or high lumbar regions; some individuals may report being free of pain; most patients can identify the specific vertebral level causing their pain; spinal movement is often restricted secondary to a vertebral fracture; anterior vertebral wedging is characteristic of this type of fracture (may present as a dowager's hump with multiple anterior wedge fractures; dowager's hump, when present, is a sign of progressing osteoporosis).

(v). Management: Heat applied to the paravertebral

musculature may decrease spasms with a subsequent decrease in pain; it is important to have these individuals avoid flexion exercises because this transmits a potentially injurious force to the vertebral body; instruction in extension exercises is usually indicated.

(c). Hip

(i). Bone composition: in the subcapital and femoral neck region, there is a higher percentage of trabecular bone; distally, into the intertrochanter region, there is a higher percentage of cortical bone.

(ii). Incidence: approximately 250,000 per year in the United States;[34] these usually occur after 65 years of age because of a combination of cortical and trabecular bone loss.

(iii). Classification: Severity (simple or comminuted); location (intracapsular [subcapital or femoral neck] or extracapsular [intertrochanteric]).

(iv). Cause: often the result of a fall in a posterior lateral direction with force transmitted through the greater trochanter of the femur; spontaneous fractures may occur and result in a fall; it is difficult to substantiate the percentage of these spontaneous fractures.

(v). Surgical considerations: (Fig. 42–5) intracapsular fractures (there is a chance that the blood supply to the femoral neck will be compromised; to avert the latent possibility of developing an avascular necrosis, the surgeon may elect to use

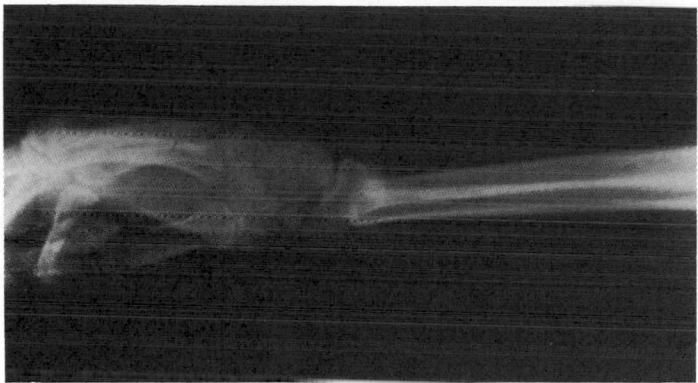

FIGURE 42–5   A radiograph showing an intracapsular fracture of a hip. (From Barth RW, Lane JM: Osteoporosis. *Orthop Clin N Am*, 1988, 29:845–858.)

a prosthesis such as an Austin-Moore); extracapsular (intertrochanteric) fractures. (The blood supply remains intact; frequently, the surgeon will elect to use a compression screw as the fixation device.)

(vi). Management guidelines: After surgical insertion of a prosthetic device (Austin-Moore), often the surgeon will allow immediate full weight bearing or weight bearing as tolerated; after surgical insertion of an internal fixation device, the patient often needs to maintain partial weight-bearing status for an average of 6 weeks to allow sufficient bony healing to occur; may need to implement total hip precautions depending on surgical approach (with anterior surgical approach avoid external rotation, extension; with lateral surgical approach avoid hip flexion beyond 90 degrees, and adduction combined with internal rotation).

(vii). Related facts: the mortality rate for the hip fracture is approximately 20%

within the first year;[34] in general, these fractures are also associated with the highest morbidity of any of the other fractures.[41]

(d). Pelvis
(i). Fractures usually remain nondisplaced and affect the superior or inferior ramus.
(ii). Are often associated with a high pain level that can persist from 6 to 8 weeks postfracture.
(iii). Individuals are usually allowed full weight bearing immediately.

(3). *Bone densitometry*
(a). Bone mass measurements can help identify and estimate those individuals at risk for fracture.[42]
(b). Plain radiography is the least sensitive method.
(c). Noninvasive radiographic and radioisotopic techniques have been developed during the past 10 years to assist in determining skeletal mass;[43,44] these techniques are accurate and safe and provide site-specific information about the quantity of bone at the time of the examination but are limited by the inability to show past or present deposits or withdrawals from the bone bank account, making sequential measurements necessary.

(i). Single-photon absorptiometry (SPA): primarily used for the assessment of cortical bone in the appendicular skeleton;[43] radioisotope iodine 125 is used, primarily on the distal radius and midshaft;[43] limitation is that SPA cannot be used on the axial skeleton.[42]

(ii). Dual-photon absorptiometry: used for assessing both cortical and trabecular bone of the spine and hip and assessing total bone mass;[42] uses a radio-

isotope that emits photons of two distinct energies;[42] has minimal side effects because of its low radiation dose;[44] is very applicable to many osteoporotic individuals because it does assess trabecular bone in high-risk areas such as hip and vertebral bodies.[42,44]

(iii). Quantitative computed tomography: only trabecular bone is measured;[44] has the benefit of excellent precision.[44]

II. Diarthrodial Joints and Aging

A. Structure

1. **Hyaline cartilage**
   a. Location: primarily on the ends of long bones.
   b. *Composition*
      (1). Eighty percent water
      (2). Twenty percent of remaining constituents include cells, primarily chondrocytes, collagen, and ground substance.[45]
   c. *Characteristics*
      (1). Porous and relatively spongelike with a pronounced capacity to absorb synovial fluid.
      (2). *Avascular*
         (a). Dependent on synovial fluid for its nutrition.[46]
         (b). Has a poor capability of repair once damaged.[47]
      (3). Healing time and metabolic rate of cartilage are very slow; cartilage healing that does occur is replaced by a fibrocartilage lacking the smooth hyaline characteristics.[47]
   d. *Mechanics*
      (1). Intermittent compression and distraction between joint surfaces must occur for adequate exchange of nutrients and waste products.[48]
      (2). There are three distinct mechanisms of this compression and distraction.[49]

(a). Weight bearing in the lower extremity and spinal joints.
(b). Intermittent contraction of muscles crossing a joint.
(c). Twisting and untwisting of a joint capsule as the joint moves toward and away from its close-packed position.
      (3). Because cartilage needs intermittent compression and distraction, immobilization causes atrophy of the cartilage, just as does prolonged compression.[50]
   e. *Degeneration*
      (1). As a joint loses its full range of motion, there is a loss of nutrition to the areas of cartilage that no longer contact one another within the joint.
      (2). Attritional changes occur in noncontacting areas of joint surfaces, such as those seen in individuals with contractures.[48]
      (3). There appears to be upper and lower limits regarding cartilage and its ability to absorb compressive forces; both underloading and overloading the joint can result in cartilage loss and damage.
      (4). These mechanical characteristics of cartilage become important when dealing with the aged population.[46]

2. **Subchondral bone**
   a. *Composition*

(1). *Surface of compact bone*
(2). *Primarily composed of trabecular bone*
    (a). Metabolically active, continually undergoing microscopic fractures and repair in response to joint loading and overloading.
    (b). Although moderate overload is effectively absorbed by the subchondral bone, an overload beyond its inherent strength results in cell and matrix damage.
        (i). Damage of sufficient intensity and duration can lead to microfracture of the subchondral bone.
        (ii). Microfracture may lead to eventual development of osteoarthritis.[51]

B. Articular cartilage loss

1. The most common cause of articular cartilage loss is degenerative joint disease, which may be the end result of severe mechanical injury to the articular cartilage with subchondral bone involvement; such articular cartilage loss may eventually lead to bone on bone.[46]
2. Three stages to the articular cartilage loss represent progressive aspects of loss and denudation.
    a. *Fasciculation: flaking of the cartilage*[46]
    (1). First stage of cartilage loss when the most superior aspect of cartilage shears off.
    (2). These cartilage flakes fall into the joint space.
    (3). This stage is undiscernible to the individual because there is no pain.
    b. *Fibrillation*[46]
    (1). With progressive degeneration, cracks or fibrillation in the cartilage occur.
    (2). This decreases the energy-absorbing capability of the cartilage, resulting in subchondral bone involvement.
    (3). The individual may become aware of joint pain during this stage because of the bone involvement.
    (4). As the cartilage continues to erode, microscopic fractures occur in the subchondral bone plate.
        (a). The subchondral bony plate thickens, decreasing the energy-absorbing capabilities of the cartilage and the subchondral

bone, leading to progressive cartilage degeneration.
        (b). Osteophytes begin forming at the joint margin, causing progressive pain.[30]
    c. *Subchondral bone involvement*
    (1). Bone and periarticular soft tissues are highly innervated; as periarticular osteophyte development continues, increasing pain may lead to restricted joint motion in an effort to inhibit pain.
    (2). As subchondral bone involvement continues, deformation of the joint will often occur.
    (3). Clinical intervention is limited at this progressive end stage; however, it is important to maintain as much joint strength and motion as possible.

C. Problems associated with aging joints

1. **Osteoarthritis**
    a. Etiology is multifactorial. One factor is the structural breakdown of the hyaline cartilage and subsequent subchondral bone involvement.[52]
    b. Occurrence: it is estimated that osteoarthritis affects 10 million people in the United States and costs $15 billion per year.[52]
    c. *Pharmacologic management*
    (1). *Nonsteroidal anti-inflammatory drugs*[52]
        (a). Do not stop progression of the disease.
        (b). Some agents may have a deleterious effect biologically on the cartilage.
    (2). *Analgesics*
        (a). Provide symptomatic relief.
        (b). Are used when symptoms are not satisfactorily managed with nonsteroidal anti-inflammatories.
    (3). More recently, conservative approaches are being advocated by some physicians who recognize the potential of developing toxicity secondary to nonsteroidal anti-inflammatories.[53]
    d. *Nonpharmacologic intervention*
    (1). Makes use of various modalities such as heat and ice, coupled with attempts to modify load patterns of the joint.

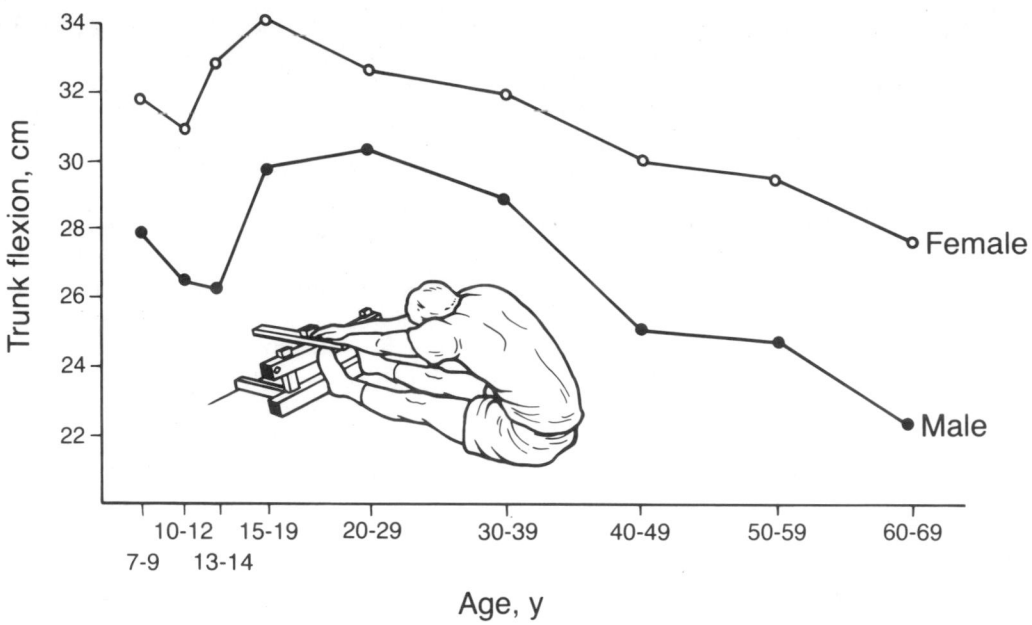

FIGURE 42–6   The decrease of flexibility with aging. (From Shephard RJ: The scientific basis of exercise prescribing for the very old. *J Am Geriat Soc,* 1990, 38(1):62–70; and *Fitness and Lifestyle in Canada.* Ottawa: Directorate of Fitness and Amateur Sport, 1983.)

(2). Recently, research projects have focused on the therapeutic effects of exercise programs for arthritic patients.[53,54]

   (a). It appears that carefully supervised exercise programs may be beneficial for persons suffering from osteoarthritis.[54]

   (b). The exercise program should be modified according to the stage of joint degeneration.

   (c). Obese people should be encouraged to lose weight because of the stress and strain on the joints.

2. **Periarticular connective tissue involvement**

  a. Includes ligaments, tendon, aponeurosis, associated joint capsule, and intramuscular connective tissue.

  b. Tissues increase in stiffness with age.[55]

   (1). Loss of extensibility with resultant loss of joint motion is one of the most clinically observable aspects of PCT involvement with aging.[55]

    (a). Through research, mostly on animals, it appears that ligaments, tendons, and joint cap-

sules increase in stiffness because of increased collagen cross-linking.[55,56]

    (b). In addition to cross-linking, there is usually an increase in the amount of collagen along with an increase in fibril size.[56]

    (c). Animal studies have also shown an age-related increase in collagen content in intramuscular tissue associated with increased muscular stiffness.[57]

   (2). Hypoactivity or decreased physical activity that seems to correlate with aging also seems to strongly correlate with joint stiffness, leading some to speculate that this age-related joint tightness can be partially or wholly prevented through activity and exercise.

   (3). Research into the effects of immobilization on periarticular tissue[58,59] verifies that the loss of extensibility in the joint capsule and related structures will decrease joint mobility; the research further indicates that this loss of joint range of motion secondary to loss of tissue extensibility can, for the most part, be prevented.[60]

(4). The need for intervention is given additional credence in that the flexibility of a typical sedentary individual decreases by 20 to 30% by the age of 70[61] (Fig. 42–6).

III. The Muscular System and Aging

A. Muscular strength

1. Individuals usually experience a general strength improvement in both isometric and dynamic strength up to and throughout the third decade of life.

2. This strength is fairly well maintained throughout the fifth decade of life.[62]

B. Disuse atrophy and aging

1. Decreases in muscle strength and muscle mass appear to be age related;[63,64] however, it is difficult to differentiate between disuse atrophy and age-related strength loss.[65]

2. In both disuse atrophy and aging, the effects are similar, resulting in loss of strength, loss of muscular endurance, and loss of muscle mass.[66]

3. It has been shown by researchers through autopsy and electromyographic studies that the number of functional motor units decreases with age;[65] factors involved include a decrease in the number of muscle fibers, a decrease in the number of functional neurons, and an alteration in neurotransmission.

4. In general, with age, there is a decrease in neurons being stimulated, with fibers responding in a slower manner.[62]

5. Aging seems to have a greater effect in strength loss in the lower extremity and back muscles than in the upper extremities.[65]

6. In aging, there will be a general decrease in muscle size from 20 to 35%.[65]
   a. The loss in gross number of muscle fibers may account for the decrease muscle in size.
   b. There is also a decrease in the size of remaining muscle fibers attributed to reduced activity and disuse atrophy.[65,67,68]
   c. Although there is a decrease in muscle size, there is no external atrophy when measuring thigh circumference;[62] a likely explanation for this morphological shift is that muscle fibers are replaced by fat and connective tissue so external atrophy is not apparent.[69]

7. In general, beginning at approximately age 60, there is a strength decline, which is markedly accelerated as the person enters their eighth decade of life.

C. Fiber-type changes

1. **Fast twitch**
   a. There seems to be a pronounced atrophy of fast-twitch fibers with disuse and aging[62,66] compared with a relative stability of slow-twitch fibers.
   b. It has been noted that fast-twitch fibers are not as detrimentally affected by immobilization as slow-twitch fibers.[67]
      (1). It is postulated that the general decline of fast-twitch fibers with aging is secondary to disuse.
      (2). Because disuse has already caused atrophy of fast-twitch fibers, immobilization will have a negligible effect on them.[70]

2. **Slow twitch**
   a. There is no prominent age-related atrophy in slow-twitch fibers.[62]
      (1). There is a morphological shift in muscle fiber composition, with an increased proportion of slow-twitch fibers compared with fast-twitch fibers.[66]
      (2). It is hypothesized that the slow-twitch fibers are recruited first in many of the activities of daily living, which are basically of a low intensity.[71]
      (3). During periods of immobilization, these slow-twitch fibers do not get their normal stimulation and, therefore, do go through a state of atrophy.[70]

b. The lack of age-related atrophy in slow-witch muscles may also be secondary to the fact the mitochondria, the principle organelles responsible for aerobic metabolism, seem to be fairly unaffected by aging.[72]

D. Positive effects of exercise

1. Strength improvements in the elderly secondary to exercise appear to be from metabolic, morphological, and neural adaptations.
   a. A great potential for improved strength in geriatric clients lies in improved neuromuscular association because strength improvement occurs out of proportion to muscle hypertrophy.[73]
   b. Adequate recovery time between episodes of exercise must be allowed to accentuate the neural association.
2. Recent research of both endurance and strengthening activities verifies the positive effect of training in aging.[66,68,71,73–77]
3. The research indicates promising results for strength improvements, even in individuals in their 70s, 80s, and 90s.[76,77]
   a. It is generally believed that once muscle fibers are lost a reverse hyperplasia does not occur.[65]
   b. There is strong evidence of hypertrophy occurring in the muscles; research shows that hypertrophy will account for perhaps up to 50% of the strength improvement; the other 50% is attributed to improvements in the neuronal connections with the muscle itself.[73]
   c. It is hypothesized that the immediate strength improvements that are seen within the first 2 weeks are due to improved neuronal connections and transmissions.[77,78]
4. There is strong evidence showing the correlation of weakness and falls in the frail elderly;[79] however, there is a need for more research showing the positive correlation between strength gains in the frail elderly and decreased falls, with increased independent functional mobility.
5. Although previous research has shown that there is greater atrophy in lower extremity and back musculature, research has also shown very favorable strength improvements when individuals engage in an upper extremity strengthening program as well. This has a very positive potential carry-over into activities of daily living.[76]

IV. Clinical Assessment and Treatment

A. Physical therapy assessment and treatment of geriatric patients

1. Intervention is multifactorial and cannot be limited to a primary musculoskeletal/medical diagnosis; the musculoskeletal/medical diagnosis is frequently limited to either disease or symptoms. The musculoskeletal/medical diagnosis may not be the sole factor contributing to functional limitation and, therefore, may not always be the primary consideration for physical therapy intervention.
2. Functional limitations related to multiple contributing factors must become the primary focus of clinical decision making with geriatric patients.

B. Considerations in clinical decision making

1. **Subjective information**
   a. Identify the patient's chief complaint.
      (1). Information will often incorporate limitations in activities of daily living that will assist in goal setting.
      (2). Information will identify the patient's primary areas of concern, which may not be limited to musculoskeletal/medical considerations.
   b. Determine the history and progression of present symptoms.
   c. Determine demographical characteristics that may contribute to functional limitations.
      (1). Consider elements of lifestyle, including previous level of function and changes in function that resulted in referral to physical therapy.
      (2). Include information on family/caregiver that may affect goals and treatment plan.
      (3). Include information on environmental factors, including barriers that

may limit the patient's ability to function at a prior level or in a prior setting.

d. Evaluate both prior and/or concurrent services related to the present referral.

e. Determine the patient's goals with respect to physical therapy intervention.

2. **Objective assessment**

a. *Musculoskeletal considerations*

(1). Determine the source of symptoms or dysfunction, including the specific structures from which the symptoms emanate.

(2). Identify predisposing or contributing factors involved in the problem.

(3). Determine the impact of musculoskeletal deficits on functional performance.

(a). Range of motion

(i). Achievement of "normal" range of motion for each joint may not be a reasonable goal for the geriatric patient on the basis of normal and pathological age-related changes.

(ii). Determine the relationship between range of motion deficits in involved joints to loss of function with respect to activities of daily living.

(b). Strength

(i). Manual muscle testing may be limited by age-related factors such as ability to assume test positions and changes in flexibility and/or muscle length.

(ii). Assessment of loss of function related to decreased strength combined with loss of range of motion and flexibility should be a primary indicator of "strength" in geriatric patients.

(c). Functional status

(i). Musculoskeletal deficits should be viewed in relationship to functional status.

(ii). Structural and functional components of postural changes should be identified.

(iii). Ability to perform functional activities of daily living, such as bed mobility, transfers, and locomotion should be assessed with respect to musculoskeletal deficits.

(iv). Gait assessment not only should identify specific deficits within the gait cycle that are related to musculoskeletal aberrations but should also incorporate functional impairment. Identify characteristics of gait related to pathology, normal age-related changes, and prior functional status; determine critical factors affecting performance (level of independence; use of assistive device; need for orthotic/prosthetic device; ability to negotiate a variety of surfaces, including carpeted surfaces, uneven terrain, and stairs; determination of weight-bearing status, where appropriate; assessment of functional parameters of gait, including such factors as distance ambulated and distance/time).

b. *Nonmusculoskeletal considerations*

(1). *Cognitive status*

(a). Evaluation must include determination of patient's alertness, mentation, and judgement.

(b). Factors such as dementia and delirium must be critically evaluated for their impact on participation in the treatment plan and goal setting.

(2). *Cardiopulmonary status*

(a). Ability to perform functional tasks may be compromised by cardiopulmonary disease or symptoms related to hypokinesis.

(b). Recognition of the contribution of cardiopulmonary deficits to decreased functional status must be incorporated into the assessment of geriatric patients with primary musculoskeletal diagnoses.

(3). *Neurological considerations*

(a). Because of age-related changes in both systems, it is frequently difficult to separate the neurological component from the musculoskeletal component when assessing strength in geriatric patients.

(b). The relationship of musculoskeletal deficits and neurological deficits as they impact on functional performance must be determined.

(4). *Sensory considerations*

(a). Changes in vision, hearing, taste, smell, and touch are known to occur with aging and may be the result of normal age-related changes or disease.

(b). Sensory changes may have a profound impact on a geriatric patient's ability to perform within the environment.

(c). Assessment of the contributions of sensory changes and environmental considerations will enhance the functional outcome of geriatric patients with musculoskeletal deficits.

(5). Pain related to musculoskeletal pathology that limits performance must be assessed.

(6). *Integument*

(a). Age-related changes must be assessed in geriatric patients to determine any relationship to the musculoskeletal diagnosis.

(b). Changes may limit or preclude the choice of modalities used to treat geriatric patients.

(c). Consideration must be given to integrity of the integument when performing transfers or other functional tasks.

(d). Integument must be assessed when making recommendations for positioning and seating for geriatric patients with primary musculoskeletal diagnoses.

c. *Special considerations*

(1). *Chronological age versus physiological age*

(a). Recognize that chronological age is frequently not the primary deterrent with respect to functional performance.

(b). Consideration must be given to the contributions of pathology and activity level (sedentary vs. active).

(2). *Pharmacological concerns*

(a). Use of prescription and over-the-counter drugs must be evaluated.

(b). Knowledge of side effects of drugs and the detrimental effects of polypharmacy on cognition and function must be incorporated into clinical decision making.

3. **Problem identification and goal setting**

a. Information from both subjective and objective assessment should be incorporated into a problem list.

b. Information must include all factors identified and not be limited to musculoskeletal considerations.

c. Problems identified should reflect functional deficits.

d. Problems should reflect lifestyle concerns.

(1). Family/caretaker support must frequently be considered with geriatric patients, especially those with increasing fraility.

(2). Locus of care must be considered during assessment and reflected in goal setting with respect to functional ability.

(a). Frequently, clinical decisions regarding locus of care are more reflective of social support than of physical performance.

(b). The ultimate goal should reflect the maximum achievable functional potential for each patient.

(3). Financial status, including Medicare reimbursement, may frequently affect access to care and must be considered during patient assessment.

4. **Implementation of physical therapy plan**

a. Plan should be reasonable, with a probability of success.

(1). Patient goals must be incorporated; unreasonable patient expectations must be tempered with appropriate patient education.

(2). Ethical concerns regarding informed consent, autonomy, and patient adherence must be addressed in implementation of treatment plan.

b. Precautions and contraindications to physical therapy treatment must be identified.
c. Specific modalities and techniques must be modified to address normal and pathological age-related changes in the musculoskeletal system as well as the other body systems.

d. A reasonable time frame for recovery should be identified.
e. Recommendations should include lifestyle modifications and strategies for prevention of further deficits.

V. Conclusions

Throughout this chapter, the detrimental aspects of aging on the musculoskeletal system have been discussed. It has become clear that many of the signs of aging, such as skeletal demineralization, osteoporosis-related fractures, loss of joint range of motion, and decline in muscular strength, are not so much directly caused by aging but rather secondary to disuse.

Considering that research is only as valuable as its application toward improving conditions, the research on musculoskeletal aging can markedly enhance the physical therapy profession. Physical therapists can profoundly and positively affect patients' lives not only in the customary rehabilitation setting but by shifting more into implementing preventive strategies. The authors strongly believe that as research is performed and presented within the profession, physical therapists have a responsibility to ensure that it is applied toward improving patient care.

Acknowledgement

Suzanne Fornataro assisted in accessing current literature and research information on musculoskeletal aspects of aging.

Clinical Decision-Making Cases

Physical Therapy Management of a Geriatric Patient with a Hip Fracture

This case study addresses the management of a geriatric patient, MH, as she recovers from a fractured hip. The case outlines goals and interventions from the initial physical therapy referral received in the acute care hospital one day after surgery and illustrates progression through a rehabilitation program carried out in a nursing facility and, ultimately, at home. The case study addresses management of factors that complicate the case, including the underlying musculoskeletal diagnoses and additional factors that may contribute to falls.

PROBLEM

MH is an 82-year-old female admitted to an acute care hospital after falling in her home. She was diagnosed as having an intertrochanteric fracture of the left hip. The x-ray examination showed intertrochanteric fracture of the left hip and osteoporosis of the left femur and thoracic spine.

HISTORY

One day before physical therapy referral, MH underwent open reduction, internal fixation (ORIF) fixed with a compression screw.

MH's medical history includes three falls in past year. She fractured her left shoulder 1 year ago as a result of a fall. She also has hypertension and angina. MH's prescribed medications include a nitroglycerin patch, chlorothiazide (Diuril), intravenous meperidine hydrochloride (Demerol), and calcium supplement.

The physical therapist consulted was to evaluate and treat MH. Weight bearing was restricted on the left lower extremity (touch-down weight bearing [TDWB] as requested by the referring orthopedic surgeon).

SUBJECTIVE ASSESSMENT

The patient's complaints include pain in the left hip, inability to walk, weakness after surgery, and nausea.

History

MH states that she fell 2 days ago in her living room when she lost her balance on standing up from a sitting position. The patient was wearing slippers. She states she was unaware that she was about to fall. She denies chest pain, dizziness, and loss of consciousness. She reports that she suffered no other injuries. Her neighbor was visiting at the time of the accident and called for an ambulance.

MH lacks a knowledge of use of assistive devices, weight-bearing status, safety factors related to transfers and ambulation, and management of left lower extremity after insertion of ORIF.

Lifestyle

The patient lives alone in a senior citizens' high-rise apartment. There are no steps to enter the building. Before this fall, MH states she was independent in all self-care activities of daily living (ADLs) and ambulated without an assistive device. MH relied on assistance from family for some housekeeping chores, grocery shopping, and transportation. Her daughter and son live nearby and are employed full time during the day.

MH describes herself as sedentary, engaging in limited physical activity.

The patient's goals are to return to her apartment with home care support, if necessary.

OBJECTIVE ASSESSMENT

Physical Examination

The patient was transported to the physical therapy department via a wheelchair. She appears lethargic, oriented to person, place, and time. Observation reveals a small-framed woman with slight forward head, rounded shoulders, and a mild kyphotic thoracic spine. She has thin, translucent skin. A Heplock® (a capped, intravenous infusion device) is in place in the dorsum of her right hand, and MH has an indwelling urinary catheter. The surgical dressing is intact on her left hip. No drainage is noted. The entire left lower extremity is moderately edematous. MH is wearing hospital slippers and long-leg antiembolus stockings, as prescribed by her orthopedic surgeon.

The patient's active range of motion (AROM) is within normal limits (WNL) except for the following: left hip flexion is 10 to 30 degrees, abduction is 0 to 7 degrees, and rotation (internal/external) is 0 degrees. Both ankles lack dorsiflexion 7 degrees from neutral. The left shoulder flexion is 0 to 145 degrees, abduction is 0 to 130 degrees, and external rotation is 0 to 60 degrees.

The patient's passive range of motion (PROM) is WNL except for the following: Left hip was not tested secondary to hip fracture 1 day post-ORIF. Both ankles lack 5 degrees from neutral secondary to Achilles tendon tightness. The left shoulder flexion is 0 to 160 degrees with bony end-feel, abduction is 0 to 140 degrees with hard, capsular end-feel, and external rotation is 0 to 65 degrees with hard capsular end-feel.

MH's strength measures 5/5 in both upper and lower extremity major muscle groups except for the following: The left hip was not tested secondary to hip fracture 1 day post-ORIF; the left knee was not tested secondary to hip fracture 1 day post-ORIF; the left shoulder scapular stabilizers are 3+/5; flexors and abductors are 3+/5 within available ROM.

The patient's neurological status includes intact sensation to superficial touch, sharp/dull, and position sense. Her reflexes measured 2+ and symmetrical knee jerk, biceps, brachioradialis, and triceps and absent ankle jerk. Her balance in sitting was normal. Balance while standing was not tested secondary to TDWB status of the left lower extremity.

The patient complained of constant pain in the left hip at 6 of 10 on pain scale (10 = severe pain, 0 = no pain). Pain increases to 8 of 10 with movement and touch-down weight bearing.

Assessment of the patient's posture included slight forward head, forward shoulders, and dorsal kyphosis.

Functional Status

The patient was able to transfer sit to and from standing from the wheelchair with moderate assistance of one individual. She was also able to pivot from the wheelchair to and from the mat with minimum assistance of one individual. MH was able to transfer sit to and from supine with moderate assistance of one individual and roll supine to and from side-lying with moderate assistance of one individual. She was unable to tolerate the prone position.

MH ambulated in parallel bars, 5 feet times two, TDWB on left lower extremity. Gait deviations included short stride length on right lower extremity and narrow base of support. The patient lacked adequate use of left upper extremity to maintain TDWB. She complained of right-hand pain with weight bearing on parallel bars.

The patient's vital signs were as follows: At rest, pulse, 72 beats per minute; blood pressure, 155/85 mm Hg; respirations, 15 breaths per minute. After ambulation, pulse, 92 beats per minute; blood pressure, 165/88 mm Hg; respirations, 20 breaths per minute.

Treatment given to the patient included gait training in parallel bars, TDWB on the left lower extremity, transfer training from wheelchair to and from stand, wheelchair to and from mat, and sitting to and from the supine position. The patient was also instructed in AROM exercises for the left hip.

ASSESSMENT/DIAGNOSIS

Problem List

Items included on the problem list include the following: dependent ambulation, TDWB status on the left lower extremity; decreased endurance for ambulation; left upper extremity fatigue; left hip pain; dependent transfers; dependent mat mobility; decreased AROM in left hip and left shoulder; decreased PROM in both ankles; decreased functional strength in the left lower extremity and left shoulder; postural changes; pain in the left hip and right hand; decreased knowledge after surgery with insertion of ORIF in the left hip. The patient was diagnosed with gait dysfunction, and impaired functional status after left intertrochanteric hip fracture with ORIF.

Summary Statement

The patient presents 1 day after ORIF of left hip secondary to a fall and fracture. She is motivated to participate in physical therapy. Factors complicating the patient's rehabilitation include left hip pain and weakness, left shoulder weakness 1 year after the fracture, pain in right hand with weight bearing resulting from Heplock®, decreased endurance secondary to cardiorespiratory status, residual effects of anesthesia, and reported sedentary lifestyle. The patient is also at risk for further falls secondary to the effects of hypertension medication and possible orthostatic hypotension, possible syncopal episode, and decreased ankle dorsiflexion.

Rehabilitation potential is fair to achieve the patient's goals of returning to her apartment safely with home care services within an acceptable length of acute care stay based on diagnosis-related group. As a result of the complicating factors identified, it is anticipated that patient will require additional rehabilitation to achieve independent function for transfers and ambulation before returning to her apartment with the limited home care services and family support available.

TREATMENT GOALS

Goals to achieve for discharge from acute care hospital are as follows:

1. The patient will ambulate 25 feet with walker, TDWB on the left lower extremity, contact guard to allow ambulation from bed to bathroom. The patient will achieve equal stride length and increase her base of support to approximate shoulder width. Vital signs will remain stable.

2. The patient will transfer sit to and from stand with contact guard of one, pivot wheelchair to and from mat with minimum assistance, sit to and from the supine position with assistance to support left lower extremity, and roll supine to and from side-lying position independently.

3. The patient will increase AROM of the left hip in supine position to 0 to 50 degrees of flexion and 0 to 20 degrees of abduction. She will also increase AROM of the left shoulder flexion 0 to 150 degrees and abduction 0 to 135 degrees. PROM of bilateral ankle dorsiflexion will increase to 0 degrees.

4. Functional use of the left upper extremity will im-

prove to enable the patient to ambulate an increased distance with an assistive device, TDWB on the left lower extremity without left upper extremity fatigue. The patient will perform postural exercises independently to correct forward head and shoulders. Pain of the left hip will decrease to 3 of 10 at rest and with TDWB ambulation to increase tolerance for ambulation. Finally, the patient will verbalize ORIF management techniques.

TREATMENT PLAN

The physical therapy plan in the acute care hospital includes the following:

1. Gait training TDWB on the left lower extremity, progressing from parallel bars to the use of a walker on level surfaces. Weight-bearing status was assigned by the orthopedic surgeon, and progression to increase weight-bearing status was not scheduled until at least 6 weeks postfracture, pending x-ray evidence of healing. Stair training was not included in the plan or goals because the patient's prior functional status did not necessitate use of stairs.

2. Transfer training sit to and from stand, pivot wheelchair to and from mat, sit to and from supine, and roll supine to and from side-lying position.

3. Therapeutic exercise: AROM exercises to the left hip and knee; strengthening exercises to the left scapular stabilizers and shoulder flexors and abductors; passive stretch to both Achilles tendons; postural exercise instruction including chin tucks, shoulder retraction, and thoracic spine extension (forward head and shoulders are a function of early osteoporosis and thoracic spine changes evident on x-ray films); strength deficits of left hip and left shoulder initially addressed with isometric exercises (the active exercises [heel slides and supine abduction exercises] used to increase ROM also serve as strengthening exercises for major hip musculature); ankle pumps to decrease swelling and actively increase Achilles tendon length; upper extremity exercise including upper body ergometer, Theraband (The Hygenic Corp), and aerobic activities to improve cardiorespiratory status and enhance endurance for achieving ambulation and transfer goals.

4. Reduce risk factors for additional falls: Refer to the physician to rule out possible syncopal episode and/or orthostatic hypotension as contributors to falls; monitor the blood pressure and radial pulse in sitting position and immediately on standing to detect positional changes, suggestive of possible orthostatic hypotension and/or dysrhythmia; educate the patient about environmental hazards through the use of a written check list that identifies potential hazards; recommend that the patient wear appropriate footwear to accommodate Achilles tendon tight-

ness, and stress the importance of continuing passive stretching exercise.

5. Pain management techniques: Ask nursing staff to provide pain medication before physical therapy sessions; request that nursing staff reposition the Heplock® to eliminate right-hand pain associated with weight-bearing on an assistive device (anticipate the Heplock® to be removed before discharge); instruct the patient to maintain TDWB status to minimize left hip pain from excessive weight bearing; provide modalities of ice or transcutaneous electrical neuromuscular stimulator to left hip to minimize pain not associated with weight bearing.

6. Patient education: Instruct patient to avoid prolonged dependent position of the left lower extremity and elevate the left lower extremity while in bed to minimize edema.

7. Recommendations to physician: referral to nutritionist to address dietary needs related to osteoporosis, hypertension, and cardiac status.

8. Comments: Anticipate nausea and lethargy to be resolved as anesthetic effects and pain medications are reduced. As patient becomes medically stable, urinary catheter will also be removed.

On discharge from the acute care hospital, this patient was transferred to a nursing facility for a short-term admission to continue her rehabilitation program.

NURSING FACILITY GOALS AND PLAN

Short-term goals were established to facilitate the long-term goal for this patient to return to her apartment with support of home care services and family. They include the following:

1. Ambulation 100 feet with walker, TDWB on left lower extremity, independently on level surfaces to ambulate throughout her apartment
2. Transfer independently supine to and from sit, and from sit to and from stand, from bed, chairs, and toilet to allow patient to return home and perform ADLs
3. Increase AROM of the left hip in supine to 0 to 70 degrees of flexion and 0 to 30 degrees of abduction
4. Increase AROM of left shoulder to 0 to 160 degrees of flexion, 0 to 140 degrees of abduction, and 0 to 65 degrees external rotation
5. Increase AROM of bilateral ankle dorsiflexion to 0 degrees

6. Decrease pain of left hip to 0 of 10 with TDWB ambulation

The physical therapy plan in the nursing facility progressed the rehabilitation program initiated in the acute care hospital.

HOME CARE GOALS AND PLANS

On discharge from the nursing facility, this patient returned to her home with home care physical therapy. The goals to be achieved to regain independent function are as follows:

1. Increase AROM of the left hip in supine position 0 to 90 degrees of flexion
2. Ambulate independently with standard cane throughout the apartment and apartment building, and begin ambulation within the community

Plan for home care includes the following:

1. Progress use of assistive device and weight-bearing status to ultimately allow patient to ambulate full weight-bearing on left lower extremity. In some situations, the therapist's clinical judgement regarding the progression of weight-bearing status may be limited by the orthopedic physician's referral. If the therapist is not limited by physician referral, clinical judgement should be based on x-ray evidence of healing, pain, and the patient's tolerance for weight bearing. The patient may not regain independent ambulation without an assistive device because of her history of falls. Ongoing assessment will determine whether use of a standard cane and appropriate footwear will adequately reduce falls. Teaching regarding the need to continue stretching exercises to maintain Achilles tendon length should be reinforced.
2. Perform detailed environmental assessment, and make recommendations regarding necessary modifications to enhance safety and decrease risk of falls caused by environmental hazards.
3. Progress therapeutic exercise program to achieve the stated goals.
4. Recommend additional home care services, including nursing services and occupational therapy, for training in personal care tasks of bathing, dressing, meal preparation, and light housekeeping chores.
5. Recommend home-delivered meals and homemaker services to assist with basic and instrumental ADLs until the patient achieves independence.

Physical Therapy Management of a Patient with Osteoarthritis

This case study addresses the course of physical therapy intervention for WM, a 68-year-old man with a diagnosis of osteoarthritis (OA) of both knees. The initial phase of the case study outlines physical therapy intervention at the time when WM was referred to outpatient physical therapy by his family physician secondary to complaints of bilateral knee pain.

Despite treatment and compliance with nonsteroidal anti-inflammatory medications, modalities, exercise, and joint protection, WM's knees continued to be painful and to limit function. This continued debility resulted in the patient undergoing an elective total knee arthroplasty 2 years later. The second phase of the case study addresses management of WM after this surgical procedure.

PART A: OUTPATIENT SETTING

The diagnosis is osteoarthritis of both knees. X-ray evidence was unavailable. Medical history includes OA and hypertension. The patient is taking nonsteroidal anti-inflammatory medication and propoxyphene napsylate and acetaminophen (Darvocet) (as needed for night pain). The physical therapy consultation is for evaluation and treatment.

SUBJECTIVE ASSESSMENT

Problem

Patient complains of intermittent bilateral knee pain, right knee greater than left knee pain.

History

The patient has had knee pain for many years, which has progressively worsened in the past 3 months. There has been occasional knee swelling. Pain increases with walking, especially initially on standing when it sometimes feels like the knees will give out. Usually the knees are more painful in the evening. WM denies morning swelling. Pain occasionally awakens him at night. He denies trauma or falls, low back pain, and paresthesias in the lower extremities. Knee pain is relieved with rest and pain medications. The patient is unable to kneel and has difficulty getting up from floor, walking long distances, and going up and down stairs. WM uses no assistive device for ambulation. He denies modality use. WM has had multiple cortisone injections over the years, most recently 2 months ago. Each time only temporary pain relief has been achieved. There is intermittent stiffness in his low back and hands, although presently he is asymptomatic. The patient has had no therapy or education for his OA in the past.

Lifestyle

The patient lives with his healthy, active wife in a two-story home with bedroom and bathroom on second floor. The stairs to the second floor have a railing. The two steps to enter the house also have a railing. The patient has been retired for 6 years as a high school mathematics teacher and football coach. He is active with walking, yard work, and babysitting his grandchildren. He does not use tobacco. WM consumes alcohol on a social level.

Patient's Goals

The patient's goals are to walk and sleep without knee pain and without pain medications. Also, he wants to be able to get down on the floor with his grandchildren.

OBJECTIVE ASSESSMENT

Physical Examination

The patient walked to the department, accompanied by his wife. He is tall and stocky. Forward head and rounded shoulders were evident. Minimally decreased lumbar lordosis is present. There is bilateral genu varus, which is greater on the right than the left. Bony hypertrophic knee changes are moderate and are greater on the right than the left. Right knee is flexed, and the patient's weight bearing is greater on left lower extremity. There is mild pes planus, which is greater on the right than the left when weight bearing and non-weight bearing.

Active range of motion (AROM) of WM's lower extremities are within normal limits (WNL) except for the following: Right knee flexion is 95 degrees, right knee extension is −15 degrees, left knee flexion is 110 degrees, and left knee extension is −10 degrees.

WM's lower extremity passive range of motion (PROM) is within normal limits except for the following: Right knee flexion is 100 degrees secondary to patellar tendon tightness and knee pain, right knee extension is −10 degrees secondary to knee pain and soft capsular tightness, left knee flexion is 115 degrees secondary to patella tendon tightness, and left knee extension is −10 degrees secondary to soft capsular tightness. Varus deformity in the right knee is measured at 10 degrees when non-weight bearing and 17 degrees when weight bearing. The varus deformity in the left knee is measured at 10 degrees when non-weight bearing and 10 degrees when weight bearing.

WM's lower extremity strength measures 5/5 except for right knee extension; which is 4/5 with minimal pain, and left knee extension, which is 4+/5 without pain.

Sensation is intact for superficial touch and position sense in the bilateral lower extremities. Reflexes are 2+ and symmetrical for bilateral knee jerk. Bilateral ankle jerk is absent. Balance while sitting and standing is normal.

The patient's pain is constant. It measures 8 of 10 when standing and walking and 2 of 10 at rest (pain scale: 0 = no pain, 10 = excruciating pain).

Patellar mobility test shows limitation in superior inferior excursion. Passively, the right patella is 50% of the left knee; bilateral crepitus is noted. Actively, there is minimal right patellar movement with a quadriceps set. On the right knee, there is evidence of moderate varus laxity with valgus stress. On the left knee, there is evidence of minimal varus laxity with valgus stress. No joint laxity is noted with anteroposterior stresses. Mild swelling is present along the medial and superior aspects of right patellar border. There is minimal tenderness in the joint spaces, which is greater medially than laterally and greater in the right knee than the left knee. Hamstring lengths are as follows: right knee, −30 degrees; left knee, −20 degrees (knee extension is measured when the patient is supine with the ipsilateral hip flexed to 90 degrees and each knee individually passively extended to end-range). According to the Thomas test, the right rectus femoris is −15 degrees, and left rectus femoris is −10 degrees. The iliotibial band is bilaterally full (measured with the patient in a side-lying position on a mat).

FUNCTIONAL STATUS

All transfers are independent with right knee held in approximately 20 degrees flexion during supine to and from sit and approximately 70 degrees flexion during sit to and from stand.

WM ambulates independently more than 100 feet without assistive device. There is decreased stance time on right, and the patient maintains the right knee in approximately 20 degrees flexion throughout gait cycle. Although the patient is independent on stairs, he does experience difficulty. He uses the hand rail and a step-over-step pattern with increased right knee pain during right lower extremity stance.

DIAGNOSIS

Problem List

Included on the patient's problem list are the following: pain in knees; deformity in knees; decreased active range of motion of bilateral knee flexion and extension; decreased passive range of motion of bilateral knee flexion and extension; decreased strength in knee extension bilaterally; shortened hamstring and quadriceps lengths bilaterally; right quadriceps lag of 5 degrees; antalgic gait when weight bearing on the right lower extremity; decreased knowledge of OA and management.

Summary Statement

The patient presented with chronic pain in the knees, which is greater in the right knee than the left knee, deformity, weakness, and swelling secondary to OA. This limits the patient's ability to kneel and play with his grandchildren, walk long distances, and walk up and down stairs. Pain interferes with his sleep. The patient is unable to manage knee problems at home because of limited knowledge. Rehabilitation potential is good to achieve patient's goals.

TREATMENT GOALS

1. Decrease right knee pain to 3 of 10 with ambulation and other weight-bearing activities.
2. Decrease right quad lag to 0 degrees.
3. Increase active range of motion in bilateral knee flexion (right knee to 105 degrees, left knee to 120 degrees).
4. Increase passive range of motion in bilateral knee flexion (right knee to 105 degrees, left knee to 120 degrees).
5. Increase passive range of motion in the bilateral knee extension to less than −5 degrees.
6. Lengthen hamstrings 15 degrees on the right and 10 degrees on the left.
7. Lengthen quadriceps 10 degrees on the right and 5 degrees on the left.
8. Perform written home exercise program independently.
9. Patient verbalizes understanding of home management of OA knees through use of modalities, compliance with exercise program, and joint protection techniques.
10. Patient ascends/descends stairs using step-to pattern when knees are painful.

TREATMENT PLAN

Examine x-ray films (or radiologist's report if films are inaccessible) of patient's knees. Characteristic progressive changes include joint space narrowing (erosion of articular cartilage), subchondral bony sclerosis (eburnation), and marginal osteophyte formation and cyst formation; x-ray films should be taken in weight-bearing and non–weight-bearing positions for anteroposterior and lateral views.

Obtain laboratory results, which are helpful to rule out other joint diseases; erythrocyte sedimentation rate (ESR) is normal in most patients with OA but may be elevated in erosive inflammatory OA. Synovial fluid is usually normal. Calcium pyrophosphate dihydrate and/or apatite crystals can be seen in many joint effusions of patients with OA.

Rule out the possibility of lumbar spine or hip dysfunction contributing to knee pain through clinical evaluation.

Implement physical therapy program two times a week for 3 to 4 weeks:

1. Apply heat modalities to reduce pain: hot packs and/or continuous wave ultrasound.
2. Use range of motion exercises and stretching for quadriceps and hamstrings, as well as trunk, hips, and ankles; these exercises improve flexibility as well as reduce stiffness from immobility. Hold each position at the joint's end-range for 5 to 10 seconds.

Caution: Do not exercise beyond the stretch to the point at which pain (or worsened pain) is felt.

3. Gait training on level surfaces and stairs. Instruct in use of standard cane to decrease pain in knees and minimize identified gait deviations.

4. Implement exercises for muscle strengthening: isometrics (involve minimal to no joint movement, cause the least rise in pressure inside the joints, the least destruction of the bone ends, and the least joint inflammation) and isotonics (require the movement of a joint; develop strength throughout the joint's full range of motion, and generally result in greater strength gains than isometrics).[77]

5. Exercise for aerobic conditioning, including use of a stationary bicycle, walking program, and therapeutic pool exercises. The intensity of exercise can be monitored by palpating the pulse and working toward a target heart rate. Target heart rate should be 60 to 75% of the maximum heart rate, which is equal to 220 − age. Example: WM is 68 years old: 220 − 68 = 152 (maximum heart rate); 152 × .6 = 91; 152 × .75 = 114; WM should work at getting his heart rate into the range of 91 to 114 beats per minute. (A more accurate calculation of maximum heart rate is to take a treadmill or cycle exercise test with electrocardiogram and blood pressure monitoring.) Caution: the formula for determining target heart rate is invalid in people taking cardiac medications, such as beta-blockers, that slow the heart rate. People in these categories should have their maximal heart rate determined by an exercise test.[80]

Education for OA and the patient's home management is as follows:

1. Provide written materials from the Arthritis Foundation regarding OA and the patient's management and allow for questions/discussion.

2. Discuss joint protection techniques of assistive device (cane and walker) for ambulation to decrease weight-bearing stresses on the knees; bracing with (neoprene) knee sleeve for joint compression to reduce pain and feeling of instability; use of soft plantar orthotics to accommodate pes planus and enhance shock absorption in the feet and knees.

3. Instruct the patient in home exercise program, initially exercising 3 to 5 days per week for three 20-minute sessions: 5 to 10 minutes for warm-up stretching, up to 10 minutes of peak intensity, and 5 to 10 minutes of cool-down stretching.

4. Provide information regarding the local swim program to continue aquatics exercise when independent.

Discharge Summary
All goals are attained within 4 weeks.

PART B: ACUTE CARE HOSPITAL SETTING

WM is a 70-year-old man with a long history of knee pain. He received a diagnosis of severe OA of the right knee. Current status: 2 days ago, he underwent right total knee replacement.

X-ray evidence (preoperatively) showed marked narrowing of medial joint space on right knee with hypertrophic bony changes throughout the knee. Medical history is as stated previously in Part A. The patient is currently taking those medications listed previously in Part A. The physical therapy consultation includes evaluation and treatment: touch-down weight bearing on the right lower extremity.

Problem
The patient complains of severe right knee pain, lightheadedness, and nausea.

SUBJECTIVE ASSESSMENT

History
The patient had been compliant with a home exercise program, including isometrics, isotonics with Theraband, stretching, knee active-assisted range of motion, and moist heat for pain. He stopped the aquatics exercise program last year and began using his cane and knee sleeve for joint protection while ambulating 6 months ago. Presently, WM denies other joint pains. This postoperative course was relatively uncomplicated. His laboratory tests taken postoperatively on Day 1 show low hematocrit and hemoglobin. The patient is knowledgeable regarding home management of OA of the knees.

Lifestyle
The patient's lifestyle is stated previously in Part A.

Patient's Goals
The patient wants to return home with his wife and be able to walk on discharge from the hospital.

OBJECTIVE ASSESSMENT

Physical Examination
WM arrived in physical therapy department via a wheelchair, accompanied by his wife. His right lower extremity was elevated and wrapped in Jones dressing. Mild swelling of right toes was evident. The patient was sleepy and pale. A Heberden's nodule (firm) on Digit 2 of the right hand and a Bouchard's nodule (soft) on Digit 3 of the left hand were noted.

Active range of motion of the lower extremities was within normal limits except for the following: Right knee flexion was 30 degrees, right knee extension was not assessed (patient was unable to extend actively), left knee flexion was 117 degrees, and left knee extension was −5 degrees.

Passive range of motion of the lower extremities was as follows: right knee flexion was not assessed. Right knee extension was −25 degrees, left knee flexion was 120 degrees (secondary to patellar tendon tightness), and left knee extension was −5 (soft capsular tightness).

The strength of the lower extremities was measured as 5/5; the right hip and knee, however, were not assessed (the patient was unable to perform straight-leg raise or short arc quad).

Sensation in the patient's right toes was intact. A dorsal pedal pulse could not be palpated on the right because of a Jones-type dressing. Radial pulse was measured at 84 beats per minute while at rest. The patient's blood pressure was 140/60 mm Hg while sitting and 130/55 on standing.

Pain is constant in the right knee. It measures 10 of 10 with movement and 6 of 10 at rest. (Pain scale: 0 = no pain; 10 = excruciating pain.)

FUNCTIONAL STATUS

The patient is able to transfer sit to and from supine with moderate assistance of one; transfer sit to and from stand with minimum assistance of one, using upper extremities; pivot wheelchair to and from mat with moderate assistance of one; and roll supine to and from side-lying position with minimum assistance of one.

Ambulation

The patient is able to ambulate in parallel bars, 25 feet × 2 with minimum assistance of one, touch-down weight bearing on the right lower extremity.

ASSESSMENT/DIAGNOSIS

Problem List

The patient's problem list includes the following: pain in right knee; dependent transfers and mat mobility; dependent ambulation; decreased endurance for ambulation; decreased active range of motion of bilateral knee flexion and extension; decreased passive range of motion of bilateral knee flexion and extension; limited knowledge of total knee arthroplasty.

Summary Statement

The patient presents 1 day after right total knee arthroplasty secondary to OA and pain. Although the patient was compliant preoperatively with his home exercise program, use of modalities, and education for joint protection techniques to remain active, OA and knee pain progressed in his right knee in the last 2 years. He has also developed Heberden's and Bouchard's nodules. WM is motivated to participate in physical therapy and is knowledgeable of the exercises

and osteoarthritic disease. Assume that lightheadedness and nausea are due to low hematocrit and hemoglobin postoperatively and will subside with autologous blood transfusions managed medically.

Rehabilitation potential is very good because of the patient's motivation and history of compliance. It is anticipated that the patient will return home on discharge from the acute care hospital.

TREATMENT GOALS

1. Transfer supine to and from sit to and from stand independently.
2. Ambulate independently more than 100 feet on level, touch-down weight-bearing right lower extremity, progressing to walker crutches.
3. Ambulate on stairs independently, touch-down weight bearing right lower extremity, with crutch and railing.
4. Increase active range of motion of right knee flexion to greater than 60 degrees and right knee extension to less than −15 degrees.
5. Increase active range of motion of left knee flexion to greater than 125 degrees.
6. Increase passive range of motion of right knee flexion to greater than 70 degrees and right knee extension to less than −10 degrees.
7. Demonstrate independence with straight-leg raise with less than a 10-degree right quadriceps lag.
8. Demonstrate at least 10 repetitions of right short arc quad with at least 1 pound on ankle.
9. Perform written home exercise program per physician's protocol independently (quadriceps sets, gluteals sets, ankle active range of motion, supine active knee flexion, straight-leg raises, and short arc quads).
10. Patient's wife verbalize understanding to remove environmental obstacles in the home before patient's discharge to home with an assistive device.

TREATMENT PLAN

Implement physical therapy program twice a day for 7 to 10 days:

1. Provide transfer training supine to and from sit to and from stand.
2. Use gait training on level with walker touch-down weight bearing of right lower extremity and progressing to crutches as patient tolerates it with respect to endurance and balance.
3. Provide gait training on stairs with crutch and rail.
4. Implement therapeutic exercises (need to consider physician protocol) including supine knee flexion with strap looped around the patient's foot for self-assisted knee flexion and sitting knee flexion.

5. Educate the patient and his wife regarding postoperative management of right knee and making home environment safe for the patient on discharge with assistive device.

The patient and his wife agree with goals/plans.

Discharge Summary (In 9 Days)

The patient attended 17 of a possible 18 physical therapy sessions, missing one because of a Doppler test, because the patient had persistent swelling around knee and an increase in pain in the posterior knee on the fourth day postoperatively.

Seven of 10 goals were attained; the status of the remaining three goals is as follows:

1. Active range of motion of right knee flexion is 55 degrees, and passive range of motion is 62 degrees secondary to persistent joint swelling and knee pain, despite patient's motivation, attempts with assisted knee flex, use of ice after exercise, and pain medications.
2. Passive range of motion of right knee extension is −15 degrees; attempts to increase passive extension were made since 5th postoperative day, with stretch applied to posterior knee soft tissue during long sit when ice was applied and patient was lying prone for 20 minutes twice a day (padding was placed superior to patella to decrease the pressure on patella).
3. The patient required contact supervision on stairs secondary to not feeling safe alone. The patient's wife was instructed on supervising him on the stairs and was safe with this.

Recommendations to Orthopedic Surgeon

Refer the patient to outpatient physical therapy to decrease right knee pain and swelling, to decrease flexion and extension contractures, and to become independent on stairs.

Summary Statement

WM attended outpatient physical therapy for 3 weeks. At discharge, flexion and extension contractures in right knee were decreased to within 10 degrees of ROM of the left knee. WM continued with a daily home exercise program and resumed his active lifestyle.

REFERENCES

1. Becker RO, Selden G: *The Body Electric: Electromagnetism and the Foundation of Life.* New York, William Morrow, 1985.
2. Kiebzak GM: Age related bone changes. *Exper Geront* 1991, 20:171–187.
3. Lanyon LE: Strain-related bone modeling and remodeling. *Top Geriatr Rehabil* 1989, 4:13–24.
4. Marcus R, Carter DR: The role of physical activity in bone mass regulation. *Adv Sport Med Fitness* 1988, 1:63.
5. Parfitt AM: Bone remodeling and bone loss: understanding the patho-physiology of osteoporosis. *Clin Obstet Gynecol* 1987; 30:789–811.
6. Lufkin EG, Dry JJ: Estrogen replacement therapy for the prevention of osteoporosis. *Am Fam Physician* 1989, 40:205–212.
7. Talbot J, Farley SM, Baylink DJ: Drug therapy for prevention and treatment of osteoporosis. *Top Geriatr Rehabil* 1989, 4(2):37–51.
8. Marcus R: Understanding and preventing osteoporosis. *Hosp Pract* 1989, 4:189–218.
9. American Dietetic Association: Position of the American Dietetic Association: Nutrition, aging and the continuum of health care. *J Am Diet Assoc* 1993, 93:80–82.
10. Felicetta JV: Age related changes in calcium metabolism. *Postgrad Med* 1989, 85–94.
11. National Research Council (US). Subcommittee on the Tenth Edition of the RDAs: *Recommended Dietary Allowances/Subcommittee on the Tenth Edition of the RDAs, Food and Nutrition Board, Commission on Life Sciences, National Research Council,* 10th ed. Washington DC, National Academy Press, 1989.
12. Heaney RP, Recker RR: Distribution of calcium absorption in middle-aged women. *Am J Clin Nutr* 1986, 43:299–305.
13. Meukman J: Osteoporosis and the elderly. *Geriartr Med* 1989, 73:1455–1470.
14. Erickson EF, Colvard DS, Berg NJ, *et al.:* Evidence of estrogen receptors in normal human osteoblast-like cells. *Science* 1988; 241:84–86.
15. Watts NB: Osteoporosis. *Am Fam Physician* 1988, 38:193–207.
16. Martin AD, Brown E: The effects of physical activity on the human skeleton. *Top Geriatr Rehabil* 1989, 4:25–35.
17. Block JE, Genant HK, Black D, *et al.:* Greater vertebral bone mineral mass in exercising young men. *West J Med* 1986, 145:39–42.
18. Wolf J: *The Law of Bone Transformation.* Berlin, A. Hirschwald, 1992.
19. Schultheis L: The mechanical control system of bone in weightless spaceflight and in aging. *Exp Gerontol* 1991, 26:203–214.
20. Jaworski ZFG, Liskova-Kiar M, Uhthoff HK, *et al.:* Effects of long term immobilization on the pattern of bone loss in older dogs. *J Bone Joint Surg* (Br) 1980, 62:104–110.
21. Dahlen N, Olsson KE: Bone mineral content and physical activity. *Acta Orthop Scand* 1974, 45:170–174.
22. Frost HK: Bone modeling and skeletal modeling errors. In *Orthopedic Lectures 4.* Springfield, IL, Charles C Thomas, 1973.
23. Stevenson JC: Pathogenesis, prevention and treatment of osteoporosis. *Obstet Gynecol* 1990, 75:36–41.
24. Uhthoff HD, Jaworski ZFG: Bone loss in response to long-term immobilization. *J Bone Joint Surg* [Br] 1978, 60:420–429.
25. Parfitt AM, Gallagher JC, Heancy RP, *et al.:* Vitamin D and bone health in the elderly. *Am J Clin Nutr* 1982, 36:1014.
26. Lindsay R: Prevention of osteoporosis. *Clin Orthop* 1987, 222:44–59.
27. Bikle DD, Genant HK, Cann C, *et al.:* Bone disease in alcohol abuse. *Am Intern Med* 1985, 103:42–48.
28. Dalen N, Feldreich AL: Osteopenia in alcoholism. *Clin Orthop* 1974, 99:201–202.

29. Aloia J, Cohn SH, Vaswani A, *et al.*: Risk factors for post-menopausal osteoporosis. *Am J Med* 1985, 78:95–100.

30. Williams AR, Weiss NS, Ure CL, *et al.*: Effects of weight, smoking and estrogen use on the risk of hip and forearm fractures in postmenopausal women. *Obstet Gynecol* 1982, 60:695–699.

31. Daniell HW: Osteoporosis of the slender smoker: vertebral compression fractures and loss of metacarpal cortex in relation to postmenopausal cigarette smoking and lack of obesity. *Arch Intern Med* 1967, 136:298–304.

32. Cummings SR, Kelsey JL, Nevitt MC, *et al.*: Epidemiology of osteoporosis and osteoporotic fractures. *Epidemiol Rev* 1985, 7:178–208.

33. Jensen J, Christiansen C, Rodbro P: Cigarette smoking, serum estrogen and bone loss during hormone replacement therapy early after menopause. *N Engl J Med* 1985, 313:973–975.

34. Barth RW, Lane JM: Osteoporosis. *Orthop Clin North Am* 1988, 19:845–858.

35. Rudy DR: Osteoporosis: overcoming a costly and debilitating disease. *Postgrad Med* 1989, 86(s):151–158.

36. Melton LJ, III, Riggs BL: Epidemiology of age related fractures. The osteoporotic syndrome: detection, prevention and treatment. In Avioli LV (ed): New York, Grune & Stratton, 1983, pp 45–72.

37. Lindsay R: Osteoporosis: an updated approach to prevention and management geriatrics. 1989, 44:45–54.

38. Thorneycroft IH: The role of estrogen replacement therapy in the prevention of osteoporosis. *Am J Obstet Gynecol* 1989, 160:1306–1310.

39. Gallagher JC: The pathogenesis of osteoporosis. *Bone Mineral* 1990, 9:215–227.

40. Dalsky GP, Stocke KS, Ehsana AA: Weight-bearing exercise training and lumbar bone mineral content in post menopausal women. *Ann Intern Med* 1988, 108:824–828.

41. Gallagher JC, Melton LJ III, Riggs BL, *et al.*: Epidemiology of fractures of the proximal femur in Rochester, Minnesota. *Clin Orthop* 1980, 150:163–171.

42. Johnston CC, Slemenda CW: Non invasive methods for quantifying bone loss of aging. *Exp Gerontol* 1990, 25:297–301.

43. Barden HS, Mazess RB: Bone densitometry of the appendicular and axial skeleton. *Top Geriatr Rehabil* 1989, 4:1–12.

44. Kimmell PL: Radiologic methods to evaluate bone mineral content. *Ann Intern Med* 1984, 100:908–911.

45. Meachim G, Stockwell RA: The Matrix. In Freeman MAR (ed): *Adult Articular Cartilage*. 1st ed. New York, Grune & Stratton, 1972.

46. Gradisar IA, Porterfield JA: Articular cartilage: structure and function. *Top Geriatr Rehabil* 1989, 4(3):1–9.

47. Mitchell J, Shephard H: The resurfacing of adult rabbit articular cartilage by multiple perforations through the subchondral bone. *J Bone Joint Surg* [Am] 1976, 58:230–233.

48. Radin EC, Paul IL: A consolidated concept of joint lubrication. *J Bone Joint Surg* [Am] 1972, 54:607–616.

49. Kessler RM: Arthrology. In Kessler RM, Hertling D (eds): *Management of Common Musculoskeletal Disorders: Physical Therapy Principles and Methods*. Philadelphia, Harper & Row, 1983.

50. Woo SL, Matthews JV, Akeson WH, *et al.*: Connective tissue response to immobility. *Arthritis Rheum* 1975, 18(3):257–264.

51. Freeman MAR: The fatigue of cartilage in the pathogenesis of osteoarthrosis. *Acta Orthop Scand* 1975, 46:323.

52. Muskowitz R: Management of osteoarthritis. *Bull Rheum Dis* 1987, 31:31–35.

53. Sager DS, Bennett RM: Individualizing the risk/benefit ratio of NSAIDS in older patients. *Geriatrics* 1992, 47(8):24–31.

54. Harkon TM, Lampman RM, Vanwell BF, *et al.*: Therapeutic value of graded aerobic exercise training in rheumatoid arthritis. *Arthritis Rheum* 1985, 28:32–39.

55. Neumann DA: Arthrokinesiological considerations in the aged adult. In Guccione AA (ed): *Geriatric Physical Therapy*. St Louis, C.V. Mosby Company, 1993.

56. Hamlin CR, Kohn RR: Determination of humans' chronological age by a study of a collagen sample. *Exp Gerontol* 1972, 7:377–379.

57. Alnaqeeb MA, Al Zaid NS, Goldspink G: Connective tissue changes and physical properties of developing an aging skeletal muscle. *J Anat* 1984, 139:677–689.

58. Akeson WH: Effects of immobilization on joints. *Clin Orthop Rel Res* 1987, 219:28–37.

59. Donatelli R, Owens-Burkhart H: Effects of immobilization on the extensibility of periarticular connective tissue. *J Orthop Sport Phys Ther* 1987, 3:67–72.

60. Akeson WH, Amiel D, Woo SL: Immobility effects on synovial joints: the pathomechanics of joint contracture. *Biorheology* 1980, 17:95.

61. Adrian MJ: Flexibility in the aging adult. In Smith EL, Serfass RC (eds): *Exercise and Aging: The Scientific Basis*. Hillside, NJ, Enslow Publishing, 1981, pp 45–58.

62. Larsson L, Grimby G, Karlsson J: Muscle strength and speed of movement in relation to age and muscle morphology. *J Appl Physiol* 1979, 46(3):451–456.

63. Clarkson PM, Kroll W, Melchionda AM: Age, isometric strength, rate of tension development & fiber type composition. *J Gerontol* 1981, 36:643–648.

64. Larsson L, Karlsson J: Isometric and dynamic endurance as a function of age and skeletal muscle characteristics. *Acta Physiol Scand* 1978, 104:129–136.

65. Wilmore JH: The aging of bone and muscle. *Clin Sports Med* 1991, 10:231–244.

66. Knortz KA: Muscle physiology applied to geriatric rehabilitation. *Top Geriatr Rehabil* 1987, 2(4):1–12.

67. Cooper RR: Alterations during immobilization and regeneration of skeletal muscle in cats. *J Bone Joint Surg* [Am] 1972, 54:919–953.

68. Aniansson A, Hedberg M, Henning G-B, *et al.*: Muscle morphology, enzyme activity and muscle strength in elderly men and women. *Clin Physiol* 1981, 1:73–86.

69. Allen TH, Anderson EC, Langham WH: Total body potassium and gross body composition in relation to age. *J Gerontol* 1960, 15:348–357.

70. Haggmark T, Jansson E, Eriksson E: Fiber type and metabolic potential of the thigh muscle in man after knee surgery and immobilization. *Int J Sports Med* 1981, 1(2):12–17.

71. Cress EM, Schultz E: Aging muscle: functional, morphologic, biochemical and regenerative capacity. *Top Geriatr Rehabil* 1985, 1(1):11–19.

72. Orlander J, Kiessling K-H, Larsson L, *et al.*: Skeletal muscle metabolism ultrastructure in relation to age in sedentary men. *Acta Physiol Scand* 1978, 104:249–261.

73. Moritani T, DeVries H: Neural factors versus hypertrophy in the time course of muscle strength gain. *Am J Phys Med* 1979, 58(3):115–130.

74. Larsson L: Physical training effects on muscle morphology in sedentary males at different ages. *Med Sci Sports Exerc* 1982, 14:203–206.

75. Shephard RJ: The scientific basis of exercise prescribing for the very old. *J Am Geriatr Soc* 1990, 38:62–70.

76. Nichols JF, Omizo DK, Peterson KK, *et al.*: Efficacy of

heavy-resistance training for active women over sixty: muscular strength, body composition and program adherence. *J Am Geriat Soc* 1993, 41:205–210.

77. Fiatarone MA, Marks EC, Ryan ND, *et al.:* High intensity strength training in nonagenarians: effects on skeletal muscle. *JAMA* 1990, 22:3029–3034.

78. Luthi JM, Howds H, Claassen H, *et al.:* Structural changes in skeletal muscle with heavy resistance exercise. *Int J Sport* Med 1986, 7:123–127.

79. Aniansson A, Zetterberg C: Impaired muscle function with aging: a background factor in the incidence of fractures of the proximal end of the femur. *Clin Orthop* 1984, 191:193–201.

80. Gordon NF: *Arthritis: Your Complete Exercise Guide.* Human Kinetics, Publishers, 1993.

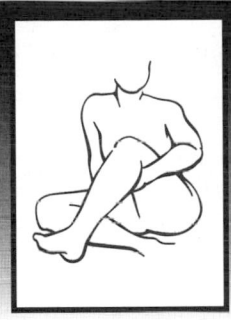

American Physical Therapy Association Code of Ethics, Guide for Professional Conduct, and Standards of Practice for Physical Therapy

Code of Ethics

Preamble

This Code of Ethics sets forth ethical principles for the physical therapy profession. Members of this profession are responsible for maintaining and promoting ethical practice. This Code of Ethics, adopted by the American Physical Therapy Association, shall be binding on physical therapists who are members of the Association.

Principle 1 Physical therapists respect the rights and dignity of all individuals.

Principle 2 Physical therapists comply with the laws and regulations governing the practice of physical therapy.

Principle 3 Physical therapists accept responsibility for the exercise of sound judgment.

Principle 4 Physical therapists maintain and promote high standards for physical therapy practice, education, and research.

Principle 5 Physical therapists seek remuneration for their services that is deserved and reasonable.

Principle 6 Physical therapists provide accurate information to the consumer about the profession and about those services they provide.

Principle 7 Physical therapists accept the responsibility to protect the public and the profession from unethical, incompetent, or illegal acts.

Principle 8 Physical therapists participate in efforts to address the health needs of the public.

Adopted by the House of Delegates June 1981
Amended June 1987
Amended June 1991
Reprinted with the permission of the American Physical Therapy Association.

American Physical Therapy Association Guide for Professional Conduct

Purpose

This Guide For Professional Conduct (Guide) is intended to serve physical therapists who are members of the American Physical Therapy Association (Association) in interpreting the *Code of Ethics* (Code) and matters of professional conduct. The Guide provides guidelines by which physical therapists may determine the propriety of their conduct. The Code and the Guide apply to all physical therapists who are Association members. These guidelines are subject to changes as the dynamics of the profession change and as new patterns of health care delivery are developed and accepted by the professional community and the public. This Guide is subject to monitoring and timely revision by the Judicial Committee of the Association.

Interpreting Ethical Principles

The interpretations expressed in this Guide are not to be considered all inclusive of situations that could evolve under a specific principle of the Code but reflect the opinions, decisions, and advice of the Judicial Committee. While the statements of ethical principles apply universally, specific circumstances determine their appropriate application. Input related to current interpretations, or situations requiring interpretation, is encouraged from Association members.

PRINCIPLE 1

Physical therapists respect the rights and dignity of all individuals.

1.1   Attitudes of Physical Therapists

A. Physical therapists shall recognize that each individual is different from all other individuals and shall respect and be responsive to those differences.

B. Physical therapists are to be guided at all times by concern for the physical, psychological, and socioeconomic welfare of those individuals entrusted to their care.

C. Physical therapists shall be responsive to and mutually supportive of colleagues and associates.

1.2   Confidential Information

A. Information relating to the physical therapist-patient relationship is confidential and may not be communicated to a third party not involved in that patient's care without the prior written consent of the patient, subject to applicable law.

B. Information derived from a component-sponsored peer review shall be held confidential by the reviewer unless written permission to release the information is obtained from the physical therapist who was reviewed.

C. Information derived from the working relationships of physical therapists shall be held confidential by all parties.

D. Information may be disclosed to appropriate authorities when it is necessary to protect the welfare of an individual or the community. Such disclosure shall be in accordance with applicable law.

PRINCIPLE 2

Physical therapists comply with the laws and regulations governing the practice of physical therapy.

2.1   Professional Practice

Physical therapists shall provide consultation, evaluation, treatment, and preventive care, in accordance with the laws and regulations of the jurisdiction(s) in which they practice.

PRINCIPLE 3

Physical therapists accept responsibility for the exercise of sound judgment.

3.1   Acceptance of Responsibility

A. Upon accepting an individual for provision of physical therapy services, physical therapists shall assume the responsibility for evaluating that individual; planning, implementing, and supervising the therapeutic program; reevaluating and changing that program; and maintaining adequate records of the case, including progress reports.

B. When the individual's needs are beyond the scope of the physical therapist's expertise, or when additional services are indicated, the individual shall be so informed and assisted in identifying a qualified provider.

C. Physical therapists shall not initiate or continue services that will not result in beneficial outcomes or are contraindicated.

D. Regardless of practice setting, physical therapists shall maintain the ability to make independent judgments.

3.2 Delegation of Responsibility

A. Physical therapists shall not delegate to a less qualified person any activity which requires the unique skill, knowledge, and judgment of the physical therapist.

B. The primary responsibility for physical therapy care rendered by supportive personnel rests with the supervising physical therapist. Adequate supervision requires, at a minimum, that a supervising physical therapist perform the following activities:

1. Designate or establish channels of written and oral communication.

2. Interpret available information concerning the individual under care.

3. Provide initial evaluation.

4. Develop plan of care, including short- and long-term goals.

5. Select and delegate appropriate tasks of plan of care.

6. Assess competence of supportive personnel to perform assigned tasks.

7. Direct and supervise supportive personnel in delegated tasks.

8. Identify and document precautions, special problems, contraindications, goals, anticipated progress, and plans for reevaluation.

9. Reevaluate, adjust plan of care when necessary, perform final evaluation, and establish follow-up plan.

3.3 Provision of Services

A. Physical therapists shall recognize the individual's freedom of choice in selection of physical therapy services.

B. Physical therapists' professional practices and their adherence to ethical principles of the Association shall take preference over business practices. Provisions of services for personal financial gain rather than for the need of the individual receiving the services are unethical.

C. When physical therapists judge that an individual will no longer benefit from their services, they shall so inform the individual receiving the services. Physical therapists shall avoid overutilization of their services.

3.4 Referral Relationships

A. In a referral situation where the referring practitioner prescribes a treatment program, alteration of that program or extension of physical therapy services beyond that program should be undertaken in consultation with the referring practitioner.

B. In a referral situation where additional service or expertise is indicated, physical therapists should recommend to the referring practitioner the referral of the individual to a qualified provider.

3.5 Practice Arrangements

A. Participation in a business, partnership, corporation, or other entity does not exempt the physical therapist, whether employer, partner, or stockholder, either individually or collectively, from the obligation of promoting and maintaining the ethical principles of the Association.

B. Physical therapists shall advise their employer(s) of any employer practice which causes a physical therapist to be in conflict with the ethical principles of the Association. Physical therapist employees shall attempt to rectify aspects of their employment which are in conflict with the ethical principles of the Association.

PRINCIPLE 4

Physical therapists maintain and promote high standards for physical therapy practice, education, and research.

4.1 Continued Education

A. Physical therapists shall participate in educational activities which enhance their basic knowledge and provide new knowledge.

B. Whenever physical therapists provide continuing education, they shall ensure that course content, objectives, and responsibilities of the instructional faculty are accurately reflected in the promotion of the course.

4.2 Review and Self Assessment

A. Physical therapists shall provide for utilization review of their services.

B. Physical therapists shall demonstrate their commitment to quality assurance by peer review and self assessment.

4.3 Research

A. Physical therapists shall support research activities that contribute knowledge for improved patient care.

B. Physical therapists engaged in research shall ensure:

1. The consent of subjects.

2. Confidentiality of the data on individual subjects and the personal identities of the subjects.

3. Well-being of all subjects in compliance with facility regulations and laws of the jurisdiction in which the research is conducted.

4. The absence of fraud and plagiarism.

5. Full disclosure of support received.

6. Appropriate acknowledgment of individuals making a contribution to the research.

C. Physical therapists shall report to appropriate authorities any acts in the conduct or presentation of research that appear unethical or illegal.

4.4 Education

A. Physical therapists shall support quality education in academic and clinical settings.

B. Physical therapists functioning in the educational role are responsible to the students, the academic institutions, and the clinical settings for promoting ethical conduct in educational activities. Whenever possible, the educator shall ensure:

1. The rights of students in the academic and clinical setting.

2. Appropriate confidentiality of personal information.

3. Professional conduct toward the student during the academic and clinical educational processes.

4. Assignment to clinical settings prepared to give the student a learning experience.

C. Clinical educators are responsible for reporting to the academic program student conduct which appears to be unethical or illegal.

PRINCIPLE 5

Physical therapists seek remuneration for their services that is deserved and reasonable.

5.1 Fiscally Sound Remuneration

A. Physical therapists shall never place their own financial interest above the welfare of individuals under their care.

B. Fees for physical therapy services should be reasonable for the service performed, considering the setting in which it is provided, practice costs in the geographic area, judgment of other organizations, and other relevant factors.

C. Physical therapists should attempt to ensure that providers, agencies, or other employers adopt physical therapy fee schedules that are reasonable and that encourage access to necessary services.

5.2 Business Practices/Fee Arrangements

A. Physical therapists shall not:

1. Directly or indirectly request, receive, or participate in the dividing, transferring, assigning, or rebating of an unearned fee.

2. Profit by means of a credit or other valuable consideration, such as an unearned commission, discount, or gratuity in connection with furnishing of physical therapy services.

B. Unless laws impose restrictions to the contrary, physical therapists who provide physical therapy services in a business entity may pool fees and moneys received. Physical therapists may divide or apportion these fees and moneys in accordance with the business agreement.

C. Physical therapists may enter into agreements with organizations to provide physical therapy services if such agreements do not violate the ethical principles of the Association.

5.3 Endorsement of Equipment or Services

A. Physical therapists shall not use influence upon individuals under their care or their families for utilization of equipment or services based upon the direct or indirect financial interest of the physical therapist in such equipment or services. Realizing that these individuals will normally rely on the physical therapists' advice, their best interest must always be maintained as well as their right of free choice relating to the use of any equipment or service. While it cannot be considered unethical for physical therapists to own or have a financial interest in equipment companies or services, they must act in accordance with the law and make full disclosure of their interest whenever such companies or services become the source of equipment or services for individuals under their care.

B. Physical therapists may be remunerated for endorsement or advertisement of equipment or services to the lay public, physical therapists, or other health professionals provided they disclose any financial interest in the production, sale, or distribution of said equipment or services.

C. In endorsing or advertising equipment or services, physical therapists shall use sound professional judgment and shall not give the appearance of Association endorsement.

5.4 Gifts and Other Considerations

A. Physical therapists shall not accept nor offer gifts or other considerations with obligatory conditions attached.

B. Physical therapists shall not accept nor offer gifts or other considerations that affect or give an objective appearance of affecting their professional judgment.

PRINCIPLE 6

Physical therapists provide accurate information to the consumer about the profession and about those services they provide.

6.1   Information about the Profession

Physical therapists shall endeavor to educate the public to an awareness of the physical therapy profession through such means as publication of articles and participation in seminars, lectures, and civic programs.

6.2   Information about Services

A. Information given to the public shall emphasize that individual problems cannot be treated without individualized evaluation and plans/programs of care.

B. Physical therapists may advertise their services to the public.

C. Physical therapists shall not use, or participate in the use of, any form of communication containing a false, plagiarized, fraudulent, misleading, deceptive, unfair, or sensational statement or claim.

D. Physical therapists shall not compensate or give anything of value to a representative of the press, radio, television, or other communication medium in anticipation of, or in return for, professional publicity in a news item.

E. A paid advertisement shall be identified as such unless it is apparent from the context that it is a paid advertisement.

PRINCIPLE 7

Physical therapists accept the responsibility to protect the public and the profession from unethical, incompetent, or illegal acts.

7.1   Consumer Protection

A. Physical therapists shall report any conduct which appears to be unethical, incompetent, or illegal.

B. Physical therapists may not participate in any arrangements in which patients are exploited due to the referring sources enhancing their personal incomes as a result of referring for, prescribing, or recommending physical therapy.

7.2   Disclosure

The physical therapist shall disclose to the patient if the referring practitioner derives compensation from the provision of physical therapy. The physical therapist shall ensure that the individual has freedom of choice in selecting a provider of physical therapy.

PRINCIPLE 8

Physical therapists participate in efforts to address the health needs of the public.

Issued by Judicial Committee of the American Physical Therapy Association
    October 1981
    Last Amended January 1993
    Reprinted with the permission of the American Physical Therapy Association, 1111 North Fairfax Street, Alexandria, VA 22314–1488.

American Physical Therapy Association Standards of Practice for Physical Therapy

Preamble

The physical therapy profession is committed to provide an optimum level of care and to strive for excellence in practice. The House of Delegates of the American Physical Therapy Association, as the responsible body representing this profession, attests to this commitment by adopting, publishing, disseminating, and promoting the application of the following *Standards of Practice for Physical Therapy*. These *Standards of Practice* are the profession's statement of conditions and performances which are essential for quality physical therapy. They provide a foundation for assessment of physical therapy practice.

Administration of the Physical Therapy Service

I. Purposes and Goals

A written statement of purposes and goals exists for the physical therapy service which reflects the needs of the individuals served, the physical therapy personnel, the facility, and the community.
- Define scope and limitation of service.
- Contain current description of purpose.
- List objectives and goals of services provided.
- Are appropriate for the population (community) served.
- Provide a mechanism for annual review.

II. Organizational Plan

A written organizational plan exists for the physical therapy service.
- Describes the interrelationships within the overall organization.
- Provides for direction of service by a physical therapist.
- Defines supervisory functions within the program/service.
- Reflects current personnel functions.

III. Policies and Procedures

Written policies and procedures, which reflect the operation of the service, exist and are consistent with the purposes and goals of the physical therapy service.
- Address pertinent information about the following:
  - Clinical education
  - Clinical research
  - Criteria for access to, initiation, and termination of care
  - Equipment maintenance
  - Fire and disaster
  - Infection control
  - Job descriptions
  - Medical emergencies
  - Patient care policies and protocols
  - Patient rights
  - Personnel-related policies
  - Position descriptions
  - Quality assurance
  - Record keeping
  - Safety
  - Staff orientation
  - Supervisory relationships
- Meet the requirements of external agencies and state law.
- Meet the requirements of the overall organization.
- Be reviewed on a regular basis.

IV. Administration

A physical therapist shall be responsible for the direction of the physical therapy service.
- Assures that the service is consistent with established purposes and goals.
- Assures that the service is provided in accordance with established policies and procedures.
- Assures compliance with local, state, and federal requirements.
- Complies with current APTA *Standards of Practice* and *Guide for Professional Conduct*.
- Reviews and updates policies and procedures as appropriate.
- Provides appropriate education, training, and review of physical therapy support personnel.

V. Staffing

The physical therapy personnel are qualified and sufficient in number to achieve the purposes and goals of the physical therapy service.
- Meets legal requirements regarding licensure and/or certification of appropriate personnel.
- Provides expertise appropriate to the case mix.
- Provides adequate staff to patient ratio.
- Provides adequate support staff to professional staff.

VI. Physical Setting

1. The physical setting is designed to provide a safe and effective environment that facilitates the achievement of the purposes and goals of the physical therapy service.
- Meets all applicable legal requirements for health and safety.
- Meets space needs appropriate for the number and type of patients served.

2. Equipment is safe and sufficient to achieve the

purposes and goals of the physical therapy service.
- Meets all applicable legal requirements for health and safety.
- Meets equipment needs appropriate for the number and type of patients served.
- Provides for routine safety inspection of equipment by a qualified individual.

VII. Fiscal Affairs

Fiscal planning and management of the physical therapy service are based upon sound accounting principles.
- Include preparation and use of a budget.
- Conform to legal requirements.
- Are accurately recorded and reported.
- Provide for optimum use of resources.
- Include a plan for audit control.
- Establish the basis for a fee schedule consistent with cost of service and within customary norms of fair and reasonable.

VIII. Quality Assurance

A written plan exists for the assessment of, and action to assure, the quality and appropriateness of the physical therapy service.
- Provides for a current written plan for assessment of the service.
- Provides evidence of ongoing review, evaluation of the service.
- Resolves identified problems.
- Is consistent with requirements of external agencies.

IX. Staff Development

A written plan exists which provides for appropriate ongoing development of staff.
- Is reflected by evidence of ongoing education or attendance at continuing education activities.

Provision of Care

X. Informed Consent

The physical therapist obtains the patient's informed consent in accordance with jurisdictional law before initiating physical therapy.

XI. Initial Evaluation

The physical therapist performs and records an initial evaluation and interprets results to determine appropriate care for the individual.
- Is initiated prior to treatment.
- Is performed by the physical therapist in a timely manner.
- Is documented, dated, and signed by the physical therapist who performed the evaluation.

- Identifies physical therapy needs of the client.
- Includes pertinent information of the following:
  - History
  - Diagnosis
  - Problem
  - Complications and precautions
  - Physical status
  - Functional status
  - Critical behavior/mentation
  - Social/environmental needs
- Provides sufficient data to establish time-related goals.
- The physical therapist shall render care within the scope of the physical therapist's education and experience. Appropriate referral to other practitioners shall be made when necessary.
- The physical therapist utilizes objective measures to establish a baseline at the time of the initial evaluation.
- Is documented, dated, and signed by the physical therapist who performed the evaluation.

XII. Plan of Care

1. The physical therapist establishes and records a plan of care for the individual based on the results of the evaluation.
- Includes realistic goals and expected outcome.
- Is based on identified needs.
- Includes effective treatment, frequency, and duration.
- Recommends appropriate coordination of care with other professionals/services.
- Is documented, dated, and signed by the physical therapist who established the plan of care.

2. The physical therapist involves the individual/significant other in the planning, implementation, and revision of the treatment program.
3. The physical therapist plans for discharge of the individual, taking into consideration goal achievement, and provides for appropriate follow-up or referral.

XIII. Treatment

1. The physical therapist provides or delegates and supervises the physical therapy treatment consistent with the results of the evaluation and plan of care.
- Is under the ongoing personal care or supervision of the physical therapist.
- Reflects that delegated responsibilities are commensurate with the qualifications of the physical therapy personnel.
- Is altered in accordance with changes in individual status.
- Is provided at a level consistent with current physical therapy practice.

2. The physical therapist records, on an ongoing basis, treatment rendered, progress, and change in status relative to the plan of care.

XIV. Reevaluation

The physical therapist reevaluates the individual and modifies the plan of care as indicated.
* Is performed by the physical therapist in a timely manner.
* Reflects that the individual's progress is reassessed relative to initial evaluation and plan of care.
* Is documented, dated, and signed by the physical therapist who performed the evaluation.

Education

XV. Professional Development

The physical therapist is responsible for his/her individual professional development and continued competence in physical therapy.

XVI. Student

The physical therapist participates in the education of physical therapy students and other student health professionals.

Research

XVII. The physical therapist utilizes research findings in practice and encourages or participates in research activities.

Community Responsibility

XVIII. The physical therapist participates in community activities to promote community health.

Legal/Ethical

XIX. Legal

The physical therapist fulfills all the legal requirements of the jurisdictions regulating the practice of physical therapy.

XX. Ethical

The physical therapist practices according to the *Code of Ethics* of the American Physical Therapy Association.

Reprinted with the permission of the American Physical Therapy Association, 1111 North Fairfax Street, Alexandria, VA 22314–1488.

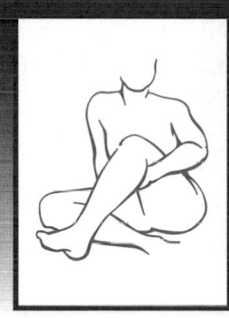

APPENDIX B

Hematology

Bleeding Time

Ivy method, 1–7 minutes (60–420 seconds).
Template method, 3–9 minutes (180–540 seconds).

Cellular Measurements of Red Cells

Average diameter = 7.3 μm (5.5–8.8 μm).
Mean corpuscular volume (MCV): Men, 80–94 fL; women, 81–99 fL (by Coulter counter).
Mean corpuscular hemoglobin (MCH): 27–32 pg.
Mean corpuscular hemoglobin concentration (MCHC): 32–36 g/dL red blood cells (32%–36%).

Clot Retraction

Begins in 1–3 hours; complete in 6–24 hours. No clot lysis in 24 hours.

Fibrinogen Split Products

Negative > 1:4 dilutions.

Fragility of Red Cells

Begins at 0.45%–0.38% sodium chloride; complete at 9.36%–0.3% sodium chloride.

Hematocrit (PCV)

Men, 40%–52% (0.4–0.52).
Women, 37%–47% (0.37–0.47).

Hemoglobin [B]

Men, 14–18 g/dL (2.09–2.79 mmol/L as Hb tetramer).
Women 12–16 g/dL (1.86–2.48 mmol/L). [S], 2–3 mg/dL.

Partial Thromboplastin Time

Activated, 25–37 seconds.

Platelets

150,000–400,000/μL (0.15–0.4 $\times$ 10^{12}/L).

Prothrombin Time

[P], 11–14.5 seconds. International Normalized Ratio (INR): [P], 2.0–3.0.

Red Blood Count (RBC)

Men, 4.5–6.2 million/μL (4.5–6.2 $\times$ 10^{12}/L).
Women, 4–5.5 million/μL (4–5.5 $\times$ 10^{12}/L).

Reticulocytes

0.2%–2% of red cells.

Sedimentation Rate

Less than 20 mm/h (Westergren); 0–10 mm/h (Wintrobe).

White Blood Count (WBC) and Differential

5000–10,000/μL (5–10 $\times$ 10^{9}/L).

Myelocytes, 0%.
Juvenile neutrophils, 0%.
Band neutrophils, 0%–5%.
Segmented neutrophils, 40%–60%.

Lymphocyte

Total, 1500–4000/μL

B cell, 5–25%.
T cell, 60%–88%.
Suppressor, 10%–43%.
Helper, 32%–66%.
H:S, >1.

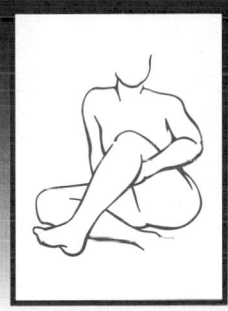

Genitourinary System: Glossary and Agencies

Glossary

1. Anuria is the absence of urine in the bladder or a urinary output of less than 50 mL/24h and indicates serious renal dysfunction that requires immediate medical intervention.
2. Burning on urination occurs in patients who have urethral irritation or bladder infections.
3. Dysuria is painful or difficult voiding.
4. Enuresis is involuntary voiding during sleep and may be physiological in patients up to 3 years of age; thereafter, it may be functional or symptomatic of obstructive disease.
5. Frequent urination describes voiding that occurs more often than seven times per day.
6. Hematuria is the presence of red blood cells in the urine and is considered a serious sign that requires medical evaluation.
7. Hesitancy is undue delay and difficulty in initiating voiding and may indicate compression of the urethra, outlet obstruction, or a neurogenic bladder.
8. Nocturia is urination that occurs more often than two times per night.
9. Oliguria is a small volume of urine output between 100 and 500 mL/24h. It may result from acute renal failure, shock dehydration, or a fluid-ion imbalance.
10. Pneumaturia is the passage of gas in urine during voiding and can be caused by fistulous connection between the bowel and bladder, rectosigmoid cancer, regional ileitis, sigmoid diverticulitis (most common), and gas-forming urinary tract infections.
11. Polyuria is a large volume of urine voided in a given time and occurs in patients with diabetes mellitus or diabetes insipidus.
12. Proteinuria is significant quantities of protein in the urine.

Agencies and Other Resources for Obtaining Information on Incontinence

The Simon Foundation
Box 815
Wilmette, IL 60091

HIP (Help for Incontinent People) Report
P.O. Box 544
Union, SC 29379

Kimberly Clark Corporation
Attn. M.L. Lennin
P.O. Box 2002
Neenah, WI 54956–9982
(For public information literature and an incontinence teaching kit)

Alliance for Aging Research
Suite 305
Washington DC 20002

Continence Restored, Inc.
785 Park Avenue
New York, NY 10021

Femina Vaginal Cones
DACOMED Corporation
1701 East 79th Street
Minneapolis, MN 55425

Section on Obstetrics and Gynecology
American Physical Therapy Association
P.O. Box 327
Alexandria, VA 22314–1488

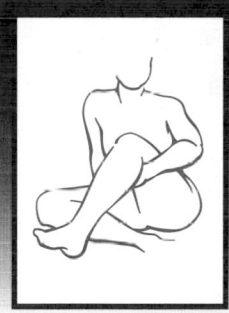

APPENDIX D

Tissue Oxygen Measurements

I. General Issues

A. Tissue oxygen measurements can provide direct, continuous, quantitative assessment of oxygen availability in the tissue. Given the relationships between wound oxygen tension and resistance to infection,[1] as well as between wound oxygen tension and promotion of healing,[1-3] it would be important to measure oxygen availability.

B. If oxygen is so important to healing and preventing infection,

> How does one accurately measure oxygen to know if it is a problem?

What is normal wound-tissue oxygen tension?

What is the evidence that problem wounds are really hypoxic?

What is the evidence that increased inspired oxygen at normobaric pressures delivers oxygen to problem wounds?

What is the evidence that oxygen is delivered to problem wounds during a course of hyperbaric oxygen treatment?

What is the optimum dose of oxygen?

II. Measuring Tissue Oxygen

A. There are a variety of techniques available to measure tissue oxygen.

1. All have some special properties and some limitations.
2. Many are not easy to use in a clinical situation.
3. Technology for the measurement of oxygen continues to develop and to be perfected.

B. Polarographic oxygen electrodes

1. These electrodes measure oxygen concentration in gases and in biological fluids and can be used to measure oxygen tension in human wounds.
2. The basic oxygen electrode consists of a cathode of moldable metal (silver, platinum, or gold) and a reference anode of silver or silver chloride.
3. The electrode is placed in an electrolyte solution, and a constant polarizing voltage from -0.6 to -0.8 volts is applied to the cathode.
4. The polarized oxygen electrode provides electrons to reduce molecular oxygen as it arrives at the electrode surface.
5. Oxygen is reduced by either a two- or four-electron reaction described by a series of equations.[4]
6. The resulting current generated is directly pro-

portional to the number of oxygen molecules in solution, and by Henry's law, to the P_{O_2} of the solution.

7. Thus, oxygen electrodes can be used to determine the oxygen tension of surrounding tissue.
8. The disadvantage of this system is that
   a. The electrode is large in size.
   b. It is limited to use in fluids and on organ surfaces.
   c. Whalen et al.[5] developed a microelectrode approximately 21 μm in diameter that could be safely inserted into tissue and cells.
   d. The technique was later refined and showed steep gradients of oxygen tension across the healing surface of experimental wounds.
9. To be reliable and accurate,
   a. The user must have experience using the equipment.
   b. The user must also be aware of the electrode properties that can result in misinterpretation of the data.
   c. The problems vary from sensor tip position, membrane characteristics, size of the cathode, temperature of the electrode, response time of the electrode, calibration of the electrode, tis-

sue damage, electromagnetic fields and transient surges in electrical power, interference of halothane and sulfhydryl groups, and drifting of the current output.

C. Transcutaneous polarographic oxygen electrodes

1. Oxygen tension of the buffer solution approximates the subject's arterial oxygen tension.
2. Clark[6] reported the development of a polarographic electrode to measure oxygen tension of the blood *in vitro* and *in vivo.*
3. Huch *et al.*[7] used the Clark electrode to develop a transcutaneous oxygen monitoring device to measure arterial oxygen tension.
4. Now, transcutaneous oxygen monitoring is commonly used in neonatology, plastic surgery, vascular surgery, anesthesiology, and hyperbaric medicine.[8–12]
5. Transcutaneous oxygen monitoring uses a large Clark polarographic electrode modified to contain a heating element and thermistor.[13]
   a. The heating element maintains a present temperature of 42°C to 45°C and is continuously monitored by the thermistor.
   b. A phosphate buffer and a potassium chloride solution are contained between the electrode surface and an oxygen-permeable membrane.
   c. The electrode is attached to the skin by an adhesive fixation ring filled with a contact solution.
   d. Heating the electrode to 42°C to 45°C transfers heat to the skin surface directly beneath the electrode, produces vasodilation of the underlying arterioles and capillary bed, increases the size of skin pores and shifts the oxyhemoglobin curve to the left, which increases blood flow, diffusion, and the release of oxygen from hemoglobin beneath the electrode.
6. The advantages of this method are that it

   is noninvasive
   is agreeable to the patient
   is simple to calibrate and use
   can be used for multiple-site sampling without cross-contamination.
7. The disadvantages are as follows:
   a. It cannot be used on thick, cornified skin.
   b. It will not adhere to the damp surface of a wound.
   c. It must be positioned on nearby viable tissue and placed carefully at certain locations of the body (*eg,* a better correlation to arterial Po_2 if found in the upper front part of the thorax).
   d. Most electrodes tend to drift and require periodic recalibration, and Po_2 values appear to vary with clinical conditions and age of the patient, with the best measurements found in newborn infants (*eg,* because of their thin skin).

   e. The transcutaneous device is designed to measure arterial, not tissue, Po_2.
   f. Where blood flow is severely compromised, oxygen utilization in skin lowers the transcutaneous reading, and the transcutaneous Po_2 does not measure a true tissue value.
   g. Transcutaneous oxygen monitoring detects major perfusion deficits when heat can no longer overcome autonomic vasoconstriction but cannot detect acute changes in human blood volume on the order of 450 cc 55.
   h. The transcutaneous oxygen monitor heats the skin, alters the physiology, and measures erroneously high values in the region of the tissue directly beneath it.

D. Tissue tonometry

1. Hunt *et al.*[14–16] developed a method of tissue tonometry based on a single, integrated value that is very effective in determining the mean oxygenation of a large area of tissue:
   a. The tonometer, a 2- to 7-cm length of Silastic tubing, is swaged to a 28-gauge cutting-tip spinal needle.
   b. The needle is passed into the skin through the subcutaneous tissue for approximately 5 cm and is then brought out through the skin again.
   c. Physiological saline is slowly perfused through the tube to allow time for tissue gases to equilibrate with the fluid in the tube.
   d. A 254-μm polarographic oxygen electrode is then inserted into the end of the tonometer for continuous measurement of oxygen tension.
   e. As an alternative, saline can be placed, allowed to equilibrate, and then collected from the tube and analyzed by standard laboratory blood gas equipment.
   f. This gives a single, integrated, mean value of extracellular fluid oxygen tension. The reading is proportional to regional blood supply, arterial oxygen tension and microvascular perfusion, and tissue oxygen tension can be read continuously for long periods. The electrode is calibrated *in situ,* and blood flow changes are calculated by the Fick principle.
   g. The advantage is the ability to analyze Co_2 and O_2 simultaneously.
   h. A major disadvantage is that this technique causes fresh trauma during initial implant and results in a transient reduction in local blood flow because of clotting and "normal" inflammation surrounding the tonometer.[17]

E. Mass spectrometer

1. The mass spectrometer is effective in measuring tissue gas tensions under normobaric and hyperbaric conditions.[18]

2. This is based on gas diffusion through a permeable membrane that is located at the tip of a flexible cannula through tubing through which gas is transported to the mass spectrometer analyzer:
   a. The inner face of the membrane is exposed to a low pressure (10–6 mm Hg), whereas the outside face is in contact with the gas to be measured.
   b. The gas molecules from the gaseous state and from solution are drawn into the evacuated space of the analyzer in quantities proportional to the partial pressures of the sample gas components.[19]
   c. Two types of membranes are commonly used: a fast-response Silastic membrane for flowing blood, and a slow-response Teflon membrane for tissue.
   d. Tissue gas molecules pass through the membrane and are drawn via tubing to the analyzer where they are separated according to molecular weight and are measured quantitatively.
3. The primary advantage of this method is that one can simultaneously analyze several tissue gases (oxygen, carbon dioxide, nitrogen, and anesthetic gases):
   a. The measurements are linear and the recordings stable, with long-term continuous monitoring possible.
   b. The system is easily converted from tissue gas monitoring to respiratory gas monitoring.
4. The primary disadvantage of mass spectrometry is that it consumes considerable oxygen from tissue in the measuring process and tends to read at artificially low levels when perfusion is poor:
   a. Because gas molecules are separated according to molecular weight, gases of similar molecular weight can be confused for each other.
   b. Response time is slow in comparison with other methods of tissue oxygen measurement. Response time is improved by reducing the length of tubing and by ensuring that there are no sharp bends that could cause molecule-to-wall collisions.
   c. Care must be taken to ensure that the tubing is gas impermeable and that the vacuum system is free of leaks.
   d. The system is also prohibitively expensive as compared with alternatives.

F. Radioactive oxygen

1. Jones et al.[20] developed the use of continuous inhalation of ^{15}O (to study the relationship between regional cerebral blood flow and oxygen utilization). Clyne et al.[21] expanded the use of the method to study blood flow and metabolism in peripheral vascular disease. ^{25}O is a radioactive isotope of oxygen that decays by positron emission with a half-life of 2.1 minutes.
   a. It is produced by a cyclotron with deuteron bombardment of nitrogen plus 1% oxygen.
   b. ^{25}O is continuously piped through small tubing to the investigation area where it is added to the breathing media in the patient's oxygen mask.
   c. After about 5–7 minutes of continuous ^{25}O inhalation, radioactivity reaches equilibrium in the tissues, principally as ^{15}O labeled water of metabolism.
   d. Accordingly, ^{15}O labeled water of metabolism at equilibrium is balanced by its disappearance from the tissues by tissue perfusion, blood flow per unit volume of tissue, and radioactive decay.
   e. Water of metabolism depends principally on the product of the oxygen extraction ratio and on the blood flow, which represents the rate of oxygen utilization.
   f. This type of scanning is relatively specialized at this time but requires less than 1 hour to perform and is conducted with the patient lying down with a gamma camera under the area of tissue under study, with ^{15}O and $C^{15}O_2$ inhaled consecutively.
   g. It takes about 5–7 minutes to reach a steady state and is followed by a 10-minute scan.

G. Optical methods to measure oxygen in biological systems

1. Bioluminescence[22] is produced by enzymatic oxidoreductions in the presence of molecular oxygen:
   a. The molecule is excited to a high-energy state.
   b. When the molecule returns to its original low-energy state, or "ground state," visible light is emitted (eg, like in the firefly).
   c. Certain molecules can be elevated to the energy-rich excited state when some of their electrons absorb a quantum of light energy.
   d. The excited molecule is usually quite unstable and returns rapidly to its ground state (accompanied by the loss of the energy originally absorbed during excitation).
   e. This loss is revealed as either heat or light.
   f. The light can then be emitted by fluorescence or phosphorescence, depending on the high-energy state of the molecule
      (1). Fluorescence results from radioactive decay of the excited singlet state.
      (2). Phosphorescence arises from radioactive decay of the excited triplet state to the ground state.
      (3). The phosphorescence lifetime is much longer than that of the fluorescence.
      (4). The lifetime of the triplet state is dependent on oxygen concentration.
      (5). The greater the oxygen concentration, the greater the probability that the ex-

cited triplet state molecule will collide with an oxygen molecule.

g. Phosphorescence probes have not usually been used to measure oxygen because the equipment is sophisticated.

   (1). Room temperature phosphorescence has been difficult to observe with oxygen present.

   (2). Since lumiphores with substantial phosphorescence at room temperature were discovered, it is more feasible to design molecules with phosphorescence intensities and lifetimes suitable for measuring oxygen at physiological temperatures and oxygen concentrations.

2. Oxygen concentration then can be measured by fiberoptic probes to which oxygen indicators with fluorescent properties are attached.

   a. The advantages are that no oxygen is consumed during the measurement process.

   b. The primary disadvantages are that the system is not yet fully refined, some of the indicators are toxic, and the response time is long.

3. In the clinical setting, optical methods would offer an improved safety factor with no electrical contact between measuring device and the patient. Also, optical devices are usually flexible and easily inserted into blood vessels.

References

1. Hunt TK, Twomey P, Zederfeldt B, *et al.*: Respiratory gas tensions and pH in healing wounds. *Am J Surg* 1967, 114:203–208.
2. Niinikoski J, Hunt TK, Dunphy JE: Oxygen supply in healing tissue. *Am J Surg* 1972, 123:247–252.
3. Silver IA: Cellular microenvironment in healing and non-healing wounds. In Hunt TK, Heppenstall RB, Pines E, *et al.* (eds): *Soft and Hard Tissue Repair.* New York, Praeger, 1984, pp 50–66.
4. Sheffield PJ: Tissue oxygen measurements. In Davis JC, Hunt TK (eds): *Problem Wounds: The Role of Oxygen.* Elsevier, New York, 1988, pp 17–52.
5. Whalen W, Riley J, Nair PL: A microelectrode for measuring intracellular Po$_2$. *J Appl Physiol* 1967, 23:798–801.
6. Clark LC Jr, Wolf R, Granger D, *et al.*: Continuous recording of blood oxygen tensions by polarography. *J Appl Physiol* 1953, 6(3):189–193.
7. Huch R, Lubgers WDW, Huch A: Quantitative continuous measurement of partial oxygen pressure on the skin of adults and newborn babies. *Pflugers Arch,* 1972, 337:185–198.
8. Hohenauer L: Transcutaneous monitoring of Po$_2$ in sick newborn babies: three years of clinical experience. In Huch A, Huch R, Lucey JF (eds): *Continuous Transcutaneous Blood Gas Monitoring.* 1979, New York, A.R. Liss, pp 375–376.
9. Serafin D, Lesesne CB, Mullen RY, *et al.*: Transcutaneous Po$_2$ monitoring for assessing viability and predicting survival of skin flaps: experimental and clinical correlations. *J Microsurg* 1981, 2(3):165–178.
10. Sheffield PJ, Workman WT: Transcutaneous tissue oxygen monitoring in patients undergoing hyperbaric oxygen therapy. In Huch R, Huch A. (eds): *Continuous Transcutaneous Blood Gas Monitoring.* New York, Marcel Dekker, 1983, pp 655–660.
11. Sheffield PJ, Workman WT: Noninvasive tissue oxygen measurements in patients administered normobaric and hyperbaric oxygen by mask. *Hyperb Oxyg Rev* 1985, 6(2):47–62.
12. Huch R, Lugbbers DW, Huch A: Quantitative continuous measurement of partial oxygen pressure on the skin of adults and newborn babies. *Pflugers Arch,* 1972, 337:285–298.
13. Gottrup F, Firmin R, Chang N, *et al.*: Continuous direct tissue oxygen tension measurement by a new method using an implantable Silastic tonometers and oxygen polarography. *Am J Surg* 1983, 14:399–403.
14. Hunt TK: Disorders of repair and their management. In Hunt TK, Dunphy JE (eds): *Fundamentals of Wound Management.* New York, Appleton-Century-Crofts, 1979, pp 68–168.
15. Kessler K, Grunewald W: Possibilities of measuring oxygen pressure fields in tissue by multiwire platinum electrodes. In Kreuzer F, Herzog H (eds): *Oxygen Pressure Recording in Gases, Fluids and Tissues.* Basel, Karger, 1969, pp 147–152.
16. Gottrup F, Firmin R, Hunt TK, *et al.*: The dynamic properties of tissue oxygen in healing flaps. *Surgery* 1984, 95(5):527–536.
17. Wells CH, Goodpasture JE, Horrigan DJ, *et al.*: Tissue gas measurements during hyperbaric oxygen exposure. In Smith G (ed): *Proceedings of the Sixth International Congress on Hyperbaric Medicine.* Aberdeen, Aberdeen University Press, 1977, pp 118–124.
18. Woldring S, Owens G, Woolford D: Blood gases: continuous in vivo recording of partial pressures by mass spectrography. *Science* 1966, 153:885–887.
19. Jones T, Chesler DA, Ter-Pogossian MM: The continuous inhalation of oxygen-15 for assessing regional oxygen extraction in the brain of man. *Br J Radiol* 1976, 49:339–343.
20. Clyne CAC, Jones T, Moss S, *et al.*: The use of radioactive oxygen to study muscle function in peripheral vascular disease. *Surg Gynecol Obstet* 1979, 149:225–228.
21. Horie T, Vanderkooi JM: Use of phosphorescence at room temperature for the study of biological molecules. *Life Chem Rep* 1984, 2:141–178.

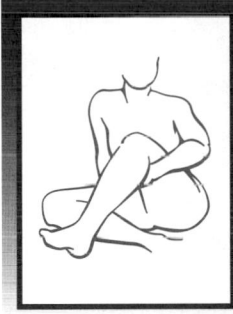

APPENDIX E

TMJ EVALUATION

NAME: AGE: PHONE:

ADDRESS: CITY: ZIP:

OCCUPATION:

1. Patient's complaint:

2. How sustained:

   Past trauma:

3. What makes your pain worse? Chewing _____   Yawning _____   Stress _____
4. What, if anything, eases your pain?

5. Does your jaw make a noise on movement?   Date _____
6. Has your jaw ever locked?   Open _____   Closed _____   Date _____
7. Do you clench or grind your teeth?
8. Is your face and mouth tired in the morning?
9. Are your teeth sore or sensitive?
10. Is it difficult to swallow?
11. Do you have a tendency to bite your cheeks, lips, or tongue while chewing or swallowing?
12. Do you have any problems or pain with your ears?   L   R
          Hearing _____   Ringing _____   Dizziness _____
13. Do you have pain in or around the eyes?   L   R
14. Do you have headaches?   (see chart)
15. Do you have any numbness?   (see chart)
16. Have you had any surgery?
17. Have you had any major dental work done?

18. Who else has seen you for this problem and what did they do?

PALPATION AND DYNAMIC FINDINGS

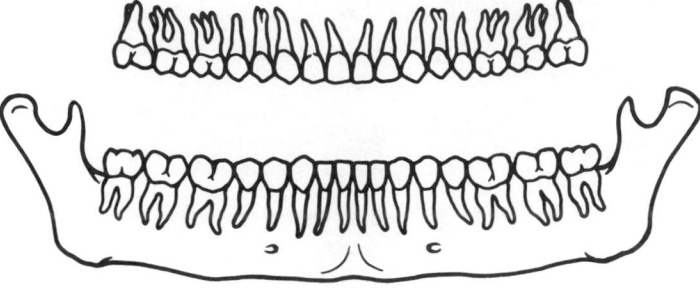

I. Resting vertical dimension

_____ mm Anteriorly

_____ mm Posteriorly

II. Condyle-Meniscus Relationship

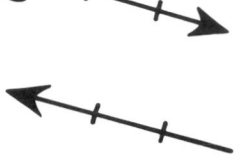

Opening click	L	R
Closing click	L	R
Force closing click	L	R
Crepitus	L	R

III. Palpation

A) Periarticular Tissue
   - External acoustic meatus

   - Anterior to tragus

	L	R
Rest -	_____	_____
Close -	_____	_____
Open -	_____	_____
Rest -	_____	_____
Close -	_____	_____
Open -	_____	_____

B) Mobility

L 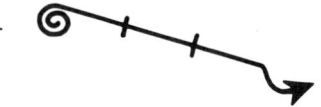   R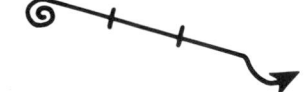

C) Muscles

1)	Temporalis	L	R
2)	Digastric	L	R
3)	Sternocleidomastoid	L	R
4)	Scaleni	L	R
5)	Mylohyoid	L	R
6)	Medial Pterygoid	L	R
7)	Masseter	L	R
8)	Lateral Pterygoid	L	R

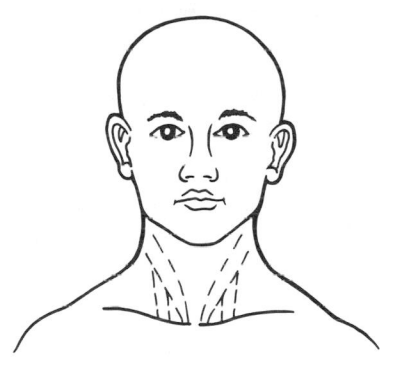
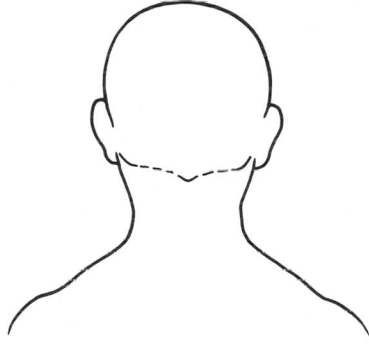
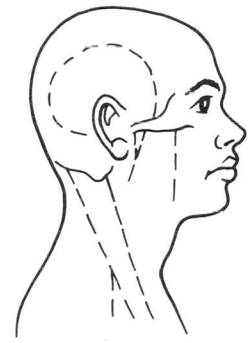
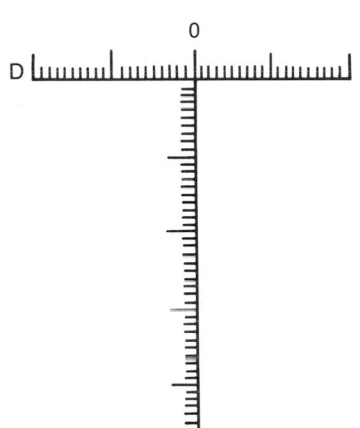
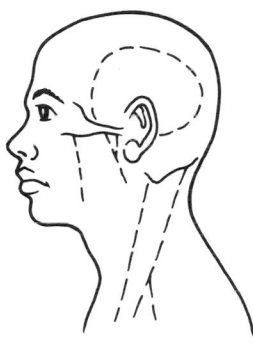
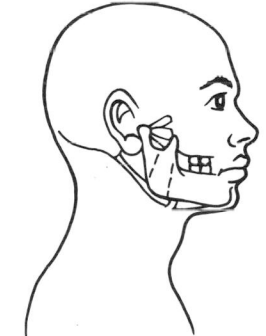
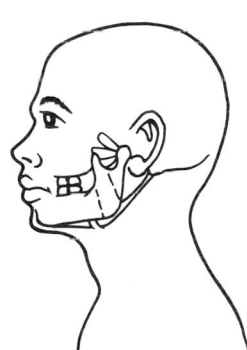

Key to functional movement

Red   = Opening
Blue   = Lateral deviation
Green = Protrusion

Respiration:

Normal diaphragmatic

Upper chest breather

Swallowing:

Hyoid movement

Tongue position

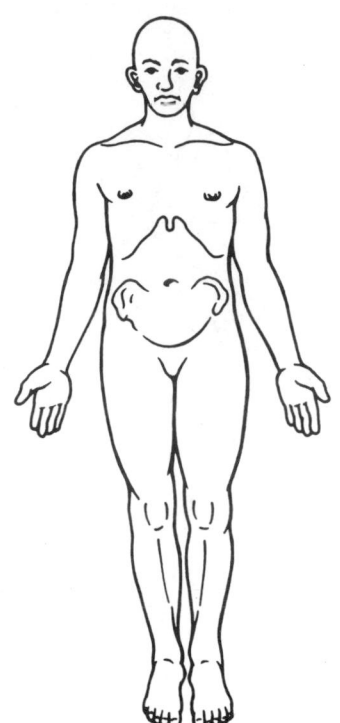 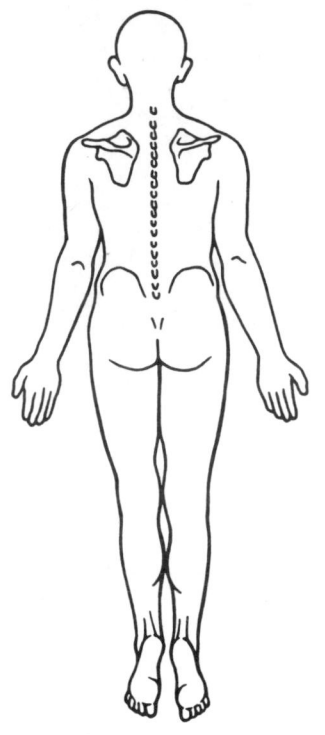

Subjective pain

Impression:

Treatment plan:

MUSCLE EXAMINATION (Pain on Palpation)

	R	L
A. Temporalis:		
1. Anterior	——	——
2. Middle	——	——
3. Posterior	——	——
B. Masseter:		
1. Origin (Zygoma)	——	——
2. Body	——	——
3. Insertion	——	——
4. Deep fibers	——	——
C. Coronoid process	——	——
D. Sternocleidomastoid:		
1. Origin (Sternum/clavicle)	——	——
2. Body	——	——
3. Insertion (Mastoid/occiput)	——	——

E. Trapezius:

    1. Body   ——— ———
    2. Insertion (Occiput)   ——— ———
    3. Middle   ——— ———

F. Posterior cervicals   ——— ———

G. Occipital area (Nuchal line)   ——— ———

H. Medial pterygoid (Internal)   ——— ———

I. Lateral pterygoid (External)   ——— ———

J. Mylohyoid   ——— ———

Other areas:

Upper back   ——— ———
Middle back   ——— ———
Lower back   ——— ———
Scapular area   ——— ———
Shoulders   ——— ———
Arms   ——— ———
Fingers   ——— ———
Chest   ——— ———
Iliac crest   ——— ———
Calves   ——— ———

TEMPOROMANDIBULAR JOINT ASSESSMENT

Part A. Patient Questionnaire/History/Symptom Assessment
Part B. Maxillofacial Evaluation (Anatomical/Neuromuscular)
Part C. Craniomandibular Evaluation
Part D. Upper Quarter Assessment (Neurological Screening)
Part E. Postural Assessment

Part A.   I. Patient Questionnaire (separate sheet to be filled out by patient)
Part A.   II. History (examiner administers)

a. General

  1. Does your pain keep you from getting to sleep easily at night? Yes _____   No _____
  2. Do you sleep on your stomach _____ side _____ back _____?
  3. Do you support your neck? Yes _____   No _____
  4. Do you wake up at night with pain? Yes _____   No _____
     If yes, where is the location of the pain? _____
     _____
  5. How do you feel in the morning? Fine _____ Stiff & sore _____ Painful _____
  6. What is the pattern of the pain during the day? _____
     _____
  7. Are there some days you have no discomfort? Yes _____   No _____
  8. Frequency_____
  9. Do you have any numbness? Yes _____   No_____   Location _____

b. Habits/Function

  1. Do you feel bite is off? _____
  2. Do you have difficulty swallowing? _____
  3. Do you grind/clench teeth? _____
  4. Do you have a habit, *ie,* pin in mouth, smoke pipe, lean hand on jaw, phone? _____
  5. Do you have joint noises? _____
  6. Has your jaw ever locked open/closed? _____
  7. Have you had orthodontic treatment? _____
  8. Do stressful situations increase pain? _____
  9. In general, rate your present stress level (0–10) _____
  10. Are you a mouth breather? _____

Part A.   III. Symptom Assessment

Verbal Questions (pain = ✔; no pain = —)

a. Pain (Rate 0–10)

	Past History	Clinical Examination Date	Date	Date	Date
Head					
Neck					
Eye(s)					
Facial muscles					
Ears					
TM joint					
Teeth					
Throat					
Upper jaw					
Lower jaw					
Mouth/tongue					
Chest					
Shoulders					
Midback					
Lower back					
Arms					
Hands					
Lower extremities					

b. Additional Symptoms (present = ✔; decreased = ↓; increased = ↑; none = —)

Symptoms	Past History	Clinical Examination Date	Date	Date	Date
Mouth/tongue burn					
Salty taste in mouth					
Copper taste in mouth					
Soreness in throat/need clear often					
Change in pitch of voice					
Ulcers					

Symptoms	Past History	Clinical Examination Date	Date	Date	Date
Swelling of gums					
Tooth temperature sensitivity					
Cavity front teeth					
Noises in ear					
Clogged, fullness in ear					
Hearing loss					
Dizziness/balance					
Postnasal drip					
Sinus congestion					
Tearing					
Light sensitivity					
Sensitivity to weather changes					
Stiffness					
Tingling, numbness, cold—where?					
Excessive fatigue					
Difficulty sleeping					
Respiratory difficulty					
Allergy to food/pollen					

Part B.   Maxillofacial Evaluation

I. Observation—anatomical

Face, *ie,* symmetry; rule of thirds; _____

_____

Nostrils, *ie,* deviated septum; patent airway; _____

_____

Upper lip _____

Lower lip _____

Mentonian groove _____

Palate _____

Lip frenulum _____

Linguinal frenulum _____

Volume of tongue _____

II. Neuromuscular (strength)

A. Lip/cheeks   R   L   Comments

    Orbicularis
    oris   ——   ——

    Buccinator   ——   ——

B. Tongue muscles

    Elevator tip _____ Dorsum _____

    Protruders _____

    Retractors _____

    Lateral deviation—right _____

    Lateral deviation—left _____

C. Masticatory muscles

    Elevators _____

    Depressors _____

    Protruders _____

    Lateral, mandible deviation—right _____

    Lateral, mandible deviation—left _____

III. Assessment/summary _____

_____

_____

Part C.   Craniomandibular Evaluation

I.   Palpation of TMJ/structures (very painful = ++; slightly painful = +; no pain = —)

    1 Pre-tragus   R _____   L _____
    2. TM ligament   R _____   L _____
    3. Intra-auricular R _____   L _____
    4. Infratemporal
       fossa (extraoral) R _____   L _____

II. Auscultation of the TMJ (Present = ✔; none = —)

    1. Crepitus   R _____   L _____
    2. Opening click   R _____   L _____
    3. Closing click   R _____   L _____
    4. Other

III. Muscle Palpation (very painful = ++; slightly painful = +; no pain = —)

	R	L
Temporalis-Ant., Med., Post.	——	——
Masseter	——	——
Digastric-Ant. Belly	——	——
Digastric-Post. Belly	——	——
Longus Colli	——	——
Suprahyoid	——	——
Infrahyoid	——	——

	R	L
SCM	——	——
Scaleni	——	——
Levator Scapula	——	——
Posterior Cervical	——	——
Medial Pterygoid	——	——
Lateral Pterygoid	——	——

IV. Additional Structural Components ENTS
Mobility Check of the Following:

1. Hyoid bone _____
2. Thyroid cartilage _____
3. Cricoid cartilage _____

V. TMJ Loading

1. Retrusive overpressure   R _____   L _____
2. Force bite left, pain   R _____   L _____
3. Force bite right, pain   R _____   L _____

VI. Balancing Interferences

1. Lateral movement   R _____   L _____
2. Protrusive movement   R _____   L _____

VII. Headaches

1. Location (circle all that apply): facial, frontal, subocciptal, temples, R/L, neck, vertex, other
   Comments: _____
2. Type of pain (circle all that apply): radiating, achy, burning, throbbing, other
   Comments: _____
3. Frequency _____
4. Duration _____

VIII.   Arthrokinematics (mandibular dynamics)

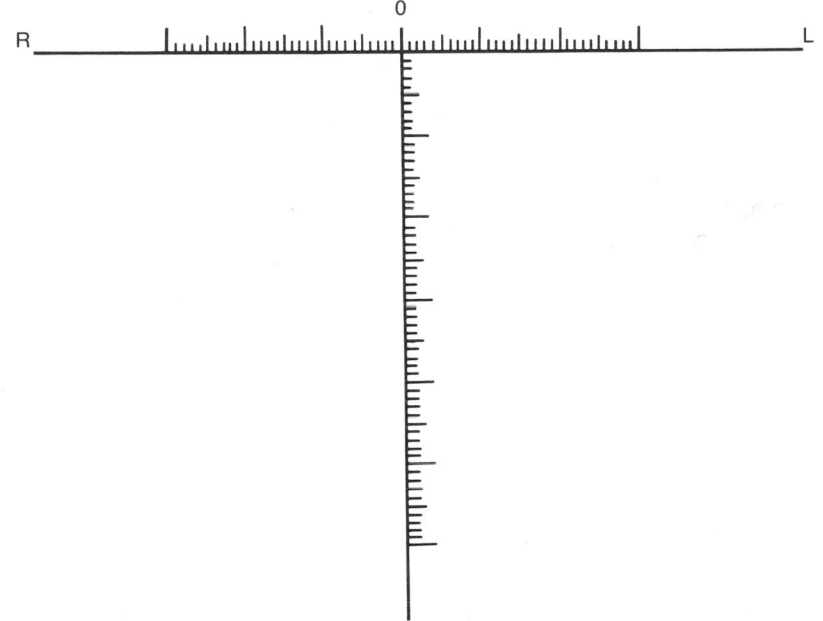

Red   = depression
Blue   = lateral deviation
Green = protrusion

Comments. _____
_____
_____

IX.   Capsular Assessment (joint play)

1. Distraction   R _____   L _____   Hyper/hypo
2. Anterior glide with distraction   R _____   L _____   Hyper/hypo
3. Lateral glide with distraction   R _____   L _____   Hyper/hypo
4. Lateral glide (pure)   R _____   L _____   Hyper/hypo

   Comments: _____
   _____
   _____

X.   Additional Findings _____
_____
_____

XI.   Craniocervical (postural evaluation) done

Yes _____   No _____

XII.   Assessment/Summary

_____
_____
_____

XIII.   Treatment Plan/Goals

_____
_____
_____

Part D.   Upper Quarter Assessment (neurological examination)

I. Nerve Root Check—Isometric Resisted Motions (pain = +; no pain = —)

	R	L		R	L
C1, C2 tk chin in			C5, C6 ± IR		
C1, C2 psh chin up			C5, C6 ± ER		
C3 lat neck			C5, C6 elbow flex		
C4 sh shrug			C7 elbow ext.		
C5 sh flex			C6, C7, wrist flex		
C6, C7, C8 sh ext.			C6, wrist flex		
C5, C6, sh abd			C7, C8 thumb ext.		
C7 sh add			T1 5th finger add		

II.   Reflexes   R   L

Biceps C5, C6   ____   ____
Triceps C7   ____   ____
Brac. rad C5, C6   ____   ____

III.   Sensation   R   L

Light touch   ____   ____
Pin prick   ____   ____

IV.   Shoulder
Gross RCM _____
Gross MMT _____

POSTURE ASSESSMENT

CORONAL VIEW

PATIENT	NORMAL(0)	MODERATE(3)	SEVERE(5)	DATE	DATE	DATE
HEAD TILT						
SHOULDER HEIGHT INFERIOR ANGLE OF SCAPULAE						
SCAPULAR HINGING						
SCOLIOSIS FUNCTIONAL STRUCTURAL						
ILIAC CRESTS TROCHANTER HEIGHT						
GENU VARUM/ VALGUM						
FOOT PRONATION SUPINATION						
			TOTAL			
			THERAPIST			

PREPARED BY: BARBARA M. BOURBON, PT, PhD
CAROL A. OATIS, PT, PhD

PHILADELPHIA INSTITUTE FOR PHYSICAL THERAPY

POSTURE ASSESSMENT

SAGITTAL VIEW

PATIENT	NORMAL(0)	MODERATE(3)	SEVERE(5)	DATE	DATE	DATE
FORWARD HEAD						
KYPHOSIS						
ROUND SHOULDERS						
LUMBAR CURVE						
ABDOMINAL PROTRUSION						
TROCHANTER ALIGNMENT						
GENU RECURVATUM ANKLE ALIGNMENT						
			TOTAL			
			THERAPIST			

PREPARED BY: BARBARA M. BOURBON, PT, PhD
CAROL A. OATIS, PT, PhD

PHILADELPHIA INSTITUTE FOR PHYSICAL THERAPY

Comments: _____

Need for detailed evaluation   Yes _____   No _____

Thoracic outlet check

V.   Assessment _____

_____

_____

_____

Examiner's
Signature _____

The posture assessment forms appear courtesy of the Philadelphia Institute for Physical Therapy.

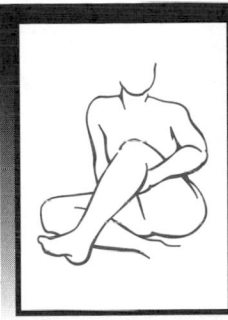

Physical Therapy Diagnosis

Table F–1. PHYSICAL THERAPY DIAGNOSIS
DIAGNOSIS: CHRONIC ANTERIOR CRUCIATE LIGAMENT LAXITY

Symptoms	Key Tests and Signs	Associated Signs	Differential Physical Therapy Diagnosis	Differential Medical Diagnosis
Knee "gives way"; true instability	*From History* Rarely complains of pain Patient describes pivot shift *From Physical Examination* + Lachmann test + Anterior drawer + Pivot shift	*Tightness* None *Weakness* Quadriceps *Postural* None	Posterior cruciate ligament injury Meniscus injury	Tumor Hematoma Fracture

Notes

High incidence of concomitant patellofemoral pain associated with anterior cruciate ligament injuries.

Usually associated with a precipitating factor that the subject can identify.

Subjects in this case are those who do not opt for surgery and prefer to rehabilitate conservatively; this will most likely cause a highly competitive athlete in a knee-demanding sport to lower his/her expectations when participating.

Can usually expect tibiofemoral joint problems (*eg*, meniscal) with increases in chronicity, especially in those patients who pivot shift commonly.

Suggested Treatments

Aggressive strengthening and endurance training of the quadriceps femoris using electrical stimulation and closed kinetic chain exercises. THE QUADRICEPS MUST BE STRENGTHENED IN A PROTECTIVE RANGE (>45 DEGREES FLEXION) OR WITH COCONTRACTION.

Consider derotational bracing.

Monitor and modify recreational and occupational activities, especially noting any incidence of pivot shifting.

Table F–2. PHYSICAL THERAPY DIAGNOSIS
DIAGNOSIS: CALF STRAIN (FIRST AND SECOND DEGREE)

Symptoms	Key Tests and Signs	Associated Signs	Differential Physical Therapy Diagnosis	Differential Medical Diagnosis
Posterior calf pain	*From History* Pain with jumping Pain with gait *From Physical Examination* Pain with stretch of gastrocsoleus Pain with gastrocsoleus resistive contraction Patient tender on calf area muscle belly	*Tightness* Gastrocsoleus *Weakness* None *Postural* None	Problem referred from the knee (meniscus)	Tumor Hematoma Fracture Reflex Sympathetic Dystrophy

Notes

Higher incidence in athletes, especially sprinters or those involved in sports that are more ballistic in nature with regard to the leg, such as basketball and tennis.
Usually associated with a precipating factor that the subject can identify.
Responds well to aggressive treatment.
Also referred to commonly as a "plantaris tear."

Suggested Treatments

Modalities (ultrasound, high-voltage pulsed monophasic current) to local area.
Stretch and strengthen conservatively.
Monitor and modify recreational and occupational activities, especially in the competitive athlete.
Deep friction massage.

Table F-3. PHYSICAL THERAPY DIAGNOSIS
DIAGNOSIS: HAMSTRING STRAIN (FIRST AND SECOND DEGREE)

Symptoms	Key Tests and Signs	Associated Signs	Differential Physical Therapy Diagnosis	Differential Medical Diagnosis
Posterior thigh pain	**From History** Pain on stairs Pain with gait **From Physical Examination** Pain with stretch of hamstrings Pain with hamstrings resistive contraction Patient tender on hamstrings belly	**Tightness** Hamstrings **Weakness** Hamstrings **Postural** None	Problem referred from the hip or back	Tumor Hematoma Fracture Reflex Sympathetic Dystrophy

Notes

Higher incidence in athletes, especially sprinters or those involved in sports that are more ballistic in nature with regard to the thigh and leg, such as basketball.
Usually associated with a precipitating factor that the subject can identify.
Responds well to aggressive treatment.
Mobilization of sacroiliac joint has a place in the management of this diagnosis, especially first-degree strain.

Suggested Treatments

Modalities (ultrasound, high-voltage pulsed monophasic current, cold whirlpool) to local area.
Stretch and strengthen conservatively.
Monitor and modify recreational and occupational activities, especially in the competitive athlete.
Mobilize the sacroiliac joint.

Table F-4. PHYSICAL THERAPY DIAGNOSIS
DIAGNOSIS: ILIOTIBIAL BAND (ITB) FRICTION SYNDROME

Symptoms	Key Tests and Signs	Associated Signs	Differential Physical Therapy Diagnosis	Differential Medical Diagnosis
Anterolateral knee pain with activities that require repetitive knee extension	**From History** Pain on stairs **From Physical Examination** + Step-down test Patient tenderness on ITB at lateral femoral condyle	**Tightness** ITB **Weakness** Quadriceps Gluteus medius **Postural** Varus knee deformity	Patellofemoral malalignment syndrome	Fractured patella Chondral fracture Dislocating patella Reflex Sympathetic Dystrophy

Notes

Higher incidence in athletes, especially runners.
Suggested in the literature to respond well to steroid injections.

Suggested Treatments

Modalities (ultrasound, high-voltage pulsed monophasic current) to ITB.
Stretch what is tight; strengthen what is weak.
Monitor and modify recreational and occupational activities, especially in the competitive athlete.

Table F–5. PHYSICAL THERAPY DIAGNOSIS
DIAGNOSIS: CHRONIC POSTERIOR CRUCIATE LIGAMENT LAXITY

Symptoms	Key Tests and Signs	Associated Signs	Differential Physical Therapy Diagnosis	Differential Medical Diagnosis
Knee pain; complaints are varied and are usually described consistent with expected sequelae from this type of injury (*eg*, meniscal)	***From History*** Rarely complains of pain unless chronic and pain is from another cause ***From Physical Examination*** + Posterior sag + Posterior drawer	***Tightness*** None ***Weakness*** Quadriceps ***Postural*** None	Anterior cruciate ligament injury Meniscus injury	Tumor Hematoma Fracture

Notes

High incidence of concomitant patellofemoral pain associated with posterior cruciate ligament injuries.

These patients do surprisingly well immediately after the injury, commonly returning to competitive sporting activities within a 1- to 2-month period after the initial injury.

Surgical options are not as clear cut as they are for the anterior cruciate ligament injury patient. Subjects in this case are those who do not opt for surgery and prefer to rehabilitate conservatively. Whether this will most likely cause a highly competitive athlete in a knee-demanding sport to lower his/her expectations when participating is still questionable.

Can usually expect tibiofemoral joint problems (*eg*, meniscal) with increases in chronicity.

Suggested Treatments

Aggressive strengthening and endurance training of quadriceps femoris using electrical stimulation and closed kinetic chain exercises.

Derotational bracing may be helpful, but this has not really been established.

Monitor and modify recreational and occupational activities, especially noting any incidence of pivot shifting.

Table F–6.   PHYSICAL THERAPY DIAGNOSIS
   DIAGNOSIS: PATELLOFEMORAL MALALIGNMENT SYNDROME

Symptoms	Key Tests and Signs	Associated Signs	Differential Physical Therapy Diagnosis	Differential Medical Diagnosis
Anterior knee pain with any activity that requires forceful knee extension	**From History** Pain on stairs "Moviegoer's syndrome" **From Physical Examination** + Step-down test	**Tightness** Hamstrings Rectus femoris ITP, iliopsoas **Weakness** Quadriceps Gluteus medius **Postural** Pronated feet Internal Rotation of the femurs Dynamic Q-angle **Other** Patellofemoral grind test Crepitus VMO weakness Inc. Q-angle	Patella Tendon tenditis Flexion contracture	Fractured patella Chondral fracture Dislocating patella Reflex Sympathetic Dystrophy

Notes

Higher incidence in adolescent females and anterior cruciate ligament postsurgical and nonsurgical patients.
Be careful not to induce patellofemoral malalignment syndrome with aggressive, open kinetic chain quadriceps exercises.

Suggested Treatments

Patellar taping or infrapatellar straps for "first-aid."
Stretch what is tight; strengthen what is weak.
Monitor and modify recreational and occupational activities, especially in the competitive athlete.
Corrective foot orthoses for severe foot deformity in active individuals.

Table F–7. PHYSICAL THERAPY DIAGNOSIS
DIAGNOSIS: PATELLAR TENDON TENDINITIS

Symptoms	Key Tests and Signs	Associated Signs	Differential Physical Therapy Diagnosis	Differential Medical Diagnosis
Anterior knee pain with any activity that requires forceful knee extension	**From History** Pain on stairs **From Physical Examination** + Step-down test Patient tenderness on patellar tendon	**Tightness** Hamstrings Rectus femoris ITP, iliopsoas **Weakness** Quadriceps Gluteus medius **Postural** Pronated feet Internal Rotation of the femurs Dynamic Q-angle **Other** Patellofemoral grind test Crepitus VMO weakness Inc. Q-angle	Petellofemoral mal-alignment syndrome	Fractured patella Chondral fracture Dislocating patella Reflex Sympathetic Dystrophy

Notes

Higher incidence in athletes or in people who have suddenly increased their activity level without proper training.
Be careful not to induce patellar tendonitis with aggressive, open kinetic chain quadriceps exercises.

Suggested Treatments

Modalities (ultrasound, high-voltage pulsed monophasic current) to patellar tendon.
Patellar taping or infrapatellar straps for "first-aid."
Stretch what is tight; strengthen what is weak.
Monitor and modify recreational and occupational activities, especially in the competitive athlete.
Corrective foot orthoses for severe foot deformity in active individuals.

Table F–8. PHYSICAL THERAPY DIAGNOSIS
DIAGNOSIS: RECTUS FEMORIS STRAIN (FIRST AND SECOND
DEGREE)

Symptoms	Key Tests and Signs	Associated Signs	Differential Physical Therapy Diagnosis	Differential Medical Diagnosis
Anterior thigh pain	*From History* Pain on stairs Pain with gait *From Physical Examination* Pain with stretch of rectus femoris Pain with rectus femoris resistive contraction Patient tender on rectus femoris muscle belly	*Tightness* Rectus femoris *Weakness* Quadriceps *Postural* None	Problem referred from the hip	Tumor Hematoma Fracture Reflex Sympathetic Dystrophy

Notes

Higher incidence in athletes, especially sprinters or those involved in sports that are more ballistic in nature with regard to the thigh and leg, such as basketball.
Usually associated with a precipating factor that the subject can identify.
Responds well to aggressive treatment.
Mobilization of sacroiliac joint may have a place in the management of this diagnosis.

Suggested Treatments

Modalities (ultrasound, high-voltage pulsed monophasic current) to local area.
Stretch and strengthen conservatively.
Monitor and modify recreational and occupational activities, especially in the competitive athlete.
Mobilize the sacroiliac joint.

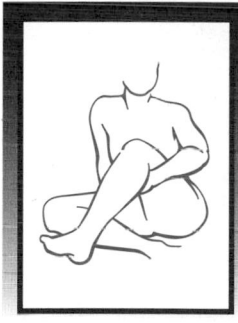

Index

Note: Page numbers in *italics* refer to illustrations. Page numbers followed by t refer to tables, and those followed by c refer to charts.

A

Abdominal oblique muscle(s), changes in, from pregnancy, 516–517, *516–517*

Abdominal splint(s), for assistance with breathing, 306

Abdominal wall, changes in, during pregnancy, 515–517, *516–517*

Abdominopelvic cavity, anatomy of, 459, *460*

Abducens nerve, testing of, 698

Abducted gait, 994

Abduction, of shoulder, in objective composite examination, 810–812, *811*

Abductor digiti minimi muscle, anatomy and biomechanics of, *1064*, 1064–1065

Abductor hallucis muscle, anatomy and biomechanics of, 1064, *1064*

Above-knee amputation (AKA), preparation of residual limb for prosthesis after, measurements for, 1126

Above-knee prostheses, 1154–1173. See also *Prosthesis (prostheses), above-knee.*

Above-knee "stubbies", for bilateral amputee, *1172*, 1173

Acantholysis, definition of, 562

Acanthosis, definition of, 562

Acanthosis nigricans, 81t, 569–570

Acceptance, as stage of grief process, 56

Accessory movement(s), of joints, assessment of, 870t

passive, definition of, 728

Accessory nerve, testing of, 699

Accommodating resistance, in isokinetics, 1022–1023

Accommodation, as learning style, 40–41

Accrediting agency(ies), for physical therapy educational programs, 4t

Ace bandage(s), for ambulation, in burn care, 655

Acetabular dysplasia, in Down's syndrome, 1253

Acetabular fracture, treatment of, 980

Acetabulum, growth and development of, 1233

Achilles tendinitis, orthosis for, 1188

Achilles tendon, 1033–1034

Acid-base balance, interpretation of, 274t

Acne, 573

ultraviolet treatment for, 647

Acoustic nerve, testing of, 699

Acquired immunodeficiency syndrome (AIDS), cutaneous manifestations of, 582–584

Acromioclavicular joint, subjective examination of, 803, *803*

Acromiohumeral joint, functional anatomy of, 795–796, *795–796*

intra-articular compressive force on, testing of, 818–820, *819–820*

Acromiohumeral space, impingement of, vs. tendinitis of supraspinatus muscle, test for, 818, *819*

Acromion, types of, 796, *796*

Actinic keratosis, 566

Actinomycin D (Cosmegen), 1273t

Active insufficiency, measurement of, 868

Active listening, 57–58

Active movement, assessment of, for examination of hips, 962

for objective examination of lumbar spine, 937–938

for objective examination of ribs, 935

for objective examination of sacroiliac joint, 940

for objective examination of thoracic spine, 933–934

for objective examination of trunk, 932

definition of, 792

posturing of extremities and, 371

spasticity and, 371

Active range of motion (AROM), assessment of, for examination of hips, 962

Active range of motion *(Continued)*

in fingers and thumbs, 866, *867–868*, 868

Activities of daily living (ADL), evaluation of, in children with cerebral palsy with spastic hemiplegia, 431

in children with cerebral palsy with spastic quadriplegia, 429

in children with hypothyroidism, 435

in children with Lesch-Nyhan syndrome, 434

in preschoolers with myotonic dystrophy, 443

training in, for patient with above-knee prosthesis, 1171–1172

for patient with below-knee prosthesis, 1152–1153

Activity, level of, in oncology patient, 72–74

guidelines for, 110t

Activity(ies), and bone growth, 1289–1290

Activity tolerance, observation of, during functional evaluation, 356t

Activity training, sequence of, in motor control/motor learning model, 369–370

Acute lymphocytic leukemia (ALL), 107–108

treatment of, 135–136

Acute myelocytic leukemia (AML), 107–108

Acute phase, of burn care, exercises for, 652–653

positioning during, 648

Acyanotic heart defect(s), 296, *297*

Addison's syndrome, 83t

Adductor hallucis muscle, anatomy and biomechanics of, 1065, *1065*

ADH (antidiuretic hormone), levels of, in cancer, 80

Adhesion(s), temporomandibular, 694, *704*, 704–705

treatment of, 712

ADL. See *Activities of daily living (ADL).*

ISBN 0-7216-3671-3

90069

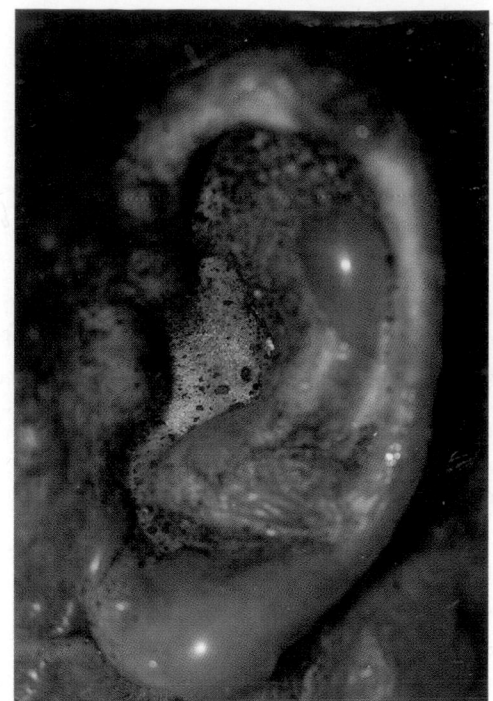

PLATE 1   A partial-thickness burn of the ear.

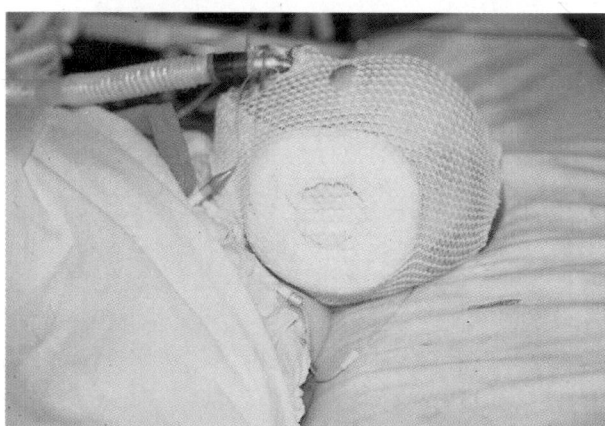

PLATE 2   A foam ear protector is in place.

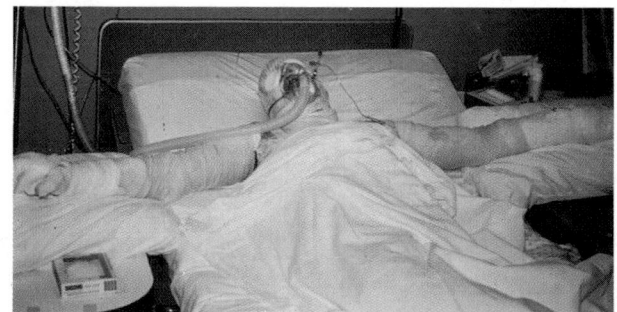

PLATE 3   Anticontracture positioning of the burn victim during the acute phase, using bedside tables and trough pillows.

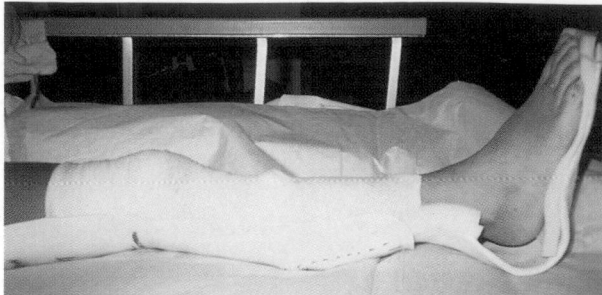

PLATE 4   An ankle-foot orthosis is combined with a knee-extension splint for protective positioning. Note that this design keeps pressure off of the heel.

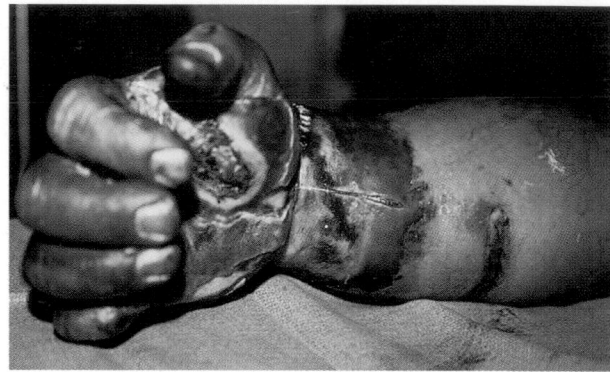

PLATE 5   An electrical burn to the hand (before surgery).

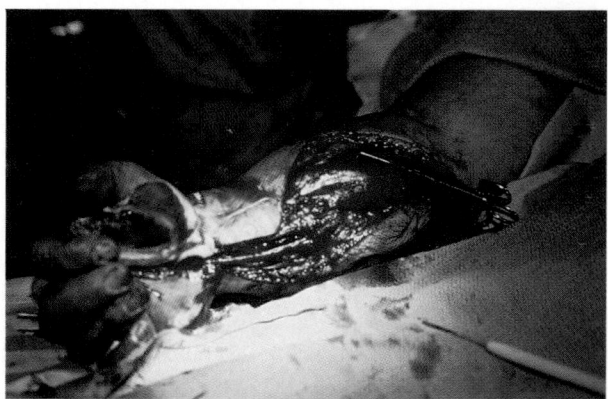

PLATE 6   An electrical burn to the hand and forearm (during surgery).

COLOR PLATES FOR CHAPTER 27